The ESC Textbook of Cardiovascular Medicine

The ESC Textbook of Cardiovascular Medicine, Second Edition is accredited by the European Board for Accreditation in Cardiology (EBAC) for external CME credits. Each reader should claim only those hours of credit that have been spent in the educational activity. EBAC works according to the quality standard of the European Accreditation Council for Continuing Medical Education (EACCME), which is an institution of the European Union of Medical Specialists (UEMS). In compliance with EBAC/EACCME guidelines, all authors of accredited chapters have disclosed or indicated potential conflicts of interest which might cause a bias in the content.

369 0160508

The ESC Textbook of Cardiovascular Medicine

SECOND EDITION

Edited by

A. John Camm

British Heart Foundation Professor of Clinical Cardiology,
Head of the Division of Cardiac and Vascular Sciences,
St. George's University of London, London, UK

Thomas F. Lüscher

Professor and Head of Cardiology,
University Hospital Zürich, Zürich, Switzerland

and

Patrick W. Serruys

Professor of Interventional Cardiology and Head of Interventional Department,
Erasmus Medical Center, Erasmus University,
Rotterdam, The Netherlands

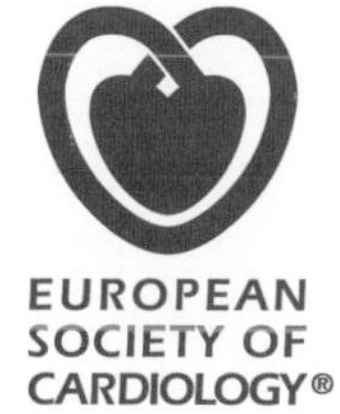

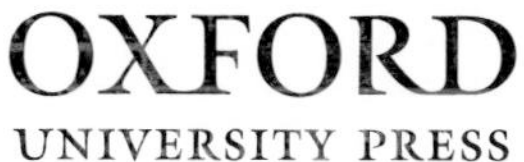

OXFORD
UNIVERSITY PRESS

Great Clarendon Street, Oxford OX2 6DP

Oxford University Press is a department of the University of Oxford.
It furthers the University's objective of excellence in research, scholarship,
and education by publishing worldwide in

Oxford New York

Auckland Cape Town Dar es Salaam Hong Kong Karachi
Kuala Lumpur Madrid Melbourne Mexico City Nairobi
New Delhi Shanghai Taipei Toronto

With offices in

Argentina Austria Brazil Chile Czech Republic France Greece
Guatemala Hungary Italy Japan Poland Portugal Singapore
South Korea Switzerland Thailand Turkey Ukraine Vietnam

Oxford is a registered trade mark of Oxford University Press
in the UK and in certain other countries

Published in the United States
by Oxford University Press Inc., New York

First edition published by Blackwell Publishing Ltd, 2006
Second edition published by Oxford University Press, 2009

British Library Cataloguing-in-Publication-Data
Data available

Library of Congress Cataloging-in-Publication-Data
Data available

Typeset by Cepha Imaging Pvt. Ltd., Bangalore, India

Printed and bound in China by

C&C Offset Printing Co., Ltd.

ISBN 978–0–19–956699–0

10 9 8 7 6 5 4 3 2

Foreword

The mission statement of the ESC is to improve the quality and quantity of lives of the European population by reducing the burden of cardiovascular disease. To fulfil its mission the ESC has taken on the responsibility of training cardiologists and disseminating knowledge through congresses, guidelines, reports, and through the publication of *The ESC Textbook of Cardiovascular Medicine*, which is now at its second edition.

We would like to take this opportunity to thank all of those who have contributed with their experience, time, and enthusiasm in order to produce this new edition, particularly the authors and editors. Their experience will be invaluable to bring the most pertinent information to our colleagues throughout Europe and around the world.

When confronted with a new project, such as the new edition of *The ESC Textbook of Cardiovascular Medicine*, a legitimate question arises: is it needed? The answer is clear: yes, it is needed.

Cardiology has in the last 50 years made incredible progress and has contributed to more than 6 out of 10 years of the lifespan increase. This is an enormous achievement, bigger than all of the other specialties combined. Despite this, cardiovascular disease is still the foremost cause of death and permanent disability in Western countries and is set to become the foremost cause of death by the year 2020. Thus, cardiology has not yet succeeded in avoiding cardiovascular mortality from occurring, it has just contributed to delaying it. Even this achievement is, of course, of paramount importance, but clearly there is still much to learn about cardiovascular disease, particularly in understanding the basic mechanism of disease, the pathophysiology, and the evolution of diagnostic methods. The explosion of diagnostic techniques combined with new biological assays, particularly those based on genomes and proteomics, do help in making more accurate and precise diagnosis, but require a unusual degree of updated knowledge, the provision of which is one of the many goals of the new edition of *The ESC Textbook of Cardiovascular Medicine*. Equally, the management of cardiology patients, from collecting their histories, to dealing with the psychological impact of ageing, to the regulatory aspects of their disease, is rapidly changing and this is discussed in depth. Sport is becoming more and more popular also as a consequence of several campaigns of prevention. Together with the problem of non-cardiac surgery in cardiac patients, these are other specific goals of the new edition. Of course, the new topics are offered in addition to an extended and comprehensive revision of all topics of the first edition according to the updated guidelines and ESC core syllabus. We are confident and proud that the second edition will become the new benchmark for cardiology in Europe and beyond.

Roberto Ferrari
President of the European Society of Cardiology
2008–2010

Michel Komajda
President Elect of the European Society of Cardiology
2008–2010

Preface

The European Society of Cardiology (ESC) has been at the forefront of establishing best practice in cardiology, and was the first cardiac professional society to publish a textbook in its field. Since its inception in 2004, *The ESC Textbook of Cardiovascular Medicine* has sold many thousands of copies, and has been translated into a number of different languages, including Polish, Turkish, and Spanish. As the science of medicine moves at a fast pace, especially in cardiovascular medicine, this second edition is a timely reminder for all physicians to remain up-to-date with the latest practice.

The ESC Textbook of Cardiovascular Medicine, Second Edition follows the cardiology training curriculum of the ESC, and is designed to be used as a text for teaching and a guide for learning. Combining the ESC guidelines, Task Force reports, and Scientific statements, the textbook is sufficiently comprehensive to inform the large majority of clinical practice in cardiovascular medicine, and to serve as the essential training tool for accreditation and re-accreditation in cardiovascular medicine within the European Union and further afield.

This new edition contains seven new chapters: physical examination and history, choice of imaging techniques, the heart and other organs, sports medicine and certification, non-cardiac surgery in cardiac patients, psychological impact of heart disease, and occupational and regulatory aspects of heart disease. We have also combined topics such as atrial fibrillation, ventricular tachycardia, acute coronary syndromes, chronic ischaemic heart disease, and heart failure that were previously covered in two chapters into one chapter. The new edition is larger than the last edition of the book, to incorporate these changes.

As in the previous edition, each chapter begins with a brief summary, and concludes with a 'Personal perspective' from the authors which outlines their view as to the 'state of the art' and the future of their subject. The contents are listed on the first page of the chapter. Each chapter is designed to provide high level information, the evidence-base from which guidelines have been derived, and, where appropriate, the major guideline recommendations.

The textbook is available both in print and online (http://esctextbook.oxfordonline.com). Purchasers of the print and online bundle can access the online material via the access codes printed at the front of this book. The online version contains all the material from the printed book, as well as extensive reference linking including via PubMed. In appropriate chapters video clips and additional images are also available online.

Purchasers with online access can also take advantage of multiple choice questions with can be used for CME/CPD accreditation, which is provided by the European Board for Accreditation in Cardiology (http://www.ebac-cme.org). Each chapter carries appropriate points of credit.

We could not have developed this textbook without the close cooperation of the Education Committee of the European Society of Cardiology. We would like to express our gratitude to those who only contributed to the first edition for their understanding. We also thank the many authors of this edition who made their contributions within the tight deadlines that were needed. Similarly we are grateful to the staff at Oxford University Press, particularly Tracey Mills, Helen Liepman, Julia Jeans, Mandy Hill, Kelly Hewinson, and Kate Wanwimolruk who worked enthusiastically and uncomplainingly to produce this new edition.

A. John Camm
Thomas F. Lüscher
Patrick W. Serruys

Contents

Contributors

Stephan Achenbach
Department of Cardiology, University of Erlangen, Erlangen, Germany.
Chapter 6

Ibrahim Akin
Department of Cardiology, Pulmonology and Intensive Care Unit, University of Rostock, Rostock, Germany.
Chapter 31

Tonje A. Aksnes
Department of Cardiology, Ullevaal University Hospital, Oslo, Norway.
Chapter 13

Stefan Anker
Department of Cardiology, Division of Applied Cachexia Research, Charite, Campus Virchow-Klinikum, Berlin, Germany.
Chapter 23

Jean-Pierre Bassand
Department of Cardiology, University Hospital Jean Minjoz, Besancon, France.
Chapter 16

Cristina Basso
Associate Professor, Cardiovascular Pathology, Department of Medical-Diagnostic Sciences and Special Therapies, University of Padua Medical School, Padua, Italy.
Chapters 20 and *32*

Jeroen J. Bax
Department of Cardiology, Leiden University Medical Center, Leiden, The Netherlands.
Chapter 3

Juan Benezet
Department of Cardiology, Fundación Jiménez Díaz – CAPIO, Madrid, Spain.
Chapter 28

Jean-Jacques Blanc
Departement de Cardiologie, Hopital de la Cavale Blanche, CHU de Brest, Brest Cedex, France.
Chapter 26

Giacomo G. Boccuzzi
Unità di Cardiologia Invasiva, Ospedale San Giovanni Bosco, Torino, Italy.
Chapter 33

Michael Böhm
Department of Cardiology, Angiology and Intensive Care Medicine, Universitätsklinikum des Saarlandes, Homburg/Saar, Germany.
Chapter 15a

Henri Bounameaux
Professor of Medicine and Director of Division of Angiology and Homeostasis, University Hospital of Geneva, Geneva, Switzerland.
Chapter 37

Pascal Bousquet
Professor of Pharmacology, Laboratoire de Neurobiologie et Pharmacologie Cardiovasculaire, Faculté de Médecine, Université de Strasbourg, Strasbourg, France.
Chapter 11

Günter Breithardt
Emeritus Professor of Medicine and Cardiology, Hospital of the University of Münster, Münster, Germany.
Chapter 30

Michele Brignole
Head of Department, Arrhythmologic Centre, Department of Cardiology, Ospedali del Tigullio, Lavagna, Italy.
Chapter 26

Harry R. Büller
Professor and Chair, Department of Vascular Medicine, University of Amsterdam, Amsterdam, The Netherlands.
Chapter 37

Paolo G. Camici
Professor of Cadiovascular Pathophysiology, Imperial College School of Medicine, Hammersmith Hospital, London, UK.
Chapters 7 and *17*

A. John Camm
British Heart Foundation Professor of Clinical Cardiology, Head of the Division of Cardiac and Vascular Sciences, St. George's University of London, London, UK.
Chapter 29

Fausto Castriota
GVM Hospitals of Care and Research, Interventional Cardio Angiology Unit, Cotignola (RA), Italy.
Chapter 36

Domenico Corrado
Professor of Cardiovascular Medicine, Department of Cardiac, Thoracic and Vascular Sciences, University of Padua, Padova, Italy.
Chapter 32

Francesco Cosentino
Division of Cardiology, 2nd Faculty of Medicine, University 'La Sapienza', Ospedale Sant'Andrea, Rome, Italy.
Chapter 14

Francisco G. Cosío
Chief Cardiology Service, Hospital Universitario de Getafe, Madrid, Spain.
Chapter 2

Filippo Crea
Professor of Cardiology, Director, Institute of Cardiology, Catholic University of the Sacred Heart, Rome, Italy.
Chapter 17

Alberto Cremonesi
GVM Hospitals of Care and Research, Interventional Cardio Angiology Unit, Cotignola (RA), Italy.
Chapter 36

Jean Dallongeville
Service d'Epidémiologie et Santé Publique, INSERM 744, Institut Pasteur de Lille, Lille, France.
Chapter 12

Werner G. Daniel
Professor of Internal Medicine, University of Erlangen, Erlangen, Germany.
Chapters 4 and 22

Estêvão Carvalho de Campos Martins
GVM Hospitals of Care and Research, Interventional Cardio Angiology Unit, Cotignola (RA), Italy.
Chapter 36

Raffaele De Caterina
Director of University Cardiology Division, Università degli, Studi di Chieti G D'Annunzio, Chieti, Italy.
Chapter 17

Pim J. de Feyter
Department of Cardiology and Radiology, Erasmus Medical Center, Erasmus University, Rotterdam, The Netherlands.
Chapter 6

John E. Deanfield
Head of Cardiothoracic Unit, Institute of Child Health, University College London, London, UK.
Chapter 10

Johan Denollet
Professor of Medical Psychology, Department of Medical Psychology and Neuropsychology, Center of Research on Psychology in Somatic diseases (CoRPS), Tilburg, The Netherlands.
Chapter 35

Carlo Di Mario
Royal Brompton Hospital & Imperial College, London, UK.
Chapter 8

Nicolas Diehm
Swiss Cardiovascular Center, Division of Clinical and Interventional Angiology, Inselspital, University of Bern, Switzerland.
Chapter 36

Hans-Christoph Diener
Department of Neurology and Stroke Center, University Hospital Essen, Germany.
Chapter 15a

Robert Dion
Head of Cardiac Surgery, ZOL–Campus St-Jan, Genk, Belgium.
Chapter 21

Lars Eckardt
Professor and Head of Department of Electrophysiology, Department of Cardiology and Angiology, University of Münster, Münster, Germany.
Chapter 30

Holger Eggebrecht
Department of Cardiology, West-German Heart Center Essen, University Duisburg-Essen, Germany.
Chapter 31

Raimund Erbel
Head of Cardiology, University of Essen, Essen, Germany.
Chapter 31

Sabine Ernst
Consultant Cardiologist, Royal Brompton and Harefield Hospital, London, UK.
Chapter 29

Robert H. Fagard
Hypertension and Cardiovascular Rehabilitation Unit, Department of Cardiovascular Diseases, Faculty of Medicine, University of Leuven, Leuven, Belgium.
Chapter 13

Gianluca Faggioli
Department of Vascular Surgery, Alma Mater Studiorum, University of Bologna, Policlinico S. Orsola-Malpighi, Bologna, Italy.
Chapter 36

Jerónimo Farré
Professor and Chairman, Department of Cardiology, Fundación Jiménez Diaz – Capio, Universidad Autonoma de Madrid, Madrid, Spain.
Chapter 28

Frank A. Flachskampf
Professor of Internal Medicine, University of Erlangen, Erlangen, Germany.
Chapters 4 and 22

Pietro Francia
Division of Cardiology, 2nd Faculty of Medicine, University 'La Sapienza', Ospedale Sant'Andrea, Rome, Italy.
Chapter 14

Nazzareno Galiè
Pulmonary Hypertension Center, Institute of Cardiology, Bologna University Hospital, Bologna, Italy.
Chapter 24

Roy Gardner
Golden Jubilee, West of Scotland Heart Centre, Glasgow, UK.
Chapter 23

Mauro Gargiulo
Department of Vascular Surgery, Alma Mater Studiorum, University of Bologna, Policlinico S. Orsola-Malpighi, Bologna, Italy.
Chapter 36

Stephan Gielen
Assistant Professor of Medicine, University of Leipzig – Heart Center, Department of Internal Medicine/ Cardiology, Leipzig, Germany.
Chapter 25

Christianne J.M. Groot
Gynaecologist/Obstetrician, Department of Obstetrics and Gynaecology, Erasmus Medical Center, Rotterdam, The Netherlands.
Chapter 33

Roger Hall
Professor of Cardiology, University of East Anglia; Consultant Cardiologist, Norfolk and Norwich University Hospital; Visiting Professor of Cardiology, Imperial College School of Medicine; Honorary Consultant Cardiologist, Hammersmith Hospital, UK.
Chapter 1

Rainer Hambrecht
Professor of Medicine, Medical Director, Klinikum Links der Weser, Department of Cardiology and Angiology, Bremen, Germany.
Chapter 25

Christian W. Hamm
Professor of Medicine and Medical Director, Kerckhoff Klinik, Heart and Thorax Center, Bad Nauheim, Germany.
Chapter 16

Axel Haverich
Head of Cardiothoracic Surgery, University of Hannover, Hannover, Germany.
Chapter 31

Otto M. Hess
Department of Cardiology, Universitätsklinik Inselspital, Bern, Switzerland.
Chapter 18

Guy R. Heyndrickx
Onze Lieve Ziekenhuis Cardiovascular Center Aalst, Belgium.
Chapter 8

Sanne Hoeks
Department of Vascular Surgery, Erasmus Medical Center, Rotterdam, The Netherlands.
Chapter 34

Stefan Hohnloser
Professor of Medicine and Cardiology, J.W. Goethe University, Department of Cardiology, Division of Clinical Electrophysiology, Frankfurt, Germany.
Chapter 30

Steve E. Humphries
Centre for the Genetics of Cardiovascular Disease, British Heart Foundation Laboratories, Rayne Building, Royal Free and University College London Medical School, London, UK.
Chapter 9

Bernard Iung
Cardiologist, Bichat Hospital, Paris, France.
Chapter 21

Graham Jackson
Honorary Consultant Cardiologist, Guy's and St Thomas' NHS Trust, London, UK.
Chapter 15c

Demosthenes G. Katritsis
Department of Cardiology, Athens Euroclinic, Athens, Greece; Cardiothoracic Centre, Guy's and St Thomas' Hospitals, London, UK.
Chapter 38

Philipp A. Kaufmann
Professor and Director of Cardiac Imaging, University Hospital Zürich, Zürich, Switzerland.
Chapter 7

Paulus Kirchhof
Professor, Department of Cardiology and Angiology, University Hospital Münster, German Atrial Fibrillation competence NETwork (AFNET), Universitätsklinikum Münster, Münster, Germany.
Chapter 29

Sverre E. Kjeldsen
Department of Cardiology, Ullevaal University Hospital, Oslo, Norway.
Chapter 13

Michel Komajda
Department of Cardiology, Pitie Salpetriere Hospital, University Pierre et Marie Curie, Paris, France.
Chapter 23

Nina Kupper
Department of Medical Psychology and Neuropsychology, Center of Research on Psychology in Somatic diseases (CoRPS), Tilburg, The Netherlands.
Chapter 35

Gaetano A. Lanza
Università Cattolica di Roma, Istituto di Cardiologia, Rome, Italy.
Chapter 17

Gregory Y.H. Lip
Professor of Cardiovascular Medicine, Haemostasis Thrombosis and Vascular Biology Unit, University Department of Medicine, City Hospital, Birmingham, UK.
Chapter 29

Massimo Lombardi
Consultant, Head Magnetic Resonance Laboratory, Institute of Clinical Physiology, National Research Council, Pisa, Italy.
Chapter 20

Giuseppe Mancia
Clinica Medica, Ospedale San Gerardo, Universita di Milano-Bicocca, Monza, Italy.
Chapter 13

Alessandra Manes
Pulmonary Hypertension Center, Institute of Cardiology, Bologna University Hospital, Bologna, Italy.
Chapter 24

Heinrich Mattle
Department of Neurology, University Hospital Bern, Bern, Switzerland.
Chapter 15a

Hercules E. Mavrakis
Senior Registrar in Cardiology, Heraklion University Hospital, Crete, Greece.
Chapter 27

William McKenna
Department of Cardiology, The Heart Hospital, London, UK.
Chapter 18

John McMurray
BHF Cardiovascular Research Centre, University of Glasgow, Glasgow, UK.
Chapter 23

Folkert J. Meijboom
Pediatric and GUCH Cardiologist, Departments of Cardiology and Pediatric Cardiology, University Medical Center Utrecht, Utrecht, The Netherlands.
Chapter 10

Linda G. Mellbin
Department of Cardiology, Karolinska University Hospital, Stockholm, Sweden.
Chapter 14

Alessandro Mezzani
Fondatione Salvatore Maugeri, Division of Cardiology, Veruno, Italy.
Chapter 25

Helge Möllmann
Kerckhoff Klinik, Heart and Thorax Center, Bad Nauheim, Germany.
Chapter 16

Laurent Monassier
Professor of Pharmacology, Laboratoire de Neurobiologie et Pharmacologie Cardiovasculaire, Faculté de Médecine, Université de Strasbourg, Strasbourg, France.
Chapter 11

Angel Moya
Department of Cardiology, Hospital General Vall d'Hebron, Barcelona, Spain.
Chapter 26

Barbara J.M. Mulder
Department of Cardiology, Academic Medical Center, Amsterdam, The Netherlands.
Chapter 10

Carlo Napolitano
Molecular Cardiology Laboratories, IRCCS Fondazione Salvatore Maugeri, Pavia, Italy; and Cardiovascular Genetics, Leon Charney Division of Cardiology, Langone Medical Center, New York University School of Medicine, New York, USA.
Chapter 9

Koen Nieman
Department of Cardiology, Erasmus Medical Center, Erasmus University, Rotterdam, The Netherlands.
Chapter 6

Christoph A. Nienaber
Head of Cardiology, Pulmonology and Intensive Care Unit, University of Rostock, Rostock, Germany.
Chapter 31

Ambrosio Núñez
Cardiology Service, Hospital Universitario de Getafe, Madrid, Spain.
Chapter 2

José Palacios
Cardiology Service, Hospital 12 de Octubre, Madrid, Spain.
Chapter 2

Agustín Pastor
Cardiology Service, Hospital Universitario de Getafe, Madrid, Spain.
Chapter 2

Susanne S. Pedersen
Associate Professor, Department of Medical Psychology and Neuropsychology, Center of Research on Psychology in Somatic diseases (CoRPS), Tilburg, The Netherlands.
Chapter 35

Antonio Pelliccia
Institute of Sports Medicine and Science, Rome, Italy.
Chapter 32

Dudley J. Pennell
Professor of Cardiology, National Heart and Lung Institute, Imperial College; and Director, Cardiovascular MR Unit, Royal Brompton Hospital, London, UK.
Chapter 5

John Pepper
Consultant Cardiac Surgeon, Royal Brompton Hospital, London, UK.
Chapter 21

Joep Perk
Professor of Health Sciences, School of Human Sciences, University of Kalmar, Kalmar, Sweden.
Chapter 12

Mark Petrie
Golden Jubilee, West of Scotland Heart Centre, Glasgow, UK.
Chapter 23

Luc Piérard
Head of Cardiology, C.H.U. Du Sart-Tilman, Université de Liège – Service De Cardiologie, Liège, Belgium.
Chapter 21

Nico H.J. Pijls
Catharina University Hospital, Eindhoven, The Netherlands.
Chapter 8

Don Poldermans
Department of Vascular Surgery, Erasmus Medical Center, Rotterdam, The Netherlands.
Chapter 34

Sanjay Prasad
Consultant Cardiologist, Cardiovascular Magnetic Resonance Unit, Royal Brompton Hospital, National Heart and Lung Institute, Imperial College London, London, UK.
Chapter 5

Francesco Prati
San Giovanni Battista Hospital, Rome, Italy.
Chapter 8

Patrizia Presbitero
Chief of Interventional Cardiology Department, Istituto Clinico Humanitas, Rozzano, Italy.
Chapter 33

Silvia G. Priori
Molecular Cardiology Laboratories, IRCCS Fondazione Salvatore Maugeri, Pavia, and Department of Cardiology University of Pavia, Pavia, Italy; and Cardiovascular Genetics, Leon Charney Division of Cardiology, Langone Medical Center, New York University School of Medicine, New York, USA.
Chapter 9

Frank E. Rademakers
Department of Cardiology, University Hospitals Leuven, Leuven, Belgium.
Chapter 5

Andrew Remppis
Department of Internal Medicine, Divisions of Nephrology and Cardiology, Ruperto-Carola University Heidelberg, Heidelberg, Germany.
Chapter 15b

Eberhard Ritz
Department of Internal Medicine, Divisions of Nephrology and Cardiology, Ruperto-Carola University Heidelberg, Heidelberg, Germany.
Chapter 15b

Jolien W. Roos-Hesselink
Cardiologist, Department of Cardiology, Erasmus Medical Center, Rotterdam, The Netherlands.
Chapter 33

Annika Rosengren
Professor, Department of Medicine, Sahlgrenska Academy/Sahlgrenska University Hospital, Gothenburg, Sweden.
Chapter 12

José M. Rubio
Director, Arrhythmia Unit, Department of Cardiology, Fundación Jiménez Díaz – CAPIO, Madrid, Spain.
Chapter 28

Frank Ruschitzka
Department of Cardiology, Center for Heart Diseases, University Hospital Zürich, Zürich, Switzerland.
Chapter 15, Chapter 15a

Lars Rydén
Department of Cardiology, Karolinska University Hospital, Stockholm.
Chapter 14

Jaume Sagristà-Sauleda
Universitat Autònoma de Barcelona, Hospital Universitari Vall d'Hebron, Barcelona, Spain.
Chapter 19

Hugo Saner
Professor of Medicine, Medical Director, Cardiovascular Prevention and Rehabilitation, Department of Cardiology, Swiss Cardiovascular Center, Inselspital, Berne, Switzerland.
Chapter 25

Irina Savelieva
Lecturer in Cardiology, Division of Cardiac and Vascular Sciences, St. George's University of London, London, UK.
Chapter 29

Sebastian M. Schellong
Head of Medical Division 2, Municipal Hospital Friedrichstadt, Dresden, Germany.
Chapter 37

Joanne D. Schuijf
Department of Cardiology, Leiden University Medical Center, Leiden, The Netherlands.
Chapter 3

Heinz-Peter Schultheiss
Professor and Director Cardiology and Pulmonology, University Hospital Benjamin Franklin, Berlin, Germany.
Chapter 18

Udo P. Sechtem
Chief, Division of Cardiology, Robert-Bosch Hospital, Stuttgart; and Associate Professor of Medicine and Cardiology, University of Tübingen, Germany.
Chapter 5

Iain Simpson
Consultant Cardiologist, Wessex Regional Cardiac Unit, Southampton University Hospital, Southampton, UK.

James Skipworth
Centre for the Genetics of Cardiovascular Disease, British Heart Foundation Laboratories, Rayne Building, Royal Free and University College London Medical School, London, UK.
Chapter 9

Jordi Soler-Soler
Professor of Cardiology, Universitat Autònoma de Barcelona, Hospital Universitari Vall d'Hebron, Barcelona, Spain.
Chapter 19

Andrea Stella
Department of Vascular Surgery, Alma Mater Studiorum, University of Bologna, Policlinico S. Orsola-Malpighi, Bologna, Italy.
Chapter 36

Richard Sutton
St Mary's Hospital and Imperial College, London, UK.
Chapter 26

Karl Swedberg
Department of Medicine, Sahlgrenska University Hospital/ Ostra, Goteborg, Sweden.
Chapter 23

Gaetano Thiene
Full Professor, Cardiovascular Pathology – Department of Medical-Diagnostic Sciences and Special Therapies, University of Padua Medical School, Padua, Italy.
Chapters 20 and 32

William D. Toff
Senior Lecturer in Cardiology, University of Leicester, Leicester, UK.
Chapter 27

S. Richard Underwood
Professor of Cardiac Imaging, National Heart and Lung Institute, Imperial College, Royal Brompton Hospital, London, UK.
Chapter 7

Alec Vahanian
Head of Cardiology, Bichat Hospital, Paris, France.
Chapter 21

Marialuisa Valente
Full Professor, Pathological Anatomy – Department of Medical-Diagnostic Sciences and Special Therapies, University of Padua Medical School, Padua, Italy.
Chapter 20

Nico R. Van de Veire
Department of Cardiology, Leiden University Medical Center, Leiden, The Netherlands.
Chapter 3

Frans Van de Werf
Professor and Head of Department of Cardiology, Gasthuisberg University Hospital, Leuven, Belgium.
Chapter 16

Panos E. Vardas
Professor of Cardiology, University of Crete and Head of the Cardiology Department, Heraklion University Hospital, Crete, Greece.
Chapter 27

Jens-Uwe Voigt
Professor of Cardiology, University of Leuven, Leuven, Belgium.
Chapter 4

Ernst E. van der Wall
Department of Cardiology, Leiden University Medical Center, Leiden, The Netherlands.
Chapter 3

Michael M. Webb-Peploe
Cardiothoracic Centre, Guy's and St Thomas' Hospitals, London, UK.
Chapter 38

Hein J.J. Wellens
Cardiovascular Research Institute Maastricht, Maastricht, The Netherlands.
Chapter 28

Robert Yates
Great Ormond Street Hospital, London, UK.
Chapter 10

Faiez Zannad
Chairman, ESC Working Group on Pharmacology and Drug Therapy; Professor of Therapeutics and Cardiology, Director, Clinical Investigation Center INSERM; Head, Heart Failure and Hypertension Unit, Department of Cardiology, CHU and University Henri Poincaré, Nancy, France.
Chapter 11

Reviewers

The editors would like to thank the reviewers who were involved with the preparation of the second edition of this textbook:

Maria João Andrade, Helmut Baumgartner, Carina Blomström Lundqvist, Kenneth Dickstein, Paul Dubach, Krzysztof J. Filipiak, Dan Gaita, Thierry Gillebert, Gilbert Habib, Hein Heidbuchel, Michael Joy, Desmond Julian, Peter Kearney, Cecilia Linde, Jose Lopez-Sendon, Hercules Mavrakis, Donato Mele, Luis Moura, Els Pieper, Claudio Rapezzi, Peta Seferovic, Sanjay Sharma, Otto Smiseth, Michal Tendera, Adam Torbicki, Renee van den Brink, Ronald Wilders.

Acknowledgement to first edition contributors

The editors would like to thank the first edition contributors whose excellent text and illustrations have been continued into this second edition:

Etienne Aliot
Maurits A. Allessie
Bert Andersson
Annalisa Angelini
Velislav N. Batchvarov
Iris Baumgartner
Antoni Bayés de Luna
Giancarlo Biamino
Carina Blomström-Lundqvist
Eric Boersma
Pedro Brugada
José A. Cabrera
Alessandro Capucci
Christian de Chillou
Harry J.G.M. Crijns
Maria Cristina Digilio
Erling Falk
Keith A.A. Fox
Kim Fox
Liv Hatle
Christopher Heeschen
Aroon Hingorani
Vibeke E. Hjortda
Roger Hullin
Pierre Jaïs
Lukas Kappenberger
Paul Kotwinski
Uwe Kühl
Christophe Leclercq
Cecilia Linde
Raymond MacAllister
Felix Mahler
Bernhard Maisch
Marek Malik
Bruno Marino
Raad H. Mohiaddin
John Morgan
Michel Noutsias
S. Bertil Olsson
Mathias Pauschinger
Henry Purcell
Henrik M. Reims
Arsen D. Ristic
Jos Roelandt
Marco Roffi
Srijita Sen-Chowdhry
Dierk Scheinert
Andrej Schmidt
Peter J. Schwartz
Christian Seiler
Mary N. Sheppard
Gerald Simonneau
Marko Turina
Patrick Vallance
William Wijns
Felix Zijlstra

Although first edition figure attributions have been carried over to the second edition it was not possible to make specific attributions to figures contributed by first edition authors.

Symbols and abbreviations

➲	cross reference
🎥	additional online material
🔗	website
(e)NOS	(endothelial) nitric oxide synthase
2D	two-dimensional
3D	three-dimensional
AACVPR	American Association of Cardiovascular Prevention and Rehabilitation
ABCD	Appropriate Blood pressure Control in Diabetes
ACC	American College of Cardiology
ACCP	American College of Chest Physicians
ACE	angiotensin-converting enzyme
ACEI	angiotensin-converting enzyme inhibitor
ACM	all-cause mortality *or* alcoholic cardiomyopathy
ACT	activated coagulation time
ADA	American Diabetes Association
ADH	antidiuretic hormone
ADP	adenosine diphosphate
AED	automated external defibrillator
AF	atrial fibrillation
AGE	advanced glycation end-product
AH	atrial–His
AHA	American Heart Association
ALAT	alanine amino transferase
ALT	alanine aminotransferase
AMDG	airport metal detector gates
AMI	acute myocardial infarction
ANP	atrial natriuretic peptide
Ao	aorta
AoA	aortic orifice area
apoB	apolipoprotein B
apoE	apolipoprotein E
aPTT	activated partial thromboplastin time
AR	aortic regurgitation
ARB	angiotensin receptor blocker
ARR	absolute risk reduction
ART	assisted reproductive technology
ARVC	arrhythmogenic right ventricular cardiomyopathy
AS	aortic stenosis
ASA	acetylsalicylic acid
AST	aspartate aminotransferase
ASD	atrial septal defect
ASF	anterosuperior fascicle
AST	aspartate aminotransferase
ATP	adenosine triphosphate
AV	atrioventricular
AVA	aortic valve area
AVN	atrioventricular node
AVNRT	atrioventricular nodal re-entrant tachycardia
AVP	arginine vasopressin
AVSD	atrioventricular septal defect
BAV	bicuspid aortic valve
BB	bundle branch/es
BIMA	bilateral internal mammary artery
BMP	bone morphogenetic protein
BNP	brain natriuretic peptide
BOLD	blood oxygen level dependent
BP	blood pressure
BPEG	British Pacing and Electrophysiology Group
bpm	beats per minute
BRS	baroreflex sensitivity
BrS	Brugada syndrome
BSA	body surface area
BUN	blood urea nitrogen
CABG	coronary artery bypass graft
CACS	coronary artery calcium scoring

CAD	coronary artery disease
CAM	cell adhesion molecule
CAPD	continuous ambulatory peritoneal dialysis
CAT	common arterial trunk
CBT	cognitive behavioural therapy
CCR	comprehensive cardiac rehabilitation
CCUS	complete or comprehensive compression ultrasound
CEA	carcinoembryonic antigen *or* carotid endarterectomy
CETP	cholesteryl ester transfer protein
CFR	coronary flow reserve
CHD	coronary heart disease
CHF	chronic heart failure
CI	cardiac index *or* confidence interval
CK	creatine kinase
CKD	chronic kidney disease
CMR	cardiac magnetic resonance
CO	cardiac output
COX	cyclo-oxygenase
CPET	cardiopulmonary exercise testing
CPK	creatine phosphokinase
CPR	cardiopulmonary resuscitation
CPVT	catecholaminergic polymorphic ventricular tachycardia
CR	cardiac rehabilitation
CRF	conventional risk factor
CRT	cardiac resynchronization therapy
cSNRT	corrected sinus node recovery time
CTPA	computed tomography pulmonary angiography
CTPH	chronic thromboembolic pulmonary hypertension
CUS	compression ultrasound
CV	cardiovascular
CVD	cardiovascular disease
CVM	cardiovascular mortality
CW	continuous-wave
CYP	cytochrome P450
DAG	dystrophin-associated glycoprotein
DCM	dilated cardiomyopathy
DES	drug-eluting stent
D_LCO	diffusion capacity for carbon monoxide
DSA	digital subtraction angiography
DSE	dobutamine stress echocardiography
DTI	direct thrombin inhibitor
DVT	deep vein thrombosis
EASD	European Association for the Study of Diabetes *or* electronic article surveillance
EBCT	electron-beam computed tomography
EBM	evidence-based medicine
ECG	electrocardiogram
ED	end-diastolic *or* Emergency Department
EDMD	Emery–Dreyfuss muscular dystrophy
EDV	end-diastolic volume
EEG	electroencephalogram
EEL	external elastic lamina
EEM	external elastic membrane
EF	ejection fraction
EHRA	European Heart Rhythm Association
ELISA	enzyme-linked immunosorbent assay
EMI	electromagnetic interference
eNOS	endothelial nitric oxide synthase
EPI	echo-planar imaging
EPO	erythropoietin
ER	European Region
ERO	effective regurgitant orifice
ES	end-systole *or* effect size
ESC	European Society of Cardiology
ESH	European Society of Hypertension
ET	endothelin
EU	Eustachian valve *or* European Union
FDCM	familial dilated cardiomyopathy
FEV_1	forced expiratory volume at 1 second
FFR	fractional flow reserve
FH	familial hypercholesterolaemia
FLAIR	fluid attenuated inversion recovery
FLASH	fast low angle shot
FPG	fasting plasma glucose
FXaI	factor Xa inhibitor
GFR	glomerular filtration rate
GIK	glucose–insulin–potassium
GORD	gastro-oesophageal reflux disease
GUCH	grown-up congenital heart
GWAS	genome-wide association study
HB	His bundle
Hb	haemoglobin
HBE	His bundle electrogram
HCM	hypertrophic cardiomyopathy
HCTZ	hydrochlorothiazide
HDL	high-density lipoprotein
HELLP	haemolysis elevated liver enzymes low platelets
HES	hypereosinophilic syndrome
HF-PEF	heart failure with preserved left ventricular ejection fraction
HHT	hereditary haemorrhagic telangiectasia
HIPA	heparin-induced platelet activation

HIT	heparin-induced thrombocytopenia
HIV	human immunodeficiency virus
HLHS	hypoplastic left heart syndrome
HMG-CoA	5-hydroxy-3-methylglutaryl-coenzyme A
HPA	hypothalamus–pituitary–adrenal
HR	hazard ratio
HRQL	health-related quality of life
HRV	heart rate variability
HV	His–ventricular
ICA	internal carotid artery
ICD	implantable cardioverter defibrillator
IEL	internal elastic lamina
IFG	impaired fasting glucose
IGT	impaired glucose tolerance
IHD	ischaemic heart disease
IMR	index of microvascular resistance
INR	international normalized ratio
IPAH	idiopathic pulmonary arterial hypertension
IPT	interpersonal therapy
ISH	International Society of Hypertension
ITT	intention to treat
IV	intravenous
IVUS	intravascular ultrasound
JLN	Jervell and Lange–Nielsen [syndrome]
JVP	jugular venous pulse
K/DOQI	Kidney Disease Outcome Quality Initiative
KCCQ	Kansas City Cardiomyopathy Questionnaire
LA	left atrium/atrial
LAA	left atrial appendage
LAD	left anterior descending
LBB	left bundle branch
LBBB	left bundle branch block
LCA	left coronary artery
LCSD	left cardiac sympathetic denervation
LCX	left circumflex coronary artery
LDL	low-density lipoprotein
LDL-C	low-density lipoprotein cholesterol
LGE	late gadolinium enhancement
LGMD	limb girdle muscular dystrophy
LIMA	left internal mammary artery
LMWH	low-molecular-weight heparin
LOE	level of evidence
LQTS	long QT syndrome
LV	left ventricle/ventricular
LVAD	left ventricular assist device
LVEDP	left ventricular filling pressure
LVEF	left ventricular ejection fraction
LVH	left ventricular hypertrophy
LVM	left ventricular mass
LVNC	left ventricular non-compaction
LVOT	left ventricular outflow tract
MA	mitral annulus
MAPCA	major aortic pulmonary collateral artery
MAPK	mitogen-activated protein kinase
MAS	multiple system atrophy
MBM	mechanism-based medicine
mcg	microgram
MDRD	Modification of Diet in Renal Disease
MDTD	maximum daily therapeutic dose
MFS	Marfan syndrome
MHC	major histocompatibility complex
MI	myocardial infarction
MIBG	meta-iodobenzylguanidine
MMP	matrix metalloproteinase
MPa	megapascal
MPA	main pulmonary artery
MPS	myocardial perfusion scintigraphy
MR	magnetic resonance
MS	metabolic syndrome
MSCT	multislice computed tomography
MTWA	microvolt T-wave alternans
MV	mitral valve
MVA	mitral valve area
MVP	mitral valve prolapse
n-3 PUFA	omega-3 polyunsaturated fatty acid
NASPE	North American Society of Pacing and Electrophysiology
NFMI	non-fatal myocardial infarction
NFS	nephrogenic systemic fibrosis
NGAL	neutrophil gelatinase-associated lipocalin
NHLBI	National Heart, Lung, and Blood Institute
NIDDK	National Institute of Diabetes and Digestive and Kidney Diseases
NM	nuclear myocardial
NNH	number needed to harm
NNT	number needed to treat
NO	nitric oxide
NOS	nitric oxide synthase
NRT	nicotine replacement therapy
NSAID	non-steroidal anti-inflammatory drug
NSTE-ACS	non-ST-elevated acute coronary syndrome
NSVT	non-sustained ventricular tachycardia
NT-proBNP	N-terminal prohormone brain natriuretic peptide

NYHA	New York Heart Association
OAC	oral anticoagulation therapy
OCT	optical coherence tomography
OFDI	optical frequency domain imaging
OGTT	oral glucose tolerance test
OH	orthostatic hypotension
OR	odds ratio
PA	pulmonary artery
PAC	premature atrial contraction
P_aCO_2	arterial carbon dioxide tension
PAD	peripheral arterial disease
PAF	pure autonomic failure
PAH	pulmonary arterial hypertension
PAI	plasminogen activator inhibitor
P_aO_2	arterial oxygen tension
PAP	pulmonary artery pressure
PAR	pulmonary arteriolar resistance
PASP	pulmonary artery systolic pressure
PAV	percutaneous aortic valvuloplasty
PCCD	progressive cardiac conduction defect
PCI	percutaneous coronary intervention
PCM	physical counter-pressure manoeuvre
PCR	polymerase chain reaction
PCW	pulmonary wedge pressure
PDA	posterior descending artery
PDE	phosphodiesterase
PDE-5	phosphodiesterase type 5
PE	pulmonary embolism
PES	programmed electrical stimulation
PET	positron emission tomography
PF	physical functioning
PFHB	progressive familial heart block
PH	pulmonary hypertension
PHQ	Patient Health Questionnaire
PI	posteroinferior fascicle
PIC	pro-inflammatory cytokine
PIH	pregnancy-induced hypertension
PISA	proximal isovelocity surface area
PKC	protein kinase C
PMC	percutaneous mitral balloon commissurotomy
PMI	point of maximal impulse or perioperative myocardial infarction
PMR	progressive muscle relaxation
PND	paroxysmal nocturnal dyspnoea
PO	per os [by mouth]
POTS	postural orthostatic tachycardia syndrome
PPCM	peripartum cardiomyopathy
PPHN	persistent pulmonary hypertension of the neonates
PSS	post-systolic shortening
PTA	percutaneous transluminal angioplasty
PTCA	percutaneous transluminal coronary angioplasty
PTEA	pulmonary thromboendarterectomy
PTFE	polytetrafluoretilene
PTH	parathyroid hormone
PTS	post-thrombotic syndrome
PTSD	post-traumatic stress disorder
PV	pressure–volume
PVD	peripheral vascular disease
PVR	pulmonary vascular resistance
PW	pulsed-wave
PWP	pulmonary wedge pressure
QTL	quantitative trait loci
RA	right atrium
RAA	renin–angiotensin–aldosterone
RAAS	renin–angiotensin–aldosterone system
RAS	renin–angiotensin system
RBB	right bundle branch
RBBB	right bundle branch block
RCA	right coronary artery
ROC	receiver operating characteristic
ROS	reactive oxygen species
RR	relative risk
RRR	relative risk reduction
rtPA	recombinant tissue plasminogen activator
RV	right ventricle/ventricular
RVA	right ventricular apex
RVOT	right ventricular outflow tract
SAECG	signal-averaged electrocardiogram
SAM	systolic anterior motion
SAQ	Seattle Angina Questionnaire
SBP	systolic blood pressure
SCD	sudden cardiac death
SES	sirolimus-eluting stents *or* socio-economic status
SF-36	Short Form Health Survey 36
SMR	standardized mortality ratio
SNP	single nucleotide polymorphism
SPECT	single photon emission computed tomography
SQTS	short QT syndrome
SR	sustained release
SR	sarcoplasmic reticulum
SSFP	steady state with free precession
SSI	steady state inactivation

SSRI	selective serotonin reuptake inhibitor
SSS	sick sinus syndrome
STEMI	ST-elevation myocardial infarction
STS	Society of Thoracic Surgeons
SV	stroke volume
SVI	stroke volume index
SVR	systemic vascular resistance
SVT	supraventricular tachycardia
TAPVC	total anomalous pulmonary venous connection
TAVI	transcatheter aortic valve implantation
TC	Takotsubo cardiomyopathy
TCA	tricyclic antidepressant
TCMP	tachycardia-induced cardiomyopathy
TCPC	total cavopulmonary connection
TDI	tissue Doppler imaging
TdP	Torsade de pointes
TE	echo time
TGA	transposition of the great arteries
TIA	transient ischaemic attack
TIMI	thrombolysis in myocardial infarction
T-LOC	transient loss of consciousness
TOE	transoesophageal echocardiography
tPA	tissue plasminogen activator
TPG	transpulmonary pressure gradient
TPR	total pulmonary resistance
TR	tricuspid regurgitation
TS	tricuspid stenosis
TSH	thyroid-stimulating hormone
TTE	transthoracic echocardiography
TTM	trans-telephonic monitoring
TWA	T-wave alternans
UFH	unfractionated heparin
VD	volume of distribution
VEGF	vascular endothelial growth factor
VF	ventricular fibrillation
VHD	valvular heart disease
VKA	vitamin K antagonist
VLDL	very-low-density lipoprotein
VPB	ventricular premature beat
VSD	ventricular septal defect
VT	ventricular tachycardia
VTE	venous thromboembolism
VVS	vasovagal syncope
WHO	World Health Organization
WPW	Wolff–Parkinson–White syndrome

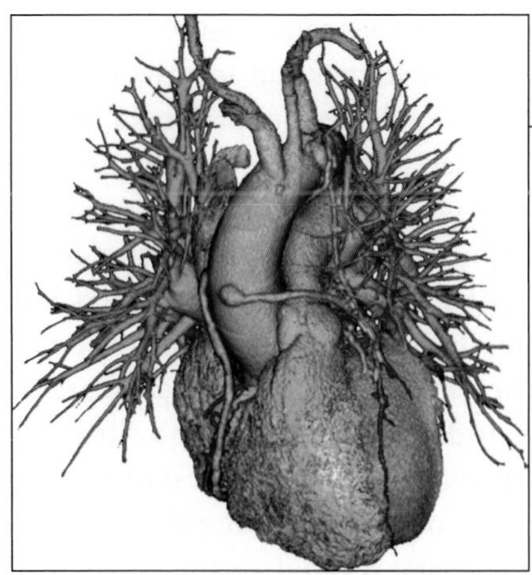

CHAPTER 1

The Cardiovascular History and Physical Examination

Roger Hall and Iain Simpson

Contents

Summary

A cardiovascular history and examination are fundamental to accurate diagnosis and the subsequent delivery of appropriate care for an individual patient. Time spent on a thorough history and examination is rarely wasted and goes beyond the gathering of basic clinical information as it is also an opportunity to put the patient at ease and build confidence in the physician's ability to provide a holistic and confidential approach to their care. This chapter covers the basics of history taking and physical examination of the cardiology patient but then takes it to a higher level by trying to analyse the strengths and weaknesses of individual signs in clinical examination and to put them into the context of common clinical scenarios. In an ideal world there would always be time for a full clinical history and examination, but clinical urgency may dictate that this is impossible or indeed, when time critical treatment needs to be delivered, it may be inappropriate. This chapter provides an insight into delivering a tailored approach in certain, common clinical situations. Skills in clinical history and examination evolve with time and experience and this chapter provides a structured approach to clinical cardiovascular history and examination which should be seen as a framework on which to build clinical experience. It also provides a hierarchical approach to the importance of certain symptoms and signs in a variety of cardiovascular conditions. Clinical history and examination has changed with modern advances in cardiology and the development of sophisticated imaging techniques. Eponymous signs beloved of the 'Old Masters of Examination' are now of historical interest but are listed in ➲ Table 1.20 for information.

Introduction

An accurate history and a careful examination are probably the least expensive and the fastest and most powerful of the tools available to a physician [1]. Their effective use requires skill and experience. It is important to recognize that it is unusual to obtain the classic history of a condition combined with all the classic physical signs. Variations in history and difficulty in eliciting physical signs need to be understood. It is always a serious mistake to massage the history and the physical signs to fit a particular diagnosis.

History

Introduction

There needs to be an awareness of potential difficulties in obtaining a clear history [2]. Patients usually, but not always, try to tell the truth, as they perceive it, to their physician who will develop an instinct for this, and must always consider whether they are misinterpreting the information given to them by the patient.

The interaction between the patient and doctor is complex and determined by many factors (➲Table 1.1). Patients with a moderate rather than good command of the language may have difficulty in expressing subtle aspects of their story and may agree to suggestions made to them by the doctor, rather than admitting they do not completely understand what is being said to them. Many patients have a poor perception of parameters such as time and distance, which are frequently important in the cardiovascular history, and rather than admit they cannot answer the question put to them will sometimes make up an answer simply to please the doctor. The way the patient presents a history will also depend on the level of their education, and the type of work that they do [3]. The doctor taking a history must not make assumptions about the patient's underlying medical knowledge. There is a tendency among doctors to slip into medical jargon which is poorly understood or completely incomprehensible to the patient. A good example is that some patients do not understand the difference between a myocardial infarction and a cerebrovascular accident and the term 'stroke' may confuse them as they are not quite sure about what it is. Similarly the patient may describe either a cardiac arrest or a myocardial infarction as 'heart attack'. This problem can sometimes be avoided if it is clear that the patient is becoming confused by asking the patient how the particular illness affected them rather than by giving it a name. The same applies to the description of symptoms. For example, a patient may use the term 'palpitation' without really understanding what it means. This aspect of history taking is discussed in more detail in the sections dealing with specific symptoms.

Table 1.1 History taking: factors that may lead to problems

Patient-based factors
Command of language (usually patient)/history via an interpreter
Patient's cultural background
Education and employment
Inaccurate perception of variables, e.g. time and distance
Underplaying/exaggeration
Responses altered by:
Alcohol
Recreational drugs
Physician-based factors
Badly structured questions
Assumptions about patient's medical knowledge
Lack of patience
Asking 'leading questions', i.e. suggesting the required answer

Particular difficulties can arise when the history is taken via an interpreter and under these circumstances much more time must be put aside and strenuous efforts made to try to establish that the doctor is being given a clear account by the patient rather than by the interpreter. There is a strong tendency for the interpreter to make up their own version of the history and deliver it to the doctor rather than asking the patient exactly what the symptoms are and describing them in detail. This may be prominent when there are major cultural differences between the doctor and the patient (and interpreter). In some situations, particularly where women do not speak the language and their husband acts as an interpreter, there may be very considerable interpretation of the history rather than the language. It may be impossible to overcome these problems, but it is important that the doctor is aware of the difficulties and how they may obscure the transmission of information (see ➲Key point 1, p. 26).

The reaction of a patient to their symptoms is often complex [4]. Florid descriptions of symptoms (e.g. 'I had seven heart attacks' when in fact there had been one myocardial infarct and some episodes of angina) may become important to the patient, particularly if the patient is validated by their illness. In addition, it becomes real to the patient with repeated re-telling of the history. Conversely, in emergency situations, particularly with young patients, there may be a major downplaying of symptoms particularly

Box 1.1 Scenario 1: downplaying symptoms—the patient who wants to go home

A 45-year-old Asian male who smokes 20 cigarettes a day arrives in the emergency department at 02.00 hours. There is a history of a heavy feeling in the central and lower chest present for 45min, but easing off before the patient arrived. The patient admits to two or three alcoholic drinks and a spicy meal at 21.00 hours the previous evening. He now maintains that his problem is 'just indigestion', but the electrocardiogram (ECG) shows some minor ST/T wave changes. Despite the protestations of the patient, the chances of an acute coronary syndrome are high and this must be excluded.

if the patient is keen to leave the emergency room and go home (➲Box 1.1). This is particularly common in young and middle-aged males who are presenting for the first time with ischaemic chest pain. Generally patients do not present as emergencies unless they or their spouse, partner, or family have been alarmed by the event which has caused them to come to hospital (see ➲Key points 2 and 3, p.26). Doctors should be extremely cautious when confronted with the patient who has arrived in the A&E department in the early hours of the morning, who does not have a lengthy past medical history, and then begins to downplay their symptoms. These patients are usually ill.

The doctor has to navigate this complex situation to obtain an accurate history and nowadays may also have the added complication of the patient having already made up their mind about aspects of their illness having consulted the Internet and often arriving in the clinic clutching printouts from their computer. It is important to allow the patient to talk rather than putting words in their mouth, but then the use of judicious direct questioning is needed to refine the history.

It can be helpful at the end of the process for the doctor to summarize the history and repeat it back to the patient and ask them whether they agree. There is always the difficulty in this situation that the patient will agree, simply because they don't want to upset the doctor, but when done carefully this process can be an extremely powerful tool for finalizing the history and eradicating errors due to misunderstanding.

The basic cardiovascular history

On rare occasions, cardiovascular disease can lead to almost any symptom; however, the most common are listed in ➲Table 1.2. The basic principles for analysing each symptom remains the same, but it is extremely important that a systematic approach is always taken (➲Table 1.3). Patients may have inaccurate perceptions of time and distance (➲Boxes 1.2 and 1.3). If a patient has a recurrence of a particular cardiovascular condition their symptoms are usually very similar on each occasion. For example, the patient who in the past experienced most of their ischaemic pain in their arm will tend to do so on another occasion, but beware, this is not always the case. One must always consider that a previous incident ascribed by the patient to the same situation was in fact different and also the diagnosis they were given may have been incorrect. Finally, a history may be so characteristic that a strong provisional diagnosis can be made over the phone (➲Box 1.4).

Table 1.2 Cardiovascular history

Past and family history
Risk factors
Employment: may be affected by the presence of cardiac problems, e.g. professional drivers, pilots, divers etc.
Chest pain ± radiation
Shortness of breath/cough
Palpitations: awareness of irregular heartbeat
'Dizziness' and unsteadiness
Syncope and falls
Fatigue
Ankle oedema (a symptom and a sign)
Less common symptoms:
Abdominal pain
Vomiting with acute MI
Polyuria associated with tachycardia
Pulsating in the neck associated with tachycardia and with tricuspid regurgitation
Abdominal swelling—ascites
Weakness of legs
Back pain

Table 1.3 Always establish some basics for all symptoms

Nature and severity of symptom
Duration of symptom:
When did it start?
How long did it last?
How often does it occur?
Precipitating and relieving factors
Similarity to previous incidents
Impact on daily life and job

Box 1.2 Scenario 2: time perception

The patient gives a history that sounds typical of angina, but states the pain lasts for 20min after they stop exercising, therefore making a clinical diagnosis of angina unlikely. Is this really long lasting pain or does the patient have an inaccurate perception of time?

Solution

Ask the patient, who has only been in your office for < 5min, 'does the pain last as long as you have been in this room?'—the patient will often realise that they have mistakenly over-emphasized the amount of time and actually the pain lasts less time than they have been in the room. They may then revise their answer

Chest pain (➲Table 1.4)

Because of the prevalence and importance of coronary disease (➲Chapters 16 and 17) inevitably there is an emphasis on determining whether or not chest pain is likely to have an ischaemic origin (➲Table 1.5). Cardiac chest pain tends to be described by doctors as being typical or atypical; the term typical referring to whether it is typical of pain usually associated with myocardial ischaemia. The nomenclature of ischaemic chest pain can be slightly confusing. Ischaemic chest pain has similar characteristics but may vary in intensity. In general, chest pain associated with myocardial infarction is the most severe pain, followed by pain associated with acute coronary syndromes (ACSs), and then pain only occurring with a precipitating factor. Ischaemic chest pain induced by precipitating factors is usually referred to as angina while pain which tends to be constant, coming on spontaneously, and often associated with an ACS, is simply referred to as ischaemic chest pain.

Typical anginal chest pain (➲Tables 1.5 and 1.6) nearly always indicates myocardial ischaemia and in the vast majority of cases this symptom occurs because of coronary artery disease. It can, however, occur in patients with normal coronary arteries as a result of aortic stenosis (➲Chapter 21) (and, occasionally, aortic regurgitation) because the increased amount of cardiac muscle makes oxygen demands that exceed the amount of oxygen that can be delivered even by the large, normal coronary arteries in many of these patients. Occasionally, anginal chest pain may be prominent in patients in whom there is a right-sided cardiac problem, such as in patients with severe pulmonary hypertension (➲Chapter 24), e.g. primary pulmonary hypertension, Eisenmenger's syndrome (➲Chapter 10), and severe mitral stenosis (➲Chapter 21) in whom blood which may have reduced oxygen content flows down the coronary arteries

Box 1.3 Scenario 3: distance perception

The patient cannot remember how far they walk before the symptoms start

Solution

Ask the patient if he or she managed to walk from the hospital car park to your clinic without stopping or take some similar example within the route they would have taken to reach your clinic.

Box 1.4 Scenario 4: using the history to be prepared for rapid action

A 65-year-old man with treated hypertension but otherwise well, returned to his car with grocery shopping. As he leant forward to put the shopping bag in to the car he felt an extremely severe burning pain in the centre of the back of his chest and fell to the ground. The pain was so severe and intense he felt that he had somehow been stabbed by a hot object from behind. An ambulance was called who found him lying on the ground, looking extremely pale and in pain but fully conscious. This history was 'phoned to the hospital by the incoming ambulance. On the basis of this story the duty cardiologist suspected a dissecting aneurysm and mobilized the cardiac surgeons. A transoesophageal echocardiogram was performed immediately he arrived in the emergency department which confirmed a type A dissecting aneurysm and he was transferred immediately to the operating theatre. He was on the operating table within 90min of the incident occurring. The surgery was successful and the patient was discharged home 10 days later.

Table 1.4 Types of chest pain

Cardiac
Angina (coronary disease)
Pericarditis
Aortic aneurysm
Non-cardiac
Pleuritic
Musculoskeletal
Gastrointestinal—particularly, oesophageal
Other

Table 1.5 Ischaemic chest pain

Location:
Central or slightly to left of centre
May be experienced anywhere between the pubis and the top of the head. Pain may be only present in the areas of radiation and not in the chest
Nature: dull, pressing, constricting (for example 'elephant sitting on chest', 'strangling')
Occasionally described as either burning or stabbing
Body language: patient may indicate that the pain has a constricting nature or may hold a clenched fist in front of their chest. This is remarkably common and indicates the constricting nature of the discomfort.
Radiation of the pain:
Common—left arm, neck, jaw
Less common—right arm (or both), back, abdomen, teeth

to a hypertrophied right ventricle (RV) which has increased demands because of the high pressure that it is generating and increased muscle to supply (RV hypertrophy). A more extreme example of this phenomenon is when there is acute right heart strain in acute massive pulmonary embolism. The combination of severe arterial desaturation and increasing RV work may lead to RV ischaemia and anginal chest pain.

Anginal chest pain rarely occurs without a precipitating factor (➲Table 1.6). Chest pain that comes on when the patient is feeling well, unstressed, and is at rest is unlikely to be cardiac chest pain. The exception is when this is the first episode of an ACS (➲Chapter 16) which would not need a precipitating factor, or if there is some underlying factor which is not unveiled by the patient's history. The two most likely circumstances are either a cardiac arrhythmia which has not produced any awareness of palpitations or change in level of consciousness, but increases cardiac work, and coronary artery spasm, although quite rare in the European population, which leads to attacks of typical anginal pain without any obvious precipitating factor. The most common precipitating factors for ischaemic chest pain are presented in ➲Table 1.6. In most situations where anginal chest pain is precipitated by increased cardiac work the pain will go away 5min or less after the precipitating factor ceases.

Table 1.6 Precipitating factors of ischaemic chest pain

None
Onset of acute coronary syndrome
Coronary spasm
Underlying arrhythmia
Exercise
Mental stress (angina may be more prolonged than with exercise):
Anxiety
Anger
Stress-induced left ventricular dysfunction ('takotsubo')
Occurs on lying down (angina decubitus) often a sign of instability
Angina occurs more easily than usual:
After meals because of blood flow needed to the gastrointestinal tract
Extremely hot or cold weather
Recent onset of anaemia
Thyrotoxicosis
Hypoxia from some other cause, e.g. onset of heart failure.

It is important to question the patient about the offset of pain as well as the onset of pain. Truly prolonged chest pain, for example after exercise, is usually not angina except in the context of an ACS. A point which may be difficult to appreciate unless the history is taken extremely carefully is that the pain may actually be occurring after exercise rather than during exercise. A common example of this is the patient who carries out some physical work, for example carrying shopping bags, arrives home and then develops chest discomfort which is in fact musculoskeletal due to the chest wall stress produced by the effort of carrying the bags. Such pain often lasts considerably longer than the normal 5min seen with angina, despite the patient resting.

More prolonged pain usually indicates the possibility of an ACS or a non-cardiac cause. An exception to this is pain occurring when patients become angry or anxious. This often has a slow offset because the sensation of anger or anxiety may take a considerable period of time to abate. Angina may sometimes be precipitated by lying flat (angina decubitus); this usually indicates severe coronary disease and is caused by the increased venous return, generated by lying flat, increasing cardiac work. There may also be associated cardiac failure with hypoxia occurring due to incipient pulmonary oedema (➲Chapter 23) when this is made worse by the patient lying flat. Pain occurring when the patient lies flat must, however, be distinguished from oesophageal pain, usually due to reflux oesophagitis. This distinction is always difficult and often impossible on clinical grounds. If the pain is instantly relieved by antacids it is probably oesophageal. The same confidence cannot be attached to relief of pain by nitroglycerine (GTN). Immediate relief does favour ischaemic chest pain, but oesophageal pain, if associated with oesophageal spasm, is also relieved by GTN (and calcium-channel blockers) (➲Table 1.7).

Angina is often described by the patient as being uncomfortable rather than painful. The patient may simply say

Table 1.7 Response of symptoms to GTN

Anginal chest pain usually resolves with GTN within 1–5min. If response takes longer the diagnosis of angina should be questioned
GTN also relieves shortness of breath (and any associated chest constriction) due to left ventricular failure by reducing venous return
May relieve pain due to any kind of smooth muscle spasm, particularly oesophageal but occasionally gallstone colic
If the patient describes the response to GTN occurring after 5–10min then it is probable this is not a response to GTN but a spontaneous resolution of the pain

they have a discomfort in their chest which is not very painful but is unpleasant, and on occasions this discomfort may be described as breathlessness. The main reason is that the constricting nature of anginal symptoms makes the patient feel that they cannot take a deep breath. This difficulty in distinguishing breathlessness from angina by the history is very common. It may be impossible to make the distinction between angina and dyspnoea clinically, but prominent tightness and difficulty taking a breath because of tightness favours angina, whereas the sensation that they are panting as though they had just run somewhere rapidly favours dyspnoea. Finally, if resting lung function and left ventricular (LV) function on echo are normal, angina becomes much more likely.

One of the most difficult situations in patients presenting with acute chest pain is the patient in whom there is a statistically low chance of serious underlying disease [5]. The classical situation would be a young woman with what appears to be typical angina. Although the chances of anginal-type symptoms described by a woman in their 20s of being due to coronary disease are low, one has to accept there are a few female patients of this age with severe coronary disease and if their condition is ignored the consequences may be serious or even fatal. Therefore, although the chances of a positive diagnosis are low, the consequences of missing it in the individual are so serious that the situation has to be treated as though it is an ACS until proved otherwise.

Chest pain in acute coronary syndrome (also see ➲ Chapter 16)

Ischaemic chest pain associated with ACSs is similar to the pain which is frequently described as 'angina' but is usually, but not always, more intense, longer lasting, as well as occurring without an obvious precipitating factor. In addition to the severity of the pain the patient may give a history of sweating, nausea, faintness, and feeling systemically more unwell than they would with straightforward exercise-induced chest pain, i.e. angina. Vomiting is not uncommon in patients with myocardial infarction.

Musculoskeletal chest pain

Pain of musculoskeletal origin occurring from around any areas of the chest is often the most difficult condition to distinguish from ischaemic chest pain, and, as with oesophageal pain, clinical distinction may be impossible. Although it may be exercise induced, some distinction can be made in taking the history by defining the precipitating factors, the duration, and localization. Musculoskeletal chest pain may have no precipitating factors or may come on during or after exercise and a history of antecedent injury or exertion should be sought. It may be made worse by breathing or by movement. It is frequently of longer duration than ischaemic chest pain and often localized to small areas of the chest; the patient may well be able to point with one finger to the site of the pain when asked where the pain is, whereas the patient who has myocardial ischaemia generally cannot identify the site of the pain as precisely and it frequently occupies an area of at least several cm^2 and often much more. Although the history may definitely make the diagnosis of musculoskeletal pain, for example episodes of very sharp pain lasting a matter of seconds, localized to a small area between the ribs, are almost never cardiac in origin, unfortunately many episodes of chest pain of musculoskeletal origin are not easily distinguished from cardiac pain and in the end it may be necessary to depend on investigations to help distinguish the pain from ischaemic cardiac pain.

Physicians frequently palpate the chest, and apply pressure to try to identify whether the pain is made worse by these manoeuvres [6]. This can be extremely helpful if the pain produced in this way is typical, but it is an approach which can be fraught with danger. A robust young cardiologist may induce pain in the chest of a frail, elderly patient which they then have difficulty distinguishing from their normal pain. In circumstances where the pain may be ischaemic pain it is not safe to dismiss it on the basis that the doctor believes that they can reproduce the pain by pressing on the chest. Finally, pain of pleuritic or pericardial origins can be made worse by pressing on the chest as this deforms the structures beneath and creates pain.

Other non-cardiac pain

Patients suffering from anxiety and/or depression often are aware of chest tightness which may sound very like angina; this may be associated with hyperventilation. It tends to be prolonged over hours, have little or no association with exercise, and indeed may be more prominent when the patient is relaxing and also often does not limit exercise. Although the history can help, it may remain difficult to be sure whether there is ischaemic heart disease. These patients often perform poorly on the treadmill and also find coronary angiography very stressful. Often stress imaging to look for ischaemia is the ideal first investigation to see if there is any evidence of ischaemia. (See ➲Key point 4, p.27.)

Pericardial pain

Pain from the pericardium (➲Chapter 19) occurs because the inflamed surfaces of the pericardium move over each other with each heartbeat and also with physical movement and respiration. The pain is nearly always extremely sharp and although may be constant it is usually made worse by moving, breathing, and by pressure over the sternum and anterior chest. Characteristically it is relieved by the patient leaning forward and sometimes this makes the diagnosis immediately recognizable when the patient is seen sitting in their bed, leaning forward over a table trying to relieve the pain.

Other cardiac pain

Pain from myocarditis may have an element of pericardial pain, but also tends to produce a deep, aching pain in the chest with some similarities to the pain occurring with ACSs, but often not as intense.

Aneurysms

Aneurysms of the thoracic aorta (➲Chapter 31) are usually painless, but if they begin to expand rapidly they may produce a non-specific chest discomfort which the patient may find hard to describe and which is difficult to diagnose. Dissecting aneurysm produces one of the most intense pains ever experienced by patients. It is often of very sudden onset and indeed the patient may believe that they have been hit in the chest or back and the pain is often described as tearing. The pain may be in the front of the body, but often in the back. The pain frequently radiates and may go down the legs and can be in the abdomen. The onset may be associated with collapse. The patient may not lose consciousness but simply falls to the ground because of the suddenness and severity of the onset of the symptoms. There may be additional truly ischaemic chest pain if the dissection has involved the origin of a coronary artery (most often the right). There may also be associated neurological symptoms if a major vessel to the head and neck has been compromised by the dissection.

Shortness of breath (dyspnoea)

The terms 'shortness of breath' and 'dyspnoea' are interchangeable. They imply that the patient has difficulty getting their breath and that this difficulty in getting breath is in some way unpleasant. This symptom must be distinguished from hyperpnoea which is increased breathing and from angina. The increased breathing associated with exercise in normal people at a moderate level is an example of hyperpnoea, but if a patient then pushes themselves beyond their limit then breathing becomes uncomfortable and the sensation can be described as being dyspnoea. Hyperpnoea does not usually feel unpleasant to the patient and is associated with conditions that lead to increased respiratory drive, e.g. the acidosis in diabetic ketoacidosis. (Also see ➲Key point 5, p.27)

The aim of the history is to begin to distinguish between the common causes of dyspnoea [7]. The most important are a cardiac cause usually associated with incipient or pre-existing left heart failure (➲Chapter 23), respiratory disease, and when there is an unreasonable demand on the normal heart and lungs. This latter situation is very often seen in patients who are severely overweight but severe anaemia leads to the same situation. In the real world patients often have more than one cause of dyspnoea. A common situation is the patient with mild heart failure secondary to ischaemic heart disease, chronic bronchitis due to smoking, and significant obesity. In such patients it is often difficult to determine how much of the dyspnoea can be attributed to each of the factors. The only way is to treat everything that is treatable and see what happens. Certain features in the history may help to distinguish the cause. Classically cardiac breathlessness is made worse by lying flat (orthopnoea) (see ➲Table 1.8). The degree of orthopnoea is usually defined by the number of pillows that the patient uses, but the physician must determine how many pillows that patient has always used. It is a change in the use of pillows that is important, rather than the actual number. Some people who have no cardiac disease like to sleep with a large number of pillows in a semi-recumbent position. Patients may also sleep sitting up because of other symptoms of which the most common is oesophageal reflux. Although

Table 1.8 Breathlessness lying flat and patients who prefer to sleep sitting up

Heart failure—orthopnoea
Angina—angina decubitus
Gastro-oesophageal reflux disease (GORD)
Lung disease—using accessory muscles and therefore sit up to fix shoulder girdle
Obesity/ascites
Pregnancy
Habit

orthopnoea points towards a cardiac cause, patients who have severe respiratory disease also find it difficult to lie flat and often tend to sit up and fix their shoulder girdle so that they can use the accessory muscles of respiration to aid their impaired respiration. Furthermore, obese patients have great difficulty lying flat because the contents of their abdomen tend to push upwards on to the diaphragm when they are lying flat. A useful line of questioning while taking the history can be to ask the patient what happens if they slip off the pillows while they are asleep. Patients with true orthopnoea tend to wake up distressed because of breathlessness, but other patients may simply continue to sleep in a flatter position than the one they started the night in.

Paroxysmal nocturnal dyspnoea

This dramatic symptom must be sought in taking the cardiovascular history and distinguished, if possible, from orthopnoea. When paroxysmal nocturnal dyspnoea (PND) occurs the patient wakes up with severe breathlessness, has to sit up and usually gets out of bed and stands up. They frequently go to the window because they believe that they can improve the situation by inhaling fresh air which they believe contains 'more oxygen'. Clearly this is not true, but the effect of standing up dramatically reduces venous return and thereby reduces right heart output and relieves pulmonary congestion. PND is a very specific symptom and indicates severe cardiac dysfunction. It may be associated with coughing which produces pink, frothy sputum. This is the stage of left heart failure just before overt pulmonary oedema (➲Chapter 23).

Cheyne–Stokes respiration

The intermittent breathing that is usually the result of a low cardiac output is really a physical sign. It is often noticed by the patient's partner during the night when breathing slows down and stops for some seconds before starting again. The patient may also be aware of it when they drift off to sleep, as the breathing slows and stops and then they wake up with a start as they begin to breathe again

Sleep apnoea

The patient is usually obese and may be plethoric and their main complaint is of somnolence during the day and they may develop heart failure as a complication. However, in common with Cheyne–Stokes respiration, the patient's partner is the best source for the history. Their sleep is ruined by their partner's loud snoring and they notice periods when breathing stops and then choking, snoring, and snorting start again

Cough

Although cough is usually regarded as a symptom denoting a respiratory origin to the patient's breathing problems, there are circumstances where coughing may point to a cardiac problem [8]. Coughing, particularly at night, may be caused by the early stages of pulmonary congestion and be a sign of impending left heart failure. Nocturnal coughing can also be a symptom either of asthma or of gastrointestinal reflux.

Palpitation(s) (cardiac arrhythmias)

Patients usually perceive cardiac arrhythmias (➲Chapters 28–30) as an awareness of their heartbeat and they may feel thumping in the chest but this may also be described as the heart racing or pounding or fluttering in the chest. This can be one of the most difficult areas in which to obtain a precise history. The history can be difficult both because the patient may be frightened by the symptoms and, furthermore, find them very difficult to describe. The age-old method of asking the patient to tap out the rhythm on the desk or on their knee is extremely helpful. Frequently patients, when asked to do so, say they are unable to reproduce the arrhythmia but if they have a demonstration from the examining doctor of the possibilities then they soon get the idea and are able to do this. The doctor can produce a variety of examples, for example rapid and regular, rapid and irregular, etc., and ask the patient to choose which most closely resembles their arrhythmia. It is also important to distinguish whether the onset of the palpitation is sudden or builds up slowly. In most cases of genuine cardiac arrhythmia the onset is extremely sudden. Theoretically, the offset should also be sudden but sometimes it is not. Although the patient may describe the classical sudden start they become used to the rhythm and the sensation of the cessation is often not as dramatic as the start. The actual offset may be sudden on the ECG tracing but the patient senses the end of the episode as a tailing off.

It is critical to establish what—if anything—precipitates the arrhythmia (➲Box 1.5). Careful questioning is required because patients may be embarrassed, e.g. symptoms during sexual intercourse, or may not have made a connection, e.g. chronic emotional stress of all types. The doctor must try to distinguish whether an arrhythmia is regular or irregular and this is often demonstrated by the tapping exercise described earlier and also to determine whether or not there are associated symptoms. In some patients there may be lightheadedness or even syncope, while in others the rapid arrhythmia may bring out myocardial ischaemia and be accompanied by ischaemic chest pain. Conversely, in a patient who has

Box 1.5 Scenario 5: palpitation triggers

A 37-year-old, slightly overweight patient complains of sudden-onset, rapid, regular palpitations occurring only while playing football and associated with dyspnoea and mild faintness. Twenty-four-hour ECG monitoring when not playing football revealed a few ectopics. The patient was reassured, but developed a similar but more prolonged episode while playing football a few months later. ECG revealed ventricular tachycardia and the patient was found to have an underlying cardiomyopathy. An ICD was implanted.

Lesson

Always use careful questioning to establish precipitating factors. Attempt to test when precipitating factors are present and continue testing until you have caught an episode. An exercise test could have been performed before reassuring the patient.

unexplained lightheadedness or syncope (➲Chapter 26) or chest pain, it is important to question the patient as to whether or not there is an associated palpitation, which could represent an arrhythmia which is causing the problem.

Perhaps the commonest symptoms are those due to ventricular or atrial ectopic beats. Patients variously describe the sensation as the heart skipping a beat or stumbling or giving a heavy thump which occurs because the post-ectopic beat is more forceful than usual as the heart has longer to fill before it occurs.

Some patients who describe palpitation are in fact describing a normal cardiac rhythm. The heartbeat may be made more forceful because of anxiety or for no obvious reason and the patient then perceives an acceleration of their normal heart rhythm. Sinus tachycardia is usually relatively slow compared with a true tachyarrhythmia, often at a rate of about 110 beats per minute. Sinus tachycardia usually builds up over a matter of some minutes and then goes off slowly and does not have a sudden onset. Like many less significant arrhythmias it may be most prominent if the patient is lying in bed on their left side; this brings the heart in contact with the chest wall. Similarly a slow regular thumping or heavy beat may occasionally occur and can be due to ventricular bigeminy or, rarely, due to sinus bradycardia.

Presyncope and syncope (also see ➲Chapter 26)

The main distinction to be made by the history is between a cardiovascular and a neurological cause (➲Table 1.9).

Table 1.9 History in syncope: cardiovascular versus neurological cause of loss of consciousness

Cardiovascular	Neurological
No warning	Warning (aura)
–	Incontinence—faecal or urinary
–	Tongue biting
Patient usually silent	Grunting and involuntary noises
Pallor + +	Often cyanosed and suffused with (particularly in tonic phase)
No movement	Convulsions (may not be particularly marked)
Afterwards: usually tired but not confused with fairly quick recovery	*Afterwards*: confusion common and a feeling of being hungover and also possible residual paralysis

This can be extremely difficult, both for the patient and for the doctor [9, 10]. Primary neurological problems often have a rotational element to them and unsteadiness and problems with balance without an associated feeling that consciousness is about to be lost. There may also be associated nausea. Cardiovascular presyncope does not usually have a rotational element, although the patient may still describe a symptom as dizziness which is really a feeling of impending loss of consciousness due to hypotension. If the patient does not notice that the room is revolving, and if they feel as though they are close to losing consciousness, then the problem is more likely to be cardiovascular. (Also see ➲Key points 6 and 7, p.27.)

Occasionally, a fall in cerebral perfusion due to a cerebrovascular cause can trigger a seizure. In a patient who complains of blacking out, it is very important to establish whether they are actually losing consciousness. Some patients may say they are blacking out, when in fact they simply feel very distant from surrounding events. Such a feelings of 'being disembodied but remaining fully conscious' is often associated with anxiety or other psychological symptoms. Another area in which confusion occurs is when the patient says they have lost consciousness when in fact they have fallen to the ground without losing consciousness. If the patient remembers hitting the ground this potential differential diagnosis has to be considered. There are a particular group of patients whose legs simply give way on them and there is no cardiovascular cause for this. These are the so-called true 'drop attacks'.

It is crucially important to discover whether there have been any eye witnesses to episodes of syncope and if so to make contact with them and question them, particularly about the onset, offset, and duration of the attack as well as the patient's colour and their behaviour, breathing pattern, and the speed of recovery. Sometimes the witness may also have taken the pulse. It may be possible, in the age of the mobile phone, to telephone the witness while the patient is actually in the clinic. In addition to trying to elicit the symptoms that may distinguish between a cardiovascular and a cerebrovascular cause, it is also necessary to establish the circumstances under which an episode of syncope occurs. This information may be helpful in making a diagnosis, particularly when the episodes occur as a result of either fear, emotion, prolonged standing, micturition, defecation, etc. (➲Box 1.6). Most of these circumstances are known to lead to a high level of vagal tone and lead on to vasovagal syncope. Such episodes are often known as 'situational'. They frequently occur in young patients without any other illness, although problems with voiding, i.e. micturition and defecation syncope, are much more likely to occur in the elderly. Such situational attacks which are vasovagal must be distinguished from the rare attack that occurs in patients particularly with the long QT syndrome, when loud noises and alarming circumstances may precipitate serious arrhythmias.

If the patient describes injury associated with syncope then this usually denotes a lack of warning and suggests a significant underlying problem and a sudden onset. A warning favours a neurological cause, particularly if this takes the form of an aura, i.e. an unusual sensation which precedes the episode of loss of consciousness. This should not be confused with a brief period of presyncope prior to a true syncopal episode. Following an episode of cardiovascular syncope, patients may feel tired, but do not usually feel particularly unwell, whereas patients who have experienced a convulsion often feel extremely unwell for a long period of time with headache, lethargy, and what they would describe as a hangover. Residual brief periods of paralysis (Todd's paralysis) are more likely to be present after a neurological event.

Occasionally patients may give a history of collapsing with syncope and then coming round after a short period and being aware of a rapid tachycardia. This may be because whatever caused the syncope also produced a tachycardia. However, more often it is because the sudden drop in cardiac output caused by the tachycardia and an unprepared dilated peripheral circulation causes a severe fall in blood pressure and syncope. Then protective constrictive reflexes raise the blood pressure despite the continuing tachycardia and the patient regains consciousness.

Oedema and ascites

Although oedema and ascites are physical signs, they are also described by patients as symptoms.

Fatigue

Fatigue is probably very common but hard to define as it has so many causes. It is most striking when a patient has a successful treatment and suddenly realizes how tired they were before. If it occurs intermittently it may have a definite underlying cause although this may be difficult to track down (➲Box 1.7).

Less common cardiological symptoms

Vomiting

Patients in the early stage of an acute myocardial infarction may vomit profusely. It may be difficult to be sure whether the stress and dehydration of the vomiting precipitates the infarction, or vice versa [11, 12].

Box 1.6 Scenario 6: effect of position

A middle-aged woman with no known cardiac problems notices a fast heartbeat at the end of eating a heavy meal in a hot restaurant. She decided that she must go to the lavatory, stands, and starts to walk to the door but loses consciousness after a few yards.

Explanation

The arrhythmia initially causes a moderate fall in cardiac output but while she is sitting the circulation can compensate. As soon as she stands up the gravitational effect on the circulation reduces the cardiac output further and loss of consciousness ensues.

Box 1.7 Scenario 7: tiredness—a difficult symptom

A 55-year-old male, who was a successful veteran cycle racer at national level, noticed that occasionally while racing he suddenly and unexpectedly ran out of energy and became tired. This caused him to slow down and abandon the race. When he did so the symptoms usually resolved within a few minutes and he felt normal again. He had no other symptoms. Holter monitoring during a cycle race showed that this loss of energy was due to the sudden occurrence of atrial flutter with 1:1 conduction. This has been cured by ablation and he is now racing successfully again.

Polyuria [13, 14]

Patients with supraventricular tachycardia (➲Chapter 28) may describe striking polyuria which starts a few minutes after the onset of an attack. This is very characteristic and is probably due to a raised intra-atrial pressure causing a release of ANP leading to natriuresis and diuresis. It is particularly common in atrial fibrillation (➲Chapter 29), and paroxysmal atrioventricular (AV) nodal re-entry tachycardia.

Fullness in the neck ± right upper quadrant abdominal pain [15]

Patients with high right atrial (RA) pressures may notice this being transmitted in to the neck as a feeling of fullness. It is particularly common in patients who have severe tricuspid regurgitation. In addition to this, venous back pressure into the liver stretches the liver capsule and causes discomfort.

Pulsation in the neck associated with tachycardia

A feeling of pulsation in the neck associated with a rapid regular tachycardia suggests an AV nodal re-entry tachycardia [16]. This is because the atrium contracts at the same time as the ventricle, i.e. when the tricuspid valve is closed and so the wave form is transmitted upward into the neck rather than forward into the RV.

Unusual noises in the chest

A very unusual but striking symptom is when the patient complains of hearing a squeaking noise in their chest, often associated with symptoms. This may occur in the context of an arrhythmia in a patient with mitral valve prolapse (➲Chapter 21) and can also be described by patients who have suddenly developed a severe degree of mitral regurgitation due to chordal rupture or when the cusp of a prosthetic tissue valve tears spontaneously.

A further example is in a patient with a mechanical valve (➲Chapter 21) in whom there is sudden cessation of clicks associated with symptoms and then the clicks resume. This is very rare, but may indicate a mechanical fault with the valve with a component sticking. When the part of the valve sticks the noises generated by the valve cease.

Using the cardiovascular history to identify danger areas

There is a high potential for harm if a serious cardiovascular diagnosis is missed and if a patient who is either in the clinic or emergency department is then sent home without further investigation. If the differential diagnosis lies between a serious cardiovascular problem, such as an ACS, and a much less serious diagnosis, such as gastrointestinal reflux, it is essential to err on the side of caution and provisionally make the more serious diagnosis while recognizing that tests must be carried out to either confirm or refute this diagnosis. Many doctors are averse to making the more serious of two potential diagnoses and have an inclination to reassure the patient unjustifiably. This is not good practice and must be resisted. It is crucial to remember that differentiation of two such diagnoses may be impossible using the history alone.

Some cardiovascular histories which require urgent attention

The patient who wants to go home

The patient in the emergency room who feels perfectly well at the time when their history is taken but has presented with an episode of chest discomfort that could well be of cardiac origin. The patient ascribes these symptoms to indigestion. The ECG is normal. This situation cannot be resolved by the history and requires a period of observation and further investigation. If the patient is in the hospital and the condition progresses, appropriate therapy, including early revascularization, can be provided or resuscitation can be given should they develop a cardiac arrest. After leaving the hospital then neither of these options is feasible and out-of-hospital resuscitation has a very low success rate. It is no disgrace to admit a patient for one night, decide the diagnosis is not myocardial ischaemia, and send the patient home. It is a disaster to send home a patient who dies because of a misinterpretation of their cardiac history.

Unexplained syncope of recent onset

A patient presents with a completely unexplained sudden blackout, usually occurring for the first time. This is a particularly difficult situation. Many of these patients will have a relatively benign cause for their symptoms, but a small number will have extremely severe underlying disease which requires immediate treatment if the patient is to survive. In such patients it is important to look for ancillary information. For example, a patient who has a massive pulmonary embolism may quickly recover after the first embolic event, but has at the time of the collapse a brief period of breathlessness and a reduced oxygen saturation if measured. These observations may have been made in the ambulance bringing the patient to hospital. It is therefore crucial in any acute patient to obtain a history from the relatives and ambulance staff, and also information from the ambulance records. Another example is the patient who has an aortic dissection with an episode of collapse, sudden pain in the back, but quick resolution so that by the time they arrive in the emergency department the patient feels perfectly well. Again it is the associated symptoms that act as the telltale for a serious underlying condition.

The patient with valvular heart disease

Intermittent symptoms of shortness of breath or episodes of presyncope or syncope in a patient with a mechanical prosthesis

These could be due to intermittent valve malfunction. This is a particularly difficult area in which to establish a diagnosis, but if a patient with a mechanical valve notices the clicks have stopped or changed in character the diagnosis of a malfunctioning valve must be seriously considered.

A patient with unexplained deterioration of valvular heart disease and non-specific symptoms

When a patient describes being generally unwell, with widespread aches and pains, weight loss, and fever, infective endocarditis must be considered. The consequences of missing it are very serious. In such patients inflammatory markers should be measured, an echocardiogram performed, and blood cultures taken if there is any suspicion of this diagnosis.

Examination

Introduction

Examination remains a key component of cardiology (➲Table 1.10). A comprehensive cardiovascular examination can be time consuming and often a rapid assessment of the patient is required, especially in acute situations. Time pressures even in an out-patient environment often make a full examination impractical. This 'scenario examination' technique can save valuable time in an acute or emergency situation. Examples of this approach are discussed later in this chapter. It is important to understanding the relevance of both the presence and the absence of particular clinical signs.

General examination

If possible, clinical examination should be performed in a quiet, warm, comfortable environment with good lighting, although clinical circumstances often dictate the need to perform an examination under suboptimal conditions. Putting the patient at ease from the outset helps examination and it is important to respect their privacy and dignity at all times.

Examination begins before the patient is settled on an examination couch and valuable insights can be gained

Table 1.10 Cardiovascular examination checklist: the essentials

Cardiovascular exam checklist	Comments
Watch patient enter the room/ get on couch	May be dyspnoeic or get pain
Correct position	45°—to see JVP
General exam	
Scars/rash	Previous surgery
Hands	Splinters/peripheral cyanosis
Face/eyes	Pallor, cyanosis, jaundice
Ocular fundi	Diabetic and hypertensive changes, endocarditis
Pulse	
Radial (both)	Feel the vessel, wall, and rhythm (catheter site)
Carotid	Best for pulse character and timing, JVP, and murmurs
Femoral	Decreased/unequal/bruit—PVD Delayed compared to radial—coarctation Catheter site
Foot pulses	PVD
Blood pressure	
Take it yourself	Use correct cuff Use point of disappearance *not* muffling as diastolic pressure Compare at different sites if dissection possible
JVP	
If invisible: ◆ Press on liver to fill JVP ◆ Sit up in case it is invisible because very high	Need good light, head turned slightly away
Normal < 4cm above sternal notch	Left usually more reliable than right JVP
	Gentle digital pressure stops pulsation
Chest	
Inspect	Scars, deformity, movement
Palpate	Body habitus has major effect on palpation and auscultation
Listen for murmurs and normal and abnormal sounds	Locate apex—feel *all over chest* for heaves, thrills etc. If necessary assess effect of: ◆ Position ◆ Respiration ◆ Exercise
Quiet environment needed	If pulse irregular compare with heart rhythm on auscultation

JVP, jugular venous pulse; PVD, peripheral vascular disease.

during general observations of gait and mobility, and associated symptoms such as breathlessness and discomfort as the patient enters the room and gets on to the couch; the presence of confusion or distress may become apparent at this stage. General observations such as height, obesity, obvious skeletal deformities such as kyphoscoliosis may also be more obvious as the patient enters the room (see ➲Key points 8 and 9, p.27).

The history should be expanded and refined during examination and if unexpected physical signs are found this may prompt further questioning of the patient. If the sign is mentioned, for example the presence of clubbing, the patient may then respond that it has been known for a long time or has been noticed by other doctors.

There are many clinical signs that might be elicited during a general physical examination which have relevance to the cardiovascular system (➲Table 1.11).

Scars from previous surgery are important especially in the unconscious or confused patient. Although a median sternotomy scar can relate to many types of cardiac surgery it may also indicate other past mediastinal problems, e.g. thymus (consider myasthenia gravis) or thyroid. A left thoracotomy scar may indicate aortic surgery, particularly previous surgery for coarctation of the aorta, and a right thoracotomy may indicate previous mitral surgery. Always look at the legs and arms for scars indicating that a vascular conduit has been harvested, strongly suggesting a previous coronary artery bypass graft. Chest scars may be due to previous lung surgery which may shift the mediastinum and with it the heart, making interpretation of physical signs more difficult.

Certain chest deformities can have cardiovascular significance. Pectus excavatum (depressed sternum) can produce a false impression of cardiomegaly by displacing the heart to the left and may also distort the RV producing an innocent murmur. Pectus excavatum and also pectus carinatum (prominent sternum) can be seen in Marfan syndrome (➲Chapter 31) [17]. In patients with cardiomegaly since early childhood the chest wall may bulge out over the enlarged heart.

Cardiovascular examination

Pulse

The rate, rhythm, pulse character, and the nature of the vessel wall can usually be assessed from the radial pulse. Although the pulse pattern may suggest a diagnosis for the underlying rhythm an ECG is always necessary for confirmation. An easily palpable radial vessel wall is usually an indication of abnormal thickening and possibly calcification, and suggests more generalized vascular disease (see ➲Key point 10, p.27).

Table 1.11 Physical signs on general examination

	Causes	**Comments**
Common signs		
Anaemia	Blood loss Infective endocarditis Hypothyroidism	Many causes of anaemia can cause sinus tachycardia, heart failure
Central cyanosis	Intracardiac or extracardiac shunting, reduced oxygen	Any situation where venous–arterial admixture occurs
Peripheral cyanosis	Vasoconstriction Low cardiac output	Can be environment dependent, e.g. Raynaud's
Corneal arcus	Aging Hyperlipidaemia	
Xanthelasma (➲Fig. 1.1)	Hyperlipidaemia	Often occur as normal variant
Splinter haemorrhages (➲Fig. 1.2)	Infective endocarditis Local trauma Vasculitis	One or two splinters may be present without disease
Tremor	Hyperthyroidism Alcohol withdrawal Drug induced	
Capillary pulsations	Severe aortic regurgitation	Quinke's sign
Rash and petechiae	Vasculitis, endocarditis, rheumatic fever	Very non-specific but extremely helpful. Often associated with arthralgia or arthropathy
Uncommon signs		
Finger clubbing (and toes)	Infective endocarditis Cyanotic congenital heart disease Idiopathic—familial	Also in lung cancer and other lung disease
Malar flush	Mitral stenosis	Also seen in systemic lupus erythematosus
Roth spots	Infective endocarditis	Retinal haemorrhage with central white spots
Janeway lesions	Infective endocarditis	Raised haemorrhagic lesions on hands and feet
Facial dysmorphism	Down, Turner, Noonan syndromes	A variety of congenital chromosomal abnormalities
Blue sclera	Pseudoxanthoma elasticum Ehlers–Danlos syndrome	Aortopathy main cardiovascular problem Most commonly occurs in osteogenesis imperfect
Cushingoid facies	Cushing's syndrome Steroid therapy	Hypertension Fluid retention
Non-pitting oedema	Hypothyroidism	
Arachnodactyly Arm span height Lens dislocation High arch palate	Marfan syndrome	Associated with aortopathy and mitral valve prolpse

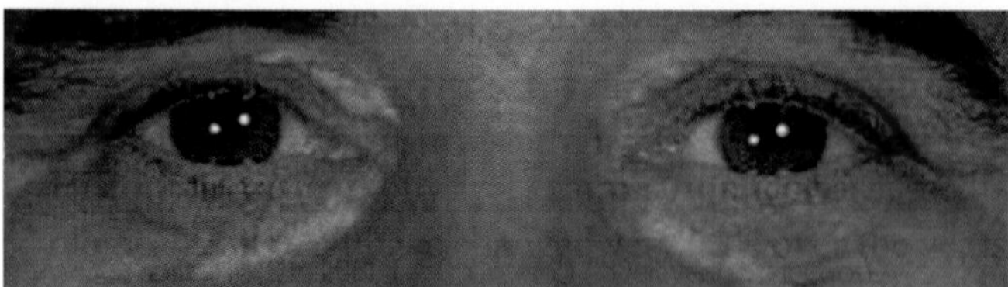

Figure 1.1 Xanthelasma. Typical appearance of xanthelasma in patient with severe hypercholesterolaemia. Note the yellowish deposits surrounding the eyes.

The character of the pulse is a valuable sign but must usually be assessed using a central pulse and the carotid is usually best although the brachial may be helpful. One exception is the collapsing pulse of severe aortic regurgitation which, although detected at the carotid, is often best appreciated by palpating the radial pulse with the arm raised above the head when the pulse acquires a very sharp tapping quality.

Some typical pulse characters are illustrated in ➲Fig. 1.3. A slow rising pulse (➲Figs. 1.3B and 1.4) is most commonly associated with significant aortic stenosis [18] (➲Chapter 21). There is a time delay to peak systolic pressure which gets later as stenosis gets worse and the pulse volume also falls. It is, however, a myth that a normal or raised systolic blood pressure *excludes* severe aortic stenosis. The LV has a remarkable ability to generate pressure which may occasionally get as high as 300mmHg. In this situation a 100mmHg gradient across the aortic valve still leaves a systolic pressure of 200mmHg! The typical slow rising pulse can be mimicked by local disease in the carotid and checking both carotids may clarify the situation. Patients can also have severe aortic stenosis without a slow rising pulse. This is because these patients are often elderly with hard sclerotic vessels which amplify the pulse pressure and mask the slow rising pulse.

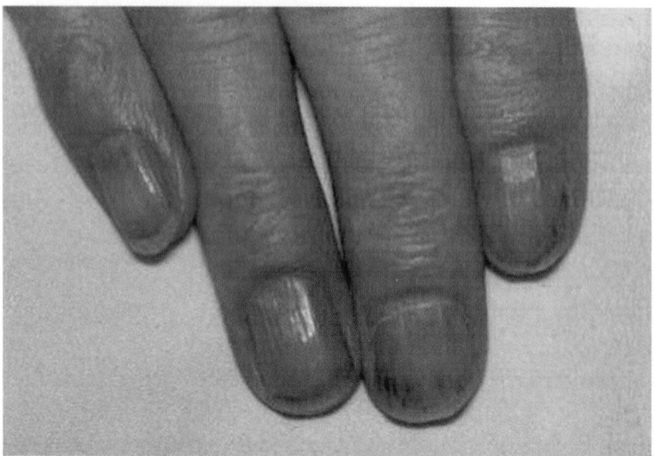

Figure 1.2 Splinter haemorrhages. Splinter haemorrhages are noted as linear haemorrhagic lesions at the distal nail bed. One or two splinters can occur in normal individuals but multiple splinters are typical of infective endocarditis or vasculitis (➲Chapter 22).

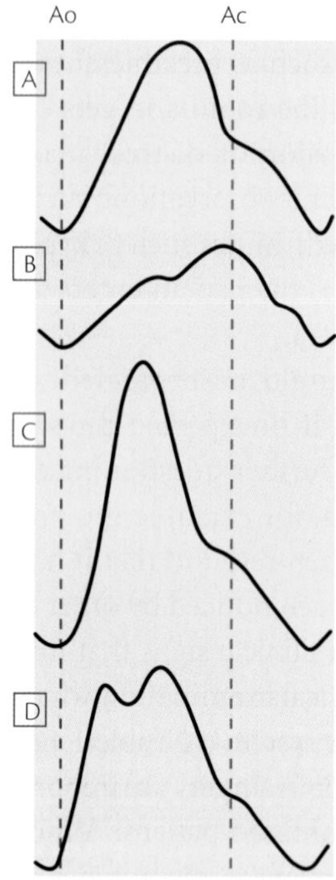

Figure 1.3 Pulse character. (A) Normal pulse. Following Ao there is a fairly rapid upstroke of the pulse to its peak, then a more gradual descent which includes an impalpable 'dicrotic notch' created as a result of aortic valve closure. (B) Slow rising pulse. The upstroke is more gradual, the peak reduced and delayed. Usually associated with aortic stenosis. (C) Collapsing pulse commonly associated with severe aortic regurgitation. There is a rapid rise in systolic and a rapid decline of pressure after the peak. (D) Bisferiens pulse. Often associated with combined aortic stenosis and regurgitation, it is characterized by twin peaks (percussion wave and tidal wave) separated by a mid-systolic dip. Ac, aortic (valve) closure; Ao, aortic (valve) opening.

➲Figs. 1.3C and 1.4 illustrate a collapsing pulse typically resulting from severe aortic regurgitation (➲Chapter 21). With each beat the LV has to eject both the forward cardiac output and the amount of blood that will leak back into the ventricle in the next early diastole. This large volume of blood is ejected forcefully into the aorta producing the sharp upstroke and then a large volume immediately falls back into the LV producing the 'collapse'. These pulse characteristics also occur in any situation when there is a large volume systolic leak from the central circulation, e.g. with a large AV fistula or an uncorrected patent ductus arteriosus (➲Chapter 10). In conditions where there is an increased cardiac output, e.g. pregnancy, fever, anaemia, Paget's disease of bone, the pulse will be of large volume and is often described as 'bounding'. The pulse in these conditions has some similarities to the collapsing pulse but there are subtle differences. The upstroke and particularly the downstroke are not as abrupt since there is not a sudden diastolic leak of blood from the central circulation

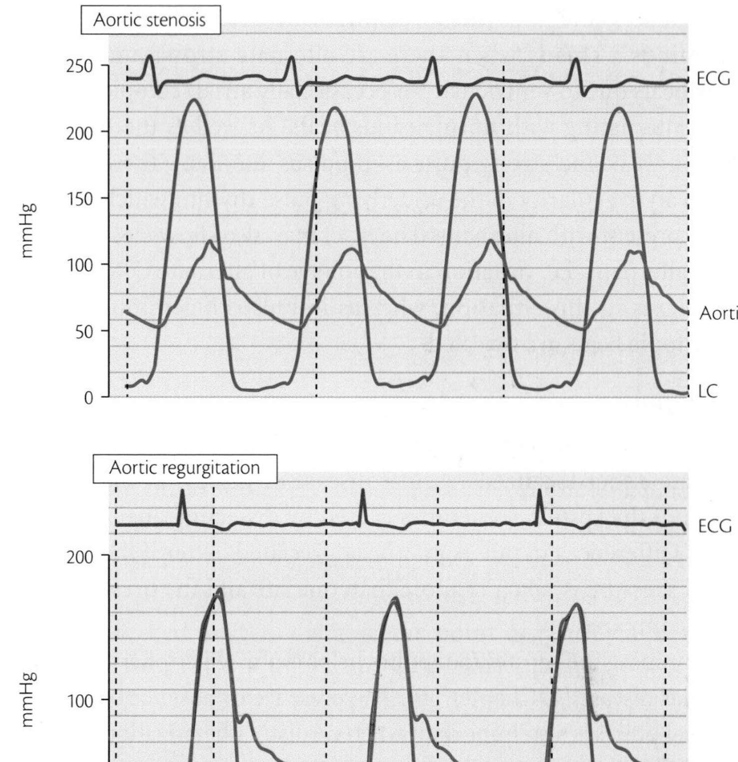

Figure 1.4 Pulse pressure waveform. Illustration of the aortic pressure waveform in aortic stenosis and aortic regurgitation compared to the simultaneous left ventricular pressure. In aortic stenosis the aortic pressure rises slowly to its peak in late systole and there is a significant systolic pressure difference between the aorta and left ventricle. In aortic regurgitation the aortic and left ventricular pressures are identical during systole but the rapid fall in aortic pressure in diastole results in a wide pulse pressure and the characteristic collapsing pulse.

Finally, ➲Fig. 1.3D illustrates the 'bisferiens' pulse which usually occurs when aortic regurgitation is combined with aortic stenosis. There are two peaks (percussion wave and tidal wave) separated by a mid-systolic dip. The bisferiens pulse is rare but very striking when it is encountered in clinical practice.

Pulsus paradoxus

Pulsus paradoxus (➲Fig. 1.5) occurs when the pulse pressure falls by > 10mmHg with each inspiration [19]. Clinically it is difficult to detect by palpation until this decrease exceeds 20mmHg. The sign is elicited and measured by slowly deflating the blood pressure cuff while listening to the blood pressure and observing the patient breathing. The commonest cause is pericardial tamponade (➲Chapter 19). The physiological mechanism is complicated but the main effect is that the heart cannot expand because of the surrounding, compressing pericardial fluid and consequently when blood is sucked into the RV by inspiration, left-sided cardiac filling from the pulmonary circulation is reduced and the output from each beat during inspiration falls. Inspiration also pulls the heart down and the globular shape of the heart becomes more cylindrical. This restricts cardiac volume further as the volume of a cylinder is smaller than that of a sphere with the same surface area. In constrictive pericarditis (➲Chapter 19) the pericardium has the same limiting effect on cardiac volume. In patients with extreme dyspnoea, e.g. due to asthma, the very striking swings in intrathoracic pressure also produce pulsus paradoxus [20].

Pulsus alternans

This is when there are alternate strong and weak pulses in a basically regular pulse. This is a sign of severely impaired LV function and may be exacerbated by the presence of

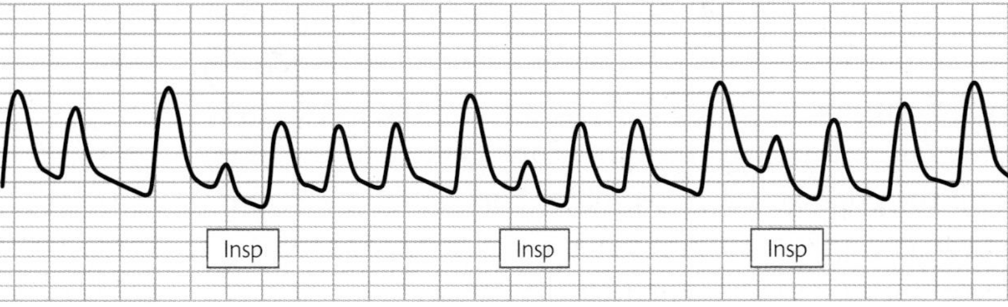

Figure 1.5 Pulsus paradoxus. Aortic pressure waveform demonstrating variation in pulse amplitude with respiration, the pressure decreasing with inspiration (insp).

hypovolaemia. It has to be distinguished from 'pulses bigeminus'. This is when there are alternate strong and weak beats due to ventricular (or occasionally atrial) ectopic beats alternating with normal sinus beats. As well as there being a weak and strong pulse as in pulsus alternans, there is also an irregularity in the underlying pulse rhythm which is not present with alternans. The ECG may also show electrical alternans, i.e. variation in the voltage of alternate QRS complexes in this situation, whereas in pulsus bigeminus the ectopic beats are revealed.

Other pulses

Differences in the volume and timing of major pulses may indicate either localized vascular disease or disease at the origin of the vessels, sometimes caused by dissecting aneurysm. Differences in pulses may be appreciated better if the blood pressure is taken in more than one site and the pressures compared.

Examining the leg and foot pulses helps evaluate peripheral vascular disease (➲Chapter 36). The presence or absence of femoral pulses is also important when cardiac catheterization is considered. In a busy clinic where it can be very time consuming to examine the femoral pulses of an elderly patient, a careful examination of the foot pulses may be a reasonable substitute. If all foot pulses (dorsalis pedis and posterior tibial on both sides) are strong and present it is very unlikely that that patient will be suffering from coarctation, particularly if they have a normal blood pressure. In the presence of hypertension the femoral pulses must be examined to exclude coarctation (➲Chapter 10), for although it is very rare for this condition to be undiagnosed in adults, occasionally patients do appear. The pulse should arrive at the femoral arteries and the radial arteries at about the same time as they are approximately the same distance from the heart. In coarctation, when there is severe obstruction at the site of coarctation the blood has to traverse collaterals and the femoral pulse is delayed.

Blood pressure

Often the blood pressures (➲Chapter 13) taken initially by the nurse are simply transferred to the notes written by the doctor, without the doctor checking them; this is bad practice. This has the disadvantage that an inaccuracy in the previous blood pressure may be perpetuated, and the blood pressure may have changed in the time between the two examinations. This is an increasing problem, especially with electronic medical records, where whole sections are often cut and pasted from one consultation to the next. With the progressively more obese population it is important to use a large cuff on big arms, otherwise there is an overestimation of blood pressure levels [21].

Jugular venous pulse (➲Table 1.12)

Assessing the jugular venous pulse (JVP) can be one of the most difficult clinical signs in cardiology [22, 23]. The JVP results from transmission of the pulsation from the internal jugular vein to the skin surface, and it is the pulsation rather than the vein itself that is visible. The two aspects of the JVP to be assessed are its level and its character (waveform). Since no valve intervenes, the pressure in the internal jugular is the same as that in the RA. The JVP is often invisible especially in obese patients. If it cannot definitely be seen, record it as 'not seen' rather than 'normal'. Engorged superficial veins may be due to kinking of the vein at the thoracic inlet and do not indicate the level of the JVP.

The JVP is examined with the patient semi-recumbent at an angle of about 45° with the patient's head partially rotated to one side. The JVP is normally just visible at or above the level of the sternal notch behind the sternal heads of the sternomastoid muscle. It is best to examine both sides of the neck when evaluating the JVP. One potential problem is that sometimes the left-sided JVP is higher than the right-sided JVP because there is some obstruction of the innominate vein as it crosses the chest which artificially raises the left JVP. If the JVP is not visible, it is useful to lie the patient flatter to accentuate a low JVP and pressing on the liver may accentuate it further. The 'hepatojugular reflex' (sometimes stated as 'reflux') does not in our experience generally contribute anything else further to the examination although some authorities believe it to be helpful in diagnosing heart failure [24]. Similarly, the pulsation of the JVP may not be visible because the top of the pulsation is above the angle of the jaw and only appears when the patient sits more upright. Pulsation from the carotid artery can be transmitted to the surface and has to be distinguished from the JVP. Firstly the waveform is often different. The carotid pulse is usually a single wave. Secondly the JVP can usually be abolished by gentle digital pressure and it is not possible to feel the pulsation with the finger while doing this, whereas

Table 1.12 Causes of an elevated JVP

Causes of an elevated JVP
Right heart failure
Right ventricular infarction
Pulmonary hypertension
Hypervolaemia
SVC compression
Tricuspid stenosis
Tricuspid regurgitation
Reduced right ventricular compliance
Pericardial constriction/tamponade

carotid pulsation is always palpable and cannot be abolished by gentle digital pressure. The one occasion when the JVP may be palpable is when there is severe tricuspid regurgitation producing a large V wave in the JVP which is caused by direct transmission of RV systolic contraction into the RA and then up the internal jugular vein. This can often be felt in the neck and may also be transmitted to the liver.

Jugular venous pulse character

The normal JVP waveform is illustrated in ➲Fig. 1.6. The 'a' wave results from an increased pressure caused by atrial contraction and is the dominant wave in the normal JVP. It is accentuated in the presence of RV hypertrophy, pulmonary hypertension, or tricuspid stenosis (➲Chapter 21) because RA contraction is powerful but lost in atrial fibrillation. It occurs just before the carotid pulse. In the normal JVP, following the 'a' wave pressure decreases (the x descent) due to atrial relaxation and RV systole which causes descent of the tricuspid valve towards the apex as a result of longitudinal shortening of the ventricle. Next comes the V wave which is due to passive filling of the RA while the tricuspid valve is closed by RV contraction. In tricuspid regurgitation, the v wave peaks earlier, is accentuated and becomes the dominant waveform (➲Fig. 1.7). This is because the 'v' wave in this situation has a completely different genesis but confusingly still carries the same name. It is due to the direct transmission of the systolic contraction of the RV into the RA and up the internal jugular rather than the passive filling of the atrium with the tricuspid valve closed. When the tricuspid valve opens, pressure falls (y descent) until continued passive filling of the atrium begins to increase venous pressure again, ending with the next atrial contraction producing the 'a' wave. Since the 'y' descent results from tricuspid valve opening it occurs after the second heart sound (S_2), a useful reference for timing of the JVP waveform. The 'y' descent becomes particularly prominent in constrictive pericarditis where venous filling of the heart is predominantly an early diastolic phenomenon. A useful sign is that the JVP elevates with inspiration (Kussmaul's sign) [25], a reversal of the normal situation where the decreased intrathoracic pressure sends blood into the chest with a resultant decrease in venous pressure in the JVP. This can also occur in some other clinical situations such as right ventricular infarction [26].

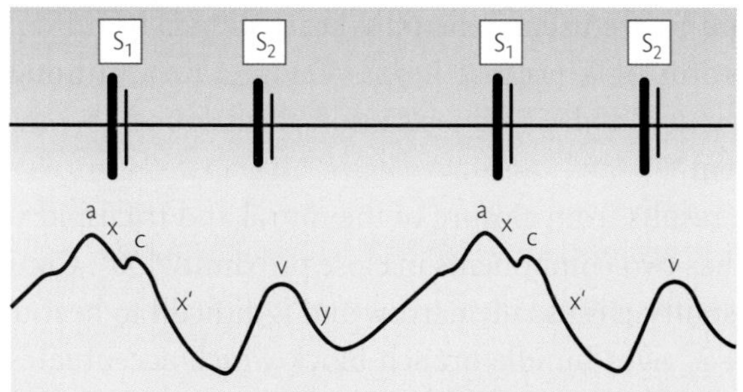

Figure 1.6 JVP Character. 'a' wave: results from an increased pressure caused by atrial contraction and is the dominant wave in the normal JVP. It is accentuated in the presence of right ventricular hypertrophy, pulmonary hypertension, or tricuspid stenosis but lost in atrial fibrillation. 'x' descent: follows the 'a' wave and is due to atrial relaxation and right ventricular systole causing descent of the tricuspid valve towards the apex as a result of longitudinal shortening of the ventricle with systolic contraction. 'c' wave: interrupts the 'x' descent as a transmitted carotid pulsation. 'v' wave: increasing pressure due to passive filling of the atrium while the tricuspid valve is closed by right ventricular systole. 'y' descent: fall in atrial pressure due to opening of the tricuspid valve; followed by passive filling of the atrium culminating in a further 'a' wave. The 'y' descent, as a result of tricuspid valve opening, occurs after the second heart sound (S_2), a useful reference for timing of the JVP waveform.

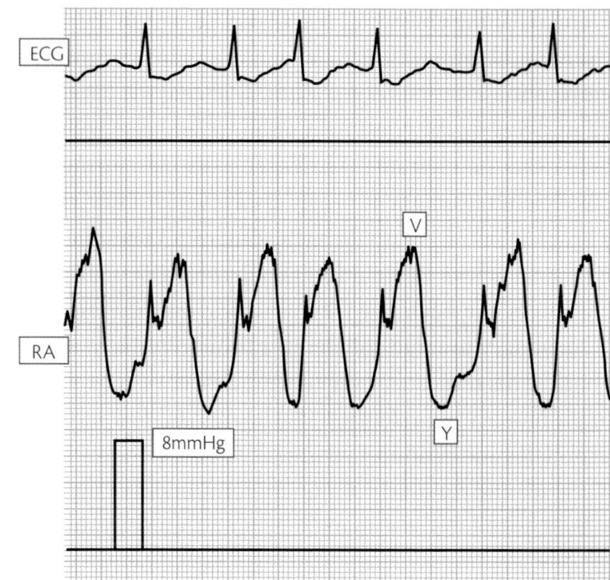

Figure 1.7 Tricuspid regurgitation. Right atrial pressure trace in tricuspid regurgitation illustrating the early, accentuated, and dominant 'v' wave.

If the RA and RV contract at the same time, as occurs intermittently with AV dissociation (e.g. complete heart block, see ➲Chapter 27), blood pumped by the atrium cannot go into the RV because the tricuspid valve is held shut by RV contraction and so shoots up the internal jugular to produce a 'cannon wave'. Cannon waves can also sometimes occur as a result of a ventricular ectopic beat that closes the tricuspid valve but is not electrically conducted to the atrium, which therefore is excited in the normal way. The resulting RA contraction shoots blood up the neck. This can also occur in patients with ventricular tachycardia without VA conduction. Regular cannon waves occur in ventricular tachycardia with intact retrograde conduction and also in AV node re-entrant tachycardia (➲Chapter 28).

Cardiac palpation

The cardiac examination always involves thorough palpation all over the front of the chest. This will pick up abnormal movement of the chest wall related to the contraction of the underlying heart, and thrills which are palpable murmurs. Abnormalities may be brought out by sitting the patient forward and feeling the chest in expiration, and also rolling the patient onto their left side. Thrills are palpable murmurs and the associated murmur is nearly always loud. They are usually best felt in the areas where the murmur is best heard. In a patient in whom coarctation (➲Chapter 10) is suspected, palpation of the back may reveal widespread diffuse pulsation secondary to large collaterals running in the muscles of the back. This indicates a very severe degree of coarctation.

In pulmonary hypertension (➲Chapter 24) the pulmonary artery dilates and produces an impulse in the second left intercostal space and the loud pulmonary component of the S_2 may also be appreciated as a sharp snapping feeling in this area.

Apical impulse (apex beat)

The lowest and most lateral position on the chest wall where a cardiac impulse can be felt is known as the apex beat. Some physicians refer to the point of maximal impulse (PMI). This can be confusing as sometimes the most laterally felt impulse is not the 'maximal impulse'. The apical impulse or apex beat is usually located in the fifth intercostal space at the level of, or just medial to the mid-clavicular line. Chest deformity, lung disease, and obesity all reduce the intensity of the apex beat or render it impalpable. In these situations, rotating the patient to a left lateral decubitus position tips the heart towards the chest wall and makes the apex beat easier to feel.

Abnormalities of the apical impulse

The most common abnormalities of the apex impulse are as follows:

- A forceful or 'thrusting' apex, either in the normal position or slightly displaced to the left. This is usually due to concentric LV hypertrophy as a result of conditions such as aortic stenosis or hypertension.
- The apical impulse may be displaced to the left and have a more diffuse heaving nature. This is usually when there is volume overload, e.g. in mitral or aortic regurgitation. A similar type of apex beat is often seen when there is severe LV dysfunction and the ventricle is enlarged. If the patient has an audible gallop rhythm this can sometimes also be palpated with a hand placed over the cardiac apex [27, 28].
- Mitral stenosis (➲Chapter 21) produces a particularly characteristic cardiac apical impulse. The apical impulse often has a sharp tapping nature. This is because the first heart sound (S_1) is loud because of forceful closure of the mitral valve and this forceful closure is transmitted to the chest wall as a 'tap'.
- Constrictive pericarditis (➲Chapter 19), which is rare in many developed countries, but common in the developing world, can produce in-drawing of the intercostal spaces during systole because the LV is tethered to the chest wall by the diseased pericardium [29].

Left parasternal (right ventricular) heave

A significantly hypertrophied and/or dilated RV will produce an abnormal impulse at the lower end of the sternum, usually to the left side. In a patient with lung disease and an abnormal RV this physical sign may be absent because the over-inflated lung acts as a cushion between the heart and the chest wall and therefore prevents the impulse being transmitted to the surface.

Auscultation

This still remains an important aspect of the clinical cardiovascular examination but auscultatory skills are decreasing with the almost universal availability of echocardiography in the developed world. Heart sounds and murmurs are often not difficult to time in the cardiac cycle but if there is doubt, palpation of the carotid pulse is extremely useful. Systolic events tend to occur at the same time as the carotid pulse since as there is only a short distance between the aortic valve and the carotid artery, the systolic pulse wave in the carotid artery occurs only a matter of milliseconds after the ejection phase of LV systole. Diastolic events occur between the palpable pulses.

Normal heart sounds

S_1 and S_2 are usually the only heart sounds heard on auscultation of a normal heart (➲Fig. 1.8A), although in young and athletic subjects a soft third sound (S_3) may be present.

S_1 results from closure of the mitral and tricuspid valves and has two components in close proximity [30]. Clinically this splitting is usually narrow and is difficult to hear unless there is right bundle branch block which accentuates this splitting by delaying the onset of RV contraction and therefore tricuspid closure. This sign has no clinical significance.

S_2 results from closure of the aortic and pulmonary valves (A_2 and P_2) [31], and is also normally split, the dominant aortic component occurring first. This splitting is usually accentuated by inspiration when right heart filling is increased and can be detected in most patients. Pulmonary hypertension (➲Chapter 24) increases the intensity of P_2 and systemic hypertension (➲Chapter 13) may make A_2 louder [32].

The splitting of the S_2 requires both the aortic and pulmonary valves to be mobile so they can contribute their

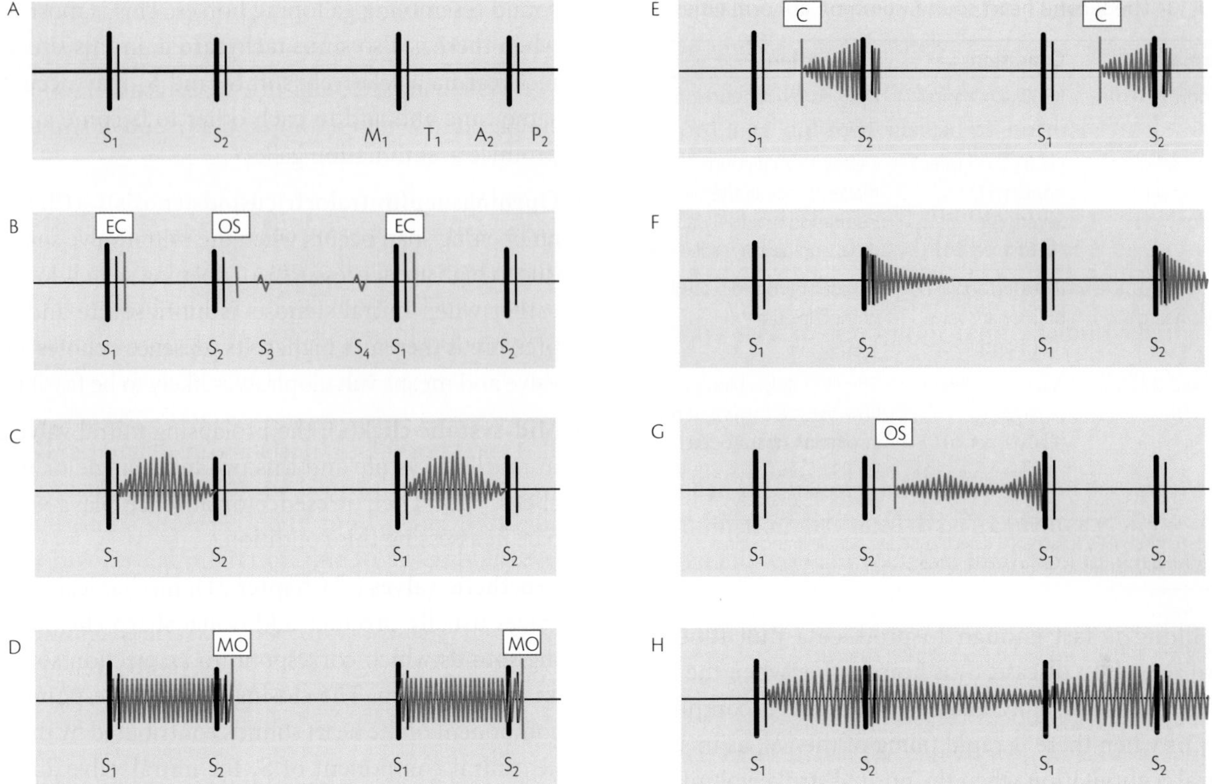

Figure 1.8 Heart sounds and murmurs. (A) Timing of normal heart sounds. S_1, first heart sound; S_2, second heart sound. S_1 has two components, mitral closure (M_1) and tricuspid closure (T_1); M_1 is louder. S_2 also has two components, due to aortic valve closure (A_2) and pulmonary valve closure (P_2) with A_2 being the louder. (B) Additional heart sounds. Third heart sound (S_3) in early diastole due to early ventricular filling. Fourth heart sound (S_4) in late diastole due to reduced ventricular compliance. EC; ejection click, (or ejection sound) an abrupt, high frequency, systolic sound associated with an abnormal (usually congenital) aortic or pulmonary valve; OS, opening snap, associated with opening of the valve in mitral stenosis. (C) Mid (ejection) systolic murmur. Typical of aortic stenosis, the murmur increases in early systole and decreases in late systole (crescendo–decrescendo pattern) and occurs only when the valve is open and ejection is occurring. As such, it starts just after S_1 and stops at S_2. (D) Pan- (holo-) systolic murmur. Typical of mitral regurgitation, the murmur intensity varies little throughout systole (plateau pattern). It starts with S_1 and continues through (and masks) S_2, stopping with mitral valve opening (MO). (E) Late systolic murmur. Typical of mitral valve prolapsed, the murmur commences in mid-late systole, often preceded by an ejection click (C). As with (D) it continues through and masks S_2, stopping with mitral valve opening. (F) Early diastolic murmur—typical of aortic or pulmonary regurgitation. It commences immediately following S_2 and decreases in intensity during diastole as the pressure difference between the respective great vessel and ventricle decreases. (G) Mid-diastolic murmur with presystolic accentuation. Typical of mitral stenosis, the murmur is a low intensity 'rumble' in mid diastole. It can be preceded by an OS when the valve is pliable and, in sinus rhythm, increases in intensity at end-diastole as a result of atrial contraction, stopping with the associated loud mitral component of S_1. (H) Continuous murmur. Murmur in systole which continues through S_2 into some or all of diastole. This results from a communication between the left- and right-sided circulations so that there is a pressure drop across the pathological structure throughout systole and diastole, hence the continuous nature of the murmur.

component. Usually the splitting widens with inspiration, mainly because blood is drawn into the right heart by negative intrathoracic pressure, increasing RV filling. It takes longer for this extra blood to be ejected thereby delaying P_2 and widening the splitting. ➲ Table 1.13 shows the commonest abnormalities of the S_2 and an illustration of wide, fixed splitting is shown in ➲ Fig. 1.9.

Further effects of respiration on auscultation

In practical terms:

- If a murmur or sound (e.g. ejection click) is made louder by inspiration it is nearly always right sided since right heart blood flow is increased in inspiration.
- If a murmur is made louder by expiration it may be left sided; however, this is not definite since expelling air from the lungs decreases the amount of air between the heart and chest walls and may increase the intensity of any event whether its source is right or left sided.

Additional heart sounds (➲Fig 1.8B)

Heart sounds other than S_1 and S_2 are usually abnormal but S_3 and an ejection sound can occur in normal subjects (➲Table 1.14).

- **S_3:** the S_3 coincides with rapid filling of the LV [33] and in fit young subjects and the athlete (usually young people), often with a slow heart rate and compliant ventricle,

Table 1.13 The second heart sound: common abnormalities

Abnormality	Condition	Explanation
Wide normal splitting	RBBB (➲Chapter 2)	Delayed RV contraction delays P_2
Reversed splitting (widening with expiration)	LBBB (➲Chapter 2) Impaired LV Severe AS (➲Chapter 21)	Delayed LV ejection makes P_2 occur after A_2. Inspiration makes P_2 late as usual and narrows splitting
Single S_2 (no split heard)	Diseased aortic or pulmonary valve (➲Chapter 21)	No sound from diseased, immobile cusp
Wide fixed splitting (➲Fig. 1.9)	ASD—moderate or large (➲Chapter 10)	The ASD allows blood to flow between atria and thus inspiration does not increase RV filling and delays P_2. Also partial RBBB delays P_2

AS, aortic stenosis; ASD, atrial septal defect; LBBB, left bundle branch block; LV, left ventricular; RBBB, right bundle branch block; RV, right ventricular.

LV filling is fast enough to produce a dull thudding third sound. In disease, S_3 is heard either when the LV is abnormal and usually dilated with reduced compliance [34] or when there is rapid filling of the LV, as in severe mitral regurgitation when the normal stroke volume and the blood regurgitated into the left atrium (LA) in the last systole returns to the LV together in early diastole.

- **Ejection sound:** an ejection sound occurs as the aortic or pulmonary valve opens and is close to S_1 and may be misinterpreted for a split S_1. Ejection sounds are sometimes heard in normal subjects but the most common cause in an asymptomatic patient is a bicuspid aortic valve (➲Chapter 21).
- **S_4:** this corresponds to atrial contraction and may be present whenever atrial contraction is powerful, usually secondary to ventricular dysfunction or hypertrophy.
- **Gallop rhythm (triple rhythm):** an additional sound combined with the normal heart sounds may produce a sound resembling galloping horses. This is most marked when there is also sinus tachycardia; in this situation of tachycardia a relatively soft S_3 and S_4 may occur at the same time and add to each other to become audible or produce a 'summation gallop'.
- **Openingsnap(mitralortricuspidstenosis)(➲Chapter21):** an opening snap occurs when the mitral valve snaps open due to high atrial pressure. An opening snap is louder and earlier when mitral stenosis is more severe and the LA pressure is therefore higher. Its presence denotes a pliable valve and means valvuloplasty is likely to be feasible.
- **Mid-systolic click(s):** the prolapsing mitral valve tenses in mid/late systole and this produces single or multiple clicks [35]. Their presence or absence plays very little part in assessing this condition.
- **Prosthetic valves (➲Chapter 21):** mechanical prosthetic valves usually produce additional sharp clicking opening sounds which correspond to an ejection sound and an opening snap. The closing sound corresponds to the component of the heart sounds contributed by that valve, i.e. mitral component of S_1 for mitral valve and aortic component of S_2 for an aortic valve. As there is normally no sound from the opening of normal heart valves, the high intensity, abrupt metallic click of mechanical valve opening produce additional opening sounds which in the case of the aortic valve has the same timing as an ejection sound, and in the case of the mitral valve occurs when an opening snap would occur. Tissue valves do not normally produce additional sounds. Both mechanical and tissue aortic valve usually causes turbulent flow and an ejection systolic murmur.
- **Pericardial knock:** in constrictive pericarditis (➲Chapter 19), a pericardial 'knock' may be heard in early diastole and is due to the high pressure atrium rapidly decompressing into a restricted LV producing an audible reverberation.

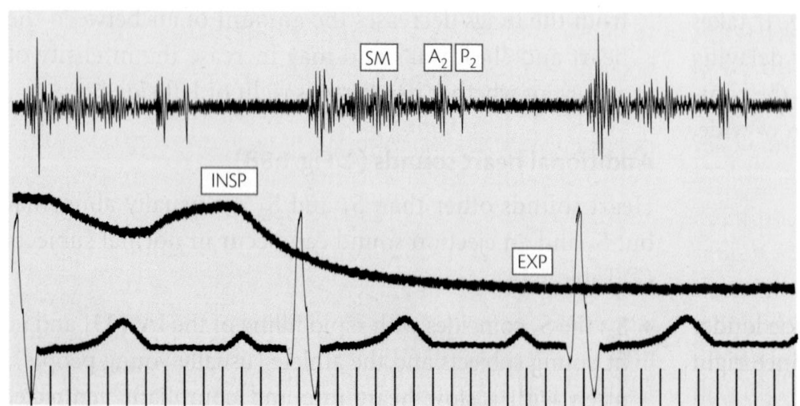

Figure 1.9 Wide, fixed splitting of the second heart sound (S_2). This illustrates that the aortic (A_2) and pulmonary (P_2) components of S_2 are widely split. Note that there is no variation in the splitting with respiration. SM, systolic murmur.

Table 1.14 Clinical implications of additional heart sounds

S_3	LV impairment or increased filling May be palpable at apex
S_4	LV impairment or hypertrophy
Gallop rhythm	The heart under stress Often palpable at apex
Ejection sound	Aortic or pulmonary valve opening suggests abnormal valve May occur in hypertension. Commonest cause bicuspid aortic valve
Opening snap	Mitral stenosis (and tricuspid stenosis—rare). High pressure opening of valve Longer the interval from the S2 the milder the mitral stenosis since it depends on LA pressure
Mechanical valve clicks	Absent or reduced sounds = *danger* Mitral valve prosthesis—gap from S_2 to opening sound is guide to LA pressure

LA, left atrial; LV, left ventricular.

Murmurs

Detecting and interpreting cardiac murmurs is difficult and needs a combination of physiological and cardiological knowledge and experience. In reality, in the developed world if a murmur is heard then it is investigated further with an echocardiogram (➲Chapter 4). Murmurs are audible vibrations produced by turbulent flow through the heart. They are described using a number of characteristics as shown in ➲Table 1.15 and the grading of murmur intensity (loudness) is described in ➲Table 1.16.

Innocent murmurs

Not all murmurs are pathological and 'innocent' murmurs are common, occurring in situations where the circulation is hyperdynamic, e.g. normal children [36], but also in pregnancy, fever, anaemia, and hyperthyroidism. It may require an echocardiogram (➲Chapter 4) to be sure that murmurs really are innocent but they are always systolic, usually soft or moderate in intensity, as well as having a musical rather than either harsh or blowing quality.

Table 1.15 Description of murmurs

Intensity (loudness)	Graded as 1–6 (or 1–4) (➲Table 1.16)
Duration	Short to long
Pattern (shape)	Crescendo, decrescendo, variable, plateau, crescendo–decrescendo
Timing	Relation to cardiac cycle, e.g. mid-systolic, ejection systolic, pansystolic, late systolic, early diastolic
Frequency	High or low pitched
Character	E.g. blowing, harsh, rasping, cooing, scraping etc.
Position	Precordial position of maximum intensity
Radiation	Precordial and other (e.g. carotids) radiation of murmur
Variation	With respiration

Table 1.16 Grading of murmur intensity

Grade 1–6	Grade 1–4	Description
1	1	Very faint murmur. Usually only heard with specialist training
2	2	Soft but easily distinguishable murmur
3	3	Loud murmur without an associated thrill (palpable murmur)
4	4	Loud murmur with barely palpable thrill
5	4	Loud murmur with easily palpable thrill
6	4	Loud murmur with thrill, and audible with stethoscope removed from chest wall

Systolic murmurs [37]

The flow of blood through or across a pathological structure generates the murmur and this flow is determined by the pressure difference on opposite sides of the responsible pathology (abnormal valve, septal defect, coarctation, etc.). The sound generated is louder when the pressure difference across the pathological structure is greater and higher velocity of flow and greater turbulence is generated. For example, ➲Fig. 1.8C illustrates the murmur generated in aortic stenosis (➲Chapter 21). The murmur does not start until ejection begins and peaks when blood flow is greatest, and consequently, as stenosis becomes more severe, the murmur peaks later in systole. The murmur stops before S2 since ejection is finished. Thus the murmur has a crescendo/decrescendo character and is contained well within the heart sounds. This type of murmur is described as an ejection murmur. The flow dependence of murmurs means that the murmur gets softer and may disappear if transvalvar flow starts to fall when a lesion is very severe and causes heart failure. Regurgitant systolic murmurs through the AV valves, e.g. mitral regurgitation [38] (➲Chapter 21), may start immediately isovolumic contraction begins (➲Fig. 1.8D), i.e. before ejection, since the leak occurs as soon as the pressure rises in the ventricle and continues up until S_2 or slightly beyond. This is because there is a continuing pressure difference between the LV and the LA during this period of time. Often the S_2 is swamped by the end of the murmur. Murmurs of this type that fill the whole of systole are described as pan- or holosytolic. Pansystolic murmurs also occur with ventricular septal defect (VSD), see ➲Chapter 10. In many patients with mitral regurgitation, however, the valve does not become incompetent until, for example, it has prolapsed and then the murmur begins in mid- or even late systole and then continues up to and slightly beyond the second heart sounds (➲Fig. 1.8E). Late systolic murmurs may have a crescendo rather similar to an ejection systolic murmur but are much later in the cycle and run into the S_2 and stop abruptly. This is easily appreciated by the experienced auscultator, particularly if the heart rate is not fast but sometimes a mid- or late systolic click is mistaken for S_2 and the murmur placed erroneously in diastole (see ➲Key point 11, p.27).

Diastolic murmurs (➲Figs. 1.8F and 1.8G)

Diastolic murmurs from the AV valves can be extremely difficult to hear. They are often very low pitched and rumbling and the inexperienced auscultator simply thinks they are ambient noise. Typically they are produced by mitral stenosis (➲Chapter 10) (and, in rare cases, tricuspid stenosis) and these conditions are becoming much less common in the developed world. A mitral diastolic murmur may be accentuated quite considerably by turning the patient on their left side and listening at the cardiac apex with the bell of the stethoscope and/or getting the patient to exercise and then listening again. Mid-diastolic murmurs are accentuated just before the next systole as blood flow across the mitral valve is increased by atrial contraction (➲Table 1.17). This presystolic accentuation usually disappears when the atrial fibrillation develops but on occasions may persist [39].

Early diastolic murmur

Early diastolic murmurs occur from regurgitation through aortic or pulmonary valves. They are decrescendo and follow the S_2. This is because the biggest pressure difference between the outflow vessel and the ventricle is at the beginning of diastole. Mild aortic regurgitation (➲Chapter 21) produces a short, soft, early diastolic murmur which is difficult to hear but this can often by elicited by leaning the patient forward and getting them to breathe out. This brings the heart closer to the chest wall and makes the regurgitation audible. Increasing intensity of the murmur tends to suggest the lesion is becoming more severe, but sometimes there is a paradoxical situation with early diastolic murmurs. When chronic aortic regurgitation is very severe the backflow into the ventricle from the aorta occurs quickly and so the murmur, although loud, is not very long. This is even more striking when there is acute aortic regurgitation due to sudden disruption of the aortic valve by endocarditis, dissecting aneurysm, or trauma. The LV immediately prior to the regurgitation developing is of normal size and the sudden torrential aortic regurgitation fills the ventricle to its full capacity almost instantaneously, and at the time slams the mitral valve shut. This leads to an extremely low cardiac output and a very short murmur [40]. The predominant signs are of a patient with cardiovascular collapse, a sinus tachycardia, and what sounds like a gallop rhythm. The experienced

Table 1.17 Important systolic murmurs: some ways of distinguishing them

Murmur	Lesion	Site	Hints
Ejection systolic	Aortic stenosis	Left upper SB—also often at apex. Radiates to carotids.	Slow rising carotid but often not obvious in the elderly. Apex if palpable forceful but not displaced Young patients' murmur preceded by an ejection click. S_2 variable and often single when the valve is heavily calcified
	Pulmonary stenosis	Right upper SB	Increases with inspiration Ejection click, delayed P_2 may be soft
	ASD		Fixed split S_2 Heaving volume-loaded RV felt at left lower SB if large shunt
	Innocent	All areas Musical quality	May just appear when cardiac output is high
Pansystolic	Mitral regurgitation	Apex and radiates to axilla	Very variable but with valvar mitral regurgitation often blowing and goes up to and into S_2. Apex heaving. May be MDM and S_3 is severe
	Tricuspid regurgitation	Left sternal border	Increase with inspiration, prominent v wave in JVP, possibly pulsatile liver. Also left parasternal heave—often also signs of pulmonary hypertension
	Ventricular septal defect	Left sternal border	Often harsh and thrill frequently present. Single S_2 with large defect.
Late systolic	Subvalvar mitral regurgitation (MVP, chordal rupture)	Apex—radiates to axilla but also may go to the back, head or neck	May be harsh and preceded by systolic click or clicks at apex. Apex heaving and an MDM and S_3 if MR severe. May be mistaken for early diastolic murmur if preceded by a late click which is mistaken for S_2
Presystolic	Mitral stenosis (and also tricuspid stenosis—very rare)	Apex to left SB	Can be difficult to time and may mistakenly be placed in systole and ascribed to mitral regurgitation. Needs meticulous timing against the carotid

ASD, atrial septal defect; SB, sternal border; MVP, mitral valve prolapse; MDM, mid-diastolic murmur.

cardiologist will immediately recognize acute severe aortic regurgitation as a possible cause of this problem and arrange suitable investigations, including immediate echocardiography. Often aortic valve surgery is lifesaving but if the condition is not recognized it will prove fatal. Pulmonary hypertension (➲Chapter 24) produces an early diastolic murmur which tends to be slightly lower pitched than the aortic murmur. The early diastolic murmur is heard at the upper left sternal border and follows the loud pulmonary component of the S_2 due to pulmonary hypertension.

Continuous murmurs

Continuous murmurs are rare in adults. They are exactly what they say they are, a murmur which continues throughout the cardiac cycle (➲Fig. 1.8H) [41]. The systolic component is usually louder than the diastolic component but the overall effect is that there is no break in the sound and the term 'machinery murmur' is extremely appropriate, as it sounds like heavy machinery working in the background. This may be due to a patent ductus arteriosus (➲Chapter 10) that has been missed in childhood, but most commonly in adults it is due to some acute communication developing between the right and left side of the heart through which flow occurs both in systole and diastole. The commonest situation is a ruptured sinus of Valsalva although infective endocarditis (➲Chapter 22) can result in arteriovenous and right/left heart communications.

Bruits and conducted murmurs in the carotids

A systolic noise over the carotids may:

1) be conducted from the heart—usually from aortic valve although anteriorly directed loud mitral murmurs may also go to the neck. The same noise will be heard in neck and chest;
2) originate from disease in the carotid in which case it is only heard in the neck.

Clearly it may be impossible to be sure if there is both carotid and valve disease or valve disease alone in situation (1).

The radiation of cardiac murmurs

The radiation of cardiac murmurs is complex and in essence any cardiac murmur from any structure can be heard anywhere in the chest. There are, however, typical areas—apical/mitral, pulmonary, aortic, and tricuspid areas, with radiation to the carotid, back, and/or axilla. It should be remembered that loud murmurs from mitral valve prolapse and ruptured chordae can radiate anywhere and can go into the neck and sound very like aortic stenosis murmurs. Furthermore, it is common for the murmur of aortic stenosis in elderly patients to be louder at the cardiac apex than it is over the aortic area, which is its classical site. This is because in elderly patients with hyperinflated lungs there is more lung between the upper part of the heart and the chest wall, i.e. around the aortic area, than there is at the cardiac apex where the heart usually remains in contact with the chest wall. Aortic murmurs that are heard only at the cardiac apex often radiate into the neck and can be heard over the carotids.

Other features of auscultation

A 'pericardial rub' is associated with pericarditis (➲Chapter 19) and is due to the inflamed visceral and parietal pericardium rubbing together with each heartbeat, producing an intermittent scratchy sound with systolic and diastolic components usually best heard with the patient recumbent, and can, on occasions, disappear when the patient sits forward, a position that also tends to relieve the discomfort of pericardial pain. Always think of the diagnosis if you see a patient leaning forward in bed.

Examination of other systems

The presence of pulmonary oedema and/or pleural effusion on chest examination is an integral part of assessing the cardiac patient, as is examination of the abdomen for ascites, splenomegaly, hepatomegaly (pulsatile and non-pulsatile), and the presence of abdominal aortic aneurysm or abdominal bruits which may indicate the presence of more extensive vascular disease or renal artery stenosis (➲Chapter 13).

Examination scenarios

Although it would be nice to have ideal conditions and unlimited time available to examine all patients in a thorough and systematic way, clinical reality is often very different and we need to tailor our examination to circumstances dictated by the clinical situation

Acute chest pain

Chest pain is the commonest reason for acute cardiac hospital admission. Performing an ECG to determine if there is ST elevation should take priority unless the patient is moribund.

ST elevation myocardial infarction (➲Table 1.18)

If a diagnosis of ST elevation myocardial infarction (STEMI) is confirmed the first priority is rapid reperfusion by thrombolysis or primary percutaneous coronary intervention. History and examination should concentrate on establishing the safety and feasibility of reperfusion and the presence of complications of acute myocardial infarction (e.g. ventricular septal defect or a ruptured papillary muscle). In patients with ST elevation alternative diagnoses

Table 1.18 Important examination points in STEMI

General examination
Responsiveness of patient
Breathing
Peripheral vasoconstriction
Sweating
Bruising/bleeding
Pulses in both arms
Aortic dissection
Blood pressure
Hypotension requiring circulatory support
Hypertension contraindicating thrombolysis
JVP
Right heart failure
Right ventricular infarction
Systolic murmur
Post-infarction ventricular septal defect
Acute mitral regurgitation
Aortic stenosis
Chest auscultation
Pulmonary oedema
Femoral pulses
Primary percutaneous coronary intervention patients
Gross neurology (in case a cerebral complication of treatment occurs)

must be considered, especially where some aspect of the history and examination does not fit well with a presumed STEMI. Pericarditis may masquerade as STEMI although the ECG is often quite different. A pericardial rub does not contribute much as it may also be secondary to an MI. The echocardiogram may show pericardial fluid in pericarditis but more importantly in the patient with a STEMI there will be reduced LV contraction in the infarcting area. A history of sudden, searing chest pain, combined with differential pulses and/or blood pressure would suggest the possibility of acute aortic dissection, including the origin of the coronary arteries.

In a patient with extreme pallor and hypotension following thrombolysis the possibility of occult bleeding should be seriously considered (clinical scenario) (see ➲Key point 12, p.27).

Non-ST elevation myocardial infarction chest pain: ?cause

If there is no ST elevation on an ECG, history and examination will be targeted at diagnosis and there will be less time pressure. More subtle aspects of cardiac examination such as the presence of a dyskinetic apex beat or a S_4 might suggest coronary artery disease whereas a raised JVP, dyspnoea, and tachycardia might point to the possibility of pulmonary embolism. The presence of a pericardial rub may suggest pericarditis alone but it is worth remembering that this can be secondary to myocardial infarction. Pain elicited by pressure on the chest can be very misleading (see ➲Key point 13, p.27).

Acute cardiovascular collapse

There is often little clinical history from the patient, and examination is crucial in pointing to the correct diagnosis and initiating potentially life-saving treatment. Do not forget to talk to the family and the ambulance crew. The clinician must examine the patient swiftly and accurately and be able to multitask, combining examination with initial treatment while assimilating all the available information from history, examination, initial investigations, and responses to initial treatment. The clinician must give both leadership and guidance to the team.

Initial examination is similar to that for a STEMI patient (➲Table 1.18). Tachycardia may result from an arrhythmia such as ventricular tachycardia or simply sinus tachycardia as a response to acute problem. Bradycardia may indicate the presence of heart block or sinus arrest and immediate external pacing may be necessary. Most acutely unwell patients will be hypotensive, but the presence of hypertension may suggest aortic dissection either because it is the underlying cause or the renal arteries are involved, pulmonary oedema, or a non-cardiac (cerebral) cause; patients with subarachnoid haemorrhage may have striking ECG changes, high blood pressures, and altered levels of consciousness. Vasodilatation suggests infection whereas vasoconstriction may suggest pump failure and different initial circulatory support requirements.

A patient with pulmonary oedema will want to sit up whereas a patient with cardiac rupture (➲Chapter 16) or tamponade or acute pulmonary embolus (➲Chapter 37) may be unable to do so because they become hypotensive. Oxygen saturation, although strictly an investigation, is a valuable part of initial examination. It can also be useful to know the early response to any treatment, such as oxygen therapy administered by paramedics prior to admission, so discussion with paramedics and examination of the paramedic charts may reveal a rapidly changing situation.

Examination is much more productive if the possible diagnoses are running through the cardiologist's mind as they examine the patient (see ➲Key point 13, p.27).

Patient with hypotension following invasive cardiac investigations or percutaneous coronary intervention

The situation that must be considered immediately is cardiac tamponade due to a perforation of a cardiac chamber or a coronary artery during the procedure. It is essential to rule this out by immediate echocardiography. The physical signs of tamponade may be present, but they may be very difficult to elicit in the acutely distressed hypotensive patient. Having said this, by far the most common cause of this problem is a vasovagal reaction, often attributable to a degree of dehydration prior to the procedure, and fear and discomfort. There is often bradycardia associated with this which will respond to atropine and in addition a quick fluid load and raising the foot of the bed will often recover the situation within a short period of time. Other possibilities are acute myocardial infarction due to an embolic event, cerebrovascular problems, retroperitoneal bleeding, and catheter-induced arterial dissection. An early ECG is an essential investigation.

Patients with multiple injuries (e.g. road traffic accident)

Major cerebral or orthopaedic injuries may seem most prominent but associated cardiac injury may be life threatening and should be considered in all patient with chest trauma. Three key areas of concern from a cardiovascular standpoint are direct traumatic injury, cardiac tamponade, and aortic transection or rupture.

Physical examination may detect cardiac tamponade and there may be missing pulses due to aortic injury. The other circulatory consequences of major trauma are more likely to be recognized with appropriate imaging (echocardiography, X-ray, or computed tomography) in response to a high level of suspicion. All patients with chest trauma need an ECG which may identify myocardial contusion or even transection of the left anterior descending coronary artery with STEMI.

Conclusion

The history and the examination are the everyday tools of the clinical cardiologist and used correctly often allow rapid diagnosis, and at other times point investigations in the correct direction from an early stage. Effective use of these tools requires thoughtful application and considerable experience. There are some golden rules:

- Listen to the patient.
- Speak to a witness.
- Record both positive and negative features of the history and examination accurately.
- If a sign cannot be elicited, e.g. a JVP cannot be seen, record it as 'not seen' instead of 'normal'.
- Tailor the history and examination to the clinical situation. In a real emergency multitasking is essential, i.e. the history must be taken while the patient is examined and while first-line resuscitative treatment is begun.
- Always seek to confirm or refute definitively the more serious of two possible diagnoses. Do not assume the less serious diagnosis is the cause of the problem and discharge the patient.
- Repeat the history and examination as appropriate. Examination may need to be frequent, e.g. in the acutely ill patient with a myocardial infarction or with endocarditis. The findings must be recorded on each occasion accurately.
- Know how reliable physical signs are (➲Table 1.19). If one of the 'top signs' is present do not be reassured by other features, e.g. the patient who feels reasonably well but has a persistent sinus tachycardia and a reduced oxygen saturation may well be on the edge of cardiovascular collapse. Young patients in particular accommodate a serious illness remarkably well until the moment when they collapse.

Table 1.19 Significance of some important physical signs

Top signs (signs that must not be ignored and are usually easy to elicit)	**Difficult signs** (often need considerable experience to detect and understand their significance)
◆ Pallor and sweating	◆ JVP level and character
◆ Hypotension	◆ Carotid pulse character
◆ Tachycardia or bradycardia	◆ Minor irregularities of the pulse
◆ Dyspnoea at rest and raised respiratory rate	◆ Subtle added heart sounds
◆ Low pulse volume	◆ Soft murmur
◆ Pulsus paradoxus	◆ Splinter haemorrhages
◆ Loud systolic murmur	
◆ Unequal pulses	
◆ Reduced oxygen saturation (cyanosis)	

Personal perspective

History taking and physical examination are basic cardiological skills that have changed very little over the years and require to be honed by frequent use. Technology, particularly in the form of echocardiography, has allowed validation of many of the auscultatory signs which are the most difficult in cardiology. Consequently the fine detail of auscultation has, to some extent, become less important as long as the echocardiogram is available. The more widespread use of small handheld echocardiography machines is likely to be a very valuable adjunct to examination for the clinician, particularly in high-volume clinics. However, all the technology in the world is no substitute for clinical experience and for being able to answer the question as to whether the patient is ill or not. The most important question is usually not 'what do the tests show?' but 'how well is the patient?'.

Table 1.20 Popular examination eponyms in cardiology

Eponym	Condition	Description
Austin Flint murmur	Aortic regurgitation	Mid-diastolic murmur due to partial closure of mitral valve by jet of aortic regurgitation
Becker's sign	Aortic regurgitation	Pulsation of the retinal vessels on fundoscopy
Broadbent's sign	Constrictive pericarditis	Intercostal indrawing during systole
Carey–Coombs murmur	Rheumatic fever	Early diastolic murmur associated with acute mitral valve inflammation
Carvallo's sign	Tricuspid regurgitation	Increasing systolic murmur intensity with inspiration
Cheyne–Stokes respiration	Heart failure	Periodic or cyclic respiration pattern
Corrigan's pulse	Aortic regurgitation	Collapsing pulse with rapid upstroke and decline, typical of aortic regurgitation
De Musset's sign	Aortic regurgitation	'Head nodding' sign in time with cardiac cycle associated with excessive pulsation from aortic regurgitation
Duroziez's sign	Aortic regurgitation	Diastolic murmur heard over femoral pulses when partly occluded below the stethoscope
Graham Steell murmur	Pulmonary regurgitation	Murmur of pulmonary regurgitation when caused by pulmonary hypertension
Janeway lesions	Infective endocarditis	Slightly raised, non-tender haemorrhagic lesions of palms of hands and/or soles of feet
Kussmaul's sign	Constrictive pericarditis	Elevation of the JVP with inspiration
Mueller's sign	Aortic regurgitation	Cyclic pulsation of the uvula in aortic regurgitation
Osler's nodes	Infective endocarditis	Small tender, purple, erythematous skin lesions due to infective emboli usually seen on fingers and toes or palms of hands/soles of feet
Quincke's sign	Aortic regurgitation	Capillary pulsation in the nail beds due to aortic regurgitation
Roth spots	Infective endocarditis	Retinal haemorrhages with central white spots, usually near the optic disc
Still's murmur	Innocent murmur	Rare but most commonly seen in children and due to vibration of normal pulmonary valve leaflets
Traube's sign	Aortic regurgitation	'Pistol shot' systolic sound in femoral arteries on auscultation

Key points

Key point 1

Let the patient talk and tell the story in their own words.

Key point 2

Use all the information available:

- Look at all ambulance records in acute patients, e.g. the ambulance crew may have observed a low oxygen saturation while the patient was in the ambulance which has resolved by the time they arrive in the hospital. They may also have detected transient hypotension, tachycardia, or bradycardia.
- Look at the nursing records.

Key point 3

Patients who present as emergencies are usually ill even if the symptoms are lessening by the time they see the doctor

Key point 4

Beware chest pain induced by chest pressure—it does not exclude cardiac chest pain. Acute musculoskeletal chest pain, severe enough to bring a patient to hospital, usually has an identifiable trigger, e.g. a fall with bruising.

Key point 5

Patients in middle and old age who have not had previous psychiatric problems do not suddenly develop hyperventilation as a cause for their symptoms. Ascribing symptoms to hyperventilation can be extremely dangerous.

Key point 6

Presyncope: most patients have had a similar feeling to cardiovascular presyncope when standing up quickly, particularly from bending or squatting on a hot day. If the patient is reminded of this they may then make the connection.

Key point 7

Palpitations and syncope:

- If there are eye witnesses speak to them.
- Rotational element to symptoms strongly suggests a neurological cause.
- Tell the patient to 'tap out' the arrhythmia.
- The patient who has unpredictable syncope and who has driven to the clinic should not be allowed to drive home.

Key point 8

Always think of these conditions during general examination: anaemia, diabetes mellitus, thyrotoxicosis, hypothyroidism, infective endocarditis

Key point 9

Observing the patient entering the consulting room and getting onto the examining couch often reveals important clinical information.

Key point 10

A persistent tachycardia in isolation may be an 'early warning sign' of circulatory stress, e.g.

- Impaired LV function.
- Pulmonary thromboembolism.

Key point 11

Severe valve lesion and little or no murmur.

- Critical aortic stenosis and low output.
- Severe paraprosthetic mitral regurgitation.
- Sudden acute aortic regurgitation, e.g. endocarditis or dissection.
- Severe mitral stenosis (occasionally).

Key point 12

Always consider possible alternative diagnoses:

- Aortic dissection.
- Coronary embolism.
- Pericarditis—thrombolysis may produce haemopericardium.
- ST elevation not new—other causes of chest pain.

Key point 13

Always consider the following in a patient with cardiovascular collapse

- Cardiac arrhythmia.
- Aortic dissection.
- Pulmonary embolism.
- Pericardial tamponade.
- Contained cardiac rupture.
- Post infarct ventricular septal defect/mitral regurgitation.
- Infective endocarditis or other form of sepsis.
- Cardiogenic shock due to myocardial infarction.
- Acute severe aortic/mitral regurgitation.
- Prosthetic valve dysfunction.

Further reading

Douglas G, Nicol F, Robertson C (eds.). *Macleod's Clinical Examination*, 11th edn., 2005. Edinburgh: Elsevier Churchill Livingstone.

Epstein O, Perkin DG, Cookson J, *et al. Clinical Examination*, 4th edn., 2008. London: Mosby Elsevier.

White PD. *Heart Disease*, 1931. New York: The Macmillan Company.

Wood P. *Diseases of the Heart and Circulation*, 1950. London: Eyre and Spottiswoode.

Online resources

The following websites are useful sources of medical images:

- http://images.google.com/
- http://www.healcentral.org/index.jsp
- http://www.images.md/users/index.asp
- http://www.omnimedicalsearch.com/images.html

For full references and multimedia materials please visit the online version of the book (http://esctextbook.oxfordonline.com).

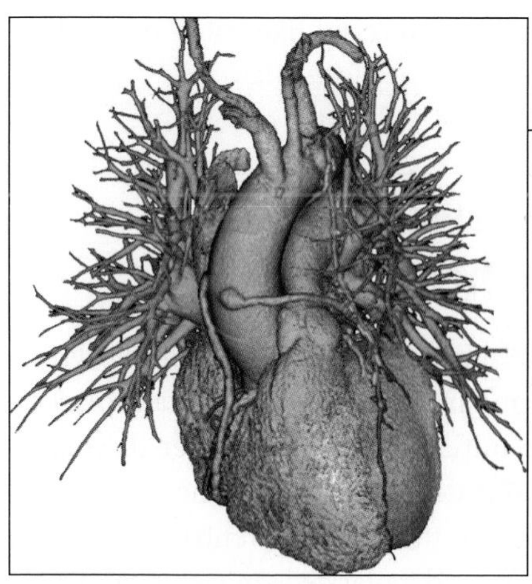

CHAPTER 2

The Electrocardiogram

Francisco G. Cosío, José Palacios, Agustín Pastor, and Ambrosio Núñez

Contents

Summary

The electrocardiogram (ECG) records electrical fields created during depolarization and repolarization of the atrial and ventricular myocardium that are referred to as vectors. The multiple leads define vector magnitude and direction in space in relation with the anatomy and the electrophysiology. The ECG does not detect activation of the specialized conduction tissues but indirect data such as changes in activation vectors and activation times may point to specific abnormalities. Atrial activation is a 'minor' portion of the ECG but the P wave can still help identify chamber enlargement and, very significantly, the mechanisms of bradycardias and tachycardias. The QRS complex, generated by ventricular activation is divided in time windows for easier analysis. Initial vectors show the direction of septal activation and the function of the left bundle branch. Abnormal negative waves pinpoint the site of myocardial infarction scars. The middle QRS vectors express the dominance of either ventricle and reflect left or right ventricular enlargement. Block of a bundle branch widens the QRS and the direction of the delayed vectors will point at the blocked branch. The ST segment and the T wave have a unique ability to show acute metabolic or inflammatory changes, and the evolution of these changes help to follow the clinical course of the disease. In its 'old age' the ECG is still an essential tool for the cardiologist, the internist, and the general practitioner, and its evaluation in the clinical context can offer information essential to make diagnostic and therapeutic decisions both cheaply and quickly.

Introduction

The ECG, with more than 100 years of history, defies time and remains one of the most popular and useful tools in modern cardiology. Decades of study have taught us to read from the ECG: heart rate and rhythm, normal or abnormal conduction through atria or ventricles, and the presence of atrial or ventricular enlargement or myocardial infarction scars can be detected. Furthermore, the repolarization contains information often leading to the diagnosis of ischaemia, myocardial stretch, pharmacological effects, electrolyte imbalance, hypothermia, or even congenital ionic channel diseases capable of producing sudden death. The ECG can detect pre-excitation in patients with a history of palpitation or syncope and, when recorded during an episode of tachycardia, it can orient the diagnosis toward supraventricular or ventricular mechanisms, thus orienting invasive diagnostic and therapeutic procedures.

The value of the ECG is magnified by recording during stress or other provocative manoeuvres, such as carotid sinus massage or tilt. Long periods of recording (Holter) may detect asymptomatic arrhythmias or document the cause of non-sustained palpitation. In addition, the ECG is also a universal 'timing' tool used in combination with echocardiographic, angiographic, or magnetic resonance studies. Granted, the information provided by the ECG is not perfectly sensitive or specific, but its easy availability, low cost, and the ease of obtaining repeated serial recordings make it an invaluable tool for the evaluation of the cardiac patient and the screening of patients for surgical procedures, high-risk activities, and competitive sports, used in combination with clinical information.

Obtaining the information contained in an ECG tracing may not be easy. Many algorithms and tables are available, but they are easy to forget or cumbersome to carry, and this information may not be easy to consult at the time of an emergency. Many ECG recorders provide automatic reading of the tracing and, even if this automatic diagnosis is not devoid of errors, it is helpful to the physician, because it may call attention to subtle abnormalities that may need consideration in the clinical context. A friendly approach to the ECG is possible using deductive interpretation, based on the anatomic position of the heart and a basic knowledge of cardiac activation mechanisms. This approach can lead the reader in the right direction immediately, leaving for later the need to qualify specificity through further tests, more reading, or repeated ECG recordings. In this chapter we will try to help the reader to develop this deductive attitude in the hope that this may help change defensive attitudes into a stimulating intellectual exercise, like most of medical practice is.

Recording the electrical activity of the heart

Heart function is intermittent in cycles, alternating systole (activation/contraction) and diastole (repolarization/relaxation). Each cycle is initiated by a pacemaker discharge, normally a spontaneous depolarization of the sinus node, which spreads throughout the atria and ventricles. As soon as a portion of the heart is depolarized, an electrical field is generated between the negative charge of the depolarized area and the positive charge of the remaining areas, and the magnitude and direction of this electrical field changes throughout activation, as the size and position of the depolarized myocardium progresses. The electrical fields thus formed are represented by vectors, a simple way to show polarity (anode at vector's head), spatial direction, and magnitude (➲Fig. 2.1) [1–7].

The site of origin of the impulse, the shape and dimensions of the heart, and the presence of specialized conduction tissues are the basic determinants of the depolarization sequence (➲Fig. 2.2). Depolarization of the atria, starting

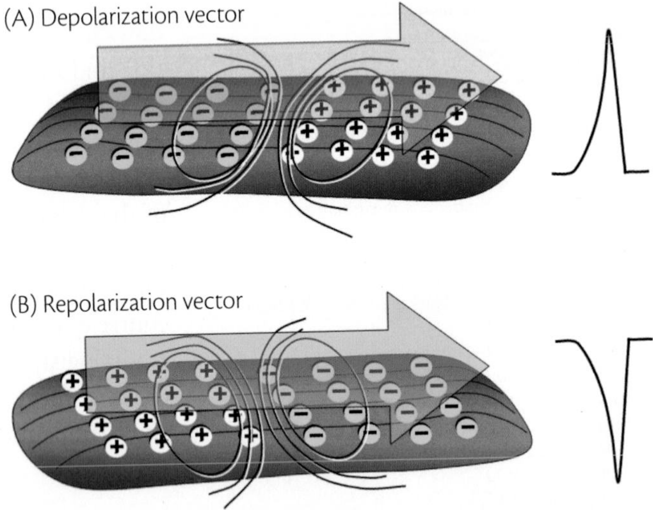

Figure 2.1 (A) Schematic representation of the genesis of electrical vectors of depolarization. On the left the myocardium is depolarized and the extracellular space becomes negatively charged. At the border between the depolarized and the polarized area an electrical field is generated that is represented by a vector. The vector head marks the anode of the electrical field. (B) The repolarization vector displays a reverse polarity (negative at the head of progression). Both vectors move in the same direction but the polarity of the wave generated at the end of the strip is negative in the repolarization vector. On the right of both A and B a simulated unipolar electrogram shows the different polarity of the recording.

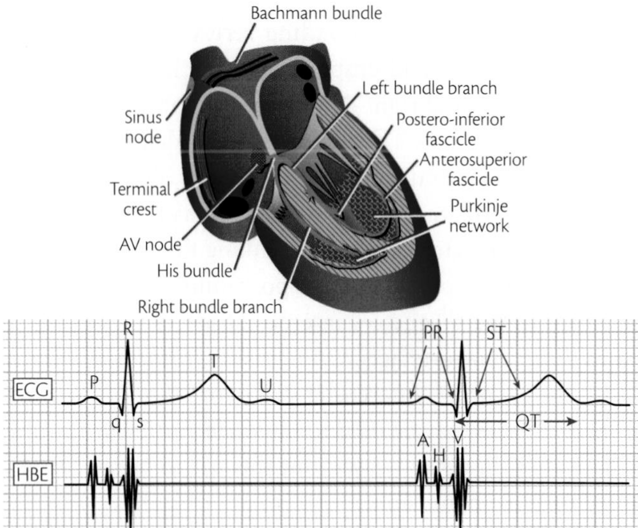

Figure 2.2 Above: schematic representation of the heart showing the endocardium and the conduction tissues. Below: schematic representation of the ECG, and the simultaneous intracardiac His bundle electrogram (HBE) filtered to show only local atrial (A), His bundle (H), and septal ventricular (V) potentials. The His bundle potential (H) is only recorded in the HBE. See text for further explanation.

at the sinus node, evolves along the surface of the relatively thin shell formed by atrial myocardium and vector sequences are relatively simple to understand. In the ventricles, the thickness of the walls and the rapid spread of activation through the subendocardial layers by the Purkinje network changes the direction of activation that now flows from endocardium to epicardium (➲Fig. 2.3). This creates opposing vectors that partially cancel each other, making the resulting vector analysis more complex and explains the voltage changes that occur in the presence of BB block (BBB) or anomalous activation.

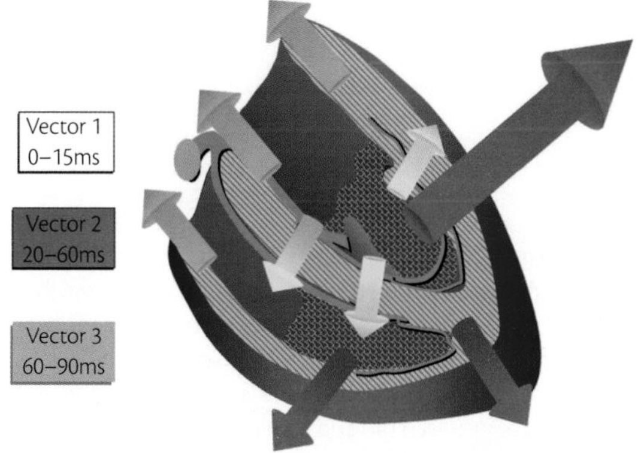

Figure 2.3 Genesis of the three main vectors of ventricular activation. In white, the three components of 'vector 1' that inscribe the 'septal' q and r waves at the beginning of the QRS. In red, the components of 'vector 2' generated by activation of the bulk of the RV and LV myocardium (note that they point in opposing directions). In magenta, activation of the basal RV, septum, and LV generating 'vector 3'. See ➲Fig. 2.2 and text for further explanation.

The ECG records from the body surface the changes in baseline potential produced by depolarization of the atria (P wave) and the ventricles (QRS complex), but the amplitude of vectors generated by the conduction tissues (atrioventricular (AV) node (N), His bundle (HB), and BB) is too small to be recorded and the study of AV conduction is based on a deductive analysis of the sequence of atrial and ventricular complexes, unless intracardiac recordings are obtained (➲Fig. 2.2) [8]. The P wave is followed by an isoelectric segment of variable length (PR) that represents conduction through the AVN, HB, and BB.

Ventricular depolarization generates a multiphasic complex that often starts with a small negative deflection (q wave) followed by a large positive deflection (R wave) and ends with another small negative deflection (s wave), therefore the denomination QRS complex (➲Fig. 2.2). The deflections are named simply following alphabetic order, and the use of upper case indicates a large deflection. The letters 'q' or 'Q' are only used for an initial negative deflection and if the initial deflection of the QRS is positive it will be named an R (or r) wave. If a QRS starts with an r wave followed with an S wave then has another positive deflection, the later is called 'r'' or 'R''.

Repolarization occurs 200–300ms after depolarization and from the ECG point of view it is a reversed process ➲Fig 2.1, where the repolarized areas now mark the anode of the electrical field, i.e. the vector head marks the cathode and the repolarization waves should, in principle, be opposite in polarity to the depolarization deflections. This is true for atrial repolarization, as the P wave is followed by a low voltage negative wave (➲Fig. 2.4). However, ventricular repolarization is different and the T wave tends to be positive where the QRS is positive. The inscription of the T wave with the same polarity as the QRS is due to a reversal of repolarization sequence that normally starts at the epicardium, where action potential duration is shorter than in the subendocardium [9].

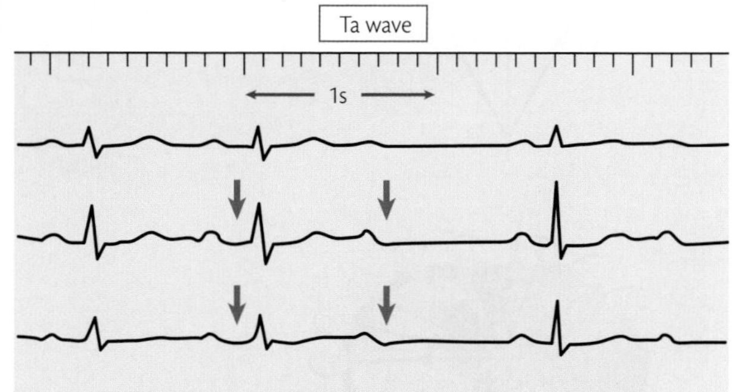

Figure 2.4 Atrial repolarization wave visible during Wenckebach block cycles (arrows) as a low voltage, negative deflection.

Recording the ECG: the leads as probes

The ECG is devised to record the sequence, direction, and magnitude of the depolarization and repolarization vectors in all three directions (supero–inferior, right–left, and antero–posterior). For this purpose, multiple 'leads' are recorded by measuring potential differences between recording electrodes in the arms and the left leg and on the anterior and left thorax, from multiple angles or perspectives (➲Fig. 2.5) [1–7]. Bipolar leads record potential differences between the arms (lead I), the right arm and the left leg (lead II), and the left arm and the left leg (lead III). Positive deflections indicate a vector direction towards the left arm in lead I and towards the left leg in leads II and III. For teaching purposes, the standard bipolar leads are considered to represent an equilateral triangle, in the centre of which originate all vectors. Vectors are recorded in each lead as orthogonal projections, and to compute vector magnitude and direction the ECG reader reverses the process, starting with the recorded deflections (➲Fig. 2.5).

Unipolar leads (V leads) record potential differences between a recording electrode and a 0 voltage reference built by linking together the arms and left leg electrodes and interposing a high resistance (Wilson's terminal). Frontal plane (limb) unipolar leads are recorded at a higher gain to compensate the low voltage caused by distance and are therefore called *augmented* (aVR, right arm; aVL, left arm; aVF, left foot). Leads I, II, and III, record vectors as projected on the lead axis (a side of the triangle) while leads aVR, aVL, and aVF record the vector projection on the axis linking the corresponding vertex with the triangle centre. The bipolar and unipolar arm and leg leads explore supero–inferior and right–left directions, only in the frontal plane (➲Fig. 2.5). The unipolar precordial leads record antero–posterior and right–left directions, defining direction in the horizontal plane. As in aVR, aVL, and aVF the vectors are projected on the axis linking the electrode with the centre of the chest. Correct positioning of the precordial leads in the 4th and 5th intercostal spaces is essential to avoid directional artefacts. On occasion, recording V1 and V2 on the 3rd or 2nd intercostal spaces or V5 and V6 on the 4th or 6th spaces may be used to illustrate particular features of activation in certain cases, but this has to be specifically noted to avoid confusion.

The direction of vectors in the frontal plane is defined in angle degrees with a positive range of 0° to +180° that starts in the left side rotating clockwise, inferiorly, and to the right and a negative range of 0 to –180° rotating counterclockwise, superiorly, and to the right (➲Fig. 2.5). The bipolar and unipolar leads axis divide this 360° range conveniently in 30° sectors, making it easier to find the lead with maximum amplitude (parallel to the vector axis) or minimum amplitude (perpendicular to the vector axis). In the horizontal plane (precordial leads), the orientation is not defined in angle degrees, but as 'rotation' in clockwise (to the left) or counterclockwise (to the right) direction (as looked at from below).

Thus, the ECG leads record the projected vectors generated by myocardial activation and the role of the ECG

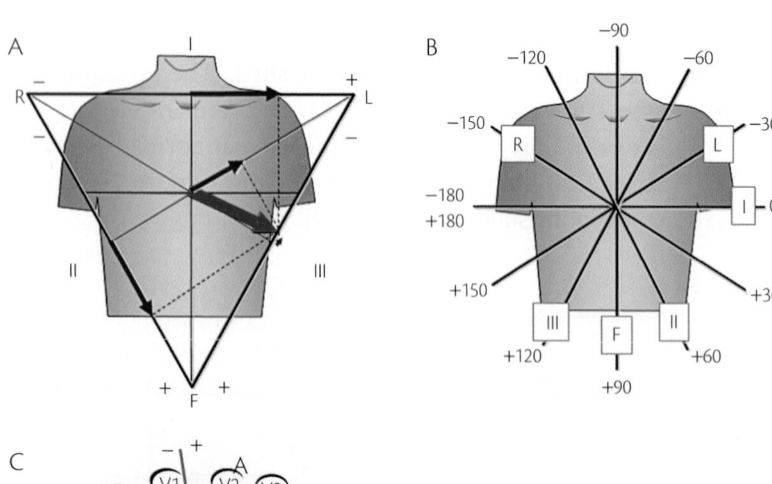

Figure 2.5 The leads as probes. Vector voltage is recorded as an orthogonal projection on each lead that allows the reader to reverse the process to deduct vector voltage and direction. A given activation vector (red) projects with different voltage depending on the angle of the lead. (A) shows the projection on a bipolar lead (III) and a unipolar lead (aVL); (B) shows the axis of the six unipolar precordial leads. (C) Vector projection on the precordial lead axis. The grey veil on the left covers the leads (V1) that will register negative potentials because it 'looks' at the vector tail. Blue arrows show the voltage projected by the activation vector on leads V2 and V6. On (A) note the cardiac vector in red has an axis close to perpendicular to lead III and clearly positive in lead I, therefore close to +30°.

reader will be to reverse the process, i.e. to deduct the size and direction of the vectors generated in all three directions of space from the deflections recorded in the multiple ECG leads. Since we are analysing the heart in its anatomic position, it is essential for the ECG reader to have a clear knowledge of the anatomic position of the different heart chambers and to be able to place the recorded vectors on (normal or abnormal) anatomy to understand their meaning.

The ECG is usually recorded at a paper speed of 25mm/s and with a voltage gain of 1cm = 1mV. Different calibrations or recording speeds can be used to highlight specific findings, but it is important to know what the recording speed and calibration are at the time of interpreting a given case in order to avoid mistakes in the evaluation of the rate, intervals duration, or voltage of the different deflections.

The anatomic position of the heart

The position of the heart chambers is more difficult to describe than the simple 'right' and 'left' designation would suggest. The right atrium (RA) is to the right of the spine, but the left atrium (LA) is in the midline, over the spine and behind (posterior to) the RA (➲Fig. 2.6). The right ventricle (RV) is in front of (anterior to) the left ventricle (LV). The left heart chambers are thus anatomically rather posterior than left, and understanding this makes it easy to understand the direction of the activation vectors, because the information provided by the ECG is anatomically accurate.

Some traditional misnomers may hinder our ability to look at the ECG intuitively [10]. The superior portion of the heart, particularly of the LV (➲Fig. 2.6) is usually called *anterior*, which creates some confusion with the true anterior part of the LV (the interventricular septum) and of the heart (the RV). The truly superior anatomic position of portions of the basal and lateral LV will help to explain ECG findings in coronary syndromes and fascicular blocks. Another significant point to note is the posterior position of the mitral ring and basal portions of the lateral LV wall which will help to explain activation in normal hearts and in pre-excitation or myocardial infarction.

Looking at leads superimposed on to chest anatomy (➲Fig. 2.5), it is easy to appreciate that I and aVL explore mainly the left lateral and superior LV walls, leads II, III, and aVF the LV and RV inferior walls, leads V1–V3 the septum and the RV free wall, and leads V4–V6 the apical and lateral LV walls. Findings such as ischaemia or infarction scars are thus localized according to the leads showing most prominently the ST, T, and QRS changes. Non-standard unipolar lead positions are occasionally used to help localize ischaemia, by placing electrodes over the right anterior thorax in a position symmetrical to the normal precordial leads to explore the RV, or beyond V6 toward the back to explore the posterior LV wall (➲Fig. 2.5).

The normal P wave and PR segment

Atrial activation starts at the high posterolateral RA, close to the superior vena cava and from there it spreads rapidly along the terminal crest and Bachmann's bundle, generating a mean activation vector pointed inferiorly and to the

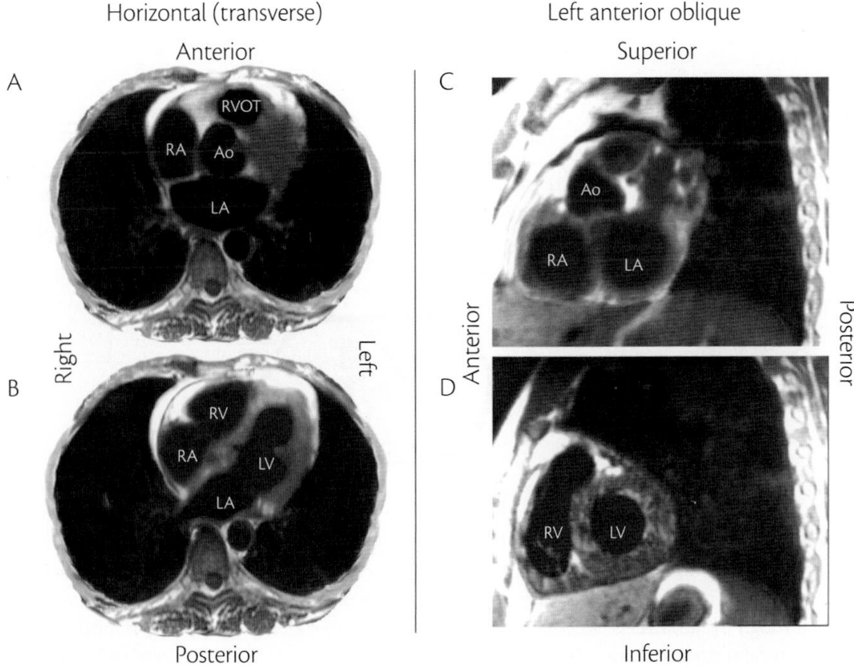

Figure 2.6 Magnetic resonance cuts of the chest showing the position of atria and ventricles. On the left, transverse (horizontal plane) cuts. On the right, left anterior oblique cuts. (A) and (C) show the LA in its midline and posterior position with the RA to its right and anteriorly. (B) and (D) show the LV is posterior to the RV. The interventricular septum is actually the anterior wall of the LV.

left (➲Fig. 2.7). P waves are normally positive in leads I, II, and aVF, negative in lead aVR, and can be flat or biphasic on lead III. The second half of activation is directed posteriorly, toward the LA, and this produces a negative terminal deflection in leads V1 and V2. In normal subjects, the origin of the sinus impulse is wide and can move from the superior to the middle or even inferior RA, changing atrial activation and P-wave morphology [11–14]. A mean P-wave frontal plane axis (âP) can be calculated obtaining the geometrical sum of positive and negative areas of the P wave in the limb leads. The normal limits of âP are between 90° and –30°.

AV conduction occurs in normal hearts only through the AVN and HB while the AV valvular rings function as electrical insulation. Slow conduction through the AVN is responsible in large part for the isoelectric PR segment recorded between P and QRS, as depolarization of the AVN, HB, and BB can not be recorded by the ECG (➲Fig. 2.2).

The normal QRS

The continuously evolving activation of the ventricles has been grouped in three time segments (vectors 1–3) as a teaching tool to ease understanding of the generation of the QRS (➲Fig. 2.3) [2, 6, 11, 15, 16]. Vector 1 (initial 12–20ms) reflects initial activation of the left side of the septum and the base of the left ventricular papillary muscles and is totally dependent of activation through the left BB (LBB) and its fascicular divisions. It is a small vector responsible for the small initial q waves in leads I, aVL, V5–V6, or in II, III, and aVF in vertical heart position (➲Figs. 2.8 and 2.9).

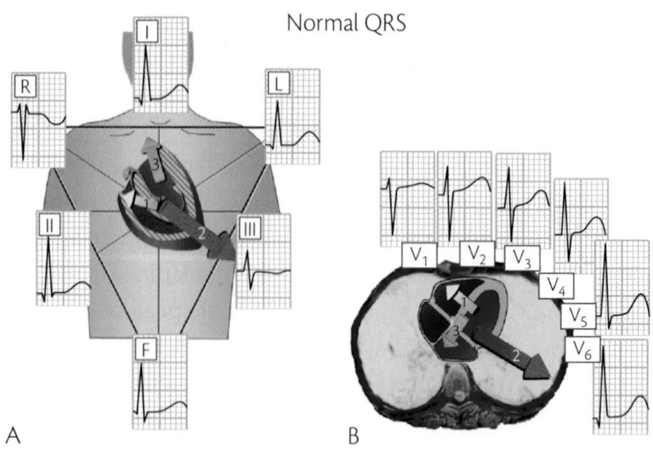

Figure 2.8 Schematic representation of the three main activation vectors and the resulting QRS complex in an intermediate-position heart. Vector 1 is grey, vector 2 is red, vector 3 magenta. ÂQRS is perpendicular to lead III which could be +30° or –150°. The positive QRS in I confirms that ÂQRS points to the left, therefore is +30°. ÂT is perpendicular to III and parallel to I (+30°).

Vector 2 (middle 20–65ms) reflects activation of the bulk of septal, RV, and LV myocardium, starting from the subendocardial Purkinje network toward the epicardium. This is a large vector, generating high voltage, sharp deflections, despite partial cancellation of voltage due to opposing vector directions (➲Figs. 2.8 and 2.9). The larger mass of the LV drives vector 2 toward the left and posteriorly with a supero–inferior direction dependent on heart position. This generates predominant R waves on leads I, aVL, and V5–V6 and S waves on leads aVR, and V1–V2. The size of R waves in each of the leads is dependent on heart position.

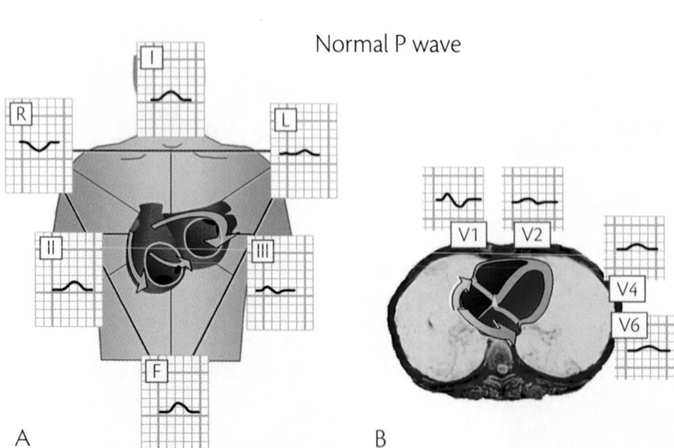

Figure 2.7 Schematic representation of the atrial chambers on the frontal and horizontal planes. A schematic recording of the P wave is shown for each lead. In green, the sinus node. Yellow arrows mark the main activation paths through the atria. ÂP is close to +40° because the P wave is clearly positive in I and close to isoelectric (slightly positive still) in III.

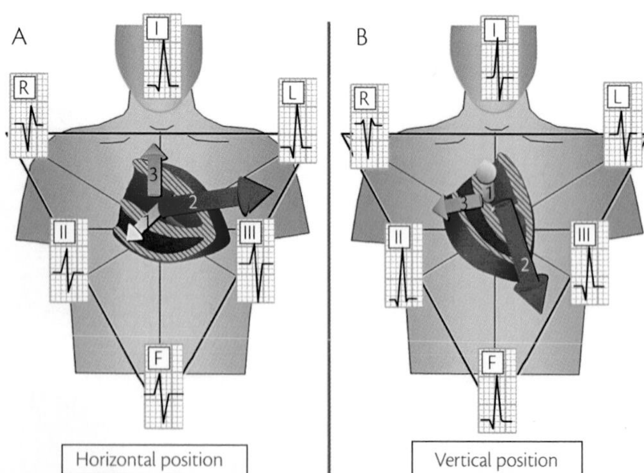

Figure 2.9 Normal variations in electrical heart position in the frontal plane. (A) Horizontal position (ÂQRS –15°). Note the most positive complex in leads I and aVL and nearly isoelectric complexes in II and aVF (slightly negative in aVF and slightly positive in II) therefore pointing between 0° and –30° (see ➲Fig. 2.5). (B) Vertical position (ÂQRS +75°). QRS is most positive in II and aVF and slightly positive in I, therefore pointing between +60° and +90°.

Vector 3 (last 65–90ms) reflects activation of the most basal part of RV, LV, and septum, including the RV outflow tract. This is normally a small vector generating slow deflections and it is directed posteriorly and superiorly, with variable right–left direction dependent on heart position (➲Figs. 2.8 and 2.9). This vector can produce s waves on leads I, II, III, or aVF or terminal slurring of the R wave in these or other leads. The activation of the RV outflow tract and terminal crest may produce an r′ on leads V1 or V2 that should not be mistaken for right BB block (RBBB) in the face of normal QRS width.

QRS voltage varies in each lead depending on the direction of the vectors, but overall QRS voltage can be abnormally low due to myocardial factors (amyloidosis, scarring), pericardial effusion, lung hyperinflation, or obesity. Low voltage in the frontal plane is present when the highest R or S wave is <5mm (0.5mV) in all the limb leads or the sum of QRS peak to peak voltage in leads I, II, and III is <15mm (1.5mV). Low voltage is present in the precordial leads when the largest R or S wave is <10mm (1.0mV) or the total QRS peak to peak voltage is <15mm (1.5mV) in all precordial leads.

Electrical position of the heart: P, QRS, and T axis

By doing a geometrical sum of all vectors of the P wave, the QRS, or the T wave we obtain a 'mean' vector for each of these deflections. Plotting the axis of these vectors gives an idea of the 'electrical' position of the heart in space that in the frontal plane is expressed as a mean axis or 'Â' in positive or negative degrees (➲Fig. 2.5). In order to calculate the mean vector it is important to take into account that areas are summed up, not only amplitudes. This is not difficult for the P or T waves (➲Figs. 2.7 and 2.8); however, the QRS complex often has multiple positive and negative deflections of which the width as well as the amplitude has to be considered.

To plot the axis, following the reverse deductive process mentioned above, it is easiest to look for the lead where the QRS is closest to isoelectric (positive areas equal to negative areas, or very small deflections in either direction), because the mean vector is perpendicular to the axis of this lead. This still marks two possible directions at 180° angles. Checking mean amplitude in another lead will solve this last question; ➲Figs. 2.5 and 2.7–2.9). The process of plotting ÂQRS can also be started by looking for the lead with the most positive direction which will be close to parallel to ÂQRS.

By obtaining a geometrical sum of positive and negative voltage *areas* of the QRS in the frontal plane (limb) leads a mean QRS axis (âQRS) can be plotted, as a rough expression of the heart position. The normal range of âQRS is between 100° and –30°, and it is influenced by body build, obesity, lung inflation, and age. Advancing age and obesity tend to shift âQRS to the left (superiorly) while lean individuals under 30 years tend to have right (inferior) âQRS (➲Fig. 2.9). In some patients, respiration changes the position of the heart enough to produce phasic changes in âQRS, usually manifest by amplitude and configuration changes in the inferior leads.

The electrical position in the horizontal plane is also variable and this will be reflected in the precordial leads as 'rotations' which are designated as 'clockwise' (to the left and posterior) or counterclockwise (to the right and anterior) as seen from below the diaphragm. The 'transitional complex' (R = S) is usually recorded in V3–V4 (➲Fig. 2.8). Counterclockwise rotation makes transitional QRS move to V2 and may have septal q waves appear as early as V4. Clockwise rotation displaces the transitional complex toward V5 and may have S waves persist in V6 (➲Fig. 2.10).

The electrical position of the heart, expressed by the axis in the frontal plane and the rotations in the horizontal plane, is determined by multiple factors, including age, body build, chest deformity or disease, chamber enlargement, myocardial infarction scars, conduction disturbances, or pre-excitation. The significance of the electrical position has to be interpreted within the clinical context.

Dextrocardia

In dextrocardia (situs inversus) all parameters of the electrical position of the heart are a mirror image to the right

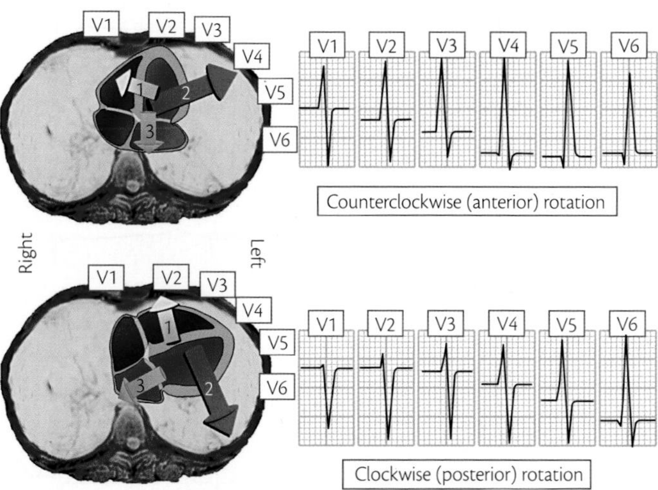

Figure 2.10 Changes in heart position on the horizontal plane. The schemas on the left show the heart on a magnetic resonance cut of the chest in an inferior look. Above: counterclockwise (anterior) rotation with the transitional complex (R = S) in V2 and septal q waves in V4. Below: clockwise (posterior) rotation with transitional complex in V5 and S waves in V6.

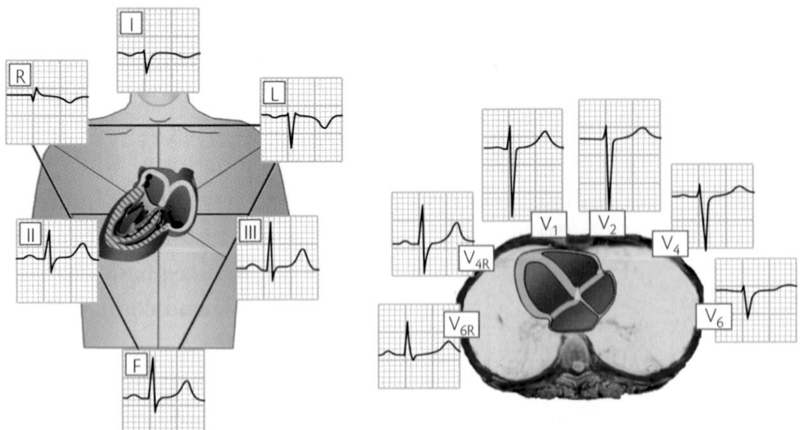

Figure 2.11 Dextrocardia. Note the mirror-image of the ECG pattern, all vectors pointing to the right. Right precordial leads record the LV vectors normally recorded in the left side.

of the midline. The P wave will be negative in lead I and the QRS axis will be shifted to the right inferior quadrant (+90 to +180). In the precordial leads the normal progression from rS to qR complexes will not happen toward V5–V6, but toward the precordial electrodes placed symmetrically on the right chest (V3R–V6R) (➲Fig. 2.11). More common than dextrocardia is having the arm electrodes switched, a situation that will mimic dextrocardia in the frontal plane, but not in the precordial leads.

Repolarization

At the end of the QRS the ECG returns to baseline where it remains for 150–200ms until the onset of the T wave which is usually slowly progressive, with a steeper return to baseline. The period between the end of the QRS and the onset of the T wave is called ST segment and the junction of the QRS and the ST segment is called 'J point'. The ST segment may be slightly elevated (0.5–1mm) in leads with large R waves and also in the right precordial leads V1–V2 with a predominant S wave. A frequent normal variant may show ST elevation ≥1mm in multiple leads called 'early repolarization'. This is often attributed to vagal tone but it may pose the differential diagnosis with pericarditis or ischaemia (➲Fig. 2.12) [17].

The T wave is normally positive in leads I, II, aVL, and V2–V6 and variable in other leads. A mean T-wave axis (âT) can be calculated on the frontal plane leads that normally will be <60° apart from âQRS. T waves can be negative in the right precordial leads (V1–V3) in children until physiological RV dominance is lost and also in normal women and in men of black African descent.

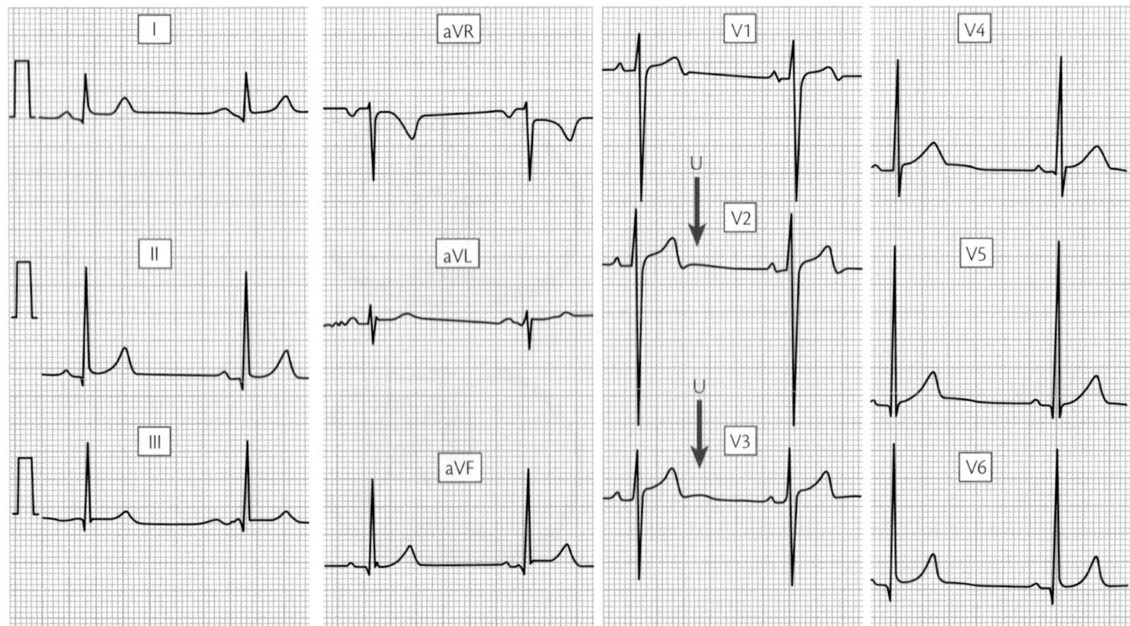

Figure 2.12 'Early repolarization' in a normal 20-year-old man. Note ST segment elevation in most leads, that was stable in time, in the absence of any cardiac symptoms. Note also high QRS voltage in inferior and precordial leads that would be suggestive of LV enlargement but is normal at this age. The blue arrows mark the normal, low voltage, U wave.

Following the end of the T wave, a low voltage, rounded deflection is often recorded, especially in the precordial leads, that is recognized as the U wave (➲Fig. 2.12). U waves are probably the expression of delayed repolarization of the slowest myocardial layers and perhaps the Purkinje network [9, 18].

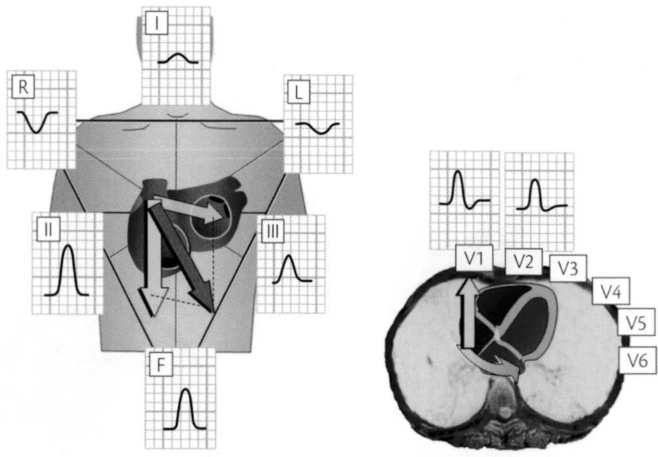

Figure 2.13 RA enlargement increases the magnitude of the vertical component of the P-wave vector and increases P-wave magnitude on the inferior leads with a peaked configuration. P wave is almost parallel to II and slightly positive in I, indicating ÂP ≈ 80º. In the horizontal plane the Increase in anteriorly directed vectors may inscribe a peaked P wave in V1–V2.

Chamber enlargement/hypertrophy

An increase in myocardial mass increases the magnitude of the vector generated during activation, changing the amplitude of the recorded deflections and often also the mean axis of activation of the involved chambers. Increased chamber volume can also increase vector magnitude [19], and that is why the term 'enlargement' is often preferred to 'hypertrophy'. Chamber enlargement can also alter myocardial conduction, by changing muscle alignment or by the appearance of interstitial fibrosis, and increased duration of activation is also common. Finally, chamber enlargement may alter repolarization by reversing the normal sequence starting in the epicardial layers, and thus cause 'secondary' ST and T changes. A normal sequence of activation is essential to make chamber enlargement criteria applicable, because conduction disturbances or ectopic rhythms may change ECG configuration in the absence of chamber enlargement [20].

Right atrial enlargement

RA enlargement will increase the initial, inferiorly directed RA activation vectors component shifting P-wave axis (âP) inferiorly (>+75°) and increasing P-wave voltage on the inferior leads II, III, and aVF (➲Figs. 2.13–2.15). There may also be an increase in amplitude of the initial positive deflection in V1 and V2 (➲Fig. 2.15). The upper limit of P-wave voltage in II, III, and aVF has been set at 0.25mV (or 2.5mm), and 0.15mV (1.5mm) in V1; however, echocardiographic studies find little correlation with RA dimensions [21, 22]. In patients with pulmonary emphysema, P wave many not reach voltage criteria, but still be prominent in relation to QRS voltage. RA enlargement does not increase P-wave duration, because RA vectors, even if delayed, will overlap with LA vectors. Criteria of RV enlargement may be better predictive of RA enlargement than P-wave changes [23].

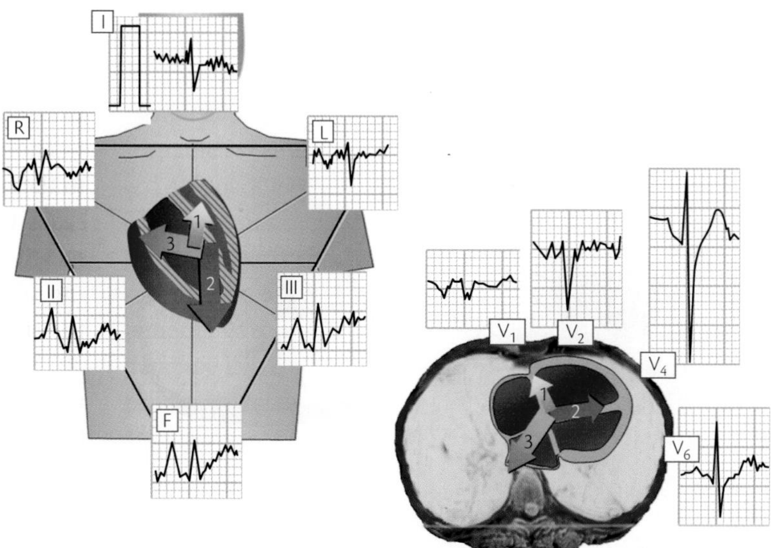

Figure 2.14 RA and RV enlargement in cor pulmonale. The P wave is peaked and tall in II, III, and aVF. QRS axis is 90º and there is clockwise rotation in the horizontal plane (S in V6). Final QRS vectors are posterior and to the right, inscribing S waves in I, V6, and V1. Respiratory muscle artefact is evident.

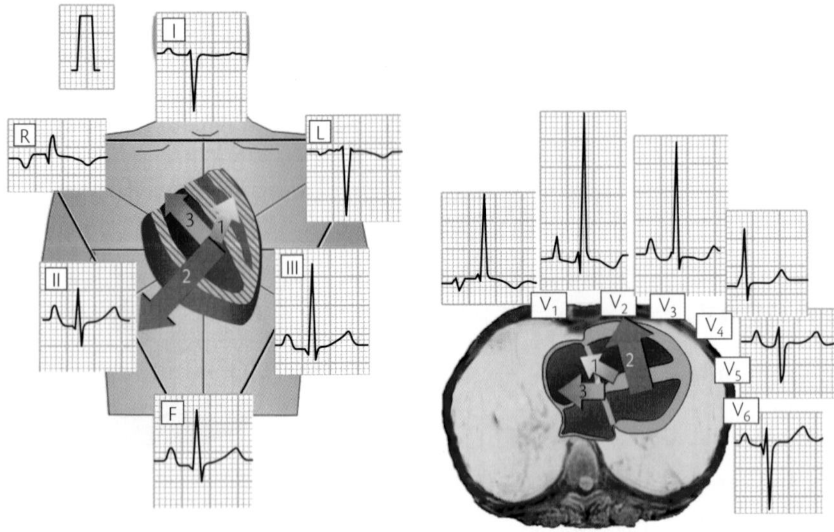

Figure 2.15 RA and RV enlargement in pulmonary valve stenosis. P wave is tall and peaked in II, aVF, and V2–V3. ÂQRS is 130° (slightly negative in aVR, slightly positive in II, and markedly negative in I). Note tall R waves in V1–V3 with S in V6.

Left atrial enlargement

LA enlargement increases the amplitude and duration of the late P-wave vectors directed to the left and posteriorly, and therefore tends to make âP horizontal and to increase P-wave duration to >100ms. The P wave often displays a double peak with an 'M' shape (➲Fig. 2.16). On V1, the posterior direction of the LA vector can produce a late negative deflection >1mm (0.1mV) in depth and >1mm (0.04s) in width. The predictive value of these criteria have been questioned [24, 25] when checked against echocardiographic atrial dimensions. One possible reason for this poor correlation could be that criteria for LA enlargement may be caused or mimicked by atrial conduction disturbances [26] and for this reason some authors prefer to talk of LA 'abnormality' rather than enlargement. The size of the terminal negative deflection in V1 has been found to correlate with LA pressure and it has been used to monitor left ventricular failure in patients with acute myocardial infarction [27, 28].

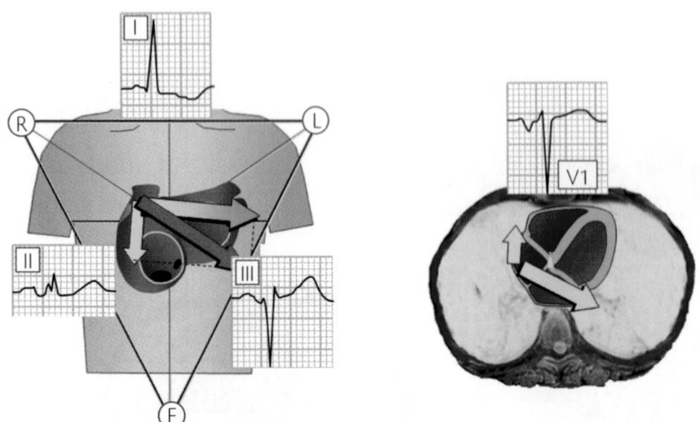

Figure 2.16 Left LA enlargement. P wave is wide and bimodal in II and there is a wide and deep negative terminal deflection in V1 produced by the posterior direction of the final vectors of the LA.

The association of RA and LA enlargement will produce a combination of findings described for each atrium, resulting in tall, broad, and often notched P waves in the limb leads, as well as large biphasic P waves in the right precordial leads.

Right ventricular enlargement

RV enlargement is difficult to diagnose because many of its signs can be produced by body build, chest pathology, lung hyperinflation, young age, or BB or fascicular blocks. On the other hand, the marked predominance of LV activation vectors makes it difficult to detect minor degrees of RV enlargement. The diagnosis of RV enlargement can not be based on strict criteria, but rather on multiple ECG findings that create a general picture leading from suspicion to clear-cut diagnosis. Signs of RA enlargement are an important confirmatory finding. Here, more than ever, it is important to interpret the ECG in the light of clinical information.

The increase in RV vector magnitude can shift âQRS to the right (inferiorly) (➲Figs. 2.14 and 2.15), but in other cases QRS axis is indeterminate, with practically equal positive and negative deflection areas in all limb leads and the salient feature is a final negative vector directed toward the right shoulder (SI, SII, SIII pattern) (➲Fig. 2.17) [29, 30]. In some cases, RV dilatation can produce clockwise rotation on the apex-to-base axis with a deep Q wave in lead III and S wave in lead I. This particular pattern is often seen in acute cor pulmonale due to pulmonary embolism (➲Chapter 37) and may pose the differential diagnosis with inferior wall myocardial infarction.

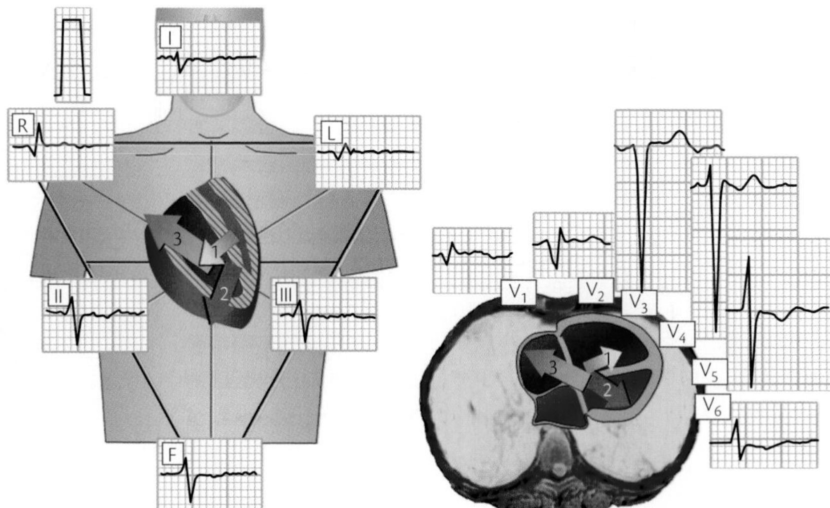

Figure 2.17 RV enlargement in cor pulmonale with atrial fibrillation. Note low voltage in the frontal plane with an indeterminate axis (r/s complexes in all leads). Late vectors point toward aVR inscribing S waves in I, II, and III. On the horizontal plane note vector 1 shifted to the left (Q waves V1–V3) and late vector 3 pointing to the right and anteriorly (R′ waves in V1–V2).

On the precordial leads (horizontal plane) there are several possible patterns of RV hypertrophy, in part determined by increased RV mass, RA and RV dilatation with posterior (clockwise) rotation, and chest anatomy and pathology. Initial r waves may decrease or disappear, mimicking an anteroseptal scar (➲Figs. 2.14 and 2.17), but the increase in anteriorly directed RV activation vectors can actually produce tall R waves (➲Fig. 2.15) or a late R′ wave (➲Fig. 2.17) in the right precordial leads. Depending on the appearance on the precordial leads, RV enlargement patterns have been classified in different types (A, B, C), but the clinical utility is limited and it is the combination of the various findings described earlier that should suggest RV enlargement.

RV hypertrophy can produce secondary repolarization changes characterized by negative asymmetric T waves, most commonly in leads III and V1–V3 (➲Fig. 2.15). However, it is not uncommon that T waves are positive in the right precordial leads (➲Fig. 2.17). Repolarization changes may be particularly acute in RV overload due to pulmonary embolism (➲Chapter 37), with ST elevation in the inferior, and/or right precordial leads, and T-wave inversion suggestive of ischaemia that can make the differential diagnosis with myocardial infarction difficult, especially when abnormal Q waves appear due to rotation (➲Fig. 2.18).

The diagnosis of RV hypertrophy has to be made with particular caution in children, particularly <1 year of age. The physiologic RV dominance in fetal life remains and a right âQRS in the frontal plane and dominant R waves with negative T waves in the right precordial leads are the rule. Negative T waves in the right precordial leads may remain for years.

RV enlargement often leads to RBBB, in which case the vector voltage and direction changes and the repolarization changes secondary to the conduction disturbance makes it very difficult to establish the diagnosis of the underlying RV enlargement.

Left ventricular enlargement

Since vector 2 is dominantly generated by LV depolarization, the main consequence of LV enlargement is an increase in QRS voltage with large R waves in leads exploring the left side of the heart (aVL, I, V5–V6) (➲Figs. 2.19 and 2.20). The right precordial leads V1–V2 can record deep S waves due to the posterior position of the LV. The increased voltage will be evident in different leads, depending on the electrical position of the heart so that voltage criteria are valid for a given lead, even in the absence of voltage criteria in other leads. Voltage criteria for the diagnosis of LV enlargement have been advanced by different authors [30–36] and the sensitivity and specificity is summarized in ➲Table 2.1. R waves of >11mm in aVL, >14mm in I, or >25mm in V5–V6, or S waves >25mm in V1–V2 have considerable specificity, although sensitivity is low. The classical Sokolov criteria (S in V1 or V2 + R in V5 or V6 ≥3.5mV (35mm)) have a lower specificity in young subjects. R- or S-wave voltage in leads V3 and V4 is less reliable, because they are recorded close to the LV apex and they are influenced markedly by anatomic variability. The scoring system proposed by Romhilt and Estes [37] includes axis deviation, ST and T changes, and signs of LA enlargement to improve diagnostic sensitivity and specificity (➲Table 2.2).

In severe LV hypertrophy due to increased afterload, as in aortic stenosis (➲Chapter 21) or hypertension (➲Chapter 13), the septal vector is often decreased or even completely lost, making the differential diagnosis difficult with septal infarction (➲Fig. 2.19). On the other hand, a pattern of 'diastolic overload' has been described in patients with ventricular septal defect or aortic insufficiency [38],

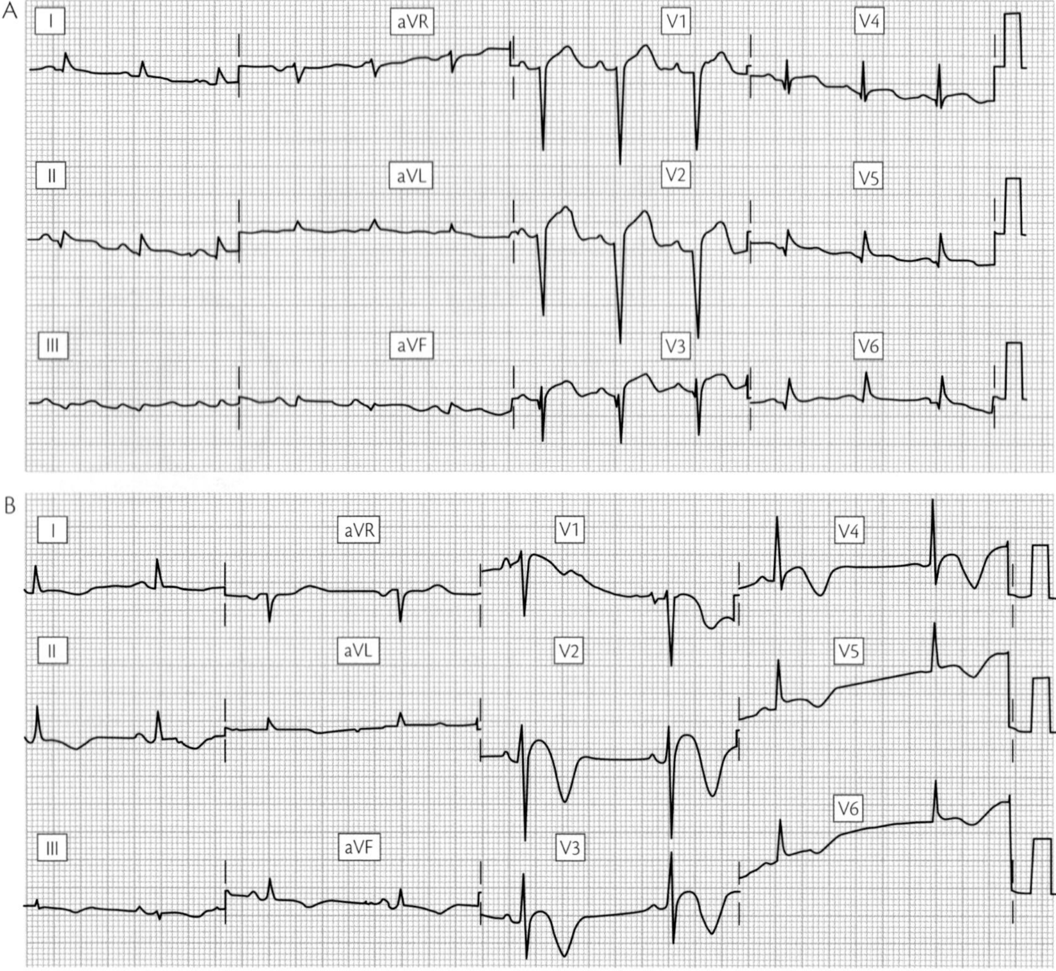

Figure 2.18 (A) Acute severe pulmonary embolism. Note QS pattern V1–V3 with ST elevation V1–V4, compatible with acute anterior myocardial infarction. There is slight ST segment elevation in II, III, and aVF. (B) Evolution after 48 hours. Note reappearance of r waves in the right precordial leads. ST segment remains elevated V1–V4. T waves have become diffusely inverted and QT interval is prolonged suggesting evolving ischaemia.

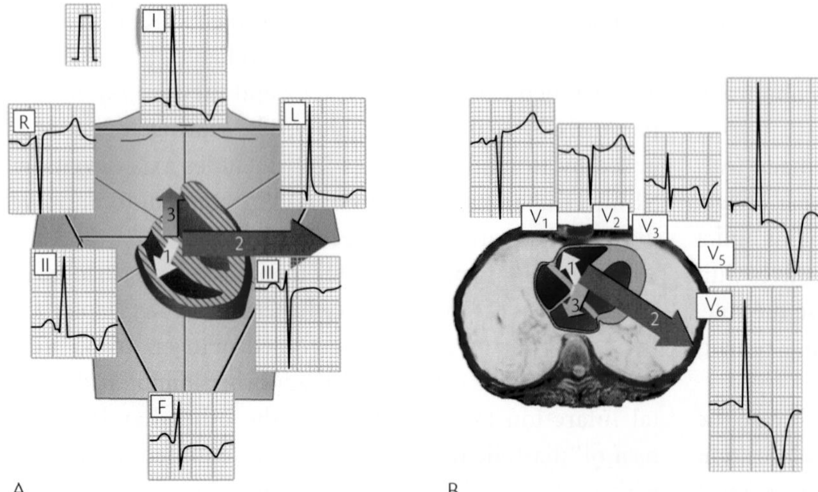

Figure 2.19 Increased vector 2 causes tall R waves or deep S waves, depending on lead direction. (A) Frontal plane leads I and aVL are most representative of LV enlargement. Vector 2 angle is drawn in this schema to show how it can be perpendicular to the axis of V5–V6 not producing tall R waves in these left precordial leads. (B) On the horizontal plane R-wave voltage tends to be high in V5–V6 and S waves deep in V1–V2.

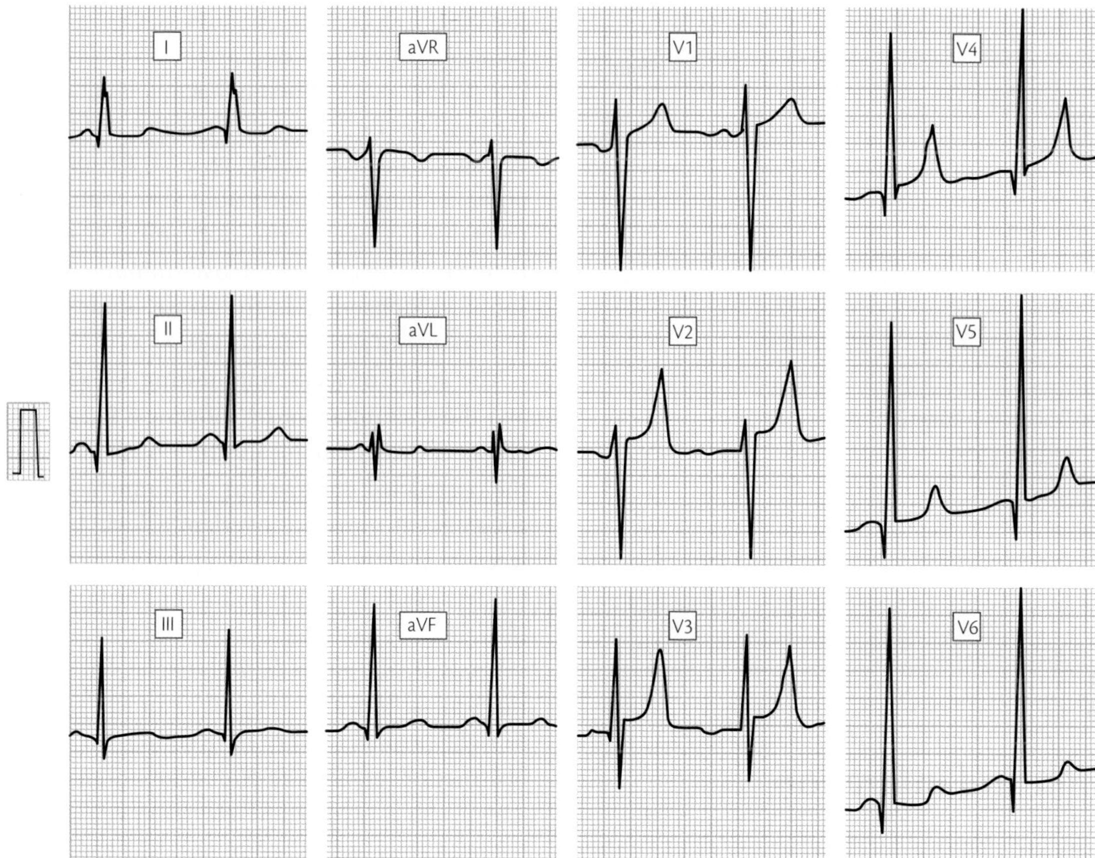

Figure 2.20 LV 'diastolic overload' pattern in a patient with severe aortic insufficiency. Note deep, narrow Q waves in V5–V6 and upright, narrow T waves.

in which the septal vector may be enhanced and T waves are upright and peaked, instead of inverted (➲Fig. 2.20). Initial q or r waves can be of very high voltage in asymmetric LV hypertrophy due to hypertrophic cardiomyopathy (➲Chapter 18).

LV hypertrophy will be often accompanied by repolarization abnormalities 'secondary' to the hypertrophy. The increased thickness of the myocardium may reverse the normal sequence of repolarization from epicardium toward the endocardium, and thus make T waves negative over the leads showing the highest R-wave voltage. Typically this is an asymmetric T wave, because the ST segment starts at the J point slightly below the isoelectric line and becomes progressively negative until merging with the T wave (➲Fig. 2.19). This has been called 'strain' pattern. It is important to know that a therapeutic level of digoxin may mimic the strain pattern.

Biventricular enlargement

This is a difficult ECG diagnosis, because when the LV is enlarged and/or hypertrophied it will be very difficult for any increased RV myocardial mass to show 'against' the potent LV depolarization vectors [30]. In the presence of signs of LV enlargement, a vertical or right axis of the QRS or a RSR pattern in V1 would suggest associated RV enlargement. Fortunately, the ECG will not bear the whole weight of the diagnosis as the clinical picture and the echocardiogram will provide the necessary information in these difficult cases.

Table 2.1 Sensitivity and specificity of LV enlargement criteria

Voltage criteria	Sensitivity (%)	Specificity (%)
R in I + S in III >25mm	10.6	100
R in aVL >7.5mm	22.5	96.5
R in aVL >11mm	10.6	100
R in aVF >200mm	1.3	99.5
S in V1+ R in V5–V6 ≥35mm	55.6	89.5
Deepest S+ tallest R >45mm V1–V6	45	93
R in V5 or V6 >26mm	25	98
R in V6 > R in V5	50	100
Combined criteria		
Romhilt and Estes	54	97

Modified with permission from Bayés de Luna A. *Clinical Electrocardiography: A Textbook*, 1993. Mount Kisko, NY: Futura.

Table 2.2 Romhilt and Estes' criteria of LV enlargement

	Points
QRS voltage (one of the following):	3
R or S ≥20mm in limb leads	
S in V1 or V2 ≥30mm	
R in V5 or V5 ≥30mm	
ST-T changes:	
Not digitalized	3
Digitalized	2
LA enlargement:	
V1 terminal P deflection ≥1mm or ≥40ms	3
Left QRS axis deviation ≥ 30°	2
QRS duration ≥90ms	1
Intrinsicoid deflection ≥50ms in V5 or V6	1
Score:	
Possible LV enlargement	4
Certain LV enlargement	≥5

Ischaemia and infarction

The ECG remains a key tool for the diagnosis of myocardial ischaemia, especially through the use of serial recordings to detect changes in repolarization and depolarization. Transient ST and T changes in relation to the clinical picture, and even in the absence of anginal symptoms, are an early and sensitive sign of myocardial ischaemia. Changes in the QRS are often permanent, but can also be transient. Directional information provided by the ECG is quite important in this setting, as it indicates the location of the ischaemia and its extension, and helps guide invasive revascularization therapy. In this section we will try to summarize a perspective of how to approach myocardial ischaemic changes from the ECG.

ST changes in ischaemia (also see ➲ Chapters 16 and 17)

When ischaemia is severe and prolonged enough (minutes), myofibres lose, at least in part, their polarized status and the ischaemic area becomes negatively charged, giving rise to ST changes that have been called lesion current, implying severe ischaemia [39–41]. The vector created by ischaemia is active only when the myocardium is repolarized (T–P segment) and paradoxically disappears during the ST segment, when all the myocardium is depolarized (➲ Figs. 2.21 and 2.22). When ischaemia is transmural, the ECG records a negative baseline potential during most of the cardiac cycle that becomes isoelectric only during the ST segment which is displayed as elevated above the baseline (➲ Fig. 2.21). When ischaemia is subendocardial, only the baseline displacement is positive and the ST segment is displayed as depressed (➲ Fig. 2.22) Changes in local action potential amplitude probably also contribute to ST segment displacement during ischaemia [39, 40]. The transient nature of ST displacement, over minutes or hours, strongly supports ischaemia as the cause, underlining again the importance of serial recordings.

The study of leads manifesting ST segment elevation and those simultaneously showing ST segment depression allows approximate localization of the ischaemic site and the obstructed coronary artery branch, although there is a significant degree of overlap. ST will be elevated in the leads facing the ischaemic epicardium and will tend to be depressed in those in the opposite side of the heart (➲ Table 2.3) [42–55].

Leads II, III, and aVF will display ST elevation in inferior wall ischaemia (➲ Figs. 2.23 and 2.24), commonly due to right coronary artery obstruction, but in other cases to obstruction of the left circumflex branch. If the apical-lateral wall is involved ST elevation will also appear in the left precordial leads V5–V6 [45]. ST depression will tend to appear in leads I and aVL when the right coronary artery is the culprit, but not if it is the left circumflex [43, 47]. Leads V1–V3 show ST depression when ischaemia involves the posterolateral wall [52, 53] (➲ Fig. 2.24). When right coronary artery obstruction is very proximal, before the origin of the lateral RV branch, RV ischaemia is often manifest by ST elevation in lead V4R (symmetrical from V4 on the right chest) [42, 51, 54]. ST depression in V5–V6

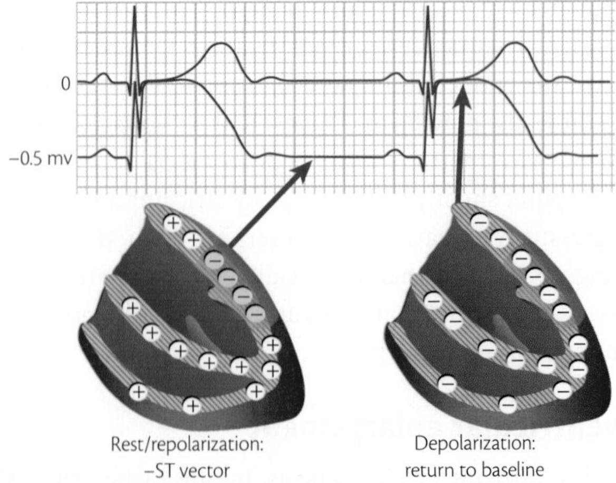

Figure 2.21 Role of localized depolarization of the ischaemic zone in the genesis of ST elevation during transmural ischaemia. Potential differences disappear after the whole myocardium has become depolarized and reappear after repolarization of the healthy myocardium.

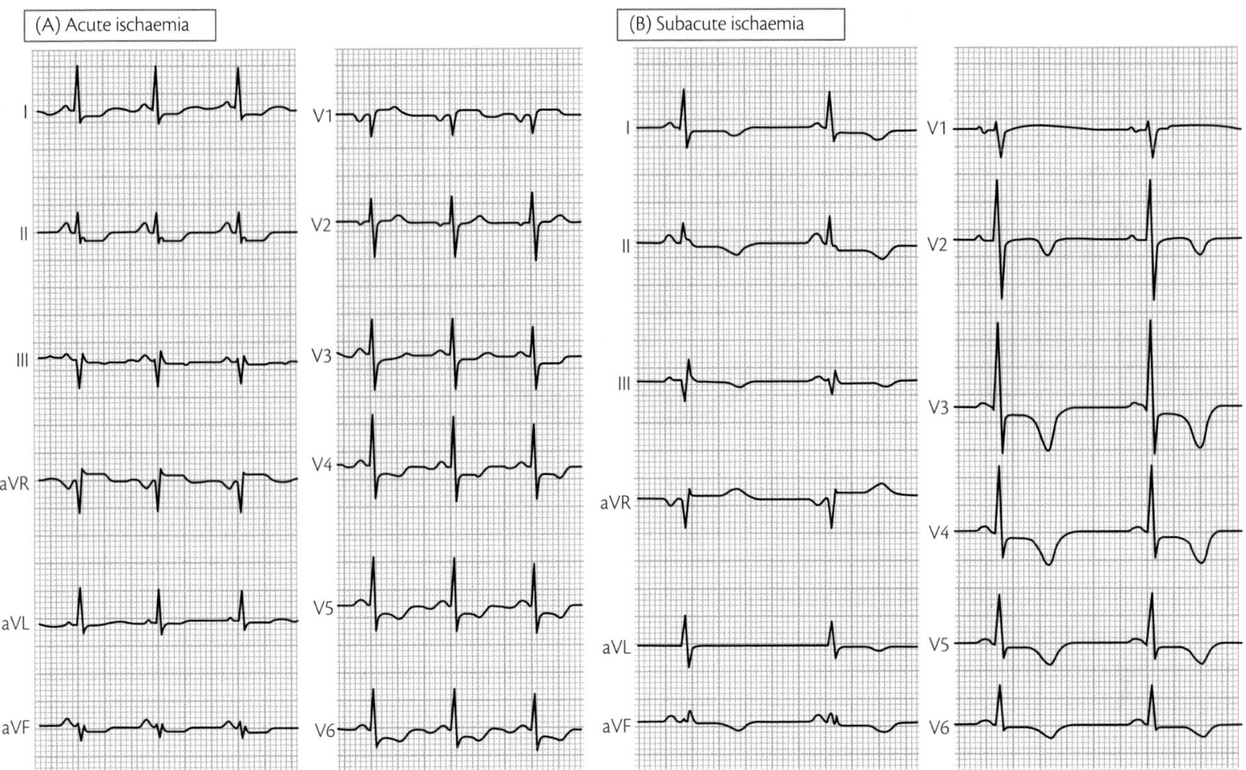

Figure 2.22 Evolution of ST segment depression to T-wave inversion in the course of acute coronary syndrome. (A) At the time of admission there is ST segment depression in I, II, aVF, and V4–V6. (B) 24 hours later, ST segment elevation is no longer present and T waves are inverted in the same leads.

associated with ST elevation in the inferior leads is an indicator of the presence of three-vessel disease [43, 53].

Obstruction of the left anterior descending branch of the left coronary artery will produce ST elevation in the right precordial leads V1–V3 that explore the septum (➲Figs. 2.25 and 2.26), and in V3–V6 if there is also antero-apical ischaemia (➲Fig. 2.25). Leads I and aVL will show ST elevation in the presence of ischaemia of the superior basal LV, and the inferior leads II, III and aVF may show ST depression as a reciprocal change (➲Figs. 2.25 and 2.27). ST depression in

Table 2.3 ST segment shift during acute ischaemia in relation to the occluded coronary artery branch

Occluded artery	V1, V3	V4, V6	I, aVL	II, III, aVF	V4R	aVR
Proximal LAD/LM	↑ ≥2mm	↓ ≥1mm	↑ ≥1mm	↓ ≥1mm		↑ ≥0.5mm
Distal LAD	↑ ≥2mm	↑ ≥1mm				
Proximal RC			↓ ≥0.5mm	↑ ≥1.5mm	↑ ≥1mm	
Distal RC	↓ ≥1mm	↑ ≥1mm	↓ ≥0.5mm	↑ ≥1.5mm		
Proximal CX	↓ ≥1mm		↑ ≥1mm			
Distal CX		↑ ≥1mm		↑ ≥1mm (III >II)		
RC occlusion + (three-vessel disease)		↓ ≥1mm		↑ ≥1mm		

CX, circumflex branch of the left coronary artery; LAD, left anterior descending branch of the left coronary artery; LM, left coronary artery main trunk; RC, right coronary artery. ↑, ST elevation. ↓, ST depression.

The values expressed indicate the relative prominence of ST deviation in each case. ST displacement may not occur in all the indicated leads or lead groups in each situation.

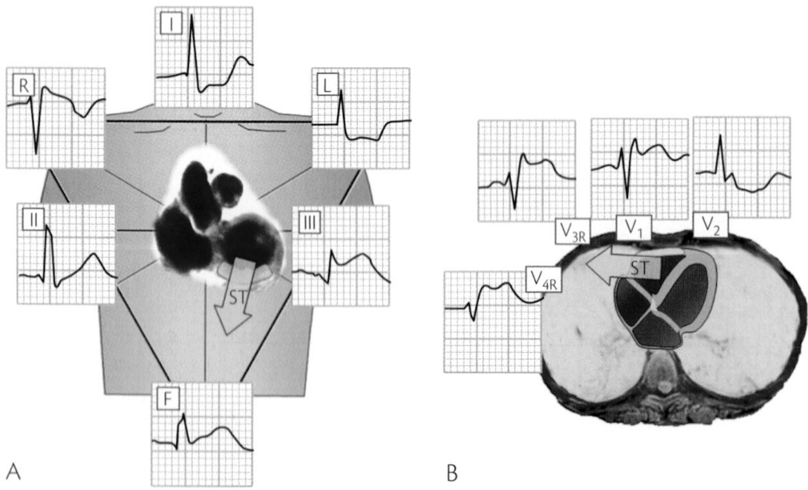

Figure 2.23 ST segment elevation in acute inferior wall myocardial infarction with RV involvement. The grey arrows mark the direction of the ST vector. Note ST elevation in III and AVF with reciprocal inversion in I aVL and V2. ST segment elevation in the right precordial leads V3R and V4R due to RV transmural ischaemia/infarction. (A) A MRI cut of the LV is shown inside the schematic thorax. The yellow zone represents the location of the inferior LV infarcted zone. (B) The horizontal plane with the anterior RV infarcted zone marked in yellow.

V5–V6 and ST elevation in aVR are additional signs of very proximal obstruction of the left anterior descending branch or the main left coronary trunk [49, 55].

Obstruction of the proximal part of the circumflex branch of the left coronary artery results in posterolateral ischaemia with ST elevation in I and aVL or ST depression in the right precordial leads V1–V3. More distal obstruction of the circumflex branch will produce ST elevation in II, III, and aVF—more marked in III than II—with or without ST elevation in V4–V6 and without ST depression in I and aVL [43, 45, 47].

Ischaemic ST segment elevation is usually transient even in myocardial infarction, and returns to baseline spontaneously after <24 hours and within minutes after myocardial reperfusion. Persistence of ST elevation beyond 24 hours is a marker of poor prognosis and the development of important segmental contraction disturbance.

ST segment depression is a common manifestation of myocardial ischaemia, both at rest or during stress/exertion (➲Fig. 2.22), although the power to localize the ischaemic area is less than in ST segment elevation. The presence of ST depression at rest is a marker [56–60] of severe coronary disease, especially in the presence of ST segment elevation in aVR [55]. Dynamic changes in minutes or hours, either spontaneously or due to treatment, increase the specificity for the diagnosis of ischaemia. ST segment displacement may disappear completely, returning to baseline, but in severe ischaemia it will often evolve to T-wave inversion in the same leads (➲Fig. 2.22).

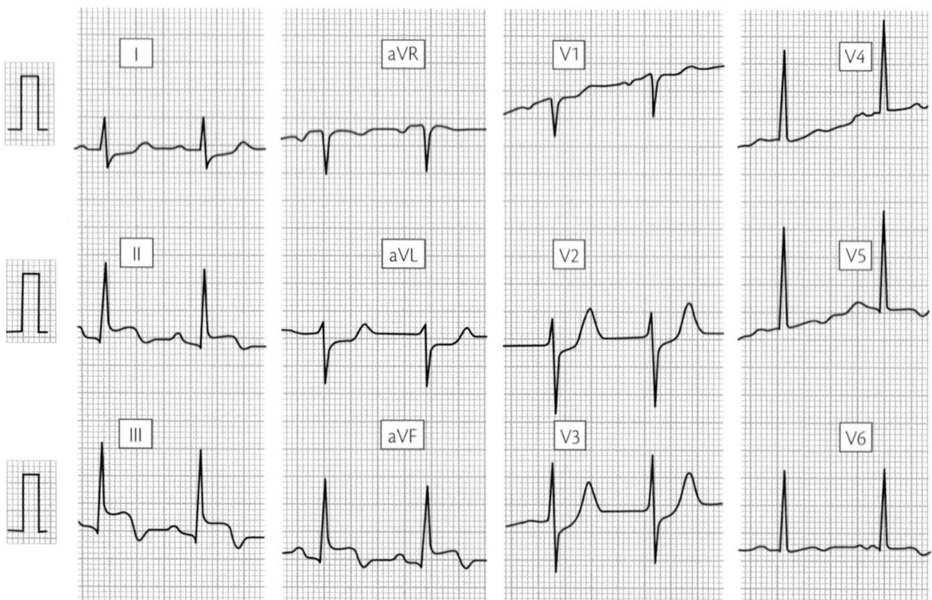

Figure 2.24 Subacute inferior wall transmural myocardial ischaemia (evolving myocardial infarction) still showing ST elevation. There is ST segment depression in aVL and V2–V3 suggesting associated posterior ischaemia with mirror image changes. T wave is negative in II, III, aVF, and V5–V6, indicating evolution of the ischaemia.

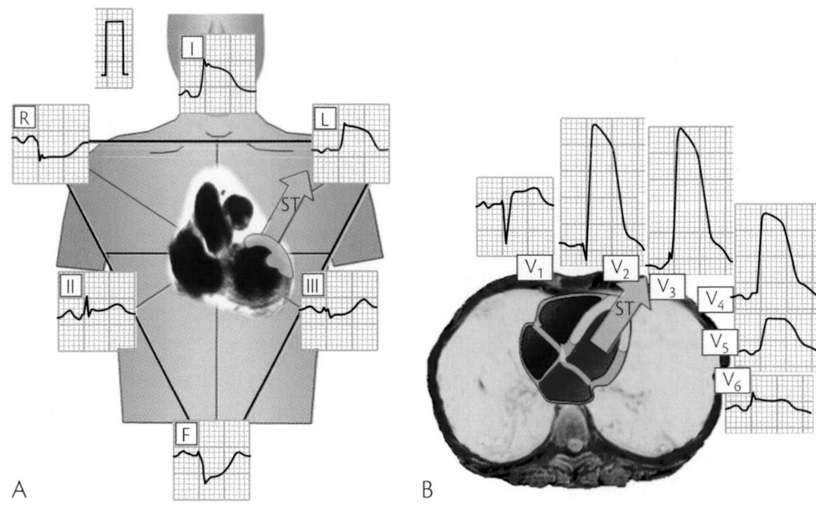

Figure 2.25 Acute anterolateral transmural ischaemia. (A) A MRI cut of the LV is shown with the ischaemic area highlighted in yellow. Note the superior position of the so called 'anterior' wall that makes it be recorded in aVL. (B) On the horizontal plane with the extensive septal and anterior-apical ischaemic area highlighted in yellow. There is ST elevation in I, aVL, and V1–V6, indicating a very large ischaemic area, probably due to a very proximal lesion in the left anterior descending branch. Note reciprocal ST depression in III and aVF. The grey arrow marks the direction of the 'ST vector'. Note the superior and inferior positions of the so called 'anterior' and 'posterior' papillary muscles.

ST segment can be persistently depressed or elevated in the absence of acute ischaemia, as in the 'early repolarization syndrome' (➲Fig. 2.12) or in some cases of pericarditis. In these cases, serial ECGs will help provide the diagnostic clues. Chronic ST elevation is common in patients with ventricular aneurysm and in these cases abnormal Q waves (see ➲QRS changes: the Q waves, p.46) will generally be present in the leads showing ST elevation. Acute pericarditis or myocarditis can produce ST segment elevation that tends to be diffuse, involving arm, leg, and precordial leads, and tends to be persistent over days. Stable ST depression <0.1mV can be seen occasionally in the left precordial leads in normal subjects, particularly women. ST segment depression can be produced by hyperventilation, especially in the presence of mitral valve prolapse [59, 60], electrolyte imbalance, and therapeutic doses of digitalis, therefore

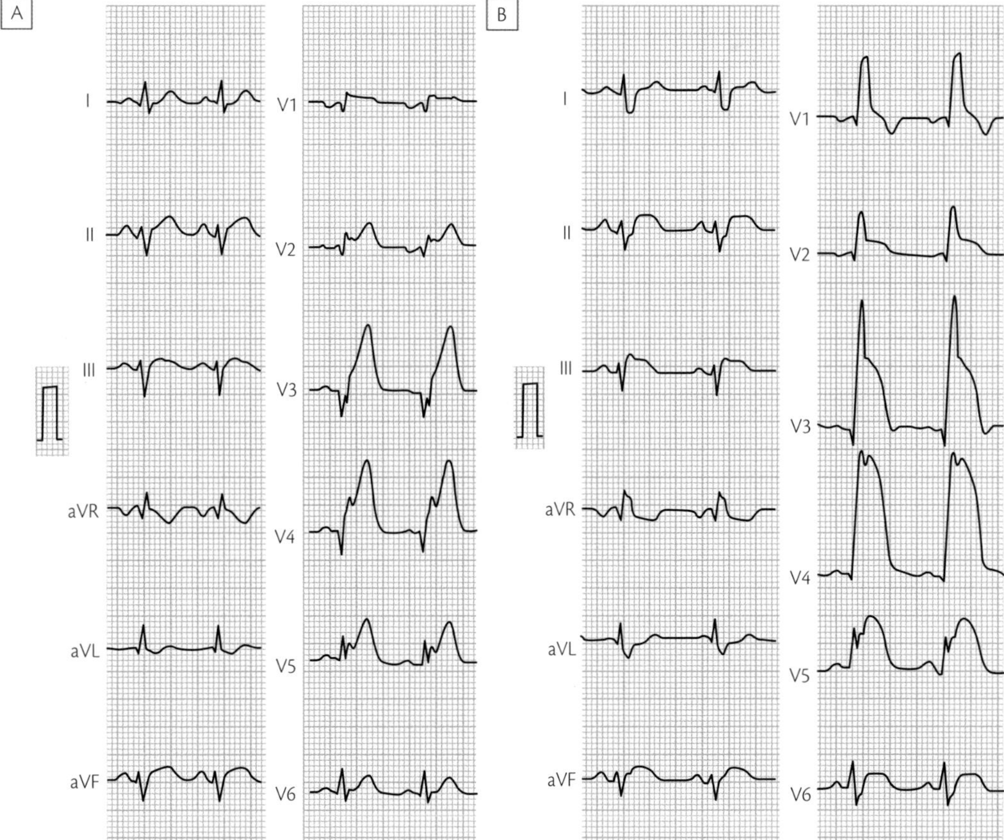

Figure 2.26 New RBBB in the course of acute anterior myocardial infarction. (A) An early tracing shows ST elevation V1–V5 indicating transmural anteroseptal ischaemia and in II, III, and aVF indicating associated inferior wall transmural ischaemia. There are abnormal Q waves already V1–V4. (B) A few hours later, ST segment elevation is increased markedly in V3–V5 and persists in II, III, and aVF. the QRS is widened with a broad R′ in V1–V3 and a broad S wave in I, diagnostic of RBBB. Note that the RBBB does not obscure the abnormal Q waves in V1–V3.

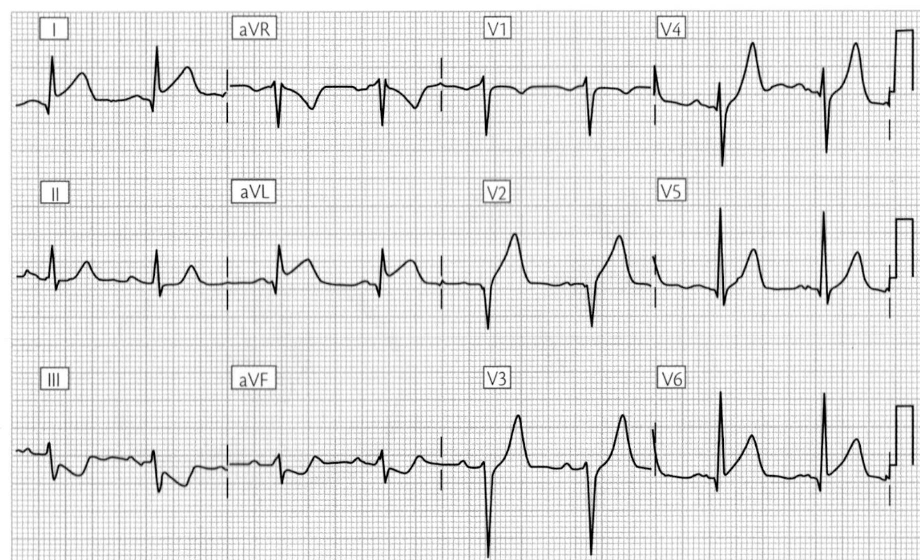

Figure 2.27 Anterolateral acute myocardial infarction. Note ST elevation in I, aVL, and V5–V6 with reciprocal, mirror-image ST depression in III and aVF. There is an abnormally broad Q wave in aVL and small or absent r waves in V2–V3 indicating high lateral and anteroseptal infarction. Note the broad-based T wave in V2–V6 associated with little ST segment shift. This is often the only ischaemic sign in the very early stages of transmural ischaemia/infarction.

making essential ECG interpretation of this finding in the light of clinical information. In patients with normal heart and coronary arteries suffering paroxysmal, narrow QRS, supraventricular tachycardia (SVT), the ST segment may become markedly depressed during the tachycardia [61].

Ischaemic T waves

A less severe degree of ischaemia than that producing ST displacement can produce negative T waves by reverting the repolarization sequence. Ischaemic T waves tend to be symmetrical, unless there is coexisting ST elevation or depression (➲Figs. 2.22 and 2.24). Extensive T-wave inversion in the precordial leads in the course of acute coronary syndrome is a marker of proximal left anterior descending branch stenosis [62] (➲Fig. 2.22). T waves are generally markers of subacute ischaemia following hours after ST segment elevation or depression in acute coronary syndromes; however, they may also be the only manifestation of ischaemia. Ischaemic T waves may persist for months or years, even in the absence of clinical symptoms. Very early transmural ischaemia often causes a broad, tall, positive T wave, before ST segment elevation develops, and this subtle change may be overlooked (➲Fig. 2.27). Subacute ischaemia may be also manifest in some cases by a peaked, tall, symmetrical T wave.

Deep negative T waves can be due to LV enlargement (strain pattern) particularly in the apical form of hypertrophic cardiomyopathy. Negative T waves may appear after an episode of SVT in patients without coronary artery disease, and may persist for days. Acute abdominal pathology or subarachnoid haemorrhages are other causes of ischaemic looking T waves. (See also ➲T-wave 'memory', p.67.)

QRS changes: the Q waves

The appearance of deep, wide Q waves has classically been the marker of myocardial necrosis. Q waves can be conceptualized as meaning the absence of R waves, i.e. the local disappearance of endocardial to epicardial activation, letting the lead exploring the area record the negative tail of vectors activating distant areas. Q waves are the sign of irreversible necrosis that usually becomes a permanent feature of the ECG after the acute episode [63] (➲Table 2.4). However, the mechanism of Q-wave generation is probably more complex, because Q waves may be transient during acute ischaemia and established Q waves may disappear spontaneously months or years after the acute event, or after surgical myocardial revascularization. Spontaneous Q-wave disappearance is more common after inferior than anterior infarction.

Table 2.4 Diagnosis of prior myocardial infarction

Any Q ≥20ms in V2–V3
QS complex in V2–V3
Q ≥30ms and ≥0.1mV or QS in any 2 of the lead groups:
I, aVL, V6
V4–V6
II, III, aVF
R ≥40ms in V1–V2 and R/S ≥1 with a concordant +T wave in the absence of conduction defect

Modified with permission from Thygesen K, Alpert JS, White HD; Joint ESC/ACCF/AHA/WHF Task Force for the redefinition of myocardial infarction. Universal definition of myocardial infarction. *Eur Heart J* 2007; **28**: 2525–38.

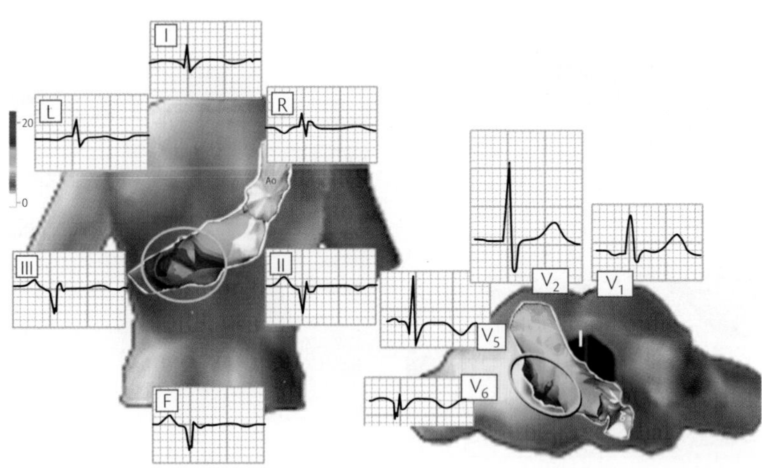

Figure 2.28 Inferior and posterior myocardial infarction in a patient with ventricular tachycardia. Magnified views of the anatomy of the LV and aorta, constructed by computer-assisted navigation (NavX™) have been superimposed to the image of the torso in the same view, in order to help establish the anatomic correlations. The colour code indicates activation times (pacing the RV), red is early, blue and violet are latest. The grey areas, surrounded by the yellow ovals, mark the precise location of the endocardial scars. Note deep Q waves in leads II, III, aVF, and V6 and dominant R waves in V1–V2. ST segment is slightly elevated in II, aVF, and V5–V6 (persistent post-infarction), and there is T wave inversion in the same leads, indicative of ischaemia.

The leads displaying Q waves localize the infarcted area, the same as ST elevation localizes the acutely ischaemic area [64]. In this way infarction may be classified as septal, anterior, inferior, lateral, inferolateral, or posterolateral.

- *Inferior wall infarction* produces Q waves most often in leads III and aVF (➲Fig. 2.28) and less often in II. An isolated Q wave in lead III is little specific, but a wide and deep Q wave in lead aVF (≥40ms and ≥25% of the R-wave height) is a more reliable sign of inferior infarction. In some cases an inferiorly directed septal vector will inscribe a small r wave in III and aVF while II shows a fully negative deflection, giving the clue to the diagnosis. It is not uncommon to find abnormal Q waves in V5–V6 in the presence of inferior infarction and then the term inferolateral infarction may be used (➲Fig. 2.28). It is possible that in some cases V5 and V6, which are placed in a relatively inferior position, may record inferior wall changes.
- *Posterior wall infarction* is diagnosed in the face of tall R waves in V1–V2 revealing loss of activation vectors in the more posterior portions of the LV posterolateral wall (➲Fig. 2.28) [65]. Posterior wall infarction is generally associated with inferior wall infarction and in the absence of this a differential diagnosis must be made with other causes of tall R waves in V1–V2 such as RV enlargement, position change (counterclockwise rotation), pre-excitation, or RBBB.
- *Septal or anteroseptal infarction* is picked-up by the right precordial leads V1–V3, because the interventricular septum is actually the anterior wall of the LV. Deep Q waves in these leads are diagnostic, but the presence of very small r waves (<20ms) in lead V2) is also quite significant in this respect (➲Figs. 2.25–2.27). LV hypertrophy (➲Fig. 2.19), LBBB (➲Fig. 2.29), or RV enlargement with clockwise rotation (➲Figs. 2.17 and 2.18) can also show Q waves or rS complexes in V1–V3 making the diagnosis of myocardial infarction uncertain in these circumstances.
- *Lateral and anterolateral infarction* is picked up by leads I and aVL, which explore the superior and lateral wall of the LV (➲Fig. 2.26). Abnormal Q waves in these leads are the clue to the diagnosis. The loss of leftward and superior vectors can produce a rightward axis shift.
- *RV infarction* does not produce abnormal Q waves in the ECG, but it usually occurs in association with inferior wall infarction. The diagnosis is made in the acute phase in the presence of ST elevation in the right precordial leads (V4R) (➲Fig. 2.23) and a clinical syndrome of low output and elevated RA pressures. The differential diagnosis must include acute cor pulmonale due to pulmonary embolism.

Abnormal Q waves can be produced by hypertrophic cardiomyopathy (➲Chapter 18), pre-excitation or LBBB, and these conditions should be ruled out before the diagnosis of old (or healed) myocardial infarction is made. On the other hand, serum markers and pathologic correlations have shown that significant necrosis can occur in the absence of Q waves, giving rise to the terms 'subendocardial' or 'non-transmural infarction', which are often called 'non-Q-wave infarction'.

The association of myocardial infarction with bundlebranch block (BBB) is common, either due to preexisting BBB or to severe ischaemia causing theconduction disturbance.(➲Fig. 2.26) [66–69].

In the presence of RBBB the diagnostic criteria for infarction do not change, because RBBB does not change the initial QRS vectors appreciably. Q waves and acute ST changes are the same as in patients with normal QRS (➲Fig. 2.26).

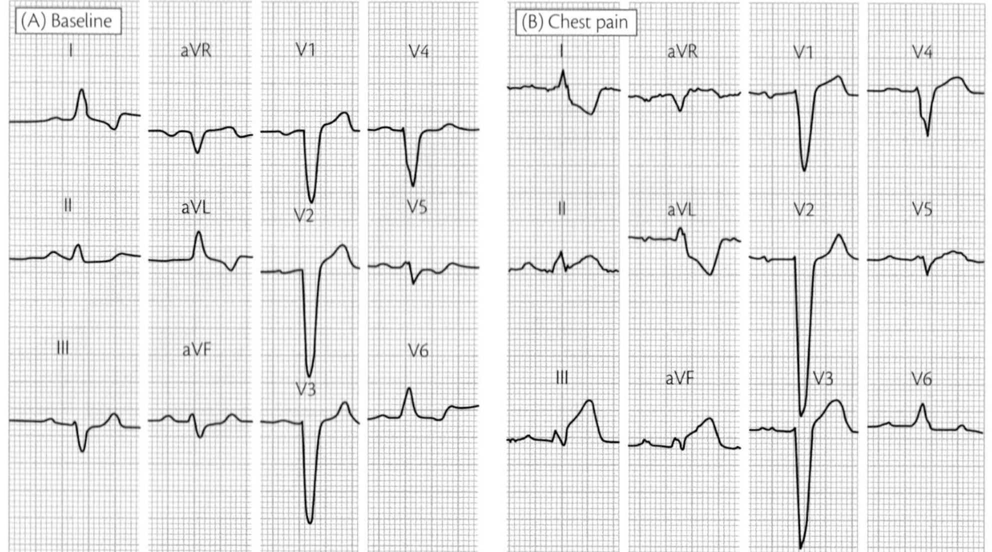

Figure 2.29 ST segment elevation during transmural inferior ischaemia in the presence of LBBB. (A) A baseline tracing before ischaemia. (B) ST elevation in leads II, III, and aVF and accentuation of ST depression in I and aVL (mirror-image change) in the course of an acute inferior wall myocardial infarction.

In the presence of LBBB, Q waves are not interpretable [70], but ST changes are still a valid marker of acute transmural ischaemia in the acute phase, especially in the inferior leads (➲Fig. 2.29) [71]. Serial tracings are necessary to confirm the ischaemic origin of the ST changes. In patients with permanent RV pacing, transient ST changes are also a valid means of diagnosing acute myocardial infarction [72].

Arrhythmias and conduction disturbances

Acute ischaemia alters myocardial automaticity and conductivity very significantly, giving rise to tachyarrhythmias based both on automatic mechanisms and re-entry. The most arrhythmogenic situation known is transmural ischaemia in the course of early acute myocardial infarction (ST elevation acute coronary syndrome) but Prinzmetal's angina due to coronary artery spasm can also produce severe arrhythmias.

Tachyarrhythmias

Atrial fibrillation (➲Chapter 29) can occur in the course of acute myocardial infarction and it is related to right coronary occlusion and LV failure [73–75]. Ventricular extrasystoles or sustained VT can be due to abnormal automaticity, re-entry, and abnormal current flow in the border zone between ischaemic and normal myocardium [76–78]. VT and ventricular fibrillation very early in the course can cause cardiac arrest in the pre-hospital phase of infarction [79]. Enhanced automaticity can produce accelerated idioventricular rhythm, a sort of 'slow VT' with rates <130 beats per minute (bpm), often well tolerated, but still considered a marker of extensive ischaemia or reperfusion [80] (➲Fig. 2.30).

Bundle branch and AV block (also see ➲Chapter 27)

Ischaemia can produce conduction disturbances related to the area irrigated by the obstructed artery. The most

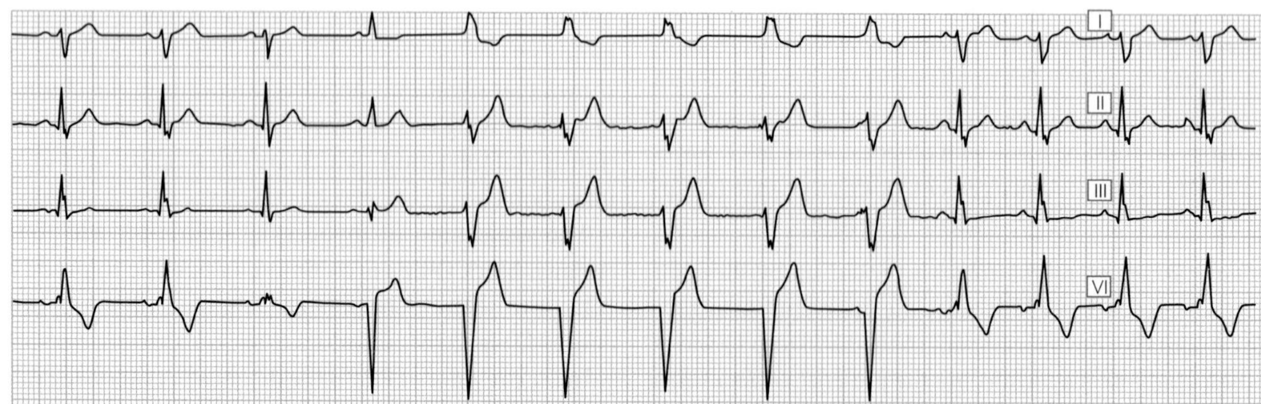

Figure 2.30 Accelerated idioventricular rhythm. Note a RBBB pattern during sinus rhythm (first two cycles). The third and fourth cycles show a shortening PR interval and a changing QRS, intermediate between the previous and the following (fusion beats). Five idioventricular beats follow, with a LBBB-like morphology and not preceded by a P wave. Finally sinus rate increases slightly and PR and QRS return to baseline.

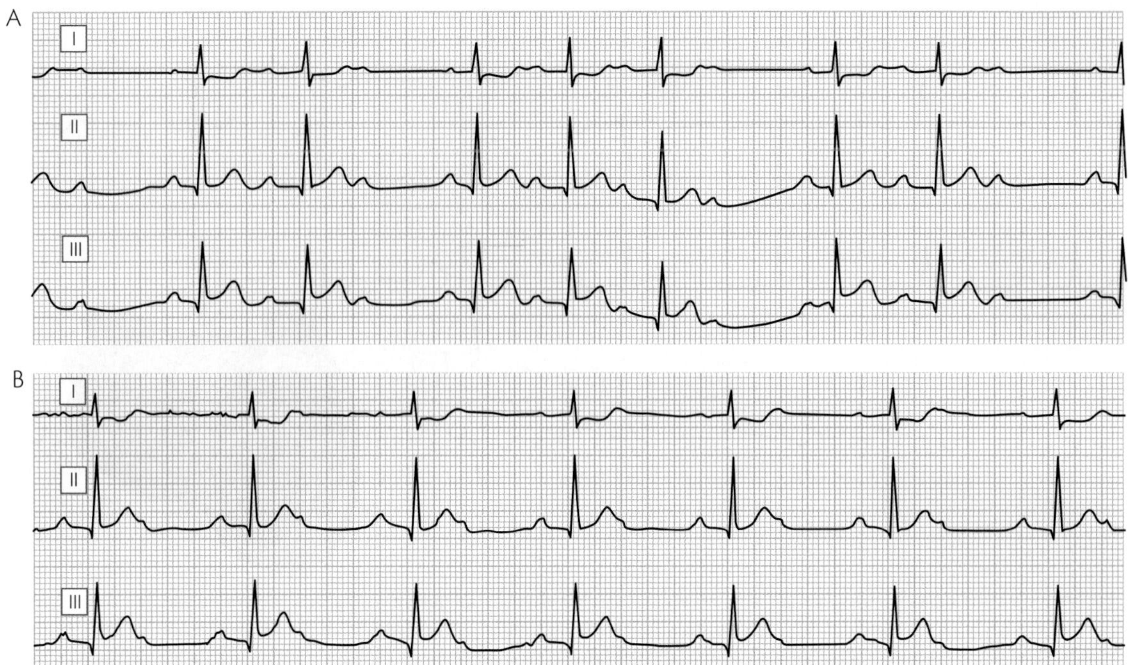

Figure 2.31 (A) Wenckebach AV block and (B) 2:1 AV block in the course of acute inferior myocardial infarction. In (A) there is progressive prolongation of the PR interval preceding the blocked P waves. Note ST elevation in II and III due to acute transmural inferior ischaemia.

common is nodal AV block in the course of acute inferior myocardial infarction [81], that can present a long PR, Wenckebach cycles, fixed 2:1 or 3:1 block, or complete AV block (➲Fig. 2.31). In all cases the QRS complex remains narrow as, even in complete block, the escape rhythm arises in the HB above the bifurcation into the BB. Escape rate is also relatively rapid and clinical and haemodynamic tolerance is usually good. Ischaemic AVN block is often relieved by atropine and by acute reperfusion by thrombolysis or angioplasty; otherwise spontaneous recovery can be quite slow, its natural course often lasting several days and occasionally up to 2 weeks [82]. Persistent complete AV block is rare and would suggest HB necrosis.

RBBB can develop in the course of acute anterior myocardial infarction when ischaemia is very extensive and involves the main septal branches of the left anterior descending artery (➲Fig. 2.26). It is associated with large ischaemic necrosis, and this is the main reason for its severe prognosis. LBBB can also occur acutely and is a sign of poor prognosis [66–68]. Second- or third-degree AV block is uncommon in this context, but has severe haemodynamic consequences because of the slow escape rate and the underlying severe myocardial damage. Temporary pacing is urgent in this situation and it can be instituted prophylactically if RBBB associates with left ASF block or PR prolongation develops. Advanced (trifascicular) block in this context is considered an indication for permanent pacemaker implantation to avoid the risk of recurrence [66, 67].

Conduction disturbances

Atrial conduction disturbances

Atrial conduction delay due to atrial dilatation or fibrosis probably contributes to the P-wave changes in atrial enlargement. Wide, notched P waves are the rule in LA enlargement and imply conduction delay, but the pattern of biphasic P waves in the inferior leads II, III, and aVF is worth highlighting for its clinical significance (➲Fig. 2.32). This pattern is due to block of conduction along Bachmann's bundle, which forces LA activation from the low septal area, around the coronary sinus ostium [14, 83]. From this low area the late atrial vectors point superiorly producing the late negative deflections in the inferior leads. Patients with Bachmann's bundle block have a high incidence of atrial flutter and fibrillation [84].

Atrioventricular conduction disturbances

Conduction in the normal AVN–HB axis can be disturbed by disease, drugs, or autonomic discharge, leading to excessive delay in AV conduction (PR prolongation) or block of the activation front at this level. PR prolongation is called

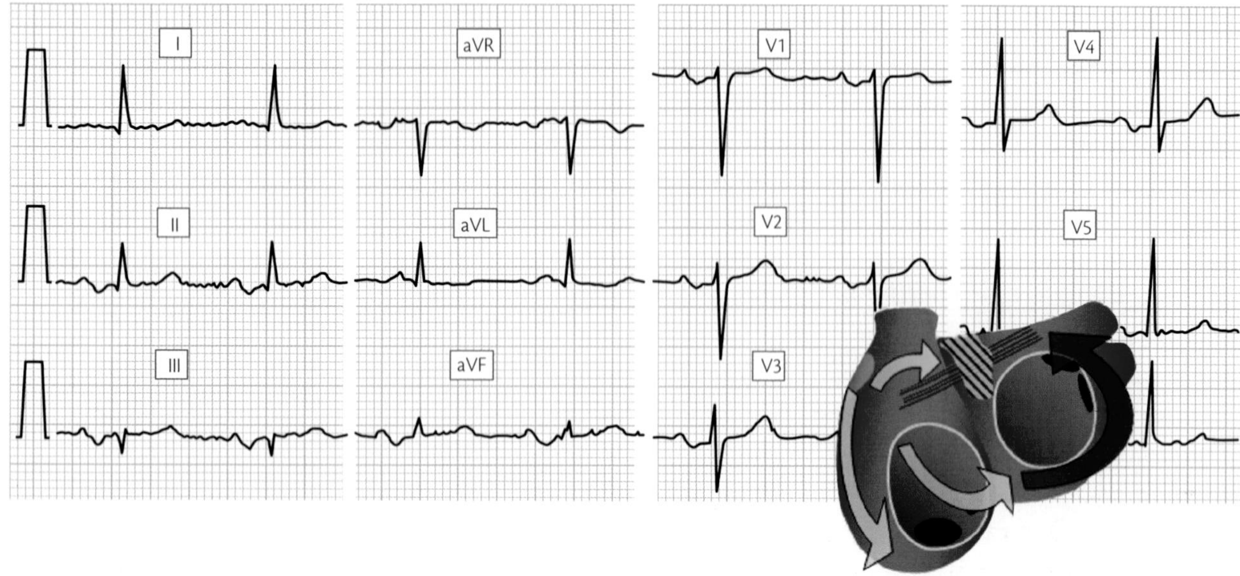

Figure 2.32 Bachmann's bundle block. The schema shows TA and LA in a left anterior oblique view. In green, the sinus node. The dashed yellow surface marks the area of block in Bachmann's bundle. Yellow arrows show normal RA activation. LA activation can not follow the normal path through the LA roof and has to start in the low septal LA and progress upward and to the left (blue arrow). Note broad biphasic P waves with a late negative deflection in II, III, AVF, and V1–V3 indicating late superior and posterior direction of atrial activation vectors.

first-degree AV block, failure to conduct of some of the P waves is called second-degree AV block, and complete failure to conduct is called third-degree (complete) AV block. AV block can occur at the AVN, at HB before its bifurcation, or at the BB. ECG and clinical manifestations differ depending on the site of block [85].

AV nodal block (also see ➲Chapter 27)

Nodal cells action potentials depend on calcium channels and exhibit decremental properties, i.e. refractory period increases and conduction velocity decreases with premature or rapid stimulation [86]. The AVN is highly responsive to vagal and adrenergic tone and is easily influenced by drugs. Vagal tone has profound effects on the AVN to the point of causing second-degree AV block during sleep in normal subjects and especially in athletes [87, 88]. On the other hand, sympathetic stimulation improves AV nodal conduction, providing the ability to conduct at fast sinus rates during exertion. The AVN can be directly affected by local pathology such as mitral ring calcification, septal abscess formation in the course of bacterial endocarditis, or surgical trauma. Beta adrenergic blocking drugs, calcium-channel blockers, digitalis, and antiarrhythmic drugs can impair AV nodal conduction [89, 90].

First-degree nodal block is an increase in conduction time through the AVN and will produce a prolonged PR interval without QRS changes. QRS width will be normal or, if BBB was present previously, it will be unchanged. The normal PR interval at rest ranges from 110–120ms in children to 220ms in the elderly, but it may be longer during sleep, due to increased vagal tone, and shorter during exertion due to decreased vagal tone and increased sympathetic tone. It is important to ensure that rhythm is normal, because PR interval may be prolonged by atrial extrasystoles or atrial tachycardia, even if it is relatively slow (<120bpm) due to decremental conduction (➲Fig. 2.33). During exercise, PR shortening occurs despite increased atrial rate, because AV nodal conduction is accelerated by the adrenergic stimulus.

Second-degree nodal block at the AVN tends to show a characteristic cyclic sequence of block of progressive lengthening of the PR interval until a P wave is blocked. This is known as Wenckebach or, less often, Mobitz type I AV block. When Wenckebach block progresses to 2:1 there is no way to know if this involves a Wenckebach mechanism unless the progression has been recorded (➲Fig. 2.31). Bedside manoeuvres can support the diagnosis of nodal block as the degree of block may increase with carotid sinus massage and decrease with leg or arm exercise, while His–Purkinje block may show the opposite response or no response.

Third-degree AV block will result in complete dissociation of atrial and ventricular rates. In the presence of atrial fibrillation this will result in regularization of the ventricular rate without change in QRS morphology. Complete nodal block may become second-degree during exercise or after atropine or catecholamine administration [86].

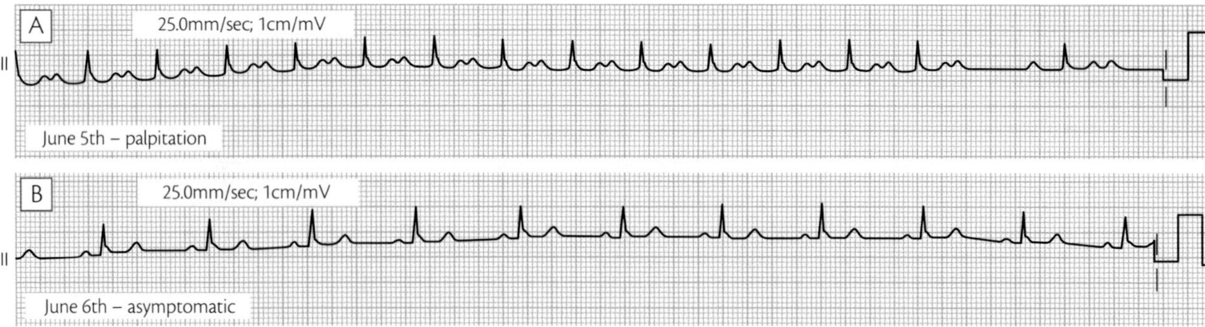

Figure 2.33 (A) PR prolongation and second-degree AV block during ectopic atrial tachycardia. (B) PR interval is normal during sinus rhythm. Note the change in P-wave configuration during tachycardia.

Intrahisian block

Block in the HB before its bifurcation is not common, but it poses an interesting differential diagnostic problem with nodal block, because the escape rhythm may be slower and symptoms more severe. Wenckebach sequences are rare, as in second-degree block occurring in the BB. Blocked P waves are not preceded by PR prolongation but occur suddenly (Mobitz II block, also called simply Mobitz block). In contrast with nodal block, intrahisian block can be precipitated by exertion, explaining some cases of exercise limitation in apparently normal subjects including a normal ECG [91, 92] (➲Fig. 2.34).

Bundle branch block (also see ➲Chapter 27)

The HB courses on the superior and basal portion of the interventricular septum, then divides in two BB, one on each side of the septum, that carry activation separately to each ventricle [93] (➲Figs. 2.2 and 2.3). The RBB follows a direct course, without branching, to the apical portion of the septal RV, then divides and spreads on the RV subendocardium forming a Purkinje network. The LBB gives a small septal branch early in its course along the middle septal LV, then divides in two main directions, reaching toward the base of the 'anterior' papillary muscle (anterior fascicle) and the base of the 'posterior' papillary muscle. Following animal experimental observations, the divisions of the LBB have been conceptualized as discrete fascicles [3]; however, in humans the divisions of LBB are rather diffuse branches, despite which the term fascicle remains in use [93]. Another significant correction is in order regarding the true anatomic position of the papillary muscles and the LBB fascicles, which is more superior than anterior and more inferior than posterior (➲Figs. 2.23 and 2.25). We will use the terms antero-superior and postero-inferior fascicles, because taking into account the anatomic position makes easier the understanding of the ECG changes produced by fascicular blocks.

Block of a BB produces a marked delay in activation of the corresponding ventricle because conduction across the interventricular septum is much slower than through the Purkinje network; therefore, QRS width becomes ≥120ms [2, 3]. Once the septum is crossed, activation re-enters the blocked branch, distal to the point of block, from where activation will follow again the normal path, unless there are more diffuse lesions in the distal branch and Purkinje network. The myocardium activated by the blocked BB 'breaks free' from the voltage cancellation occurring in normal activation and the delayed vectors show an abnormally large voltage in the absence of chamber enlargement. The direction of the delayed activation vectors is marked by the anatomic position of each ventricle: the RV anterior and to the right, and the LV posterior and to the left (➲Fig. 2.6).

Although we refer to the BB in this section, it is known that the Purkinje fibres pertaining to each branch may already be packed separately in the HB itself so that BBB patterns may be due to HB lesions. In these cases pacing the distal HB may normalize the QRS complex, making the BBB disappear [94].

Right bundle branch block

RBBB results in little change in the initial QRS vectors, which still arise normally from the LBB. Vector 1 is unchanged and changes in vector 2 are minor. Delayed RV activation is inscribed as an abnormally large, slow vector 3 directed to the right and anteriorly [1–7, 15]. As a consequence, there are wide, slurred S waves in I, aVL, and V5–V6 and wide R′ in V1–V2 (➲Figs. 2.26 and 2.35). In some cases the QRS complex is totally positive in V1 with a notch in the upstroke of the R wave. In uncomplicated RBBB, QRS axis in the frontal plane is generally indeterminate, i.e. not clearly defined, with positive and negative deflections in all leads (➲Fig. 2.35). It is always possible to calculate a mean axis, but in RBBB the bulk of the QRS is formed by two main vectors with very different directions and the calculated axis does not represent a predominant direction of activation

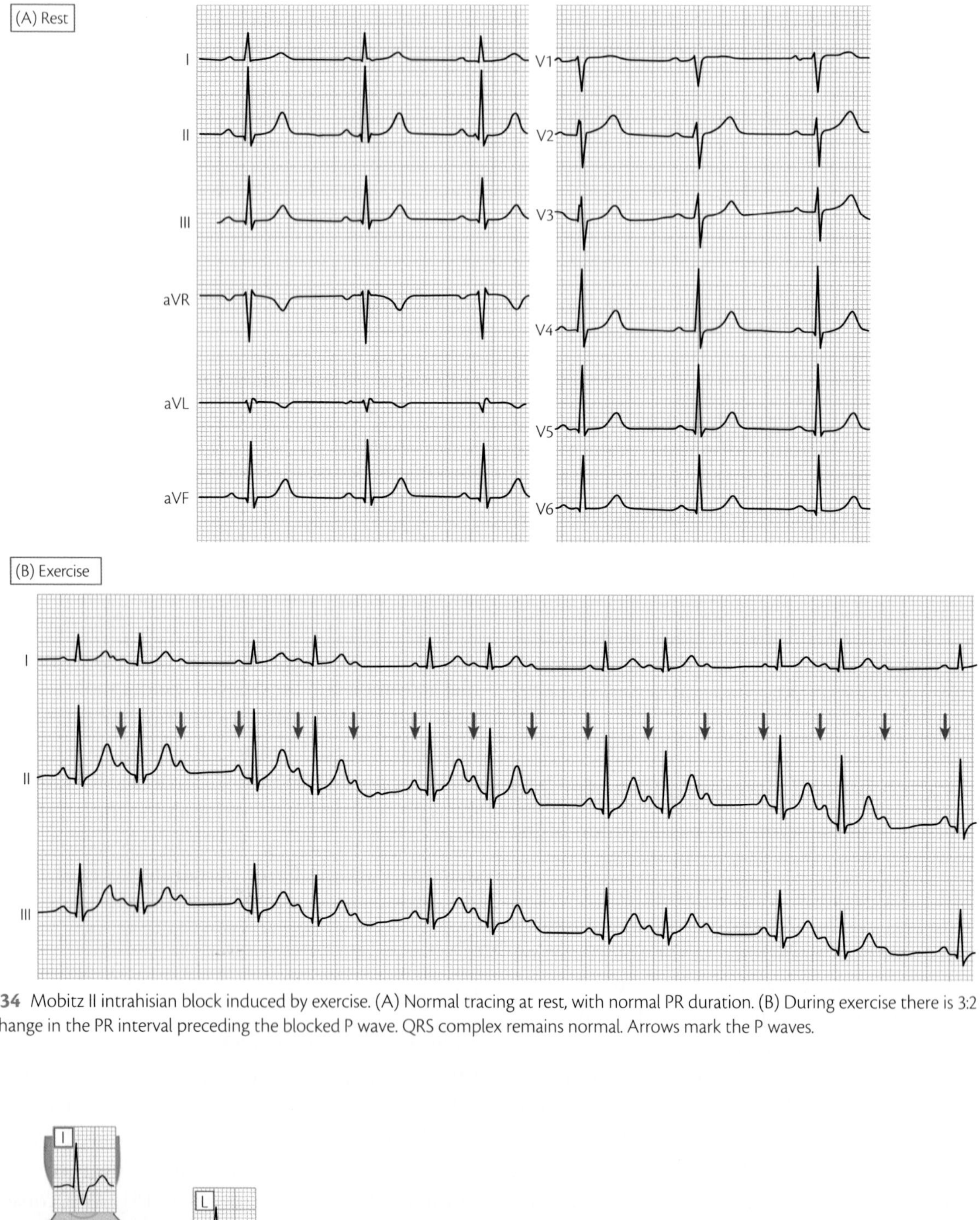

(A) Rest

(B) Exercise

Figure 2.34 Mobitz II intrahisian block induced by exercise. (A) Normal tracing at rest, with normal PR duration. (B) During exercise there is 3:2 AV block without change in the PR interval preceding the blocked P wave. QRS complex remains normal. Arrows mark the P waves.

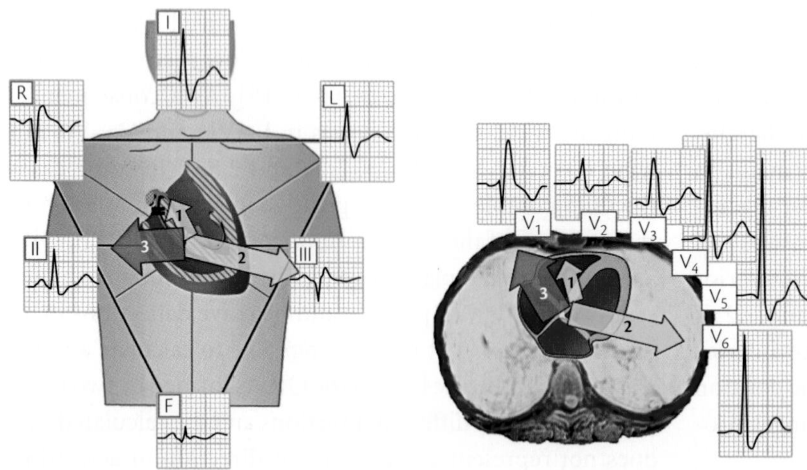

Figure 2.35 QRS changes in RBBB explained by vectorial changes. Vectors 1 and 2 (yellow) maintain a normal direction but RV activation delay generates a large, delayed vector 3 (red) directed to the right and anteriorly.

in this plane. When the RBBB pattern is present but the QRS does not quite measure 120ms in width this is called incomplete RBBB [95].

Change in RV activation causes a change in repolarization (secondary changes) and the T wave is negative where the delayed vectors are positive, especially V1–V2. The T wave is asymmetric, as the ST segment slopes progressively down from the J point (➲ Fig. 2.35). The predominant R wave in V1 and V2 and the secondary ST and T-wave changes would be suggestive of RV enlargement, but in the presence of RBBB this diagnosis can not be made by these criteria, because the block itself will alter both R-wave voltage and ST and T configuration.

RBBB appears not to be necessarily related to structural heart disease and by itself, as an isolated finding, does not carry an adverse prognostic significance, although a higher incidence of heart block can be observed in long follow-up observations [95–99].

Left bundle branch block

Contrary to RBBB, LBBB changes the whole QRS. Activation starts in the septal RV then propagates across the interventricular septum to re-enter the LBB and Purkinje system of the LV [100–103]. The initial septal q wave is lost [104] and the predominant vectors are directed to the left and posteriorly inscribing broad, notched R waves in I, aVL, and V5–V6 (➲ Figs. 2.29 and 2.36). Initial r waves are small or absent in the right precordial leads where configuration is rS or QS. Configuration of the QRS in the other leads depends on the QRS axis, which is variable. The QRS complex is widened to ≥120ms but it may be much wider depending on the presence of added intraventricular conduction disturbances (muscle fibrosis, Purkinje network damage). In some cases with delay, but not complete block of the LBB, the same QRS changes are present with a QRS width <120ms, a pattern called incomplete LBBB. In the presence of LBBB the diagnosis of associated LV enlargement or old myocardial infarction becomes practically impossible [70, 105, 106].

In LBBB, secondary ST and T-wave changes occur over the leads showing predominant R waves (I, aVL, V5-6), with the same asymmetric T-wave inversion described in RBBB (➲ Figs. 2.29 and 2.36).

LBBB is associated with cardiovascular disease in a higher proportion than RBB, and is also a long-term predictor of heart block. In patients with congestive heart failure LBBB is a sign of adverse prognosis [96–99].

Fascicular blocks

The concept of left fascicular block (or hemiblock) was a significant step forward in the study of the mechanisms and progression of AV block because it helped detect the presence of LBB involvement in the presence of RBB (bifascicular block) [3, 107]. Initial enthusiasm with this view led to the implantation of prophylactic pacemakers in many cases of bifascicular block, a strategy that was later found unjustified in the absence of frank trifascicular block [108–110]. The hemiblocks were initially defined in experiments with dogs, where the LBB appears to bifurcate into two rather well-defined fascicles. In humans, the LBB seems to fan out over the septal LV rather than to bifurcate into two well-defined fascicles [93], but the fascicular block patterns are still applicable, although not necessarily implying discrete lesions of a single, well-defined fascicle.

The main effect of a fascicular block is a delay in activation of the myocardium dependent on the affected fascicle which, as in BBB, will then generate more prominent vectors [3, 106]. Delay is not very prominent (≤20ms) because the Purkinje network carries activation rapidly from the normal fascicle to the blocked fascicle distal to the point

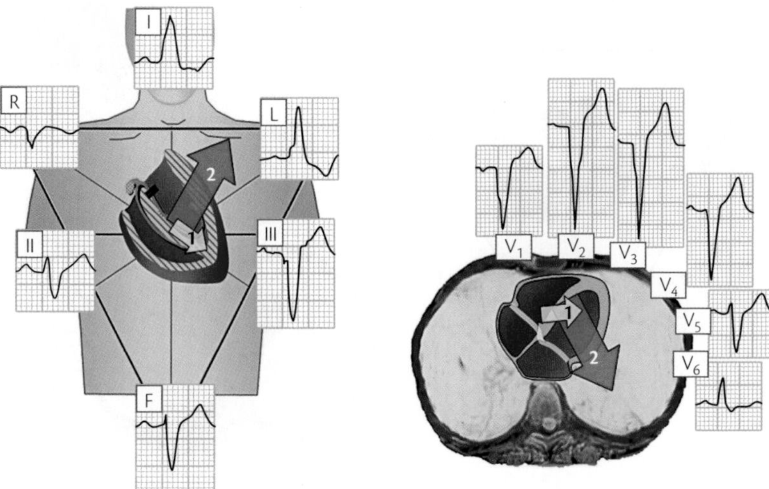

Figure 2.36 LBBB mimicking anteroseptal myocardial infarction. As in Fig. 2.52 the initial vectors are absent and there are no septal q waves in I, aVL and V6. In this case r waves are completely absent V1–V3 where QS complexes are recorded. QRS axis in the frontal plane is left (−45°).

of block. Hemiblocks thus produce minor QRS widening to ≤110ms but the QRS axis shifts markedly toward the blocked area. The initial vectors are also affected by hemiblocks. Understanding the anatomic position helps explain the direction of the axis shift.

Left antero-superior hemiblock

Block of the antero-superior fascicle (ASF) shifts the initial (0–20ms) vectors inferiorly and to the right because early activation at the base of the anterosuperior papillary muscle is absent [3]. As a consequence, q waves are recorded in I and aVL and r waves in II, III, and aVF. The inferior shift may be marked enough to inscribe small q waves in the right precordial leads, which are recorded in a relatively high position in the 4th intercostal space (➲Fig. 2.37). The hallmark of ASF block is a QRS axis between –45° and –60°, due to a shift of vector 2 markedly to the left and superiorly [111]. QRS configuration is qR in I and aVL and rS in II, III, and aVF. The precordial leads most often display an apparent clockwise rotation with S waves in V5 and V6, as if terminal QRS vectors were shifted to the right; however, this is not confirmed in the absence of an S wave in leads I and aVL. The explanation for these S waves in V5-V6 is the marked superior direction of vector 2, which can actually point away from V5 and V6, despite a leftward direction (➲Fig. 2.37). Recording V5 and V6 from the 4th intercostal space, instead of its normal position in the 5th space, decreases S-wave amplitude or makes it disappear. QRS width is mildly increased to ≤110ms and there may be some terminal slurring. There are no secondary ST or T changes attributable to left anterosuperior hemiblock.

The differential diagnosis of ASF block includes real clockwise rotation, either due to RV enlargement, or positional changes, as in chest deformity. The presence of prominent S waves in leads I and aVL is the feature that marks clockwise rotation and allows the differentiation. The clinical meaning of an isolated ASF block is minimal, even in the presence of a prolonged HV interval [112].

Postero-inferior hemiblock

Isolated block of the postero-inferior fascicle (PIF) is rare, and it is more commonly observed in association with RBBB. The clinical experience with PIF block is very limited and this ECG diagnosis has to be supported, more than ever, by clinical data [3, 106]. The hallmark of PIF block is a rightward shift of âQRS to between +100° and +120° and this can be observed in normal subjects, particularly at young age, or in the presence of RV enlargement or chest deformity, and all of these circumstances have to be ruled out before the diagnosis of PIF block is made.

PIF block produces QRS changes that are almost a mirror image of ASF block (➲Fig. 2.38). Initial activation vectors (vector 1) are shifted superiorly, because the inferior component normally generated by activation at the base of the postero-inferior papillary muscle is absent. This is reflected by the presence of q waves in the inferior leads II, III, and aVF. Delay in activation of the postero-inferior wall of the LV shifts vector 2 inferiorly and to the right, and this is

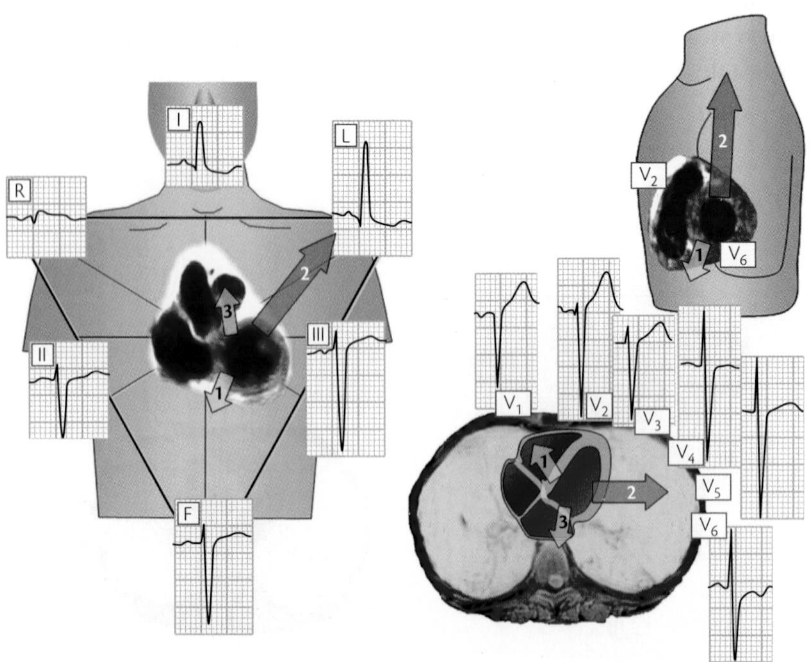

Figure 2.37 Schematic and ECG representation of changes produced by left ASF block. The thorax is represented in frontal (A), horizontal (B), and left lateral (C) views. Magnetic resonance cuts of the heart have been included in the schematic representations of the thorax to show the anatomic position (B). The shifted vector 2, determining QRS axis, is in red. Note in the left lateral view how the relatively high recording position of V1 and V2 may cause the recording of an initial q wave even with an anteriorly directed vector 1 (yellow). Note also in this view that the superiorly directed vector 2 can be recorded as negative in V6 due to its relatively inferior location. For further explanation see text.

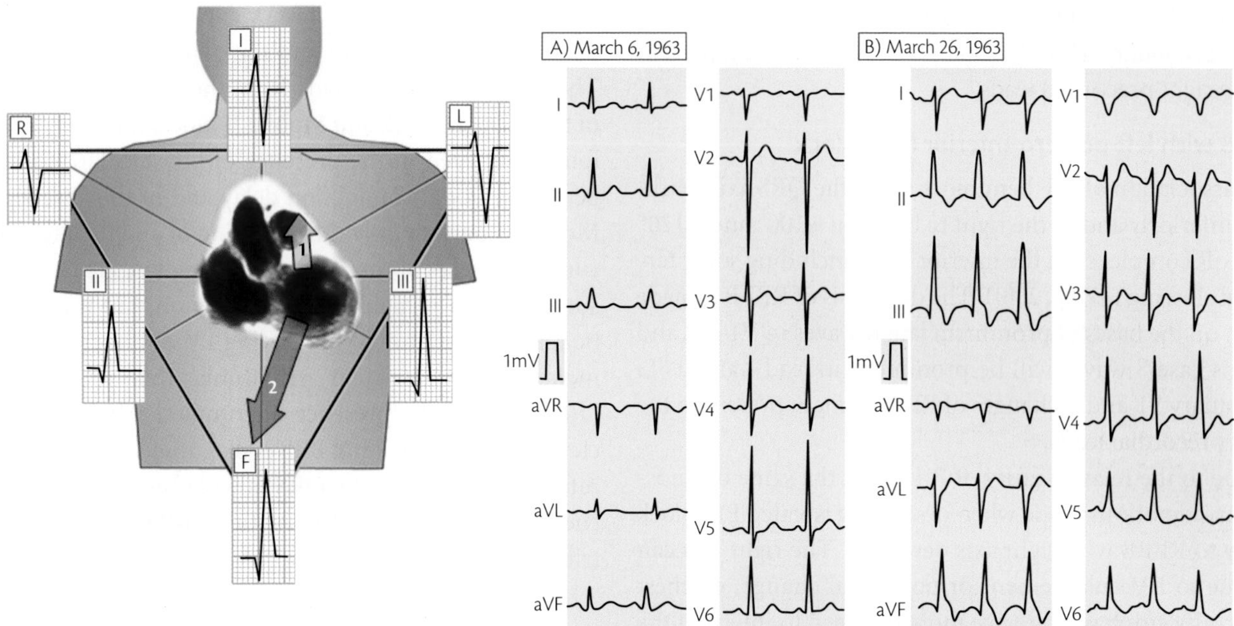

Figure 2.38 Left postero-inferior hemiblock in the course of acute inferior myocardial infarction. (A) shows a normal ECG taken days before the acute episode; (B) shows ST segment elevation in II, III, and aVF with beginning T-wave inversion and a QRS axis shift to +100° which was completely reversible after the acute episode. The drawing shows the shifts in vectors 1 and 2 produced by left PIF block.

responsible for the rightward âQRS shift and the appearance of qR complexes in II, III, and aVF. There are no particular changes in the precordial leads.

Bifascicular blocks

The diagnosis of bifascicular block is made mainly on the bases of marked axis shifts in the presence of RBBB. Final S waves may be absent in lead I and the diagnosis of RBBB will be mainly based on the presence of late, anteriorly directed vectors, inscribing late prominent R waves in the right precordial leads V1 and V2.

RBBB with left antero-superior hemiblock

While uncomplicated RBBB tends to show an undetermined axis in the frontal plane, the association of a ASF block creates a clear superior (left) axis shift, to between –45° and –60° with rS complexes in the inferior leads, that may show terminal slurring representing the more marked RV activation delay produced by the RBBB (➲ Fig. 2.39). QRS width will be ≥120ms. Lead I may still show an S wave also due to the RV delay, but in some cases lead I may show a qR configuration, resembling LBBB. This particular pattern is called masquerading RBBB, because it looks like

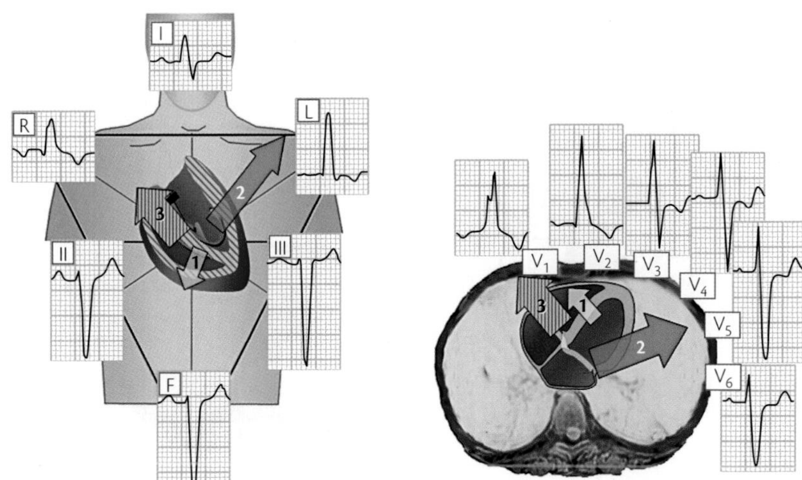

Figure 2.39 Schematic representation of the vector changes in RBBB and associated left ASF block. Upward directed vector 2, due to left ASF block is red. The delayed vector 3 produced by RBBB is dashed. For explanation see text.

LBBB in the frontal plane leads and RBBB in the precordial leads. Secondary ST and T changes of RBBB remain present in the right precordial leads.

RBBB with left postero-inferior hemiblock

The association of PIF hemiblock shifts the QRS axis markedly inferiorly and to the right to between +100° and +120° with qR complexes in the inferior leads including some terminal slurring (➲Fig. 2.40). The diagnosis of RBBB is made again on the bases of prominent late R waves in V1–V2 and in this case S waves will be prominent in lead I and aVL. Secondary ST and T changes of RBBB remain present in the right precordial leads.

Due to the relative rarity of PIF block the same diagnostic considerations made when describing isolated PIF block apply to RBBB with right axis deviation. The right axis can be due to RV enlargement or positional change, or chest deformity emphasizing once more the need to interpret the ECG in the light of clinical information. The association of RBB and PIF block implies very severe conduction disease and is often associated with paroxysmal AV block.

Bilateral bundle branch block and trifascicular block

A pattern of BBB may be due to a marked delay in conduction through a branch and this slow conduction can be put in evidence if the contralateral branch is blocked or delayed further. When this happens RBBB and LBBB patterns alternate and this alternation is accompanied by PR segment alternation (➲Fig. 2.41). Alternating BBB implies a severe disturbance of the His–Purkinje axis and a high risk of advanced-degree AV block. As in intrahisian block, a latent conduction disturbance in the contralateral branch can be put in evidence by an exercise test [91, 92].

Trifascicular block is the AV block due to conduction disturbances in the RBB and the two fascicles of the LBB. The diagnosis can be made from the ECG in the presence of bifascicular block and Mobitz II block; however, PR prolongation, even in the presence of bifascicular block, can be due to nodal conduction delay and in the absence of a Mobitz II pattern only the recording of an HV interval can confirm a delay of the only conducting fascicle. The risk of sudden death is high in this population, but it appears to be related more to the underlying LV dysfunction and the incidence of ventricular arrhythmias than to heart block [108–110]. In the presence of complete AV block, trifascicular block or bilateral BBB is diagnosed when the escape rate is ≤35bpm and the QRS is wide, suggesting idioventricular escape rhythm. Alternating BBB is another form of trifascicular block.

Pre-excitation (also see ➲ Chapter 28)

Wolff, Parkinson, and White (WPW) defined a syndrome of short PR segment with wide QRS complex usually associated with a history of tachycardia that is related to the presence of anomalous or accessory AV connections. Normally the AVN–HB axis is the only structure to connect atria and ventricles electrically, while in the WPW syndrome one or more accessory connections are present that cross the AV junctions, through the AV valve rings, the AV septum,or the coronary sinus and its branches. Anatomical and electrical connection of atrial and ventricular myocardium is free early in fetal life but it normally disappears by the third month when the fibrous cardiac skeleton which insulates them from one another, is formed, leaving the AVN and HB as the only electrical connection. Accessory connections

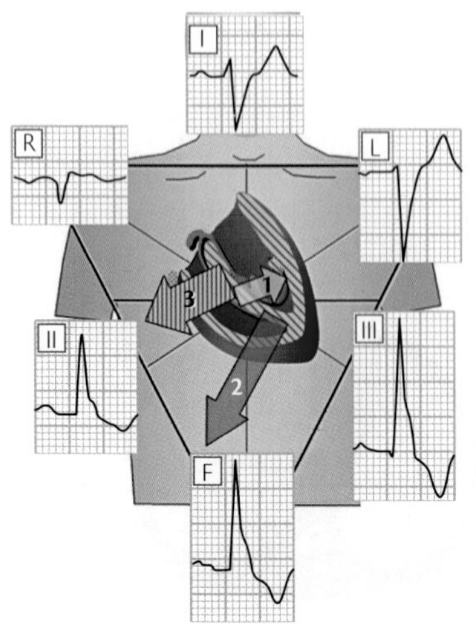

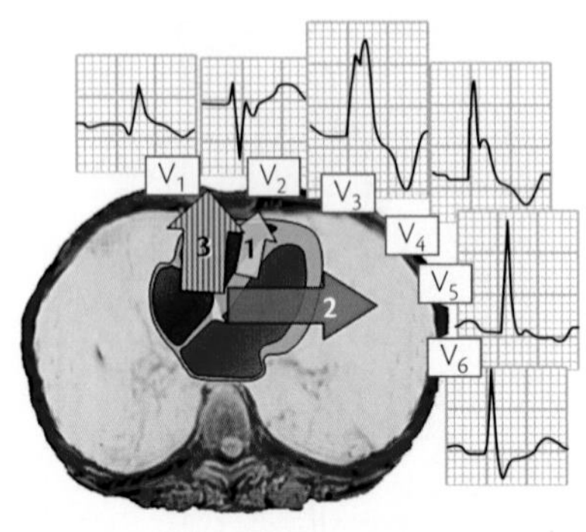

Figure 2.40 RBBB with associated left PIF block. Note the marked right axis shift in the frontal plane. The patient had Mobitz II AV block and syncope.

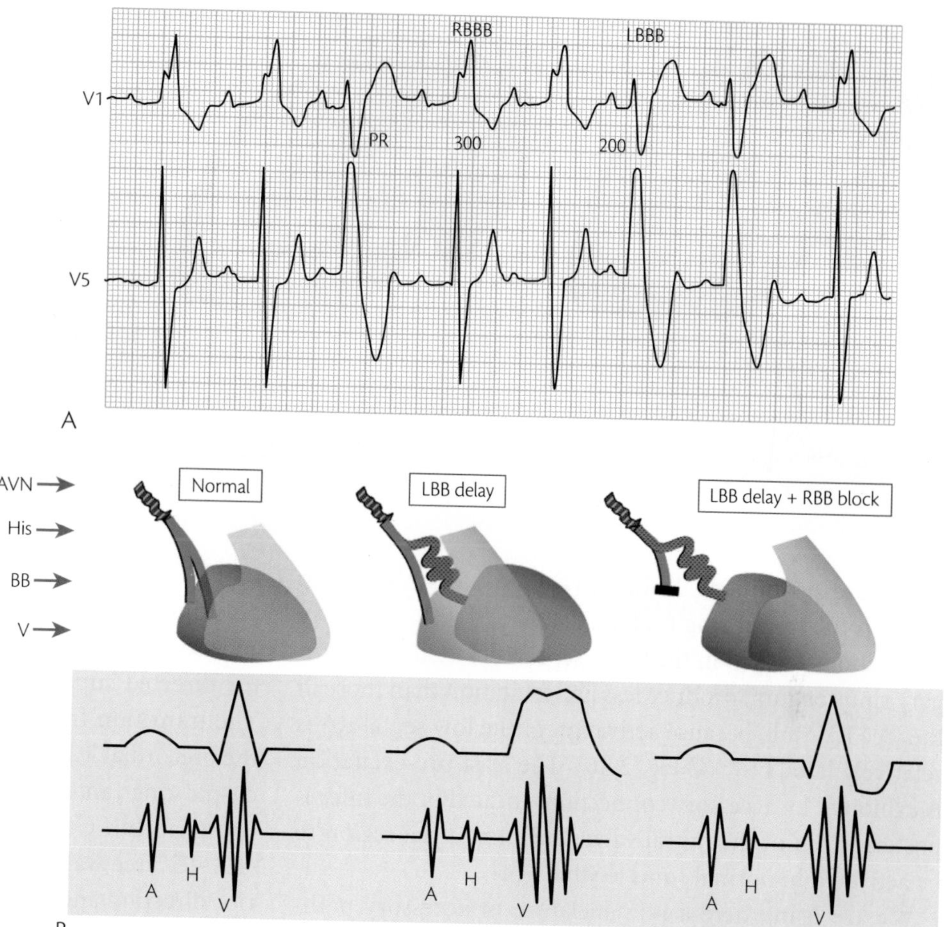

Figure 2.41 Bilateral, alternating BBB. (A) Leads V1 and V5 showing alternatively RBBB and LBBB patterns. Note the change in PR interval with the change in BBB. (B) The mechanism of alternating BBB implies delayed conduction through one BB and intermittent block in the other. The LBBB pattern is produced by conduction delay, not total block, and when the RBB is blocked the LBB conducts with a marked delay, prolonging the PR (and HV) interval and producing a RBBB pattern in the QRS.

(or accessory pathways) are gaps in this electrical insulation allowing AV conduction (antegrade), ventriculo-atrial (VA) (retrograde) conduction, or both [113]. The consequences can be a pre-excitation pattern in the ECG, re-entrant tachycardias with normal QRS, re-entrant tachycardias with a wide QRS, and high ventricular rate with a wide QRS in the presence of atrial flutter or fibrillation, possibly leading to ventricular fibrillation.

Delta wave and ECG localization of accessory connections

When the accessory connection is capable of AV conduction, this is usually faster than AVN conduction and the QRS in sinus rhythm is the result of fusion of normal activation and earlier ('pre-excited') activation through the accessory connection [114, 115]. This is true even in intermittent pre-excitation, because conduction is not decremental in the common form of accessory connections. The pre-excited myocardium is activated before AVN–HB delay ends and therefore the PR segment is filled with a slow, early QRS deflection called delta (Δ) wave for its triangular appearance (➲Fig. 2.42). The late portions of the QRS inscribe sharper deflections, as it depends on activation though the normal conduction tissues. The QRS is widened but, in contrast with BB blocks where QRS slurring appears in the mid or late QRS, in WPW syndrome it occurs in the early portions, shortening the PR interval.

QRS widening and the prominence of the pre-excited Δ wave vary with the proximity of the accessory connection to the sinus node and the duration of the AV nodal delay. AVN delay varies in different individuals and with changes in autonomic tone or drug effects and a shorter AVN conduction time increases the proportion of normally activated myocardium and decreases the size of the Δ wave. Conversely, connections closer to the sinus node start ventricular pre-excitation earlier and activate a larger myocardial mass, therefore producing shorter PR intervals and more prominent Δ waves (➲Fig. 2.42). For a given AV nodal delay, accessory connections located in the anterior and superior tricuspid ring produce shorter PR intervals

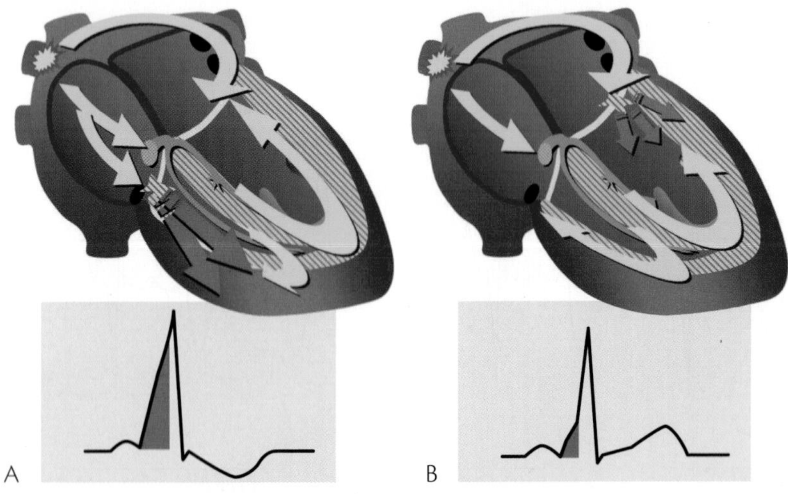

Figure 2.42 Mechanism of fusion (Δ waves) in WPW syndrome. Pre-excited activation through the accessory connection (red arrows) depends on the distance from the sinus node to the accessory connection. An accessory connection at the tricuspid ring (A) provokes rapid activation of the RV, a short PR segment, and a large Δ wave. An accessory connection in the mitral ring (B) starts activating the LV later and produces a longer (even normal) PR segment and a smaller Δ wave. Activation through the AVN–HB axis is more dominant in LA–LV connections and the QRS looks more normal.

and more prominent Δ waves (➲Figs. 2.42–2.44) than those in the mitral ring (➲Figs. 2.42 and 2.45). Accessory connections located in the lower septum, close to the coronary sinus ostium, produce less pre-excitation than those in the free RV wall, because activation of the low septal RA is relatively late [116] (➲Fig. 2.46). The least pre-excitation is exhibited by accessory connections located in the infero-posterior rim of the mitral valve, the latest atrial region to be activated in normal sinus rhythm [14].

We are using here a nomenclature of accessory pathways that is faithful to their true anatomic location [10], but the WPW literature uses a different terminology that originated in the operating room, that calls 'posterior' the inferior part of the tricuspid and mitral rings and interatrial septum [117, 118]. The use of an anatomic nomenclature makes ECG interpretation more intuitive and deductive. It can be understood intuitively that accessory connections located in the high portions of the AV junctions, be it right (➲Fig. 2.44) or left (➲Fig. 2.45), will generate a vector pointing inferiorly and so will the QRS axis. Conversely, accessory connections located inferiorly will produce a vector directed superiorly and a superior axis (➲Fig. 2.46). The transition from negative to positive QRS complex in the precordial leads helps localize the connection in the tricuspid ring (anteriorly), the septal area, or the mitral ring (posteriorly). Connections in the anterior tricuspid ring (RA–RV free wall) generate a vector with a marked posterior direction and the QRS complex is predominantly negative V1 through V3–V4 (➲Fig. 2.43). Connections located in the septal area will generate a less posterior vector and the QRS complex will be positive in V2 or V3 (➲Figs. 2.44 and 2.46) and those in the posterior mitral ring will make positive QRS complexes V1–V3 (➲ Fig. 2.45).

A number of algorithms have been published to help localize the ventricular insertion of the accessory connections by the ECG pattern [118–120]. All of them depend on

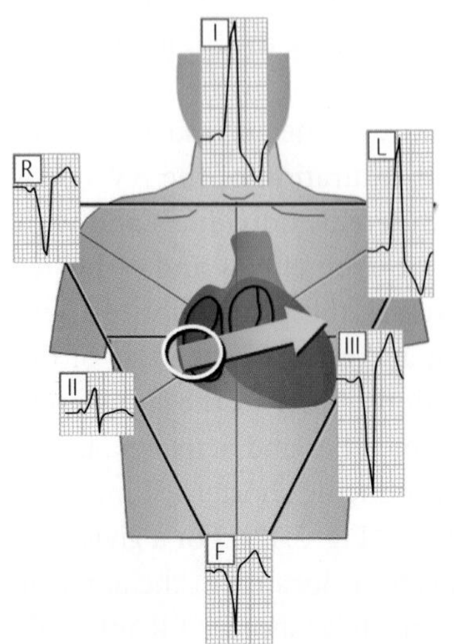

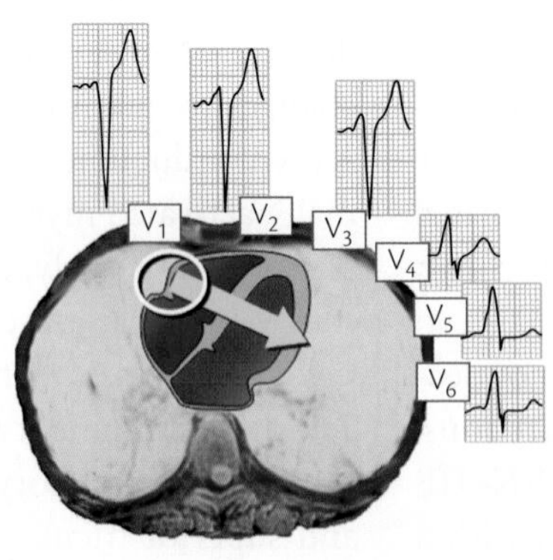

Figure 2.43 Marked pre-excitation due to an accessory connection located in the anterior tricuspid ring (white ring). Note the very short PR interval and the widening and slurring of the QRS with sharp deflections only in the latest portions. A mid-position in the supero-inferior direction is suggested by the nearly horizontal axis in the frontal plane. The posterior direction in the horizontal plane is reflected in predominantly negative QRS complexes V1–V3. This position is called 'right lateral' in the prevalent surgical terminology.

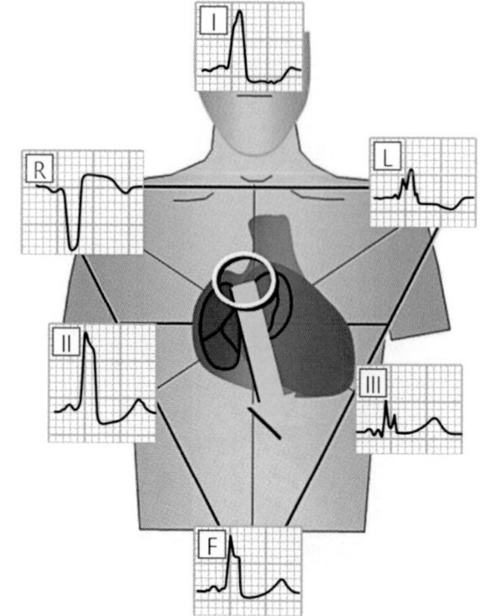

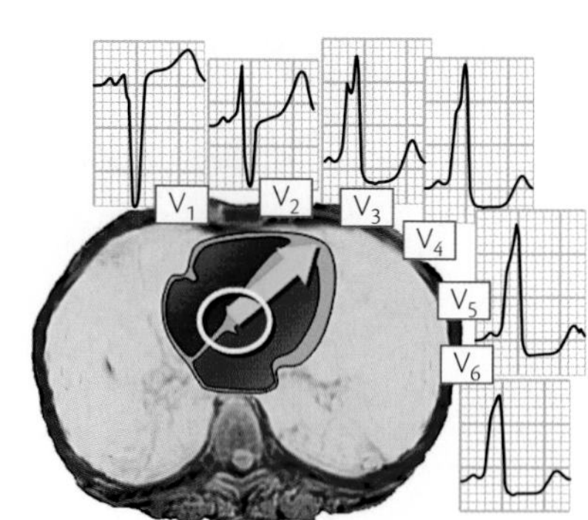

Figure 2.44 Marked pre-excitation due to an accessory connection located in the high tricuspid ring, close to the HB. Note marked pre-excitation as in ➲Fig. 2.65, however, the QRS axis is now inferior due to the high position of the connection. On the horizontal plane the intermediate position of the connection in the anterior-posterior direction determines a less posterior vector and QRS complexes are clearly positive in V3. This position is called 'anteroseptal' in the prevalent surgical terminology.

the presence of marked pre-excitation for accuracy because when there is little pre-excitation, as in the presence of little AVN delay, it becomes difficult to determine the location of the connections. When connections are multiple, the diagnosis can be very difficult and the diagnosis can sometimes be suspected only by the changing pre-excitation patterns during sinus rhythm or during atrial fibrillation or the transition from orthodromic to antidromic tachycardia (see ➲Orthodromic tachycardia, p.59 and Antidromic tachycardia, p.60) [121, 122].

WPW syndrome can be mimicked by abnormal intraventricular conduction in hypertrophic cardiomyopathy, that can cause initial QRS slurring, like a Δ wave, with or without a short PR interval, in the absence of accessory connections [123]. A short PR with a normal QRS complex can be a sign of fast conduction through the AVN, a condition that is not by itself associated with tachycardias [124].

Orthodromic tachycardia

Orthodromic tachycardia is the most common clinical manifestation of WPW syndrome. Its mechanism is re-entry (circular activation) with sequential atrial and ventricular participation (➲Fig. 2.47) where activation jumps from ventricle to atrium (retrograde, VA conduction) through the accessory connection and returns to the ventricles through the AVN–HB axis. The QRS is normal during tachycardia (narrow QRS tachycardia) because the accessory connection is used for VA conduction, not for AV conduction [125–128]. The P wave may be recorded superposed to the ST segment with an RP interval shorter than

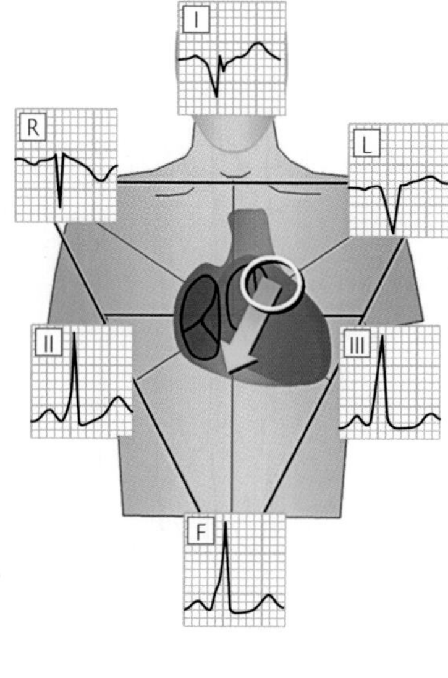

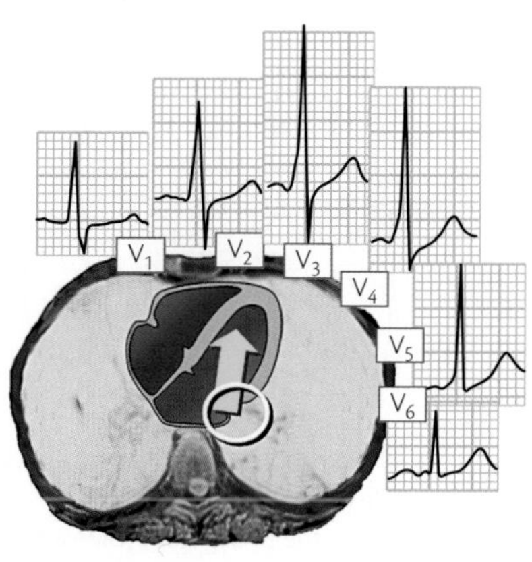

Figure 2.45 Lesser degree of pre-excitation in an accessory connection located in the posterior-superior portion of the mitral ring. Note the borderline-normal PR interval and a smaller Δ wave than in ➲Figs. 2.65 and 2.66. The position of the connection determines a QRS axis inferior and to the right in the frontal plane and predominant R waves in the right precordial leads (V21–V4). This position is called 'left anterolateral' in the prevalent surgical terminology.

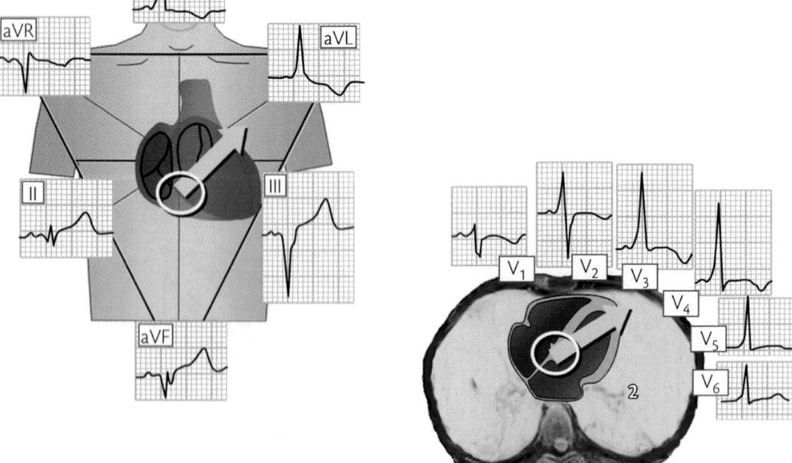

Figure 2.46 Less prominent degree of pre-excitation in a low paraseptal accessory connection. The superior QRS axis in the frontal plane indicates the inferior location of the connection. As in ➲Fig. 2.66 the horizontal plane shows an intermediate direction of the vectors (QRS clearly positive in V3), typical of septal connections. This position is called 'posteroseptal' in the prevalent surgical terminology.

the PR. Orthodromic tachycardia is perfectly regular and the rate can be from 160 to >200bpm. Rate-dependent BBB can occur during orthodromic tachycardia, posing the differential diagnosis with VT or pre-excited tachycardia.

Antidromic tachycardia

Antidromic tachycardia is due also to a macro-re-entrant circuit with atrial and ventricular participation, but in the opposite direction than orthodromic tachycardia. Retrograde VA conduction uses the HB–AVN axis and antegrade AV conduction the accessory connection (➲Fig. 2.48). The tachycardia is regular, the QRS is fully pre-excited (wide QRS tachycardia), and the rate is similar to orthodromic tachycardia [129, 130]. Antidromic tachycardia is much less common than orthodromic tachycardia, probably because AVN conduction is slower in the orthodromic direction, which facilitates re-entry. Antidromic tachycardia can occur with accessory pathways capable only of AV conduction,

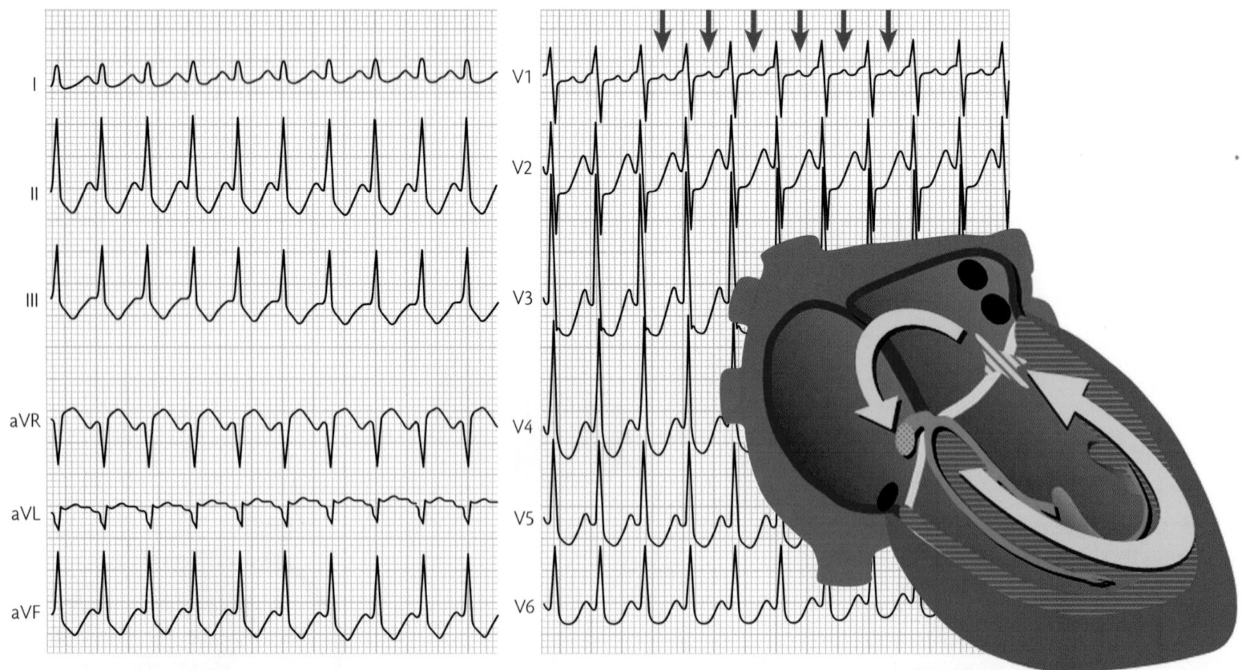

Figure 2.47 Orthodromic tachycardia in WPW syndrome. The accessory pathway is the retrograde (VA) arm of the tachycardia and the AVN–HB axis the antegrade (AV) limb. Ventricular activation is normal and the QRS loses the Δ wave and becomes normal (narrow QRS tachycardia). The P wave can often be seen on the ST segment (blue arrows).

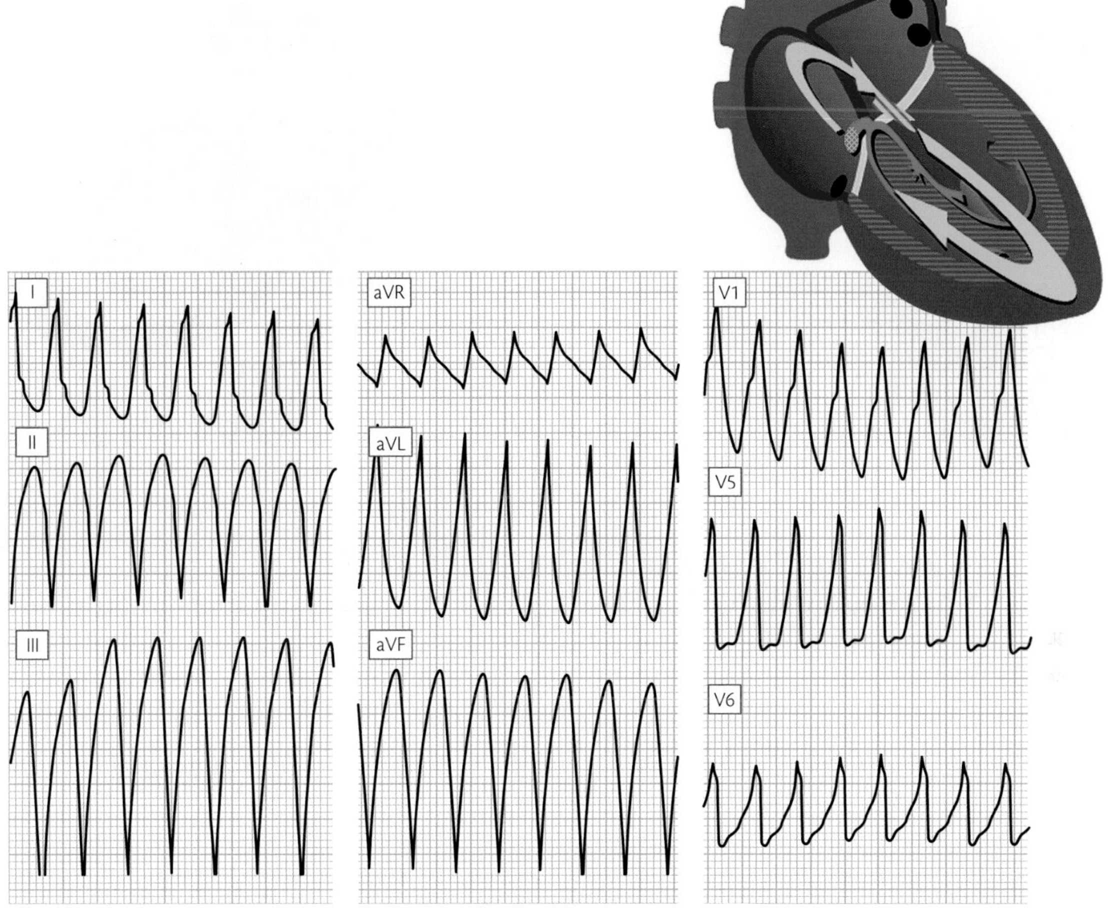

Figure 2.48 Antidromic tachycardia in a 23-year-old man with an inferior paraseptal accessory connection. See text for explanation.

therefore in the absence of episodes of orthodromic tachycardia [131, 132] and it is more common in cases with multiple accessory connections, when the tachycardia circuit can use one of the connections for retrograde (VA) conduction [121, 122].

Pre-excited atrial flutter and fibrillation

Pre-excited atrial flutter occurs when the refractory period of the accessory connection is short enough to conduct at the fast flutter rates [129]. The QRS complex is fully pre-excited, as in antidromic tachycardia and ventricular rate is regular at ≥250bpm.

Pre-excited atrial fibrillation can also be conducted at rapid rates through an accessory conduction with a short refractory period, ventricular rate reaching up to 300bpm in bursts. Ventricular rate is irregular and the QRS complex is wide, fully pre-excited, but occasional conduction through the AVN–HB axis can produce a narrow QRS or fusion beats [128, 132, 133] (➲Fig. 2.49).

The diagnosis of pre-excited atrial flutter or fibrillation is crucial because digoxin and verapamil, often used to control rate in atrial flutter and fibrillation, are contraindicated. The fast ventricular rates in these pre-excited atrial arrhythmias can induce ventricular fibrillation and sudden death in patients with WPW syndrome [134].

Accessory connections without pre-excitation

Some accessory connections with the usual rapid conduction properties are capable only of retrograde (VA) conduction and can not be detected in the ECG in sinus rhythm, but can still cause orthodromic tachycardias [135, 136]. The presence of the accessory connection can be suspected during tachycardia by the recording of a retrograde P wave on the ST segment [126, 127] (➲Fig. 2.47), but in many cases precise diagnosis can only be made during electrophysiological study.

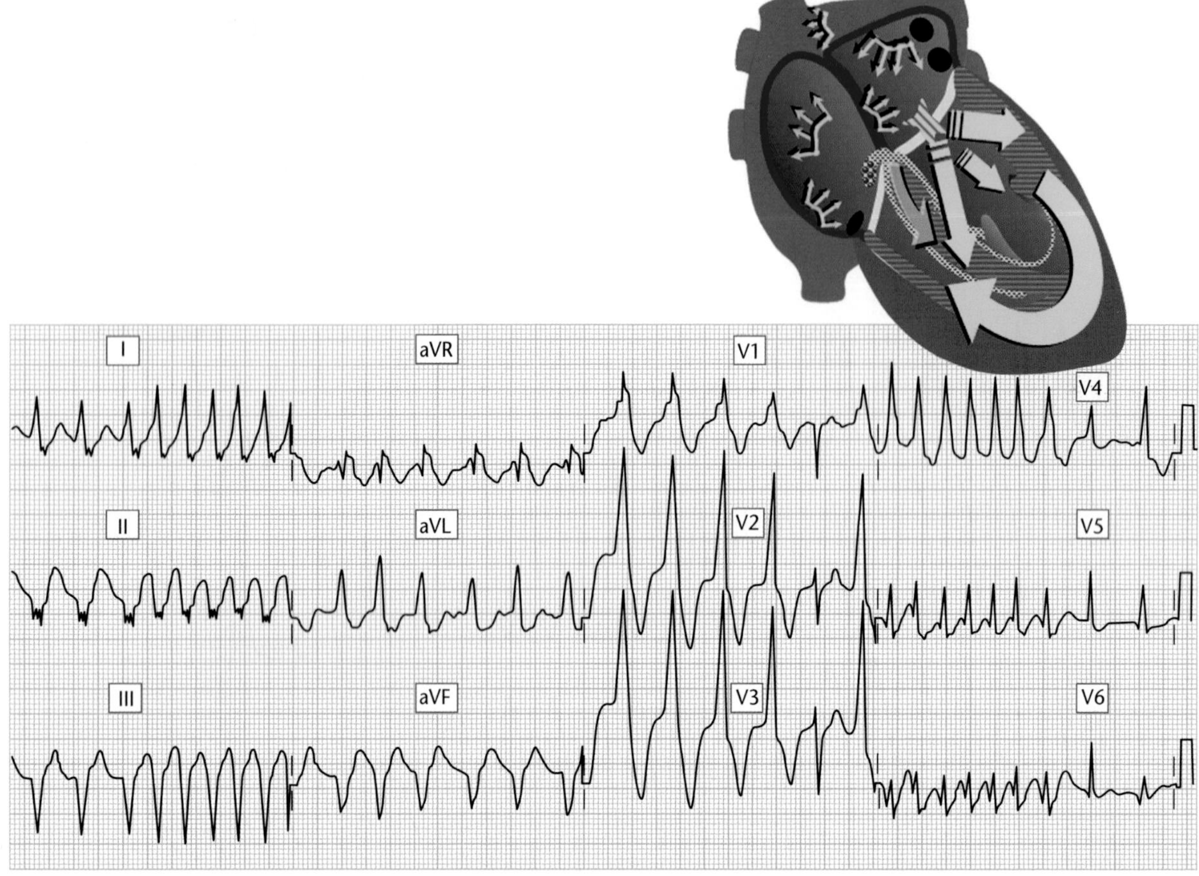

Figure 2.49 Pre-excited atrial fibrillation in a patient with a left inferior accessory connection. Note the wide QRS complexes with irregular rate reaching 280–300bpm in short bursts. The precordial leads show some normally conducted QRS complexes and one fusion beat (last of the tracing on the right).

Some atypical accessory connections show only retrograde (VA) conduction with decremental properties, similar to the AVN. The atrial insertion is usually located around the coronary sinus ostium and the ventricular connection is probably in the basal RV. These 'slow' connections cause incessant orthodromic tachycardias with negative P waves preceding the QRS with a normal PR interval [137, 138] (➲Fig. 2.50). The differential diagnosis with atypical nodal tachycardias can be difficult, even in the electrophysiology laboratory. The incessant character of the tachycardia can cause a cardiomyopathy in children.

An unusual form of accessory connection with slow AV conduction has been called 'Mahaim pre-excitation' in the belief that the slow conduction was due to insertion of the accessory connection in the AVN [114, 115]. It is known today that these connections represent an accessory AVN–HB structure in the RV free wall (anterior tricuspid ring) that can insert in the RBB, instead of the basal ventricular wall [139, 140] (➲Fig. 2.51). Pre-excitation is minimal or absent at baseline, due to slow AV conduction through the accessory connection. Antidromic tachycardias are typical of this type of connections, with a wide QRS with typical LBB configuration, due to the insertion of the accessory HB in the RBB [140, 141] (➲Fig. 2.51). Retrograde (VA) conduction is generally absent in these connections, therefore they do not cause orthodromic tachycardias.

Primary repolarization disturbances

The QT interval

QT interval, measured from the onset of the QRS complex to the end of the T wave is taken to represent action potential duration, an important parameter in arrhythmias related to triggered activity. The relationship between QT interval and action potential duration can not be very direct, because action potential duration differs very significantly across the ventricular myocardium depth [9], but still the QT interval is capable of reflecting the presence of excessive prolongation and the risk of arrhythmias related to it. Prolongation of phase 2 of the action potential increases calcium entry in the cell making it unstable with

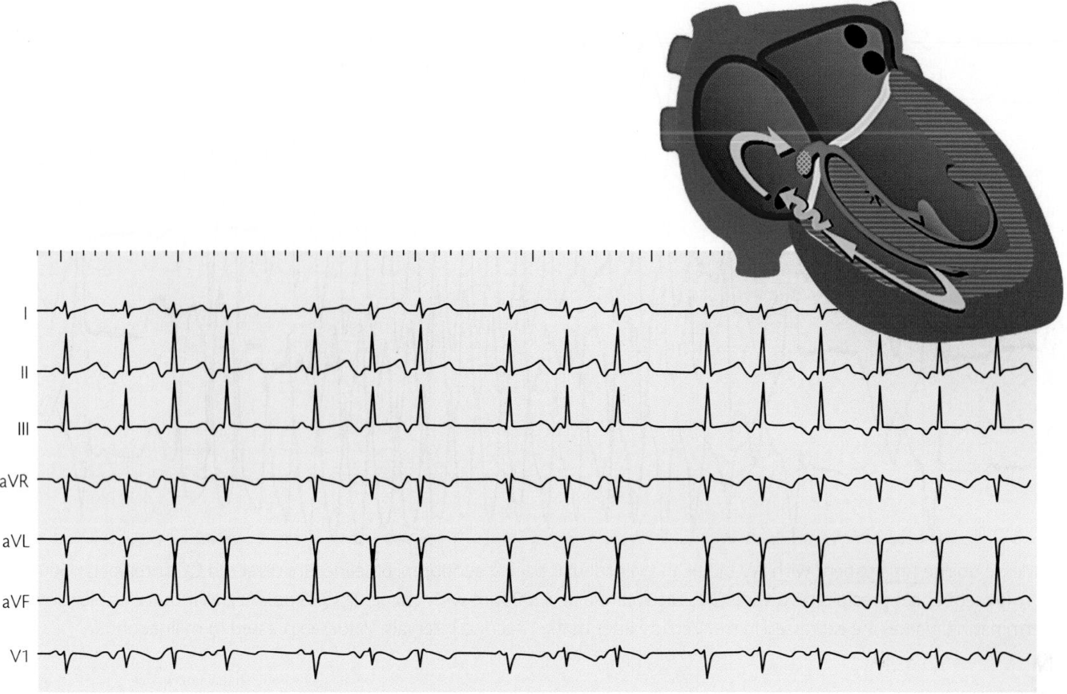

Figure 2.50 Incessant tachycardia ('Coumel type') due to an accessory AV connection with exclusive retrograde slow conduction. Note the constant termination and reinitiation cycles of the tachycardia, even at rest. Time marks (top) are 0.1s and 1s.

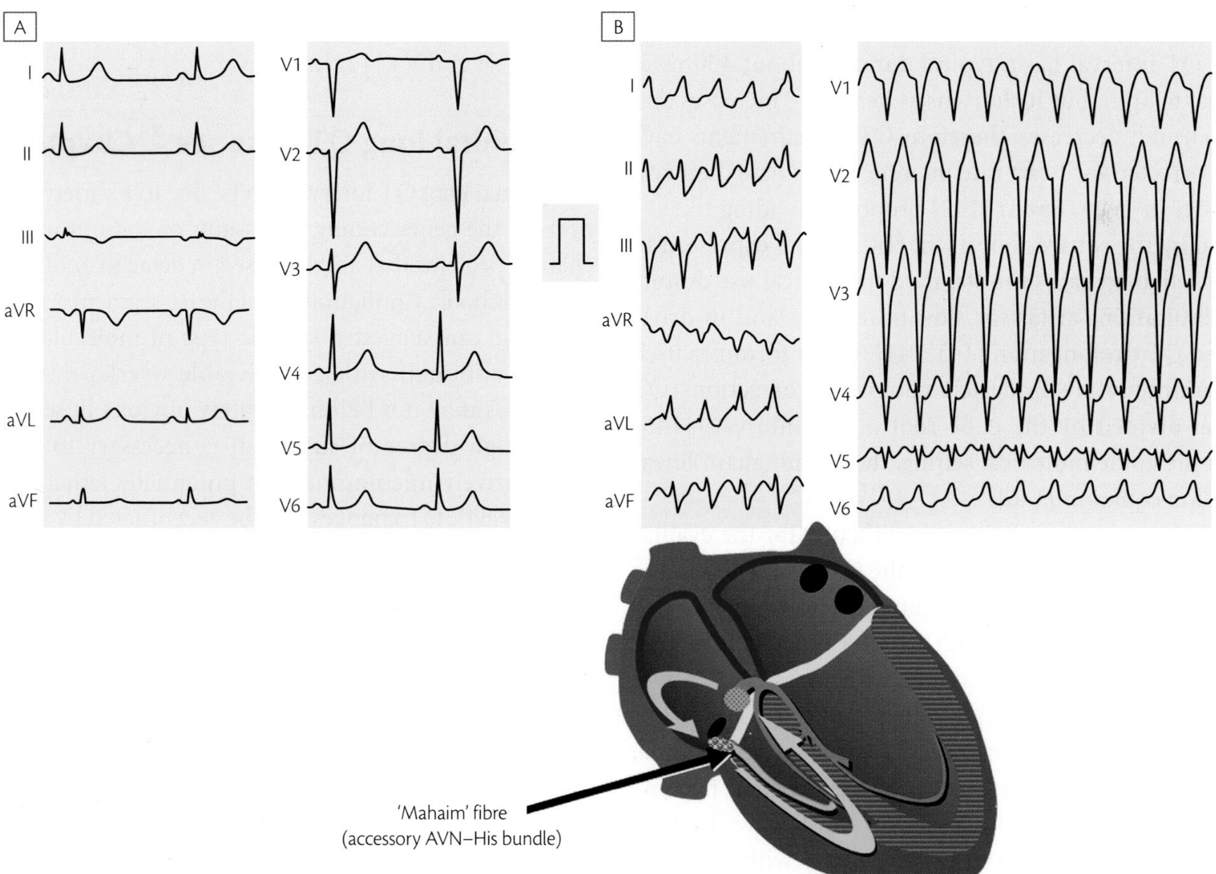

Figure 2.51 Accessory AVN–HB ('Mahaim') pre-excitation. (A) Shows the baseline ECG with a normal PR and no Δ waves; (B) shows the same patient during antidromic tachycardia with the typical LBBB QRS morphology.

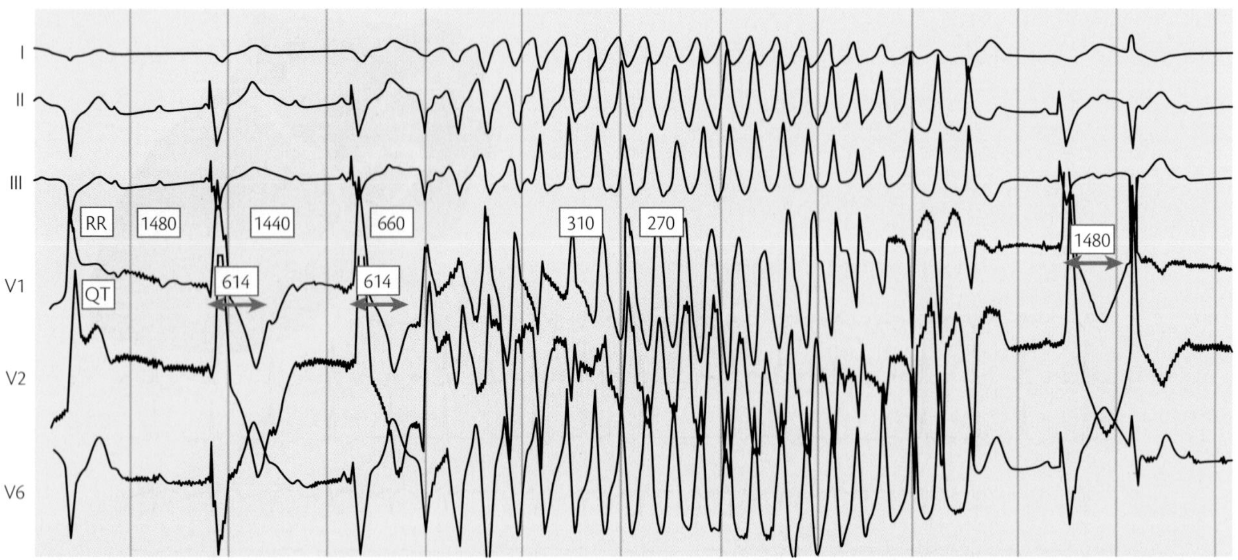

Figure 2.52 Torsade de pointes in a patient with AV block and ventricular pacing at 40bpm. Baseline, uncorrected QT interval is >600ms. An extrasystole at 660ms (long–short RR sequence) precipitates a wide QRS tachycardia at >200bpm with changing QRS polarity, as if there was 'torsion' of the QRS. The tachycardia is self terminating. Values are expressed in ms. Vertical lines mark 1-second intervals. Values expressed in milliseconds.

membrane voltage oscillations that can cause repetitive firing, the worst consequence of which is the polymorphic tachycardia known as 'torsade de pointes' that may appear in patients with very long QT intervals, particularly after long–short sequences of the RR intervals (➲Fig. 2.52).

The QT interval has a typical duration about 400ms at a rate of 60bpm, but it shortens as heart rate increases and lengthens if it decreases; therefore, QT measurements have to be corrected for heart rate in order to evaluate their real meaning. In 1920, Bazett [142] proposed dividing the QT interval by the square root of the RR interval expressed in seconds, that remains the standard for clinical use despite some limitations at fast or slow heart rates and in drug-induced QT prolongation [143, 144]. Other formulas used less commonly are Fridericia cube-root correction (QT interval divided by the cube root of RR interval) [145] and in the epidemiological setting, the Framingham linear regression equation [146].

Rate correction is not the only difficulty for the evaluation of QT intervals. The onset of the QT is easy enough to mark, at the onset of the QRS complex, however, the end of the T wave may be difficult to determine, as it merges smoothly with the baseline or even with a U wave. U waves are generally of low enough voltage not to pose a problem, but in some circumstances, such as hypokalaemia, ischaemia, or antiarrhythmic drug effects they may become prominent, merging with the end of the T wave, making very difficult to measure the QT interval with certainty (➲Fig. 2.53). Still another problem is the 'dispersion' (different values) of QT interval throughout the different ECG leads, which makes it uncertain in what lead it should be measured. It is recommended that QT interval be measured on a standard 12-lead ECG at 25mm/s paper speed and 10mm/mV amplitude. The mean of 3–5 cycles in leads II, V5, or V6 (the longest) should be taken [146]. Others suggest V3 and V4 [147].

Congenital long QT (also see ➲Chapter 9)

Congenital long QT interval can be due to a variety of mutations in the genes coding potassium or sodium membrane channel proteins that are discussed in detail in another chapter of this book. Configuration of the ST segment and T-wave ensemble can suggest a specific type of molecular abnormality, although with considerable overlap [148, 149]. Diagnosis may not be immediately obvious in some cases and a high degree of suspicion is necessary to diagnose this relatively uncommon, but potentially lethal problem (➲Fig. 2.54). QT changes may be accentuated by slow rates in some cases, but a lack of shortening during exercise or under catecholamine infusion may be the clue in others.

Congenital short QT (also see ➲Chapter 9)

Recent observations have shown a relationship between unexplained sudden death and a short QT interval in the ECG [150, 151]. There are no precise limits with an established predictive value, but QT is <360ms and typically ≤320ms. ST segment is practically absent in the precordial leads and T waves are symmetrical and peaked. Short QT is related to syncope, sudden death, and a higher incidence

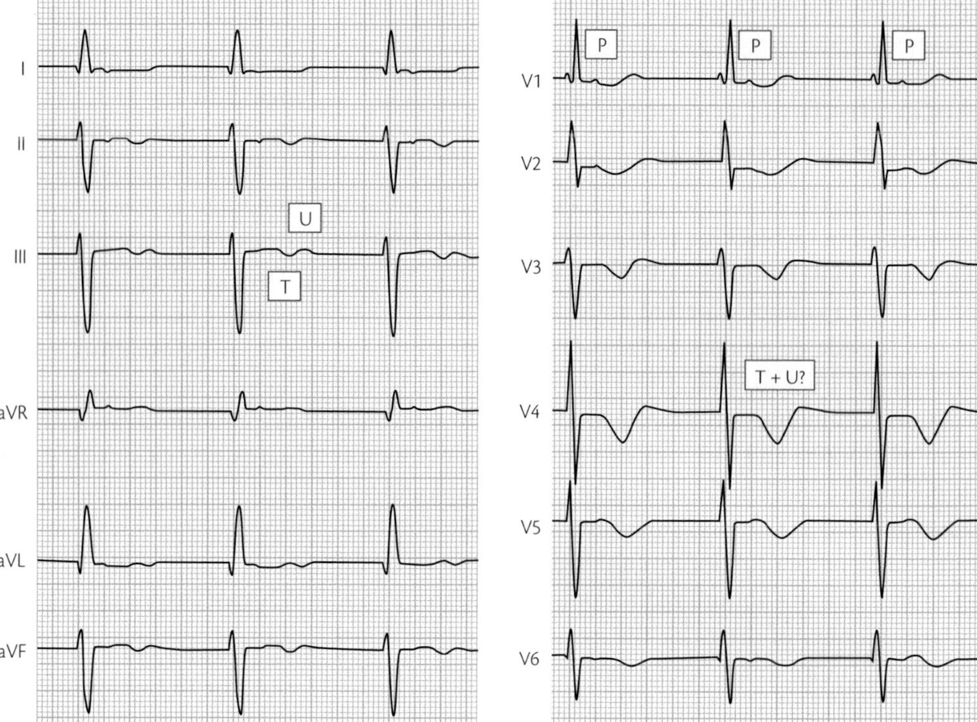

Figure 2.53 Difficult delimitation of the QT interval. There is a slow junctional rhythm, the P wave inscribed on the ST segment. The QRS shows incomplete RBBB and ASF block. The U wave is prominent in the limb leads. The apparent negative T wave in V2–V6 probably includes a U wave.

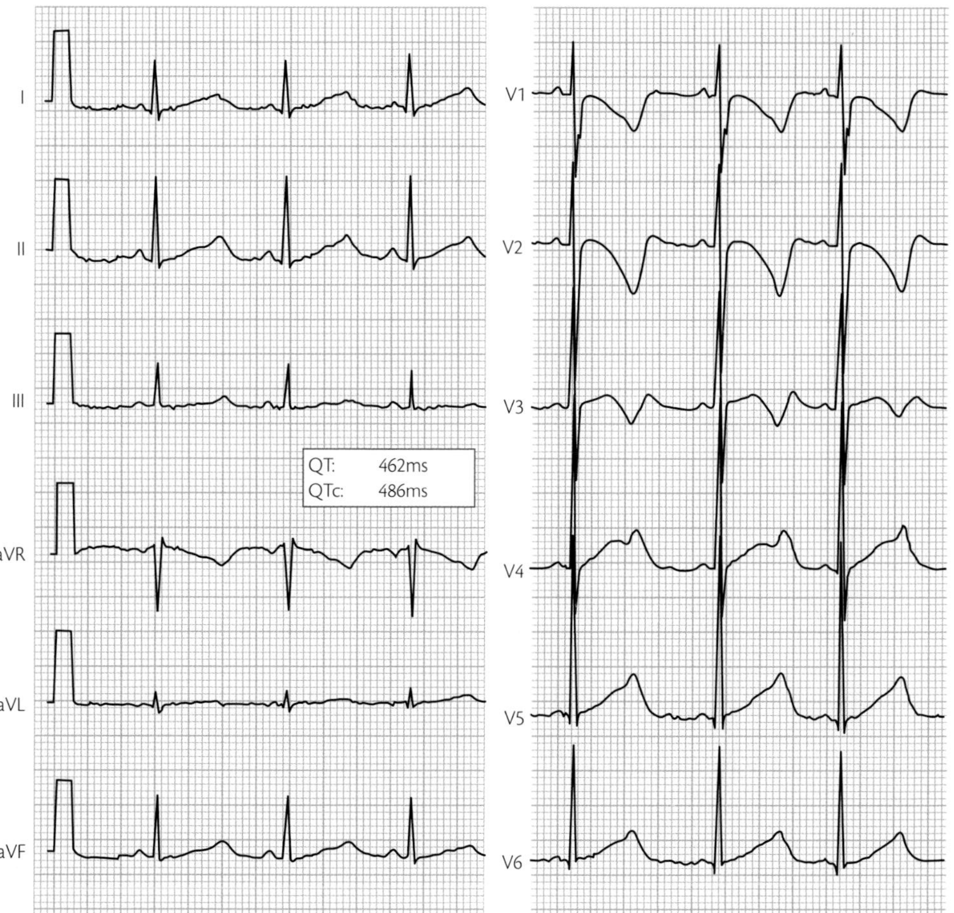

Figure 2.54 Congenital long QT syndrome (type 2). This was the asymptomatic 9-year-old son of a woman who had suffered cardiac arrest. Note the very long QT but also the double peaked T wave characteristic of this variant of the syndrome.

of atrial fibrillation. A genetic basis can be found in some cases [152].

Antiarrhythmic and other drugs (also see ➲Chapter 28)

Some antiarrhythmic drugs are designed to prolong repolarization by blocking potassium membrane channels, such as sotalol, ibutilide, dofetilide, or azimilide, and QT prolongation is to be expected at therapeutic doses, with a risk of torsade de pointes. Serial measurements of the QT interval are used to limit arrhythmogenesis, with a limit <500ms. Quinidine and procainamide are also potassium channel blockers and can prolong QT and produce torsade de pointes. Amiodarone blocks potassium channels and produces marked QT prolongation but torsade de pointes is rare with its administration, even at high doses, therefore QT measurements are not utilized to control amiodarone dose. A large number of drugs for the treatment of non-cardiac conditions (antibiotics, antihistamines, psychotropic) can produce QT prolongation and ventricular arrhythmias in a susceptible population [153, 154]. The problem is so widespread that there are continuously updated databases that can be accessed through the Internet (for examples see ➲Online resources, p.82). Serial ECGs should be obtained when using drugs with this side effect.

Digitalis shortens QT and produces characteristic repolarization changes with depression of the ST segment and decreased T-wave voltage or even T-wave inversion that can pose the differential diagnosis with ischaemia (➲Fig. 2.55).

Electrolyte disturbances

Changes in serum potassium concentration influence markedly the ECG [149]. Hypokalaemia tends to prolong the QT, flattens the T wave, and makes U waves prominent. Hyperkalaemia can produce peaked T waves when mild, but if severe, with potassium levels above 7mmol/L, sinus arrest, AV block, severe QRS widening, and VT may develop (➲Fig. 2.56). It is very important to recognize these changes because rapid treatment of hyperkalaemia can be life saving. Acidosis may accompany and mimic hyperkalaemia, while alkalosis does the same with hypokalaemia. Hypomagnesaemia is often associated with hypokalaemia in patients treated with diuretics or in special situations such as enteric fistula. Severe atrial and ventricular arrhythmias can occur in this situation, related to triggered activity.

Hypothermia

Hypothermia due to accidental exposure to low temperatures or to therapeutic intervention can result in marked prolongation of the PR interval and QT interval. QRS widening can occur with the appearance of a characteristic slow terminal QRS deflection known as an Osborn wave or J wave (➲ Fig. 2.57).

Brugada syndrome (also see ➲Chapter 9)

Brugada and Brugada [156] described an association of sudden death, in the absence of long QT or structural heart disease in patients with a peculiar ECG with a RBBB pattern

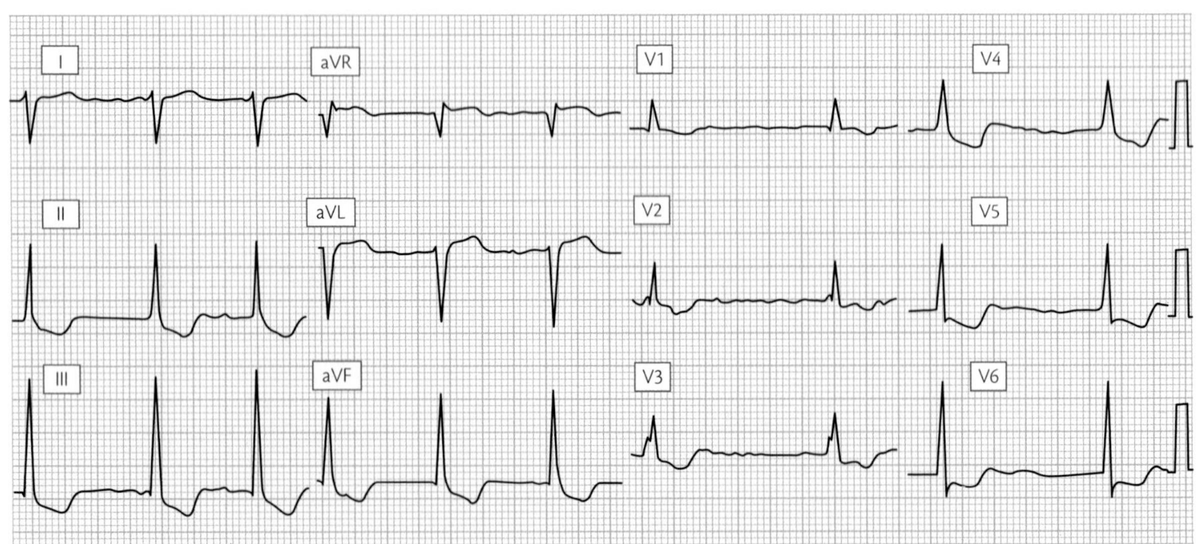

Figure 2.55 Typical coved ST depression due to digitalis effect at therapeutic doses. There are no regular P waves, but irregular oscillation of the baseline and irregular ventricular rate typical of atrial fibrillation The right axis deviation (≈+130°) and dominant R waves V1–V3 are due to RV enlargement. The patient had mitral stenosis with moderate pulmonary hypertension.

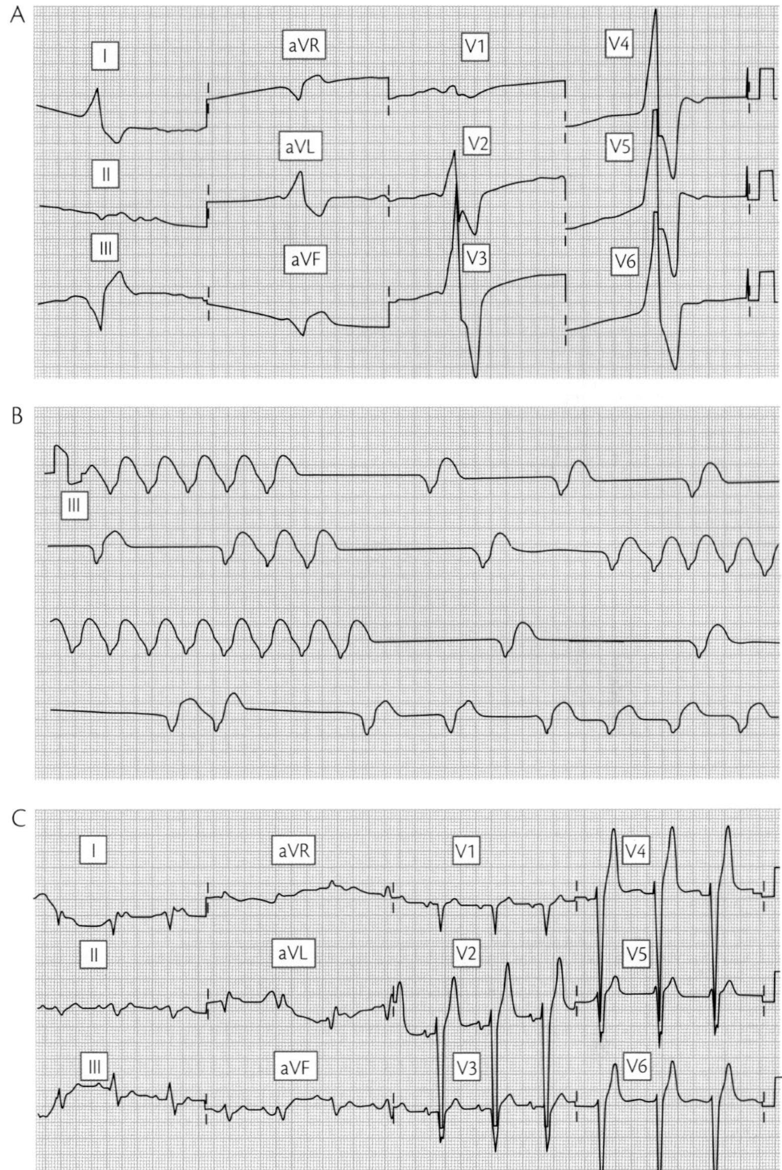

Figure 2.56 ECG changes in severe hyperkalemia (8mmol/L). A complete AV block with idioventricular rhythm at 27bpm. (B) Runs of ventricular tachycardia alternating with idioventricular rhythm. (C) After intravenous Ca^{2+} gluconate rhythm is sinus with normal PR interval, intraventricular conduction disturbance (QRS = 120ms) related to anterolateral wall scar (note QR complex in aVL, QS in V3, and Q in aVL).

and persistent ST elevation in leads V1–V2 (➲Fig. 2.58). In about one-quarter of the cases an abnormality in sodium channels is detected, but most cases are still unexplained [157]. The management of asymptomatic cases with the characteristic ECG changes is subject to debate, because the incidence of arrhythmias is very low; nevertheless, the diagnosis of Brugada syndrome is important even in this situation, in order to avoid antiarrhythmic drugs that could precipitate ventricular arrhythmias, and to perform special follow-up to detect an initial incidence of syncopal episodes or ventricular arrhythmias indicative of a potentially poor prognosis [158].

The typical Brugada ECG shows a very characteristic ST elevation with upward convexity, leading to a negative T wave in leads V1 and V2 (type 1 ECG; ➲Fig. 2.58). The pattern can be accentuated in some cases by recording these leads from the 3rd and 2nd intercostal spaces, instead of the standard 4th space level. In other cases, the ST shows an upward concavity, often difficult to differentiate from normal variants. The administration of intravenous class I antiarrhythmic drugs (ajmaline, flecainide) can convert the ECG from type II to type I, revealing the syndrome in symptomatic patients. AV conduction disturbances (prolonged PR and HV intervals) or atrial fibrillation can occur.

T-wave 'memory'

When LBBB is intermittent, return to normal QRS may be accompanied by persistent negative T waves for hours

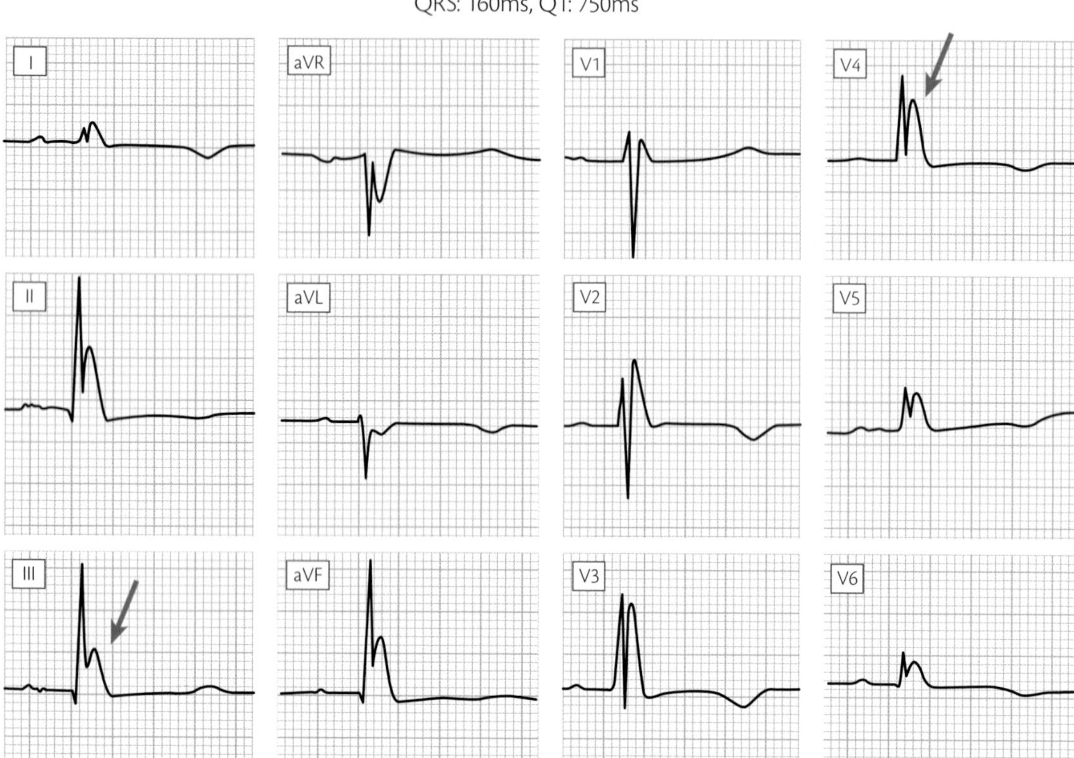

Figure 2.57 ECG changes in hypothermia after cold weather exposure in an alcoholic subject. Note PR prolongation to 260ms, QRS widening to 150ms with a very prominent J 'Osborn' wave (red arrows) and marked QT prolongation to 750ms.

or days, suggestive of ischaemia (➲Fig. 2.59) [159]. These changes can be due to persistence of the repolarization sequence changes secondary to abnormal activation and can be observed also after ventricular pacing [160] or WPW catheter ablation [161]. This electrical phenomenon is known as T-wave 'memory'.

Pericarditis and pericardial effusion

Pericardial disease can change the ECG by the inflammatory changes in the subepicardial layers of the myocardium and by the accumulation of fluid in the pericardial space. Arrhythmias are rare unless there is frank myocarditis [162].

Acute pericarditis (also see ➲Chapter 19)

Acute 'benign' pericarditis, manifested clinically by chest pain in many cases, produces ST elevation and T-wave inversion in the ECG that will often pose the differential diagnosis with acute coronary syndromes. The most typical manifestation of acute pericarditis is ST segment elevation but, in contrast with most acute coronary syndromes, where ST elevation is localized in some leads and there may be ST depression in other leads, in acute pericarditis ST elevation is present in most leads at the same time, with the exception of aVR that shows mirror-image ST depression [163] (➲Fig. 2.60). An interesting additional feature is PR segment depression in relation to the T-P interval, which is considered typical of pericarditis [164, 165]. The time course of ST elevation is also different from acute coronary syndromes, because ST elevation tends to persist for days, rather than hours. This diffuse ST elevation can be mimicked very closely by normal subjects with an early repolarization pattern, making it again necessary to obtain clinical information [166]. In doubtful cases, the time course of the ST shift will give the clue, as it will be stable in early repolarization but will tend to change in days in pericarditis. ST elevation can be followed by T-wave inversion similar to ischaemic T waves, and again the time course for this change is slow, evolving in days, and there are no QRS changes. T-wave inversion can sometimes persist for weeks or months [167].

Pericardial effusion (also see ➲Chapter 19)

Pericardial effusion decreases QRS voltage in all leads and if the effusion is large enough it may allow a swinging motion

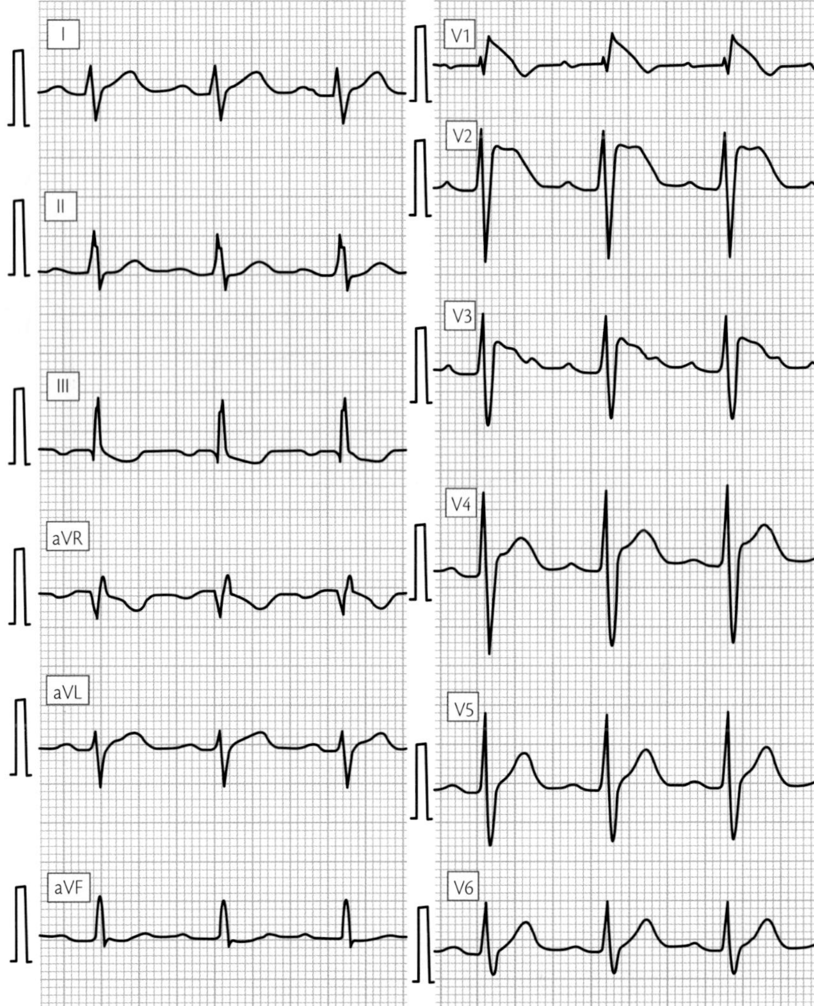

Figure 2.58 Typical Brugada syndrome ECG ('type 1'). Note r' and down sloping ST elevation in V1–V3. PR interval is borderline prolonged (220ms).

of the heart that changes QRS voltage in alternating beats [168] (➲Fig. 2.61). This phenomenon is called electrical alternans and has no relationship to paradoxical pulse. The largest pericardial effusions are not related to acute pericarditis, therefore low voltage and electrical alternans are not usually related to diffuse ST elevation as in acute pericarditis.

An approach to ECG reading

The non-initiated physician or student may feel frustrated by the ease with which an experienced cardiologist extracts information from an ECG, making it look like a magic process; however, the reality is that reading an ECG is a systematic process within the reach of every physician. Experience simply allows applying the method more rapidly.

Reading the ECG starts by checking the rhythm for the normal sequence of P waves, each followed by a QRS with a PR >110 and <220ms. If there are more P waves than QRS, or if QRS rate is >100bpm or <40bpm, P and QRS duration should be measured to ensure that there is no gross abnormality in atrial and ventricular conduction. If the QRS is >110ms the PR interval should be checked again to rule out pre-excitation. If there is AV block or a tachycardia, analysis of the ECG should be made in relation with the mechanism of the arrhythmia. If rate is very slow, P and QRS are wide and PR and QT are long, recording speed should be checked to be 25mm/s because a recording speed of 50mm/s can mimic all these changes in a normal subject.

When sinus rhythm and normal intervals are confirmed, detailed analysis can start by checking P-wave axis, then P-wave voltage in the inferior leads and duration and depth of a negative terminal deflection in V1. If P-wave duration is >100ms check for notching or a negative terminal deflection in II, III, or aVF, as indicators of atrial conduction disturbances or LA enlargement. If the P wave is negative in lead I and âQRS is shifted to the right (>+90°), this may be a case of dextrocardia, but more frequently the position of the arm electrodes may be inverted (aVR in the left arm, aVL

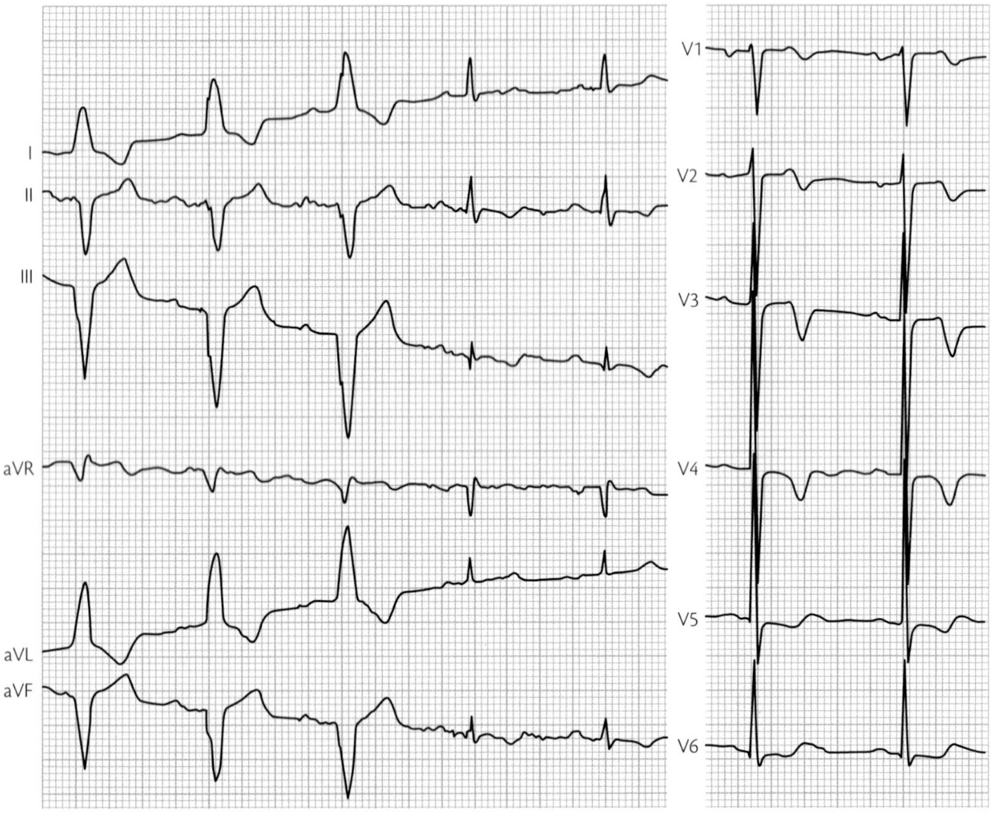

Figure 2.59 T-wave inversion due to T-wave 'memory' in a patient with intermittent LBBB. The limb leads show typical LBBB spontaneously changing to a normal QRS but with T-wave inversion in multiple arm and precordial leads.

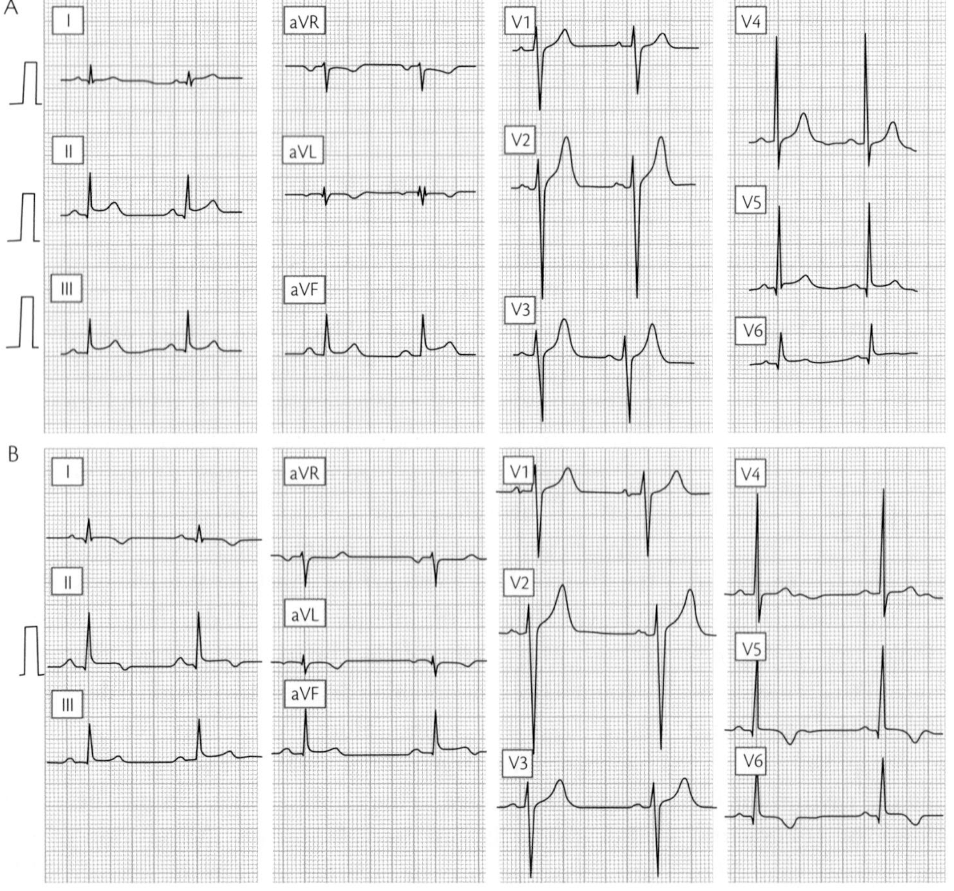

Figure 2.60 Evolving ST and T changes in acute pericarditis. (A) Shows an ECG recorded hours after the onset of symptoms with diffuse ST segment elevation; (B) shows the ECG 2 days later with persisting ST elevation but new T-wave inversion in multiple leads. There have been no QRS changes.

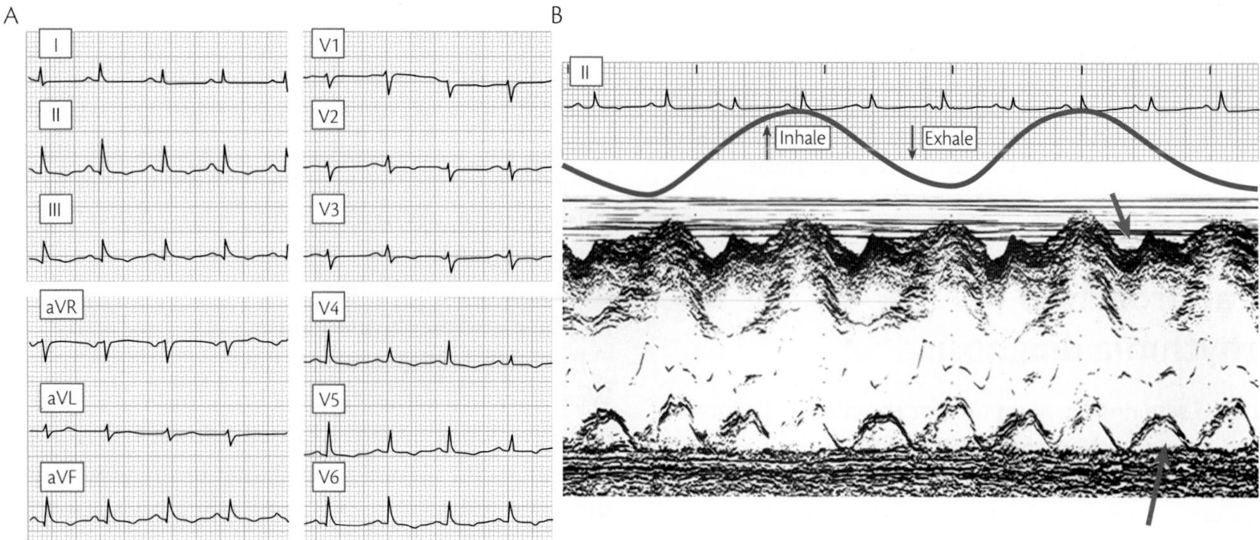

Figure 2.61 Electrical alternans in large pericardial effusion. (A) Shows the 12-lead ECG with marked low voltage with alternation of QRS amplitude; (B) shows the M mode echocardiogram and the ECG (lead II). Note the eco-free spaces anterior and posterior to the ventricles (red arrows). The green line marks respiration cycles. Note that QRS amplitude alternation is not related to respiration, but to position changes (swinging) of the heart in the pericardium. Note the absence of ST elevation. T wave is diffusely inverted.

in the right arm). Naturally, dextrocardia can be ruled out if the precordial leads show normal progression from rS to qR from V1 to V6, because in dextrocardia there will be low voltage rS complexes in the left precordial leads.

The next step may be plotting electrical position of the ventricles both in the frontal plane (limb leads) and the horizontal plane (precordial leads). The ÂQRS will give a general idea of normality or of deviations that can point toward chamber hypertrophy, conduction disturbances (fascicular blocks), infarction scars, or even chest anomalies, such as deformity, pneumothorax, or pleural effusion. Clinical information is essential, as discordance between âQRS and body build may raise an alert. On the precordial leads the normal position will show a transition from predominantly negative to predominantly positive QRS in V3 or V4. Rotations are designated as looked at from below the diaphragm, so that predominantly positive QRS in V1 or V2 is called counterclockwise rotation and predominantly negative complex in V5 or V6 is called clockwise rotation. Rotation may not be more than a position change, but it does call attention to possible problems, as mentioned earlier.

The detailed analysis of the QRS starts by confirming the presence of normal q waves in leads I, aVL, and V6 indicating normal septal activation. The lack of a 'septal q wave' is an abnormal finding that may be due to LBB conduction disturbances, LV hypertrophy, septal myocardial infarction, or pre-excitation. If Q waves are deep and wide myocardial infarction, pre-excitation (the PR segment will be double-checked) or cardiomyopathy may be present. QRS voltage in leads I, aVL, V1–V2, and V5–V6 will be measured to test for LV enlargement, keeping in mind that if the QRS is wide high voltage may be due to LBBB or pre-excitation. The presence of high R waves in V1–V2 will suggest RV hypertrophy or posterior infarction. However, if the QRS is ≥120ms they will be more likely due to RBBB or pre-excitation.

The final step will be checking repolarization. T-wave axis should be between 0–90°, and a clearly negative T wave in I or aVF it raises the possibility of ischaemia, ventricular hypertrophy with strain, BBB, pre-excitation, electrolyte imbalance, or drug effects. When T-wave axis is borderline, it is useful to check the angle between T and QRS axis which normally should be ≤60°. In the precordial leads, T waves are usually positive in V2–V6. However, negative T waves V1–V3 may not be abnormal, depending on the age, sex, race, and clinical situation of the patient, which again becomes essential to make an interpretation. A not uncommon cause of negative T waves in V1 and V2 is incorrect placement of the electrodes in the 2nd intercostal space instead of the 4th. This mistake can become important if one is looking at serial ECGs under suspicion of ischaemia. The ST segments should be examined for upward or downward deviation, be it diffuse or localized, and any deviation should be analysed together with other findings.

You should make a note of the findings at each one of these steps, because an unexpected finding is sometimes the clue to a diagnosis. This systematic look at the ECG is particularly important when a very prominent finding is obvious right away, such as a marked ST segment elevation suggestive of acute coronary syndrome. The elevation could be due to an idioventricular rhythm, or acute pulmonary embolus, or pericarditis, and axis deviation, low voltage, or lack of P waves would give away the real diagnosis.

An approach to arrhythmia diagnosis

The ECG remains the main tool for the clinical diagnosis of arrhythmias and the recording of an ECG during a symptomatic episode is often the critical step in the diagnosis, leading to effective treatment. It is essential that a full 12-lead ECG is obtained at this time, if the patient's situation permits. This emergency recording should be treasured and all measures should be taken to prevent its loss. Urgent analysis of the tracing may not yield all the information that an expert may be able to obtain with a more careful study. Arrhythmias are discussed in depth in different chapters of this book and here we will just give some general suggestions as to how to approach the diagnosis of an abnormal rhythm on the ECG.

Bradycardias

Sick sinus syndrome is often manifest episodically and after repeated Holter recordings an ECG during a symptomatic episode may give the clue to the diagnosis. It is important to have a good recording of the P waves in order to distinguish sinus pauses or sinus arrest from AV block as pacemaker indications vary significantly between them. Carotid sinus massage on the one hand and exercise on the other may help disclose the mechanism of the bradycardia.

It is important to recognize the limits of normal rhythm. We mentioned earlier that the limit for bradycardia often quoted as 50bpm has to be carried to lower values, always in the light of the clinical context, that include oscillations in sinus rate related to respiration (respiratory sinus arrhythmia) (➲Fig. 2.62A) or changes in P-wave axis due to variation in the point of exit of the impulse from the sinus node. The P wave can become negative in the inferior leads or even change from positive to negative along the recording (➲Fig. 2.62B).

Tachycardias

The tachycardia limit is generally set at 100bpm, but patients with increased sympathetic tone due to heart

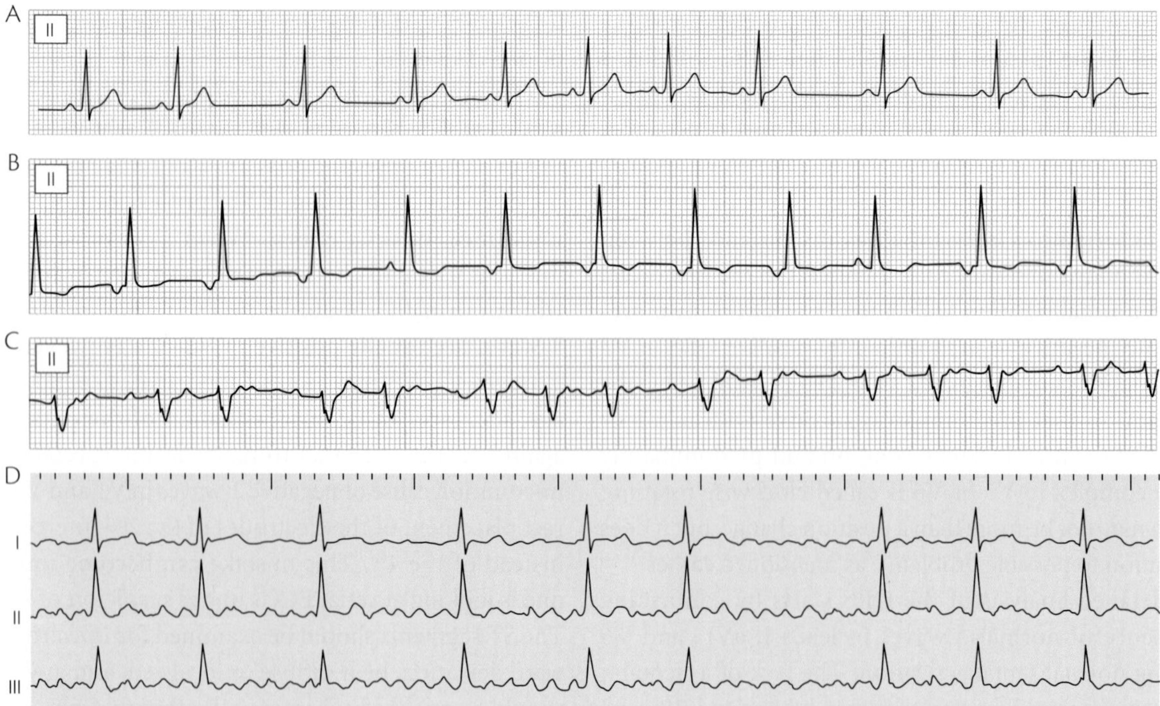

Figure 2.62 Sinus and supraventricular rhythms with narrow QRS. (A) Normal sinus respiratory arrhythmia. P wave does not change, but rate accelerates during inspiration. (B) Migratory atrial pacemaker. P wave turns from negative to positive with some intermediate configurations (5th P wave from the left). Rate is slightly faster when P wave is positive. (C) Atrial tachycardia at a rate of 140bpm with variable AV conduction causing an irregular ventricular rate. Note isoelectric intervals between P waves. Continuation of the tachycardia despite AV block confirms a localization of the tachycardia mechanism to the atria. (D) Atrial fibrillation; atrial waves are completely irregular with no stable baseline. Time marks on the top of tracing D are 0.1s and 1s.

failure, anaemia, fever, even nervousness, may have normal sinus rhythm above that level. Sinus tachycardia may pose the differential diagnosis with focal atrial tachycardia, which may slow rates, close to 100bpm. Changes in P-wave configuration relative to previous or subsequent recordings in sinus rhythm are helpful to confirm ectopic atrial tachycardia (➲Fig. 2.33).

A very simple separation in narrow (<120ms) QRS tachycardia versus wide (>120ms) QRS tachycardia will help avoid important mistakes in management. Most tachycardias with a narrow QRS have a supraventricular mechanism (➲Figs. 2.33, 2.47, 2.50, 2.62, and 2.63). On the other hand, practically all tachycardias with ventricular mechanisms will fit the broad QRS tachycardia group, with the only exception of some unusual VTs of septal origin, but in this case the QRS will still be different from the QRS in sinus rhythm. Wide QRS tachycardias will include some of supraventricular origin where ventricular activation is delayed by pre-existing or rate-dependent BBB, but it also includes all the more dangerous mechanisms, i.e. VT, pre-excited atrial tachycardia, flutter or fibrillation, and antidromic tachycardia in the WPW syndrome (➲Figs. 2.48, 2.49, and 2.51).

Narrow QRS tachycardias

The three main mechanisms of narrow QRS tachycardia are atrial, nodal, or accessory connection related.

Atrial tachycardia flutter and fibrillation

Atrial tachycardias will be clearly set apart when AV block occurs without tachycardia interruption (➲Figs. 2.33, 2.62C and 2.63). Atrial tachycardia or atrial flutter are classically separated by rate criteria (cut-off = 240–250bpm) but this simple classification will give no clue of the real mechanism (macro-re-entrant versus focal) in patients with structural heart disease, especially if there is a history of cardiac surgery. A typical saw-tooth pattern of the atrial waves is diagnostic of typical atrial flutter with a RA circuit (➲Fig. 2.63). It is very important to separate the regularity or irregularity of the atrial and ventricular rhythms because atrial tachycardia and flutter may result in an irregular ventricular rate on the bases of irregular conduction at the AVN (➲Figs. 2.33, 2.62C, and 2.63), and this should not be mistaken for the irregularity in atrial fibrillation, where the atrial waves are also irregular (➲Fig. 2.62D). Interventions directed at blocking the AVN often help make the diagnosis. In atrial tachycardia carotid

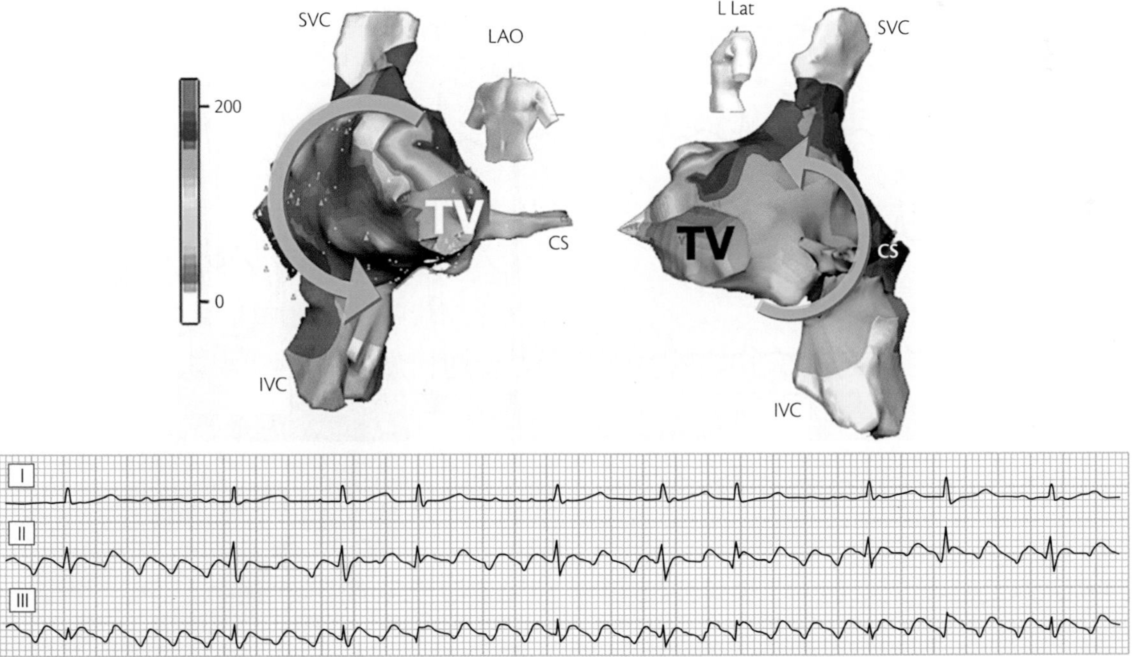

Figure 2.63 Activation sequence and ECG pattern of typical atrial flutter. Top, two views of the colour-coded activation sequence on a virtual anatomic cast of the RA constructed by means of computer-assisted navigation. Yellow arrows mark the direction of activation around the tricuspid valve (TV), descending the anterior wall and ascending the septal wall (white is earliest, following red, yellow, green, and blue, then meeting white again on the superior RA wall. This up–down sequence is reflected by the wide positive–negative deflections in the inferior leads II and III, a characteristic appearance of typical (common) atrial flutter. Note the irregular ventricular rate in the face of perfectly regular atrial deflections.

sinus massage or adenosine may produce AV block and reveal the underlying atrial tachycardia mechanism.

Nodal and orthodromic tachycardias

Intranodal re-entry and AV orthodromic tachycardia using an accessory pathway produce an ECG with regular tachycardia and normal QRS complex, unless functional, rate-dependent BBB develops (➲Figs. 2.47, 2.50, and 2.64). The P wave is generally hard to distinguish during the tachycardia. In nodal tachycardia, the P wave is inscribed simultaneously with the QRS and can be identified sometimes as an apparent r′ wave in V1 [126, 127] (➲Fig. 2.64). In the usual form of orthodromic tachycardia, the P wave occurs over the ST segment and can be difficult to distinguish from the onset of the T wave (➲ Fig. 2.47). In atypical cases of either mechanism with a long interval between the QRS and the following P wave (Rp >PR), the P wave can be well identified [169, 170] (➲Fig. 2.50). Carotid sinus massage or adenosine administration interrupts AV nodal and orthodromic tachycardia, because conduction through the AVN is an essential part of the mechanism.

Wide QRS complex tachycardias

The ECG with a broad QRS tachycardia poses a difficult diagnostic problem, including the possibility of an imminent cardiac arrest if the rhythm is VT and it degenerates into ventricular fibrillation. The clinical context here may be misleading because VT can be rather well tolerated, even in the presence of structural heart disease, and many a VT has been diagnosed as SVT because the patient was conscious and the systolic blood pressure was measurable in a range of 90–110mmHg. SVT can show a wide QRS when there is rate-dependent BBB, but also when there is AV conduction via an accessory pathway and the administration of intravenous digitalis or verapamil (even amiodarone) in patients with a pre-excited atrial flutter or fibrillation or with VT can be disastrous.

Pre-excited tachycardias in patients with WPW syndrome were described earlier (see ➲Pre-excitation, p.56). Previous knowledge of the baseline ECG, including the diagnosis of pre-excitation is of great help. A QRS pattern of typical BBB can be suggestive of SVT with aberrant conduction; however, such a pattern can be present in VT due to BB re-entry and in pre-excited tachycardias due to slow conducting accessory connections. A previous history of myocardial infarction or cardiomyopathy should make the diagnosis of VT most probable.

Interventions directed at slowing or blocking conduction through the AV node, such as vagal manoeuvres can be of help if ventricular rate is slowed or the tachycardia is interrupted, but they may not be effective in an acute situation. The intravenous injection of adenosine or adenosine triphosphate (ATP) is a more powerful intervention and the lack of effect on the tachycardia would support a ventricular origin

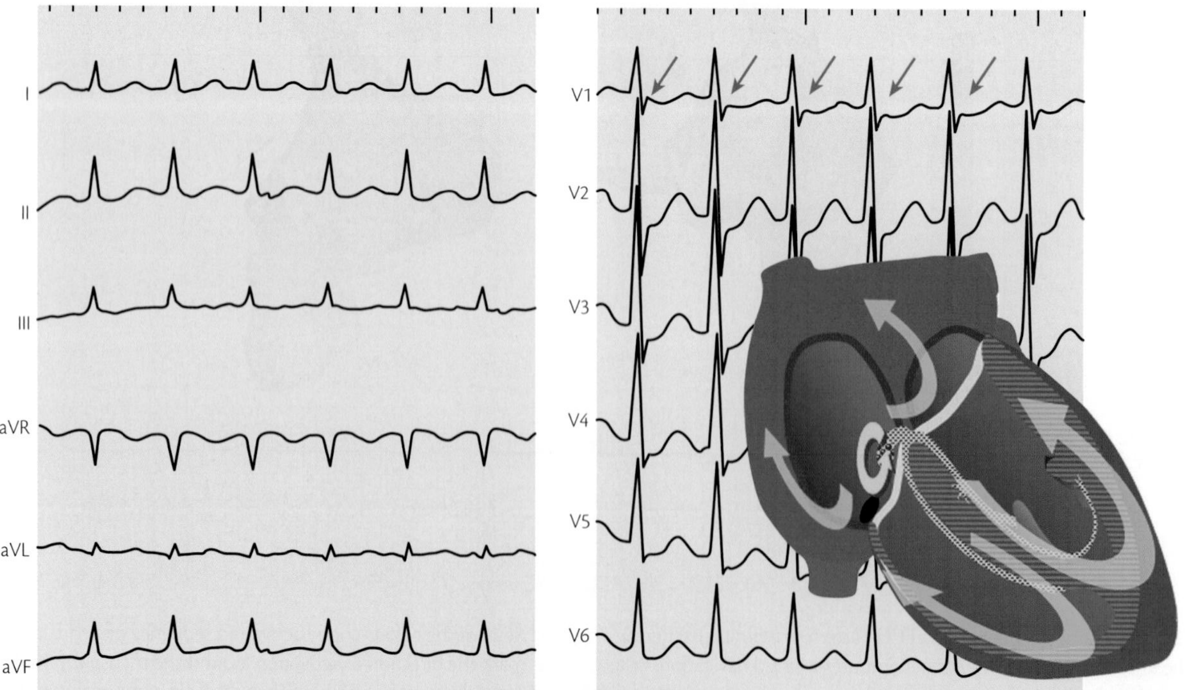

Figure 2.64 Intranodal re-entrant tachycardia. The re-entry circuit is localized in the immediate vicinity of the AVN (yellow circular arrow). Ventricular activation is normal, making a narrow QRS. Atrial activation is reversed. The P wave can be seen as an apparent r′ in V1 (red arrows). Time marks (top) are 0.1s and 1s.

or pre-excited atrial tachycardia or flutter. Cardioversion may be needed to solve the clinical problem, but in this case the tachycardia should be thoroughly documented in a full 12-lead ECG to be able to compare later with the baseline tracings and reach a diagnosis in retrospect.

Ventricular tachycardia

In sustained monomorphic VT the mechanism can be focal or macro-re-entrant but in both cases activation starts in some point of the ventricular myocardium. Activation spreads slowly because it does not follow the normal activation path and the QRS becomes wide and aberrant. The mechanism of VT is totally independent of the atria and the tachycardia can continue in the presence of VA dissociation. The ECG of VT is characterized by a wide, aberrant QRS complex and an atrial rate dissociated from ventricular rate (➲Fig. 2.65). In some cases, VA conduction can be 1:1 and the diagnosis will depend on the QRS morphology, especially comparing with QRS morphology in sinus rhythm. Ventricular rate is usually perfectly regular; however, VA dissociation may allow occasional AV conduction of a sinus impulse through the AVN–HB axis, producing 'fusion' of activation from the VT and the sinus impulse. These fusion beats are advanced with respect to the VT rate and are narrower (➲Fig. 2.65).

A QRS width ≥140ms, a RBBB morphology with âQRS between −30° and −180°, an Rr complex in V1 (double peaked R wave with a larger first peak), a LBBB morphology with a Q wave in V6, an RS complex in V1 with an interval between the R peak and the S trough ≥100ms, or the presence of 'concordant' QRS complexes (all positive or all negative) V1–V6, or the lack of RS complexes V1–V6 have been proposed criteria, among others. Unfortunately, the sensitivity and specificity are low, especially when the baseline ECG is not known [171, 172]. In VT where activation starts in the interventricular septum, the QRS complex can be relatively narrow because the activation system is activated early, thus shortening ventricular activation time.

Short bursts of VT from 3 cycles to several seconds' duration are a common manifestation of severe myocardial involvement in heart disease, but in some cases they manifest focal activity in normal hearts. Non-sustained VT is often irregular, especially at the onset and before termination. Some VTs are precipitated by exercise and require

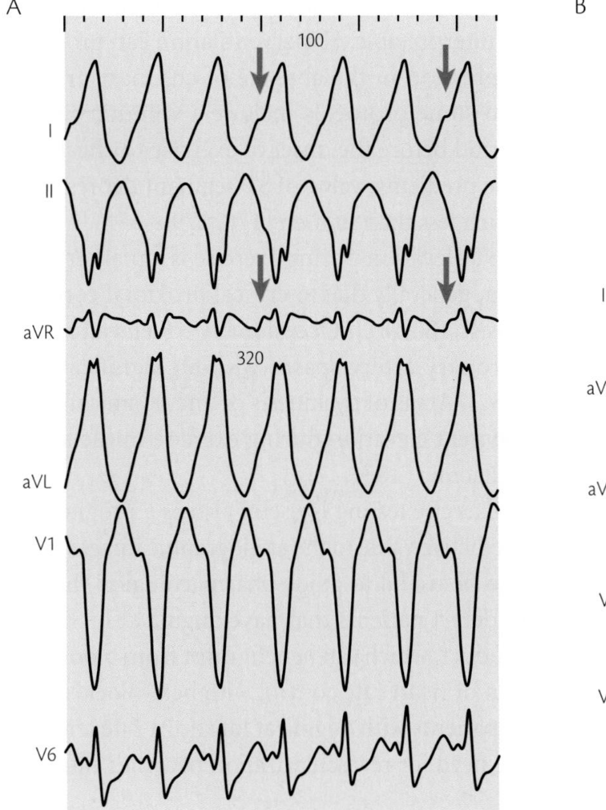

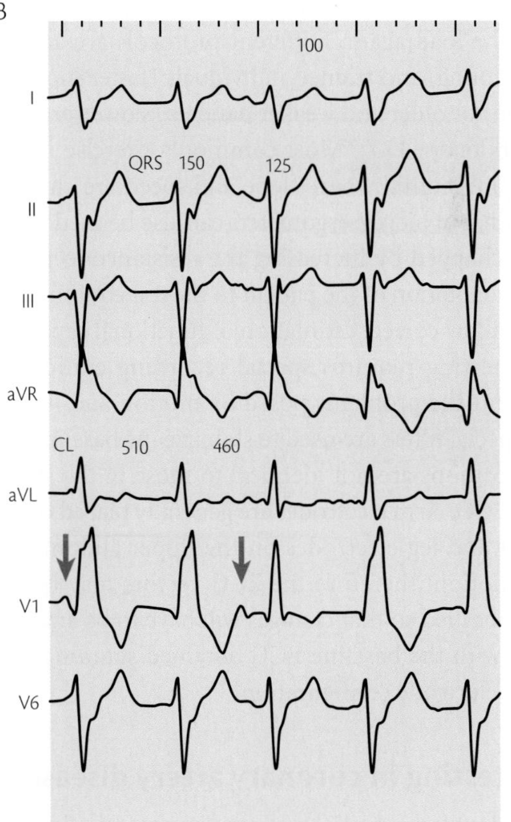

Figure 2.65 Different ECG manifestations of VT. (A) Post-infarction VT with 3:1 VA conduction. The deflection pointed by the red arrow marks P waves at a rate 1/3 the ventricular rate. (B) Idiopathic 'fascicular' VT with AV dissociation and sinus captures producing fusion beats. Red arrows mark P waves independent of TV rate. The third QRS complex is narrower and advanced because the P wave has conducted through the AVN–HB axis, capturing part of the ventricles (fusion beat). Time marks (top) are 100ms and 500ms.

a stress test. Polymorphic tachycardias in the context of the long QT interval or ischaemia have been described in the corresponding sections of this chapter.

Stress ECG

Stress ECG was devised in the 1960s to improve the diagnostic sensitivity of the resting ECG in patients with coronary artery disease by reproducing the circumstances that most often cause angina (see ➲Chapter 25). Exercise increases sympathetic tone and decreases parasympathetic tone, increasing heart rate and blood pressure, the main determinants of myocardial oxygen consumption (MVO_2). Exercise can also precipitate arrhythmias or AV block and exercise testing has become a very useful tool in the evaluation of patients with chest pain, dyspnoea, or syncope precipitated by exertion. In patients with severe heart disease, such as aortic stenosis, or with unstable angina, exercise testing should be avoided or, if considered essential for diagnosis, it should be performed with special precautions.

Exercise is performed according to progressive protocols that allow a warm-up period and progressively increase exercise load allowing a 2–3min stabilization period before increasing the load again. Different protocols are applied for strong, young, and trained individuals (faster increases in work load) or older and weaker patients (slower progression of workload) [173]. Most commonly exercise is performed on a treadmill where slope and speed are changed every 2–3min, but bicycle ergometers can also be used where the load is changed by increasing the resistance to pedalling. Good adaptation of the patient to the test equipment is essential to allow correct estimation of functional capacity.

Exercise testing requires special recording equipment to circumvent the problems posed by motion and muscle artefacts. Special filters are used to stabilize the baseline and electrode positions are not identical to those in the standard resting ECG. Arm electrodes are generally placed on the upper chest and leg electrodes on the upper abdomen to minimize motion, therefore the ECG vectors may be significantly modified so that changes will have to be analysed comparing with the baseline ECG obtained standing with the exercise electrode configuration.

Exercise testing in coronary artery disease

The simple 'double product' (heart rate (bpm) × systolic blood pressure) is linearly related to MVO_2, allowing estimation of coronary artery flow reserve [174, 175]. Besides increasing oxygen demand, exercise produces distal vasodilatation in areas irrigated by both normal and stenotic arteries producing a 'steal' phenomenon that shifts collateral flow supplying the compromised territories at rest to the normally irrigated areas, now in demand during exercise. Exercise testing thus allows a controlled reproduction of the mechanism of myocardial ischaemia and an estimation of coronary flow reserve.

The most reliable sign of ischaemia is ST segment depression with a horizontal (flat) configuration from the end of the QRS (J point) to the onset of the T wave (➲Fig. 2.66). T wave may also become inverted, but isolated T-wave inversion is not a reliable sign of ischaemia. To increase specificity a cut-off point of –1.5mm (–0.15mV) is generally required. Even ST depression may have a low predictive value in women or in subjects with baseline ST segment depression due to drugs (digitalis) or LV overload (hypertension). Obtaining multiple ECG leads does not help localize the ischaemic area according to ST depression [176].

Ischaemic ST depression should be differentiated from the rapidly up-sloping depression occurring in normal subjects at high heart rates, that becomes isoelectric in <80ms [177] (➲Fig. 2.66). This normal J-point depression is attributed to an atrial repolarization (Ta) wave. In the presence of ST and T changes secondary to hypertrophy, BBB or pre-excitation ST changes during exercise become uninterpretable. Hyperventilation can produce ST segment depression in the absence of coronary artery disease [59] and some protocols include a voluntary hyperventilation period before the onset of exercise to check this possibility. The predictive value of ST segment depression in women is much less than in men [178, 179].

ST elevation during exercise is a marker of severe ischaemia, generally due to critical proximal coronary artery stenosis [180,181]. Occasionally ST elevation may be due to coronary artery spasm without significant fixed stenosis [182]. Areas of dyskinesis or aneurysm can also produce ST segment elevation during exercise in the absence of severe ischaemia [183].

Exercise testing is useful also as a prognostic tool, adding predictive value to the angiographic images [184, 185]. It can also be useful to guide pharmacological therapy by helping to detect patients that have angina at high levels of double product, which can benefit most from blood pressure reduction or heart rate control with beta-blockers or other drugs. In patients with angina at low heart rate and blood pressure, the need for revascularization becomes equally obvious.

Stress ECG in other cardiac conditions

The changes in autonomic tone provoked by exercise can have a significant influence in heart rhythm, as discussed

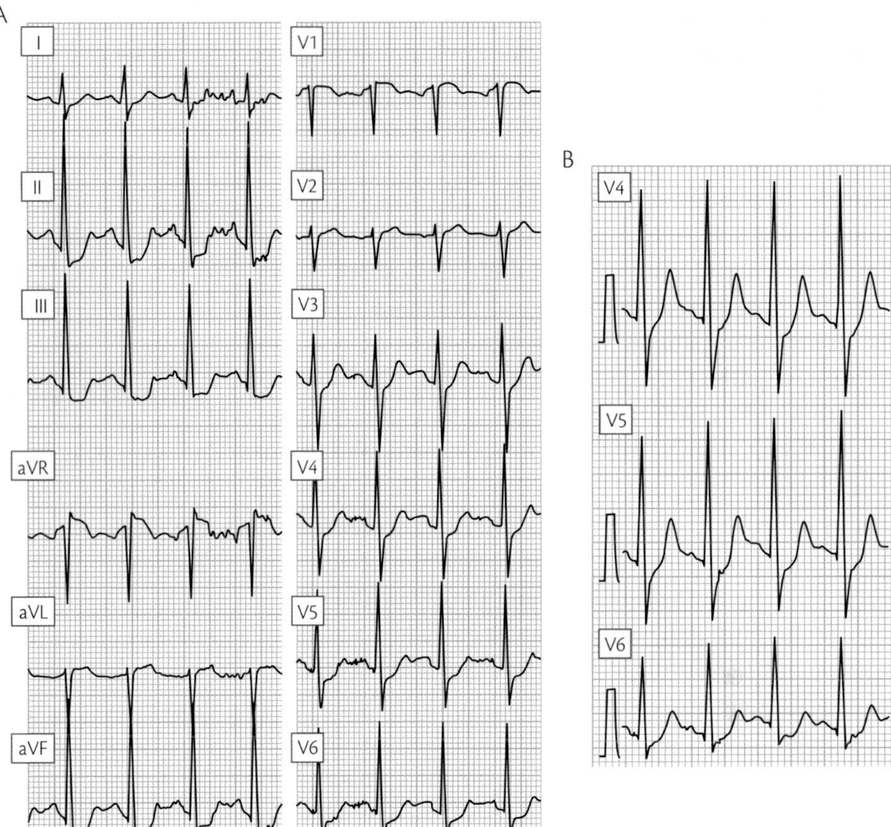

Figure 2.66 (A) Ischaemic response to exercise. Note the flat ST segment depression in II, III, and aVF and slightly up-sloping depressed ST in V5–V6 that remains depressed at 80ms from the J point. (B) Normal ST segment depression in V5–V6 due to Ta wave. Note that ST segment is isoelectric 80ms after the J point.

earlier. Nodal AV block can improve or disappear during exertion, while AV block at the His bundle or bundle branches (trifascicular) can be precipitated by exercise, thus explaining symptoms such as dyspnoea or syncope during exercise (➲Fig. 2.34). Atrial and ventricular arrhythmias due to focal discharge and some re-entrant tachycardias due to accessory pathways (Coumel's incessant tachycardia; ➲Fig. 2.50) can also be precipitated by exercise, allowing the diagnosis leading to effective treatment. In patients with persistent atrial fibrillation the exercise test can help to adjust ventricular rate control during effort. In patients with WPW syndrome, exercise testing has been used to estimate the refractory period of the accessory connection, in an effort to evaluate the risk of rapid AV conduction in the event of atrial fibrillation, but the predictive value is less than optimal and this indication has practically disappeared in the era of catheter ablation.

Ambulatory ECG monitoring

The development of small tape recorders in the 1970s and 1980s made recording the ECG during prolonged periods of time possible, including normal activity. As in exercise testing, special electrode settings and signal filtering are necessary. A limited number of electrodes facilitates patients' acceptance and ability to perform normal activities. The recordings are analyzed off-line with automated detection algorithms that facilitate the review of large amount of data. Despite some limitations due to the appearance of motion artefacts, electrode disconnection and occasional difficulty to identify P waves, Holter monitoring (named after its inventor, Dr. Norman J. Holter) has become an essential tool in cardiology to study ECG changes occurring during activity. The main application is in the study of syncope or palpitations, but it can also reveal ischaemia in the form of ST segment displacement, either in the presence or in the absence of symptoms [186].

Holter recordings have been essential to improve our understanding of the normal limits of heart rhythm and rate. We know, thanks to Holter recordings, that resting sinus rate can go down to 30–35bpm during rest or sleep in some normal subjects, especially in those of young age or with athletic training, simply on the bases of high vagal tone. Vagal tone can also be responsible for the appearance of second-degree Wenckebach block during sleep in athletes and also in elderly people without heart disease or functional limitation.

In patients with documented paroxysmal sustained arrhythmias that are candidates for antiarrhythmic drugs, the 24-hour Holter ECG will reveal the underlying sinus rhythm, alerting about possible underlying bradycardia or AV conduction disturbance. In patients with episodes of atrial fibrillation or flutter, Holter ECG may reveal frequent atrial ectopy as a possible underlying mechanism. In the absence of symptoms, Holter ECG can be used to detect non-sustained ventricular arrhythmias as a prognostic indicator in patients with coronary artery disease and cardiomyopathies. In patients with congenital long QT syndrome, the changes in autonomic tone and heart rate throughout day and night help to appreciate the extremes and circumstances of QT prolongation. Heart rate variability can also be measured in Holter ECG recordings, as a prognostic sign. When arrhythmic episodes occur during the recording the sympathetic and parasympathetic tone before and during the episode can be evaluated.

Holter ECG recordings have some limitations at the time of documenting QRS morphology during arrhythmias. Some new devices can record multiple leads and compose a '12-lead ECG' that mimics the standard ECG, but the number of electrodes to paste on the patient is large and inconvenient and, as with the exercise test, some differences in lead direction remain. Another limitation is the duration of the recording, which makes it difficult to document most paroxysmal arrhythmias which have less than a daily incidence. For the evaluation of asymptomatic atrial fibrillation it has been shown that continuous 7-day recordings improve the yield over 1-day recordings, but still do not reveal the full incidence.

Implantable loop recorder

Implantable ECG recorders with a loop-type memory are capable of recording and storing one ECG lead for minutes before and after an event detected either clinically or by automatic detection algorithms. The duration of battery life has been extended up to 3 years in recent devices, allowing extended monitoring periods. The device is a few millimetres thick and about 5cm long and can be implanted subcutaneously on the area of the precordium that shows the best P and QRS deflections, with no intracardiac leads. Bradycardia- and tachycardia-related causes of syncope can be revealed in most cases after a few weeks or months of monitoring [187] (➲ Fig. 2.67). The recording of a single lead poses obvious limitations, including transient loss of adequate voltage, poor recognition of the P waves, and lack of precise information on QRS morphology. However, QRS duration can be estimated in most cases, helping to separate narrow QRS from wide QRS tachycardias. Difficult identification of P waves makes recognition of atrial fibrillation episodes even more difficult, and these may have to be diagnosed through changes in QRS rate and regularity. Despite these limitations the implantable loop recorder is the present-day gold standard for the diagnosis of syncope in patients with and without structural heart disease.

Computer analysis of the ECG

A number of computer-assisted techniques have been applied to the ECG in order to expand its applications in the clinical field. Efforts have been directed at the detection of arrhythmogenic substrates and modulators through analysis of high-gain recordings of the QRS to detect abnormal, delayed activation, RR interval variability as a marker of autonomic tone, and micro T-wave voltage alternation as a sign of repolarization instability. These techniques have offered valuable new insights in the mechanisms of arrhythmias and can help to define a high-risk patient population. However, clinical applicability remains in question, due to the low positive predictive value for arrhythmic events [188].

Signal-averaged ECG

The limitations of the ECG to record low-voltage intracardiac activity can be circumvented by the signal-averaged (SA) ECG, a special recording technique that allows elimination of background noise in very high-amplification recordings. The more commonly used time-domain technique utilizes a very high amplification gain (× 10–100), digital high-frequency sampling (1000–10000Hz), and high pass filtering (25–100Hz, commonly 40Hz). In order to improve signal-to-noise ratio, hundreds of QRS complexes are averaged. Orthogonal leads X, Y, and Z are integrated into a single QRS (filtered and averaged) vector magnitude [189].

Low-voltage deflections preceding or following the high-voltage QRS can be evaluated in the 'time domain' analysis. Early on the technique was used to record the HB potential non-invasively [190]. However, this was soon abandoned and interest turned to the detection of abnormal low-voltage potentials following the QRS that were related to late activation of diseased myocardium with arrhythmogenic potential after myocardial infarction [191, 192]. The detection of late potentials by SAECG and total filtered-averaged QRS duration were found to predict arrhythmic events and total mortality after myocardial infarction and, although it

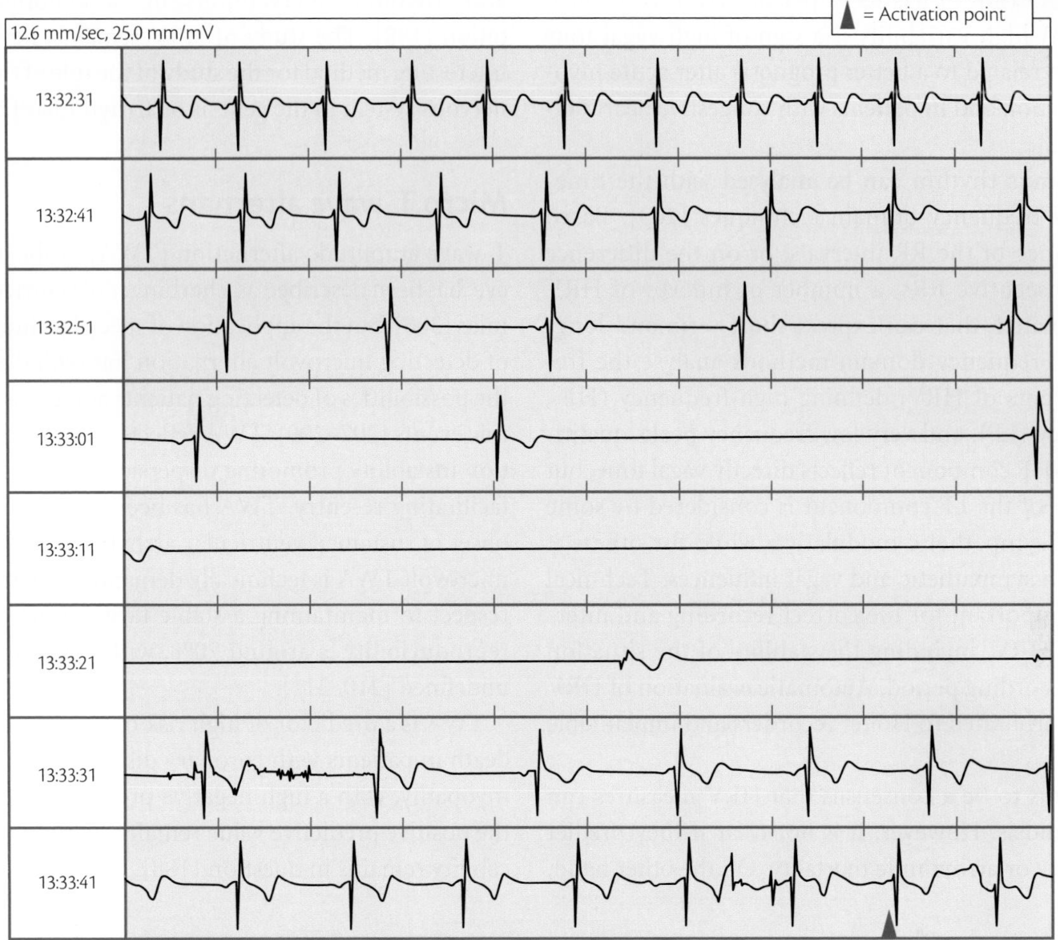

Figure 2.67 Recording of the mechanism of a syncopal episode retrieved by telemetry from an implanted loop recorder. A continuous recording of a single lead is displayed. Time is recorded on the left column. QRS and P waves are clearly identified. At 20s into the recording, sinus pauses start to appear, leading to a maximum 15-s cardiac standstill interrupted by an escape beat. Sinus rhythm recovers after 30s. Time marks are 1s.

showed a high negative predictive value, the positive predictive value was low. Late potentials were most closely related to the inducibility of VT, but were less commonly detected in patients resuscitated from sudden death [193]. The widespread application of pharmacologic and interventional reperfusion strategies in acute coronary syndromes has decreased the incidence and has lowered even further their utility as a prognostic indicator [194, 195].

The prognostic value of SAECG in dilated cardiomyopathy appears to be even less than in coronary artery disease [196]. SAECG can be used to detect RVs cardiomyopathy [197] and it has been related to the incidence of arrhythmias in Brugada syndrome [198].

More recently, the SAECG has been applied to the exploration of the arrhythmogenic substrate in patients with atrial fibrillation. The application of SAECG to the P wave needs a special technique to trigger the averaging on the P wave and at the same time discard P waves of different morphologies due to sinus node pacemaker migration or ectopic atrial activation. P-wave duration measured by SAECG has been related to atrial fibrillation recurrence [199]. Some data suggest that late low-voltage atrial potentials could represent arrhythmogenic substrates in the pulmonary veins [200].

Heart rate variability

The importance of the autonomic nervous system in the genesis of arrhythmias is well known, although not completely understood. Research in the 1980s showed that patients with acute myocardial infarction could suffer a decrease in baroreflex sensitivity that was related to a poor prognosis. Interest in autonomic activity led to its evaluation through the variations in sinus node rate induced mainly by vagal reflexes, including respiratory sinus arrhythmia. It is important to realize that vagal and sympathetic tone are quite variable from rest to exercise and a number of other factors can change them, therefore measurement of heart rate variability (HRV) has to be performed in controlled conditions. A high variability is a sign of high vagal tone and has been related to a better prognosis after acute myocardial infarction and in patients with congestive heart failure [201, 202].

HRV in sinus rhythm can be analysed with the time-domain and frequency-domain techniques [203]. Based on the variance of the RR intervals, or on the difference between consecutive RRs, a number of indexes of HRV can be calculated, that can express short-term and long-term HRV. Frequency-domain methods analyse the frequency contents of HRV, defining high frequency (HF), low frequency (LF), and very low frequency peaks quantitatively. The HF component reflects directly vagal tone, but the meaning of the LF component is considered by some a marker of sympathetic modulation while for others it includes both sympathetic and vagal influences. Technical aspects are important for the correct recording and interpretation of HRV, including the stability of the situation during the recording period. Automatic evaluation of HRV has been incorporated to Holter recorders and implantable devices.

There seems to be a consensus that HRV measures can predict prognosis. However, it is not clear if they predict total mortality or arrhythmic mortality. On the other hand, the positive predictive power for events is too low to orient antiarrhythmic interventions such as defibrillator implantation [188]. The study of HRV remains, nevertheless, an interesting method for the study of the role of the autonomic nervous system in the genesis of arrhythmias [204, 205].

Micro T-wave alternans

T-wave amplitude alternation (TWA) visible to the naked eye, has been described as a harbinger of ventricular arrhythmias [206], but the application of special techniques capable of detecting microvolt alternation has rekindled interest in the possibilities of detecting patients at high risk of arrhythmic events [207–209]. TWA reflects rate-related repolarization instability promoting dispersion of repolarization and facilitating re-entry. TWA has been shown to precede the onset of sustained ventricular arrhythmias. The analysis of microvolt TWA is technically demanding, particularly with respect to maintaining a stable target heart rate, and the reproducibility is around 70%, with many tests remained undefined [210, 211].

TWA is a predictor of high risk of arrhythmic events and death in patients with coronary disease and dilated cardiomyopathy, with a high negative predictive value; however, the positive predictive value remains low and clinical applicability remains in question [188].

Personal perspective

The ECG is not getting old. It is now a small part of the diagnostic means available to the cardiologist, and we rely more on imaging and biochemical markers to support many diagnoses. However, the ECG remains irreplaceable for the first-line diagnosis of ischaemic, electrical, and metabolic processes involving the heart, as well as a timing and monitoring tool. Nothing can reveal changes in ischaemia or rhythm so instantly and nothing can guide therapy or acute conditions at the bedside so effectively and efficiently.

In the 1960s, too much was demanded of the ECG, as little else was available at the bedside to the cardiologist. Today, many more diagnostic means are available and this, rather than making the ECG obsolete, has consolidated its value. No sound clinical decision can be made in cardiology without a look at the ECG. ECG changes are better interpreted when viewed with all the other new diagnostic information. Also serum markers and imaging are better focused by looking at the ECG. In fact, the ECG is a necessary tool for all internists, general practitioners, and emergency specialists. Unfortunately, the ECG seems arcane to those used to quick decisions made on visible images. The ECG demands deductive power, and this is frustrating to many a busy physician.

Chronic monitoring will be a very important field in the near future. Implantable devices (pacemakers and defibrillators) have already shown the importance of recording events in digital memory banks for patients with ventricular arrhythmias. As the challenge has turned to atrial arrhythmias, long-term monitoring has become a necessary step to understand the real depths of the problem. New implantable or non-implantable devices will be necessary and they will introduce significant changes in our data base and our therapeutic strategies. The ECG will be at the core of it again.

An essential role of individual cardiologists and cardiological societies in regard to the ECG is to maintain a constant teaching line to make the non-cardiologists feel comfortable with the ECG. Recordings could be made easier, eliminating cumbersome cables by using telemetry transmission. Some bright mind could devise an easy way to place the electrodes accurately in a minimum of time. Computer analysis could be improved to facilitate analysis of arrhythmias. Hospitals should offer on-line interpretation services by cardiologists to assist emergency teams working out of hospital. But still we should make a strong effort to help all physicians feel comfortable with ECG interpretation, and conscious of the irreplaceable value that ECG recording makes in the acute situation. We should be able to make the essentials clear and understandable, intuitive, and easy to learn and use. The real challenge is to ensure that ECG reading is stimulating and fun. We have tried here to take some steps in that direction. Much more will have to be done.

Further reading

Anderson JL, Adams CD, Antman EM, et al. ACC/AHA guidelines for the management of patients with unstable angina/non-ST-segment elevation myocardial infarction. *J Am Coll Cardiol* 2007; **50**: e1–e157.

Antman EM, Hand M, Armstrong PW, *et al.* Focused update of the ACC/AHA 2004 guidelines for the management of patients with ST-elevation myocardial infarction. *J Am Coll Cardiol* 2008; **51**: 210–47.

Blomström-Lundqvist C, Scheinman MM, Aliot EM, *et al.* ACC/AHA/ESC guidelines for the management of patients with supraventricular arrhythmias—executive summary: A report of the American College of Cardiology/American Heart Association Task Force on Practice Guidelines and the European Society of Cardiology Committee for Practice Guidelines (Writing Committee to Develop Guidelines for the Management of Patients With Supraventricular Arrhythmias). *Circulation* 2003; **108**: 1871–909.

Breithardt G, Cain ME, El-Sherif N, *et al.* Standards for analysis of ventricular late potentials using high resolution electrocardiography. A statement by a Task Force Committee between the European Society of Cardiology, the American Heart Association and the American College of Cardiology. *J Am Coll Cardiol* 1991; **17**: 999–1006.

Brignole M, Vardas P, Hoffman E, *et al.* Indications for the use of diagnostic implantable and external ECG loop recorders. *Europace* 2009; **11**: 671–87.

Crawford MH, Bernstein SJ, Deedwania PC, *et al.* ACC/AHA guidelines for ambulatory electrocardiography: executive summary and recommendations: a report of the American College of Cardiology/American Heart Association Task Force on Practice Guidelines (Committee to Revise the Guidelines for Ambulatory Electrocardiography). *Circulation* 1999; **100**: 886–93.

Drew BJ, Califf RM, Funk M, *et al.* Practice standards for electrocardiographic monitoring in hospital settings: An American Heart Association scientific statement from the Councils on Cardiovascular Nursing, Clinical Cardiology, and Cardiovascular Disease in the Young: Endorsed by the International Society of Computerized Electrocardiology and the American Association of Critical-Care Nurses. *Circulation* 2004; **110**: 2721–46.

Gibbons RJ, Balady GJ, Bricker JT, *et al.* ACC/AHA 2002 guideline update for exercise testing: summary article: A report of the American College of Cardiology/American Heart Association Task Force on Practice Guidelines (Committee to Update the 1997 Exercise Testing Guidelines). *Circulation* 2002; **106**: 1883–92.

Goldberger JJ, Cain ME, Hohnloser SH, *et al.* American Heart Association/American College of Cardiology Foundation/ Heart Rhythm Society. Scientific statement on non-invasive risk stratification techniques for identifying patients at risk for sudden cardiac death. *J Am Coll Cardiol 2008*; **14**: 1179–99.

Hancock EW, Deal BJ, Mirvis DM, *et al.* AHA/ACCF/HRS Recommendations for the Standardization and Interpretation of the Electrocardiogram: Part V: Electrocardiogram Changes Associated With Cardiac Chamber Hypertrophy: A Scientific Statement From the American Heart Association Electrocardiography and Arrhythmias Committee, Council on Clinical Cardiology; the American College of Cardiology Foundation; and the Heart Rhythm Society: Endorsed by the International Society for Computerized Electrocardiology. *Circulation* 2009; **119**: e251–e261.

Kligfield P, Gettes LS, Bailey JJ, *et al.* AHA/ACC/HRS scientific statement. Recommendations for the standardization and interpretation of the electrocardiogram. Part I: The electrocardiogram and its technology. a scientific statement from the American Heart Association Electrocardiography and Arrhythmias Committee, Council on Clinical Cardiology; the American College of Cardiology Foundation; and the Heart Rhythm Society: Endorsed by the International Society for Computerized Electrocardiology. *Circulation* 2007; **115**: 1306–24.

Laks MM, Arzbaecher R, Bailey JJ, *et al.* Recommendations for safe current limits for electrocardiographs: a statement for healthcare professionals from the Committee on Electrocardiography, American Heart Association. *Circulation* 1996; **93**: 837–9.

Mason JW, Hancock EW, Gettes LS. AHA/ACC/HRS scientific statement. Recommendations for the standardization and interpretation of the electrocardiogram. Part II: Electrocardiography diagnostic statement list. a scientific statement from the American Heart Association Electrocardiography and Arrhythmias Committee, Council on Clinical Cardiology; the American College of Cardiology Foundation; and the Heart Rhythm Society: Endorsed by the International Society for Computerized Electrocardiology. *Circulation* 2007; **115**: 1325–32.

Mieres JH, Shaw LJ, Arai A, *et al.* Role of noninvasive testing in the clinical evaluation of women with suspected coronary artery disease: Consensus statement from the Cardiac Imaging Committee, Council on Clinical Cardiology, and the Cardiovascular Imaging and Intervention Committee, Council on Cardiovascular Radiology and Intervention, American Heart Association. *Circulation* 2005; **111**: 682–96.

Rautaharju PM, Surawicz B, GettesLS. AHA/ACCF/HRS Recommendations for the Standardization and Interpretation of the Electrocardiogram: Part IV: The ST Segment, T and U Waves, and the QT Interval: A Scientific Statement From the American Heart Association Electrocardiography and Arrhythmias Committee, Council on Clinical Cardiology; the American College of Cardiology Foundation; and the Heart Rhythm Society: Endorsed by the International Society for Computerized Electrocardiology. *Circulation* 2009; **119**: e241–e250.

Schlant RC, Adolph RJ, DiMarco JP, *et al.* Guidelines for electrocardiography. A report of the American College of Cardiology/American Heart Association Task Force on Assessment of Diagnostic and Therapeutic Cardiovascular Procedures (Committee on Electrocardiography). *J Am Coll Cardiol* 1992; **19**: 473–81.

Surawicz B, Childers R, Deal BJ, *et al.* Recommendations for the Standardization and Interpretation of the Electrocardiogram: Part III: Intraventricular Conduction Disturbances: A Scientific Statement From the American Heart Association Electrocardiography and Arrhythmias Committee, Council on Clinical Cardiology; the American College of Cardiology Foundation; and the Heart Rhythm Society: Endorsed by the International Society for Computerized Electrocardiology. *Circulation* 2009; **119**: e235–e240.

Task Force of the European Society of Cardiology and the North American Society of Pacing Electrophysiology. Heart rate variability: standards of measurement, physiological interpretation, and clinical use. *Circulation* 1996; **93**: 1043–65.

Thygesen K, Alpert JS, White HD; Joint ESC/ACCF/AHA/WHF Task Force for the redefinition of myocardial infarction. Universal definition of myocardial infarction. *Eur Heart J* 2007; **28**: 2525–38.

Van de Werf F, Bax J, Betriu A, *et al.* Management of acute myocardial infarction in patients presenting with persistent ST-segment elevation: The Task Force on the management of ST-segment elevation acute myocardial infarction of the European Society of Cardiology. *Eur Heart J* 2008; **29**: 2909–45.

Wagner GS, Macfarlane P, Wellens H, *et al.* AHA/ACCF/HRS Recommendations for the Standardization and Interpretation of the Electrocardiogram: Part VI: Acute Ischemia/Infarction: A Scientific Statement From the American Heart Association Electrocardiography and Arrhythmias Committee, Council on Clinical Cardiology; the American College of Cardiology Foundation; and the Heart Rhythm Society: Endorsed by the International Society for Computerized Electrocardiology. *Circulation* 2009; **119**: e262–e270.

Online resources

- Arizona CERT: Center for Education and Research on Therapeutics: http://www.azcert.org
- Cardiac Arrhythmias Research and Education Foundation, Inc.: http://www.longqt.org
- Sudden Arrhythmia Death Syndromes (SADS) Foundation: http://www.sads.org

➲ For full references and multimedia materials please visit the online version of the book (http://esctextbook.oxfordonline.com).

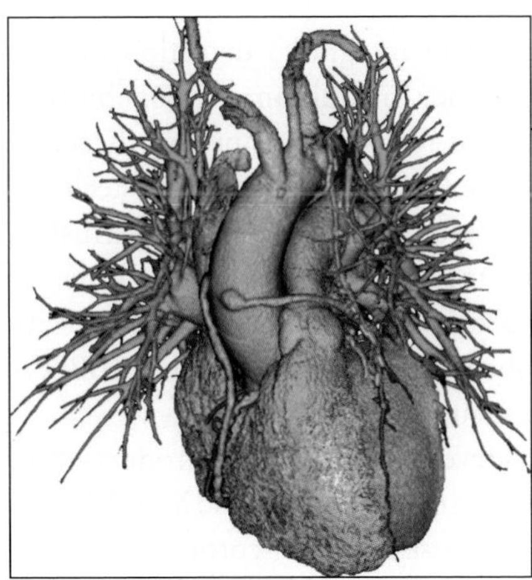

CHAPTER 3

Choice of Imaging Techniques

Joanne D. Schuijf, Nico R. Van de Veire, Ernst E. van der Wall, and Jeroen J. Bax

Contents

Summary

Cardiovascular non-invasive imaging has become an important component in the diagnosis and guidance of therapy in patients with cardiovascular disease.

At present, the four main non-invasive imaging techniques are echocardiography, nuclear imaging with single photon emission computed tomography and positron emission tomography, magnetic resonance imaging, and multi-slice computed tomography. All of these non-invasive imaging modalities have witnessed a rapid technological development and allow visualization of virtually all aspects of the cardiovascular system. While their increased use may potentially improve diagnosis and therapeutic decision making, it has simultaneously led to uncertainty as to which technique should be used when, and in which patient.

The aim of this chapter is to provide some examples on how to integrate the various imaging modalities in the management of patients. Two specific disease states, namely the patient with stable chest pain suspected for coronary artery disease presenting at outpatient clinic, and the patient with chronic heart failure, are used as examples. While the proposed approaches and algorithms are not meant to represent guidelines, they may serve as an illustration for the potential implementation of the various imaging techniques in diagnostic and therapeutic decision-making processes.

Introduction

Cardiovascular non-invasive imaging has become an important component in the diagnosis and guidance of therapy in patients with cardiovascular disease. Currently, the four main non-invasive imaging techniques are echocardiography, nuclear imaging with single photon emission computed tomography (SPECT) and positron emission tomography (PET), cardiac magnetic resonance imaging (CMR), and multi-slice computed tomography (MSCT). The applications of these different modalities are discussed in detail elsewhere in this textbook.

Over recent years, each of these modalities has witnessed a rapid technological development. All of the techniques can presently provide integrated information on myocardial function and perfusion, whereas in the past the techniques could provide most information on either perfusion or function. Traditionally, echocardiography provides the most comprehensive anatomic and functional information of the heart, including the pericardium, myocardium, and heart valves.

Recently, echocardiography (➲Chapter 4) has developed in the direction of (real-time) three-dimensional (3D) imaging, which provides extremely valuable information on cardiac structures, and also has improved accuracy of assessment of left ventricular (LV) volumes and ejection fraction. With 3D imaging, superior information on valvular pathology is possible, particularly information on mitral valve anatomy, which is extremely useful for cardiac surgeons in planning mitral valve surgery.

Another important development in echocardiography is the use of intravenous contrast. With contrast administration substantially improved LV endocardial delineation is possible, with superior detection of wall motion, LV volumes, and ejection fraction, and also identification of cardiac tumours and thrombi (see ➲Chapter 4). With the use of contrast it has also become possible to evaluate myocardial perfusion and myocardial viability. Together, these components have resulted in the integrated assessment of cardiac anatomy as well as cardiac function. For practical reasons, echocardiography is the most often used non-invasive imaging technique in clinical cardiology.

Nuclear cardiology is mainly a non-anatomical but rather functional imaging technique, and detailed information on myocardial perfusion (ischaemia) and viability (and scar) can be obtained (see ➲Chapter 7). The technique has also developed substantially over recent years. The major breakthrough was the feasibility of electrocardiogram (ECG)-gated imaging, permitting the expansion from assessment of myocardial perfusion to integrated detection of perfusion and cardiac function. In addition, the possibility of attenuation correction has resulted in improved detection of coronary artery disease (CAD). PET is the only technology that can provide absolute quantification on perfusion, aerobic and anaerobic metabolism, and cardiac innervation. In particular, cardiac innervation assessment with 123-iodine meta-iodobenzylguanidine (MIBG) and SPECT has attracted a lot of attention.

Another important development is the introduction of hybrid imaging; integration of PET/SPECT and MSCT equipment provides integrated assessment of coronary anatomy and cardiac perfusion (ischaemia). This again illustrates the development in the direction of more comprehensive imaging to integrate anatomy and function (see ➲Chapter 7).

MSCT is the most recently developed technique and is mainly used for evaluation of the coronary arteries. The technique is excellent for excluding significant coronary artery stenoses, and software for precise quantification of stenosis severity is being developed. In addition, coronary calcium can be detected, and the so-called coronary calcium score adequately reflects the total atherosclerotic burden of the coronary arteries (see ➲Chapter 6). However, with the use of contrast, non-calcified plaques can also be detected. Moreover, information on LV volumes and ejection fraction can be obtained as well. MSCT provides excellent information on anatomy of other cardiac structures, includes valves, cardiac veins, etc.

With the introduction of hybrid imaging, as already mentioned, integrated information on coronary anatomy and perfusion can be obtained. The disadvantage of both nuclear imaging and MSCT is the radiation associated with these procedures, although recent innovations have resulted in significant reductions in radiation dose.

The remaining technique is CMR. This technique provides excellent information on cardiac structures (anatomy), similar to echocardiography but with extremely high resolution, particularly regarding the pericardium/myocardium and valves. Non-invasive coronary angiography is also possible, although image quality is lower as compared to MSCT (see ➲Chapter 5). In addition, functional information can be obtained including perfusion (ischaemia), LV volumes, and ejection fraction, but also haemodynamic information on stenotic or leaking valves. Contrast-enhanced CMR has resulted in better tissue characterization, including improved detection of fibrosis and scar tissue. Recent introduction of 3-Tesla magnets and new contrast agents will contribute to further refinements in imaging with CMR.

Accordingly, all techniques have developed rapidly over the past decade and virtually all aspects of the cardiovascular system can be visualized with non-invasive tools. This has resulted in an increased implementation of cardiovascular imaging in clinical patient management. Consequently, improved diagnosis and therapeutic decision making has become possible. But at the same time, clinicians have become confused about which imaging techniques to use when, with the potential disadvantage of 'over-using' the imaging techniques.

When selecting imaging techniques in a particular patient, various issues need to be considered. The main questions are:

- 'Which cardiovascular disease is considered?'
- 'What information on that disease is needed for clinical management in this particular patient?'

In turn, this depends on:

- 'What are the characteristics of this particular patient?'

To that end, several factors have to be considered, i.e. the pre-test likelihood of disease, and also in which setting the patient presents (acute presentation at emergency room; stable, elective presentation at outpatient clinic; elective presentation at the heart failure clinic; hospitalized at the cardiac care unit; etc.).

Consequently the following question arises:

- 'Which imaging technique can provide the required information in this particular patient?'

Frequently, different techniques can provide the requested information; it is therefore also important to consider the local availability, expertise, and experience with the individual imaging techniques.

Two specific disease states (the patient with stable chest pain suspected for CAD presenting at outpatient clinic, and the patient with chronic heart failure) will be used as examples to illustrate these issues. How imaging can help and provide information in these two patient categories will be discussed in the next sections. It is important to realize that these are examples, and the proposed approaches and algorithms are not guidelines, but rather are meant to illustrate the potential implementation of imaging techniques in the diagnosis and therapeutic decision-making process of these patients.

The patient with stable chest pain presenting at the outpatient clinic

Considering the patient presenting to the outpatient clinic with stable chest pain, the disease that has to be primarily considered is CAD (➲Chapter 17). The information needed on that disease includes the presence of atherosclerosis and the presence of ischaemia. The choice of the imaging approach depends on the patient characteristics, and in this particular scenario (stable chest pain, outpatient clinic), the pre-test likelihood of CAD is important. In patients with low to intermediate pre-test likelihood, the question is mainly whether CAD is present (since then medical therapy is needed). These patients may therefore first be referred for atherosclerosis imaging. In contrast, in patients with intermediate to high pre-test likelihood of CAD (or known CAD), the main question is whether there is ischaemia (since then invasive angiography and revascularization should be considered). In these patients, therefore, ischaemia imaging may be preferred.

The patient with low to intermediate pre-test likelihood of CAD

In patients with a relatively low pre-test likelihood of CAD, the ability to accurately rule out CAD is preferred. To accurately rule out CAD, imaging should be targeting detection of atherosclerosis and not ischaemia, since absence of atherosclerosis indicates no CAD, whereas absence of ischaemia can still mean CAD (atherosclerosis without ischaemia).

Henneman and colleagues recently demonstrated in 340 patients without a history of CAD that the ability to sufficiently rule out any CAD was related to pre-test likelihood [1]. While the value of atherosclerosis imaging was limited in patients with high pre-test likelihood, the technique was capable to rule out atherosclerosis in a considerable proportion of patients with respectively low (58%) and intermediate (33%) pre-test likelihood of CAD [1]. Similarly, Meijboom and colleagues demonstrated that the diagnostic performance of atherosclerosis testing is highly influenced by the pre-test likelihood of CAD [2]. In 254 patients, the post-test probability of CAD after atherosclerosis assessment with MSCT was directly related to pre-test probability. The authors revealed that following a negative MSCT study, post-test probability was reduced to 0% in those patients with low and intermediate pre-test likelihood of CAD. In contrast, the post-test probability remained fairly high (17%) in patients with high pre-test likelihood of CAD, despite a negative test result. Accordingly, the clinical utility of atherosclerosis imaging appears to be highest in patients in whom the likelihood of significant stenosis and subsequent need for revascularization is relatively low but knowledge of coronary anatomy is still preferred for further management (medical therapy or not) [3].

Atherosclerosis imaging can be performed with both CMR and CT-based techniques, which will be discussed in more detail in Chapters 5 and 6. Briefly, two distinct approaches are available, namely non-invasive assessment of coronary calcium and direct non-invasive coronary angiography.

Coronary artery calcium scoring (CACS) is a relatively simple technique that uses the presence of coronary calcium deposits as a marker for CAD. Electron-beam computed tomography (EBCT) has been predominantly used during the past 15 years, but CACS can also be performed with MSCT. The Agatston score is used to express the extent of calcifications in the coronary arteries [4]. A score of 0 indicates absence of coronary calcium, suggesting a very low likelihood of CAD (although not zero since sometimes non-calcified lesions are present); scores >1000 indicate severe atherosclerosis, with also a high likelihood of coronary artery stenoses. Importantly, one should remember that no linear relationship exists between CACS and the presence and severity of luminal narrowing. Also, non-calcified atherosclerosis is not visualized, and significant CAD may be present in the absence of coronary calcium.

CACS is most useful in risk stratification [5]. In large cohorts of asymptomatic individuals with high-risk profiles for CAD, CACS provided incremental information over baseline clinical characteristics and effectively differentiated patients with a low or high risk for future cardiac events.

The second approach is non-invasive coronary angiography which can be performed with CMR, EBCT, and MSCT. This approach integrates visualization of atherosclerosis and assessment of luminal stenosis. MSCT is most often used for non-invasive angiography; the technique has a good sensitivity and specificity (in the range of 90–95%), but its particular strength is the high negative predictive value (>95%) [6]. Indeed, a normal MSCT angiogram (i.e. absence of calcium or non-calcified lesions) virtually rules out the presence of CAD. An example of a patient without CAD on MSCT angiography is provided in ➲Fig. 3.1. Drawbacks however, include the radiation dose as well as its inability to precisely grade the degree of luminal narrowing, resulting in frequent overestimation of stenosis. In addition, no information on the haemodynamic significance of the lesion is obtained [6]. Accordingly, further testing by means of functional techniques may be necessary to determine the need for invasive coronary angiography and revascularization [7]. The particular advantages of CACS and non-invasive angiography are summarized in ➲Table 3.1.

In clinical scenarios where detailed information on the presence and location of luminal narrowing is preferred, the benefits of MSCT as compared to CACS will outweigh its limitations, which include the higher radiation dose and need for contrast administration. However, in some patients such as asymptomatic patients with an elevated risk profile, it may be sufficient to establish the presence and extent of atherosclerosis, in order to determine the intensity of risk factor modification. In these patients, in whom no evident indication for possible revascularization exists, use of CACS may be preferred. At the same time however, it is important to realize that at present no data are available that demonstrate that changes in management based on detection of subclinical atherosclerosis on either CACS or MSCT angiography result in improved outcome. Accordingly, screening for atherosclerosis in the general asymptomatic population seems at present not justified.

The patient with intermediate to high pre-test likelihood of CAD or known CAD

In patients with intermediate to high pre-test likelihood of CAD (or known CAD), the clinical question is whether ischaemia is present. The ability of stress imaging techniques to define both severity and location of ischaemia represents an important advantage over both exercise ECG testing (➲Chapters 2 and 25) and atherosclerosis imaging, and may help to decide when invasive angiography and potential revascularization should be considered. Indeed, observational data have indicated a clear survival benefit of coronary revascularization over medical therapy in case of moderate to severe ischaemia [8]. In combination with clinical characteristics such as symptoms, the presence and extent of ischaemia therefore remains an essential guide for further referral to invasive coronary angiography and revascularization [9].

Accordingly, in patients with high pre-test likelihood or known CAD and more typical symptoms (in whom the clinical question is: is there a need for invasive angiography and revascularization?) ischaemia testing is preferred. While symptomatic patients with high pre-test likelihood of CAD could potentially proceed directly to invasive angiography, cost-effectiveness studies have shown that initial imaging for ischaemia (followed by selective invasive coronary angiography only in those with abnormal or high risk studies) may be preferred over direct referral to invasive coronary angiography [10, 11]

Various imaging techniques are available to detect ischaemia, including nuclear perfusion imaging and stress echocardiography (or CMR). These techniques are based on demonstration of stress-induced wall motion or perfusion abnormalities, indicative of ischaemia.

Nuclear perfusion imaging employs radioactive tracers to assess myocardial perfusion during stress and at rest, yielding sensitivities and specificities of approximately 90% for

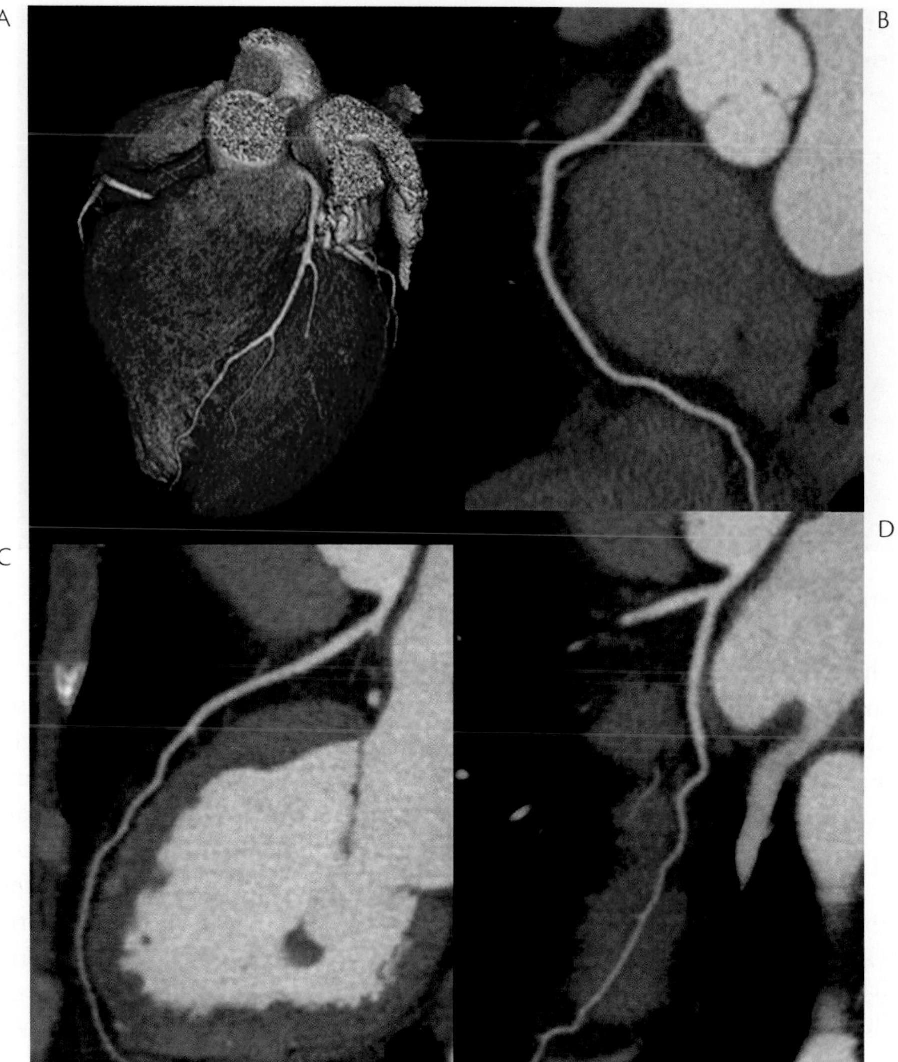

Figure 3.1 Ruling out atherosclerosis with MSCT coronary angiography. A 46-year-old female presented to the outpatient cardiology clinic for evaluation of atypical complaints in combination with a positive family history for CAD (father sudden cardiac death at age 39 years, brother non-fatal myocardial infarction at age 46 years). 320-slice MSCT was performed showing normal coronary arteries. (A) 3D volume rendered reconstruction. (B) Curved multiplanar reconstruction of the right coronary artery. (C) Curved multiplanar reconstruction of the left anterior descending coronary artery. (D) Curved multiplanar reconstruction of the left circumflex coronary artery. The patient was reassured and discharged from further cardiac evaluation.

Table 3.1 Comparative advantages of atherosclerosis imaging techniques

Advantages of calcium scoring (with EBCT or MSCT)
High technical success rate
Low radiation dose
No contrast agent required
Validated and reproducible quantification
Reliable rule out of CAD in asymptomatic patients
Extensive prognostic data supporting value in risk stratification of asymptomatic patients
Advantages of coronary angiography with MSCT
Assessment of degree of stenosis
Identification of both non-calcified and calcified plaque
Higher diagnostic accuracy for significant CAD
Reliable rule out of CAD in both asymptomatic and symptomatic patients

CAD, coronary artery disease; EBCT, electron beam computed tomography, MSCT: multi-slice computed tomography.

detection of CAD [12] (see also ➲Chapter 7). An example of a patient with evidence of ischaemia (obtained by SPECT perfusion imaging) is provided in ➲Fig. 3.2. Nuclear imaging is performed with either SPECT or PET systems; the main advantage of PET over SPECT is the higher resolution and the fact that it allows absolute quantification of perfusion. In addition to perfusion imaging, the introduction of ECG-gated SPECT and PET imaging has permitted for assessment of wall motion.

Stress echocardiography detects wall motion at rest and during stress, yielding sensitivities and specificities in the range of 80–84% for detection of CAD [13]. In addition to wall motion imaging, the introduction of intravenous contrast agents has permitted assessment of perfusion.

With CMR, pharmacological stress is applied as physical exercise is difficult in the scanner. Similar to echocardiography, wall motion can be assessed, and first-pass imaging of contrast agents permits assessment of perfusion.

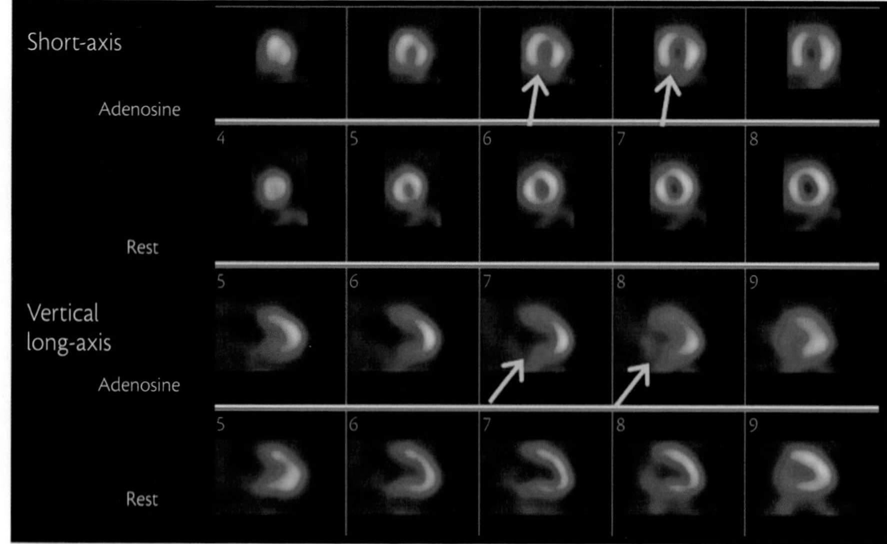

Figure 3.2 Identification of ischaemia with stress–rest myocardial perfusion imaging. A 58-year-old male presented to the outpatient clinic with stable chest pain complaints and an elevated risk profile for CAD. The patient was referred for ischaemia imaging. SPECT myocardial perfusion imaging revealed a large perfusion abnormality during adenosine stress which resolved during rest, indicating the presence of ischaemia. The patient was subsequently referred for invasive coronary angiography in combination with revascularization.

The sensitivity and specificity to detect CAD are in the range of 84–89% and 84% for perfusion and wall motion CMR [13].

Imaging approach to the patient with stable chest pain

In the patient presenting to the outpatient clinic with stable chest pain, the pre-test likelihood and history of CAD determines which imaging approach is chosen. ➲Fig. 3.3 illustrates a potential imaging approach in patients with low to intermediate pre-test likelihood. In these patients, initial evaluation is performed by means of atherosclerosis imaging. As already described, the presence of atherosclerosis can be assessed by both CACS and non-invasive angiography. While each technique has its particular advantages and disadvantages (➲Table 3.1), it remains to be fully elucidated which technique may be preferred. Nevertheless, in symptomatic patients, it is anticipated that angiography may be favoured as it provides more comprehensive information, including the presence of non-calcified plaque as well as more detailed information on the location and severity of disease.

Based on the findings of atherosclerosis imaging, (➲Chapter 17) patients can then be stratified into:

- having no atherosclerosis;
- having atherosclerosis but without obstructive luminal narrowing (degree of luminal stenosis <40%);
- having atherosclerosis of borderline severity (degree of luminal stenosis between 40–70%);
- having severe atherosclerosis with luminal narrowing >70% or left main and/or three-vessel involvement.

In patients in whom atherosclerosis imaging revealed borderline stenoses (luminal narrowing between 40–70%), their physiological relevance and thus management remains uncertain. Additional ischaemia testing is therefore required in order to determine the optimal therapeutic strategy. As described earlier, several modalities are available for this purpose with more or less similar diagnostic accuracies. Accordingly, the local availability and expertise are likely to determine which particular technique is used.

Since the pre-test likelihood of CAD is low to intermediate, atherosclerosis imaging will rule out CAD in a large proportion of patients. These patients can then be reassured and discharged from intensive medical therapy and close monitoring. In contrast, patients with evidence of atherosclerosis yet without obstructive stenosis (luminal narrowing <40%), may benefit from initiation or increased intensity of anti-atherosclerotic therapy. However, as obstructive lesions are absent no further imaging by means of ischaemia testing or invasive angiography is required at this stage. In those patients with atherosclerosis of borderline severity (degree of luminal stenosis between 40–70%), the results of ischaemia imaging will determine further management. If the ischaemia test is normal, there is no indication for invasive coronary angiography and possible revascularization. However, the patient still has confirmed atherosclerosis and may benefit from (increased) medical therapy. On the other hand, if ischaemia is identified, the patient may indeed be referred for invasive coronary angiography and possible revascularization. Similarly, if atherosclerosis imaging has revealed severe atherosclerosis, direct referral to invasive coronary angiography may be preferred.

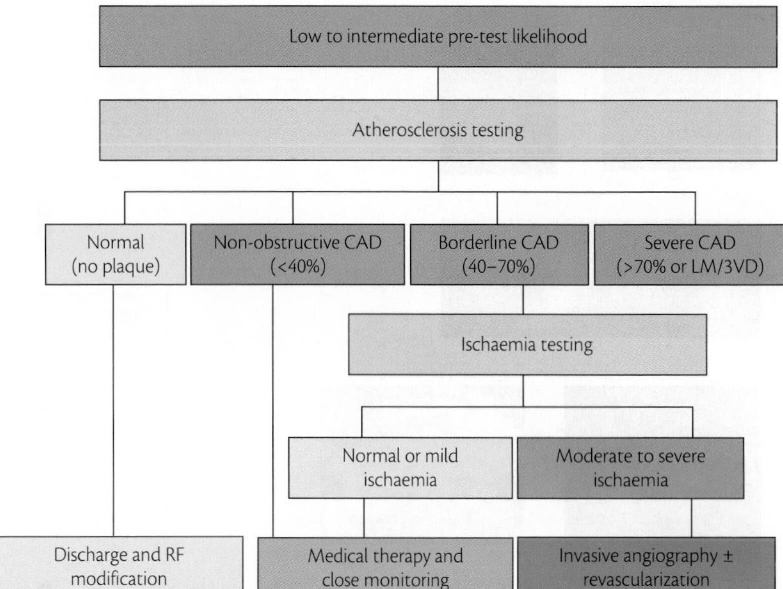

Figure 3.3 Potential algorithm for sequential imaging of anatomy and function for diagnosis and management of CAD in patients with a low to intermediate pre-test likelihood for CAD. A low to intermediate pre-test likelihood favours initial imaging of atherosclerosis, as the prevalence of CAD and thus the proportion of patients potentially requiring revascularization will be low. CAD, coronary artery disease; LM, left main coronary artery; RF, risk factor; VD, vessel-disease.

In patients with relatively higher pre-test likelihood of CAD (intermediate to high) or established CAD, an imaging approach directed towards detection of ischaemia may be preferred. This approach is illustrated in ➲Fig. 3.4. In these patients, atherosclerosis testing has limited value since (extensive) atherosclerosis is either known or anticipated. Accordingly, the presence and extent of ischaemia dictates further management. In a substantial proportion of patients, ischaemia will indeed be identified, resulting in referral to invasive coronary angiography and possible revascularization. In those patients without ischaemia, the likelihood of atherosclerosis remains high. Accordingly, intense medical therapy and close monitoring remains indicated.

The patient with chronic heart failure

The approach to the chronic heart failure patient (➲Chapter 23) is very different from the approach to the stable chest pain patient at the outpatient clinic. Heart failure is a complex disease state and careful assessment of underlying aetiology is needed in order to determine the optimal therapeutic management for the individual patient. A practical approach using different steps is shown in ➲Fig. 3.5 and the potential role of the imaging techniques is highlighted for the different steps. The information that imaging provides at each step will form the basis for the components of the final therapy for the heart failure patient; the therapy is focused at:

- Should revascularization be performed or medical therapy?
- Should LV restoration or LV aneurysmectomy be performed?
- Is mitral valve repair needed?
- Is cardiac resynchronization therapy needed (possibly with an implantable cardioverter defibrillator (ICD))?

The aetiology underlying heart failure

The first step in the diagnostic work-up of every heart failure patient is to determine whether CAD is the underlying

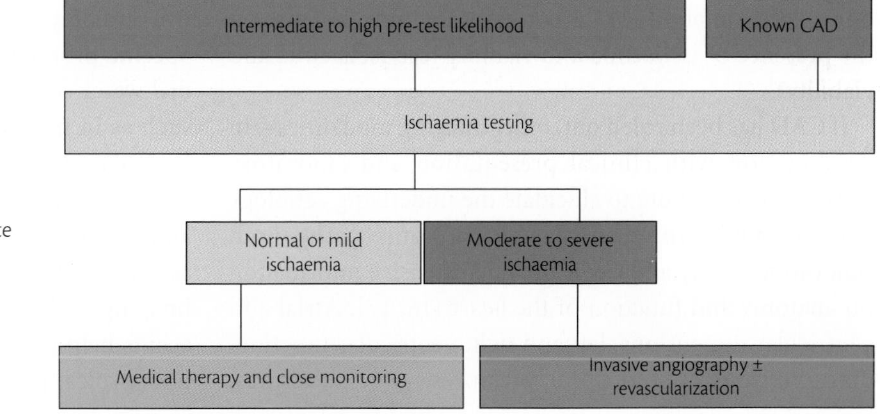

Figure 3.4 Potential algorithm for sequential imaging of anatomy and function for diagnosis and management of CAD in patients with an intermediate to high pre-test likelihood for CAD or known CAD. An intermediate to high pre-test likelihood or the presence of known CAD favours initial imaging of ischaemia, as the prevalence of CAD and thus the proportion of patients potentially requiring revascularization will be high.

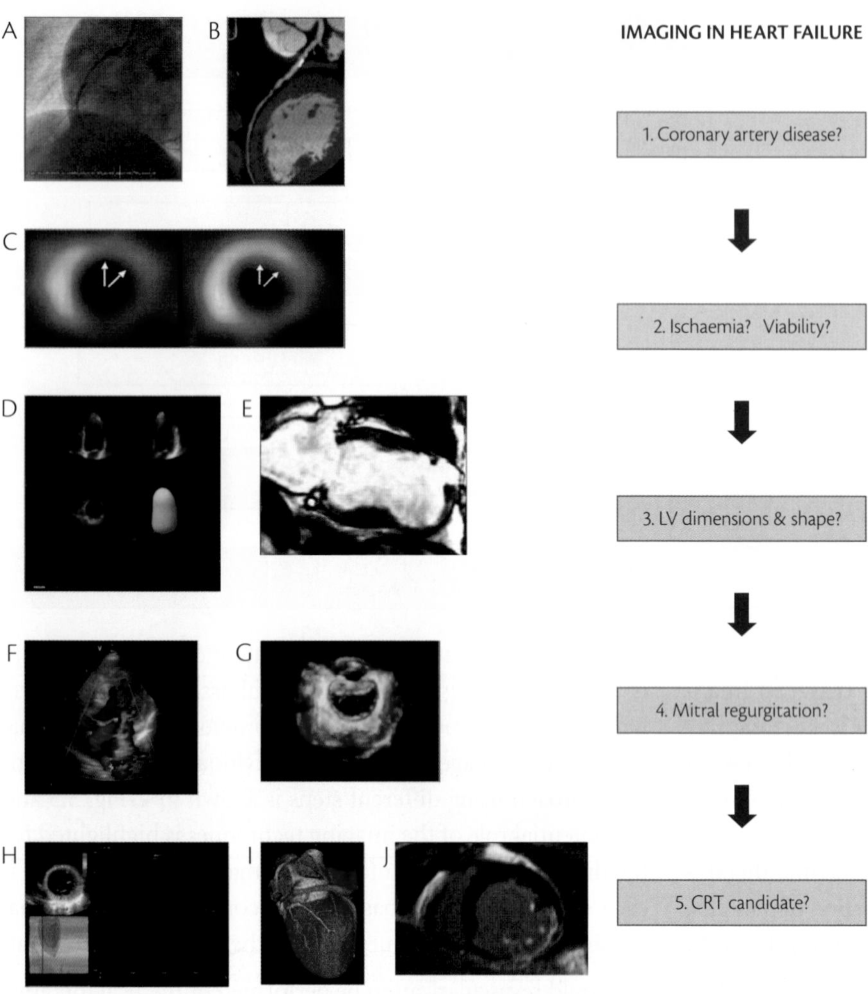

Figure 3.5 Proposed algorithm for the implementation of cardiac imaging modalities in heart failure patients to guide diagnosis and treatment. First, CAD has to be confirmed or excluded with invasive coronary angiography (A) or possibly MSCT (B). In patients with ischaemic cardiomyopathy, ischaemia and viability need to be detected with nuclear imaging (C), dobutamine stress echocardiography, or CMR. LV dimensions and function can be quantified with all available imaging modalities; in this example, three-dimensional echocardiography is used (D). The LV shape can be evaluated with echocardiography or CMR (E). Presence and severity of mitral regurgitation can be evaluated with echocardiography (F). Three-dimensional transoesophageal echocardiography is useful to determine the underlying mechanism of mitral regurgitation (G). Finally, to support the use of cardiac resynchronization therapy (CRT), intraventricular dyssynchrony can be quantified with echocardiography (H), venous anatomy visualized with MSCT (I), and viable tissue determined with CMR or nuclear imaging (J).

aetiology, since this is the most prevalent cause of heart failure. Invasive coronary angiography remains the first-choice technique to determine the presence, location, and extent of coronary artery lesions, and percutaneous coronary intervention can be performed if needed [14]. Recently, MSCT has emerged as an alternative technique and excellent diagnostic accuracy has been reported in patients with suspected CAD, although not much data are available in heart failure patients [15]. If CAD is present, the option of revascularization should be considered; this depends not only on the suitability of the coronary anatomy, but also on the presence of ischaemia and viability (see Ischaemia and viability).

If CAD has been ruled out, other imaging modalities—in combination with clinical presentation and laboratory tests—can contribute to elucidate the underlying aetiology of heart failure. In non-ischaemic cardiomyopathy, both echocardiography and CMR provide extensive information on anatomy and function of the heart [16, 17]. Atrial and ventricular dimensions, left and right ventricular function, diastolic function and filling pressures, valve structures, myocardial appearance, and pericardial effusion, can all be evaluated with echocardiography and CMR [16, 17] (see also ➲Chapters 4 and 5). The use of intravenous contrast during echocardiography can facilitate the evaluation of ventricular structures such as trabeculations in non-compaction cardiomyopathy and right ventricular crypts and aneurysms in arrhythmogenic right ventricular cardiomyopathy (➲Chapters 9 and 18) (➲Fig. 3.6; 🎥3.1–3.4) [18]. With CMR, t1- and t2- weighted turbo-spin sequences are useful to assess the pericardium if the clinical question is constrictive cardiomyopathy versus restrictive cardiomyopathy [17]. Specific protocols are used to identify increased myocardial water content, indicating oedema and inflammation, such as in myocarditis and cardiac sarcoidosis. CMR has a unique role in the assessment of heart failure caused by iron overload. If haemochromatosis is suspected, the degree and distribution of myocardial iron can be simultaneously assessed and followed during therapy from myocardial t2* imaging. Administration of gadolinium-based contrast agents help to detect myocardial fibrosis and scar formation; typical patterns of contrast-enhancement may help

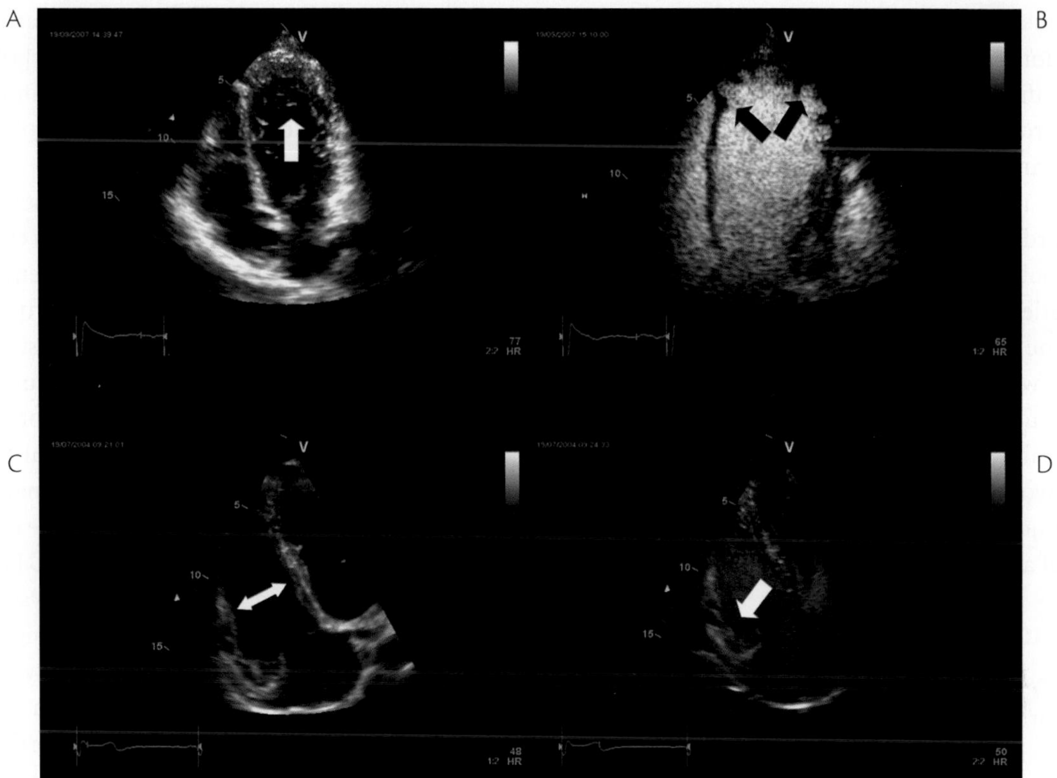

Figure 3.6 (A) Heavy trabeculations in the LV apex (white arrow) are suspected on this two-dimensional echocardiogram. (B) The use of intravenous contrast shows the endocardial layer with trabeculations and deep recesses (black arrows) confirming non-compaction cardiomyopathy. (C) Conventional echocardiography shows marked dilatation of the right ventricle (white arrow). (D) Intravenous contrast demonstrated small aneurysms in the basal part of the right ventricle (white arrow) suggestive for arrhythmogenic right ventricular cardiomyopathy. Also see 3.1–3.4

to determine the aetiology of non-ischaemic cardiomyopathy. In summary, the first step in the diagnostic process of the heart failure patient is to confirm or exclude CAD using invasive coronary angiography or possibly MSCT. In non-ischaemic cardiomyopathy, echocardiography and CMR provide a wealth of information to arrive at a diagnosis, supporting the therapeutic decision-making process.

Ischaemia and viability

Once CAD has been confirmed, further imaging is needed to document ischaemia and viability to determine therapeutic management; in particular whether revascularization is useful. Accordingly, detection of ischaemia is needed, and various techniques are available including nuclear imaging, stress echocardiography, or CMR. These techniques have similar diagnostic performance and technique choice depends on local availability and expertise.

Moreover, whether LV dysfunction is caused by scar tissue or dysfunctional but viable myocardium (hibernation or repetitive stunning) needs to be determined [19]. Recovery of function after revascularization will not occur when LV dysfunction is caused by scar tissue, but improvement of LV function may occur after revascularization in patients with viable myocardium. The most frequently used techniques to assess viability include nuclear imaging, echocardiography, and CMR (Table 3.2). Using these modalities, viability can be detected in >50% of patients with LV dysfunction.

Table 3.2 Characteristics of viable myocardium detected by different imaging modalities

Imaging modality	Viability marker
Nuclear imaging	
SPECT using ^{201}Tl	Perfusion, cell membrane integrity
SPECT using ^{99m} Tc-labelled tracers	Perfusion, cell membrane integrity, intact mitochondria
PET or SPECT with F-18 FDG	Glucose utilization
Echocardiography	
Low-dose dobutamine infusion	Contractile reserve
Intravenous contrast agents	Perfusion
CMR	
Low-dose dobutamine infusion	Contractile reserve
Intravenous contrast agents	Scar tissue

F-18 FDG: F-18 fluorodeoxyglucose; ^{99m}Tc, technetium-99m; ^{201}Tl, thallium-201.

Adapted with permission from Schinkel AF, Poldermans D, Elhendy A, *et al.* Assessment of myocardial viability in patients with heart failure. *J Nucl Med* 2007; **48**: 1135–46.

All techniques have a fairly high sensitivity for the prediction of functional recovery after revascularization (>80%), whereas specificity was lower (65–75%), indicating that viable myocardium may not always improve in function post-revascularization [20]. However, from a prognostic point of view, it has been demonstrated that patients with viable myocardium who are treated medically have a high event rate. Pooled data from 24 prognostic studies (including >3000 patients) using various viability techniques illustrated that the annual death rate of patients with viable myocardium who underwent revascularization was 3.2% as compared to 16% in patients with viability who were treated medically. These data strongly suggest that patients with viable myocardium need to undergo revascularization. Which technique is used for assessment of viability depends again on local availability and expertise.

The size and shape of the left ventricle

LV dimensions offer important prognostic information in the heart failure patient. The major predictor of long-term survival following myocardial infarction is the functional status of the LV. Several studies have shown that LV end-systolic volume has greater predictive value for survival than LV end-diastolic volume or LV ejection fraction. LV dimensions and function are also relevant for the choice of therapy. For example, the likelihood of functional recovery after revascularization is not only determined by the presence of viability but also by the size of the LV. When the LV is too dilated, improvement of function is not likely to occur post-revascularization even in the presence of viable myocardium [21].

LV volumes and ejection fraction are also taken into account to determine the need and timing of surgery in heart failure patients with valvular disease [22]. Moreover, a reduction in LV ejection fraction is mandatory for implantation of an ICD or biventricular pacemaker (see Is cardiac resynchronization therapy with or without ICD needed?) (➲Chapter 23) [23].

For the assessment of LV volumes and ejection fraction several imaging modalities can be used. Echocardiography, due to its non-invasive nature and availability, is particularly useful for repeated measurements over time (e.g. to evaluate effect of therapy and document possible LV reverse remodelling). Visual estimation of LV ejection fraction has important limitations and depends on highly-trained expert interpretation for accuracy. Quantitative, objective measurements of LV systolic function, such as the bi-plane method of discs, should become the standard practice [24]. With the recent introduction of 3D echocardiography, more reliable assessment of LV volumes and LV ejection fraction is possible (➲Fig. 3.7). The use of intravenous contrast for LV endocardial border opacification can improve the accuracy of echocardiography even further [18]. The other imaging modalities (gated SPECT, CMR, and MSCT) can also provide reliable information on LV volumes and LV ejection fraction.

When structural heart disease progresses into clinical heart failure, LV size increases, becomes less elliptical, more spherical, and LV ejection fraction will eventually decline (LV remodelling). Surgical resection of dysfunctional myocardium and/or scar tissue can reduce LV size and restore normal geometry [25]. With the increasing use of LV aneurysmectomy and LV restoration, precise information on the presence, location, and extent of the LV aneurysm is needed. Echocardiography is the first choice examination; suboptimal image quality can be improved by the use of intravenous contrast agents. CMR is a valid alternative (➲Fig. 3.8). CMR allows a precise delineation between aneurysm, non-viable and viable myocardium by combining resting images (providing information on LV end-diastolic wall thickness), dobutamine CMR (providing information on contractile reserve), and contrast-enhanced CMR (providing information on scar tissue). Based on the imaging information, surgical aneurysmectomy can be planned.

Mitral regurgitation

To distinguish regurgitation caused by a primary (organic) problem of the mitral valve itself from a secondary (functional) mitral regurgitation, echocardiography is the first-choice imaging modality. Heart failure patients with LV systolic dysfunction frequently develop mitral regurgitation as a consequence of LV remodelling (➲Chapter 23). The pathophysiological mechanism involves enlargement of the LV cavity with increased sphericity resulting in systolic retraction of the mitral leaflets (with reduced leaflet coaptation) and mitral valve annular dilatation. Moderate to severe mitral regurgitation is noted in up to 50% of patients with dilated cardiomyopathy (➲Chapter 18) and presence and severity are negative prognostic markers in heart failure patients [26]. Worsening of mitral regurgitation after isolated coronary artery bypass grafting (CABG) has been demonstrated and is associated with reduced long-term survival. Therefore, in case of severe mitral regurgitation, mitral valve surgery should be performed at the time of CABG. A comprehensive echocardiographic evaluation of the LV shape and the geometry of the mitral valve is necessary to understand the mechanism of regurgitation, which determines the surgical options. For the anatomical evaluation of the mitral valve, transoesophageal echocardiography provides additional information. In case of organic disease,

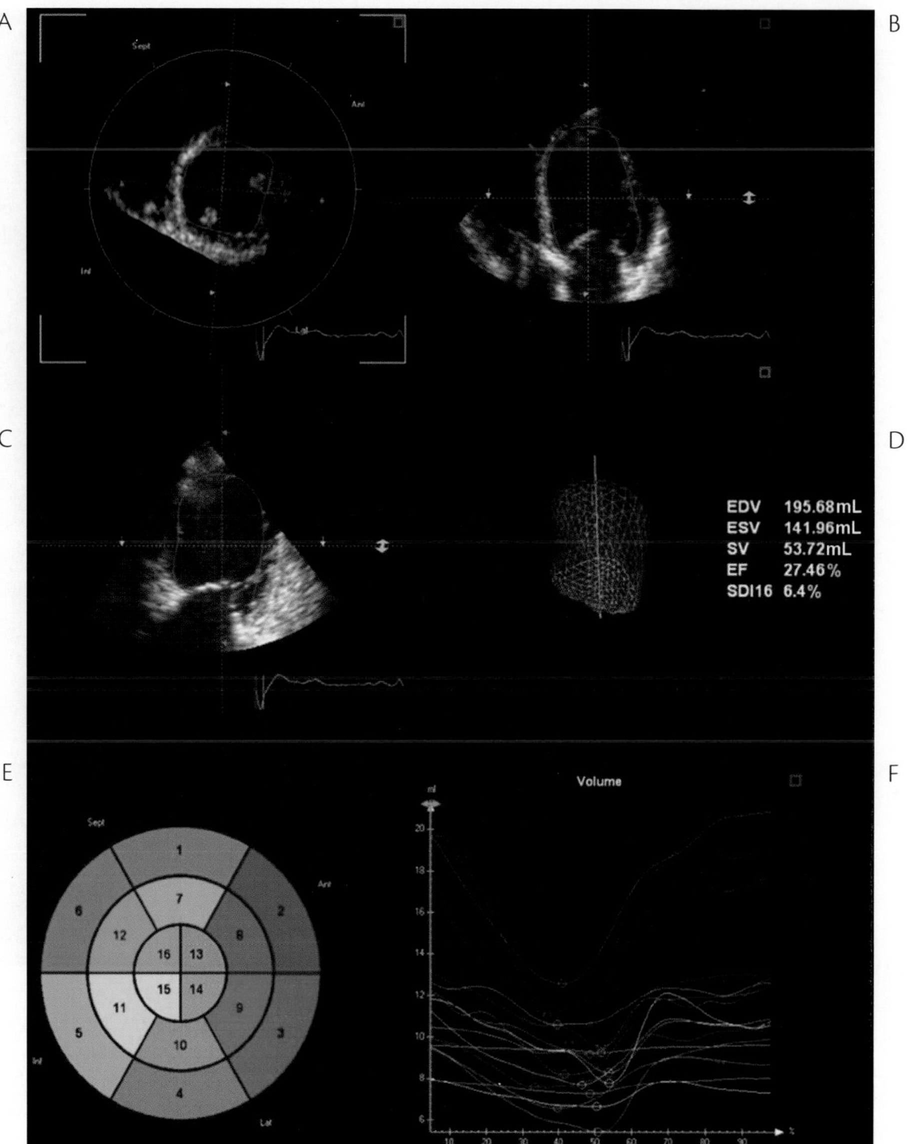

Figure 3.7 A real-time three-dimensional echocardiographic dataset is used to trace the endocardium of the LV in three orthogonal planes, (A), (B), and (C). The software generates a LV volume and calculates end-diastolic volume (EDV), end-systolic volume (ESV), stroke volume (SV), and ejection fraction (EF) (D). A 16-segment model (E) is used to calculate time-volume curves (F). From the dispersion of time to minimal volume of each LV segment (16 segments), a systolic dyssynchrony index (SDI 16, (D)) can be calculated.

the exact mechanism (Barlow, flail leaflet, prolapse) and location (which leaflet and scallop) can be determined. Mitral annulus diameter, leaflet coaptation height, displacement of papillary muscles, and leaflet motion are important points when surgery is considered in heart failure patients. The new 3D echocardiographic technologies in particular can provide this information (➲Fig. 3.9A; 3.5).

Mitral valve anatomy and adjacent structures can also be assessed with MSCT. This could be of particular use for the selection of heart failure patients for a percutaneous approach of mitral valve annuloplasty. During this procedure a device is inserted in the coronary sinus and inflated. A potential problem is when the circumflex coronary artery courses between the coronary sinus and mitral annulus, and this was indeed demonstrated in a significant percentage of patients using MSCT imaging [27]. Moreover, the coronary sinus is located along the left atrial wall in the majority of patients, rather than along the mitral valve annulus.

The next step is quantification of mitral regurgitation; using colour Doppler echocardiography, mitral regurgitation can be assessed by the 'eyeball method', and graded in a categorical, semi-quantitative sense (mild, moderate, or severe). The colour Doppler jet area is sensitive to driving pressures, equipment settings, and left atrial size, and it has been recommended to quantify mitral regurgitation with methods such as vena contracta width, stroke volume calculations, and proximal isovelocity surface area (PISA) [28]. From the latter methods, regurgitant volume and effective regurgitant orifice (ERO) area can be calculated; the novel 3D technology will further improve accuracy (➲Fig. 3.9B). It has been shown that quantification of mitral regurgitation provides major information for risk stratification and

A

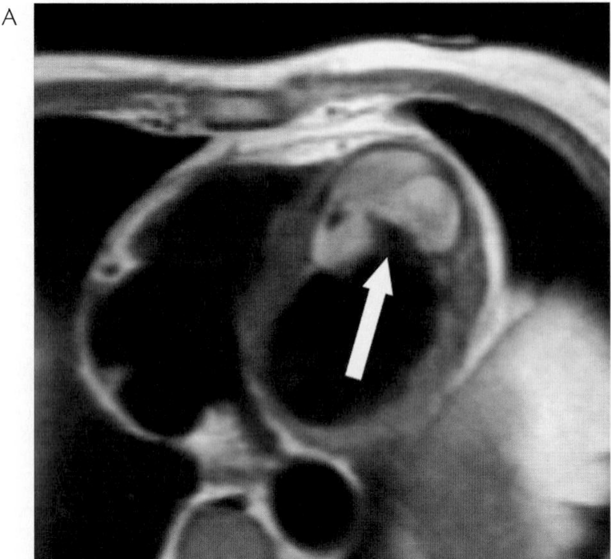

B

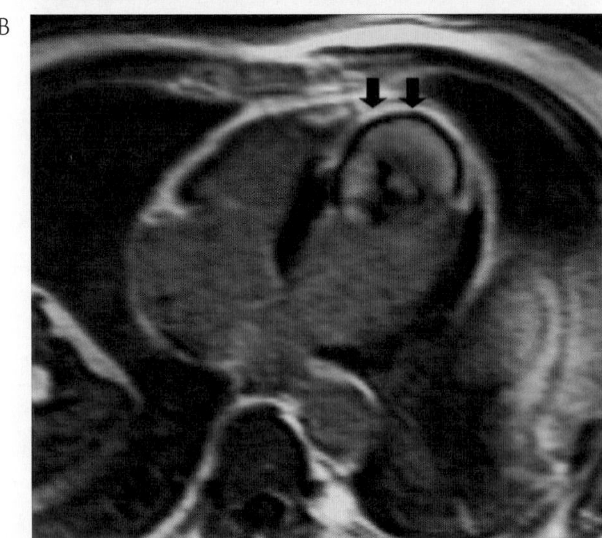

Figure 3.8 (A) Apical left ventricular aneurysm with thrombus formation (white arrow) can be identified on this CMR image of a patient with a history of anterior myocardial infarction. (B) With the use of contrast-enhanced imaging, the non-viable scar can be recognized as white tissue (black arrows); the black ring underlying the white (scar) tissue demonstrates the presence of thrombus formation.

A

B

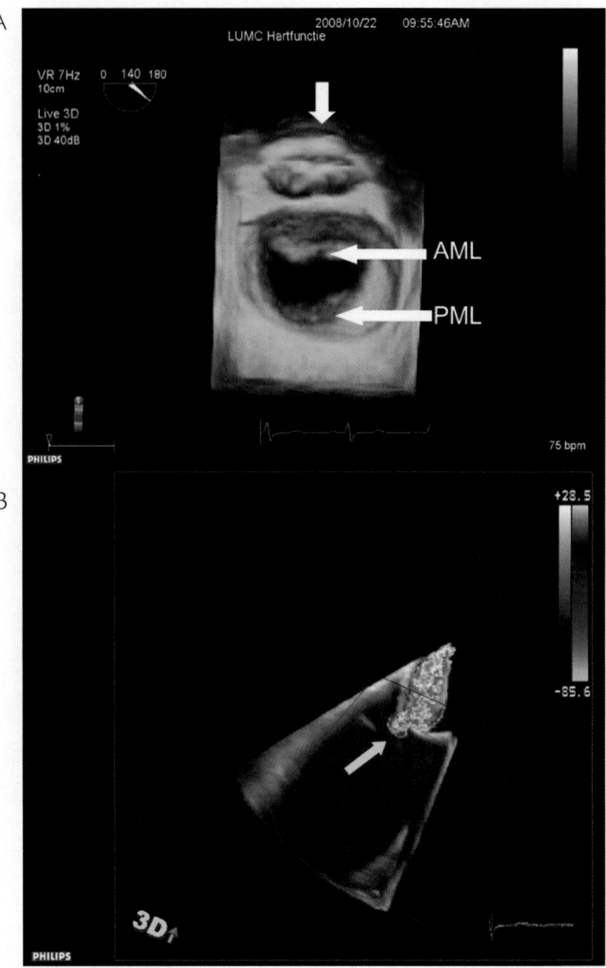

Figure 3.9 (A) Real-time three-dimensional transoesophageal image showing the anterior (AML) and posterior mitral valve (PML) leaflets from the surgeon's view. Also note the sclerotic aortic valve (white arrow). (B) Illustration of a significant mitral regurgitation using 3D transoesophageal echocardiography with colour flow imaging. Also see 3.5.

clinical decision making [29]. Besides the quantification of the regurgitation, other echocardiographic parameters should also be considered when judging the severity of mitral regurgitation including LV size, diastolic function, left atrial size, and pulmonary artery pressures. Besides echocardiography, CMR can also be used to quantify the severity of mitral regurgitation. Recently, a new method for quantifying the transvalvular flow through the mitral valve based on three-directional velocity-encoded CMR was validated [30].

Accordingly, imaging is needed to determine the presence, aetiology, and severity of mitral regurgitation, which in turn decides on the planning of surgical procedures.

Is cardiac resynchronization therapy with or without ICD needed?

Selected patients with heart failure and reduced LV function benefit from either ICD and/or cardiac resynchronization therapy (CRT). According to the guidelines, a cut-off value for LV ejection fraction is used (among other criteria) to select candidates for ICD and/or CRT [23] (➲Chapter 23). Imaging is thus needed to provide the LV ejection fraction in these patients, and all imaging modalities can provide this information (see earlier sections).

With CRT, it has been shown that 30–40% of patients do not respond to therapy, and additional criteria (beyond heart failure New York Heart Association (NYHA) class III–IV, LV ejection fraction <35% and QRS duration >120ms) are needed. In order to improve the response rate of patients treated with CRT, imaging can provide information on mechanical dyssynchrony, viability, and cardiac venous anatomy [31]. Implementation of these parameters may eventually improve patient response. Mechanical dyssynchrony refers to differences in timing of activation between the right and the left ventricle (interventricular dyssynchrony) or between the LV segments (intraventricular dyssynchrony). Various echocardiographic methods and parameters have been proposed to quantify dyssynchrony including conventional pulsed-wave Doppler, M-mode echocardiography, and tissue Doppler imaging (TDI) (➲Fig. 3.10A) [32]. In numerous non-randomized single-centre studies, intraventricular dyssynchrony before CRT implantation was important to predict CRT response in terms of improvement in symptoms, functional capacity, and LV reverse remodelling [33]. There is however no consensus on which parameter to use in clinical practice, and modest accuracy to predict outcome was reported in the first multicentre trial [34]. It was evident that the community needs better training in assessment of cardiac dyssynchrony (as reflected in the modest inter- and intra-observer agreement for echo measurements of dyssynchrony), but also more accurate techniques are needed for dyssynchrony assessment. Novel techniques such as speckle-tracking (to analyze radial strain; ➲Fig. 3.10B), and 3D echocardiography (to analyze cardiac dyssynchrony; ➲Fig. 3.7D) have shown

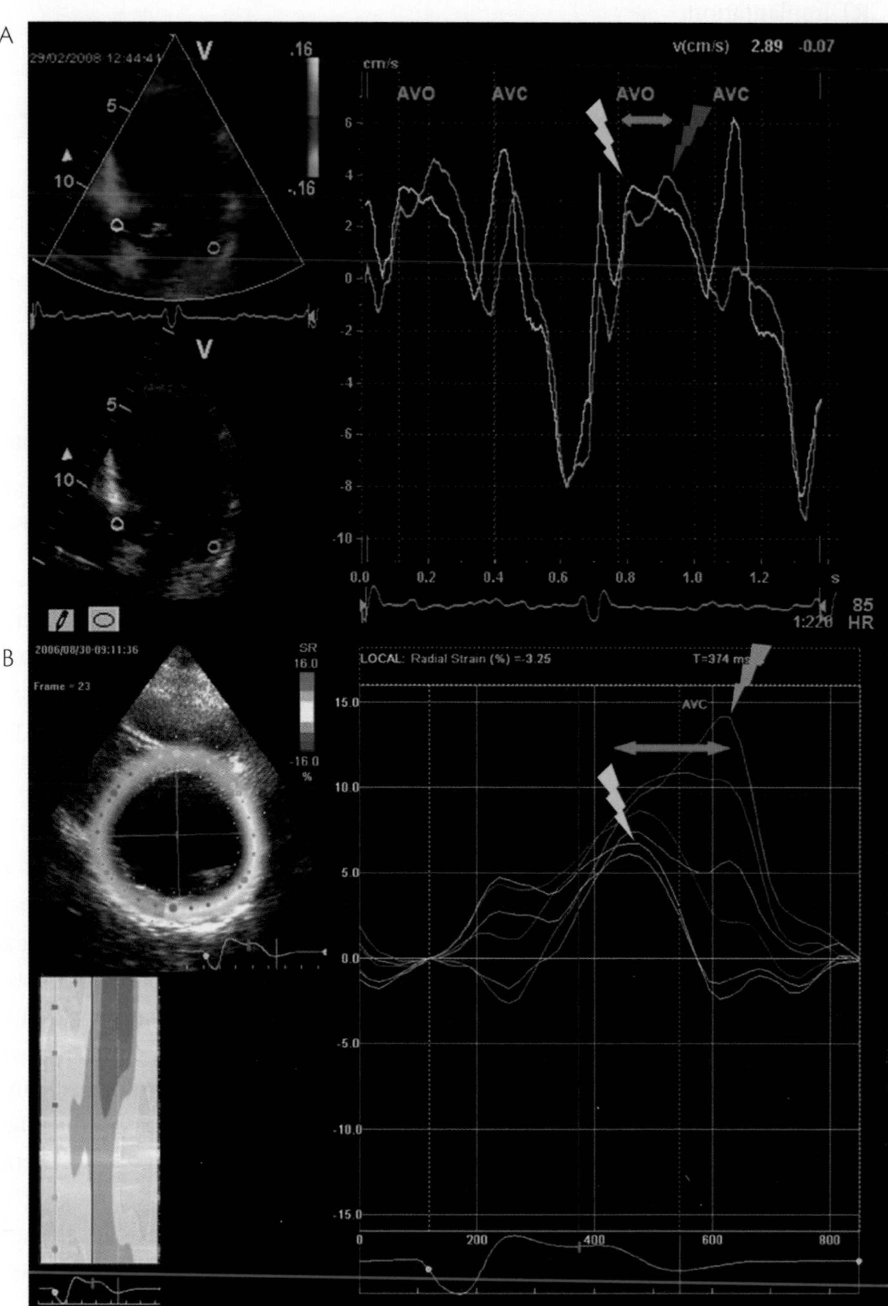

Figure 3.10 (A) Myocardial velocity curves of the septum (yellow) and lateral (green) myocardial wall derived from colour-coded tissue Doppler imaging. There is a significant difference between the peak myocardial systolic velocities of the septum and lateral wall (>65ms) indicating significant intra-ventricular dyssynchrony. (B) Radial strain curves derived from speckle tracking of a LV short-axis standard two-dimensional echocardiogram. There is a significant time delay (>130ms) between the anteroseptal (yellow) and posterior (pink) segments indicating significant intra-ventricular dyssynchrony.

promising preliminary results to predict CRT response [35, 36]. These techniques also allow identification of the area of latest mechanical activation; it has been shown that pacing of this area is probably needed for best response to CRT, and thus this area may be used for LV lead positioning [37]. In that respect, information on venous anatomy is important, and this can be provided by MSCT. In the absence of veins in the area of latest mechanical activation, transvenous LV lead implantation may be avoided and surgical implantation may be preferred. Generally, cardiac veins are widely distributed, but after large infarctions, cardiac veins tend to be absent in the infarct zone; accordingly, these patients may be considered for imaging of venous anatomy prior to CRT implantation.

Imaging of scar tissue in the LV is also important; it has been shown that patients with scar tissue in the region of the LV pacing lead or large amounts of scar tissue in general do not respond to CRT. All imaging techniques can provide information on scar tissue, but CMR may be preferred, since the high spatial resolution permits for differentiation of transmural and subendocardial scar tissue.

In summary, for optimal prediction of response to CRT, additional information beyond classic selection criteria is probably needed. This can be obtained by multi-modality imaging, integrating information on dyssynchrony, area of latest activation, viability, and venous anatomy (➲Fig. 3.11).

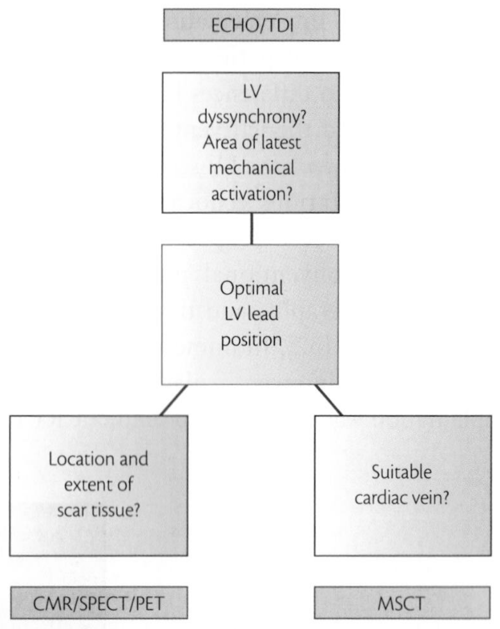

Figure 3.11 Cardiac imaging can provide additional information beyond classic selection criteria to improve CRT response. Presence of intraventricular dyssynchrony as well as site of latest activation can be assessed with echocardiography including tissue Doppler imaging (TDI). For evaluation of extent and location of scar tissue and viable myocardium, nuclear imaging or CMR can be used, whereas MSCT can be of value evaluating venous anatomy before LV lead implantation.

Which imaging technique in which patient?

The proposed five-step approach permits comprehensive assessment of the heart failure patient. In these patients, imaging will provide information on:

- aetiology of heart failure (coronary artery disease or not);
- the presence of ischaemia and viability;
- the size and shape of the LV;
- the presence and severity of mitral regurgitation;
- the need for ICD and cardiac resynchronization therapy.

Based on this comprehensive assessment, it will be possible to tailor therapy to the individual heart failure patient. It is important to realize that heart failure is such a complex disease that precise assessment is needed to provide the best therapy for each patient.

Personal perspective

The current chapter is not all encompassing regarding imaging techniques and does not provide guidelines, but rather aims to provide some practical examples on how to integrate the various imaging modalities in the management of patients. It is the task of every practising clinician to design algorithms to integrate imaging in the management of patient groups with specific cardiovascular diseases (e.g. development of appropriateness criteria), but at the same time to keep a close eye on the needs of the individual patient. Also, the concept of 'randomized controlled trials' and 'evidence-based medicine' will be difficult to apply to the use of imaging techniques considering the rapid developments and continuous changes in this particular field. How would one in the current times evaluate a patient without echocardiography? Rather, good clinical practice based on the view of a good and well-informed clinician may guide the selection and integration of imaging techniques in daily practice.

Finally, as mentioned several times in this chapter, various imaging techniques provide similar information and local availability, experience, and expertise may influence which technique is used.

Further reading

Greenland P, Bonow RO, Brundage BH, *et al.* ACCF/AHA 2007 clinical expert consensus document on coronary artery calcium scoring by computed tomography in global cardiovascular risk assessment and in evaluation of patients with chest pain: a report of the American College of Cardiology Foundation Clinical Expert Consensus Task Force (ACCF/AHA Writing Committee to Update the 2000 Expert Consensus Document on Electron Beam Computed Tomography) developed in collaboration with the Society of Atherosclerosis Imaging and Prevention and the Society of Cardiovascular Computed Tomography. *J Am Coll Cardiol* 2007; **49**: 378–402.

Hendel RC, Patel MR, Kramer CM, *et al.* ACCF/ACR/SCCT/SCMR/ASNC/NASCI/SCAI/SIR 2006 appropriateness criteria for cardiac computed tomography and cardiac magnetic resonance imaging: a report of the American College of Cardiology Foundation Quality Strategic Directions Committee Appropriateness Criteria Working Group, American College of Radiology, Society of Cardiovascular Computed Tomography, Society for Cardiovascular Magnetic Resonance, American Society of Nuclear Cardiology, North American Society for Cardiac Imaging, Society for Cardiovascular Angiography and Interventions, and Society of Interventional Radiology. *J Am Coll Cardiol* 2006; **48**: 1475–97.

Kirkpatrick JN, Vannan MA, Narula J, *et al.* Echocardiography in heart failure: applications, utility, and new horizons. *J Am Coll Cardiol* 2007; **50**: 381–96.

O'Hanlon R, Prasad SK, Pennell DJ. Evaluation of nonischemic cardiomyopathies using cardiovascular magnetic resonance. *J Nucl Cardiol* 2008; **15**: 400–16.

Schroeder S, Achenbach S, Bengel F, *et al.* Cardiac computed tomography: indications, applications, limitations, and training requirements: report of a Writing Group deployed by the Working Group Nuclear Cardiology and Cardiac CT of the European Society of Cardiology and the European Council of Nuclear Cardiology. *Eur Heart J* 2008; **29**: 531–56.

Ypenburg C, Westenberg JJ, Bleeker GB, *et al.* Noninvasive imaging in cardiac resynchronization therapy – part 1: selection of patients. *Pacing Clin Electrophysiol* 2008; **31**: 1475–99.

Additional online material

- 3.1 Suspicion of heavy trabeculations in the left ventricular apex on two-dimensional echocardiography.
- 3.2 Intravenous contrast shows the endocardial layer with trabeculations and deep recesses confirming non-compaction cardiomyopathy.
- 3.3 Conventional echocardiography showing marked dilatation of the right ventricle.
- 3.4 Intravenous contrast demonstrating small aneurysms in the basal part of the right ventricle suggestive of arrhythmogenic right ventricular cardiomyopathy.
- 3.5 Example of a three-dimensional transoesophageal echocardiographic dataset illustrating prolapse of both mitral leaflets.

For full references and multimedia materials please visit the online version of the book (http://esctextbook.oxfordonline.com).

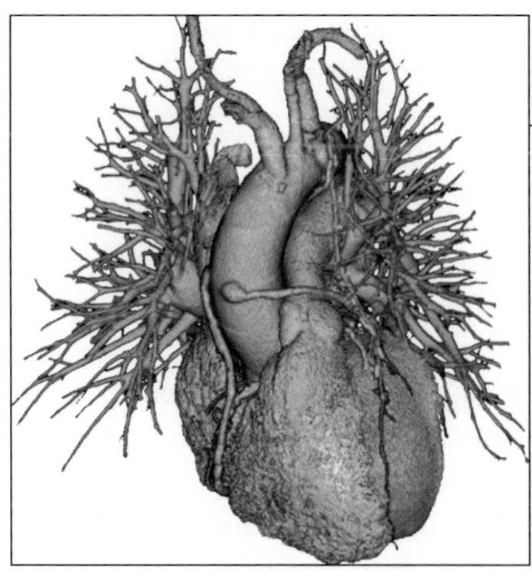

CHAPTER 4

Cardiac Ultrasound

Frank A. Flachskampf, Jens-Uwe Voigt, and Werner G. Daniel

Contents

Summary

Cardiac ultrasound, or echocardiography, is by far the most extensively used imaging modality for the diagnosis of cardiovascular disease. Two- and three-dimensional real-time echocardiography provide comprehensive cardiac morphology at very high spatial (with good images, <1mm) and temporal (>100 frames/s) resolution. Moreover, Doppler and speckle tracking techniques are able to measure the local velocity of blood flow and of the myocardium throughout the heart, thus allowing blood flow analysis in valvular lesions (stenosis or regurgitation) and shunt lesions, as well as analysis of motion and deformation of the myocardium, enabling detection of functional abnormalities, e.g. in the presence of ischaemia or cardiomyopathy. Echocardiography is non-invasive and devoid of ionizing radiation; the hardware is mobile and ideal for bedside use. For special purposes, ultrasound imaging can also be performed semi-invasively via the oesophagus or invasively via the vessels. Further refinements include its application during stress, in particular to elicit an ischaemic myocardial response, and with right and left heart contrast. Because of its ubiquitous availability, lack of untoward biologic effects, relatively low cost, and unparalleled diagnostic power, it is the first-line imaging approach in cardiology and indicated in practically all cardiovascular diseases.

Physical and technical principles of echocardiography

Principles of echocardiographic imaging and velocity assessment by Doppler and speckle tracking

Sound is an audible pressure wave which transmits pressure energy through media such as air or water. As a wave, it can be characterized by the parameters wavelength λ (in length units, e.g. mm or μm), frequency f (in 1/s, or Hz), and velocity of propagation c (in m/s; ➲Fig. 4.1); these parameters have the relation:

$$c = f \times \lambda$$

Sound waves with frequencies above the audible range (>20,000Hz) are denominated ultrasound. The velocity of sound in water is 1540m/s, much faster than in air, and this velocity is assumed when ultrasound travels in biologic tissue. Diagnostic ultrasound utilizes frequencies typically in the range of 2–7MHz (1MHz = 10^6Hz), with corresponding wavelengths of 0.8–0.2mm; intravascular ultrasound catheters use frequencies up to 40MHz (➲Table 4.1). The energy of a sound wave is characterized as ultrasound intensity per unit area (in W/cm^2) where the area is positioned orthogonal to the propagation direction of the sound wave. Diagnostic ultrasound machines are set to operate at sound intensities

Table 4.1 Typical diagnostic ultrasound frequencies

Audible sound: <20kHz (1kHz = 10^3Hz)
Transthoracic echocardiography: 2–3MHz (1MHz = 10^6Hz)
Transoesophageal echocardiography: 5–7MHz
Intravascular ultrasound: 40MHz
Acoustic microscopy: 100–1000MHz

which are considered biologically safe. Since intensity is not easy to measure in tissue, a surrogate parameter of ultrasound intensity is mandatorily displayed on echo machines, the 'Mechanical Index'. This is the dimensionless ratio of peak rarefactional pressure (in megapascal, MPa) divided by the square root of the carrier frequency (in MHz), which should not exceed the value of 2 for diagnostic purposes.

When ultrasound is transmitted through tissue, several interactions take place:

- Pressure energy is dissipated (mainly into heat), and the intensity of ultrasound decreases with progressive distance from the ultrasound source; this process is called attenuation and increases with ultrasound frequency. Thus, lower frequencies suffer less attenuation per travelled distance unit and are more suitable to image deep structures than higher frequencies.
- When ultrasound strikes the interface between media of different acoustic properties, several interactions are possible (➲Fig. 4.2): if the media are acoustically very

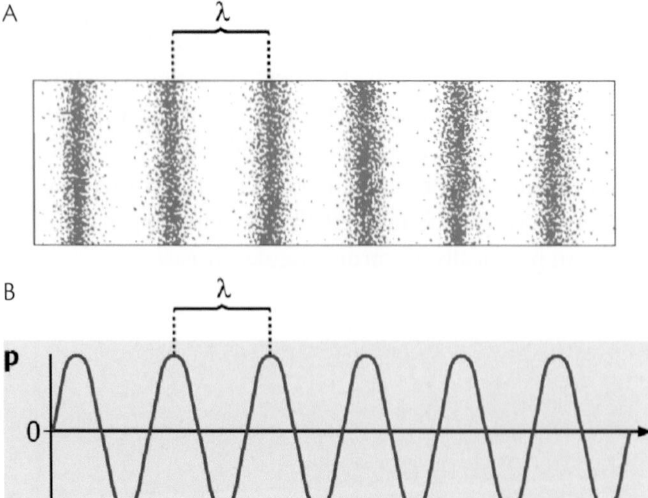

Figure 4.1 Schematic representation of a sound wave. Top image: zones of compression (high pressure) and of rarefaction (low pressure) alternate; the distance between two pressure peaks is one wavelength (λ). Lower image: the course of pressure (on the y-axis) over distance (on the x-axis) can be represented as a sine wave. A similar wave would represent pressure over time at a fixed location; the time interval of two pressure peaks would be 1/f with f for frequency. Modified with permission from Weyman AE. *Principles and Practice of Echocardiography*, 2nd edn., 1994. Philadelphia, PA: Lea & Febiger.

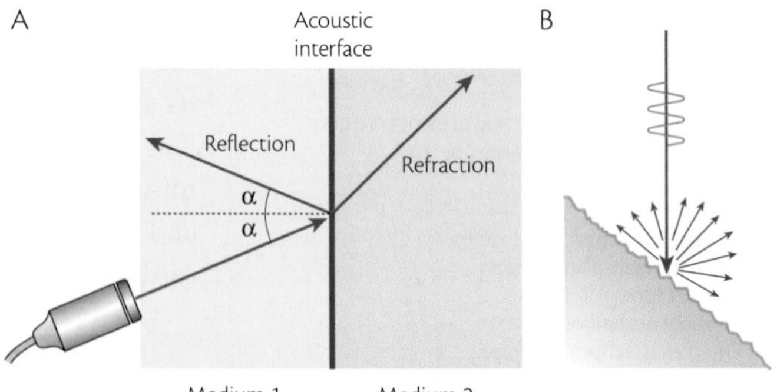

Figure 4.2 Reflexion, refraction, and scattering of sound. All of these processes take place when ultrasound interacts with tissue. (A) If a sound wave hits a large interface where acoustic impedances suddenly changes (a reflector), sound is partially reflected in a direction which depends on the angle of incidence. The amount of reflected energy increases with increasing difference in acoustic impedances of the two media forming the interface. Another part of the sound wave energy proceeds into the second medium, but the direction of propagation is changed. This is called refraction. (B) If the reflector size is in the range of the sound wave's wavelength or the interface is 'rough' (left), sound is redirected in all directions, a process called scattering. Note that some sound energy is cast back in the direction of the original source of the sound wave. Reproduced with permission from Flachskampf FA. *Kursbuch Echokardiographie*, 4th edn., 2008. Stuttgart: Thieme.

different, like air and water (technically, this difference is quantified as 'acoustic impedance'), reflection occurs, meaning that the ultrasound is not transmitted further but sent back from the interface at an angle depending on the angle of incidence. Reflection can be total or partial. If the interface (the 'reflector') is small, i.e. of a size comparable with the wavelength of the sound, a process called scattering occurs, where instead of unidirectional reflection ultrasound is redirected into many directions ('scattered'). In the body, all of these sound–tissue interactions can occur, with a multitude of tissue reflectors creating complex wave interactions which form the basis for the 'echo texture' or 'speckle pattern' of a tissue.

- Passage of ultrasound through tissue creates a subtle distortion of the waveform which can be understood as the addition of 'harmonic frequencies' (double, thrice, etc., the original transmitted frequency) to the original 'fundamental' frequency. These 'harmonics', while weak in intensity, can be extracted from the reflected ultrasound signal and are used in ultrasound imaging to improve signal-to-noise ratio, since they are less prone to near-field artefacts and other factors detrimental to image quality.
- When a sound wave is reflected by a moving reflector, the reflected wave undergoes a shift in frequency which is proportional to the reflector's velocity relative to the ultrasound source. This effect, named after the Austrian physicist Christian Doppler, allows measurement of the velocity of moving blood or tissue in the heart by analyzing the frequency shift Δf of reflected ultrasound. The relation involved, the 'Doppler equation', is

$$\Delta f = 2 \times f \times v/c$$

where f is the carrier frequency emitted by the transducer, c the velocity of sound propagation in tissue, and v the velocity of the moving reflector (towards or away from the transducer). The velocity v of the moving reflector relative to the sound source (in practice, the transducer)

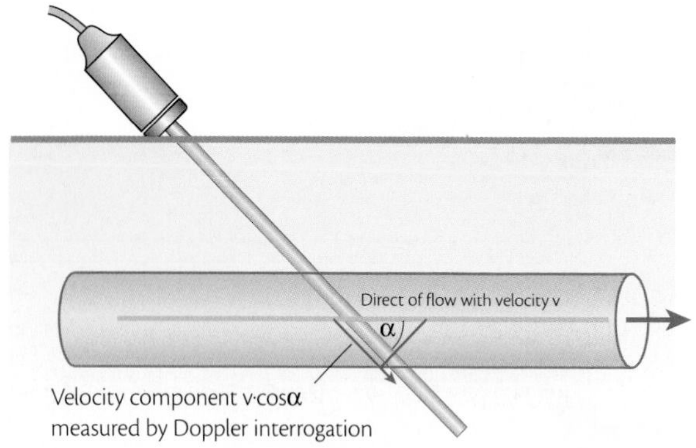

Figure 4.3 Angle dependency of Doppler interrogation of flow velocity. If the interrogating ultrasound beam and the direction of blood flow are at an angle α, the velocity calculated from the Doppler shift vDOPP only represents the magnitude of the partial vector parallel to the ultrasound beam. Thus, non-coaxial velocities are underestimated. Adapted with permission from Flachskampf FA. *Kursbuch Echokardiographie*, 4th edn., 2008. Stuttgart: Thieme.

can therefore be calculated from the frequency shift and the known velocity of sound in tissue. However, the calculated velocity depends on the angle in which the velocity vector is oriented compared to the ultrasound beam (➲Fig. 4.3). Since only the velocity towards or away from the transducer is calculated correctly from the Doppler equation, velocities not aligned with the ultrasound beam will be measured falsely too low. The measured velocity vDOPP differs from the true velocity vTRUE by

$$\text{vDOPP} = \text{vTRUE} \times \cos\alpha$$

where α is the angle between true velocity vector and ultrasound beam direction. Importantly, Doppler measurement of velocities works for both the very weak, but comparatively fast-moving reflections from blood (typical normal velocities <1.5m/s) and the strong, comparatively slow-moving reflections from heart tissue, especially the myocardium (typical normal velocities <15cm/s; ➲Fig. 4.4). Blood flow Doppler and tissue Doppler signals can be selectively recorded and displayed by appropriate use of electronic filters and thresholds.

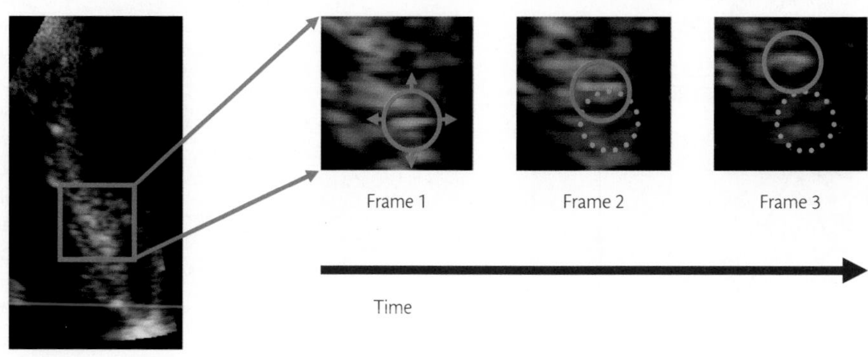

Figure 4.4 Principle of speckle tracking: features of the image are detected and tracked frame by frame. From the measured displacement of the features and the known frame rate, amplitude and direction within the image plane can be calculated, and from these velocity and deformation parameters of the myocardium can be derived.

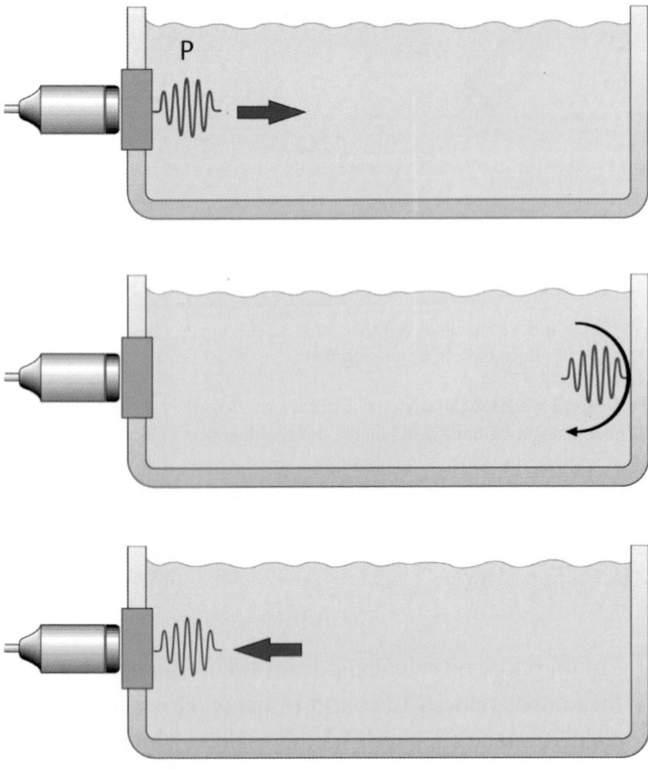

Figure 4.5 Principle of depth measurement by pulsed ultrasound. In this schematic example, the pulse P, a short ultrasound wave train generated by a short burst of activity of the transducer, is reflected by the wall of the container at the far right and returns to the transducer after a measurable time interval T. Since sound propagation velocity c is known, this allows calculation of the distance of the reflector as c × T/2. Modified with permission from Weyman AE. *Principles and Practice of Echocardiography*, 2nd edn., 1994. Philadelphia, PA: Lea & Febiger.

- Measurements of blood flow velocity are crucial in the assessment of valvular disease, allowing detection and (semi-)quantitation of valvular stenosis, stroke volume, regurgitation, shunts, and others. Tissue velocities, on the other hand, contain information on myocardial function which can be further refined by analyzing regional deformation. Recently, measurement of velocities in tissue by a different technique has become available, so-called 'speckle tracking', where tissue texture ('speckle') patterns are tracked from two-dimensional frame to two-dimensional frame, yielding the translation of a given set of reflectors from one frame to the next, thus also allowing calculation of motion and velocity (➲Fig. 4.4). This technique, while still in its infancy, is angle-independent and may in the future be extended to blood velocity measurements.

Technical equipment for echocardiography

In echo machines, focused ultrasound is emitted from a transducer, an instrument containing an array of piezoelectric elements ('crystals'), which transform electromagnetic waves into ultrasound waves and vice versa. The ultrasound transducer both generates and receives ultrasound waves. Echocardiography uses ultrasound pulses, meaning that ultrasound emission occurs during a very short period, followed by a period in which the transducer is 'listening' to returning, reflected ultrasound. Since the speed of sound is known, the amount of time that it takes for an ultrasound pulse to strike a reflector in the tissue and to return to the transducer defines the distance of this reflector from the transducer (➲Fig. 4.5). This principle allows the construction of images. One piezoelectric element or crystal can only generate a one-dimensional representation of reflectors along the direction of the emitted ultrasound wave. This is the principle of the oldest form of echocardiography, the M-mode (M for motion, if displayed over time), which nowadays is still often used for linear measurements (➲Fig. 4.6). The typical two-dimensional echocardiographic image today is generated by

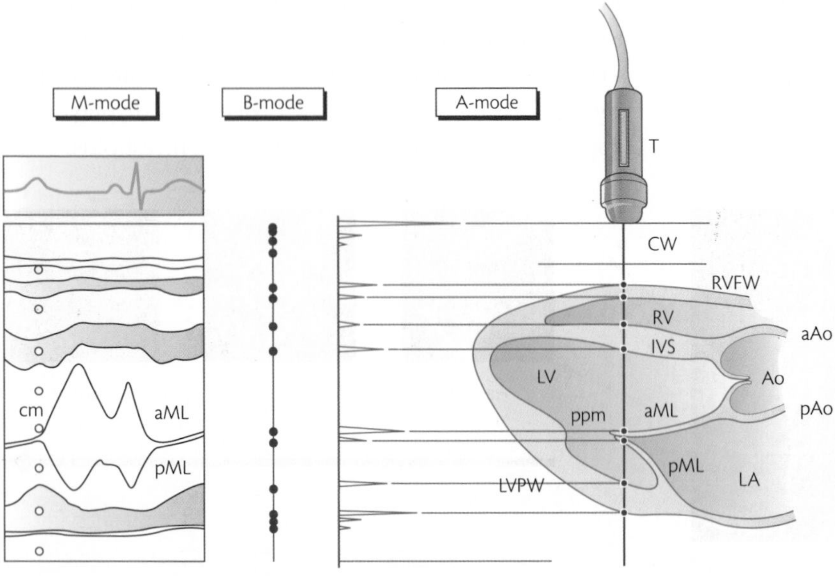

Figure 4.6 Schematic diagram showing the creation of the M-mode echocardiogram. A long-axis cross-section of the heart from base to apex with cardiac structures is shown. The single sound beam produced by the transducer (T) on the chest wall (CW) is aimed so that it traverses from anterior to posterior: right ventricular free wall (RVFW), right ventricle (RV), interventricular septum (IVS), left ventricular cavity (LV), anterior and posterior mitral valve leaflets (aML and pML) and the posterior wall (LVPW). The echoes originating from the structure boundaries can be represented in three types of oscilloscope display: A-mode, B-mode and M-mode. Ao, aorta; LA, left atrium; aAo and pAo, anterior and posterior aortic wall; ppm, posteromedial papillary muscle.

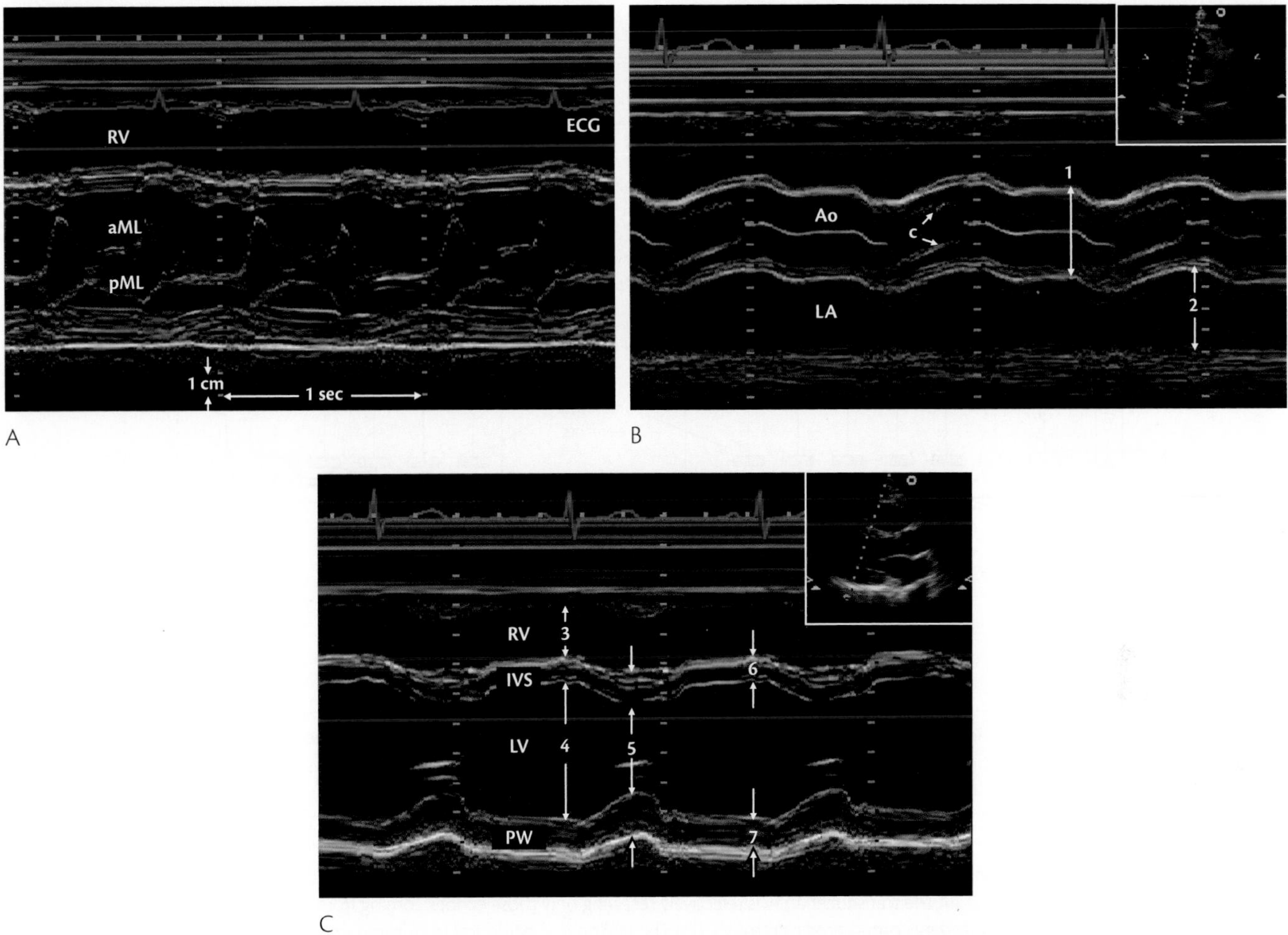

Figure 4.7 (A) M-mode registration of a normal subject showing the structures discussed in ➲ Fig. 4.6. The anterior mitral valve leaflet moves anteriorly and the posterior leaflet posteriorly with less excursion but a similar pattern. The recording speed is 50mm/s. The calibration scale of depth is in centimetres from top to bottom and time in seconds from left to right. (B) Two-dimensional reference image shows the cursor indicating the direction of the sampling sound beam in the short-axis view through the base of the aorta and aortic valve. The aorta (Ao) is seen as two parallel structures moving in an anterior direction in systole. The aortic valve cusps (c) are open in systole and are seen as a single echo when closed in diastole, with the same motion as the aortic walls. The left atrium (LA) is posterior to the aorta. Arrows 1 and 2 indicate the landmarks for diameter measurements. (C) M-mode registration of the left ventricle (LV) at the tips of the mitral valve leaflets showing inward motion of the interventricular septum (IVS) and posterior wall (PW) in systole. The cursor in the two-dimensional image shows the direction of the sampling sound beam. The arrows indicate landmarks for diameter measurements of the right ventricle (RV) (3), left ventricular end-diastolic diameter (4), left ventricular end-systolic diameter (5), interventricular septal thickness (6), and posterior wall thickness (7). (Courtesy of J. Roelandt and R. Erbel).

a multitude of near-simultaneously firing crystals, a 'two-dimensional array' of typically 64–96 elements. This allows steering the resulting ultrasound beam electronically so that an image sector is created successively, which provides an accurate tomographic image of the scanned structure, i.e. the heart (➲ Figs. 4.7–4.9). The electromagnetic waveforms generated by the piezoelectric elements of the transducer in response to the received ultrasound echoes are called the radiofrequency signal; these waveforms are digitally processed in several steps (envelope detection, compression, scan conversion) to finally generate digital images in the DICOM (Digital Images and Communication in Medicine) format, which is adhered to by all manufacturers (for more detail see [1, 2]). All of this happens fast enough to allow creation of real-time tomographic images of the heart at frame rates >100/s, a temporal resolution unmatched by any other cardiac imaging modality.

Currently in early clinical use are transthoracic and transoesophageal transducers generating three-dimensional images from two-dimensional piezoelectric element arrays ('matrix arrays' of several thousand single elements), which capture a whole three-dimensional, pyramidal data set (also called 'volume data set') in real time. This data set can be sliced and cropped off-line at will, similar to data sets from other tomographic techniques such as magnetic resonance or computed tomography (➲ Fig. 4.10; 🎥 4.1).

Besides morphologic imaging, echocardiography provides data on motion of cardiac structures and derived parameters.

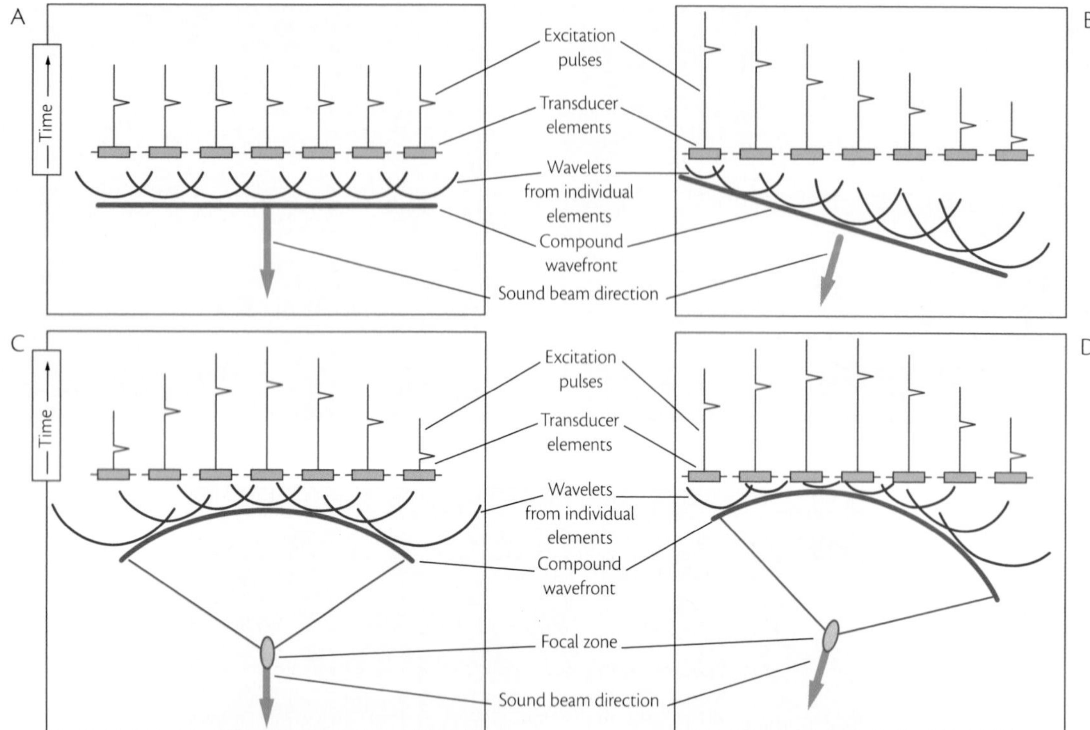

Figure 4.8 The concept of electronic beam steering. (A) Seven elements of a phased-array transducer firing simultaneously. A short distance from the transducer the individual wavelets from each of the elements merge to produce a compound wavefront, which creates a sound beam in the direction perpendicular to the transducer face. (B) The elements are now fired in sequence but are all used to create a single sound beam. When the individual wavelets merge to form a compound wavefront, it is not perpendicular and the sound beam travels away at an angle. Varying the excitation sequence allows rapid steering of a sound beam in any direction through a sector. (C) Electronic beam focusing is realized by exciting the peripheral elements first and the centre element last (cylindrical time-gated excitation). In addition to focusing the transmitted sound beam, it is also possible to focus the returning signals so that at any one instant the transducer array is selectively receiving only those echoes coming from a specified beam direction and depth (dynamic receive focusing). This requires very complicated electronics. (D) The principle of cylindrical time-gated excitation can be used to steer and focus sound beams in any direction during both transmission and reception.

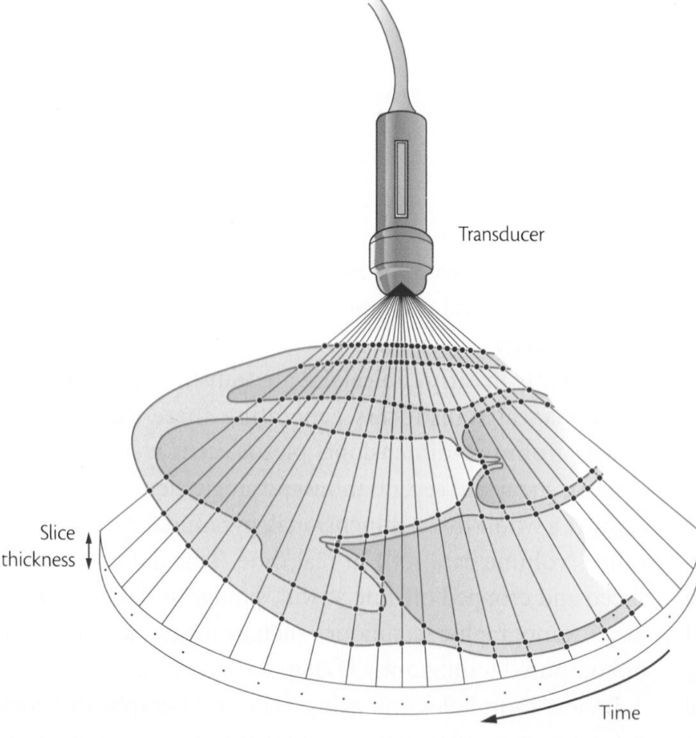

Figure 4.9 How a two-dimensional image of the heart is created. The ultrasound beam is electronically steered through a sector arc of 80° at a uniform speed at an imaging rate of 25/s. The radial scan line data from the transducer are converted into a digital memory matrix (scan converter), which can be frozen and displayed in the horizontal TV/video format. A cursor can be moved over the image to select a scan line to produce an M-mode recording (see ➲ Figs 4.6 and 4.7).

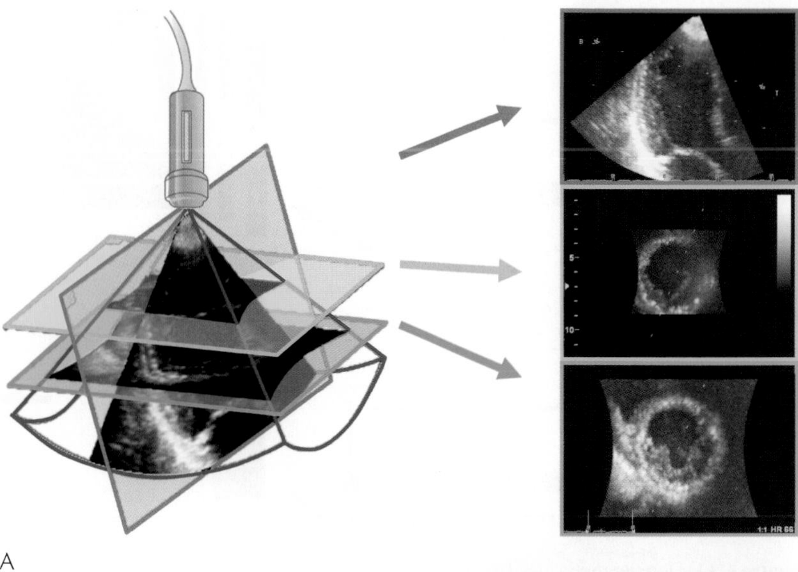

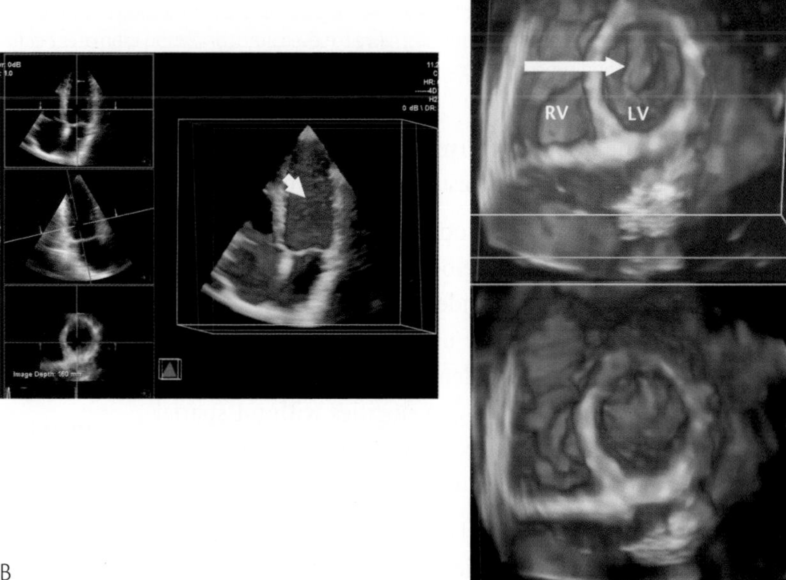

Figure 4.10 (A) Three-dimensional echocardiography. Instead of a single image plane as in two-dimensional echocardiography, a three-dimensional 'volume data set' is acquired during scanning. Different post-processing options allow visualization of the data afterwards. In this example, one basal (red rectangle) and one apical (yellow rectangle) short-axis view of the left ventricle as well as an apical long axis (red rectangle) are reconstructed from one and the same apically recorded three-dimensional volume data set. (B) Left, four-chamber view-like cut of data set; note the corrugated left ventricular endocardium in the 'depth' of the image (small arrow), which would not be visible on a two-dimensional image. Right, example of short-axis views of the left ventricle extracted from the three-dimensional data set. Arrow points at anterior mitral leaflet, which is open in the upper image and closed in the lower image. Also see 4.1.

Doppler echocardiography of blood flow velocity is of paramount importance in echocardiography for functional information, especially in valvular heart disease, shunt lesions, and for the assessment of left ventricular filling. At the core of Doppler measurements is the calculation of motion velocity of a reflector from the Doppler shift of the reflected signal; this calculation is performed by a Fourier type analysis called the fast Fourier transform, which is applied to the returning Doppler shifted ultrasound data (for more detail see [1]). The Doppler shift typically is within the audible range and can be displayed as sound by the echo machine. Note that all Doppler measurements are angle dependent such that only the velocity component parallel to the ultrasound beam is correctly measured, while velocities oblique or orthogonal to the ultrasound beam are reduced by cosine α. For measuring and displaying blood flow velocity, three Doppler modalities are used (➲Fig. 4.11):

- Pulsed-wave (PW) Doppler, which allows local interrogation of a flow field by placing a sample volume into a blood filled space, e.g. the left ventricular outflow tract. Blood flow velocities are displayed over time in a so-called spectral display with velocity on the y-axis and time (parallel to an ECG signal) on the x-axis. The integral of this curve is the velocity-time integral (unit cm). PW Doppler is limited in the maximal velocity (towards or away from the transducer) which it can unambiguously display, typically in the range of 1–2m/s; this velocity is termed the Nyquist velocity or limit. Above this velocity

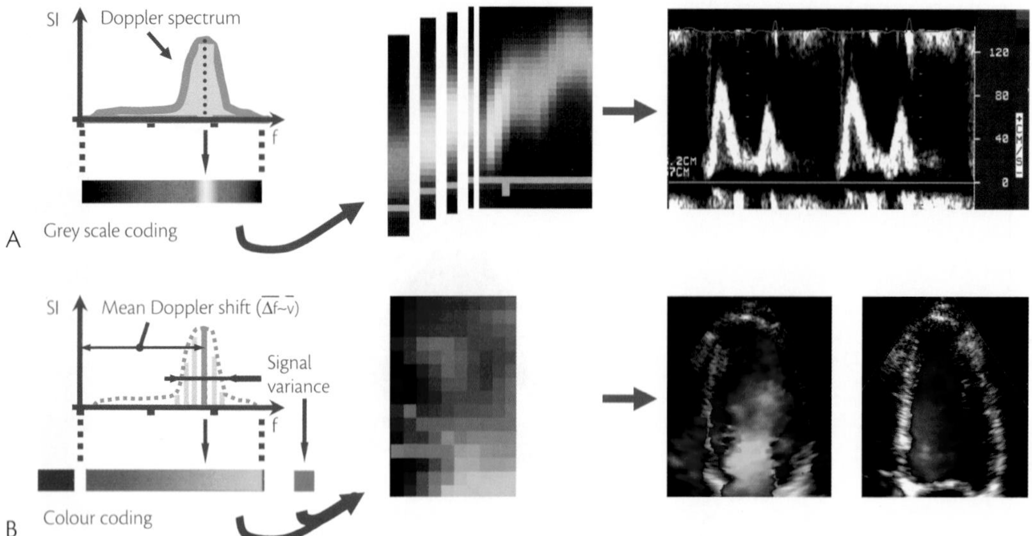

Figure 4.11 Doppler modalities. (A) Spectral Doppler analyzes the frequency shift of the echo from one sample volume position (pulsed wave Doppler, PW) or continuously and, thus, along the entire ultrasound beam (continuous wave Doppler, CW) by the 'fast Fourier transform'. The resulting spectrum of Doppler shifts is coded in shades of grey (left). If these spectra, which represent only one point in time, are added and displayed next to each other (middle), the spectral curve becomes visible (right). (B) Colour Doppler uses an autocorrelation method to estimate velocities in a great number of sample volumes in real time. Only a mean Doppler shift is obtained, calculated from five to seven autocorrelation estimates per frame and sample volume. The mean Doppler shift is then colour coded in red and blue and superimposed on the image. A high variance between the estimates is regarded as turbulence and colour coded in green.

a measurement ambiguity termed 'aliasing' occurs, which precludes unequivocally measuring higher velocities.

- Continuous-wave (CW) Doppler, which allows interrogation of blood flow velocities of all magnitudes. However, it does not allow identification of the location where they occur along the ultrasound beam. CW and PW Doppler thus are complementary, the former allowing identification of very high velocities without spatial resolution, the latter limited in velocity resolution but providing good spatial resolution.
- Colour Doppler mapping. This is a form of parametric imaging where flow velocities are coded by colours and the colour map overlaid on two- or three-dimensional images. Conventionally, red colour codes flow velocities towards the transducer and blue colour velocities away from the transducer. The velocities coded in colours are derived from multiple PW-like Doppler interrogations by a simplified analysis technique called autocorrelation.

The most important applications of blood flow velocity analysis are:

- Calculation of (maximal and mean) gradient (Δ p) across stenotic or regurgitant orifices from instantaneous velocity (v) by the simplified Bernoulli equation:

$$\Delta p = 4 \times v^2$$

and of stenotic or regurgitant orifice areas by formulae based on the conservation of mass. In spite of some limitations, this allows assessment of severity of valvular stenoses, calculation of systolic right ventricular pressure from tricuspid regurgitation, (semi-) quantitation of regurgitation severity, and other measurements.

- Visualization of regurgitant jets and of shunt lesions by colour Doppler.
- Assessment of left ventricular filling and qualitative estimation of filling pressures.

The Doppler analysis of the high-amplitude, low-velocity signals from cardiac tissue is called tissue Doppler. It is used mainly to examine myocardial function (➲Fig. 4.12). The longitudinal (apex-to-base) motion velocities of the basal segments of the left ventricle give information on global left ventricular systolic and diastolic function. Moreover, the rate of regional deformation ('strain rate', in 1/s or Hz) can be calculated from spatial velocity gradients and, by integration of strain rate over time, deformation ('strain', in per cent) itself can be computed. This deformation takes place as shortening and lengthening of the myocardium in a longitudinal direction from apical views and of thickening and thinning in a short-axis direction in parasternal views. The advantage of deformation data over velocity data lies in their truly local character, while tissue velocities are always influenced by adjacent tissue ('tethering') and translation movements (see ➲Stress echocardiography, p.112 and Left ventricular function, p.116 for more detail). Recently, deformation has also been calculated by speckle tracking of the

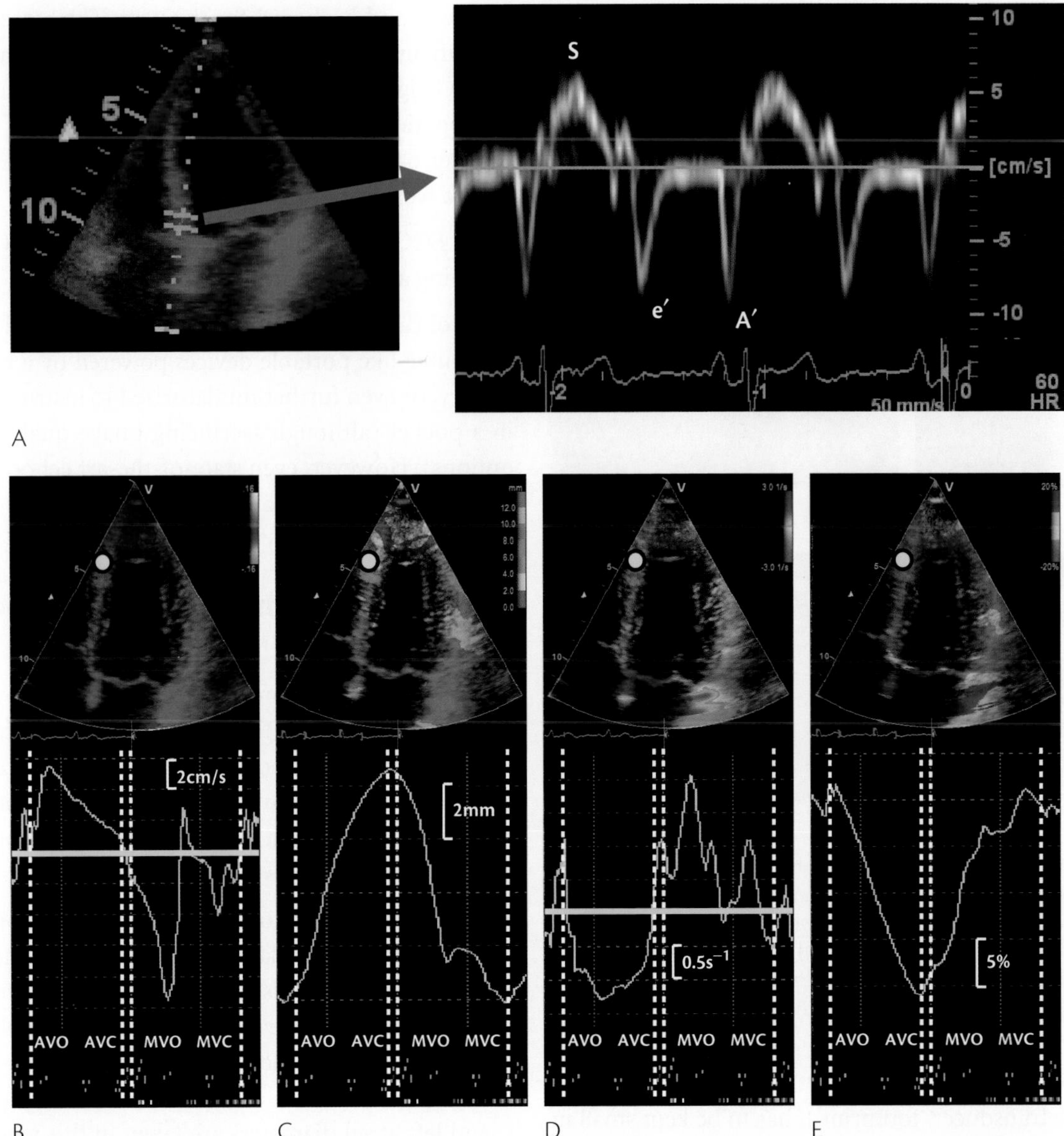

Figure 4.12 The Doppler-based tissue velocity and deformation modalities. (A) Principle of PW tissue Doppler. The myocardial velocity is measured by placing a PW Doppler sample volume in the myocardium (here: the basal septum in the four-chamber view, see tissue colour Doppler still frame on the left) while the echocardiography machine is set to tissue Doppler mode. The typical waves of the spectral tissue Doppler display are termed S for the systolic peak velocity, e′ for the early diastolic and A′ for the late diastolic velocity. (B) Velocity, (C) motion, (D) strain rate, and (D) strain recordings from the septal wall (see yellow circle for position of sample volume) of a healthy subject. The top row shows the colour Doppler maps of the respective parameters in the apical four-chamber view. The bottom row shows (normal) curves of the different parameters. ECG signal for timing; AVO, AVC, MVO, MVC denote aortic and mitral valve opening and closure, respectively.

myocardium, which is not Doppler based and thus angle independent. This technique allows measurement of regional tissue velocity, deformation, and deformation rate in all directions. Tissue velocity, strain, and strain rate can be displayed either in velocity over time graphs or as colour maps.

The echo machine

Echocardiography machines today are fully digital devices and consist essentially of the following elements (➲Fig. 4.13):

- Transducers. The typical transthoracic transducer operates with 'broad-band' frequency, i.e. with a range of frequencies and uses at least partially the harmonic frequencies of the reflected ultrasound to generate imaging information. It is able to produce M-mode and two-dimensional imaging, as well as incorporating all Doppler modalities (blood flow as well as tissue Doppler). The transducer surface emitting the ultrasound, which is in contact with the patient during the echocardiography

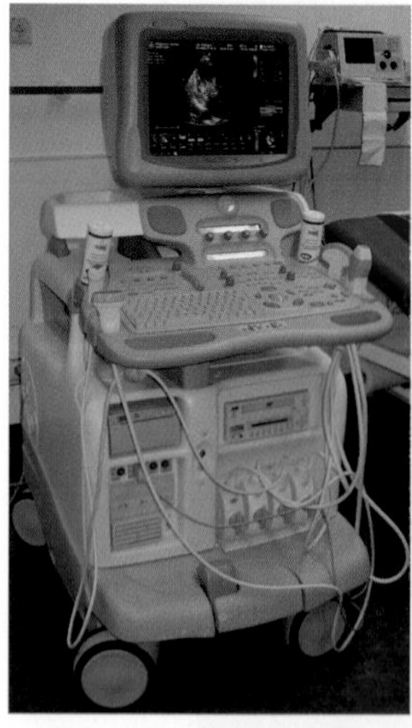
A

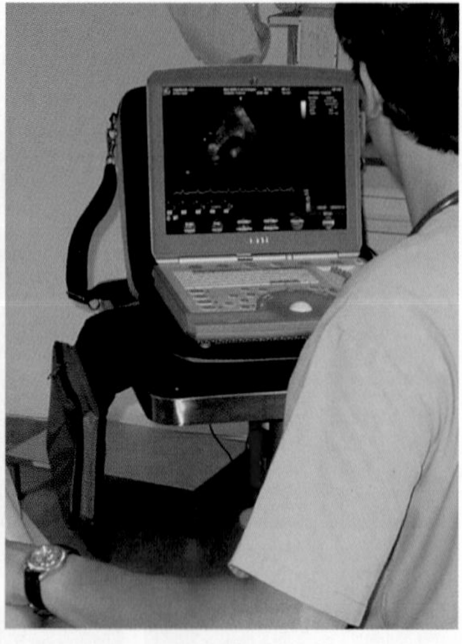
B

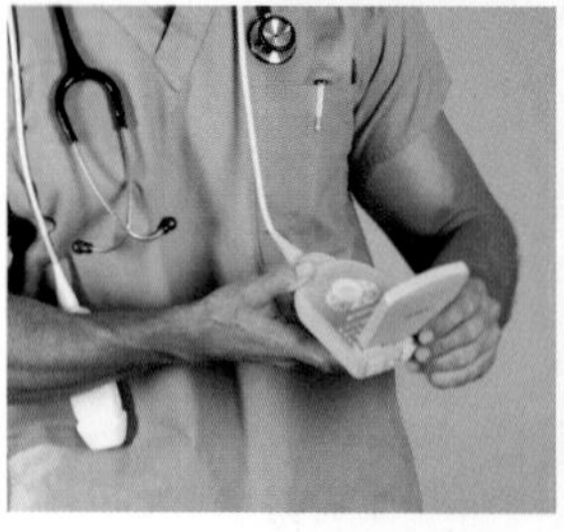
C

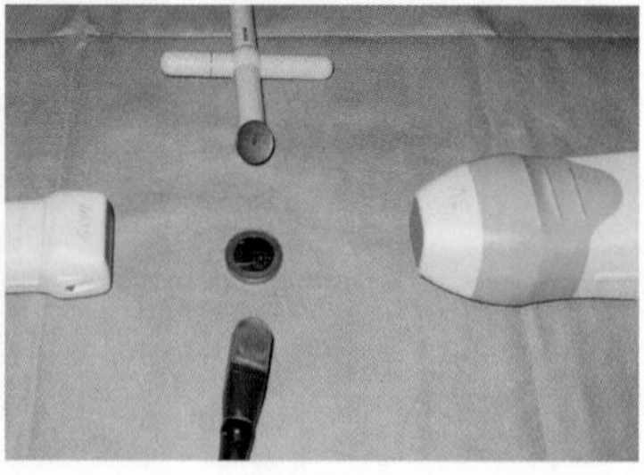
D

Figure 4.13 The diversity of echocardiographic equipment. (A) State-of-the-art echocardiography machine with screen, controls, keyboard, several transducers, video recorder and printer, and wheels. (B) Laptop-type echo machine. (C) Palmtop-type echo machine. (D) Transducers with €1 coin for size comparison: left, standard transthoracic transducer, right, transthoracic 3D matrix array, transducer, bottom, standard 2D transoesophageal probe tip, top, dedicated CW Doppler probe.

exam (the transducer 'footprint'), has to be kept small in order to fit into the intercostal spaces. Separate, dedicated three-dimensional transducers or small probes exclusively for CW Doppler are also in use. Inside a transducer lies a stacked array of piezoelectric crystals which transform ultrasound waves into electromagnetic waves. Focusing of the ultrasound beam, crucial for image quality, is achieved by acoustic lenses and electronic measures. Ultrasound gel is necessary to achieve acoustic coupling between the transducer surface and the skin of the patient.

- A computer to process the electromagnetic waveforms arriving from the transducer and generating images, graphs, and other displays.
- Digital storage capacity (hard disk) and/or interfaces to export digital data to a network and remote mass storage or to removable storage devices such as magneto-optical discs; in addition, most machines still have hard-copy printers and video recorders.
- Screen and keyboard for the user. The screen is usually configurable and contains the image sector as well as an ECG signal for timing, a clock, and identification data for patient and hospital. Detailed analysis of images and other data is often performed off-line after acquisition on a workstation.
- An ECG cable to provide a single-lead ECG signal for timing and monitoring purposes.

All of this equipment can now be condensed into laptop computer-like portable devices powered by a rechargeable battery, or even further miniaturized to instruments that fit in a pocket (although sacrificing image quality and some options). However, even state-of-the-art echocardiography machines have wheels and can be rolled to the bedside of an intensive or emergency care patient.

Transthoracic echocardiography and the standard exam

Echocardiography is routinely performed as a transthoracic exam. In the course of this exam, several 'echocardiography windows' are utilized to give the transducer access to heart. These echocardiography windows vary from person to person somewhat in location and therefore are only broadly defined (➲Fig. 4.14; 🎥 4.2–4.7). They include

- A parasternal window, at the left sternal border, with the patient in a left lateral decubitus position; important views (cross-sections) are the parasternal long-axis view of the left ventricle and several parasternal short-axis views of left ventricle and basal cardiac structures; linear measurements such as left ventricular diameters, aortic and left atrial diameters are taken in this view, either by M-mode or from two-dimensional images.
- An apical window, in the region of the apical cardiac impulse, with the patient in the left lateral decubitus position slightly reclined to their back; typical views are the apical four-chamber, two-chamber, and the long-axis views.
- A subcostal window at the subxyphoidal angle beneath the ribcage, with the patient lying on their back; subcostal four-chamber views, as well as long-axis and short-axis views can be obtained.
- A suprasternal window at the suprasternal notch, with the patient on their back with their head angled backwards. This window is insufficient in many patients. The thoracic aorta, especially the aortic arch, can be visualized from here.
- A right parasternal window is sometimes used for Doppler interrogation of the aortic valve.

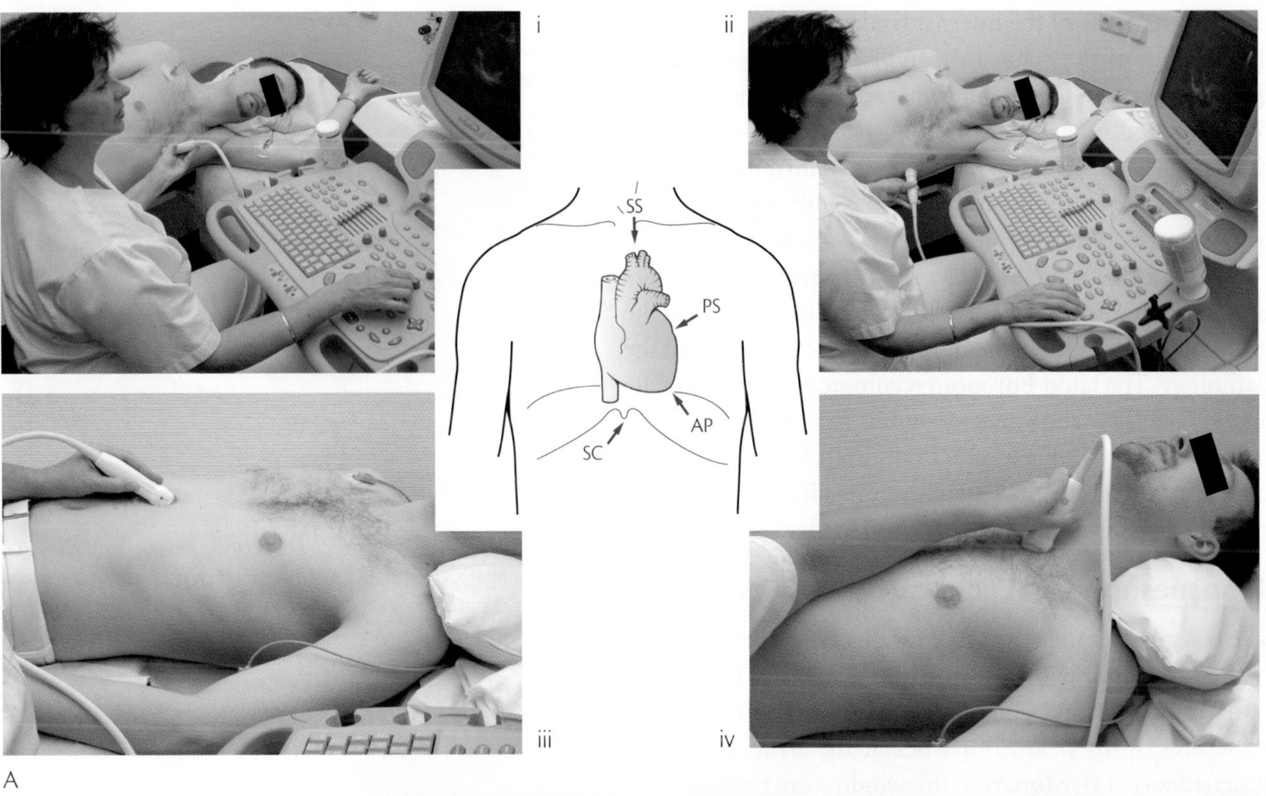

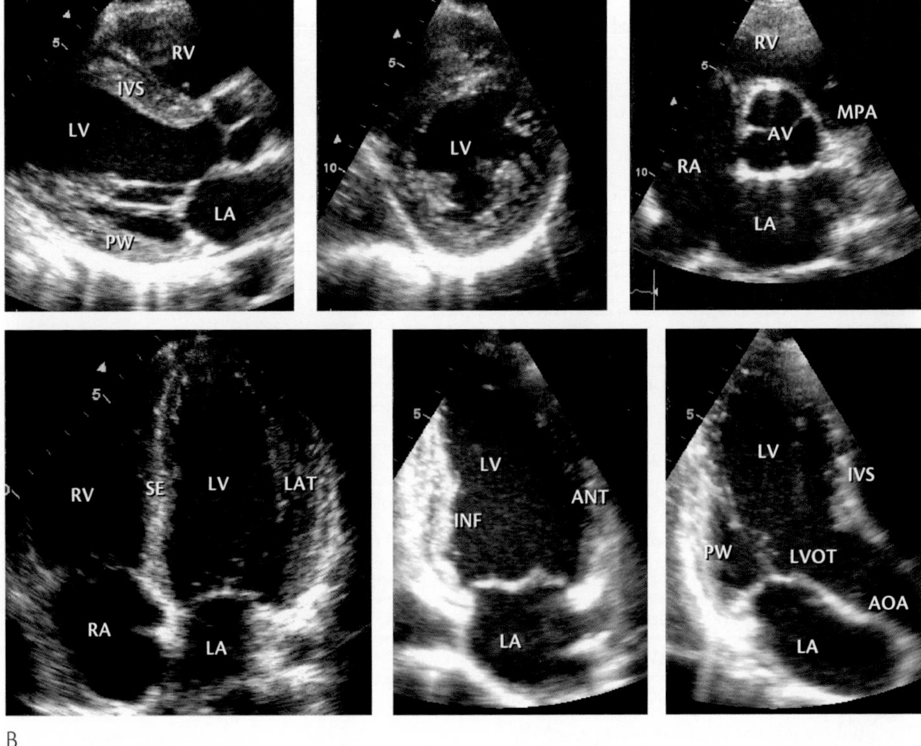

Figure 4.14 (A) Routinely used echocardiographic windows: i) parasternal (PS); ii) apical (AP); iii) subcostal (SC); iv) suprasternal (SS). Note different patient positioning for each window. (Courtesy of J. Roelandt and R. Erbel). (B) Selection of normal standard echocardiographic views. Top row, left: parasternal long-axis view, middle: parasternal short-axis view at mid-papillary muscle level, right: parasternal short-axis view at aortic valve level. Bottom row, left: apical four-chamber view, middle: apical two-chamber view, right: apical long-axis view. AOA ascending aorta; AW anterior wall; INF inferior wall; IVS anterior ventricular septum; LA left atrium; LAT lateral wall; LV left ventricle; LVOT left ventricular outflow tract; MPA main pulmonary artery; PW posterior wall; RA right atrium; RV right ventricle; SE (inferior) septum. Also see 4.2–4.7.

The examiner sits at the right or left side of the patient, with one hand holding the transducer and the other hand operating the control settings, while concentrating on the screen of the echocardiography machine. It is important to understand that the standard views and signals obtained during an echocardiography examination are largely defined by internal landmarks, e.g. for the apical four-chamber view the visualization of a maximal long axis of the left ventricle with maximal diameter of the mitral and tricuspid annulus; the external location and position of the transducer follows the requirements of the internal landmarks, not vice versa. The quality of the echocardiography recordings depends both on patient and examiner characteristics. Patients with hyperinflated lungs (e.g. suffering from obstructive lung disease or on a ventilator), with chest deformities, or very obese patients are difficult to examine, although in practically all patients at least one window is usable.

The sequence and typical elements of a standard echocardiography exam are given in ➲Table 4.2. The duration of the exam depends on the difficulty of image generation and the pathology. The latest European recommendations stipulate an average time allowance of 30min per exam, including report writing [3]. Each echo exam must be recorded permanently, preferentially digitally or on videotape, with representative recordings from all acquired views.

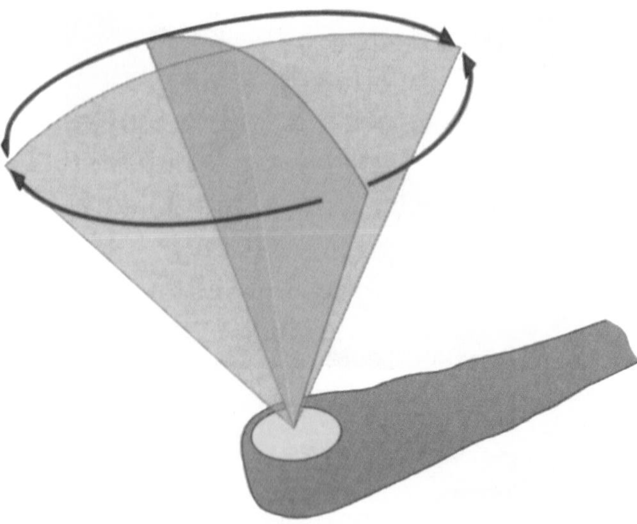

Figure 4.15 Schematic drawing of operating mode of a multiplane transoesophageal transducer. Internal rotation of the transducer allows changing the imaging planes through an arc of 180°. Modified with permission from Roelandt JRTC, Thomson IR, Vletter WB, *et al.* Multiplane transesophageal echocardiography: latest evolution in an imaging revolution. *J Am Soc Echo* 1992; **5**: 361–7.

Transoesophageal echocardiography

The oesophagus and the gastric fundus provide an echocardiography window on the heart unobstructed by lung or bone interposition, which is in close proximity to basal structures of the heart, in particular the atria, and to the thoracic aorta [4]. Moreover, this window can be used when

Table 4.2 Sequence and typical elements of a standard echocardiography exam

View	Data type
Parasternal long-axis view of the LV (2D + colour Doppler + M-mode)[a]	Loop
Parasternal short-axis view at aortic valve level (2D + colour Doppler + M-mode)[a]	Loop
Parasternal short-axis view at mitral valve level (2D)[a]	Loop
Parasternal short-axis view at mid-papillary level (2D)	Loop
Parasternal RV inflow-tract view (2D + colour Doppler)[a]	Loop
Parasternal RV outflow-tract view (2D + colour Doppler)[a]	Loop
Apical four-chamber view (2D + colour Doppler)[a]	Loop
Apical five-chamber view (2D + colour Doppler)[a]	Loop
Apical two-chamber view (2D + colour Doppler)[a]	Loop
Apical long-axis view (2D + colour Doppler)[a]	Loop
Subcostal four-chamber view (2D + colour Doppler)[a] atrial septum	Loop
Subcostal-inferior vena cava collapse during inspiration or sniff (+M-mode)	Loop
Suprasternal long-axis view of the aortic arch (2D + colour Doppler)[a,b]	Loop
Transmitral velocities (PW Doppler)	Spectral Doppler (still frame)
LV outflow tract velocities (PW Doppler)	Spectral Doppler (still frame)
Transaortic/outflow tract velocities (CW Doppler)	Spectral Doppler (still frame)
Tricuspid regurgitant velocities (CW Doppler)	Spectral Doppler (still frame)
Transpulmonary velocities (PW Doppler)	Spectral Doppler (still frame)
Tissue Doppler on mitral annulus (septal, lateral velocities)	Spectral Doppler (still frame)

[a]Doppler studies with colour-flow imaging may be performed at the end of the grey-scale (B-mode) imaging. M-mode optional in still frames and not necessary in both long- and short-axis views.

[b]In adults this projection may not always be required.

LV, left ventricle; 2D, two dimensional echocardiography; PW, pulsed-wave Doppler; CW, continuous-wave Doppler.

Reproduced with permission from Evangelista A, Flachskampf F, Lancellotti P, *et al.* European Association of Echocardiography. European Association of Echocardiography recommendations for standardization of performance, digital storage and reporting of echocardiographic studies. *Eur J Echocardiogr* 2008; **9**: 438–48.

access to the classic transthoracic windows is not available, e.g. during cardiac surgery. Transoesophageal echocardiography (TOE) is performed via an endoscopic probe with a transducer incorporated in its tip (➲Figs. 4.13 and 4.15). The tip can be flexed mechanically in different directions, and the transducer itself can be electrically rotated through a 180 degree arc to provide all possible cross-sectional plane orientations within a conical volume which has its tip at the transducer centre (➲Fig. 4.16; [5, 6]). Transoesophageal transducers, due to the proximity to cardiac structures, can be operated at higher frequencies than transthoracic transducers, typically 5–7MHz. They can be equipped with all echocardiography modalities, including, recently, real-time three-dimensional imaging. The transoesophageal examination requires informed consent from the patient, since there is discomfort and a very small risk of oesophageal or pharyngeal perforation involved (~1:10,000), especially in the presence of tumours, diverticula, or strictures, as well as risks from sedation [7]. The patient is kept fasting for at least 4 hours. Under provisional light sedation and topical anaesthesia, the probe is passed blindly with active swallowing into the oesophagus and the gastric fundus.

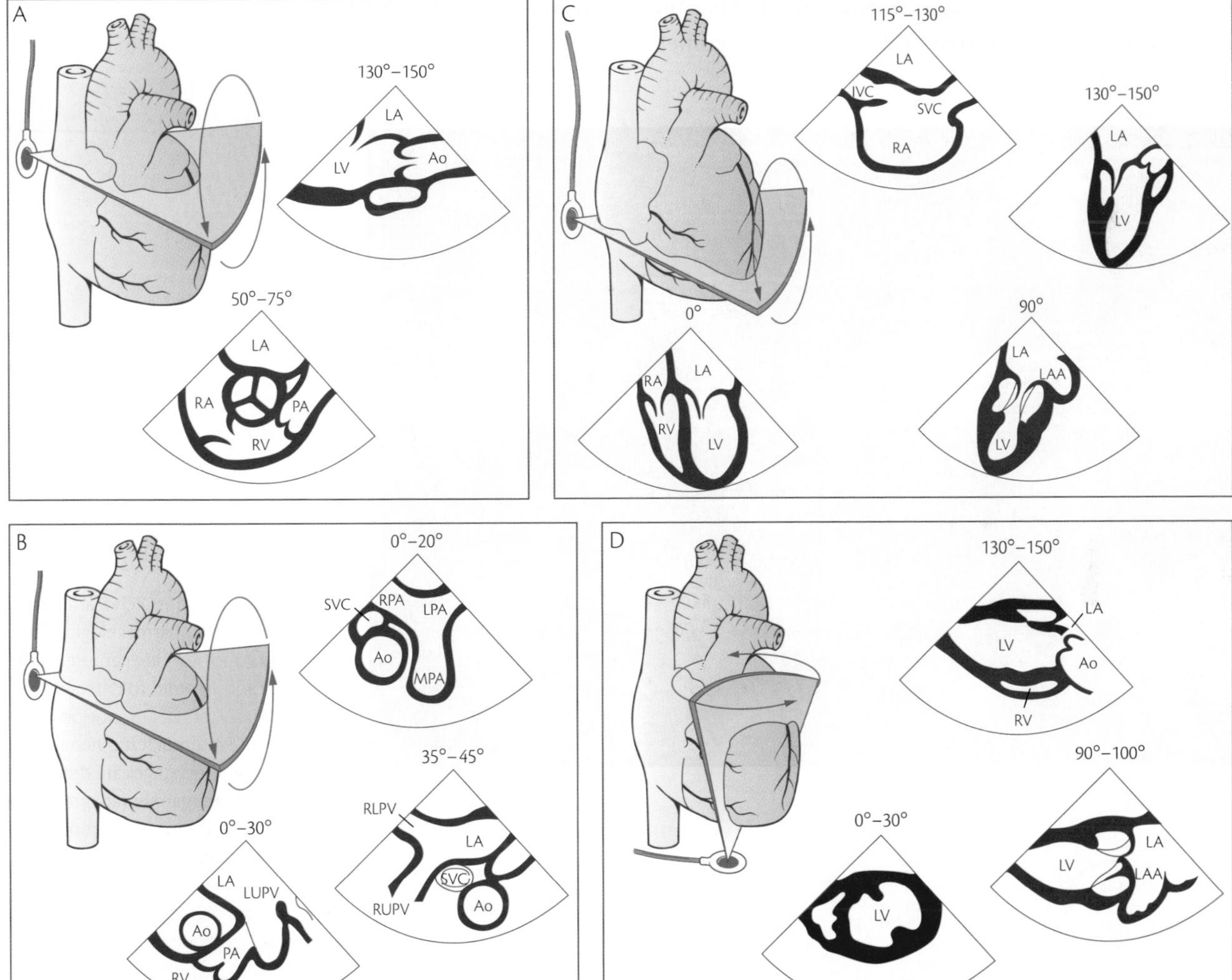

Figure 4.16 Typical TOE probe positions and views. Positioning of the scanning plane is indicated on the display screen: 0° indicates the transverse view, which is orthogonal to the probe, 90° shows a longitudinal view and 180° is the mirror image of 0°. (A) Upper transoesophageal views of the aortic valve in long-axis (130–150°) and short-axis (50–75°) views. (B) Upper transoesophageal views of the great vessels and atrial appendage (counter-clockwise): transverse view of the left atrial appendage and the left upper pulmonary vein (0–30°); intermediate view of ascending aorta, left atrium and right pulmonary veins (35–45°); and, with anterioflexion of the probe, transverse view of the ascending aorta, superior vena cava and main pulmonary artery with its bifurcation are obtained (0–20°). (C) Lower-middle transoesophageal views with exemplary cross-sections corresponding to (counter-clockwise) the four-chamber view of the left ventricle. From this transducer location, right heart structures can be visualized. A right atrial longitudinal view is visualized at 115–130°. (D) Transgastric views with exemplary cross-sections corresponding to (counter-clockwise) transgastric short-axis view at mid-papillary level, transgastric two-chamber view and transgastric long-axis view of the left ventricle after passing the left liver lobe. AO, ascending aorta; IVC, inferior vena cava; LA, left atrium; LAA, left atrial appendage; LV, left ventricle; LPA, left pulmonary artery; LUPV, left upper pulmonary vein; MPA, main pulmonary artery; RA, right atrium; RPA, right pulmonary artery; RLPV, right lower pulmonary vein; RUPV, right upper pulmonary vein; RV, right ventricle; SVC, superior vena cava.

TOE has been well demonstrated to provide higher diagnostic accuracy than transthoracic echocardiography (TTE) in the diagnosis of infective endocarditis, prosthetic valve dysfunction, cardiac sources of embolism (particularly left atrial and left atrial appendage thrombi), aortic dissection, and other diseases.

Stress echocardiography

Ischaemia

While echocardiography is not able to consistently visualize the coronary arteries directly, its ability to identify stress-inducible ischaemia by detecting new wall motion abnormalities under stress is well established. The most common stress forms are treadmill or bicycle ergometer exercise, dobutamine infusion (in incremental doses up to 40mcg/kg/min and additional 0.25mg atropine doses up to a total of 1mg), and dipyridamole infusion [8]. Digital baseline and stress cine-loops of the left ventricle in several views are carefully compared side by side to detect new or worsening wall motion abnormalities (➲Fig. 4.17). (For details of wall motion analysis see ➲Systolic function, p.116.) If a sufficient level of stress is achieved (generally defined by achieving a 'submaximal' target heart rate of 85% × (220 – age)), the test can be considered valid and has a sensitivity and specificity of 80–90% compared to angiographic detection of >50% diameter stenoses of the major coronary arteries [8]. Overall, the diagnostic accuracy of stress echocardiography is very similar to tomographic

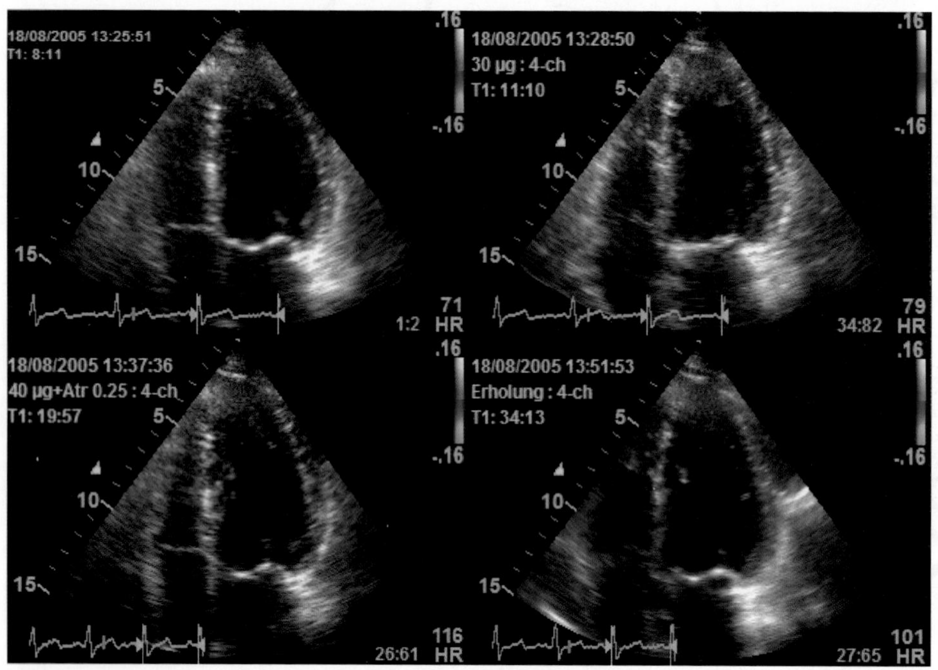

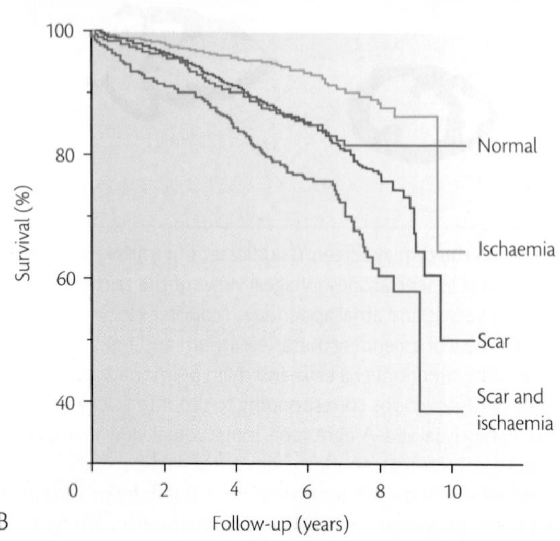

Figure 4.17 (A) Stress echocardiography. During physical or pharmacological stress, cineloops of the heart are captured and digitally stored. In order to detect subtle wall motion abnormalities, cineloops of the same view (here: apical four-chamber view) from different stress stages are displayed in a synchronized manner (adapted replay speed) side-by-side. In this example, apical four-chamber view loops at rest (top left), at 30mcg/kg/min dobutamine infusion (top right), and 40mcg/kg/min dobutamine infusion and additional atropine (peak stress; bottom left), and at recovery are displayed. Note different heart rates in the right lower corner of each loop. (B) Survival of 5375 patients undergoing treadmill exercise stress echocardiography according to results of the test: normal; presence of scar; presence of ischaemia; presence of scar and ischaemia combined. Reproduced with permission from Marwick TH, Case C, Vasey C, *et al.* Prediction of mortality by exercise echocardiography. A strategy for combination with the Duke treadmill score. *Circulation* 2001; **103**: 2566–71.

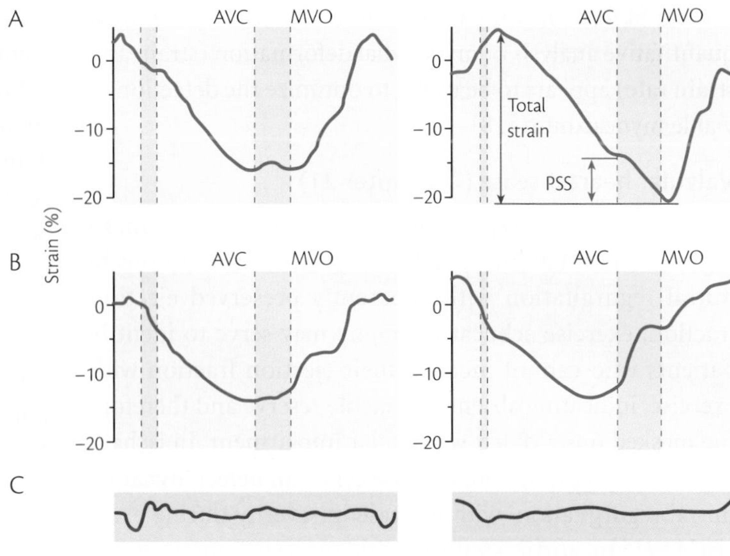

Figure 4.18 Use of strain analysis in dobutamine stress echocardiography. Longitudinal strain curves at baseline (left) and at peak stress (right). (A) Stress-induced ischaemia during a dobutamine stress echocardiogram results in a reduced regional systolic strain and the development of post-systolic shortening (PSS). The total strain may remain constant. (B) In normally perfused regions, the longitudinal strain profile hardly changes during a stress test. (C) ECG. AVC, aortic valve closure; MVO, mitral valve opening. Modified and reproduced with permission from Voigt JU, Exner B, Schmiedehausen K, *et al.* Strain rate imaging during dobutamine stress echocardiography provides objective evidence of inducible ischemia. *Circulation* 2003; **107**: 2120–6.

nuclear perfusion scanning (single photon emission computed tomography, SPECT), in most head-to-head comparisons with minor advantages in specificity for stress echocardiography and in sensitivity for nuclear imaging.

A negative stress echocardiogram is an excellent predictor of a low annual mortality of ≤1% [9,10]; see ➲Fig. 4.17. Similarly, stress echocardiography has excellent negative predictive value for peri-operative adverse events in the setting of non-cardiac surgery [11].

If image quality is insufficient, application of left heart echocardiographic contrast improves wall motion assessment and observer variability. Tissue Doppler parameters such as peak systolic velocities and magnitude and timing of systolic strain may also aid in the diagnosis of ischaemia ([12]; ➲Fig. 4.18). Especially with pharmacologic stress (dobutamine and dipyridamole), care has to be taken to immediately recognize and treat life-threatening complications such as ventricular arrhythmias, hypotension, and others, estimated to occur in approximately 0.3–0.7% of tests [8]. Thus, proper training and emergency equipment are mandatory.

Coronary flow reserve in the left anterior descending artery may be evaluated by TOE [13], visualizing the proximal segment of the artery, or by transthoracic Doppler interrogation of the peripheral left anterior descending artery [14]. Evaluation of other coronary arteries is less established.

Compared to competing imaging modalities used for evaluating coronary artery disease, stress echocardiography has very substantial advantages:

- No radiation as in nuclear imaging or cardiac computed tomography exists, nor are contrast media of any kind routinely necessary.
- No restrictions as to the presence of pacemakers or underlying heart rhythm exist.
- Stress echocardiography can be performed almost anywhere, if necessary with portable equipment.
- Stress echocardiography directly detects the functional effects of myocardial ischaemia, not a perfusion imbalance (as in nuclear imaging) or the presence of coronary stenoses (as in cardiac computed tomography).
- Stress echocardiography costs are far lower than with any other technique.

On the other hand, stress echocardiography is very dependent on an experienced, well-trained operator, probably more so than other imaging techniques. Inter-observer variability, in spite of decreasing over recent years due to improved equipment and standardized protocols, remains the Achilles heel [15, 16].

Viability

Under low-dose dobutamine and also low-dose exercise, functionally impaired, but viable (hibernating or stunned) myocardium may improve its function. This can be detected by comparison of baseline and stress images and predicts recovery of function, which occurs after revascularization in the case of hibernating myocardium and spontaneously in stunned myocardium. In many cases, there is a 'biphasic response', where the myocardium first improves contraction under low-dose dobutamine (<20mcg/kg/min) and then at higher dosage again deteriorates, signalling an ischaemic response at the higher stress level. Dobutamine stress echocardiography has shown slightly lower sensitivity (70–80%) and higher specificity (80–90%) for the presence of dysfunctional but viable (hibernating) myocardium than nuclear SPECT in comparative studies [17]. The additional quantitative analysis of myocardial deformation (strain and strain rate) appears to be useful to optimize the detection of viable myocardium [18].

Valvular heart disease (➲Chapter 21)

Stress echocardiography can aid clinical decision making in some situations in valvular heart disease. In severe mitral regurgitation with apparently preserved ejection fraction, exercise echocardiography may serve to identify patients who cannot increase their ejection fraction with exercise, indicating absent contractile reserve and therefore the masked onset of left ventricular impairment. In ischaemic mitral regurgitation, exercise echo can detect 'dynamic mitral regurgitation' with increase in severity during exercise [19]. In aortic stenosis with severely impaired left ventricular function and low transvalvular gradient, low-dose dobutamine stress echocardiography may be useful to confirm whether aortic stenosis is really severe or only apparently so due to a low stroke volume.

Contrast echocardiography

Echocardiography typically does not need the application of contrast agents to image cardiac structures. In some instances (e.g. ventilated or very obese patients), however, delineation of the border between blood and tissue, especially the endocardial border of the left ventricle, is insufficient for diagnostic purposes. In this case, left heart contrast agents, which consist of gas-filled small lipid-shell spheres with a diameter similar or smaller than red blood cells, can be intravenously injected as a bolus or infusion (➲Fig. 4.19). The gas-shell interface provides bright ultrasound reflection, which first lights up the right heart chambers and after pulmonary passage appears in the left atrium and finally in the left ventricle. Left heart contrast has proven value for improving the delineation of the left ventricular endocardial border, thus aiding in the calculation of left ventricular volumes or the identification of wall motion abnormalities.

Moreover, left heart contrast also enters the coronary circulation and thus increases the reflectivity of the myocardium. It has therefore been used as an equivalent of nuclear perfusion tracers, especially with vasodilatory drugs like adenosine [20, 21]. Quantitative assessment of myocardial brightness and measurement of myocardial refilling kinetics after 'destructive' high-energy ultrasound pulses have been shown to allow quantitative inferences about vascular volume and perfusion rate. The interpretation of myocardial perfusion studies with echocardiographic contrast, however, remains difficult and cannot yet be regarded as clinical routine.

Apart from the commercially available left heart contrast media, ordinary intravenous liquids, especially agitated blood-saline mixtures, can be used to increase the visibility of right heart structures as well as Doppler signals. These microbubbles do not appreciably cross the lungs and therefore do not or only minimally show up in the left atrium or ventricle after intravenous injection. Right heart contrast is frequently used to detect small atrial shunts, e.g. patent foramen ovale, especially after a Valsalva manoeuvre, by directly observing the passage of microbubbles from the right to left atrium via the atrial septum (see ➲Cardiogenic embolism, p.142).

Three-dimensional echocardiography

After initial experimentation with three-dimensional reconstruction from spatially registered two-dimensional planes, the engineering of so-called 'matrix transducers' with up to approximately 3000 separate piezoelectric elements now allows real-time acquisition of a pyramidal 'volume data set', which contains the entire heart or parts thereof. Theoretically, acquisition of such 'volume data' throughout a single heartbeat for example from an apical window could provide all morphological data, and at least partially also blood flow data. The data set could then be sliced in any

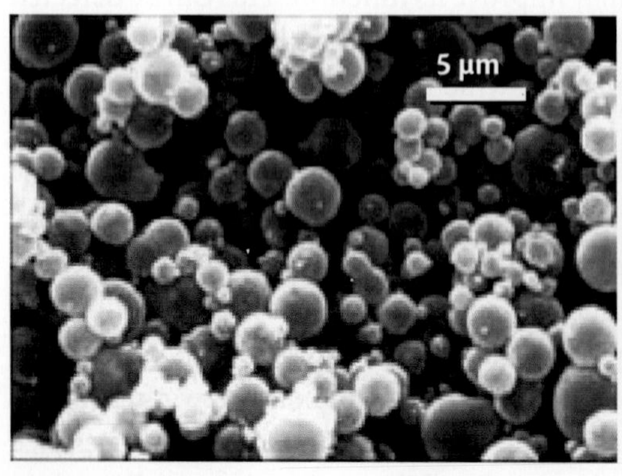

A

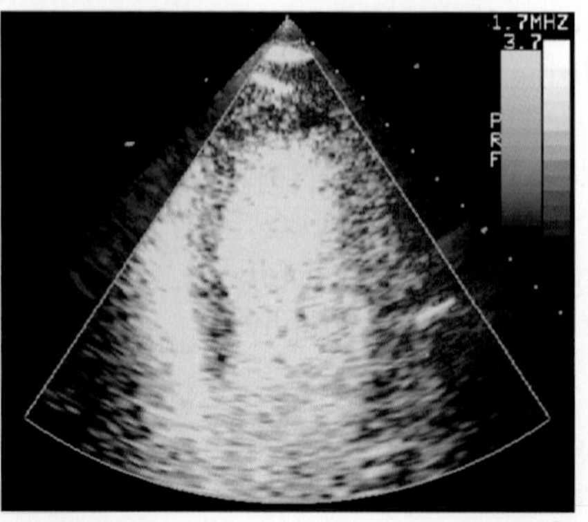

B

Figure 4.19 Left heart contrast echocardiography. (A) Microbubbles consist of a stabilizing shell (albumine, fatty acids, or phospholipids) and are filled with an inert gas or air. Intravenous injection results in a strong opacification of the heart chambers and, partially, of the myocardium (B).

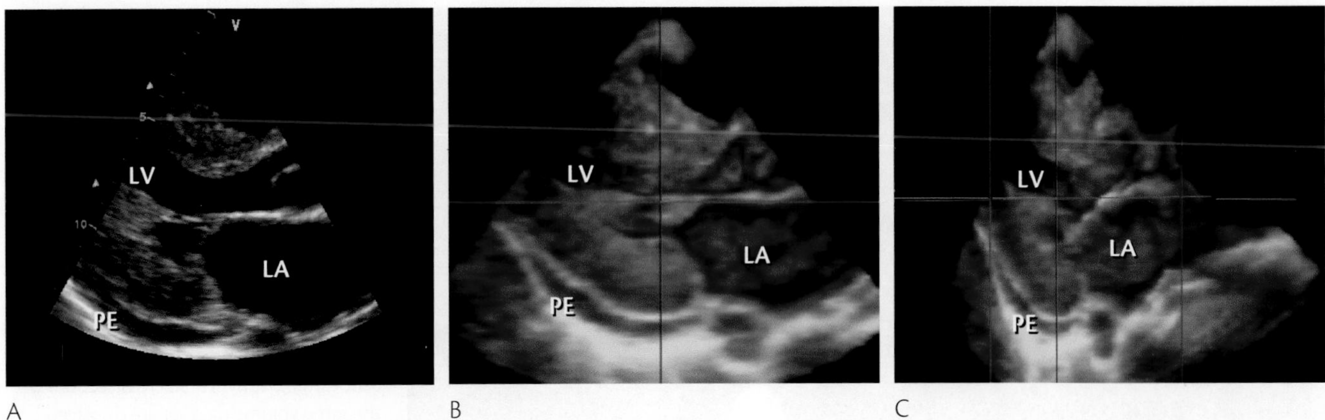

Figure 4.20 Two-dimensional (A) and three-dimensional images (B and C) of left ventricle in a patient with amyloidosis (note increased wall thickness). Parasternal images. While the three-dimensional image in (B) closely resembles the two-dimensional parasternal long axis, the same data set can be rotated to enable a view from the left atrium through the mitral valve into the left ventricle (C). LA left atrium; LV left ventricle; PE pericardial effusion. Also see 4.8 and 4.9.

way desired to display the morphology (➲Fig. 4.20; 4.8 and 4.9). In practice, most transducers still need several heart beats to acquire the morphological data and additional heartbeats for colour Doppler acquisition. The main drawback, however, at present is the still considerably inferior spatial and temporal resolution of three-dimensional transducers compared to two-dimensional transducers, which preclude their use for routine purposes. Nevertheless, some applications of three-dimensional echocardiography are emerging which presently already provide a net benefit over conventional two-dimensional imaging [22]. They exploit two unique three-dimensional imagery features: the ability to accurately visualize irregular cavities, e.g. the aneurysmal left ventricle, or the ability to display morphological data in en-face views which are difficult or impossible to obtain by two-dimensional echocardiography. In short, these applications are:

- Calculation of left and right ventricular volumes and ejection fraction. Three-dimensional echocardiography data provide volume calculations free of the geometric assumptions which are inherent in two-dimensional algorithms, such as Simpson's rule for volume calculation (➲Fig. 4.21). Provided image quality is sufficient, end-systolic and end-diastolic ventricular volumes as well as mass can be calculated with an accuracy and reproducibility similar to magnetic resonance tomography. Current three-dimensional software packages incorporate tools to at least partially obviate manually drawing ventricular endocardial contours, thus speeding up the analysis of volumes. Furthermore, segmental inward motion of left ventricular endocardium can be conveniently quantified and assessed with regard to synchrony or dyssynchrony.
- Morphologic analysis of rheumatic and degenerative mitral valve disease (➲Chapter 21). Properly three-dimensional-aligned short-axis views of mitral stenosis allow accurate planimetry [23], and the location of segmental mitral prolapse or flail is nicely displayed on 'surgeon's view' images from a left atrial perspective [24].
- En-face views of the atrial septum, especially of atrial septal defects (➲Chapter 10)and occluder devices (➲Fig. 4.22; 4.10 and 4.11).

Other techniques and developments

Hand-held devices of laptop or palmtop computer size became available during the last decade, allowing echocardiography examinations to be performed in practically all environments (see ➲Fig. 4.13). While quality and number of diagnostic modalities are reduced compared to state-of-the-art machines, these devices are often not inferior to a good 'big' echocardiography machine from 10–15 years ago. As a rule, the skills of the echocardiographer are more important than the sophistication of the machine.

Intracoronary ultrasound is covered in ➲Chapter 8 of this book. Another form of intravascular and intracardiac ultrasound are disposable, 10 French (3.3mm diameter) ultrasound catheters (AcuNav®) with an integrated 5–10MHz transducer tip that can be introduced in the great vessels. They have been used for imaging in aortic stenting, atrial catheter ablation procedures, and other applications.

Cardiac ultrasound also has emerging therapeutic applications: with hand-held, high-intensity, focused ultrasound catheters, surgical epicardial ablation of atrial fibrillation (➲Chapter 29) has been performed [25]. Catheter-based ultrasound thrombolysis has been evaluated in patients, and preliminary animal experience exists with

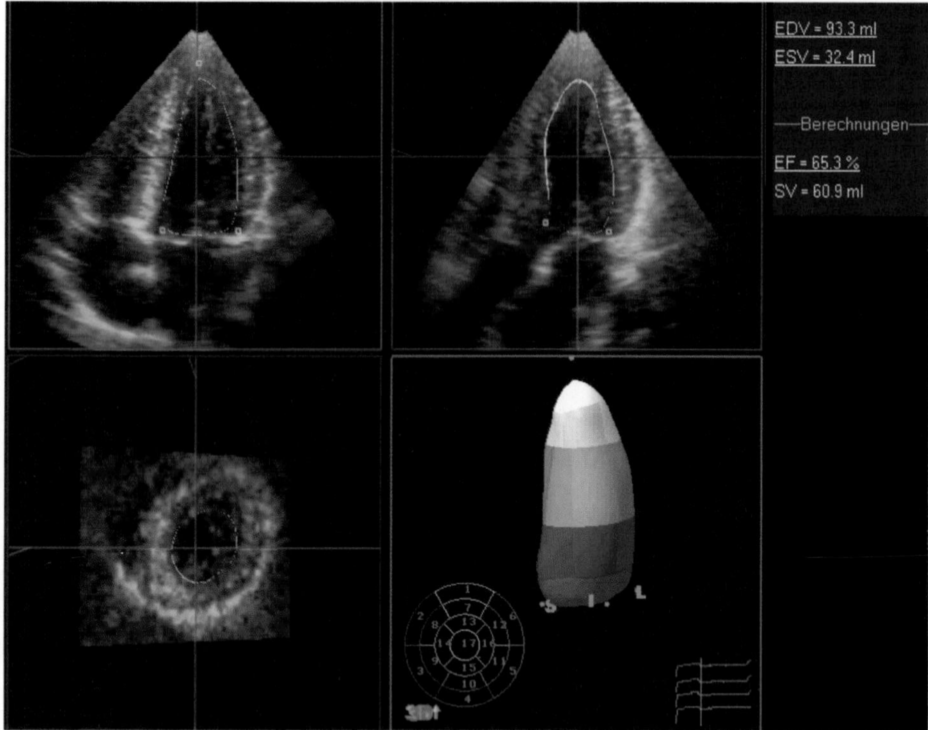

Figure 4.21 Left ventricular volume calculation by three-dimensional echocardiography. Three cross-sections of the same volume data set are displayed, with largely automatically traced endocardial borders throughout the cardiac cycle. With modest user input, accurate end-systolic and end-diastolic volumes, ejection fraction, and stroke volume are calculated from the full dataset, obviating any geometrical assumptions. Clockwise, apical four-chamber view, apical long-axis view, and a short-axis view of the left ventricle; bottom right, reconstructed model of left ventricular cavity.

transcutaneous ultrasound in experimentally induced myocardial infarction [26, 27].

Specific cardiovascular structures

Left ventricle

Left ventricular function

The assessment of left ventricular function probably represents the most frequent request from an echocardiography exam. Conceptually, it has become customary to separate systolic or pump function (which can be further subdivided into global and regional systolic function) from diastolic function, which relates to the left ventricular diastolic pressure volume relationship. The most widely accepted parameter of global systolic function is ejection fraction, which is a relatively crude parameter which may fail to reflect early and subtle disturbances of systolic function. On the other hand, there is a large group of patients suffering from symptoms of heart failure, although ejection fraction is preserved, especially in the presence of hypertension (➲Chapter 13) and left ventricular hypertrophy (➲Chapter 18). Such a constellation has been termed 'heart failure with normal ejection fraction' [34]. Echocardiography can provide—beyond the detection of hypertrophy—an estimate of elevated filling pressures in these patients, thus validating the diagnosis of heart failure with normal ejection fraction.

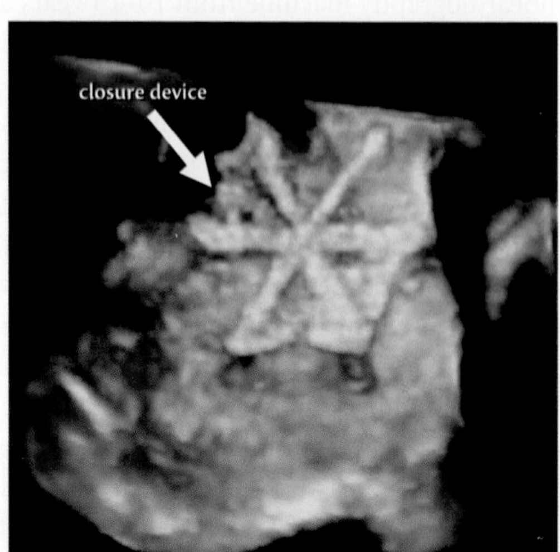

Figure 4.22 En face view by transoesophageal three-dimensional echocardiography of a closure device for a patent foramen ovale *in situ* in the atrial septum. Also see 🎥 4.10 and 4.11.

Systolic function

Global systolic function is evaluated in the following ways [28]:

- Ejection fraction (EF) is calculated from end-diastolic and end-systolic left ventricular volumes. It may be visually estimated from several cross-sections, or preferentially measured by tracing the left ventricle in end-diastole and end-systole in the four-chamber view (monoplane EF), or additionally in the two-chamber view (biplane EF), enabling the calculation of left ventricular volumes and EF by the modified Simpson's rule method (summation of discs; ➲Fig. 4.23). If three-dimensional echo is available, volumes can be calculated from the full 'volume data

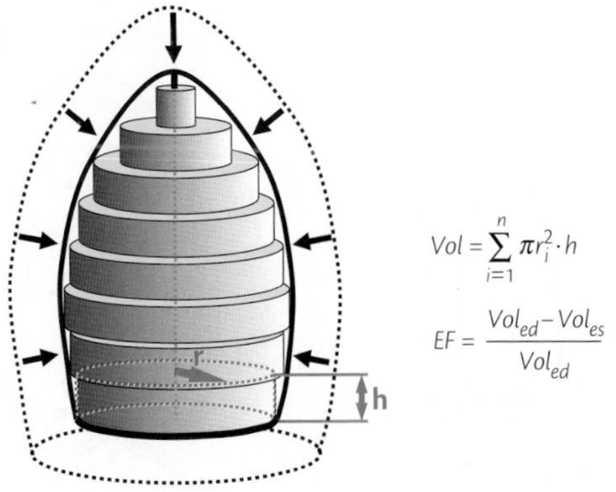

Two-dimensional measurements for calculations using the biplane method of discs, in the apical four-chamber (A4C) and apical two-chamber (A2C) views at end diastole (LV EDD) and at end-systole (LV ESD).

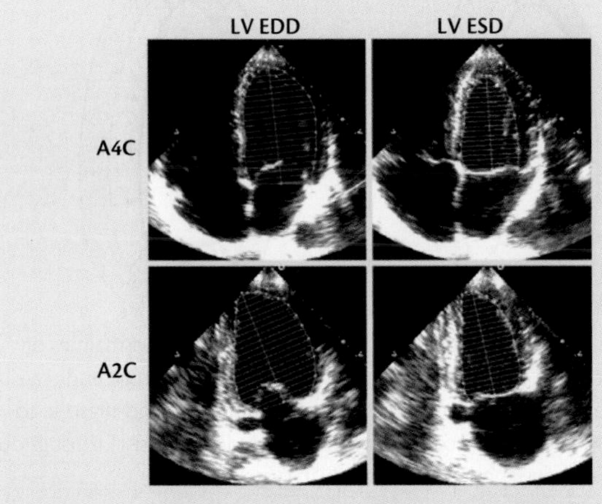

Ejection fraction = (EDV – ESV)/EDV

WOMEN and MEN

Two-dimensional method	Reference range	Mildly abnormal	Moderately abnormal	Severely abnormal
LV diastolic volume/BSA (mL/m^2)	35–75	76–86	87–96	≥97
LV systolic volume/BSA (mL/m^2)	12–30	31–36	37–42	≥43
Ejection fraction (%)	≥55	45–54	30–44	<30

B

Figure 4.23 (A) Calculation of LV volume and ejection fraction by the modified Simpson's rule. The ventricle is manually delineated. The method assumes rotational symmetry. Thus, the ventricular volume can be assumed to be equal the added volumes of the cylinders which fit into the delineated border. If systolic and diastolic volumes are estimated in this way, stroke volume and ejection fraction can be calculated. (B) Example of left ventricular biplane volume and ejection calculation, with normal values. Reproduced with permission from Lang R, Bierig M, Devereux R, *et al.* Recommendations for Chamber Quantification. A report from the American Society of Echocardiography's Nomenclature and Standards Committee, the Task Force on Chamber Quantification, and the European Association of Echocardiography. *Eur J Echocardiogr* 2006; **7**: 79–108.

set' without any geometric assumptions (see ➲Fig. 4.21). The latter method can be considered the gold-standard and correlates very well with magnetic resonance volumes, although echo volumes are systematically smaller than volumes calculated by magnetic resonance or from X-ray ventriculograms. The reason lies in the different recognition of the irregular trabeculated endocardial border with these methods.

- End-systolic (LVESD) and end-diastolic (LVDD) left ventricular short axis diameters (by M-mode or by two-dimensional echo measured from a parasternal long-axis view, see ➲Fig. 4.7) and the shortening fraction (LVEDD – LVESD)/LVEDD are the oldest quantitative parameters of global left ventricular function. However, they only take into account wall motion at the base of the left ventricle.
- The systolic excursion of the atrioventricular plane of the left ventricular, i.e. the apical displacement of the mitral annulus during systole, can serve as a measure of global systolic function. It is normally >12mm.
- On tissue Doppler recordings from the mitral annular region of the septal and lateral wall in the apical four-chamber view, peak systolic longitudinal velocities are normally >5cm/s. Strain values averaged over all left ventricular segments ('global strain') may also be used to evaluate left ventricular function.
- Physical exercise can be used to elicit contractile reserve measured as an increase in ejection fraction. Lack of contractile reserve implies beginning impairment of systolic function even if resting ejection fraction is still within normal range.

Regional systolic function is mainly evaluated visually in a 16-segment model of the left ventricle, where the individual segments can be assigned to typical coronary perfusion territories (➲Fig. 4.24).,Each segment then is visually assigned normokinetic, hypokinetic, akinetic, dyskinetic, or aneurysmatic wall motion (➲Fig. 4.25). This grading can be semi-quantified by a 'wall motion score' of 1–4. Such wall motion scores can be displayed in maps of the left ventricle, e.g. bull's eyes plots, and their average (sum of all wall motion scores divided by number of scored segments), the wall motion score index, can be used as a measure of global systolic function.

Deformation imaging provides truly regional strain and strain rate values and seems to be particularly useful when using speckle-tracking based techniques ('two-dimensional strain', 'velocity vector imaging'). Due to considerable variation even in normals it is difficult, however, to define wall motion abnormalities quantitatively.

Diastolic function: assessment of filling pressures

Practically all patients with impaired global systolic function have elevated filling pressures and hence impaired diastolic function. If heart failure symptoms occur in the presence of preserved ejection fraction, several echocardiographic

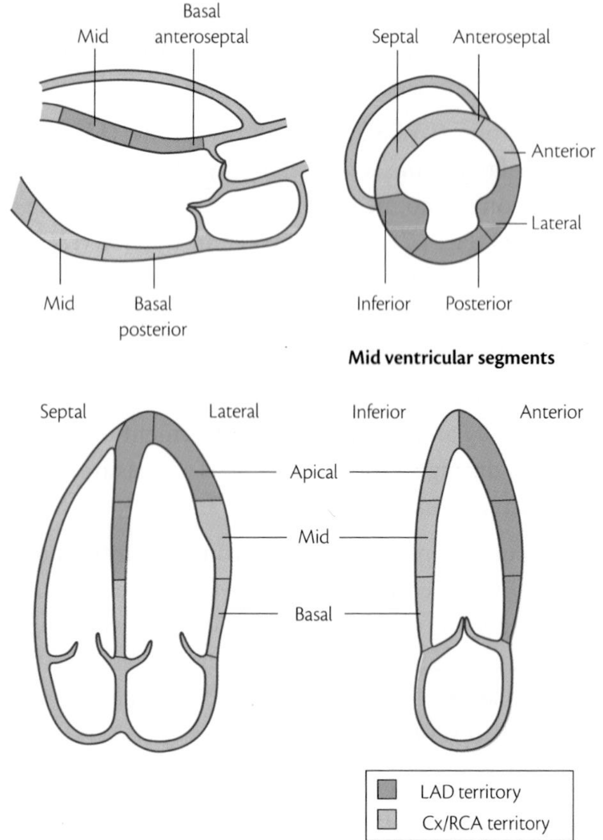

Figure 4.24 Left ventricular 16-segment model and assignment to anterior (left anterior descending) and posterior perfusion territories (circumflex and right coronary artery). Reproduced, with permission, from Flachskampf FA. *Kursbuch Echokardiographie*, 4th edn., 2008. Stuttgart: Thieme.

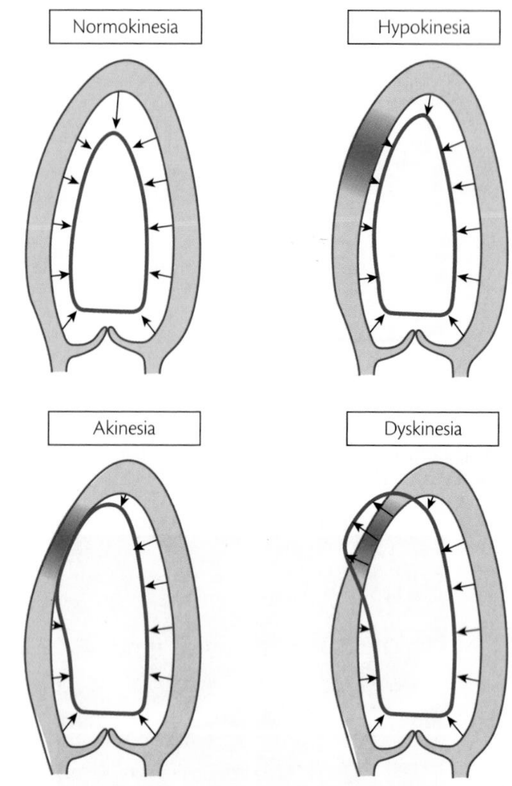

Figure 4.25 Schematic representation of wall motion abnormalities of the left ventricle. The innermost contour shows the endsystolic endocardial border, while the arrows depict endocardial motion from end-diastole to end-systole. In aneurysm (not shown), outward bulging persists throughout diastole, while in dyskinesia it occurs only in systole.

parameters should be evaluated and integrated to arrive at an assessment of filling pressures ([29,30]; ➲Figs. 4.26–4.28):

- The size of the left atrium (see ➲Left atrium, p.123). A normal left atrial size (≤34mL/m^2) excludes chronic elevation of left ventricular filling pressures. However, the left atrium also enlarges in other conditions, e.g. atrial fibrillation (➲Chapter 29).
- The ratio E/e′ (E, the peak transmitral early diastolic flow velocity, divided by e′, peak early diastolic mitral annular tissue velocities averaged from the septal and lateral mitral annular region). A ratio <8 largely excludes elevated filling pressures, while a ratio ≥15 largely proves substantially elevated filling pressures. Between these values, other parameters have to be used to evaluate filling pressures. These include a longer duration of the retrograde pulmonary atrial wave than of the transmitral A wave (➲Fig. 4.28), reduction in pulmonary systolic forward flow, a delay in the onset of e′ with relation to E, and others.
- A restrictive transmitral flow pattern (peak E >2 × peak A wave velocity and E wave deceleration time <150ms; ➲Fig. 4.27c) represents an ominous sign with severely

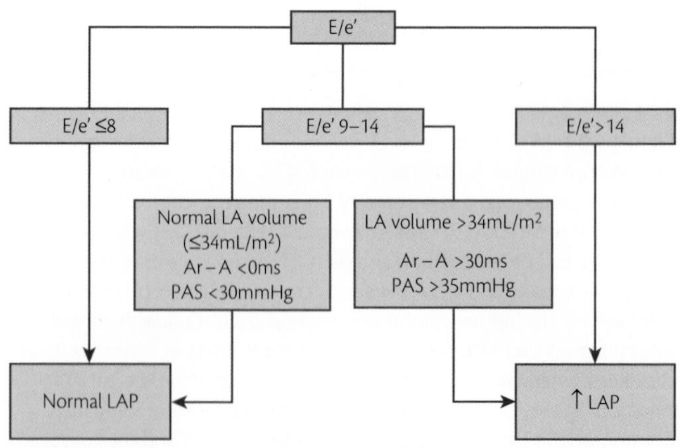

Figure 4.26 Algorithm for estimation of left ventricular filling pressures in patients with normal ejection fraction. See text for details. Ar, duration of reverse pulmonary venous wave; A, duration of transmitral A wave; LA, left atrium; PAS, systolic pulmonary artery pressure (estimated from tricuspid regurgitation). Modified and reproduced with permission from Nagueh SF, Appleton CP, Gillebert TC, *et al.* Recommendations for the evaluation of left ventricular diastolic function by echocardiography. *Eur J Echocardiogr* 2009; **10**: 165–93

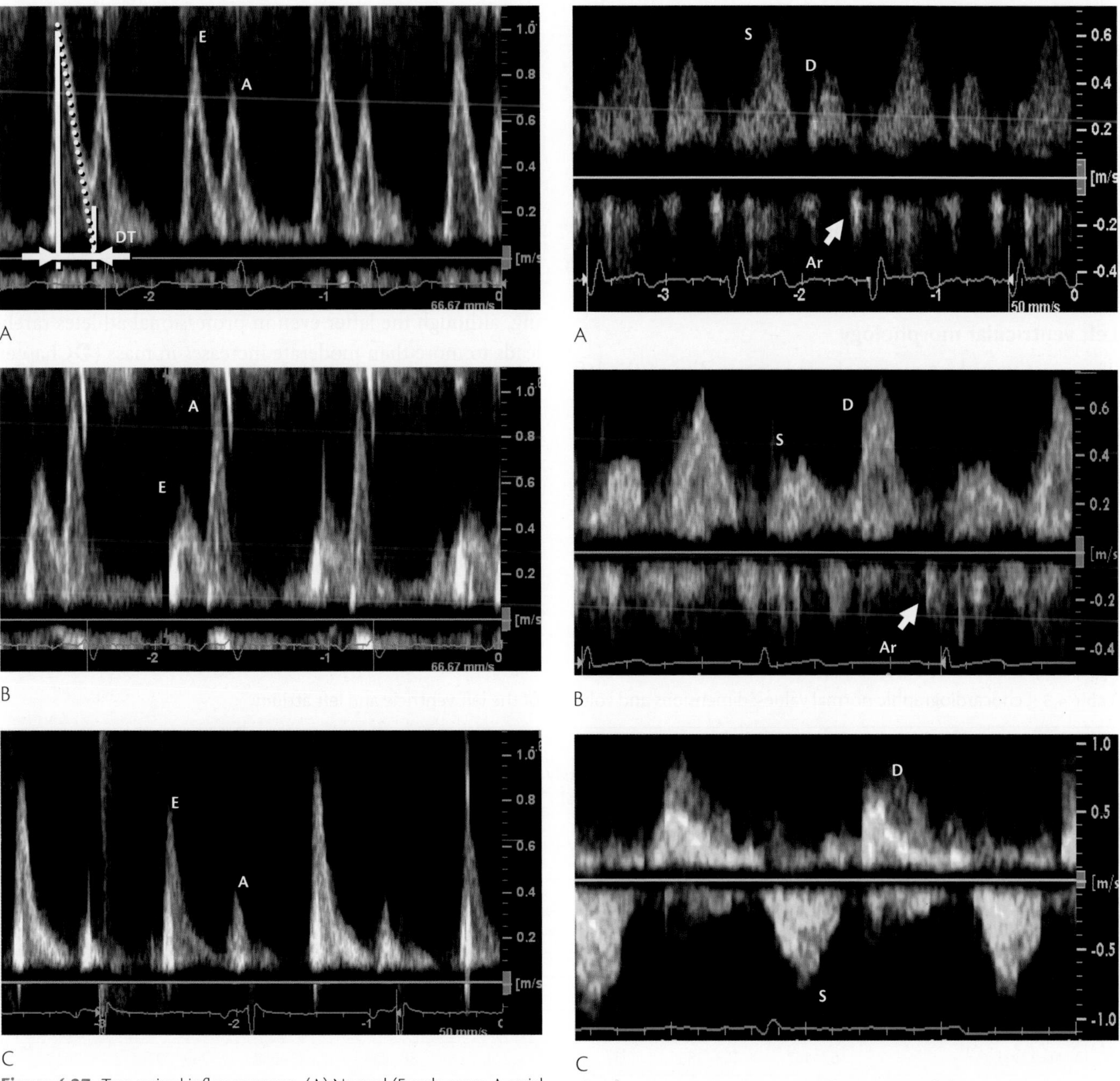

Figure 4.27 Transmitral inflow patterns. (A) Normal (E early wave, A atrial wave). E wave deceleration time is indicated as time from peak E wave to end of the E wave. (B) Pattern of 'impaired relaxation'. This pattern of E <A is frequent with left ventricular hypertrophy and other myocardial diseases. It is normal in middle or advanced age and can also be found if atrial pressure is low. (C) 'Restrictive pattern' with peak E more than double of peak A velocity and short E wave deceleration time (<150ms). This pattern is indicative of high filling pressures and severe left ventricular disease, but can also occur in constrictive pericarditis and in young healthy persons due to very vigorous early diastolic relaxation of the left ventricle.

Figure 4.28 Pulmonary venous inflow patterns. (A) Normal pattern. There is a systolic (S) and diastolic (D) forward (i.e. into the left atrium) wave and a small retrograde wave (Ar) due to atrial contraction. (B) Increased left atrial pressure. There is a reduction in the S wave compared to the D wave. (C) Severely elevated left atrial pressure, with prominent systolic flow reversal and fusion of the reverse S wave with the Ar wave. This pattern occurs with severe mitral regurgitation or otherwise severely elevated left atrial pressure.

impaired prognosis; however, this is usually accompanied by systolic dysfunction. Isovolumic relaxation time, a highly preload-dependent time interval measured from cessation of aortic flow to onset of transmitral inflow, is severely shortened (<60ms). A pseudo-restrictive pattern may be observed in young, perfectly healthy individuals due to very vigorous relaxation.

- A transmitral flow pattern with E <A peak velocities is very frequent (➲ Fig. 4.27b). Isovolumic relaxation is prolonged (>100ms). It can be considered normal in patients >60 years, although some researchers view this as an expression of a genuine age-related diastolic dysfunction. It has been termed the pattern of 'impaired relaxation', although this implies a diagnosis impossible to conclusively make by echocardiography alone. The pattern excludes, however, substantially elevated filling pressures, since these would increase peak E wave. If E/e′ is also intermediate, a 'diastolic stress test' by exercise and measurement of transmitral flow and tissue Doppler parameters may show or exclude an exercise-induced substantial increase in filling pressures [31].

Left ventricular morphology

The most prevalent morphologic abnormality of the left ventricle is an increase in mass (left ventricular hypertrophy). Left ventricular mass (LVM, in g) is mostly calculated from left ventricular wall and cavity diameters, provided that no major scar or localized hypertrophy is present, by the formula:

$$LVM + 0.8[1.04(LVEDD + PWEDD + SEDD)^3 - LVEDD^3] + 0.6$$

where LVEDD is end-diastolic left ventricular diameter, PWEDD end-diastolic posterior wall thickness, and SEDD end-diastolic septal thickness (all in cm). For normal values see ➲Table 4.3. Left ventricular mass can be determined more precisely from three-dimensional echocardiography. The aetiology of hypertrophy cannot be inferred directly from echocardiography; in the absence of hypertension, hypertrophy may be due to aortic stenosis (➲Chapter 21), hypertrophic cardiomyopathy (➲Chapter 18), infiltrative cardiomyopathy (➲Chapter 18), or exercise training, although the latter even in professional athletes rarely leads to more than moderate increases in mass (➲Chapter 32). Moderate hypertrophy initially is accompanied by a transmitral filling pattern featuring a reduced ratio of the transmitral peak E and A velocities (the maximal velocities of early and late transmitral diastolic inflow, compare ➲Fig. 4.27), which has been termed the 'impaired relaxation pattern'. However, this pattern also may be mimicked by decreased preload, high heart rate, and increasing age, and therefore does not necessarily imply functional

Table 4.3 Echocardiographic normal values: dimensions and volumes of the left ventricle and left atrium

	Women				Men			
	Reference range	Mildly abnormal	Moderately abnormal	Severely abnormal	Reference range	Mildly abnormal	Moderately abnormal	Severely abnormal
LV dimension								
LV diastolic diameter	3.9–5.3	5.4–5.7	5.8–6.1	≥6.2	4.2–5.9	6.0–6.3	6.4–6.8	≥6.9
LV volume								
LV diastolic volume (ml)	56–104	105–117	118–130	≥131	67–155	156–178	179–201	≥201
LV diastolic volume/BSA (ml/m^2)	35–75	76-86	87-96	≥97	35–75	76–86	87–96	≥97
LV systolic volume (ml)	19–49	50–59	60–69	≥70	22–58	59–70	71–82	≥83
LV systolic volume/BSA (ml/m^2)	12–30	31–36	37–42	≥43	12–30	31–36	37–42	≥43
LV mass (g)	67–162	163–186	187–210	≥211	88–224	225–258	259–292	≥293
LV mass/BSA (g/m^2)	43–95	96–108	109–121	≥122	49–115	116–131	132–148	≥149
LV mass/height (g/m)	41–99	100–115	116–128	≥129	52–126	127–144	145–162	≥163
LV mass/height (g/m)$^{2.7}$	18–44	45–51	52–58	≥59	20–48	49–55	56–63	≥64
Relative wall thickness (cm)	0.22–0.42	0.43–0.47	0.48–0.52	≥0.53	0.24–0.42	0.43–0.46	0.47–0.51	≥0.52
Septal thickness (cm)	0.6–0.9	1.0–1.2	1.3–1.5	≥1.6	0.6–1.0	1.1–1.3	1.4–1.6	≥1.7
Posterior wall thickness (cm)	0.6–0.9	1.0–1.2	1.3–1.5	≥1.6	0.6–1.0	1.1–1.3	1.4–1.6	≥1.7
Atrial dimensions								
LA diameter (cm)	2.7–3.8	3.9–4.2	4.3–4.6	≥4.7	3.0–4.0	4.1–4.6	4.7–5.2	≥5.2
Atrial volumes								
LA volume (ml)	22–52	53–62	63–72	≥73	18–58	59–68	69–78	≥79
LA volumes/BSA (ml/m^2)	22 ± 6	29–33	34–39	≥40	22 ± 6	29–33	34–39	≥40

LA, left atrium; LV, left ventricle.

Reproduced with permission from Lang R, Bierig M, Devereux R, *et al.* Recommendations for Chamber Quantification. A report from the American Society of Echocardiography's Nomenclature and Standards Committee, the Task Force on Chamber Quantification, and the European Association of Echocardiography. *Eur J Echocardiogr* 2006; **7**: 79–108.

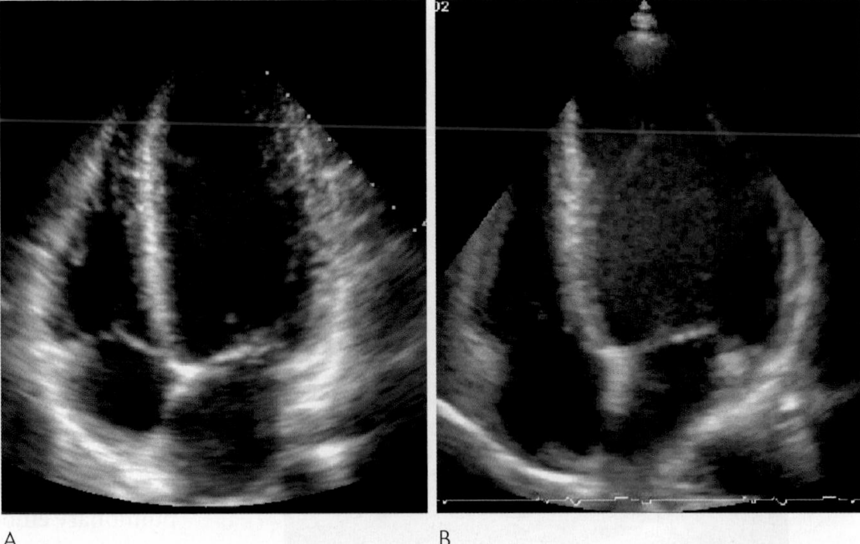

Figure 4.29 Left ventricular remodelling. Apical four-chamber views of same patient: (A) shortly after anterior infarction, (B) 1 year after infarction. Note enlargement (both images have the same scale), relative increase in width of left ventricle (spherical remodelling), and spontaneous echocardiographic contrast in the cavity after 1 year. Also see 4.12 and 13.

myocardial impairment. Significant left ventricular hypertrophy forces the circulation to increase filling pressures to maintain stroke volume, leading to increased, left atrial size, and increasing pressures lead to 'pseudonormalization' of the decreased E/A ratio, which can be unmasked by a Valsalva manoeuvre, or by the finding of an increased E/e′.

In response to a loss of contractile function (e.g. after a large myocardial infarction) the left ventricle enlarges—a process termed left ventricular remodelling (➔Fig. 4.29; 4.12 and 4.13). Severely enlarged left ventricles change their shape from conical to spheroid, which leads to eccentric displacement of the papillary muscles and functional mitral regurgitation. In severely dilated and hypocontractile left ventricles, thrombi may be present, especially at the apex, and spontaneous echocardiographic contrast may be visible in the cavity. This is a pattern of swirling, smoke-like echoes often detectable in regions of low blood velocity and ascribed to aggregated red blood cells ('rouleaux'), indicating a thrombogenic milieu. Aneurysms are wall motion abnormalities with a persistent systolic and diastolic bulging and usually represent large infarct scars (➔Fig. 4.30; 4.14). Such aneurysms have thin, often echo-dense walls and lack contraction. They may contain thrombus. An important differential diagnosis is the left ventricular pseudoaneurysm (➔Fig. 4.31; 4.15). This is the result of a contained myocardial free wall rupture, mostly due to myocardial infarction, although traumatic pseudoaneurysms occur. Characteristics of a pseudoaneurysm include an abrupt thinning of the left ventricular wall at the border and often a relatively narrow 'neck', which is smaller in diameter than the largest diameter of the pseudoaneurysm. There may be paradoxical flow into the pseudoaneurysm in systole and out in diastole. For other regional wall motion abnormalities, see ➔Stress echocardiography, p.112. Another 'mechanical' complication of myocardial infarction is ischaemic ventricular septal defect (➔Chapter 16), which is located in the muscular portion of the septum. The hallmark of this complication is a systolic high-velocity blood jet in the right ventricle representing left-to-right shunt; the peak velocity reflects the systolic pressure difference between left and right ventricle. The morphologic defect may be difficult to clearly delineate on two-dimensional images alone. For congenital ventricular septal defect, see ➔Chapter 10.

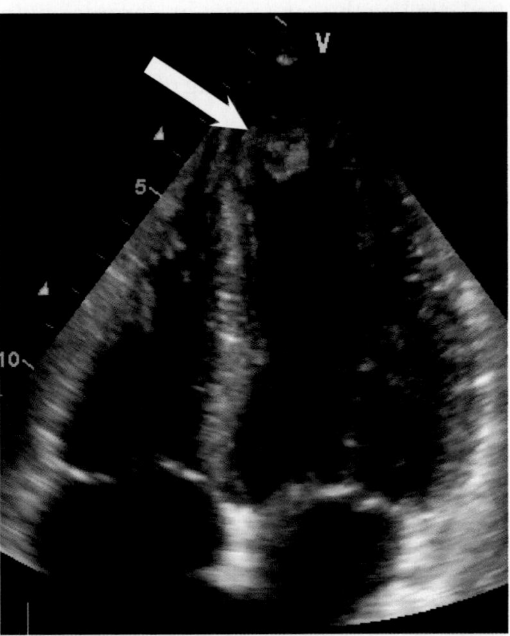

Figure 4.30 Left ventricular apical akinesia with thrombus (arrow) due to an anterior myocardial infarction. Apical four-chamber view. Also see 4.14.

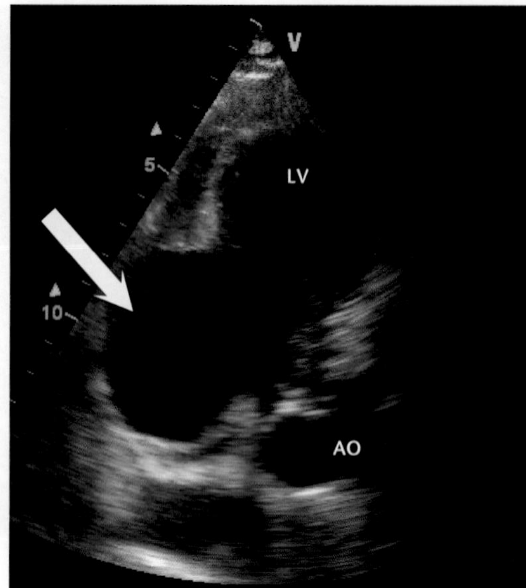

Figure 4.31 Infero-posterior pseudoaneurysm (arrow) of left ventricle (LV) after inferior infarction. Note the 'neck' of the pseudoaneurysm, which is narrower than its largest diameter. AO, ascending aorta. Also see 4.15.

Right ventricle

Although the right ventricle can be imaged well by echocardiography, assessment is hampered by its very irregular shape. Three-dimensional echocardiography provides the most complete and definitive possibility of assessing volumes and right ventricle EF, but is often limited by impaired image quality. Size and function therefore are usually assessed in a qualitative way. Impaired pump function most frequently is due to right ventricular infarction, cardiomyopathy, or (acute or chronic) pulmonary hypertension (➲Chapter 24). Longitudinal tissue Doppler velocities and deformation imaging of the right ventricular free wall have been reported to be helpful to quantify right ventricular function.

An important aspect of right ventricle function is the maximal right ventricular systolic pressure, which corresponds, in the absence of pulmonary stenosis (➲Chapters 10 and 21), to systolic pulmonary pressure. If tricuspid regurgitation is present, this value can be assessed by calculating the peak systolic gradient between right ventricle and right atrium. To this gradient an estimate of mean right atrial pressure may be added, e.g. from physical examination of the patient or by judging presence and extent of inspiratory collapse of the inferior vena cava. The estimation of peak systolic right ventricle pressure is extremely helpful to assess presence and degree of pulmonary hypertension, e.g. in pulmonary embolism (➲Chapter 37).

In chronic pulmonary hypertension (➲Fig. 4.32), the right ventricle enlarges and hypertrophies (end-diastolic free-wall thickness >5mm). Tricuspid regurgitation is usually present. Right ventricle function varies, but very often is impaired. The interventricular septum is shifted to the left ventricle. This is appreciable especially in short axis-views, where the septum, which normally is convex to the right ventricle side, becomes straight, giving the left ventricular cross-section the shape of a 'D' instead of an 'O'. In acute pulmonary hypertension due to pulmonary embolism, the right ventricle also enlarges and is functionally impaired (except in mild pulmonary embolism). In massive pulmonary embolism, the right ventricle is acutely overloaded and dilated, with substantial tricuspid regurgitation. Systolic pulmonary pressure is elevated, but due to acute right ventricle failure often only moderately so. In some cases, transit thrombi may be seen in the right heart or lodged in the main pulmonary artery or its main branches.

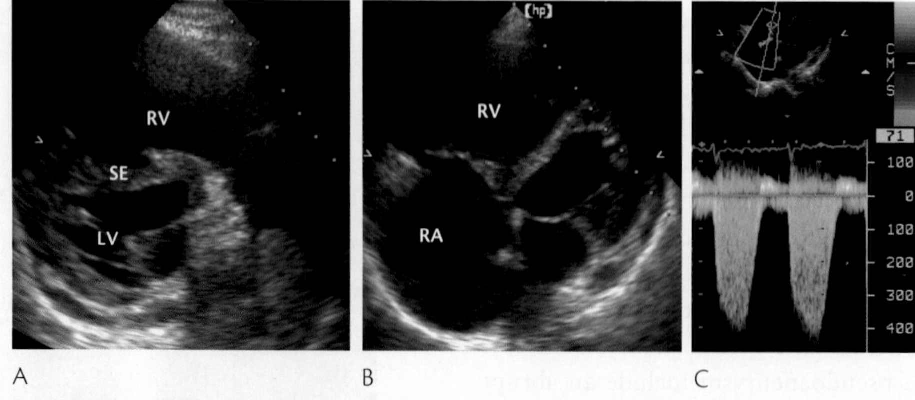

Figure 4.32 Chronic severe pulmonary hypertension. The size of right ventricle (RV) and atrium (RA) far exceeds that of left ventricle and atrium. (A) Parasternal short-axis view with displacement of ventricular septum (SE) to the left ventricle, creating the 'D sign' as opposed to the normal circular shape of the left ventricle in short-axis views. (B) Modified apical four-chamber view. (C) Peak tricuspid regurgitant velocity (right) is 420cm/s, which by the simplified Bernoulli equation amounts to a ventriculo-atrial pressure gradient of 71mmHg. To estimate peak systolic RV and pulmonary artery pressure, an estimate of right atrial pressure can be added to that value.

Paradoxical embolism at the atrial level through a patent foramen ovale is a well recognized complication in these circumstances. Because of the ease of diagnosing severe pulmonary embolism by the findings of right ventricular enlargement and dilatation together with elevated pulmonary pressures, emergency echocardiography should be performed as quickly as possible in these patients to guide management.

Arrhythmogenic right ventricle cardiomyopathy (➲Chapters 9 and 30) is a rare disease echocardiographically characterized by enlargement of the right ventricle and dyskinetic areas especially in the proximity of the tricuspid annulus, the apex, and the outflow tract of the right ventricle (➲Fig. 4.33; 4.16). The diagnosis is not easy and many patients do not have conspicuous right ventricle abnormalities on echocardiography. For congenital heart disease affecting the right ventricle, see ➲Chapter 10.

Left atrium and pulmonary veins

Left atrial function can conceptually be separated into three elements:

- a conduit function, passively conveying blood during diastole from pulmonary veins to the left ventricle;
- a reservoir function, accumulating blood during ventricular systole; and
- a booster pump function, ejecting blood by atrial contraction.

The best parameter of left atrial size is systolic left atrial volume, measured by monoplane or biplane modified Simpson's rule (summation of discs; ➲Fig. 4.34). The antero-posterior diameter of the left atrium (from parasternal views or M-mode) is a less reliable measure of size. Enlargement occurs in the following situations:

- increase in left ventricular diastolic filling pressures (impaired left ventricular function);
- mitral valve regurgitation or stenosis (➲Chapter 21);
- atrial fibrillation (➲Chapter 29);
- atrial septal defect (➲Chapter 10);
- dilatation of the right atrium.

In atrial fibrillation and flutter of >24–48 hours, the left atrial appendage becomes a predilection site for the formation of spontaneous echocardiographic contrast (see ➲Left ventricular morphology, p.120) and thrombi (➲Fig. 4.35; 4.17). Inspection for thrombi, especially of the left atrial appendage, is a classic domain of TOE, which should be performed before cardioversion of atrial fibrillation or flutter unless the patient has been thoroughly anticoagulated for 4–6 weeks. The occurrence of thrombi in the body of the left atrium is rarer, but well known in mitral stenosis (usually also with atrial fibrillation).

The left and right upper pulmonary veins are well assessable by TOE, while the lower veins are more difficult to visualize. Pulmonary venous inflow patterns (compare ➲Fig. 4.28) change in response to elevation in left atrial pressure, the

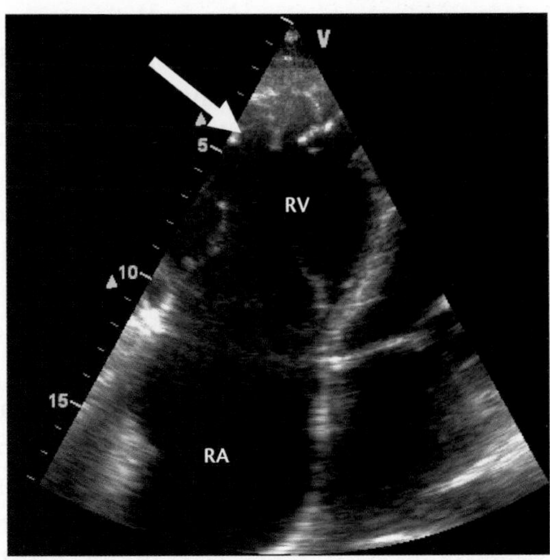

Figure 4.33 Arrhythmogenic cardiomyopathy of the right ventricle. Note enlarged right ventricle with aneurysmatic zones at the apex (arrow). Also see 4.16.

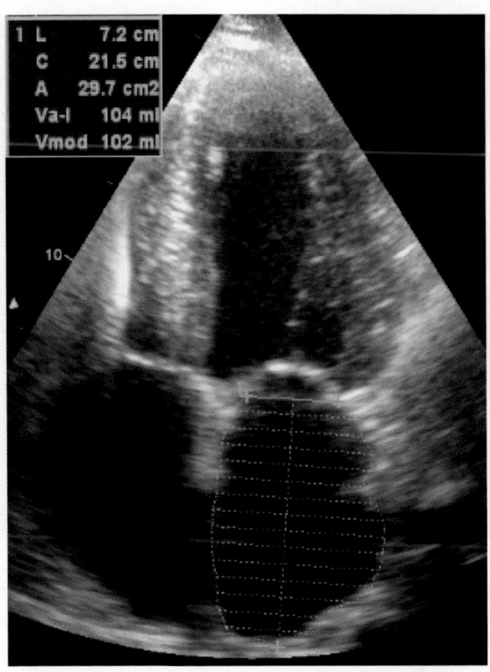

Figure 4.34 Left atrial volume calculation by summation of discs (modified Simpson's rule) in the apical four-chamber view derived from planimetry of the left atrium in end-systole. The left atrial volume is markedly elevated (102mL). Note marked left ventricular hypertrophy.

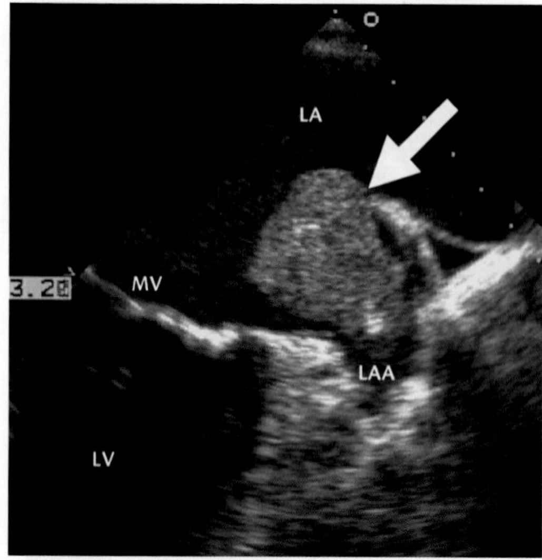

Figure 4.35 Uncommonly large thrombus (arrow) in the left atrial appendage (LAA) in a patient with atrial fibrillation. Transoesophageal image; LA left atrium; LV, left ventricle; MV mitral valve. Also see 🎥 4.17.

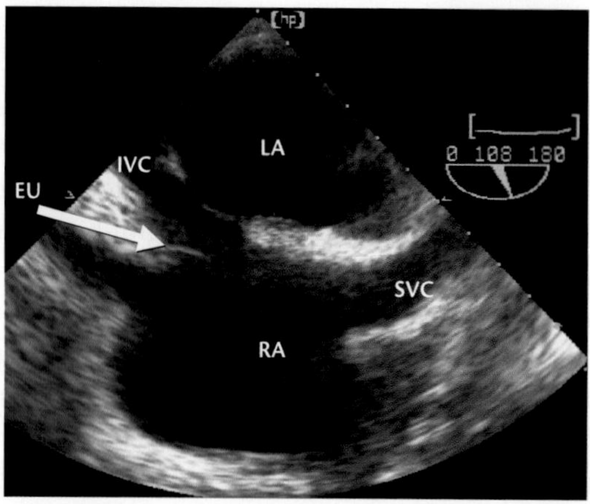

Figure 4.36 Sagittal transoesophageal view of the right atrium at 108° rotation. EU, Eustachian valve; IVC, inferior vena cava; LA, left atrium; RA, right atrium; SVC, superior vena cava. Note thin part of atrial septum, the fossa ovalis, between left and right atrium. Also see 🎥 4.18.

presence of atrial fibrillation (in both conditions, the systolic wave decreases), and the severity of mitral regurgitation, where systolic reversal of pulmonary venous inflow indicates severe regurgitation. For congenital heart disease affecting the pulmonary veins, see ➲Chapter 10.

Right atrium, atrial septum, and caval veins

Enlargement of the right atrium usually parallels left atrial enlargement, e.g. in atrial fibrillation. Tricuspid regurgitation is a frequent cause of right atrial enlargement. The orifices and proximal portions of the caval veins can be appreciated from subcostal views and particularly well by the transoesophageal sagittal view (➲Fig. 4.36; 🎥 4.18). At the orifice of the inferior caval vein, the Eustachian valve is detectable, a structure of variable prominence, which may extend into the right atrium as a 'Chiari network' (a fenestrated membrane). Both structures are remnants of a valve of the embryonic sinus venosus. Pacemaker and implantable cardioverter/defibrillator electrodes, as well as central venous catheters are visible in the superior vena cava and right atrium, and may give origin to thrombi or endocarditic vegetations (➲Chapter 22), besides causing or increasing tricuspid regurgitation.

The atrial septum is constituted by ontogenetically different components. It may contain several types of defects, the most frequent of which is the secundum defect, which occurs in the area of the fossa ovalis and may be multiple (see ➲Chapter 10). Atrial septal defects lead to predominant left-to-right shunting, dilatation of both atria, pulmonary congestion, increase in transtricuspid velocities, and enlargement of the right ventricle. The presence of an atrial septal defect can be ascertained directly by detecting a defect in the membrane (by transthoracic, or, in particular with sinus venosus defects, by TOE) and by spectral and colour flow Doppler showing cyclic left-to-right shunting (in the absence of right atrial pressure elevation). If a shunt is present, there is also regularly at least a small right-to-left shunt, which can be proven by injecting intravenously a bolus of agitated intravenous infusion solution or blood and detecting the bubbles crossing the atrial septum to appear in the left atrium. Approximately one-fourth of the adult population has a patent foramen ovale, which constitutes another potential source of right-to-left-shunting across the fossa ovalis portion of the atrial septum. This slit-like orifice, most of the time kept shut by higher left atrial than right atrial pressure, may open during a Valsalva manoeuvre or in other instances of right atrial pressure elevation—most importantly in acute pulmonary embolism. By injection of right heart contrast, especially during TOE, and performance of a Valsalva manoeuvre, patent foramen ovale can be echocardiographically diagnosed or excluded (cf. ➲Fig. 4.61). Closure devices, such as the Amplatzer device, for secundum atrial septal defects or patent foramen ovale, can be conveniently monitored during implantation by TOE (compare ➲Fig. 4.22) (➲Chapter 10). On follow-up, they should be inspected for residual shunt and thrombus formation.

Frequent atrial septal anomalies are lipomatous hypertrophy of the septum, a benign condition which characteristically spares the fossa ovalis region, and atrial septal aneurysm, often defined as a deviation of the thin portion of the membranous atrial septum from the interatrial midline of 1cm or more to either side or both sides. This abnormality occurs in 1–2% of the population, is better diagnosed by TOE than TTE, and often coexists with atrial septal defect, septal fenestrations, and patent foramen ovale; an association with unexplained ischaemic neurologic events has been noted in the literature.

Cardiac valves

Assessment of valvular heart disease (➲Chapter 21) is one of the prime strengths of echocardiography [32]. Morphologically, pathologic thickening, calcification, abnormal masses (e.g. fibroelastoma), excessive or restricted mobility, functional integrity, and congenital malformations (e.g. bicuspid aortic valve) can be detected. In infective endocarditis (➲Chapter 22), new mobile mass lesions (vegetations) attached to the valve can be detected, and abscess formation in the perivalvular tissue may be observed, especially in valvular prostheses. Further sequelae of endocarditis are fistulae, perforations, or the formation of mitral pseudoaneurysms (see also ➲Chapter 21).

Functionally, valvular dysfunction can be divided into stenosis and regurgitation. Stenotic lesions are assessed morphologically by noting reduced mobility, thickening, and calcification of valvular leaflets. In the mitral, and to a lesser degree, the aortic valve, direct planimetry of the stenotic orifice area is possible [33]. Doppler echocardiography allows calculation of maximal and mean transvalvular gradients from the simplified Bernoulli equation. The continuity equation (an expression of the conservation of mass) especially in the aortic valve permits calculation of a stenotic orifice area from stroke volume and maximal transvalvular velocities; this principle is also applicable to other valves. In the mitral valve, an estimate of stenotic valve area can be derived from the rate of decrease of the diastolic transmitral gradient, expressed as pressure half-time.

Valve regurgitation (see ➲Table 4.4) manifests itself morphologically as incomplete leaflet closure due to leaflet prolapse or a flail leaflet, due to annular dilatation (in the mitral, aortic, and tricuspid valve), due to defects, e.g. in bacterial endocarditis (➲Chapter 22), or other reasons (➲Fig. 4.37). By colour Doppler, regurgitant jets are seen in the receiving chamber of the regurgitation. The overall

Table 4.4 Echocardiographic criteria for the definition of severe native valvular regurgitation: an integrative approach

	AR	MR	TR
Specific signs of severe regurgitation	Central jet, width ≥65% of LVOT[a] Vena contracta >0.6 cm[a]	Vena contracta width ≥0.7cm with large central MR jet (area >40% of LA) or with a wall improving jet of any size, swirling in LA[a] Large flow convergence[b] Sytolic reversal in pulmonary veins Prominent flail MV or ruptured papillary muscle	Vena contracta width >0.7cm in echo Large flow convergence[b] Systolic reversal in the hepatic veins
Supportive signs	Pressure half-time <200ms Holodiastolic aortic flow reversal in descending aorta Moderate or greater LV enlagement[d]	Dense, triangular CW, Doppler MR jet E-wave dominant mitral inflow (E > 1.2m/s)[c] Enlarged LV and LA size[e] (particularly when normal LV function is present)	Dense, triangular CW TR signal with early peak Inferior cava dilatation and respiratory diameter variation ≤50% Prominent transtricuspid E-wave, especially if >1m/s
Quantitative parameters			
R Vol, mL/beat	≥60	≥60	
RF, %	≥50	≥50	
ERO, cm^2	≥0.30	≥0.40	

AR = aortic regurgitation, CW = continuous wave, ERO = effective regurgitation orifice area, LA = left atrium, LV = left ventricle, LVOT = LV outflow tract, MR = mitral regurgitation, MS = mitral stenosis, MV = mitral valve, R Vol = regurgitation volume, RA = right atrium, RF = regurgitant fraction, RV = right ventricle, TR = tricuspid regurgitation.

[a] At a Nyquist limit of 50–60 cm/s.

[b] Large flow convergence defined as flow convergence radius ≥0.9 cm for central jets with a baseline shift at a Nyquist of 40 cm/s; cut-offs for eccentric jets are higher and should be angled correctly.

[c] Usually above 50 years of age or in conditions of impaired relaxation, in the absence of MS or other causes of elevated LA pressure.

[d] In the absence of other aetiologies of LV dilatation.

[e] In the absence of other aetiologies of LV and LA dilatation and acute MR.

Reproduced with permission from Zoghbi WA, Enriquez-Sarano M, Foster E, *et al.* American Society of Echocardiography: recommendations for evaluation of the severity of native valvular regurgitation with two-dimensional and Doppler echocardiography: A report from the American Society of Echocardiography's Nomenclature and Standards Committee and The Task Force on Valvular Regurgitation, developed in conjunction with the American College of Cardiology Echocardiography Committee, The Cardiac Imaging Committee, Council on Clinical Cardiology, The American Heart Association, and the European Society of Cardiology Working Group on Echocardiography. *Eur J Echocardiogr* 2003; **4**: 237–61.

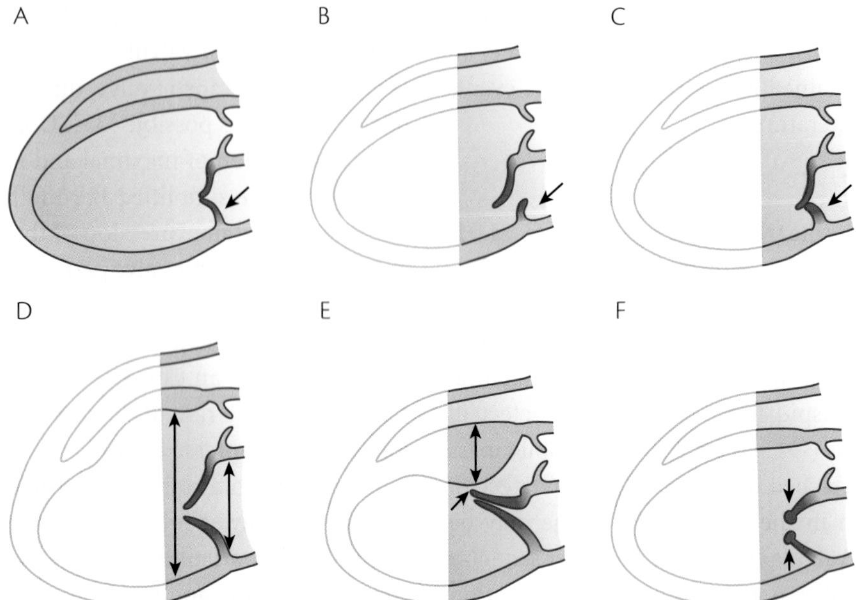

Figure 4.37 Schematic illustrations of typical mitral pathomorphologies in the parasternal long-axis view. (A) Posterior leaflet prolapse (arrow; systolic frame). (B) Posterior leaflet flail (arrow; systolic frame). (C) Thickening and stiffening (restricted motion) of posterior leaflet (arrow; systolic frame). (D) Functional regurgitation due to left ventricular dilatation. Note lack of closure of leaflet tips and displacement of leaflets into the left ventricle ('tenting'; systolic frame). (E) Systolic anterior motion (arrow) in hypertrophic obstructive cardiomyopathy. Note increased septal thickness (double arrow). Systolic frame. (F) Mitral stenosis with doming (diastolic frame). Arrows indicate the reduced opening amplitude of the thickened leaflet tips.

size of these jets is loosely related to the severity of regurgitation, but also to many other factors and thus alone is not sufficient to grade severity in more than mild regurgitation. Additional Doppler-based methods to evaluate the severity of regurgitation include (➲Fig. 4.38):

- The proximal jet width ('vena contracta') immediately after passage of the valve, which is related to the size of the regurgitant orifice.
- The proximal convergence zone ('proximal isovelocity surface area', or PISA), which at least theoretically allows calculation of regurgitant flow rate, regurgitant volume, regurgitant fraction, and regurgitant orifice area, and practically is very helpful in distinguishing moderate and severe regurgitation. This method is based on the assumption of concentric hemispheres of fluid of differing flow velocity in the upstream chamber, which are centred around the regurgitant orifice, upon which the regurgitant flow converges. By a combination of colour Doppler and CW-Doppler parameters of regurgitation severity, most importantly regurgitant orifice area (in cm^2), are calculated. In spite of many limitations inherent in the theoretical basic assumptions of the method, it works relatively well if image quality is sufficient.
- The inflow pattern of the receiving chamber (pulmonary venous flow in mitral regurgitation and hepatic vein flow in tricuspid regurgitation).
- Others (see sections on individual valves).

Importantly, evaluation of the severity of regurgitation should never be based on a single number or parameter but on an 'integrative approach' (see ➲Table 4.4) synthesizing all available morphologic, Doppler, and ultimately, clinical information [34].

Mitral valve

The normal mitral valve opens quickly and completely in early diastole, with thin and pliable leaflets. The normal diastolic transmitral flow pattern is characterized by an early diastolic E wave, in response to rapid left ventricular pressure fall due to relaxation in early diastole, and a late diastolic A wave due to atrial contraction (after the P wave of the ECG; see ➲Figs. 4.27 and 4.28). For changes of the transmitral inflow profile due to elevation of left ventricular filling pressures, see ➲Left ventricular function, p.116. In long-standing hypertension and in advanced age, calcification of the mitral annulus—in particular posteriorly—is frequent.

Mitral stenosis (➲Chapter 21) is almost always rheumatic and produces the characteristic 'doming' appearance of the leaflets in diastole (➲Figs. 4.37 and 4.39; 🎥 4.19 and 4.20). The stenotic orifice area is best planimetered by two- or three-dimensional echocardiography. If this is not possible due to image quality, the next best method to assess orifice area A in cm^2 is by the empirical formula A = 220/PHT,

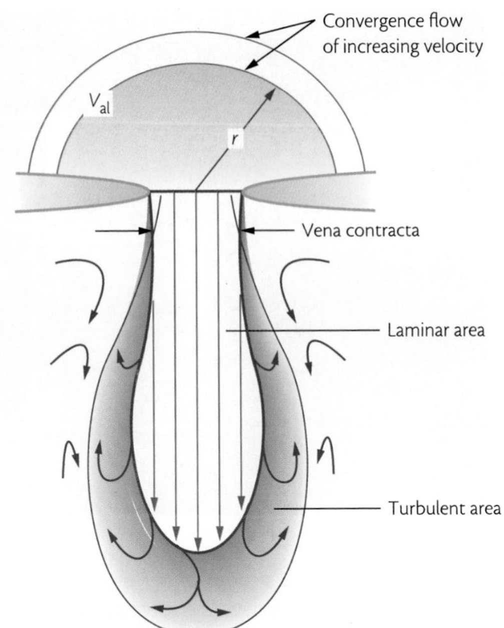

Figure 4.38 The principle of the proximal isovelocity surface area (PISA) method and vena contracta measurement for regurgitant volume measurement. The vena contracta or narrowest extent of the regurgitant jet as it passes through the effective regurgitant orifice correlates well with the severity of regurgitation. This method assumes that the regurgitant orifice does not alter in shape or size during regurgitation. As blood flow accelerates towards the regurgitant orifice, concentric hemispheres rings of isovelocity regions are produced and visualized with colour Doppler. The smallest hemisphere nearest the regurgitant orifice has the highest velocity. The PISA radius (*r*) is the radial distance between this aliasing contour (V_{al}) and the centre of the regurgitant orifice. The regurgitant jet area consists of the laminar area with the highest velocities and a turbulent area caused by entrainment of stagnant blood volume.

where PHT is the pressure half-time in ms measured from the CW Doppler transmitral flow profile. This method is based on the observation that the early diastolic transmitral pressure gradient decay depends on mitral orifice area, declining rapidly with larger orifice areas and slower with smaller orifice areas. The mean diastolic transmitral gradient (by CW Doppler), although strongly heart rate dependent and affected by concomitant mitral regurgitation, is a further useful measure of severity.

Mitral regurgitation (➲Chapter 21) is very frequent. Minimal or mild regurgitation, especially in early systole, occurs in many apparently healthy individuals. More severe mitral regurgitation is either organic (e.g. mitral valve prolapse) or functional (e.g. in the impaired and dilated left ventricle; see ➲Chapter 21). The mechanism can usually be identified by careful echocardiographic examination of the valve (➲Fig. 4.37; ➲Table 4.4). The most important degenerative mechanisms are prolapse and flail (➲Figs. 4.40 and 4.41; 🎥 4.21 and 4.22); these terms are often used interchangeably, but in prolapse proper it is the body of the leaflet that is most prominently displaced beyond the leaflet coaptation point into the left atrium in systole, while in mitral flail leaflet it is the tip of the leaflet that moves farthest into the left atrium due to disruption of its subvalvular support (chordal rupture), invariably leading to substantial regurgitation. In functional mitral regurgitation the underlying cause is impaired regional or global left ventricular function, while the valvular apparatus itself is intact (➲Fig. 4.42). However, due to displacement of the papillary muscles the leaflets are pulled into the left ventricle during systole and prevented from closing. This occurs both with global dilatation of the left ventricle (dilated or ischaemic cardiomyopathy) or with regional posterior/inferior wall motion abnormalities. The typical configuration of functional mitral regurgitation is a structurally intact valve, the leaflets of which in systole are entirely on the ventricular side of the mitral annulus, with the closure line at a distance from the line connecting the insertion of the leaflets. This appearance has been termed 'tenting' and is characteristic for functional mitral regurgitation. In ischaemic mitral regurgitation, it has been shown that under exercise stress, the regurgitant orifice area of mitral valves may increase, which is a negative prognostic marker [19, 35]. This increase is not due to acute ischaemia, but instead to non-ischaemic changes in ventricular and valvular geometry under stress. On the other hand, acute ischaemic regurgitation also may occur, either by acute ischaemic dilatation of the left ventricle or as a complication of myocardial infarction, by rupture of papillary muscle (usually partial rupture of the posteromedial papillary muscle) or of chordae.

While for the diagnosis of mild mitral regurgitation the observation of a small colour Doppler jet is sufficient, differentiation of moderate or large severity, besides appreciation of mitral valve and left ventricular morphology (e.g. presence of a flail leaflet or of marked tethering of the leaflets with a dilated left ventricle), often necessitates analysis of proximal jet width, proximal convergence zone, pulmonary venous flow, and sometimes further parameters. The best appreciation of regional morphologic alterations of the mitral valve, especially of prolapse or flail, is obtained by TOE. Morphologic changes are often expressed in Carpentier's nomenclature with regard to mechanism (excessive/restricted leaflet mobility and others) and location (P1–P3 for posterior leaflet scallops, A1–A3 for anterior leaflet scallops) of the regurgitant lesion. This is important for preoperative planning of reconstructive versus replacement surgery, as well as intraoperatively to check the success of reconstructive surgery, and should be performed routinely

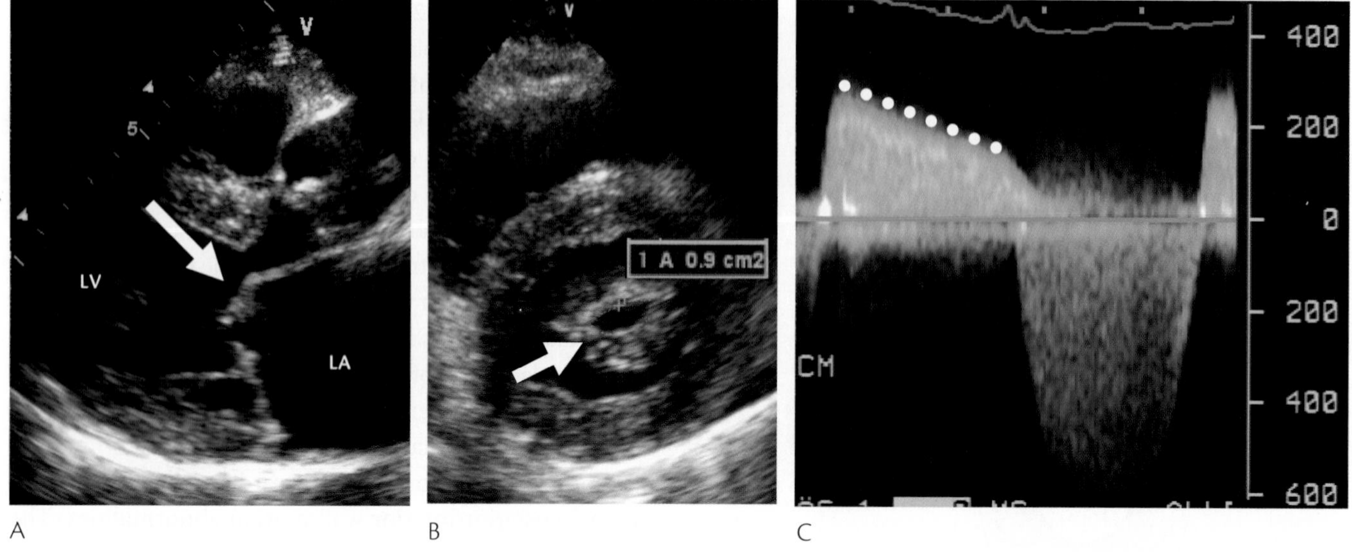

A B C

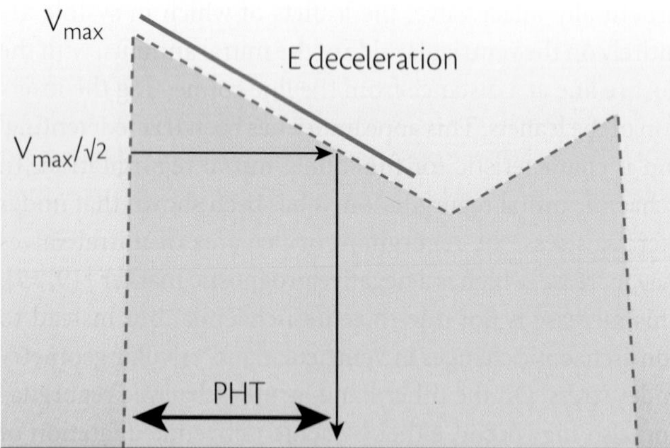

D

Figure 4.39 (A) Rheumatic mitral stenosis with diastolic doming of the leaflets (arrow), parasternal long-axis view. The patient is in atrial fibrillation. LA, left atrium; LV, left ventricle. Note enlarged left atrium. There is also rheumatic aortic valve disease. Also see 4.19. (B) Mitral valve planimetry in the parasternal short-axis view. The stenotic orifice area (arrow) is 0.9cm^2. (C) CW Doppler recording of transmitral flow in combined rheumatic mitral stenosis and regurgitation. The scale is in cm/s. The deceleration slope of the diastolic flow profile is marked with a white dotted line; from this slope, pressure half-time is calculated as the time interval from peak transmitral pressure gradient at the onset of diastole to decrease of the gradient to one half of its initial value. Because the instantaneous gradient is proportional to the square of the flow velocity, this corresponds to a decay from the initial maximal transmitral flow velocity v_{max} to $v_{max}/\sqrt{2}$. Note also systolic profile of mitral regurgitation with a peak regurgitant velocity of 6m/s, corresponding to a systolic peak pressure difference between left ventricle and left atrium of 144mmHg. (D) Schematic drawing explaining the calculation of pressure half-time. Also see 4.20.

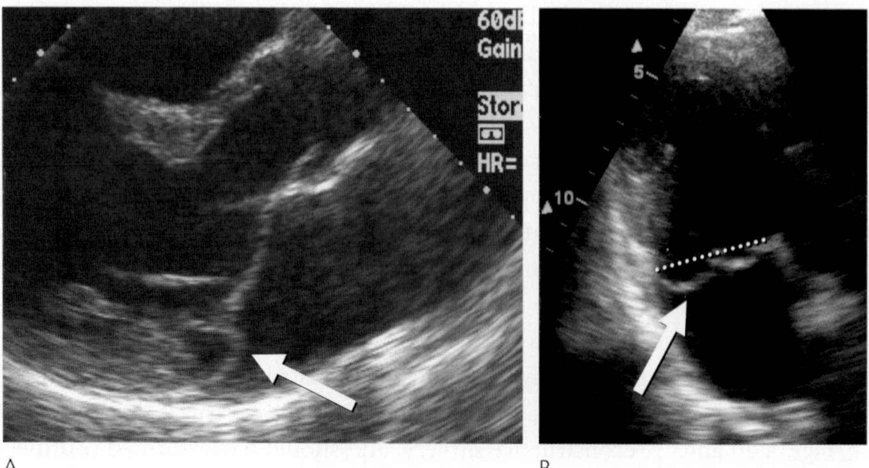

A B

Figure 4.40 Mitral valve prolapse involving both leaflets. (A) Parasternal long-axis view; (B) apical long-axis view, with the level of the mitral annulus marked by a dotted line.

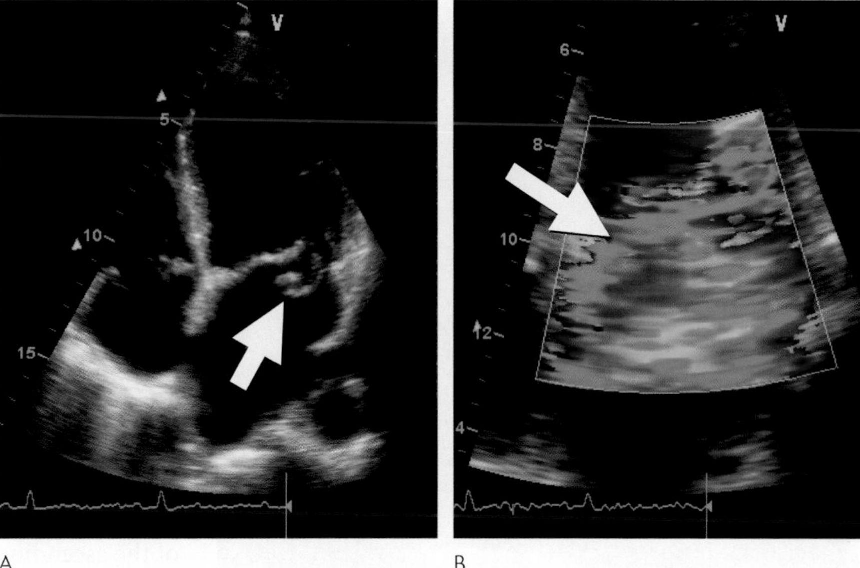

Figure 4.41 Posterior mitral flail leaflet (arrow) in the apical four-chamber view (A) and corresponding colour Doppler representation (B) of severe mitral regurgitant jet directed to the opposite side (arrow). Also see 4.21 and 4.22.

during mitral valve repair. Mitral valve endocarditis may induce regurgitation of all degrees by perforation or rupture of mitral structures (see ➲Chapter 22).

Several congenital malformations of the mitral valve exist (e.g., stenosis, cleft). Hypertrophic obstructive cardiomyopathy is frequently associated with valvular malformations and with moderate or severe mitral regurgitation. Mitral valve endocarditis is characterized by the attachment of vegetations, most frequently to the atrial side of the leaflets and annulus, mitral regurgitation, and sometimes development of a mitral pseudoaneurysm. Restriction of valvular leaflet mobility, leading to progressive regurgitation, occurs in carcinoid syndrome and has been reported as a side effect of drugs such as dexfenfluramine (an appetite suppressant) and pergolide (a dopamine agonist), an effect which seems to be mediated by the release of serotonin.

Aortic valve (➲Chapter 22)

The aortic valve is normally tricuspid. About 0.5% of the population have a congenitally bicuspid valve, which is prone to degeneration and the development of combined aortic regurgitation and stenosis (➲Fig. 4.43; 4.23). Furthermore, these patients are at an increased risk of aortic dissection. Bicuspid valves normally can be detected during

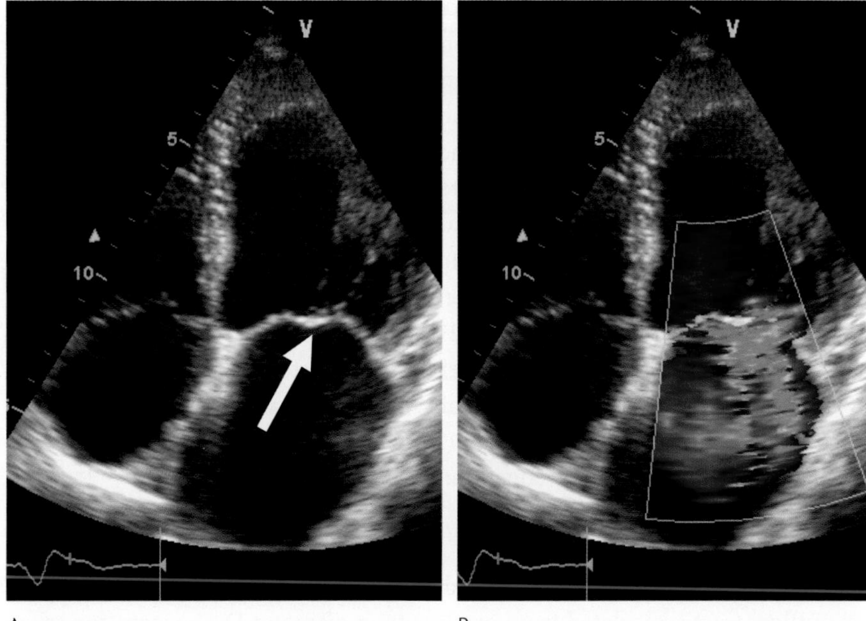

Figure 4.42 (A) Functional (ischaemic) mitral regurgitation in a patient with ischaemic cardiomyopathy. Note tenting of the mitral valve (arrow) due to eccentric pull of the papillary muscles. (B) Colour Doppler of mitral regurgitation.

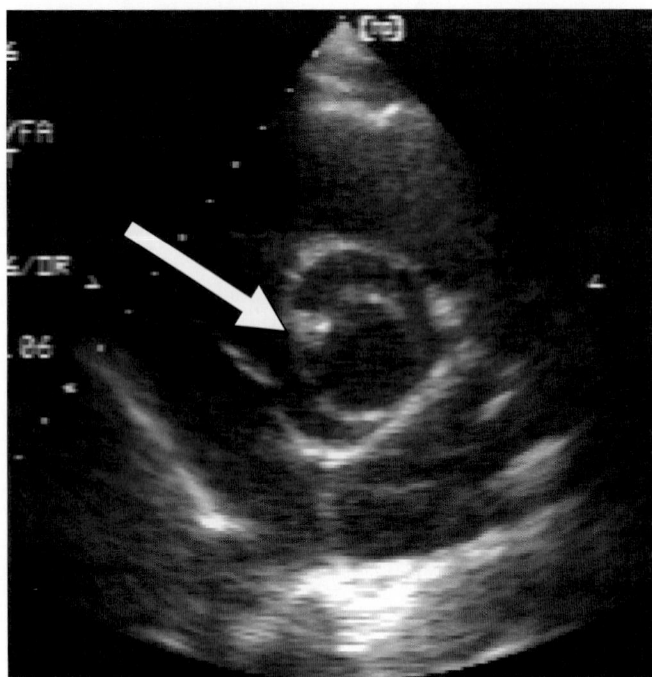

Figure 4.43 Typical aspect of congenitally bicuspid aortic valve in the parasternal short-axis view. The arrow points at the circular shape of the opened valve. Also see 4.23.

a routine echocardiographic examination. In advanced age and in long-standing hypertension, the aortic valve frequently develops focal sclerosis without significant obstruction. Minimal aortic regurgitation is common, especially in the elderly.

Aortic stenosis (➲Chapter 22)is the most frequent severe valvular heart disease requiring surgical treatment in our populations. The disease begins with focal sclerosis, becoming diffuse and leading to severe thickening, immobility, and calcification of the leaflets. These characteristics are well appreciated by echocardiography. Even aortic valve sclerosis, which involves only small increments in flow velocity (<2.5m/s peak velocity), entails a distinctly impaired cardiovascular prognosis. Severe aortic valve stenosis, defined as orifice area <1.0cm^2 or, indexed to body surface area, <0.6cm^2/m^2, requires careful scrutiny for symptoms or deterioration of left ventricular function, which both constitute indications for valve replacement (see ➲Chapter 21). The most important parameters to characterize the severity of aortic stenosis by echocardiography are the maximal and mean transvalvular gradient and the aortic orifice area (AoA), which usually is calculated by the continuity equation:

$$AoA = A_{LVOT} \times VTI_{LVOT}/VTI_{CW}$$

where A_{LVOT} is the cross-sectional area of the left ventricular outflow tract (calculated from outflow tract diameter D as $\pi \times D^2/4$), VTI_{LVOT} is the time velocity integral of systolic flow in the outflow tract (measured by PW Doppler), and VTI_{CW} is the time velocity integral of trans-stenotic flow measured by CW Doppler (➲Fig. 4.44; 4.24 and 4.25). Sometimes, especially with TOE, the stenotic orifice area can be planimetered directly. Importantly, the orifice area does not depend on stroke volume and therefore is the only reliable parameter in the presence of an impaired left ventricular function.

In some cases of severely impaired left ventricular function with questionably severe aortic stenosis, a dobutamine stress echocardiogram may provide additional functional and prognostic information.

Aortic regurgitation is the most difficult valvular lesion to grade by echocardiography. It may be due to dilatation of the ascending aorta (e.g. in Marfan's syndrome), calcific disease of the valve, bacterial endocarditis, degenerative changes such as prolapse, rheumatic disease, and others. The severity of regurgitation may be semiquantitatively estimated by (see ➲Fig. 4.45; 4.26; and ➲Table 4.4):

- assessment of valve morphology and the degree of dilatation of the left ventricle;
- comparing the proximal jet diameter of the regurgitant jet to the diameter of the outflow in the parasternal long-axis view tract (≥65% indicating severe regurgitation);
- calculating the pressure half-time of the regurgitant flow signal on CW Doppler (<250ms being typical for severe regurgitation);
- recording a holodiastolic reverse flow signal from the descending aorta (from the suprasternal window), with end-diastolic velocities approximately >16cm/s indicating severe regurgitation.

An important part of the evaluation of moderate and severe aortic regurgitation is 1) the assessment of left ventricular function (diameters and ejection fraction); and 2) the assessment of the ascending aorta, especially as to diameter (see [32] and ➲Chapter 21).

Signs of aortic valve endocarditis include vegetations, new aortic regurgitation, structural defects of aortic leaflets, and tissue invasion leading to para-aortic abscess formation and fistulae, e.g. from the aortic outflow tract to the left atrium. Such complications are especially well identified by TOE [36].

Tricuspid valve

Intrinsic diseases of the tricuspid valve are relatively rare, except for tricuspid endocarditis, which occurs mainly in

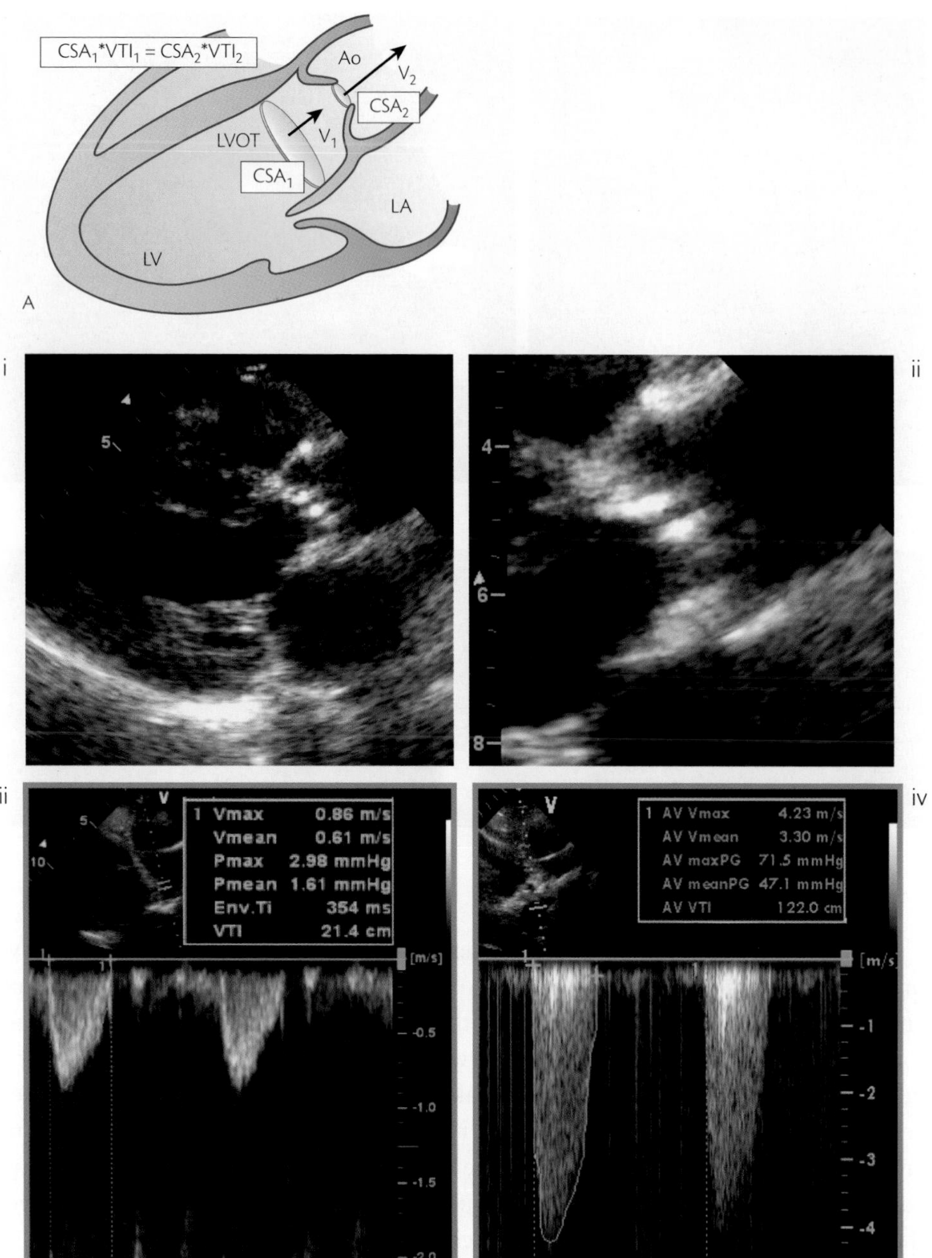

Figure 4.44 (A) The principle of the continuity equation. Conservation of mass dictates that the product of cross-sectional area (CSA) and averaged flow velocity or flow velocity integral (v) is equal at each cross-section of a tube, which is expressed by the continuity equation in the left upper corner of the image. Stenotic aortic area is calculated by solving the equation for CSA_2. (B) Application example of the continuity equation in severe aortic stenosis. i) parasternal long-axis view of aortic stenosis (arrow); note concentric left ventricular hypertrophy. ii) zoom of aortic valve with measurement of left ventricular outflow tract diameter D at the aortic annulus level (2cm). iii) PW Doppler recording of left ventricular outflow tract velocities and velocity time integral (VTI_{LVOT}). iv) CW Doppler recording of transaortic velocities and velocity time integral (VTI_{AS}). By the continuity equation, aortic valve area (A) is calculated as $A = \pi \times (D^2/4) \times VTI_{LVOT}/VTI_{AS}$, which here results in 0.6cm² (severe). Also see 4.24 and 4.25.

drug addicts and patients with long-standing disease necessitating the insertion of in-dwelling central catheters and ports. Pacemaker endocarditis may also extend to the tricuspid valve. Other structural tricuspid valve diseases are rheumatic fever, carcinoid heart disease, iatrogenic injury e.g. due to right ventricular biopsy, and others (see ➲Chapter 10 for Ebstein's disease).

Tricuspid stenosis is very rare and usually accompanies rheumatic mitral valve disease. A mean transtricuspid gradient from CW Doppler >5mmHg is regarded as clinically relevant.

Trace or mild tricuspid regurgitation is almost universally present and should not be regarded as a disease. Moderate or severe tricuspid regurgitation (➲Fig. 4.46; 4.27; see ➲Table 4.4), except in the presence of a pacemaker/defibrillator electrode or in the course of infective endocarditis, almost always is the consequence of a dilatation of the right ventricle—most frequently due to pulmonary hypertension. Further causes to consider in functional tricuspid regurgitation are atrial fibrillation, a left-to-right shunt (see ➲Chapter 10), or primary right ventricular diseases (e.g. right ventricular infarction or cardiomyopathy).

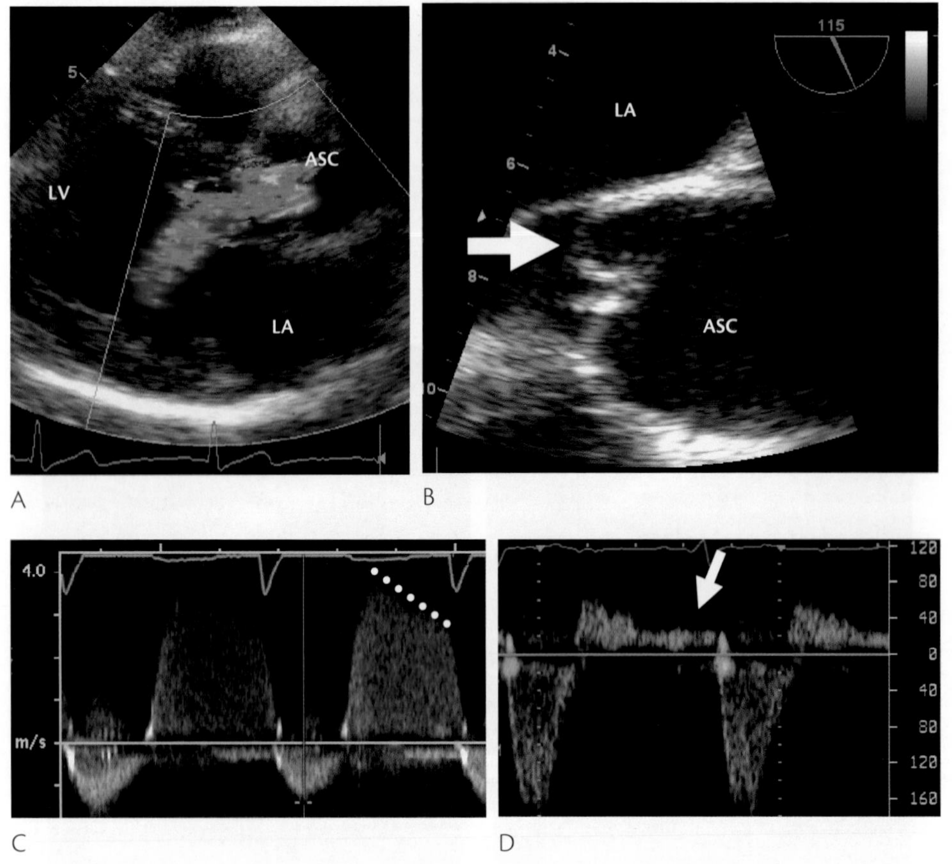

Figure 4.45 Aortic regurgitation. (A) Parasternal long-axis view showing regurgitant jet (in diastole) filling the complete left ventricular outflow tract. (B) Transoesophageal magnified long-axis view of aortic valve showing prolapse of the acoronary aortic cusp (arrow). (C) CW Doppler signal of aortic regurgitation. Diastolic velocity decay, from which pressure half-time can be measured, is marked by the white line. (D) Suprasternal PW Doppler recording of descending aortic flow, showing substantial holodiastolic flow reversal (arrow points to reversal persisting until end-diastole). ASC, ascending aorta; LA left atrium; LV left ventricle. Also see 4.26.

Severe tricuspid regurgitation can be identified by a large proximal convergence zone, a broad proximal jet width, and dilatation of the inferior vena cava with absent inspiratory collapse and reversal of systolic forward flow in the hepatic veins (see ➲Table 4.4). The peak regurgitant jet velocity is used to estimate peak systolic right ventricular, and thus pulmonary artery pressure. Since the gradient calculated from the simplified Bernoulli equation represents the peak pressure difference between right ventricle and right atrium, to arrive at an estimate of absolute right ventricular or pulmonary pressure, the systolic right atrial pressure must be added. This may be accomplished by adding for the right atrial pressure either a constant (usually 10mmHg) or estimating right atrial pressure from jugular vein filling, respiratory variation in the diameter of the inferior vena cava, or hepatic vein flow pattern. Many laboratories, however, choose to only report the pressure gradient itself.

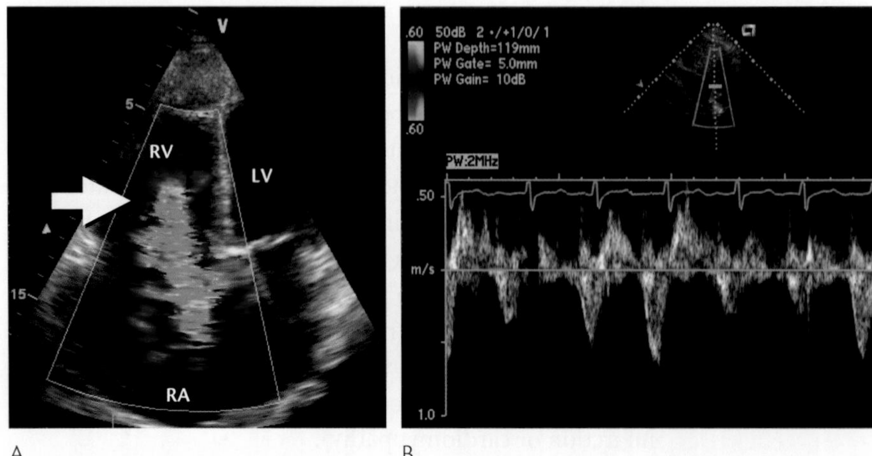

Figure 4.46 Severe tricuspid regurgitation. (A) Colour Doppler recording in the apical four-chamber view. Note large proximal convergence zone. (B) PW Doppler of hepatic venous flow; note systolic flow reversal as a sign of severe tricuspid regurgitation. RA right atrium; RV right ventricle. Also see 4.27.

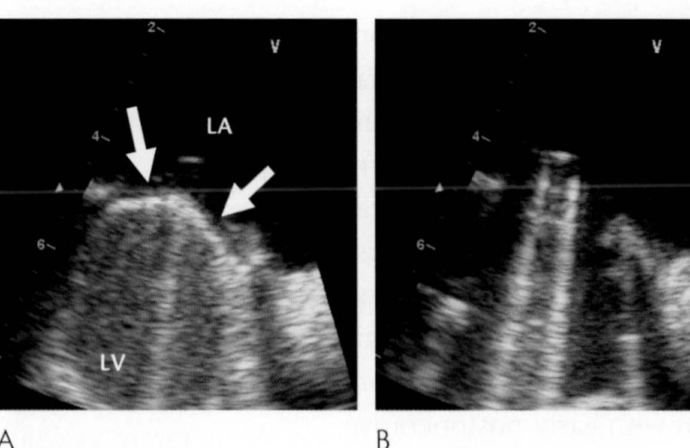

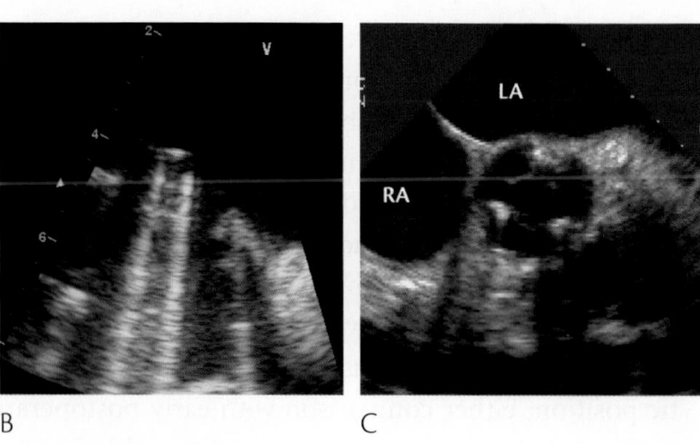

Figure 4.47 Mechanical bileaflet prosthesis in the mitral position with closed (A) and opened (B) discs (arrows); transoesophageal images. (C) Bioprosthesis in the aortic position in a transoesophageal short-axis view. LA left atrium; LV left ventricle; RA right atrium. Also see 4.28.

Pulmonary valve

The pulmonary valve is not well visualized either by TTE or TOE. Pulmonary stenosis (➲Chapter 10) is almost always congenital, and may be present with subvalvular, valvular, and supravalvular components in complex congenital heart disease such as Fallot's tetralogy (see ➲Chapter 10). Minimal pulmonary regurgitation is an almost universal finding even in apparently healthy individuals. More severe degrees of pulmonary regurgitation are graded by the degree of right ventricular dilatation, shortened pressure half-time of the regurgitant CW Doppler signal (<100ms indicating severe regurgitation; [37]), and cessation of regurgitation before the end of diastole.

Prosthetic valves

Valve replacement is performed by inserting biologic or mechanical prostheses (see also ➲Chapter 21). Non-biologic material of the prostheses impairs imaging by artefacts and acoustic shadowing, so that the examination is more difficult than that of native valves. TOE should be performed whenever there is a suspicion of prosthetic malfunction or endocarditis.

Prostheses differ by their design and valve mechanism. Accordingly, they present differing echocardiographic characteristics:

- Homografts or the native pulmonary valve transposed to the aortic position after a Ross procedure practically are indistinguishable from native valves.
- Porcine or bovine biological prostheses are relatively well imaged, including their leaflets (➲Fig. 4.47; 4.28). They undergo a degenerative process over time with thickening, calcification, and increasing leaflet tissue rigidity, as well as increasing regurgitation. Tears in the leaflets of degenerated bioprostheses can lead to sudden massive regurgitation. Biological prostheses have relatively minor transvalvular gradients (➲Table 4.5) and almost always at least mild transvalvular regurgitation.
- Mechanical prostheses nowadays are most often of the bileaflet type. The two leaflets or discs of such prostheses are mostly visualizable in the mitral position (➲Fig. 4.47; 4.28), but often impossible to evaluate in the aortic position, even by TOE. These prostheses in the aortic position may have considerable transvalvular gradients despite normal mechanical function, especially if the valve size is small (19–21) and the aorta is narrow. Maximal velocities >4m/s are not rare in these conditions. The reason may be pressure recovery, which is a phenomenon due to localized high pressure gradients occurring in these prostheses due to their geometric design [38]. These pressure gradients are picked up by CW interrogation; however, they are larger than the 'net' gradient between left ventricle

Table 4.5 Echocardiographic normal values: blood flow and tissue Doppler (adapted from [1, 52, 53])

Peak transvalvular and transprosthetic blood flow velocities (m/s). Data for prostheses are averaged over a range of sizes, except for mechanical aortic prostheses	
Aortic valve	1.0–1.7
Mitral valve	0.6–1.3
Tricuspid valve	0.3–0.7
Pulmonary valve	0.6–0.9
Stented bioprostheses in the aortic position	2.8 ± 0.4
Mechanical prostheses in the aortic position: tilting disc	1.9 ± 0.2 to 3.3 ± 0.6
Mechanical prostheses in the aortic position: bileaflet	1.9 ± 0.3 to 3.1 ± 0.4
Stented bioprostheses in the mitral position	1.0 ± 0.3
Mechanical prostheses in the mitral position: tilting disc	1.3 ± 0.3
Mechanical prostheses in the mitral position: bileaflet	0.9 ± 0.2
Peak longitudinal tissue velocities (cm/s) in left ventricular basal septum by pulsed Doppler (from 54–56)	
S wave	8.0 ± 2cm/s (<40 years) to 7.1 ± 1.3cm/s (> 70 years)
e′ wave	10.1 ± 2.6 (<45 years) to 6.2 ± 1.7 (>74 years)

and ascending aorta, thereby leading to 'overestimation' of the net gradient. Unfortunately, a high transvalvular pressure gradient created by a true dysfunction, e.g. pannus or thrombus, is indistinguishable from a high pressure gradient generated by the design of the valve; the two gradients do not necessarily add, because in the case of prosthetic obstruction the 'in-built' gradient may be decreased [39]. Thus, in bileaflet valves (and also in other mechanical valves) with high transvalvular gradients in the aortic position, either comparison with early postoperative gradients (when the prosthesis was presumably intact) or fluoroscopy or cardiac computer tomography should be performed to exactly delineate leaflet mobility.

Several typical complications of valvular prostheses must be searched for and evaluated whenever a patient with a prosthetic valve is examined echocardiographically. These include:

- Obstruction: due to thrombus, pannus (sterile tissue ingrowth), or, rarely, vegetation growth in mechanical valves; in biological prostheses, degenerative changes may lead to obstruction. The severity of obstruction is graded in accordance with assessment of stenosis in native valves. For the problem of high gradients across aortic mechanical prostheses, see earlier discussion.
- Regurgitation: transvalvular and paravalvular regurgitation occurs. Transvalvular regurgitation of minor degree is present in mechanical prostheses by design [40]; prosthetic dysfunction, e.g. by a thrombotically fixed disc, may lead to more severe regurgitation, and catastrophic regurgitation follows embolization of a disc. Paravalvular regurgitation is frequent and often minor. It should be ascertained whether it was present immediately after operation or appeared later, which would raise the question of endocarditis. Large paravalvular leaks leading to rocking of the whole prostheses are termed dehiscence and are associated with severe regurgitation. Three-dimensional TOE appears to be especially useful for the assessment of size of paravalvular leaks.
- Prosthetic endocarditis: valve prostheses are prone to infections. Typically, the infection manifests as vegetations attached to the prosthetic ring, and abscesses may develop in the immediate proximity of the prosthetic ring. This is best appreciated by TOE. Vegetations may also originate from the leaflets of biological prostheses. More rarely, vegetations may be attached to the discs of a mechanical prosthesis (see also ➲Chapter 21).

Pericardium

The posterior pericardium is the brightest structure in the far field of parasternal echocardiographic cross-sections of the heart. The anterior pericardium is less echogenic. Pericardial fat is relatively frequent in elder patients and has an echo-lucent, but not echo-free appearance. Pericardial effusion, which is echo-free in the acute stage, can be seen in all views if circular. Small effusions are best appreciated from the subcostal window with the patient supine. The haemodynamic impact of a pericardial effusion should be examined by looking for compression of a cardiac chamber, in circular pericardial effusion the right atrium, since its inner pressure level is lowest of all chambers (➲Figs. 4.48 and 4.49; 🎥 4.29–4.31), and the right ventricle. In rare cases of localized pericardial effusions (e.g. postoperatively) other chambers may be compressed first. The constriction created by external compression of the heart chambers leads to an exaggeration of respiratory variation of inflow and outflow patterns of the ventricles, similar to constrictive pericarditis: mitral inflow decreases with inspiration, as does aortic stroke volume, while tricuspid inflow increases (➲Chapter 19). A >25% decrease in peak transmitral E wave velocity with

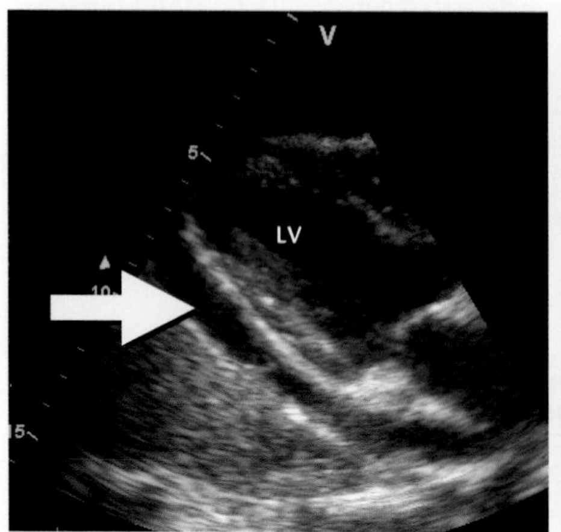

A

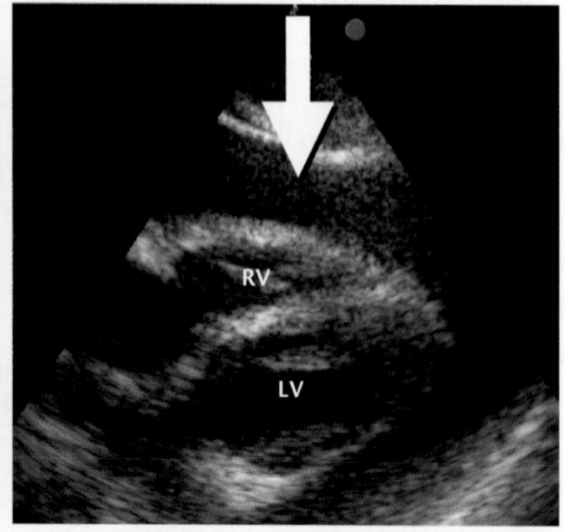

B

Figure 4.48 Pericardial effusions. (A) Parasternal long-axis view and modest effusion (arrow). (B) Large effusion viewed from subcostal view. The arrow indicates the direction of advancement of puncture needle if pericardial tap is performed. Also see 🎥 4.29 and 4.30.

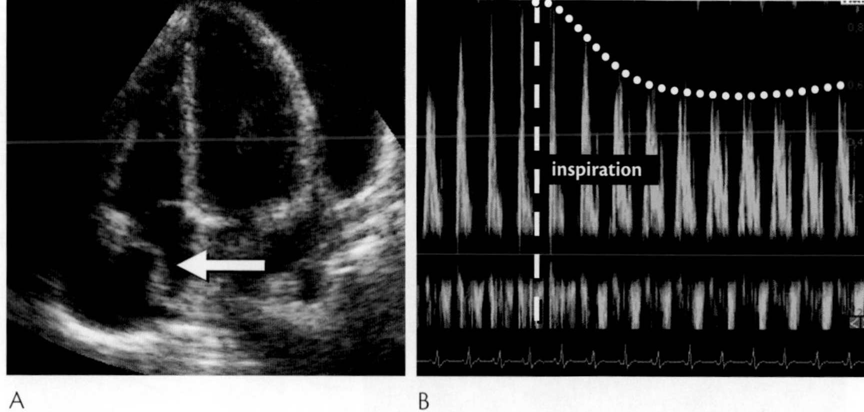

Figure 4.49 Pericardial tamponade. (A) Apical four-chamber view with large circular effusion and compression of right atrium. (B) PW Doppler recording of transmitral flow at low sweep speed, showing inspiratory decrease in peak transmitral velocities. Also see 4.31.

inspiration is considered a sign of pericardial tamponade. A 'paradoxical' septal shift to the left in early diastole, created by the increase in transtricuspid flow, is also observed. In expiration, these changes are reversed.

To prepare pericardial puncture, the subcostal view is useful to determine the location, angle, and depth of the puncture (Fig. 4.49; 4.31). After puncture, the location of the tip of the needle or of a catheter introduced in the pericardial space may be confirmed by injecting an agitated infusion solution, which will create a bright contrast echocardiogram.

Constrictive pericarditis (see Chapter 19) is not easy to diagnose by echocardiography. Thickened (>5mm), calcified pericardium may be apparent, but often is not. The ventricles are of normal size, while the atria are enlarged. A paradoxical septal motion is almost universally present. Left and right ventricular systolic function is mostly unimpaired. The inspiratory decrease in transmitral flow and increase in transtricuspid flow, very similar to tamponade, is present in clear-cut cases. Sometimes, however, this sign is blunted by massive diuretic therapy. The transmitral flow in the typical case exhibits a tall, short E wave with short deceleration time ('restrictive pattern'). E/e′ in this disease should not be used to predict the left ventricular filling pressures.

Tumours

Myxoma is by far the most frequent originary cardiac tumour (see Chapter 20). It typically has an irregular shape, with possible calcifications and echo-lucent regions, and is mobile. Embolic complications are relatively frequent. The most frequent attachment point is the left side of the atrial septum in the fossa ovalis region. The tumour may prolapse through the mitral valve into the left ventricle during diastole (Fig. 4.50) and obstruct left ventricular inflow. Other locations occur (right atrium, left ventricle). Fibroelastomas arise from valvular tissue, mostly from the aortic valve, but they also occur on other valves. Like myxomas, they may embolize. Typical appearance and location make the diagnosis of these two tumour types very likely, but ultimately it is impossible to predict histology from echocardiographic data. Metastatic tumours often cause pericardial effusions.

Aorta

The ascending aorta can be seen over its first few centimetres from the parasternal long-axis view. Access to the aortic arch is provided by the suprasternal window, which, however, is often obstructed in elderly or emphysematous individuals. A much more complete evaluation of the thoracic aorta is possible by TOE, where almost the entire course is visible except for a 'blind spot' created by tracheal and left bronchial interposition at the distal ascending aorta and proximal arch. Dilatation and aneurysms, atheromatous disease, plaque-adherent thrombi, and aortic dissection or intramural haematoma can be diagnosed by TOE (see Chapter 31).

- Aortic diameters. At the aortic root, several diameters can be measured. The first and usually smallest is the diameter of the aortic annulus. A few millimetres distally, at the sinuses of Valsalva, the diameter is considerably larger. At the transition from sinuses to ascending aorta, the 'sinotubular junction', the normal aorta becomes narrower again, although it is still wider than at the annulus. In Marfan's syndrome, the sinotubular junction typically is effaced, and the aorta dilates immediately distal to the aortic valve in a funnel-like shape. Normal values are given in Fig. 4.51.
- Atheromatosis is mainly observed in the descending aorta and the arch. Sometimes, mobile thrombi may be noted which may embolize.
- Aortic dissection (Chapter 31) is diagnosed by identifying the pathognomonic dissection membrane, a thin, undulating membrane ('intimal flap') separating true and

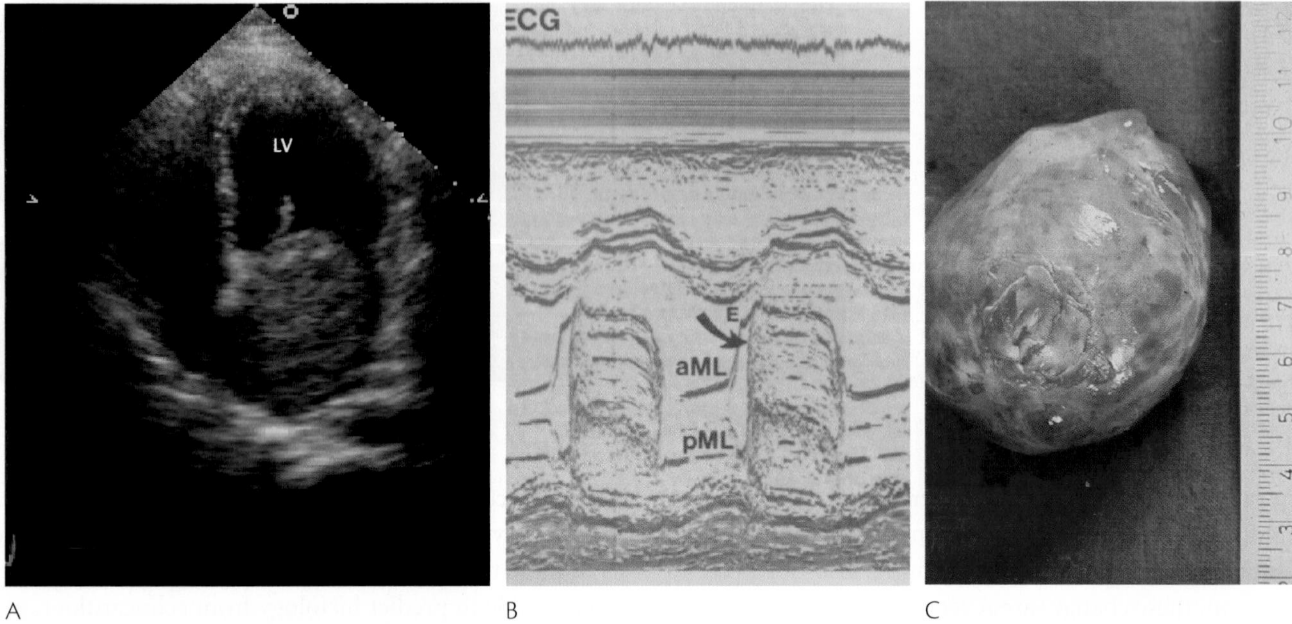

Figure 4.50 (A) Apical four-chamber view shows a large myxoma prolapsing into the mitral orifice in diastole. LV, left ventricle. (B) M-mode recording shows the tumour in the mitral orifice (arrow). Note that there is an interval between mitral valve (aML and pML) opening and diastolic prolapse of the tumour corresponding to the tumour plop heard on auscultation. Ventricular filling takes place during this short interval. (C) Anatomical specimen showing the excised attachment of the tumour to the interatrial septum.

false lumen (➲Fig. 4.52). Entry and re-entry sites may be identified by two-dimensional echocardiography and colour flow Doppler. The false lumen typically is larger, has slower flow (often spontaneous contrast or even thrombosis is present), and is convex towards the higher-pressurized, but smaller true lumen. The site of the intimal rupture and the extent of the dissection are crucial for identification of the type of dissection and thus prognosis and management. Typical concomitant signs of type A dissections (involving the ascending aorta) are aortic regurgitation and pericardial haemorrhage, portending imminent lethal tamponade. A special form of dissection is aortic intramural haematoma, which manifests as thickening of the aortic wall (➲Fig. 4.53; 🎥 4.32).

An emerging role for TOE and intravascular ultrasound is to provide imaging support for the interventional

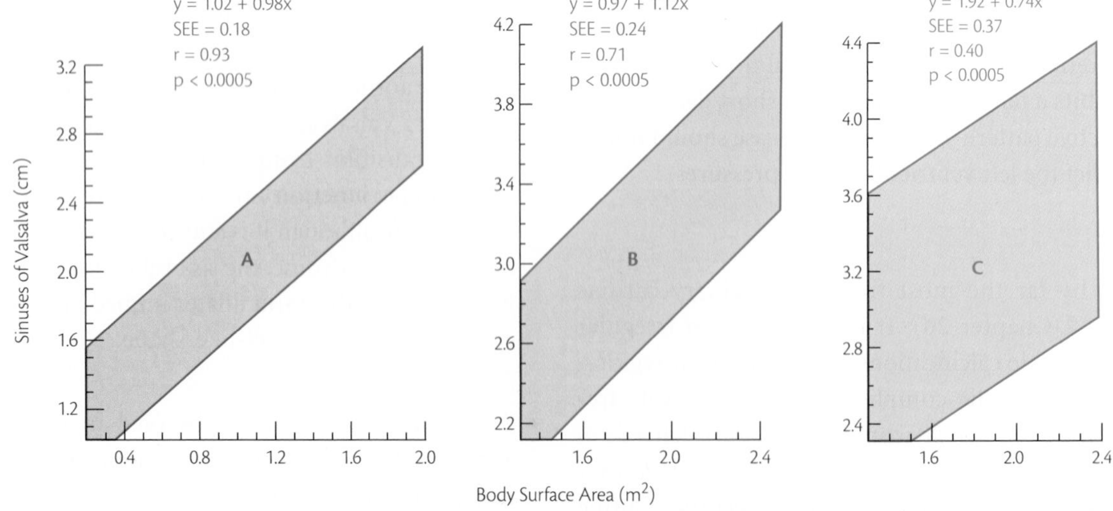

Figure 4.51 Normal range of aortic diameters at the sinuses of Valsalva (95% confidence intervals; (A) <20 years; (B) 20–39; (C) ≥40 years). Reproduced with permission from Lang R, Bierig M, Devereux R, *et al.* Recommendations for Chamber Quantification. A report from the American Society of Echocardiography's Nomenclature and Standards Committee, the Task Force on Chamber Quantification, and the European Association of Echocardiography. *Eur J Echocardiogr* 2006; **7** : 79–108.

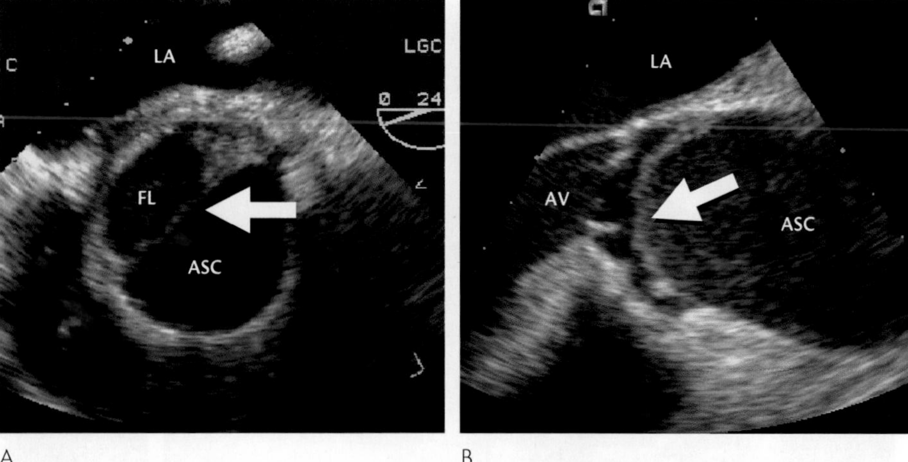

Figure 4.52 Aortic dissection of the ascending aorta (ASC; arrows point to intimal flap). (A) Transoesophageal short-axis view of a dissection with spontaneous contrast and beginning thrombosis of the false lumen (FL). (B) Transoesophageal long-axis view of a dissection of the ascending aorta.

treatment of type III dissections with stents, where stent location, coverage of dissection, leaks, and other questions may be addressed by ultrasound imaging.

Pulmonary artery

The main pulmonary artery and the right pulmonary artery are reasonably well visualized from transthoracic parasternal and subcostal views and by TOE. Dilatation or the detection of thrombotic material is important in the evaluation of patients with suspected acute or chronic pulmonary hypertension.

Key echocardiographic features of frequent diseases and clinical scenarios

Coronary artery disease (➲Chapters 16 and 17)

The coronaries are only marginally visualized by echocardiography; the ostia of the left and right coronary are frequently identifiable, especially by TOE (see ➲Fig. 4.53; 🎥 4.32), and the left main stem as well as the very proximal segments of the left anterior descending and sometimes the circumflex artery may be visualized by TOE. With transthoracic transducers, some centres have been able to visualize the distal left anterior descending by colour Doppler in 90% of patients or more, allowing measurement of flow velocity and—by performing a vasodilator stress test—to determine the coronary flow reserve of this artery [14]. Moreover, myocardial contrast echocardiography allows in principle to evaluate regional myocardial blood volume and flow reserve (see ➲Contrast echocardiography, p.114). Nevertheless, at present these techniques are not widely used.

The most important sign of coronary artery disease (CAD) is therefore the impairment of regional wall motion of the left (and rarely, right) ventricle as a consequence of previous ischaemia. For this purpose, the regional function of the left ventricle is visually evaluated (see ➲Left ventricle, p.116). Objective evaluation of regional myocardial function by quantitative parameters can be achieved using tissue velocity and deformation data (see ➲Figs. 4.12 and 4.18). However, longitudinal myocardial velocities have location-specific normal values and are subject to the influence of neighbouring regions ('tethering') and are therefore difficult to use in particular when evaluating mild or moderate wall motion abnormalities. The greatest promise at presents seems to lie in regional strain and strain rate measurement, preferably based on speckle tracking algorithms

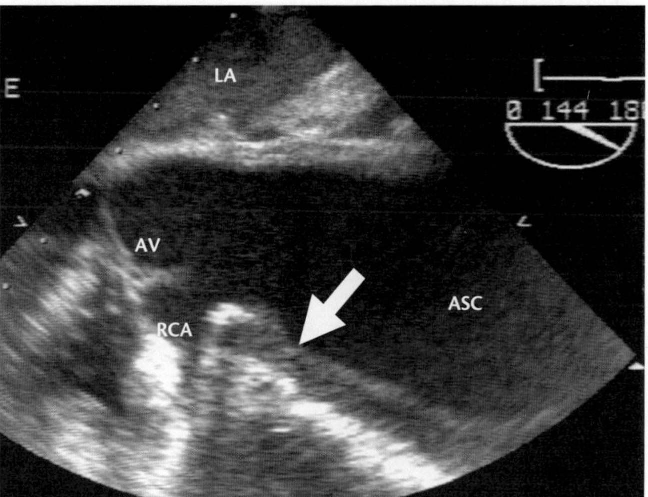

Figure 4.53 Intramural haematoma (arrow) of ascending aorta. Note thickened aortic wall starting at the take-off of the right coronary artery (RCA). Transoesophageal long-axis view. AV, aortic valve. (Courtesy of J. Roelandt and R. Erbel.) Also see 🎥 4.32.

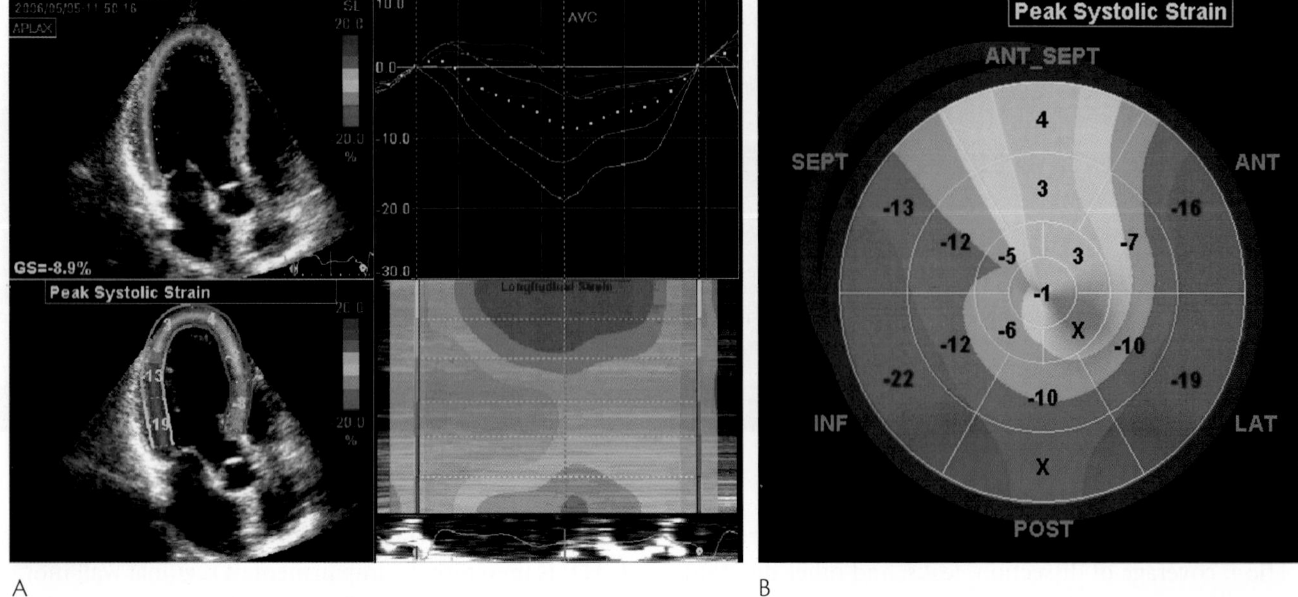

Figure 4.54 'Two-dimensional strain' imaging using speckle tracking. Velocity and deformation parameters can be estimated in any direction within the image plane. (A) Colour-coded longitudinal strain is superimposed on an apical three-chamber view (top left). End-systolic strain is displayed per segment (bottom left). Strain curves and curved M-mode display of strain allow evaluation of the temporal course of regional deformation (top and bottom right). (B) Bull's eye view of the left ventricle with colour coded segmental endsystolic strain values obtained from the three apical views. The infarcted region is clearly visualized. Segmental systolic strain values are displayed. X denotes a segment not scored. Also see 4.33 and 4.34.

('two-dimensional strain'; Fig. 4.54; 4.33 and 4.34). The detection of regional wall motion abnormalities at rest is not specific for CAD; cardiomyopathies, myocarditis, and other diseases may also lead to regionally variable wall motion abnormalities. On the other hand, even diffusely reduced wall motion may be due to multivessel coronary disease or post-infarct remodelling.

Stress-inducible myocardial ischaemia can be diagnosed by stress echocardiography (see Stress echocardiography, p.112). Viability of dysfunctional myocardium due to reduced coronary perfusion or non-transmural infarction is detectable by pharmacologic or exercise stress tests. Aneurysmal wall motion abnormality, marked thinning, and increased myocardial reflectivity are signs of myocardial scar.

Acute myocardial ischaemia during an acute coronary syndrome manifests on echocardiography as an acute wall motion abnormality in the perfusion territory of the affected vessel with a severity ranging from hypokinesia to dyskinesia. This is also detectable by deformation imaging (strain and strain rate; Fig. 4.55). Acute echocardiography in the early evaluation of a suspected acute coronary syndrome, e.g. in the presence of inconclusive ECG changes and before confirmation or exclusion of the diagnosis by biomarkers, therefore is extremely useful to

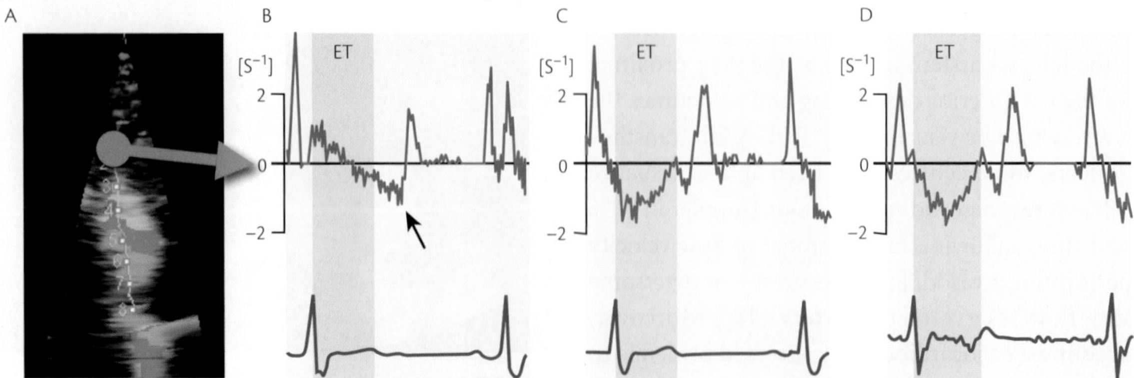

Figure 4.55 (A) Strain rate in acute septal myocardial infarction. (B) On admission to the emergency room, the septum shows positive longitudinal strain rate (lengthening) during ejection time (ET), indicating systolic stretching of this myocardial region. Note the marked post-systolic shortening (arrow). (C) 1 day after successful acute coronary intervention, the strain rate curve has normalized. (D) Normal curve pattern 2 weeks after the event.

confirm or refute the presence and extent of ischaemia. Besides, it quickly provides critical information on potential confounding diseases such as pulmonary embolism, aortic dissection, and others. However, small wall motion abnormalities, especially in the circumflex perfusion territory, may elude echocardiographic diagnosis.

In the setting of a myocardial infarction, echocardiography provides data crucial for management and prognosis:

- site and extent of wall motion abnormalities, left and right ventricular systolic function and volumes, and increase in filling pressures;
- presence, mechanism, and severity of mitral regurgitation;
- presence of thrombi;
- presence of infarct complications such as papillary muscle rupture, ventricular septal defect, pseudoaneurysm (contained myocardial rupture), pericardial effusion.

Thus, every patient with a suspected or proven acute coronary syndrome should undergo echocardiography as quickly as it can be offered. In the subacute stage, stress echocardiography for ischaemia and/or viability is often helpful to determine further management in terms of coronary revascularization.

Hypertension

The echocardiographic hallmark of hypertension (➲Chapter 13) is an increase in left ventricular mass, which is called left ventricular hypertrophy. In hypertension, several patterns of change in left ventricular morphology have been described, depending on the relation of end-diastolic wall thickness and end-diastolic left ventricular cavity diameter. The most frequent type pattern is eccentric hypertrophy, implying an increased left ventricular mass (indexed to body surface area) together with an increased left ventricular end-diastolic diameter. Concentric hypertrophy (increased indexed left ventricular mass together with a normal or decreased left ventricular diameter), carries the worst prognosis as to cardiovascular adverse events [41].

As discussed in the section on the left ventricle, left ventricular hypertrophy is frequently associated with characteristic changes of diastolic filling pressures, either at rest or during exercise. Furthermore, long standing hypertension is commonly accompanied by aortic valve sclerosis and mitral valve calcification, left atrial dilatation, aortic dilatation, and aortic atheromatosis.

Cardiomyopathies, myocarditis, and the transplanted heart

Dilated cardiomyopathy (➲Chapter 18) is characterized by dilatation and functional impairment—both systolic and diastolic—of the left ventricle, and in some cases also of the right ventricle (➲Fig. 4.56). Parameters of systolic function, most prominently EF, are decreased, and parameters of diastolic function indicate elevated filling pressures. The presence of a 'restrictive' transmitral filling pattern (see ➲Fig. 4.26c), which cannot be reversed by therapy, independently from EF implies particularly elevated filling pressures, severe myocardial disease, and impaired prognosis. Almost universally, mitral regurgitation is present with the configuration of functional regurgitation (see ➲Mitral valve, p.126). Peak tricuspid regurgitation velocity usually identifies elevated right ventricular systolic pressure. In severe left ventricular dilatation, spontaneous echocardiographic contrast and left ventricular or left atrial thrombi are frequently seen. Early impairment of systolic and diastolic function may be detected by reduced longitudinal systolic and early diastolic myocardial velocities on tissue Doppler before EF

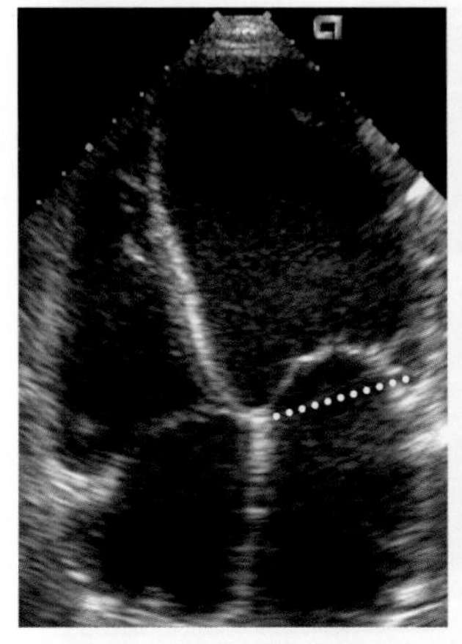
A

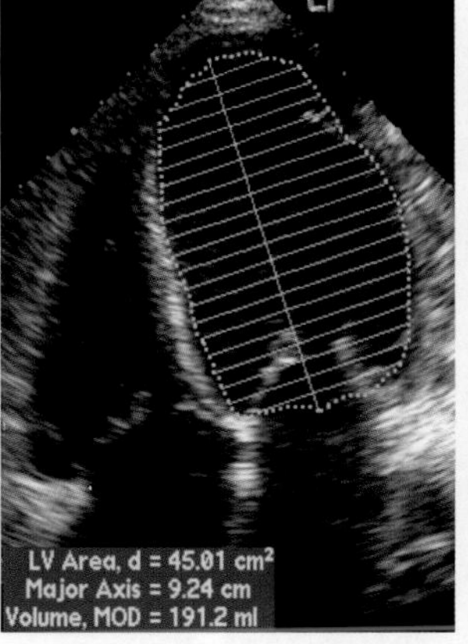

B

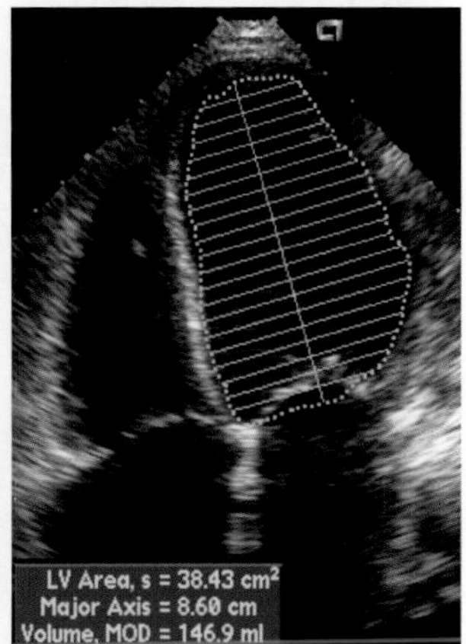

C

Figure 4.56 Dilated cardiomyopathy. (A) All heart chambers are enlarged. Note mitral 'tenting' due to eccentric pull of papillary muscles with apposition of the leaflets displaced into the left ventricle. The dotted line marks the level of the mitral annulus. (B) and (C) Calculation of left ventricular volumes and ejection fraction by modified Simpson's rule (in this case, monoplane from planimetry of the left ventricle in end-systole and end-diastole). End-systolic volume: 147mL; end-diastolic volume: 191mL; ejection fraction 23% (severely reduced).

becomes noticeably reduced [42]. Similar changes are seen in the toxic, dose-dependent cardiomyopathy induced by chemotherapy, in particular by anthrachinolones (doxorubicin and daunorubicin); see also ➲Heart failure, p.141.

Hypertrophic cardiomyopathy (➲Chapter 18) is often asymptomatic and is diagnosed by echocardiography based on increased wall thicknesses and increased left ventricular mass in the absence of hypertension. The location of increased wall thickness is very variable and may occur anywhere in the left ventricle, although the ventricular septum is most frequently involved. A subgroup of patients—usually with greatly increased septal thickness—develops obstruction to systolic ejection in the outflow tract. The mechanism of hypertrophic obstructive cardiomyopathy or 'subaortic stenosis' is believed to be a combination of increased basal septal thickness and structural changes of the mitral valve leading to systolic anterior motion (SAM) of the mitral valve in systole, a phenomenon most likely due to redundant mitral leaflet tissue being dragged or sucked into the outflow tract by vigorous ejection (➲Fig. 4.57). The result is a late peaking systolic gradient occurring in the outflow tract, which is highly variable depending on load conditions, sympathetic drive, and other factors; provocative manoeuvres include exercise or the application of nitroglycerin. The CW Doppler spectrum typically is dagger-shaped with a late systolic peak; peak velocities may exceed 5m/s, but also may be barely elevated. This so-called 'dynamic obstruction' may also generate a mid-systolic closure movement of the aortic valve and a deceleration in mid-systolic septal tissue velocities. Similar to dilated cardiomyopathy, myocardial tissue Doppler shows reduced myocardial systolic and early diastolic peak velocities in patients with hypertrophic cardiomyopathy, although ejection fraction in these patients is usually in the high normal range. Moreover, genetic carriers of the disease without manifest hypertrophy may also be identifiable based on reduced tissue velocities [43, 44]. Furthermore, deformation parameters have been shown to be useful in distinguishing hypertrophic cardiomyopathy from hypertensive hypertrophy [45].

Echocardiography has an important further role in the follow-up of these patients under therapy and has been reported to be useful for planning of transcutaneous septal alcohol ablation by performing intracoronary echocardiographic-contrast injections into the septal branch targeted for alcohol ablation to delineate the corresponding perfusion territory [46].

Restrictive cardiomyopathy (➲Chapter 18), of which cardiac amyloidosis is the most prominent form, is characterized by diffusely thickened walls (including the right ventricular wall and sometimes even the valve leaflets), a highly reflective myocardial texture (so-called 'granular sparkling'), the very frequent presence of small pericardial effusions, enlarged atria, and signs of increased filling pressures even if EF is still preserved (➲Fig. 4.58). In the end stage, the patients uniformly develop the 'restrictive pattern' of transmitral filling (see ➲Fig. 4.26), portending a very grave prognosis. Tissue Doppler velocities, as well as regional deformation parameters, are impaired already early in the course of the disease. Another, rarer infiltrative form of hypertrophic cardiomyopathy is Fabry disease, which shows very variable patterns of hypertrophy which are less diffuse than in amyloidosis. Myocardial deformation parameters such as myocardial velocities, peak systolic strain, and strain rate are reduced, and the effect of causal treatment by substitution of beta-galactosidase may be documented by these parameters [47, 48].

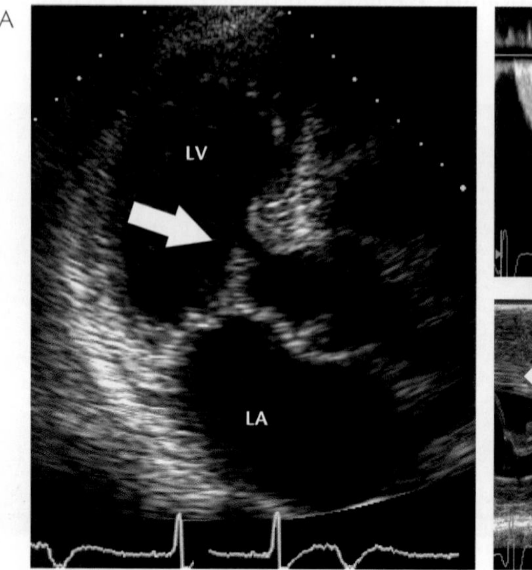

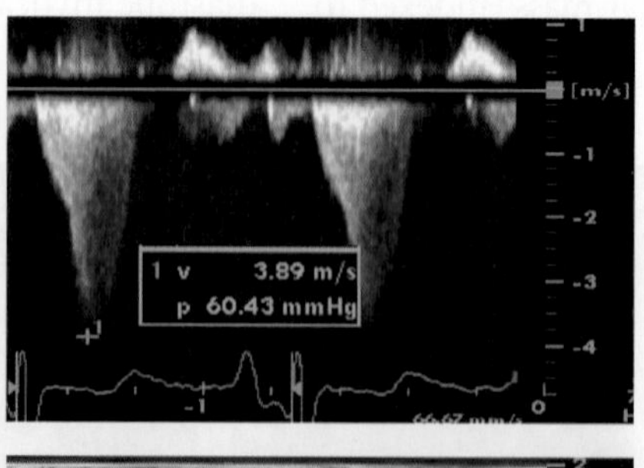

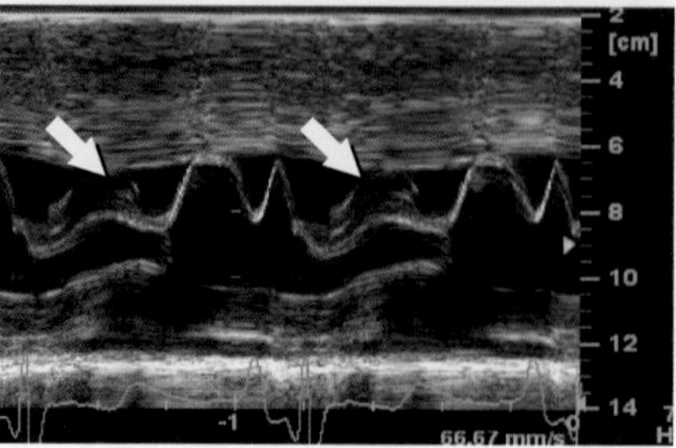

Figure 4.57 Hypertrophic obstructive cardiomyopathy. (A) Apical long-axis view in mid-systole, showing systolic anterior motion of the mitral valve (arrow) leading almost to septal contact of the anterior leaflet tip. (B) CW Doppler signal of left ventricular outflow tract velocities with a characteristic late systolic peak velocity of 389cm/s (60mmHg). (C) M-mode recording showing systolic anterior motion of the mitral valve (arrows). Note massively thickened septum.

Another cardiomyopathy that may mimic hypertrophic cardiomyopathy is left ventricular non-compaction. This is a cardiomyopathy characterized by a two-layered left ventricular wall structure with a heavily trabecularized inner layer (the non-compacted layer) showing prominent intertrabecular spaces and a thickness at least twice as large as the compacted outer layer [49]. For arrhythmogenic right ventricular cardiomyopathy see ➲Right ventricle, p.122.

Myocarditis is a difficult diagnosis short of myocardial biopsy evidence, and echocardiography contributes only modestly. There may be diffuse or regional wall motion abnormalities of all degrees (except for dyskinesia and aneurysms, which, however, uniquely do occur in tropical Chagas disease). Sometimes, a pericardial effusion is present, implying perimyocarditis. Tissue oedema may be present and manifest as increased wall thickness. Unfortunately, all these signs are highly unspecific, and magnetic resonance imaging is clearly superior for this indication.

After heart transplantation, there are several typical characteristics of the transplanted heart:

- The right ventricle is enlarged, there is tricuspid regurgitation of varying degree, and especially early postoperatively, significant pulmonary hypertension can be inferred from peak tricuspid regurgitant velocity.
- The atria are enlarged and the anastomosis between the grafted atria and the remnant of the host atria is often visible as a slight indentation in the atrial walls.
- Transmitral flow profiles often show the influence of competing rhythms of graft and host components of the atrium.
- Diagnosis of rejection, the holy grail of echo in the transplanted patient, has proven elusive. The hallmark of severe rejection is impairment in systolic left and right ventricular function. Milder forms of rejection however are difficult to diagnose. Pericardial effusion, increased wall thickness, and signs of elevated filling pressures—particularly decreased E wave deceleration and shortened isovolumic relaxation period—may be indicative. Good predictive value has been reported from single centres by intra-individual follow-up of tissue velocity and deformation parameters.

Heart failure

All patients with heart failure (➲Chapter 23) should be evaluated by echocardiography [50]. To validate and refine the diagnosis of heart failure, this may include:

- Assessment of left ventricular systolic and diastolic function, including estimation of filling pressures. The latter is

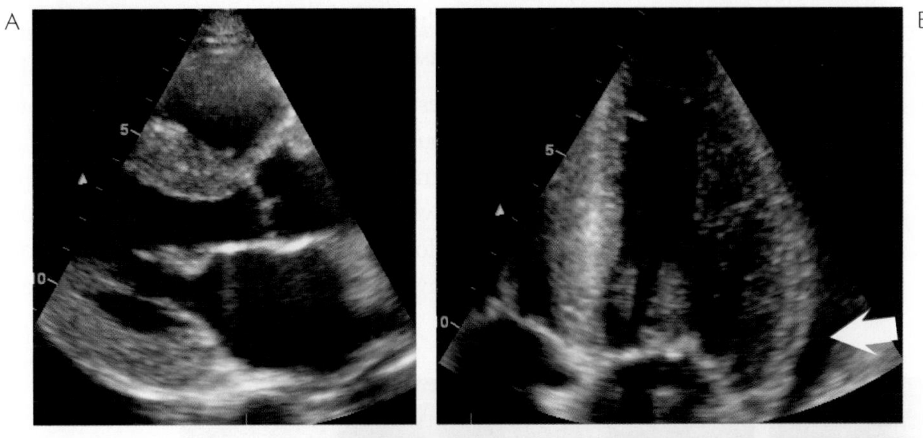

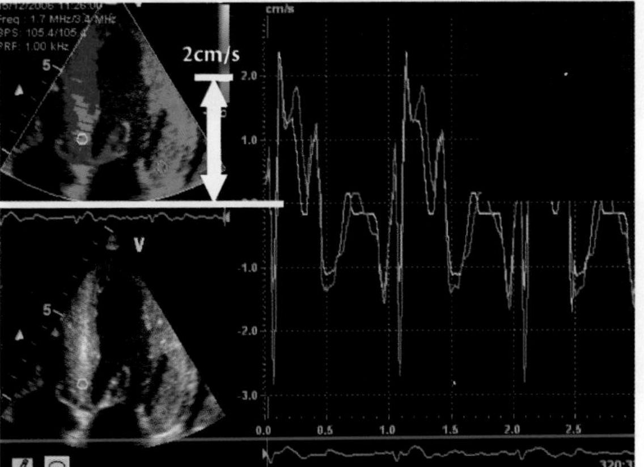

Figure 4.58 Restrictive cardiomyopathy (amyloidosis). (A) Parasternal long axis; (B) magnified apical four-chamber view. Note massive thickening of left ventricular walls with bright echo texture ('granular sparkling'), and pericardial effusion (arrow). (C) Reduced systolic and early diastolic longitudinal tissue velocities from basal septum and basal lateral wall (note scale).

especially important in patients with preserved EF, where the diagnosis of heart failure is less obvious than in patients with depressed EF (see ➲Left ventricle, p.116). The assessment includes evaluation of right ventricular function and estimation of right ventricular systolic pressure.

- Evaluation of concomitant valvular heart disease, in particular mitral regurgitation. Mitral regurgitation is almost uniformly present in severe left ventricular dilatation, but such functional mitral regurgitation must be distinguished from primary mitral regurgitation as the cause for left ventricular failure.
- Assessment for the presence of a cardiomyopathy, myocarditis, or constrictive pericarditis.

Echocardiography also plays a critical role in identifying candidates for therapies and procedures which may reverse, ameliorate, or prognostically improve heart failure. The most important issues are:

- Measurement of EF to identify candidates for implantable defibrillator therapy (EF <35%).
- Diagnosis of hibernating myocardium with the potential to improve function after revascularization. Hibernating, i.e. dysfunctional, but viable myocardial regions can be identified by dobutamine or exercise stress echocardiography (see ➲Stress echocardiography valve, p.112). The identification of hibernating myocardium predicts improvement of EF and prognosis after revascularization.
- Identification of candidates for cardiac resynchronization therapy (CRT; see ➲Chapter 22). Although so far the selection of CRT candidates by echocardiography criteria has not been proven to discriminate well between potential responders and non-responders, and criteria for identifying CRT-responsive left ventricular dyssynchrony continue to evolve [51], several parameters seem to have at least moderate predictive value (➲Figs. 4.59 and 4.60):
  - the interventricular delay, measured as the delay of onset of left ventricular ejection versus the onset of right ventricular ejection (measured from PW-Doppler of pulmonary and aortic flow), considered to be significant >40ms;
  - the differences in the time that it takes myocardial longitudinal systolic velocities to reach their systolic maximum ('time to peak') in the basal or mid segments of the left ventricle, in particular comparing septal to lateral wall segments (with a delay >65ms considered predictive);
  - differences in timing of systolic strain on longitudinal, radial, or circumferential strain of different wall segments;
  - differences in timing of maximal contraction of wall segments as calculated from three-dimensional volume sets.

Cardiogenic embolism

The search for a cardiac source of embolism is a frequent indication for echocardiography, in particular TOE, due to its well established higher yield than TTE in identifying potential sources of cardiac embolism. The following principal pathologies should be systematically sought:

- Atrial thrombi, in particular thrombi of the left atrial appendage (see ➲Fig. 4.35; 4.17) (➲Chapter 29). This structure is known to harbour thrombi in >10% of patients with non-valvular atrial fibrillation (➲Chapter 29). Even in the absence of demonstrating a thrombus, TOE can detect a thrombogenic environment as evidenced by spontaneous echocardiographic contrast and <25cm/s peak flow velocities in the appendage.

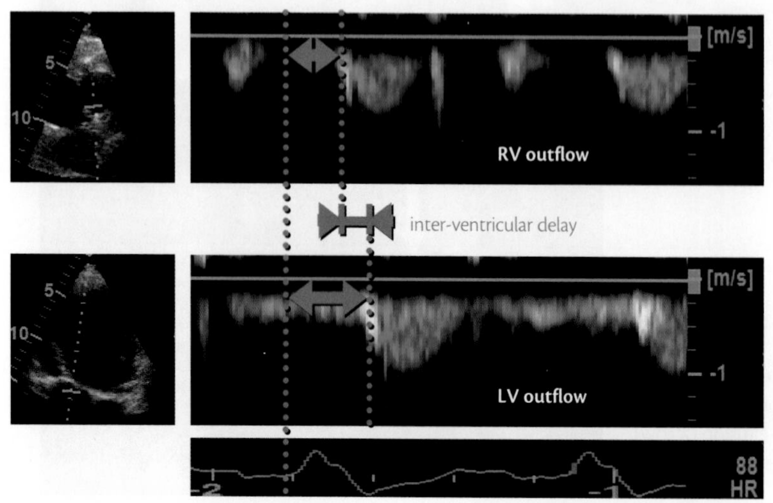

Figure 4.59 Evaluation of patients in heart failure who are candidates for cardiac resynchronization therapy: inter-ventricular delay. The onset of ejection of the right and left ventricle is measured against the ECG (e.g. onset QRS). The difference between both measurements is a marker of interventricular asynchrony, with a difference of >40ms considered a predictor of response to resynchronization.

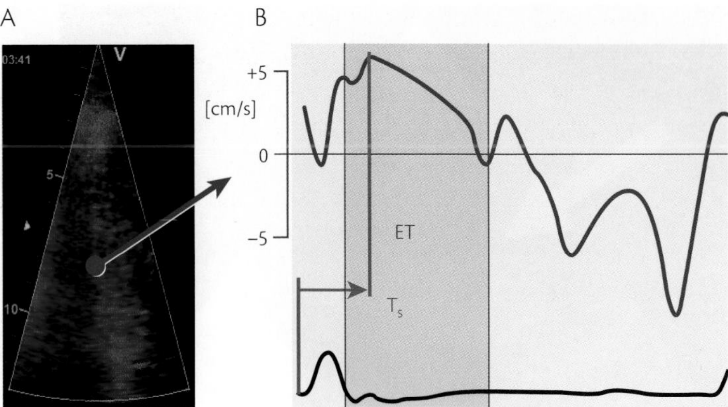

Figure 4.60 Evaluation of patients in heart failure who are candidates for cardiac resynchronization therapy: intra-ventricular asynchrony identified by tissue velocity curves. Time to peak systolic tissue velocity (Ts) is measured either with PW or from high frame rate colour tissue Doppler (as in the case shown) as the interval between onset of QRS and peak positive velocity during ejection time (ET). A difference in the time to peak systolic velocity between septal and lateral basal or mid segments > 65ms is a widely used criterion of significant intraventricular asynchrony.

- Infective endocarditis. Again, TOE has a higher sensitivity in detecting small vegetations than TTE. The risk of embolization from vegetations correlates with their size and mobility, and decreases with elapsed time under antibiotic treatment and with increasing echo-density. See also ➲Chapter 22.
- Left ventricular thrombi occur in areas of large and severe wall motion abnormalities of the left ventricle, whether of ischaemic or cardiomyopathic origin (see ➲Fig. 4.30; 🎥 4.14). TOE has no advantage in detecting left ventricular thrombi.
- Tumours, e.g. myxoma or fibroelastoma, best diagnosed or excluded by TOE (➲Chapter 20).
- Atrial septal defect (➲Chapter 10) or patent foramen ovale (see ➲Right atrium, atrial septum, and caval veins, p.124; ➲Fig. 4.60) as the gate for paradoxical embolism. Through this frequent anomaly, thrombi may cross from the right to the left atrium if a permanent or even transient right-to-left pressure gradient occurs, causing paradoxical embolism to the brain and other organs. While this demonstrably is not infrequent in the context of severe pulmonary embolism, the true significance of this mechanism in cryptogenic embolism remains questionable. An association with unexplained neurologic events has been reported especially for the combination of patent foramen ovale and atrial septal aneurysm.
- Aortic atheromatosis with superimposed thrombi of the arch, ascending aorta, or proximal portions of the descending aorta (➲Fig. 4.61; 🎥 4.35). This is chiefly the domain of TOE, although large thrombi may be detectable from the suprasternal notch (➲Fig. 4.62; 🎥 4.36).

Emergency echocardiography

In all patients with acute, life-threatening cardiovascular disease, echocardiography provides timely, crucial information and can be performed with today's highly portable equipment virtually anywhere inside and outside the hospital. These exams have to be short and focused. As an example, in a patient with unexplained sudden severe hypotension, the following potential mechanisms should be quickly evaluated:

- impaired left ventricular function with a large severe wall motion abnormality (e.g. acute myocardial infarction);
- massive pulmonary embolism with an enlarged and hypokinetic right ventricle, usually with elevated right ventricular systolic pressure as detectable by the almost invariably present tricuspid regurgitation;

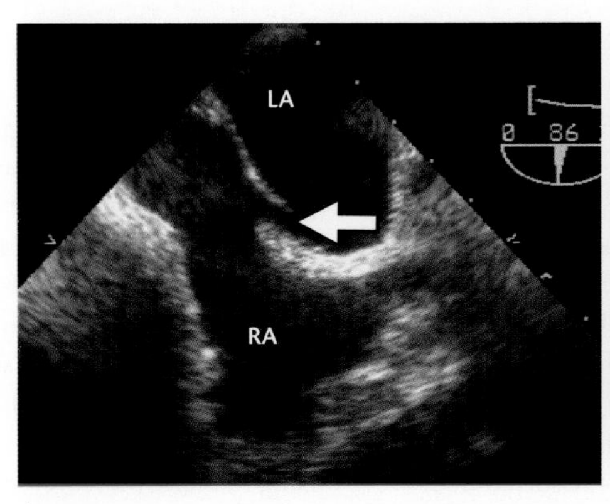

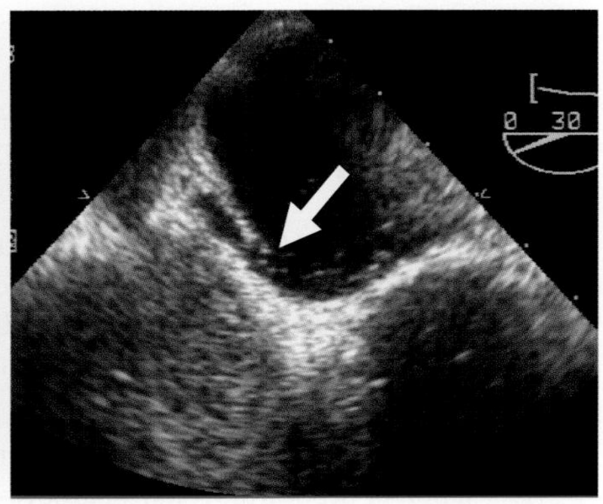

Figure 4.61 Detection of patent foramen ovale by transoesophageal echocardiography with right heart contrast (e.g. agitated saline-blood mixture). (A) View of left (LA) and right atrium (RA) before contrast injection. The arrow points to the patent foramen ovale. (B) Contrast injection, with passage of a few bubbles from right to left atrium across the atrial septum through the patent foramen ovale (arrow). Also see 🎥 4.35.

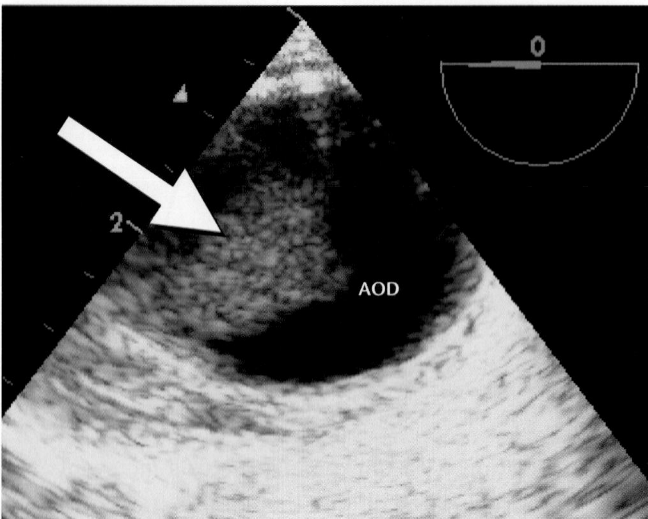

Figure 4.62 Mobile thrombus (arrow) in the descending aorta (AOD). Transoesophageal short-axis view. Also see 4.36.

- pericardial tamponade;
- infarct complications: right heart infarction, papillary muscle rupture with severe mitral regurgitation, ventricular septal defect, myocardial free wall rupture with tamponade;
- acute severe aortic or mitral regurgitation due to infective endocarditis or aortic dissection;
- decompensated aortic stenosis;
- acute aortic dissection or rupture (mostly necessitates TOE).

Intraoperative and interventional echocardiography

Intraoperative TOE is mainly used to check the results of valvular heart surgery, in particular after mitral valve repair. Detection of persistent moderate or severe mitral regurgitation allows to re-operate before the sternum is closed; other complications such as new wall motion abnormalities due to damage to the circumflex artery, new systolic anterior motion of the mitral valve, and others can be detected in a timely way. A clinical benefit of intraoperative TOE has also been seen in other valvular and also revascularization procedures. Direct application of the echocardiographic transducer in a sterile pouch on the aorta may help to detect calcified sites and thus guide aortic cannulation.

During device closure of patent foramen ovale or atrial septal defect, or during percutaneous valve procedures (e.g. percutaneous aortic valve replacement), TOE can be used in the sedated patient in the catheterization laboratory to guide the procedure, detect complications, and check the final results (see Fig. 4.22; 4.10 and 4.11).

Personal perspective

The wealth of morphologic and functional information obtained by echocardiography will keep this technique at the centre of patient evaluation in the foreseeable future, although competing imaging modalities will continue to carve out niches according to their specific strengths. Perhaps surprisingly, echocardiographic techniques and modalities continue to evolve and improve, and therefore have expanded into new territory such as the early diagnosis of clinically inapparent myocardial disease, the exact calculation of cavity volumes from three-dimensional datasets, the estimation of left ventricular filling pressures, and others. It is likely that three-dimensional echocardiography in the long run will supersede two-dimensional echocardiography not only for the evaluation of morphology, but also for blood flow and myocardial deformation analysis. In this context, speckle tracking as a teschnique to detect motion may come to play a similar or larger role than classic Doppler analysis.

Further reading

Baumgartner H, Hung H, Bermejo J, *et al.* Echocardiographic Assessment of Valve Stenosis: EAE/ASE Recommendations for Clinical Practice. *Eur J Echocardiogr* 2009; **10**:1–25.

Daniel WG, Mügge A. Transesophageal echocardiography. *N Engl JMed* 1995; **332**:1268–79.

Evangelista A, Flachskampf F, Lancellotti P, *et al.* European Association of Echocardiography. European Association of Echocardiography recommendations for standardization of performance, digital storage and reporting of echocardiographic studies. *Eur J Echocardiogr* 2008; **9**:438–48.

Flachskampf FA, Decoodt P, Fraser AG, *et al.* Recommendations for performing transesophageal echocardiography. *Eur J Echocardiogr* 2001; **2**:8–21.

Hung J, Lang R, Flachskampf F, *et al.* 3D echocardiography: a review of the current status and future directions. *J Am Soc Echocardiogr* 2007; **20**:213–33. An update of this paper will appear in 2009.

Lang R, Bierig M, Devereux R, *et al.* Recommendations for Chamber Quantification. A report from the American

Society of Echocardiography's Nomenclature and Standards Committee, the Task Force on Chamber Quantification, and the European Association of Echocardiography. *Eur J Echocardiogr* 2006; **7**: 79–108.

Nagueh SF, Appleton CP, Gillebert TC, *et al.* Recommendations for the evaluation of left ventricular diastolic function by echocardiography. *Eur J Echocardiogr* 2009; **10**: 165–93.

Paulus WJ, Tschope C, Sanderson JE, *et al.* How to diagnose diastolic heart failure: a consensus statement on the diagnosis of heart failure with normal left ventricular ejection fraction by the Heart Failure and Echocardiography Associations of the European Society of Cardiology. *Eur Heart J* 2007; **28**: 2539–50.

Sicari R, Nihoyannopoulos P, Evangelista A, *et al.* European Association of Echocardiography. Stress echocardiography expert consensus statement: European Association of Echocardiography (EAE) (a registered branch of the ESC). *Eur J Echocardiogr* 2008; **9**: 415–37.

Vahanian A, Baumgartner H, Bax J, *et al.* Guidelines on the management of valvular heart disease: The Task Force on the Management of Valvular Heart Disease of the European Society of Cardiology. *Eur Heart J* 2007; **28**: 230–68.

Zoghbi WA, Enriquez-Sarano M, Foster E, *et al.* American Society of Echocardiography: recommendations for evaluation of the severity of native valvular regurgitation with two-dimensional and Doppler echocardiography: A report from the American Society of Echocardiography's Nomenclature and Standards Committee and The Task Force on Valvular Regurgitation, developed in conjunction with the American College of Cardiology Echocardiography Committee, The Cardiac Imaging Committee, Council on Clinical Cardiology, The American Heart Association, and the European Society of Cardiology Working Group on Echocardiography. *Eur J Echocardiogr* 2003; **4**: 237–61.

Additional online material

- 4.1 Three-dimensional echocardiography.
- 4.2 Parasternal long-axis view.
- 4.3 Parasternal short-axis view at papillary muscle level.
- 4.4 Parasternal short-axis view at aortic valve level.
- 4.5 Apical four-chamber view.
- 4.6 Apical two-chamber view.
- 4.7 Apical long-axis view.
- 4.8 Cardiac amyloidosis (1).
- 4.9 Cardiac amyloidosis (2).
- 4.10 Transoesophageal three-dimensional echo during interventional closure of an open foramen ovale (1).
- 4.11 Transoesophageal three-dimensional echo during interventional closure of an open foramen ovale (2).
- 4.12 Left ventricular remodelling (1).
- 4.13 Left ventricular remodelling (2).
- 4.14 Left ventricular thrombus.
- 4.15 Left ventricular pseudoaneurysm.
- 4.16 Arrhythmogenic cardiomyopathy of the right ventricle.
- 4.17 Thrombus in the left atrial appendage.
- 4.18 Sagittal transoesophageal view of the right atrium.
- 4.19 Mitral stenosis (1).
- 4.20 Mitral stenosis (2).
- 4.21 Degenerative mitral regurgitation (1).
- 4.22 Degenerative mitral regurgitation (2).
- 4.23 Bicuspid aortic valve.
- 4.24 Aortic stenosis (1).
- 4.25 Aortic stenosis (2).
- 4.26 Aortic valve prolapse.
- 4.27 Severe tricuspid regurgitation.
- 4.28 Mechanical bileaflet mitral prosthesis.
- 4.29 Pericardial effusion.
- 4.30 Pericardial tamponade (1).
- 4.31 Pericardial tamponade (2).
- 4.32 Intramural haematoma of ascending aorta.
- 4.33 Large anteroseptal wall motion abnormality after myocardial infarction (1).
- 4.34 Large anteroseptal wall motion abnormality after myocardial infarction (2).
- 4.35 Detection of patent foramen ovale by transoesophageal echocardiography with right heart contrast.
- 4.36 Thrombus in the descending aorta.

For full references and multimedia materials please visit the online version of the book (http://esctextbook.oxfordonline.com).

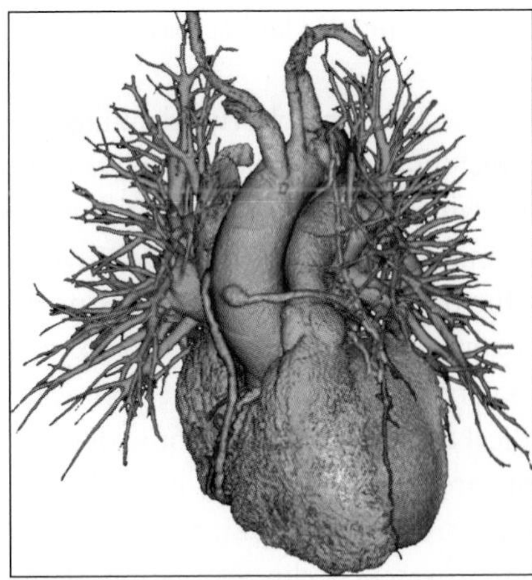

CHAPTER 5

Cardiovascular Magnetic Resonance

Dudley J. Pennell, Udo P. Sechtem, Sanjay Prasad, and Frank E. Rademakers

Contents

Summary

This chapter summarizes the contemporary clinical role of cardiovascular magnetic resonance (CMR) in clinical cardiology. Techniques are described which can be applied widely in the cardiovascular system, and these include assessment of anatomy and function, blood flow, ventricular volumes and mass, myocardial abnormality, and the response to stress.

The longest established indications for CMR are anatomical, including the great vessels, congenital heart disease, pericardium, and cardiac masses, but more recently increasing importance has been placed on assessment of myocardial abnormality. This has opened up new avenues of infarction and viability assessment in coronary artery disease, and phenotyping in cardiomyopathy with distinct distribution patterns of abnormality. The prognostic value of myocardial fibrosis in these settings is now under investigation.

CMR is also becoming more widely used to assess ischaemia, particularly with stress ventriculography and myocardial perfusion imaging. Both techniques have substantial clinical application, and the avoidance of X-ray exposure for high resolution myocardial perfusion imaging is very attractive. Coronary imaging is currently still limited to assessing the course of anomalous coronaries, for which it is ideally suited. Work in acute coronary syndromes has been promising with new techniques to assess areas at risk, as has the visualization of vessel wall changes for the earliest detection of atherosclerosis. Finally, interventional CMR continues to develop, but the question of whether MR might or might not replace X-ray based techniques remains an open long-term question.

Basic principles

This technical introduction to CMR aims to facilitate understanding but greater detail is available elsewhere [1]. Magnetic resonance (MR) depends on the interaction between some atomic nuclei and radiowaves in the presence of a magnetic field. In clinical practice, imaging is almost exclusively performed using hydrogen-1, which is abundant in water and fat. A small excess number of hydrogen nuclei align to the magnetic field, and can be excited by a radiowave at a resonant frequency (63MHz with a 1.5 Tesla scanner). After the excitation pulse, the net magnetization decays (*relaxation*) and releases energy as a radio signal (used to form an *echo*). Sophisticated techniques convert these echoes into images which therefore represent a spatially resolved map of radio signals. Tissue contrast depends on the delay from excitation to signal read out (*echo time; TE*) and the time between radiowave pulses (*repeat time; TR*). Two relaxation processes occur and are known as *T1* and *T2*, and these vary widely between different tissues. A CMR scanner has a magnet which is superconducting, *gradients* which are driven by pulses of electricity and provide extra temporary magnetic fields, a *radiofrequency transmitter and receiver* connected to *radio coils* to transmit and receive the radio signals, and a *computer*. Images are formed by using the electrocardiogram (ECG) as a trigger.

A scanner requires coordination of action of many individual processes to produce images and the controlling 'orchestral score' is known as a scanning *sequence*. Sequence components include *preparation pulses* (generates contrast between tissues), *excitation pulses* (localizes the excitation area), *gradient and magnetic field pulses* (formation of the imaging echo), and *signal read-out* (data collection). *Spin echo* sequences give anatomical images with black blood, and *gradient echo* sequences give cines. The *inversion recovery* pre-pulse is valuable for infarct imaging by yielding high T1 contrast. The signal read-out for CMR is usually fast to allow breath-hold imaging, and the faster schemes include fast low angle shot (FLASH), steady state with free precession (SSFP), spiral, and echo-planar imaging (EPI). *Velocity mapping* displays each pixel in the image as a velocity rather than a signal magnitude, and this is used to measure velocity and flow by integration over time of the product of mean velocity in a vessel and its cross-sectional area. For coronary CMR, *navigator echoes* are used to correct respiratory motion during long acquisitions by diaphragm monitoring. CMR *angiography* visualizes the vessel lumen after intravenous injection of a *gadolinium*-based MR contrast agent. A sequence called *tagging* measures myocardial contraction from the distortion of a magnetic grid laid across the image in diastole.

The safety of CMR is excellent and clearly advantageous compared with X-ray techniques. However, problems can occur with MR. Items which are ferromagnetic may be strongly attracted to the magnet, become projectile, and have the potential to strike the patient. The more obvious problem items include scissors, injection pumps, and oxygen cylinders and strict safety protocols must be followed. A second issue is medical implants and electronic devices. Most metallic implants are MR compatible, including all prosthetic cardiac valves, coronary stents [2], and orthopaedic implants. Some cerebrovascular clips can be problematic, and specialist neurological advice is required in these patients. The high magnetic field may interfere with electronics devices such as pacemakers and cardioverter defibrillators. In addition, pacing wires can couple to the radiofrequency waves and heat significantly. These devices are a strong relative contraindication for CMR, although recent reports have shown MR in patients with pacemakers to be safe under special circumstances [3], and approved MR compatible pacemakers have been developed which have completed clinical trials.

Volumes and function

CMR is highly accurate and reproducible to determine the parameters that are used to characterize cardiac function such as ventricular volumes, ejection fraction, ventricular mass, and great vessel flow. CMR is independent of acoustic windows which may limit echocardiography, and acquires images in contiguous parallel planes making data analysis consistent and free from errors caused by plane overlap, which may be a source of significant error for two-dimensional echocardiography. The reproducibility of CMR is significantly better than that of echocardiography which makes it the ideal tool for serial examination of patients over time [4, 5] and this also minimizes the sample size for studies of the effects of drugs on cardiac function in heart failure or hypertension.

Although it is possible to determine ventricular volumes with CMR using the area length technique which is often used in echocardiography, the more commonly used three-dimensional technique is preferred because geometric assumptions are not necessary. From the stack of short-axis images, the volumes and left ventricular (LV) mass are determined by planimetry for each slice and summed for the entire ventricle (Simpson's rule; ➲Fig. 5.1).

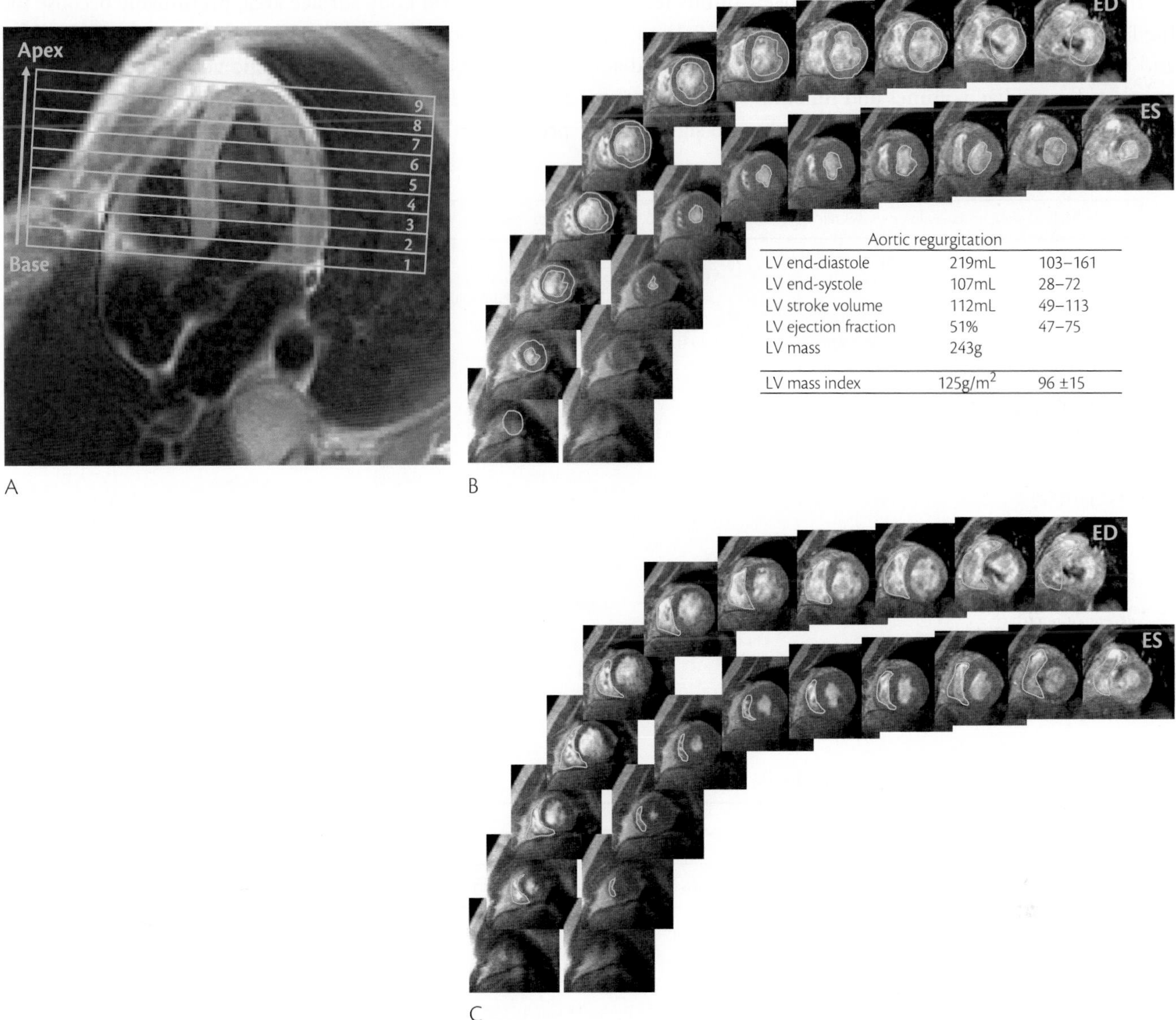

Figure 5.1 CMR technique for measuring ventricular volumes. (A) The horizontal long-axis plane is used to plane a series of contiguous short-axis cuts which start at the base of the left ventricle (LV) and right ventricle (RV) with slice 1. In this normal subject, nine slices were needed to encompass the ventricles to the apex. (B) The LV short-axis cuts are shown from a patient with chronic aortic regurgitation, where 11 end-diastolic (ED) slices were needed to cover the ventricles. Planimetry of the epicardial and endocardial contours at ED and the endocardial contours at end-systole (ES) are shown. The contours are added to derive volumes. ED volume (EDV) is derived from the endocardial contours at ED, and likewise for ES volume (ESV). Myocardial volume is derived from the difference in the ED epicardial and endocardial contours, and converted to LV mass by multiplying by the density of myocardium (1.05g/cm^2). Stroke volume is calculated as EDV – ESV. Ejection fraction (EF) is calculated as SV/EDV. The results in this patient show high volumes (normal values shown on right for this patient), and a borderline low EF with LV hypertrophy; (C) The contours used to calculate RV volumes are shown.

Semiautomatic techniques are available which minimize the analysis time, and make automatic corrections for valve plane descent towards the apex between diastole and systole. As quantitative information on the functional capacity of both ventricles is necessary in most patients, the short-axis approach is routinely used in most CMR centres as it covers both ventricles in a single imaging stack. As the right ventricle (RV) has a more irregular shape than the LV, Simpson's rule additions are the only reasonable approach for quantifying RV volumes. In patients with diseases mainly related to the RV therefore, CMR is often very useful.

The high fidelity of the ventricular volumes measurements by CMR allows correction to non-cardiac factors which affect the normal values of the measurements. These include body surface area (which acts as the simplest approximation to lean body mass), gender, and age.

Normalized values and graphs have been published for the left (➲Fig. 5.2) and right ventricle (➲Fig. 5.3) [6, 7] and these show significant effects of all three non-cardiac variables for cardiac volumes and function, with the main exception of the ejection fraction which has no significant dependence on body surface area, presumably because the effects of body habitus are cancelled out by equal effects on end-diastolic and end-systolic volumes. The normalized values for normal cardiac volumes and function have proved particularly useful in the assessment of the early

Males: Left ventricular volumes, systolic function and mass (absolute and indexed to body surface area) by age decile (mean, 95% confidence interval)

Males	20–29 years	30–39 years	40–49 years	50–59 years	60–69 years	70–79 years
			Absolute values			
EDV [mL] SD 21	167	163	159	154	150	146
	(126, 208)	(121, 204)	(117, 200)	(113, 196)	(109, 191)	(105, 187)
ESV [mL] SD 11	58	56	54	51	49	47
	(35, 80)	(33, 78)	(31, 76)	(29, 74)	(27, 72)	(25, 70)
SV [mL] SD 14	109	107	105	103	101	99
	(81, 137)	(79, 135)	(77, 133)	(75, 131)	(73, 129)	(71, 127)
EF [%] SD 4.5	65	66	66	67	67	68
	(57, 74)	(57, 74)	(58, 75)	(58, 76)	(58, 76)	(59, 77)
Mass [g] SD 20	148	147	146	146	145	144
	(109, 186)	(109, 185)	(108, 185)	(107, 184)	(107, 183)	(106, 183)
			Indexed to body surface area (BSA)			
EDV/BSA [mL/m²] SD 9.0	86	83	81	79	77	75
	(68, 103)	(66, 101)	(64, 99)	(62, 97)	(60, 95)	(58, 93)
ESV/BSA [mL/m²] SD 5.5	30	29	27	26	25	24
	(19, 41)	(18, 39)	(17, 38)	(15, 37)	(14, 36)	(13, 35)
SV/BSA [mL/m²] SD 6.1	56	55	54	53	52	51
	(44, 68)	(43, 67)	(42, 66)	(41, 65)	(40, 64)	(39, 63)
Mass/BSA [g/m²] SD 8.5	76	75	75	74	73	73
	(59, 93)	(59, 92)	(58, 91)	(57, 91)	(57, 90)	(56, 89)

EDV, End-Diastolic Volume; ESV, End-Systolic Volume; SV, Stroke Volume; EF, Ejection Fraction; BSA, Body Surface Area; SD, Standard Deviation.

A

Females: Left ventricular volumes, systolic function and mass (absolute and indexed to body surface area) by age decile (mean, 95% confidence interval)

Females	20–29 years	30–39 years	40–49 years	50–59 years	60–69 years	70–79 years
			Absolute values			
EDV [mL] SD 21	139	135	130	126	122	118
	(99, 179)	(94, 175)	(90, 171)	(86, 166)	(82, 162)	(77, 158)
ESV [mL] SD 9.5	48	45	43	41	39	36
	(229, 66)	(27, 64)	(25, 62)	(22, 59)	(20, 57)	(18, 55)
SV [mL] SD 14	91	89	87	85	83	81
	(63, 119)	(61, 117)	(59, 115)	(57, 113)	(56, 111)	(54, 109)
EF [%] SD 4.6	66	66	67	68	69	69
	(56, 75)	(57, 75)	(58, 76)	(59, 77)	(60, 78)	(60, 78)
Mass [g] SD 18	105	106	107	108	109	110
	(69, 141)	(70, 142)	(71, 143)	(72, 144)	(73, 145)	(74, 146)
			Indexed to body surface area			
EDV/BSA [mL/m²] SD 8.7	82	79	76	73	70	67
	(65, 99)	(62, 96)	(59, 93)	(56, 90)	(53, 87)	(50, 84)
ESV/BSA [mL/m²] SD 4.7	28	27	25	24	22	21
	(19, 37)	(17, 36)	(16, 34)	(14, 33)	(13, 31)	(12, 30)
SV/BSA [mL/m²] SD 6.2	54	53	51	50	48	47
	(42, 66)	(40, 65)	(39, 63)	(37, 62)	(36, 60)	(34, 59)
Mass/BSA [g/m²] SD 7.5	62	62	63	63	63	63
	(47, 77)	(47, 77)	(48, 77)	(48, 78)	(48, 78)	(49, 78)

EDV, End-Diastolic Volume; ESV, End-Systolic Volume; SV, Stroke Volume; EF, Ejection Fraction; BSA, Body Surface Area; SD, Standard Deviation.

B

Figure 5.2 Normal values for left ventricular (LV) volumes, mass, and function derived from CMR. (A) Table showing normal values per age decile for males. (B) Table showing normal values per age decile for females.

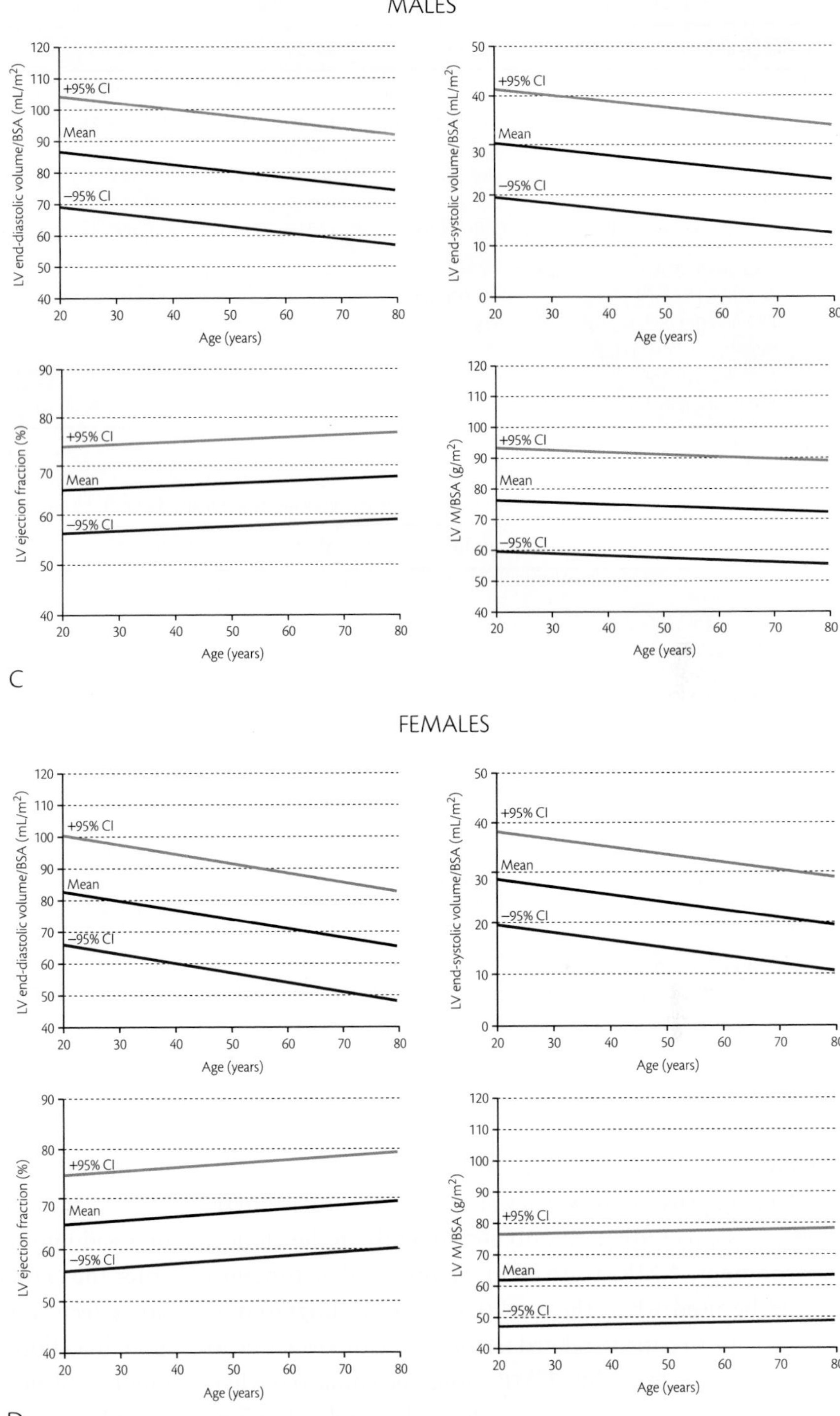

Figure 5.2 *(cont'd)* (C) Graphs showing normal indexed values for LV parameters with regression lines (mean and upper/lower 95% confidence intervals) for males. (D) Graphs showing normal indexed values for LV parameters with regression lines (mean and upper/lower 95% confidence intervals) for females. Data reproduced from Maceira AM, Prasad SK, Khan M, *et al.* Normalized left ventricular systolic and diastolic function by steady state free precession cardiovascular magnetic resonance. *J Cardiovasc Magn Reson* 2006; **8**: 417–26.

stages of cardiomyopathy and the longitudinal follow up of patients with heart failure, both to assess progression and the effects of treatment.

Assessment of regional wall motion is greatly facilitated by the high quality images acquired in most patients using SSFP cines. Wall motion abnormalities are better seen and with greater confidence compared with echocardiography [8]. Important parameters such as regional wall thickness and regional wall thickening can be derived. Nevertheless, image quality depends on the ability of the patient to breath-hold, and the absence of poorly controlled cardiac rhythms. Using myocardial tagging techniques, the deformation of the tagging grid provide estimates of myocardial strain, torsion, and shear (➲Fig. 5.4). It has been suggested that a two-dimensional strain analysis may be better than measuring wall thickening in order to distinguish between

Males: RV volumes, systolic function and mass (absolute and normalized to BSA) by age decile (mean, 95% confidence interval)

Age (years)	20–29	30–39	40–49	50–59	60–69	70–79
Absolute values						
EDV [mL] SD 25.4	177 (127, 227)	171 (121, 221)	166 (116, 216)	160 (111, 210)	155 (105, 205)	150 (100, 200)
ESV [mL] SD 15.2	68 (38, 98)	64 (34, 94)	59 (29, 89)	55 (25, 85)	50 (20, 80)	46 (16, 76)
SV [mL] SD 17.4	108 (74, 143)	108 (74, 142)	107 (73, 141)	106 (72, 140)	105 (71, 139)	104 (70, 138)
EF [%] SD 6.5	61 (48, 74)	63 (50, 76)	65 (52, 77)	66 (53, 79)	68 (55, 81)	70 (57, 83)
Mass [g] SD 14.4	70 (42, 99)	69 (40, 97)	67 (39, 95)	65 (37, 94)	63 (35, 92)	62 (33, 90)
Normalized to BSA						
EDV/BSA [mL/m^2] SD 11.7	91 (68, 114)	88 (65, 111)	85 (62, 108)	82 (59, 105)	79 (56, 101)	75 (52, 98)
ESV/BSA [mL/m^2] SD 7.4	35 (21, 50)	33 (18, 47)	30 (16, 45)	28 (13, 42)	25 (11, 40)	23 (8, 37)
SV/BSA [mL/m^2] SD 8.2	56 (40, 72)	55 (39, 71)	55 (39, 71)	54 (38, 70)	53 (37, 69)	52 (36, 69)
EF/BSA (%/m^2) SD 4	32 (24, 40)	32 (25, 40)	33 (25, 41)	34 (26, 42)	35 (27, 42)	35 (27, 43)
Mass/BSA [g/m^2] SD 6.8	36 (23, 50)	35 (22, 49)	34 (21, 48)	33 (20, 46)	32 (19, 45)	31 (18, 44)

A

Females: RV volumes, systolic function and mass (absolute and normalized to BSA) by age decile (mean, 95% confidence interval)

Age (years)	20–29	30–39	40–49	50–59	60–69	70–79
Absolute values						
EDV [mL] SD 21.6	142 (100, 184)	136 (94, 178)	130 (87, 172)	124 (81, 166)	117 (75, 160)	111 (69, 153)
ESV [mL] SD 13.3	55 (29, 82)	51 (25, 77)	46 (20, 72)	42 (15, 68)	37 (11, 63)	32 (6, 58)
SV [mL] SD 13.1	87 (61, 112)	85 (59, 111)	84 (58, 109)	82 (56, 108)	80 (55, 106)	79 (53, 105)
EF [%] SD 6	61 (49, 73)	63 (51, 75)	65 (53, 77)	67 (55, 79)	69 (57, 81)	71 (59, 83)
Mass [g] SD 10.6	54 (33, 74)	51 (31, 72)	49 (28, 70)	47 (26, 68)	45 (24, 66)	43 (22, 63)
Normalized to BSA						
EDV/BSA [mL/m^2] SD 9.4	84 (65, 102)	80 (61, 98)	76 (57, 94)	72 (53, 90)	68 (49, 86)	64 (45, 82)
ESV/BSA [mL/m^2] SD 6.6	32 (20, 45)	30 (17, 43)	27 (14, 40)	24 (11, 37)	21 (8, 34)	19 (6, 32)
SV/BSA [mL/m^2] SD 6.1	51 (39, 63)	50 (38, 62)	49 (37, 61)	48 (36, 60)	46 (34, 58)	45 (33, 57)
EF/BSA [%/m^2] SD 5.2	37 (27, 47)	38 (27, 48)	38 (28, 49)	39 (29, 49)	40 (30, 50)	41 (31, 51)
Mass/BSA [g/m^2] SD 5.2	32 (22, 42)	30 (20, 40)	29 (19, 39)	27 (17, 37)	26 (16, 36)	24 (14, 35)

B

Figure 5.3 Normal values for right ventricular (RV) volumes, mass, and function derived from CMR. (A) Table showing normal values per age decile for males. (B) Table showing normal values per age decile for females. (*Continued* p. 153.)

dysfunctional and normal myocardium. Although myocardial tagging provides new ways of looking at cardiac physiology, it is currently used only infrequently in the clinical environment. CMR assessment of myocardial function should be used when the quality of echocardiography is reduced due to patient-related factors [9]. Moreover, due to its superior image quality, CMR should be employed when there is a discrepancy between echocardiographic findings and the overall clinical scenario.

Myocardial infarction and viability

Infarction

Myocardial infarction (➲Chapter 16) can be detected with very high sensitivity using a CMR technique known as late gadolinium enhancement (LGE) (➲Fig. 5.5). This is performed 10 or more minutes after the intravenous injection of a gadolinium MR contrast agent. These contrast agents enter the extracellular space and, due to kinetic and partition effects, are concentrated in infarcted myocardium late after injection, where the extracellular space is expanded due to cell necrosis (acute infarction) or fibrotic replacement (chronic infarction) [10]. By using an inversion recovery sequence, the signal intensity of normal myocardium is driven to zero by adjusting the inversion time, and this leads to high signal in infarcted areas which have a shorter T1 due to gadolinium accumulation. Thus CMR gives a near histological in vivo depiction of myocardial abnormality (➲Fig. 5.6). Regions within the perfusion bed of an occluded coronary artery which are underperfused but are not necrotic do not enhance. Some acute infarcts have a central dark zone in the area of LGE which represents microvascular obstruction,

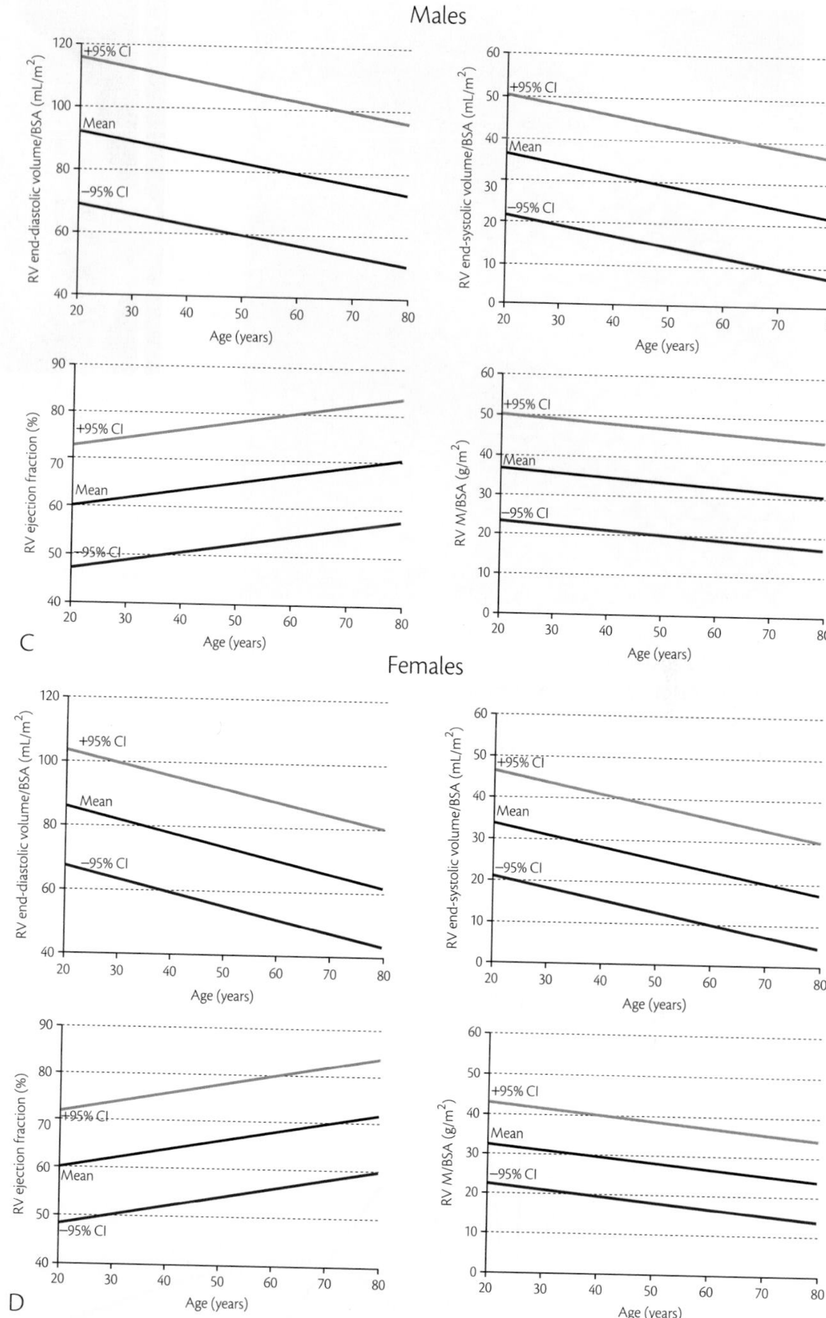

Figure 5.3 *(cont'd)* (C) graphs showing normal indexed values for RV parameters with regression lines (mean and upper/lower 95% confidence intervals) for males. (D) graphs showing normal indexed values for RV parameters with regression lines (mean and upper/lower 95% confidence intervals) for females. Reproduced with permission from Maceira AM, Prasad SK, Khan M, *et al.* Reference right ventricular systolic and diastolic function normalized to age, gender and body surface area from steady-state free precession cardiovascular magnetic resonance. *Eur Heart J* 2006; **27**: 2879–88.

where gadolinium penetration is very slow being limited by diffusion (➲Fig. 5.7). Infarcts with microvascular obstruction are associated with a poorer prognosis, as an independent predictor over and above the ejection fraction [11]. The area of microvascular obstruction slowly shrinks over weeks and is not seen in chronic infarctions. The area of LGE (infarction) also shrinks substantially over time, both in volume and transmural extent. This occurs due to scar formation with involution and hypertrophy of the adjacent and overlying myocardium. As CMR provides high spatial resolution, it has a high interstudy reproducibility. This, combined with being non-invasive, makes CMR the ideal tool to study acute infarction, healing, and remodelling in vivo in humans. In the chronic stage of myocardial infarction, the scar is still clearly visualized by LGE although the signal intensity is reduced because of a lower extracellular space than during the acute phase. LGE CMR is significantly more sensitive for infarction detection than perfusion SPECT (➲Fig. 5.8) [12].

Using LGE CMR, previously unsuspected myocardial infarctions have been found commonly in 70-year-old

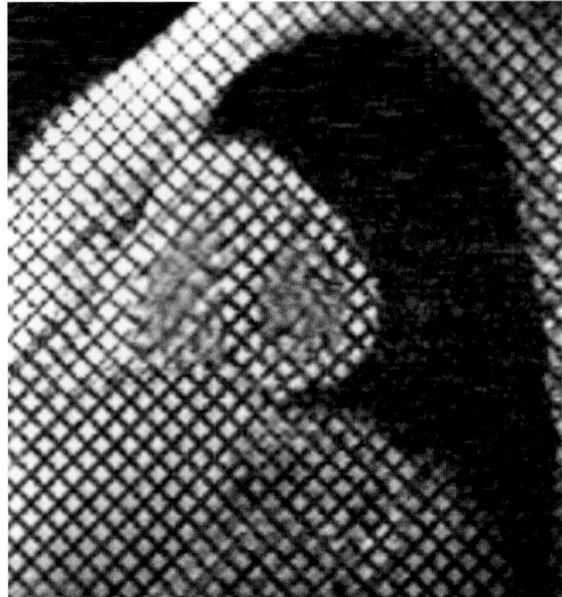

Figure 5.4 CMR tagging. A grid of magnetic lines is applied across the images at end-diastole which appear dark on the cine images. Stationary tissue shows no deformation of the lines, but in the heart the lines deform through the cardiac cycle to a maximum at end-systole. By measuring the intersection points of the lines, myocardial strain can be calculated and used as an observer-independent assessment of contractility.

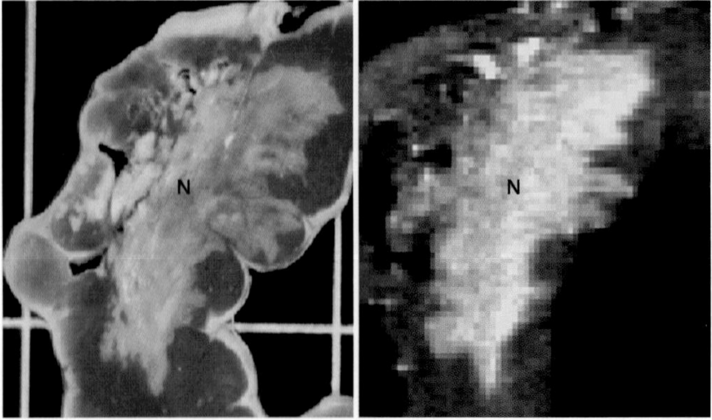

Figure 5.6 Comparison of triphenyltetrazolium chloride (TTC) stained slice of the left ventricle (left) with ex vivo high-resolution contrast enhanced MR image (right) showing necrotic myocardium (N) as pale non-stained tissue (left) and high signal intensity area (right). Note the detailed correspondence between the two images. Adapted from Kim RJ, Fieno DS, Parrish TB, *et al.* Relationship of MRI delayed contrast enhancement to irreversible injury, infarct age, and contractile function. *Circulation* 1999; **100**: 1992–2002.

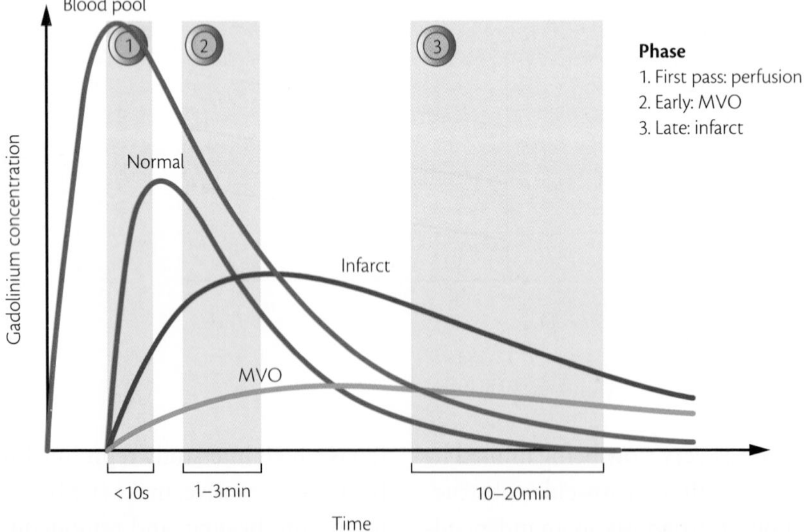

Figure 5.5 The use of intravenous gadolinium for CMR in detecting pathology depends on the time after injection that the images are taken. The bolus of gadolinium is given at time point 0, and the red line indicates gadolinium concentration in the blood (for clarity recirculation has been omitted). After a short delay, gadolinium enters the coronary arteries and the first pass through the myocardium is shown as the blue line. At this time, ultrafast CMR can be used to measure myocardial perfusion (phase 1). After 1–3min, early gadolinium enhancement imaging can be performed: at this time, the lowest gadolinium concentration is in avascular areas such as in microvascular obstruction (MVO, orange line) in acute infarction; however, thrombus also is very well shown by this technique, and both appear very dark on the images (phase 2). When MVO is present, it is surrounded by infarction, which is bright on the late gadolinium enhancement images taken after 10–20min, when gadolinium is in highest concentration in infarcted areas (blue line, phase 3) or in cardiomyopathies in those areas of expanded extracellular space due to fibrosis or infiltration. The times given are for illustration of the principles and are dependent on the dose of gadolinium given and other factors.

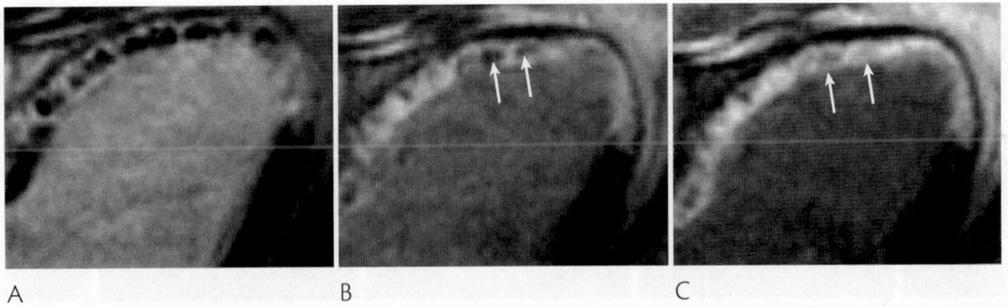

Figure 5.7 Patient 5 days after primary percutaneous transluminal coronary angioplasty plus stenting of the left anterior descending coronary artery for anterior myocardial infarction. Temporal changes in signal intensity after 0.2mmol/kg gadolinium administered intravenously. There is hypoenhancement of the infarcted area at 2min (A) indicating microvascular obstruction. At 15min (B) there is some slow contrast wash-in into areas with milder damage from surrounding regions with intact microcirculation. At 30min (C) there is even some contrast wash-in in areas showing hypoenhancement at 15min (arrows in B and C). Segments with dark zones within the enhanced areas at delayed imaging have poor function in the acute stage of infarction with a very low likelihood of improvement at follow-up. Adapted with permission from Beek AM, Kühl HP, Bondarenko O, *et al.* Delayed contrast-enhanced magnetic resonance imaging for the prediction of regional functional improvement after acute myocardial infarction. *J Am Coll Cardiol* 2003; **42**: 895–901.

subjects. Such subjects represent a high-risk group for future cardiovascular events [13]. Following heart transplantation, LGE CMR identifies silent myocardial infarction in apparently event-free patients, indicating the presence of transplant coronary artery disease (CAD) and the need for intensified medical intervention [14]. In patients with complex percutaneous coronary interventions with subsequent troponin elevation, CMR shows the location of the associated necrosis and distinguishes between embolic and side-branch related complications.

CMR can also depict the regional reduction in wall thickness and wall thickening associated with myocardial infarcts. The degree of abnormal systolic function is, however, only a poor indicator of the degree of infarct transmurality. Myocardial stunning contributes to the observed loss of regional systolic function and it is not possible to distinguish this influence from the contractile dysfunction caused by infarct scar when using deformation imaging alone.

Viability

Accurate prediction of recovery of function following revascularization has been achieved with low dose dobutamine CMR, with similar results to positron emission tomography (PET). However, LGE CMR also allows the assessment of viable myocardium. Areas surrounding an infarct which do not enhance are composed of viable myocardium (➲Fig. 5.9). The transmural extent of scarring is closely related to the likelihood of recovery of function after revascularization and also to recovery of ejection fraction [15]. Studies suggest that a significant improvement in ejection fraction after successful revascularization occurs when 20% of the myocardium is hibernating, although significant improvements in regional wall function may of course be seen with smaller areas of hibernating myocardium. Low-dose dobutamine stress CMR may be more sensitive in predicting recovery of function however [16]. This is not surprising as the dobutamine assisted test simulates the effects of revascularization. The main problem with late gadolinium enhanced CMR is its reduced specificity in predicting the absence of recovery in non-transmural scars. The inability of non-transmural scar to recover function after adequate revascularization is poorly understood. One of the factors involved may be that recovery of function may require more time than the usual 3 months, which is the normal period after revascularization at which recovery function is studied. Moreover, coronary revascularization may be incomplete, particularly in patients with extensive atherosclerosis and diffuse disease. Whatever CMR technique is used for assessing myocardial viability, it is appropriate to view viability as a continuum. There is no single cut-off value for predicting functional improvement. Instead, one should base the clinical expectation of recovery on the extent of transmurality of the infarcts in a particular region. If >50% of the myocardium is infarcted, the probability of no recovery following revascularization is approximately 90% (negative predictive value) (➲Fig. 5.10) [15]. On the other hand, segments without scar have an 80% likelihood (positive predictive value) of recovery [15]. LGE CMR can also predict the effect of beta-receptor blocking agents in patients with severely reduced LV function. For larger scars, the improvement achieved by beta-blockade diminishes [17].

Ischaemia detection

The presence and extent of myocardial ischaemia are important determinants of the prognosis of patients with coronary heart disease (➲Chapter 17). CMR uses functional and

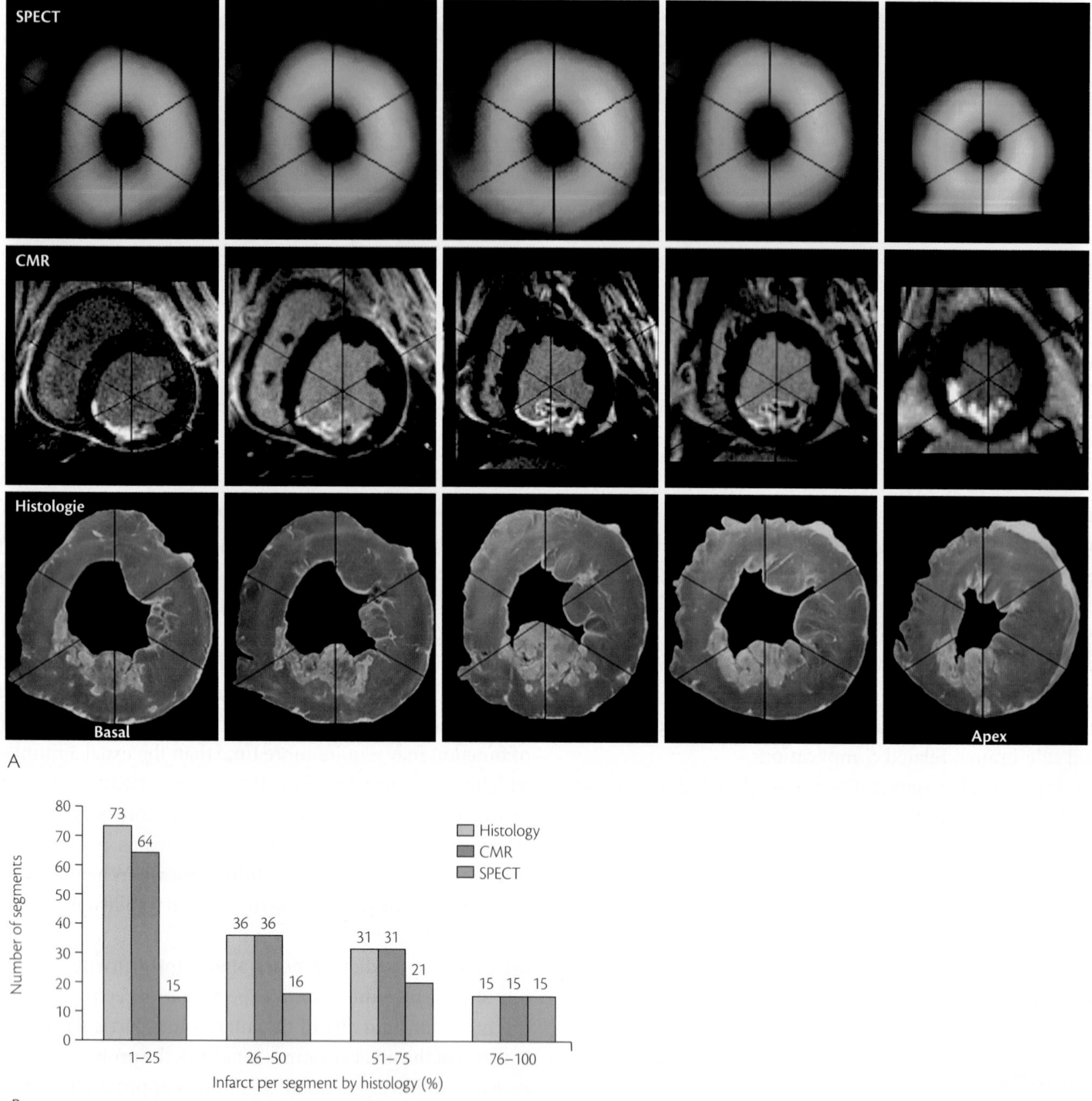

Figure 5.8 (A) Comparison of CMR and myocardial perfusion SPECT for detection of myocardial infarction in animals. The lower row shows the sliced experimentally induced infarct with TTC staining. The ex vivo gadolinium images (middle row) show excellent correspondence with the TTC gold standard, but perfusion SPECT (upper row) fails to identify the small infarcted areas. (B) The graph relates the number of segments seen by each technique against the transmural extent of the infarction in quartiles. The light orange bar shows the results of histology, and comparison with the CMR (blue bar) is excellent. However, the proportion of missed infarct segments by scintigraphy (dark orange bar) increases as the infarcted segments become more subendocardial. Reproduced with permission from Wagner A, Mahrholdt H, Holly TA, *et al.* Contrast-enhanced MRI and routine single photon emission computed tomography (SPECT) perfusion imaging for detection of subendocardial myocardial infarcts: an imaging study. *Lancet* 2003; **361**: 374–9.

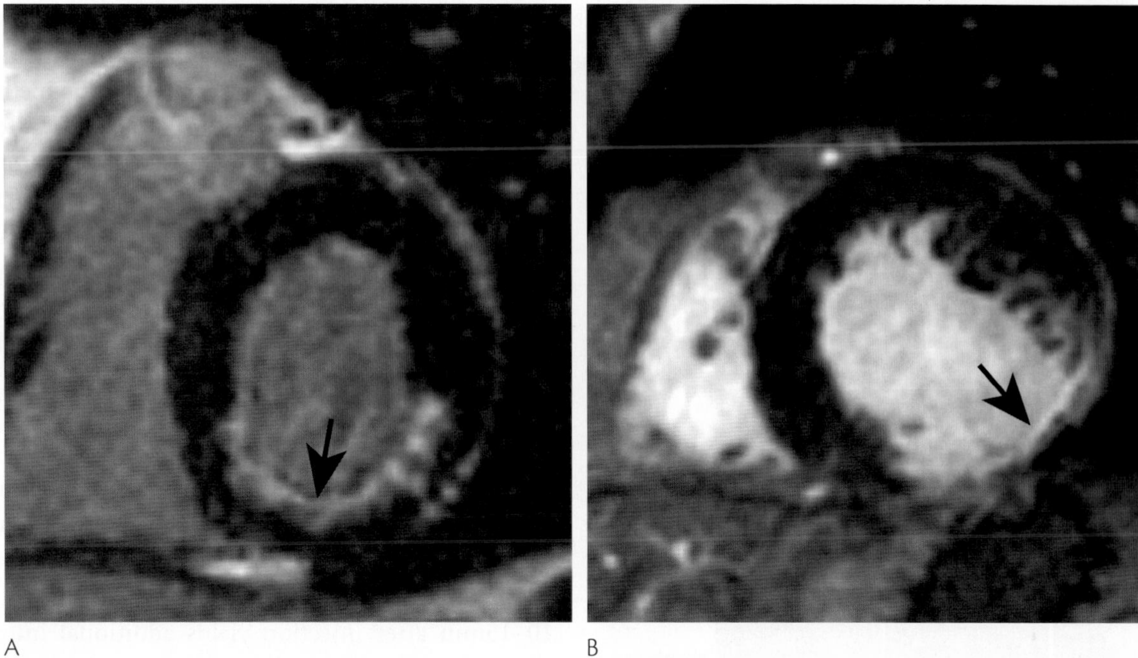

Figure 5.9 (A) Non-transmural inferolateral myocardial infarction with plenty of viable tissue surrounding the subendocardial zone of late gadolinium enhancement (arrow). (B) Mostly transmural myocardial infarction with transmural late gadolinium enhancement (arrow).

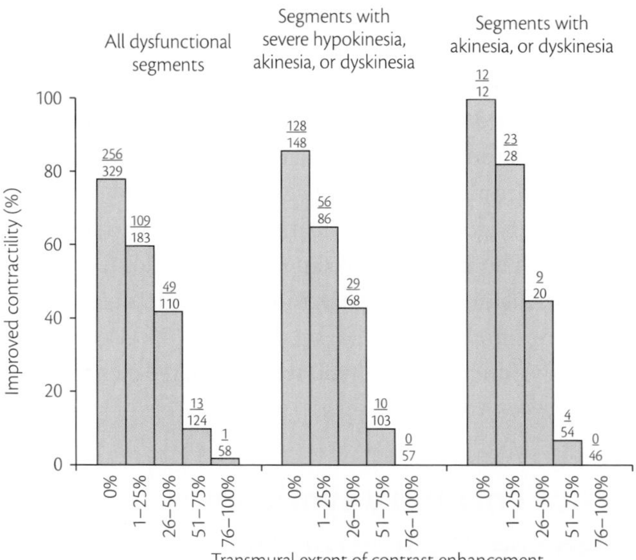

Figure 5.10 Relation between the transmural extent of late gadolinium enhancement before revascularization and the likelihood of improved contractility after revascularization. Irrespective of the degree of segmental wall motion abnormality there is an inverse relation between the transmural extent of late enhancement and the likelihood of improvement in contractility. Adapted with permission from Kim RJ, Wu E, Rafael A, *et al.* The use of contrast-enhanced magnetic resonance imaging to identify reversible myocardial dysfunction. *N Engl J Med* 2000; **343**: 1445–53.

perfusion imaging with different stressors to investigate ischaemia, both for diagnostic and prognostic purposes [18].

Dobutamine stress

Dobutamine stress CMR uses the same protocol as stress echocardiography with increasing doses of dobutamine and the addition of atropine to reach the target heart rate [19]. Induction of new regional wall motion abnormalities (based on the 17-segment model) is assessed on three short-axis and three long-axis cines, acquired at rest and during each stage of the study. Images are reviewed in real-time to stop the test when ischaemia occurs. In a recent meta-analysis overall sensitivity was 83% and specificity 86%, compared to invasive angiography (➲Chapter 8) [20]. Results are very similar to echocardiography (➲Chapter 4), provided the image quality on echocardiography is good; otherwise dobutamine CMR is superior and is the preferred method (➲Fig. 5.11). As with nuclear techniques (➲Chapter 7), normal stress CMR indicates a low event rate, and increasing amounts of ischaemia indicates an increased risk [21, 22]. Ischaemia by stress CMR has also been used for the assessment of increased preoperative risk. Stress CMR can also quantify wall motion (wall thickening) to reduce observer variability. The most advanced method is tagging, which allows the calculation of myocardial strain, yielding increased sensitivity, but larger trials and faster post-processing are needed for

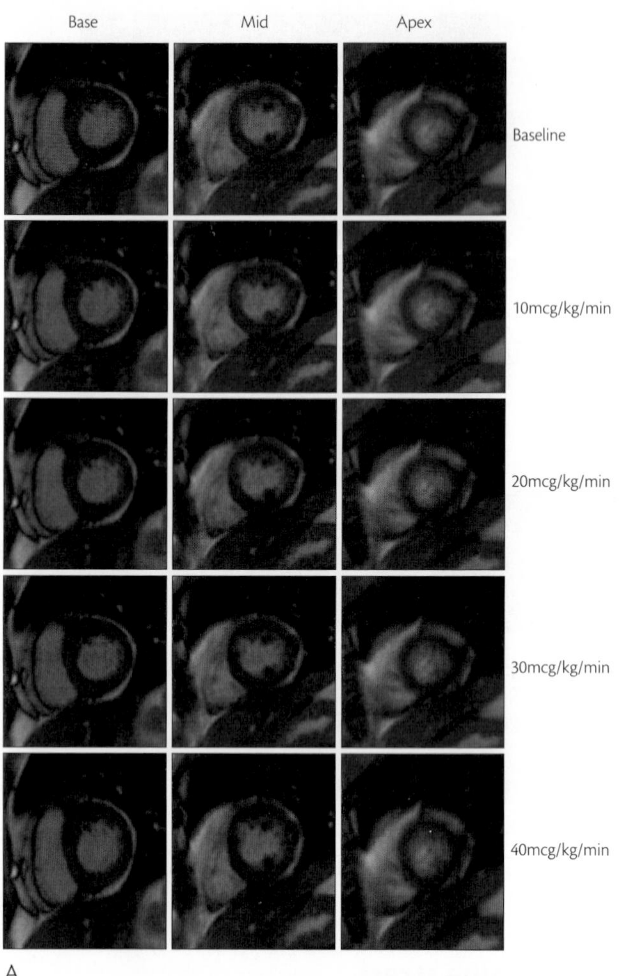

Figure 5.11 Dobutamine wall motion. (A) Normal dobutamine CMR stress study with end-systolic images at three levels (base, mid, and apex) at rest, 10, 20, 30, and 40mcg/kg/min dobutamine. (*Continued*, p. 159.)

clinical application [23]. Dobutamine stress CMR has been shown to be safe in large patient cohorts [24].

Myocardial perfusion

Myocardial perfusion is studied at rest and during infusion of adenosine by measuring the first-pass signal changes in the myocardium after intravenous injection of a fast bolus of a gadolinium contrast agent. Typically three short-axis slices are imaged per cardiac cycle, allowing a full segmental perfusion analysis [25]. Areas of reduced perfusion are visualized as having persistent low signal and in CAD always involve the subendocardium (extent of ischaemia) with variable transmural extension (severity of ischaemia). Although the resting study is not absolutely required for interpretation, it helps to identify endocardial artefacts and to calculate regional myocardial perfusion reserve. Given the high spatial resolution of CMR, abnormalities in endocardial perfusion can be studied separately, yielding a higher sensitivity. Analysis of perfusion is qualitative (visual), semi-quantitative using the upslope methodology, or quantitative [26], using the deconvolution method optimally in combination with a form of dual-bolus technique which captures the arterial input function. The latter permits the calculation of absolute perfusion in mL/mg/min. Perfusion measured by CMR and microspheres in validation experiments shows a good linear relationship, which does not suffer from roll-off at higher perfusion rates that is seen with the nuclear tracers thallium and technetium MIBI or tetrofosmin. This means that perfusion CMR is more sensitive for identifying moderate coronary stenoses (➲Fig. 5.12).

After a period of technical development to optimize perfusion sequences, the technique is now stable and usable in CAD and ischaemia due to epicardial or microvascular perfusion abnormalities (➲Fig. 5.13) [27–29]. LGE imaging 10–15min after injection yields additional information about infarction/scar and the differentiation of peri-infarct ischaemia.

A CMR technique which does not require gadolinium contrast or ultrafast imaging has also been described and this is called T2* blood oxygen level dependent (BOLD) [30]. However, the sensitivity of T2* to perfusion change may be quite low and its clinical role is not yet defined.

Using invasive coronary angiography (➲Chapter 8) as the gold standard (with the implicit problem of comparing anatomical and functional parameters), CMR perfusion performs very well from the diagnostic perspective. There is also high agreement with PET and single photon emission computed tomography (SPECT). For prognosis, both in the acute (emergency room, acute coronary syndromes) [31] and chronic setting, absence of perfusion abnormalities carries a very good prognostic implication with a low event rate [32]. The non-invasive and non-radiation context of CMR perfusion allows the pathophysiologic investigation of less common entities like syndrome X [33, 34], microvascular dysfunction, and hypertrophy-related ischaemia.

Acute coronary syndromes (also see ➲Chapter 16)

In an attempt to identify faster and more accurately those patients with chest pain who present with true unstable coronary syndromes to the emergency room, CMR has been used to depict the abnormalities of wall motion, perfusion, and infarct enhancement potentially associated with acute coronary chest pain. When performed at rest within

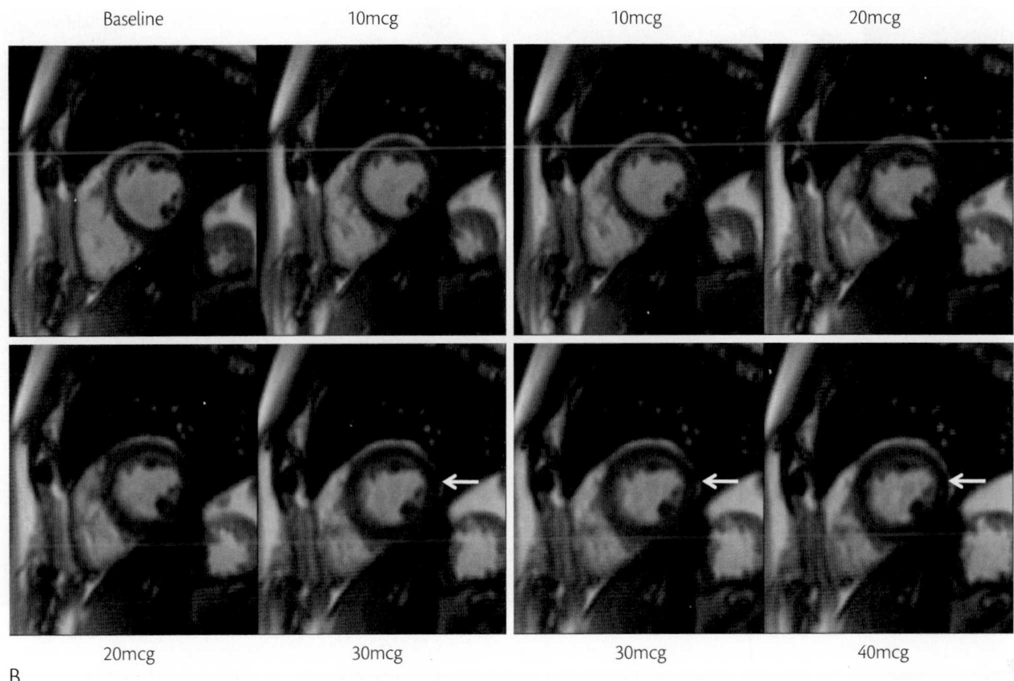

Figure 5.11 (*cont'd*) (B) Abnormal response in the basal slice (arrowed) during increasing doses of dobutamine with lateral wall hypokinesia at 30 and 40mcg/kg/min.

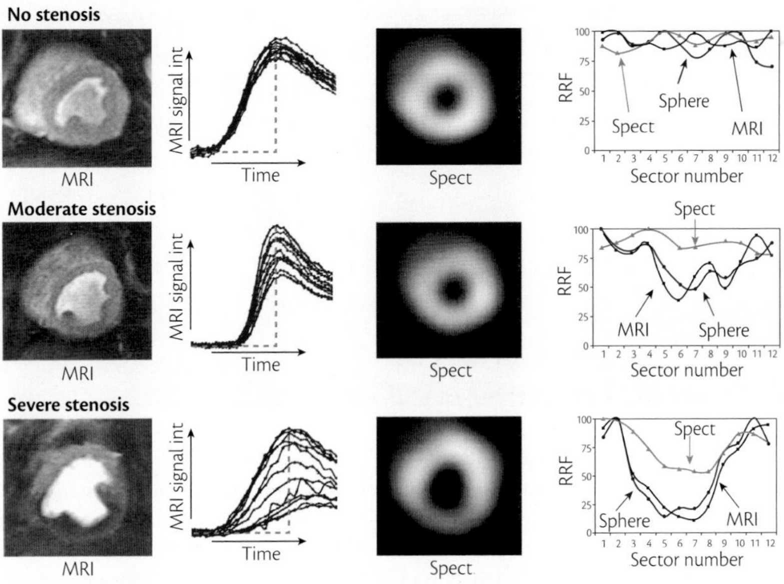

Figure 5.12 In this experimental study, perfusion measured using SPECT and CMR is compared with the gold standard, microspheres. CMR perfusion images are in the first column, quantitative signal intensity curves at different depths through the myocardium of these CMR maps are in the second column. SPECT images are in the third column, and the quantitative perfusion traces from the three techniques are in the right column. The top row represents the results in basal condition with normal perfusion. The middle row is with a limited stenosis and the bottom row shows the results with a severe stenosis. With its higher spatial resolution, CMR shows the gradual decrease in transmural perfusion, starting at the endocardium and progressing towards the epicardium with increasing severity of stenosis. SPECT, with a more limited spatial resolution, only shows a perfusion deficit with the severe pronounced stenosis. In the quantitative analysis, CMR perfusion closely followed the microsphere results, while SPECT was less sensitive. Adapted from Lee DC, Simonetti OP, Harris KR, *et al.* Magnetic resonance versus radionuclide pharmacological stress perfusion imaging for flow-limiting stenoses of varying severity. *Circulation* 2004; **110**: 58–65.

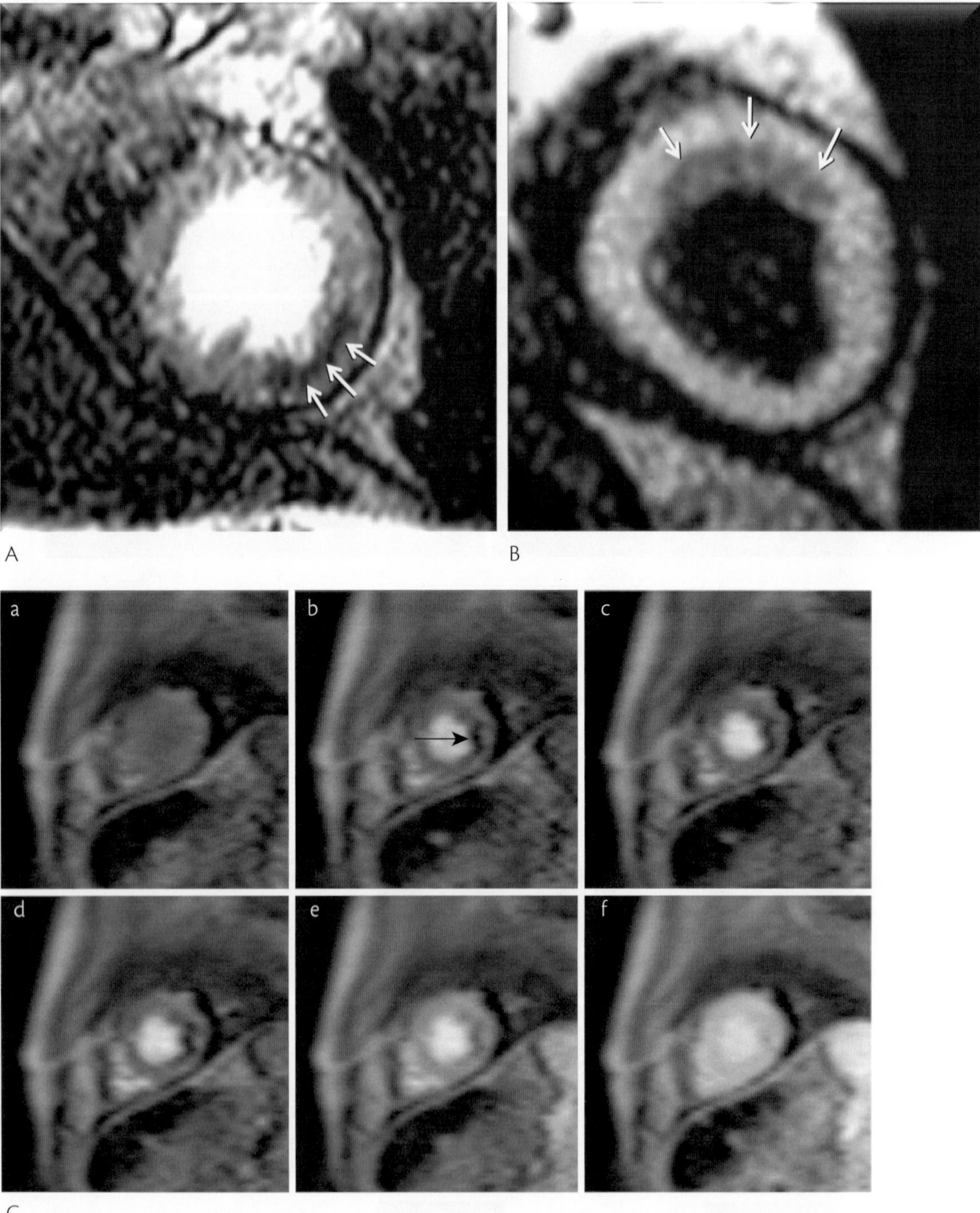

Figure 5.13 Perfusion CMR scan. (A) Near transmural perfusion deficit leaving only a small epicardial rim of normal myocardium in a patient with 99% left circumflex stenosis (arrows). (B) Near transmural perfusion deficit in the anterior wall in a patient with a 75% stenosis in the left anterior descending artery (arrows). (C) CMR perfusion artefact (arrow) in a series of images of a single slice, which in this case is most pronounced in the lateral wall. These artefacts are sequence related, appear at the time of contrast arrival in the LV cavity, and are due to differences in relaxivity and susceptibility at the edges of the blood pool/myocardium. They are usually darker than the non-enhanced myocardium and rapidly decrease in severity with disappearance during contrast washout in ventricular cavity but have a possible reappearance during second pass; they are most pronounced in basal part/septum/papillary muscles. These artefacts are becoming less intense and less frequent with improved perfusion sequence design.

12 hours of presentation, the sensitivity and specificity for detecting acute coronary syndromes was 84% and 85% respectively by CMR which was more sensitive than when ECG criteria for ischaemia (➲Chapters 2 and 16), peak troponin I, or the TIMI risk score were used [35]. CMR was also more specific than an abnormal ECG [35].

Current European Society of Cardiology (ESC) guidelines recommend coronary angiography in patients with acute coronary syndromes and intermediate risk features [36]. However, low-risk patients and those presenting late after symptom onset require a stress test for inducible ischaemia before discharge for further decision making. CMR (comprehensive analysis imaging of myocardial function, perfusion, viability, and coronary anatomy) is well suited for this purpose (➲Fig. 5.14) with a sensitivity of 96% at a specificity of 83% for detecting >70% stenosis at invasive coronary angiography [37]. In patients after ST-elevation myocardial infarction, adenosine perfusion CMR can be safely performed and is significantly more sensitive (86% vs. 48%) and more specific (100% vs. 50%) than exercise ECG stress testing for detecting significant coronary stenosis [38]. CMR is able to identify residual inducible ischaemia in the infarct-related artery territory in patients with smaller infarcts and less transmurality of infarction [38]. In patients presenting to the emergency department with chest pain but a normal troponin and no ECG changes indicative of acute ischaemia, a normal CMR perfusion adenosine stress test identifies those without subsequent diagnosis of CAD or an adverse outcome [39]. Moreover, those with significant CAD (defined as coronary artery stenosis ≥50% on angiography, abnormal correlative stress test, new myocardial infarction, or death within 1 year) can be identified with a sensitivity of 100%. Addition of T2-weighted imaging (detection of oedema associated with ACS) and wall motion imaging may further increase the accuracy of identifying those in need of invasive coronary angiography [40].

Some patients presenting acutely with chest pain have an elevated troponin but normal coronary arteries. CMR has incremental diagnostic value in these patients identifying the cause of troponin elevation in two-thirds of patients. The most common cause seems to be myocarditis in half the population, whereas myocardial infarction (possibly related to plaque rupture or coronary vasospasm) and dilated cardiomyopathy are less commonly found [41].

In patients presenting with acute MI and a history of chronic infarction it may be clinically difficult to identify the site of acute MI. T2-weighted CMR offers the unique possibility of performing this difficult task, as acute MI is characterized by increased tissue oedema whereas chronic MI lacks this feature [42]. Both types of MI, however, may exhibit LGE. T2-weighted imaging may also be employed to measure the extent of tissue salvaged by coronary intervention, by subtracting the infarct size from the original area at risk [43].

CMR is also helpful in detecting small, acute MIs such as those associated with coronary interventions [44]. After more extensive acute infarctions, CMR can depict large aneurysms and pseudo-aneurysms well, and ventricular thrombi are detected with higher accuracy than by echocardiography using an early gadolinium enhancement technique [45]. This has consequences in patients after MI because thrombi mandate oral anticoagulation therapy for several months.

Coronary arteries

Although CMR angiography is an accepted technique for the visualization of arteries and veins throughout the body, its use in the coronary circulation is hampered by the inherent technical difficulties associated with imaging small, tortuous vessels on the curved surface of a continuously moving object [46]. The optimal spatial and temporal resolution, as present in conventional invasive coronary angiography, for the visualization of coronary vessels cannot be achieved by conventional CMR sequences, so a number of special techniques are used. To reduce blurring, coronary imaging is performed during the diastole, when motion is most limited (this timing is obtained from a high temporal resolution cine sequence); to image the tortuous vessels, a three-dimensional volume is acquired with a MR angiography sequence; to minimize cardiac displacement from respiratory movement, diaphragmatic monitoring (called navigator echoes) and gating is used; to increase the spatial or temporal resolution parallel imaging is performed; and to improve contrast, pre-pulses are used to suppress fat and non-coronary artery tissues (T2 preparation). If navigators are unavailable or navigator efficiency is low due to a variable breathing pattern, breath-hold techniques can be used as an alternative to navigator gating. Good imaging results can be obtained in experienced hands using advanced sequences (➲Fig. 5.15), and whole heart sequences have shown considerable promise recently (➲Fig. 5.16). In the future, MR contrast agents may contribute to improved signal from the coronary lumen [47], and higher field magnets may also be useful as well as improvements in the gating algorithms and higher multiple receiver channel coils [48].

With the current limitations, coronary CMR cannot replace conventional invasive coronary angiography and its

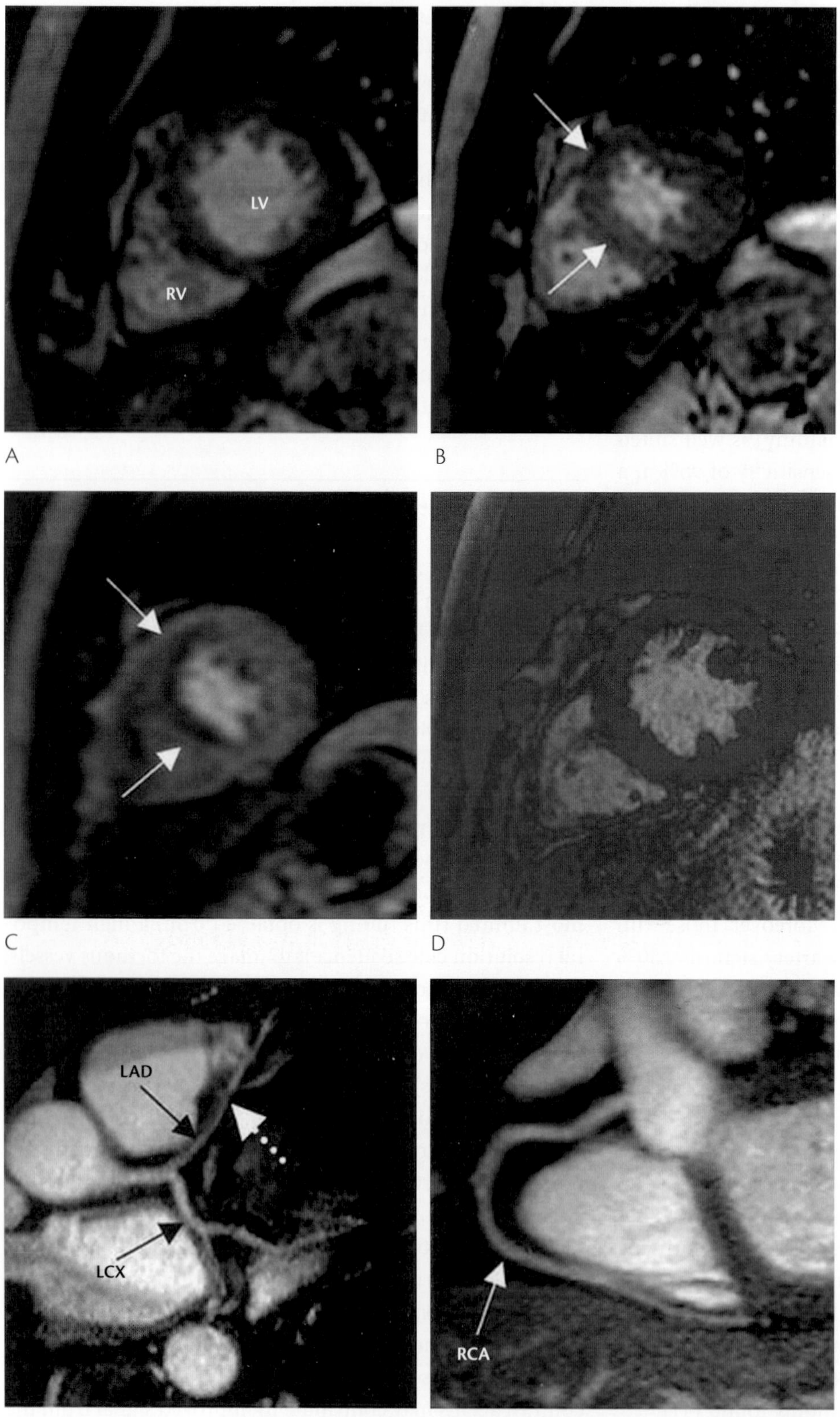

Figure 5.14 CMR findings in a 49-year-old male patient presenting with anterolateral ST-segment depression and a troponin I level of 0.2mg/L. Cine images demonstrate anteroseptal hypokinesia (diastolic frame at midventricular level in (A), systolic frame in (B), white arrows). Stress perfusion imaging (C) shows an anteroseptal perfusion defect. Late contrast-enhanced images (D) show no late gadolinium enhancement, indicating that the entire myocardium is viable. Coronary CMR shows a lesion in the mid-left anterior descending coronary artery (LAD) (E, dotted arrow), with normal left circumflex coronary artery (LCX) and right coronary artery (RCA) (F). The combined CMR analysis thus suggested significant coronary artery disease with a stenosis of the LAD and a large area of viable myocardium at ischaemic risk. X-ray angiography confirmed a proximal high-grade lesion in the LAD with a normal LCX and RCA. LV left ventricle; RV right ventricle. Modified with permission from Plein S, Greenwood JP, Ridgway JP, *et al.* Assessment of non-ST-segment elevation acute coronary syndromes with cardiac magnetic resonance imaging. *J Am Coll Cardiol* 2004; **44**: 2173–81.

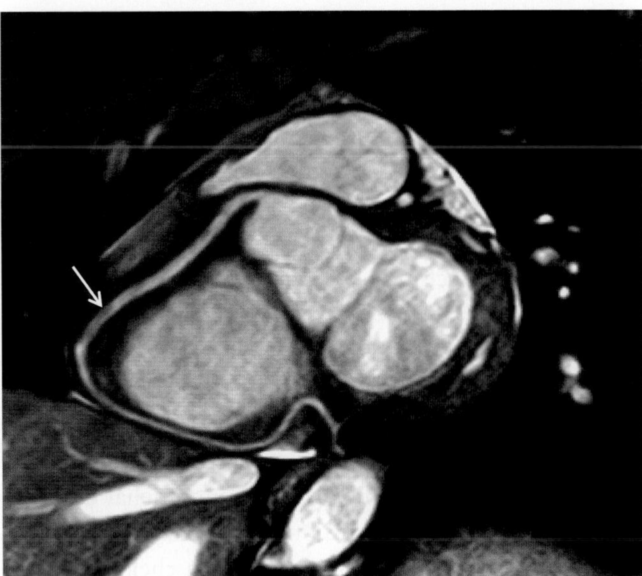

Figure 5.15 State-of-the-art three-dimensional CMR coronary image. This reconstructed image shows the normal right coronary artery (arrow), coursing in the AV groove and progressing over the inferior aspect of the heart.

performance is lower than coronary CTA [49]. There are encouraging clinical results showing a high negative predictive value for left main stem or three-vessel disease [50], and technical improvements have led to higher sensitivities and better accuracy, but these results were often obtained in single centres with highly experienced operators [51]. In everyday clinical practice, coronary MRA is not ready for reliable determination of the location and extent of coronary stenotic disease. On the other hand, coronary CMR has proven clinically valuable in congenital abnormalities of the coronary tree with abnormal origin and course of the proximal artery [52]. Here, the three-dimensional tomographic nature of coronary CMR gives superior results to projection conventional coronary angiography for the relation of the proximal coronary artery to the aortic root and pulmonary trunk. Since this diagnostic question is often relevant in children and young adults—where the impact of radiation is most relevant—CMR is a first-line technique. Bypass grafts can also be visualized confidently with CMR allowing the exclusion of graft occlusion but the exact morphology of the connection with the native circulation (often the location of pathology) is frequently difficult to

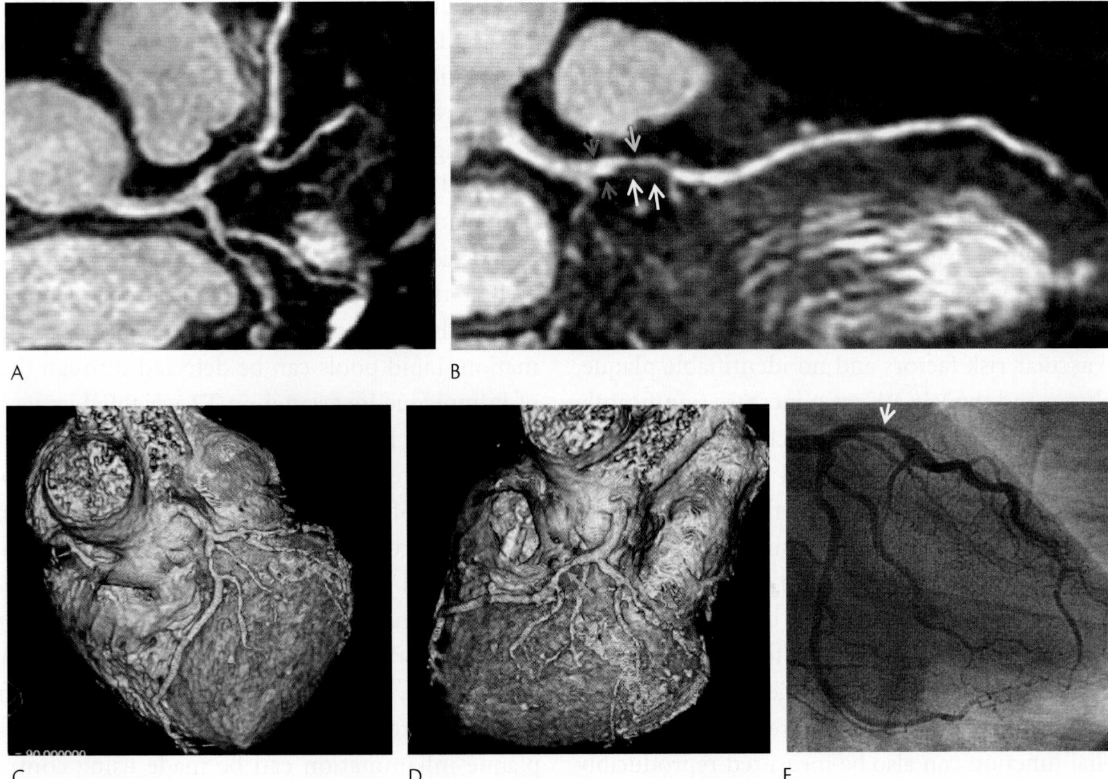

Figure 5.16 Whole heart coronary CMR. (A) and (B) show curved multiplanar reconstruction of the left coronary artery, focusing on a narrowing in the proximal left anterior descending artery (red arrows) with an eccentric lesion (white arrows), and the narrow lumen (yellow arrow). (C) and (D) show the volume rendering of this whole heart and the LAD stenosis (blue arrows). (E) The catheter X-ray coronary angiography showing the stenosis (white arrow). Images courtesy of Dr Hajime Sakuma, Matsusaka Central Hospital, Mie, Japan.

visualize accurately. Here, the use of flow reserve measurements can be helpful [53]. Inflammatory diseases of the coronary arteries giving rise to aneurysm formation can be visualized and followed over time to judge evolution with treatment [54]. Documenting the location and composition of obstructive and non-obstructive coronary plaques holds potential for CMR [55, 56] but remains technically very challenging and not currently clinically relevant.

Vessel wall

CMR can directly assess atherosclerosis, both for atheroma (the development of focal arterial plaque with lipid components) and sclerosis (the generalized thickening of the arterial wall). This is currently most easily accomplished in the carotid arteries, because the artery is superficial and surface coils allow high spatial resolution, although work has also been done in the aorta and the peripheral arteries, and, to a lesser extent, the coronaries. CMR can also assess arterial function, most importantly the endothelial function, but also arterial distensibility and pulse wave velocity.

CMR measures arterial sclerosis by simply assessing the total arterial wall volume. Typically, multiple contiguous cross-sectional slices of the carotid artery above and below the bifurcation are acquired (multiple single two-dimensional slices, multiple thin three-dimensional slabs, or a single thick three-dimensional slab) using T1-weighted images with blood signal suppression. The difference in each image slice between the outer and inner vessel boundary is summed to obtain the total vessel volume. The wall volume can be normalized to overall vessel size (which relates to body size) using division by the outer wall volume, yielding the wall to outer wall (W/OW) ratio. In normals without cardiovascular risk factors and no identifiable plaque, the wall volume and the W/OW ratio increase significantly with age (➲Fig. 5.17), indicating that sclerosis is an inevitable consequence of ageing [57]. Wall volume measurement is highly reproducible and allows the demonstration of regression of atherosclerosis (combined sclerosis and plaque) with statin treatment [58]. The coronary wall has also been imaged directly using black blood techniques, and there may be particular advantage to performing this using 3 Tesla scanners taking advantage of the increased signal and resolution of the high field strength.

Endothelial function can also be measured reproducibly by CMR using stimuli which cause arterial vasodilation, such as flow mediated dilation (endothelium dependent) and glyceryl trinitrate (endothelium independent). Flow-mediated dilation of the brachial artery is assessed by forearm cuff-occlusion for a standard time period followed by release, which induces increased endothelial shear, the release of nitric oxide, and arterial dilation [59]. The use of CMR allows area measurement of the vessel which has advantages over the diameter measurement made by ultrasound. Validation studies have been performed in humans using invasive techniques, and repeated measurements by CMR appear to have greater reproducibility than by ultrasound, suggesting smaller sample sizes for trials using CMR [59]. An additional advantage of CMR is that flow changes can also be measured directly in response to the standard stimuli. Alterations in endothelial function have been demonstrated in smokers, and endothelial dysfunction in patients with transfusional iron loading has shown to be fully corrected with aggressive iron chelation. Most recently, coronary endothelial function has been assessed by high-resolution cross sectional CMR of the response to GTN vasodilation. Arterial function can also be assessed using CMR by measuring compliance in the ascending aorta (change of aortic volume in a slice normalized to pulse pressure) and pulse wave velocity (rate of propagation of the flow wave around the aortic arch in m/s). These age dependent measures are abnormal in early atherosclerosis, and predict cardiac events.

CMR is also used to directly assess atheroma, with characterization of size and constituents of arterial plaque. This is achieved using a variety of characterization techniques, including a combination of T1, T2, and proton density-weighted images, and contrast agents [60]. The most important plaque components are those which are linked to prognosis via the propensity to plaque rupture, and these include the presence of lipid pool in the plaque, the thickness of the fibrous cap, and the presence of plaque inflammation. Lipid pools can be detected through the presence of intraplaque low signal on T2-weighted images, which is greater on T1 weighting. Newer contrast agents based on fluorine have also been used to identify lipid pools. The fibrous cap of the arterial plaque is seen as a continuous line on the surface of the plaque, and this is reduced in thickness or disrupted in patients with cerebrovascular events [61]. Thrombus may also be visible in the plaque or on the surface of a disrupted fibrous plaque as a high signal area in T1 imaging, because of signal enhancement from haemoglobin breakdown products. Finally, an assessment of plaque inflammation can be made using contrast agents based on iron oxide, which are taken up by activated plaque macrophages. These cells are found in vulnerable plaque, and ingestion of iron causes identifiable signal loss within

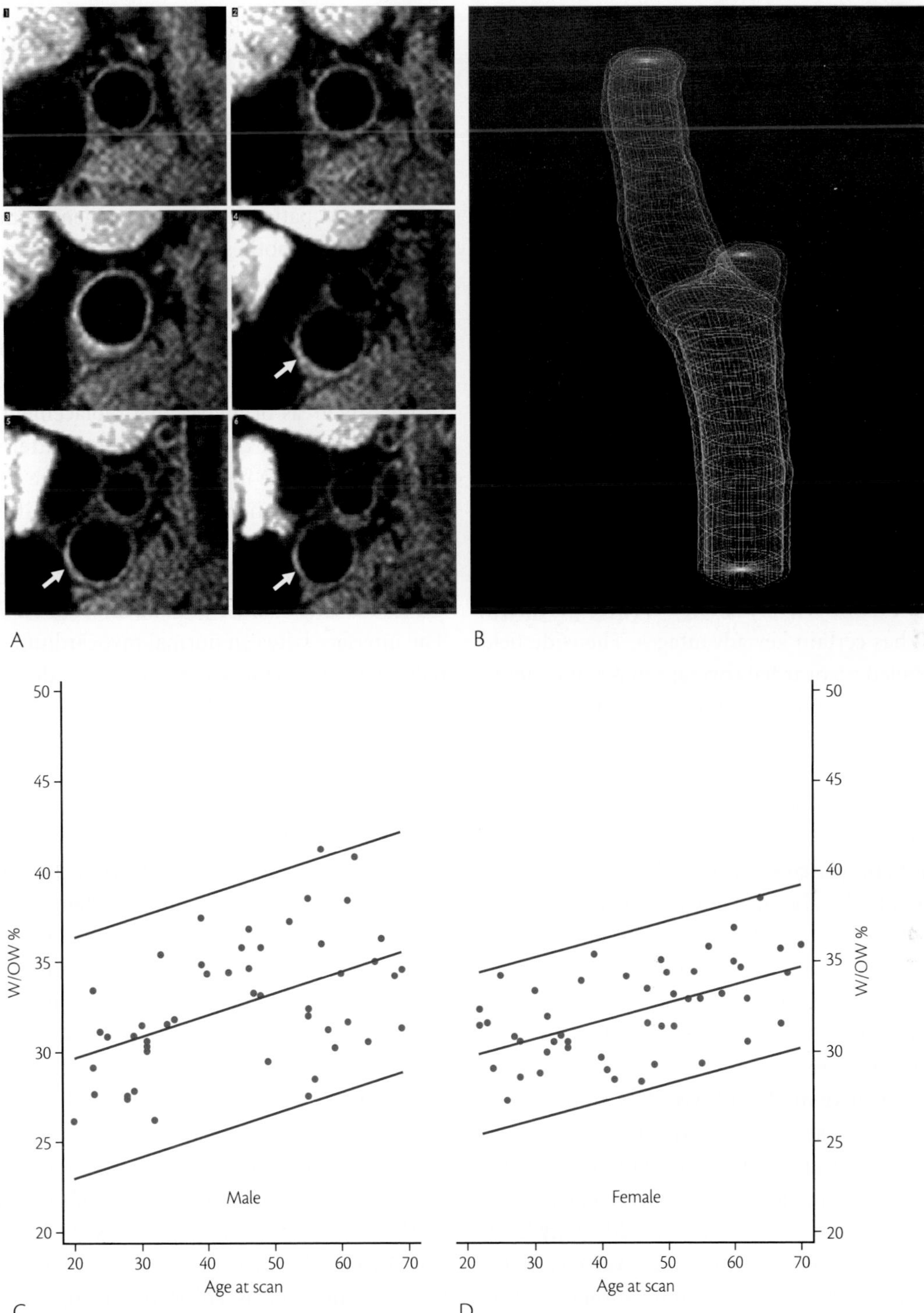

Figure 5.17 Carotid wall imaging by CMR. (A) T1-weighted fast spin-echo images acquired perpendicular to a normal right carotid artery with a slice thickness of 2mm, with in-plane resolution of 0.43 × 0.43mm. Images 1–3 show the common carotid and images 4–6 show the bifurcation into internal carotid artery (white arrows) and external carotid artery (truncated). (B) Computer modelled three-dimensional reconstruction of the carotid artery in a normal subject showing the adventitial and luminal surfaces. (C) and (D) Graphs of carotid wall volume normalized to total vessel volume (W/OW ratio) plotted against age with regression line and upper and lower 95% confidence intervals in males (C) and females (D). Reproduced from Keenan NG, Locca D, Roughton M, *et al.* Magnetic resonance of carotid artery aging in healthy subjects. *Atherosclerosis*, in press.

plaque. CMR can also image coronary plaque although this remains at the limits of current resolution.

Cardiomyopathy

Hypertrophic cardiomyopathy (also see ➲Chapter 18)

The diagnosis of hypertrophic cardiomyopathy (HCM) is usually made clinically by the combination of an abnormal ECG and echocardiography findings of LV hypertrophy in the absence of underlying hypertension or aortic stenosis. Whilst this is a reasonable pathway, there are limitations including certain segments such as the apex and lateral wall being difficult to visualize on echocardiography. In addition, a challenging area is the grey-zone cohort of patients where LV wall thickness is around 14mm so that the clinical question of whether this is a response to mild hypertension or a result of a sarcomeric mutation becomes pertinent, and here CMR has certain key advantages. The wide field of view and detailed myocardial coverage makes it easier to identify areas of regional hypertrophy than echocardiography, and this is particularly true for the basal regions [62]. There is excellent natural subendocardial resolution so that accurate measurement of wall thickness and LV mass can be performed [63, 64].

Thus CMR is mainly used diagnostically when the results from echocardiography are inconclusive, such as in apical hypertrophy [65]. The 'inverted spade' configuration is typical of the apical variant, and is diagnosed on the basis of disproportionate apical wall thickening relative to other segments. As such, wall thickness at the apex does not have to exceed 15mm. Also, recent work suggests that LV mass index is a more sensitive marker of risk of death than peak wall thickness. Other features of HCM can also be shown including the demonstration of small cavity dimensions, hyperdynamic resting function, and RV involvement [66]. Obstruction in the outflow tract or at the mid-cavity level, and systolic anterior motion of the mitral valve can also be identified. The latter is due to a combination of factors and is often associated with some degree of mitral regurgitation. The accuracy of CMR for the phenotypic determination of HCM may also be helpful for screening of relatives of probands.

A number of other CMR techniques may also be helpful, although their place in clinical practice is not yet established. One feature of myopathic hypertrophy is impaired contraction and this can be quantified using CMR tagging. In HCM, tagging shows abnormal strain, shear, and torsion in dysfunctional hypertrophic areas. This may prove to have value in differentiating HCM from hypertrophy due to exercise or hypertension. Another feature of myopathic heart is a bioenergetic defect in high-energy phosphate compounds such as adenosine triphosphate (ATP), which can be detected using complex CMR spectroscopic methods in HCM patients with varying genetic mutations. This suggests the hypothesis that inefficient energy utilization may be the underlying substrate for HCM [67].

Finally, autopsy data confirms that patients with HCM have a high incidence of patchy or mid-wall fibrosis. Whilst this has often been diagnosed in vivo by biopsy, LGE is able to identify areas of myocardial replacement fibrosis non-invasively [68]. A common benign pattern of enhancement occurs at the insertion points of the RV into the LV. However, some patients have extensive LGE. Usually this is in the region of maximal wall thickening but not uniquely so. A link has been shown between the extent of LGE and the risk of heart failure or sudden death (➲Fig. 5.18) [69]. The interface between normal myocardium and scar tissue represents a focus for re-entrant tachycardia. The presence of fibrosis also impacts on both systolic and diastolic function. It is not yet known whether LGE in HCM is an independent risk factor in comparison with other established parameters and this is an area of much interest. Recent data has confirmed a correlation between the presence of late enhancement and the subsequent detection of arrhythmia [70]. It also appears to be an independent predictor for the occurrence of new onset atrial fibrillation (AF). At present it cannot be used clinically to guide implantable cardioverter defibrillator (ICD) therapy but our understanding is likely to evolve over the next few years. LGE also occurs in therapeutic septal myocardial infarction. This is useful for localizing and assessing the transmural extent of the infarction to assess procedural success. Stress perfusion CMR can be used to demonstrate microvascular dysfunction which correlates with wall thickness and fibrosis and may be a marker of early-stage disease processes [71].

CMR has also proved useful in other causes of hypertrophy which act as HCM phenocopies, which form a differential diagnosis in HCM. About 4% of HCM patients have Fabry's disease [72] in which alpha-galactosidase is deficient, causing accumulation of glycosphingolipid GB3 in myocytes and endothelium. CMR typically shows basal lateral wall LGE in these patients [73] which has been related to increased myocyte vacuolation as well as fibrosis, although the cause for this distribution is not known. It may be due to an increase in wall stress in these regions. It is however, useful to guide diagnosis and raise the suspicion for a

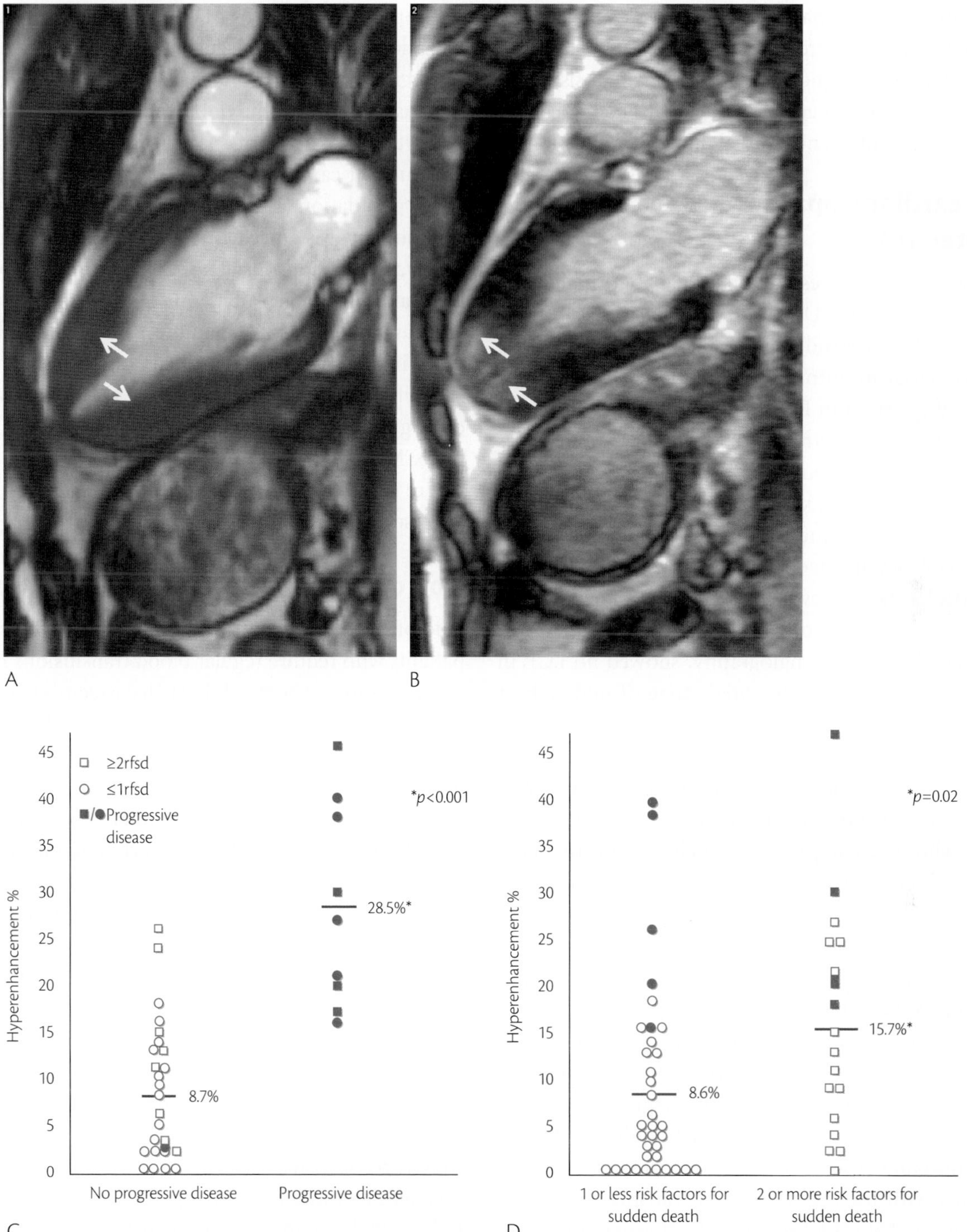

Figure 5.18 Hypertrophic cardiomyopathy. (A) Gradient-echo vertical long-axis view of left ventricle in apical HCM. The apical hypertrophy is well seen (arrows). (B) Late gadolinium enhancement shows fibrosis at the apex (bright signal arrowed). (C) Association between likelihood of having progressive left ventricular dilation and the extent of late gadolinium enhancement: patients with progressive disease have significantly greater amounts of fibrosis. (D) Association between the amount of late gadolinium enhancement and risk factors for sudden cardiac death: patients with two or more risk factors are likely to have greater amounts of fibrosis. Reproduced with permission from Moon JC, McKenna WJ, McCrohon JA, *et al.* Toward clinical risk assessment in hypertrophic cardiomyopathy with gadolinium cardiovascular magnetic resonance. *J Am Coll Cardiol* 2003; **41**: 1561–7.

HCM phenocopy. CMR has been used to assess the efficacy of enzyme replacement treatment in Fabry's disease [74]. Another differential diagnosis is cardiac amyloidosis which shows a different pattern again, with global subendocardial LGE due to preferential endocardial amyloid deposition.

Dilated cardiomyopathy (also see ➲Chapter 18)

CMR shows and quantifies the functional abnormalities in dilated cardiomyopathy (DCM) for both ventricles. Because CMR has excellent reproducibility, changes over time can be used for serial monitoring of function. However, the main clinical question in DCM is the differentiation from CAD. This may not be straightforward and many centres routinely perform coronary angiography as a gold standard. Both conditions can show regional thinning and wall motion abnormalities due to increased wall stress. Also, there is variable RV involvement in the two conditions.

LGE CMR has been shown to be useful as a non-invasive alternative [75]. A study of patients labelled as DCM following normal coronary angiography, showed no LGE in 59%, and patchy or circumferential striae of mid-wall or subepicardial enhancement sparing the subendocardium in 28% (➲Fig. 5.19). In all these cases, CMR correctly identified that MI was not the cause of ventricular dysfunction. Also of significant interest was the final group of 13% of patients in whom LGE was present which was indistinguishable from infarction. This suggests that these patients were incorrectly assigned the clinical label of DCM following 'normal' coronary angiography, probably due to coronary recanalization post-infarction and untreated ventricular remodelling. When it is also considered that bystander coronary stenosis may occur in patients with true DCM which has not resulted in infarction, the use of coronary angiography as a gold standard for diagnosis of DCM appears flawed. CMR is useful to distinguish bystander from attributable disease where infarction is seen and corresponds with the experiences of transplant pathologists who often note the presence of extensive infarction in patients labelled as a DCM and with unobstructed coronaries. These findings have been replicated by other groups showing an important potential application in the work-up of patients with heart failure and no evidence of CAD, as well as an alternative to coronary angiography in the diagnostic workup of DCM or as a gatekeeper.

The mid-wall LGE identified in DCM patients is similar to the fibrosis found in these patients at post-mortem. This has not previously been identified in vivo. The presence of mid-wall fibrosis appears to be an important predictor of the combined endpoint of all-cause mortality and hospitalization for a cardiovascular event. In two recent studies, it was independent of more conventional markers of risk such as LV ejection fraction. Mid-wall fibrosis was also an important predictor of sustained ventricular tachycardia and sudden cardiac death. In a recent study of high risk DCM population (EF <35%, pre-ICD implantation), mid-wall fibrosis was a predictor of the composite endpoint of cardiac death, appropriate ICD firing, and hospitalization for heart failure, even after adjustment for LV volume index and functional class. The amount of myocardial enhancement in DCM can be quantified, and has shown to correlate with the likelihood of inducible ventricular tachycardia during electrophysiological testing [76–79] The prognosis in DCM has also been assessed using CMR spectroscopy, where a low phosphocreatine to ATP ratio predicts an adverse outcome [80].

Iron overload (siderotic) cardiomyopathy

Siderotic cardiomyopathy (➲Chapter 18) occurs mainly in patients who require regular blood transfusions for chronic anaemia, most importantly beta-thalassaemia major. It is rare in hereditary haemochromatosis, where body iron overload occurs from dysfunction of one or more of a number of iron homeostatic mechanisms, which result in chronic increased intestinal iron absorption. The human body has no mechanism for the excretion of iron, which therefore accumulates initially in the tissues as ferritin, which is the very large iron storage molecule configured from 45 subunits as a hollow sphere which can contain about 4500 iron atoms. This normal storage capacity becomes overwhelmed with advancing overload, which promotes the formation of haemosiderin. Haemosiderin is a ferritin breakdown product which exists in its main form as ferrihydrite, which is ferromagnetic and can be detected by CMR. Organ dysfunction and oxidative cellular damage occur due to the presence of free labile iron, which creates reactive oxygen species that damage cell and organelle membranes, and impairs mitochondrial function. In beta-thalassaemia major, heart failure from myocardial siderosis is the cause of death in 70% of patients [81].

Conventional clinical management of thalassaemia has been based on measurements of blood ferritin and liver iron levels—which reflect total body iron—but these are not ideal because they are poor surrogate measures for the target lethal organ, which is the heart [82]. The direct measurement of cardiac iron clinically has been difficult, and myocardial biopsy has rarely been used because of the risk of complications and sampling error due to inhomogeneous myocardial iron distribution at the microscopic level [83].

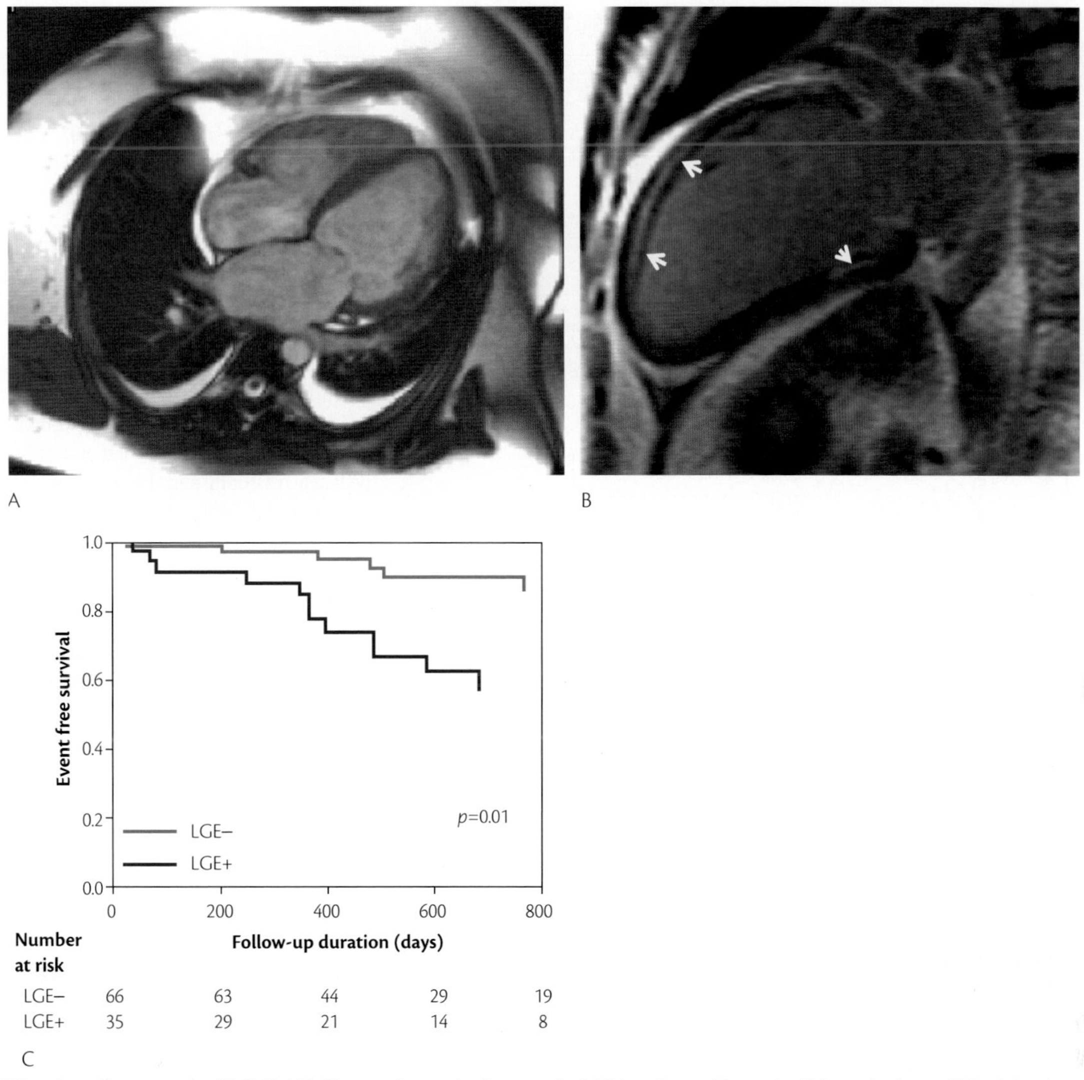

Figure 5.19 Dilated cardiomyopathy (DCM). (A) Cine gradient echo image of a DCM patient with marked biventricular and biatrial enlargement. (B) Late gadolinium enhancement (LGE) showing mid-wall fibrosis of both the anterior and inferior walls (arrows). (C) Patients with DCM and fibrosis on LGE (blue line) have a greater likelihood of adverse outcomes such as all-cause mortality and unplanned cardiovascular hospitalization, compared to those patients with no demonstrable fibrosis (red line). Reproduced with permission from Assomull RG, Prasad SK, Lyne J, *et al.* Cardiovascular magnetic resonance, fibrosis, and prognosis in dilated cardiomyopathy. *J Am Coll Cardiol* 2006; **48**: 1977–85.

Recently however, it has shown that the myocardial relaxation parameter T2* measured by CMR can be used to assess iron in the heart [84], based on the microscopic disturbance of magnetic field caused by microparticulate haemosiderin. The T2* technique can now be completed in a single breath-hold of 15s [85], and is very reproducible [86, 87] making it cost-effective even in countries with limited resources which have a high incidence of haemoglobinopathy, such as Thailand where abnormal allele frequencies can reach 50%. The normal myocardial T2* is 40ms, and normal subjects have never been shown to have a myocardial T2* of <20ms. Therefore values <20ms indicate myocardial siderosis. The severity of myocardial siderosis correlates with LV dysfunction (➲Fig. 5.20), and increased volumes and mass typical of remodelling in heart failure [84]. Follow-up studies have shown that a very high proportion of patients with decompensated heart failure have a myocardial T2* of <10ms at presentation, and therefore this is used a threshold to define severe myocardial iron loading. Liver and heart iron can be very discrepant [84], making clinical management using direct heart iron measurement essential. This explains the high toll of myocardial dysfunction and death that has occurred in the past using other measures to guide treatment. A number of studies across the world have shown that myocardial siderosis occurs at a frequency of ~50%, which indicates that all patients require direct myocardial iron assessment for assessment of risk [88–91].

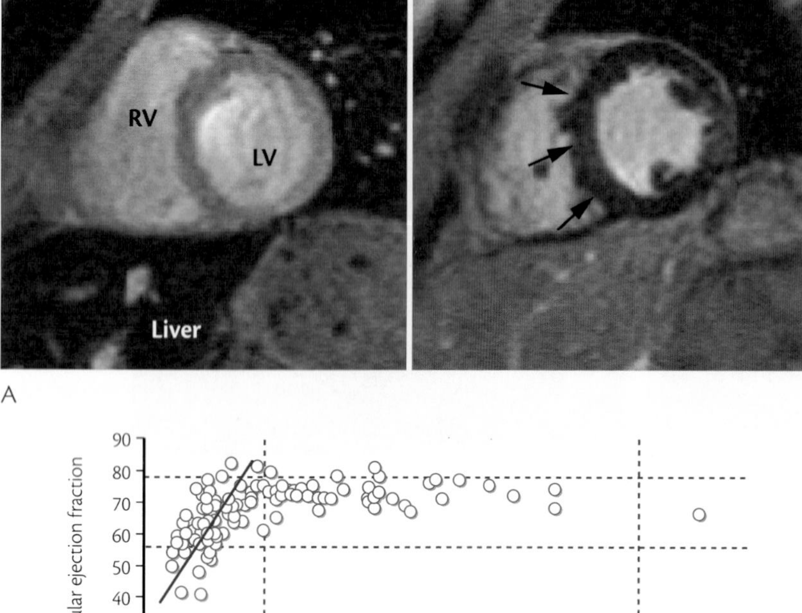

Figure 5.20 T2* CMR in iron overload cardiomyopathy. The upper panel left shows an iron loaded liver (dark) but normal myocardial signal. If a liver biopsy was performed this would suggest iron loading, and chelation therapy might be increased with the risk of significant side effects. The upper panel right shows a counter example, where the liver is normal, but the heart is iron loaded (arrows). If a liver biopsy were performed on this patient, it would be falsely reassuring and the patient would be at risk of cardiac complications. The inter-organ disparity in iron loading explains why heart failure is the biggest cause of mortality in thalassemia patients. The lower graph shows the relation between myocardial T2* and the ejection fraction. The normal myocardial T2* is >20ms, and this is associated with a normal ejection fraction, but below this the ejection fraction falls with iron toxicity. Reproduced with permission from Anderson LJ, Holden S, Davies B, *et al.* Cardiovascular T2* (T2 star) magnetic resonance for the early diagnosis of myocardial iron overload. *Eur Heart J* 2001; **22**: 2171–9.

Although asymptomatic LV dysfunction appears common in thalassaemia, it is difficult to detect with conventional measures of ejection fraction, because the entire population ejection fraction is shifted up by 6–8% because of high cardiac output resulting from chronic anaemia [92]. This results in underdiagnosis of early dysfunction. Measures of diastolic function have not proven to be more helpful [93]. Decompensated myocardial siderosis can be reversed using iron chelation, but very intensive treatment is required for patients who develop heart failure [94], as mortality is high once decompensation occurs as intramyocardial iron release can become uncontrollable. The oral chelator deferiprone accesses myocardial iron preferentially compared with the established subcutaneous injected drug deferoxamine, and may stabilize mitochondrial iron levels, and therefore is widely used when myocardial siderosis is identified [95]. The combination of both drugs is often used in patients with severe myocardial iron loading [96, 97]. Use of these treatment protocols has been associated with a 71% reduction in cardiac deaths in thalassaemia patients in the UK since it was introduced in 1999 [98], and marked reductions in cardiac mortality have also been shown in Italy [99] and Cyprus [100].

Arrhythmogenic right ventricular cardiomyopathy (also see ➲Chapters 9 and 18)

The RV is difficult to visualize by echocardiography partly because of its crescentic shape wrapped around the LV, and the proximity to the sternum. While the bulk of changes in this condition occur in the RV, the LV is also affected in at least 25% of cases. This reflects the underlying genetic abnormalities that result in structural changes to the intercellular desmosome, which is important for structural integrity. Both structural and functional abnormalities of the RV are well seen by CMR and therefore it is used in expert centres for the investigation of arrhythmogenic right ventricular cardiomyopathy (ARVC). CMR assists in locating diagnostic criteria for ARVC including the presence of regional wall motion abnormalities, increased volumes, morphological abnormalities, fibrofatty infiltration, and LV involvement (➲Fig. 5.21). Follow up of RV volumes over time can be helpful as the condition is progressive and it can present in the early concealed phase. Scan interpretation is not straightforward however, because the RV has

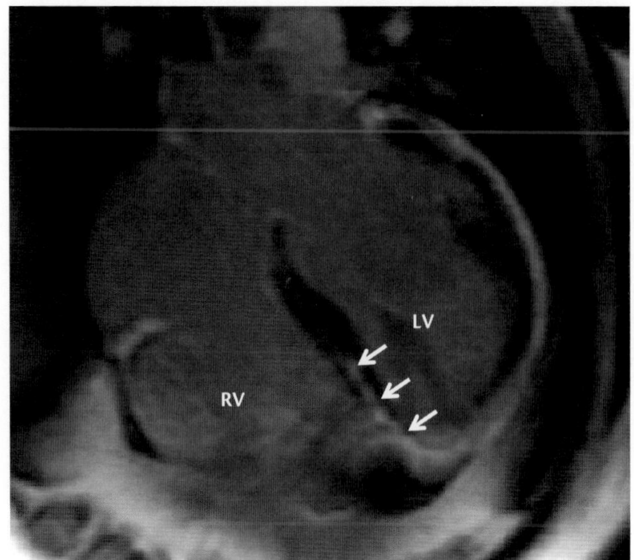

Figure 5.21 Arrhythmogenic right ventricular cardiomyopathy (ARVC). The patient has dilated right (RV) and left (LV) ventricles and a confirmed causative genotype for desmosomal abnormality. On this late gadolinium image, there is mid-wall enhancement of the septum particularly towards the apex (arrows) showing that LV involvement occurs in this condition.

significant variation of normality, including hypokinesia at the moderator band insertion, variable trabeculation, and epicardial fat deposits which may mask the normal thin RV myocardium except in the best quality images. Fatty infiltration can also occur in circumstances other than ARVC. Recent work in genotyped populations demonstrates the role of LGE to detect fibrous replacement in both the RV and LV. Identifying LGE in the RV is difficult because it is a thin structure, and it can be difficult to confidently distinguish fatty changes from the late enhancement. Care should be taken not to over-interpret findings such as increased RV trabeculation, which have a low specificity. T1-weighted spin-echo imaging has conventionally been used, but it is now known to have low sensitivity and low reproducibility, and in many institutions it is no longer routinely performed. It might prove useful if combined with fat-suppression imaging, which allows signal from fat to be reduced, and leaves the normal RV myocardium better seen and fatty infiltration as dark areas. There is no doubt about the value of CMR in ARVC, but more work needs to be done in this area, and an improved understanding of the underlying condition in important. It is clear that any evaluation must still be based in conjunction with Taskforce criteria. Prospective studies are also looking at the predictive value of CMR to identify those at risk of sudden cardiac death [101, 102] (➲Chapters 9 and 30).

Myocardial sarcoidosis

Sarcoidosis of the heart (➲Chapter 18) is seen in about 25% of autopsy hearts in sarcoid patients with established extra-cardiac involvement, but demonstrating this *in vivo* can be challenging [103]. While endomyocardial biopsy is often considered to be the diagnostic gold standard, its accuracy is low (<20%) due to sampling error, as cardiac involvement is usually patchy and mainly affects the LV. The areas most commonly affected are the LV lateral wall, papillary muscles, RV subendocardial surface, and RV free wall although any segment can be affected. It is a well-recognized cause of sudden death in patients with sarcoidosis. The clinical diagnosis is difficult, although changes in the ECG can be indicative. LGE CMR has been used to show myocardial abnormalities in presumed areas of fibrosis in sarcoidosis [104]. T2-weighted sequences show potential in identifying areas of active myocardial inflammation. Further work is required to assess the value of CMR as an indication for steroid treatment, and serial monitoring [105].

Myocardial amyloidosis

In myocardial amyloidosis (➲Chapter 18) CMR can show the features of restrictive cardiomyopathy such as in amyloidosis, with diastolic dysfunction, ventricular hypertrophy, and interatrial septum thickening [106]. The distinction from other forms of LV hypertrophy can be difficult in the early stages. On cine images, important clues are that there is a concentric pattern of hypertrophy and unlike HCM, long-axis function and radial thickening are poor. Pericardial and pleural effusions may be seen in conjunction with the LV hypertrophy, and this is less common with HCM or hypertension. Amyloid infiltration is seen using LGE [107], which is typically a global subendocardial pattern that results from dominant interstitial expansion of the endocardial layer with amyloid protein (➲Fig. 5.22). However, patchy amyloid deposition has also been seen. A very characteristic finding is a dark blood pool which is caused by abnormal gadolinium handling kinetics, and this results in difficulty nulling normal myocardium. In one study, the LGE pattern had a sensitivity of 80% and a specificity of 94% versus the gold standard of endomyocardial biopsy, indicating that this non-invasive technique alone has major potential in this condition [108]. At present, pending further outcome studies, CMR is used to direct rather than confirm the diagnosis.

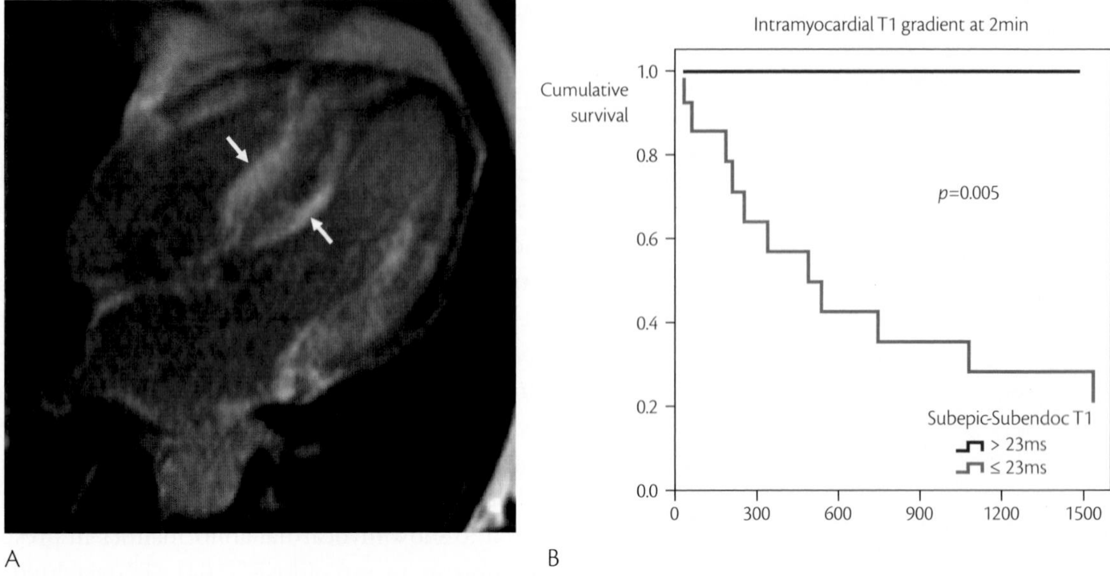

Figure 5.22 Cardiac amyloidosis. (A) Late gadolinium enhancement image in the four-chamber view shows the characteristic pattern for cardiac amyloid infiltration. There is a circumferential pattern of late enhancement associated with a dark blood pool. A 'zebra-stripe' pattern is often seen with greater enhancement of the LV and RV subendocardium (asterisks) relative to the epicardium. Enhancement reflects the severity of myocardial amyloid loading, and commonly starts in the endocardium. (B) Once enhancement also affects the epicardium, the myocardial amyloid burden is greater, and this can be measured as the transmural difference in T1 within 2min after gadolinium. The dark line (transmural T1 difference <23ms) shows that such patients have a far worse prognosis Reproduced with permission from Maceira AM, Prasad SK, Hawkins PN, *et al.* Cardiovascular magnetic resonance and prognosis in cardiac amyloidosis. *J Cardiovasc Magn Reson* 2008; **10**: 54.

Myocardial non-compaction

Non-compaction (➲Chapter 18) is a disorder of embryonic endomyocardial development in which the myocardium fails to compact properly and deep clefts occur in the LV. The marked trabeculation typically involves the lateral wall and apex, with deep intertrabecular recesses and a relatively thin epicardial layer. There is much controversy over how to make the precise diagnosis and as a consequence, data on the prevalence and incidence of the condition is unclear. It is associated with progressive dysfunction, arrhythmias, and systemic embolism. The diagnosis can be made by echocardiography, but CMR depicts the abnormality well with comprehensive ventricular coverage if there is limited involvement, and underlying fibrosis can be shown with LGE [109, 110].

Myocarditis

The clinical diagnosis of myocarditis (➲Chapter 18) is often difficult and may mimic infarction. CMR can be very useful in this diagnosis. Focal increase of myocardial signal is seen in acute myocarditis with T1-weighted spin echo imaging at 1–2min after gadolinium injection. Global myocardial enhancement relative to skeletal muscle may be increased [111]. The relative enhancement falls over time and is predictive of long-term ventricular function. T2-weighted spin-echo imaging can show high signal either globally or more focally if imaging is performed during the acute phase. LGE CMR has also been shown to be abnormal in the acute phase, particularly in the epicardial portion of the lateral wall (➲Fig. 5.23) [112], and subsequently this may develop into patchy chronic fibrosis. LGE representative of areas of myocardial injury has been shown in 95% of cases with histopathology confirmation. Characteristic patterns of LGE in the septal mid-wall or subepicardial lateral wall were seen. The location of enhancement was shown to be specific for the underlying viral pathogen and may potentially help guide where to perform a myocardial biopsy. The presence of LGE in the septum and the total amount of late enhancement have been shown to be strong predictors of adverse ventricular remodelling at follow-up [113]. Myocarditis has been shown to be a common differential diagnosis of patients presenting with acute chest pain but normal coronary arteries [114].

Valvular heart disease

Echo Doppler is the first-line technique for the diagnosis and follow-up of valvular disorders (➲Chapter 21), but can be challenging and sometimes nearly impossible in patients with poor echo windows. In these patients CMR

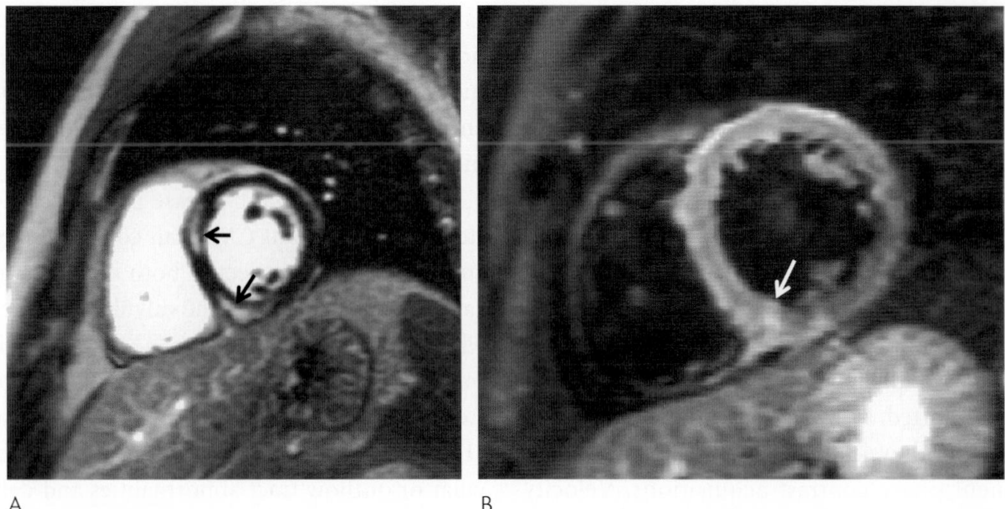

Figure 5.23 Myocarditis. (A) Late gadolinium enhancement study shows mid-wall enhancement of the septum and part of the inferior wall (arrows). (B) On T2-weighted STIR imaging, there is increased signal in the inferoseptal wall consistent with oedema and active inflammation.

is a valid alternative (➲Fig. 5.24) [115]. In selected patients, CMR offers the added value of quantifying the severity of the lesion, of reproducibly quantifying the impact on ventricular morphology and function, and of evaluating prognosis with respect to timing of surgical or pharmacologic treatment by using LGE imaging. Associated pathology can also be evaluated more easily with CMR than with echocardiography. SSFP cine sequences are primarily used for studying ventricular and valvular morphology and function. Turbulence of flow resulting from stenosis or

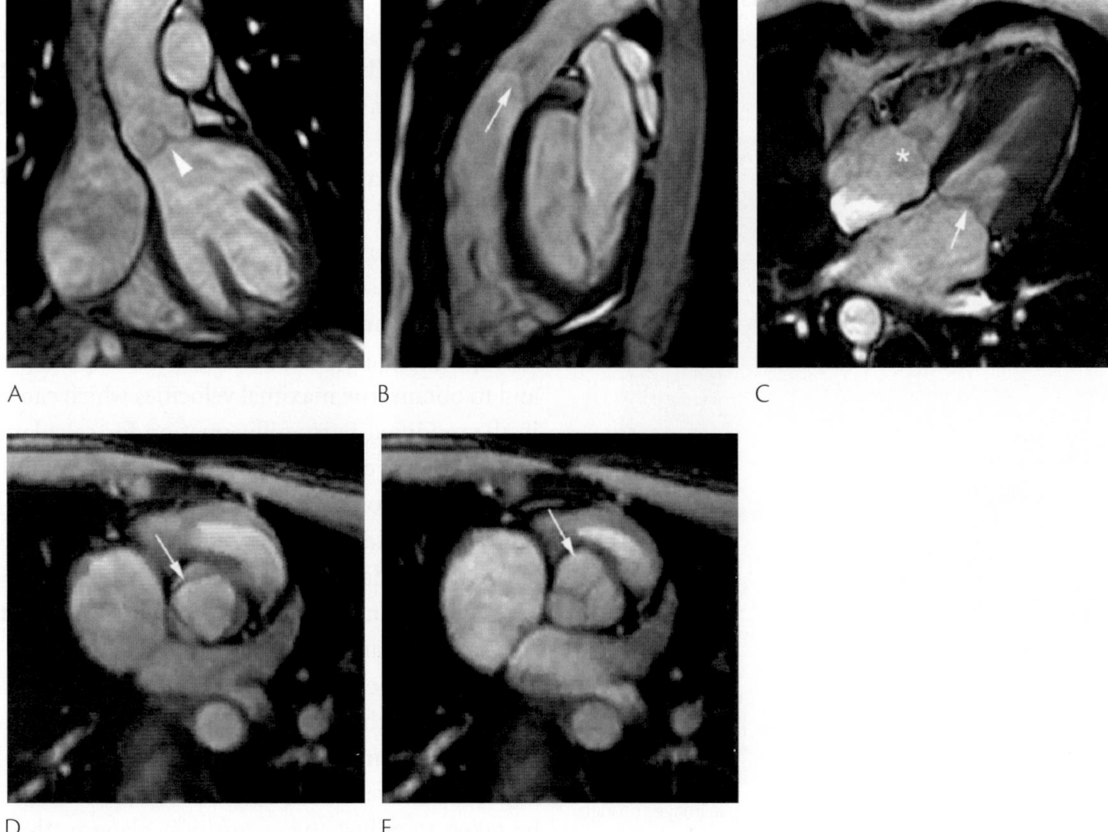

Figure 5.24 Appearances of normal valves by CMR. (A) Aortic valve; (B) pulmonary valve; (C) mitral (arrow) and tricuspid (asterisk) valves; (D) the aortic valve open in systole in a transverse plane (arrow); (E) aortic valve closed in diastole (arrow).

regurgitation causes signal loss on cine sequences allowing ready identification of the abnormality. The size and extension of the signal loss, however, is only a semi-quantitative measure for lesion severity because of the influence of haemodynamics, shape of the valve, and parameters of the sequence, just as in colour flow mapping in echo Doppler. Imaging perpendicular to the stenotic valve with thin, adjacent slices enables the planimetry of the stenotic area (➲Fig. 5.25). Through-plane motion, signal voids due to turbulence or calcification, and distorted valve morphology may interfere with this measurement, but overall good results have been reported. Multiple SSFP cines, parallel and perpendicular to the flow jets, permit optimal alignment for the subsequent phase contrast acquisitions. Velocity mapping permits the quantification of peak and mean flow velocities (m/s) (as with Doppler which can be used in the Bernouilli equation) as well as volume flow (mL/s) at multiple sites in the heart [116]. Integration of volume flow over time provides the stroke volume, as well as antegrade and retrograde flow volumes. Combining such measurements with each other and with the stroke volumes from LV and RV enables the calculation of gradients, resistance, valve area, regurgitant volumes, and fraction. The impact of valvular dysfunction can be reliably and reproducibly followed over time by measuring myocardial mass, cavity volumes, and shape. End-systolic volume

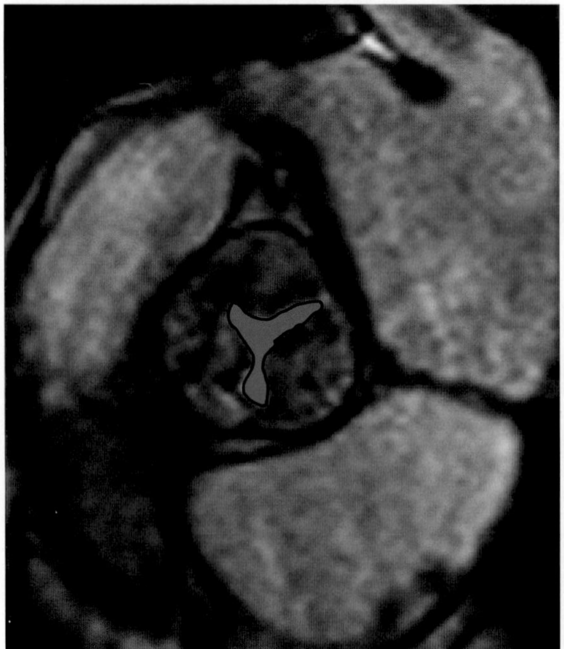

Figure 5.25 Valve planimetry in aortic stenosis. Transverse image through the narrowest part of a stenosed aortic valve, showing automated tracing of the narrowed valve, providing an area of 1.2cm^2.

(among others) has been shown to be an important prognostic factor. Automated tracking of valve through-plane motion may in the future improve the reliability of velocity encoded measurements and make CMR the optimal technique to quantify valvular dysfunction.

Overall, regurgitant disease is more easily studied than stenotic disease, but CMR can contribute in nearly all circumstances with respect to both intrinsic valve characterization and the impact of the valvular dysfunction. The valve where CMR could constitute the first line of investigation is pulmonary valve dysfunction, for both regurgitation and stenosis, certainly in the setting of congenital heart disease [117]. CMR can quantify the different aspects of the valvular or outflow tract abnormalities and define the impact on the right heart and the pulmonary circulation. In aortic valve pathology, aortic regurgitation can be quantified by measuring retrograde diastolic flow immediately above the valve and below the coronary ostia (➲Fig. 5.26) [118]. By dividing retrograde by antegrade flow volume, the regurgitant fraction is obtained. Associated pathology such as coarctation can be identified and quantified. When echocardiography cannot provide the required information [119], aortic stenosis can be studied by direct measurement of valve area on SSFP sequences [120], and by calculation of the gradient on phase-contrast studies [121, 122]. A similar approach is less obvious for the mitral valve: quantification of mitral insufficiency is less consistent due to the larger, less circular mitral ring area and the three-dimensional motion of the valve [123]. Eccentric jets can also cause problems. Measuring the difference between stroke volume, obtained from cavity measurements, and antegrade flow in the aorta is therefore a more reliable technique. For stenosis assessment, both in-plane and through-plane velocity measurements can be used, but in both instances multiple parallel planes are required to optimize alignment and to obtain true maximal velocities which can be inserted in the modified Bernouilli equation for calculation of gradients and valve area with the continuity equation. Also for tricuspid pathology, CMR constitutes a second-line alternative to echocardiography, especially in Ebstein's anomaly where the displacement and malformation of the valve, the severity of regurgitation, and the function of the remaining right ventricular cavity can be studied.

It is safe to perform CMR in all prosthetic valves although the metal in the prostheses causes focal artefacts which can obscure small jets [124]. Quantification of valvular regurgitation remains possible, but even more care has to be taken to adjust the acquisition plane to the motion of the valve. Endocarditis lesions can be visualized if they do

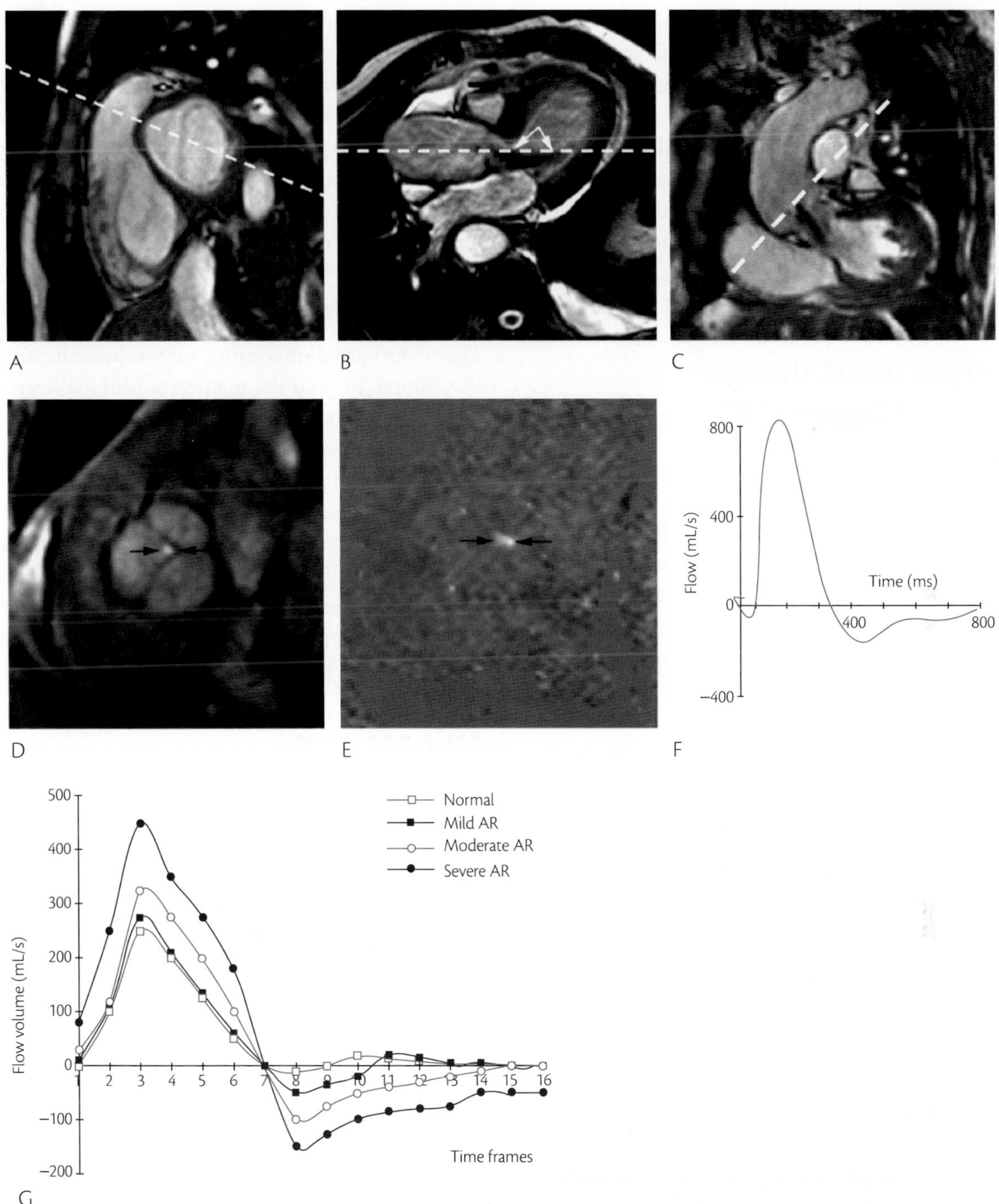

Figure 5.26 Quantification of aortic regurgitation showing the method of acquisition of the correct imaging plane. (A) Basal short-axis cut, with the dashed line showing the oblique plane through the left ventricular outflow tract. (B) left ventricular outflow tract view obtained from image (A). The dashed line is placed through the jet of aortic regurgitation. (C) Oblique coronal view obtained from image (B). The dashed line shows the oblique plane used to generate the following velocity map. (D) The jet of aortic regurgitation is seen as a white dot in the cine image (arrows). (E) The corresponding velocity map. (F) The quantitative flow across the valve during the cardiac cycle. The positive flow is the forward flow during systole, the negative flow is the regurgitation during diastole. (G) Both the forward and backward flow increase with increasing severity of regurgitation. The ratio of reverse and forward flow is the regurgitant fraction.

not show a rapid, erratic motion pattern which makes them 'invisible' on gated sequences but typically echocardiography is preferred. Real-time CMR may make imaging of endocarditis lesions more reliable.

Overall, in valve disease, CMR is a valid alternative when echocardiographic quality is suboptimal and can be the technique of choice in pulmonary valve disease and for individual patient follow-up with respect to volumes and mass [125].

Congenital heart disease (also see ➲Chapter 10)

Congenital heart disease is a major indication for CMR. The three-dimensional character of CMR, together with the ability to quantify local flow and therefore shunts, the absence of radiation, and the difficulties of using echocardiography post-surgery, have all contributed to its successful use [126]. Patients often need serial scans and the avoidance of undergoing invasive tests as well as minimizing exposure to ionizing radiation have been major advantages of CMR. In addition, the wide field of view is essential in identifying both individual abnormalities and their wider significance, as well as excluding concurrent defects. There is no routine need for contrast agents. Within one study, anatomy, function, and flow can be assessed. The full spectrum of CMR sequences is used in congenital heart disease: SSFP sequences for overall anatomy and function (LV, RV, and atrial volumes, stroke volumes and ejection fraction, myocardial mass); spin-echo for morphologic details, T2 imaging for tissue characterization; velocity mapping of local flow and for valvular function (aorta, pulmonary artery, caval veins, pulmonary veins, grafts, and conduits, valve planes); and gadolinium angiography for three-dimensional representation of the great vessels and complex anatomy [126, 127]. Fibrosis detection is also developing important application in congenital disease. The use of three-dimensional coronary imaging gives diagnostic information on anomalous coronary anatomy.

Viscero-atrial situs

The viscero-atrial situs (situs, solitus, inversus, ambiguous) (➲Chapter 10) and the malposition of the heart (dextrocardia) can be more easily obtained with CMR since the technique offers a large field of view which includes the surrounding structures—including the abdomen—and identification of the different chambers from morphologic and functional characteristics. A full set of images in the three orthogonal planes (transverse, sagittal, coronal) is the basis for this analysis. Depending on the anomalies observed, further images, taken in oblique planes, can be combined with functional imaging.

Atria and veins

Atrial septal defect (➲Chapter 10), can usually be visualized with echocardiography (especially transoesophageal echo) but the impact on the circulation (shunt quantification [127], RV dilatation and function) is better evaluated with CMR (➲Fig. 5.27). By measuring the flow in the ascending aorta and in the pulmonary artery the shunt flow and fraction can easily be determined. RV dimensions and function are notoriously difficult to evaluate with echo; CMR can

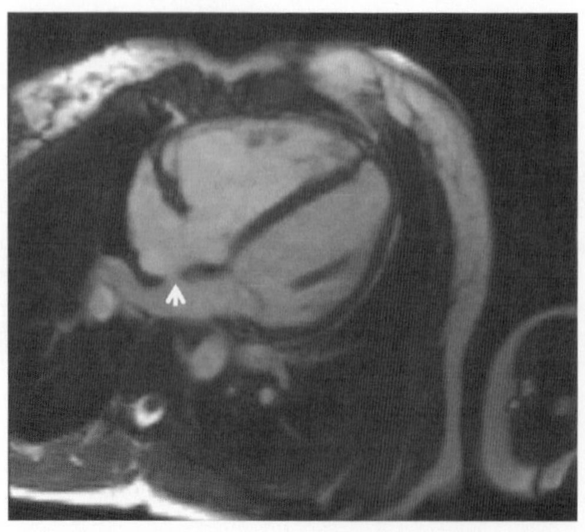

A

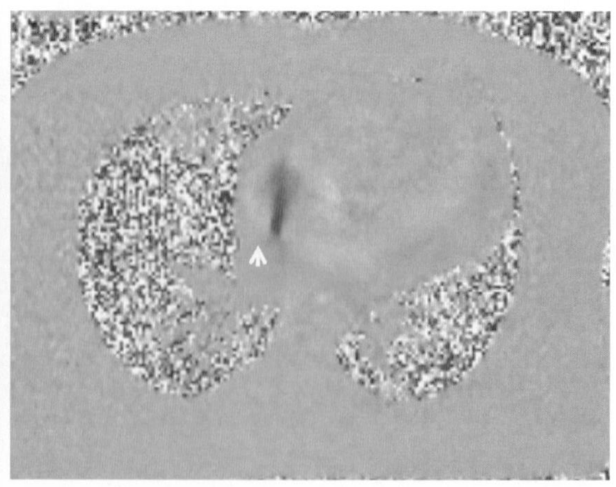

B

Figure 5.27 Atrial septal defect. (A) A four-chamber view with atrial secondum defect arrowed. (B) A flow map demonstrating left-to-right shunt across the defect (arrow).

quantify volumes, ejection fraction, and pulmonary valve flow. The location of an atrial septal defect from the AV groove and pulmonary veins can be established. Partial anomalous pulmonary venous return can be difficult to detect even with transoesophageal echocardiography. CMR visualizes well the (sometimes very variable) morphology of the pulmonary veins but can also measure the flow in the aberrant vein, calculate the shunt fraction, and show the abnormal connection [128]. Systemic venous abnormalities or variants can be visualized with contiguous two-dimensional scanning or three-dimensional volume acquisitions (left superior vena cava, interrupted inferior vena cava). After surgery, for example, repair for transposition of the great arteries, the reconstructed venous conduits and baffles may become obstructed and stenotic, and the morphology and degree of stenosis can be measured from cine and flow imaging. Work is underway to evaluate three-dimensional real-time imaging to facilitate intervention.

Atrioventricular connections

CMR can be used to identify atria and ventricles using characteristic morphologic features, allowing the demonstration of discordant atrioventricular connections (➲Chapter 10). Abnormal morphology or function of the valves (straddling, atresia, regurgitation, stenosis) can be visualized. A reliable quantification of ventricular volumes and function can be used for surgical decisions (repair versus Fontan). The use of three-dimensional anatomy can help guide both surgical and electrophysiological therapeutic strategies.

Ventricles

Complex ventricular anomalies (➲Chapter 10) (tetralogy of Fallot, univentricular hearts, valve atresia) can be depicted with CMR and the shunt fraction and morphologic and haemodynamic consequences can be quantified. This can help in treatment decisions. Ventricular septal defects can be visualized (jet on cine images) and the shunt quantified, but it is mainly in complex lesions (double outlet) where CMR proves superior to echocardiography. Increasingly, there is interest in the diagnostic and prognostic value of fibrosis detection. Recent work has shown that this can be used to predict adverse remodelling and a greater likelihood of poor exercise capacity.

Valves

While direct depiction of valves is less good with CMR compared to echocardiography (➲Chapter 4), its main importance lies in the quantification of regurgitation and the impact on the receiving chamber, especially for the RV. An example is pulmonary regurgitation after patch surgery for tetralogy of Fallot, where it is clinically difficult to decide on the appropriate timing for valve replacement [129].

Great arteries and conduits

Coarctation of the aorta (➲Chapters 10 and 31) is the most common anomaly of the thoracic aorta. CMR can visualize the lesion itself and also the collateral circulation. By comparing flow before the coarctation and at the level of the diaphragm, the collateral circulation can be quantified and used to judge the success of invasive treatment. Common complications of coarctation repair such as recoarctation, aneurysm repair can be identified. Secondary changes such as LV hypertrophy may also be seen. Work is underway to detect early changes to coronary flow and brachial endothelial function. Other abnormalities of the aorta (double aortic arch, aneurysm of the sinus of Valsalva, dilatation in Marfan (➲Chapter 31) and Ehler–Danlos syndromes) can be followed over time. Patent ductus arteriosus can be easily seen with echo in newborns but in older patients CMR can be more reliable. Abnormalities of the pulmonary circulation in patients with reduced pulmonary artery flow or systemic to pulmonary collaterals, as well as pulmonary anomalies can be shown with CMR. Comparing flow in the right and left pulmonary artery and comparing these to systemic return flow can help in evaluation the severity of the lesions and the options for therapy. Also after intravascular or surgical treatment CMR can be useful to evaluate the effects and evolution (to stenosis) of the intervention.

Postoperative follow-up

CMR is very helpful after surgery for complex anomalies since the echocardiographic quality is often degraded and a need exists for a quantitative technique which can reliably follow volumes, function, and morphology over time. This is especially true for conduits and for the RV which is often overloaded as it functions as the systemic ventricle or due to pulmonary insufficiency [130].

Tetralogy of Fallot

Tetralogy of Fallot (➲Chapter 10) is one of the commonest forms of congenital heart disease (➲Fig. 5.28). At presentation four usual features are seen including (1) mal-alignment ventricular septal defect (VSD); (2) subvalvar (infundibular) and valvar pulmonary stenosis; (3) overriding aorta; and (4) right ventricular hypertrophy. However, within this cohort there is a wide range of presentations and individual variation ranging from tetralogy of Fallot with pulmonary

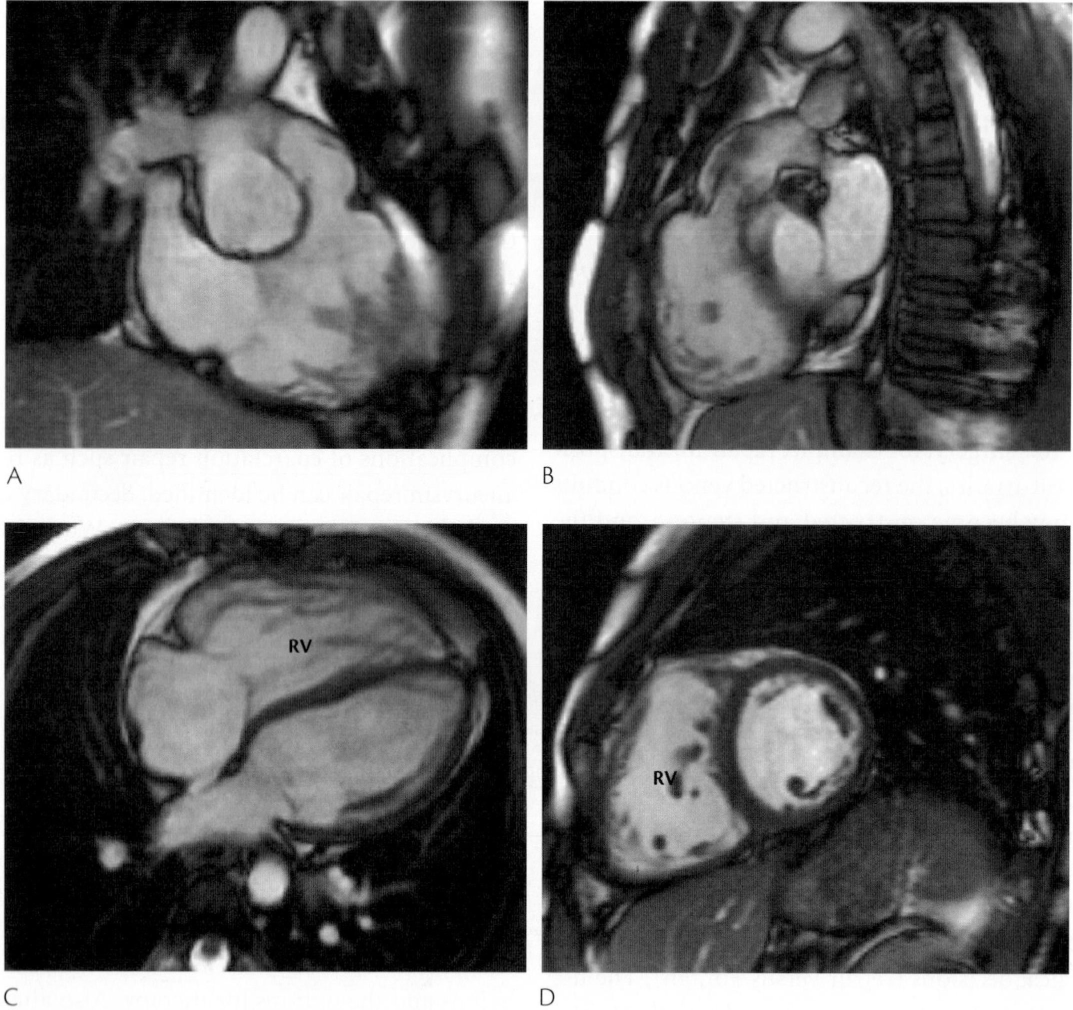

Figure 5.28 Tetralogy of Fallot after repair. (A) Right ventricular (RV) outflow tract view. (B) RV outflow tract cross-cut view demonstrating turbulent flow. (C) Four-chamber view showing RV dilation. (D) Short-axis cut showing RV dilatation.

atresia and multiple aortopulmonary collateral vessels to tetralogy of Fallot with only mild pulmonary stenosis. In adults, most patients will have undergone surgical repair at the time of presentation. Increasingly, most patients undergo repair at an early age. However not infrequently patients will be encountered who have undergone some form of previous or current palliation such as a procedure to supplement pulmonary blood flow with later definitive repair. CMR is useful to assess the quality of repair and degree of pulmonary regurgitation/ recurrent stenosis. RV dilatation and hypertrophy are important markers of disease severity. Tricuspid regurgitation may also be noted [131].

Coronary arteries

CMR is the technique of choice for the diagnosis of congenital coronary abnormalities (➲Chapter 10). It can show the abnormal origin of the artery but also the course with respect to aorta and pulmonary artery which is important for risk and surgical planning in congenital heart disease.

Transposition of great arteries

Usually in the adult, most patients will have undergone repair at the time of presentation. Initially patients underwent some form of atrial level switch but subsequently, the move has been to arterial switch operations. Important features to identify are systemic RV failure in the atrial switch patients. This may be augmented by systemic AV valve regurgitation. Baffle obstruction may also occur and can be more difficult to detect. CMR is useful through the multiplanar cine format options and flow maps in the plane of interest. The frequency of serial evaluation will be guided by the severity of observed lesions.

Comparison to other modalities

Echocardiography usually remains the technique of choice in newborns and young infants, since image quality is usually very good and CMR would require sedation or anaesthesia. On the other hand, in older infants, adolescents and adults, in complex pathology and after surgery, CMR is often useful. In the latter two conditions, the full advantage of CMR becomes evident offering unlimited image planes, irrespective of scar or lung interposition and the capability of localized flow measurements for the evaluation of shunts, stenoses, and valve lesions. The CMR information may allow cardiac catheterization to be avoided, significantly shortened, or reserved for interventional procedures. For follow-up, CMR usually offers all the necessary information and cumulative radiation can be avoided [132, 133] (➲Chapter 3).

Great vessels (also see ➲Chapter 31)

CMR has become the primary imaging modality for assessment of great vessel disease. Gadolinium enhanced CMR angiography generates high resolution three-dimensional angiograms and velocity mapping provides reliable measurements of blood flow. The most common indications for performing CMR in aortic disease (➲Chapter 31) are to depict or follow aneurysms (➲Fig. 5.29) or dissections. Although CMR angiography shows the size, extent, and shape of aneurysms, additional use of black-blood (fast spin-echo) and LGE imaging is needed for depiction of the vascular wall and peri-aortic soft tissue. Image acquisition in at least two planes is helpful in order to optimally identify the typical features of arteritis [134], perivalvular abscesses, and mycotic aneurysms or post-surgical infections. CMR is well suited to identify the presence of thrombus [135] and distinguish it from slow flow in a patent lumen in dilated and especially dissected aortas (➲Fig. 5.30). Care is required when using CMR following stent placement in the aorta, as artefacts are introduced by the metal. These are more prominent in SSFP images than in turbo spin-echo images.

CMR has a high accuracy in diagnosing and excluding aortic dissection [136] and the entire aorta can be imaged within 15min. Therefore, even in cases with acute disease, CMR is competitive with more commonly used techniques

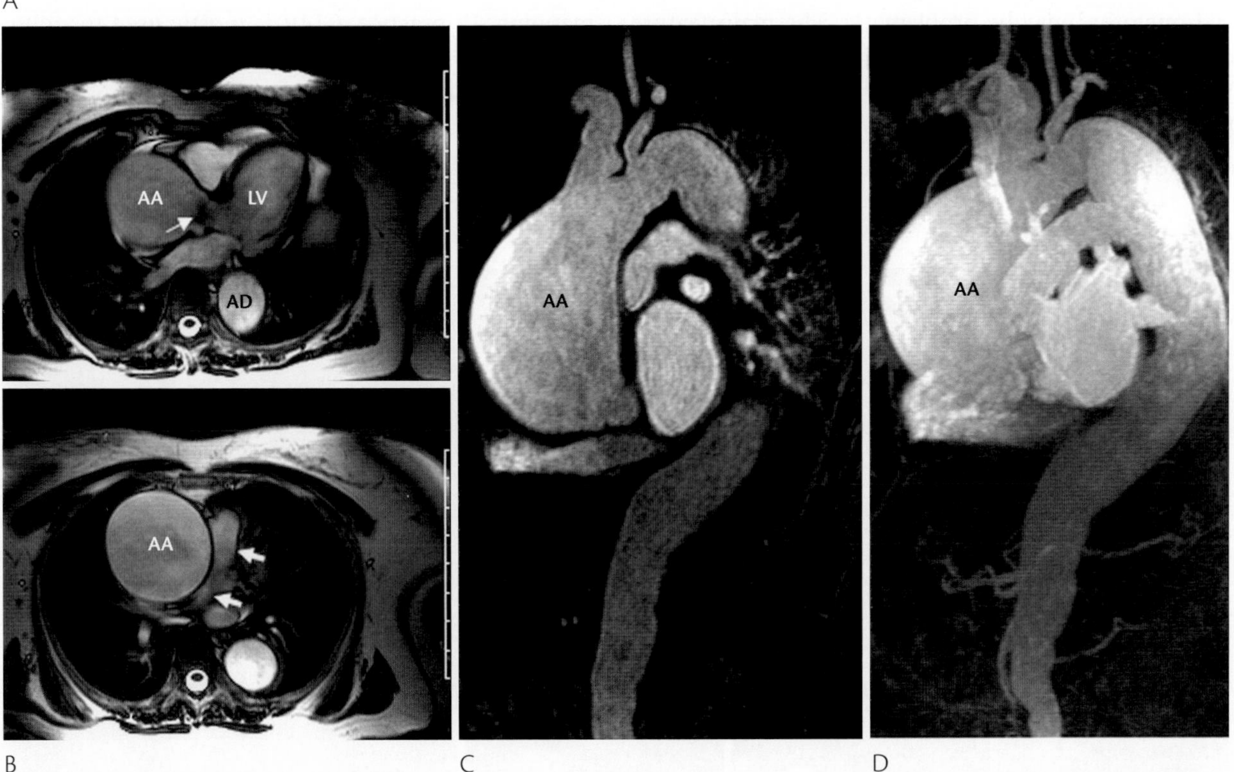

Figure 5.29 Comprehensive CMR depiction of an aneurysm of the ascending aorta (AA) in a patient with aortic regurgitation. AD, descending aorta, LV, left ventricle. (A) SSFP sequence, transverse section. Systolic turbulence, extending into the aorta (small white arrow). The aneurysm begins immediately superior to the sinus of Valsalva. (B) SSFP sequence, transverse section at the largest diameter of the aorta at the level of pulmonary artery. The AA should be orthogonally sectioned in order to provide reliable measurements. In oval shaped aortas the smaller diameter needs to be taken for treatment decisions. (C) Single slice of a stack of slices acquired for three-dimensional angiography reconstruction. (D) Three-dimensional aortography provides comprehensive information about the vessel lumen and its branches. However, neither the wall nor its surrounding can be reliably assessed in this way.

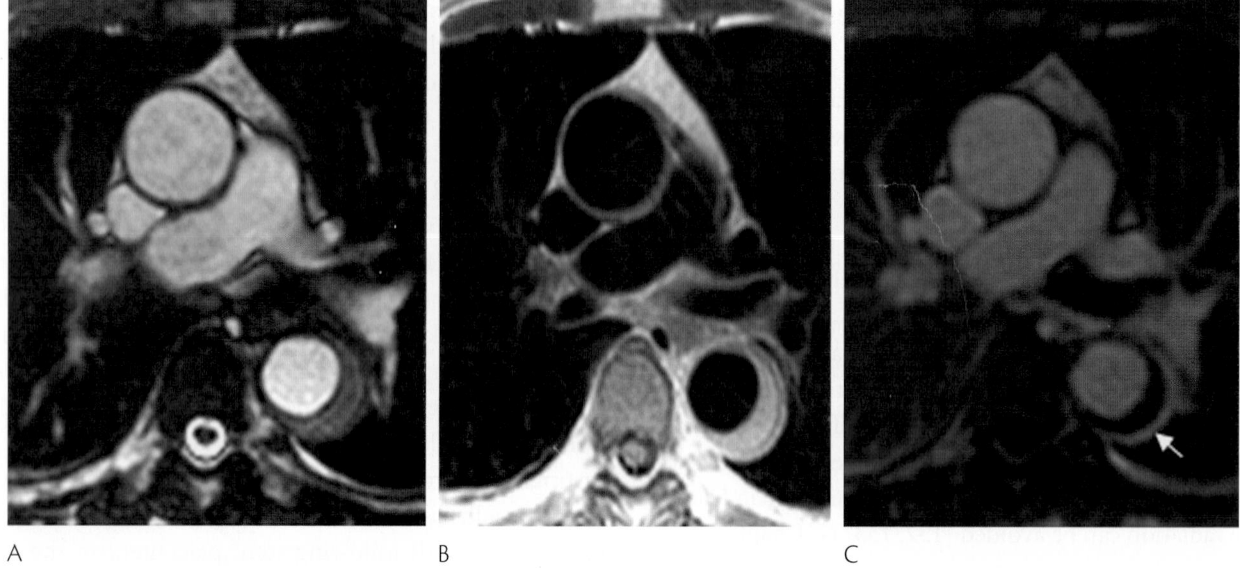

Figure 5.30 Intramural haematoma of the descending aorta. Transverse sections. (A) Cine SSFP sequence clearly shows abnormality in the descending aorta. (B) HASTE pulse sequence (black blood sequence)—intramural haematoma has high signal intensity. (C) Gradient echo pulse sequence with inversion pulse following gadolinium injection. Intraluminal thrombus has low signal intensity and can be differentiated from the aortic wall. There is no flowing blood within the false lumen but enhancement of parts of the aortic wall (small white arrow).

such as computed tomography (CT) and transoesophageal echocardiography. Patient monitoring in the magnet is straightforward but 24-hour magnet availability with experienced operators may be problematic. The main feature of aortic dissection is the presence of an intraluminal intimal flap which is easily demonstrated using transverse cine CMR (➲Fig. 5.31). Gadolinium CMR angiography may provide additional information regarding branch vessel involvement. The presence of pericardial effusions and the function of the aortic valve can also be depicted and quantification of aortic regurgitation is possible using velocity mapping. In practice, CMR is mostly used for follow-up or in patients with chronic disease. This is because CMR is free from ionizing radiation, MR contrast agents are not nephrotoxic (nephrogenic systemic fibrosis only occurs in patients with severe renal failure), and serial measurements

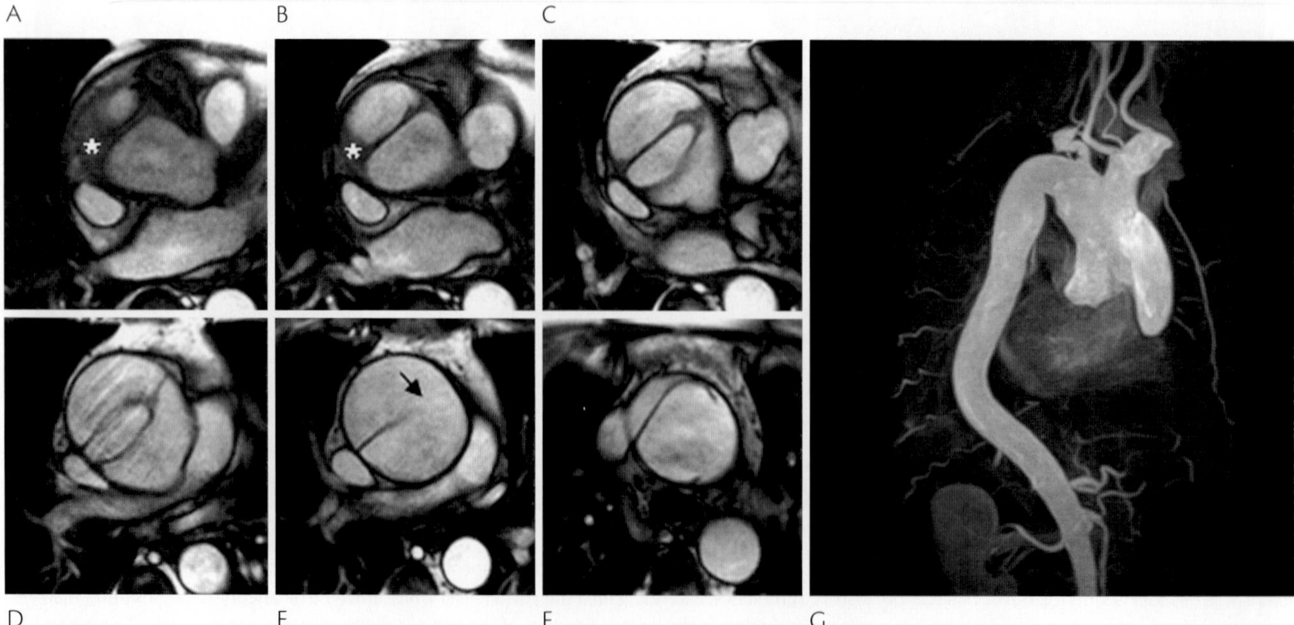

Figure 5.31 Patient with chronic aortic dissection and a complex dissecting membrane. Transverse cine images (A)–(E) show the aortic root from caudal to cranial. There is some thrombus (*) in the false lumen. The true lumen is surrounded by two compartments of false lumen. There is a large entry (small black arrow) in (E). The three-dimensional angiogram (G) does not reveal the internal geometry of the dissection.

at pre-defined landmarks are more reliably performed than from transoesophageal echocardiography.

Intramural haematoma is characterized by the presence of a false lumen without blood flow. The likely mechanism is intramural haemorrhage resulting from leaking vasa vasorum. Black-blood pulse sequences such as spin-echo sequences with T1 weighting are especially useful for depicting the bright crescentic thickening of the aortic wall (➲Fig. 5.32). Another acute aortic syndrome is the penetrating aortic ulcer which occurs predominantly in the elderly with diffuse and severe forms of atherosclerosis but may also be associated with bacterial infection (➲Fig. 5.33). Atherosclerotic ulcers can lead to large aneurysms which may need placement of endovascular stent-grafts. Such ulcers can be distinguished from small and benign ulcers by using both black-blood CMR and angiography.

CMR is also useful for depicting the pulmonary vasculature and may be a useful adjunct to functional CMR of right heart abnormalities. However, pulmonary MR angiography still requires relatively long breath-holds which may not always be possible especially in this patient population. Nevertheless, in patients with contraindications to iodinated contrast agents, CMR detects and excludes pulmonary emboli with good sensitivity and specificity [137]. In most other patients, CT remains the technique of choice for this clinical question.

Pericardium (also see ➲Chapter 19)

CMR is able to depict the pericardium and the pericardial space with high spatial resolution. It is thus clinically helpful in patients with suspected pericardial disease in whom echocardiography may provide suboptimal image quality. Moreover, pericardial thickness can be accurately determined which may be difficult with echocardiography. When compared to CT, CMR has the disadvantage of a longer examination time and inferior image quality in very

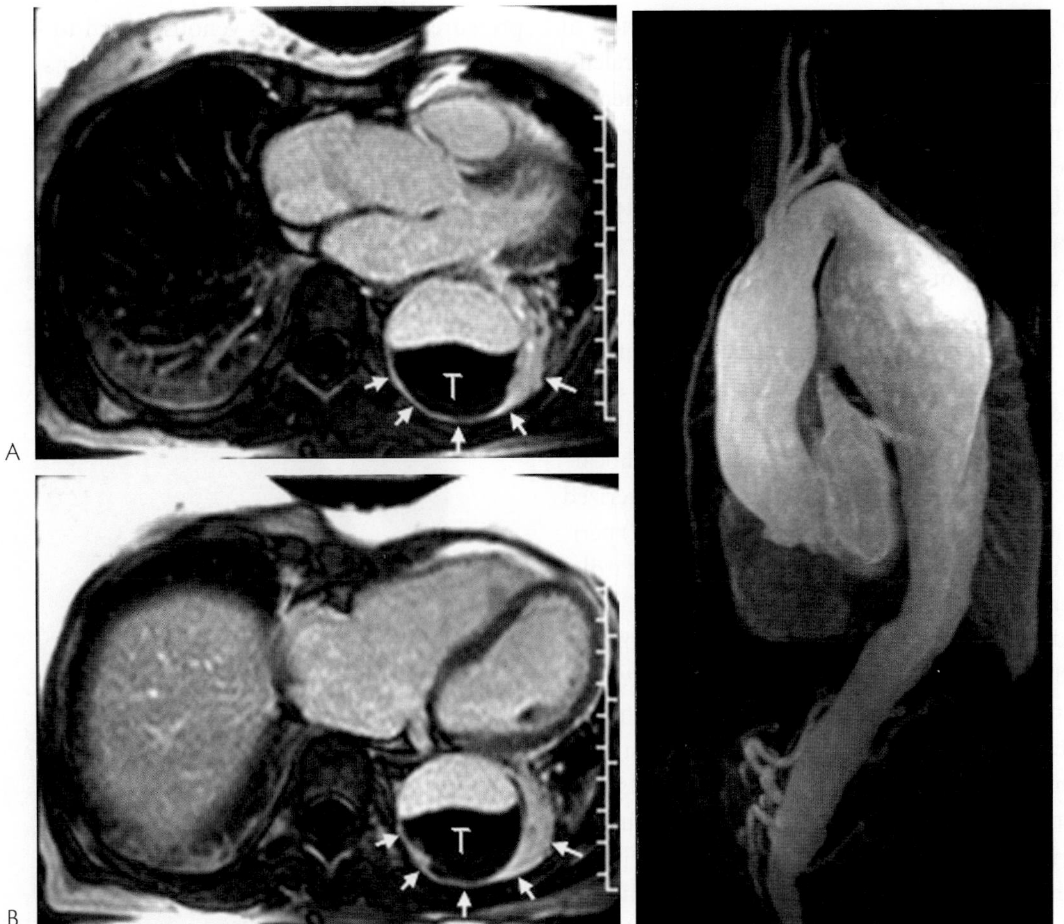

Figure 5.32 Aortic pathology in a 64-year-old woman with giant cell arteritis. (A) and (B) Transverse sections of the thorax. There is extensive thrombus (T) in the descending aorta well depicted on these CMR images taken 10min after gadolinium injection, with optimization to null thrombus not myocardium. The wall of the aorta enhances (small arrows) as a sign of ongoing aortitis. (C) The three-dimensional MR aortogram shows the extent of aneurismal dilatation but is not helpful to identify details of the underlying pathology.

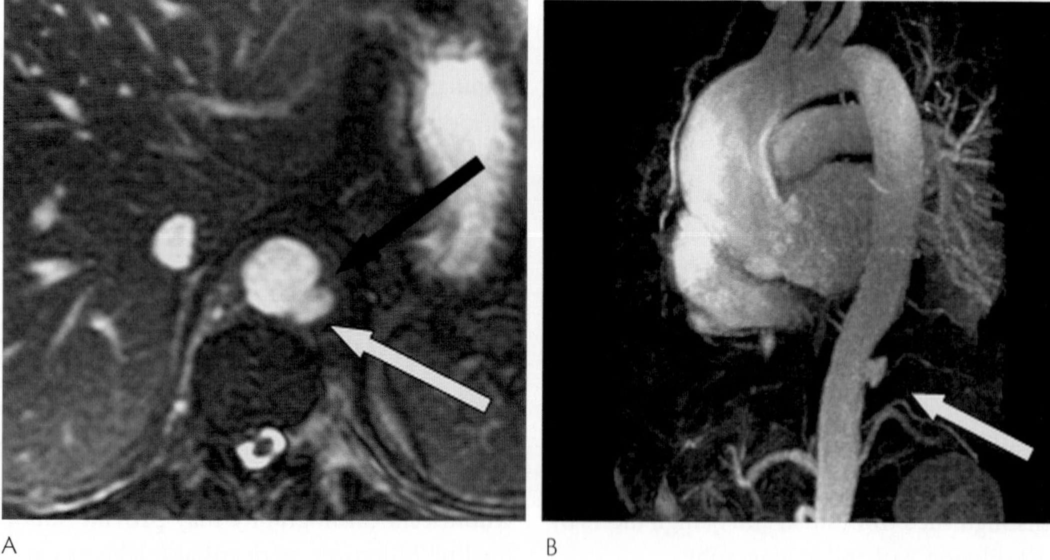

Figure 5.33 Penetrating aortic ulcer near the thoracoabdominal junction. Clinical presentation of the patient was with abdominal pain and fever. Blood culture showed *Salmonella* spp. White arrows: lumen of the ulcer. Black arrow on surrounding haematoma. (A) SSFP pulse sequence, transverse section. (B) Three-dimensional MR angiography.

sick patients who have poorly controlled atrial fibrillation or are unable to hold their breath for a longer period of time. CMR is also inferior in depicting pericardial calcification. However, CMR provides a functional assessment of the abnormalities associated with pericardial disease and this may make CMR the preferred technique in difficult cases.

As pericardial fluid is depicted as a high signal intensity space between the epicardium and the fibrous pericardium, even small quantities of pericardial fluid can be reliably detected. This may be important in patients with infectious pericarditis and myocarditis with pericardial involvement. Although systematic comparisons are lacking, the sensitivity and the confidence for detecting especially inferior localized effusions may be better for CMR than for echocardiography. Acute pericardial inflammation is characterized by both early and LGE (➲Fig. 5.34) of the (thickened) pericardium. Similar to the situation in chronic myocardial infarction, pericardial scar will show LGE only.

In order to distinguish between restrictive cardiomyopathy (➲Chapter 18) and constrictive pericarditis (➲Chapter 19), reliable measurements of pericardial thickness are important. CMR is highly accurate in distinguishing between these two clinical entities, although it is limited in patients who develop constrictive pericarditis following cardiac surgery when the pericardium may have normal thickness [138]. Another helpful feature to distinguish restrictive cardiomyopathy from constrictive pericarditis is that CMR identifies amyloid heart disease—one of the most common causes of restrictive cardiomyopathy. A useful technique to differentiate constriction from restriction is real-time in the short-axis plane, during respiration. Inspiration lowers intrathoracic pressure which increases venous return to the RV, and in constriction this causes the interventricular septum to bulge into the LV. CMR is also helpful to identify pericardial cysts (➲Fig. 5.35) and distinguish them from other tumours. It is also possible to identify a rare pericardial abnormality,

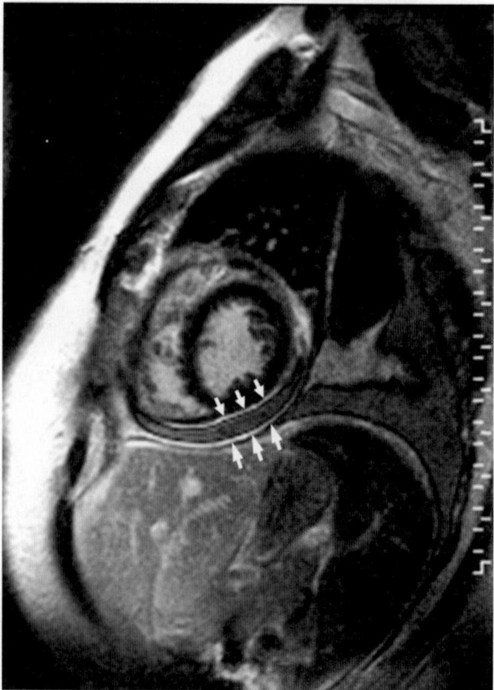

Figure 5.34 Patient with pericarditis of 3 weeks' duration and signs of right heart failure. There is partially organized fluid between the pericardial layers (white arrows) which enhance on this short-axis late gadolinium enhancement image.

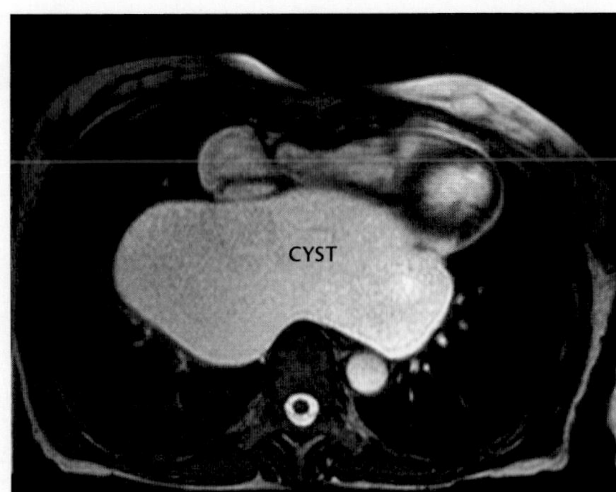

Figure 5.35 Unusual pericardial cyst. High signal intensity within the cavity in the cine images is indicative of fluid and further tissue differentiation is possible using T1- and T2-weighted pulse sequences (not shown). Fluid was drained using CT guidance.

absence of the pericardium, or partial absence of the pericardium, by the unusual position of the heart.

Tumours and masses

Intracardiac tumours (➲Chapter 20) and masses are relatively uncommon, and the clinical challenge is to determine whether surgical intervention or a conservative approach is required. Chest X-ray and echocardiography are the first-line imaging techniques to visualize cardiac tumours and masses, but CMR is useful to obtain more detailed information on the relation of the mass to the surrounding tissue and organs (extension, mobility, infiltration, vascular relation) and for tissue characterization, both of which can help to better plan treatment [139]. Simple visualization of a mass is usually done with the cine SSFP sequences. Important diagnostic features are whether the mass is well formed or irregular, if a stalk is present, whether single or multiple, and whether there is invasion of tissue planes (including transvenous extension). Tissue characterization requires T1- and T2-weighed spin-echo imaging, fat suppression, and gadolinium studies including first pass, early enhancement, and late enhancement for interpreting vascularity, necrosis, or thrombus formation, and fibrosis or expansion of the interstitial space. It is not uncommon for the mass to have a mixed composition including thrombus or a necrotic core. Together with the location of the tumour (right heart more malignant), its size, homogeneity, and extension in surrounding tissues (malignancy), the presence of pleural and pericardial effusion (malignant, metastatic), and tumour vascularity (benign tumours have low perfusion except for haemangiomas and myxomas) allows

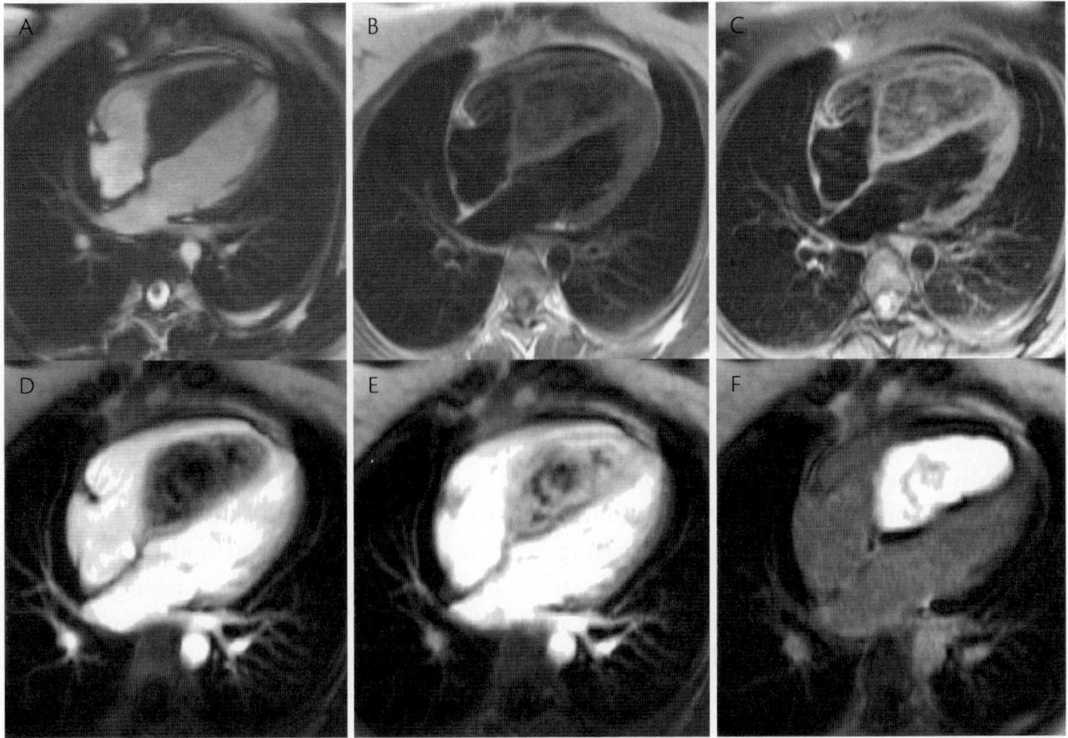

Figure 5.36 Myocardial fibroma in the interventricular septum. (A) Cine image showing very thick septum. (B) T1-weighted image showing low signal intensity of the mass. (C) T2-weighted image showing low signal intensity of the mass. (D) and (E) Perfusion images show relatively low perfusion to the mass. (F) Late gadolinium enhancement images show intense enhancement. These images show the typical signal characteristics of a fibroma.

for a good, but not perfect, characterization of the mass. Furthermore, the haemodynamic and functional effects of the tumour can be quantified, including any concurrent valvular disease or leaflet infiltration. Malignant tumours of the heart often have a characteristic panoply of diagnostic features.

Heart masses are more likely to be benign (75%) than malignant (25%), and thrombi should not be forgotten, particularly in the setting of infarction, arrhythmia, cardiomyopathy, and RV cannulae. Some normal variants also need to be recognized, including lipomatous atrial hypertrophy, false tendons, and an enlarged crista terminalis. The commonest benign tumours are myxoma and lipoma in adults, but in children a wider range of tumours is seen (fibroma, ➲Fig. 5.36; rhabdomyoma) sometimes associated with genetic syndromes (hamartoma in tuberous sclerosis). The commonest malignant tumours are metastases (e.g. melanoma) which are more common at post-mortem than usually thought, direct invasion (lung cancer), and primary tumours (angiosarcoma). Angiosarcoma is very well characterized by CMR because of intense perfusion, usually located in the anterior atrioventricular groove, with local pericardial extension, and central necrosis (➲Fig. 5.37).

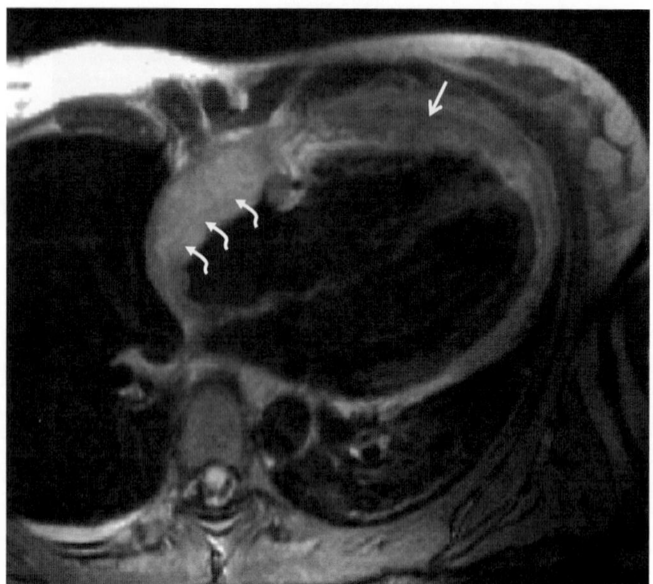

Figure 5.37 Angiosarcoma. T2-weighted four-chamber image showing a large mass around the anterior aspect of the right atrium and the anterior atrioventricular groove (curved arrows), which shows evidence of tumour infiltration of the right atrial wall. A pericardial effusion (straight arrow) is present.

Personal perspective

CMR has rapidly developed in recent years and now fulfils an indispensable role in major cardiac centres in the investigation and management of cardiovascular disease. Currently, the most frequent clinical referrals are in cardiomyopathy, arterial angiography (non-coronary), congenital heart disease, and the assessment of ischaemia, viability, and infarction. However, there are two other generic sources of clinical referral which come into the scope of 'unusual or uncertain cardiovascular pathologies', and 'suboptimal results from other imaging techniques'.

The role of CMR in cardiomyopathy has exploded in the last 5 years, as the ability to image myocardial interstitial abnormality in high resolution using LGE imaging, has become widely clinically appreciated. Pathologists now refer to this technique as 'in vivo pathology' as detail can now be seen in life which before could only be seen at post-mortem. Myocardial fibrosis is the end pathway of a number of pathologies, but the pattern of distribution is telling. In addition, there is growing evidence of the link between the presence and extent of fibrosis and future clinical events, and careful studies in this area may lead to significant changes in clinical practice in coming years.

The role of CMR in CAD is also expanding but more slowly. This is due to three main reasons: conventional techniques are well entrenched clinically; there is limited availability of dedicated CMR scanners, CMR expertise, and appropriate reimbursement; and publication of larger multicentre clinical trials with outcomes analysis is needed. The exception, as noted earlier, is the use of LGE to identify infarction. This new high-resolution technique has made significant contributions to our understanding of infarction and viability because the circumferential and transmural extent of necrosis and scar can be imaged in vivo for the first time. Thus, not only is CMR now the most sensitive clinical method for detection of infarction—other than cardiac enzymes in the acute phase—but the presence of stunning and hibernation and therefore the likelihood of functional recovery can be directly determined. This technique has shown fascinating results in the identification of unidentified infarction in the elderly population, with a strong association between such infarcts and future cardiac events. In CAD, the next area for significant clinical application by CMR is perfusion imaging. The advantages include high resolution, lack of radiation burden, quantitative analysis of perfusion, and a fast procedure time for the patient (approximately 30min). The optimal imaging sequence and clinical protocol needs to be finalized but will come in the near future.

The future for CMR is bright, because no other technology offers a comparable combination of safety, high resolution, image quality, and versatility. The incorporation of CMR into cardiology training programmes recognizes the importance of this new technology for trainees and established cardiologists.

Further reading

Gerber BL, Raman SV, Nayak K, *et al.* Myocardial first-pass perfusion cardiovascular magnetic resonance: history, theory, and current state of the art. *J Cardiovasc Magn Reson* 2008; **10**: 18.

Hendel RC, Patel MR, Kramer CM, *et al.* ACCF/ACR/SCCT/SCMR/ASNC/NASCI/SCAI/SIR 2006 appropriateness criteria for cardiac computed tomography and cardiac magnetic resonance imaging: a report of the American College of Cardiology Foundation Quality Strategic Directions Committee Appropriateness Criteria Working Group, American College of Radiology, Society of Cardiovascular Computed Tomography, Society for Cardiovascular Magnetic Resonance, American Society of Nuclear Cardiology, North American Society for Cardiac Imaging, Society for Cardiovascular Angiography and Interventions, and Society of Interventional Radiology. *J Am Coll Cardiol* 2006; **48**: 1475–97.

Kim RJ, Wu E, Rafael A, *et al.* The use of contrast-enhanced magnetic resonance imaging to identify reversible myocardial dysfunction. *N Engl J Med* 2000; **343**: 1445–53.

Kim RJ, de Roos A, Fleck E, Higgins CB, Pohost GM, Prince M, Manning WJ; Society for Cardiovascular Magnetic Resonance (SCMR) Clinical Practice Committee. Guidelines for training in cardiovascular magnetic resonance (CMR). *J Cardiovasc Magn Reson* 2007; **9**: 3–4.

Kramer CM, Budoff MJ, Fayad ZA, *et al.* ACCF/AHA 2007 clinical competence statement on vascular imaging with computed tomography and magnetic resonance: a report of the American College of Cardiology Foundation/American Heart Association/American College of Physicians Task Force on Clinical Competence and Training: developed in collaboration with the Society of Atherosclerosis Imaging and Prevention, the Society for Cardiovascular Angiography and Interventions, the Society of Cardiovascular Computed Tomography, the Society for Cardiovascular Magnetic Resonance, and the Society for Vascular Medicine and Biology. *Circulation* 2007; **116**: 1318–35.

Manning WJ, Pennell DJ. *Cardiovascular magnetic resonance*, 2002. Philadelphia, PA: Churchill Livingstone.

Pennell DJ, Sechtem UP, Higgins CB, *et al.* Clinical indications for cardiovascular magnetic resonance (CMR): Consensus panel report. *Eur Heart J* 2004; **25**: 1940–65.

➲ For full references and multimedia materials please visit the online version of the book (http://esctextbook.oxfordonline.com).

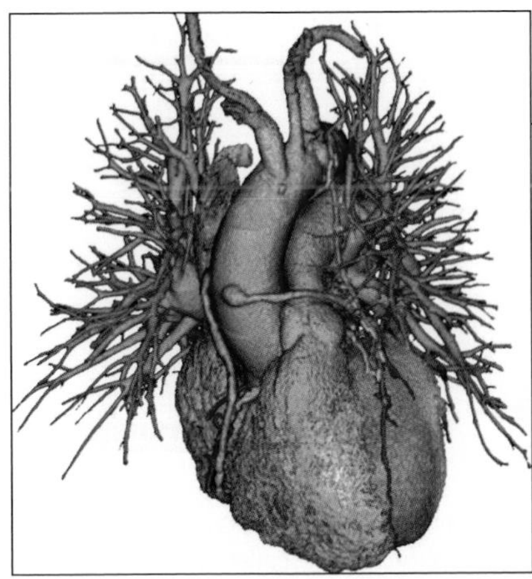

CHAPTER 6

Cardiovascular Computed Tomography

Pim J. de Feyter , Stephan Achenbach, and Koen Nieman

Contents

Summary

Non-contrast-enhanced computed tomography (CT) coronary calcium imaging is predictive of adverse coronary events, independently and beyond that of traditional risk factors, because calcium is a marker of the presence of coronary atherosclerosis.

Contrast-enhanced CT coronary angiography is a reliable non-invasive diagnostic modality to rule out the presence of significant obstructive coronary artery disease in patients with low-to-intermediate pretest risk of CAD and stable heart rhythm. CT-coronary imaging of non-obstructive atherosclerotic disease of the coronary wall offers the opportunity to evaluate early manifestations of coronary atherosclerosis. Severe coronary calcifications and irregular heart rhythm significantly limit the evaluation of CT-coronary images while the relatively high radiation exposure is of concern. CT imaging for pulmonary embolism and acute aortic dissection is highly accurate and may be considered the first-choice diagnostic option. CT imaging of great thoracic vessels, for cardiac function, heart valves, cardiac tumours and thrombi, or pericardial disease is feasible but the non-radiation diagnostic modalities echocardiography or cardiac magnetic resonance (CMR) imaging should be considered as first diagnostic options.

Introduction

The development of X-ray CT in the 1970s is considered one of the greatest advances in diagnostic imaging because of its ability to non-invasively image the internal structures in the body with unprecedented accuracy. No other modality allows scanning of large body regions with comparable spatial resolution and contrast within such a short scan time. The high spatial and tissue resolution of CT can be achieved because the collimated X-ray beam is transmitted selectively through a specific cross-section which minimizes superimposition of structures above and below a specific cross-section (slice) while this also reduces X-ray scatter and improves image contrast. Finally, CT makes use of refined detectors that can measure small differences in contrast resolution (to <0.1 per cent). In 1995, contrast-enhanced electron beam CT (EBCT) coronary angiography was first described [1] and in subsequent evaluations was demonstrated to permit non-invasive detection of haemodynamically relevant coronary artery stenoses with moderate reliability.

'Spiral' or 'helical' CT—which combines continuous rotation of the x-ray tube with continuous movement of the patient table along the z-axis—was introduced in the 1990s and, unlike EBCT, this technique has undergone such extremely rapid development that it has in the past few years emerged as a reliable, non-invasive cardiovascular imaging technique.

Basics of computed tomography

CT is an imaging modality that uses roentgen to create cross-sectional images. Photons are emitted by the roentgen tube and collimated into a fan or cone-shaped beam to pass from one side of the gantry through an object within the gantry (➲Fig. 6.1).

After partial absorption and dispersion, the remaining photons are collected and quantified by detectors on the opposite side of the scanner (➲Fig. 6.2). The attenuation profile produced by the combined detectors is a result of the summed attenuation by the tissues. By collecting a large number of attenuation profiles from different rotational angles the regional contribution to the roentgen attenuation throughout a cross-sectional plane can be calculated. The minimal number of profiles required to perform this computation are acquired over a 180°-rotation of the roentgen tube and detectors. From the attenuation measurements

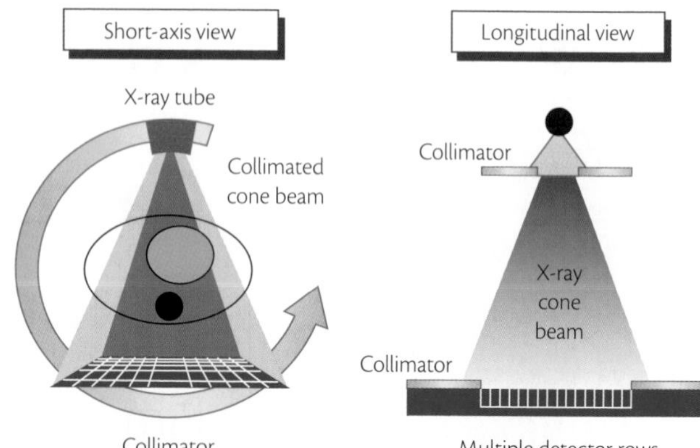

Figure 6.1 MDCT scanner geometry. The rotating X-ray tube produces a collimated cone beam, which passes through the patient within the gantry. Attenuated X-rays are collected by multiple rows of detectors.

CT numbers, expressed in Hounsfield units (HU), can be calculated:

$$\text{CT number (HU)} = \frac{\mu_{tissue} - \mu_{water}}{\mu_{water}} \times 1000$$

where μ_{tissue} represents the attenuation value of tissue and μ_{water} the attenuation value of water. By definition, water has a CT number of 0HU, air (absent attenuation) has a

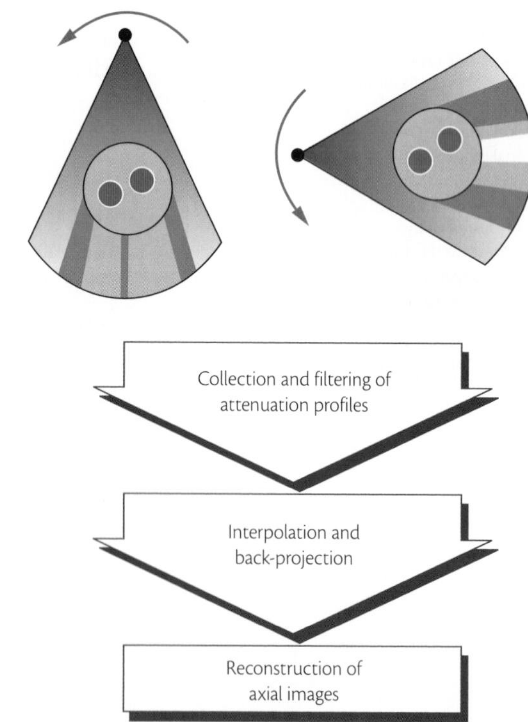

Figure 6.2 Principle of CT. Multiple attenuation profiles from different angles are acquired during a 180°-rotation of the X-ray tube and detector system. In case of spiral CT, the projection profiles are interpolated in the longitudinal axis, to create complete data sets (profiles) at each plane position. Using back-projection reconstruction algorithms, axial images are created from the interpolated projection profiles.

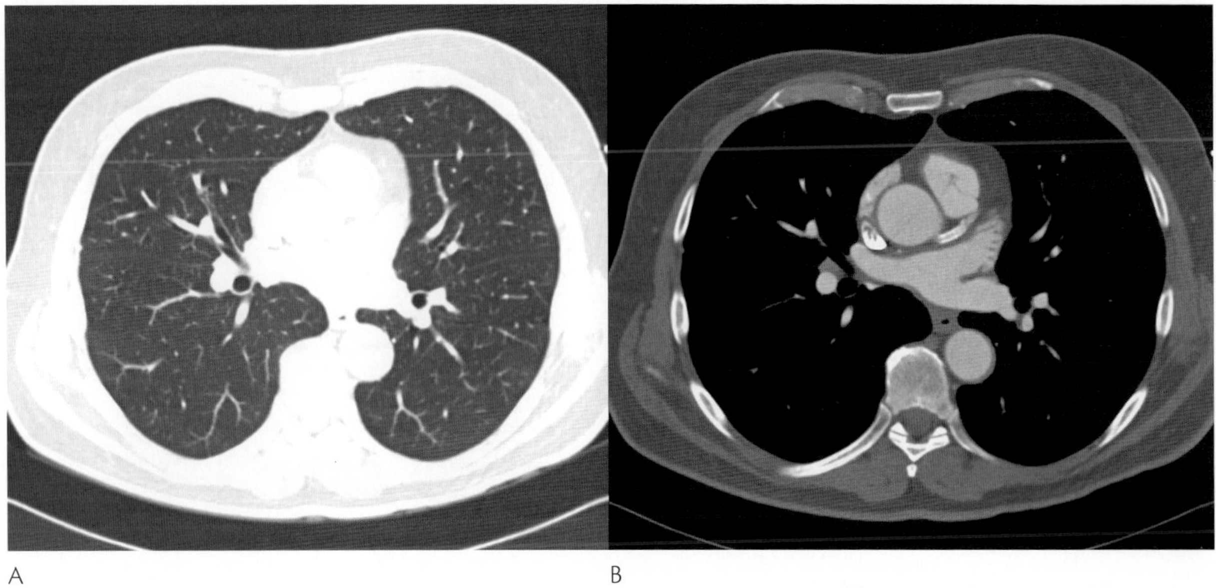

Figure 6.3 Axial CT image of the chest. Axial images of the thorax at the level of the origin of the left main coronary artery. The same image is displayed using a 'lung' window (used for evaluation of lung parenchyma, left panel) and a 'cardiac' window (used for evaluation of cardiac structures, right panel). The image is displayed as if looking from the patient's feet upwards.

CT number of –1000 HU. Bone as well as metal (highly attenuating) have CT numbers >1000HU and will generally be displayed as white; tissues with low attenuation, such as air and lungs as black. Soft tissues have CT values up to 150HU; fat tissue has CT numbers below 0. Contrast-enhanced blood should have a CT number between 200–500HU. Within a matrix of predefined size (512 × 512 or 1024 × 1024) each image element (pixel) represents the average attenuation at that location, which can be displayed using a grey scale. Because the human eye can only differentiate a limited number of shades of grey, the window settings can be selected to display and differentiate the structures of interest (➲Fig. 6.3).

Cardiac computed tomography

ECG-synchronization

Imaging of the small, tortuous, and continuously moving coronary arteries challenges the technical boundaries of current CT technology. Images need to be acquired fast enough to freeze coronary motion, while the entire scan needs to be performed within the time of a comfortable breath-hold. High spatial resolution is needed to detect and semi-quantify obstructive coronary artery disease. Contrast, by intravenous injection of X-ray contrast medium, needs to be created between the blood and the surrounding tissues, which would otherwise have similar attenuation characteristics.

The longitudinal range of current 64-slice CT systems is insufficient to scan the entire heart at once. Therefore CT data need to be acquired over several heart cycles. To obtain phase-consistent images the acquisition of data or the reconstruction of images needs to be synchronized to the heart rhythm. Basically there are two ways to scan the beating heart. Using the ECG-triggered, sequential mode (step-and-shoot mode), scanning is triggered by the ECG, with timing based on the previous heart cycles during a preselected and expectedly motion-sparse phase of the heart cycle (➲Fig. 6.4). After image acquisition the table is moved to the next position for the next scan. ECG-gated spiral CT combines continuous table movement with continuous data acquisition (➲Fig. 6.5). Based on the simultaneously recorded ECG, images are reconstructed using phase-consistent spiral CT data (➲Fig. 6.6). Because of the ability to reconstruct

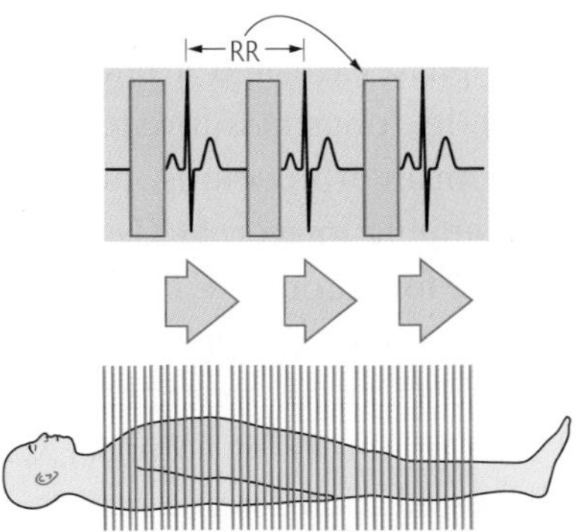

Figure 6.4 Prospectively ECG-triggered sequential CT acquisition mode. Scanning takes place while the table remains stationary. The acquisition is triggered by the ECG. Timing of the acquisition can be selected by the operator, and is based on the length of the previous heart cycles when a relative delay (as a percentage of the R-to-R interval) is used. The patient is moved incrementally between successive acquisitions.

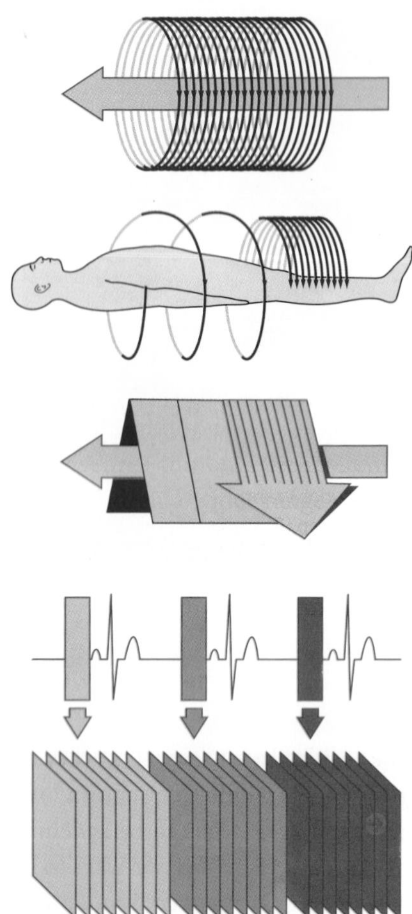

Figure 6.5 ECG-gated spiral CT acquisition mode. Uninterrupted propagation of the patient on the table through the gantry during continuous scanning creates a helical or spiral-shaped tube-detector trajectory from the patient's perspective. Conventional spiral scan protocols perform continuous, overlapped scanning that allows image reconstruction during any cardiac phase. Using the recorded ECG, isocardiophasic raw spiral CT data is extracted for reconstruction of axial images during a specific cardiac phase. Contrary to sequential CT, these images can be reconstructed at an arbitrary (overlapping) increment, improving the longitudinal image quality.

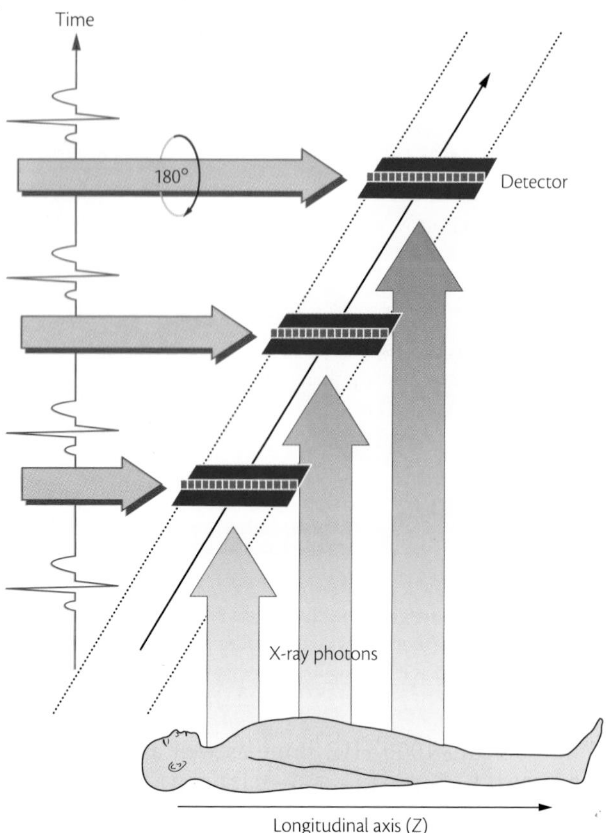

Figure 6.6 ECG-gated spiral CT data acquisition. Graph depicting the longitudinal position (x-axis) of the detector unit in time (and ECG, y-axis). While data is acquired more or less continuously, only data acquired during a selectable interval (≈150–200ms, while the tube-detector unit completes a 180°-rotation) is used for reconstruction of a CT coronary angiogram. The longitudinal position of the detectors needs to overlap between consecutive heart cycles to guarantee availability of data at any plane position during any cardiac phase. This requires slow table propagation, overlapping sampling and results in a considerable radiation exposure. Because the longitudinal position of the detectors changes, also during the short reconstruction interval, some form of data interpolation is necessary to reconstruct axial slices.

different cardiac phases (to find a phase with minimal motion artefacts), its robustness towards rhythm irregularities or ECG misinterpretations, and the ability to reconstruct overlapping images, ECG-gated spiral CT is the preferred mode for coronary CT. The consequence of continuous data acquisition during spiral CT is a relatively high radiation dose which has generated renewed interest in sequential scan protocols for coronary CTA, that are associated with less radiation dose.

Images acquired or reconstructed during the relatively motion-sparse phase of mid diastole are generally least affected by motion artefacts. End-systolic images may be useful in patients with a fast or irregular heart rate, particularly to assess the right coronary artery.

Technical scanner performance

Current state-of-the-art multidetector CT (MDCT) scanners are able to simultaneously acquire 64 channels of data, which has significantly shortened the scan time, and the breath-hold, to 10s or less. CT systems with as many as 320 detectors have become available, which can scan the entire heart without the need for table movement during the scan.

Contrast between the blood and the vessel wall and other surrounding tissue is achieved by intravenous injection of a high-attenuating iodine-based contrast medium. To time the scan with contrast enhancement either a test bolus injection can be performed to determine the contrast transit time, or the scan can be triggered after starting the bolus injection by contrast enhancement in the aorta using a monitor

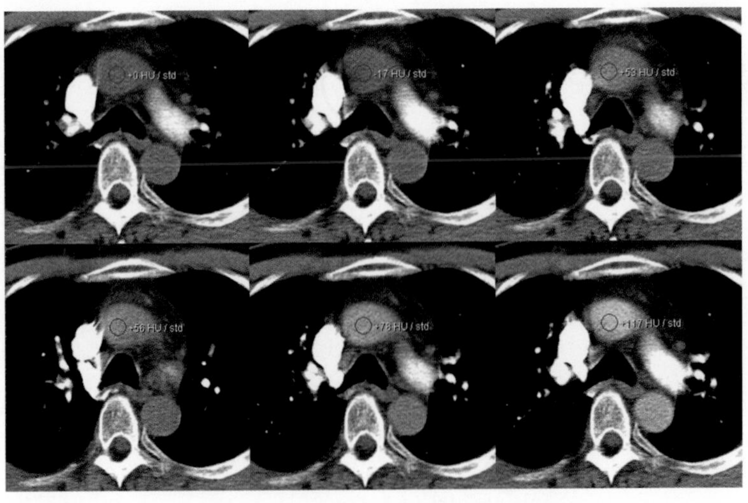

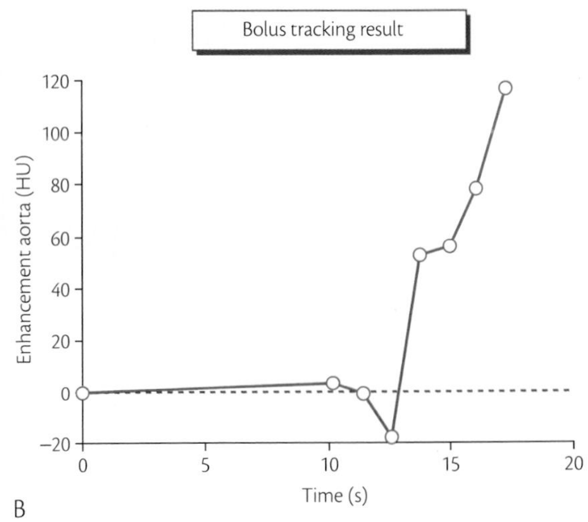

A B

Figure 6.7 Contrast bolus tracking. Scanning can be synchronized to contrast-enhancement of the cardiac vasculature using a bolus tracking technique. After injection of contrast, axial images are acquired at a regular interval at the level of the ascending aorta. Arrival of contrast (enhancement) is measured using a so-called *region of interest* placed within the aorta. After a preset threshold (e.g. a 100HU attenuation increment) has been reached the scan sequence, including table positioning and breath-hold command, is automatically initiated.

scan (➲Fig. 6.7). A saline bolus can be injected after the contrast to flush forward lingering contrast material.

To avoid motion blurring the temporal resolution, comparable to the shutter time of a photo camera, needs to be as short as possible. Using partial scan reconstruction algorithms the minimal amount of projections needed for image reconstruction are acquired during an approximately 180°-scanner rotation (➲Fig. 6.8). The rotation time of the scanner (330–420ms) therefore directly affects the temporal resolution (165–210ms). Dual-source CT scanners are equipped with two tube-detector combinations at an angle of 90°, enabling the scanner to acquire all projections during a 90°-, instead of a 180°-rotation. Multisegmental reconstruction algorithms combine data from consecutive heart cycles to improve the effective temporal resolution. Effectiveness is variable depending on the relation between the instant heart rate and the scanner rotation time and requires each section to be scanned during at least two heart cycles. In clinical practice, motion artefacts, which occur mostly in patients with a fast heart rate, are minimized by administration of beta-blockers, or other medication that slows the heart rate, before the CT scan.

The spatial resolution, or the ability to differentiate small structures, depends on many factors, including the CT hardware (focal spot size, gantry geometry, detector quality, and dimensions), the scan protocol, and reconstruction parameters, but is also affected by other aspects of image quality, including contrast enhancement, image noise, and motion artefacts. The width of the detector rows varies between 0.5–0.7mm, although often slightly thicker, but overlapping slices are reconstructed to reduce image noise. Under optimal conditions the spatial resolution of current CT technology is approximately 0.5mm in three dimensions. Smaller voxels (3-dimensional image elements) can be created without necessarily improving spatial resolution (optical versus digital zoom). The appearance of the images is further influenced by the filtering (kernels) used during reconstruction, resulting in smoother or sharper (but noisier) images.

Although the capabilities of current CT systems are impressive, one should not forget that despite its non-invasive advantages the spatial resolution, temporal resolution and contrast-to-noise of CT is still inferior to invasive, selective coronary angiography (➲Chapter 8).

Radiation and contrast media issues

CT is a roentgen-based technology and cannot be performed without exposing the patient to (potentially) harmful radiation; because of the equal distribution of radiation deterministic effects (skin erythema) are rare. Most relevant in cardiac CT are stochastic effects, where cell modification could result in cancer or genetic effects. These effects are dose related, arguably without a minimal threshold.

The principle parameter of absorbed dose, i.e. the amount of energy absorbed per unit mass, is the CT dose index (CTDI), which can be measured by an ionization chamber along the z-axis during a single tube rotation. The weighted CTDI (CTDIw) can be calculated to account for

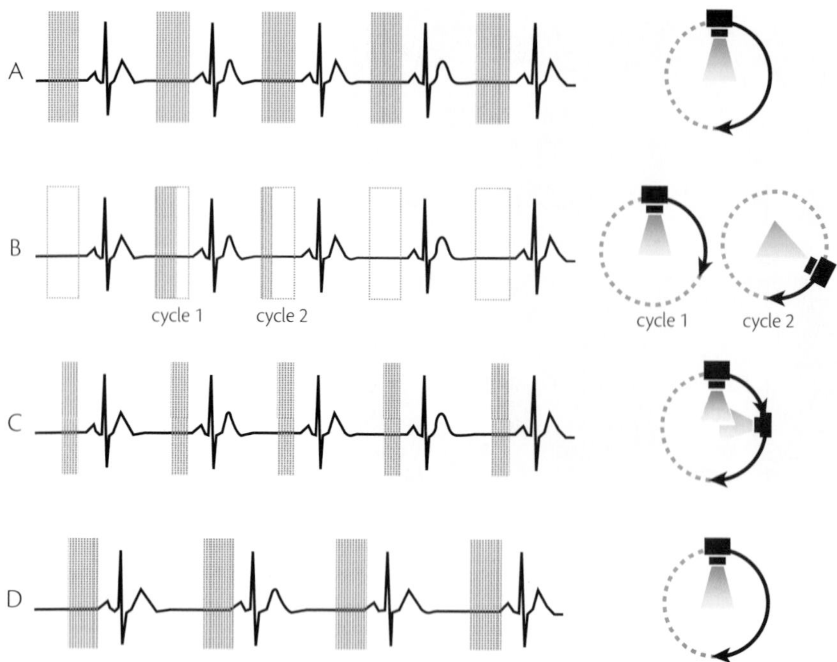

Figure 6.8 Temporal resolution and image reconstruction algorithms. Using partial scan algorithms, the required attenuation profiles to reconstruct an image are acquired during a (approximately) 180°-rotation. The temporal resolution (approximate exposure time) of the scanner is therefore directly affected by the rotation speed of the system (A). Multi-segmental reconstruction algorithms combine data from two or more heart cycles to reconstruct images with an improved (effective) temporal resolution (B). A 90° variation between the positions of the tube between two heart cycles will provide optimal effect and reduce the effective reconstruction window by half. An identical position or 180° variation between heart cycles will allow for no improvement of temporal resolution. The (two-segment) algorithm requires that each plane position is scanned during at least two heart cycles (instead of one), necessitating a fast heart rate or a slow table feed. Dual-source CT is equipped with two tube-detector units at a 90° angle (C). Instead of a 180°-rotation, only a 90°-rotation is needed, which improves the temporal resolution by a factor 2. Heart rate modulation (by beta blockers) prolongs the heart cycle and the mid-diastolic phase, which improves the relative temporal resolution (D).

non-homogeneous distribution of the CTDI within the body; the volume CTDI (CTDIvol) accounts for the fact that generally CT scans involve adjacent or overlapping acquisitions. To determine the radiation dose of an entire scan the dose-length product (DLP, mGy·cm) can be calculated by multiplying the $CTDI_{vol}$ by the scan length. The damage or risk of a CT scan depends on the susceptibility of the organs or body region exposed to the X-ray. The effective dose (E, mSv) reflects the risk of harm of a given dose to a specific body region, and can be calculated by multiplying the DLP by a conversion coefficient (*k*), representing that specific body region. For thoracic CT:

$$E\ (\text{mSv}) = 0.017 \times \text{DLP}$$

ECG-gated spiral CT is associated with a relative high radiation dose, the result of overlapped scanning to guarantee availability of CT data throughout the cardiac cycle [2]. Additionally, the thin detector collimation and fast scanner rotation require a high photon flux to avoid excessive image noise. Concerns about the potential adverse effects of cardiac CT have motivated manufacturers and operators to reduce the radiation dose, preferably without compromised diagnostic performance. Technical innovations to reduce dose include ECG-triggered tube output modulation for spiral CT protocols (➲Fig. 6.9), automatic adaptation of the tube output based on anatomy and overall attenuation, heart rate dependent table advancement to avoid oversampling, as well as a reintroduction of ECG-triggered sequential CT scanning (➲Fig. 6.4). According to the ALARA principle (as low as reasonably possible) the operator has the obligation to strive for maximum diagnostic accuracy (not maximum aesthetic quality) at the lowest possible dose. Individualized dose-saving modifications of scan protocols include lowering tube voltage (100kV instead of 120kV) and tube current (mA) when the size of the patient allows it, and a tighter scan range to avoid redundant scanning above and below the heart. However, the most important first step remains confirmation that the test is needed and appropriate with consideration of alternative diagnostics.

With the development of more powerful CT systems the radiation dose of cardiac CT has gradually increased from <10mSv with 4-detector CT to 15–20mSv with 64-detector CT. With earlier mentioned measures the dose

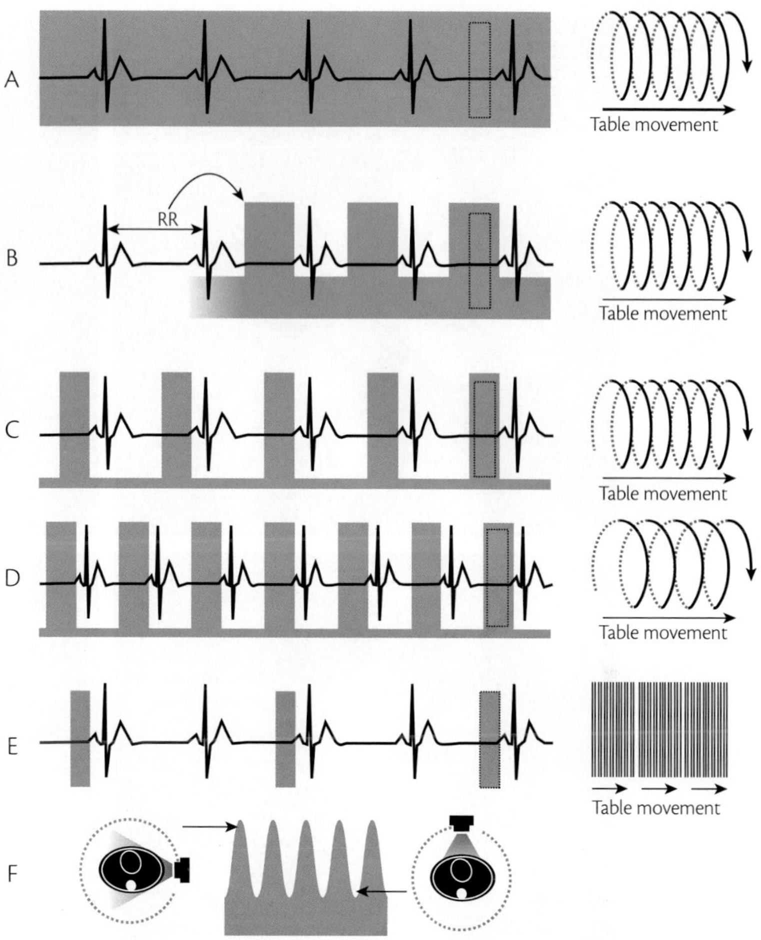

Figure 6.9 Dose-saving techniques. Conventional ECG-gated spiral CT protocols involved continuous scanning throughout the cardiac cycle resulting in a considerable radiation dose (A). Prospectively ECG-triggered roentgen tube modulation (ECG-pulsing) can be used to reduce the roentgen output during cardiac phases that are unlikely to contribute to angiographic image interpretation (B). Triggered by the ECG with timing based on previous heart cycles the tube current is turned to a low level (≈20%) that still allows for functional reconstructions of the cardiac cavities. The period of full exposure is wide enough to allow for reconstruction of different phases. By shortening the period of full exposure with further tube output reduction for the remainder additional dose saving can be accomplished (C). Systems with a variable table speed can increase the table speed (pitch) and reduce dose in patients with a faster heart rate (D). During ECG-triggered sequential CT scanning roentgen is only emitted during the acquisition of axial slices (E). Anatomy-based roentgen tube modulation allows for tube current variation based on the amount of tissue reflected in the global attenuation of the roentgen beam. This can be accomplished in an angular (in-plane) direction by reducing the current during anteroposterior acquisition, as opposed to acquisition in a lateral direction (F), as well as in a longitudinal direction.

can be lowered to 5–10mSv, depending on patient characteristics, namely size and heart rhythm [3], and available dose saving innovations on the CT system. ECG-triggered sequential imaging in selected patients can bring the radiation dose even below 5mSv [4]. For comparison, the yearly radiation exposure from natural sources varies between 2–4mSv depending on location. Radiation exposure during conventional angiography varies around 4–5mSv.

The use of contrast medium is associated with a low risk of contrast nephropathy and intolerance, but nevertheless CT investigations should be avoided in patients with renal dysfunction

Image evaluation

The result of the reconstruction process is a large stack of overlapping slices (>200), representing the contrast-enhanced heart and coronary arteries during a specific cardiac phase (➲Fig. 6.10; 6.1), which are considered the source images and the basis for all further assessments. However, to facilitate evaluation of this large amount of data various 2-dimensional and 3-dimensional image reconstruction and post-processing applications have been developed, including multiplanar reformation (MPR), maximum intensity projection (MIP), and volume rendering (VR) (➲Fig. 6.11; 6.2). Maximum-intensity projections, which display the highest densities within a thin slab allow assessment of longer vessel segments and are particularly useful to evaluate side branches. Three-dimensional reconstructions are attractive means to present and communicate findings, but are generally not used for initial assessment of the CT angiogram, particularly in the presence of calcifications and stents. The diagnostic advantage of these advanced image reconstruction techniques over evaluation of the axial source images has not been shown, and suspected lesions on 2- or 3-dimensional image reconstructions will require confirmation on the original source images (➲Fig. 6.12).

Stenosis severity can be graded semi-quantitatively, for example as occluded, severe (70–99%), moderate (50–70%), and mild (<50%). Stenosis can also be quantified using (semi-) automated software, although correlation between quantitative CT and quantitative angiography is variable in non-selected populations.

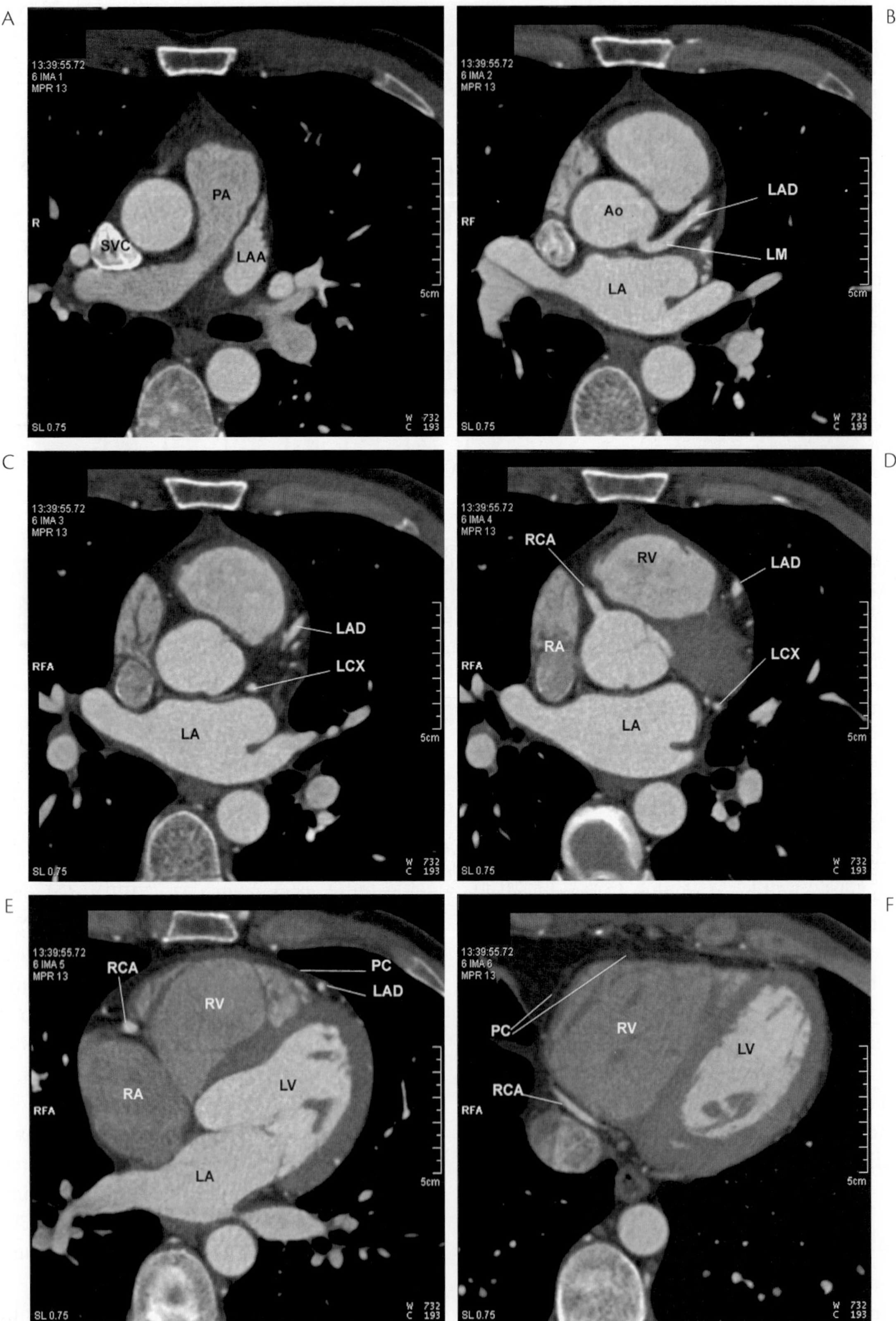

Figure 6.10 Cross-sectional CT anatomy of the heart. Typical axial images of the heart acquired by contrast-enhanced MDCT. From a set of 250, six axial images were selected to demonstrate typical cardiac anatomy on CT (A–F). CT images are displayed as if looking from below. The right side is indicated (R), the sternum is in the top of the image. Ao, ascending aorta; CS, coronary sinus; LA, left atrium; LAA, left atrial appendage; LAD, left anterior descending coronary artery; LCX, left circumflex coronary artery; LM, left main coronary artery; LV, left ventricle; PA, pulmonary artery; PC, pericardium; RA, right atrium; RCA, right coronary artery; RV, right ventricle. Also see 6.1

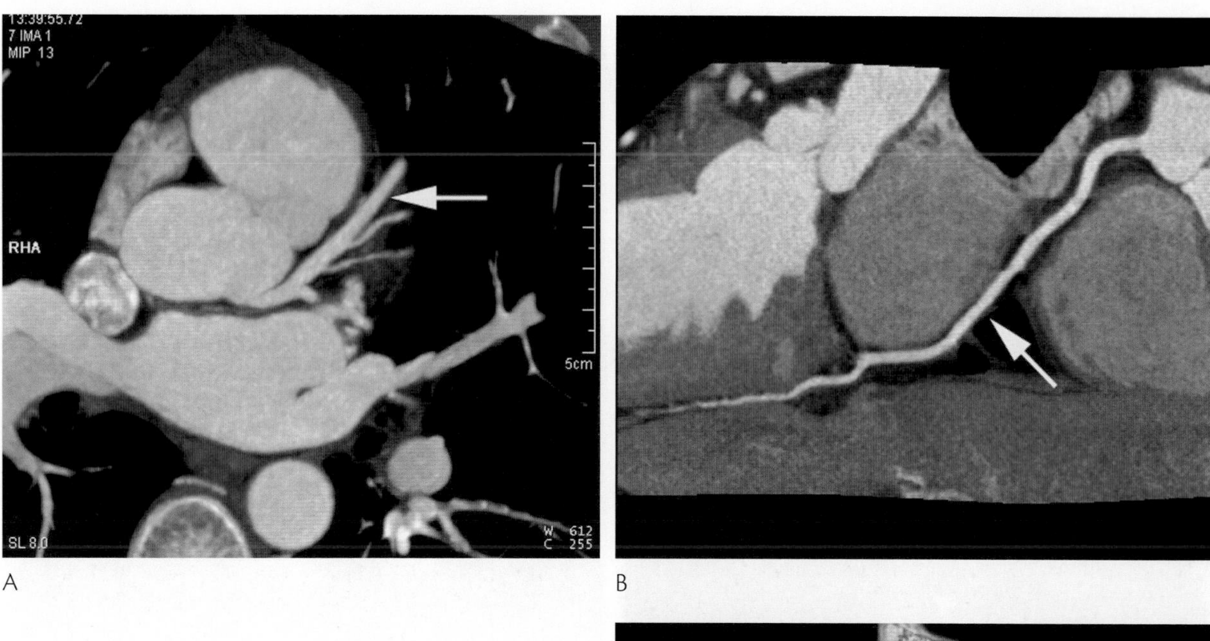

A

B

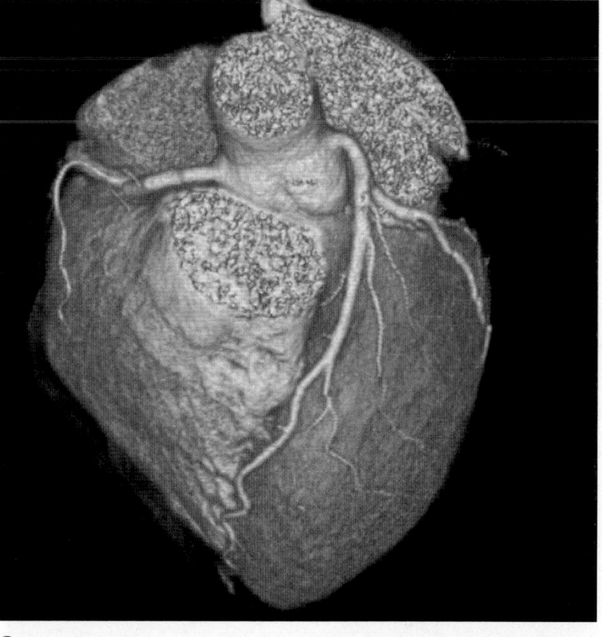

C

Figure 6.11 Secondary image reconstruction and postprocessing. Secondary reconstruction techniques to display the same MDCT data set as in Fig. 6.10. (A) Thin-slab maximum intensity projection (MIP) at the same level as 4.8, panel B. Within an 8-mm slab only the highest CT-numbers (generally contrast-enhanced blood, or metal and calcifications) are displayed which allows for evaluation of longer vessel segments and small side branches. MIP is less suited for severely calcified vessels or stents. Also see 6.2. (B) Curved reconstructions following the course of a vessel can display an entire coronary branch in a single plane, in this case the right coronary artery. (C) 3-D volume rendered reconstruction of the heart and coronary arteries (superior, left anterior-oblique view) provides an overview of coronary anatomy and its relation to cardiac anatomy (➲ Fig. 6.10).

Clinical applications of cardiac computed tomography

Coronary artery calcification

CT is a highly sensitive, non-invasive diagnostic modality to determine the presence of coronary calcium, because calcium has a high X-ray attenuation value (high CT number). Tissue within the vessel wall with a CT number of 130HU or more is defined as calcified (➲ Fig. 6.13).

Initially, calcium detection had been performed with EBCT using a non-enhanced, ECG-triggered sequential CT technique [5]. Recently MDCT has emerged as an alternative modality. The traditional method to quantify coronary calcification is the 'Agatston score' [5]. The Agatston score is derived from the area of a calcified lesion and the maximum CT attenuation within that lesion. Alternative quantification methods include assessment of the calcified volume (e.g. in mm^3) and of the mass of calcium (e.g. in mg) [6, 7]. In spite of potential advantages of these newer quantification methods, especially with regards to variability and independence from scanner type, no clinical studies of significant size have used these latter algorithms and all published studies demonstrating the predictive value of calcium are based on the Agatston score.

The presence of coronary calcium is invariably associated to coronary atherosclerosis and the amount of coronary

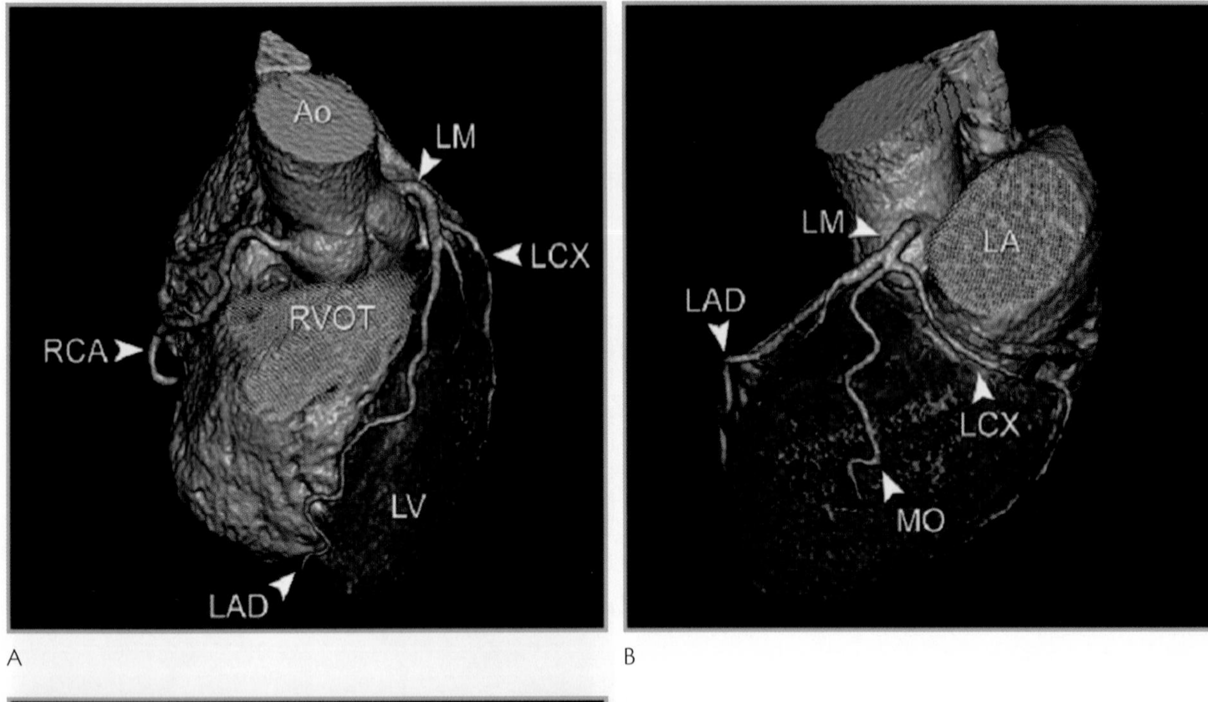

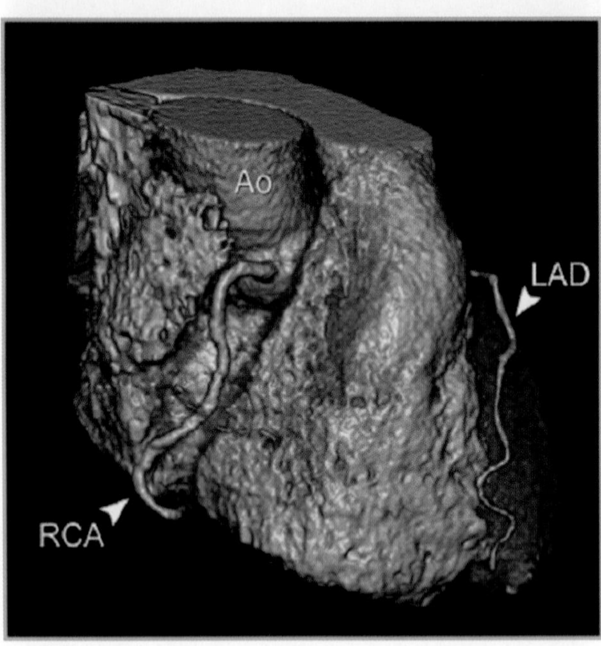

Figure 6.12 3-D volume rendered reconstruction. (A) Superior left-anterior view showing the left and right coronary artery. (B) Left lateral view showing the left coronary artery. (C) Right lateral view of the right coronary artery. Ao, aorta; LA, left atrium; LAD, left anterior descending; LCX, left circumflex; LM, left main; LV, left ventricle; MO, marginal obtuse branch; RCA, right coronary artery; RVOT, right ventricular outflow tract.

calcium correlates to the histological 'total coronary plaque burden' [8]. A high coronary calcium score, in particular when adjusted for age and gender, is predictive of coronary adverse events, independent and beyond the predictive value of traditional risk factors in men and women who are white, black, Hispanic, or Chinese (➲Tables 6.1 and 6.2) [9–12]. The absence of coronary calcium virtually rules out the presence of coronary atherosclerosis and is associated with a very low risk of adverse coronary events. However in younger patients a non-calcified plaque may be related to acute chest pain (➲Table 6.3).

Coronary calcium scanning cannot be recommended as a screening method for the unselected general population, but may play a role in selected individuals at intermediate risk of coronary events where a high calcium score may promote these individuals to a high risk group in need of a more aggressive risk-factor modification [10].

Assessment of coronary stenoses

The rapid evolution of scanner technology from 4-slice technology around the year 2000 to 64-slice CT (which was

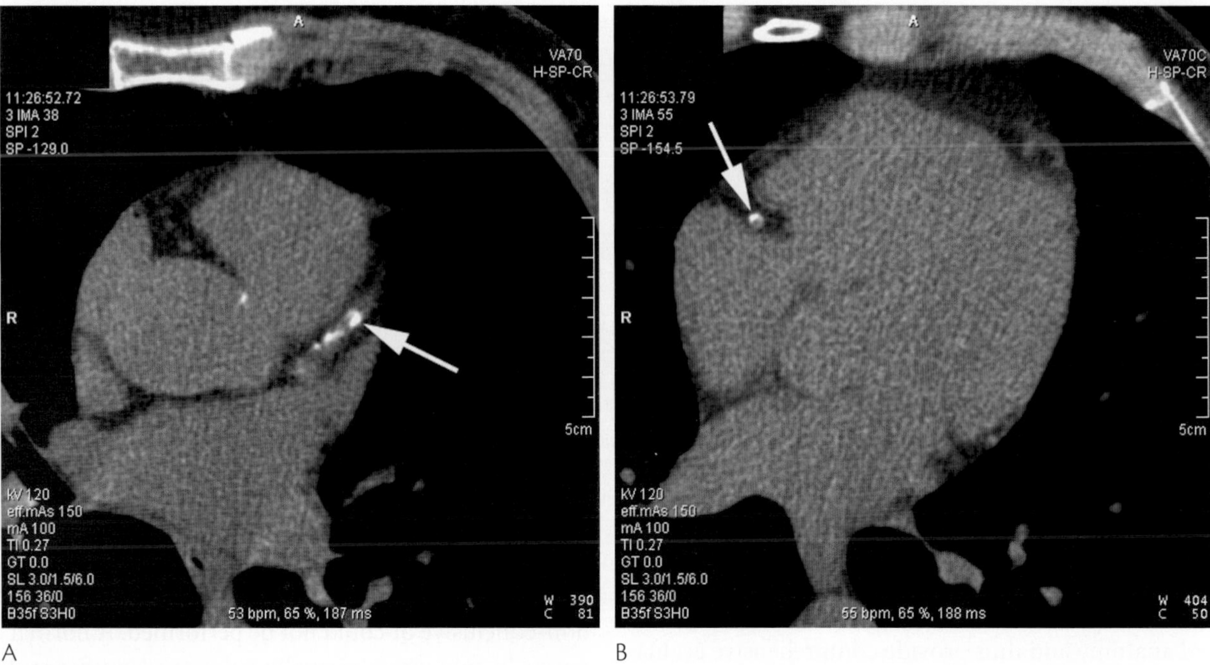

Figure 6.13 Visualization of coronary calcification by CT. Non-contrast enhanced MDCT scan (16 × 0.75mm collimation, 370ms rotation, retrospective ECG gating) to visualize coronary calcifications. (A) Calcification of the proximal left anterior descending artery (arrow). (B) Calcification of the mid right coronary artery (arrow).

introduced in the year 2005) brought about a substantial increase in image quality and accuracy of visualizing the coronary arteries and detecting coronary artery stenoses (➲Figs. 6.14, 6.15, and 6.16). Sixty-four-slice CT currently is considered to be the 'technology standard' for CT coronary angiography [13–19]. The diagnostic performance is presented in ➲Table 6.4. Several factors substantially impact on image quality—and diagnostic accuracy—of coronary CT angiography with 64-slice CT systems. High body weight can lead to excessive image noise and severe coronary calcification can render the arteries unevaluable due to partial volume effects and blooming artefacts. High heart rates are often associated with impaired image quality and to achieve sufficient image quality, the heart rate should be <65bpm [14]. Newer technology, such as the Dual Source CT systems which have higher temporal resolution are less affected by heart rate (➲Table 6.4) [15–19]. Larger studies allowing more detailed analyses better illustrate the diagnostic capabilities of coronary CT angiography in the setting of suspected coronary artery disease. Meijboom *et al.* demonstrated that coronary CT angiography performs best in patients with a low-to-intermediate clinical likelihood of coronary artery stenoses, while accuracy is substantially lower in high-risk patients most likely due to the more challenging conditions for imaging (➲Table 6.5) [20]. Two multi-centre trials of patients with suspected coronary artery stenoses studied by 64-slice CT confirmed the high sensitivity and very high negative predictive value (99%) of coronary CT angiography to identify patients with at least one significant coronary artery stenosis (94%) [21, 22]. However, specificity was only 48% to 83%, indicating a tendency of coronary angiography to overestimate stenosis severity, which in very low risk patient groups, may lead to an unacceptable number of false-positive diagnoses. Furthermore, comparisons between coronary CT angiography, invasive angiography, and stress perfusion imaging have demonstrated that CT allows to rule out coronary stenoses and myocardial ischaemia very reliably, but even

Table 6.1 Value of calcium score to predict death or myocardial infarction or all-cause mortality

	N	Mean age	F-up years	Comparator calcium score	Calcium score	RRR	Event
Shaw [9]	10,377	53 v ± 0.1	5	<10	>10	≈4.0	All-cause mortality
Greenland [10]	30,854	wide range	3-5	0 to <10	>10	4.3	Cardiac death or MI
Budoff [11]	25,253	56 ± 11	7	0	>0	1.7	All-cause mortality

RRR = relative risk ratio

Table 6.2 Predictive value of calcium score: number of subjects 25,253; age 56 ± 11; F-up 6.8 years; all-cause deaths 510 (2%)

Calc. score	N individuals (%)	RRR	Adjusted RR
0	11,064 (44)	–	–
1–10	3567 (14)	2.6	1.5
11–100	5033 (20)	6.7	3.6
101–400	3177 (13)	13	3.9
401–1000	1469 (6)	23	6.2
>1000	965 (4)	38	9.4

RRR, relative risk ratio
Adjusted RR: adjusted for risk factors and age

pronounced atherosclerotic changes and stenoses seen on CT do not reliably predict the presence of ischaemia as identified by perfusion imaging [23]. Recently hybrid single photon emission computed tomography (SPECT)-CT or PET-CT scanners permit the possibility to integrate function and anatomy and thus provide comprehensive evaluation of a coronary lesion.

It has been shown that a coronary CT angiogram negative for coronary artery stenoses allows the identification of individuals with a very favourable clinical outcome, with low rates of death and revascularization, even if stress testing suggested the presence of ischaemia [23–25].

Coronary CT angiography can safely and effectively rule out coronary artery stenoses in patients, with acute chest pain and low risk of CAD (negative enzymes and no ECG changes) and it has been demonstrated that the clinical course during 1 year follow-up of patients who are discharged based on a 'negative' coronary CT angiogram is benign [26–28].

Currently, no guidelines on the clinical application of coronary CT angiography in symptomatic patients exist. However, consensus is that coronary CT angiography is of clinical value to rule out coronary stenoses and avoid invasive coronary angiography in patients who are symptomatic, at low-intermediate risk of actually having coronary artery stenoses, in particular when a stress test was non-conclusive or could not be performed. A normal coronary CT angiogram virtually rules out significant disease of the epicardial coronary branches (➲Table 6.6). A positive CT-scan is moderately reliable and depending on the severity of chest pain, the extent of CAD (LM, 3VD), the amount of coronary calcification and presence of an intermediate lesion further downstream stress testing to assess the presence of objective ischaemia or direct referral to invasive coronary angiography is recommended. However, it is important to consider that only data sets of high image quality yield reliable diagnostic results. Coronary CT angiography should therefore only performed with adequate technology—currently state-of-the-art 64-slice CT—in experienced centres, with sufficient expertise to score the CT-scan, and in patients in whom good image quality can be expected [14, 29, 30]. Screening for coronary disease in asymptomatic patients is not recommended.

Table 6.3 Significance of coronary calcium

Absent	Present
Presence of atherosclerosis unlikely	Presence of atherosclerosis
Low likelihood of severe luminal narrowing	Higher amount of calcium increases the likelihood of obstructions, which, however, is not site-specific
Nearly always normal coronary angiogram But younger patients with acute coronary syndrome may have non-calcified plaques	Total amount of calcium correlates with total plaque burden but still severely underestimates the amount of histologic plaque burden
Low risk of cardiovascular event (2–5 years)	High calcium adjusted for age and gender is associated with higher likelihood of cardiac adverse event (in the next 2–5 years)

Table 6.4 Sensitivity and specificity for detection of coronary artery stenoses by 64-slice CT-scanners of CT

	Sensitivity (%)	Specificity (%)	PPV (%)	NPV (%)
Per 64-slice CT 13				
Per segment	86	96	83	96.5
Per patient	97.5	91	93.5	96.5
Dual-source CT [15–18]				
Per segment	93	96	78	98
Per patient	98	87	89	97

NPV, negative predictive value; PPV, positive predictive value.

Coronary anomalies

Cross-sectional MDCT imaging, especially in combination with two- and three-dimensional image reconstruction techniques, permits an accurate assessment of the aberrant

Table 6.5 Diagnostic performance of 64-slice CT depending on the clinical pre-test likelihood of coronary artery disease in 254 patients [20]

Pre-test probability*	N	Sensitivity (%)	Specificity (%)	PPV (%)	NPV (%)
High	105	98	74	93	89
Intermediate	83	100	84	80	100
Low	66	100	93	75	100

NPV, negative predictive value; PPV, positive predictive value.
*Estimated with the Duke Clinical Risk Score.

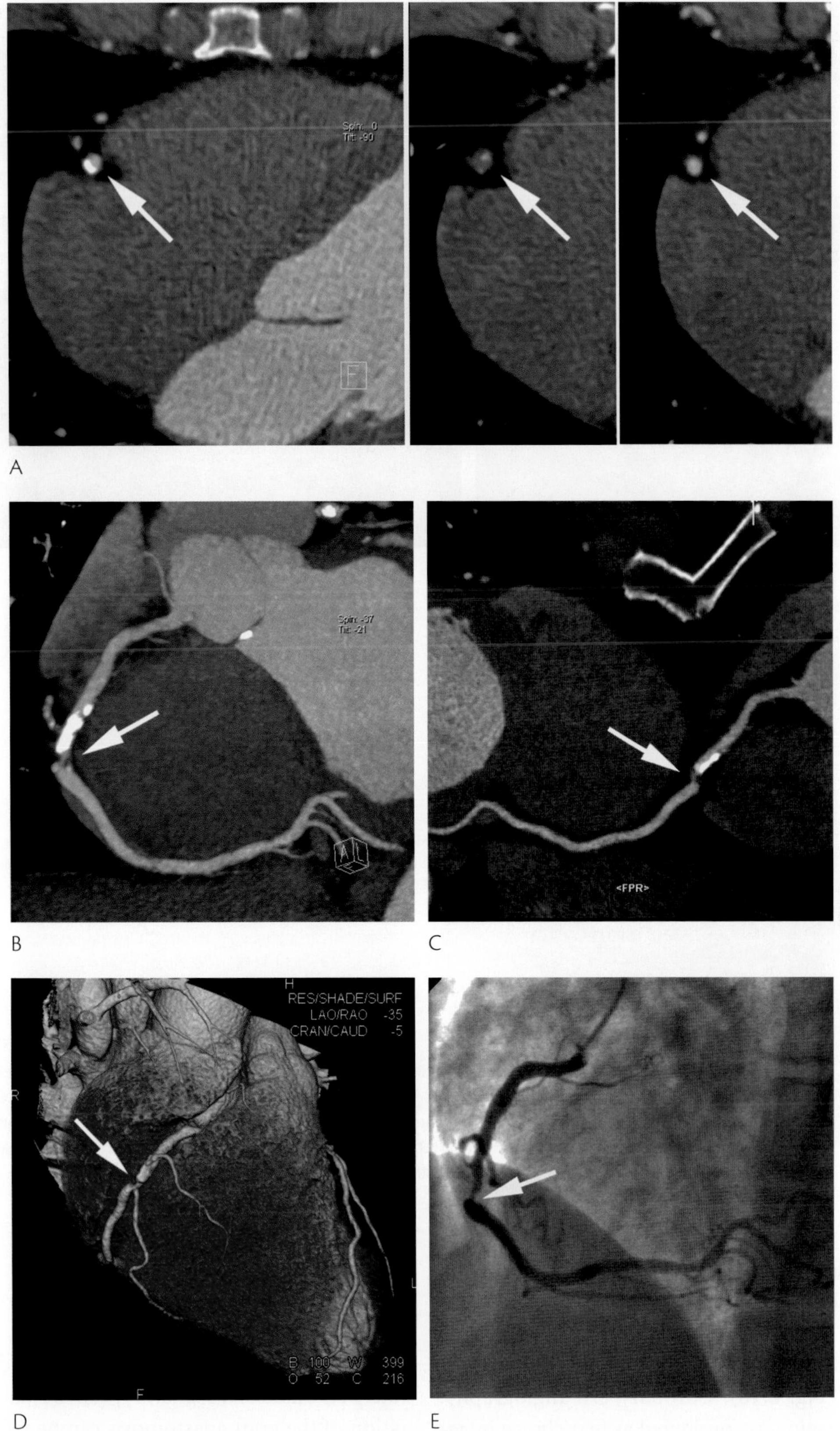

Figure 6.14 Visualization of coronary artery stenosis by contrast-enhanced dual source CT. (A) Cross-sectional images of the right coronary artery at three consecutive levels are shown (arrows). While the topmost image (left) shows some calcification and a contrast-enhanced lumen, the next slice (middle) does not show any contrast-enhanced lumen. A few mm further distal (right), the lumen is again contrast-enhanced. (B) Maximum intensity projection in an oblique plane that shows a long segment of the right coronary artery. The stenosis is clearly visible (arrow). (C) Curved multiplanar reconstruction which displays the right coronary artery along its centreline. Again, the short, concentric stenosis is clearly visible (arrow). (D) 3-D reconstruction, also showing the stenosis (arrow). (E) Corresponding invasive coronary angiogram (arrow = stenosis).

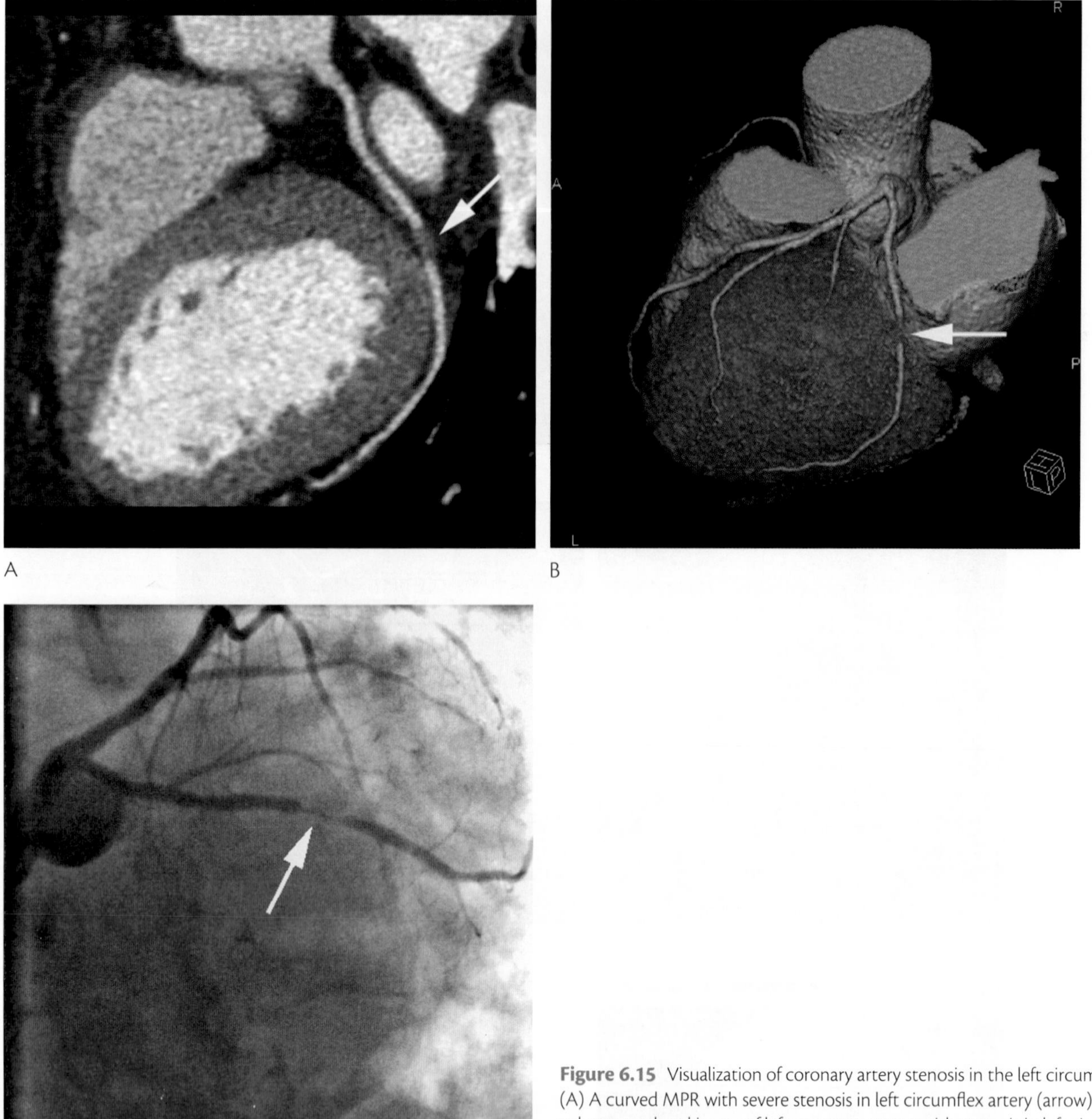

Figure 6.15 Visualization of coronary artery stenosis in the left circumflex artery. (A) A curved MPR with severe stenosis in left circumflex artery (arrow). (B) The volume-rendered image of left coronary system with stenosis in left circumflex artery (arrow). (C) Corresponding diagnostic invasive coronary angiogram with severe stenosis in the left circumflex artery (arrow).

origin and course of anomalous coronary arteries (➲Figs. 6.17 and 6.18) [31, 32]. An anomalous course of one of the coronary arteries between the pulmonary outflow tract and aorta has been associated with myocardial ischaemia and sudden death (➲Fig. 6.18). Coronary CT angiography, along with MR imaging, is considered as first choice imaging modality in suspected coronary anomalies (➲Table 6.6) [14, 29, 30]. Since the patients are often young, special efforts should be undertaken to use low radiation exposure protocols for data acquisition.

Bypass grafts

Because of their relatively large diameter size and modest motion grafts are well assessable by CT. Both patency or occlusion, as well as graft stenosis can be determined accurately (➲Table 6.7; Fig. 6.19)] [33–39], although interpretation of the graft anastomosis can be affected by residual motion and metal artefacts caused by vascular clips [37]. Angiographic assessment of patients with previous bypass graft surgery should also include the native coronary arteries, including the distal coronary run-offs. Due to advanced

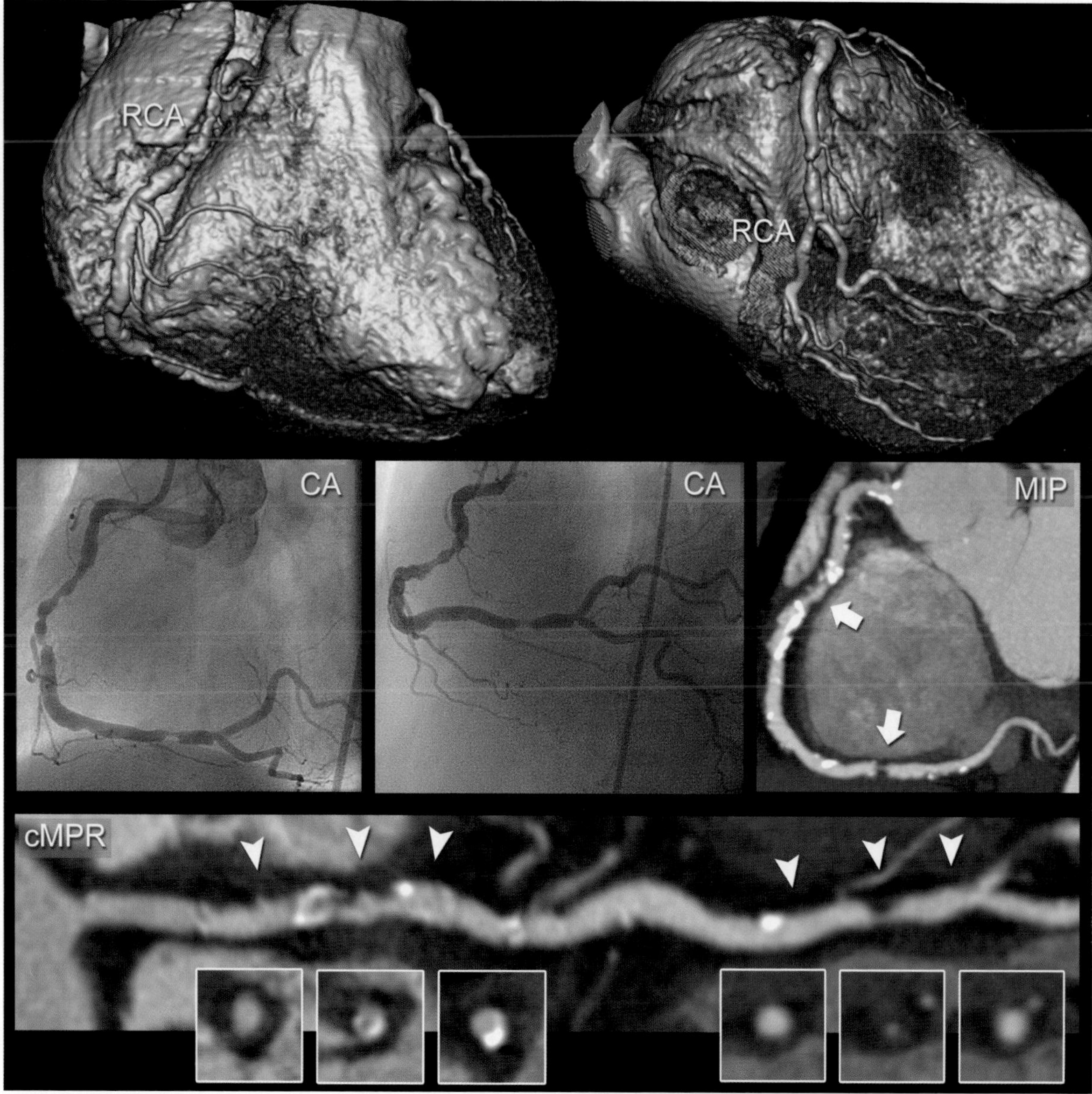

Figure 6.16 Visualization of stenoses in the right coronary artery. CT coronary angiogram and corresponding conventional angiogram (CA) of a right coronary artery. Volume rendered CT images (coloured images) show the presence of a large, dominant RCA. Detailed maximum intensity projected and curved multiplanar reconstructed CT images reveal the presence of 2 significant lesions; One long significant lesion located at the mid RCA, another short significant lesion located at the distal RCA. Cross-sectional CT images (inlays) show the presence of both non-calcified and calcified plaque tissue within the proximal stenosis, whereas exclusively non-calcified plaque tissue is visualized within the more distal stenosis. The presence of two significant lesions was confirmed on the diagnostic conventional angiogram. CA, conventional angiogram; cMPR, curved multiplanar reconstructed image; MIP, maximum intensity projection; RCA, right coronary artery.

atherosclerotic disease, these vessels are often calcified and more difficult to assess by CT, compared to patients without previous bypass surgery [34, 35, 38]. In addition to the lack of information regarding myocardial ischaemia, which is particularly important in these patients, this limits the application of CT to situations where catheter angiography (of the grafts) is technically challenging or not desired (aortic valve endocarditis), or when only the grafts are of interest.

Coronary stents

Metal coronary stents cause blooming artefacts, as a result of limited spatial resolution and filtering, which increases the apparent size of the stent struts on CT [40]. Beam hardening artefacts, combined with residual cardiac motion artefacts, further complicate the interpretation of the lumen within the small coronary stent. The severity and extent of the artefacts depends on the stent material and the strut thickness (➲ Fig. 6.20) [41]. Stents without use of

Table 6.6 Indications for coronary CT angiography according to 'appropriateness criteria' published by a group of professional societies in 2006 [29]

Detection of CAD with prior test results—evaluation of chest pain syndrome
Uninterpretable or equivocal stress test result (exercise, perfusion, or stress echo)
Detection of CAD: symptomatic—evaluation of chest pain syndrome
Intermediate pre-test probability of CAD, ECG uninterpretable or unable to exercise
Detection of CAD: symptomatic—acute chest pain
Intermediate pre-test probability of CAD, no ECG changes and serial enzymes negative
Evaluation of coronary arteries in patients with new onset heart failure to assess etiology
Evaluation of suspected coronary anomalies

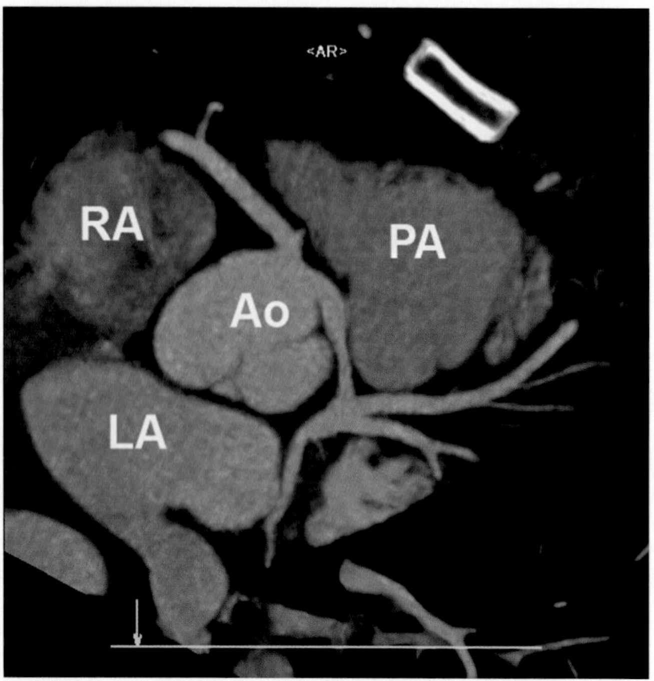

Figure 6.18 Coronary anomaly visualized in a 2-D reconstruction by contrast-enhanced CT angiography. The left main coronary artery arises from the right sinus of valsalva and passess between the aorta (Ao) and pulmonary artery (PA) to the left (LA, left atrium, RA, right atrium). This anomaly is considered malignant.

metal alloys are becoming available. Stent patency or complete occlusion can often be determined by CT (➲Fig. 6.21). Particularly for smaller stents (<3.5mm) and bifurcation stenting assessment of moderate in stent stenosis is less reliable [40–47]. Although routine use of CT after coronary stenting is generally discouraged, it may be of use for follow-up of larger single stents in the proximal coronary arteries, particularly the left main [47] or grafts, provided that good image quality can be achieved.

Coronary plaque imaging

Coronary CT angiography allows for detection and, to a certain extent, the characterization of non-stenotic, non-calcified coronary atherosclerotic plaque (➲Fig. 6.22). In comparison to IVUS, accuracy for detecting non-calcified plaque has been found to be approximately 80–90% [48–50]. Accurate classification of plaque composition by coronary CTA is not possible in clinical routine. The average CT attenuation within 'fibrous' plaques is higher than within 'lipid-rich' plaques (mean attenuation values of 91–116HU versus 47–71HU) [50–54]. However, individual density measurements are widely distributed with significant overlap between plaque types. Additionally measurements are affected by the surrounding tissues, in particular the contrast density of the coronary lumen [55]. CT-plaque imaging may contribute to the identification of plaques at high risk of rupture and subsequent acute coronary syndrome (➲Fig. 6.23). Few small studies have retrospectively analyzed CT plaque characteristics by CT in patients after acute coronary syndromes. They found a higher percentage of non-calcified plaque, more positive remodelling, and a higher frequency of very low CT attenuation (<30HU) in lesions responsible for acute cardiac events as compared to stable lesions [56–58]. However, CT plaque analysis was performed *after* the acute coronary event and plaque rupture with subsequent thrombus formation may have contributed to the CT appearance of these lesions, raising doubts about the actual characteristics of the plaque before rupture.

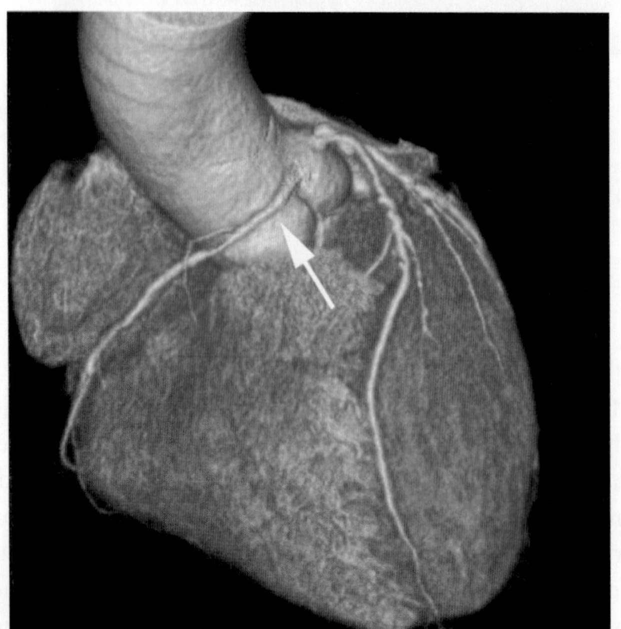

Figure 6.17 Visualization of anomalous coronary artery. The right coronary artery originates from the left coronary cusp (arrow).

Table 6.7 Diagnostic performance of 64-slice CT after coronary bypass graft surgery

		Bypass grafts			Coronary arteries*		
	N	Excluded (%)	Sensitivity (%)	Specificity (%)	Excluded (%)	Sensitivity (%)	Specificity (%)
Pache [33]	31	–	98	89%			
Ropers [34]	50	–	100	97	9	86	90
Malagutti [35]	52	–	99	96	–	96	88
Meyer [36]	138	–	97	97			
Jabara [37]	50	1	100	100			
Onuma [38]	53	5	100	91	9	93	95
Feuchtner [39]	41	–	95	95			

Diagnostic performance for detection of >50% stenosis, including total occlusion, with catheter coronary angiography as reference.

*Distal coronary run-offs and non-grafted coronary branches.

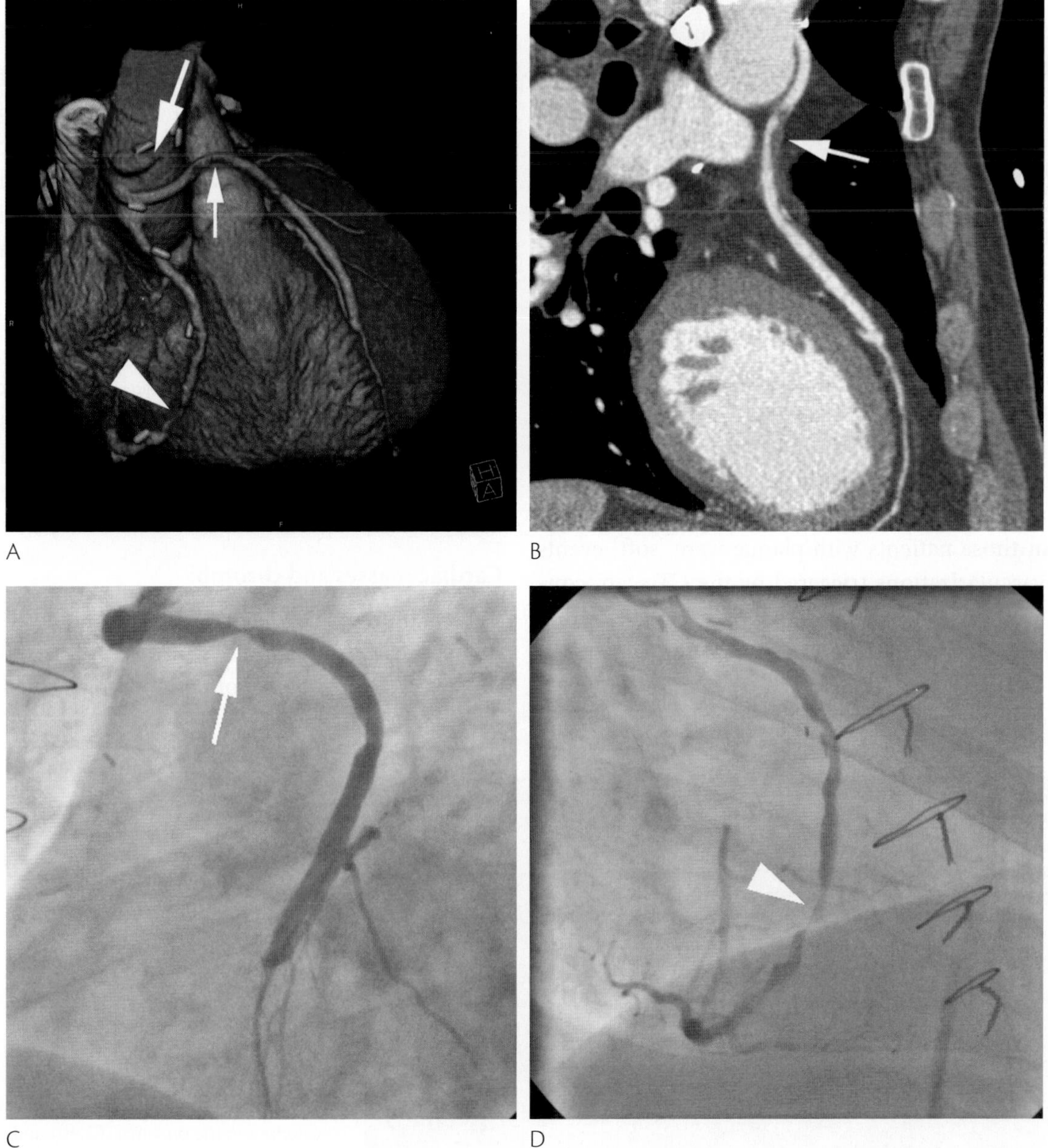

Figure 6.19 Bypass graft imaging. 3-D reconstructed CT angiogram of a patient with three venous bypass grafts (A). The graft to the left circumflex artery, with the most cranial anastomosis to the aorta, is occluded (large arrow). The second graft to the left anterior descending artery is stenosed (small arrow, B), confirmed by catheter angiography (C). Third graft to the right coronary artery is also significantly stenosed (D).

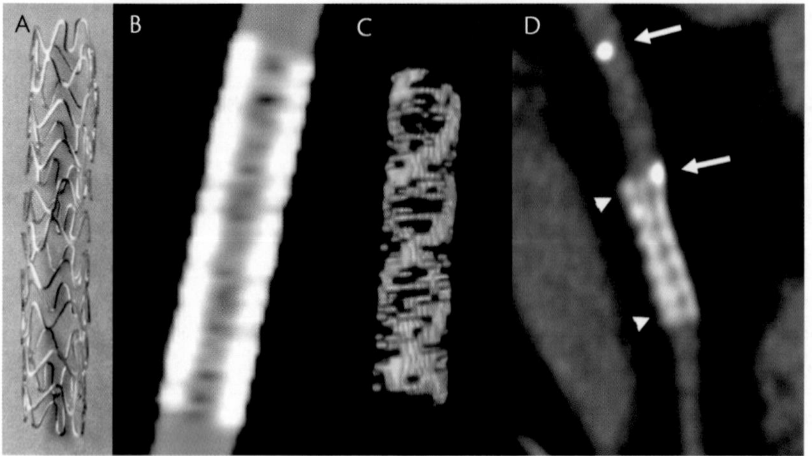

Figure 6.20 Stent imaging. A stationary 4.0 x 15mm stent (Crossflex, Cordis; panel A) within a contrast-filled tube was scanned using a high 0.5-mm collimation. The multiplanar reformation shows the enlarged appearance of the thin struts on CT, which is caused by limited spatial resolution as well as filtering. (B) Varying strut density creates the appearance of a double helix on the 3-D volume rendered image. (C) Compared to a conventional, metal stent (arrow heads), a poly-lactic acid, bioabsorbable stent (BVS, Abbott Vascular) is radiolucent and invisible on CT, except for the two metal markers at the proximal and distal end (arrows).

Prospective trials concerning the value of non-calcified atherosclerotic plaques seen in coronary CT angiography to predict future cardiovascular events are scarce. One analysis of 100 patients with suspected coronary disease who were followed for 16 months after coronary CT angiography demonstrated a higher cardiovascular event rate in patients with non-obstructive plaque detected by MDCT as compared to individuals without any plaque [59]. Another retrospective analysis of 1127 chest-pain patients found increased total mortality in patients who had more than five coronary segments affected by plaque (whether calcified or non-calcified) as compared to individuals with less than five involved segments [24]. Only one study prospectively followed 1000 middle-aged asymptomatic individuals after coronary CT angiography and, since all events that occurred in those patients with plaque were 'soft' events such as revascularizations triggered by the CT scan, concluded that coronary CT angiography is not a useful tool to contribute to risk stratification in individuals without chest pain [60].

Cardiac and pericardial abnormalities

Due to its capability for high-resolution imaging of the entire heart and high contrast between the contrast-enhanced blood pool and surrounding tissues, cardiac CT permits assessment of cardiac morphology with high image quality. It can thus theoretically be applied in numerous clinical situations calling for accurate visualization of cardiac morphology. However, CT imaging is associated with radiation exposure and in most cases requires iodinated contrast agent. Therefore, morphology of the heart and pericardium is usually assessed by echocardiography or CMR imaging. All the same, CT can serve as a second-choice technique and provide accurate information on cardiac morphology and pathology if echocardiography and CMR cannot be performed with satisfactory image quality.

Cardiac masses and thrombi

Cardiac tumours (➲Chapter 20). appear on CT as contrast filling defects or deformities of the contrast-filled cardiac cavities or as thickening, often inhomogeneous, of the soft

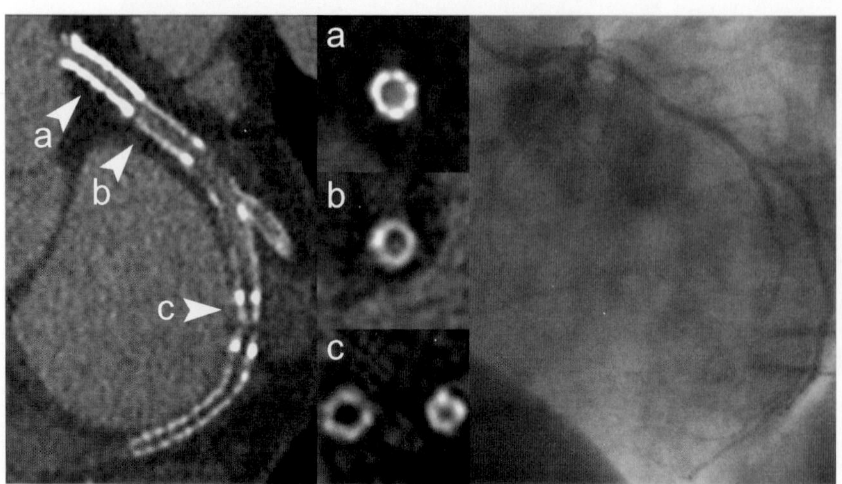

Figure 6.21 Coronary stent imaging. Curved multiplanar reformation (left) of the left main trunk (LM) and left circumflex branch (LCX) after extensive stenting, with cross-sectional views at three levels showing a patent stent in the LM (a), in-stent restenosis in the proximal LCX (b), and occlusion of the mid-portion of the LCX (c), as well as a patent stent in a marginal branch, confirmed by catheter angiography (right panel).

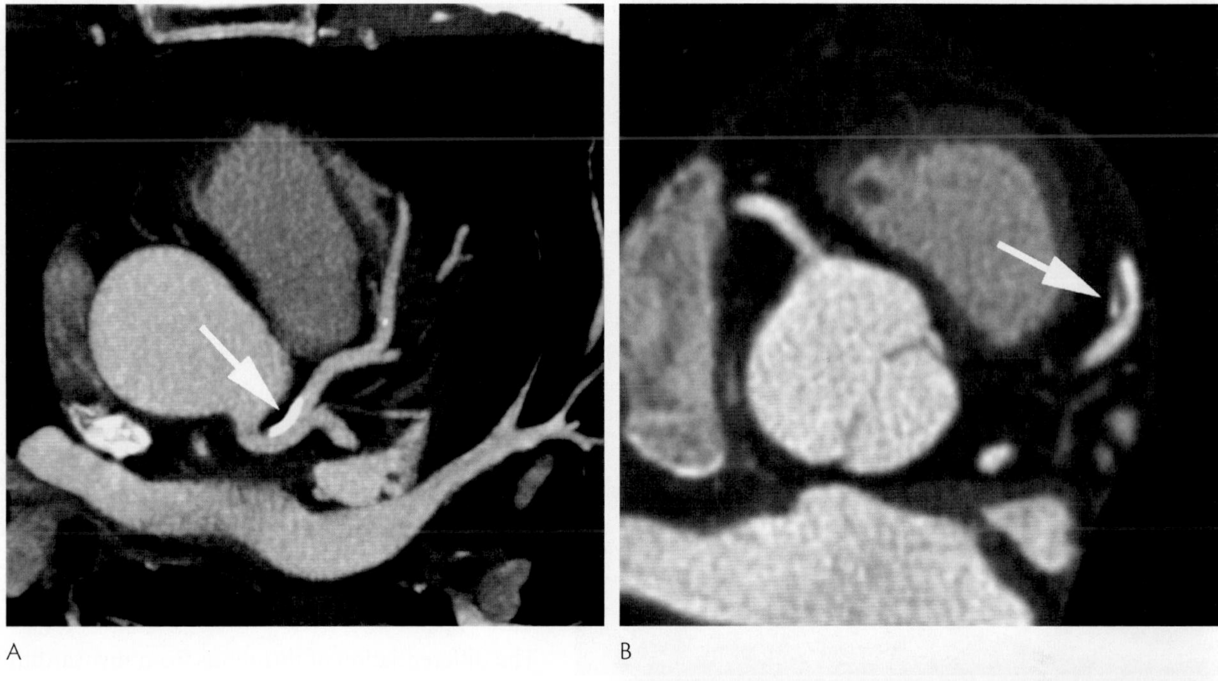

C

Figure 6.22 Visualization of coronary atherosclerotic plaque. Different plaque types visualized by 16-slice MDCT (370ms rotation, 16 × 0.75mm collimation) after intravenous injection of contrast agent. (A) Completely calcified plaque of the proximal left anterior descending coronary artery (arrow). (B) Partly calcified plaque of the proximal left anterior descending coronary artery (arrow). (C) Non-calcified plaque of the proximal left anterior descending coronary artery (arrow).

cardiac tissue (e.g. myocardium or pericardium). CT has limited capabilities for soft-tissue characterization and exact delineation of tumours that infiltrate or are immediately adjacent to the myocardium can therefore be difficult [61]. However, the presence of calcium (e.g. in myxomas), can sometimes be diagnostically helpful and can easily be established or ruled out by CT.

Similar to tumours, intra-cardiac thrombi are depicted as contrast-filling defects within the opacified cardiac chambers. Thrombi may be solitary or multiple and may be sessile, pedunculated, or laminar in shape. Atrial thrombi, mostly located within the left atrial appendage, are the most frequently occurring cardiac thrombi and will appear as a filling defect (➲ Fig. 6.24) (see ➲ Chapter 29). However, it has to be considered that poor atrial function as in atrial fibrillation may result in poor opacification of the atrial appendage after injection of contrast, even in the absence of thrombus.

Thrombi within the left ventricle are usually located adjacent to infarcted myocardium with associated wall motion abnormalities and are frequently seen after anterior wall myocardial infarction (➲ Fig. 6.25) (see ➲ Chapter 16).

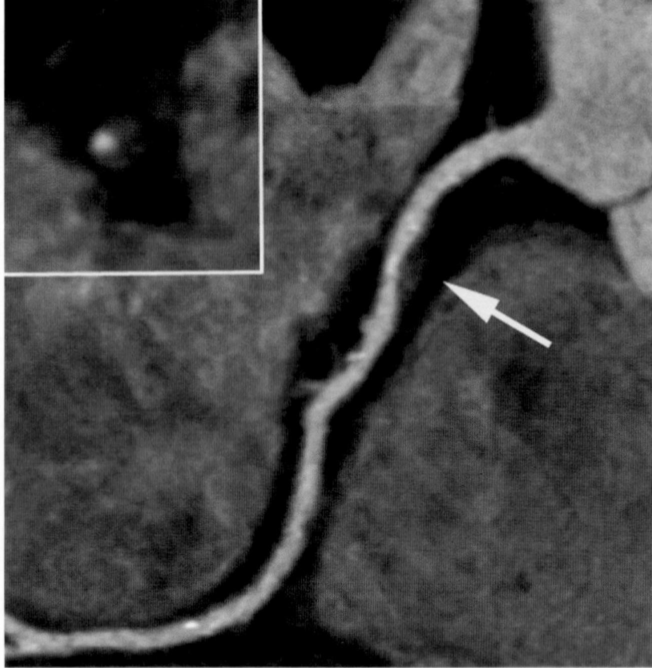

A

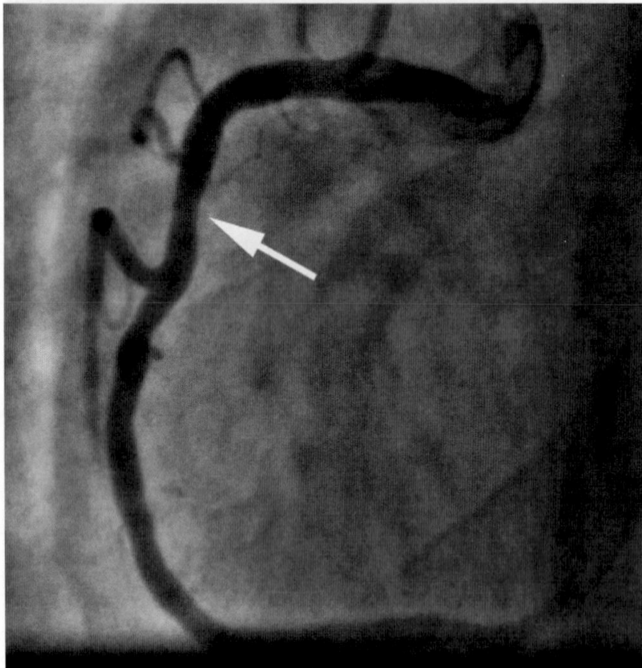

B

Figure 6.23 Coronary atherosclerotic plaque with little luminal stenosis, but substantial positive remodelling. (A) Coronary CT angiography, showing a non-calcified plaque with positive remodelling in the proximal right coronary artery (arrow). The insert shows a cross-section of this plaque. (B) Invasive coronary angiogram. There is only very mild luminal stenosis at the site of the artherosclerotic lesion (arrow).

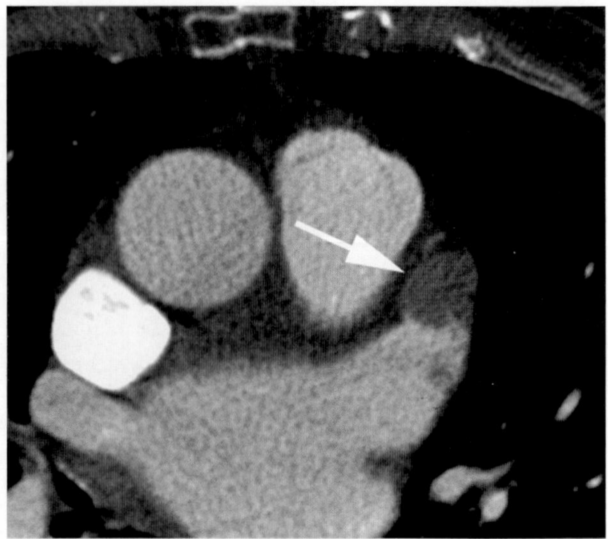

Figure 6.24 Visualization of atrial thrombus. A filling defect is shown in the left atrial appendage (arrow).

The differentiation of thrombus from myocardium and papillary muscle may be difficult. Older thrombi can be calcified.

Pericardial abnormalities

In CT images, the pericardium can usually be appreciated on the anterior face of the heart. It is delineated as a thin structure of soft-tissue density, adjacent to mediastinal fat ventrally and epicardial fat dorsally. The thickness of normal pericardium is 1–2mm, but inferiorly, at the insertion of the pericardium to the diaphragm, it thickens to 3–4mm [62].

Pericardial abnormalities include thickening and calcification of the pericardium, pericardial effusion, and localized pericardial masses or intrapericardial tumours. Pericardial thickening may be localized or general. It may

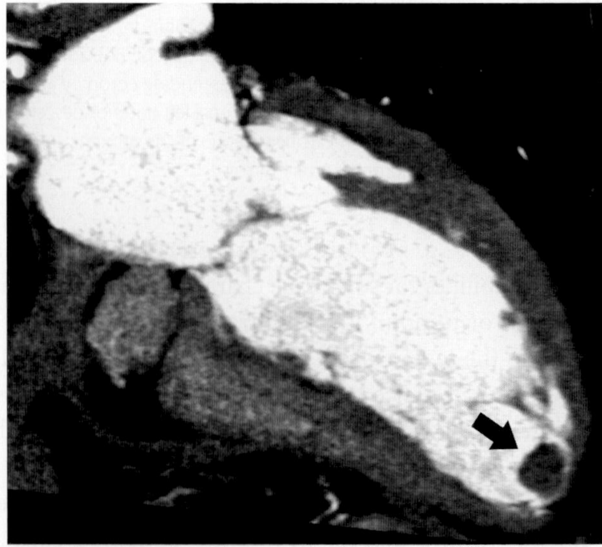

Figure 6.25 Visualization of a ventricular thrombus. Thrombus at the apex of the left ventricle (arrow).

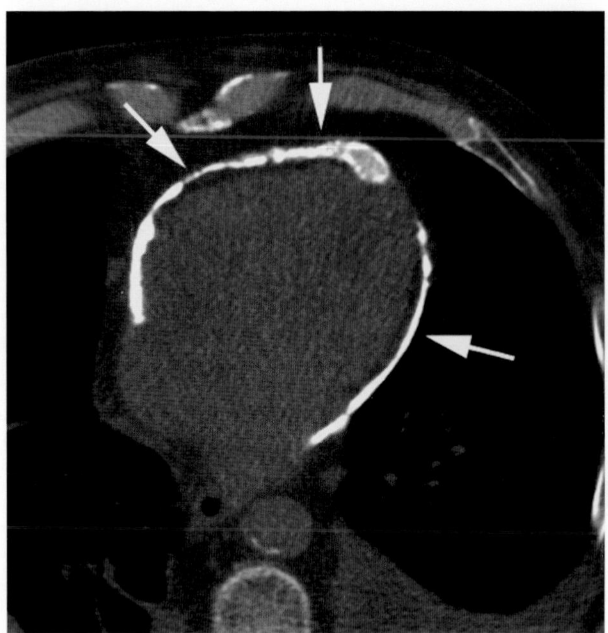

Figure 6.26 Visualization of pericardial calcification. Thickened pericardium with severe calcifications (arrows).

involve both parietal and visceral pericardium and sometimes the myocardium. However, the presence of pericardial thickening by itself is no proof of haemodynamically relevant pericardial constriction. The detection of pericardial calcification can be helpful in this context (➲Fig. 6.26). Pericardial effusion usually accumulates in the caudal portion of the pericardium and appears as a density dorsal to the left ventricular myocardium. As the effusion increases it will extend to the ventral surface of the right atrium and ventricle. Post-operative pericardial effusions can be localized, e.g. adjacent to the right atrium. Pericardial cysts appear as a round or oval mass usually in the right pericardiophrenic angle (➲Fig. 6.27). The cysts are filled with fluid that has a CT density similar to water. Breast and lung carcinoma can metastasize to the pericardium.

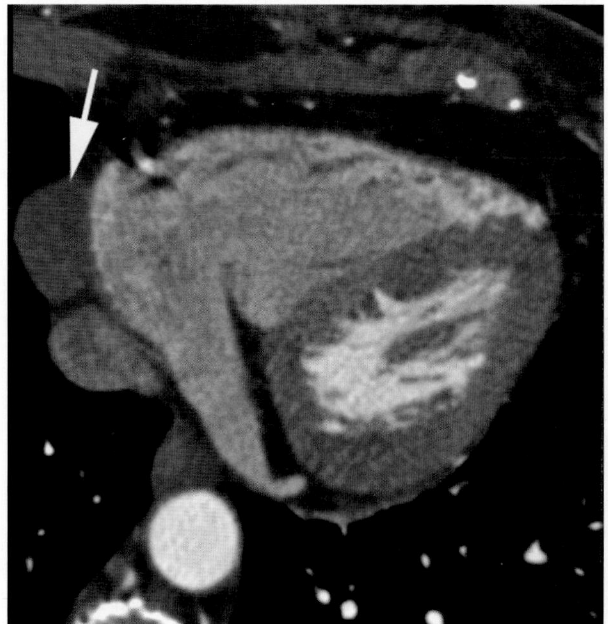

Figure 6.27 Visualization of pericardial cyst. Pericardial cyst in the right costophrenic angle (arrow).

Great vessels

Since the great vessels are subject to cardiac and respiratory motion, the high imaging speed of modern CT scanners, its high spatial resolution, and high contrast between vessel lumen and surrounding tissue have made contrast-enhanced MDCT an important, reliable, clinical diagnostic modality in evaluating the great vessels of the thorax. ECG-gating is infrequently used for thoracic CT imaging.

Thoracic aortic aneurysm

Aneurysms of the aorta (➲Chapter 31) are caused by degeneration of the media. This is most frequently seen in atherosclerotic disease but also as a consequence of Marfan syndrome, cystic medial necrosis, trauma, poststenotic dilatation, or infectious-mycotic diseases.

Aneurysms can be divided into true aneurysms and false aneurysms. A true aneurysm involves all wall layers, is often associated with atherosclerosis, and is usually fusiform in shape (➲Fig. 6.28). False aneurysms consist of a perforation or penetration of the intima and media of the vessel wall, and are contained by adventia and perivascular tissue (➲Fig. 6.29). They are often saccular in shape, have a narrow neck, and are associated with trauma or infection. Thoracic aneurysms are often filled with mural thrombi and long-standing aneurysms may be calcified. On CT, aneurysms are seen as (localized) increases of the aortic diameter.

Aortic dissection

A dissection (➲Chapter 31) is caused by a tear within the intimal layer of the artery with subsequent development and antegrade propagation of a false lumen tracking along the media. There can also be retrograde extension of a dissection with involvement of the aortic valve. The false lumen is often large in diameter and may end blindly or re-enter into the true lumen. The false lumen may become occluded by thrombus or may remain patent. Dissections are usually associated with hypertension or Marfan syndrome (➲Chapter 31). They can be classified according to the De Bakey or Stanford classifications, which both differentiate involvement of the ascending aorta (De Bakey I and II, Stanford A), which constitutes a surgical emergency and serious prognosis, from dissections limited to the descending aorta (De Bakey III, Stanford B)

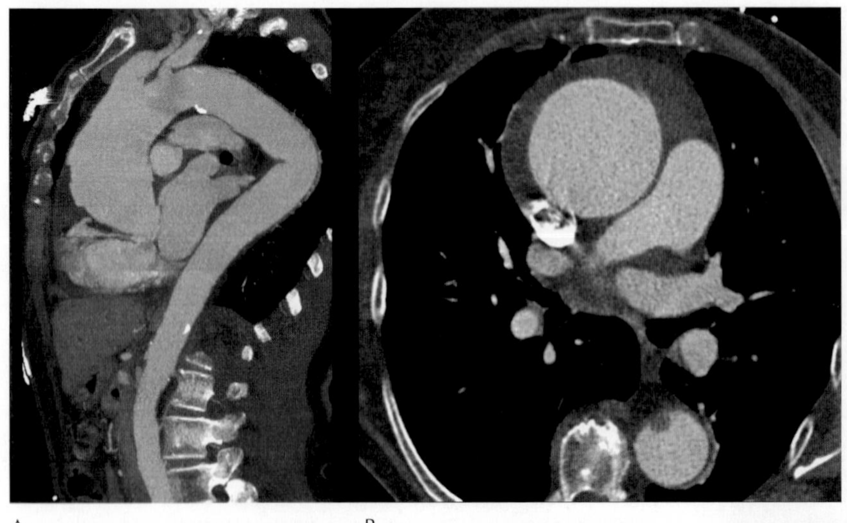

Figure 6.28 Visualization of aneurysm of the aorta. Aneurysmatic dilatation of the ascending aorta (A). An axial image at the level of the aortic arch (B) reveals a significant difference in lumen diameter between the ascending and descending aorta. A significant amount of fluid in the pericardial space is surrounding the ascending aorta (arrowheads).

which in the absence of complications is best treated medically and has a relatively good prognosis.

On CT, a dissection can be recognized by the presence of an intimal flap separating the true and false lumen (➲Fig. 6.30). More indirect CT signs of dissection include inward displacement of intimal calcification by the false lumen, differential contrast opacification between the true and false lumen, presence of (unenhanced) thrombus in the false lumen, thickening of the aortic wall, and, potentially, pericardial effusion.

Pulmonary emboli

CT scanning has been demonstrated to provide high diagnostic accuracy for the detection of pulmonary embolism (➲Chapter 37). Pulmonary emboli on CT are shown as obstruction or filling defects of the contrast-enhanced common pulmonary artery, right or left pulmonary arteries, or their side-branches (➲Fig. 6.31). Pulmonary emboli are usually bilateral [45]. CT-angiography is now considered the method of first choice for suspected pulmonary embolism in routine clinical practice [63].

Evaluation of acute chest pain

Coronary calcium scanning and coronary CT angiography have been investigated to improve the triage of patients with acute chest pain in the emergency ward. A negative calcium scan, or the absence of obstructive or non-obstructive plaque on CTA in patients with acute rest chest pain at low risk (no ECG changes or enzyme elevations), practically rules out an acute coronary syndrome, and has an excellent short and long term prognosis [64–68]. Exclusion of an acute coronary syndrome, a pulmonary embolism or aortic dissection, all life-threatening conditions associated with acute chest pain, by a single CT scan

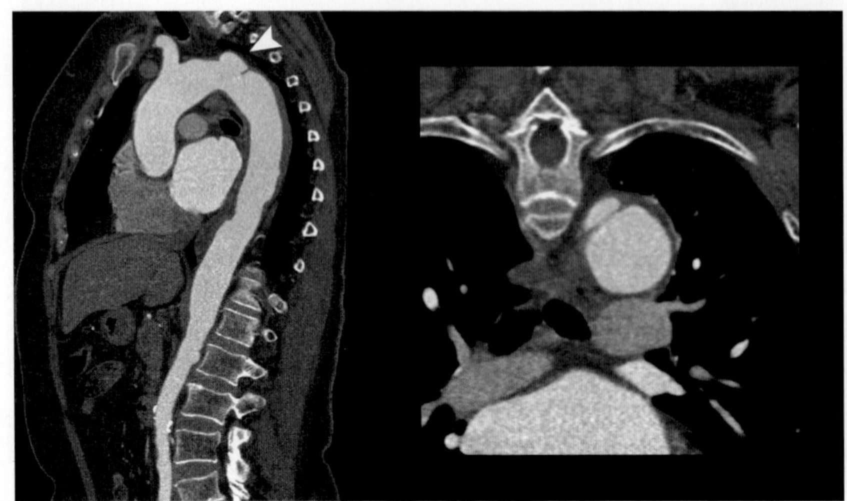

Figure 6.29 Visualization of aneurysm of the aorta. Small saccular aneurysm at the level of the aortic arch (arrowhead, A). The small neck and the location are easily appreciated on the para-coronal plane. The cross-section of the aortic arch shows the eccentric configuration of the aneurysm (B).

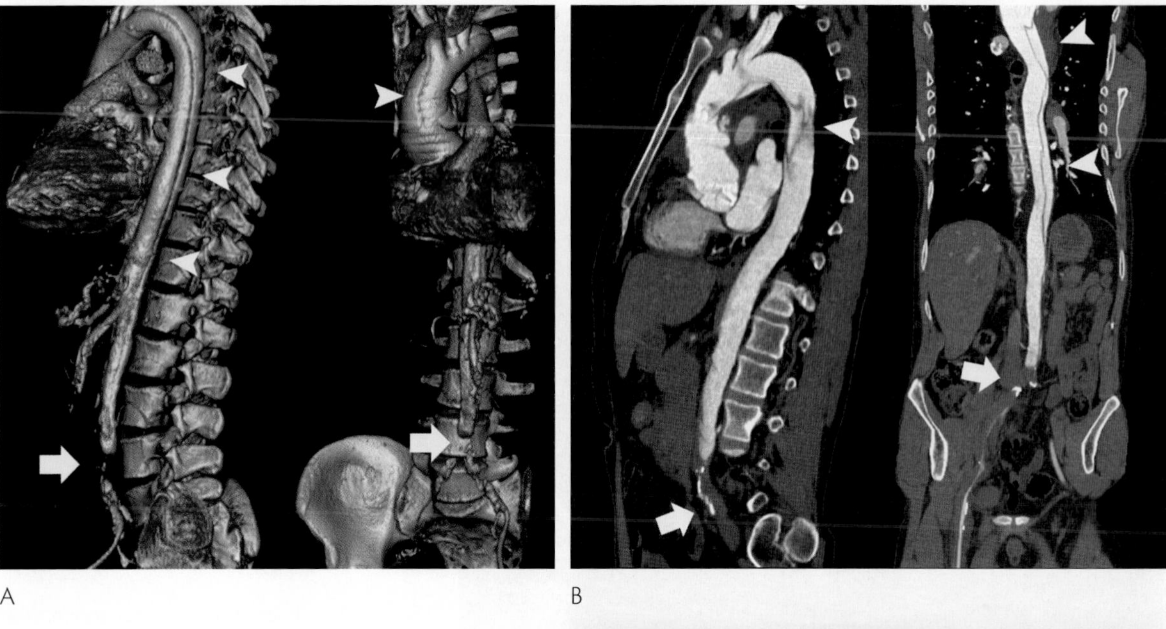

A

B

C

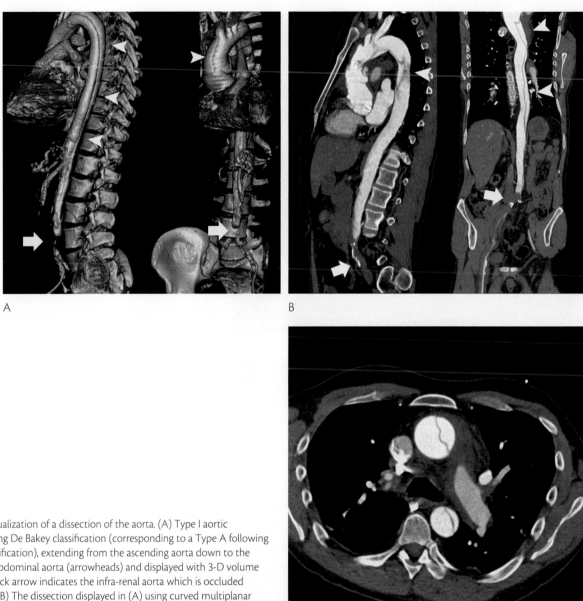

Figure 6.30 Visualization of a dissection of the aorta. (A) Type I aortic dissection following De Bakey classification (corresponding to a Type A following the Stanford classification), extending from the ascending aorta down to the descending and abdominal aorta (arrowheads) and displayed with 3-D volume rendering. The thick arrow indicates the infra-renal aorta which is occluded at the Carrefour. (B) The dissection displayed in (A) using curved multiplanar reformations along the central-lumen line of the aorta. The infra-renal aorta is occluded (thick arrow) and longitudinal calcification is also visible. (C) Para-axial plane through the thorax showing the dissection. The intimal flap is evident both in the ascending and descending aorta (arrows).

is technically feasible. Because of the longer scan range and required enhancement of both the pulmonary arteries and coronary arteries, it is associated with a significantly higher contrast medium and radiation dose. In clinical practice one of these conditions is generally more suspected than the others, in which case a dedicated (CT) examination is recommended in favour of the so-called triple rule-out scan. Nevertheless, non-cardiac disease responsible for the complaints may be detected on a CT intended to exclude coronary artery disease.

Functional imaging with computed tomography

If data are acquired throughout the entire cardiac cycle, images can be reconstructed during multiple cardiac phases, which allows for assessment of global and regional contractile function. Despite a relatively modest temporal resolution, global left ventricular function by CT correlates well with echocardiography and CMR imaging [69]. New scanning protocols that dramatically reduce radiation exposure do not provide

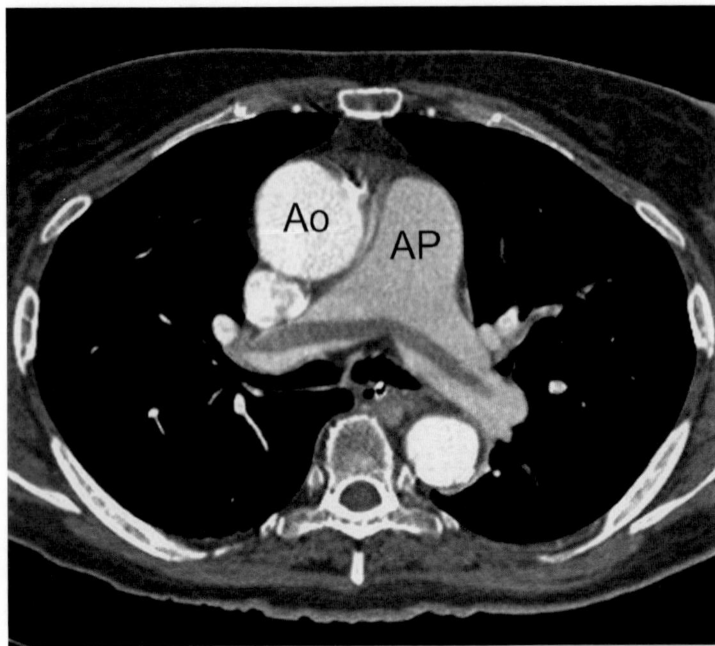

Figure 6.31 Visualization of pulmonary embolism. Large pulmonary embolism at the level of the bifurcation of the pulmonary artery.

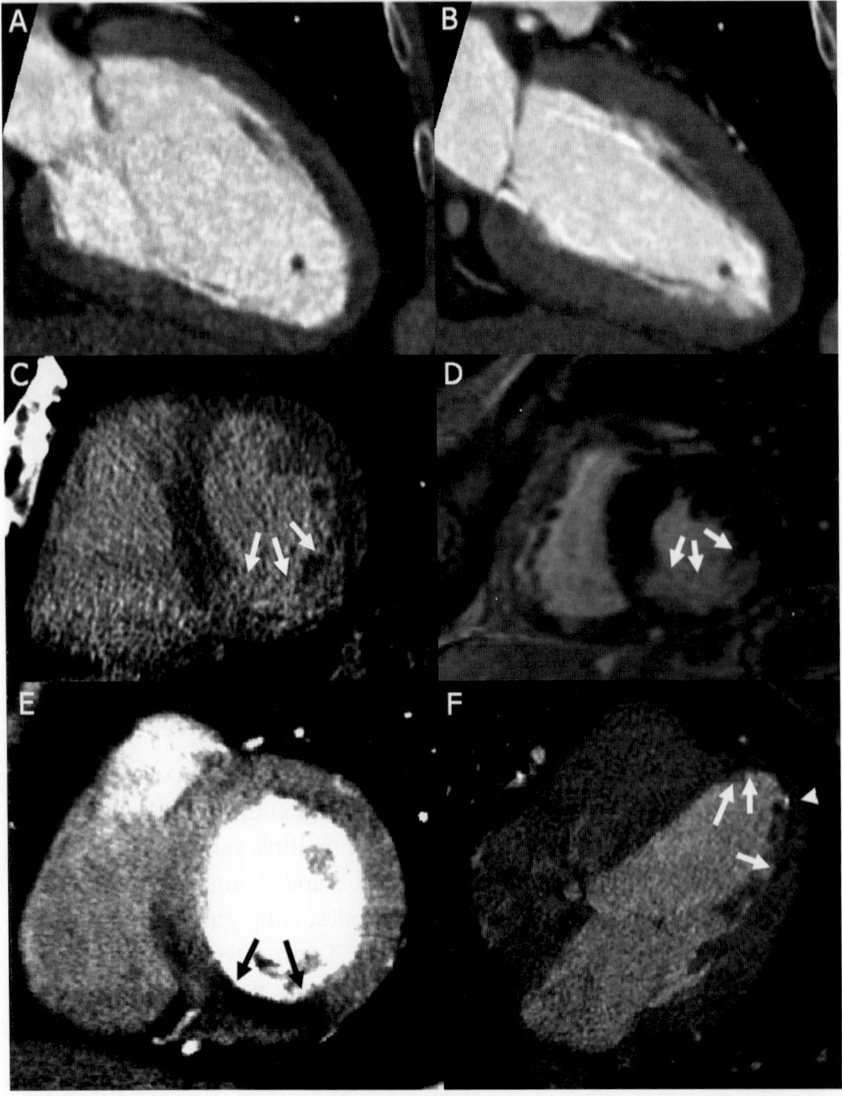

Figure 6.32 Myocardial imaging. End-diastolic (A) and end-systolic reconstructions (B) can be used to assess global ventricular function. Delayed hyperenhancement (arrows) by CT (C) and MRI (D) in a case of acute (reperfused) myocardial infarction of the inferior wall. Myocardial hypo-enhancement (arrows) of the inferior wall by CT immediately after contrast injection by CT in a patient shortly after reperfused myocardial infarction (E). Wall thinning and very low attenuation (arrows) of the (endocardial) anterior wall, as well as some calcium deposition (arrow head) in a patient who suffered an anterior myocardial infarction in the past (F). Also see 6.3–6.7.

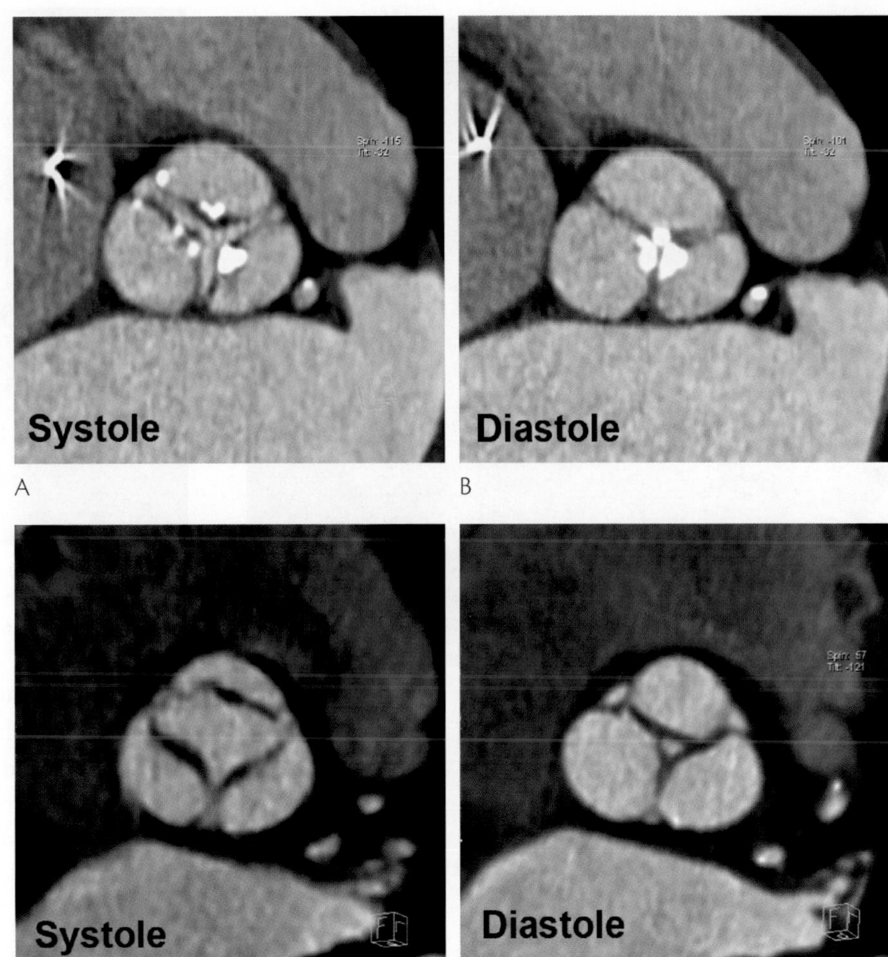

Figure 6.33 Imaging of the aortic valve by contrast-enhanced CT angiography after injection of contrast agent. (A, B) Patient with aortic valve stenosis. A tricuspid valve with a moderate amount of calcification is seen. Closure in diastole is complete, but the orifice remains small (here: $1.1cm^2$) in systole. (C, D) Patient with aortic valve regurgitation. Opening is slightly impaired in systole (orifice area: $2.4cm^2$), while in diastole, a small central area of regurgitation remains. The valve leaflets are thickened as often seen in aortic regurgitation. Also see 6.8 and 6.9.

information on LV function. The myocardium on contrast-enhanced CT angiograms may show hypoenhancement due to decreased myocardial perfusion in case of prior myocardial infarction or severe ischaemia (➲Fig. 6.32; 6.3–6.7). Heterogeneous myocardial enhancement may also be caused by motion and beam hardening artefacts. To complement the angiographic information of CT angiography, use of myocardial perfusion imaging after pharmacological stress to detect ischaemia is being investigated [70]. Long after myocardial infarction wall thinning, calcifications or very low myocardial attenuation as a result of replacement by fat tissue, may be detected [71]. Similar to CMR imaging, delayed enhancement may be demonstrated after myocardial infarction or other forms of myocardial injury [72]. Due to its superior image quality without the need for roentgen or iodine contrast media, CMR imaging remains the preferred technique for the detection of (chronic) myocardial infarction.

Computed tomography for valve disease

- CT imaging can provide morphological information regarding the aortic and mitral valves (➲Fig. 6.33; 6.8 and 6.9).
- The orifice area in aortic valve stenosis can be measured accurately by MDCT [73–77] The high spatial resolution of CT sometimes is advantageous for assessing perivalvular morphology, such as abscesses or dehiscence after surgical repair for endocarditis, which may be difficult to demonstrate by echocardiography or MR imaging due to artefacts caused by valve prostheses (➲Fig. 6.34; 6.10).
- Functional information, such as flow velocities and pressure gradient, cannot be determined by CT. Right-sided heart valves are difficult to visualize by CT, due to the lower and often inhomogeneous contrast in the right-sided cavities, but adjustment of scanning protocols can ensure contrast opacification in both ventricles and allow quantification of RV ejection fraction.
- CT imaging may have a role for cardiac assessment in preparation for valvular surgery and percutaneous aortic valve replacement.
- Coronary CT angiography can reliably rule out coronary artery stenoses in patients scheduled for valvular surgery [78–80].

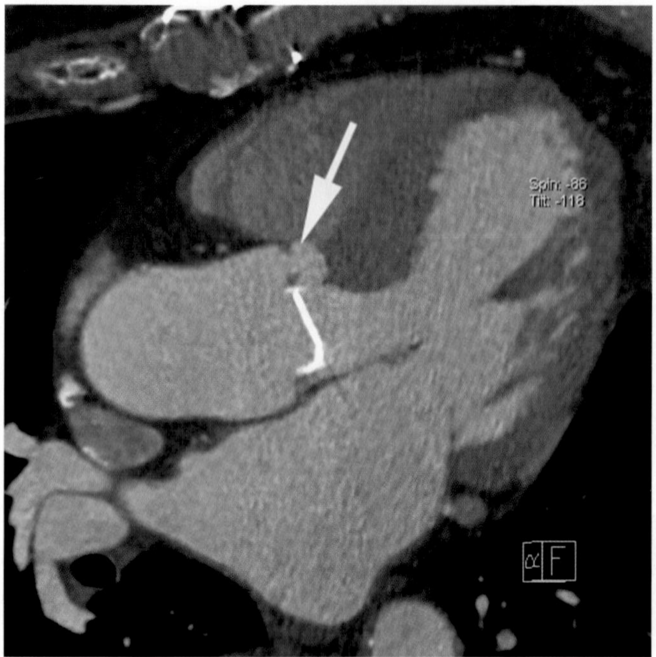

Figure 6.34 Visualization of a paravalvular leakage in a patient after aortic valve replacement (arrow). Modern prosthetic valves typically cause very little artefact in CT imaging. Also see 6.10.

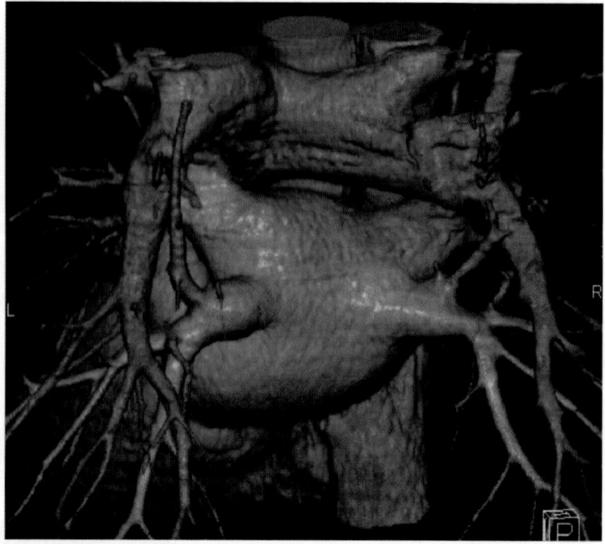

Figure 6.35 Pulmonary vein imaging. 3-D volume rendered CT angiogram with a posterior view on the left atrium and the pulmonary veins, as well as the pulmonary arteries above.

Cardiac computed tomography in electrophysiology

In preparation for pulmonary vein isolation, detailed information concerning atrial and pulmonary vein anatomy and size, and oesophagus localization behind the left atrium potentially improves efficiency and safety of the procedure (➲Fig. 6.35). CT without ECG-gating will often suffice, particularly during atrial fibrillation. By integrating the CT images into the electro-magnetic mapping system during ablation procedures, navigation of catheters and registration of ablation lesions can be performed using the individual anatomy, although coregistration of the catheter position into the CT images is limited by cardiac and respiratory motion [81]. Postprocedural stenosis or thrombosis of a pulmonary vein can be identified with CT [82].

Imaging of the venous system of the heart can be helpful prior to implantation of a biventricular pacemaker. By imaging the availability, location, and size of the individual cardiac veins the options for left ventricular lead placement are displayed [83, 84]. Challenging take-off angles of the venous side branch, variant sinus anatomy, and rudimentary valvular structures (Thebesian valves) at the sinus orifice may also be important. Image quality of coronary CT scans may be affected by the presence of pacemaker wires (➲Chapter 27), particularly near the distal electrodes and particularly in case of ICD coils (➲Chapter 30).

Cardiac computed tomography for complex congenital heart disease

Usually patients with complex congenital heart disease (➲Chapter 10) are young and CT-associated radiation doses are highly undesirable due to stochastic effects; therefore, MR examination is considered the first choice method. However MR imaging may be contraindicated in patients with a pacemaker, ICD or severe claustrophobia. In these cases cardiac CT may provide accurate anatomical information including the right ventricle (after adjustment of scanning protocol) of these complex congenital abnormalities, but CT does not offer flow information [85].

Personal perspective

Spiral CT coronary angiography is a highly sensitive diagnostic modality to rule out the presence of significant obstructive coronary atherosclerosis, but at its current stage of development cannot (yet) replace selective conventional coronary angiography that is vital to plan either catheter-based or surgical revascularization of coronary artery stenoses and serve as road map for catheter-based coronary diagnostic modalities such as intra-coronary ultrasound virtual histology, optical coherence tomography, spectroscopy, or thermography. Replacement of invasive coronary angiography by spiral CT coronary angiography requires improvement in temporal resolution (faster tube rotation, two or more X-ray tubes, non-mechanical X-ray steering) and spatial resolution (improved detector technology, which should not come at the price of increased radiation exposure). Current issues with spiral CT coronary angiography—such as calcification, atrial fibrillation, and relatively high radiation exposure—should be addressed by new technical advances and CT-protocols that may be expected to occur in the foreseeable future. The clinical role of spiral CT to detect or exclude coronary artery stenoses with respect to other non-invasive modalities (stress echo ECG, stress echo, SPECT) need to be established in comparative studies that should include cost-effectiveness analysis. Coronary atherosclerosis imaging (calcific and non-clacific plaques) studies are needed to further assess their role in prediction, prevention, and cost-effectiveness of coronary artery disease in asymptomatic subjects.

Further reading

Bluemke DA, Achenbach S, Budoff M, *et al.* Noninvasive coronary artery imaging: magnetic resonance angiography and multidetector computed tomography angiography: a scientific statement from the American Heart Association Committee on Cardiovascular Imaging and Intervention of the Council on Cardiovascular Radiology and Intervention, and the Councils on Clinical Cardiology and Cardiovascular Disease in the Young. *Circulation* 2008; **118**: 586–606.

Greenland P, Bonow RO, Brundage BH, *et al.* Clinical Expert Consensus Document on Coronary Artery Calcium Scoring by Computed Tomography in Global Cardiovascular Risk Assessment and in Evaluation of Patients With Chest Pain. A Report of the American College of Cardiology Foundation Clinical Expert Consensus Task Force (ACCF/AHA Writing Committee to Update the 2000 Expert Consensus Document on Electron Beam Computed Tomography) Developed in Collaboration With the Society of Atherosclerosis Imaging and Prevention and the Society of Cardiovascular Computed Tomography. *Circulation* 2007; **115**: 402–26.

Hendel RC, Patel MR, Kramer CM, *et al.* ACCF/ACR/SCCT/SCMR/ASNC/NASCI/SCAI/SIR 2006 appropriateness criteria for cardiac computed tomography and cardiac magnetic resonance imaging: a report of the American College of Cardiology Foundation Quality Strategic Directions Committee Appropriateness Criteria Working Group, American College of Radiology, Society of Cardiovascular Computed Tomography, Society for Cardiovascular Magnetic Resonance, American Society of Nuclear Cardiology, North American Society for Cardiac Imaging, Society for Cardiovascular Angiography and Interventions, and Society of Interventional Radiology. *J Am Coll Cardiol* 2006; **48**: 1475–97.

Schroeder S, Achenbach S, Bengel F, *et al.* Cardiac computed tomography: indications, applications, limitations, and training requirements: Report of a Writing Group deployed by the Working Group Nuclear Cardiology and Cardiac CT of the European Society of Cardiology and the European Council of Nuclear Cardiology. *Eur Heart J* 2008; **29**: 531–56.

Additional online material

- 6.1 Cross-sectional computed tomography anatomy of the heart.
- 6.2 Volume rendered reconstruction of the heart and coronary arteries.
- 6.3 Three-chamber view.
- 6.4 Four-chamber view.
- 6.5 Two-chamber view.
- 6.6 Short-axis, left ventricle post inferior myocardial infarction.
- 6.7 Four-dimensional computed tomography angiogram.
- 6.8 Aortic stenosis.
- 6.9 Aortic regurgitation.
- 6.10 Prosthetic aortic valve.

➲ For full references and multimedia materials please visit the online version of the book (http://esctextbook.oxfordonline.com).

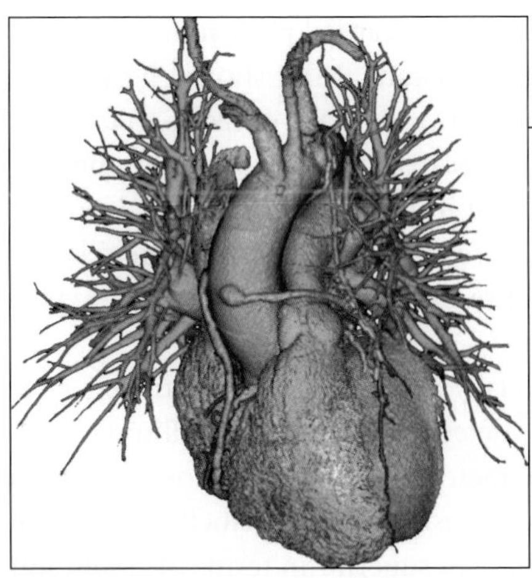

CHAPTER 7

Nuclear Cardiology

Philipp A. Kaufmann, Paolo G. Camici, and S. Richard Underwood

Contents

Summary

Non-invasive images of the myocardium that reflect myocardial perfusion can be obtained either by using conventional nuclear medicine radiopharmaceuticals and cameras or by positron emission tomography (PET). Myocardial perfusion scintigraphy (MPS) with thallium-201 and/or technetium (Tc)-99m-labelled sestamibi and tetrofosmin, in combination with single photon emission computed tomography (SPECT), is a robust and well validated technique for the identification of myocardial ischaemia and infarction with high sensitivity and specificity. 99mTc-labelled myocardial perfusion agents have a high-count density which enables acquisition of electrocardiogram-gated images. Spatial and temporal changes in activity during the cardiac cycle reflect regional myocardial motion and thickening and this technique allows left ventricular volume, ejection fraction, and myocardial motion and thickening to be measured in addition to the information on perfusion. Since the main feature of an acute coronary syndrome is reduced myocardial perfusion, MPS can provide important diagnostic and prognostic information in the emergency department and allows patient stratification in the post-infarction phase. PET provides absolute measurement of myocardial blood flow and has enabled the demonstration of coronary microvascular dysfunction. This has highlighted the potential contribution of the microcirculation to myocardial ischaemia in patients with angiographically normal coronary arteries. Both SPECT and PET are invaluable tools for the identification of viable myocardium in patients with coronary artery disease and congestive heart failure. The constant technological developments of non-invasive cardiac imaging over the past years, including the advent of hybrid nuclear and computer tomography (CT) scanners now allow image fusion of CT coronary angiography and nuclear imaging which can be achieved by using hybrid scanners or software fusion of data sets obtained from stand-alone scanners. Although the potential of such comprehensive non-invasive coronary artery disease assessment appears great, the clinical impact of this tool remains to be established.

Diagnosis of coronary artery disease

Chronic chest pain

Sensitivity and specificity

A range of investigations is normally used in patients with suspected coronary artery disease (CAD), the simplest 'investigation' being the history. Typical angina is a good indicator of myocardial ischaemia and abolition of symptoms is the primary aim of treatment. Symptoms however can be indeterminate and they do not indicate the site or extent of underlying ischaemia. It is therefore often helpful to proceed to further investigations to aid the diagnosis and guide future management. MPS is a robust, non-invasive, and widely available method of assessing regional myocardial perfusion, and has an obvious role in the clinical setting. Many studies have assessed the sensitivity and specificity of this technique for the detection of CAD—coronary arteriography usually being used as the standard by which the accuracy of scintigraphy is judged. The wisdom of this approach can be debated, but at least the arteriogram provides a universal standard for coronary anatomy even if it is less suited to assess coronary arterial function. Published figures for sensitivity and specificity of MPS vary widely and depend upon the characteristics of the population studied (gender, presenting symptoms, medication, previous infarction, etc.), the imaging technique used (planar or SPECT, qualitative or semi-quantitative analysis), and the experience of the centre. Using modern techniques with tomographic imaging good accuracy can be achieved with sensitivity and specificity as high as 91% and 87%, respectively [1]. This is significantly better than exercise electrocardiography for which a large meta-analysis has shown sensitivity of 68% and specificity 77%.

It is reasonable to ask therefore whether MPS should not replace exercise electrocardiography (➲Chapter 25) in patients with suspected CAD. Several factors militate against this. The most important is the relative availability of the two techniques, but radiation burden and cost are also relevant. Although the cost of myocardial perfusion imaging (MPI) is higher than that of the exercise electrocardiogram (ECG) this is more than outweighed by its greater effectiveness [2]. Studies of cost-effectiveness have shown significant advantages for strategies of investigation using MPS, with savings in total diagnostic and management costs over two years in the region of 20% in centres routinely using scintigraphy.

Many centres use a staged approach with the exercise ECG being the initial stress test and MPS next if the likelihood of disease is indeterminate after the exercise ECG, or if further information on myocardial perfusion is required to assist management decisions. MPS should be the initial investigation in patients who are unlikely to exercise adequately, in women (because of the very high number of false-positive ECGs), and if the exercise ECG will be uninterpretable because of resting abnormalities such as left bundle branch block, pre-excitation, left ventricular hypertrophy, or drug effects.

The three commercially available perfusion tracers have equal accuracy for the detection of CA [3]. Thallium (^{201}Tl) has better uptake characteristics and, in theory, provides defects with greater contrast, but ^{99m}Tc-labelled sestamibi and tetrofosmin images are superior in terms of resolution and susceptibility to attenuation artefact. The net effect of these technical differences in clinical practice is negligible, but the technetium tracers are preferred in obese patients or when ECG-gating is required. In fact, ECG-gating can aid the distinction between artefact and perfusion defect (➲ Fig. 7.1) and can increase confidence in reporting [4].

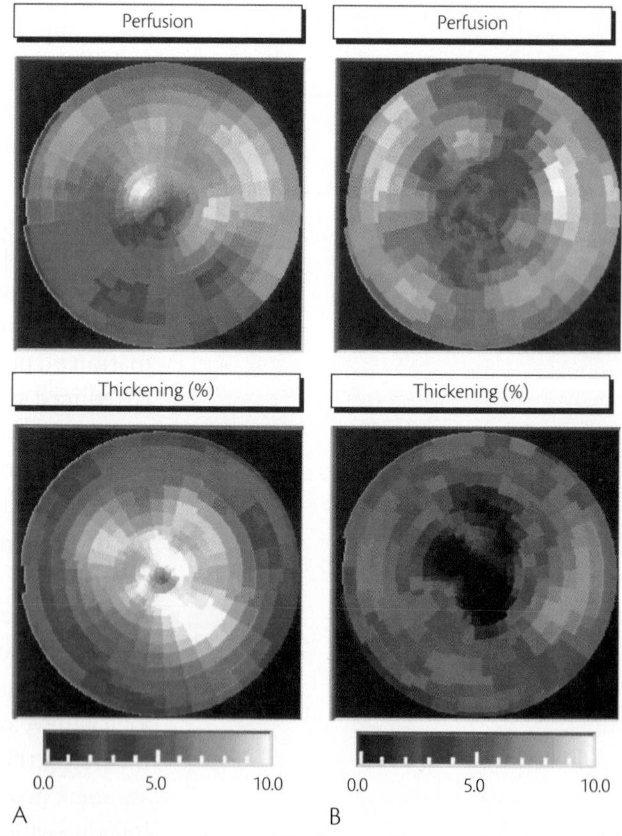

Figure 7.1 Polar map of a normalized rest perfusion scan (upper panels) with the corresponding map representing the thickening assessed by gated SPECT (lower panels). (A) Example of a patient with fixed inferoseptal perfusion defect but normal thickening, identifying the perfusion defect as an attenuation artefact. (B) Example of a patient with fixed apical perfusion defect with congruent decreased wall thickening, confirming that the perfusion defect is a scar.

Attenuation correction is another technique that can reduce artefact although it is controversial whether this can be achieved without loss of sensitivity and attenuation correction is not used routinely in most centres.

Attenuation correction

Soft-tissue attenuation in the chest produces regional inhomogeneities in the normal pattern of tracer uptake and is one of the most frequent causes of artefact in MPS. Attenuation refers to the combined effects of photoelectric absorption and Compton scattering. The former occurs, when a photon interacts with an orbital electron in the tissue and the total energy of the photon is lost. The latter indicates interaction of a photon in the patient prior to detection, which makes the photon change direction. If patient positioning for rest and stress acquisition is kept constant, soft-tissue attenuation appears as a fixed defect. The resulting uncertainty in differentiating between a fixed defect due to attenuation artefact and myocardial infarction can reduce the specificity of the test for detecting CAD. Several methods of non-uniform attenuation correction are now available commercially, albeit with variable clinical success. Most of these methods use attenuation maps based on radionuclide line sources. Recently, however, the use of CT attenuation correction has been introduced and established for SPECT (➲ Fig. 7.2) as well as for quantitative myocardial perfusion measurement with PET. The transmission scan can by CT can be acquired in a much shorter time and with higher quality than can be obtained from a conventional radionuclide transmission scan, because CT achieves a far higher spatial resolution and higher photon flux. It has been shown that the respiration-dependent change in attenuation maps to correct SPECT is a possible drawback of CT-based attenuation correction. The attenuation map obtained with the lower resolution X-ray-based CT data of hybrid SPECT with low-end CT systems represent an average over many breathing cycles, similar to the attenuation maps acquired with Germanium sources in conventional PET scanners. By contrast, data acquisition with a modern multislice CT scanner occurs within fractions of a breath-hold. As a consequence, even slight misalignments may have a large adverse impact on image quality. Therefore, careful

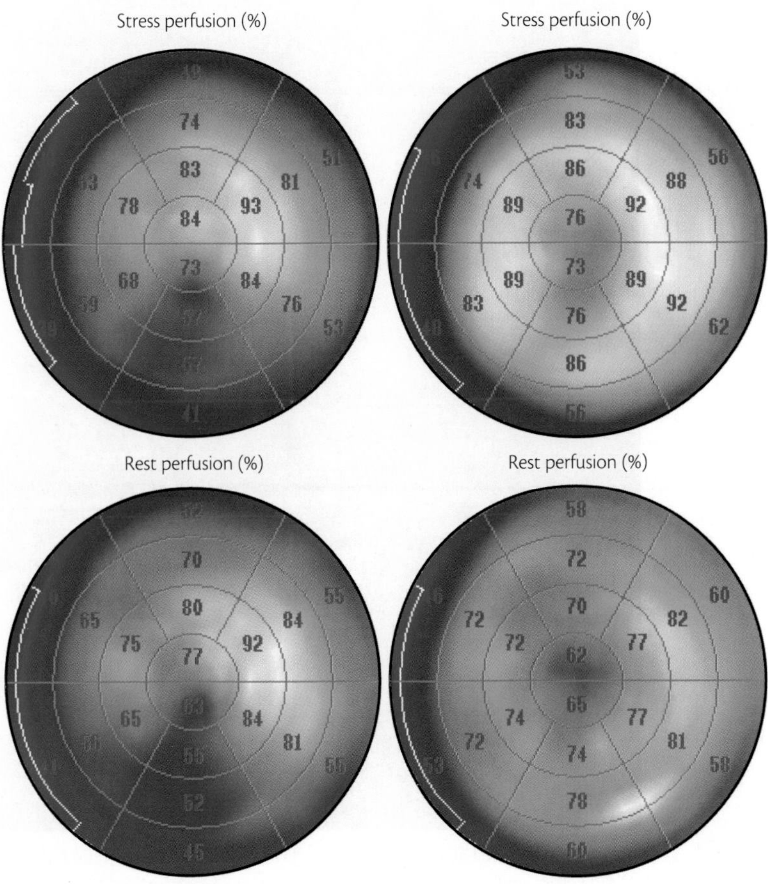

Figure 7.2 Polar map of a normalized stress (upper panels) and corresponding rest perfusion scan (lower panels) of an obese male patient with normal coronary arteries. (A) There appears to be a fixed inferior defect in the images without attenuation correction. (B) After attenuation correction with a CT (using a hybrid SPECT-CT scanner) perfusion appears normal, indicating that the inferior defect was due to attenuation.

verification of alignment and meticulous manual correction for any misalignment is important (➲ Fig. 7.3). Under this condition CT yields good results. Although several studies of attenuation-corrected SPECT have demonstrated improved specificity with no change in overall sensitivity, attenuation correction is not yet widely used. The relative capabilities of gated SPECT and attenuation correction to improve diagnostic specificity are still uncertain. The fact that from most vendors SPECT/CT scanners, combining a multihead gamma camera with a CT facility, are now available will contribute to more widespread use and increase in knowledge about the clinical validity of X-ray-based CT attenuation correction.

ECG-gated SPECT

^{99m}Tc-labelled myocardial perfusion agents are valid alternatives to ^{201}Tl for the assessment of CAD. Their high-count density has enabled acquisition of ECG-gated SPECT studies. ECG-gating represents a great step forward in the evolution of functional myocardial imaging as it allows simultaneous assessment of resting ventricular function and either stress or rest perfusion. Due to the limited resolution of MPS with SPECT it is not possible to assess the left ventricular wall thickness by geometric methods. Because ^{99m}Tc-labelled tracer (tetrofosmin and sestamibi) distribution in the myocardium is stable, spatial and temporal changes in activity during the cardiac cycle

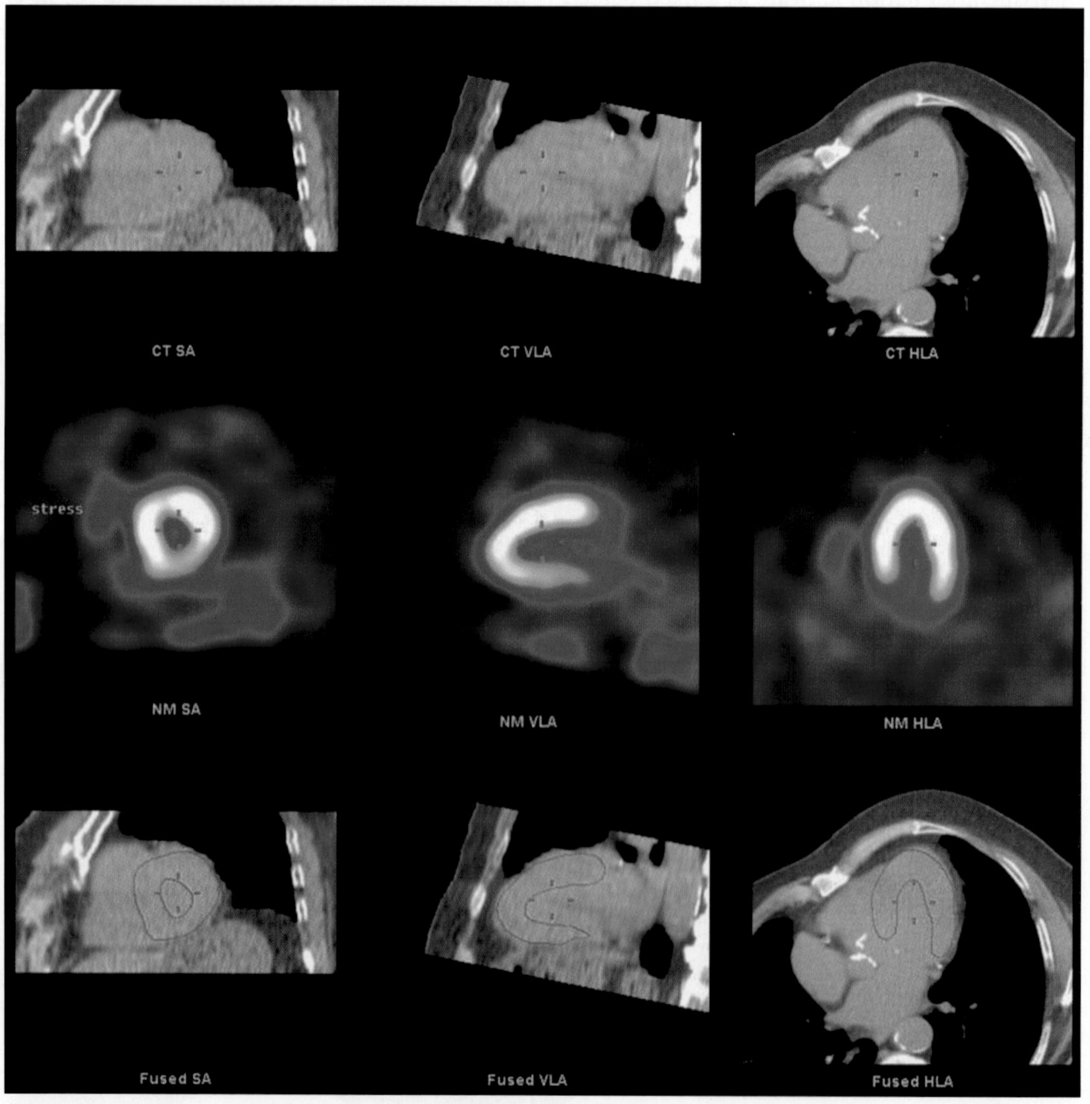

Figure 7.3 Short axis (SA) as well as vertical (VLA) and horizontal long axis (HLA) of native CT images are fused with the non-corrected nuclear myocardial (NM) SPECT images to check the alignment of the coregistration. Misalignment needs to be corrected manually by adjusting CT images to best match SPECT images.

reflect regional myocardial motion. An increase in regional myocardial activity from diastole to systole is proportional to wall thickening. Thus, in addition to perfusion data, gated SPECT offers the potential to measure left ventricular volume, ejection fraction, and myocardial motion and thickening [5].

A precise and reliable assessment of left ventricular function and LV dimensions is prognostically important in most cardiac diseases. Quantifying the degree and extent of left ventricular function offers an objective risk stratification and selection of therapeutic strategy and allows for the sequential follow-up of the therapeutic response. Prerequisites for successful ECG triggering allowing quantification of left ventricular volumes and function are adequate count density (low-dose protocols may not provide valid numbers and should not be triggered for clinical use) and a fairly regular heart rhythm (atrial fibrillation, sinus arrhythmia, frequent premature beats, intermittent pacing etc. are conditions that may render appropriate triggering impossible). The ECG lead should be carefully chosen so that the R wave is a marker of end-diastole and the R wave must be positive in most triggering systems. The cardiac cycle is usually divided into eight, and sometimes into sixteen intervals (frames, bins). The lower frame rate results in a slight underestimation of the ejection fraction by about four units. Sixteen intervals provide better determination of ejection fraction and end-systolic volume (enhanced temporal resolution) and offers some information on the diastolic function while eight intervals might provide a better assessment of regional wall motion (due to enhanced signal-to-noise ratio of gated SPECT images) and is probably the most frequently used protocol. Commercially available, widely used, standardized, and well established software solutions can be used for automated detection of endocardial and epicardial contours reliably and without user intervention. These fully automatic methods of measuring left ventricular function (➲ Fig. 7.4) have been extensively validated against a variety of techniques, such as equilibrium and first-pass radionuclide ventriculography, X-ray contrast ventriculography, magnetic resonance imaging, and two-dimensional echocardiography. Wall motion analysis aids the distinction between attenuation artefact and true perfusion abnormality because infarcted myocardium is unlikely to move or thicken normally and hence reporting confidence is increased and additional prognostic information is obtained. It appears that wall thickening is the best parameter derived from gated SPECT (and superior to wall motion alone) [4], which increases test specificity for CAD assessment by allowing better differentiation of scars from attenuation artefacts when interpreting the cause of fixed defects (see ➲ Fig. 7.1). Recently, phase analysis of gated SPECT MPI has been introduced and shown to compare well to tissue Doppler imaging for the assessment of left ventricular dyssynchrony. The latter is an important predictor of response to cardiac resynchronization therapy (CRT). Information on left ventricular dyssynchrony can be provided by gated SPECT with phase analysis of regional maximal count changes throughout the cardiac cycle, which tracks the onset of wall thickening [6]. This method may play a major role in the near future for predicting response to CRT in heart failure patients.

Positron emission tomography

The most commonly used radiopharmaceuticals for PET imaging of myocardial perfusion are ^{15}O-water, ^{13}N-ammonia, and rubidium-82 (^{82}Rb). For the latter two tracers, sensitivities between 83–100% for the detection of CAD have been reported with specificities between 73–100%.

^{13}N-ammonia and ^{15}O-water are the most commonly used PET tracers for the quantification of regional myocardial perfusion. They have similar half-lives of 10min and 2min respectively and so they both require an on-site cyclotron, which limits their widespread use. ^{15}O-water is superior to ^{13}N-ammonia as a perfusion tracer because it is metabolically inert and it diffuses freely across capillary and sarcolemmal membranes. It equilibrates rapidly between the vascular and extravascular spaces and its myocardial uptake varies linearly with perfusion over a wide range. But ^{15}O-water has an important shortcoming compared with ^{13}N-ammonia: it does not accumulate in myocardial cells and it does not therefore provide images for clinical use. In contrast, ^{13}N-ammonia accumulates in myocardial cells and provides high quality images of perfusion (➲ Fig. 7.5). Therefore, it is the preferred tracer for clinical use provided that a cyclotron is available. The problem of attenuation correction has been solved for PET by using external ^{68}Ge or X-rays sources as recently established in the hybrid PET/CT scanners [7].

The main advantages of ^{82}Rb are its short half-life of 78s and the fact that it is readily produced at the point of use by a ^{82}Rb generator without the need for a cyclotron. Although several methods of quantifying regional myocardial perfusion using ^{82}Rb have been described, their accuracy is limited by the dependence of myocardial extraction of this tracer on perfusion and on the metabolic state of the myocardium. The high energy of the positron emitted (3.15MeV) also reduces resolution of the images because of

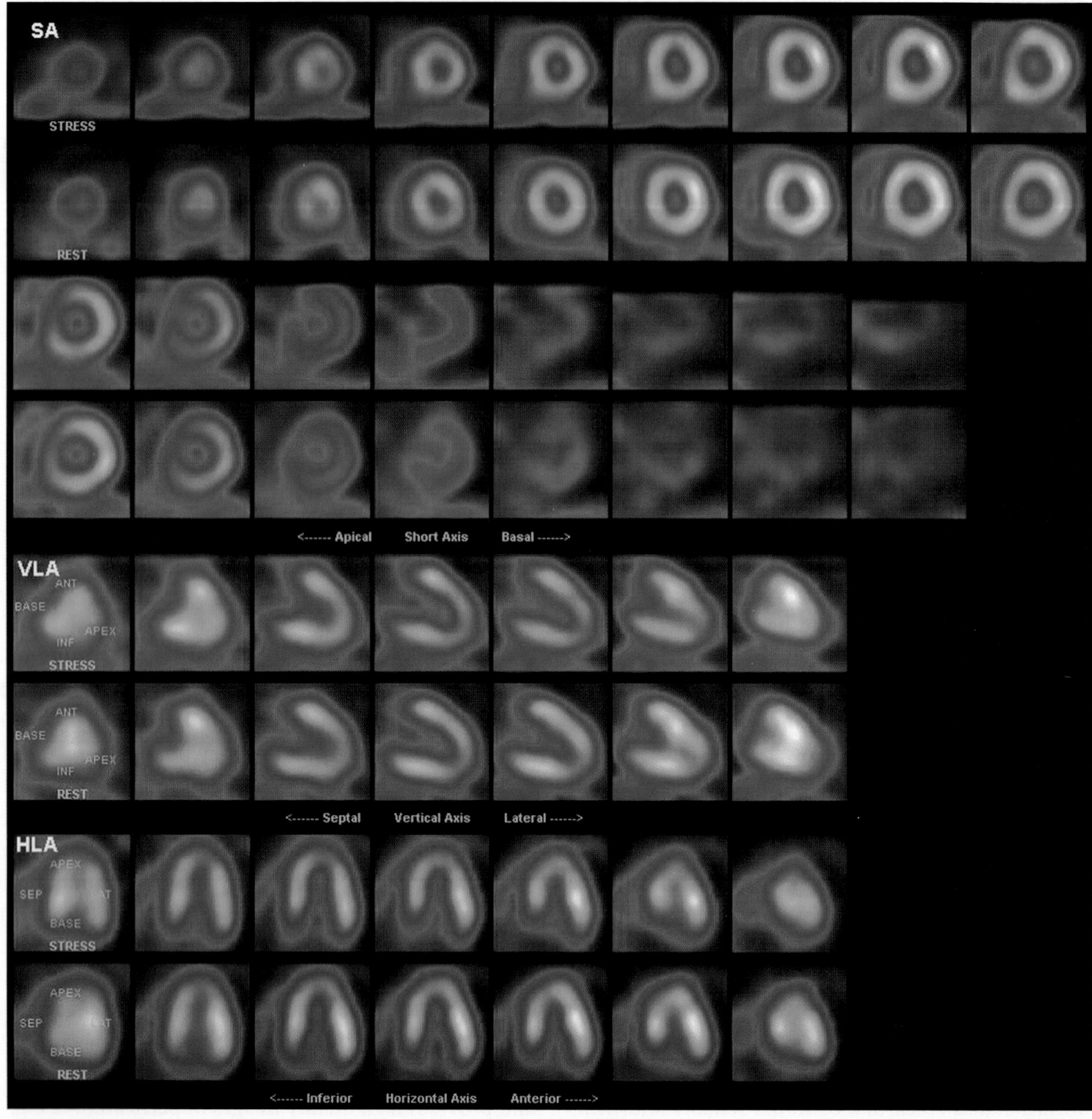

A

Figure 7.4 (A – C) Example from a female patient with normal coronary arteries and normal myocardial perfusion at rest and at stress assessed with ^{99m}Tc-labelled tetrofosmin. (A) The top four rows contain short-axis (SA) slices (stress and rest), the lower four rows represent the vertical- (VLA) and horizontal (HLA) long-axis slices. All slices show normal perfusion without defect. (*Continued*, p. 221.)

the long track of the positron before annihilation with an electron. Nevertheless, ^{82}Rb is now widely used in the USA while this tracer has had no commercial success in Europe so far. The fact that the prognostic value of PET perfusion scanning with ^{82}Rb has been fully established may help to increase its acceptance in Europe. This in turn may help to increase the use of perfusion PET, as with the widespread use of oncology PET scanning the availability of PET scanners has substantially improved [8]. Myocardial perfusion scanning with ^{82}Rb and PET has several advantages over conventional SPECT. It is possible to perform a complete stress and rest study within about 30min, aiding patient comfort and throughput. This straightforward ^{82}Rb protocol compares favourably with cardiac ^{99m}Tc SPECT, as the latter generally is a multistage procedure which may take half a day or may require acquisitions on two separate days.

Because of the higher resolution of PET and its integrated attenuation correction, accuracy for the detection of CAD is thought to be superior to SPECT although only a

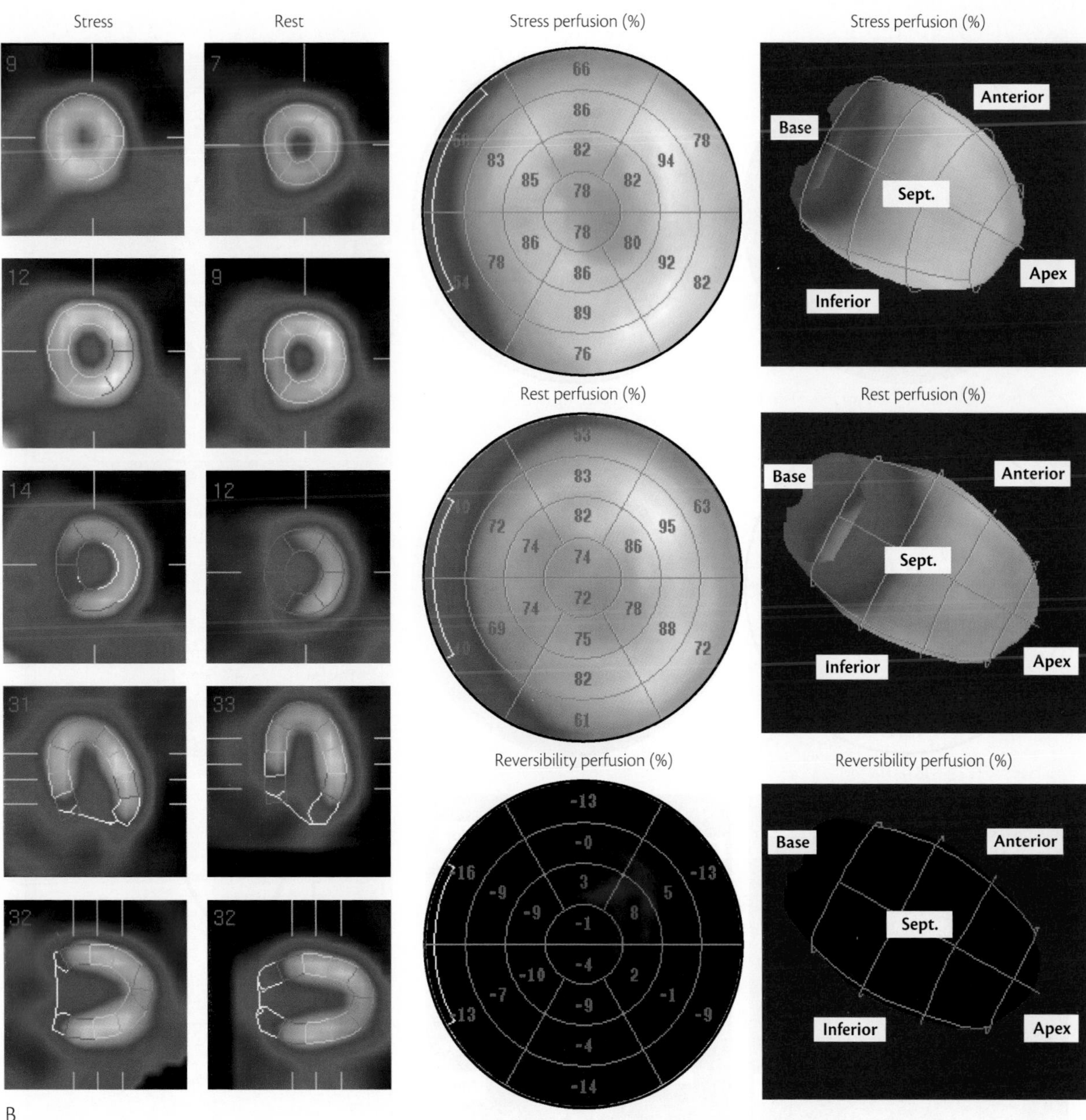

Figure 7.4 (*cont'd*) (B) Right: polar plots and three-dimensional view of the perfusion scan indicating normal perfusion at rest and at stress. Left: the apical, mid-ventricular and basal short-axis slices illustrate the location of the radial-search boundaries. The mid-ventricular vertical and horizontal long-axis slice images illustrate the placement of the apical and basal slice selections. (*Continued*, p. 222.)

small number of studies have directly compared the techniques [3] and it is not known if its higher cost outweighs its greater accuracy. In complex conditions of coronary disease where there may be no normal reference segment such as in multi-vessel disease or coronary microcirculatory dysfunction PET is a preferred tool (➲ Fig. 7.6) and has been recently proven to be of great value for clinical decision-making and to be cost effective [9]. Quantification may allow the demonstration of endothelial dysfunction before an anatomical stenosis is apparent and it has had a great impact on our understanding of the pathophysiology of coronary disease [10]. In daily clinical routine, however, quantification of absolute myocardial perfusion for CAD assessment has played a minor role, as its added value on top of MPI remains to be elucidated. This may be achieved in the near future due to the fact that availability of PET devices has much increased mostly due to the widespread use in oncology.

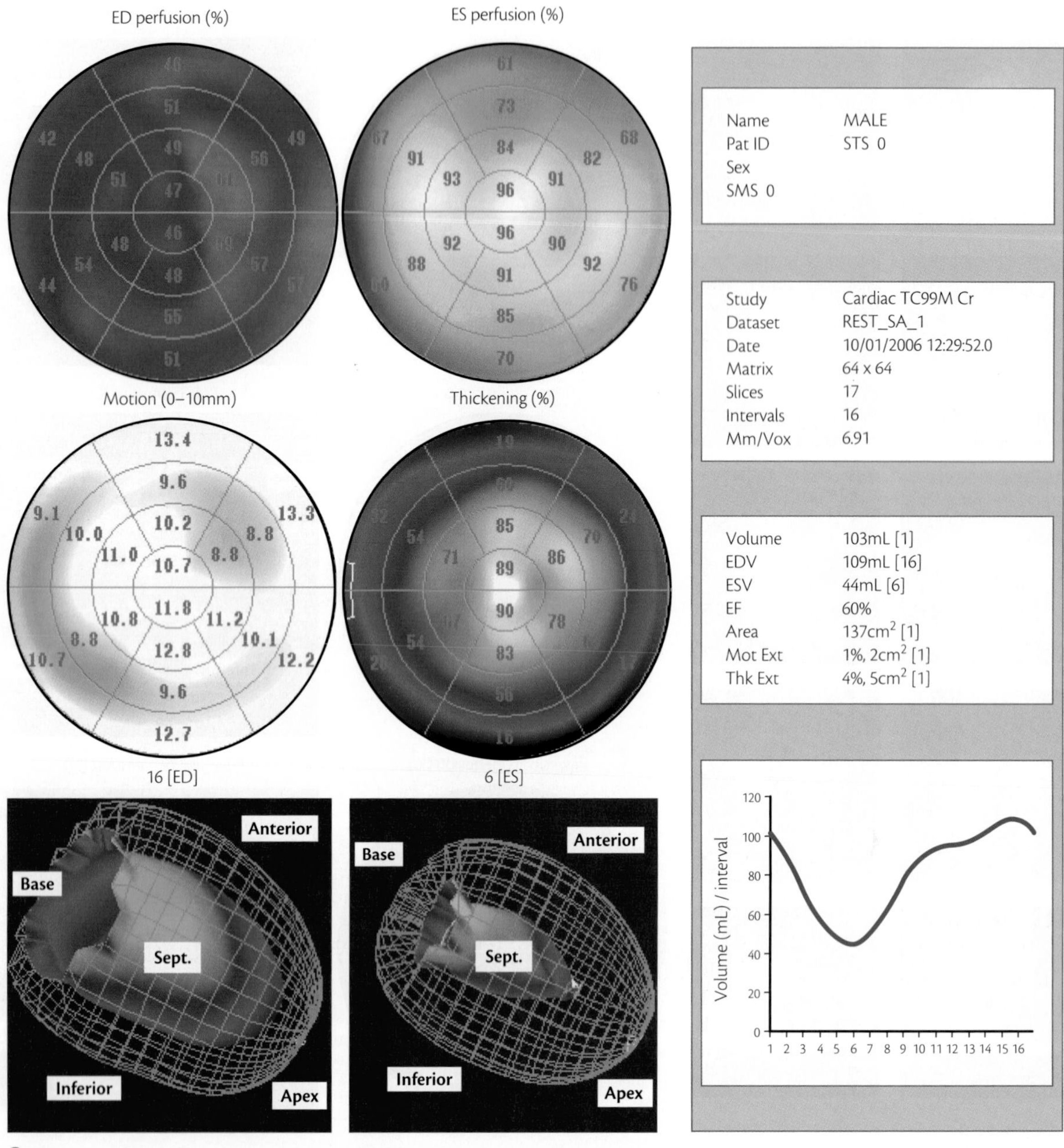

Figure 7.4 (*cont'd*) (C). Quantitative gated SPECT analysis (normal female patient). Left ventricular ejection fraction (LVEF) is 84%: in patients with end-systolic LV volume <15mL EF is often overestimated. Nevertheless there is quantitative proof of normal LV wall motion and thickening, with a summed wall motion (SMS) and summed wall thickening score (STS) of 0. The LV time–volume curve shows excellent diastolic function (rapid filling due to rapid relaxation in the early diastolic time and second peak filling due to atrial contraction in the late diastolic phase).

Hybrid imaging

An ideal non-invasive technique for the diagnosis of CAD should provide complementary information on coronary artery anatomy and pathophysiologic lesion severity. This is usually achieved by mental superposition of the information from coronary angiography with that from nuclear MPI. However, standardized myocardial distribution territories correspond in only 50–60% to the real anatomy coronary tree. Multislice X-ray computed tomography (MSCT) has emerged as a valuable alternative to conventional angiography with excellent accuracy in selected patients [11].

The combined use of two data sets both equally contributing to image information is the generally preferred definition of hybrid imaging. By contrast, in the setting of MPI with X-ray based attenuation correction the CT part of the

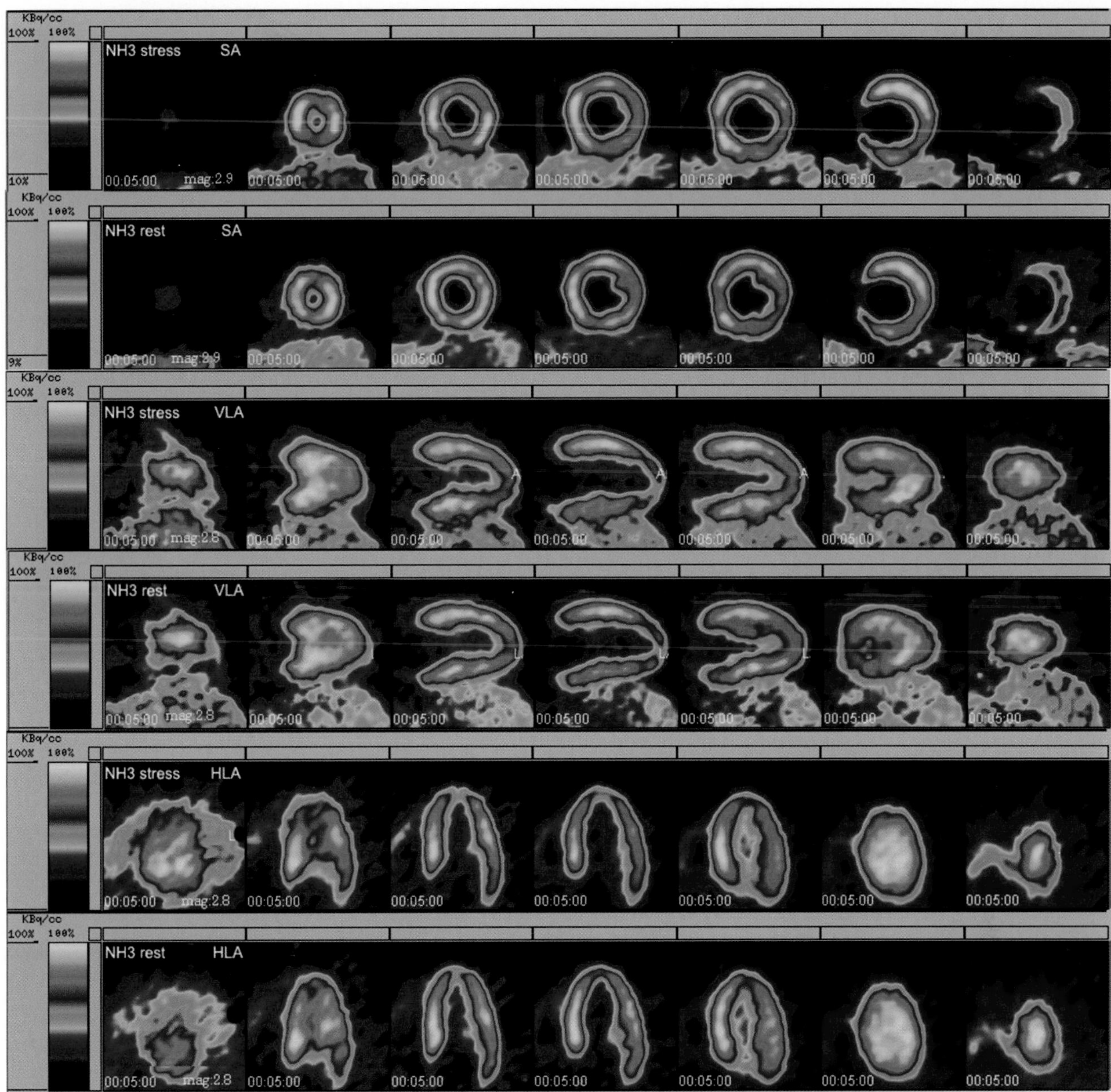

Figure 7.5 PET perfusion scan using ^{13}N-ammonia as perfusion tracer. Short axis (SA), vertical (VLA) and horizontal long axis (HLA) indicate normal perfusion during adenosine stress as well as at rest.

imaging does not provide added anatomical or functional information, but is merely used to improve image quality of the other modality (SPECT or PET). If CT is solely used for attenuation correction of MPI acquired in a PET/CT scanner, the term hybrid imaging should probably not be used as attenuation correction with 68Ge sources used in the previous generation of PET scanners provided the same information as parametric maps obtained from low-dose CT, but this was not perceived as hybrid imaging due to the lack of topographic image information. Furthermore, the term 'hybrid imaging' does not seem appropriate for side-by-side analysis of MPI and CT images, but it has rather been suggested to be used in describing any combination of structural and functional information beyond that of attenuation correction.

The advent of hybrid scanners which are an integration of SPECT or PET with CT reflect the growing interest for the fusion of image data sets from nuclear and CT. Combined with the advancements in fast-processing software for three-dimensional reconstructions, this has allowed initial promising attempts of purely non-invasive CAD assessment directly relating individual myocardial wall territories to the subtending coronary artery by use of SPECT and CT or PET and CT [12].

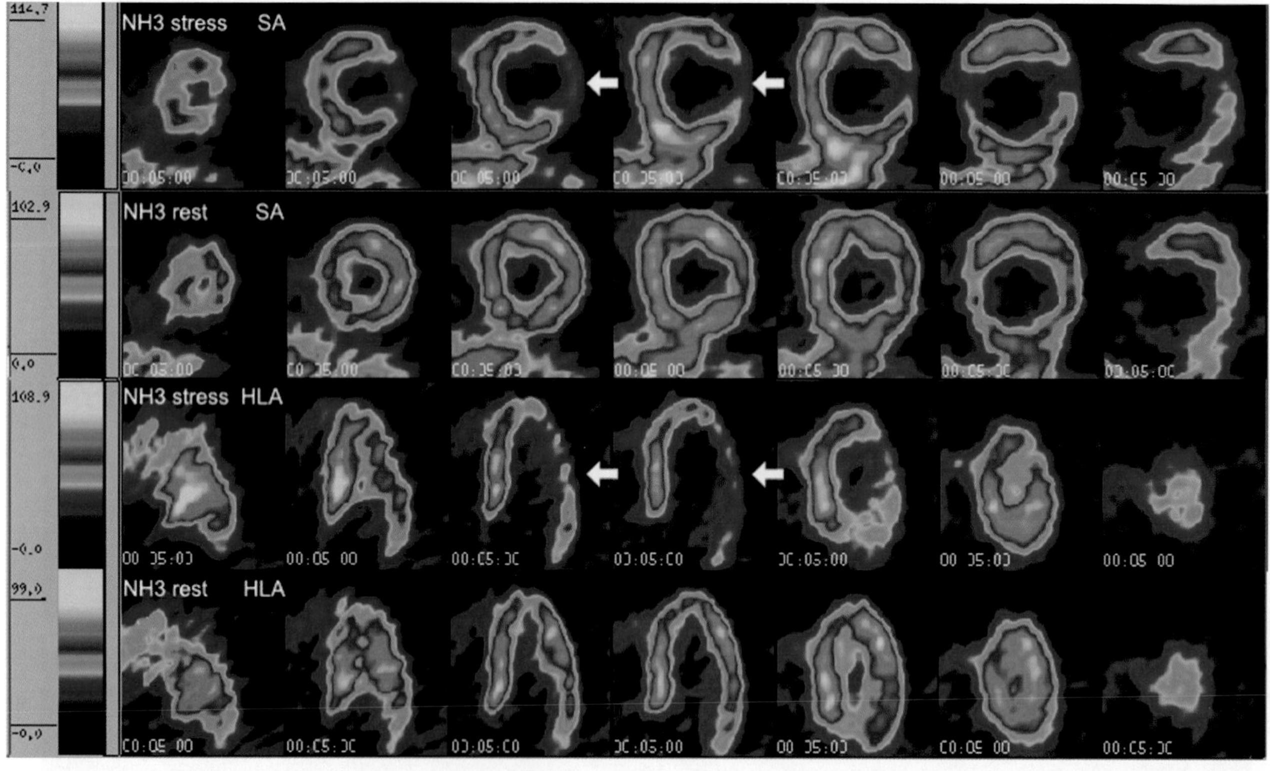

A

Segment	Flow (rest) (mL/min/mL)	Flow (adenosine) (mL/min/mL)	CFR (Norm >2.0)	Flow difference
Septum	0.662	1.891	2.86	1.23
Apex sep	0.657	1.888	2.87	1.23
Mid sep-i	0.746	2.265	3.04	1.52
Mid sep-a	0.618	2.001	3.24	1.38
Basal sep-i	0.706	1.563	2.21	0.86
Basal sep-a	0.592	1.857	3.14	1.27
Anterior	0.515	1.322	2.57	0.81
Apex ant	0.477	1.046	2.19	0.57
Mid ant	0.539	1.232	2.29	0.69
Basal ant	0.515	1.504	2.29	0.99
Lateral	0.557	0.634	1.14	0.08
Apex lat	0.503	0.543	1.08	0.04
Mid lateral	0.632	0.413	0.65	−0.22
Basal lat	0.527	0.831	1.58	0.30
Inferior	0.544	1.861	3.42	1.32
Apex inf	0.562	1.468	2.61	0.91
Mid inf-p	0.512	1.119	2.19	0.61
mid inf-i	0.626	2.562	4.09	1.94
Basal inf-p	0.508	1.851	3.64	1.34
Basal inf-i	0.506	1.996	3.94	1.49
Global	0.561	1.407	2.51	0.85

B

Figure 7.6 (A) Short axis (SA, upper rows) and horizontal long axis cuts (HLA) of PET perfusion scan with ^{13}N-ammonia from a patient with suspected coronary artery disease. The images show a defect in the left ventricular lateral wall that becomes evident during adenosine stress. Blunted hyperaemic response cannot be distinguished from decrease in absolute flow (potentially induced by a steal phenomenon). (B) Quantification of myocardial blood flow reveals absolute decrease in blood flow during adenosine stress, indicating that steal phenomena may be involved. Coronary angiography confirmed subtotal occlusion of the left circumflex coronary artery. Ant, anterior; CFR, coronary flow reserve; inf, inferior; lat, lateral; sep-a, septal anterior; sep-i, septal-inferior.

The increasing interest in cardiac fusion imaging after establishing its clinical feasibility is currently raising the question of its clinical usefulness, which has been confirmed in early preliminary studies [13]. Such evaluation seems pertinent, as the integration of SPECT or PET devices and high-end CT scanners into hybrid scanners will promote the combined use of both techniques in the same patient. Alternatively, however, software solutions for fusion of SPECT or PET information with CT coronary angiography may allow the combination of image sets obtained on separate non-integrated stand-alone scanners. This can be achieved using commercially available software, which has been recently validated [14] (➲ Fig. 7.7). It reliably allows superposition of myocardial segments depicted by SPECT onto cardiac CT anatomy, resulting in an easily interpretable panoramic view of the heart, integrating the high-resolution three-dimensional information of the coronary arteries with the functional information of the SPECT perfusion image. This may facilitate a comprehensive non-invasive assessment of CAD yielding complementary information on a coronary lesion and its pathophysiologic relevance.

Despite many technical advances in invasive coronary angiography, the definition of functionally relevant coronary stenoses by purely morpho-anatomical criteria remains controversial. Although it is generally accepted that a coronary stenosis >50% may start to be haemodynamically relevant, many factors that cannot be fully explored by coronary angiography (including both invasive and CT angiography) will eventually determine whether a given lesion produces stress-induced ischaemia or not. The current approach to mentally match angiographic findings with the SPECT perfusion images faces many difficulties as the planar projections of coronary angiograms and axial slice-by-slice display of SPECT images may lead to inaccurate allocation of the coronary lesion to its subtended myocardial territory (➲ Fig. 7.8). Although fusion of invasive coronary angiography with SPECT has repeatedly been attempted, the warping and three-dimensional unification to force a planar two-dimensional angiogram into a fusion with a three-dimensional perfusion scan data set proved technically unsatisfying. In addition, such an approach would not allow non-invasive preplanning of the intervention as the information on the coronary anatomy is obtained by invasive coronary angiography, when rapid decision making during an ongoing procedure should not be slowed and delayed by the need of time consuming offline analysis. This may explain why such techniques which do not allow careful non-invasive planning of the elective intervention have not been adopted into daily clinical routine.

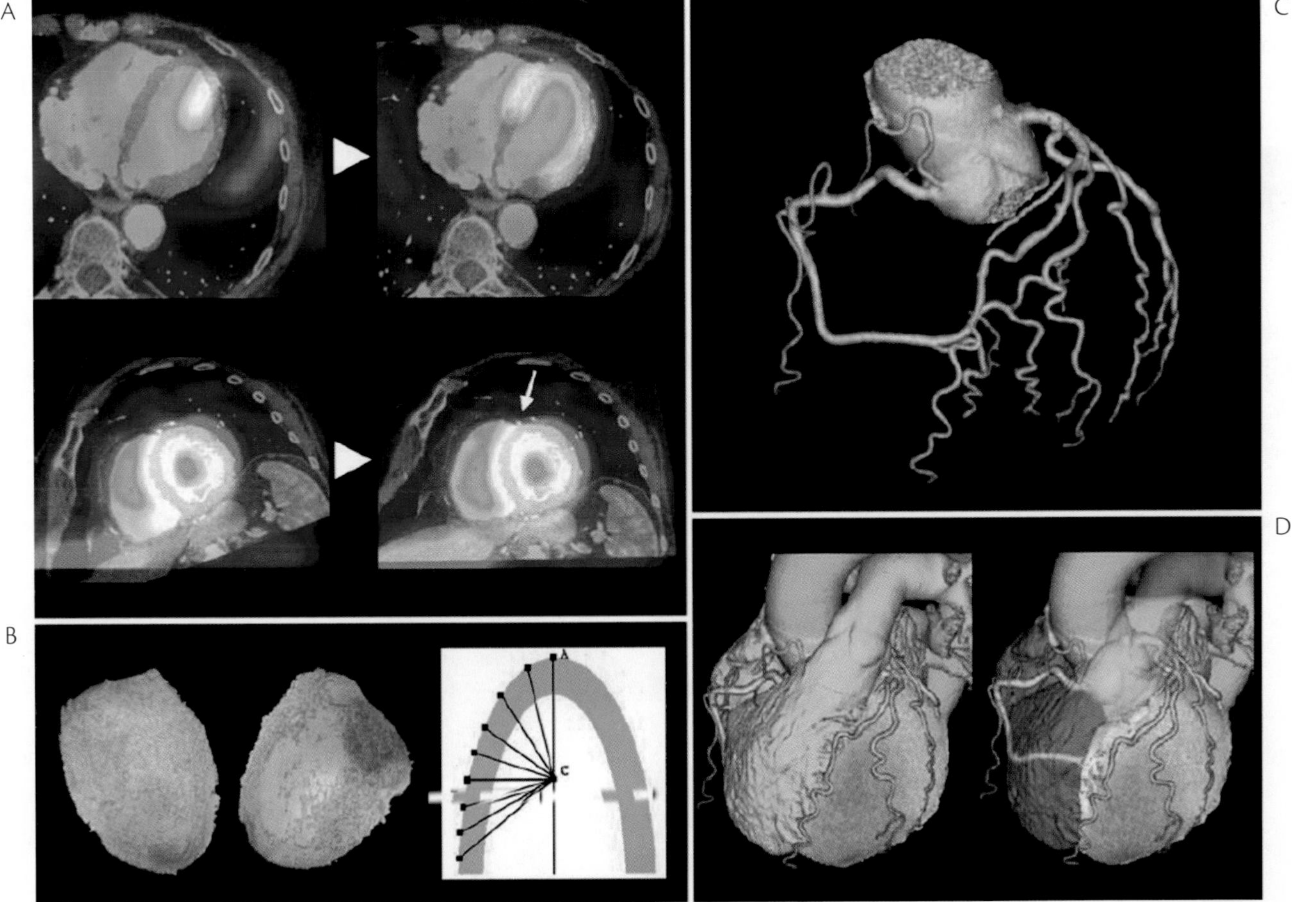

Figure 7.7 Illustration of the main software fusion process including (A) image coregistration; (B) epicardial contour detection; (C) coronary artery segmentation; and (D) three-dimensional volume rendered fusion. Reproduced with permission from Gaemperli O, Schepis T, Kalff V, *et al.* Validation of a new cardiac image fusion software for three-dimensional integration of myocardial perfusion SPECT and stand-alone 64-slice CT angiography. *Eur J Nucl Med Mol Imaging* 2007; **34**: 1097–106.

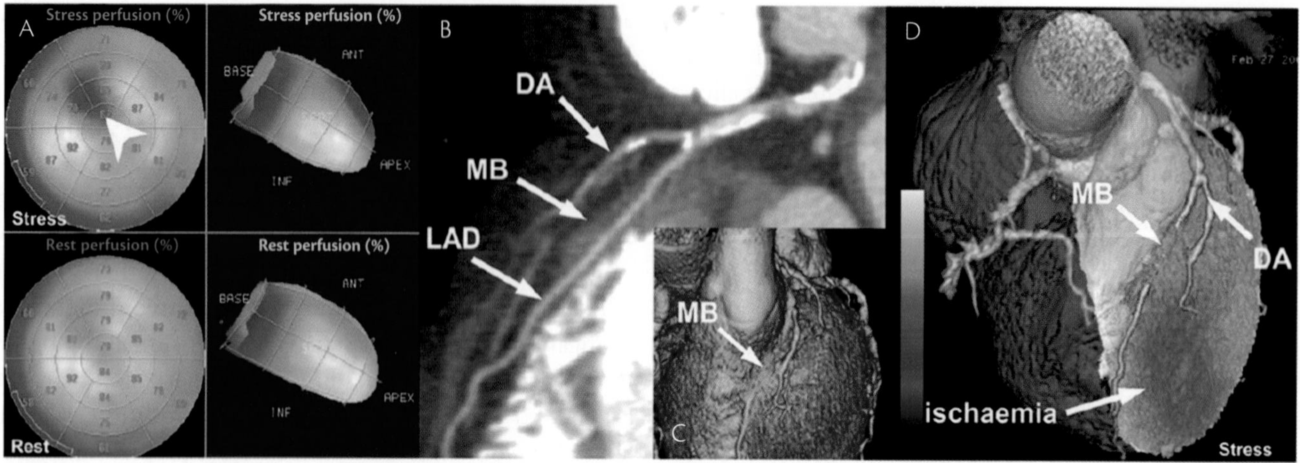

Figure 7.8 (A) Perfusion polar maps at stress (dobutamine stress) and rest show reversible anteroseptal perfusion defect. (B and C) 64-slice CT angiography reveales myocardial bridging (MB) of midventricular left anterior descending artery (LAD) of >2cm length and calcified plaque at origin of first diagonal branch (DA). (D) Fused 3-dimensional SPECT/CT images allocate reversible perfusion defect to DA, whereas MB seems to be haemodynamically insignificant. Reproduced with permission from Gaemperli O, Schepis T, Valenta I, *et al.* Cardiac image fusion from stand-alone SPECT and CT: clinical experience. *J Nucl Med* 2007; **48**: 696–703.

The continuing rapid evolution of CT angiography suggests that, when combined with perfusion imaging, it has the potential to be implemented into clinical practice. This may further help to reduce the frequency of unnecessary angioplasty and stent placement as it should allow evidence driven intervention targeting relevant lesions only (➲ Fig. 7.9).

First clinical results appear encouraging, supporting that hybrid images offer superior diagnostic information with regard to identification of the culprit vessel with the haemodynamic relevant lesion and increase diagnostic confidence for categorizing intermediate lesions and equivocal perfusion defects. Thus, the greatest added

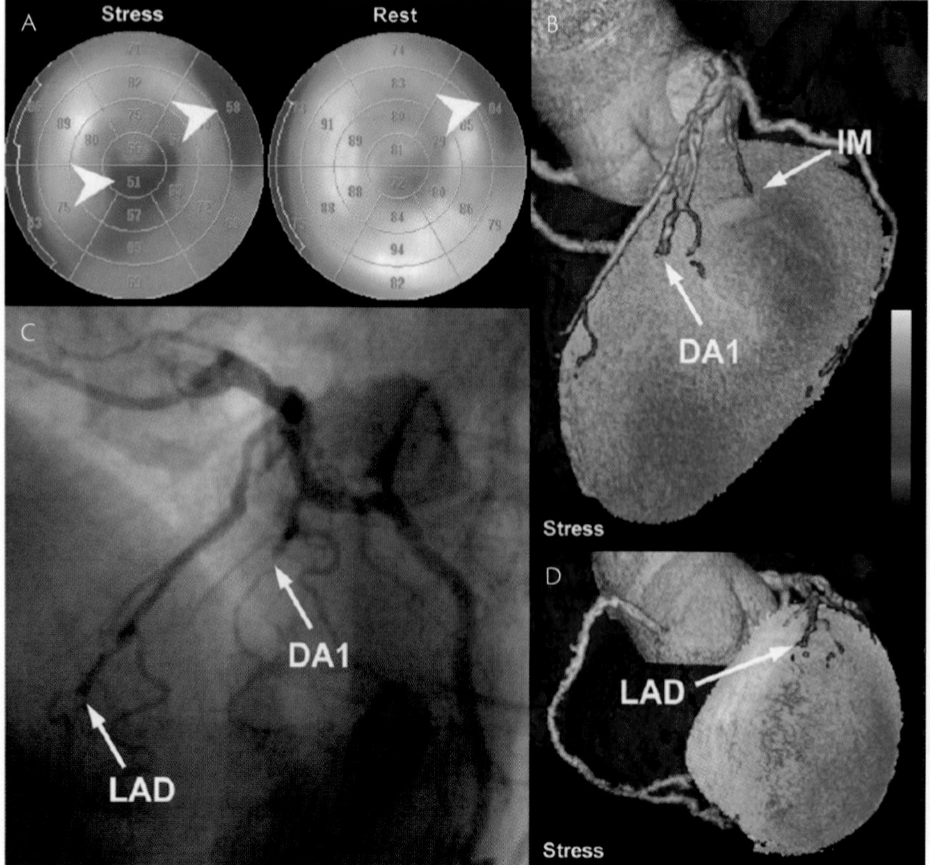

Figure 7.9 (A) Stress and rest perfusion polar maps of SPECT study with mixed basal anterolateral defect and reversible inferoapical perfusion defect (arrowheads). (B) and (D) Fused SPECT/CT images reveal total occlusion of LAD and subtotal occlusion of first diagonal branch (DA1), which are confirmed by conventional coronary angiography (C). Anterolateral perfusion defect is caused by lesion of partially calcified small intermediary branch (IM). However, this vessel is not well visualized by coronary angiography. Reproduced with permission from Gaemperli O, Schepis T, Valenta I, *et al.* Cardiac image fusion from stand-alone SPECT and CT: clinical experience. *J Nucl Med* 2007; **48**: 696–703.

value seems to be firm exclusion of haemodynamic relevance of coronary abnormalities seen on CT angiography. Results from a first multicentre study underline the value of a combined functional and anatomical approach even without hybrid imaging showing that this combination allows improved risk stratification [15]. The clinical usefulness in terms of impact on treatment strategy and subsequently on outcome by hybrid imaging remains, however, to be determined in long-term studies. Similarly, it remains uncertain at this point whether hybrid scanners offer advantages over software fusion of data sets obtained from different scanners, as by either way one can obtain hybrid images (➲ Fig. 7.10). The discrepancy between emission from SPECT and CT transmission scan times determines that high-end CT facilities constituting the CT component of hybrid cardiac scanners will be blocked by long emission scan time and is therefore forced to operate at low capacity. On the other hand, a combined device may fit into one room, needs one operating team, and does not require positioning of the patient into two different scanners. The development of ultrafast SPECT scanners allowing substantially shorter acquisition time may shift the balance towards hybrid scanners in the future.

Acute coronary syndromes (➲Chapter 16)

Chest pain unit

The majority of patients presenting to emergency departments with chest pain are admitted because the initial clinical examination, ECG results, and cardiac enzyme levels are insufficient to exclude an acute coronary syndrome, although most patients without obvious ECG changes do not have an acute syndrome. Conversely, a substantial minority of patients who are discharged from the emergency department have undetected acute ischaemia and an adverse outcome. Because the main feature of an acute coronary syndrome is reduced myocardial perfusion, MPS in the emergency department can provide important diagnostic and prognostic information. It has not been used widely because of the logistical problems of providing an acute radionuclide imaging service, but several studies have now shown the effectiveness and cost-effectiveness of MPS in the acute setting, especially when the resting ECG is not diagnostic of myocardial ischaemia. A resting perfusion defect has a high positive predictive value for acute infarction in patients without a history of previous myocardial infarction, particularly if it is associated with a wall motion abnormality on gated imaging, and these patients should be admitted to the coronary care unit. Conversely, a normal perfusion scan excludes acute infarction and exercise ECG or stress MPS can be the next diagnostic steps. If the perfusion tracer can be injected during chest pain, a normal perfusion scan excludes a cardiac cause and allows the patient to be discharged. In patients with symptoms suggestive of an acute coronary syndrome, acute MPS reduces unnecessary hospital admission without reducing appropriate admission of patients with a genuine acute coronary syndrome [16]. The sensitivity of acute rest MPS for the diagnosis of myocardial infarction is high very early after the onset of ischaemia, in contrast to serum enzyme markers, which require several hours to become clearly abnormal. Patients discharged with normal MPS have a very low likelihood of future cardiac events whereas patients with abnormal scans are at higher risk [17].

An intriguing option in patients with acute chest pain that has settled is to perform SPECT with free fatty acids (e.g. ^{123}I-(p-iodophenyl)-3-(R,S)methyl-pentadecanoic

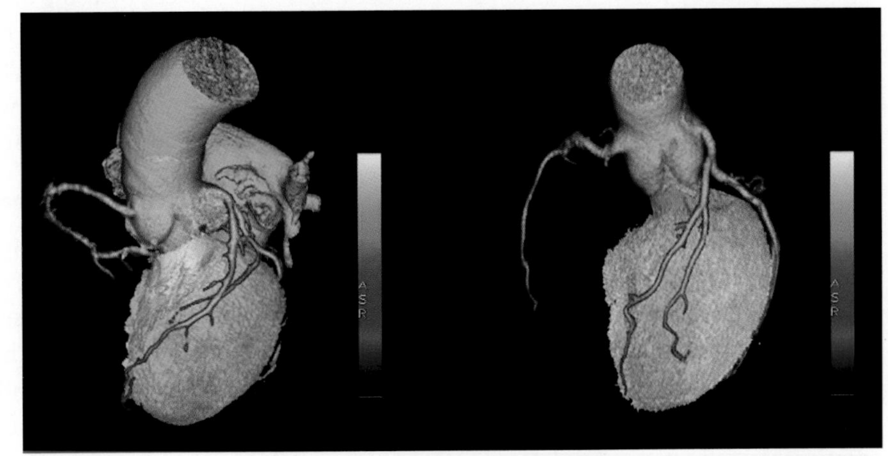

Figure 7.10 Hybrid images combining information on cardiac and coronary anatomy with that on perfusion can be obtained either on a hybrid scanner or by using software fusion of separately acquired datasets from two scanners. (A) Hybrid cardiac image obtained on a hybrid PET/CT scanner (GE healthcare) using ^{13}N-ammonia for perfusion. (B) Hybrid image obtained by fusing a SPECT MPI from a gamma camera (Ventry) with a CT angiography obtained on a standalone 64-slice CT (both GE Healthcare). Image quality is identical and the two images cannot be distinguished although providing comparable or even equivalent information. Perfusion was assessed in both patients during adenosine stress.

acid [BMIPP]) since fatty acid metabolism is reduced for some time after acute ischaemia has resolved. This 'metabolic memory' might allow diagnosis for up to 24 hours after ischaemic chest pain and the theory is proven in principle although it has not been widely applied.

Risk assessment after myocardial infarction

Because the prognosis of ST segment elevation myocardial infarction (STEMI) is determined by left ventricular ejection fraction (LVEF), infarct size, and residual viable myocardium, radionuclide techniques provide important information that aids patient management. MPS provides additional prognostic information over clinical factors and LVEF and coronary angiography may not provide prognostic information beyond this. MPS with vasodilator stress allows risk to be assessed safely 2–5 days after infarction and is superior to early sub-maximal exercise testing. Even when used a few weeks after infarction MPS.

Patients with small, fixed perfusion defects have a good prognosis, and are unlikely to benefit from invasive investigation and revascularization. Conversely, patients with MPS markers of high risk can be referred for coronary angiography and possible revascularization, although the superiority of revascularization over medical therapy has not been established in this setting. Although primary percutaneous coronary intervention is the treatment of choice in STEMI, it is not currently available in all centres and some patients present too late for alternative thrombolysis. When this is the case MPS is very helpful for risk stratification and a large prospective randomized trial (INSPIRE—AdenosINE Sestamibi SPECT Post InfaRction Evaluation) using gated SPECT MPS and adenosine stress has determined the value of MPS to assess risk [18] and to guide subsequent therapeutic decision making in clinically stable patients early after acute myocardial infarction [19]. The INSPIRE results establish that the perfusion variables obtained by MPS, i.e. total and ischaemic perfusion defect size, improve the precision for assessing risk beyond that provided by the Thrombolysis In Myocardial Infarction (TIMI) risk score alone or when combined with LVEF. The cornerstone of risk stratification in stable survivors of an acute myocardial infarction is rapid discrimination of patients at high risk who might benefit from coronary revascularization from low-risk patients for whom medical therapy and early hospital discharge is appropriate. The INSPIRE trial proved that this goal can be achieved using MPS. In the interventional part of the trial confined to high-risk patients, both intensive medical therapy and revascularization produced comparable reductions (and frequently elimination) of both total and ischaemic perfusion defect sizes on follow-up scans. This resulted in no difference between the two groups with regards to total cardiac events, cardiac death, and reinfarction. In hospitals without cardiac catheterization facilities, MPS can identify those patients who do not require transfer to another facility for cardiac catheterization and can be discharged safely at an early date. In unstable angina and non-STEMI an early invasive strategy is recommended for patients with indicators of high risk and no serious comorbidities and this can be assessed by exercise ECG and by MPS. MPS is particularly useful for risk assessment of unstable angina once stabilized.

Specific patient populations

The exercise ECG has moderate specificity for the detection of CAD in the absence of resting repolarization abnormalities, left ventricular hypertrophy, and if patients are not treated with digoxin. Thus, when the resting ECG is normal and the likelihood of CAD from clinical assessment is low (for instance <25%) a stepwise strategy is appropriate with an exercise ECG as the initial diagnostic test. When the likelihood of CAD is very low (for instance <10%) then the best strategy will be reassurance without any provocative testing. If the resting ECG is abnormal or the likelihood of CAD is >25% then MPS may be the better initial test on grounds of cost-effectiveness [2].

Women

The exercise ECG has lower specificity for the detection of CAD in women than in men and so MPS is a better diagnostic test even at lower likelihoods of disease. Pharmacological stress MPS is particularly valuable in women who are unable to exercise maximally. Although perfusion images are susceptible to breast attenuation artefacts, specificity can be maintained with awareness of the potential for artefacts, by using of ^{99m}Tc perfusion tracers rather than ^{201}Tl, and employing ECG-gating and attenuation correction. Sensitivity of MPS is similar in men and women. PET perfusion imaging, when available, may be an additional way of avoiding attenuation artefacts.

Normal ECG, unable to exercise

Patients unable to exercise because of physical limitations such as arthritis, amputations, peripheral vascular disease, or pulmonary disease should undergo MPS with pharmacological stress as the initial diagnostic test. Inability to exercise is itself an adverse prognostic indicator, presumably because of the increased incidence of CAD, and this should be borne in mind when interpreting MPS in these subjects.

Conduction abnormality (➲Chapter 27)

Patients with conduction abnormalities such as left bundle branch block, bifascicular block, and paced rhythms may have inducible and fixed perfusion abnormalities on MPS even in the absence of underlying CAD, particularly when imaged during exercise or dobutamine stress (➲ Fig. 7.11). Similar defects are much less common in patients with right bundle branch block although they can occur. These defects most commonly are confined to the septum although they can be more extensive. The causes of these defects in patients with conduction abnormalities are still uncertain and likely to be multifactorial, but they generally reflect true perfusion heterogeneities related to delayed septal relaxation and shorter diastolic perfusion time, or possibly to reduced regional afterload and hence reduced myocardial oxygen demand. Fixed defects may be due to reduced myocardial thickening or they may result from an underlying myocardial abnormality such as cardiomyopathy.

The specificity of MPS for the detection of CAD is therefore reduced in these patients when dynamic exercise is used, but specificity is maintained using vasodilator stress if the heart rate does not increase significantly. In practice, when there is a diagnostic problem in a patient with left bundle branch block or paced rhythm, MPS should be performed with adenosine or dipyridamole without additional exercise. A normal study excludes underlying coronary obstruction but an abnormal study may be less helpful diagnostically.

Type 2 diabetes (➲Chapter 14)

Myocardial ischaemia in patients with type 2 diabetes is often asymptomatic and frequently in an advanced stage when it becomes clinically manifest. Once coronary artery disease is symptomatic in diabetes, it is associated with a morbidity and mortality significantly higher than in patients without diabetes. In a large study in patients with type 2 diabetes (DIAD—Detection of Ischemia in Asymptomatic Diabetics trial) silent ischaemia was found in more than one in five asymptomatic patients [20]. In the follow-up a resolution of ischaemia occurred in the majority of these patients [21]. These unexpected results highlight the importance of studying whether a strategy of screening for inducible ischaemia impacts on clinical outcomes in such patients. So far it remains unclear whether the observed resolution of ischaemia which was associated with an intensification of the medical treatment was causally related to initial screening.

Prognosis of coronary artery disease

Beyond diagnosis, the most valuable contribution that MPS can make to the management of known or suspected CAD is to assess the likelihood of a future coronary event such as myocardial infarction or coronary death. Prognosis is strongly influenced by the extent and severity of inducible perfusion defects and this can guide the need for further invasive investigation and revascularization. MPS is a more powerful prognostic indicator than clinical assessment, the exercise ECG, and coronary angiography, and provides incremental prognostic value even once the other tests have been performed.

The most important variables that predict the likelihood of future events are the extent and depth of the inducible perfusion abnormality. The relative value of the fixed component of a stress defect is unclear, but it is likely that left ventricular function is the best indicator of prognosis in

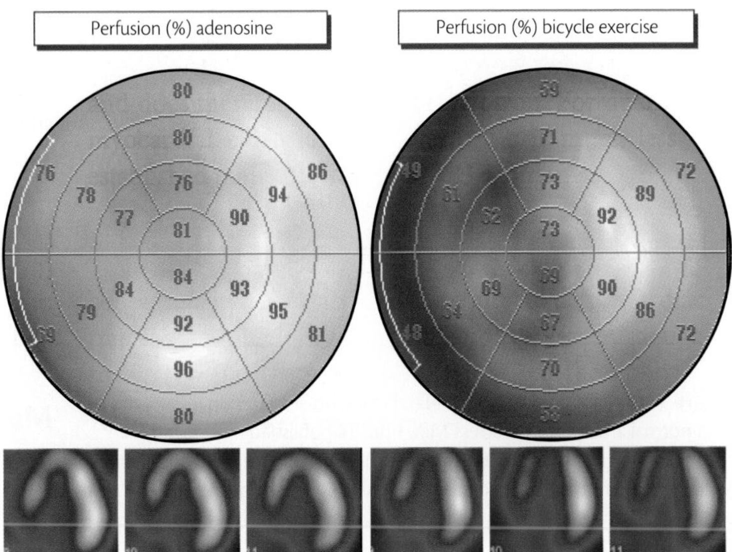

Figure 7.11 Polar maps of two perfusion scans, obtained using different stressors, in the same patient with left bundle branch block. During adenosine stress (left) perfusion is homogenous while during bicycle exercise stress (right) there is reduced septal perfusion despite normal coronary arteries.

patients with predominantly fixed defects. Thus, the patient with extensive ischaemia is at high risk of a coronary event and sudden death irrespective of the presence of infarction, and the patient without ischaemia, but with a fixed defect is only at risk if the defect leads to significantly impaired function. Additional markers of risk are increased lung uptake on stress thallium images, since this indicates raised pulmonary capillary pressure either at rest or in response to stress, and ventricular dilation that is greater in stress thallium images than at rest. Transient ischaemic dilation can also be seen with technetium imaging and it may be the result of extensive sub-endocardial ischaemia giving the impression of cavity dilation.

In patients with known or suspected CAD, a normal perfusion scan is very valuable because it indicates a likelihood of coronary events of <1% per year [22], a rate that is lower than that in an asymptomatic population (➲ Fig. 7.12). Thus whether non-obstructive CAD is present or not, further investigation can be avoided. This negative predictive value is independent of the imaging agent and technique, the method of stress, the population studied, and the clinical setting. Exercise radionuclide ventriculography has also been used to assess prognosis because abnormal regional contraction is an early manifestation of inducible ischaemia. Stress LVEF provides more information than resting LVEF since it reflects the extent of both infarction and transient ischaemia. However, the comparative prognostic value of perfusion imaging and exercise ventriculography has not been fully assessed, although it has been suggested that knowledge of rest and stress LVEF from resting gated MPS and stress first-pass ventriculography provides additional prognostic information compared with the perfusion information alone.

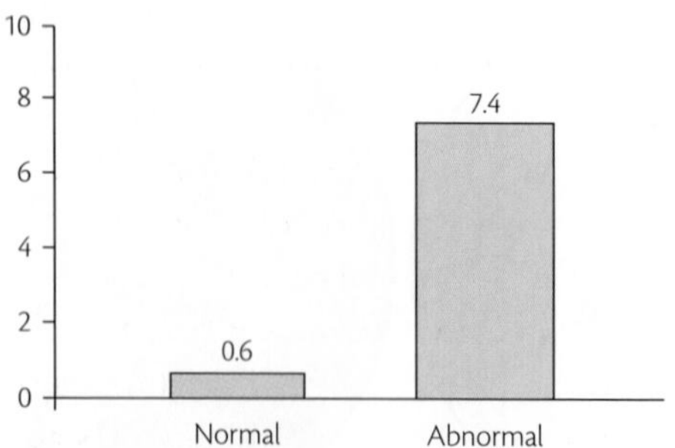

Figure 7.12 Rate of death or non-fatal myocardial infarction in patients with normal and abnormal stress MPS from 14 published reports comprising more than 12,000 patients. Reproduced with permission from Iskander S, Iskandrian AE. Risk assessment using single-photon emission computed tomographic technetium-99m sestamibi imaging. *J Am Coll Cardiol* 1998; **32**:57–62.

Preoperative risk assessment (➲ Chapter 34)

A common clinical problem is that of assessing cardiac risk in patients that require non-cardiac surgery. In this as in other clinical settings, MPS provides useful information although these patients are generally at low cardiac risk and the predictive value of a normal perfusion study is greater than that of an abnormal study. Whether investigation beyond simple clinical assessment is required should be based upon the urgency of the surgery and its own cardiac risk, the risk factors of the individual, and his or her exercise tolerance. Patients with only minor clinical predictors (age >70 years, abnormal resting ECG, history of stroke or hypertension) who require low- (endoscopic or superficial procedures, cataract surgery, and breast surgery) to moderate-risk surgery (carotid endarterectomy, head and neck surgery, intraperitoneal and intrathoracic surgery, orthopaedic surgery, and prostate surgery), are not at high risk and do not require further investigation. Patients with intermediate clinical predictors (stable angina, prior infarction, treated heart failure or diabetes) or with minor predictors and impaired exercise tolerance need further assessment if they are to undergo moderate- or high-risk surgery. Patients at high clinical risk (recent infarction or unstable angina, decompensated heart failure, or significant arrhythmias) require investigation even for low-risk surgery.

For patients who are able to exercise, further investigation normally means exercise ECG, but if the resting ECG is abnormal or in patients who are unable to exercise, MPS should be used instead. If further testing suggests a low risk, then surgery can proceed as planned. If it suggests a high risk then the need for coronary angiography and revascularization is determined by the clinical setting. In general terms, revascularization should not be performed if it would not have been performed in the absence of surgery since the risk of revascularization may still exceed the risk of non-cardiac surgery. In patients at intermediate risk after further testing, the best strategy is uncertain but aggressive medical management at the time of surgery rather than revascularization is preferred. This medical management involves rigorous control of pain, fluid balance, and coagulation state after surgery, as well as preoperative beta-blockade and possibly perioperative nitrate infusion.

Management of myocardial revascularization (➲ Chapter 17)

MPS can be valuable both before and after myocardial revascularization, either by angioplasty or bypass surgery.

Neither procedure should be undertaken without objective evidence of ischaemia, and perfusion imaging is often the most reliable way of obtaining this information and of ensuring that angioplasty is targeted at the culprit lesion [23]. It has an excellent negative predictive value for predicting restenosis and clinical events after angioplasty, and this can be particularly helpful in patients with recurrent, but atypical, symptoms. Routine MPS after angioplasty in the absence of symptoms is not common, although it can sometimes be useful as a new baseline in case symptoms recur. It can however be justified routinely in patients with impaired left ventricular function, proximal disease of the left anterior descending coronary artery and multivessel disease, suboptimal results of angioplasty, diabetes, and those with occupations requiring low coronary risk. If MPS is performed after angioplasty, then it should ideally be performed at least 6 weeks after the procedure since perfusion abnormalities can persist for some time even with a good anatomical result. Possible exceptions to this are patients with high-risk anatomy who can benefit from earlier imaging.

As with angioplasty, patients who are asymptomatic after bypass surgery do not routinely undergo perfusion imaging, although it can be helpful as a baseline for future management since revascularization is not infrequently incomplete. More commonly it is used for follow-up and it can be used roughly 5 years after surgery to guard against silent progression of prognostically important disease. Patients with symptoms after surgery may certainly benefit from MPS and the algorithms to be used are very similar to those in the diagnostic setting.

Myocardial infarction (➲Chapter 16)

Infarct detection

The diagnosis of acute myocardial infarction is normally made from the clinical history, the ECG, and from cardiac enzymes. In most cases these provide a conclusive answer but the diagnosis can be unclear in those seen late after the onset of chest pain, those with a conduction abnormality or pacemaker, those with perioperative infarction, and those in whom right ventricular infarction is a possibility. Nuclear techniques may then be helpful.

A number of radiopharmaceuticals have an affinity for acutely necrotic myocardium. Imaging of ^{99m}Tc-pyrophosphate has a sensitivity of at least 85% for the detection of acute infarction when performed 1–3 days after the event. Specificity is lower because uptake may occur in areas of old infarction or aneurysm, and also in areas of subclinical myocardial damage after unstable angina. Persistent blood pool activity or activity in bone and skeletal muscles can also cause difficulties, although these may be overcome by tomographic acquisition. In clinical practice, the technique is not used commonly, but it can be helpful in cases of doubt.

Imaging with antimyosin antibodies labelled with indium has also been used and it has both high sensitivity and specificity. A multicentre trial of 492 patients showed sensitivities of 94% in Q-wave infarction and 84% in non-Q-wave infarction. Specificity was 93% in patients with chest pain but no infarction and there was focal uptake in 48% of patients with unstable angina suggesting sub-clinical infarction [24]. Despite this, the long time that is required after injection to obtain images limits its use for the early detection of infarction. This is also a drawback when using this compound for the detection of myocarditis and transplant rejection.

Myocardial salvage

Because ^{99m}Tc labelled perfusion agents (MIBI and tetrofosmin) do not redistribute, they can be used in acute infarction to demonstrate the territory at risk before thrombolysis or acute angioplasty, and to assess the amount of myocardial salvage. The tracer is injected immediately before intervention and imaging can be performed several hours later once the intervention is complete and the clinical situation is stable. The defect will then correspond to the territory at risk and repeat injection and imaging several days later will show the actual extent of infarction. This is not a technique that can guide the need for intervention but it has been used in a number of clinical trials to assess the effect of acute intervention and to compare different regimens of thrombolysis on infarct size.

Management after infarction

An important aspect of clinical management after infarction is to identify patients at high risk of further events such as re-infarction or death, and hopefully to intervene in order to prevent these events. Clinical indicators of high risk in the acute phase include hypotension, left ventricular failure, and malignant arrhythmias and these patients are candidates for early coronary angiography. After the acute phase however, prognosis is related to the degree of left ventricular dysfunction and the extent and severity of residual ischaemia, and radionuclide imaging can assess both objectively. LVEF at the time of discharge or 10–14 days after infarction is a strong predictor of mortality, and patients with impaired function in particular can benefit from MPS to assess whether viable but jeopardized myocardium remains in the infarct zone and whether remote territories may also be jeopardized by ischaemia.

Heart failure: myocardial viability and hibernation

The term'viable' is an umbrella term that includes several different subtypes of myocardium. One of these is hibernating myocardium, which is chronically dysfunctional but still viable myocardium that recovers function after coronary revascularization. For many years the functional sequelae of chronic CAD were considered to be irreversible and amenable only to palliative therapy. For example, akinesis on the left ventriculogram implied infarcted myocardium or scar. We now know that chronic left ventricular dysfunction in patients with CAD is not necessarily irreversible and areas of akinetic myocardium have frequently been observed to improve in function after revascularisation.

In 1978 Diamond *et al.* [25] suggested the possibility that 'ischaemic non-infarcted myocardium can exist in a state of function hibernation'. Several years later Rahimtoola [26] popularized the concept of hibernating myocardium and noted 'there is a prolonged subacute or chronic stage of myocardial ischaemia that is frequently not accompanied by pain and in which myocardial contractility and metabolism and ventricular function are reduced to match the reduced blood supply'. It is now known that perfusion is not always significantly reduced at rest in myocardial hibernation, but the debate on whether resting myocardial blood flow to hibernating myocardium is reduced or not has attracted a lot of interest and, undoubtedly, has contributed significantly to stimulate new research on heart failure patients with coronary artery disease. Although the debate is not over yet, some of the initial paradigms have been shown to be incorrect while new pathophysiological concepts have emerged. Clinically, the concept of hibernation has made a significant contribution to our understanding and management of patients with advanced ischaemic left ventricular dysfunction. Failure to identify and rescue hibernating myocardium may lead to loss of viable myocytes, progressive deterioration of heart failure, and death. A number of imaging techniques have been used to detect viable myocardium and to characterize it as hibernating.

Positron emission tomography

Initial studies indicated that myocardial hibernation and infarction could be distinguished by a combination of PET perfusion imaging using ^{13}N-ammonia and metabolic imaging using the glucose analogue ^{18}F-fluorodeoxyglucose (FDG) after an oral glucose load. Regions with a concordant reduction in both ^{13}N-ammonia and FDG uptake ('perfusion-metabolism match', ➲ Fig. 7.13) were predominantly infarcted, whereas regions with reduced ^{13}N-ammonia uptake but preserved or increased FDG uptake ('perfusion-metabolism mismatch', ➲ Fig. 7.13) were hibernating [27]. Myocardial FDG uptake, however, depends on many factors such as dietary state, cardiac workload, insulin sensitivity, sympathetic drive, and the presence and severity of ischaemia. These factors lead to variable FDG uptake in the fasted or glucose-loaded state and complicate image interpretation.

Semi-quantitative and quantitative analyses of FDG uptake improve the detection of viable myocardium but require standardization of imaging conditions particularly with regard to myocardial glucose uptake. Many patients with CAD are insulin resistant and have poor FDG image quality after an oral glucose load. Myocardial glucose metabolism can therefore be standardized using the hyperinsulinaemic euglycaemic clamp, essentially the simultaneous infusion of insulin and glucose acting on the tissue as a metabolic challenge and stimulating maximal FDG uptake [28]. This allows absolute values of glucose metabolism to be measured (μmol/g/min) and aids comparisons between different subjects and centres (➲ Fig. 7.14). To determine the threshold value above which the best prediction of improvement in functional class of at least one grade could be obtained, in a prospective study in 24 patients undergoing coronary revascularization, a receiver-operator-characteristic curve (ROC) was constructed. According to this analysis the optimal operating point on the curve (point of best compromise between sensitivity and specificity) was at the absolute threshold of FDG uptake of 0.25μmol/g/min (where the gold standard was the evidence of functional recovery at follow up) [29]. By comparing FDG images obtained under these conditions with regional wall motion from another imaging technique, the need for a simultaneous perfusion tracer is avoided.

In summary, clinically there is now wide consensus on the importance of identifying and treating hibernating myocardium in patients with coronary artery disease and heart failure. Although randomized studies are needed before a definitive influence on clinical practice is achieved, the contribution of the existing experimental studies is compelling.

Single photon tracers

The disadvantage of PET is that it is not widely available. Thallium provides information on both myocardial perfusion and viability and has been widely used for identifying myocardial hibernation. Because redistribution can

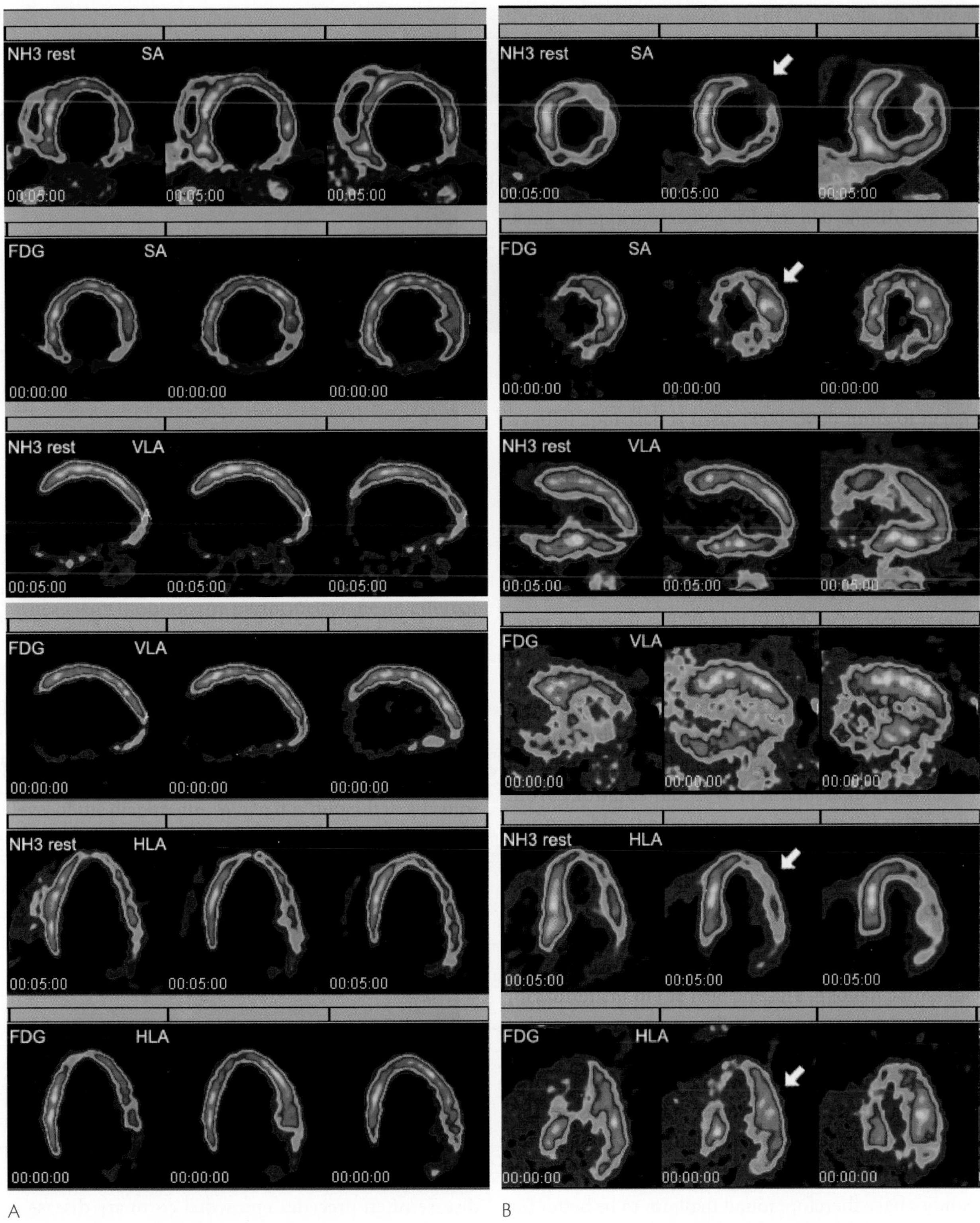

Figure 7.13 Short axis (SA), vertical long axis (VLA) and horizontal long axis (HLA) tomograms of ^{13}N-ammonia (NH3) perfusion at rest and ^{18}F-fluorodeoxy-glucose (FDG) metabolism. (A) Matched inferior defect of perfusion and metabolism indicating infarction without viable myocardium. (B) Antero-lateral defect of perfusion with preserved FDG uptake indicating viable tissue. The mismatch of perfusion and metabolism indicates hibernating myocardium (white arrow).

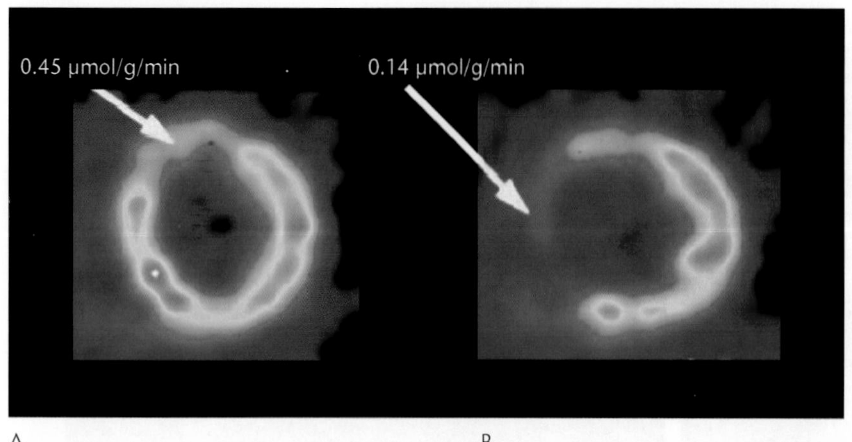

Figure 7.14 Quantitative images of myocardial ^{18}F-fluorodeoxy-glucose (FDG) uptake. (A) The anterior wall is viable with FDG uptake above the threshold of 0.25μmol/g/min. (B) The septum does not contain clinically significant viable myocardium.

be slow or incomplete in regions of reduced perfusion, the usual stress/redistribution protocol can underestimate myocardial viability and additional steps to ensure complete assessment of viability are required. These include late redistribution imaging at 8–24 hours after stress injection, re-injection of tracer at rest after redistribution imaging, and a resting injection on a separate day with both early and delayed imaging.

In any of these viability images, the amount of viable myocardium is proportional to the amount of tracer uptake relative to a normal area. A common threshold for defining clinically significant viability is 50% of maximal uptake although the best threshold may be higher. In addition to detecting viable myocardium in an area of akinesis it is important to demonstrate inducible ischaemia before diagnosing hibernation since hibernation is an ischaemic syndrome.

MIBI and tetrofosmin have also been used for the detection of viable and hibernating myocardium. In theory these tracers may underestimate viability in areas with reduced resting perfusion because they are combined tracers of viability and perfusion without the property of redistribution that allows viability to be assessed independently. This results in a high positive but low negative predictive value. Some studies have therefore found thallium to be better for the assessment of viability but others have found them to provide comparable information. It does appear though that if the tracers are given under the cover of intravenous or sublingual nitrates, then resting perfusion is improved and the technetium tracers may be used as markers of viability.

ECG-gated SPECT

An important problem in studies of hibernation is that viability and function are often assessed from different techniques, and it can be difficult to be sure that the same myocardial segments are being compared. Thus, the ideal technique should combine information on viability, perfusion, and function in a single image, and ECG-gated technetium MPS is very helpful. In regions of previous infarction with reduced tracer uptake, the assessment is more difficult, but this is not a major limitation since these areas contain little viable myocardium and may not benefit from revascularization.

Microvascular disease (➲ Chapter 17)

Until recently, ischaemic heart disease was primarily thought to be caused by disease of large vessels, particularly the conduit coronary arteries. However, it is now clear that abnormalities of the coronary microcirculation may contribute to the generation of ischaemia even in the absence of demonstrable disease of the large epicardial arteries. Microvascular disease often precedes epicardial coronary disease and its extent may have independent prognostic value.

Myocardial perfusion reserve is the ratio of myocardial perfusion during maximal coronary vasodilation and at baseline. It is an integrated measure of flow through the epicardial coronary arteries and perfusion through the microcirculation and it can be used to assess the function of

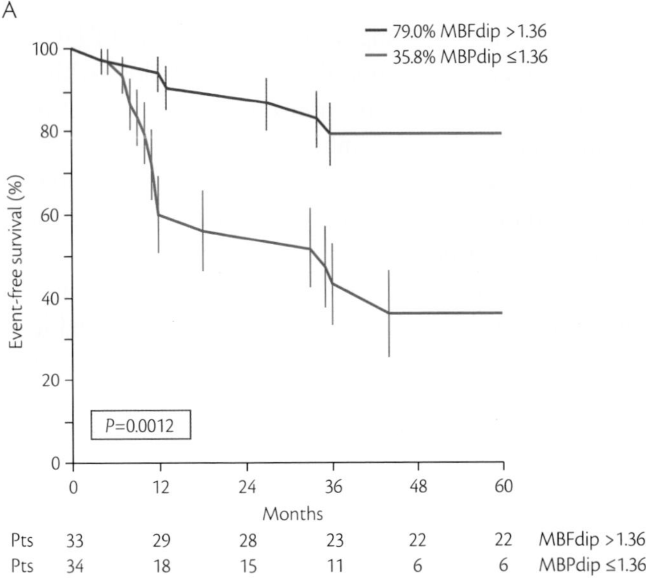

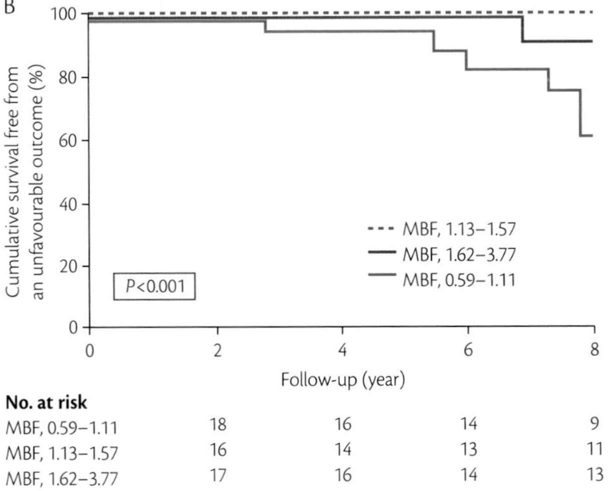

Figure 7.15 Kaplan–Meier event-free survival curves over 5 years in patients with dilated (A) and hypertrophic cardiomyopathy (A). Event-free survival is lowest in those patients with a severely blunted blood flow response to dipyridamole. Reproduced with permission from Cecchi F, Olivotto I, Gistri R, *et al.* Coronary microvascular dysfunction and prognosis in hypertrophic cardiomyopathy. *N Engl J Med* 2003; **349**: 1027–35. Neglia D, Michelassi C, Trivieri MG, *et al.* Prognostic role of myocardial blood flow impairment in idiopathic left ventricular dysfunction. *Circulation* 2002; **105**: 186–93.

the coronary circulation as a whole. An abnormal perfusion reserve can be due to narrowing of the epicardial coronary arteries or, in the absence of angiographically demonstrable atherosclerotic disease, may reflect dysfunction of the coronary microcirculation. The latter can be caused by structural (e.g. vascular remodelling with reduced lumen to wall ratio) or functional (e.g. vasoconstriction) changes, which may involve neurohumoral factors and/or endothelial dysfunction. Furthermore, an abnormal perfusion reserve may also reflect changes in coronary and/or systemic haemodynamics as well as changes in extravascular coronary resistance (e.g. increased intramyocardial pressure).

The coronary microcirculation cannot be imaged directly in man in vivo. The resistance vessels in the coronary circulation are not generally visible on angiography and are too small to be catheterized selectively. Instead, indirect parameters such as myocardial perfusion and perfusion reserve can be used since, in the absence of coronary stenoses, they provide an index of microvascular function.

PET can be used to measure both absolute myocardial perfusion and perfusion reserve and microvascular dysfunction has been demonstrated in patients with hypercholesterolaemia, hypertension, diabetes, and smoking. The measurements can also be used as surrogate endpoints to assess the effectiveness of therapeutic interventions such as alpha- and beta-adrenoreceptor blockade [30], lipid-lowering, antioxidants [31], cardiovascular conditioning, and coronary angioplasty. They also provide prognostic information [32, 33] and microvascular dysfunction assessed by PET is an independent predictor of long-term outcome and cardiovascular death in patients with hypertrophic and dilated cardiomyopathies (➲ Fig. 7.15). The best established flow tracers are ^{15}O-water and ^{13}N-ammonia. The short half-lives (2min and 9.8min, respectively) require an on-site cyclotron for the use of these isotopes. As an alternative, ^{68}Rb has been introduced, which is a generator product and does therefore not need a cyclotron. For quantifying myocardial perfusion, however, ^{68}Rb is much less well established than ^{15}O-water and ^{13}N-ammonia.

Personal perspective

The first nuclear cardiology examinations were performed as early as 1927, when Blumgart and Weiss measured circulation times by intravenously injected radon gas. The next milestone followed in 1965 when Anger and colleagues first demonstrated the ability to define cardiac transit with a single-crystal scintillation camera. Although the 1970s and the early 1980s witnessed the onset of quantification of planar and tomographic imaging with SPECT and later with PET, it was only two decades ago that the prognostic applications of stress radionuclide imaging modalities were defined and pharmacologic stress imaging protocols were validated. In the 1990s, the role of nuclear imaging in the assessment of myocardial viability was established. Since then, nuclear cardiology has become an important cornerstone of cardiovascular evaluation in daily clinical routine. Myocardial perfusion study is a well-established, non-invasive technique with a large body of evidence to support its effectiveness in the diagnosis and management of angina and myocardial infarction. Nuclear cardiology procedures are an integral part of many clinical guidelines for the investigation and management of angina and myocardial infarction.

In recent years, advances in imaging technologies have allowed integration of CT into PET and SPECT scanners. With this, hybrid imaging with SPECT/CT and PET/CT has emerged as a new tool of nuclear cardiology which now allows comprehensive non-invasive assessment of coronary artery disease combining information on both anatomy, i.e. coronary stenosis by CT coronary angiography, and function, i.e. pathophysiological relevance of a lesion by stress perfusion imaging.

The combination of new biologically derived radiopharmaceuticals and further refinements in imaging technologies may result in new clinical applications for diagnosis, functional characterization (plaque vulnerability), and prognosis as well as evaluation of therapeutic strategies.

Further reading

Hendel RC, Berman DS, Di Carli MF, *et al.* ACCF/ASNC/ACR/AHA/ASE/SCCT/SCMR/SNM 2009 appropriate use criteria for cardiac radionuclide imaging: a report of the American College of Cardiology Foundation Appropriate Use Criteria Task Force, the American Society of Nuclear Cardiology, the American College of Radiology, the American Heart Association, the American Society of Echocardiography, the Society of Cardiovascular Computed Tomography, the Society for Cardiovascular Magnetic Resonance, and the Society of Nuclear Medicine. Endorsed by the American College of Emergency Physicians. *J Am Coll Cardiol* 2009; **53**: 2201–29.

Hesse B, Tagil K, Cuocolo A, *et al.* EANM/ESC procedural guidelines for myocardial perfusion imaging in nuclear cardiology. *Eur J Nucl Med Mol Imaging* 2005; **32**: 855–97.

Hesse B, Lindhardt TB, Acampa W, *et al.* EANM/ESC guidelines for radionuclide imaging of cardiac function. *Eur J Nucl Med* 2008; **35**: 851–5.

Kaufmann PA. Cardiac hybrid imaging: state-of-the-art. *Ann Nucl Med* 2009; **23**: 325–31.

Underwood SR, Anagnostopoulos C, Cerqueria MD, *et al.* Myocardial perfusion scintigraphy: the evidence. *Eur J Nucl Med* 2004; **31**: 261–91.

Underwood SR, Bax JJ, vom Dahl J, *et al.* Imaging techniques for the assessment of myocardial hibernation. Report of a study group of the European Society of Cardiology. *Eur Heart J* 2004; **25**: 815–36.

➲ **For full references and multimedia materials please visit the online version of the book (http://esctextbook.oxfordonline.com).**

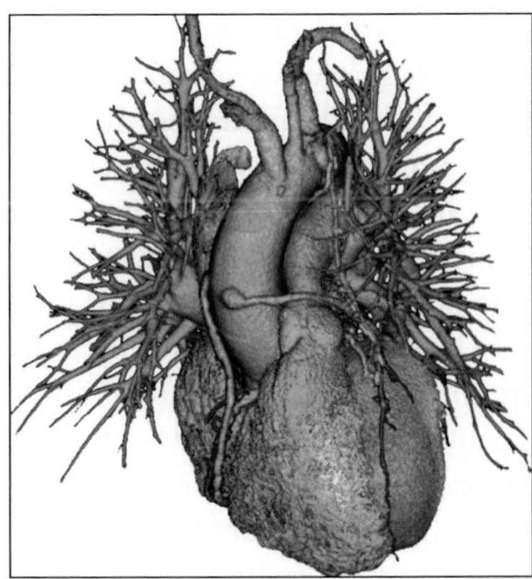

CHAPTER 8

Invasive Imaging and Haemodynamics

Carlo Di Mario, Guy R. Heyndrickx, Francesco Prati, and Nico H.J. Pijls

Contents

Summary

Direct catheter-based measurements of saturation and pressure in the various cardiac cavities allows full characterization of patient haemodynamics, including presence of intracardiac shunts, valve gradients and areas, and pulmonary and vascular resistances. The most important invasive haemodynamic assessment in today's practice, however, is now performed in the coronary arteries using microsensor-tipped guidewires able to measure post-stenotic pressure. When measured after maximal vasodilation, fractional flow reserve offers reliable individual characterization of coronary lesions. Results from large randomized long-term studies have shown that this technique can be safely used to defer interventions in single vessel disease and to target only functionally significant lesions in multivessel disease.

The diffuse practice of performing angioplasty immediately after diagnostic catheterization requires streamlined individualized coronary angiographic studies unfolding the relevant coronary segments in the projections that will optimally guide the angioplasty procedure. Tomographic high resolution images can be obtained with intravascular ultrasound (IVUS) or optical coherence tomography (OCT). The former does not require replacement of blood with crystalloids and measures the full thickness of the vessel wall encroachment (vessel or external elastic membrane diameter and area). IVUS has revolutionized our approach to stent deployment which became more aggressive using higher pressures for stent deployment or post-dilatation. However, convincing data on improved prognosis is still lacking for stent implantation, with the exception of non-randomized or small-scale studies in left main disease or small vessels and long lesions. OCT is limited by low penetration and the need to replace blood but has greater resolution compared with IVUS. At present, the main application is in the detection and quantification of malapposition and strut coverage. The clinical relevance of these findings is still under debate because no correlations are available between those parameters and long-term outcome after stenting.

Introduction

Therapeutic decisions in cardiology are crucially determined by invasive circulatory imaging and haemodynamics, which are essential for understanding the pathophysiological and diagnostic aspects of cardiovascular disease. This is related to the fact that the cardiovascular system can be elegantly conceptualized using mechanical laws and the basic dimensions of mass (M), length (L), time (t), and temperature. Invasive examination allows the most direct determination of parameters derived from these dimensions, such as volume (L^3), force ($F = M \times$ acceleration), pressure (F/L^2), and flow (L^3/t), i.e. variables that permit the exact description of the forces generated by the different cardiac chambers. Thus, assessment of the haemodynamics of the circulation enables one to grasp the system's function, whereas invasive imaging depicts its structure in terms of lumen size, arterial branch lengths, branching patterns, etc. Accordingly, the goal of this chapter is to provide practical suggestions on how to become familiar with invasive techniques, how haemodynamic variables are obtained invasively, and how the structure of the coronary artery tree is visualized. Finally, the epidemiologically important issue of coronary artery haemodynamics, including the relevance of coronary atherosclerotic lesions, is also discussed.

Percutaneous techniques of cardiac catheterization

Invasive assessment of cardiac haemodynamics and coronary physiology and imaging needs temporary vascular access. Today, arterial puncture (femoral, brachial, radial, axillary) to access the left heart and coronary arteries has mostly replaced arterial denudation techniques. The radial approach is still gaining in popularity and acceptance. Similarly, venous puncture (femoral, brachial, internal jugular vein, subclavian) to access the right heart (or the left heart through trans-septal puncture) is currently favoured over antecubital vein denudation.

Right side of the heart

Following local anaesthesia, the femoral vein is punctured before the common femoral artery is catheterized, and the sheath introduced by the Seldinger technique [1]. Using a 6F Swan–Ganz catheter allows a mostly easy passage to the pulmonary artery with low risk of injury to the right-heart chambers. To advance the catheter from the femoral vein to the pulmonary artery, the tip of the catheter is advanced from the lower right atrium by clockwise rotation over the tricuspid orifice, and then advanced into the right ventricle. To reach the pulmonary artery, the catheter must be slightly withdrawn so that its tip lies horizontally and just to the left of the spine. Clockwise rotation then causes the tip of the catheter to point upwards towards the right ventricular outflow tract. The catheter should only be advanced when it is in this position in order to minimize the risk of arrhythmia and injury to the right ventricular wall. If these manoeuvres fail to gain access to the pulmonary artery due to enlarged right-heart chambers, the catheter may be withdrawn to the right atrium and formed into a large 'reverse loop' by catching the tip in a hepatic vein and advancing the catheter quickly into the right atrium. This allows the tip of the catheter to advance through the tricuspid valve in an upward position. The catheter should then cross the pulmonary valve and advance to a pulmonary wedge position without difficulty. If the pulmonary valve cannot be passed, a guidewire can be employed to facilitate positioning in the pulmonary artery. Once in the pulmonary wedge position, measurements of pressure and blood oxygen saturation are recorded. Following measurement of the wedge pressure, the catheter is withdrawn into the proximal pulmonary artery, into the right ventricle and then into the right atrium, with corresponding recordings of pressure and oxygen saturation. Unsuspected anatomical abnormalities encountered during right-heart catheterization include passage across a patent foramen ovale into the left atrium (➲Fig. 8.1), a persistent left superior vena cava, a patent ductus arteriosus, or an anomalous pulmonary vein (➲Fig. 8.2).

Access to the right heart through the internal jugular vein is often used when only right heart catheterization is performed. The key point for a successful puncture is correct identification of anatomical landmarks. To puncture the right internal jugular vein, the high anterior approach is recommended whereby the puncture site is at the top of the triangle formed by the two heads of the sternocleidomastoid muscle and the clavicle. Alternatively, ultrasound guidance puncture has been proposed when this triangle is difficult to localize as is the case in obese or short-necked patients.

Left side of the heart

The common femoral artery is punctured as follows: the three middle fingers of the left hand palpate the pulse and the skin is pierced with the needle three finger-breadths below the inguinal ligament [2]. The radiological identification of the

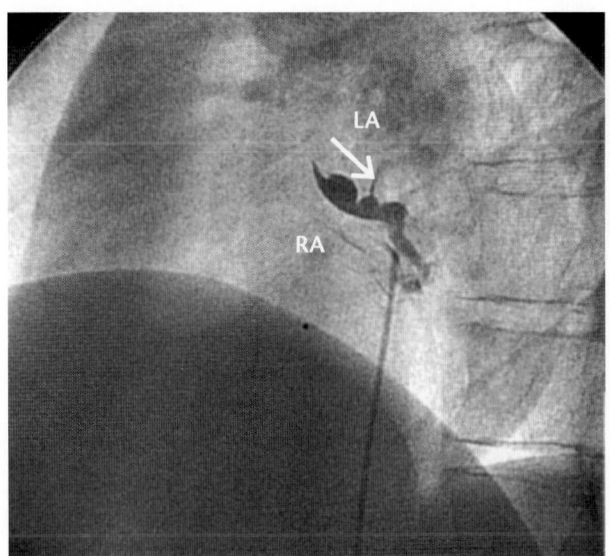

Figure 8.1 Patent foramen ovale. Imaging (lateral view) using radiographic contrast medium of the interatrial septum ('tunnel' between septum primum and septum secundum) with a small jet (arrow) between the right atrium (RA) and left atrium (LA).

femoral head with the puncture performed at the junction of the upper third and lower two-thirds results in higher puncture sites than the standard technique but avoids puncture below the femoral bifurcation and possibly reduces vascular complications. After puncture of the artery, a 0.89-mm (0.035-inch) J-guidewire should be advanced carefully into the needle. It should move freely up the aorta and be placed at the level of the diaphragm. When it is difficult to advance

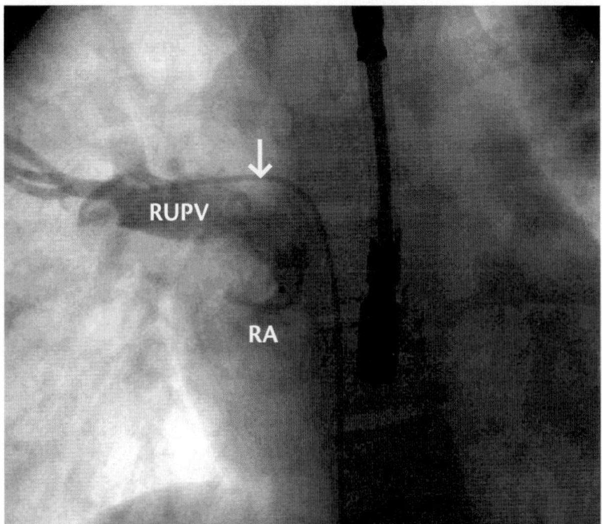

Figure 8.2 Anomalous right upper pulmonary venous return. Injection of contrast material via a multipurpose catheter (arrow) inserted in the right upper pulmonary vein (RUPV). The catheter is introduced in the right femoral vein. The contrast is filling the right atrium (RA).

the guidewire close to the tip of the needle, the wire should be withdrawn to ascertain that forceful arterial flow is still present; if not, the needle should be removed and the groin compressed for 5min. Problems that can be encountered in advancing the guidewire include severe arterial tortuosity, stenosis, occlusion (➲Fig. 8.3) or dissection. Left heart catheterization via the femoral approach is performed using an appropriately sized vascular sheath (we use 4–5F for diagnostic coronary angiography, 5–8F for percutaneous coronary interventions). The sheath is introduced via the guidewire and flushed with heparinized saline.

For routine diagnostic coronary angiography, intravenous bolus administration of unfractionated heparin is not required but for long diagnostic procedures or when a radial approach is used, 3000–5000 units of heparin are normally administered.

All left-heart catheters are exchanged via the guidewire, which is positioned with its tip at the level of the diaphragm. The pigtail catheter for left ventricular (LV) pressure measurements and angiography can be easily advanced across the aortic valve in the absence of aortic stenosis. If the latter is present, a 0.89-mm (0.035-inch) straight guidewire is employed to cross the valve, with its soft tip leading and pointing towards the stenotic valve and with the pigtail catheter pulled back into the ascending aorta by about 4–5cm. In this position, the wire tip usually quivers in the systolic jet. The pigtail catheter remains fixed and the guidewire is moved towards the valve in attempts to cross it. If this is not possible, the process can be repeated using a Judkins right coronary catheter or a left Amplatz or Feldman catheter, which allow better targeting of the valve opening than the pigtail catheter. When the guidewire has crossed the valve, it should be placed in the left ventricle, with a loop to minimize the risk of injury to the left ventricle. Accurate measurement of the true pressure gradient across the stenotic valve requires simultaneous pressure measurements in the left ventricle and in the ascending aorta just above the valves. This is best achieved using a double lumen pigtail catheter rather than relying on the peripheral arterial pressure measured through the arterial sheath (even if one size larger than the catheter) based on the knowledge that the pulse pressure continues to increase as far as the third generation of arteries (e.g. femoral artery) (➲Fig. 8.4)

Despite the ease in measuring the aortic gradient using echo Doppler, these measurements may be less accurate in situations of aortic stenosis with low gradients and low cardiac output (CO). A careful attempt to cross the stenotic valve should always be made in these patients to ascertain the exact gradient and valve orifice.

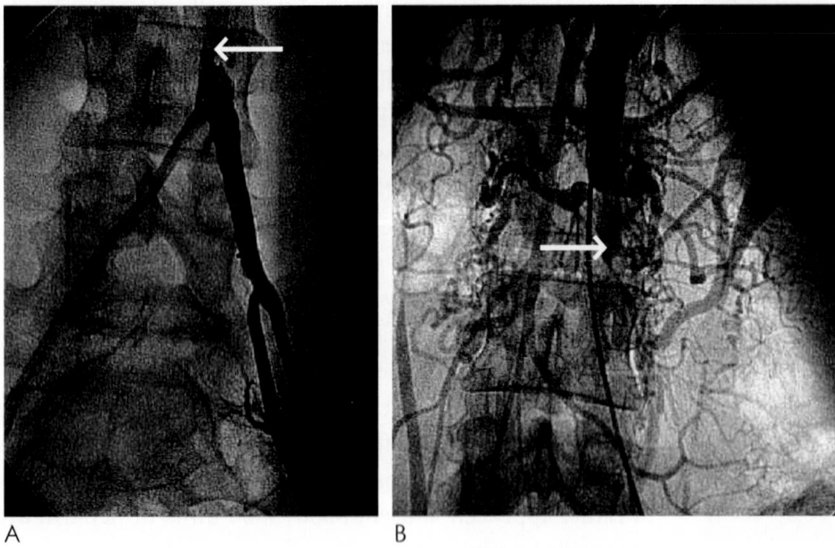

Figure 8.3 Chronic occlusion of the abdominal aorta immediately proximal to the iliac artery bifurcation (arrows). (A) Contrast injection from the left superficial femoral artey. (B) Contrast injection from the thoracic aorta descendens: imaging of multiple corkscrew-like collateral arteries bypassing the occlusion.

Relative contraindications for left heart catheterization via the femoral artery include occlusive peripheral vascular disease (➲Fig. 8.3), extreme iliac tortuosity, aortic abdominal aneurysm, femoral graft surgery, and gross obesity. In these instances catheterization of the radial artery carries a great number of advantages: superficial location, easy access, better control of haemostasis, and comfort for the patient. A growing number of operators prefer the radial puncture as first-line approach because this minimizes the bleeding risk and allows an easy external compression, avoiding closure devices and prolonged hospital stay. Some specific precautions such as the performance of the

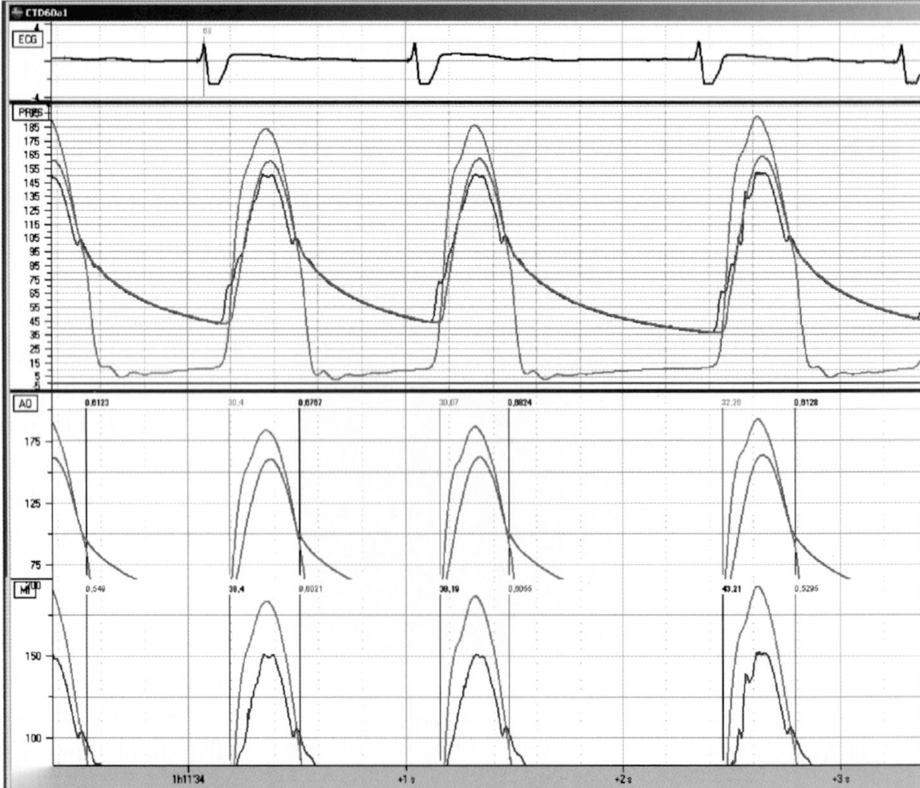

Figure 8.4 (Top panel) Simultaneous LV pressure (red), central aortic pressure (blue) and femoral artery pressure (green) tracings in a patient with aortic valvular stenosis demonstrating that the pressure gradient between LV and peripheral femoral artery underestimates the true aortic valve gradient. Lower panel) Beat to beat analysis of the peak gradient and aortic valve area using the peripheral femoral artery pressure versus the central aortic pressure. Values preceding the tracings: peak gradient (mmHg); values following the tracings: aortic valve area (mm^2).

Allen test to ensure the presence of adequate ulnar collaterals and the use of vasodilators to counteract potential arterial spasm are required. Since the anatomical approach to the coronary arteries is slightly different when approaching from the right radial artery, different curves of catheters are also available. Successful use of the ulnar artery has also been described.

Haemodynamic measurements during cardiac catheterization

Pressure measurements

An important goal of cardiac catheterization is precise assessment of pressure waves generated by the different cardiac chambers. Pressure is equal to force per unit area (in dynes/cm^2), force being transmitted through fluid as a wave. Considered as a complex periodic waveform, the pressure wave can be subdivided into a series of sine waves of variable amplitude and cycle frequency, whereby the sine wave frequency is expressed as harmonics or multiples of the fundamental frequency of the composite wave. This is important practically because an ideal pressure recording system must respond with identical amplitude for a given input throughout the range of frequencies contained within the pressure wave. The sensitivity of such an instrument can be defined as the amplitude ratio of the recorded (output) to the input signal. Its frequency response is the ratio between output and input amplitude over a range of frequencies of the input signal. A stiff as opposed to a flabby pressure-sensing membrane renders the recording instrument less sensitive but more frequency responsive. The useful frequency response of commonly used pressure measurement systems is <20 cycles/s (1 cycle/s corresponds to a heart rate of 60 beats per minute, bpm). For example, the dicrotic notch of the aortic pressure curve contains frequencies >10 cycles/s. The natural frequency of a sensing membrane and how it determines the degree of damping (by friction) is another important feature of the instrument, because its dynamic response is largely determined by them. The amplitude of an output signal tends to be augmented as the frequency of the input signal approaches the natural frequency of the membrane. In this situation, the sensing membrane begins to vibrate with increasing energy, i.e. it resonates. Damping dissipates the energy of the oscillating membrane, and optimal damping dissipates the energy gradually such that there is a constant output/input amplitude ratio. Optimally, the system must be set up to have the highest possible natural frequency and optimal damping: the former is directly proportional to the size of the catheter system, and inversely related to the length of the catheter plus tubing and to the square root of the catheter and tubing compliance and the fluid density filling the system. Damping is introduced into the system by filling the tubing with a viscous medium. If more accurate pressure measurements are required, for example to study small changes in absolute pressure during the diastolic events or to measure rate of pressure changes during contraction and relaxation, high-fidelity solid-state pressure transducers mounted on the tip of the catheter are available. The frequency response of these systems are far superior (>200 cycles/s) than those of fluid-filled catheters and therefore suitable for precise measurements of contractility and active myocardial relaxation.

Blood oxygen measurement and flow and shunt calculations

According to the Fick principle [3], the total uptake or consumption of a substance by an organ is the product of the blood flow to that organ and the arteriovenous concentration difference of the substance. Since measurements of flow, particularly CO, is of central importance in invasive cardiology, the determination of blood oxygen is similarly pivotal, since CO is most often calculated on the basis of the Fick oxygen method:

$$\text{Cardiac output (CO)} = \frac{\text{oxygen consumption}}{\text{arteriovenous oxygen difference}}$$

Oxygen consumption is measured directly by a polarographic method or the Douglas bag method. Alternatively, oxygen consumption can be predicted on the basis of the patient's body surface area corrected for age and gender. Thus it is assumed that resting oxygen consumption is 125mL/m^2, or 110mL/m^2 for older patients. Assumed versus directly obtained values for oxygen consumption are likely to introduce errors of >10% [4].

The arteriovenous oxygen difference is determined on the basis of blood sampling from appropriately positioned catheters in the left ventricle and the pulmonary artery. The oxygen content of the arterial and venous blood samples is the product of the measured oxygen saturation (per cent) and the oxygen-carrying capacity (in millilitres of oxygen per litre of blood). The former can be determined by reflectance oximetry of heparinized blood, which measures the percentage of haemoglobin present as oxyhaemoglobin. Oxygen-carrying capacity is approximated by multiplying the patient's haemoglobin (in grams per litre) by 1.36 (i.e. millilitres of oxygen per gram of haemoglobin).

Detection and localization of an intracardiac shunt can be easily performed using blood oxygen saturation as the indicator, which is obtained at many different sites within and close to the heart (i.e. 'oximetry run'; (➲Figs. 8.5 and 8.6)) [5]. Quantification of the shunt is based on measurements of pulmonary (Q_p, l/min) and systemic (Q_s) CO as outlined in (➲Table 8.1).

$$Q_p = \text{oxygen consumption}/(\text{pulmonary venous oxygen content} - \text{pulmonary arterial oxygen content})$$

$$Q_s = \text{oxygen consumption}/(\text{systemic arterial oxygen content} - \text{mixed venous oxygen content})$$

The key to measuring Q_s in the presence of an intracardiac shunt is that the mixed venous oxygen content must be obtained in the chamber immediately proximal to the shunt.

Catheterization protocol

➲Table 8.2 indicates the different steps of a complete right and left haemodynamic assessment. Pressure recordings and data acquisition during right and left heart catheterization should adhere to a strict protocol. After positioning a flotation catheter (Swan-Ganz) into the right atrium and a pigtail catheter in the ascending aorta at the level of the aortic valves the steps described in Table 8.2 must be performed.

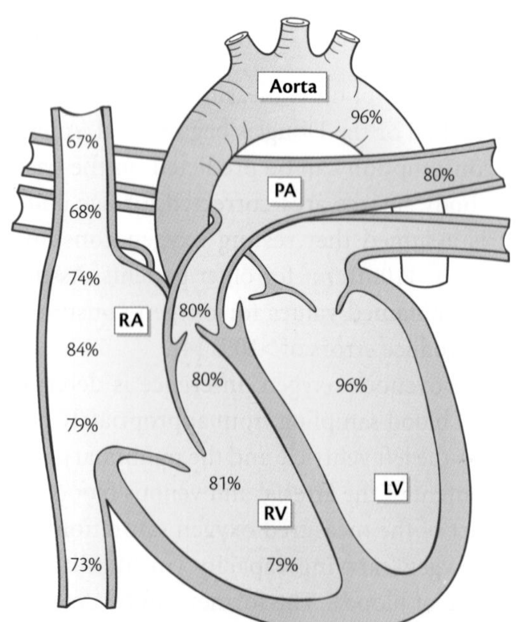

Figure 8.5 'Oximetry run' with multiple intracardiac oxygen saturation values in a patient with atrial septal defect. The 'step-up' detected in the right atrium (RA) identifies a left-to-right shunt at this location. LV, left ventricle; PA, pulmonary artery; RV, right ventricle.

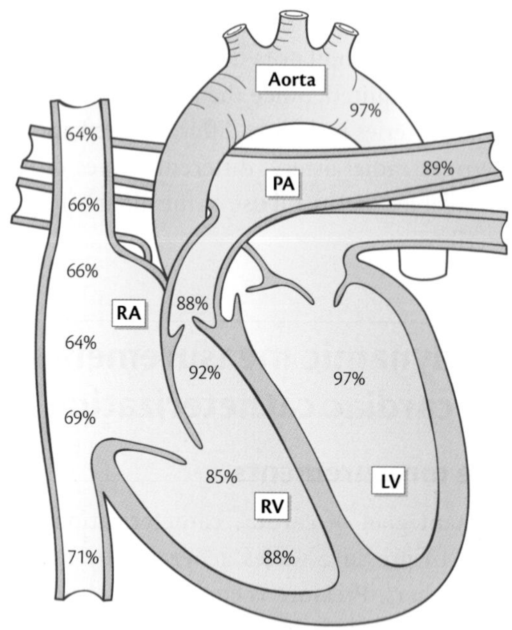

Figure 8.6 'Oximetry run' with multiple intracardiac oxygen saturation values in a patient with ventricular septal defect. The 'step-up' detected in the right ventricle (RV) identifies a left-to-right shunt at this location. LV, left ventricle; PA, pulmonary artery; RA, right atrium.

Additional sites for pressure measurements and blood sampling are needed in certain pathological conditions (e.g., congenital heart disease). ➲Table 8.3 tabulates the normal range of pressures, oxygen saturations, and oxygen volume. ➲Table 8.4 reports the most commonly used formulas to calculate derived haemodynamic parameters.

Physiological stress test during catheterization

Haemodynamic data recorded during heart catheterization are often within normal limits even in the presence of severe heart disease. Therefore several interventions have been advocated during heart catheterization to more closely correlate symptoms with haemodynamic measurements:

Tests used to challenge myocardial function or unmask valvular heart conditions

- **Dynamic exercise**: this is usually performed on a bicycle device mounted on the catheterization table. Simultaneous recordings of heart rate, pressures in the left and right heart together with blood sampling for oxygen measurements and CO measurements are performed at rest and during peak exercise level. Changes in CO will usually predict a normal response. The Dexter index

Table 8.1 Shunt detection and calculation

$$\text{PBF (L/min)} = \frac{O_2\text{ consumption (mL/min)}}{\text{P venous } O_2 \text{ content (mL/L)} - \text{P arterial } O_2 \text{ content (mL/L)}}$$

$$\text{SBF (L/min)} = \frac{O_2\text{ consumption (mL/min)}}{\text{Systemic arterial } O_2 \text{ content (mL/L)} - \text{mixed venous } O_2 \text{ content (mL/L)}}$$

$$\text{L-to-R shunt (L/min)} = \text{PBF} - \text{SBF}$$

Bidirectional shunt

$$\text{L-to-R shunt (L/min)} = \frac{\text{PBF (mixed venous } O_2 \text{ content} - \text{PA } O_2 \text{ content}}{\text{(mixed venous } O_2 \text{ content} - \text{PV } O_2 \text{ content}}$$

$$\text{R-to-L shunt (L/min)} = \frac{\text{PBF (PV } O_2 \text{ content} - \text{BA } O_2 \text{ content) (PA } O_2 \text{ content} - \text{PV } O_2 \text{ content)}}{\text{(BA } O_2 \text{ content} - \text{mixed venous } O_2 \text{ content) (mixed venous } O_2 \text{ content} - \text{PV } O_2 \text{ content)}}$$

BA, brachial artery; PA, pulmonary arterial; PBF, pulmonary blood flow; PV, pulmonary venous; SBF, systemic blood flow.

(measured cardiac index (CI) during exercise divided by the predicted CI) should be >1. In addition, changes in heart rate and blood pressure, changes in LV filling pressures, as well as volumes and valvular gradients are all useful in categorizing the haemodynamic responses.

- **Isometric exercise**: an isometric exercise test uses a handgrip device to activate a group of skeletal muscle to increase oxygen consumption. Again, intracardiac pressure measurements, oxygen consumption, and ventricular function data are recorded at rest and during isometric contraction.

Table 8.2 Catheterization protocol for a complete right and left haemodynamic assessment

Step 1 Record phasic and mean pressure in right atrium and aorta
Step 2 Withdraw simultaneously blood samples from right atrium and aorta for oxygen saturation measurements
Step 3 Advance the Swan–Ganz catheter sequentially into the right ventricle and pulmonary artery for pressure measurements and blood samples for oxygen saturation measurements
Step 4 Measure cardiac output using the triple lumen thermodilution catheter (Swan–Ganz)
Step 5 Advance the Swan–Ganz catheter to pulmonary wedge pressure and cross the aortic valve with the pigtail catheter for simultaneous recordings of left ventricular end-diastolic pressure and pulmonary wedge pressure (same scale)
Step 6 Deflate the balloon and pull the Swan-Ganz catheter back towards the pulmonary artery
Step 7 Record simultaneous left ventricle pressure and femoral artery pressure (through the arterial sheath) or aortic pressure (via double lumen catheter)
Step 8 After left ventriculography (if needed) pull back from the left ventricle into the aorta.

- **Volume loading**: rapid infusion of 500mL of saline over 3min is a challenge to the ventricle and can often unmask underlying pathological conditions such as constrictive pericarditis and restrictive haemodynamic conditions, especially when patients have been extensively treated with diuretics.
- **Pharmacologic stress**: administration of nitroglycerine will relieve myocardial ischaemia and improve ventricular function through a potent reduction of preload and afterload. Infusion of dobutamine, an inotropic agent, may mimic exercise and increase oxygen consumption which may unmask underlying obstructive coronary artery disease.

Tests used to challenge the coronary vascular bed

- **Cold pressure test**: immersion of the hand and forearm in ice will elicit an alpha-adrenergic response characterized by an increase in heart rate, systolic and mean arterial

Table 8.3 Normal pressure ranges (mmHg), oxygen saturations (%), and oxygen volume percentages in resting conditions

	S	D	Mean	O_2 sat	O_2 volume %
RA			5	75	15
RV	24	4		75	15
PA	24	10	15	75	15
PCW			12		
LV	120	12		95	19
LA			12	95	19
Ao	120	80		95	19

Ao: aorta; LV, left ventricle; LA: left atrium; PA, pulmonary artery; PCW, pulmonary wedge pressure; RA, right atrium; RV, right ventricle.

Table 8.4 Calculations for haemodynamic measurements

$$\text{CO (L/min)} = \frac{O_2 \text{ consumption (mL/min)}}{\text{AV} - O_2 \text{ difference (mL } O_2\text{/100mL blood)} \times 100}$$

$$\text{CI (L/min/m}^2\text{)} = \frac{\text{CO (L/min)}}{\text{BSA (m}^2\text{)}}$$

$$\text{SV (mL/beat)} = \frac{\text{CO (mL/min)}}{\text{HR (bpm)}}$$

$$\text{SVI (mL/beat/m}^2\text{)} = \frac{\text{SV (mL/beat)}}{\text{BSA (m}^2\text{)}}$$

$$\text{SW (g.m)} = \text{Mean LV systolic pressure} - \text{mean LV diastolic pressure} \times \text{SV.0.0144}$$

$$\text{PAR (units)} = \frac{\text{Mean PA pressure} - \text{mean LA pressure (or PCW)}}{\text{CO}}$$

$$\text{TPR} = \frac{\text{Mean PA pressure}}{\text{CO}}$$

$$\text{SVR} = \frac{\text{Mean arterial pressure} - \text{mean RA pressure}}{\text{CO}}$$

Conversion to metric units (dynes.s.cm^{-5}): SVR, PAR, TPR units × 80.

bpm, beats per minute; BSA, body surface area; CI, cardiac index; CO, cardiac output; HR, heart rate; LA, left atrial; LV, left ventricular; PA, pulmonary artery; PAR, pulmonary arteriolar resistance; SVR, systemic vascular resistance; SV, stroke volume; SVI, stroke volume index; SW, stroke work; TPR, total pulmonary resistance.

blood pressure, and CO. While in normal individuals this stress will elicit an increase in coronary flow and decrease in coronary vascular resistance, in patients with underlying coronary atherosclerosis it may cause coronary vasoconstriction, and a decrease in regional coronary flow resulting in changes in regional LV function.

- **Hyperventilation**: may be used to provoke coronary spasm. Increased deep breathing for 5min is associated with an increase in heart rate, oxygen consumption, arteriovenous oxygen difference and arterial pH, and a decrease in arterial PCO_2 and arterial pressure.
- **Pharmacologic stress**: ergonovine, in sequential doses of 0.02, 0.08, 0.2mg IV with 3-min intervals, is used to provoke coronary vasospasm. Diffuse reduction in coronary diameter, often asymptomatic, is a normal response. Focal narrowing of a coronary artery associated with clinical symptoms and electrocardiogram (ECG) changes and relieved with IV nitrates is considered a positive test.

Ventricular volumes

Quantitative information on ventricular dimension, area, and wall thickness derived from LV cineangiography allows assessment of ventricular volume, ejection fraction, mass, and wall stress (together with pressure measurement). Ventriculograms are usually recorded at 30–60 frames/s, and radiographic contrast agent is injected in adults at rates of 10–15mL/s for a total volume of 30–50mL. For the calculation of LV volume, the outermost margin of visible radiographic contrast is traced. Volume (V) is computed using long-axis (L) and short-axis (S) measurements (V = [frac16] πLS^2) or area–length measurements ($V = 8A^2/3\pi L$) using an ellipsoid approximation for ventricular shape. Alternatively, techniques based on Simpson's rule, which is independent of assumptions regarding ventricular shape, may be used. Correction has to be made for magnification of the ventricular image onto the image intensifier.

Pressure–volume loop

Variations in pressure and volume occurring during the cardiac cycle are integrated in the pressure–volume diagram (PV) (➲Fig. 8.7). This instantaneous relationship between changes in intraventricular pressure and changes in volume throughout the cardiac cycle is a powerful tool to study and comprehend the performance of the left ventricle. For a long time these measurements were confined to the realm of research laboratories. However, since the development of the conductance catheter by Baan and colleagues, continuous on-line measurements of LV volume and pressure offer today the possibility to assess LV function in patients during catheterization in great detail [6]. Analysis of these PV loops permits distinction of the different phases of the cardiac cycle, and enables recording of the parameters of ventricular performance, systolic and diastolic function.

Vascular resistance

Calculations of vascular resistance are usually applied to the pulmonary circulation (normal value 67 ± 30 dynes/s/cm^{-5}) and systemic circulation (normal value 1170 ± 270 dynes/s/cm^{-5}). Vascular resistance (R) is determined on the basis of Ohm's law ($R = \Delta P/Q$), where Q is the CO and ΔP is the pressure gradient across the pulmonary circulation (mean pulmonary artery pressure – mean left atrial pressure) or across the systemic circulation (mean aortic pressure – mean central venous pressure). The mentioned equations yield arbitrary resistance units (also called hybrid resistance units or Wood units in mmHg/L/min), and for conversion to metric units expressed in dynes/s/cm^{-5}, a factor of 80 has to be used.

Valve area calculations

As valvular stenosis develops, the valve orifice poses progressively greater resistance to flow across the opening, resulting in a pressure drop across the valve. Greater flow across the valve yields greater pressure gradient. These qualitative relationships, Torricelli's law describing flow

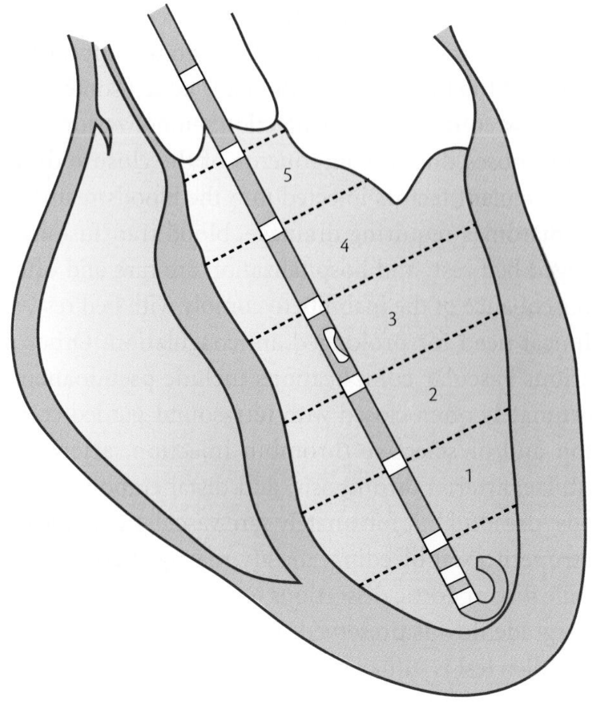

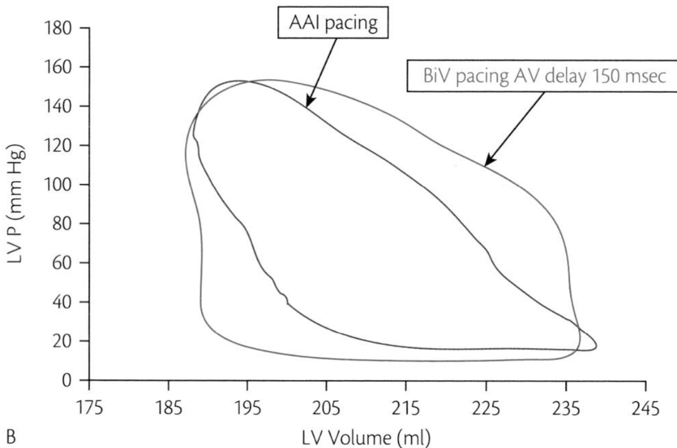

Figure 8.7 (A) Positioning of a pressure-conductance catheter mounted with multiple electrodes (usually 12) in the ventricle. Two electrodes (one proximal and one distal) generate an intracavity electrical field. The other electrodes are measuring in pairs, several segmental conductance signals representing instantaneous volumes of corresponding slices which are then converted to absolute volumes. Reproduced with permission from Steendijk P, Tulner SAF, Wiemer M, *et al.* Pressure–volume measurements by conductance catheter during cardiac resynchronization therapy. *Eur Heart J* Suppl 2004; **6**: D35–D42. (B) Example of a pressure–volume loop derived from the conductance catheter in a patient with LV asynchrony during atrial pacing (blue) and during biventricular pacing (red). Parameters derived from the pressure–volume loop are: SBP, systolic blood pressure; $P_{end\ syst,}$ end systolic pressure; DBP, diastolic blood pressure; EDP, end diastolic blood pressure; LAP, left atrial pressure; ESV, end systolic volume; EDV, end diastolic volume; SV, stroke volume. Derived parameters: ejection fraction, dP/dt_{max}, peak ejection rate, $dP/dt_{min,}$ $dP/dt_{max,}$ relaxation time constant(τ).

across a round orifice ($A = Q/VC_C$) and the relationship between flow velocity and pressure drop ($V = C_v(2g\Delta P)^{1/2}$), form the basis of the calculation of valvular orifice area (A) using cardiac pressure (ΔP; (➲ Figs. 8.8 and 8.9)) and flow (Q) measurements [7]:

$$A = Q/C_v C_C (2g\Delta P)^{1/2}$$

where C_C and C_v are a coefficient of orifice contraction and a coefficient of velocity correcting for energy loss as pressure energy is converted to kinetic energy, respectively; and g is acceleration due to gravity (980cm/s^2). In the case of aortic valve area (AVA) and mitral valve area (MVA), the following specific formulae can be used:

$$\text{AVA} = (\text{cardiac output/systolic ejection period} \times \text{heart rate})/44.3\Delta P^{1/2}$$

$$\text{MVA} = (\text{cardiac output/diastolic filling period} \times \text{heart rate})/37.7\Delta P^{1/2}$$

Invasive imaging techniques and coronary morphology

Coronary angiography

Consent for the procedure, risks and benefits of angiography

Although the techniques of angiography and angioplasty should only be performed by qualified and dedicated

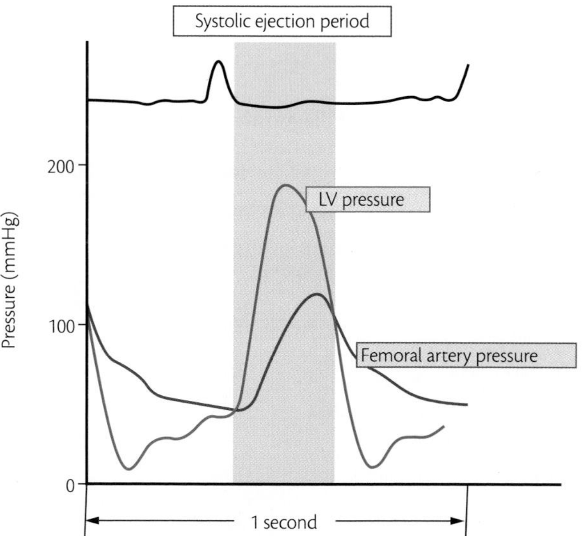

Figure 8.8 Simultaneous ECG, left ventricular (LV) and femoral artery pressure recordings in a patient with aortic stenosis and insufficiency. During the systolic ejection period, there is a marked pressure gradient. At end-diastole, aortic regurgitation leads to pressure equilibration of systemic arterial and left ventricular pressure.

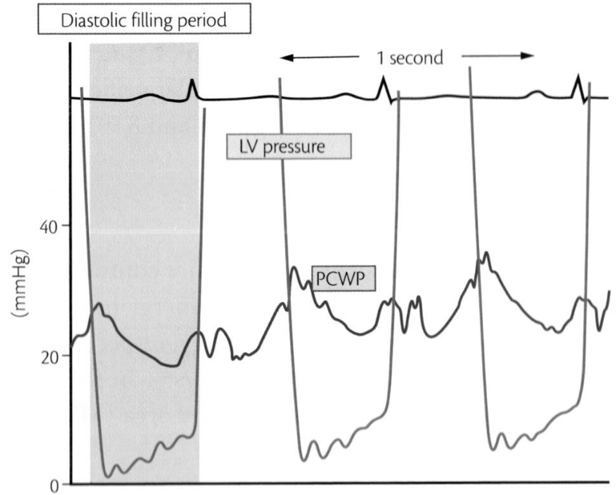

Figure 8.9 Simultaneous ECG, left ventricular (LV) and pulmonary capillary wedge pressure (PCWP) recordings in a patient with mitral stenosis indicated by the severe pressure gradient during the diastolic filling period.

operators, every cardiologist treating adult patients must be aware of the indications, risks, and potential benefits of this procedure. ➲Table 8.5 indicates the complications in a general population but the data are too old to reflect practices such as the radial approach or the use of new contrast agents [8]. These figures are a good indication for average patients but they must be individualized for morbid obesity, diabetes, peripheral vascular disease, and poor LV function. The most frequent complications of angiography occur at the catheter entry site. The 2–5% incidence currently quoted is based on a series using a femoral approach before the use of 4F and 5F catheters. Closure devices have reduced the time to ambulation, increased patient comfort, and shortened the hospital stay, but do not appear to have modified the bleeding risk and have added some rare specific new complications (infection, embolization, or arterial stenoses due to components of the closure device or procoagulant factors injected into the bloodstream). Large haematomas requiring drainage, blood transfusions, prolonged bed rest, and hospitalization are rare and often the consequence of the inability to comply with bed rest, or the clinical need for prolonged anticoagulation. Other more serious vascular complications include pseudoaneurysm, fortunately often closed with ultrasound-guided compression and/or selective thrombin injection, arteriovenous fistulae, arterial thrombosis, and distal embolization. The most dreadful but fortunately rare vascular complication is retroperitoneal bleeding, mostly managed conservatively, while iliac or aortic dissections tend to seal spontaneously if antegrade flow is preserved. For radial procedures a negative Allen test is sufficient to exclude critical hand ischaemia even in cases of total radial occlusion (1–4% of patients). Large haematomas are rare but very painful and possibly in need of surgical decompression. They are easily avoidable with careful wire manipulation during initial cannulation, with fluoroscopy used for all polymer coated wires and subsequent catheter exchanges over long (300 cm) guidewires, and with frequent controls of the compression bandage in the first hours post-catheterization. The frequency of serious complications, such as death, myocardial infarction, or cerebrovascular accident with permanent damage, is very low (0.1–0.2%). Myocardial infarction is often due to catheter-induced ostial damage due to pre-existing severe pathology or the presence of unstable plaques at risk of embolization and can potentially be treated with angioplasty and stenting. Stroke is the consequence of thromboembolism due to thrombi in the access sheath or the catheter, dislodgement of plaques from the iliac vessels or aorta, calcium from the aortic valve, or thrombi in the left ventricle. Meticulous attention to catheter flushing and atraumatic wire-lead insertion can reduce but not eliminate the risk, whilst there is no evidence that systemic heparinization is required for diagnostic catheterization. Death can be the direct consequence of infarction, stroke, or cardiac and vascular perforation but can also be induced by late complications of prolonged hospitalizations triggered by relatively minor complications such as bleeding events and renal dysfunction. A clear explanation of other more frequent albeit minor and promptly controlled adverse effects helps the patient to accept them without unnecessary stress. Reactions to the contrast medium (nausea, vomiting, rash)

Table 8.5 Complications of diagnostic angiography

	Incidence (per 1000)	
Death	1.0–1.5	Cumulative incidence 1.5–2.5
Myocardial infarction	1.0–2.0	
Neurological events		
Permanent	1.0–5.0	
Transient deficit	3.0–5.0	
Ventricular fibrillation/tachycardia requiring defibrillation	1.0–2.0	
Vascular/bleeding complications		
Requiring surgery or late US-guided compression or thrombin injection	10–20	
Managed conservatively	10–50	

US, ultrasound.

are very rare and the amount of contrast used for a diagnostic angiogram cannot induce permanent renal damage unless a severe previous dysfunction was present. Bradycardia and hypotension develop because of periprocedural vasovagal reactions, prevented by generous sedation, liberal local anaesthesia, reassurance, and appropriate filling with intravenous fluids. Other major arrhythmias (ventricular fibrillation and tachycardias, supraventricular arrhythmias) can be induced by catheter damping, excessively prolonged injection, or mechanical stimulation.

Catheter selection and manipulation

Improvements in catheter technology have allowed the flow rate obtained with old 8F (1F = 0.33mm) diagnostic catheters to be achieved with 6F thin-walled catheters and satisfactory coronary opacification with 4F and 5F diagnostic catheters. Newly developed automatic injectors with adjustable increases in injection pressure have the potential to allow more consistent homogeneous opacification of large left coronary arteries through 4–5F catheters. Preshaped catheters (e.g. Judkins, Amplatz) can be used for injection of both coronary vessels, not only via the femoral and left radial or brachial approach but also the right radial/brachial approach. A reduction in pressure with ventricularization (low diastolic values) of the pressure waveform indicates that the catheter is obstructing flow. This may be caused by the presence of a true ostial stenosis, by the small size of the coronary ostium, or by deep engagement of the catheter beyond the left main or first curve of the right coronary artery, often causing ostial spasm. Injection of intracoronary nitrates and gentle test injections with careful withdrawal of the catheter can identify and solve these various problems. It is very important not to start the injection before the angiographic acquisition in order to identify calcifications or late staining of contrast. Contrast injection should be sufficiently rapid and large to fully replace the epicardial vascular volume and avoid the phenomenon of streaming or incomplete visualization. When the proximal coronary segments are fully opacified, the prolongation of injection offers no diagnostic advantage, increases the contrast volume used, and carries potential risks in vessels with a large epicardial volume and slow flow, such as vein grafts. On the other hand, angiographic acquisition should be prolonged to allow visualization of the distal vessels, identification of thrombolysis in myocardial infarction (TIMI) flow, and characterization of type of dissection (with/without persistence of contrast at the end of the injection). An important determinant of injection duration is the need to visualize collaterals for occluded vessels, which also means adjustment of the view to include the recipient vessel in the image.

Left coronary artery

Cannulation

Selection of coronary catheters should aim at an optimal coaxial atraumatic intubation of the coronary artery and should be based on the size of the aortic root. In the majority of cases standard 4.0 Judkins catheters can be used. If it is known from previous invasive or non-invasive examination that there is an enlarged ascending aorta, a 4.5 or 5.0 left Judkins catheter should be preferred. Smaller sizes, 3.5 or 3.0 Judkins, can be a first choice in small females or for right radial approaches.

The optimal view for engaging both the right and left coronary arteries is the left anterior oblique view where the ostium is not covered by the aorta (➲Fig. 8.10). The left

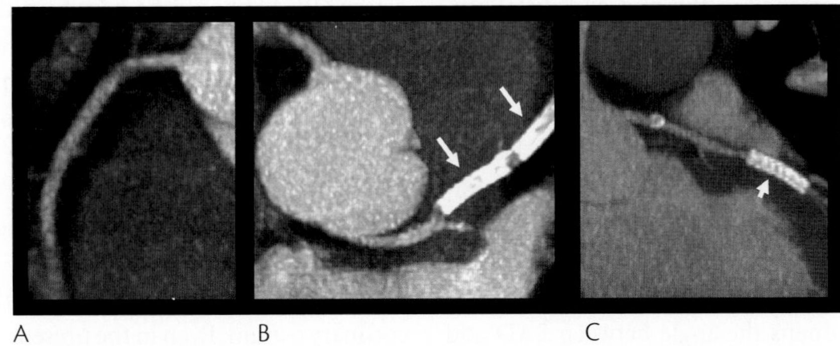

Figure 8.10 Multislice computerized tomography (B) shows the origin of both coronary ostia in an axial view simulating an angiographic spider view (note the two stents in the proximal left anterior descending artery, arrows). The two multiplanar reconstructions on the right and left delineate the ostium of the right coronary artery (A) and left coronary artery (C) with a stent easily visible in the left circumflex artery (arrow). If cannulation of the arteries is performed using an anteroposterior view, a common mistake repeatedly performed, injections in the aortic root will never catch the position and level of the coronary ostia. It is also intuitive that the left catheter will often directly cannulate the left coronary ostium while anterior rotation is required to engage the right coronary ostium.

coronary artery requires only minimal catheter manipulation; the J-tipped 0.89-mm (0.035-inch) wire is atraumatically advanced to the level of the aortic valve and the tip of the previously flushed Judkins catheter is opened as low as possible pointing to the left coronary ostium. When retrograde bleeding ensures the catheter has been purged of air, a pressure line is connected and a test injection performed, often showing that the catheter is already engaged or is located immediately below or in front of the ostium. In the latter case, gentle withdrawal of the catheter tip (helped by asking the patient to take a deep breath) will allow engagement of the catheter tip in most cases. If the tip of the catheter immediately closes in the ascending aorta, prolonged attempts with the same catheter should be avoided and rapid switching to a larger catheter is probably advantageous in terms of time lost and contrast used. When it is known that the coronary ostia are in an unusual position (aortic valve disease, Marfan syndrome, congenital heart disease), it is probably worthwhile performing an aortic angiogram in the left anterior oblique view in order to guide catheter selection, since this may require unusual shapes (e.g. left Judkins 6.0 or left Amplatz 2.0 and 3.0).

Optimal views (➲ Fig. 8.11)

The main advantage of the so-called spider view (left 40–55°, caudal 25–40°) is to delineate the branching of the left main coronary artery from the aorta and its bifurcation into the left anterior descending (LAD) and left circumflex (LCX) arteries (or trifurcation if an intermediate branch is present). For this reason it is better to acquire this view first in order to exclude this most fearsome lesion location, at risk of plaque disruption during catheter injection and which may require an urgent surgical approach. The LAD artery is greatly foreshortened in the mid and distal segments in this view but stenosis of the proximal segment or of the ostium of the first diagonal branch is often optimally shown. The LCX artery, on the other hand, is optimally opened in its proximal and mid segments. The classical 30–40° right view is limited by the frequent superimposition of the proximal LAD and LCX. A smaller angulation to the right (10–20°) avoids superimposition of the catheter and the spine and, combined with relatively skewed caudal angulations (30–40°), opens the angle between LAD and LCX (and intermediate branch, if present) sufficiently to obtain optimal images of the proximal and mid segment of the LCX and bifurcation of its marginal branches. The image is of more limited interest for the proximal and mid LAD because of the frequent superimposition of diagonal and septal branches but remains the most important view for the distal LAD. Skewed cranial views (40° or more), with 5–10° angulation to the right to avoid superimposition of the catheter and the vertebral spine, elongate the proximal and mid LAD and open the bifurcation of the proximal diagonal branches which run to the right, clearly distinguished from the septal branches which run to the left of the screen. The segments that are foreshortened in this view are the distal LAD and the proximal LCX but this view is also ideal for visualizing the distal posterolateral branches of the LCX and, in the 15–20% of cases with left dominance or codominance, the left posterior descending artery (PDA).

In the left cranial view (30–45° left, 25–40° cranial) the LAD is further elongated by asking the patient to take a deep breath and maintain breath-holding during injection. The cranial view also offers optimal views of the mid and distal segments of the LCX, and is especially useful in the presence of a dominant LCX. The lateral view is far from standard in modern coronary angiography because the additional value of this view is quite limited, only providing excellent visualization of the mid/distal LAD around the apex, information which is at most complementary to right caudal views. Occasionally, however, eccentric short lesions of the proximal and mid segment of the LAD might be covered by septal or diagonal branches in all the conventional previously reported views and can be better visualized in the lateral projection, sometimes using variable cranial or caudal angulations to ensure no superimposition from the diagnostic catheter and side branches.

Right coronary artery

Cannulation

Catheter selection for cannulation of the right coronary artery (RCA) should be based on the same policy as for the left coronary artery, taking into account the size of the aortic root. In the left anterior oblique or lateral view, the catheter must be rotated to point to the left of the screen and this is better achieved when the rotation is performed during a slow pull-back motion of the catheter from the right coronary sinus. Breath-holding after a deep inspiration may facilitate this manoeuvre. In 10–15% of cases a high origin of the RCA complicates the search for the right coronary ostium. Even in the presence of a hypoplastic non-dominant RCA, selective injection is still required because small proximal branches can be an important source of collaterals for occluded vessels. It is often possible to obtain a semi-selective injection with the Judkins catheter that will further guide catheter selection. A multipurpose catheter

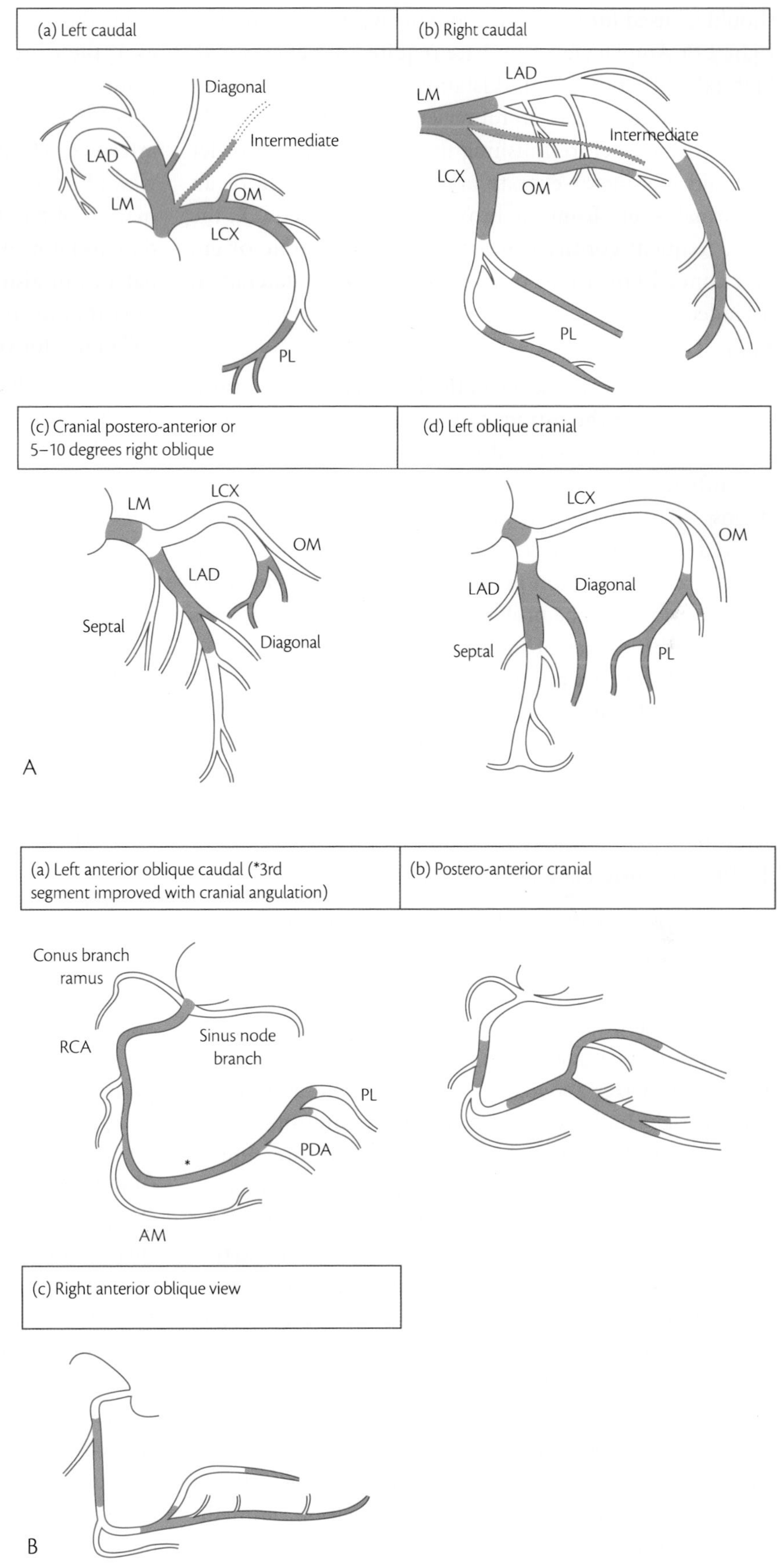

Figure 8.11 The most frequent angiographic projections: their relative merits in the visualization of different coronary segments are indicated. Filled segments indicate the segments optimally visualized.

should be used for downward-looking RCAs, and Amplatz right 2 or Amplatz left 1 or 2 are required in patients with high take-off and/or with dilatation of the coronary sinus and ascending aorta. Careful review of the images should be performed before finishing the examination in order to avoid missing a separate origin from the aorta or an abnormal origin from the proximal RCA of the LCX, the most frequent coronary anomaly, or the separate origin of a conus branch that provides important collaterals to occluded arteries.

Optimal views

The RCA has few branches in the first, second, and third segments (from the ostium to the crux cordis) and often two views (left anterior and right anterior oblique views) are sufficient to identify all stenoses, including eccentric stenoses. The lateral view might be ideal for assessment of the mid segment of the artery and may occasionally be used as a working projection for occlusions in this segment or stent positioning. The problems with these standard views lie in the difficulties of interpretation in the presence of stenoses at the crux cordis or at the ostia of the PDA and posterolateral branches. Cranial angulation (30°) of the left anterior view is often sufficient to solve diagnostic questions but many operators prefer to use as a routine view a cranial (30°) posteroanterior view of the RCA, which clearly delineates the region of the crux cordis and possible lesions of the PDA or posterolateral branches.

Venous bypass grafts and left internal mammary artery

Aortic anastomoses of radial arteries or venous grafts are rarely indicated by radio-opaque markers positioned at the time of operation (a neglected practice in cardiac surgery), but can often be visualized in the left anterior oblique view a few centimetres above the ostium of the RCA by dragging the right Judkins catheter along the right profile of the ascending aorta. Although the position and direction of aortic anastomoses is influenced by the surgical technique, in general the anastomosis for the RCA tends to be the lowest and to have a more vertical origin from the aorta, so that selective cannulation may require the use of a multipurpose catheter. Grafts for the marginal or diagonal branches often require catheter rotation and occasionally catheters with a longer tip (right or left Amplatz 1 and 2, left coronary bypass catheters) are required. Instead of wasting a large amount of contrast in locating the ostium, it can be cost-effective to perform an aortogram with the pigtail catheter slightly above the usual supravalvular position, immediately above the level of the RCA, in order to ascertain at least the number of open grafts. A limitation is obviously the inability to detect grafts with extremely slow flow; however, these are often identified because of the presence of contrast staining in cases of recent occlusion.

For the left mammary artery, the origin of the subclavian arteries can be more easily engaged in a left anterior oblique view (40–60°). Complete visualization of the internal mammary is of paramount importance because it is crucial not only to know whether the left internal mammary artery is patent but also to exclude the presence of distal stenoses (anastomotic or in the distal native vessels) and to visualize collaterals for other occluded vessels. The selective visualization of the mammary artery is more easily achieved with a specially designed catheter, which has a longer tip than the classical right Judkins catheter. In case of failure, other types of modified left internal mammary catheter with a hook-like shape can be tested. Selective engagement is often made difficult by the presence of severe tortuosity of the proximal subclavian artery, which makes manipulation of the left internal mammary catheter very difficult. The problems are greater for the right internal mammary artery because of the more tortuous track from the ascending aorta. A power injection through 6F large-lumen diagnostic or guide catheters can occasionally avoid the troubles and risks of a true superselective injection of the internal mammary arteries in very tortuous and frail subclavian vessels, reducing brachial flow with a pressure cuff inflated around the arm. Alternatively, a radial approach (more often left as the left mammary is most frequently used) can be the safest solution if multiple attempts from the groin remain unsuccessful.

The distal anastomosis of the mammary artery is often optimally displayed in the lateral view, which is also ideal for excluding adhesion of the left internal mammary to the sternum, a condition that may increase the risk of surgical reintervention with median sternotomy.

Angiographic report

Coronary angiography requires a report indicating the vascular access site, type and size of catheters used, type and total amount of contrast, allergic reactions or other procedural complications, closure devices, aortic pressure, and heart rate and rhythm before and after the procedure. After having described the type of dominance and possible anomalies of origin and location, each individual coronary segment (from the left main to three segments for the LAD and RCA, two for the LCX plus the main diagonal, intermediate, marginal, and posterolateral branches) and the presence of a lesion must be indicated, with description of the characteristics as indicated in ➲Table 8.6. While the

Table 8.6 Qualitative definitions of angiographic lesions

Eccentric: luminal edge in outer one-quarter of the normal lumen
Irregular: ulceration, aneurysm or saw-tooth pattern
Discrete: estimated lesion length <10mm
Tubular: estimated lesion length 10–20mm
Diffuse: estimated lesion length ≥20mm
Ostial: within 3mm from origin
Angulated: ≥45° angle between centre-line of proximal and distal segments
Bifurcational: branch ≥1.5mm involving the lesion
Calcified: readily apparent densities within the vessel wall at the site of the lesion
Functionally occluded (99% diameter stenosis): antegrade flow TIMI 1
Totally occluded (100% diameter stenosis): antegrade flow TIMI 0 with/without opacification from collaterals
Thrombotic: intraluminal filling defect separated from the vessel wall in two views (with or without contrast staining)
Type A (ACC/AHA): discrete, concentric, non-angulated, readily accessible, regular, non-calcified or minimally calcified, non-occlusive, non-ostial, non-bifurcational, non-thrombotic lesion
Type B: tubular, eccentric, with two ≥75% bends proximal to the stenosis, angulated (but less than 90°), irregular, calcific, occluded (functional or >3 months), ostial, bifurcational (side branch accessible for wire protection), thrombotic lesion
Type C: diffuse, three ≥75° bends in the proximal segment, angulated (≥90°), occluded >3 months old or unknown duration), bifurcational (side branch non-accessible), degenerated vein graft

terms 'irregular' and 'mild' can be used to describe stenoses of <30% and 30–50%, stenoses of 50% or greater require attempts at visual estimation of severity based on comparison with the closest normal-looking reference segment. The presence of thrombus and irregularities of stenosis contour are often more subjective, although the presence of multiple unfavourable characteristics (graded ABC in the ACC/AHA Task Force definitions [9]) is still predictive of immediate success and complications.

Besides the pressure measurements, in the angiographic report the operator must indicate the semi-quantitative estimate of LV cavity size and the presence and type of wall motion abnormality (from normal to hypokinetic, akinetic, or dyskinetic). Five regions should be reported for the right anterior oblique view and two for the left anterior oblique view (➲Fig. 8.12). The presence of thrombi or other filling defects and abnormalities in shape must also be reported.

Mitral insufficiency is graded 1–4 according to the presence and amount of regurgitant flow (➲Table 8.7) and, for the most severe levels, also allows delineation of the contours of the left atrial cavity. Obviously, the size of the LV and, especially, left atrial cavity, the acuteness of the process, the position of the catheter and rate and volume injected may modify this semi-quantitative assessment, which remains subjective, although the distinction between non-surgical (grade 1 and 2) and possible surgical (grade 3 and 4) severity is clear in most patients. Whilst angiography is not the easiest technique for defining absolute volumes, relative changes such as LV ejection fraction must be regularly measured using the quantitative packages all digital systems offer.

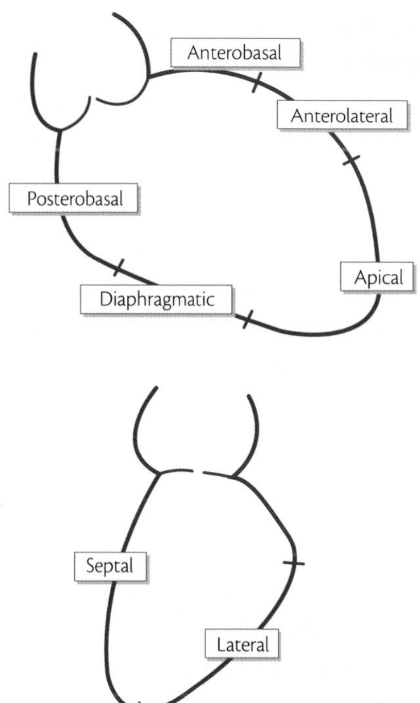

Figure 8.12 Regional wall motion during left ventriculography as assessed in the right and left oblique views.

Table 8.7 Semi-quantitative classification of mitral regurgitation

Trivial (grade 1 or 1+/4+): contrast material enters the left atrium during systole without filling the entire atrial cavity and is cleared in the subsequent beat
Mild (grade 2 or 2+/4+): contrast opacification of the left atrium is less dense than the opacification of the left ventricle but contrast is not cleared with each beat
Moderate/severe (grade 3 or 3+/4+): opacification of the left atrium is as dense as the opacification of the left venticle
Severe (grade 4 or 4+/4+): opacification of the left atrium greater than that of the left ventricle and/or complete atrial filling in one systole and/or contrast opacifies the pulmonary veins

Angiography in heart valve diseases and cardiomyopathies

The progress of echocardiography has made angiography redundant for the evaluation of many valvular disorders and cardiomyopathies. When the severity of valve disease requires surgical replacement or repair, coronary angiography is required in all candidates >40 years of age (or younger if multiple risk factors or anginal symptoms are present). While no other acquisitions or injections in heart cavities are strictly necessary, in the absence of severe haemodynamic compromise or renal impairment, left ventriculography is recommended for all patients with mitral valve disease and aortic insufficiency. Besides confirming the presence and severity of mitral regurgitation or indirect signs of mitral stenosis, the examination will define the presence and pattern of LV dysfunction. For aortic stenosis, crossing the valve when the need for valve replacement is already unequivocally confirmed by symptoms and non-invasive tests is not recommended. If, however, there is any doubt concerning the accuracy and reproducibility of the Doppler flow velocity measurement, the additional minimal risk of embolization and perforation while crossing a stenotic and calcific aortic valve becomes clinically acceptable. Once the gradient is measured, for left ventriculography it is recommended that a pigtail catheter for injection is advanced over a 0.89-mm (0.035-inch) J-tipped 260-cm wire. Occasionally, when pressure measurements in the right heart are required to better define the severity of mitral valve stenosis and pulmonary hypertension, injection of the right ventricle can offer additional data to confirm presence and severity of right ventricular dilatation and tricuspid regurgitation. In the laevophase, after having delineated the size of the arterial and venous pulmonary tree and circulation time, the dilatation of the left atrium and abnormal movement of the mitral cusps can be observed. In patients with aortic valve disease, the presence and severity of calcifications of the aortic cusps and ascending aorta, number of cusps and deformity of cusp opening, and presence of a pre-shaped aortic jet can be judged from both left ventriculography and aortography. The semi-quantitative assessment of the degree of aortic dilatation, the severity of aortic insufficiency (➲Table 8.8), and the description of irregularities and calcifications of the aortic wall are other key features to describe in a patient with aortic valve disease, hypertension, or Marfan syndrome. The use of a pigtail with radiopaque markers 1cm apart is preferred when the patient is under consideration for aortic root replacement or transcatheter implantation of an aortic valve.

Table 8.8 Semi-quantitative classification of aortic regurgitation

Trivial (grade 1 or 1+/4+): contrast visible in the left ventricle, without reaching the apex, clears during each heart beat
Mild (grade 2 or 2+/4+): contrast opacification less dense than that of the ascending which does not clear during a single heart beat
Moderate/severe (grade 3 or 3+/4+): opacification of the left ventricle as intense as that of the ascending aorta
Severe (grade 4 or 4+/4+): opacification of the left ventricle more intense than that of the ascending aorta and/or full left ventricular cavity opacified in one beat

Intracoronary ultrasound imaging

When IVUS was introduced 20 years ago, the pioneers of this technique believed it could replace angiography in the same way that endoscopic techniques have replaced conventional radiological assessment in gastroenterology. There are a number of reasons why this has not happened.

1) Unlike endoscopy, the technique does not stand alone, since it requires fluoroscopy and contrast injection to advance the IVUS probe.
2) Complete IVUS examination of all the major coronary vessels and their branches including the distal segments is cumbersome and requires expert image interpretation.
3) IVUS allows detection of angiographically silent atherosclerotic changes, but no new methods of focal plaque stabilization have been developed to justify routine application of this additional diagnostic method.
4) Despite the fact that the fundamental insights derived from IVUS had a dramatic impact in the improvement of our techniques of percutaneous revascularization, starting from high pressure stent deployment, no large randomized studies have convincingly shown clinical benefit over angiographic guidance alone

Image acquisition

Miniaturized flexible intracoronary ultrasound probes generate high-resolution cross-sectional images by spinning a single piezoelectric crystal at 360 degrees or by activating in sequence multiple (64) transducer elements (➲Fig. 8.13). The catheter produced by Boston-Scientific, Natick, MS, USA (Atlantis Pro) has a central frequency of 40MHz, a short Monorail at the tip with a very low crossing profile of 0.22 inch. The larger diameter of the shaft, required for saline flushing during catheter preparation and to

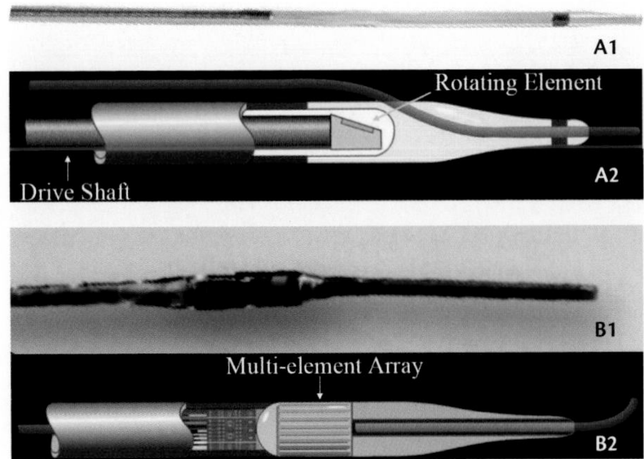

Figure 8.13 (A1–A2) Magnified photograph of the tip and schematics of a mechanical single element intravascular ultrasound (IVUS) catheter. Please note that the imaging cable moves inside a stationary transparent tube. (B1–B2) Magnified photograph of the tip and schematics of a multi element IVUS catheter.

accommodate the rotating cable, makes the profile compatible only with 6F guiding catheters. Volcano Therapeutics, Rancho Cordova, CA, USA has pioneered solid state IVUS technology and with its EagleEye Gold catheter of a uniform 2.9mm profile is the only system compatible with 5F guiding catheters. It is available for insertion as an over-the-wire catheter or with a normal monorail length with the imaging site very close to the distal tip. This system is preferable for IVUS guidance of a distal entry in a chronic total occlusion where the catheter has to be introduced into the false lumen (➲Fig. 8.14). In order to improve resolution, the same company has also developed a 45MHz catheter (Revolution), 3.2F in diameter, with mechanical characteristics similar to the Atlantis catheter. Larger probes with lower frequencies to improve penetration (10–15MHz) are used for intracardiac or intravascular examination of peripheral arteries but their use is illustrated with the specific technique of application. To add a third dimension (length) to the tomographic representation of the vessel wall, the catheter (in multi-element array systems) or the inner driving cable of the ultrasound crystal (in mechanical probes) is connected to a pull-back system, regulated at speeds between 0.5 and 2mm/s. Some investigators prefer the greater resolution and dynamic range that a mechanical system with a single large crystal (centre frequency 40 or 45MHz) can offer and consider favourably the unusual modality of imaging through a steady distal sheath that remains in position during the IVUS examination, with accurate pull-back allowed by the absence of friction against the vessel wall (➲Table 8.9). The safety of the technique was investigated in the first years after introduction [10], when stiffer and larger probes were available. These studies showed that the main complications were spasm, dissection, and thrombosis and that they occurred almost exclusively before or after angioplasty. More interestingly, no difference was observed in the mean diameter of arteries of heart transplant recipients repeatedly instrumented with ultrasound probes when compared with matched controls who had no IVUS examinations [11].

Image interpretation

Measurements

A truly normal intima is beyond the axial resolution of IVUS which, even at 40–45MHz, is >70μm *in vivo*. However, in most patients treated for coronary artery disease, almost all the sites explored in the coronaries will exhibit enough intimal thickening, due to ageing or early atherosclerotic changes, to separate it from the underlying adventitia. The acoustic interface between the intima surrounded by the echo-poor muscular media and the intensely bright collagen and elastic fibres of the adventitia induces an appearance often described as 'three-layered' or 'target-like'.

➲Table 8.10 indicates the main measurements offered by ultrasound. Both the European Society of Cardiology [12] and the American College of Cardiology [13] provide guidelines regarding common nomenclature and methods of qualitative and quantitative analysis of IVUS images. The most obvious measurement available with a technique that provides a circumferential image of the vessel is area, with the external contour drawn at the leading edge of the surrounding structures (➲Fig. 8.15). The area of the lumen and the area within the external elastic membrane (EEM), also called total vessel area, are the two most important dimensions and their difference provides the area of the intima–media complex. After treatment, stent area can also be measured and this is equivalent to the lumen area immediately after deployment unless a strut is not apposed to the vessel wall, or there is plaque prolapse narrowing the lumen. In the era before the advent of drug-eluting stents (DES), weeks and months after stent deployment a rim of tissue of variable thickness constantly covered the stent struts, allowing easy definition of the neointimal area, calculated as the difference between stent area and lumen area at follow-up. The anti-proliferative effect of DES often reduces intimal coverage to a thickness beyond the resolution capabilities of ultrasound.

Linear measurements are also possible with ultrasound and are required when IVUS is used to size devices for vessel dilatation, such as balloons and stents. Unfortunately, the vessel lumen and, especially, the area inside the EEM are rarely truly circular because plaques mostly grow

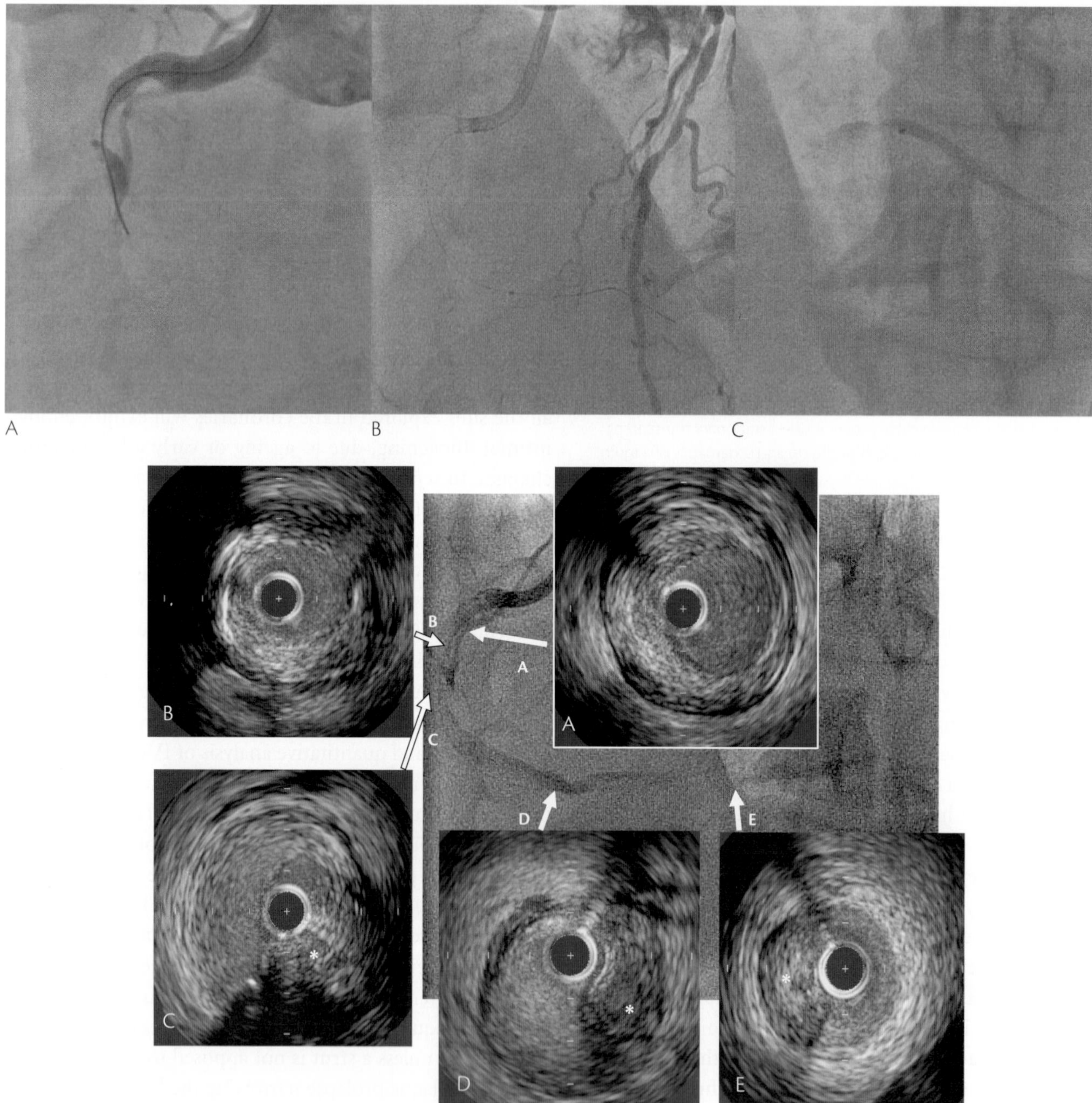

Figure 8.14 Panel 1: (A) Total occlusion of the mid RCA. (B) A polymer-coated wire is easily advanced into the occlusion, supported by an over-the-wire (OTW) balloon. Contralateral injection suggests that the position of the distal wire is extraluminal. (C) Injection after wire removal through the OTW balloon confirms the subintimal position with a cul-de-sac at the end of a large dissection. Further manipulation of an additional wire under conventional angiographic guidance was unable to reach the distal true lumen. Panel 2: five intravascular ultrasound (IVUS) cross-sections from proximal to distal (A – E) are indicated by arrows in the angiographic image. (A) and (B) are positioned in the proximal segment, proximal to the occlusion and the dissection. (C – E) are at various levels without the large dissection. Asterisks indicate the compressed false lumen.

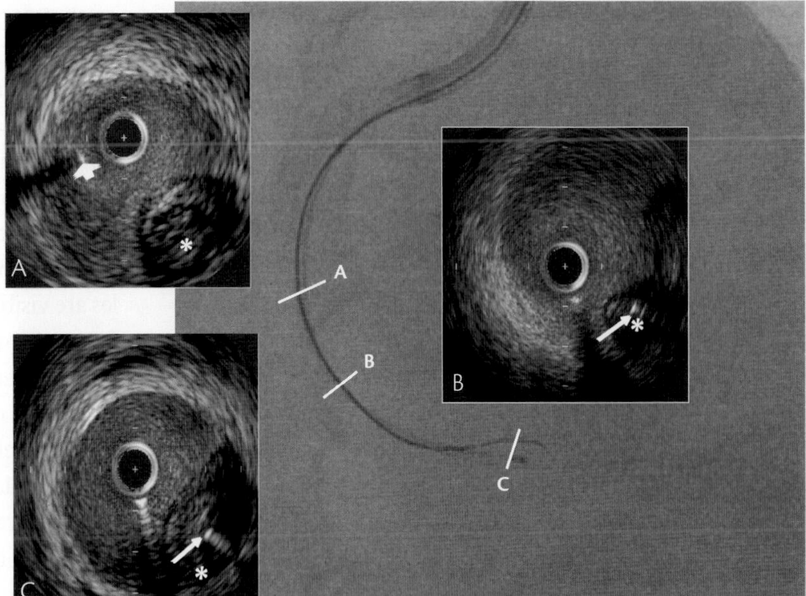

Figure 8.14 *(cont'd)* Panel 3: three IVUS cross-sections from proximal to distal (A –C) clearly show the position of the wire with respect to the collapsed true lumen (*). In (A) the wire, indicated by an arrowhead, is clearly in the dissection. In (B) and (C) the wire, indicated by a thin arrow, has been advanced into the true lumen under guidance of the IVUS catheter, initially position at the end of the true lumen to assess the correct direction required to penetrate the proximal cap and subsequently advanced more distal to confirm the persistent intraluminal position. An excellent result was achieved with ballooning and multiple stents along the intraluminal wire.

eccentrically or because the probe is not perfectly aligned with the long axis of the vessel, generating an oblique cut of the vessel. Two linear measurements are normally required for each cross-sectional image: minimal and maximal diameter. Minimal and maximal plaque thickness are also used to provide an index of plaque eccentricity (➲Fig. 8.15). In clinical practice, area and linear measurements are rarely taken in more than two or three locations, corresponding to the minimal lumen area before angioplasty or after balloon dilatation and the minimal stent area after stenting and to one-two reference sites proximal and/or distal outside the stenotic segment or the stent (➲Fig. 8.16). This last site is more subjective, although a cross-section with the largest area and/or the smallest plaque burden within 5–10mm of the margins of the stenotic segment or stent edge is often used. Because of vessel tapering, an average of the proximal and distal reference can offer a better estimate of the lesion severity and type of remodelling present within the stenotic segment. The comparison between vessel area in the stenosis and at a reference site allows calculation of the remodelling index. The positive remodelling described by Glagov in pathology studies has been confirmed in vivo and shown to be present in most sites with early atherosclerotic changes and critical stenoses. More rarely, the IVUS measurements are consistent with the presence of negative remodelling, either as a spontaneous process or as a consequence of shrinkage promoted by angioplasty (➲Fig. 8.17). In research applications, serial IVUS examinations are performed to obtain a reliable assessment of the biological processes of restenosis or progression of atherosclerosis. More reliable results are obtained averaging the lumen, stent and/or vessel area measurements over a certain length, with longitudinal measurements determined by steady pull-back at known speed during examination. This allows reproducible measurements of volumes from multiple equidistant cross-sections (Simpson's rule) or by the interpolation of longitudinal and cross-sectional contours [14]. Unfortunately, the lack of sharp contours between lumen and intima and, especially, between intima–media and adventitia often precludes a fully automated contour detection.

Qualitative assessment

The echo-intensity of the different plaque components in the image varies according to the system settings and requires a standard intensity for comparison. The adventitia, relatively spared by the disease process, offers a natural site for comparison of the different components of the atherosclerotic plaque, which are rarely homogeneous and often contain various elements of different echo-reflectivity (➲Fig. 8.18). Plaques as bright, or brighter than the adventitia are often referred to as 'fibrous' unless they induce acoustic shadowing and reverberations, specific landmarks of the presence of calcium (➲Fig. 8.19).

Calcification, detected with greater sensitivity than with angiography, can be located within the plaque, from superficial subendothelial calcium speckles to deep deposits at the base of the plaque, and can be quantified based on their circumferential extension, measured in degrees or quadrants, and length. Plaques with low echo-reflectivity are often described as 'soft', a very inappropriate term since most of these plaques are far from mechanically pliable

Table 8.9 Protocol of intravascular ultrasound image acquisition

Before imaging
Connection of the ultrasound catheter with the imaging console
Patient demographics and vessel examined entered
For mechanical transducer accurate flashing with a small syringe
Connect the catheter/handle to the motorized pullback system set to 0.5mm/s
Activate and test that an image is generated before insertion
Inject 0.1–0.3mg of nitroglycerine or 1–3mg of isosorbide dinitrate according to blood pressure and risk of spasm
During imaging
For electronic catheters, before intracoronary insertion withdraw the guiding catheter, obtain an image immediately outside the coronary ostium, and subtract the ring down artefact
Advance the catheter distal to the segment of interest
Optimize the ultrasound setting (depth and gain) and start digital acquisition/mechanical pullback
Check ECG and pressure during pullback to rule out prolonged ischaemia, especially during pre-dilatation imaging
Complete the pullback, in general waiting until the catheter reaches the coronary ostium or is withdrawn inside the guiding catheter
Avoid stopping the mechanical pullback and rather recall the cross-sections of interest from the digital archive after the acquisition has been completed
Re-insert the catheter for acquisition of the images in a segment of interest only if there are doubts in image interpretation (e.g. if there is a need to use saline flushing in a specific segment to confirm the presence of ulcerated plaques, dissections, lumen/intima border in the presence of slow flow, etc., or contrast injection to identify the location of a given cross-section along the vessel)
After imaging
Flush the ultrasound catheter (in particular for mechanical probes) and clean it
Reposition the catheter ready for a new pull-back
Identify and perform measurements (diameter and areas) of the most important cross sections (usually reference segment, proximal and/or distal or both, minimal cross-sectional area within the lesion or minimal cross-sectional stent area of other segments of interest (➲Fig. 8.16)
Allow longitudinal display of the image after longitudinal reconstruction (long view) and measure the length of the segment of interest (e.g. length of segment to be stented)
Store the images in a DICOM digital format in the same server and with the same identification name of the DICOM angiographic images
Prepare a report including measurements and qualitative image interpretation

and include histological components as dyshomogeneous as fibrofatty tissue, thrombus, and neointima inside stents (➲Fig. 8.20).

Other qualitative characteristics include the presence of plaque disruption, spontaneous or after angioplasty. Niches, ulcers, spontaneous dissections with thrombi, often associated with positive pathological remodelling and frequently multifocal, are the pathognomonic changes described in unstable syndromes (➲Fig. 8.17) [15]. Rupture, dissections, mural haematomas were the end result of angioplasty before stenting and are now confined to the stent edges in most cases. In the stent era other qualitative characteristics concern the relationship between struts and vessel wall. Strut malapposition can be detected when blood speckles are visible between stent and wall. These changes are rather frequent immediately after stent deployment unless a consistent attempt is made to use IVUS to size the balloons for final stent expansion. At follow-up, only IVUS examination immediately after deployment can distinguish between persistent malapposition, present from the time of deployment, and acquired malapposition, possibly a more worrisome phenomenon related to positive remodelling, lysis of thrombus, or toxic vascular effects of the antiproliferative drug.

Prestenotic atherosclerosis

Patients with angina or silent myocardial ischaemia dismissed as 'false positive' or 'possible vasospastic angina' [16] or 'cryptogenic' myocardial infarction because of the presence of a normal or near-normal coronary angiograms show atherosclerotic changes at IVUS in the majority of cases, suggesting more aggressive treatment of the risk factors in order to tackle both disease progression and impaired coronary vasomotor activity. The new challenge for treatment of coronary artery disease is the detection of plaques not yet impairing flow but at risk of rapid progression and destabilization. 'Vulnerable' plaques are typically characterized by a thin fibrous cap infiltrated by inflammatory cells and a large superficial lipid pool within a positively remodelled plaque [17, 18]. The application of radio frequency analysis (virtual histology, VH) to IVUS backscatter enhances characterization of plaque components [19]. Still, not all episodes of unstable angina and infarction are caused by 'vulnerable' plaques (erosion, protruding calcium, ischaemia secondary to increased demand), and the resolution and qualitative interpretation of IVUS is insufficient to precisely measure the fibrous cap or detect macrophages. Results of the PROSPECT trial (Providing Regional Observation to Study Predictors of Events in the Coronary Tree) will be soon presented and will be helpful to determine the likelihood of plaques with different IVUS-VH morphology, of causing disease progression and acute clinical events.

Recent data however emphasize that the relation between plaque burden, plaque composition, and prognosis is complex. In the IBIS-1 study (Integrated Biomarker and Imaging Study) VH was applied to relate temporal changes in plaque

Table 8.10 Intracoronary ultrasound measurements in common use

Measurement	Units	Definition	Comments
Lumen area	mm^2	Area inside the intimal leading edge	If separation between intima and lumen is unclear because of lumen irregularities (ulcus within plaques of dissections) or because of slow flow, injection of saline may facilitate contour detection. Ideally do not perform measurement during saline infusion (increased lumen because of higher pressure, and different speed of ultrasound in saline than in blood)
EEM area (total vessel area)	mm^2	Area inside the leading edge of the adventitia	Do not trace if >90° of vessel circumference not visible because of shadowing or attentuation
Stent area	mm^2	Area inside the stent struts	Stented area corresponds to lumen area unless a strut is not apposed to the vessel wall (under-expansion or localized aneurysm) or there is plaque prolapse
Plaque plus media area	mm^2	Difference between EEM area and lumen area in a corresponding cross-section	Not detectable if obscured by the presence of superficial calcium or stent struts
In-stent neointimal area	mm^2	Difference between stent area and lumen area images in images acquired late after stent development	Can be missed because of very poor echogenicity of the intimal areas, difficult to distinguish from the lumen, especially in cases of subocclusive restenosis or because (drug-eluting) stent is reduced to a micrometric rim of thickening below the threshold of measurement with ultrasound
Percentage plaque area	%	Percentage of EEM area occupied by plaque and calculated as: (EEM area – lumen area) / EEM area × 100	
Percentage neointimal area	%	(Stent area – lumen area) / stent area × 100	
Plaque eccentricity index		Measurement of plaque eccentricity calculated as the ratio between minimal and maximal plaque plus media thickness	1 indicates concentric plaque, <1 indicates increasing plaque eccentricity. *NB* American authors tend to use the reverse index, with larger numbers indicating progressively greater eccentricity
In-stent lumen volume	mm^3	Lumen volume inside the stent segment calculated with multiple equispaced area measurements and Simpson's rule or with automatic contour detection of multiple cross-sectional and longitudinal contours	Immediately after stent deployment, area should be equal to stent volume
Stent volume	mm^3	Volume inside the stent	Easily calculated because of the bright stent landmarks
Neointimal stent volume	mm^3	Difference between stent volume and lumen volume inside the stent	More difficult to assess with drug-eluting stents because of the extremely thin rim of intimal hyperplasia
Percentage intimal volume in-stent	%	(Stent area – lumen area) / stent area × 100	Ideal biological indicator of intimal proliferation inside a stent

EEM, external elastic membrane.

composition and volume, and circulating biomarkers [20]. After 6 months, an overall decrease in biomarkers levels was not coupled with changes in IVUS-VH plaque size or composition.

IVUS is an accepted gold standard for validating other tomographic non-invasive imaging modalities which still have much lower resolution such as cardiac magnetic resonance imaging and high-resolution 64-slice electron beam computed tomography. Three-dimensional reconstruction of IVUS cross-sections generates a volume of plaque in a given segment, identified by reliable anatomical markers (side branches, aortic anastomosis), and has become the technique of choice for the assessment of progression/regression of coronary atherosclerosis and comparison of the effects of different drug regimens. Allograft vasculopathy is another field now of potential application. In donor-related coronary atherosclerosis, IVUS often shows spectacular regression after heart transplantation. Both the early development of atherosclerotic changes (>0.5mm thickness in the first year post transplant) and its progression in serial studies carry a negative

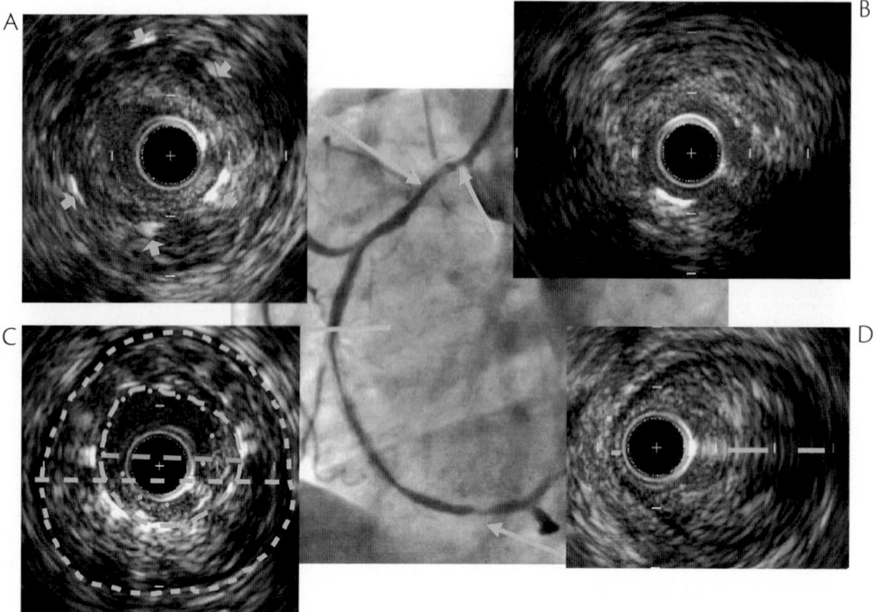

Figure 8.15 Four intravascular ultrasound cross-sectional images corresponding to the positions indicated in the left anterior oblique angiographic image of a right coronary artery in a patient with diffuse restenosis 3 months after multiple stents were implanted from the ostium to the mid segment. (A) Gross under-expansion and diffuse hyperplasia within the stent indicated by the bright dots/strips (arrowheads). (B) In this cross-section at the level of the vessel ostium the absence of stents is obvious, with restenosis probably due to recoil of the large concentric lesion not covered during the initial procedure. (C) Lumen (inner dotted line), stent (dashed lines around circumference and across maximal diameter) and vessel (external elastic membrane, EEM) area (outer dotted line around circumference and across maximal diameter). Using the 1-mm divisions of the calibration grid, it is apparent that the stent diameter is 2.3mm compared with an EEM diameter of 4.5mm. (D) Distal stenosis: the extreme eccentricity (0.2mm minimal plaque thickness, 1.9mm maximal plaque thickness) cannot be fully appreciated with angiography.

prognostic value. IVUS can also be used to monitor the effect of drugs to prevent or delay coronary vasculopathy.

Lesions of intermediate severity

The superiority of IVUS over angiography for detecting coronary stenoses that are difficult to assess in multiple views allows its use in the study of lesions of questionable severity. The threshold of absolute cross-sectional area most frequently used to determine whether interventions must be carried out is 3.5–4.0mm^2 in epicardial native coronary arteries [21]. The threshold for the left main coronary artery is more controversial, but most operators would treat lesions with a MLCSA <6.0mm^2. Absolute areas >6.9mm^2 (or 2.8mm diameter) has recently been shown to be associated with a normal fractional flow reserve (FFR) and a good 3-year prognosis when left untreated [22]. The presence of a good correlation with FFR does not mean that IVUS, in the absence of longitudinal studies confirming its good prognostic value, can replace pressure measurements to assess lesion severity. Conceptually, it is obvious that a lumen area of <4.0mm^2 has a completely different functional relevance in a proximal LAD than in a diagonal branch. Still, for assessment of stenoses in main vessels when the operator feels there is high likelihood treatment is required, IVUS is a potential alternative because it offers the additional value of measuring the proximal and distal reference lumen diameter, to assess presence, size, and characteristics of the plaque, to visualize the relationship of the lesion with other branches, especially for ostial and bifurcational lesions, and to demonstrate the type of remodelling, all important factors to guide the angioplasty procedure (➲Fig. 8.20).

Guidance of coronary interventions

The wealth of data accumulated in the attempt to demonstrate the usefulness of IVUS for guiding balloon angioplasty and atherectomy is now obsolete because of the universal use of coronary stenting. Nevertheless, it is obvious from trials such as PICTURE [23] and CLOUT [24] that IVUS is the most sensitive technique for detecting dissection after balloon dilatation and for determining the most appropriate balloon size to safely achieve a large lumen gain. Other trials showing the equivalence of IVUS-guided coronary angioplasty and stenting are only of historical interest. Stenting was the main promoter of the use of ultrasound in the interventional community [25]. The frequent detection of incomplete stent expansion and apposition when stent size was selected angiographically and stents were expanded at nominal balloon pressures were associated with

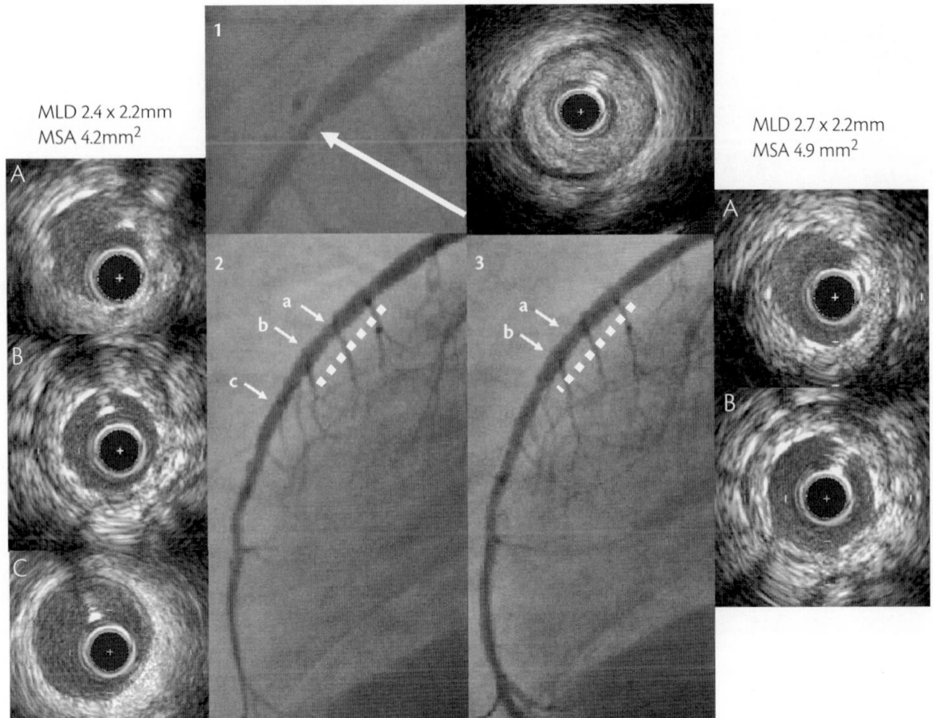

Figure 8.16 Angiographic images and corresponding cross-sectional images of a short lesion of the mid-LAD before and after intravascular ultrasound (IVUS)-guided stent expansion. Panel 1 on top indicates the pre-intervention angiogram and the corresponding IVUS image. Note that there is almost no lumen around the ultrasound catheter because of a large concentric plaque with no calcium but a high echoreflectivity matching the echoreflectivity of the adventitia. Panel 2 on the left indicates the angiographic result after implantation (dotted line on the panel) of a 2.5mm x 13mm sirolimus eluting Cypher® stent at 18 Atm. The mild residual under expansion observed angiographically is confirmed with ultrasound which shows in (a) an area and minimal diameter far smaller than the distal reference area/diameters (5.9mm^2, 2.9 x 2.6mm), shown in (c). Panel 3 on the right shows the angiographic result after further expansion with a short (8mm) 3.0mm non-compliant balloon at 24 Atm. The measurements at the site of the minimal cross-sectional area in (a) indicate a moderate further expansion, with a final area approaching the distal reference area, while the image in (b) shows better compression of the highly resistant fibrous plaque compared with the corresponding image on the left panel.

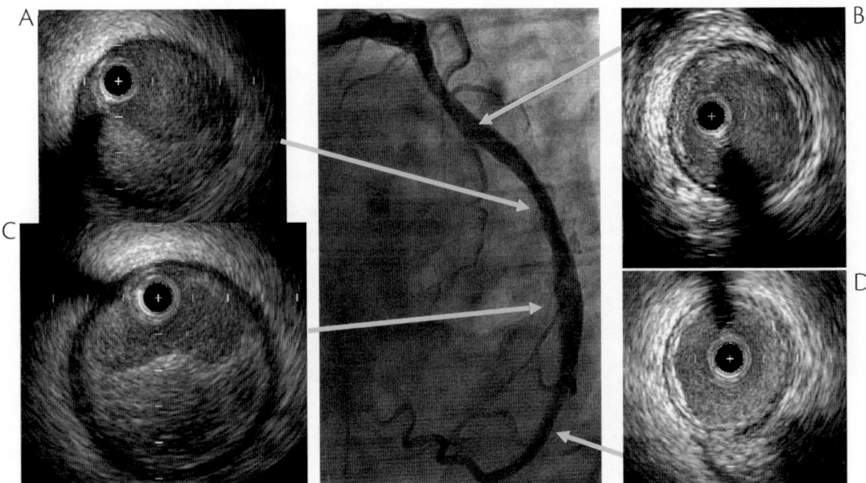

Figure 8.17 Four intravascular ultrasound cross-sectional images corresponding to the positions indicated in the left anterior oblique angiographic image of a left circumflex artery in a patient with recent ST-elevation lateral myocardial infarction 3 days after thrombolysis. The absence of severe residual stenosis is confirmed by ultrasound, which shows extreme positive remodelling when the cross-sections at the level of the culprit lesion (A and C) are compared with the proximal (B) and distal (D) reference cross-sections, where only a concentric rim of fibrous plaque is observed. Note that the eccentric plaque in (A) has a much lower echogenicity than the surrounding adventitia and that the inhomogeneous texture of the plaque in (C) is due to plaque rupture with channels communicating with the lumen inside the plaque. The absence of regular concavity of the intimal edge suggests recent thrombosis.

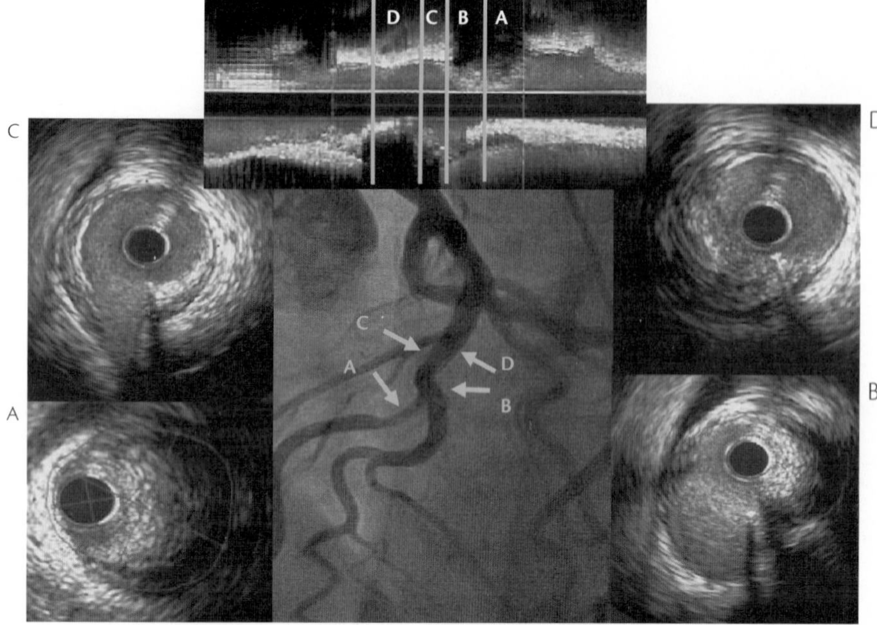

Figure 8.18 Four intravascular ultrasound cross-sectional images corresponding to the positions indicated in the cranial left anterior oblique angiographic image of a left anterior descending coronary artery in a patient with a lesion immediately distal to the bifurcation of a large diagonal branch. The heterogeneous plaque composition and involvement of the main vessel proximal to the bifurcation are clearly displayed in the longitudinal reconstruction of the multiple images acquired during pull-back. (A) Main subocclusive eccentric fibrotic lesion with no lumen around the ultrasound catheter. (B) Cross-section at the origin of the diagonal branch (below) shows normal intima in the branch but a large eccentric plaque opposite the bifurcation. More proximally (C) a fibrous concentric plaque is observed, with a large inhomogeneous eccentric plaque in (D) at a level which appears angiographically normal.

greater frequency of subacute stent thrombosis and restenosis. The rationale for the development of the technique of high-pressure stent implantation is derived from IVUS observations and was universally accepted during stenting procedures, also by operators sceptical about IVUS. Multiple randomized trials have shown the efficacy of adequate double antiplatelet treatment without ultrasound guidance in reducing subacute stent thrombosis to 1–1.5% in discrete lesions suitable for stenting. Larger lumen areas obtained with IVUS guided upsizing of the balloons used were consistently associated with lower restenosis rates. Randomized studies and meta-analyses on the ability of IVUS to reduce restenosis after stenting have given conflicting results, with no advantage shown in the largest randomized trial [26].

The use of antiproliferative stent coatings to reduce intimal hyperplasia has had a significant impact in modern

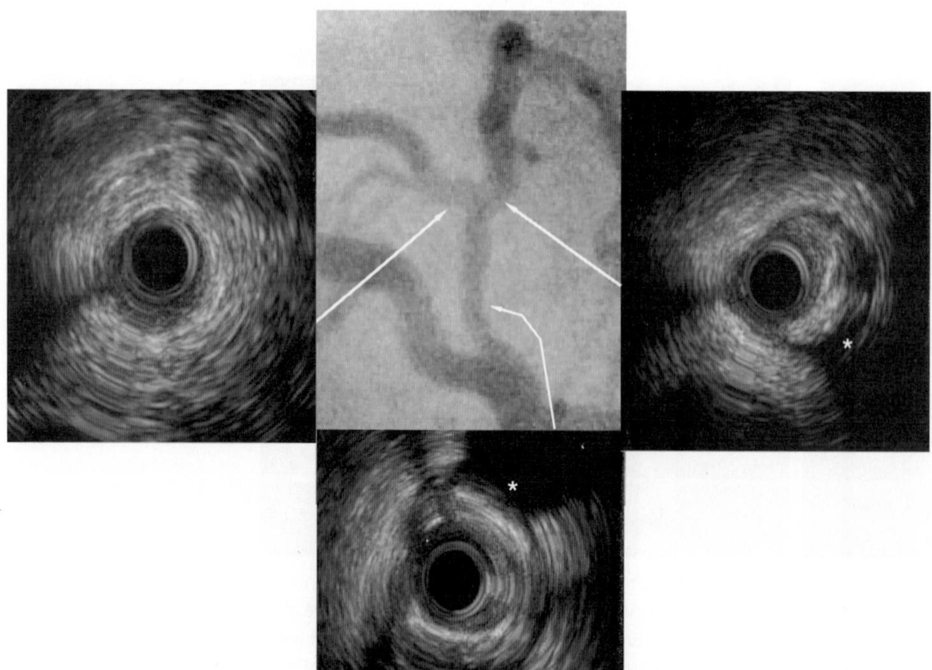

Figure 8.19 Panel 1: angiographic image in a skewed 'spider' (left caudal) view shows a lesion in a large diagonal branch involving two bifurcation branches of this vessel. The corresponding ultrasound images in the proximal diagonal and at the ostium of the distal branches indicate severe plaque accumulation and calcification (shadowing marked by asterisks) with a vessel (EEM) diameter ranging from 3.2mm in the proximal diagonal to 2.3 and 2.8mm in the two distal branches.

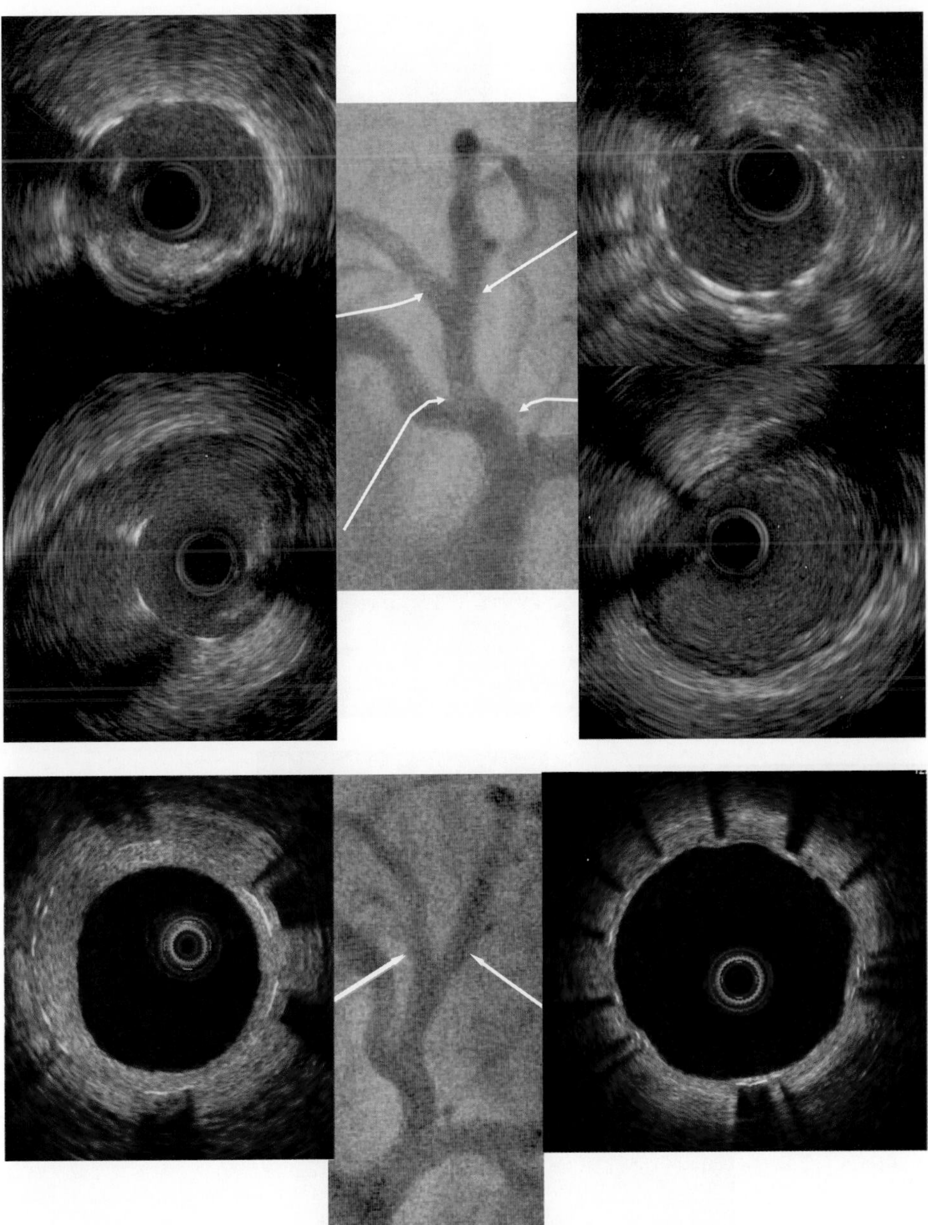

Figure 8.19 *(cont'd)* Panel 2: based on the pre-intervention intravascular ultrasound (IVUS) images, after cutting balloon dilatation with a 2.5mm balloon, a modified culotte technique is applied using a Tryton bare metal stent (19mm) mounted on a tapered balloon (3.5mm proximal and 2.5mm distal) and a 3.0 x 23mm sirolimus eluting Cypher® stent overlapping the proximal Tryton stent in the proximal vessel. The result after final post-expansion with kissing balloon dilatation (2.5 and 3.0mm balloons at 12 Atm) show good expansion in the larger of the two branches (upper right IVUS image), incomplete eccentric expansion at the ostium of the smaller of the two branches (upper left IVUS image), good deployment up to the diagonal ostium of the stent, with minimal strut protrusion into the LAD (lower left IVUS image), and moderate eccentric plaque with deep calcium in the proximal unstented LAD (lower right panel). Panel 3: elective angiographic control 7 months after stenting, showing a persistently good angiographic result with mild narrowing in the smaller of the branches where a bare metal stent was deployed. The corresponding optical coherence tomography images in both branches indicate minimal thickness and diffuse uniform coverage of the Cypher® stent and more evident asymmetric intimal proliferation in the bare metal stent, still non functionally significant.

interventional cardiology and profoundly modified the technique of stent implantation. Measurements of percentage neointimal volume obstruction with IVUS in large multicentre randomized trials have confirmed a consistent reduction of in-stent hyperplasia in comparison with conventional stenting [27]. This has led to a less compulsive attempt to achieve proper stent expansion. Still, stent under-expansion is associated with more frequent restenosis and stent failure, with a lower threshold of absolute minimal lumen cross-sectional area within the stent than in the bare metal stent era [28, 29]. Recent data confirmed that stent under expansion is the most common mechanism of restenosis after DES implantation [30, 31]. In a large study of 550 patients with 670 native coronary artery lesions treated with Cypher stents, IVUS cut-offs that best predicted angiographic restenosis were an MLCSA of 5.5mm^2 and a stent length of 40mm [32].

Late stent thrombosis is a rare but feared complication of DES. IVUS has been used in the attempt of identifying the features that increase the risk of thrombosis. Some studies focused on the relationship between malapposition and thrombosis [33–36]. Acute malapposition after DES was revealed by IVUS more frequently than in bare metal stents [27, 33, 34]. Late-acquired malapposition after DES,

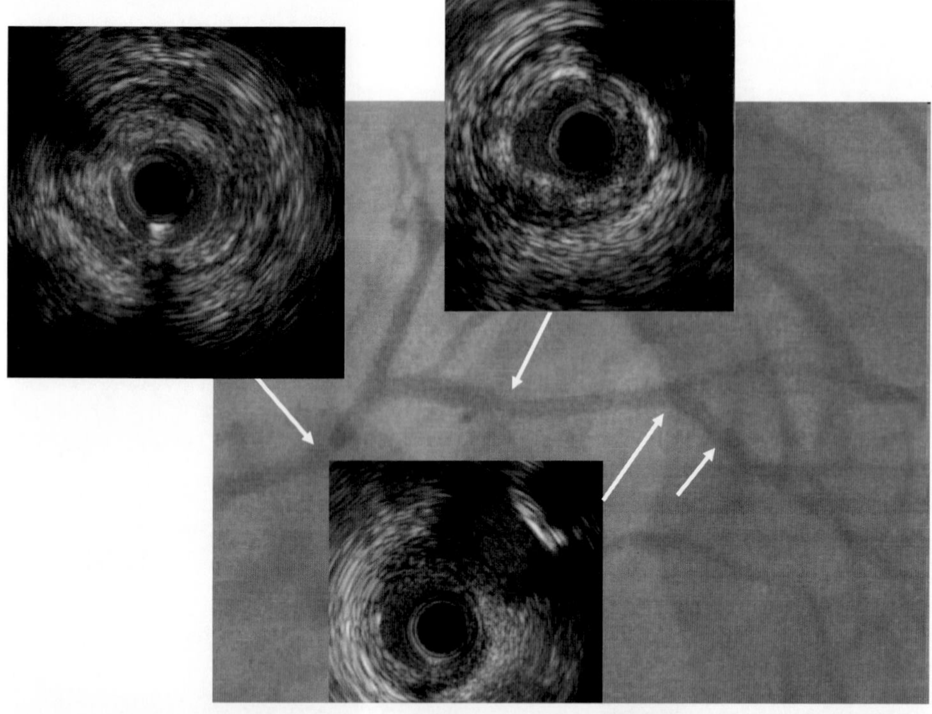

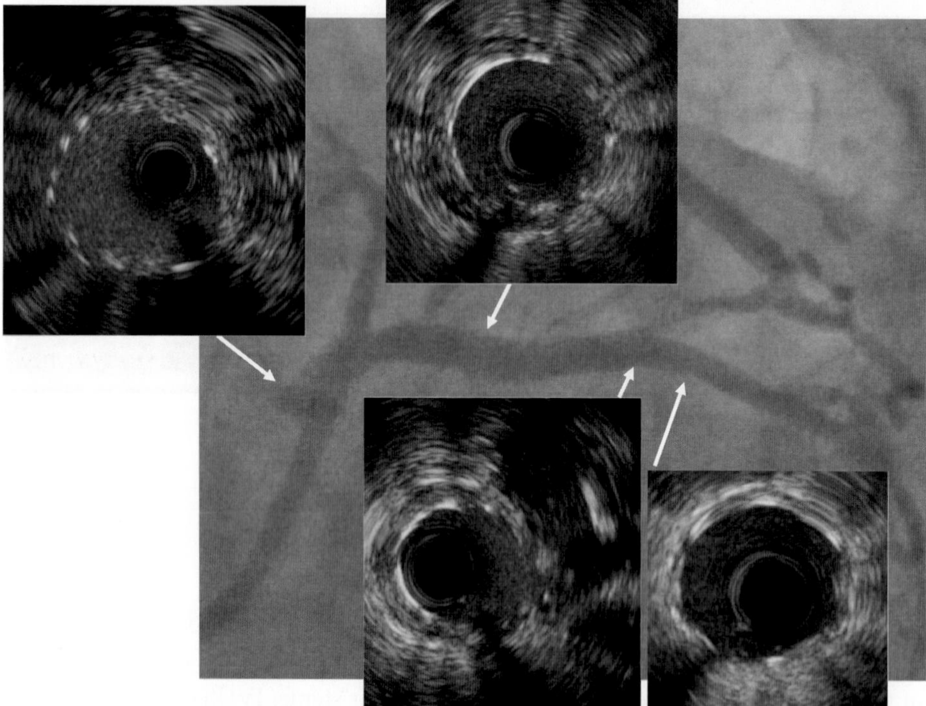

Figure 8.20 Panel 1: angiographic image in a 'spider' (left caudal) view ishowing an ostial lesion in the left main coronary artery and the mid left circumflex, with difficult visualization of the distal vessel because of competitive flow via a vein graft for a marginal branch with severe proximal stenosis. The severity and length of disease is well demonstrated with pre-intervention intravascular ultrasound (IVUS) showing severe concentric non-calcific stenosis of the left main coronary artery (upper right IVUS image), severe stenosis of the mid-left circumflex (LCX) with an eccentric calcific plaque (upper left IVUS image) extending up to the origin of the obtuse marginal branch (lower left IVUS image). The normal appearance of the distal LCX (lower left panel) offers a good distal reference segment. Panel 2: based on the length of the diseased segment in the motorized pre-intervention IVUS run and the vessel (EEM) diameter in the various location explored, three Everolimus® eluting stents are expanded to 3mm in the distal LCX (right lower IVUS image), 3.5mm at very high pressure in the more resistant lesion of the proximal LCX (upper right IVUS image) and LCX bifurcation (lower right IVUS image), 4.0mm in the left main with kissing balloon dilatation for the left anterior descending artery where a patent mammary is implanted downstream (upper left IVUS image). Please note that partial protrusion into the aorta is unavoidable to obtain full ostial coverage in ostial lesions of the left main and right coronary arteries.

a phenomenon related to regional vessel positive remodelling, was less common than acute malapposition as it was observed in <13% of patients [33, 34].

When to use IVUS

With in-stent restenosis dramatically reduced to single figures in most lesion subsets, edge restenosis has become a more frequent cause of treatment failure. Ultrasound can be used to optimize the selection of the length and the precise placement of the stent, thus avoiding leaving segments of severe plaque accumulation or dissection uncovered.

As under expansion is the main cause of DES failure [35, 36], in the presence of long lesions or calcified vessels or in segments of difficult angiographic assessment (ostia or bifurcations), ultrasound is the best technique to properly assess expansion. Full lesion coverage is also very difficult to confirm with only angiography (➲Fig. 8.18). The application of these concepts potentially will improve clinical results in the presence of an IVUS-guided approach of DES deployment, as pointed out by a recent study comparing the clinical outcomes of 884 patients having an IVUS-guided strategy with the outcomes of a propensity-score matched population undergoing an angiographic guided approach. Patients undergoing IVUS-guided DES implantation had, at 30 days and at 12 months, a significantly lower rate of definite stent thrombosis and a favourable trend of lower target lesion revascularization [38]. Despite the uncertainty on the clinical significance of malapposition, it is intuitive that a complete apposition of equispaced stent struts is not only important for reducing thrombogenicity but also allows the stent to uniformly deliver the antiproliferative drug where needed [37]. Incomplete apposition cannot be assessed with angiography, and is in large vessels, bifurcation lesions and long lesions in tapering vessels a frequent phenomenon, possibly explaining some of the failures of DES. These considerations may explain the mortality reduction observed after 3 years in the patients treated with left main stenoses under IVUS guidance in the unpublished MAIN-COMPARE IVUS Registry.

For restenoses after both conventional bare metal stents and DES, treatment is currently performed with the use of DES. Knowledge of the initial mechanism of restenosis (under-expansion, hyperplasia, incomplete lesion coverage) (➲Fig. 8.15) is important for selecting the proper length and diameter of stent to be deployed and for guiding its expansion.

Optical coherence tomography

Physical principles and image acquisition

OCT is a novel imaging modality that is capable of visualizing vessel anatomy at a resolution around ten times greater than IVUS due to the much shorter wavelength of the imaging light [39].

Current OCT images are obtained via 0.019 in imaging wires containing optical fibres, at a peak wavelength in the 1280–1350nm band, that enables a 10–15μ tissue axial resolution. Images are then displayed using a log false colour scale, at 20 frames/s and 200 lines/frame. These parameters have been further improved with the use of frequency domain OCT which allows acquisition of 100 frames/s and 500 lines/frame, allowing a more rapid pull-back and a wider field of view with maintained or improved image quality [40].The superb resolution of OCT is obtained at the expense of a limited tissue penetration, which is the main limitation of OCT. Penetration is dependent on tissue characteristics and is between 0.5–1.5mm of imaging depth; it is minimal in presence of thrombus, poor for superficial necrotic lipid pools, higher for calcific components, and maximal for fibrous tissues [41–43] (➲Fig. 8.21).

The main obstacle to the widespread application of OCT imaging in clinical practice is the need for a bloodless field, which requires clearing or flushing of blood from the lumen. In the occlusive technique, coronary blood flow is stopped by inflating a proximal occlusion balloon and a crystalloid solution, usually Ringer's lactate, is flushed through the end-hole of the balloon catheter at a flow rate of 0.5–1.0mL/s [44]. In the non-occlusive technique, pull-back is performed during infusion of iodinated contrast through the guiding catheter at an infusion rate between

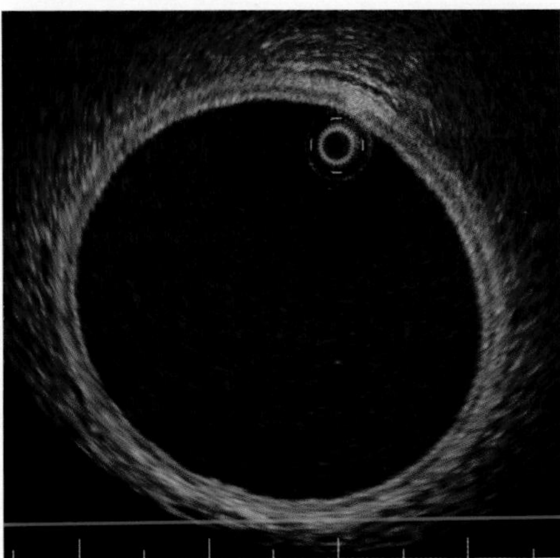

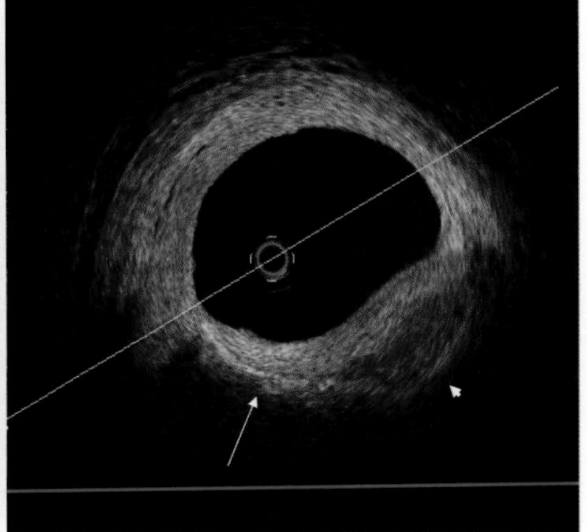

Figure 8.21 Left panel: normal three layer appearance in a 31-year-old female patient can be appreciated, with the muscular media being shown as a low signal layer comprised between internal and external lamina. Right panel: eccentric coronary plaque with fibrous (arrow) and calcific (arrow-head) components. Note that outer wall is shown only between 9 and 2 o'clock, where only minor hyperplasia is present.

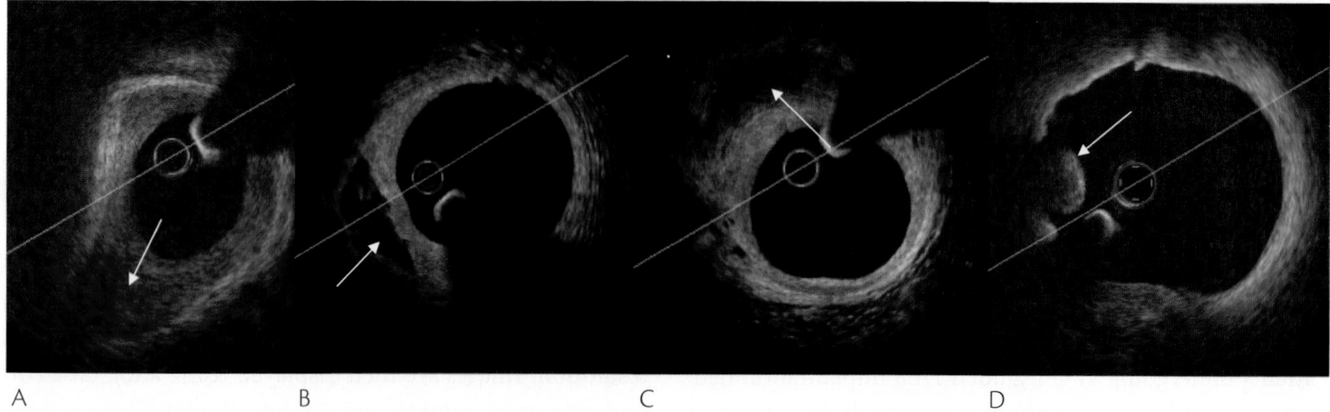

Figure 8.22 Examples (arrows) of fibrotic (A), calcific (B), lipid-rich (C) plaque components and of protruding thrombus (D).

1cc/s and 3cc/s. Iodixanol-320, Visipaque®, GE Health Care, Ireland is often preferred because of its high viscosity, minimizing artefacts due to blood mixing, and its low arrhythmogenicity [45–47].

Normal coronary morphology and atherosclerosis

In normal vessels and at sites with mild intimal thickening, not exceeding 1–1.5mm, the coronary artery wall appears as a three-layer structure in OCT images. The media is seen as a dark band delimited by the internal elastic lamina (IEL) and external elastic lamina (EEL). Despite their minimal thickness (<6μm) IEL and the EEL generates a 20-μm rich band that can be visualized by OCT. The adventitia is a signal-rich, heterogeneously texted outer layer (➲ Fig. 8.21).

Unfortunately, because of its limited tissue penetration (1–1.5mm), OCT does not appear to be suited to study vessel remodelling or to visualize the deeper components of thick plaques, which are well addressed by IVUS.

Qualitative definitions

Calcifications within plaques are identified by the presence of well-delineated, low back-scattering heterogeneous regions (➲ Fig. 8.22). Fibrous plaques consist of homogeneous high back-scattering areas (➲ Fig. 8.22). Necrotic lipid pools are less well-delineated than calcifications and exhibit lower signal density and more heterogeneous back-scattering than fibrous plaques. There is a strong contrast between lipid-rich cores and fibrous regions within OCT images. Therefore, lipid pools most often appear as diffusely-bordered, signal-poor regions (lipid pools) with overlying signal-rich bands, corresponding to fibrous caps [48–50] (➲ Fig. 8.22). In the majority of lesions, lipid pool thickness cannot be measured because of insufficient OCT imaging penetration but the thickness of the subendothelial fibrous cap delineating superficial lipid pools can be measured by OCT [48–51]. Pathological studies of plaques leading to fatal events have established 65μm as the threshold of fibrous cap thickness that best identifies vulnerable lesions so that this value is often adopted as the cut-off threshold for identifying thin capped atheromas prone to rupture *in vivo*.

Thrombi are identified as masses protruding into the vessel lumen discontinuous from the surface of the vessel wall. Red thrombi are characterized by high-backscattering protrusions with signal-free shadowing. White thrombi appear as signal-rich, low-backscattering billowing projections protruding into the lumen [51] (➲ Figs. 8.22 and 8.23A).

OCT has the potential to identify inflammatory cells such as clusters of macrophages, seen as bands of high reflectivity in OCT images. When macrophages are located in a plaque with a lipid pool, macrophage streaks appear within the fibrous cap covering the lipid pool [53].

Acute plaque ulceration or rupture can be detected by OCT as a ruptured fibrous cap that connects the lumen with the lipid pool (➲ Figs. 8.22 and 8.23B).These ulcerated or ruptured plaques may occur with a superimposed thrombus and this can impair the visualization of the underlying rupture [54, 55].

Optical coherence tomography for assessment of coronary interventions

Poor penetration limits the practical value of OCT for pre-intervention imaging, making this technique less suitable than IVUS for sizing balloons and stents. Still lumen area, with the exception of the largest vessels, can be easily detected with OCT. Potentially, all the considerations made before to determine when treatment is warranted and when the lumen inside the stent matches the proximal and distal

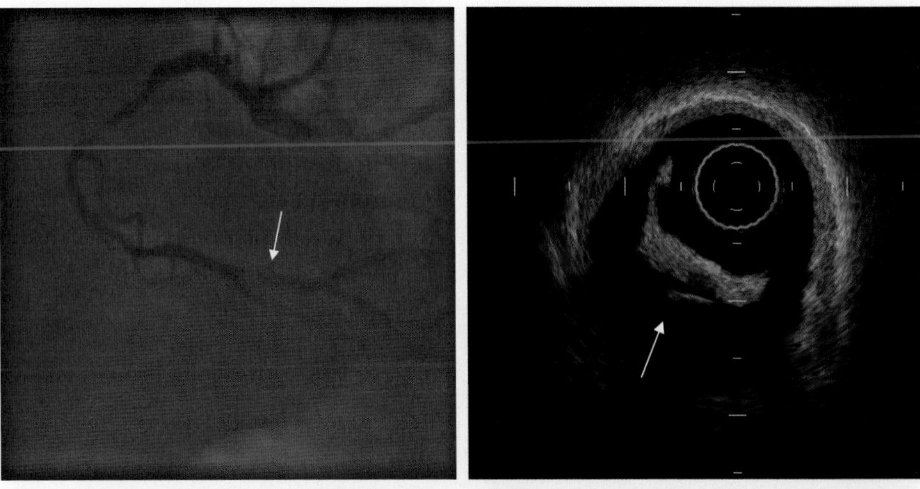

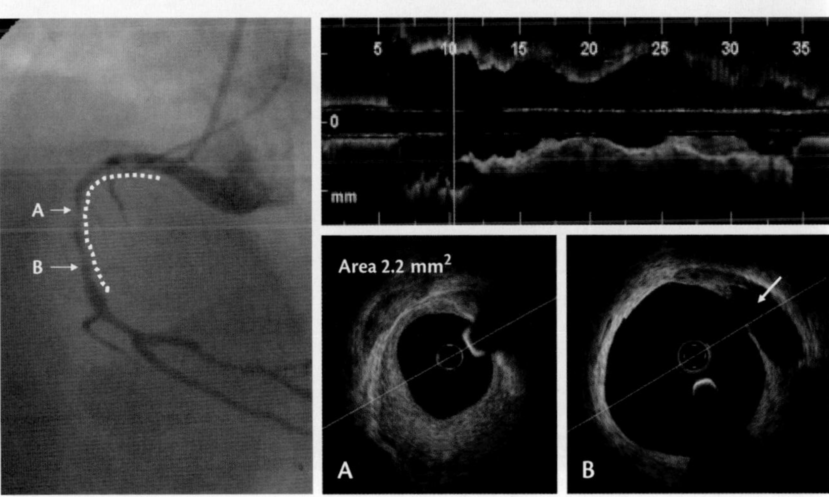

Figure 8.23 Panel 1: culprit lesion in a distal right coronary artery (arrow in the angiographic image). In the corresponding optical coherence tomography image an intraluminal thrombus is indicated by an arrow. Panel 2: more proximal lesions shown in the same artery during a motorized pull-back at 3mm/s during contrast injection. From the longitudinal image (upper right) it is obvious that >30mm of vessels have been successfully visualized during a single pull-back, covering the entire segment delineated by the dotted line in the angiographic image. In the segment marked with A in the angiographic image, a stable lesion with smooth contours is observed (A). More distally, the arrow in the corresponding optical coherence tomography image (B) indicates an ulcerated plaque, with a large cavity in communication with the vessel lumen.

lumen can be repeated for OCT. The exquisite sensitivity in detecting dissections, including thin flaps created by wire passage of no clinical relevance, is sometimes confusing for beginners but the sharp contours facilitate measurements and avoid the need of the long training required for interpretation of IVUS images. The main limitation of the technique is the complexity of performing repeated examinations, especially when the cumbersome occlusion balloon method is used. OCT images acquired during contrast flush via the guiding catheter have facilitated acquisition but it is unthinkable that multiple passages are performed when 30–40mL of contrast are required per acquisition and the wire must be exchanged several times using an over-the-wire dedicated catheter. The very fast acquisition of the new development of optical frequency domain analysis, allows acquisition with a catheter-based probe during few seconds of flushing, possibly with saline. When available, this may ensure that optical based imaging is used to replace, at least in part, IVUS for guidance of coronary interventions.

The real value of OCT is the superior ability to study apposition and intimal coverage after stent implantation. Struts are seen as dense strips because metal, unlike calcium, cannot be penetrated by OCT (➲Fig. 8.24 and 8.25). Although the intima immediately below the strut cannot be seen, the artefacts around struts are much less prominent than with ultrasound and the relationship between strut and surrounding intima can be studied. Struts often appear as protruding from the intima but the physical thickness of the strut must be considered to judge apposition [56]. Thinner stent struts have been shown to have fewer protruding or unapposed struts than thicker stent struts [57] but no longitudinal observations correlating these findings with late coverage or clinical events are available at this stage.

A number of OCT results after implantation of DES have been reported [58–64] (➲Figs. 8.19 and 8.26). Takano and colleagues undertook OCT examination at 3 months and 2 years following SES implantation in 21 patients [58, 59]. The thickness of tissue at 2 years was greater than that

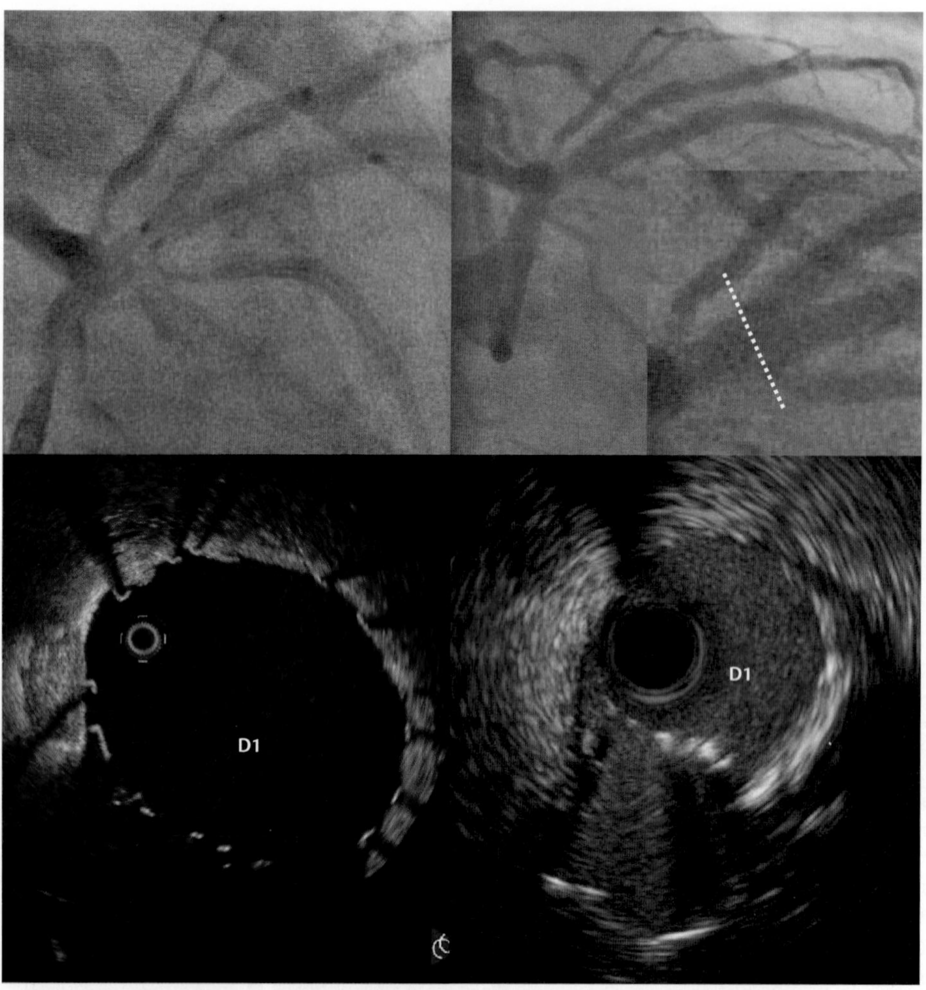

Figure 8.24 Simultaneous kissing stent implantation for a bifurcation lesion of the left anterior descending artery and first diagonal branch (D1). The two stents before the deployment are shown in the left upper panel, with the result in the right upper panel where a magnified image indicates the position of the corresponding optical coherence tomography (lower left) and intravascular ultrasound (lower right) cross-sections. Please note the much better identification with optical coherence tomography of the two-strut layer forming the neo-carina in the middle of the lumen typical of the implantation technique used.

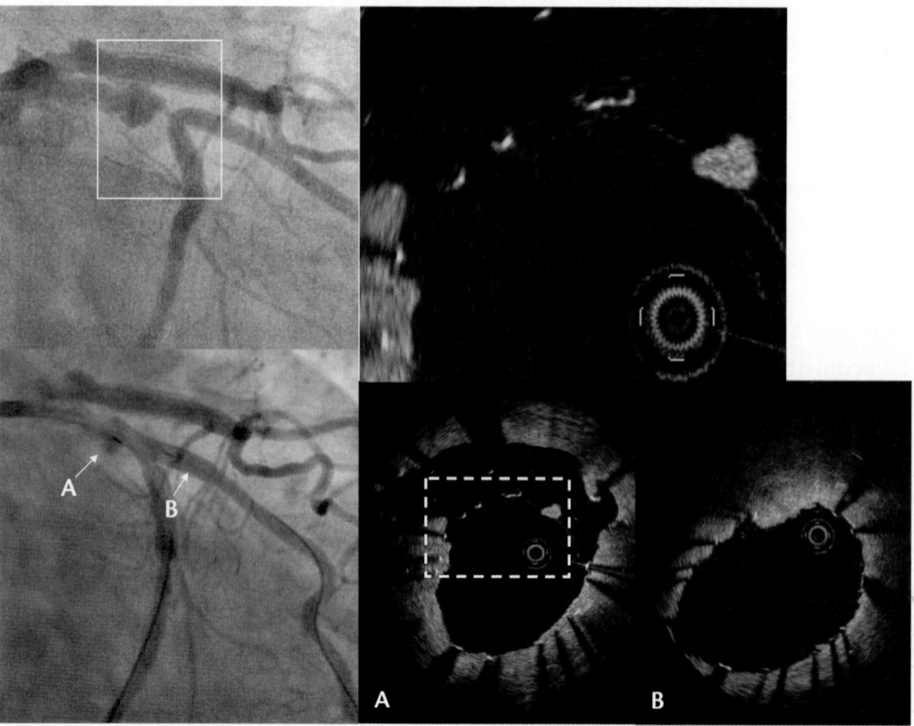

Figure 8.25 Upper left angiogram shows a severe edge restenosis distal to a focal aneurysm 14 months after implantation of a sirolimus eluting stent (Cypher®). The optical coherence tomography image (position A) obtained after implantation of a bare metal stent more distal (position B) indicates late acquired malappostion of the struts due to positive wall remodelling. The magnified area marked with a dotted square in A shows, from right to left, a stent strut covered by redundant soft tissue (organized thrombus?), three unapposed and still uncovered struts, one apposed strut with a thin rim of intimal coverage.

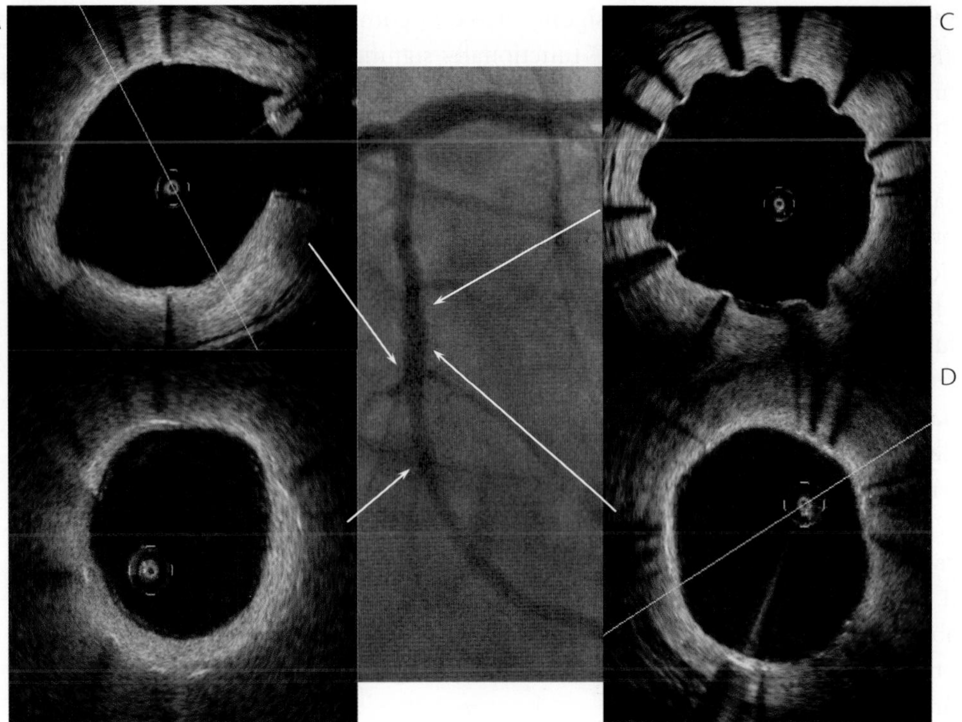

Figure 8.26 Angiographic and optical coherence tomography result 8 months after implantation of a 33mm long Cypher® stent in a small left circumflex. The angiographic image shows good result throughout the stent segment. The optical coherence tomography images show alternation of cross-sections with moderate hyperplasia (B), minimal intimal coverage (D), mainly uncovered and still partially protruding struts (C). Please note in (A) a strut at the ostium of a side-branch covered by a redundant intimal layer (at 2 o'clock).

at 3 months (71 ± 93μm versus 29 ± 41μm, respectively; p <0.001). Frequency of struts with no visible coverage was lower in the 2-year group compared to the 3-month group (5% versus 15%, respectively; p <0.001), with a prevalence of patients with uncovered struts between 3 months and 2 years falling from 95% to 81%, respectively. Matsumoto and colleagues examined 57 sirolimus-eluting stents (SES) in 34 patients at 6 months after implantation and found the median tissue thickness to be 52.5μm with 89% of struts covered and 11% exposed [60]. These and other [61] studies are limited by the small sample size and by the fact the population consisted almost exclusively of single short SES because of the limitations of the balloon occlusive technique used for OCT image acquisition.

Recently, results from a randomized trial of OCT in long lesions requiring overlap stenting were presented [63]. In 22 patients receiving SES, 6% of all struts had no visible coverage at 6 month follow-up. In a substudy of LEADERS [63], 407 out of 6476 struts were uncovered among patients allocated to SES, which corresponds to approximately 6% while the percentage dropped to 2% in lesions treated with the new thinned strut BioMatrix® stent eluting biolimus via a biodegradable coating. Similar low percentages of uncovered stents were reported at 13 months in a larger trial after paclitaxel-eluting stent implantation during primary PCI for acute myocardial infarction [64]. OCT observations are at variance with the much higher prevalence of absent or incomplete endothelialization from pathology observations which, as expected in such a highly negatively selected group, are characterized by high incidence of persistent naked struts and infiltrates [65–67]. The presence or absence of neointimal coverage is limited by the resolution of OCT. Struts scored as uncovered might have a very thin lining of tissue (<10μm), though the biological protection offered by such a thin coverage is debatable. Conversely, OCT evidence of early tissue coverage days after DES implantation has been reported but fibrin and no endothelium was observed in the corresponding histology. The absence of longitudinal studies correlating intimal coverage of DES and late stent thrombosis is the main limitation of all OCT studies late after stenting at this stage.

Functional assessment of the coronary circulation

Coronary angiography continues to play a pivotal role in invasive imaging of the coronary arteries. Despite rapid developments in non-invasive imaging, the temporal and spatial resolution of coronary angiography is still unsurpassed and it will remain the road map for cardiologic interventionalists and cardiac surgeons to perform revascularization. Nevertheless, it has been recognized for many years that coronary angiography is of limited value to define the functional significance of a coronary artery stenosis. In this respect, 'functionally significant' means 'haemodynamically significant', or 'associated with inducible ischaemia' in case of stress.

It is important to emphasize that in coronary artery disease, the most important factor related to outcome is the presence and extent of inducible ischaemia [68, 69]. A functionally significant stenosis generally causes anginal complaints and is associated with impaired outcome. Therefore, functionally significant stenoses should be revascularized, if technically possible [70]. On the other hand, if a stenosis has no functional significance, it will not cause angina by definition and the outcome of medical treatment is excellent with an infarction and mortality rate of <1% per year [71]. Therefore, for decision making in the interventional catheterization laboratory with respect to revascularization, it is of paramount importance to be informed about the ability of a stenosis to induce reversible ischaemia. Or in other words: to assess if a stenosis is functionally significant or not.

Although in many patients with single vessel disease, non-invasive testing is a suitable methodology to be informed about the potentially ischaemic nature of a stenosis, in multivessel disease it is often very difficult to judge which out of several lesions are 'functional significant' (associated with reversible ischaemia) and should be stented; and vice versa which stenoses could better be left alone and treated medically [72].

Both exercise testing, MIBI SPECT, and other classical non-invasive tests often indicate ischaemia in patients with multivessel disease but fail to distinguish the specific ischaemic territories and responsible stenoses.

FFR is a very accurate and lesion-specific index to indicate if a particular stenosis or coronary segment can be held responsible for ischaemia or not [73, 74]. It has been shown that deferring stenting in a FFR-negative stenosis is safe and associated with excellent long-term outcome. Vice versa, it has also been shown that revascularization of a FFR-positive stenosis is associated with significant decrease of ischaemia and improved outcome [71, 72, 75].

Definition of fractional flow reserve

FFR is defined as the ratio of maximum blood flow in a stenotic artery to maximum blood flow if the same artery was normal. Stated in another way, maximum flow in the presence of the stenosis is expressed as a fraction of maximum flow in the hypothetical case that the epicardial artery would be completely normal. It may be clear that FFR is a

Table 8.11 Simplified theoretical explanation illustrating how a ratio of two flows can be derived from a ratio of two pressures provided these pressures are recorded during maximal hyperaemia

1. Fractional flow reserve is the ratio of hyperaemic myocardial flow in the stenotic territory (Q_S^{max}) to normal hyperaemic myocardial flow (Q_N^{max}) $FFR = \frac{Q_S^{max}}{Q_N^{max}}$ (empiric definition)
2. Since the flow (Q) is the ratio of the pressure (P) difference across the coronary system divided by its resistance (R), (Q) can be substituted as following: $FFR = \frac{(P_d - P_v)/R_S^{max}}{(P_a - P_v)/R_N^{max}}$
3. Since the measurement are obtained under maximal hyperemia resistances are minimal and therefore equal, and thus they cancel out; $FFR = \frac{(P_d - P_v)}{(P_a - P_v)}$
4. Inaddition P_v is negligible as compared to P_a or P_d, therefore, $FFR = \frac{P_d}{P_a}$ (practical measurement)

P_a, aortic pressure; P_d, distal coronary pressure; P_v, venous pressure; Q_N^{max}: hyperaemic myocardial blood flow in the normal territory; Q_S^{max}, hyperaemic myocardial blood flow in the stenotic territory; R_N^{max}, hyperaemic myocardial resistance in the normal territory R_S^{max}, hyperaemic myocardial resistance in the stenotic territory.

ratio of two flows: the maximum myocardial flow in the stenotic territory divided by the maximum myocardial flow in the same territory in the normal case. The ratio of the two flows is expressed as the ratio of two pressures, which can be easily measured by a pressure wire and the guiding catheter respectively. The concept of FFR is explained in ➲Table 8.11 and ➲Fig. 8.27.

FFR has a direct clinical equivalent: FFR of 0.60 means that the maximum blood flow (and oxygen supply) to the myocardial distribution of the respective artery, only reaches 60% of what it would be if that artery were completely normal. An increase to 0.90 after stenting, indicates that maximum blood supply has now increased by 50%.

So, FFR is linearly related to maximum blood flow and its normal value is 1.0, irrespective of the patient, artery, blood pressure, etc.

Practical aspects of fractional flow reserve measurements

Catheters

Generally, guiding catheters are used when measuring FFR. The use of diagnostic catheters is technically feasible. Yet, due to higher levels of friction hampering wire manipulation, the

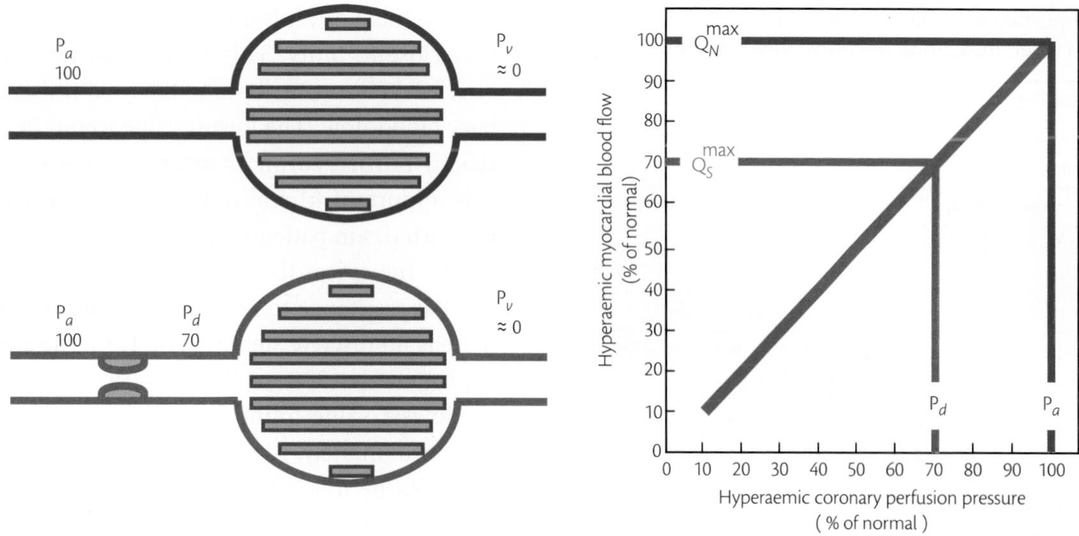

Figure 8.27 Concept of fractional flow reserve measurements. When no epicardial stenosis is present (black lines) the driving pressure P_a determines a normal (100%) maximal myocardial blood flow. In case of stenosis responsible for a hyperaemic pressure gradient of 30mmHg (red lines), the driving pressure will no longer be 100mmHg but 70mmHg (P_d). Since the relationship between driving pressure and myocardial blood flow is linear during maximal hyperaemia, myocardial blood flow will only reach 70% of its normal value. This numerical example shows how a ratio of two pressures (P_d/P_a) corresponds to a ratio of two flows (Q_S^{max} / Q_N^{max}). It also illustrates how important it is to induce maximal hyperaemia.

smaller internal calibre interfering with pressure measurements, and the inability to perform ad hoc percutaneous coronary intervention (PCI) by using diagnostic catheters, the use of guiding catheters is recommended.

Wires

Measuring intra-coronary pressure requires the use of a specific solid-state sensor mounted on a floppy-tipped guide wire. In mainstream practice two such systems exist, namely the PressureWire® (RadiMedical Systems Inc, Uppsala, Sweden) and the WaveWire® (Volcano Inc, Rancho Cordova, CA). The sensor is located at the junction between the 3-cm-long radiopaque tip and the remainder of the wire. The last generations of these 0.014 inch wires have similar handling characteristics to most standard angioplasty guide wires. Before introducing the sensor into the vessel to be studied, the pressures recorded by the sensor and by the guiding catheter should be equalized.

The pressure wire has to be connected to an interface (Analyzer® or Combomap®) which offers the possibility to record the registrations and shows FFR immediately.

Recently, a 'wireless' pressure wire has been introduced (Aeris-wire®, RadiMedical Systems Inc). This wire does not need to be connected to an interface anymore. Its pressure signal is transmitted wirelessly and displayed together with the aortic pressure on the normal haemodynamic monitoring system of the catheterization laboratory, greatly facilitating use of coronary pressure.

Anticoagulation

As soon as any device is advanced into the coronary tree, the use of the same anticoagulation regimens as routinely used during a PCI procedure is recommended: heparin adjusted to weight, validated by a monitored activated coagulation time (ACT) of at least 250s, or a fixed number of units per time and/or body weight, in accordance to the local routine.

Hyperaemic stimuli

FFR, by definition, represents an index of maximum blood flow. Therefore, it is absolutely essential to induce maximal vasodilatation of the two compartments of the coronary circulation (epicardial or 'conductance arteries' and the microvasculature or 'resistance arteries'). The pharmacological options for inducing hyperaemia are summarized in ➲Table 8.12 [76–78].

A bolus of 200mcg isosorbide dinitrate, (or any other form of intra-coronary nitrates) allows the abolition of any form of epicardial vasoconstriction.

Microvascular vasodilation is equally paramount for the calculation of FFR. To gauge pressure differences at rest does not offer a definitive measure. It cannot be emphasized strongly enough that there is no such thing as a 'baseline FFR'. Even when the resting pressure gradient is large it is recommended to induce hyperaemia because it allows evaluation of the residual resistance reserve. An example of

Table 8.12 Importance of epicardial and microvascular vasodilatation when measuring fractional flow reserve

Epicardial vasodilation	
Isosorbide dinitrate: at least 200mcg IC bolus, at least 30s before the first measurements	
Microvascular vasodilation	
Adenosine or ATP IC	At least 40mcg IC bolus in RCA, 40–80mcg in LCA
Papaverine IC	10–12mg in the RCA, 15–20mg in the LCA
Adenosine or ATP IV	140mcg/kg/min (preferably through a central venous e.g. femoral line)

ATP, adenosine triphosphate; IC, intracoronary; IV, intravenously, LCA, left coronary artery; RCA, right coronary artery.

a typical coronary pressure tracing during the administration of intravenous adenosine is shown in ➲Fig. 8.28.

Special features of fractional flow reserve

FFR has a number of unique characteristics that make this index particularly suitable for functional assessment of coronary stenoses and clinical decision making in the catheterization laboratory.

- **FFR has a theoretical normal value of 1 for every patient, for every artery, and for every myocardial bed.** An unequivocally normal value is easy to refer to but is generally rare in clinical medicine. So, this is a unique advantage of FFR. Since in a normal epicardial coronary artery there is virtually no decline in pressure, not even during maximal hyperaemia [79], it is obvious that P_d/P_a will equal or be very close to unity. This means that normal epicardial arteries do not contribute to the total resistance to coronary blood flow. The lowest value found in a total of 65 strictly normal coronary arteries was 0.94 [79, 80]. Yet it is important to realize that in normal-looking coronary arteries in patients with proven atherosclerosis elsewhere, the epicardial coronary arteries may contribute to total resistance to coronary blood flow even though there is no discrete stenosis visible on the angiogram. In approximately 50% of these arteries, FFR is lower than the lowest value found in strictly normal individuals. In approximately 10% of atherosclerotic arteries, FFR will even be lower than the ischaemic threshold [79]. Practically speaking, this finding implies that myocardial ischaemia might be present in atherosclerotic patients in the absence of discrete stenoses.

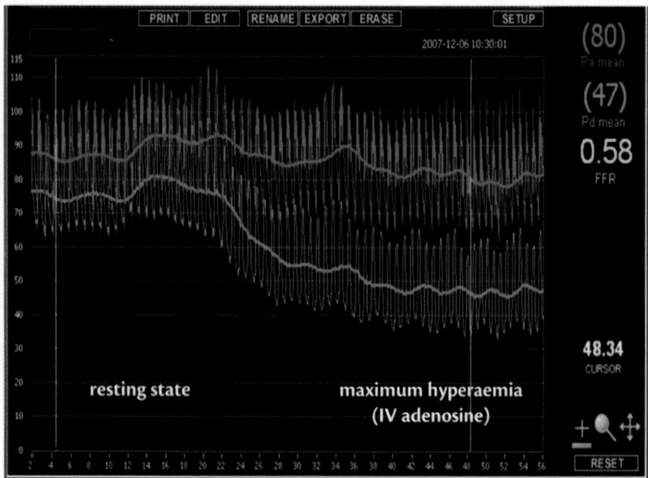

Figure 8.28 Typical example of simultaneous aortic pressure (P_a) and distal coronary pressure (P_d) recordings at rest and during maximal steady-state hyperaemia as induced by an intravenous infusion of adenosine. Fractional flow reserve is simply calculated as the ratio between distal coronary pressure and aortic pressure during steady state maximum hyperaemia.

- **FFR has a well-defined cut-off value with a narrow 'grey zone' between 0.75 and 0.80.** Cut-off or threshold values are values that distinguish ischaemic from non-ischaemic levels for a given measurement. To enable adequate clinical decision making in individual patients it is paramount that any level of uncertainty is reduced to a minimum. Stenoses with an FFR <0.75 are almost invariably able to induce myocardial ischaemia; while stenoses with a FFR >0.80 are almost never associated with exercise-induced ischaemia. This means that the 'grey zone' for FFR (between 0.75–0.80) spans over <10% of the entire range of FFR values.
- FFR in fact is the only index of ischaemia which has been validated versus a true gold standard [81]. Over the last few years, many studies have been performed examining the grey zone and in all these studies invariably a best cut-off value between 0.75–0.80 was found in many subsets of patients including left main disease, diabetes, multivessel disease, previous infarction, etc.

  So, the practical lesson is that in a stenosis with FFR ≤0.75, stenting is always justified (if technically feasible) whereas in a stenosis with FFR >0.80, stenting can be safely deferred and optimum medical treatment is sufficient. Between 0.76–0.80, sound clinical judgment (taking into account the character of complaints, results of non-invasive tests if available, and the fact if a gradient is focal or diffuse), should balance the final decision.

- **FFR is not influenced by systemic haemodynamics.** In the catheterization laboratory systemic pressure, heart rate, and LV contractility are prone to change. In contrast to many other indices measured in the catheterization laboratory, changes in systemic haemodynamics do not influence the value of FFR in a given coronary stenosis [82]. In addition, *FFR measurements are extremely reproducible* [83]. This is due not only to the fact that aortic and distal coronary pressures are measured simultaneously, but also to the extraordinary capability of the microvasculature to repeatedly vasodilate to exactly the same extent. These characteristics contribute to the accuracy of the method and to the trust in its value for clinical decision making.

- **FFR takes into account the contribution of collaterals.** Whether myocardial flow is provided antegradely by the epicardial artery or retrogradely through collaterals, does not really matter for the myocardium. Distal coronary pressure during maximal hyperaemia reflects both antegrade and retrograde flow according to their respective contribution [73, 80]. This holds for the stenoses *supplied* by collaterals but also for stenosed arteries *providing* collaterals to another more critically diseased vessel. ➲ Fig. 8.29 shows the influence on the FFR measurements of left to right collaterals.
- **FFR specifically relates the severity of the stenosis to the mass of tissue to be perfused: 'normalization for perfusion area'.** The larger the myocardial mass subtended by a vessel, the larger the hyperaemic flow, and in turn, the larger the gradient and the lower the FFR for a given stenosis. This explains why a stenosis with a minimal cross sectional area of $4mm^2$ has totally different haemodynamic significance in the proximal LAD versus the second marginal branch. It also means that the haemodynamic significance of a particular stenosis may change if the perfusion territory changes (such as is the case after myocardial infarction). These changes are also accounted for by FFR (see ➲ Fractional flow reserve after myocardial infarction, p.274).
- **FFR has unequalled spatial resolution.** The exact position of the sensor in the coronary tree can be monitored under fluoroscopy, and documented angiographically. Pulling back the sensor under maximal hyperaemia gives the operator an instantaneous assessment of the abnormal resistance of the arterial segment located between the guide catheter and the sensor. While other functional tests reach a 'per patient' accuracy (exercise ECG) or, at best, a 'per vessel' accuracy (myocardial perfusion imaging or stress echo/MRI), FFR reaches a 'per segment' accuracy with a spatial resolution of a few millimetres.

Application of fractional flow reserve in different lesion subset

Fractional flow reserve in angiographically intermediate stenoses

Cardiologists have a large glossary to describe coronary narrowings with uncertain functional consequences: mild

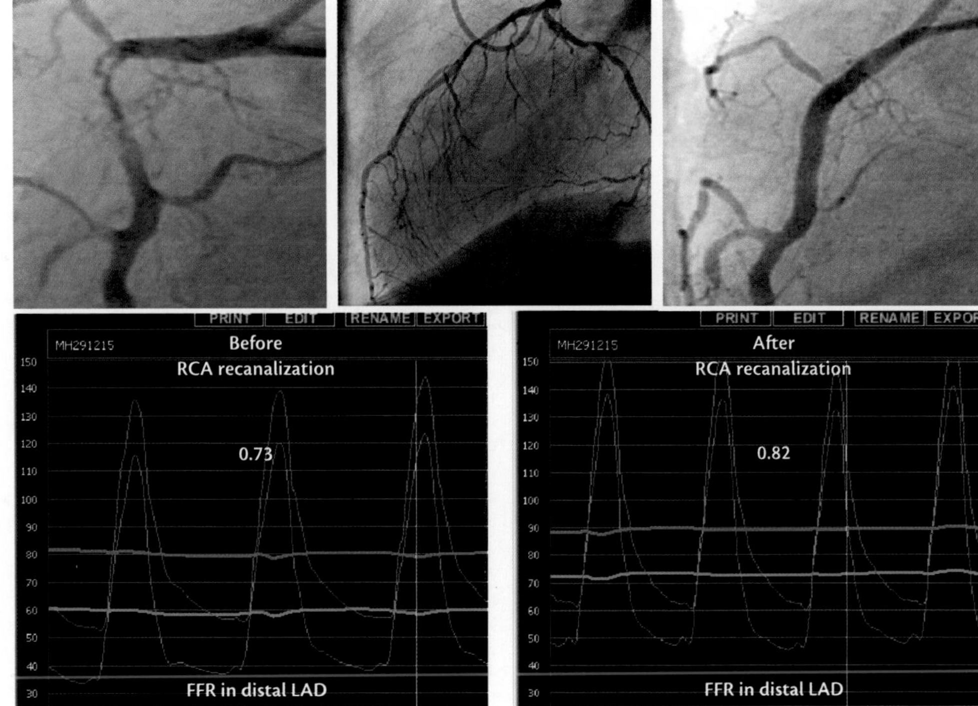

Figure 8.29 Example of the influence of collaterals on fractional flow reserve (FFR) measurements in a 76-year-old man with a critical stenosis in the proximal right coronary artery (RCA) (A) and collaterals supplied by the left coronary artery (LCA) (B). The FFR in the distal left anterior descending artery (LAD) was measured first before recanalization of the RCA ((A) and (D)) and after recanalization of the RCA ((C) and (E)). When antegrade flow was restored in the RCA, the LAD had no longer to supply blood to the territory of the RCA. Therefore, hyperaemic flow in the LAD was lower than before and the FFR increased from 0.73 to 0.82. This example also illustrates the relationship between FFR and the myocardial mass supplied by the artery: the larger the myocardial mass, the larger hyperaemic flow, the lower the FFR for a given stenosis.

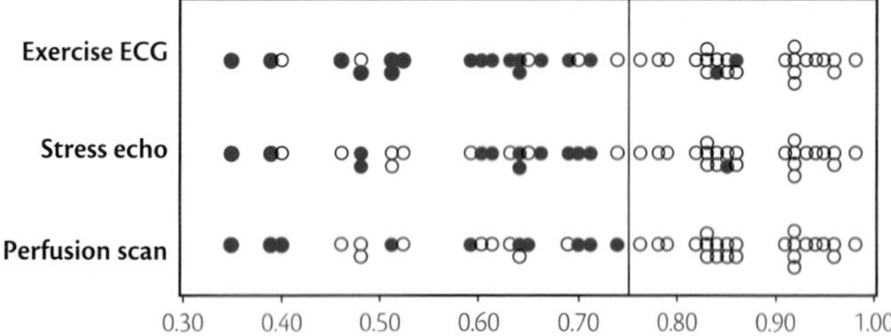

Figure 8.30 Plots of the fractional flow reserve (FFR) in 45 patients with an angiographically intermediate stenosis according to the results of non-invasive testing. The hollow circles represent negative tests. The black dots represent positive tests. Tests were considered positive only if they were positive before revascularization *and* reversed to negative after revascularization. Among the 21 patients with an FFR <0.75, only four showed concordant results of non-invasive tests [14].

to moderate stenoses, dubious lesions, intermediate stenoses, non-flow limiting, non-significant stenoses. The multiplicity of these denominations betrays the inaccuracy of methods to assess those lesions. One of the standard indications for FFR is the precise assessment of the functional consequences of a given coronary stenosis with unclear haemodynamic significance [81]. In a study of 45 patients with angiographically dubious stenoses it was shown that FFR has a much larger accuracy in distinguishing haemodynamically significant stenoses than exercise ECG, myocardial perfusion scintigraphy, and stress echocardiography taken separately. This was shown using a so-called sequential Bayesian approach, providing proof that FFR can indeed be considered as a true gold standard [81].

Furthermore, results of non-invasive tests are often contradictory which renders appropriate clinical decision making difficult (➲Fig. 8.30). In addition, the clinical outcome of patients in whom PCI is deferred because FFR indicated no haemodynamically significant stenosis, is very favourable. In such a population the risk of cardiac death or myocardial infarction is approximately 1% per year, and this risk is not decreased by PCI [71]. These results strongly support the use of FFR measurements as a guide for decision making about the need for revascularization in 'intermediate' lesions. ➲Fig. 8.31 illustrates how two angiographically similar stenoses may have a completely different haemodynamic severity. One of them should be revascularized, the other not. Based solely on the angiogram, the decision should be identical in both cases, which would lead to an inappropriate interventional decision in one of these patients.

Fractional flow reserve in left main stenosis

The presence of a significant stenosis in the left main stem is of critical prognostic importance [84]. Conversely, revascularization of a non-significant stenosis in the left main may lead to atresia of the conduits, especially when internal mammary arteries are used [85]. Furthermore, the left main is among the most difficult segments to assess by angiography [86]. Non-invasive testing is often non-contributive in patients with a left main stenosis. Perfusion defects are often seen in only one vascular territory especially when the right coronary artery is significantly

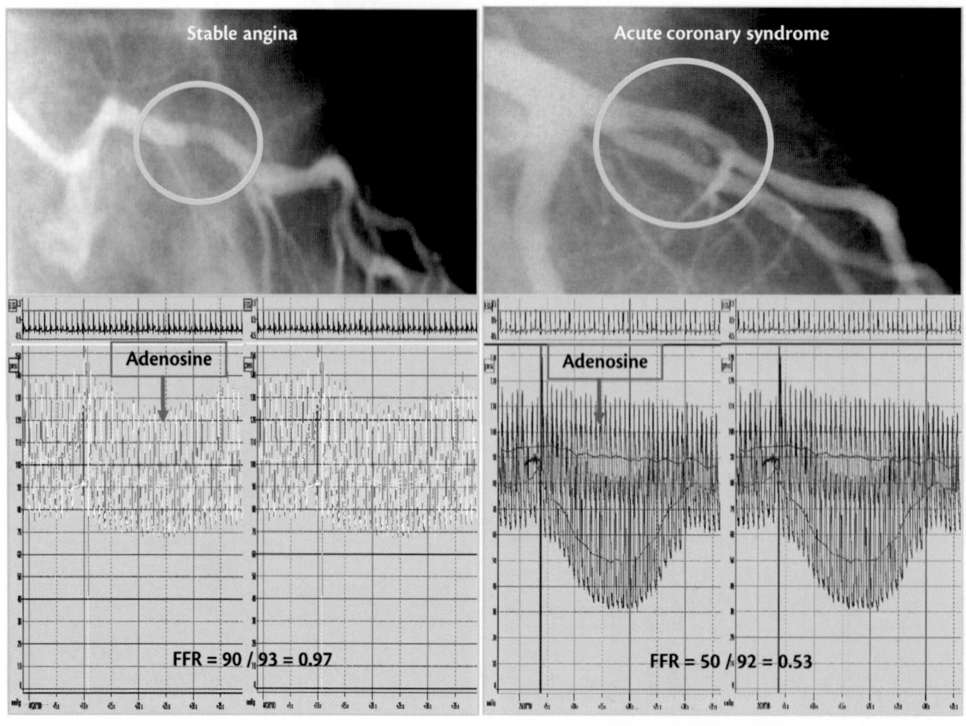

Figure 8.31 Example of two patients presenting with different clinical syndromes, and in whom an angiographically similar stenosis is found in the proximal left anterior descending coronary artery. In the left example the lesion has no haemodynamic significance and does not need any form of mechanical revascularization. In the right example the stenosis is haemodynamically very significant and deserves percutaneous coronary intervention.

diseased [87]. In addition, tracer uptake may be reduced in all vascular territories ('balanced' ischaemia) giving rise to false negative studies [88]. Several studies have shown that FFR could be used safely in left main stenosis and that the decision not to operate on left main stenosis with an FFR larger than 0.75 is safe [89–91]. In addition, angiographic assessments of left main lesions with an FFR <0.75 were no different from those with an FFR >0.75 further reinforcing the importance of physiological parameters in case of doubt. Therefore, patients with an intermediate left main stenosis deserve physiologic assessment before blindly taking a decision about the need for revascularization. Two examples shown in ➲ Fig. 8.32 illustrate how FFR measurements in the left main may drastically influence the type of treatment in these patients.

Left main disease is rarely isolated. When tight stenoses are present in the LAD or in the LCX the presence of these lesions will tend to increase the FFR measured across the left main. The influence of a LAD/LCX lesion on the FFR value of the left main will depend on the severity of this distal stenosis but, even more, on the vascular territory supplied by this distal stenosis. For example, if the distal stenosis is in the proximal LAD, its presence will markedly impact the stenosis in the left main. If the distal stenosis is located in a small second marginal branch, its influence on the left main stenosis will be minimal (➲ Fig. 8.33).

Fractional flow reserve in multivessel disease

Patients with multivessel disease actually represent a very heterogeneous population. Their anatomical features (number of lesions, location, and respective degree of complexity) may vary tremendously and have major implications for the revascularization strategy. Moreover, there is often a large discrepancy between the anatomic description and the actual physiologic severity of each stenosis. For example, a patient may have 'three vessel disease' based on the angiogram, but actually have only two haemodynamically significant stenoses. And vice versa a patient can angiographically be considered as one vessel disease of the RCA but actually have a haemodynamically significant stenosis of the left main. ➲ Fig. 8.34 shows a typical example of a patient in whom the RCA and the LCX are critically narrowed and in whom the mid-LAD shows a mild stenosis. Myocardial perfusion imaging showed a reversible perfusion defect in the inferolateral segments and a normal flow distribution in the segments supplied by the LAD. In contrast, FFR shows that all three vessels are significantly narrowed but to a different extent. And by nuclear scintigraphy, the significant defect in the anterior wall is masked by the more severe defects in the other areas. This has a major implication as far as revascularization is concerned. FFR-guided revascularization strategies in patients with multivessel disease were very encouraging [92–94]. Tailoring the revascularization according to the functional

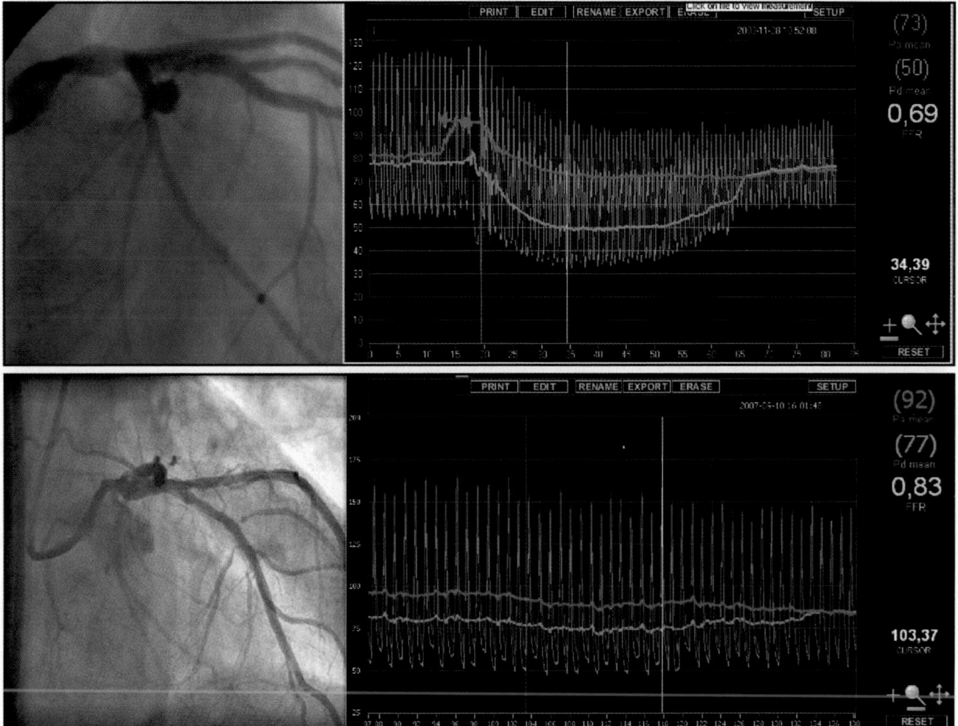

Figure 8.32 Example of two patients in whom fractional flow reserve (FFR) measurements in an 'intermediate' ostial left main stenosis changed the therapeutic strategy. The first (upper panel) represents a 67-year-old man with massive mitral regurgitation who was assessed for minimally invasive (port access) mitral valvuloplasty. The coronary angiogram showed an 'intermediate' ostial left main stenosis. The FFR of the left main stenosis was 0.69. Accordingly, this patient underwent conventional coronary artery bypass grafting and mitral valvuloplasty *via* a median sternotomy. The second (lower panel) represents an 89-year-old man with critical aortic stenosis, referred for aortic valve replacement and bypass surgery because of the presence of an ostial left main stenosis. FFR of the left main stem was 0.83. Accordingly, only a percutaneous aortic valve implantation was performed.

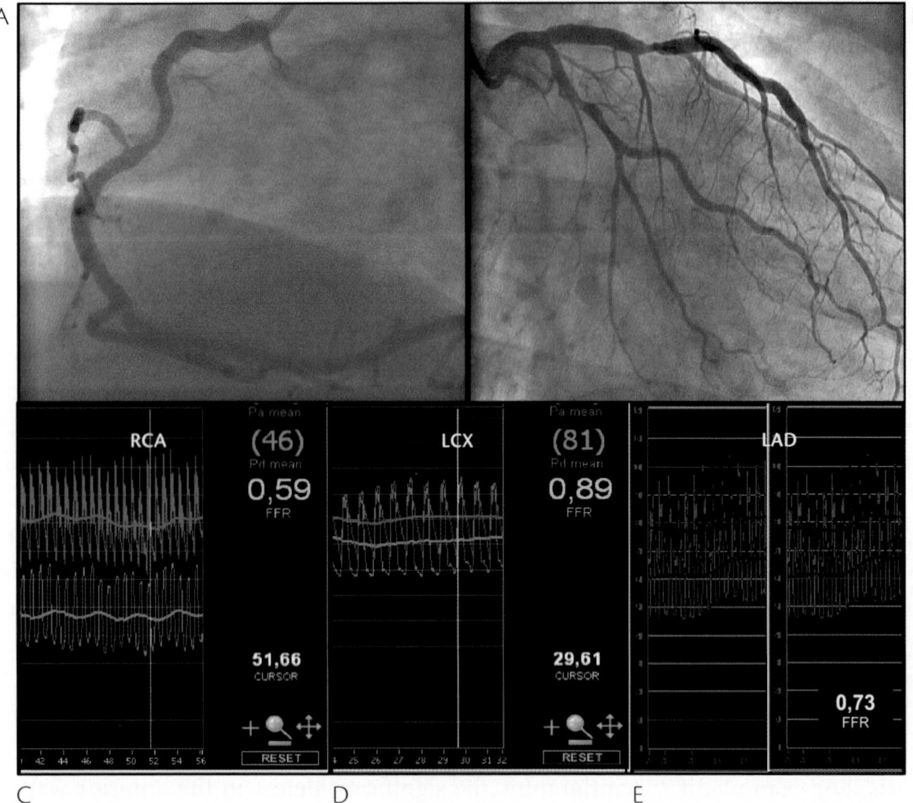

Figure 8.33 Patient with multivessel disease admitted for percutaneous coronary intervention of the LCX. Non-invasive exercise testing was positive. Except for the angiographically (apparently) severe lesion in the left circumflex artery (LCX), mild to moderate stenoses are present in the right coronary artery (RCA) and mid-left anterior descending artery (LAD) artery. Coronary pressure measurement changes the strategy completely: It is not the LCX which causes complaints and the positive exercise test, but the RCA and LAD artery. Both were stented subsequently and the LCX was left unstented.

significance of the stenoses rather than on their mere angiographic appearance decreased costs and avoided the need for surgical revascularization [92]. Recently, incontrovertible proof for the benefit of FFR-guided multivessel PCI compared to standard angiography was provided in the large randomized multicentre FAME study [75, 95]. In that study, it was demonstrated that all types of adverse events were decreased by 30% in the first year after PCI in multivessel disease, when guided by FFR. This was achieved at a lower cost and without prolonging the interventional procedure, whereas angina in FFR-guided patients was relieved at least as effectively (see ➲Optimum treatment of multivessel disease, p.276).

Fractional flow reserve after myocardial infarction

After a myocardial infarction, previously viable tissue is partially replaced by scar tissue. Therefore, the total mass of viable myocardium supplied by a given stenosis in an infarct-related artery will tend to decrease [96]. By definition, hyperaemic flow and thus hyperaemic gradient will both decrease as well. Assuming that the morphology of the stenosis remains identical, FFR must therefore increase. This does not mean that FFR underestimates lesion severity after myocardial infarction. It simply illustrates the relationship that exists between flow, pressure gradient, and myocardial mass. And conversely illustrates that the mere morphology of a stenotic segment does not necessarily reflect its functional importance. This principle is illustrated in ➲Fig. 8.35. Recent data confirm that the hyperaemic myocardial resistance in viable myocardium within the infarcted area remains normal [97]. This further supports the application of the established FFR cut-off value in the setting of partially infarcted territories. In the acute phase of myocardial infarction, FFR is neither reliable nor useful to assess the culprit lesions and the ECG trumps any other investigation. From 5 days after the infarction, FFR can be used as regular to indicate residual ischaemia of the infarct-related or remote arteries.

Earlier data had suggested that microvascular function would be abnormal in regions remote from a recent myocardial infarction [98, 99]. However, more recent work taking into account distal coronary pressure indicates that hyperaemic resistance is normal in those remote segments [100]. These data support the use of FFR to evaluate stenoses remote from a recent myocardial infarction.

Fractional flow reserve in diffuse disease

Histopathology studies, and, more recently, intravascular ultrasound, have shown that atherosclerosis is diffuse in nature and that a discrete stenosis in an otherwise normal artery is actually rare. The concept of a focal lesion is a mainly angiographic description but does not

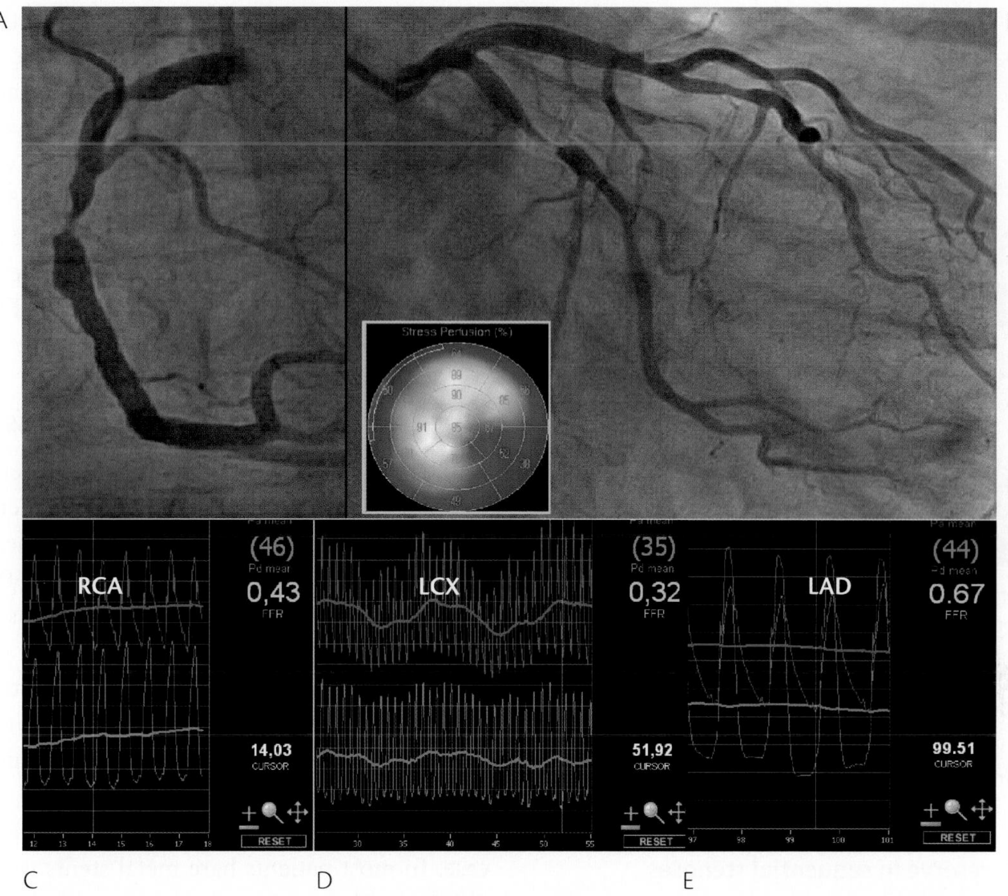

Figure 8.34 69-year-old man with severe angina. Myocardial perfusion imaging (MPI) showed a reversible defect in the inferolateral segments. From the angiogram it is obvious that the right coronary artery (RCA) and the left circumflex artery (LCX) are significantly narrowed (no pressure measurements are needed!). However, the mid-left anterior descending artery (LAD) stenosis, considered 'non-significant' on the angiogram, appears to be haemodynamically significant. This LAD stenosis was undetected by MPI because the uptake of tracer is markedly worse in the LCX territory than in the LAD territory.

reflect pathology. Until recently, it was believed that when no focal narrowing of >50% was seen at the angiogram, no abnormal resistance was present in the epicardial artery. It was therefore assumed that distal pressure was normal and thus that 'diffuse mild disease without focal stenosis' could not cause myocardial ischaemia. This paradigm has recently been shifted: the presence of diffuse disease is often associated with a progressive decrease in coronary pressure and flow and this cannot be clearly assessed from the angiogram [79, 100]. In contrast, this decline in pressure correlates with the total atherosclerotic burden [101]. In approximately 10% of patients this abnormal epicardial resistance may be responsible for reversible myocardial ischaemia. In these patients chest pain is often considered non-coronary because no single focal stenosis is found, and the myocardial perfusion imaging is wrongly considered false positive [102, 103]. Such diffuse disease and its haemodynamic impact should always be kept in mind when performing functional measurements. In a large multicentre registry of 750 patients FFR was obtained after technically successful stenting. A post-PCI FFR value of <0.9 was still present in almost one-third of patients (despite absence of a gradient across the stent), reflecting diffuse disease, and was associated with a poor clinical outcome [104]. The only way to demonstrate the haemodynamic impact of diffuse disease is to perform a careful pull-back manoeuvre of the

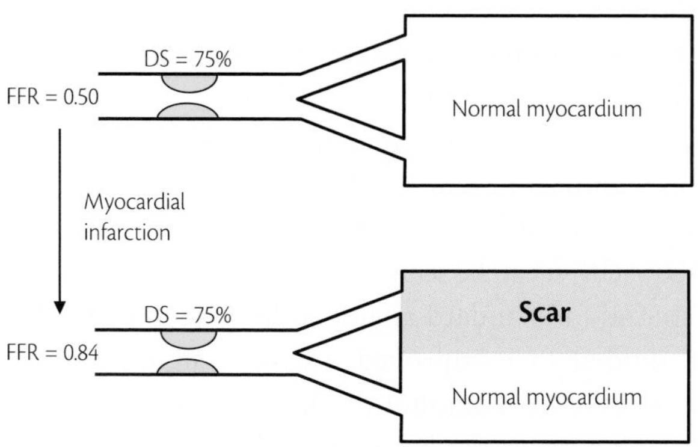

Figure 8.35 Schematic representation of the relationship between fractional flow reserve and myocardial mass before and after myocardial infarction. See text for details.

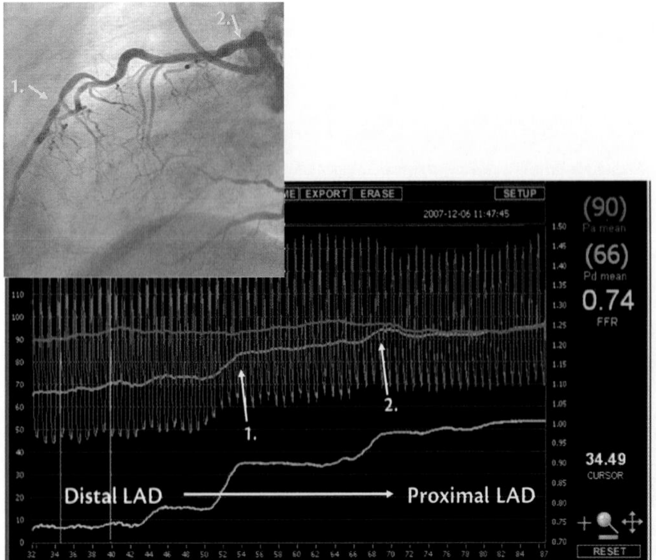

Figure 8.36 Hyperaemic pressure pull-back recording in a diffusely diseased left anterior descending artery (LAD) artery with superimposed focal lesions. The pressure recording nicely shows that all the disease in the LAD summed together is responsible for inducible ischaemia (fractional flow reserve 0.74) and indicates exactly the origin of the gradient (arrows).

pressure sensor under steady-state maximal hyperaemia (➲Fig. 8.36).

Fractional flow reserve in sequential stenoses

When several stenoses are present in the same artery, the concept and the clinical value of FFR is still valid to assess the effect of all stenoses together. Yet, it is important to realize in such cases that each of several stenoses will influence hyperaemic blood flow and therefore FFR across the other one. The influence of the distal lesion on the proximal is more important than the reverse. Theoretically the FFR can be calculated for each stenosis individually [105, 106]. However, this is neither practical nor easy to perform and therefore of little use in the catheterization laboratory. Practically, as for diffuse disease, a pull-back manoeuvre under maximal hyperaemia is the best way to appreciate the exact location and physiological significance of sequential stenoses and to guide the interventional procedure step-by-step.

Fractional flow reserve in bifurcation lesions

Overlapping of vessel segments as well as radiographic artefacts render bifurcation stenoses particularly difficult to evaluate at angiography, while PCI of bifurcations is often more challenging than for regular stenoses. The principle of FFR-guided PCI applies in bifurcation lesions even though clinical outcome data are currently limited. Two recent studies by Koo and colleagues [107, 108] used FFR in the setting of bifurcation stenting. The results of these studies can be summarized as follows: (1) after stenting the main branch, the ostium of the side branch often looks 'pinched'. Yet such stenoses are grossly overestimated by angiography: none of these ostial lesions with a diameter stenosis <75%, were found to have an FFR below 0.75; (2) when kissing balloon dilation was performed only in ostial stenoses with an FFR <0.75, the FFR at 6 months was >0.75 in 95% of cases. These studies favour an approach in bifurcation lesions with stenting the main branch and kissing balloon thereafter if FFR of the side branch is <0.75.

Optimum treatment of multivessel disease

In the last years, three large studies have been performed to examine the best possible treatment of patients with multivessel coronary artery disease. In these studies the respective value of optimum medical treatment only, PCI in addition to medical treatment, and coronary bypass surgery were investigated [95,109, 110].

These studies were the COURAGE study, SYNTAX study, and FAME study [95, 109, 110]. In the COURAGE study, optimum medical treatment only and PCI in addition to medical treatment were investigated in patients with multivessel disease and moderately severe coronary disease. In most patients bare metal stents were used. In the SYNTAX–3VD study, only patients with three vessel disease were included and only DES stents were used. The degree of disease was more severe than in the COURAGE trial and in these patients standard angiographic guided PCI with drug-eluting stents only, was compared to bypass surgery. In the FAME study, also in patients with mainly three vessel disease but excluding left main stenosis, standard angiography-guided PCI with drug-eluting stents was compared to FFR-guided multivessel PCI with drug-eluting stents. The SYNTAX-3VD and FAME study had wider inclusion criteria, including unstable patients and NSTEMI, decreased LV function, and the FAME study also included patients with previous PCI.

The most important results of these three studies are presented in ➲Fig. 8.37.

Although the baseline characteristics of the studies were slightly different (with the angiographically most complex disease in SYNTAX and least complex disease in COURAGE) it can be seen that outcome was comparable in all studies for standard angiography-guided PCI, whereas FFR-guided PCI improved outcome significantly. Not only was the total amount of MACE significantly reduced by routine measurement of FFR, but also the mortality and occurrence of myocardial infarction. In ➲Fig. 8.37 it can also be observed that multivessel PCI guided by FFR

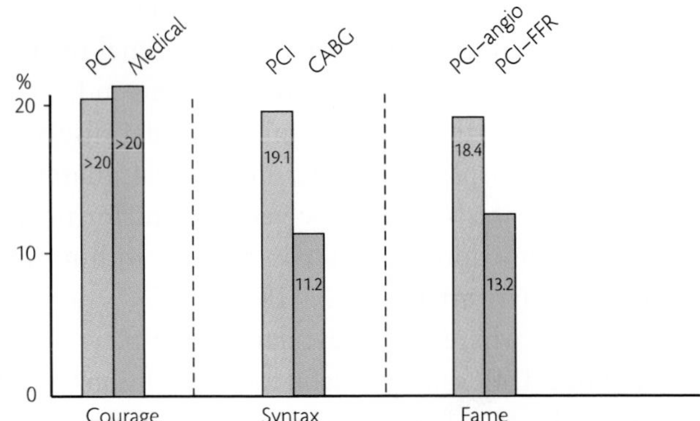

Figure 8.37 Major adverse event rate (death from all causes, myocardial infarction, and (repeated) revascularization) in the COURAGE study, SYNTAX-3VD study, and FAME study. It is clear that in patients with multivessel coronary disease, fractional flow reserve-guided percutaneous coronary intervention (PCI) is superior to standard angiography-guided PCI but also to optimal medical treatment. Moreover, in many patients fractional flow reserve (FFR) guided PCI can be considered as an excellent alternative for coronary artery bypass grafting. Also with respect to CCS-class at follow-up, FFR-guided PCI yielded the best outcome. Note: the exact MACE rate in the COURAGE trial at 1 year has not been published to our knowledge, but from published data a MACE rate exceeding 20% can be deduced [75, 109, 110].

is superior to optimum medical treatment and yields results comparable to coronary artery bypass graft surgery in many patients.

Therefore, it is expected that the indications for performing PCI will further extend when guided by FFR measurements, and that more patients, previously treated by medical treatment alone or by CABG, will be better candidates for sophisticated PCI guided by FFR measurements.

Pitfalls and limitations of fractional flow reserve

There are several pitfalls related to FFR measurement and a few clinical situations where it is not reliable and should not be applied. The most important of these is acute ST-elevation myocardial infarction (STEMI). During primary PCI for acute myocardial infarction, the combination of the symptoms, ECG, and angiogram usually makes it possible to determine the culprit lesion in the majority of cases. In addition, thrombus embolization, myocardial stunning, acute ischaemic microvascular dysfunction, and other factors make obtaining complete microvascular vasodilation unlikely. Therefore, FFR measurement makes no sense in the setting of acute STEMI.

When a couple of days has passed (usually 5 days is taken as sufficient), FFR can be applied as in routine practice. It is still a point of discussion whether FFR can be applied during primary PCI to assess the haemodynamic severity of remote lesions.

From the technical point of view, there are several pitfalls to watch out for when performing an FFR measurement. The two most important pitfalls are submaximal hyperaemia (underestimating the stenosis severity) and pitfalls related to the guiding catheter. Such situations can be easily recognized and avoided, once the operator has some experience with FFR.

For a more in-dept discussion of pitfalls, we refer to several excellent reviews in the literature [103, 111].

Finally, there are a number of physiologic reasons why FFR can be high despite an apparently tight stenosis. This is further explained in ➲Table 8.13.

Other methods for functional assessment of the coronary circulation

Doppler wire measurements

Before guidewire-based coronary pressure measurements were possible, Doppler wires were available to measure coronary flow velocity and classic coronary flow reserve (CFR) [112]. Because of the intrinsic shortcomings of coronary flow reserve, such as dependence on baseline flow almost never present in the catheterization laboratory, absence of a normal value, dependence on blood pressure and heart rate, age dependency, and non-specificity with respect to

Table 8.13 Reasons of non-ischaemic fractional flow reserve despite an apparently tight stenosis

Physiologic explanations
Stenosis haemodynamically non-significant despite angiographic appearance
Small perfusion territory, old myocardial infarction, little viable tissue, small vessel
Abundant collaterals
Severe microvascular disease (rarely affecting FFR)
Interpretation explanations
Other culprit lesion
Diffuse disease rather than focal stenosis (make pull-back recording)
Chest pain of non-cardiac origin
Technical explanations
Insufficient hyperaemia (check system and solution; or use other stimulus)
Guiding catheter related pitfall (deep engagement, small ostium, sideholes)
Electrical drift (pull sensor back to ostium to check and equalize)
Actual false negative FFR
Acute phase of ST-elevation myocardial infarction (STEMI)
Severe left ventricular hypertrophy
Exercise-induced spasm

the epicardial coronary artery, its use for practical decision making has faded. Doppler measurements in combination with pressure measurements have been used to define combined indexes which can be useful especially for microvascular dysfunction [113]. However, those applications are more sophisticated and scientific and not often performed in routine clinical practice.

Coronary thermodilution

The sensor on the PressureWire® (Radi Medical Systems Inc.), can also be used as a thermistor and coronary thermodilution measurements have been performed [114, 115]. In that way, thermodilution-based CFR could be calculated and was applied in several studies. However, the shortcomings of thermodilution CFR are similar to those of Doppler CFR and other methodologies for CFR measurement. The advantage of thermodilution CFR is that it can be more easily combined with pressure measurement because only a single sensor is necessary. Comparative studies in animals showed somewhat better results for thermo-CFR measurements than for Doppler-CFR, when compared to electromagnetic flow measurement as the gold standard [116].

Index of microvascular resistance

Of more clinical importance is the index of microvascular resistance (IMR), introduced by Fearon and colleagues [117]. It is also derived from coronary pressure and hyperaemic temperature measurement. Because it uses only mean transit time during maximum hyperaemia, it is not dependant on baseline blood flow as is the case for CFR. Because hyperaemic blood flow is inversely proportional to hyperaemic mean transit time, the product of distal pressure and mean transit time can be used as an index of minimal microvascular resistance. It has been shown that this index corresponds well with the degree of microvascular disease in patients after transplant and after myocardial infarction. Moreover, IMR was shown to be very specific for microvascular (dys)function, especially in patients with normal epicardial coronary arteries [117, 118].

In situations where microvascular disease plays a predominant role, IMR can be a useful tool in addition to FFR. It addresses the microcirculation specifically, whereas FFR addresses the epicardial conduit.

Thermodilution-based absolute blood flow

More recently, measurement of absolute blood flow has been described using a continuous thermodilution technique [119]. Because those measurements are performed during hyperaemia and can be performed during a steady-state infusion of saline, in preliminary studies accuracy and reproducibility was high. However, because absolute blood flow as a number has little significance without knowing the extent of the distribution area, the value of these measurements is mainly limited to comparison of blood flow within one patient at different points of times (e.g. before and after intervention, before and after long-lasting lipid-lowering treatment, during follow-up of transplant patients, before and after stem cell therapy, etc.).

Although the technique in itself is sound and well validated, the instrumentation is not trivial and therefore this methodology is limited so far to investigational purposes in scientific orientated catheterization laboratories [119].

Personal perspective

Therapeutic decisions in cardiology have been crucially determined by invasive circulatory imaging and haemodynamics in the last decades. They have been essential for understanding pathophysiological and diagnostic aspects of cardiovascular disease and indispensable to the development of modern surgical and percutaneous treatment in coronary artery disease and valve disease. In the most recent years, with a trend going to continue in the future, non-invasive diagnostic techniques have replaced the classical invasive methods both for haemodynamics and imaging. A diagnostic catheterization in a patient with severe valve disease is far from being routine with the exception of patients with possible coronary artery disease before surgery or in patients treated with percutaneous mitral balloon valvuloplasty or transcatheter aortic valve implantation. The rapid growth of this last procedure, still limited to high-risk surgical candidates but possibly going to wider applications soon, and the development of methods of percutaneous repair of mitral insufficiency, may lead to a new interest for techniques such as retrograde crossing of a stenotic aortic valve or trans-septal puncture to probe the left atrium. Coronary angioplasty is critically dependent on a focused acquisition of high quality angiographic images. Rotational acquisition and three-dimensional reconstruction may limit contrast injection and facilitate the selection of an optimal working view for angioplasty. For optimal stent expansion and better procedure planning, intravascular ultrasound is a great practical help and its use is likely to increase when working in segments of less predictable anatomical characteristics, such as in left main coronary artery disease.

Similarly, diagnostic coronary angiography, one of the most successful and widely applied procedures ever introduced in medicine, is going to be progressively replaced by non-invasive methods of coronary imaging. Faster scanners have made multislice CT coronary angiography a valid alternative to invasive coronary angiography in patients at low or intermediate risk of disease. Even with better image quality and reduced radiation doses, however, multislice CT will never replace invasive coronary angiography because this technique can provide immediate diagnosis and simultaneously offer access for subsequent percutaneous revascularization in patients with acute coronary syndromes. Also in stable syndromes artefacts due to calcium and inherent lower resolution of multislice CT often require an invasive angiographic confirmation, with FFR used with increasing frequency to avoid treatment of haemodynamically non-significant stable plaques. The real challenge for invasive diagnostic techniques is the identification of vulnerable plaques in patients at high risk, a growing population with the current epidemics of diabetes and possibly better identified with the use of biomarkers and genetic characterization. Percutaneous coronary angioplasty is a late response in the natural history of atherosclerosis targeting well-developed flow-limiting lesions. If new safe and cost-effective methods develop to stabilize vulnerable plaques, their identification becomes of paramount importance. The non-invasive techniques proposed are unlikely to ever reach sufficient resolution to identify early atherosclerotic changes with the exception of calcium deposition and intimal thickening. Also conventional angiography has the same limitation but additional information can come from concomitant intracoronary high resolution imaging with optical coherence tomography.

Further reading

Baim D (ed). *Grossman's Cardiac Catheterization, Angiography and Intervention*, 7th edn, 2006. Philadelphia, PA: Lippincott William & Wilkins.

Moliterno DJ, Mukherjee D, Sketch MH, Jr., *et al.* (eds.). CathSAP 3. Cardiac Catheterization and Interventional Cardiology Self-Assessment Program. Book 2: Cardiovascular anatomy and physiology. [CD-ROM] ACC/SCAI, 2008.

Di Mario C, Gorge G, Peters R, *et al.* Clinical application and image interpretation in intracoronary ultrasound. Study Group on Intracoronary Imaging of the Working Group of Coronary Circulation and of the Subgroup on Intravascular Ultrasound of the Working Group of Echocardiography of the European Society of Cardiology. *Eur Heart J* 1998; **19**: 207–29.

Di Mario C, Barlis P, Dangas G (eds.). *Textbook of Interventional Cardiology*, in press. Wiley.

Mintz GS, Nissen SE, Anderson WD, *et al.* American College of Cardiology Clinical Expert Consensus Document on Standards for Acquisition, Measurement and Reporting of Intravascular Ultrasound Studies (IVUS). A report of the American College of Cardiology Task Force on Clinical Expert Consensus Documents. *J Am Coll Cardiol* 2001; **37**: 1478–92.

Pijls NHJ, Bruyne B, Peels K, *et al.* Measurement of fractional flow reserve to assess the functional severity of coronary artery stenoses. *N Engl J Med* 1996; **334**: 1703–8.

Prati F, Regar E, Mintz G, *et al.* Expert review. Methodology, terminology and clinical application of OCT. Physical principles, methodology of image acquisition and clinical application for assessment of coronary arteries and atherosclerosis. *Eur Heart J* 2009; in press.

Silber SP, Albertsson P, Fernandez-Avilès F, *et al.* Guidelines for percutaneous coronary interventions. *Eur Heart J* 2005; **26**: 804–47.

Tonino PA, De Bruyne B, Pijls NH, *et al.*; FAME Study Investigators. Fractional flow reserve vs angiography for guiding percutaneous coronary interventions. *N Engl J Med* 2009; **360**: 213–24.

Vahanian A, Baumgartner H, Bax J, *et al.* Management of valvular heart disease. *Eur Heart J* 2007; **28**: 230–68.

➲ For full references and multimedia materials please visit the online version of the book (http://esctextbook.oxfordonline.com).

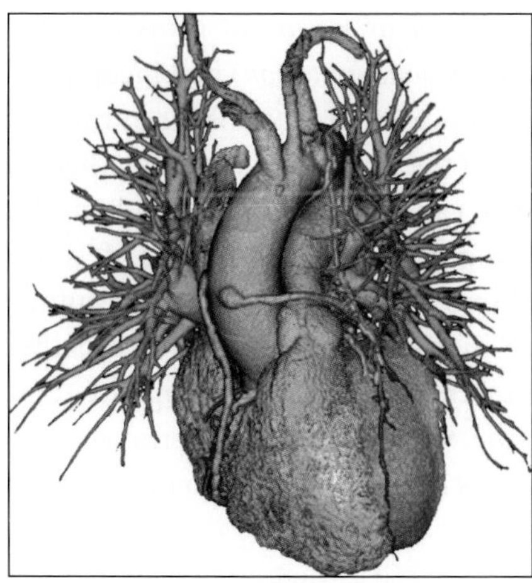

CHAPTER 9

Genetics of Cardiovascular Diseases

Silvia G. Priori, Carlo Napolitano, Steve E. Humphries, and James Skipworth

Contents

Summary

Since the identification of the basis of the human genome, molecular genetics has progressively entered into many fields of medicine. Cardiovascular medicine does not represent an exception to this rule. The unravelling of the molecular determinants of cardiovascular diseases took off from studies of the so-called 'monogenic' diseases that provided evidence showing that the genes/proteins involved in genetic diseases of the heart belong to three major functional classes: 1) structural; 2) electrical; 3) regulatory.

It is clear that mutations in structural proteins are associated with structural cardiomyopathies (dilated cardiomyopathy, hypertrophic cardiomyopathy, and arrhythmogenic right ventricular cardiomyopathy, etc.), while proteins underlying cardiac excitability are predominantly associated with inherited arrhythmogenic disorders (long QT syndrome, catecholaminergic tachycardia, Brugada syndrome, etc.). Finally, regulatory proteins (chaperones, second messengers, signal transduction proteins) may be associated either with structural involvement or with arrhythmias in a normal heart. Furthermore it is also clear that, with few exceptions, all monogenic diseases of the heart are characterized by remarkable 'two-way' heterogeneity: 1) The same clinical phenotype may be caused by different genes/mutations. 2) The same gene and, in some instances, even the same mutation, can cause different clinical phenotypes.

In parallel with this growing recognition of heterogeneity we are also learning how to get the best from the results of genetic testing to tailor and individualize risk stratification and therapy. Genotype-driven clinical management is therefore progressively entering the clinical practice.

Another major line of research in the field of genetics of cardiovascular diseases is represented by investigations aimed at discovering the genetic determinants of complex traits such as coronary artery disease and hypertension. These conditions recognize both environmental and genetic components. The latter is clearly supported by the evidence of familial predisposition. However, such genetic predisposition is usually polygenic and only rarely results from a single gene mutation. The 'two ways' in this case are represented by the 'initial' conditions, coded in the genotype, and by the exposure to environmental agents over time.

This chapter will review the current understanding of genetic determinants of cardiovascular diseases spanning monogenic to polygenic disorders, and will highlight the genetic heterogeneity and the mechanisms leading from gene mutation to clinical phenotype.

Mendelian monogenic human diseases: an overview

Monogenic diseases result from modifications in a single gene occurring in all cells of the body. Though relatively rare, they affect millions of people worldwide. Scientists currently estimate that >10,000 human diseases are known to be monogenic. Pure genetic diseases are caused by a single error in a single gene in the human DNA.

Monogenic diseases are inherited as dominant or recessive traits with five major inheritance patterns (see ➲Box 9.1 for a list of common genetic terms):

- **Autosomal dominant**: all chromosomes with the exception of X and Y can be affected. One mutated allele is sufficient to cause the phenotype. The chance of transmission to the offspring is 50% and both males and females can be affected.
- **Autosomal recessive**: only the homozygote is clinically affected (two mutated alleles must be present) while the heterozygote is defined as a 'healthy carrier' or shows very mild or absent signs of the disease. The chance of receiving two defective alleles/genes (one from the mother and one from the father) is 25%. Fifty per cent of the offspring will receive only one defective allele (heterozygotes) and 25% will receive two normal alleles (homozygotes).
- **X-linked dominant**: both males and females can be affected but no male-to-male transmission is possible and an affected male has 100% chance of transmitting the disease to daughters. Female-to-female transmission of the defective allele has a 50% chance.
- **X-linked recessive**: heterozygous females are healthy carriers and 50% of their sons are clinically affected. No female-to-female transmission of the disease is possible but 50% of daughters are silent carriers. Affected males will generate unaffected males and heterozygous unaffected females (healthy carriers).
- **Matrilineal transmission:** this refers to diseases caused by mitochondrial DNA. Since mitochondria are only present in oocytes and not in sperm, only females may transmit the disease to the offspring.

Besides the 'textbook' definition of 'monogenic disorders', it is important to considerer that the clinical manifestations of these diseases may significantly vary from one patient to the other even in the presence of the same genetic defect. In technical terms, this phenomenon is due to the variable expressivity (*the extent to which a genetic disease or condition is expressed in an individual. Expressivity is demonstrated by variations in the strength or nature of traits amongst individuals with the same genetic mutation*) and incomplete penetrance (i.e. the presence of <1 ratio between carriers of a given gene defect and the number of clinically affected individuals). Penetrance can also be time-dependent: the phenotype becomes progressively worse during life since the organ damage induced by the defective gene accumulates. This is the case in hypertrophic cardiomyopathy, arrhythmogenic right ventricular cardiomyopathy, and dilated cardiomyopathy where disease penetrance may reach 100% when patients live long enough to manifest the symptoms.

An emerging line of research is that aiming to identify the genetic determinants of such variable expressivity and variable penetrance. Investigators are specifically seeking to identify the association between common genetic variants (single nucleotide polymorphisms, SNPs) and the clinical manifestations. Indeed, it is evident that besides the primary (pathogenetic) mutation, which is per se necessary and sufficient to cause a disease, SNPs (that per se are neither sufficient nor necessary to cause a disease) exert their role by attenuating or worsening the clinical presentation of monogenic disorders. The role of SNPs is briefly outlined in this chapter for hypertrophic cardiomyopathy and inherited arrhythmogenic diseases where many data are available.

It is important to highlight the concept that despite the heterogeneity of substrates and clinical expressivity, genetic testing has a direct impact on clinical practice: it allows an accurate diagnosis including the silent carriers (i.e. pre-symptomatic diagnosis). Furthermore, in selected diseases the identification of a mutation has major importance for risk stratification and the treatment of patients. Unfortunately, in some instances the genetic heterogeneity is so great that it is virtually impossible to set up comprehensive genetic testing strategies based on the currently available technologies. ➲Table 9.1 summarizes the clinical value of genetic testing in different monogenic diseases.

Monogenic diseases with myocardial involvement

Hypertrophic cardiomyopathy

Clinical presentation and management

Hypertrophic cardiomyopathy (HCM) (➲Chapter 18) is diagnosed when left ventricular hypertrophy (typically asymmetric in distribution) is evident in the absence of cardiac or

Box 9.1 Commonly utilized genetic terms

- **Allele**: the alternative forms of a gene; any one of several mutational forms of a gene.
- **Alu repetitive sequence**: the most common dispersed repeated DNA sequence in the human genome, accounting for 5% of human DNA. The name is derived from the fact that these sequences are cleaved by the restriction endonuclease *Alu*.
- **Autosome**: a nuclear chromosome other than the X- and Y-chromosomes.
- **Baysian analysis**: a mathematical method to further refine recurrence risk, taking into account other known factors.
- **Carrier**: an individual heterozygous for a single recessive gene.
- **Chromosome**: in the eukaryotic nucleus, one of the threadlike structures consisting of chromatin; carries genetic information arranged in a linear sequence.
- **Contiguous genes**: genes physically close on a chromosome that, when acting together, express a phenotype.
- **Deletion**: the loss of a segment of the genetic material from a chromosome.
- **Dominant**: alleles that determine the phenotype displayed in a heterozygote with another (recessive) allele. Seen when an 'affected' parent passes the disease to, on average, 50% of their children, e.g. familial hypercholesterolaemia (FH) and hypertrophic cardiomyopathy (HCM).
- **Exon**: the portions of a gene which encodes for part of a protein. Usually genes have multiple exons that together form the so-called 'coding sequence', i.e. the DNA part that encodes for a protein. The remaining sequences of a gene have regulatory (or unknown) functions.
- **Founder effect**: seen where a rare disease reaches high frequency in a particular population that has recently expanded by immigration, e.g. FH in the Afrikaner group in South Africa.
- **Genetic linkage map**: a chromosome map showing the relative positions of the known genes on the chromosomes of a given species.
- **Genetic screening**: testing groups of individuals to identify defective genes capable of causing hereditary conditions.
- **Genetic variation**: the phenotypic variance of a trait in a population attributed to genetic heterogeneity.
- **Genome**: all of the genes carried by a single gamete; the DNA content of a human individual, which includes all 44 autosomes, two sex chromosomes, and the mitochondrial DNA.
- **Genome-wide scan**: analysis of (a representative subset) of all the common genetic variation across the whole genome in a single experiment. Allows novel gene loci to be identified. Uses commercially available 'chips' containing large numbers of single nucleotide polymorphisms (SNPs) (now >1,000,000) spaced along all chromosomes. Can be used to compare SNP allele frequency between cases and controls or in association studies with traits such as plasma cholesterol etc.
- **Genotype**: genetic constitution of an organism.
- **Hardy–Weinberg law**: the concept that both gene frequencies and genotype frequencies will remain constant from generation to generation in an infinitely large, interbreeding population in which mating is at random and there is no selection, migration, or mutation.
- **Heterozygote**: having two alleles that are different for a given gene.
- **Homozygote**: having identical alleles at one or more loci in homologous chromosome segments.
- **Housekeeping genes**: those genes expressed in all cells because they provide functions needed for sustenance of all cell types.
- **Incomplete penetrance**: the gene for a condition is present, but not obviously expressed in all individuals in a family with the gene.
- **Intron**: a segment of DNA (between exons) that is transcribed into nuclear RNA, but is removed in the subsequent processing into mRNA.
- **Linkage**: the greater association in inheritance of two or more non-allelic genes than is to be expected from independent assortment; genes are linked because they reside on the same chromosome.
- **Locus**: the specific place on a chromosome where a gene is located.
- **Lod score**: logarithm of the odd score; a measure of the likelihood of two loci being within a measurable distance of each other.

(Continued)

Box 9.1 (*Continued*) Commonly utilized genetic terms

- **Mutation**: process by which genes undergo a structural change.
- **Missense mutation:** a mutation in which a codon is changed to that encoding a different amino acid, resulting in a protein product with altered (usually detrimental) function.
- **Nonsense mutation**: a mutation in which a codon is changed to a stop codon, resulting in a truncated protein product.
- **Phenotype**: observable characteristics of an organism produced by the organism's genotype interacting with the environment.
- **Polymorphism**: a DNA sequence variant present in the general population at a frequency of >1%, e.g. the common apolipoprotein (Apo) E variants, ApoE3, E2, E4.
- **Rare variant**: a DNA sequence variant present in the general population at a frequency of <1%, e.g. any of the mutations causing FH or HCM in European populations.
- **Recessive**: a gene that is phenotypically manifest *only* in the homozygous state but is masked in the presence of a dominant allele. Seen when 'healthy' carrier parents have an affected child, e.g. cystic fibrosis.
- **Recombination**: the natural process of breaking and rejoining DNA strands to produce new combinations of genes and, thus, generate genetic variation. Gene crossover during meiosis.
- **Single nucleotide polymorphism (SNP)**: a DNA sequence variation occurring when a single nucleotide (A, T, C, or G) in the genome (or other shared sequence) differs between members of a species (or between paired chromosomes in an individual).
- **Trait**: any detectable phenotypic property of an organism.
- **Transcription**: the formation by RNA polymerase of an RNA molecule from a DNA template by complementary base pairing. Occurs in the nucleus of eukaryotic cells.
- **Translation**: the formation of a polypeptide chain in the specific amino acid sequence directed by the genetic information carried by mRNA. Occurs in the cytoplasm of eukaryotic cells on ribosomes.
- **Translocation**: a chromosome aberration which results in a change in position of a chromosomal segment within the genome, but does not change the total number of genes present.
- **Transgenic organism**: one into which a cloned genetic material has been experimentally transferred, a subset of these foreign gene express themselves in their offspring.

systemic conditions (e.g. hypertension or aortic stenosis), that could potentially induce hypertrophy of the magnitude observed. The disease is characterized histologically by myocyte disarray and hypertrophy, interstitial fibrosis, and thickening of the media of the intramural coronary arteries. The severity of the phenotype is largely heterogeneous and hypertrophy preferentially involves the interventricular septum. Most patients have remarkable regional variations in the extent of hypertrophy (➲Chapter 18).

The clinical presentation and management of HCM is characterized by incomplete and time-dependent penetrance. However, sudden death may be the first manifestation of the

Table 9.1 Clinical applicability of genetic testing in monogenic cardiac diseases*

Disease	Success rate	Identification of silent carriers/diagnosis	Reproductive risk assessment	Prognosis	Therapy
MFS	80–90%	+	+	–	–
HCM	60–65%	+	+	+/–	–
LQTS	60–65%	+	+	+	+
CPVT	50%	+	+	+/–	–
NS	40%	+	+	–	–
BrS	20%	+	+	–	–
ARVC	<10%	+	+	–	–
DCM	NA	+	+	–	–

* Only conditions in which consistent epidemiological data are available have been listed. ARVC, arrhythmogenic right ventricular cardiomyopathy; BrS, Brugada syndrome; CPVT, catecholaminergic polymorphic ventricular tachycardia; DCM, dilated cardiomyopathy; HCM, hypertrophic cardiomyopathy; LQTS, long QT syndrome; MFS, Marfan syndrome; NA, not applicable, NS, Noonan syndrome.

disease in some cases [1]. Therefore, risk stratification represents a crucial step for correct clinical management.

Beta-blockers, amiodarone, and calcium antagonists might be considered the most effective pharmacological treatment although the data are observational and there are no controlled comparative trials available. Besides secondary prophylaxis, implantable cardioverter defibrillator (ICD) implant for primary prevention of sudden death can be considered in patients with one or more major risk factors.

The guidelines for diagnosis and management of HCM are outlined in a joint consensus document of the American College of Cardiology and European Society of Cardiology [1] and are available online (see ➲Online resources, p.312).

Genetic bases

Since the discovery of the first locus for familial HCM (1989) and the first mutations involving the MYH7-encoded beta myosin heavy chain (1990) the understanding of HCM genetics has grown impressively. Most cases of HCM are transmitted as an autosomal dominant trait while other uncommon variants are inherited as autosomal recessive, X-linked, or mitochondrial disorders. Currently at least 21 genes encoding various sarcomeric, calcium-handling, and mitochondrial proteins have been identified (➲Table 9.2). Mutations in the HCM genes also cause some of the milder forms of ventricular hypertrophy in the elderly, which are usually considered as acquired conditions [2]. The prevalence of HCM is estimated to be 1 per 500, making HCM one of the most prevalent genetic diseases.

Table 9.2 Risk stratification in hypertrophic cardiomyopathy

Major risk factors	Minor risk factors
Previous cardiac arrest	Atrial fibrillation
Spontaneous sustained or non-sustained VT	Myocardial ischaemia
Unexplained syncope	LV outflow obstruction
LV wall or septum thickness ≥ 30mm	High-risk mutation
Lack of increase or fall in blood pressure during exercise	Involvement in competitive sports

LV, left ventricular; VT, ventricular tachycardia.

Modified from with permission from Maron BJ, McKenna WJ, Danielson GK, *et al.* American College of Cardiology/European Society of Cardiology Clinical Expert Consensus Document on Hypertrophic Cardiomyopathy: A report of the American College of Cardiology Foundation Task Force on Clinical Expert Consensus Documents and the European Society of Cardiology Committee for Practice Guidelines. *Eur Heart J* 2003 **24**: 1965–991.

An altered function of proteins of the cardiac sarcomere is the most frequent cause of HCM (➲Fig. 9.1). In such instances, myocardial hypertrophy is the only phenotype ('pure' HCM). Non-sarcomeric proteins have also been associated with HCM in a minority of cases. These variants usually show additional phenotypes such as abnormal conduction pathways (Wolff–Parkinson–White), sensorineural deafness, neurological and neurogenic muscular atrophy, trunk hypotonia, and encephalopathy.

Pathophysiology

The general scheme for HCM pathophysiology is that of a disorder of contractile function. In this context, hypertrophy represents an adaptation to the inability to generate

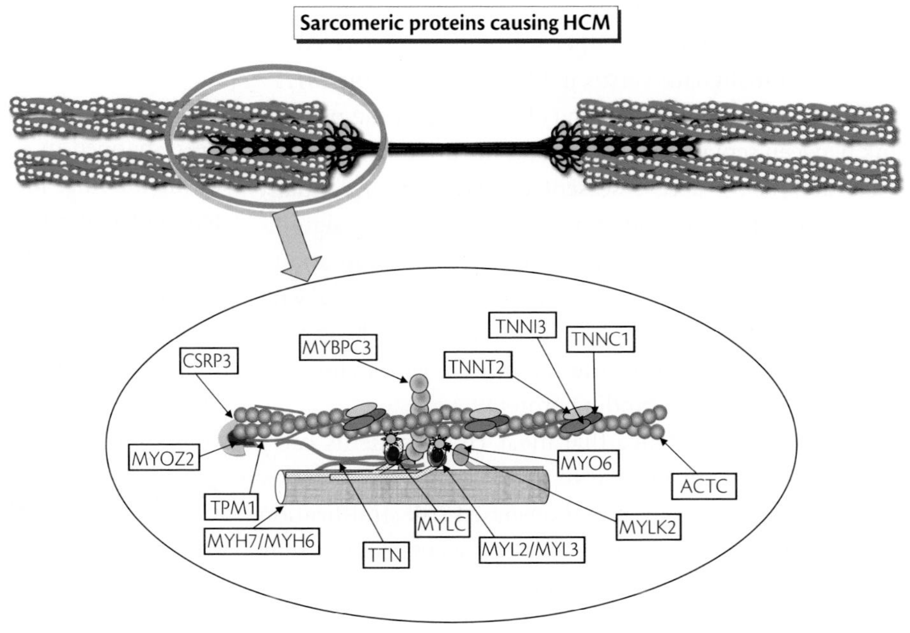

Figure 9.1 Schematic representation of a cardiac muscle sarcomere. The circled cartoon represents the area in which myosin–actin interaction take place. Most of the key proteins involved in the HCM pathogenesis take part in this macromolecular complex. ➲See Table 9.3 for gene symbols.

sufficient contractile strength to maintain adequate cardiac output. Fibroblast proliferation (fibrosis) and tissue disarray are the result of such adaptive modifications.

Functional expression studies of mutant sarcomeric proteins show a variety of abnormalities, spanning defects in myofibril formation, altered ATPase activity, Ca^{2+} sensitivity, and impaired actin–myosin interaction.

In vitro studies have shown that mutant sarcomeres are usually incorporated in the myofibril, but assembly abnormalities (reduced incorporation efficiency and accelerated disruption/catabolism) may occur. Whether the myocardial disarray observed at the clinical level may be a direct consequence of mutant protein mis-incorporation and/or mis-folding has not yet been definitely established.

The globular (head) domain of beta-myosin heavy chain is the site of actin binding and the region of ATP utilization (hydrolysis). *MYH7* mutations may alter the actin-dependent ATPase activity by disrupting the actin–myosin interaction. Several experimental studies also suggest that at least some HCM mutations increase the calcium sensitivity of the contractile apparatus. In addition, functional studies from muscle biopsies in humans and in mouse models of HCM demonstrate a depressed shortening velocity and power, and increased Ca^{2+} mobilization. These phenomena may represent the initial signal for myocardial compensatory hypertrophy [3].

Genotype–phenotype correlation

HCM is characterized by a wide spectrum of clinical phenotypes. Therefore, the attempt to derive prognostic information based on the specific defect is an attractive perspective. It has been suggested that *MHY7* mutations are often associated with a worse prognosis and severe hypertrophy while *TNNT2* mutations present with mild hypertrophy but increased risk of SCD [4]. Other authors have suggested the presence of malignant versus mild mutations in the *MHY7* gene [5, 6]. Another interesting observation is the possible link between septal morphology and the underlying genetic substrate [7, 8]: a reverse septal curve is preferentially associated with myofilament mutations while a sigmoidal septum is more frequently found in Z-disc mutations. Furthermore, reverse septum morphology is associated with higher probability of successful identification of the genetic defect upon screening of the sarcomeric genes (myosin, troponin, and myosin binding protein C).

However, the evidence that most HCM patients carry mutations that are unique to their family has recently challenged the idea of a mutation-based risk stratification scheme, since such genotype–phenotype correlations may only apply to a small subset of patients. Furthermore, the spectrum of clinical presentation is so wide, that one single genetic factor is probably not enough to fully explain the clinical presentation, and modifiers (both environmental and genetic) play a significant role.

Clinical applicability of genetic testing in HCM

The molecular epidemiology of HCM has been systematically addressed [9] by screening the entire open reading frame of nine HCM genes in 197 probands (*MYH7, MYBPC3, TNNI3, TNNT2, MYL2, MYL3, TPM1, ACTC, TNNC1*). Approximately 63% of these patients have been successfully genotyped. Interestingly, two genes, *MYH7* and *MYBPC3*, made up 82% of genotyped patients, while troponin T and troponin I, were present in 6.5% of probands. Therefore, >90% of HCM patients with an identifiable mutation may be detected by the analysis of only four out of the 21 known genes. Similarly to what has been identified in the case of long QT syndrome, approximately 5% of patients present with more than one genetic defect (on the same or on two different genes), therefore genetic testing of all genes has to be completed in all patients even if a first genetic defect has been found.

Genetic modifiers in HCM

Identification of 'modifier genes' is an attractive possibility for the improvement of genotype-based risk stratification. Genetic modifiers are represented by frequent genetic variants in the population that are neither sufficient nor necessary to cause the disease but they can worsen or attenuate the phenotype. Hints for the existence and clinical relevance of genetic modifiers in HCM have been brought to light [6, 10, 11] (➲Table 9.3). Other authors have suggested that modifiers can be located either in known HCM genes [12] or in other situations such as the renin–angiotensin–aldosterone pathways. Recently, four modifier loci on 3q26.2, 10p13, 17q24, and 16q12.2 (73cM) have been mapped in a large family with HCM. The effect size of the modifier loci ranged from approximately 8g shift in left ventricular mass for 10p13 locus heterozygosity up to approximately 90g for 3q26.2 locus homozygosity for the uncommon allele (➲Table 9.3) [11].

Despite their early stage, these studies suggest that the clinical course of HCM may be influenced by additional genetic factors. In the future this approach may allow individualized risk profiling by elucidation of a series of genetic variables.

Dilated cardiomyopathy

Dilated cardiomyopathy (DCM (➲Chapter 18)) is a myocardial disease characterized by dilatation and impaired

Table 9.3 Genetic causes of hypertrophic cardiomyopathy

Locus name	Gene symbol	Phenotype	Inheritance	Chromosomal locus	Protein	Estimated prevalence (*)	OMIM ID
CMH1	*MYH7*	HCM	AD	14q12	Beta-myosin heavy chain	35–45%	192600
CMH2	*TNNT2*	HCM*	AD	1q32	Cardiac troponin T	5–10%	115195
CMH3	*TPM1*	HCM*	AD	15q22.1	Alpha tropomyosin	1–5%	115196
CMH4	*MYBPC3*	HCM*	AD	11p11.2	Cardiac myosin-binding protein C	20–50%	115197
CMH6	*PRKAG2*	HCM, WPW	AD	7q36	AMP-az\ctivated protein kinase	<1%	600858
CMH7	*TNNI3*	HCM*	AD	19q12.2–q13.2	Cardiac troponin I	1–5%	191044
CMH8	*MYL3*	HCM	AD	3p21	Cardiac essential myosin light chain	1–51%	608751
CMH9	*TTN*	HCM*	AD	2q31	Titin	<1%	590040
CMH10	*MYL2*	HCM	AD	12q23–24.3	Cardiac regulatory myosin light chain	<1%	160781 and 608758
CMH11	*ACTC*	HCM*	AD	15q14	Actin	<1%	102540
CMH12	*CSRP3*	HCM	AD	11p15.1	Cysteine and glycine rich protein 3	@1%	612124
–	*MYOZ2*	HCM	AD	4q26–q27	Myozenin 2	Unknown/rare	605602
–	*TNNC1*	HCM	AD	3p21.3–14.3	Cardiac troponin C	0.4%	191040
–	*MYH6*	HCM	AD	14q12	Alpha-myosin heavy chain	<1%	160710
–	*MYLK2*	HCM	AD	20q13.3	Myosin light chain kinase 2	Unknown/rare	606566
–	*MTTI***	HCM*	Matrilineal	Mitochondrial DNA	tRNA isoleucine and tRNA glycine	Unknown/rare	590045
–	*MTTH***	HCM*	Matrilineal	Mitochondrial DNA	tRNA histidine	Unknown/rare	
–	*MYO6*	HCM, deafness	AD	6q13	Myosin VI	Unknown/rare	606346
–	*NDUFV2*	HCM, encephalopathy	–	18p11.3–11.2	NADH dehydrogenase ubiquinone flavoprotein 2	Unknown/rare	600532
GSDIIb#	*LAMP2***	HCM, muscle weakness, mental retardation, glycogen storage	XD	Xq24	Lysosome-associated membrane protein-2	Unknown/rare	300257
Fabry disease	*GLA*	HCM, isolated or with Fabry phenotype	XD	Xq22	Alpha-galactosidase-A	Unknown/rare	301500

AD, autosomal dominant; CM, cardiomyopathy; WPW, Wolf–Parkinson–White syndrome; XD, X-linked dominant; XR, X recessive.

* associated with both hypertrophic and dilated cardiomyopathy; ** Danon disease; # GSDIIb, glycogen storage disease IIb.

contractile function of the heart. The aetiology of DCM is multifactorial, and many different clinical conditions can lead to the phenotype. Ventricular dilatation may result as the consequence of different causes ranging from myocarditis due to viral infections, coronary artery disease, and systemic diseases (➲Chapter 18). The most frequent forms of DCM are those secondary to ischaemic and valvular heart disease. In some instances, no aetiologic factor can be identified and the disease is defined as 'idiopathic'. Idiopathic DCM may occur in sporadic as well in familial forms (FDCM). FDCM may frequently present with associated cardiac (conduction delays, bradycardia, atrioventricular and intraventricular conduction delay) or extra-cardiac (skeletal muscle dystrophy, myopathy, deafness, mental retardation, endocrine system abnormalities, granulocytopaenia) phenotypes [13].

Clinical presentation

The cardiac manifestations, risk stratification, and management of DCM are discussed in Chapter 23, Heart Failure.

Genetic bases and pathophysiology

The list of DCM genes has increased substantially over the last 10 years (➲Table 9.4) and the genetic heterogeneity is impressive. Furthermore, understanding of multiple pathogenetic mechanisms has advanced. In general, genetically determined DCM is related to malfunction of proteins controlling the mechanical resistance of myocardial cells or the tightness of cell-to-cell junctions. Therefore, the mechanism is reasonably apparent in the case of structural proteins (cytoskeletal and adherens junction) or contractile proteins. On the other hand, the pathogenesis of some rare genetic variants of DCM remains less clear.

The most frequent pattern of inheritance is autosomal dominant, but autosomal recessive, matrilineal, and X-linked transmissions have also been reported.

With some exceptions, six major groups of molecules are involved:

1) nuclear envelope and nuclear lamina proteins;
2) sarcomeric proteins;
3) cytoskeletal proteins;
4) adherens junction proteins;
5) mitochondrial DNA;
6) ion channels.

Nuclear envelope and nuclear lamina proteins

Five proteins of the nuclear structure have been associated with DCM: lamin A/C (which causes the most frequent autosomal dominant variant) emerin, thymopoietin, and presenilin 1 and 2 (➲Fig. 9.2).

The most frequent DCM variant due to nuclear envelope mutations is that linked with *LMNA* mutation, also called autosomal dominant Emery–Dreyfuss muscular dystrophy (EDMD). The *LMNA* gene encodes two proteins of the nuclear lamina: lamins A and C. Lamins form dimers through their rod domain and interact with chromatin and with other key proteins of the inner nuclear membrane. More than 60 known *LMNA/C* mutations may not only cause DCM and EDMD but, according to more recent data, also other allelic phenotypes: partial lipodystrophy, Charcot–Marie–Tooth disease, limb girdle muscular dystrophy (LGMD), partial lipodystrophy, mandibulosacral dysplasia, increased plasma leptin levels. The association of DCM with conduction defects is a typical feature of the *LMNA* mutation and it represents an indication for genetic testing in all patients with this phenotype.

Dilatation and conduction defects are the typical cardiac features of EMDM that may present with or without skeletal muscle abnormalities. In heart, the specific localization of emerin to desmosomes and adherens fascia could account for the characteristic conduction defects described in patients with EDMD. Since emerin is a ubiquitous protein the existence of alterations limited to skeletal and cardiac muscle remains difficult to explain.

Table 9.4 Modifier genes in hypertrophic cardiomyopathy

Gene/variant	Gene product	Clinical variable	Result	Number of patients	Reference
ACE: D allele	Angiotensin-converting enzyme	Cardiac hypertrophy	HCM 0.69 Not affected: 0.57	100	Marian 1993 [14]
		SCD	0.74 (high incidence SCD) 0.55 (low incidence SCD)		
AGT	Angiotensinogen	LVMI	Not significant	108	Brugada *et al.* 1997 [15]
AT1a	Angiotensin II receptor 1a	LVMI	Not significant		
END1:AA and AG alleles	Endothelin 1	LVMI	Accounts for 7.3% of the variability of the LVMI		
TNF-α: G308A allele	Tumour necrosis factor	LVMI	Accounts for 6% of variability	142	Patel *et al.* 2000 [16]
IL-6: G174C allele	Interleukin-6	LVMI	Not significant		
IGF2: G829A allele	Insulin-like growth factor-2	LVMI	Not significant		
TGFβ1: C509T	Transforming growth factor beta-1	LVMI	Not significant		
CTP11β2: T344C	Aldosterone synthase	LVMI	Not significant		
Chromosomal loci 3q26.2, 10p13, 17q24	Unknown	LVMI	Increase of left ventricular mass from 8 to 90g	100 (members of the same MYBPC3 family)	Daw *et al.* 2007 [11]

LVMI, left ventricular mass index; SCD, sudden cardiac death.

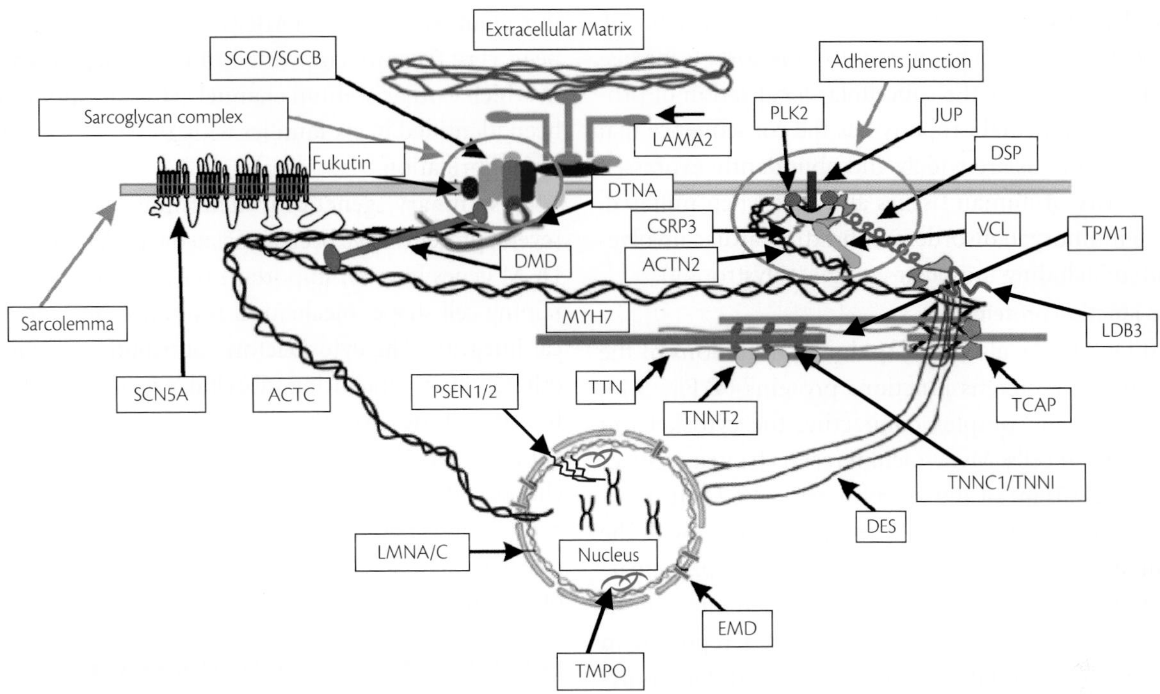

Figure 9.2 Structural proteins associated with inherited dilated cardiomyopathy. Four groups of proteins are identified: cytoskeletal proteins, sarcoglycan complex proteins, nuclear envelope proteins, adherens junction proteins. See text for details.

The pathogenesis of DCM linked to the other nuclear proteins is still obscure. It is interesting to note that presenilin 1 and 2 are highly expressed in the central nervous system and they primarily cause Alzheimer disease, which in some cases, for still unknown reasons, is associated with the DCM phenotype.

Sarcomeric proteins

Mutations in sarcomeric proteins have been often associated with DCM, thus suggesting pathophysiological similarities between DCM and HCM.

The first identified gene in this group is cardiac actin. Actin, by linking the sarcomere with the cytoskeletal apparatus, is involved in force generation as well as in force transmission. As a consequence it has been considered a rational candidate for both diseases, and mutations have been identified by Olson and colleagues [17] and confirmed by other authors despite the low prevalence of actin mutations in DCM [3]. Other typical HCM genes associated with DCM are *MYH7* (cardiac myosin heavy chain) *TNNT2* (troponin T), *TNNC1* (troponin C), *TPM1* (tropomyosin 1), *ACTN2* (alpha-actinin), and *TNNI3* (troponin I) (➲Figs. 9.1 and 9.2).

The reason why different mutations in the same gene recapitulate two different phenotypes (DCM and HCM) has still to be elucidated. Interestingly, the knock-in mouse model of DCM-cardiac myosin heavy chain mutation shows impaired contractility while the HCM-associated mutations are usually associated with an enhanced function [18]. In the clinic it is not infrequent to observe HCM patients who progress to DCM, therefore, some cases of DCM may represent a final stage of HCM. Therefore it is possible to hypothesize differential clinical manifestations associated with 'loss of function' and 'gain of function' sarcomeric proteins.

An additional sarcomeric protein causing DCM but not HCM is telethonin (*TCAP* gene), which is probably a very rare cause of cardiac dilatation and heart failure. Telethonin is a sarcomeric protein that localizes to the Z-discs of skeletal and cardiac muscle where it acts as a molecular 'ruler' for the assembly of the sarcomere by providing spatially defined binding sites for other sarcomeric proteins (19).

Cytosleletal proteins

Several, cytoskeletal protein-encoding genes are known to cause DCM (➲Fig. 9.2; Table 9.4). Desmin and dystrophin are those that appear to be most frequently involved. Desmin encircles the Z-discs and it connects adjacent myofibrils. It also forms a link between actin and the dystrophin–sarcoglycan complex [20]. Therefore, desmin attaches and stabilizes the sarcomere. Dystrophin is a large cytoskeletal protein, which is part of the dystrophin-associated glycoprotein (DAG) complex. The DAG complex includes dystroglycan, sarcoglycan, syntrophin complex, and caveolin. The DAG complex forms a transmembrane link between the extracellular matrix and the intracellular cytoskeleton [21].

Cytoskeletal proteins create a kind of framework deputed: (1) to serve as cellular 'backbone'; (2) to allow force transmission; and (3) to convey the subcellular localization of proteins. This fundamental property has the consequence that cytoskeletal proteins are widely and abundantly expressed in the majority of human tissues and that when mutated, they cause multiorgan disorders with extra-cardiac involvement (often including muscular weakness/dystrophy).

Adherens junction proteins

Inherited DCM may also develop due to mutations of the genes encoding adherens junctions proteins (➲Fig. 9.2), a macromolecular complex connecting the cytoskeleton with the adjacent cells. Metavinculin results from a cardiac-specific splice variant of the vinculin gene (*VCL*). It interacts with alpha-actinin to anchor the cytoskeleton with the sarcolemma at the adherens junction level, thus participating in the cell-to-cell adhesion process. Altered interactions between metavinculin and actin have been reported in patients with VCL mutations. There are anecdotal reports of additional genes (*DSP* and *CSRP3*) but their epidemiological relevance is not known at the present time.

Mitochondrial DNA

Evidence of a mitochondrial form of DCM initially came from two cases of early-onset fatal DCM associated with the presence of large deletions of mitochondrial DNA [22]. Other reports followed and mutations in mitochondrial DNA encoding for histidine tRNA [23] and isoleucine tRNA [24] were identified. Interestingly, both mitochondrial DNA genes have also been implicated in HCM. Mitochondrial DNA defects cause very complex phenotypes with multiorgan involvement including deafness, focal glomerulosclerosis, and epilepsy. The pathophysiological mechanisms leading from these mutations to the clinical phenotype are largely unknown but there are likely to involve energetic substrate production.

Other variants

A mutation in the *TAZ* gene in a family with a malignant form of myopathy co-segregating with an X-linked pattern has been reported [25]. This finding indicates that Barth syndrome and this DCM variant are allelic diseases. *TAZ* is expressed at high levels in cardiac and skeletal muscle and encodes an alternatively spliced protein called tafazzin, which has no known similarities to other proteins and unknown function. Another *TAZ* allelic disease is left ventricular non-compaction (LVNC) (see ➲Left ventricular non-compaction, p.290).

Additional genes that may cause rare instances of DCM have been reported. These genetic variants not only involve structures devoted to force transmission control (*DSP*), chaperone-like proteins (*CRYAB*), but also transmembrane ion channel subunits (*ABCC9*). This latter finding has been very recently confirmed in two independent studies in which cardiac sodium channel (*SCN5A*) mutations have been identified in six families with DCM, heart failure, and atrial fibrillation.

In summary, genetically determined abnormalities of several proteins have been associated with DCM. Most of the DCM genes have an important physiological role in maintaining cell shape, mechanical resistance, and morphological integrity. The cytoskeleton contributes substantially to cell stability by anchoring subcellular structures and it is also linked with desmosomes, thus participating in cell-to-cell adhesion function. Sarcomeric proteins, and possibly mitochondrial DNA, may cause DCM by an impairment of force generation capabilities. Given the important physiological role of DCM-related genes, it is not surprising that mutations often cause severe phenotypes with multiorgan involvement.

Left ventricular non-compaction

LVNC is due to an arrest of myocardial morphogenesis (➲Chapter 18). The disorder is characterized by a hypertrophic left ventricle with deep trabeculations and poor systolic function, with or without associated left ventricular dilatation. In some cases, the right ventricle is also affected. LVNC may be an isolated disorder or associated with congenital heart anomalies such as ventricular septal defects, pulmonary stenosis, and atrial septal defects. LVNC becomes clinically overt at any time from infancy through adolescence and the clinical course of the disease is often severe with a progressive worsening of contractile function. Three genes causing LVNC are known: 1) alpha-dystrobrevin (*DTNA*), a protein participating in the dystrophin-associated complex [26]; 2) cypher/*ZASP*, a gene encoding for a component of the Z-line in both skeletal and cardiac muscle, participating in assembly and targeting of cytoskeletal proteins [27]; 3) *TAZ*, a gene with unknown function also causing X-linked DCM [26]. These genetic abnormalities suggest that the pathophysiology of LVNC is similar to that of DCM, associated with cytoskeletal proteins mutations.

Arrhythmogenic right ventricular cardiomyopathy

Clinical presentation and management

Arrhythmogenic right ventricular cardiomyopathy (ARVC (➲Chapter 18)) is a predominantly autosomal dominant disease characterized by myocardial degeneration and fibro-fatty infiltration of the right ventricular free wall, the subtricuspid region, and the outflow tract (➲Chapter 30). A rare autosomal recessive variant (Naxos disease) characterized by typical myocardial involvement, palmar keratosis, and woolly hair has been also described.

Syncope and sudden death due to ventricular arrhythmias, often precipitated by intense physical activity, are the typical manifestation of ARVC. Conversely, the cases progressing to heart failure are rare. Diagnosis is based on morphological/structural signs (right ventricular dilatation, adipose tissue infiltration, and kinetic abnormalities), and electrocardiographic signs (T-wave inversion in leads V1–V3, epsilon waves, and late potentials) (➲Fig. 9.3). Major and minor diagnostic criteria have been defined by a task force of the European Society of Cardiology [28] (➲Table 9.5). These criteria are clinically useful although it should be emphasized that due to incomplete penetrance (clearly demonstrated after the identification of ARVC genes), several patients may present 'borderline' or non-conclusive diagnosis despite harbouring pathogenetic ARVC mutation. Indeed, the clinical picture may include: (1) a subclinical phase without symptoms and with ventricular fibrillation being the first presentation; (2) development of the typical morphological abnormalities only at later stages; (3) severe structural deterioration (right ventricular or biventricular) causing pump failure requiring cardiac transplant in rare instances.

ARVC is a relevant cause of sudden death in the young [29]. Patients usually present with palpitations and/or syncope, often before overt right ventricular abnormalities become detectable. Ventricular arrhythmias are of right ventricular origin (both right ventricular outflow tract and right ventricular apex morphology) and differential diagnosis with idiopathic right ventricular outflow tract tachycardia (a benign condition) is important, although often difficult.

Few risk factors have been identified in ARVC although it has to be emphasized that epidemiological data in large cohorts are still not available: young age, 'malignant' family history, QRS dispersion ≥ 40ms, T-wave inversion beyond V1, left ventricular involvement, documented ventricular tachycardia (VT), syncope, or previous cardiac arrest [30, 31]. On the other hand, inducibility at programmed electrical stimulation does not predict future events [1].

Pharmacological therapy for ARVC includes, as primary choices, beta blockers, sotalol, and amiodarone. ICD is indicated in all patients with a previous cardiac arrest and it can be considered for primary prophylaxis in all high-risk patients. Sotalol and amiodarone are also indicated for high-risk patients when ICD implantation is not feasible [1]. Finally, catheter ablation can be considered in patients with recurrent VT despite pharmacological therapy, although the rate of recurrence is not negligible [1].

Genetic bases and pathophysiology

ARVC primarily affects the desmosomal proteins that constitute the mechanical junctions between myocardial cells. The elucidation of genes underlying autosomal dominant ARVC has grown dramatically after the discovery of mutations in the plakophilin-2 gene (*PKP2*) encoding for a desmosomal protein, which is involved in 30–40% of cases [32]. Desmoplakin (*DSP*) and plakoglobin (*JUP*) are also associated with ARVC in rare instances and they both are constitutive proteins of the desmosomes. Several additional chromosomal loci linked to ARVC for whom the corresponding gene has not been identified yet are also known (see Gene Connection for the Heart database at http://www.fsm.it/cardmoc/).

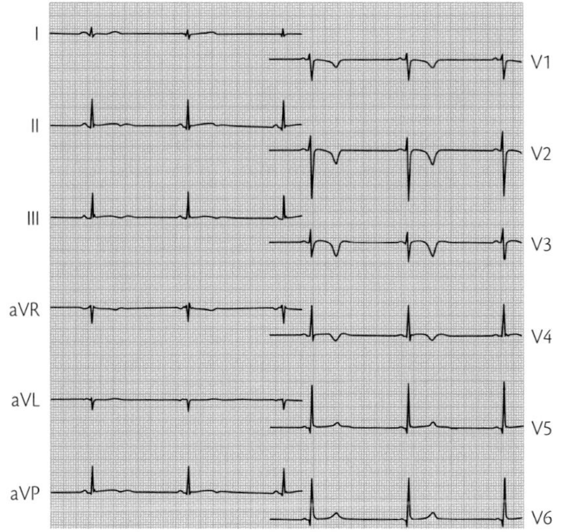

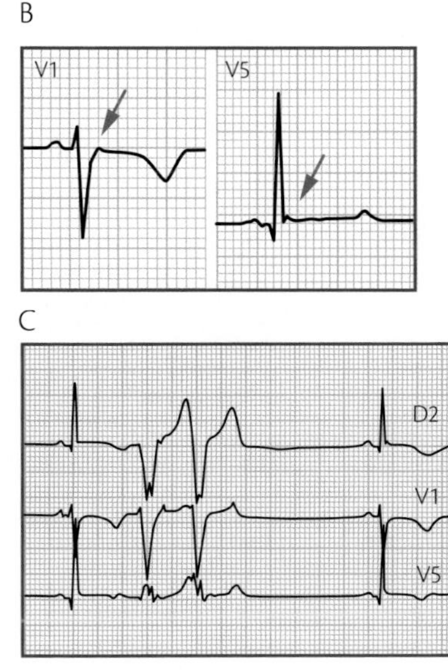

Figure 9.3 Electrocardiogram in a patient with ARVC. T-wave inversion in precordial leads (A) and epsilon waves (B) are the most typical features although not always present. Ventricular arrhythmias have a LBBB-like morphology indicating the right ventricular origin.

Table 9.5 Genetic loci and genes involved in DCM

Locus name	Gene symbol	Functional class	Phenotype	Inheritance	Chromosomal locus	Protein	OMIM ID
CMD1A and LGMD1B	*LMNA**	Nuclear envelope/ lamina	DCM with conduction defects, limb-girdle muscular dystrophy	AD	1q21.2	Lamin A/C	115200 and 159001 and 607920
CMD1B	Unknown		DCM	AD	9q13	–	600884
CMD1C	*LDB3*	Cytoskeleton/protein clustering	DCM	AD	10q21-q23	Lim domain binding 3	601493
CMD1D	*TNNT2*†	Contractile system	DCM**	AD	1q32	Cardiac troponin T	601494
CMD1E	*SCN5A*	Ion channel	DCM, conduction defect, sinus node dysfunction	AD	3p25-p22	Cardiac sodium channel gene	601154
CMD1F or LDMD1E	*LAMA2*	Cytoskeleton/ extracellular matrix	DCM, conduction defect, limb-girdle muscular dystrophy	AD	6q23	Laminin alpha-2	602067
CMD1G	*TTN****	Cytoskeleton	DCM/HCM	AD	2q24.3	Titin	604145
CMD1H	Unknown		DCM with conduction defect	AD	2q14-q22	–	604288
CMD1I	*DES*	Cytoskeleton	DCM with skeletal myopathy#	AD	2q35	Desmin	604765
CMD1K	Unknown		DCM	AD	6q12-q16	–	605582
CMD1J	*EYA4*	Development	DCM with sensorineural deafness	AR	6q23-q24	–	605362
CMD1L or LGMD1F	*SGCD*	Cytoskeleton/adherens junction	DCM, limb-girdle muscular dystrophy	AD	5q33	Delta-sarcoglycan	606685
CMD1M	*CSRP3*	Adherens junction	DCM	AD	11p15.1	Cysteine- and glycine-rich protein-3	600824
CMD1N	*TCAP*	Contractile system	DCM, limb-girdle muscular dystrophy	AD	17q12	Telethonin	607487
CMD1O	*ABCC9*	K(ATP) channel regulator	DCM with ventricular tachycardia	AD	12p12.1	ATP-binding cassette subfamily C	608569
CMD1P	*PLN*	Calcium handling/ contractile system			6q22.1	Phospholamban	
CMD1Q	Unknown		DCM		7q22.3-q31.1		
CMD1S	*MYH7*	Contractile system	DCM	AD	14q12	Cardiac myosin heavy chain	115200 and 160760
CMD1R	*ACTC*	Contractile system/ cytoskeleton	DCM	AD	15q14	Cardiac actin	102540
CMD1T	*TMPO*	Nuclear envelope/ lamina	DCM	AD	12q22	Thymopoietin	188380
CMD1U	*PSEN1*	Nuclear envelope/ lamina, cellular transport	DCM Alzheimer disease	AD	14q24.3	Presenilin 1	104311
CMD1V	*PSEN2*	Nuclear envelope/ lamina, cellular transport/growth	DCM Alzheimer disease	AD	1q31-q42	Presenilin 2	600759
CMD1X	*Fukutin*	Cytoskeleton/ extracellular matrix	DCM, limb-girdle muscular dystrophy	AD	9q31	Fukutin	607440
CMD1Y	*TPM1*	Contractile system	DCM/HCM	AD	15q22.1	Tropomyosin 1	191010
CMD1Z	*TNNC1*	Contractile system	DCM	AD	3p21.3–p14.3	Troponin C	191040

(Continued)

Table 9.5 (*Continued*) Genetic loci and genes involved in DCM

Locus name	Gene symbol	Functional class	Phenotype	Inheritance	Chromosomal locus	Protein	OMIM ID
CMD1AA	*ACTN2*	Contractile system/ cytoskeleton	DCM	AD	1q42–43	Alpha-actinin	102573
CMD2A	*TNNI3*	Contractile system	DCM/HCM	AR	19q13.4	Troponin I	191044
EDMD1	*EMD*	Nuclear envelope/ lamina	DCM, AV block, myopathy	XR	Xq28	Emerin	310300
CMD3B-XLCM	*DMD*	Cytoskeleton	DCM	XD	Xp21.2	Dystrophin	302045
CMD3A	*TAZ (G4.5)*	Cytoskeleton	DCM/HCM, skeletal myopathy	XR	Xq28	Tafazzin	300069 and 302060
DSP	*DCWHK*	Adherens junction	DCM, Carvajal syndrome	AR	6p24	Desmoplakin	605676
CMD1W	*VCL*	Adherens junction	DCM	–	10q22.1–q23	Metavinculin	193065
–	*MTTH*	–	DCM/HCM	matrilinear	mtDNA	tRNA-histidine	590040
–	*TRMI*	–	DCM/HCM, encephalopathy	matrilinear	mtDNA	tRNA-isoleucine	510000
LVNC1	*DTNA*	Cytoskeleton/ extracellular matrix	DCM, left ventricular non-compaction	AD	18q12.1–q12.2	Alpha-dystrobrevin	601239
LVNC	*LDB3*	Cytoskeleton	DCM, left ventricular non-compaction	AD	10q22.2–q23.3	Z-band alternatively spliced protein	605906

AD, autosomal dominant; AR, autosomal recessive; AV, atrioventricular; XD, X-linked dominant; XR, X-linked recessive.

* also causing familial partial lipodystrophy and mandibuloacral dysplasia; **probably the most frequent variant so far identified; *** also causing and tibial muscular dystrophy (600334); # also causing isolated distal muscle myopathy without DCM; †identified also in left ventricular non-compaction patients.

On the basis of the available data, the molecular pathogenesis of ARVC is that of a mutation-dependent impaired mechanical coupling or desmosome disruption, followed by remodelling of the intercalated discs. This would result in the delocalization and nuclear localization of plakoglobin and in effects at cellular signal transduction. Reduced tolerance to mechanical stretch ultimately leads to apoptosis and fibrofatty infiltration. This substrate creates the conditions for slowing and inhomogeneous electrical conduction leading to re-entrant arrhythmias. The prevalent right ventricular localization of ARVC is explained by the natural lower tolerance of the right ventricle to mechanical stretch as it is a low-pressure chamber with thin walls. It is important to emphasize, however, that ARVC can also involve the left ventricle in particularly severe cases.

Marfan syndrome

Clinical presentation and diagnosis

Marfan syndrome (MFS) (➲Chapter 31) affects mainly the skeletal apparatus, the eyes, and the cardiovascular system (➲Chapter 31). Skeletal abnormalities include: increased height; disproportionately long limbs and digits; anterior chest deformity; mild to moderate joint laxity; and vertebral column deformity (scoliosis and thoracic lordosis) [33]. Myopia, increased axial orbital length, corneal flatness, and subluxation of the lenses (ectopia lentis) are ocular findings. At the cardiovascular level, mitral valve prolapse, mitral regurgitation, dilatation of the aortic root, and aortic regurgitation have been reported [33]. The major life-threatening cardiovascular complication is aneurysm of the aorta and aortic dissection, which represent the major cause of mortality and morbidity [33].

The mean age of death for overt MFS is 45 years, but survival is affected by gender with males having a worse prognosis. Diagnostic criteria for MFS have been published pointing to the need for the application of strict rules, especially for relatives, in order to avoid over-diagnosis [34]. MFS is usually treated with beta-blockers and surgery, when indicated, to correct aortic dilatation.

Genetic bases and pathophysiology

MFS presents with highly variable expression, but complete non-penetrance (silent gene carriers) has not been definitively documented. In the pre-genetic era, consistent deficiency of elastin-associated microfibrillar fibres was also shown, and directed attention toward fibrillin, a glycoprotein of the microfibrillar component of the elastic fibre system. When MFS was mapped to chromosome 15, the fibrillin gene (*FBN1*) was immediately identified as a strong candidate. In 1991 [35] the first *FBN1* mutation in a patient with MFS was reported. This finding was subsequently confirmed by several groups and it is now evident that *FBN1* accounts for the vast majority of MFS with >300 mutations published in the last decade. A second locus on 3p25–p24.2 was mapped in 1994 but the corresponding gene has not yet been identified [36]. The pathophysiology of fibrillin-linked MFS is characterized by an abnormal metabolism of this protein. Mutated fibrillin subunits appear to exert a dominant-negative effect on the wild type subunits thus inhibiting the correct polymerization of collagen fibres. Other *in vitro* assays have suggested that, while synthesis and secretion of the polypeptides is unaffected, mutated polypeptides are significantly more susceptible to proteolytic degradation as compared with their wild type counterparts. Genetic screening of *FBN1* leads to the identification of a pathogenetic mutation in the majority of cases (see ➲Table 9.1).

Genetic disorders in the structurally normal heart

This group of diseases typically occurs in the absence of morphological abnormalities of the heart. They are also called 'primary electrical disorders' or 'inherited arrhythmogenic diseases' since their primary manifestation is a cardiac arrhythmia (➲Fig. 9.4) (➲Chapter 30). A peculiar electrocardiographic phenotype, which is a marker of electrical instability, is often recognized. Common symptoms are syncope and sudden death due to ventricular fibrillation. Beta-blockers are effective in some instances (e.g. long QT syndrome, catecholaminergic tachycardia) but the ICD is the only option for high-risk patients in some cases. Therefore risk stratification is very important. ESC/AHA guidelines for therapy and risk assessment were published in 2006 [1] and are available online (see ➲Online resources, p.312). The common denominator is the abnormality of proteins controlling the excitability of myocardial cells. In recent years, mounting evidence has highlighted the concept that allelic variants (i.e. two or more phenotypes caused by mutations in the same gene) are the rule rather than the exception in these conditions. As an example, the *KCNQ1* gene causes the LQT1 variant of long QT syndrome, the SQT2 variant of short QT syndrome, and familial atrial fibrillation (➲Table 9.6).

Long QT syndrome

Clinical presentation

The congenital long QT syndrome (LQTS) (➲Chapter 30) is characterized by abnormally prolonged QT interval leading to life-threatening arrhythmias in the presence of a structurally normal heart [37]. The mean age of onset of symptoms, (syncope or sudden death) is 12 years and earlier onset is usually associated with a more severe form of the disease. The estimated prevalence of this disorder is between 1:7000 and 1:3000. However, given that 10–35% of LQTS patients presents with a normal QTc interval and that 3–4% of probands inherit two independent mutations from non-consanguineous parents [37, 38], it is likely that the actual prevalence is higher.

Two major phenotypic variants were originally described in the early 1960s: one autosomal dominant (Romano–Ward syndrome) and one rare autosomal recessive (Jervell and Lange–Nielsen syndrome, JLN), also presenting with sensorineural deafness (➲Chapter 30).

Affected patients have abnormally prolonged repolarization (QT interval on the surface electrocardiogram, ECG),

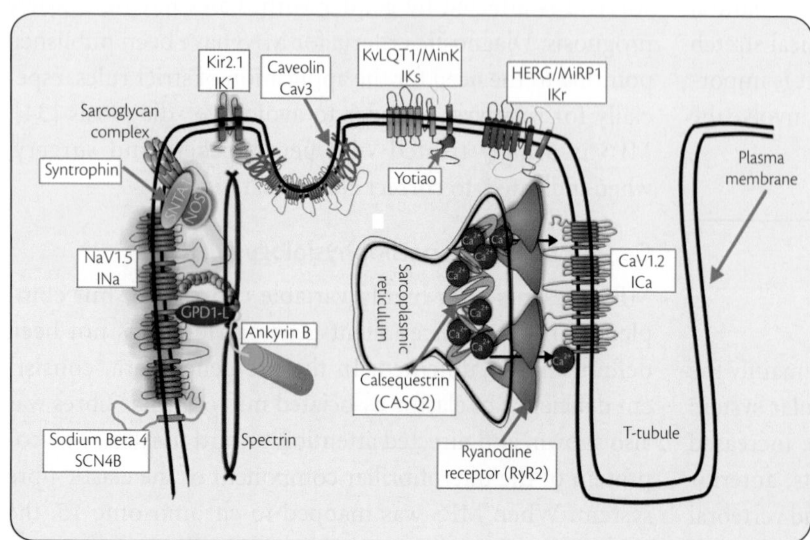

Figure 9.4 Cartoon showing the proteins involved in the pathogenesis of monogenic diseases causing arrhythmias and sudden death in the structurally normal heart. The relevant proteins are highlighted with white boxes.

Table 9.6 Diagnostic criteria for ARVC

	Major	Minor
Family history	Familial disease confirmed at necropsy or surgery	Family history of premature sudden death (age <35 years) due to suspected ARVC
ECG	Epsilon waves or localized prolongation (>110ms) of QRS complex in right precordial leads (V1–V3)	Late potentials on signal-averaged ECG
		Inverted T-waves in right precordial leads (V2 and V3) in people aged >12 years
		Sustained or non-sustained left bundle branch block-type ventricular tachycardia documented on ECG, or Holter monitoring, or during exercise testing; frequent ventricular extrasystoles (>1000/24 hours on Holter monitoring)
Right ventricular dysfunction	Severe dilatation and reduction of RV ejection fraction with no or mild LV involvement; localized RV aneurysms (akinetic or dyskinetic areas with diastolic bulging); severe segmental dilatation of RV	Mild global RV dilatation or ejection fraction reduction with normal LV; mild segmental dilatation of RV; regional RV hypokinesia
Histology	Fibrofatty replacement of myocardium on endomyocardial biopsy	

The diagnosis of ARVC is achieved in the presence of two major criteria, or one major plus two minor, or four minor criteria from different groups.

ECG, electrocardiogram; LV, left ventricular; RV, right ventricular.

Reproduced with permission from McKenna WJ, Thiene G, Nava A, *et al.* Diagnosis of arrhythmogenic right ventricular dysplasia/cardiomyopathy. Task Force of the Working Group Myocardial and Pericardial Disease of the European Society of Cardiology and of the Scientific Council on Cardiomyopathies of the International Society and Federation of Cardiology. *Br Heart J* 1994; **71**: 215–18.

abnormal T-wave morphology, and life-threatening cardiac arrhythmias. Cardiac events are often precipitated by physical or emotional stress but in a small subset cardiac events occur at rest [39]. This observation constitutes the basis for the effectiveness of beta-blockers that are the cornerstone of therapy in the LQTS. For patients unresponsive to this approach, ICD and/or cardiac sympathetic denervation have been applied. Accordingly, locus-specific risk stratification for therapeutic management has been proposed.

Genetic bases and pathophysiology

The number of genes that may cause QT prolongation and cardiac arrhythmias is continuously expanding. Interestingly several LQTS variants incorporate phenotypes other than QT prolongation, arrhythmias, and SCD. Furthermore, while LQTS was initially thought to be a pure cardiac channelopathy, it is now clear that non-ion channel-encoding genes may cause the disease. On the other hand, the concept that LQTS genes ultimately affect ionic currents, either directly (ion channel mutations) or indirectly (chaperones and other modulators), still holds true.

Mutations in potassium channel genes such as *KCNQ1* (LQT1) and *KCNH2* (LQT2) and in the sodium channel gene *SCN5A* (LQT3) were the first genetic causes of LQTS to be identified. The LQT1–3 variants constitute >90% of LQTS patients with identified mutation [38] and therefore large cohorts of individuals affected by the three variants of the disease have been made available for genotype–phenotype correlation studies.

At present, 12 LQTS genes have been identified (➲Table 9.6; Fig. 9.4). Some of these genes (encoding proteins ankyrin B, caveolin-3, A-kinase anchoring proteins, and syntrophin) cause LQTS by altering the intracellular protein localization, the ion channels gating, the response to the sympathetic stimulation, or nytrosylation of ion channels [41–43]. Other genes cause extracardiac abnormalities. As an example, *CACNA1C* mutation causes Timothy syndrome, a highly lethal and rare variant that associates long QT, ventricular arrhythmias with congenital defects (patent foramen ovale, tetralogy of Fallot), developmental disorders, autism, and facial dysmorphisms. *KCNJ2* mutations cause Andersen syndrome: prolonged QT, arrhythmias, periodic paralysis, and facial dysmorphisms (➲Table 9.6).

Risk stratification and therapy

In the last few years several studies have outlined the distinguishing features of the three most common autosomal dominant variants of LQTS (LQT1, LQT2, LQT3). Genotype–phenotype correlation for the remaining genes can often be reconciled to the abnormality of the final 'target ion current' (➲Table 9.7).

Locus-specific repolarization morphology and locus-specific triggers for cardiac events have been described [44]. LQT1 patients usually develop symptoms during physical activity (➲Fig. 9.5); conversely, LQT3 patients tend to experience events at rest (➲Fig. 9.5). Auditory stimuli and

Table 9.7 Genetic loci and genes causing arrhythmogenic diseases

Gene symbol	Locus name	Chromosomal locus	Inheritance	Protein	Functional effect	Phenotype
KCNQ1	LQT1	11p15.5	AD	I_{Ks} potassium channel alpha subunit (KvLQT1)	Loss of function	Long QT
	JLN1		AR		Loss of function	Long QT, deafness
	SQT2		AD		Gain of function	Short QT
	AF1		AD		Gain of function	Atrial fibrillation
KCNH2	LQT2	7q35–q36	AD	I_{Kr} potassium channel alpha subunit (HERG)	Loss of function	Long QT
	SQT1		AD		Gain of function	Short QT
	AF2		AD		Gain of function	Atrial fibrillation
SCN5A	LQT3	3p21	AD	Cardiac sodium channel alpha subunit (Nav 1.5)	Gain of function	Long QT
	BrS1		AD		Loss of function	Brugada syndrome
	AF3		AD		Loss of function	Atrial fibrillation
	PCCD		AD		Loss of function	Conduction defect/blocks
	SSS		AD		Loss of function	Sick sinus syndrome
*KCNJ2**	AND/ LQT7	17q23.1–q24.2	AD	I_{K1} potassium channel (Kir2.1)	Loss of function	Long QT, potassium sensitive periodic paralysis, dysmorphic features
	SQT3		AD		Gain of function	Short QT
	AF4		AD		Gain of function	Atrial fibrillation
KCNE1	LQT5	21q22.1–q22.2	AD	I_{Ks} potassium channel beta subunit (MinK)	Loss of function	Long QT
	JLN2		AR		Loss of function	Long QT, deafness
	AF5		AD		Gain of function	Atrial fibrillation
*ANK2**	LQT4	4q25–q27	AD	Ankyrin B, anchoring protein	Loss of function	Long QT, atrial fibrillation
KCNE2	LQT6	21q22.1–q22.2	AD	I_{Kr} potassium channel beta subunit (MiRP)	Loss of function	Long QT
	AF6		AD		Gain of function	
CACNA1C	TS/LQT8	12p13.3	AD/mosaicism	Calcium channel alpha subunit	Gain of function	Timothy syndrome: long QT, syndactyly, septal defect, patent foramen ovale
	BrS3		AD		Loss of function	Brugada syndrome with short QT
CACNB2B	BrS4	10p12	AD	Calcium channel beta subunit	Gain of function	Brugada syndrome with short QT
Cav3	LQT9	3p24	AD	Caveolin	Gain of function of sodium current	Long QT
SCNb4	LQT10	11q23.3	AD	Sodium channel beta subunit	Gain of function of sodium current	Long QT
AKAP9 (yotiao)	LQT11	7q21–q22	AD	A-kinase-anchoring protein	Reduced IKs current due to loss of camp sensitivity	Long QT
SNTA1	LQT12	20q11.2	AD	alpha1-syntrophin	Increased sodium current due to S-nitrosylation of SCN5A	Long QT syndrome
GPD1-L	BrS2	3p22.3	AD	glycerol-3-phosphate dehydrogenase 1-like	Reduced sodium current	Brugada syndrome
RyR2	CPVT1	1q42–43	AD	Cardiac ryanodine receptor	Diastolic calcium release	Catecholaminergic tachycardia
CASQ2	CPVT2	1p13.3–p11	AR	Cardiac calsequestrin	Diastolic calcium release	Catecholaminergic tachycardia

AD, autosomal dominant; AR, autosomal recessive;

* may cause CPVT phenocopy.

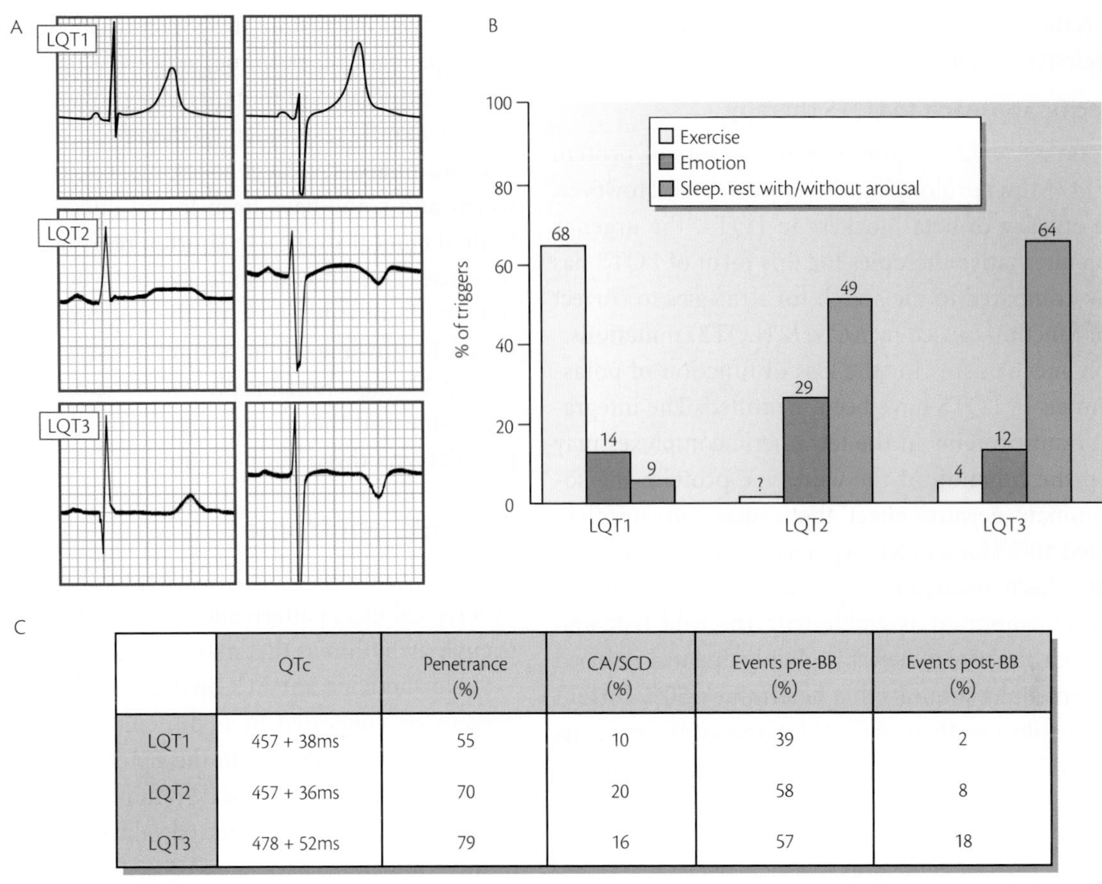

	QTc	Penetrance (%)	CA/SCD (%)	Events pre-BB (%)	Events post-BB (%)
LQT1	457 + 38ms	55	10	39	2
LQT2	457 + 36ms	70	20	58	8
LQT3	478 + 52ms	79	16	57	18

Figure 9.5 Genotype–phenotype correlation in the long QT syndrome: repolarization morphology, event rate, triggers and response to beta-blocker therapy in the three most frequent genetic variants: LQT1, LQT2, and LQT3.

arousal are relatively specific triggers for LQT2 patients while swimming is a predisposing setting for cardiac events in LQT1 patients [44].

Clinically relevant differences exist in terms of cardiac event rate, morphology of repolarization, and response to therapy (➲Fig. 9.5). Locus-specific differences of the natural history of LQTS have also been demonstrated and allow genotype-based risk stratification [44]. A QTc interval >500ms, and a LQT2 or LQT3 genotype determines the worst prognosis. Gender differentially modulates the outcome according to the underlying genetic defect: the LQT3 males and LQT2 females are the highest-risk subgroups.

In 2004 data were reported on the response to therapy in the large LQTS cohort that are followed at the Maugeri Foundation in Italy. LQT1 patients showed an excellent response to beta-blocker therapy as 90% of them remained free from syncope and cardiac arrest after 5.4 years of mean follow up, and showed a total mortality rate of 1% [45]. Few LQT1 patients treated with beta-blockers required additional therapy such as the implant of defibrillators (ICD) or left cardiac sympathetic denervation (LCSD). Interestingly, it has been reported that lack of compliance is the most important cause of events occurring during antiadrenergic treatment in LQT1 [46].

By means of multivariate analysis we also identified the predictors of events during antiadrenergic therapy:

1) the presence of a QTc interval >500ms;
2) the occurrence of a life-threatening arrhythmic event before age 7 years;
3) being affected by the LQT2 orLQT3 variants.

Carriers of a *KCNH2* or *SCN5A* mutation have a 2.81 and 4.00 relative risk of arrhythmic events on beta-blockers as compared with LQT1, respectively [45]. According to the ACC/AHA/ESC 2006 guidelines [1], the use of the ICD in the primary prevention of cardiac arrest has a Class IIb indication in LQT2 and LQT3 patients with QTc >500ms. Since the ICD dose not prevent the occurrence of arrhythmias, and given the young age of the patients, its implant is more prone to complications related to lead fracture and inappropriate shocks, the search for therapeutic alternatives represents a priority.

Gene-specific approach to LQTS therapy

KCNQ1 and *KCNH2* mutations lead to a loss of protein function [47] thus prolonging the QT interval. However, given the efficacy of beta-blockers in LQT1, the urgency to develop alternative therapies for this form of LQTS has been weak compared to the search for strategies to correct the loss of function caused by *KCNH2* (LQT2) mutations.

Multiple mechanisms for the loss of function of potassium channels in LQTS have been identified. The integration of mutant proteins in the tetrameric complexes may impact on the function of the wild type protein: the so-called 'dominant negative effect' that causes a greater than the expected 50% (for a heterozygous condition) reduction of current. Alternatively, mutations may lead to truncated proteins that cannot co-assemble with the wild type and therefore their functional defect is mainly due to a reduced production of alpha subunits that determine a 50% current reduction (haplo-insufficiency) [47]. Some of the mutants do not affect functional properties of channels but, rather, they interfere with the localization of the protein in the membrane: this behaviour is often referred to as 'defective intracellular trafficking' [48, 49].

The evidence that conductance of *KCNH2* channels is directly related to extracellular [K^+], prompted the use of potassium supplements that, by increasing extracellular [K^+], could enhance IKr current and at least partially compensate for the mutation [50]. This approach proved useful in small clinical trials [50, 51]. Oral potassium supplements are effective in reducing repolarization abnormalities in LQT2 but unfortunately no data demonstrate that they can also reduce the risk of cardiac events.

Several strategies to rescue the defective trafficking of LQT2 mutants were explored in the last 10 years [52, 53], but the compounds tested so far are either toxic or they block the target channel, thus losing therapeutic efficacy.

In the case of the LQT3 variant (gain-of-function mutations in the *SCN5A* gene), sodium-channel blockers have used. Unfortunately, not all the LQT3 patients respond favourably to this treatment. The clinical response to mexiletine in LQT3 (both in terms of QT duration and cardiac events) depends upon the specific biophysical properties of the mutant channel (different mutations = different biophysical properties). Specifically, the analysis of the current/voltage relationship of the channel shows that if the mutation induces a negative shift of the steady state inactivation (SSI) (i.e. less current is available at any given membrane voltage), the treatment with mexiletine is predicted to be effective. Interesting the SSI shift parallels the EC50 for use-dependent block of mexiletine (➲Fig. 9.6) [54]. Thus, *in vitro* expression of mutants may provide useful information to identify responders to therapy.

In summary, several gene-specific compounds have been tested and some have been found effective *in vitro* or in limited clinical studies, to shorten repolarization. Whether their use can be useful clinically, and whether they will also reduce life-threatening arrhythmias, remains to be established. Meanwhile it is important to emphasize that the role of beta-blockers remains pivotal in the management of this syndrome and these drugs are the first-line treatment for patients with this clinical diagnosis.

Brugada syndrome

Brugada syndrome (BrS) (➲Chapter 30) is characterized by a typical ECG pattern and a risk of life-threatening ventricular arrhythmias that may lead to sudden death.

Since the aberrant ECG pattern can be intermittently present or concealed, it is difficult to estimate the true prevalence of the disease in the general population [55]. A recent meta-analysis of the current literature on prevalence of the Brugada pattern reported values between 0.12– 0.2% of the population. Type 2 and 3 ECGs, which are *not* diagnostic of BrS, were much more prevalent: 0.6% (SG Priori, personal communication). Undoubtedly, for reasons that

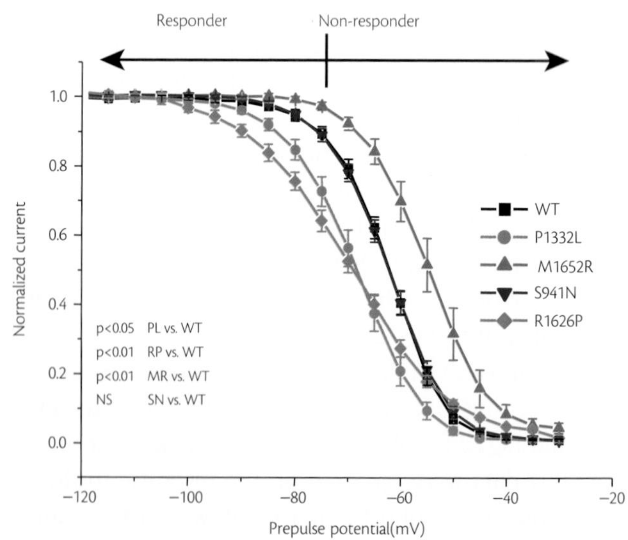

Figure 9.6 *In vitro* expression of LQT3 (SCN5A) mutants permits prediction of the response to mexiletine therapy based on the analysis of the steady state inactivation (SSI). A negative shift (green lines) is associated with favourable clinical effect on QT cans symptoms. Reproduced from Ruan Y, Liu N, Bloise R, *et al.* Gating properties of SCN5A mutations and the response to mexiletine in long-QT syndrome type 3 patients. *Circulation* 2007; **116**: 1137–44.

remain elusive, the disease is either more prevalent or more penetrant in eastern countries (mainly in Southeast Asia), where prevalence may be as high as 3% of the population [56]. A genetic modifier recently identified (Asian-specific haplotype in the *SCN5A* promoter region) may play a role in worsening the phenotype [57].

Clinical presentation

Electrocardiographic criteria for BrS have been defined [58]: a type 1 ECG is considered diagnostic and it includes ST segment elevation of ≥2mm, with a 'coved morphology' associated with incomplete or complete right bundle branch block followed by a negative T wave; types 2 and 3 are considered inconclusive (➲Fig. 9.7).

A type 1 ECG may occur spontaneously or it may be induced by pharmacological testing with class IC sodium-channel blockers (ajmaline 1mg/kg; flecainide 2mg/kg). Such drug testing is indicated in patients presenting with a type 2 or type 3 ECG. It is important to recognize that BrS is characterized by incomplete penetrance and that the sensitivity of these criteria in the identification of affected individuals remains undefined, and it is certainly lower than 100%; research estimates a sensitivity of 77% in the subgroup of patients carrying a mutation in the *SCN5A* gene [59]. Therefore, the diagnosis of BrS may be challenging in some patients.

The ECG pattern in BrS fluctuates over time and the use of 12-lead Holter monitoring may help to detect the presence of a spontaneous type 1 ECG. The ECG pattern is also influenced by the position of the leads being more evident when the V1 and V2 leads are positioned one intercostal space higher. Recent data [60] suggest that patients with a diagnostic ECG with high lead positioning (in either the second or third intercostal space) have a prognosis similar to that of individuals with a type 1 ECG recorded using the standard position. Unfortunately, the sensitivity and specificity of the diagnosis established with this configuration is unknown. Therefore, it is premature to provide robust guidelines for ECG recording in BrS patients.

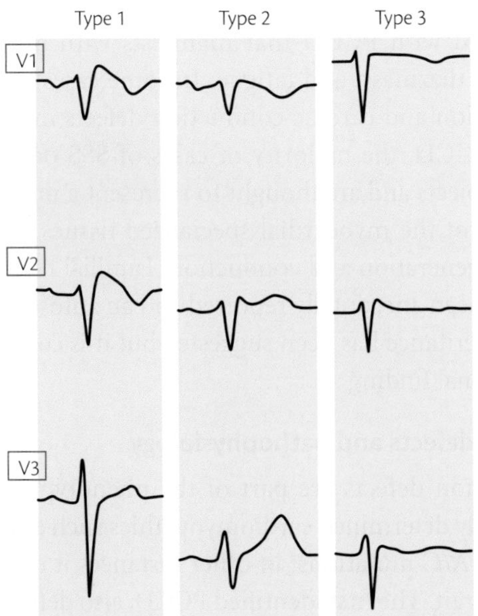

Figure 9.7 Electrocardiogram in Brugada syndrome. Only type 1 is considered diagnostic for the disease.

The age of onset of clinical manifestations (syncope or cardiac arrest) is the third to fourth decade of life. BrS is seldom diagnosed in children and teenagers but, when present, the manifestations appear similar to those of adults [61]. Cardiac events typically occur during sleep or at rest [62] and are facilitated by fever, drugs (especially tricyclic antidepressant and class I antiarrhythmic agents), and lavish meals especially in the evening. As a general rule it should be considered that electrocardiographic manifestations of BrS can be modulated by autonomic interventions: vagal activation worsen while adrenergic stimuli usually improves the manifestations [63].

The incidence of cardiac events (cardiac arrest, ICD shocks) is in the range of 8–12% from birth to 45 years of age [64, 65]. Recent pooled data from 1500 patients with a mean observation time after diagnosis of 32 months, report a 10% event rate including syncope, SCD, and ICD shocks [66]. The disease is inherited as an autosomal dominant trait but there is a striking male to female ratio of 8:1 of clinical manifestations.

Genetic basis and pathophysiology

Four Brugada syndrome genes have been identified (see ➲Table 9.7).

The first gene for BrS is *SCN5A*, which was identified in 1998. *SCN5A* accounts for approximately 20–25% of cases [65]. Several mutations with a spectrum of biophysical consequences have been identified by *in vitro* expression but the common final pathway is that of a loss of sodium current [47]. Interestingly, *SCN5A* mutations in BrS patients are also associated with a high incidence of atrioventricular block and conduction defect [67]. Some authors have suggested that the most prevalent phenotype of *SCN5A* mutations is not BrS (which is characterized by a high degree of incomplete penetrance) but a progressive conduction defect [67]. The presence of a conduction block in a BrS patient is significantly associated with an increased probability of SCN5A mutation [68].

More recently, three additional genes have been reported. *GPD1-L* (glycerol-3-phosphate dehydrogenase

1-like) has been mapped in a previously identified BrS locus (3p22–25) and mutations have been identified in a few patients [69]. *GPD1-L* is a dimer involved in the glycerol phosphate shuttle transfers electrons from cytosolic NADH to the mitochondrial transport chain. Although the molecular mechanism is not yet fully understood, *in vitro* expression studies demonstrated that *GPD1-L* mutations may cause BrS by reducing Na^+ channel trafficking to the plasma membrane. *GPD1-L* mutations in BrS are likely to be infrequent.

More recently, cardiac calcium channel mutations have been associated with BrS. Antzelevitch and colleagues have reported mutations in both alpha (*CACNA1C*) and beta (*CACNB2B*) subunits in families with a typical BrS ECG and short repolarization (QTc interval <360ms) [70]. In both cases the electrophysiological effect is loss of ICa current during the plateau phase of the cardiac action potential.

Although these latter findings have significantly improved the knowledge on the genetic determinants of BrS, the incidence of the novel variants is unknown and therefore it is too early to include such genes in the routine testing for BrS.

Risk stratification and therapy

Since no effective pharmacological treatment has so far proven effective for BrS patients, the implant of an ICD is currently the only available option. Therefore, risk stratification is an important issue for BrS management.

Available evidence attributes the highest risk to patients with a spontaneously abnormal ECG and a history of syncope (➲Fig. 9.8). Patients showing a spontaneous ECG pattern (i.e. no drug challenge required for diagnosis) are at intermediate risk for cardiac events [65]. In a recent

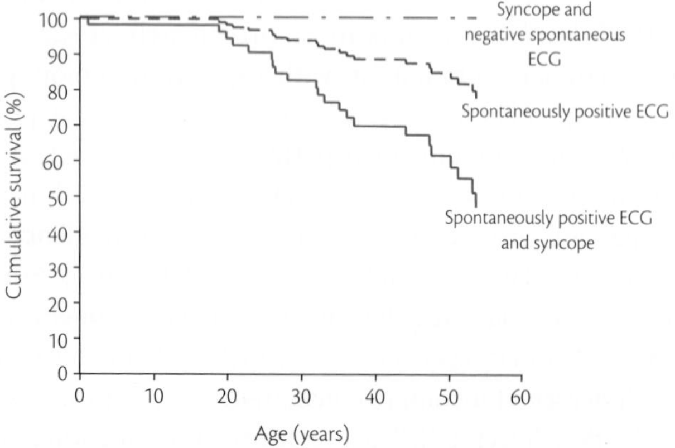

Figure 9.8 Natural history of Brugada syndrome according to clinical presentation. Patients with history of syncope and spontaneous type 1 ECG pattern have the worse outcome. Reproduced from Priori SG, Napolitano C, Gasparini M, *et al.* Natural history of Brugada syndrome. Insights for risk stratification and management. *Circulation* 2002; **105**: 1342–7.

analysis on paediatric patients (mean age 8 ± 4 years), fever represented the most important precipitating factor for arrhythmic events, and, as in the adult population, the risk of arrhythmic events was higher in previously symptomatic patients and in those displaying a spontaneous type I ECG [71]. Familial SCD and the presence of a *SCN5A* mutation are not significant predictors of events, although in clinical practice, multiple SCD events in a family may become an argument for ICD implant for primary prophylaxis. The usefulness of programmed electrical stimulation (PES) in the identification of high-risk patients is less certain and it has been challenged by a recent meta-analysis [67]. ICD therapy is obviously indicated in all cases for secondary prevention of ventricular fibrillation.

Progressive cardiac conduction defect and sick sinus syndrome

Clinical presentation

Progressive cardiac conduction defect (PCCD) is a common disorder, especially in the older population. It is characterized by progressive slowing of cardiac conduction through the His–Purkinje system with right or left bundle branch block and widening of the QRS complex. In many cases the conduction block generates long pauses and severe bradycardia that may cause dizziness and syncope. PCCD is a major cause of pacemaker implantation. In the majority of cases, it develops as a sporadic trait and is a degenerative disease that occurs with ageing. However, in other instances familial cases have been reported, suggesting a genetic predisposition.

Sick sinus syndrome (SSS) is a disorder phenotypically associated with PCCD that manifests with bradycardia, syncope, dizziness, and fatigue. In some cases, sinus node dysfunction and cardiac conduction defects may co-exist. As for PCCD, the majority of cases of SSS occur among older subjects and are thought to represent a manifestation of aging of the myocardial specialized tissues controlling rhythm generation and conduction. Familial recurrence of SSS has been anecdotally reported and an autosomal dominant inheritance has been suggested but it is considered an 'exceptional finding'.

Genetic defects and pathophysiology

Conduction defects are part of the phenotype of several genetically determined cardiomyopathies such as DCM due to lamin A/C mutations; in other instances it occurs as an isolated trait. The first identified PCCD, also defined as progressive familial heart block (PFHB) locus, maps to 19q13.3 with an autosomal dominant inheritance. The linkage with this region was subsequently confirmed by other authors but the corresponding gene is yet to be identified. Conversely, by candidate gene screening, after the exclusion of the 19q linkage, another group [72] described two families with conduction defects and identified in both a mutation in the *SCN5A* gene. *In vitro* assays suggest a loss of function effect [47]. It is now clear that the SCN5A-dependent conduction defect is tightly linked with SCN5A-Brugada syndrome and distinction between these phenotypes is often difficult.

In 2003, Benson and colleagues [73] described five affected children from three kindreds with congenital SSS, and identified compound heterozygosity for six distinct mutations in the *SCN5A* gene. Two of these mutations had previously been associated with BrS. Heterozygous carriers were asymptomatic, but showed subclinical cardiac conduction disease, particularly first-degree heart block, suggesting a close relationship between PCCD and SSS. These data support an autosomal recessive pattern. As for PCCD, *in vitro* expression of the SSS mutation is consistent with a loss of function. Few other mutations have been reported subsequently. Another cause of sinus node dysfunction and bradycardia has been identified in the cardiac pacemaker channel HCN4 [74].

Atrial fibrillation

Clinical presentation

Atrial fibrillation is the most common sustained arrhythmia encountered in clinical practice (➲Chapter 29). It is a frequent cause of embolic stroke, accounting for approximately 75,000 strokes per year in the USA and leading to more hospital admissions than any other arrhythmia. In the majority of cases, atrial fibrillation is an acquired disorder but, in 3–31% of cases no underlying cardiovascular disease can be detected and in some of them a familial inheritance is evident [75].

Genetic bases and pathophysiology

After the initial identification of a *KCNQ1* gain-of-function mutation in a family with atrial fibrillation [76], there is growing evidence to show that several cardiac ion channels may indeed create a vulnerable substrate for the development of this arrhythmia (➲Table 9.7; Fig. 9.4). Mutations have been found both in familial atrial fibrillation and in cases of lone atrial fibrillation (isolated AF in a structurally normal heart). (Also see ➲Chapter 29.)

Ion channel genes associated with AF are: *KCNQ1, KCNE1, KCNE2, KCNH2, SCN5A, KCNJ2, CACNA1C,* and *KCNA5* [75]. All genes so far identified in AF, with the exception of *KCNA5*, are gain of function and have the final effect of reducing action potential duration and refractory period. Of note, the same genes are expressed both in atria and ventricles and they also cause other cardiac channelopathies with a similar gain of function effect. The reasons that some mutations cause atrial fibrillation while others cause short QT syndrome or BrS are yet to be elucidated.

Short QT syndrome

Clinical presentation

Short QT syndrome (SQTS) is an arrhythmogenic disorder in the structurally normal heart which is primarily characterized by short repolarization [77] (➲Chapter 30). Syncope and sudden death, usually occurring at rest, are the common manifestation of this disorder. Unlike other inherited arrhythmogenic disorders, it appears that syncope is less frequent and that the majority of symptomatic patients manifest cardiac arrest as the initial manifestation [78]. Atrial fibrillation is also frequently reported in SQTS. Although SQTS has been recognized as a clinical entity for several years, only very few patients have been described, thus leaving open several issues concerning diagnosis, natural history, and treatment.

The reported SQTS cases present a QTc <320–325ms). A peculiar ST–T-wave pattern is also observed [78, 79]: narrow and peaked T wave (hyperkalaemic-like) with no detectable ST segment, or relatively normal ST with an accelerated descending T-wave limb (➲Fig. 9.9).

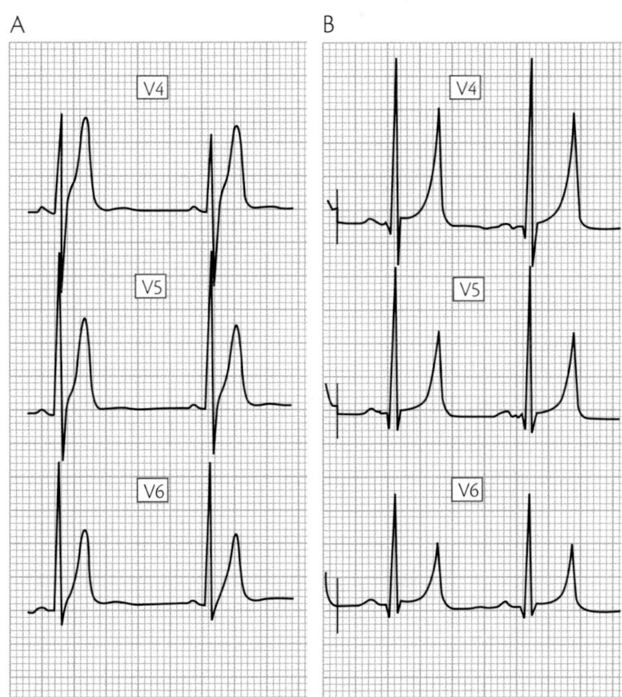

Figure 9.9 Morphology of repolarization in the short QT syndrome. (A) Tall and peaked but regular T wave with absent ST segment in a patient with KCNH2 (*SQTS1*) mutation. (B) Normal ST segment and ascending limb followed but very sharp descending limb associated with KCNJ2 (*SQTS3*).

The definition of a QT cut off for diagnosis remains blurred. Based on the published data it appears that diagnosis can be reasonably suspected when the QTc interval is <340–350ms. QT adaptation to heart rate changes is impaired. Therefore, the QT nterval should be always measured at heart rates around 60 beats per minute (bpm) to avoid bias introduced by the Bazett QT correction formula.

Genetic bases and pathophysiology

Gain-of-function mutations in three cardiac ion channels may cause SQTS: *KCNH2* [80], *KCNQ1* [81], and *KCNJ2* [79]. These genes also cause LQTS with an opposite mechanism. Thus, SQTS and LQTS are allelic diseases. More recently, mutations of the cardiac L-type calcium channel gene alpha and beta subunit (*CACNA1C* and *CACNB2*, respectively), responsible for shortening of the QT interval in families characterized by SCD, atrial fibrillation, and a Brugada type 1 ECG pattern, have been reported. Furthermore, given the pathogenetic similarities, it is important to consider that Brugada syndrome, atrial fibrillation, and SQTS may have substantial overlap in some patients.

Catecholaminergic polymorphic ventricular tachycardia

Catecholaminergic polymorphic ventricular tachycardia or CPVT was described by Reid in 1975 and Coumel and colleagues in 1978 [82, 83] as a disorder characterized by VT syncope and sudden death occurring in familial or in sporadic cases in the absence of structural abnormalities of the heart and in the absence of any ECG abnormality (➲Chapter 30). In the last few years, CPVT has attracted the interest of several investigators and the disease is now a well-characterized clinical entity.

Clinical presentation

The resting ECG of CPVT patients is unremarkable with the exception of a sinus bradycardia reported in some patients; atrioventricular conduction is within normal limits and no significant abnormalities are identified on the signal averaged ECG.

Physical activity or acute emotions are the specific triggers for arrhythmias. During graded exercise stress testing, ventricular and supraventricular arrhythmias appear at 90–100bpm and the complexity of the arrhythmia progressively worsens with increase in workload. If the patients continue to exercise, the duration of runs of VT progressively increases and the arrhythmia may become sustained. A 180° alternating QRS axis on a beat-to-beat basis—so-called bi-directional VT—is often the distinguishing presentation of CPVT-related arrhythmia, although polymorphic VT is observed in some cases. Supraventricular tachycardia and atrial fibrillation are also a relatively common finding (➲Fig. 9.10).

Epidemiological data from a CPVT registry, which includes one of the largest cohorts worldwide, show that up to 60% of patients experience at least one cardiac event up to age 40 and that 30% of such events are cardiac arrest or CPVT-related sudden deaths. Therefore, CPVT is a malignant disorder requiring careful management and follow up. Beta-blockers (nadolol 1–2mg/kg/day metoprolol 2–4mg/kg/day) are often effective in controlling exercise-induced arrhythmias. The reproducibility of arrhythmias makes exercise stress very useful for titration of dosage during follow-up. However, in a subset of patients, acute emotion represents a more powerful trigger than exercise. Thus, Holter monitoring is also an important tool for diagnosis and management. Beta blocker therapy (at maximally tolerated dosages) does not afford complete protection in 29% of patients [84]. Since no additional drugs with ascertained effectiveness are available, the implant of an ICD

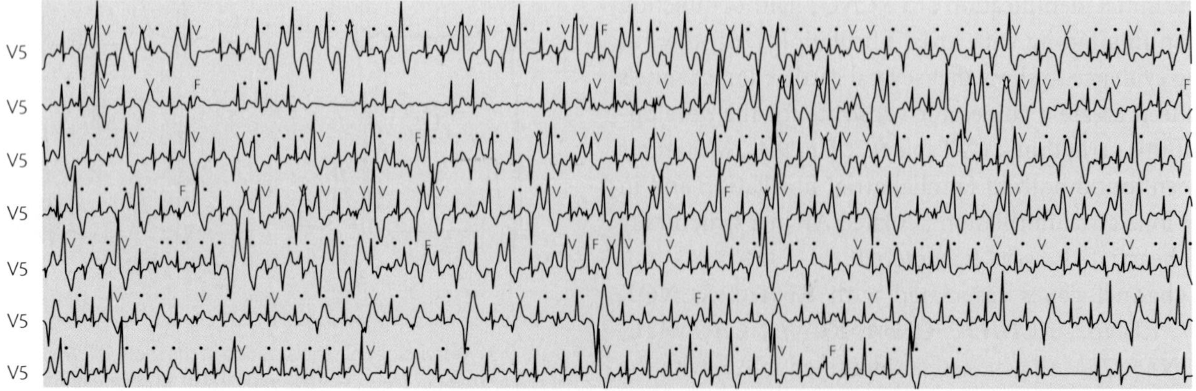

Figure 9.10 Arrhythmias in catecholaminergic polymorphic ventricular tachycardia. The ECG shows the typical bidirectional VT and the presence of supraventricular arrhythmias during exercise.

is indicated [1]. Anecdotal reports suggest that calcium-channel blocker might provide additional protection but these data require confirmation in larger cohorts.

Genetic bases and pathophysiology

Genes and loci associated with the CPVT phenotype are reported in ➲Table 9.7. Based on genetic linkage mapping, molecular screening identified *RyR2* mutations in four CPVT families thus demonstrating that *RyR2* is the gene for autosomal dominant CPVT [85]. The involvement of the cardiac ryanodine receptor as a cause of CPVT was subsequently confirmed by several other investigators during the last 6 years (see Gene Connection for the Heart database at http://www.fsm.it/cardmoc). A recent analysis of published *RyR2* mutations showed that they tend to cluster in 25 exons encoding four discrete domains of the RYR2 protein: domain I (amino acid (AA) 77–466), II (AA 2246–2534), III (AA 3778–4201), and IV (AA 4497–4959), (DI–DIV). These clusters are made by amino acid sequences highly conserved through species and among RyR isoforms [86] and are thought to be functionally important.

Soon after the identification of the *RyR2* mutations in the autosomal dominant CPVT, Lahat and colleagues. mapped the recessive variant on chromosome 1p23–21 and subsequently identified one mutation in the cardiac calsequestrin gene (*CASQ2*) [87]. CASQ2 is a Ca^{2+}-binding protein localized in the terminal cisternae of the sarcoplasmic reticulum. Calsequestrin together with triadin and junctin belongs to the RyR2 macromolecular complex that regulates sarcoplasmic Ca^{2+} release in cardiac myocytes. Available data show that *CASQ2* mutations are present in approximately 2% of CPVT patients.

The biophysical consequences of *RyR2* and *CASQ2* mutations have been widely studied *in vitro* and in transgenic models [88–91]. Overall, despite the existence of multiple functional abnormalities, the final common consequence of *RyR2* mutations is that of increased diastolic Ca^{2+} release from the sarcoplasmic reticulum (SR) that facilitates the development of after-depolarizations and triggered arrhythmias (➲Fig. 9.11).

Additional loci and CPVT phenocopies

In 2007, a novel recessive CPVT locus was mapped to the short arm of chromosome 7 (7p14–22) with a maximal multipoint LOD score of 3.17 at marker D7S493 [92]. The study was carried out in a single pedigree with a high level of consanguinity, three sudden death cases at a young age (10 years) and one living subject presenting with stress-induced ventricular arrhythmias. Interestingly the available clinical evidence suggested that this CPVT variant may be associated with QT interval prolongation (480–490ms). Unfortunately, candidate gene screening in the 25cM critical region did not lead to the identification of pathogenetic mutations in several analyzed genes (*SP4*, *FKBP9*, *FKBP14*, *PDE1C*, and *TBX20*).

Ankyrin 2 (*ANK2*) has been implicated in different arrhythmogenic syndromes starting in 2003 when it was associated with the LQT4 variant of LQTS. More recently, a group of patients characterized by a broad range of 'adrenergically mediated arrhythmias' was screened on *ANK2*,

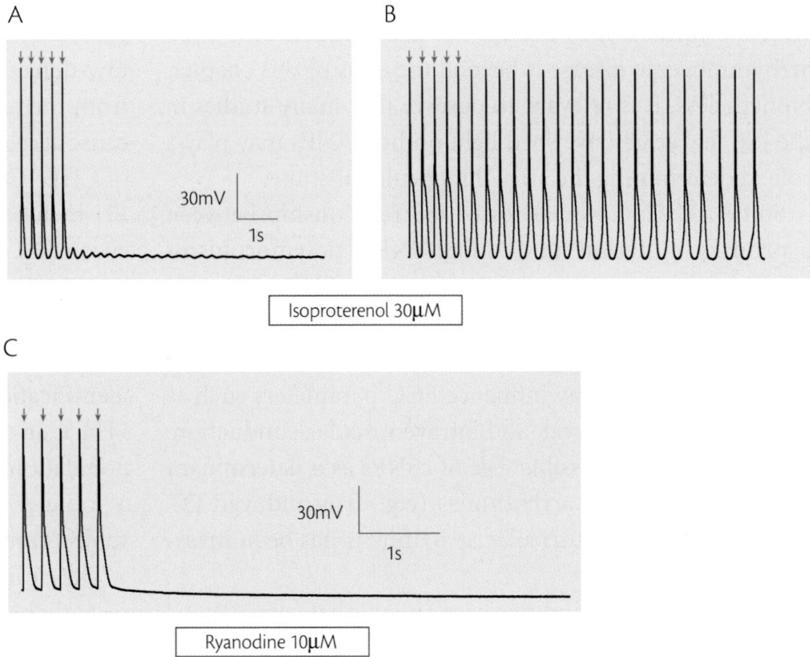

Figure 9.11 Delayed afterdepolarizations (DADs) (A) and triggered activity (TA) (B) elicited by adrenergic stimulation in a myocyte isolated from transgenic mouse harbouring the *RyR2* R4496C mutation found in several CPVT patients. RyR2 block with ryanodine inhibits both DAD and TA. Arrows indicate paced beats.

including CPVT patients without mutations on *RyR2* or *CASQ2*. In one patient presenting with adrenergically mediated bi-directional VT [93], an ankyrin mutation was identified. Functional assay showed that the mutation caused a loss of expression and miss-localization of the Na/K ATPase, Na/Ca exchanger and InsP3 (inositol 3-phosphate) receptor.

The yield of *ANK2* screening in patients with CPVT is still undefined (but it is likely that it is very low); therefore, the clinical applicability of such testing is unknown.

A possible phenotypic overlap may also exist between CPVT and Andersen–Tawil syndrome (ATS or LQT7) (➲Table 9.7). The latter is an inherited arrhythmogenic disorder caused by mutations in the *KCNJ2* gene (also defined as LQT7). ATS is characterized by cardiac (QT prolongation, prominent U waves) and extracardiac (facial dysmorphisms, periodic paralysis), phenotypes. However, some ATS patients may present atypical manifestations including mild or absent QT interval prolongation [94], and bidirectional VT with evidence of an adrenergic trigger. We have recently reported evidence that *KCNJ2* mutations associated with a CPVT phenotype induce delayed after-depolarization and triggered activity when expressed *in vitro* [95].

It is presently unclear whether patients with clinical manifestations that overlap with CPVT also have a severe prognosis, such as the one observed in *RyR2* and *CASQ2* genotyped CPVT patients, or whether they have the more benign outcome typical of ATS patients.

Genetic modifiers in inherited arrhythmogenic disorders

A detailed analysis of the all the genomic variants associated with the variability of the clinical presentation of a given arrhythmogenic disease is beyond the aims of this chapter. Nonetheless, it is relevant to observe that many studies in the last few years have shed light on how SNPs may play a role in determining the arrhythmogenic substrate.

Some studies have addressed the relationship between a primary mutation and coding SNPs (polymorphisms occurring in the coding region of a gene, cSNPs) [96, 97]. Other investigators have shown that common cSNPs, or SNPs occurring in the promoter region or causing alternative gene splicing, may influence ECG parameters such as QT interval, PR interval, and intraventricular conduction. Furthermore, the possible role of cSNPs as a determinant of risk for acquired arrhythmias (e.g. drug-induced QT prolongation and ventricular arrhythmias has been investigated [98, 99].

Other interesting findings have shown that even genetic variants in non-ion channel genes, such as the *NOS1AP* [100] can significantly affect cardiac repolarization in the general population.

Overall, these studies clearly highlight the concept that the individual-specific genetic background has an influence on the electrophysiological substrate. The practical consequence, in terms of the amount of SNP-attributable risk, is still to be precisely defined, but once the full picture is available it will become possible to individualize the risk stratification based on a panel of critical genetic variants.

Polygenic diseases: genetic aspects of coronary artery disease

Introduction

Coronary heart disease (CHD) has a complex, multifactorial aetiology (➲Chapters 16 and 17). That CHD has a familial basis is well recognized by clinicians and borne out by the scientific evidence. However, genetic predisposition is usually polygenic and only rarely does CHD result from a single gene mutation; rather, as shown in ➲Fig. 9.12, disease develops as a consequence of two-way interactions between the 'initial' conditions—coded in the genotype—and exposures to environmental agents over time.

A monogenic cause of CHD: familial hypercholesterolaemia

The clinical characteristics and genetic determinants of familial hypercholesterolaemia (FH) have been reviewed recently [101]. FH is an autosomal co-dominant disorder caused by mutations that directly affect the rate at which low-density lipoprotein-cholesterol (LDL-C) is cleared from the blood. The subsequent elevated levels of LDL-C cause accelerated atherosclerosis resulting in increased risk of CHD. Clinical CHD typically manifests in heterozygous FH men between the ages of 30–50 years, and in heterozygous FH women between 50–70 years [102]. FH is present in 5–10% of individuals who develop CHD under the age of 55 years. Since lipid-lowering drug therapy with statins substantially reduces coronary morbidity and mortality, identification of affected individuals is crucially important. FH has an estimated prevalence of roughly 1:500 in outbred populations (but may be higher in countries where there is a 'founder' effect), but currently the vast majority of these subjects are undiagnosed.

The clear benefits of statin treatment in FH patients have recently been documented [103] by estimating the standardized mortality ratio (SMR), compared to the population

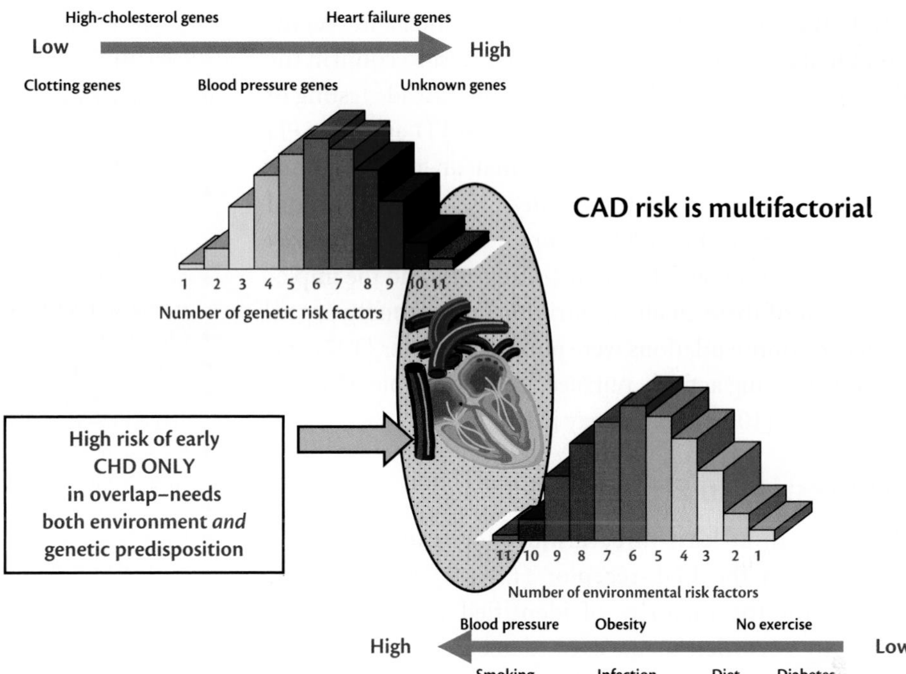

Figure 9.12 Model for gene–environment interaction in the development of premature coronary heart disease.

in England and Wales, in 3382 FH patients (1650 men) in the UK FH register. SMRs were calculated before and from 1 January 1992 as representing the pre- and post-statin era. Overall, CHD mortality fell significantly by 37% from a 3.4 to a 2.1-fold excess, and, as shown in ➲Fig. 9.13, primary prevention resulted in a 48% reduction in CHD mortality from a two-fold excess to none, with a smaller reduction of nearly 25% in patients with established disease. In the post-statin period, all-cause mortality was essentially the same as in the general population, mainly due to a 37% lower risk of fatal cancer (probably due to the lower smoking rate in FH patients). The results emphasize the major importance of early identification of FH and the clear benefit of treatment with statins.

Recently, evidence-based guidelines for the identification and management of FH have been published in the UK [104, 105]. These show that it is cost-effective to treat FH patients with high-potency statins to achieve at least a

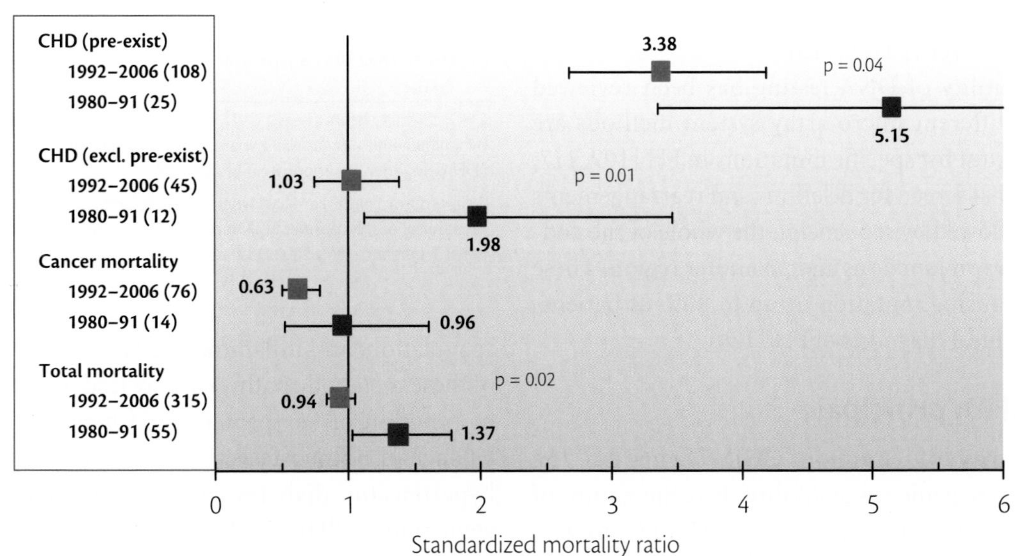

Figure 9.13 Standardized mortality ratio (SMR) in 3382 FH patients (1650 men) in the UK FH register followed prospectively between 1980–2006 for 46,580 person-years. In patients aged 20–79 years there were 370 deaths, including 190 from CHD and 90 from cancer. SMRs were calculated before and from 1 January 1992 as representing the pre- and post-statin era. Data from Neil A, Cooper J, Betteridge J, *et al.* Reductions in all-cause, cancer, and coronary mortality in statin-treated patients with heterozygous familial hypercholesterolaemia: a prospective registry study. *Eur Heart J* 2008; **29**: 2625–33.S

50% reduction in LDL-C levels from baseline, and recommend that all patients be offered a DNA test to confirm the diagnosis and to help with the systematic cascade testing of relatives. This is because LDL-C levels in FH and non-FH subjects overlap considerably, so that an unambiguous diagnosis cannot be made in many cases, based on lipid measures [106] will be 100% accurate using DNA. The key recommendations are shown in ➲Table 9.8, and the implementation of these in all countries is now strongly urged. Similar recommendations were published earlier [107] and are already being actively pursued in, for example, Holland [108], Spain [109], and Norway [110].

DNA testing in FH patients

Mutations in at least three distinct loci cause FH [97]. Mutations in the LDL-receptor (LDL-R) gene (*LDLR*) account for the majority of identified mutations, and >1000 are recorded in the UCL database [111]. FH can also be caused by mutations in the gene for apolipoprotein B (*APOB*), the major protein component of the LDL-cholesterol particle, and the ligand for the removal of the LDL by the LDL-R. One particular mutation (commonly called R3500Q) in the gene occurs commonly in European subjects [101], although the frequency is lower in Southern Europe. The most recently identified gene for FH codes for protein convertase subtilisin/kexin type 9 (*PCSK9*), which is an enzyme involved in degrading the LDL-R protein in the lysosome of the cell and preventing it recycling [101]. One common gain-of-function mutation (p.D374Y) in the *PCSK9* gene has been identified [112–114] which occurs in the UK in ~2% of FH patients and carriers of this mutation tend to have very severe CHD [115].

The clinical utility of DNA testing has been reviewed [116]. Several different micro-array system methods are now available to test for specific mutations in FH [109, 117, 118] and those that screen for deletions and rearrangements [119]. This is followed by sequencing the whole of the coding exons and intron junctions and promoter region. These detect the FH-causing mutation in up to 80% of patients with a strong clinical diagnosis of FH [120].

Table 9.8 Key priorities for diagnosis and management of familial hypercholesterolaemia

Recommendations
◆ Consider the diagnosis of FH in adults with total cholesterol >7.5mmol/L or LDL-C >5.2mmol/L
◆ Do not use risk algorithms, such as Framingham/SCORE/HEART SCORE (or other risk estimation algorithms) to estimate the CHD risk in FH patients
◆ Because of their high CHD risk, patients with FH should be aggressively treated with statins at a young age, in an experienced lipid clinic setting
◆ Lifestyle advice should be offered and supported
◆ Active testing to identify affected relatives should be performed
◆ For optimal diagnostic and management results, both phenotypic and genotypic diagnosis should be used
◆ Because of their high CHD risk, patients with FCH should be treated with lipid-lowering therapy and life-style advice
◆ Testing to identify affected relatives is likely to be beneficial
◆ Once secondary causes have been ruled out, patients with a virtual absence of HDL must undergo careful physical examination for the clinical hallmarks of certain HDL deficiency syndromes
◆ Family studies should be performed
◆ Prevention of CVD in these patients should have the aim of the avoidance and treatment of additional risk factors
◆ For individuals with a family history of early CHD (defined as evidence of CVD or CHD in a first-degree male relative <55 years and female relative >65 years) their Framingham estimated risk should be multiplied by 1.5, and other modifiable risk factors including blood lipids, blood pressure, and body mass index treated accordingly.
◆ Risk factor screening should be carried out in the first-degree relatives of any patient developing coronary disease before 55 years in men and 65 years in women
Family history
◆ The importance of a family history of CHD has been established, and is included as a risk factor in some risk prediction algorithms (e.g. PROCAM)
DNA-based tests for risk prediction
◆ In subjects in the general population, DNA-based tests do not, at the present time, add significantly to diagnostic utility or patient management, over-and-above the use of measures of established CHD risk factors

CHD, coronary heart disease; CVD, cardiovascular disease; FCH, familial combined hyperlipidaemia; FH, familial hypercholesterolaemia; HDL, high-density lipoprotein LDH-C, low-density lipoprotein-cholesterol.

Adapted from NICE. Familial Hypercholesterolaemia, 2008. NICE: London; Wierzbicki, AS, Humphries SE, Minhas, R. Familial hypercholesterolaemia: summary of NICE guidance. *BMJ* 2008; **337**: a1095.

Polygenic CHD: principals

The vast majority of common CHD occurs on the background of polygenic susceptibility. It is the nature of polygenic disease that any single variant will only provide a small or modest contribution to risk. At the molecular level, atherosclerosis is a time-dependent, multistep process involving the interaction of many different key biochemical pathways. These include lipoprotein metabolism, coagulation, and inflammation [121]. Gene variants in any of these metabolic pathways may lead to altered production or function of key proteins and hence upset the delicate balance of homeostasis. Intermediate phenotypes such as hypertension, diabetes, and obesity, themselves all polygenic traits, will interact to modulate risk.

Furthermore, environmental risks such as smoking, sedentary lifestyle, and high-calorie diets are not simply additive with genetic risk. Gene–environment interactions are critically important, and, as shown in ➲Fig. 9.13, it is believed that only in subjects with a genetic predisposition, who also adopt a high-risk environment, will premature CHD develop. Thus, a polymorphism may have a modest (or negligible) effect on CHD risk in individuals who have a low environmental risk, but a major effect in a particular environment. Gene–gene interactions are also likely to be important, although relatively little is understood about these in the context of CHD.

Genetic determinants of CHD phenotypes

For many measurable traits (phenotypes) there is good evidence for a relatively strongly genetic contribution to the determination of levels, which is usually estimated by 'heritability'. For apoproteins and lipid traits, heritability varies between 40–60% [122], meaning that genetic factors are determining around half of the between-individual differences and environmental factors the remainder. For C-reactive protein heritability is rather lower [123] and for fibrinogen it is lower still [124], reflecting the fact that they are acute phase proteins and levels are greatly influenced by factors such as infection, malignancy, or auto-immune disease.

Plasma Lp(a) is a factor where levels are remarkably stable within an individual over time, and heritability is reported to be >90% [125]. Variability at the locus coding for the Apo(a) gene itself accounts for almost all of the variance of plasma Lp(a) in normal populations [126]. The relevance of this is that a recent meta-analysis reported that levels of Lp(a) in the top tertile was associated with a 1.6-fold greater risk of CHD [26], an effect which is of similar magnitude as smoking, and thus the Apo(a) gene would appear to be a major genetic factor for CHD. In support of this, a common SNP in the *LPA* gene has a replicated effect on CHD risk (hazard ratio = 1.62) [128]. Measuring Lp(a) is a relevant 'genetic' factor to add in clinical management of high risk patients.

The candidate gene approach and meta-analyses to identify risk alleles

There has been an exponential increase in the number of CHD candidate gene studies over the past 15 years. However, the lack of consistent reproducibility of candidate gene alleles and their association with CHD risk and intermediate traits, has introduced an element of doubt into the field of genetic epidemiology. Much of this stems from the approach of studying one SNP, studies which lack power and may be subject to population stratification [129]. The tagging SNP approach and haplotype analysis aimed at covering maximum variability of the gene has gone some way to overcome this. However, the absence of robustness of these associations is concerning, and meta-analyses provide the possibility of more robust odds ratios, although once again there is often evidence of between-study heterogeneity, and always the problem of publication bias. Over the past year there have been several new meta-analyses published and these are presented in ➲Table 9.9.

Table 9.9 List of gene variants with published meta-analysis on CAD risk and >2000 cases. Where several analyses have been conducted on the same gene variant only the latest reference is shown

Gene (SNP)	Risk genotype	No. of studies (no. of cases)	Size of the effect (95%CI)	Reference
AT1R (1166A>C)	C+	27 (10,180)	1.13 (1.04–1.23)	Ntzani *et al.* 2007 [137]
MMP3 (5A/6A)	5A+	8 (3655)	1.26 (1.11–1.4)	Abilleira *et al.* 2006 [138]
MMP9 (1562C>T)	T+	5 (4817)	1.11 (1.0–1.3)	Abilleira *et al.* 2006 [138]
APOE ε2, ε3, ε4	ε2+ ε4+	121 (37,850)	0.8 (0.70–0.90) 1.06 (0.99–1.13)	Bennet *et al.* 2007 [130]
LTA (10G>A)	A+	7 (10,996)	1.09 (1.02–1.16)	Clarke *et al.* 2006 [139]
LPL (N291S)	S+	21 (1203)	1.48 (1.09–2.00)	Hu *et al.* 2006 [140]
AGT (T174M) (M235T)	M+ T+	43 (13478)	1.07 (0.93–1.22) 1.11 (1.03–1.19)	Xu *et al.* 2007 [141]
F5 (1691G>A) *F7* (10976G>A) *F2* (20210G>A) *PAI1* (4G/5G) *GP1A* (807C>T) *GP1BA* (5T>C) *GP3A* (1565 C>T)	A+ A+ A+ 5G+ T+ C+ T+	60 (15,704) 24 (7444) 40 (11,625) 37 (11,763) 15 (6414) 14 (6652) 43 (16,984)	1.17 (1.08–1.28) 0.97 (0.91–1.04) 1.31 (1.12–1.52) 1.06 (1.02–1.10) 1.02 (0.97–1.08) 1.05 (0.96–1.13) 1.03 (0.98–1.07)	Ye *et al.* 2006 [142]
IL6 (174G>C)	C+	8 (4799)	1.12 (0.97-1.29)	Sie *et al.* 2006 [143]
F13 (V34L)	L+	12 (8743)	0.79 (0.66–0.93)	Shafey *et al.* 2007 [144]

One of the best studied genes codes for a plasma apolipoprotein called ApoE. The common *APOE* allele is called E3, and there are two variants, E4 and E2 (allele frequency in Europeans roughly 0.15 and 0.07 respectively). The sequence changes in the gene alter two charged amino acids, which affect plasma clearance of the protein and the cholesterol-rich lipoproteins carrying them. The consequence of this is that, as shown in ➲Fig. 9.14, there is a strong and consistent impact on plasma lipid levels (E2 lowering and E4 raising), which translates into a modest E2 lower and E4 higher impact on CHD risk [130].

Gene–environment interaction and risk prediction

Since it is now well-accepted that atherosclerosis and CHD develop as a result of the interplay between the environment adopted by an individual and their genetic predisposition, any genetic test to predict CHD must include such interactions in the algorithm. From a mechanistic viewpoint such interaction suggests that, at the molecular level, the effect or by-product of the environmental insult modifies the molecular function of the product of the gene under observation.

As an example, smoking is associated with a twofold lifetime risk of CHD, but anecdotally some smokers develop disease early while some appear relatively protected. Several studies have reported that subjects carrying the *APOEε4* allele who were smokers had a particularly high CHD risk compared to *APOEε4* never smokers, while risk was also low in *APOEε4* ex-smokers, supporting the benefit of smoking cessation [131]. Although not all published studies have confirmed this interaction, a re-analysis [132] of a large case–control study showed that compared with *APOEε3/ε3* never smokers, *APOEε4* smokers had significantly higher risk of CHD, with a greater than additive interaction between genotype and smoking on risk. Re-analysis of the Framingham Offspring data also supports this greater than additive interaction between *APOEε4* and smoking on risk [133], and in the large prospective Whitehall-II study in the UK, where smoking prevalence is low (<15%) the ε4 was not associated with a significant effect on CHD risk [134]. These data suggest that carrying the *APOEε4* allele does not significantly increase risk of cardiovascular disease *unless* the subject is a smoker. If this interaction can be confirmed, clearly, any *APOE* genetic test result estimating risk in the absence of information about smoking will be misleading.

Use of meta-analyses risk estimates in combination

As shown in ➲Table 9.9, as well as *APOE*, several variants appear to be associated with statistically robust, although rather modest, effects on risk. Although these data seem encouraging, based as they are on the combined results from many studies, they need to be interpreted with some caution. Several analyses have looked separately at the results from the smaller studies and found a much larger risk estimate than in the larger studies [135]. This suggests the problem of publication bias, in which small studies where a statistically significant result were obtained have been published, while in those where the result was not significant, the data have not appeared in the literature. The result of this would be that these meta-analyses estimates

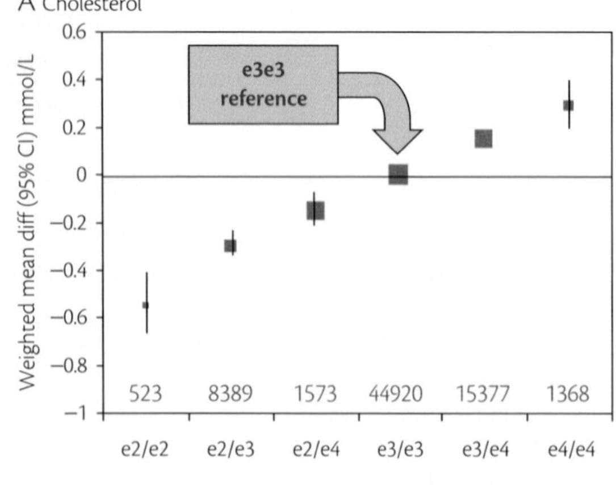

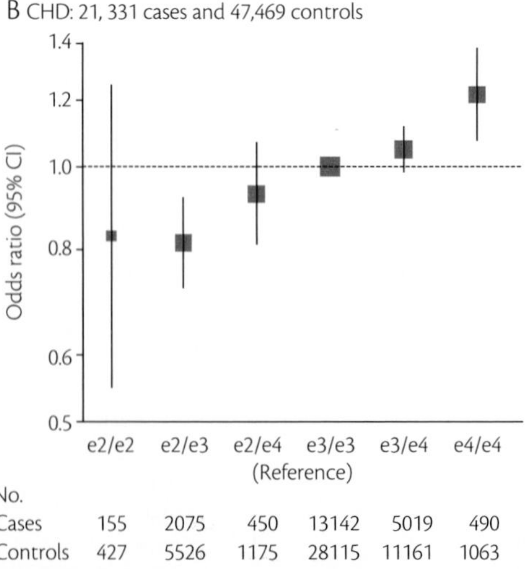

Figure 9.14 Meta analysis of ApoE genotype effect on plasma lipids and CHD risk. For each study the non-smokers with the genotype ε3ε3 are set as the reference group. Adapted with permission from Bennet AM, Di Angelantonio E, Zheng Y, *et al.* Association of apolipoprotein E genotypes with lipid levels and coronary risk. *JAMA* 2007; **298**: 1300–11.

in ➲Table 9.7 may actually be inflated, with the true value being smaller if data were available from all studies.

Although the meta-analysis risk estimates for each gene variant are modest they may still have some clinical value if they can be combined in developing a genetic risk profile. Thus, to develop useful genetic tests will require the *simultaneous study of many genes* and to understand how their effects add up and interact. The threshold of a single genotype significantly improving CHD risk prediction is unlikely to be crossed partly because the effect associated with any single SNP is relatively modest (in the range 1.12–1.73, see ➲Table 9.9), and partly because the number of individuals carrying the risk genotype is low. However, when several independent, confirmed CHD risk SNPs are combined, a greater proportion of subjects will be carrying *any* risk genotype, and many individuals will, by chance, carry more than one risk allele (since they are inherited independently) and effects on risk are likely to be additive. As an example, the potential utility of 11 SNPs in ten candidate genes (*APOB, eNOS, APOE, ACE, PAI1, MTHFR, GPIIb-IIIa, PON1, LPL*, and *CETP*), has been examined, using the predicted risk estimates from meta-analysis. As shown in ➲Fig. 9.15a [136], based on published allele frequencies, ~18% of the general population would be expected to carry less than three risk alleles, approximately 50% would carry three or four risk alleles, 8.3% would have six, and 3% have seven or more risk alleles. Compared to those with three or four risk-associated genotypes, those with six, and seven or more alleles had a significantly higher risk mean odds ratio (OR) of CHD, 1.70 (95% confidence intervals (CI) 1.14–2.25) and 4.51 (95% CI 2.89–7.04), respectively, while those with two and fewer would be significantly protected. Taking into account age and the risk alleles carried, the mean 10-year probability for developing CHD for a 55-year-old man was calculated to be 16% (8.6–24.8%) with nearly 1 in 5 having >20% risk. These results are encouraging and suggest that in combination, common SNPs of modest impact on risk will have clinical utility, but whether this particular group of 11 SNPs will do so, and whether or not this will be over and above the effect of CRFs requires further experimental evidence.

Novel CHD genes

Recently, three genome-wide association studies (GWASs), one led by the Icelandic company DeCode, one led by a Canadian-based group, and one from the UK Wellcome Trust Case–Control Consortium, all identified a single region on chromosome 9p21.3 associated with CHD or myocardial infarction risk [145–147]. Because of the size of the studies (in combination >10,000 cases and 20,000 controls), the level of statistical certainty is large (e.g. $p < 10^{-20}$), and the replication in a number of independent studies means that this finding cannot be in any doubt. Interestingly SNPs in this region have also been associated with type 2 diabetes [147] and with risk of abdominal aortic aneurysm [148, 149], suggesting a unifying underlying mechanism for these three diseases. Because of the high frequency of the 'risk' allele (~50% of subjects are carriers, with ~23% having two copies), and because of the size of the effect, this SNP has been estimated to have a population attributable risk (PAF) of 20% for myocardial infarction [145]. This implies that if the effect of this allele could be removed from the population the incidence of myocardial infarction would be reduced by 20%. The identification of

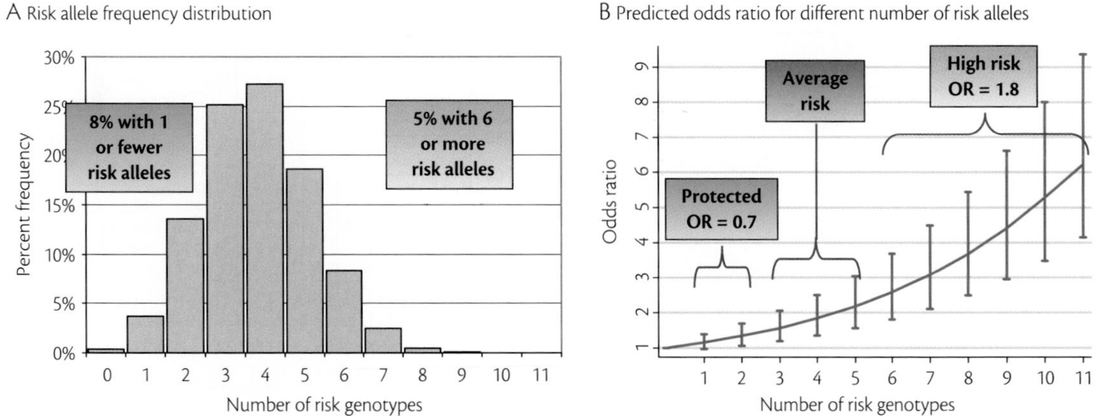

Figure 9.15 Risk alleles in coronary heart disease. (A) Frequency distribution of number of individuals with different number of 'risk' allele SNPs, based on their reported frequency in Caucasian populations (assuming independent segregation). (B) Frequency-adjusted odds ratios of coronary heart disease for different number of risk alleles carried, with 95% confidence intervals. Calculated from reported risk estimates and assuming additive effects on risk. Data from Drenos F, Whittaker JC, Humphries SE. The use of meta-analysis risk estimates for candidate genes in combination to predict coronary heart disease risk. *Ann Hum Genet* 2007; **71**: 611–19.

this locus as being associated with CHD risk thus identifies a novel and potentially highly important new causal pathway for investigation and the development of therapeutic approaches that will complement current risk-reducing modalities.

So far, the mechanism by which DNA variants in this region of chromosome 9 increase risk of CHD is unclear. Furthermore, none of the genotypes used in the three studies were associated with any of the usual CHD risk factors, such as increased blood pressure or lipid levels. The chromosomal 9 region has relatively few identified genes, but the most likely candidates are a cluster consisting of *CDKN2A-ARF-CDKN2B*, which are all involved in cell-cycle control. This locus is often deleted in malignant tumours, but also plays a role in cell proliferation, senescence, and apoptosis, all features implicated in atherogenesis. Although no sequence changes that directly alter the *function* of these proteins were identified by any of the recent publications, it is possible that DNA changes which alter the *level of expression* of these key proteins may be important. This would then influence the ability of cells in the vascular system to continue to proliferate (for example, endothelial, smooth muscle cells, or monocyte-macrophage-foam cells in the lesion), and as a consequence lead to senescence and apoptosis, causing plaque progression or rupture.

So will a SNP like this have clinical utility? Case–control studies are efficient for gene discovery, yet they provide limited information on predictive utility, which require prospective studies. The possibility that addition of chromosome 9p21.3 genotype improves risk stratification for future CHD events, over and above that of CRFs, such as cholesterol, triglycerides, blood pressure, age, and smoking, has been examined and the data is shown in ➲Fig. 9.16. The lead SNP from the GWASs (rs10757274 A>G (frequency G = 0.48) was genotyped in the Northwick Park Heart Study-II of 2742 middle-aged men, with 270 CHD events over 15 years prospective study [150]. As shown in ➲Fig. 9.16A, the association with CHD was confirmed, (hazard ratio in GG compared to AA men of 1.60 (1.12–2.28)) and a population attributable frequency of 26.2%. The potential utility of this SNP in identifying men at high CHD risk was examined. As shown in ➲Fig. 9.16B, of the NPHS-II men, 157 had a baseline CRF score of ≥23, giving them a predicted 10-year CHD risk of >20%, which would qualify them for statin use under Joint British Society (JBS) guidelines. Of this group 33 men went on to have a CHD event (event rate of 21%). However, there were 55 men with a score of <23 using CRFs, but whose score was >23 when rs10757274 genotype was added, and in this group 12 CHD events were observed in follow-up (event rate = 22%). The mean cholesterol levels at baseline in these two groups were 6.73mmol/L and 6.78mmol/L, respectively, and based on the expected benefit of reducing their individual cholesterol levels to the JBS2 target of 4.0mmol/L, a similar number of CHD events would be prevented in both groups (9.1 vs. 8.5 prevented/100 treated, p>0.5).

Thus, while no single SNP by itself will have clinical utility, several other common potentially useful SNPs in novel genes have been identified by the GWASs [151] and if confirmed, their use, in combination with the chromosome 9 SNP and the meta-analysis SNPs would be very likely to have clinical utility.

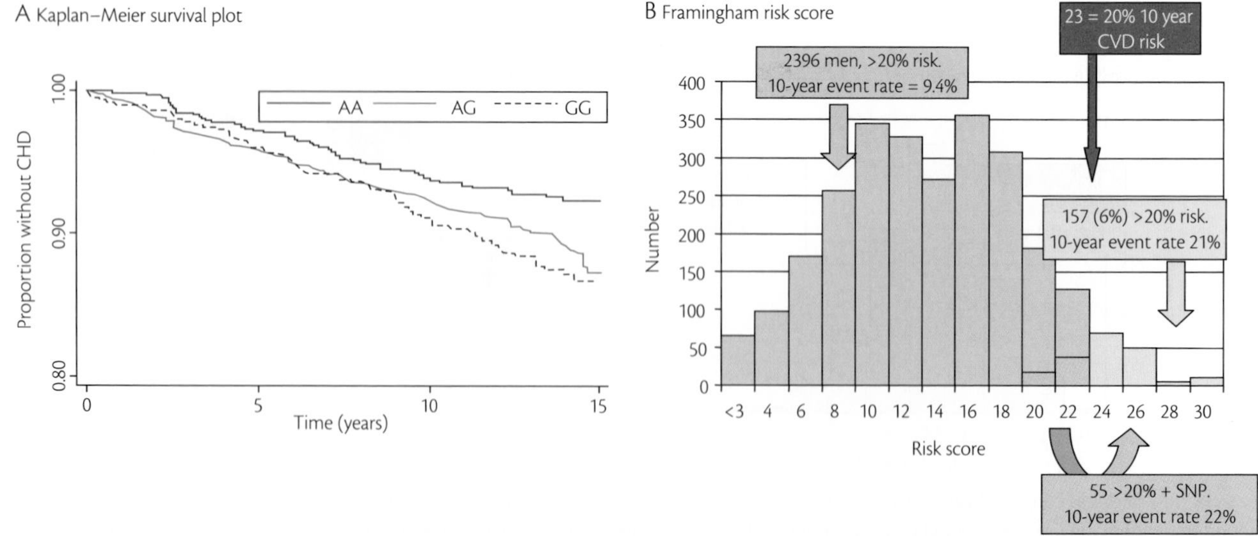

Figure 9.16 Clinical utility of chromosome 9 SNP. (A) Kaplan–Meier survival plot for the chromosome 9 SNP rs10757274 A>G in NPHS-II men. (B) Framingham risk score. Data from Talmud PJ, Cooper JA, Palmen J, *et al.* Chromosome 9p21.3 coronary heart disease locus genotype and prospective risk of CHD in healthy middle-aged men. *Clin Chem* 2008; **54**: 467–74.

Hypertension (➲Chapter 13)

Polygenic hypertension: principles

The numerous factors that determine arterial blood pressure (BP)—cardiac output, systemic vascular resistance, circulating volume [152, 153], and renal control of fluid and electrolyte balance [152, 154, 155]—are regulated by various neurocrine, endocrine, paracrine, and autocrine factors [152] (➲Chapter 13). This complex disease mechanism has led to approaches aiming at identification of genes responsible for BP regulation, susceptibility to end-organ damage, and susceptibility to dietary and environmental factors [156, 157].

Twin studies suggest that >30% of BP variability may be attributable to genetic variation. However, in rare patients with Mendelian forms of arterial hypertension, a single abnormality can increase BP significantly [158, 159] but in the majority of individuals, multiple genes contribute to hypertension in a polygenic fashion, such that any single variant probably has only a minimal effect on BP.

Genetic determinants of hypertension phenotypes

Mendelian forms

The characterization of genetic variations within families affected by monogenic forms of hypertension, has led to the identification of specific mutations that lead to hyper- (or hypo-) tension [158, 160–163]. Many of these mutations have been found to directly influence renal electrolyte and fluid balance, but these rare abnormalities account for <1% of all cases of hypertension.

Candidate-gene linkage studies

The investigation of biological pathways of interest has focused mainly upon polymorphic markers in the renin–angiotensin system, adrenergic pathways, metabolism-related, and vascular-related genes. Candidate gene selection in such approaches has been based largely upon the understanding of the molecular action of the encoded protein. However, a lack of consistent results and a failure to provide a strong, consistent association with hypertension [164, 165] suggests that there are limitations to this approach, such as reliance on pre-existing mechanistic hypotheses, insufficient power, and inappropriate choice of candidate genes.

Candidate-gene association studies

Most candidate-gene association studies for the investigation of hypertension have involved case–control comparisons of 300–500 hypertensive subjects with an equal number of control subjects. Candidate genes are again selected on the basis of a mechanistic understanding of a particular protein in BP regulation. These studies have generally yielded weak levels of statistical significance that are difficult to replicate in alternate populations [166]. Genome-wide association approaches may allow the identification of novel genes and mechanisms involved in hypertension and BP regulation.

Genome-scanning linkage studies

Thousands of microsatellite markers and microchips, containing up to 500,000 SNPs have recently become commercially available, and have been used to identify >100 BP-related quantitative trait loci (QTL). Indeed, some human chromosomes, specifically 1, 2, 3, 17, and 18, contain multiple QTLs for BP-related phenotypes (often with overlapping confidence intervals), thus illustrating that any single genomic region has only a modest effect upon susceptibility to hypertension.

The Wellcome Trust Case Control Consortium (WTCCC) recently performed a genomewide association study on approximately 2000 individuals and 3000 controls. No significant associations were found with hypertensive phenotypes, although this may be due to the fact that many of the controls were also hypertensive. The small effect of each genomic region on susceptibility to hypertension means that such a study is probably under-powered to identify any yet to be discovered genes [147].

Personal perspective

So how soon is this new genetic information likely to become useful in cardiology? It is clear that DNA tests should be used now to help identify relatives in monogenic situations like HCM and FH. It is also highly likely that in 2–3 years' time we will have a panel of DNA tests that will have clinical utility in risk stratification over and above the classical risk factors currently used in risk algorithms. Thus, in the future, a patient could be booked for a clinic visit in 2–3 weeks and sent a mouthwash tube to be returned to the laboratory immediately, so that genetic information would be available for discussion. This sample could easily be tested for 20–100 different mutations and, with falling costs and high throughput, costs in the range of €25–€60 are achievable.

In parallel, resequencing technologies (e.g. DNA resequencing chip) will allow screening of hundreds of different SNPs that have been progressively recognized to confer risk for the onset of complex traits. Knowing in advance of being at high or low risk of developing conditions like coronary artery disease or hypertension may remarkably improve not only the outcomes (by allowing the establishment of preventive treatments/lifestyle changes) but also the use of resources allocated to healthcare.

Another ambitious goal made conceivable by the detailed understanding of the molecular pathways to cardiovascular diseases is the development of more effective therapies to directly target those pathways. Two approaches are being followed: (1) to use/develop chemicals (drugs) that can specifically and selectively target the consequence of a genetic variant (as an example, this is the case in gene-specific therapy of inherited arrhythmogenic diseases) and (2) to directly modify the abnormal genetic substrate (gene therapy). This latter objective can be achieved either by correcting the mutation by substitution with healthy copies of the gene or by modulating the expression of other genes (up-regulation or down-regulation) to specifically counteract the effects of the genetic mutations. Many investigators are actively working in this field and predictably the goal of genetic therapy will be achieved in the future, allowing us to overcome the limitations of traditional drug therapies.

Further reading

Ashrafian H, Watkins H. Reviews of translational medicine and genomics in cardiovascular disease: new disease taxonomy and therapeutic implications cardiomyopathies: therapeutics based on molecular phenotype. *J Am Coll Cardiol* 2007; **49**: 1251–64.

Graham I, Atar D, Borch-Johnsen K, *et al.* European guidelines on cardiovascular disease prevention in clinical practice: full text. Fourth Joint Task Force of the European Society of Cardiology and other societies on cardiovascular disease prevention in clinical practice (constituted by representatives of nine societies and by invited experts). *Eur J Cardiovasc Prev Rehabil* 2007; **14**(Suppl.2): S1–S113.

Hamsten A, Eriksson P. Identifying the susceptibility genes for coronary artery disease: from hyperbole through doubt to cautious optimism. *J Intern Med* 2008; **263**: 538–52.

Liu N, Ruan Y, Priori SG. Catecholaminergic polymorphic ventricular tachycardia. *Prog Cardiovasc Dis* 2008; **51**: 23–30.

Marian AJ. Genetic determinants of cardiac hypertrophy. *Curr Opin Cardiol* 2008; **23**: 199–205.

Priori SG, Napolitano C. Role of genetic analyses in cardiology: part I: Mendelian diseases: cardiac channelopathies. *Circulation* 2006; **113**: 1130–5.

Priori SG, Napolitano C, Cerrone M. Experimental therapy of genetic arrhythmias: disease-specific pharmacology. *Handb Exp Pharmacol* 2006; **171**: 267–86.

Roberts R. Genetics of premature myocardial infarction. *Curr Atheroscler Rep* 2008; **10**: 186–93.

Watkins H, Ashrafian H, McKenna WJ. The genetics of hypertrophic cardiomyopathy: Teare redux. *Heart* 2008; **94**: 1264–8.

Zipes DP, Camm AJ, Borggrefe M, *et al.* ACC/AHA/ESC 2006 guidelines for management of patients with ventricular arrhythmias and the prevention of sudden cardiac death–executive summary: A report of the American College of Cardiology/American Heart Association Task Force and the European Society of Cardiology Committee for Practice Guidelines (Writing Committee to Develop Guidelines for Management of Patients with Ventricular Arrhythmias and the Prevention of Sudden Cardiac Death) Developed in collaboration with the European Heart Rhythm Association and the Heart Rhythm Society. *Eur Heart J* 2006; **27**: 2099–140.

Online resources

- The guidelines for diagnosis and management of HCM are outlined in a joint consensus document of the American College of Cardiology and European Society of Cardiology: http://www.escardio.org/guidelines-surveys/esc-guidelines/Pages/ventricular-arrhythmias-and-prevention-sudden-cardiac-death.aspx
- Gene Connection for the Heart database: http://www.fsm.it/cardmoc/

➲ For full references and multimedia materials please visit the online version of the book (http://esctextbook.oxfordonline.com).

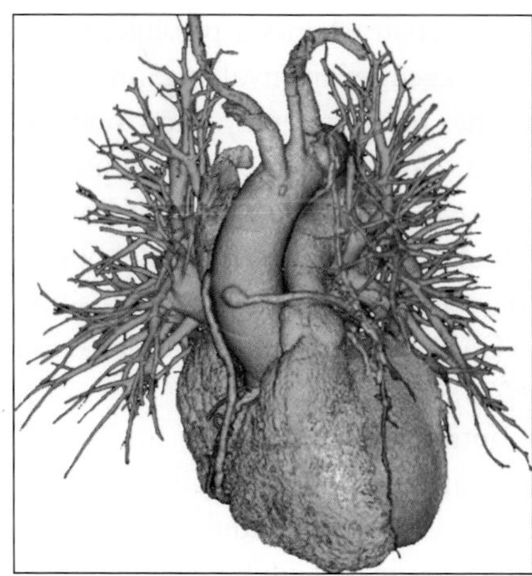

CHAPTER 10

Congenital Heart Disease in Children and Adults

John E. Deanfield, Robert Yates, Folkert J. Meijboom, and Barbara J.M. Mulder

Contents

Summary

This chapter describes the enormous progress that has been made in the diagnosis, investigation, and management of patients with congenital cardiac malformations, who are seen with increasing frequency in adult cardiac practice. Management of these often challenging patients has become an important 'subspecialty' of adult cardiology, but appropriate systems for care delivery have not yet been developed in most countries. Nomenclature, aetiology, and incidence are considered as well as common presenting features. Investigative strategies are then reviewed as these have evolved rapidly in the last two decades, with a shift from invasive to non-invasive protocols involving echocardiography, magnetic resonance imaging and computed tomography. Modern treatment approaches have also developed considerably and now involve both surgery and interventional catheterization, often as part of a 'hybrid' lifetime strategy for management of the congenital malformation.

In the second half of the chapter, the most important congenital cardiac malformations are described individually, with discussion on morphology, pathophysiology, early presentation, investigation, natural history, management, and late outcome. The information on these individual lesions should be invaluable to the practising cardiologist involved in the care of patients with congenital heart disease (CHD), and, in particular, inform on when referral to a specialist centre is appropriate. It is essential for those involved in the care of adults with CHD to understand the childhood phase of the various malformations. Similarly, paediatric cardiologists and allied professionals can only improve management if they are familiar with long-term results of the various treatment strategies undertaken in childhood.

Introduction

A congenital cardiac malformation complicates approximately 8 per 1000 live births [1]. In the last 60 years, advances in diagnosis as well as in medical and surgical treatment in the neonatal period have transformed the outlook for even the most complex of malformations. As a result, it is now expected that >90% of all children with CHD will reach adulthood. Consequently, there will soon be more adults than children with congenital cardiac malformations [2]. Accurate long-term survival data are still lacking, but in the UK it has been estimated that there is an annual increase of 1600 adults with congenital cardiac malformations and 800 patients annually require specialist follow-up [3]. In Europe, the number of adults with CHD is presently estimated to be around 1.2 million. These numbers will continue to rise due to ongoing advances in surgery and cardiac care [4]. Adult physicians are thus increasingly likely to encounter patients with a range of these complex conditions who will need ongoing surveillance and often further medical or surgical intervention [5]. With improving outcome prospects, the goals of treatment have shifted from merely improving survival during childhood towards 'lifetime management' aimed at optimizing life expectancy and quality of life.

There have been a number of important trends in the management of congenital cardiac malformations. Invasive diagnostic techniques, based on cardiac catheterization, have often been replaced by the rapidly improving non-invasive modalities. In the 1980s, cross-sectional echocardiography revolutionized investigation, with enormous outcome benefits. Further evolution is continuing in the current era, with cross-sectional imaging by cardiac magnetic resonance (CMR) imaging and CT, permitting three-dimensional reconstruction and accurate definition of both anatomy and physiology. In parallel with a shift away from cardiac catheterization for diagnosis, there has been a spectacular increase in the range and number of therapeutic catheterization procedures [6]. Paediatric cardiology has led the way in this area and progress shows no signs of slowing. For example, the recent successful implantation of stent-mounted tissue valves in the pulmonary position should lead to new opportunities for treatment of other cardiac valves in children and adults with both congenital and acquired pathology [7]. Often, a treatment plan that integrates surgery and interventional catheterization is required and this 'hybrid' approach can be tailored towards lifetime management [8]. Reduced morbidity and mortality has also been achieved with treatment directed towards primary neonatal repair whenever possible, rather than the performance of staged repair involving initial palliative procedures. This has been driven by improvements in neonatal management, as well as in cardiopulmonary bypass, together with increasing confidence instilled by the successful introduction of new corrective neonatal operations, such as the arterial switch operation for transposition of the great arteries (TGA) (see ➲Complete transposition of the great arteries, p.358).

New investment in optimization of care of adults with CHD is important as many will have conditions which are unfamiliar even to the experienced adult cardiologist. Appropriate transition to designated adult CHD units will ensure continuity of the excellent care provided during childhood [9].

There is a compelling need for education and increased awareness of CHD among adult cardiologists. This chapter aims to cover the field of congenital cardiac malformations by describing the aetiology, presentation, principles of investigation, modern treatment approaches and outcomes, as well as providing more detailed accounts of the common individual malformations which are seen in adult practice. Cardiologists treating adults with CHD must also have an understanding of the presentation and management issues during childhood, and key issues during both paediatric and adult care are described. We have excluded conditions such as bicuspid aortic valve and mitral valve prolapse, which are covered in other chapters. Furthermore, more information on conditions that may complicate congenital cardiac malformations, such as heart failure and arrhythmia, can be found elsewhere in the text.

Nomenclature

The almost infinite number of complex cardiac congenital malformations requires the development of a consistent, easily comprehensible approach to nomenclature that is based on observation rather than on assumptions about development. This has largely been achieved with the sequential segmental approach. Initially proposed by van Praagh and co-workers [10] in the 1960s and subsequently revised by Anderson and colleagues [11], this approach analyses malformed hearts on the basis of their atrial, ventricular and great arterial components as well as the connections between these segments and the abnormalities associated with them. It avoids the use of embryological terms such as 'endocardial cushion defect' to describe congenital cardiac malformations. The very rapid progress of molecular genetics and its application to cardiac development has dispelled many previously accepted embryological assumptions, often rendering such descriptive terms both incorrect and confusing.

The starting point for this system of nomenclature is the identification of atrial arrangement or situs. This is most accurately determined by examination of the atrial appendages as these are the most distinct morphological features of the atrium. Since all hearts have two atrial appendages, there are four possible combinations: usual (situs solitus), mirror image (situs inversus), and isomerism of the right or left appendages. Anatomical inspection of the appendages is rarely possible and therefore inference about atrial arrangement is usually based on echocardiographic findings. The most important of these is examination of the great vessels at the level of the diaphragm in the abdomen (➲ Fig. 10.1).

The atria connect to the ventricles via the atrioventricular valves. The 'type' of connection describes what flows into what, being either concordant (right atrium to right

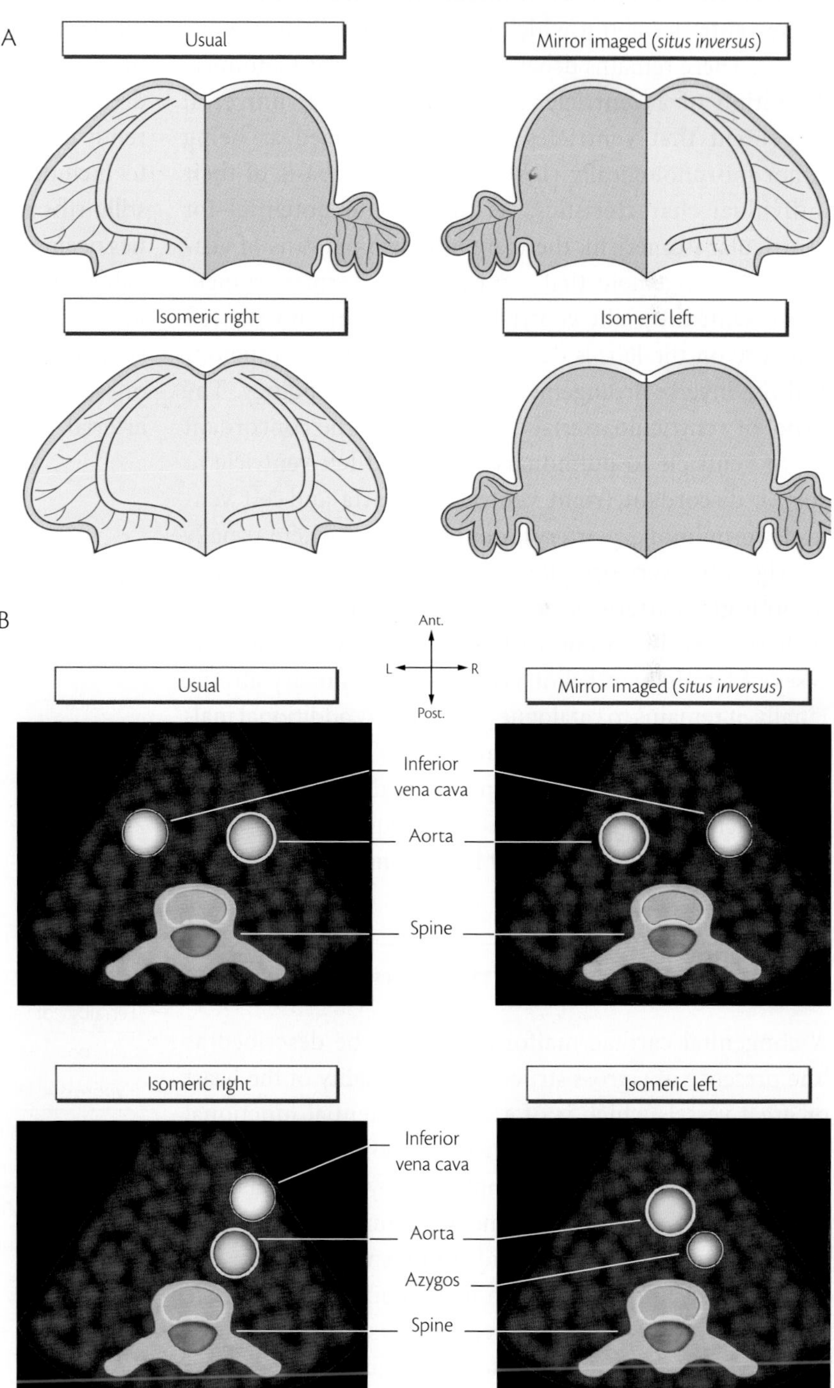

Figure 10.1 (A) Possible atrial arrangements. (B) Schematic representation of echocardiographic images of the great vessels at the level of the diaphragm associated with usual atrial arrangement, mirror-image arrangement as well as right and left atrial isomerism.

ventricle and left atrium to left ventricle), discordant (right atrium to left ventricle and left atrium to right ventricle) or ambiguous when the atrial appendages are isomeric. The 'mode' of atrioventricular connection addresses the structural make-up of the connecting segments and includes a description about the nature of the valve or valves. Valves may be perforate, imperforate, or absent. However, the atrioventricular junction could be guarded by a single atrioventricular valve as in absent right or left connection; equally, there may be two separate valves, or a common atrioventricular valve as in double-inlet left ventricle. It is the ventricles about which there is generally least consensus. There remains debate about the precise anatomical definition of a ventricle, but there is almost universal agreement that ventricles can be recognized as being either morphologically right or left on the basis of their individual characteristics. As there is no potential for ventricular isomerism, there are only two patterns of ventricular arrangement that can exist. The normal arrangement, with the right ventricle on the right and the left ventricle on the left, is described as 'right hand' topology and the inverse arrangement as 'left hand' topology. The 'type' of ventriculoarterial connection can be concordant (right ventricle to pulmonary artery and left ventricle to aorta), discordant (right ventricle to aorta and left ventricle to pulmonary artery), double outlet (where usually the right, but very occasionally the left ventricle gives rise to both great arteries), or solitary outlet from the heart, such as occurs in common arterial trunk (CAT) or in many cases of tetralogy of Fallot (ToF) with pulmonary atresia. Finally, it remains to catalogue precisely any additional malformations both within the heart itself as well as within the great vessels. Description of any isolated malformation is incomplete without first undertaking sequential segmental analysis of the heart in which it is contained [11].

Epidemiology and incidence

A congenital cardiac malformation can be described as 'the presence of a gross structural abnormality of the heart or great vessels which is of actual or potential functional significance [12]. According to this definition, between 0.5–0.8% of live births are complicated by a cardiovascular malformation, but this fails to include a number of common abnormalities such as bicuspid non-stenotic aortic valve or mitral valve prolapse, which may significantly influence the true incidence. Furthermore, some less common abnormalities may remain undetected throughout life, such as a persistent left-sided superior caval vein draining to the coronary sinus. Ascertainment of the incidence of CHD may provide vital information on the aetiology of congenital cardiac malformations and can also be used in the planning of appropriate healthcare resources (➲Table 10.1).

The 'incidence' of congenital cardiac malformations is the number of children born with congenital cardiac malformations relative to the total number of births over a given period, usually a calendar year. Defining the denominator in such a rate has a significant influence as there are major differences between rates based on live births compared with those based on conception. For a measure of the true 'incidence' of congenital cardiac malformations, it would be necessary to have accurate information about all children with congenital cardiac malformations, which is currently underestimated. In addition, calculations would need to include congenital cardiac malformations detected in stillbirths and aborted fetuses, in which cardiac abnormalities occur up to 10 times more frequently than in live-born babies. Accurate data on the incidence of individual congenital cardiac malformations are also lacking. In many series, small ventral septal defects (VSDs) were either not detected or were actively excluded and few studies include patent arterial ducts in preterm infants. Furthermore, selection

Table 10.1 Median and interquartile range (%) of congenital cardiac lesions in newborn infants obtained from 34 studies involving 26,904 patients

	Median	25th–75th
Ventricular septal defect	32.0	27.1–42.3
Patent arterial duct	6.8	5.2–11.0
Atrial septal defect	7.5	6.2–10.8
Atrioventricular septal defect	3.8	2.8–5.2
Pulmonary stenosis	7.0	5.2–8.8
Aortic stenosis	3.9	2.7–5.8
Coarctation of the aorta	4.8	3.6–5.7
Transposition of the great arteries	4.4	3.5–5.4
Tetralogy of Fallot	5.2	3.8–7.6
Common arterial trunk	1.4	0.6–1.7
Hypoplastic left heart syndrome	2.8	1.6–3.4
Hypoplastic right heart syndrome	2.2	1.5–3.2
Double-inlet ventricle	1.5	0.8–1.9
Double-outlet right ventricle	1.8	1.0–3.0
Total anomalous pulmonary venous connection	1.0	0.6–1.9
Others	10.0	7.6–14.6

Adapted with permission from Hoffmann J. Incidence, mortality and natural history. In Anderson RH, Baker EJ, Macartney F, *et al.* (eds.). *Paediatic Cardiology*, 2002. London: Churchill Livingstone, pp. 111–39.

of both the study population and the source of data will affect reported incidence. The most often quoted incidence of CHD of 8 per 1000 live births, is based on the studies presented in ➲Table 10.1. This is a compilation of a large number of series over many years. Over the last 5–7 years, a substantial drop in the incidence of CHD diagnosed at birth has been noticed in several countries, with the reported incidence dropping as low as 4 per 1000 live births. Together with the reduction in the number of pregnancies in many Western countries, this has led to a significant reduction of the number of babies born with a congenital cardiac malformation. The cause of this phenomenon remains speculative and it is also unclear whether it will be transient or will persist. If it persists, it will have large effects on the organization of healthcare for children with CHD.

Congenital cardiac malformations often occur in association with extracardiac abnormalities, which may be multiple. The additional burden of such abnormalities may have an unexpectedly high adverse effect on mortality compared with that of the individual abnormalities in isolation. About 30% of children with both cardiac and extracardiac malformations have an identifiable syndrome. Further details of such syndromes can be obtained from a genetic database, such as the London Medical Database for Dysmorphology (see ➲Online resources, p.364). Of all congenital heart defects, approximately 60% are diagnosed in the first year of life. During childhood, 30% of heart defects are detected and 10% of all lesions are only diagnosed in adult life.

A large proportion of CHD (>40%), diagnosed at birth or in the neonatal period disappears completely ('cured' spontaneously) during follow-up. This includes most small VSDs [13]. In the era before effective cardiac intervention, up to 85% of the patients died before adulthood, usually in the first year of life. This made CHD the most important cause of infant mortality. Nowadays, >90% of all patients with CHD survive beyond adolescence. The life expectancy of patients with simple congenital cardiac malformations is now similar or only slightly less than that of the general population, but the survival of patients with more complex malformations remains substantially shorter [14]. Despite the increased survival, late complications occur frequently and morbidity in these patients appears to be substantial. Nearly all patients have residual cardiac problems of varying degrees of severity and most require lifelong cardiological follow-up [15]. Many patients need one or more reoperations or percutaneous interventions. Arrhythmias occur especially frequently with increasing age. Few data on long-term outcome are currently available for many of the complex malformations. The notion that CHD is increasing in adulthood is still rather new to many cardiologists. This emphasizes the need for education and organization of an effective clinical service.

Aetiology and prevention

The rapid progress of cytogenetics offers the prospect of improved understanding of the role of inherited and environmental factors and their interaction on the development of congenital cardiac malformations [16–18]. Environmental factors are rare, but important and potentially preventable. Congenital rubella is now less common in European populations and maternal diabetes, alcohol ingestion and possibly drugs are the most important external adverse influences on cardiac development [19, 20]. Major chromosomal abnormalities can cause syndromes, of which congenital cardiac malformations play an important part. Trisomy 21 (Down syndrome) and Turner syndrome (XO) are classic examples. Other important syndromes include Edwards syndrome (trisomy 18) and Patau syndrome (trisomy 13).

In several other syndromes associated with congenital cardiac malformations, such as Williams syndrome, a specific microdeletion has been established, blurring the distinction with major chromosomal abnormalities. The most important example is the 22q11 deletion, which emerged as the basis of DiGeorge syndrome in the late 1980s. A European study of almost 600 patients with 22q11 deletion showed that 75% had a ventricular outflow abnormality, emphasizing the importance for understanding of cardiac development as well as patient management. Alagille syndrome is another example where a causative gene defect, loss of *jagged-1* on chromosome 20p12, is associated with peripheral pulmonary stenosis [21].

The traditional view that the majority of congenital cardiac malformations are not genetic but multifactorial in origin is probably incorrect, and it appears likely that an increasing number of specific point mutations associated with cardiac malformations will be described (such as those already identified for Noonan syndrome, Marfan syndrome, Ellis–van Creveld syndrome, and Holt–Oram syndrome and abnormalities of laterality [22, 23].

Understanding the aetiology and genetic basis for congenital cardiac malformations has practical implications for counselling. Risks of sibling recurrence have been difficult to define, often due to selection bias and limited phenotyping and only recently has the opportunity arisen to assess recurrence risk in offspring of mothers and fathers who themselves have congenital cardiac malformations.

In a large UK multicentre study, the overall recurrence risk was 4.5%, which is significantly higher than the risk for siblings. Interestingly, the rate was higher in the offspring of affected females [24]. Preventative strategies for congenital cardiac malformations are still in their infancy. Physicians should always emphasize the importance of avoiding alcohol and drugs from the time pregnancy is planned. The increased availability of screening for major chromosomal abnormalities, which has become faster and more accurate, should permit the identification of affected fetuses at risk of congenital cardiac malformations. Fetal echocardiography, which can now reliably identify major malformations from as early as 14 weeks' gestation, does not provide true 'prevention opportunities' but does enable informed decisions to be made regarding continuation of pregnancy in the presence of cardiac malformations.

Fetal circulation

Much of the information about the fetal circulation has been derived from animal studies. Increasingly sophisticated, non-invasive, ultrasound assessment of the human fetal circulation has both confirmed these early data from animal studies and at the same time has demonstrated important differences in the human fetus [25, 26].

Fetal circulatory pathways

In contrast to the normal postnatal circulation, in the fetus, the systemic and pulmonary circulations exist in parallel (➲Fig. 10.2). Prenatal survival is possible with even major structural cardiovascular malformations, provided that either the right or left ventricle is able to pump blood derived from the great veins into the fetal aorta. In the fetus, oxygenated blood returns from the placenta via the umbilical vein to the inferior caval vein, either through the portal system or through the venous duct. A proportion of this relatively high oxygenated inferior caval vein blood entering the right atrium is directed across the oval foramen to the left atrium. The output of the left ventricle is directed predominantly towards the developing brain. Superior caval vein blood enters the right atrium and the majority will enter the right ventricle

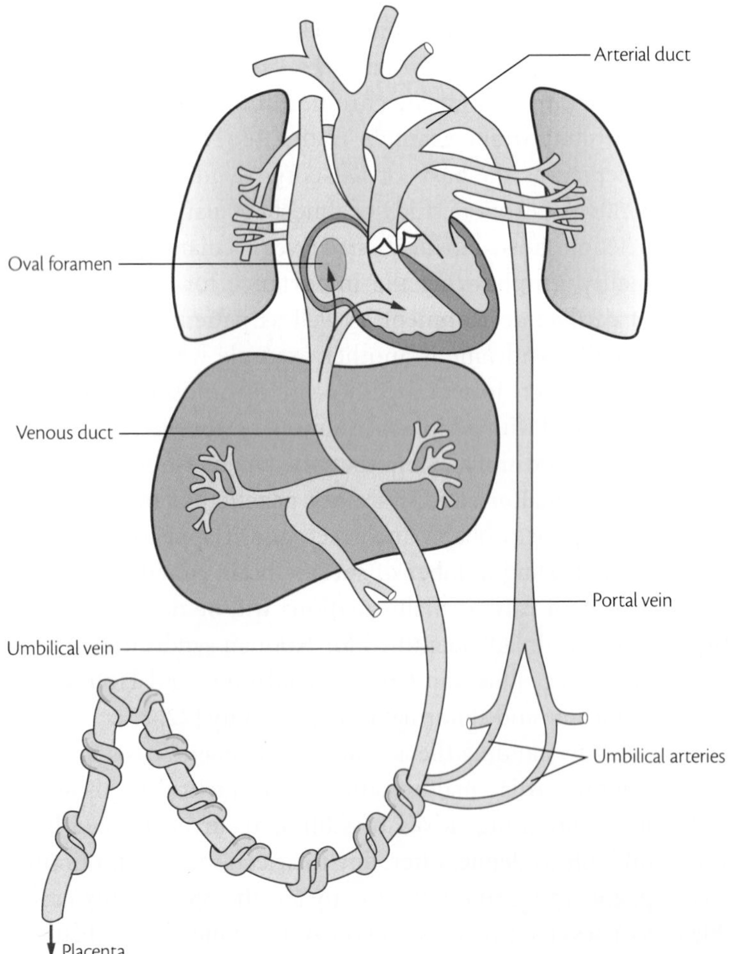

Figure 10.2 Schematic representation of the fetal circulation demonstrating sites of shunting, including venous duct, patent oval foramen and patent arterial duct. The venous duct acts as a regulator allowing variable amounts of blood to bypass the hepatic circulation according to the metabolic demands of the fetus.

via the tricuspid valve. Almost all of the right ventricular output will be directed through the arterial duct into the systemic circulation, bypassing the high resistance pulmonary circulation. The proportion of pulmonary blood flow changes with gestation, with an increase during the third trimester. Just as in postnatal hearts, the fetal pulmonary vascular bed is reactive. Fetal pulmonary blood flow can be increased by pulmonary vasodilator agents (such as oxygen) administered to the mother [27]. As pregnancy progresses, the effective cardiac output increases to a maximum of approximately 250mL/kg/min by term, with the right ventricle contributing 55% and the left ventricle 45% of the fetal cardiac output. Of the combined output, 65% returns to the placenta and 35% to the fetal organs and tissues [28].

Function of the fetal heart

Compared with the adult heart, there are differences both within the fetal heart itself and between the physiological environment during fetal and postnatal life, which explain many of the observations of fetal cardiac function. The expression of contractile proteins and collagen types in the fetal heart is different from the postnatal pattern [29]. Therefore, the immature fetal heart is both less compliant and less able to generate contractile force for the same degree of stretch [30]. Advancing gestation allows maturation of excitation–contraction coupling as well as increasing autonomic innervation [31]. Such findings contribute to a blunted Starling curve in the fetus. However, it has been shown that external constraints around the heart in the fetus, including the fluid-filled lungs and rigid chest wall, are equally important [32].

Circulation and changes at birth

With birth, there is a shift from a circulation 'in parallel' to one 'in series', as well as a marked increase in cardiac output from both ventricles. At term, the cardiac output from each ventricle approximately equals the combined cardiac output from both ventricles in the immediately preterm fetus. With inspiration, there is a rapid fall in pulmonary vascular resistance, as lung expansion allows new vessels to open and existing vessels to enlarge. Reduced resistance and decreased pulmonary artery pressures increase pulmonary blood flow. Simultaneously, the lower-resistance placental circulation is removed from the systemic circulation as the cord is cut. The sudden increase in oxygen tension produced by breathing alters local prostaglandin synthesis, resulting in a constriction of both the arterial and venous ducts. For most neonates, functional closure of the arterial duct occurs within 24–72 hours and anatomical closure is complete by 1–2 weeks [33]. The oval foramen and venous duct may remain patent for some time after birth, with the potential to allow shunting after birth. This can mask the signs of underlying structural congenital cardiovascular malformations, such as infracardiac total anomalous pulmonary venous drainage or, occasionally, TGA. The oval foramen is functionally closed in the majority of cases by the third month of life.

Pathophysiology

Without prompt recognition, accurate diagnosis and appropriate treatment, about one-third of all babies with congenital cardiac malformations will die within the first 2 months of life. Cardiac failure and cyanosis are the principal signs in infants but there is a temporal progression in the presentation of congenital cardiac malformations (➲Table 10.2). The majority of patients present in infancy, but some will present in childhood and adolescence or even during adult life. Typical presentations include cardiac murmurs, abnormal heart rate, absent pulses or hypertension, fits, faints and funny turns, chest pain, and airway obstruction.

Cardiac failure

While many of the mechanisms of cardiac failure are common to all ages, the pathophysiology in CHD may be different and may vary with age. In newborns, early heart failure usually results from left heart obstructive lesions, sustained tachyarrhythmias, primary myocardial dysfunction, or large arteriovenous malformations [34]. Neonatal heart failure presents with rapid onset of circulatory collapse but poor feeding, failure to thrive, and respiratory distress are the most frequent symptoms in infancy. Additional findings include tachycardia with a gallop rhythm, cardiac murmurs, hepatomegaly, poor colour, and excessive perspiration. As heart failure is most frequently caused by either unobstructed communication between the right and left sides of the heart or myocardial dysfunction involving both ventricles, a distinction between right and left heart failure is less meaningful than in the adult population. Beyond the newborn period, lesions causing a large left-to-right shunt are the most common cause of heart failure, usually becoming manifest when the neonatal pulmonary vascular resistance falls. Presentation is hastened and frequently more severe when lesions occur in combination (e.g. VSD and patent ductus arteriosus (PDA)).

Table 10.2 Causes of common presenting manifestations of cardiac disease in early infancy

Heart failure
Hypoplastic left heart syndrome
Coarctation of the aorta
Critical aortic stenosis
Arteriovenous fistula
Patent arterial duct
Atrioventricular septal defect
Large ventricular septal defect
Unobstructed total anomalous pulmonary venous connection
Anomalous origin of left coronary artery from pulmonary artery
Cyanosis
Transposition of the great arteries with or without ventricular septal defect
Severe tetralogy of Fallot or pulmonary atresia with ventricular septal defect (pulmonary atresia with intact ventricular septum)
Critical pulmonary stenosis
Common arterial trunk
Functionally univentricular heart
Ebstein's anomaly
Total anomalous pulmonary venous connection
Abnormal heart rate
Supraventricular tachycardia
Complete heart block
Atrial or ventricular extrasystoles
Murmurs
Innocent, functional
Patent arterial duct
Pulmonary stenosis
Atrial septal defect
Ventricular septal defect
Atrioventricular septal defect
Atrioventricular valve regurgitation
Arteriovenous fistula

Cardiac failure rarely presents for the first time beyond infancy, except in association with primary myocardial dysfunction. Increasingly, however, cardiac failure is a feature of adolescents and adults with complex CHD, particularly those with single ventricle circulations or repairs which result in the right ventricle supporting the systemic circulation (e.g. intra-atrial repair of TGA). Palliative systemic to pulmonary shunts relieve cyanosis at the cost of a chronic increase in ventricular work. After the Fontan operation, the systemic ventricle may become in-coordinate and fail due to a different mechanism, involving 'preload deprivation' [35]. Understanding the determinants of cardiac failure in adults with such complex hearts needs to improve in order to guide appropriate management.

Cyanosis (➲Table 10.3)

Detection of cyanosis depends not only on arterial oxygen saturation but also on haemoglobin concentration, making clinical assessment inherently inaccurate. Cyanosis, in association with congenital cardiovascular malformations, is produced by three principal mechanisms which may coexist. The commonest is obstruction to pulmonary blood flow, associated with a right-to-left shunt. Cyanosis is also evident when there are discordant ventriculoarterial connections (complete transposition) with adverse streaming of blood through the heart. The third haemodynamic basis for cyanosis is common mixing of blood, which may occur at atrial, ventricular, or great artery level (the mixed systemic and pulmonary venous return is distributed to both pulmonary

Table 10.3 Medical complications of chronic cyanosis

Haematological
↑ Red cell mass
↑ Red cell turnover
↑ Viscosity
Haemostasis
↓ Platelet count
↓ Platelet function
Clotting factor deficiency
Metabolic
↑ Urate production
Calcium bilirubinate gallstones
Renal
↓ Glomerular filtration rate
↓ Creatinine
Proteinuria
↓ Urate clearance
Orthopaedic
Hypertrophic osteoarthropathy
Scoliosis
Skin
Clubbing
Acne
Infection
Cerebral abscess

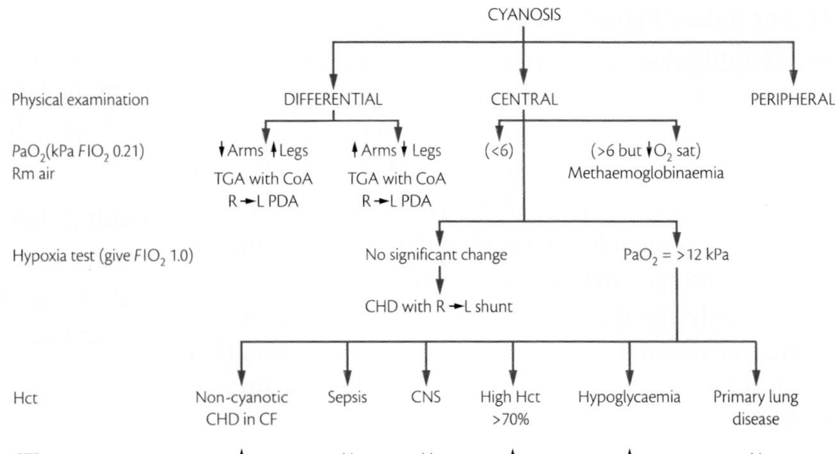

Figure 10.3 Algorithm for the evaluation of cyanotic infants. CHD, congenital heart disease; CNS, central nervous system; CoA, coarctation of the aorta; Hct, haematocrit; L, left; N, normal; R, right; PDA, patent ductus arteriosus; TGA, transposition of the great arteries.

artery and aorta). The algorithm in ➲Fig. 10.3 provides assistance in decision making. In patients with congenital cardiovascular malformations, a distinction should be made into those with cyanosis associated with reduced pulmonary blood flow and those with cyanosis and increased pulmonary blood flow. In those with reduced pulmonary blood flow, obstruction may occur at tricuspid valve, right ventricular, pulmonary valve, or pulmonary artery level and there is an obligatory communication within the heart, allowing shunting of the blood returning via the systemic veins from the right to the left side of the heart.

Examples of this include ToF, pulmonary atresia (with or without VSD) and tricuspid atresia. Patients with cyanosis and normal or increased pulmonary blood flow will most frequently have complete transposition or, less commonly, a complete mixing situation. Mixing at atrial level occurs in total anomalous pulmonary venous connection (TAPVC) and at ventricular level in hearts with a functionally single ventricle. A CAT provides an example of mixing at the level of the great arteries. Common mixing may occur with decreased or increased pulmonary blood flow, dependent on the degree of pulmonary outflow obstruction. Cyanosis and cardiac failure may coexist where there is common mixing and unobstructed pulmonary blood flow.

Long-term cyanosis is associated with a number of well recognized sequelae, which include impaired growth and delayed physical development in the child [36]. Mental development, however, is rarely affected. Finger clubbing and polycythaemia are responses to chronic hypoxaemia, as are renal dysfunction, hyperuricaemia, and acne. The incidence of cerebral abscess appears to be related to arterial saturation and occurs in older children or adults [37]. This diagnosis should be considered in any patient with a cyanotic congenital cardiovascular malformation, who presents with fever and neurological signs. Haemoptysis, results from the enlargement of the bronchial collateral circulation, and in association with pulmonary vascular obstructive disease.

Other presentations

Heart murmur

In later infancy and in older children, heart murmurs are the most common presenting manifestation of congenital cardiac malformations. Up to 1% of newborns will have a cardiac murmur in the first few days of life, but most innocent murmurs will have disappeared by the end of the first year of life [38]. Beyond infancy, a clearly detectable murmur in a child warrants referral for paediatric cardiac assessment. Persisting innocent murmurs are almost always systolic, very localized, and occur in children who are otherwise well from a cardiovascular point of view.

Abnormal heart rate

Specific rhythm disturbances are discussed elsewhere but in brief, older children and adults may present with paroxysmal tachycardia (as palpitations) or persistent tachycardia, most commonly, due to supraventricular tachycardia or much less commonly due to ventricular tachycardia. Infrequently, children will present with sustained bradycardia secondary to complete heart block (either congenital or acquired as part of the natural history of a congenital malformation). In both brady- and tachyarrhythmias, the rhythm disturbance may or may not be associated with an underlying structural cardiovascular malformation and this has an important impact on management and outcome. As children with treated CHD survive to adolescence and adulthood, arrhythmias are becoming an increasingly encountered and difficult management problem. Optimal treatment requires a thorough understanding of both the electrophysiological abnormalities and of the underlying haemodynamics, as treatment approaches may differ considerably from those in patients with structurally normal hearts.

Absent pulses/hypertension

The identification of hypertension at routine examination should prompt a search for femoral pulses in all patients. Mild to moderate coarctation may not cause symptoms in infancy and signs may only become evident only when the pace of somatic growth exceeds the growth of the narrowed segment. Treatment for coarctation in childhood (surgical or interventional) may alleviate associated hypertension initially only for it to reappear years later, even in the absence of recoarctation [39]. Coarctation is a condition which on occasion is still diagnosed for the first time in adulthood.

Fits, faints, and funny turns

In children, 'anoxic seizures' may result in a primary cerebral event which is associated with transient asystole and a normal underlying cardiac conduction system. In adolescents and adults with CHD, syncope is rare but should be investigated promptly and thoroughly as it may be due to a sustained cardiac arrhythmia and be a marker of risk of sudden death. Both atrial and ventricular tachycardias are more common after repair of complex anomalies and may cause syncope.

Chest pain

This frequently encountered complaint is very rarely associated with an underlying structural cardiovascular malformation in the young. Angina pectoris may occur in association with a coronary artery abnormality, including an ostial abnormality or an anomalous left coronary artery from the pulmonary artery, as well as in hypertrophic obstructive cardiomyopathy and severe aortic outflow obstruction. It may also occur in patients with right ventricular hypertension. Almost always, there are baseline abnormalities of the electrocardiogram (ECG) to suggest underlying disease.

Airway obstruction

This uncommon mode of presentation in infancy is usually associated with inspiratory stridor or difficulty in swallowing. When associated with a structural cardiac malformation, the manifestations are most frequently caused by a vascular ring, such as a double aortic arch or a pulmonary artery sling. In the newborn period, major airway obstruction can be an important manifestation of the absent pulmonary valve syndrome [40].

Abnormal chest radiograph

An abnormal cardiac contour is an unusual presentation for a haemodynamically significant congenital cardiac malformation, except when there is isolated cardiomegaly. Occasionally, a routine chest radiograph may reveal previously undetected abnormalities of cardiac position, size, or shape, which may be associated with structural cardiac malformations.

Adult presentation

The large majority of patients with congenital heart malformations will have presented before reaching adult life. Indeed, in many, the definitive treatment (by surgery or increasingly by interventional catheterization) will have already been undertaken. In some, however, the first presentation may be to the adult cardiologist. This is more common in countries with less well-developed paediatric care, but with increasing immigration, patients with even complex underlying malformations may be seen in developed countries. Late referral may be associated with much more advanced complications including cyanosis, heart failure, pulmonary vascular disease, and arrhythmia.

In some situations, the first adult presentation is the result of a new symptom as part of the natural history of the malformation, or the result of a complication such as infective endocarditis or a paradoxical embolism. For example, adults with atrial septal defects (ASDs) may present for the first time, with dyspnoea and palpitation (usually due to atrial arrhythmia). Those with relatively minor malformations may remain undetected until the development of an acquired cardiac problem which exacerbates symptoms. Patients with small secundum ASDs may become symptomatic for the first time after the age of 40 years, with an increase in left-to-right shunting caused by change in left ventricular dynamics secondary to hypertension or coronary disease. Patients with VSD can become symptomatic as a result of new aortic regurgitation or when cyanosis develops due to pulmonary vascular disease. Alternatively, abnormal findings at routine medical examination for insurance employment or other reasons such as pregnancy, may uncover an undetected congenital malformation. Well-recognized examples are hypertension in coarctation or an abnormal chest X-ray and ECG in congenitally corrected transposition.

Investigation

Strategies for investigation of anatomy and physiology in patients with congenital cardiac malformations are changing rapidly, with a shift away from invasive to non-invasive modalities. This is particularly true in neonates and small infants, where cross-sectional echocardiography has almost eliminated the need for diagnostic cardiac catheterization [41]. In adults, cross-sectional techniques such as CMR imaging and CT are able to provide physiological and three-dimensional anatomical information and their use during long-term follow-up is increasing rapidly [42].

Chest radiography

Chest radiography provides valuable information about the physiological consequences of congenital cardiac malformations. This includes pulmonary plethora associated with a large VSD or oligaemia associated with severe ToF. Cardiac position and size, side of the aortic arch, associated bony abnormalities, and visceral situs can also be assessed. Chest radiography is less valuable in newborns or during early infancy, as a normal appearance can still be associated with a severe congenital cardiac malformation. The chest radiograph is readily available and cheap, but its diagnostic role has diminished since cross-sectional echocardiography has become available.

Electrocardiography

The ECG is one of the earliest tests applied to the investigation of patients with suspected congenital cardiac malformations. Abnormal electrocardiographic findings are common, but are very rarely specific enough to provide a precise diagnosis. Exceptions in the newborn include the dominance of left ventricular forces seen in tricuspid atresia, the abnormally large P wave with prolonged PR interval, and bundle branch block pattern associated with Ebstein's malformation, and the left-axis deviation with reversed septal depolarization characteristic of congenitally corrected transposition. However, the ECG remains a vital diagnostic tool in the evaluation of all arrhythmias, which occur frequently, and are sometimes asymptomatic, in adult patients. Many patients with a congenital cardiac malformation have been operated upon in childhood and have bundle branch block as a result. If, later in life, a tachycardia develops, it can be difficult to discriminate between a ventricular tachycardia and a supraventricular tachycardia with a pre-existing wide QRS. Like the chest radiograph, the ECG is readily available and inexpensive.

Blood gas analysis

In combination with other investigations, assessment of blood gases in the newborn and in infancy is one of the most commonly used means of distinguishing cardiac from non-cardiac causes of cyanosis. A hyperoxic test in the newborn may assist in identifying patients who have a duct-dependent cardiovascular malformation and may be helpful when there is no immediate access to cross-sectional echocardiography. In adults, blood gases at rest and during exercise may be used to detect the presence of right–to-left shunts or to assess the severity and direction of intra-cardiac shunts.

Cross-sectional echocardiography

Cross-sectional echocardiography, together with Doppler studies, has revolutionized the practice of congenital cardiology over the last two decades. Its non-invasive, immediate and portable nature makes it ideally suited to the investigation of even the smallest children. It can define structure and function, which can also be quantified. Increasingly, echocardiography is also playing a role during cardiac catheterization and surgery. There are however some limitations. Whilst imaging windows are almost universally excellent in infants and small children, with growth and after multiple operations, transthoracic windows deteriorate significantly in older patients. A transoesophageal approach may therefore be required. Imaging of the intracranial structures is usually excellent, but extracardiac structures such as the great vessels and abnormalities around the heart may be difficult to see. At present, most information is obtained in a two-dimensional format, and three-dimensional echocardiography still has a limited clinical role. With this technique, it is easier to understand and show anatomy of abnormal valves and other intracranial structures and assessment of left ventricular function may be more reliable with three-dimensional than with two-dimensional echocardiography [43, 44].

There is continuing progress in this area, which will impact on the investigation of patients with congenital cardiac malformations. Additional functional information can be obtained using techniques such as Doppler tissue imaging and its derivatives as well as colour kinesis [45]. The former may assist assessment of ventricular diastolic performance, which has been notoriously difficult to study. The use of contrast echocardiography and perfusion imaging may provide further functional information [46]. Stress echocardiography has had a limited role, but may be useful for assessment of myocardial perfusion in patients after operations such as the arterial switch [47]. Intracardiac echocardiography (ICE) is useful for percutaneous interventions, particularly ASD closure [48]. Anaesthesia is not required with this mode of imaging, an advantage compared to the transoesophageal approach traditionally used during ASD closure. Cross-sectional echocardiography is increasingly being complemented by additional imaging modalities, such as CMR imaging and CT.

Cardiac catheterization and angiography

Diagnostic cardiac catheterization and angiography were for many years the principal means of evaluation of patients with congenital cardiovascular malformations. Measurement of oxygen saturation and pressures enables calculation of intracardiac shunts, gradients, flows, and resistances. Anatomy and function with high resolution, particularly excellent edge detection, is obtained by angiography. Much of this diagnostic information can now be obtained less invasively. Cardiac catheterization in small children carries a small but definite risk, particularly when they are unwell, and almost inevitably requires general anaesthesia. This will influence cardiac physiology and the relevance of measurements obtained. Current diagnostic indications for catheterization and angiography include assessment of pulmonary vascular resistance in patients with suspected or established pulmonary vascular obstructive disease, imaging of the coronary arteries, which should be performed preoperatively in all patients >40 years who are referred for cardiac surgery, and evaluation of extracardiac vessels such as aortopulmonary collateral arteries. Increasingly, invasive procedures are being performed for interventional purposes, with classical diagnostic information obtained during these procedures used to evaluate the success of treatment (see later sections).

Cardiac magnetic resonance imaging and computed tomography

See ➲ Figs. 10.4 and 10.5; 🎥 10.1.

CMR of the heart and great vessels is becoming commonplace in the assessment of adults with congenital cardiac malformations and is playing an increasing role in the evaluation of neonates, infants, and younger children [49]. Multislice computed tomography (CT) is also able to provide cross-sectional imaging. The indications for cardiovascular CMR include evaluation of right ventricular to pulmonary artery conduits, aortic pathology, anomalous coronary arteries, and complex congenital cardiac malformations, where understanding of three-dimensional information is essential. Cardiovascular CMR in children <8 years of age is usually performed under general anaesthesia, but with the development of faster sequences, breath-holding may become less of a necessity and CMR data may be acquired more easily during sedation. With the newly designed 'open' CMR, paediatric patients can be imaged within the comforting reach of a parent or nurse, thus eliminating anxiety or claustrophobic tendencies. Moreover, the extra large bore of the open magnets comfortably provides enough room to image patients weighing up to 450 pounds (approximately 204 kg).

Imaging sequences can be broadly divided into:

- 'black-blood' spin-echo images, where signal from blood is nulled and thus not seen (accurate anatomical imaging);
- 'white-blood' gradient echo or steady-state free precession (SSFP) images, where signal from blood is returned for anatomical and cine imaging;
- phase contrast imaging, where velocity information is encoded for quantification of vascular flow;
- contrast-enhanced MR angiography, where non-ECG-gated three-dimensional data are acquired after gadolinium contrast has been administered for thoracic vascular imaging.

As volumetric measurements are much more reproducible than those obtained using echocardiography, CMR is increasingly proving useful in serial assessment of cardiac chamber structure and function as part of natural history or intervention studies [50].

Multidetector CT enables acquisition of volumes of CT data that can be reformatted in any imaging plane. Multidetector CT images of the entire thorax can be acquired in 3–10s depending on the size of the subject. Using iodinated contrast agents, CT angiography can now be rapidly performed and three-dimensional reconstruction aids considerably in the appreciation of complex cardiovascular anatomy. Cardiac CT images of the intracardiac anatomy that are not ECG-triggered or -gated are often blurred and of limited value. ECG-gated multi-slice CT, however, facilitates imaging of cardiac anatomy and function with outstanding quality. The spatial resolution of the modern scanners is so good that CT imaging of coronary arteries is becoming an alternative to coronary angiography. The speed at which CT images can be acquired means that imaging in young children can be performed unsedated with 'feed and wrap', or with sedation, and general anaesthesia is rarely required. Furthermore, imaging of cardiac anatomy and function has become possible in patients with an irregular heart rhythm, as in atrial fibrillation. However, a 64-slice CT-scan exposes a patient to a high radiation dose of approximately 20–25mSv. The latest developments, dual source CT and 256+ CT scans, have demonstrated the potential to reduce significantly radiation exposure to approximately 3–5mSv.

As compared with CT, CMR is currently superior for acquisition of information on intracardiac anatomy, ventricular function, and vascular flow quantification, whereas CT may be performed without general anaesthesia and may provide information on airways and lung parenchyma that is not obtained by CMR. CT may also be used to

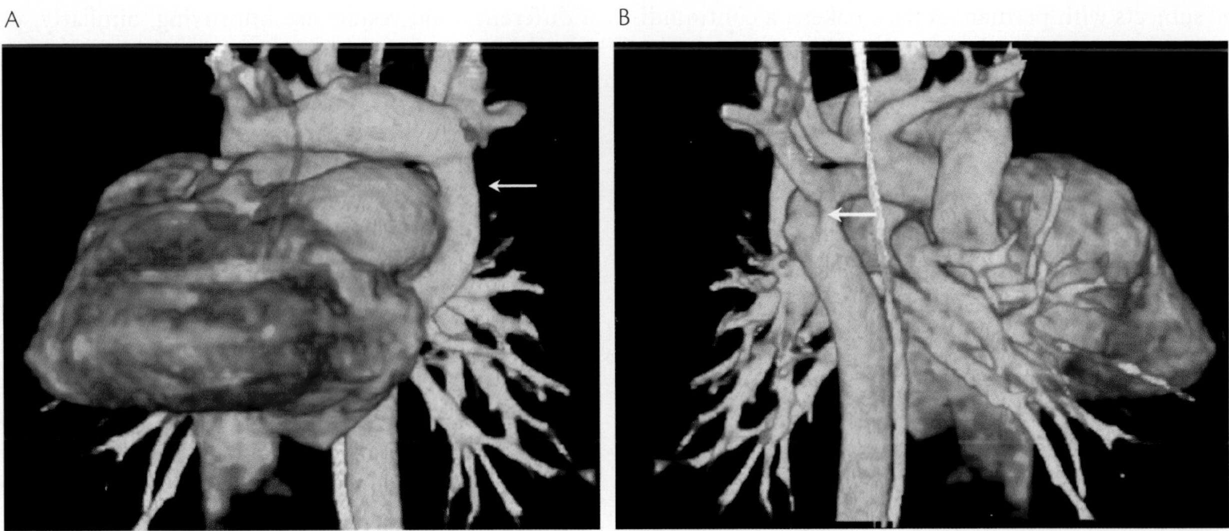

Figure 10.4 Multislice three-dimensional reconstruction of complex cardiac lesion with dextrocardia, functional univentricular heart, supracardiac total anomalous pulmonary venous drainage and anterior aorta with coarctation. (A) Arrow shows ascending vertical vein on the left side entering into dilated innominate vein. (B) From posterior aspect, arrow shows aortic coarctation just distal to the left subclavian artery. Entering into the superior aspect of the right atrium is a dilated superior caval vein.

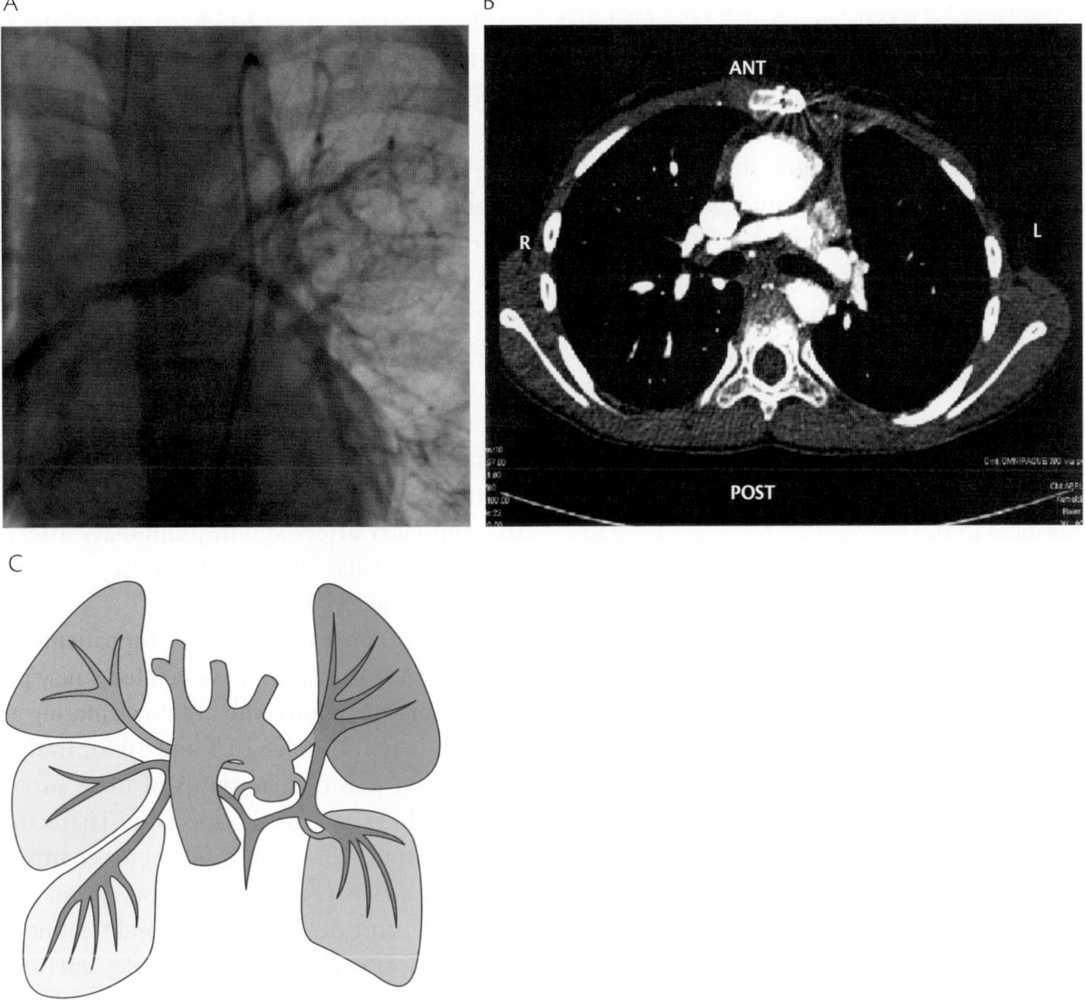

Figure 10.5 Investigations in a patient with pulmonary atresia, ventricular septal defect and multifocal pulmonary blood supply. (A) Angiography with injection into collateral vessel supplying left upper lobe with retrograde filling of central pulmonary artery confluence. (B) Axial CT scan demonstrating anterior aorta with confluent pulmonary arteries. (C) Schematic representation of pulmonary blood supply depicting dual supply to left upper and lower lobes, as well as confluent small central pulmonary arteries (blue) with supply to right upper lobe being derived exclusively from an aorto-pulmonary collateral artery (red).

image subjects with permanent pacemakers, a contraindication to CMR. CT is currently used for evaluation of aortic pathology (in particular the aortic arch and vascular rings, pulmonary artery, and pulmonary venous anatomy), but this is a rapidly changing area and the indications are likely to increase considerably. In contrast to CMR, CT can show calcifications. This is useful in the evaluation of vascular pathology and in the assessment of valves. Presently, CT is more widely available and therefore more often used in acute situations, for example when an aortic dissection is suspected. For assessment of the anatomy of intracardiac structures, especially of delicate and fast moving structures like valves, echo remains superior to both CT and CMR.

Management

Medical

With exceptions, medical management for congenital cardiac malformations is largely supportive (e.g. for heart failure) and significant structural abnormalities usually require interventional treatment. The pathophysiology of cardiac and respiratory dysfunction is different from that of the failing normal adult circulation, so that extrapolation from the results of adult cardiac studies is not always easy. For example the impact of angiotensin-converting enzyme (ACE) inhibitors in Fontan or Mustard/Senning circulations has proved disappointing [51, 52]. A few specific medical treatments target the disease and its consequences more directly. For example, maintenance of ductal patency with prostaglandin infusion and use of nitric oxide, phosphodiestase inhibitors and endothelium antagonists for pulmonary hypertension have been important advances [53].

The electrophysiological consequences of congenital cardiac malformations are key issues for treatment, especially during long-term follow-up. The principles of arrhythmia diagnosis and management are the same as in normally formed hearts, but risk stratification, investigation, and choice of treatment are often very different. The onset of arrhythmia may be the first sign of haemodynamic decompensation. Furthermore, the risk of arrhythmia may be much greater in the presence of the abnormal underlying circulation (e.g. atrial flutter in a Mustard/Senning patient with right ventricular dysfunction and venous pathway narrowing) [54]. The complex anatomy and basis for arrhythmia makes interventional electrophysiology more challenging and the results are generally worse [55]. However, improved mapping and catheter design has made a difference and results are improving. Similarly, pacing is more demanding in patients with congenital cardiac malformations, due to the size and anatomy of the heart. Pacemaker therapy for heart failure in CHD is challenging, but can be very rewarding [56, 57].

Resynchronization protocols developed for heart failure, in patients with normal cardiac morphology, are being applied to those with congenitally malformed hearts. Little evidence based medicine is however currently available to define indications and outcomes [58, 59]. Similarly, indications for implantation of defibrillators in patients with CHD have not yet been established [60]. Markers of risk for serious arrhythmia and sudden death remain difficult and there are substantially more problems with lead placement, ECG recognition algorithms, and inappropriate shocks in patients with CHD [61, 62].

Surgical

Continuing improvement in surgical results for congenital cardiac malformations has been one of the triumphs of modern cardiology. Conditions which even 20 years ago were considered virtually untreatable, for example hypoplastic left heart syndrome (HLHS), now have very acceptable childhood mortality [63]. This has been achieved through accurate diagnosis, better preoperative and postoperative management, improvements in anaesthesia and cardiopulmonary bypass, together with increasing surgical skill and confidence. Intraoperative transoesophageal echocardiography has also played a role in ensuring adequate repair. There has been a major shift from the early approach of palliation with later repair towards primary repair from the time of diagnosis. This has reduced anatomical distortion from palliative surgery (e.g. systemic to pulmonary artery shunt, pulmonary artery band), the decline in cardiac function before repair, and the overall risk of treatment.

Improved surgical results, even for patients with the most complex malformations, have created a new population of adolescents and adults who are now entering adult cardiac practice [64] (➲Tables 10.4 and 10.5). Evaluation of the cardiac and non-cardiac status of these survivors is now a major obligation for the specialty. There are, for example, important concerns about neurocognitive problems in HLHS survivors of the Norwood approach, which may influence future decision making and treatment [65].

The majority (about 75%) of adolescents and adults will have had multiple previous operations, but still require further surgery. This may be required: in (1) patients who have not been diagnosed or considered severe enough in

Table 10.4 Common congenital heart defects compatible with survival to adult life without surgery or interventional catheterization

Mild pulmonary valve stenosis
Peripheral pulmonary stenosis
Bicuspid aortic valve
Mild subaortic stenosis
Mild supravalvar aortic stenosis
Small atrial septal defect
Small ventricular septal defect
Small patent ductus arteriosus
Mitral valve prolapse
Ostium primum atrial septal defect (atrioventricular septal defect)
Marfan syndrome
Ebstein's anomaly
Corrected transposition (atrioventricular/ventriculo-arterial discordance)
Balanced complex lesions (e.g. double-inlet ventricle with pulmonary stenosis)
Defects with pulmonary vascular obstructive disease (Eisenmenger's syndrome)

childhood; (2) those with prior palliation; and (3) those with prior repair and residual or new haemodynamic complications (see ➲Table 10.6). Surgical practice in this population is different from conventional adult cardiac surgery, providing a strong case for concentration of resources into specialist units for both treatment and training [2, 64]. Reopening a sternal incision in such patients is a potentially hazardous undertaking, especially if the right ventricle or a

Table 10.5 Common congenital heart defects surviving to adult life after surgery/interventional catheterization

Aortic valve disease, valvotomy or replacement
Pulmonary stenosis, valvotomy
Tetralogy of Fallot
Atrial septal defect
Ventricular septal defect
Atrioventricular septal defect
Transposition of the great arteries, atrial redirection
Complex transposition of the great arteries
Total anomalous pulmonary venous connection
Pulmonary atresia/ventricular septal defect
Fontan operation for complex congenital heart disease
Ebstein's anomaly
Coarctation of the aorta
Mitral valve disease

Table 10.6 Indications for reoperation in adults with congenital heart disease

Inevitable reoperation after definitive repair: prosthetic valves, extracardiac conduits placed at an early age that become of inadequate size because of body growth
Residual defects after definitive repair: ventricular septal defect after tetralogy of Fallot and left atrioventricular valve
New/recurrent defects after definitive repair: subaortic stenosis, restenosis of aortic valve, pulmonary regurgitation in tetralogy of Fallot
Staged repair of complex defects: pulmonary atresia with ventricular septal defect
Unexpected complications: infective endocarditis
Heart/heart–lung transplantation for uncorrectable congenital heart disease
Patient operated on for congenital heart disease with new acquired heart disease: coronary disease

conduit is in close proximity. The establishment of cardiopulmonary bypass by femoral cannulation may be required. There are often multiple collaterals in the cyanotic patient and abnormalities of myocardial function and the pulmonary bed together with comorbidity (e.g. kyphoscoliosis) are frequently present. Careful preoperative planning, by all the professionals involved in treatment, is vital for all stages of the intervention, including myocardial protection, anaesthesia, and blood salvage techniques. The risk:benefit ratio for these complex operations is often difficult to assess and to communicate with patients and their families.

Even relatively minor non-cardiac surgery may carry a high risk in patients with complex congenital cardiac malformations as a result of haemodynamic instability, hypotension, hypovolaemia, and endocarditis. Careful preoperative planning and intraoperative monitoring is therefore vital if disasters are to be avoided [66].

Despite the success of intervention for congenital cardiac malformations, in a proportion of children and adults, cardiopulmonary function declines sufficiently for transplantation to be considered the only option. While this group is challenging because of previous surgery, comorbidity, pulmonary vascular problems, and occasionally anatomical difficulties, results for paediatric and adult congenital transplantation have improved in specialist centres (➲Fig. 10.6) [67]. Despite this, the worsening donor situation means that many patients will never receive a transplant unless viable alternatives such as long-term mechanical support or xenotransplantation become available [68].

Interventional catheterization

There has been a spectacular increase in the number and range of interventional catheter techniques for

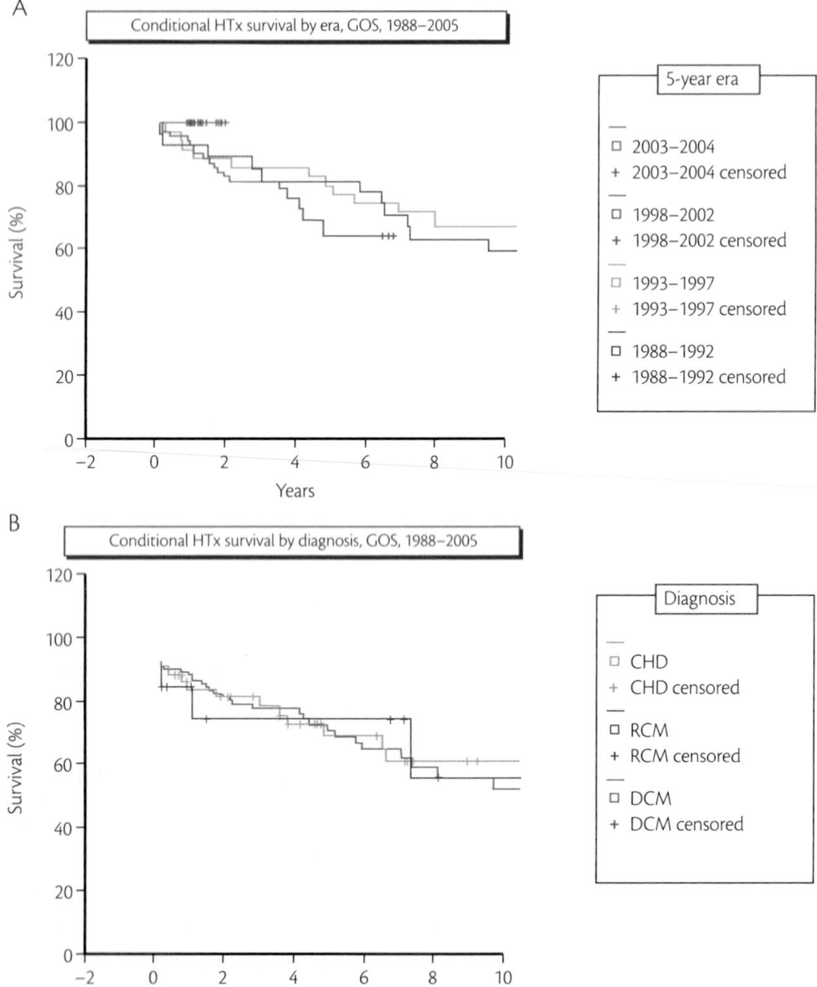

Figure 10.6 (A) Transplantation outcome by era. (B) Transplantation outcome by diagnosis.

congenital cardiac malformations, which has coincided with the decline in indications for diagnostic catheterization (➲Fig. 10.7). For many years, it has been possible to relieve obstructive lesions with balloon dilatation and more recently stenting. New opportunities have arisen to replace regurgitant and/or stenotic cardiac valves without surgery, as well as to close not only patent arterial ducts and ASDs but also VSDs [7, 69–72]. The range of therapeutic procedures that can be performed without surgery is likely to increase, as even 'stitching' becomes possible using catheter techniques. In some situations, interventional catheterization has become the clear treatment of choice over surgery (e.g. pulmonary stenosis, closure of patent arterial duct). However, in the majority, no clear evidence of superiority has been demonstrated in clinical trials. The decision to perform an interventional catheter procedure should therefore undergo the same process of multidisciplinary peer review as for surgery. Treatment of congenital cardiac malformations can often best be achieved by a collaborative approach involving both interventional catheterization and surgery. The management of aortopulmonary collaterals in ToF with pulmonary atresia is an example. Lesions accessible to the interventionalist are often challenging to the surgeon (e.g. peripheral pulmonary stenosis) and vice versa (e.g. non-valve outflow obstruction). In the near future, three-dimensional imaging, by transoesophageal echo or CMR, during interventional catheterization should refine many of these procedures. Interventional catheterization is cheaper than surgery, less dependent on infrastructure, and can be performed in a broader range of units. However, any specialized programme treating congenital cardiac malformations should have expertise in both approaches.

Grown-up congenital heart disease

Recognition of the needs of the increasing population of adults with congenital cardiac malformations has prompted

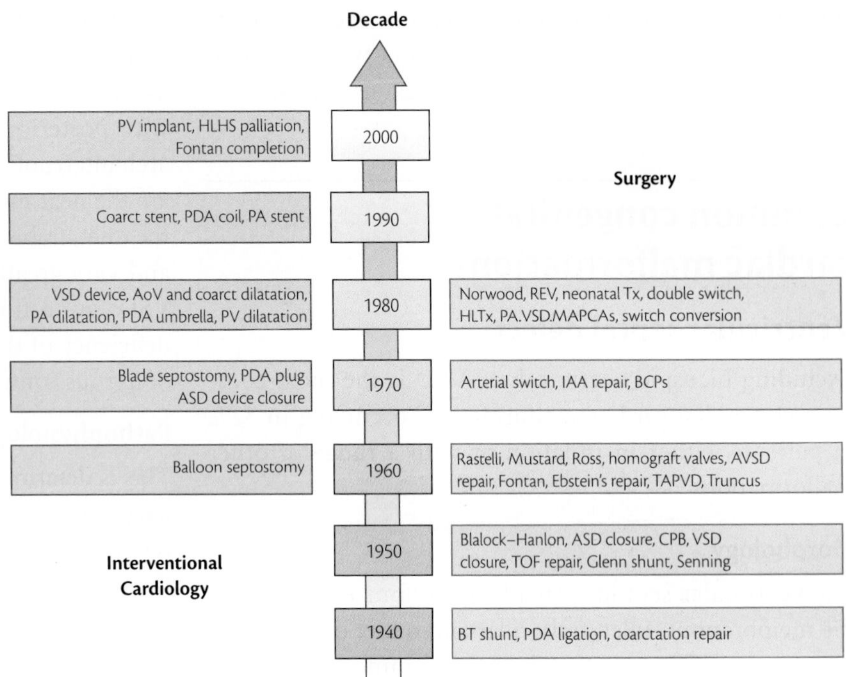

Figure 10.7 Advances in interventional cardiac catheterization according to era compared with surgical advances during the same periods. PV, percutaneous venous; HLH, hypoplastic left heart syndrome; PDA, patent ductus arteriosus; PA, pulmonary artery; VSD, ventricular septal defect; AoV, aortic valve; REV, reparation a l'étage ventriculaire; Tx, transplant; HLTx, heart and lung transplant; MAPCA's, major aortic pulmonary collateral arteries; IAA, interrupted aortic arch; BCPS, bidirectional cavopulmonary shunt; AVSD, atrioventricular septal defect; TAPVD, total anomalous pulmonary venous drainage; CPB, cardiopulmonary bypass; BT, blalock taussig. With kind permission of Phillip Moore MD, Clinical Professor of Paediatrics, Director, Congenital Cardiac Catheterization Program.

the publication of several strategic documents, including the ESC Taskforce Report on grown-up CHD [2]. This set out principles for care delivery, involving specialists and other practitioners, as well as educational and training requirements. Implementation of a hierarchical system of care based on specialist units with appropriate transition from paediatrics will ensure continued excellence of care past childhood, provide feedback of late results to refine early treatment, and drive forward progress in 'lifetime' management of congenital cardiac malformations [9]. While generally accepted, implementation of this type of care delivery model has been slow in most countries. The establishment of specialist centres with trained staff and facilities is the first step. This should provide expert care in adults to match that which has been delivered during childhood and most adults with CHD should be seen at least once in such a specialist referral centre. For the more complex conditions, lifelong follow-up in the specialist centre is required. For others, shared care with a regional unit and primary care is appropriate. Close collaboration between tertiary centres, local hospitals, and primary care with each having specific tasks and responsibilities, is mandatory. Regional facilities are crucial for support of acute complications, such as heart failure and arrhythmia.

Non-cardiac problems are common in the adult population and often a multi-disciplinary approach in the specialist centre is required, involving different experts (e.g. obstetrics and gynaecology, rheumatology, orthopaedics, neurology, haematology, genetics). The grown-up congenital heart (GUCH) population have numerous anxieties about their past treatment, current status, and future prospects. Specialist nurses, psychologists, and social workers are a key part of the GUCH clinical team [73, 74].

Patients are confronted by issues of education, employment, sports, contraception, pregnancy, and insurance, and are often discriminated against in daily life (➲Table 10.7). One of the roles of the GUCH clinical team is to act as an advocate for their patient over these important 'life issues'. Over the next few years, informed 'evidence-based' recommendations on all these issues should become possible and guidelines are being published from several international societies. The ESC Task Force report on Grown-up Congenital Heart Disease, periodically updated, provides

Table 10.7 Non-cardiac issues in grown-up congenital heart disease

Intellectual development
Psychosocial development
Employment
Insurance (medical)
Mortgage (life)
Contraception
Pregnancy
Exercise/sports
Air travel

consensus advice on the follow-up and management of the individual conditions that adult cardiologists will encounter with increasing frequency over the next few years.

Common congenital cardiac malformations

Ventricular septal defect

Excluding bicuspid aortic valves, VSD is the most common congenital cardiac malformation, occurring in 32% of patients, either in isolation or with a range of other malformations.

Morphology

The ventricular septum is made up of four components: the membranous, inlet, trabecular and outlet or infundibular septum (➲ Fig. 10.8). The most common defects are perimembranous, and these may be further classified according to their extension into adjacent areas (e.g. inlet or outlet). Outlet defects can be subdivided into those with anterior deviation of the outlet septum (as in ToF, associated with aortic override) (🎥 10.2) and those with posterior deviation (as seen associated with aortic arch interruption). VSDs with an entirely muscular margin are the next most common type. These may be situated in the inlet, trabecular, apical or anterior parts of the septum, and vary greatly in size, shape, and number. Subarterial VSDs are a further important type, in which there is a deficiency of the infundibular septum resulting in an area of fibrous continuity between the semilunar valves.

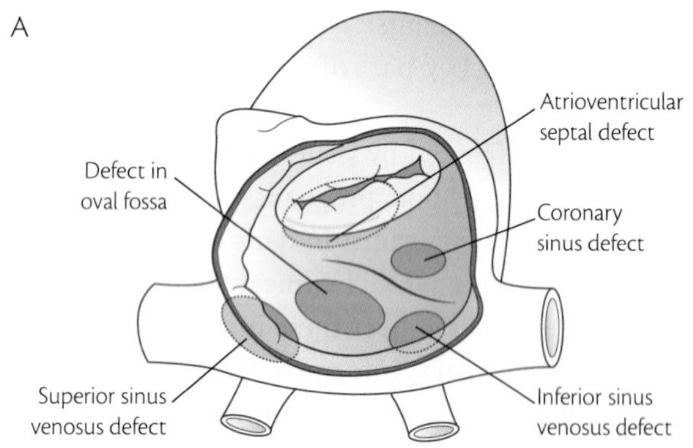

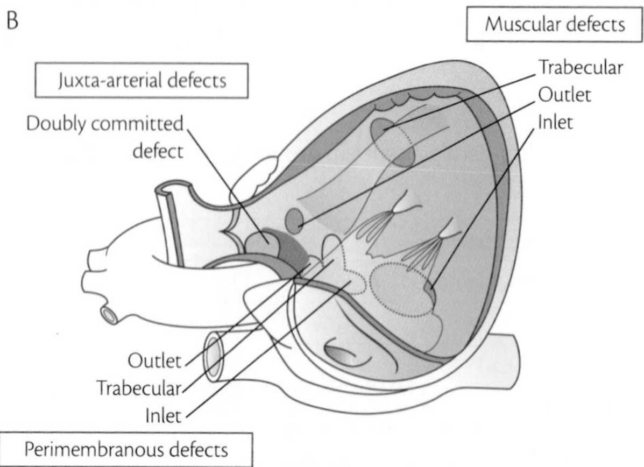

Figure 10.8 (A) Schematic representation of the various sites of atrial communication seen within the atrial septum. (B) Schematic representation of the various sites of ventricular communication seen within the ventricular septum.

Pathophysiology

This is determined by the size of the VSD and the pulmonary vascular resistance relative to the systemic vascular resistance, which determines the magnitude and direction of flow through the defect. A small VSD with a high resistance to flow results in a small left-to-right shunt and minimal haemodynamic disturbance. A large defect results in a large left-to-right shunt if there is no pulmonary outflow tract obstruction, pulmonary vascular resistance is low and systemic vascular resistance is high. When the systemic vascular resistance is higher than normal, e.g. in the presence of an aortic coarctation, or when a left ventricular outflow tract obstruction exists in the form of a valvular, sub-, or supravalvar aortic stenosis, the left-to-right shunt will increase. Typically, beyond infancy, as pulmonary vascular resistance starts to rise as a consequence of pulmonary vascular disease, the size of the shunt falls. Eventually the direction of the shunt may reverse when the pulmonary vascular resistance will become higher than the systemic vascular resistance.

Diagnosis

The clinical presentation, chest radiograph and ECG findings associated with VSDs of different sizes are shown in ➲ Table 10.8.

Echocardiography

This provides an accurate and reliable method of interrogating the ventricular septum using a combination of imaging planes. The size of the defect and its relationship to adjacent structures within the heart can be documented. This is very important, since the course of conduction tissue differs in the various types of VSD. Doppler study yields useful haemodynamic data about the shunt and its direction. Colour flow techniques can demonstrate very small defects that are often not visible on two-dimensional imaging and occasionally not audible on auscultation. The search for additional abnormalities is important, especially atrioventricular valve straddling, aortic valve

Table 10.8 Clinical findings in ventricular septal defect

Size	Very small	Small	Moderate	Large	With PVOD (Eisenmenger)
Thrill	No	Yes	Yes	No	No
Murmur and site	ESM at LSE	PSM loud LSE → apex	PSM, LSE → apex with mitral MDM	ESM at upper LSE and mitral MDM	None or soft ESM
Apex	Normal	Normal	LV+	LV+, RV+	RV++, palpable PA
S_2	Normal	Normal	Obscured by mitral	S_2 single with ↑P_2	Single loud palpable P_2
ECG	Normal	Normal	LV+, LA+, LAD	LV+, LA+, RV+	RV+, RA++, RAD
Chest X-ray	Normal	Normal	↑CTR, plethora	↑CTR, plethora, prominent PAs	↑CTR, large central PAs, no plethora

CTR, cardiothoracic ratio; ESM, ejection systolic murmur; LA, left atrium; LAD, left axis deviation; LSE, left sternal edge; LV, left ventricle; MDM, mid-diastolic edge; P_2, pulmonary component of second heart sound; PA, pulmonary artery; PSM, pan-systolic murmur; PVOD, pulmonary vascular obstructive disease; RAD, right axis deviation; RV, right ventricle; S_2, second heart sound.

prolapse, right ventricular outflow tract obstruction, and aortic coarctation.

Cardiac catheterization

The role of cardiac catheterization is now limited to evaluation of pulmonary vascular resistance in a small proportion of patients. Transcatheter VSD closure is feasible in selected patients, but the relatively high prevalence of atrioventricular block—caused by mechanical pressure of the closing device on the adjacent His bundle—has made this approach suitable in only a small number of patients [75–77].

Natural history

The majority of VSDs are small and do not require intervention. It is impossible to determine the proportion that close spontaneously, but it may be as high as 80%, usually within the first few years of life. Even larger VSDs can become smaller, but complete closure is less common. Cardiac failure occurs in infants with a large VSD, often from the first few weeks of life. This is due to the predominant flow towards pulmonary circulation in the presence of a larger VSD and low pulmonary resistance. Early closure may be required. Unoperated patients are at risk of developing pulmonary vascular obstructive disease, which may be progressive and irreversible by 1 year of age and very occasionally earlier. These patients with Eisenmenger's syndrome usually survive into adult life but have a reduced life expectancy [78, 79].

A small number of patients present in later childhood, adolescence, or adulthood with small to moderate left-to-right shunts, normal pulmonary vascular resistance, and left ventricular volume overload and dilatation. They are likely to benefit from VSD closure. A small proportion of infants develop a midventricular or subpulmonary stenosis and become cyanosed and a further cohort (about 1% in the Western world) develop aortic regurgitation, most frequently associated with subarterial or perimembranous defects [80]. Usually, right coronary prolapse develops and this may actually close the VSD but cause aortic regurgitation that may progress rapidly. Infective endocarditis is an important cause of morbidity and mortality in VSD (1–2 per 1000 patient-years or 10% incidence by 70 years) and is unrelated to the size of the defect [79].

Management

Medical management of heart failure is required in symptomatic neonates. The mainstay is diuretic treatment. The role, if any, of digoxin or ACE-inhibitors is very limited. Surgical closure is usually performed within the first few months of life. Banding of the pulmonary trunk was often performed as palliation for infants with a VSD and a large shunt in the early days of cardiac surgery. It is now reserved for multiple VSDs, very large defects in very small children or when significant contraindications to cardiopulmonary bypass are present. In childhood, it is rare for VSD closure to be required over 1 year of age. Recently, closure of both muscular and perimembranous VSDs has been performed by interventional catheterization, obviating the need for surgery (10.3 and 10.4) [81]. This is clearly attractive for families, but a comparison of results between this approach and surgery is not yet available. After initial enthusiasm, many programmes have stopped closing perimembranous defects because the risk of developing an atrioventricular block seems much higher than with surgical closure [75, 76].

Small restrictive VSDs, without left ventricular volume overload or increased right-sided pressures, appear benign into adult life and closure is only indicated if infective endocarditis or aortic regurgitation develop. However, all these patients should have lifelong follow-up, since as a result of alterations of left ventricular haemodynamic properties (such as elevated systolic and diastolic pressures) that are inherent to ageing, the left-to-right shunt can increase to such an extent that closure may be indicated. Following closure of VSD, most patients have normal exercise capacity patterns and should be encouraged to lead normal lives. In the modern era, postoperative heart block is very uncommon, as are tachyarrhythmias. Unfortunately, patients with established pulmonary vascular obstructive disease and Eisenmenger's syndrome are still seen. They suffer the consequences of cyanosis and progressive exercise intolerance. Death usually occurs by 50 years, although life expectancy can be prolonged by careful medical management, especially avoidance of unnecessary, even minor, medical or surgical procedures [82]. Patients with chronic hypoxaemia, like patients with Eisenmenger's syndrome, need an increased number of red blood cells (expressed as a high haematocrit) for adequate oxygen transport capacity to body tissues. This is a physiologic compensation mechanism and not, like in diseases like idiopathic erythrocytosis or polycythaemia vera, a risk in itself that should be treated. Regular exchange transfusions, until recently often advocated to keep the haematocrit below a certain level (often 0.65l/L) are contraindicated and should be limited to patients who have symptoms due to the high haematocrit. These can be notoriously difficult to differentiate from another often-encountered problem: iron deficiency which occurs especially in patients who undergo regular venesection, It should be treated as it can lead to abnormal erythrocytes deformability, increasing the risk for cerebrovascular accidents. Regular monitoring of the iron status of a patient with Eisenmenger's syndrome and considering iron supplementation before the effects of the deficiency are seen in the red blood count, is now considered best practice nowadays. Oral contraceptives and pregnancy in these patients are contraindicated as the latter carries an unacceptably high risk [83].

Long-term outcome

Adults with successful VSD closure and normal pulmonary artery pressure, with no associated lesions do very well and do not require specialist follow-up. There is no reason to restrict activity and pregnancy can proceed normally.

Atrial septal defect

Defects in the atrial septum are common and comprise 7% of all congenital cardiac malformations. They can occur at a variety of sites and this affects approach to management (➲Fig. 10.8):

- ostium secundum defect;
- sinus venosus defect (superior and inferior);
- ostium primum defect;
- coronary sinus defect.

Morphology

ASDs most frequently involve the oval fossa. Secundum defects occur as a result of a deficiency of the flap valve tissue of the oval foramen, so that the flap valve does not completely cover the oval fossa or there are fenestrations within the flap valve tissue (🎥 10.5). Secundum ASDs may be multiple. Sinus venosus defects occur either high up in the atrial septum, when they are described as superior sinus venosus defects, or more uncommonly low down in the atrium septum astride the entry of the inferior caval vein into the right atrium. Superior sinus venosus defects are very frequently associated with anomalous drainage of the right-sided pulmonary veins into the right atrium adjacent to the entrance of the superior caval vein. Ostium primum defects are more appropriately considered as a form of atrioventricular septal defect (AVSD) and are described below. The most uncommon form of intra-atrial communication occurs between the left and right atrium at the level of the coronary sinus. ASDs may occur in isolation but they are also often found as part of more complex congenital structural cardiac malformations.

Pathophysiology

Reversal of the direction of shunt across the atrial septum starts to occur following the transition from the fetal to the postnatal circulation. In the presence of persisting interatrial communication, the shunt from left to right increases as pulmonary vascular resistance falls, right ventricular compliance increases and left ventricular compliance decreases. Increased flow over the pulmonary and tricuspid valves causes audible murmurs. Pulmonary vascular resistance in infants and older children remains low in the presence of an ASD and the volume load is well tolerated despite a pulmonary to systemic flow ratio, which may be as high as 3:1. In late childhood and in adults, increasing right atrial and right ventricular dilatation predispose to the development of arrhythmias, which may not necessarily resolve with closure of the defect [82].

Diagnosis

Clinical

Most ASDs in childhood are identified during cross-sectional echocardiography following the detection of an asymptomatic cardiac murmur. Symptoms, if present, are usually minor and include an increase in frequency of chest infections, mild exercise intolerance, and failure to thrive. Atrial arrhythmias, pulmonary hypertension, and the development of pulmonary vascular disease are exceedingly uncommon in childhood. These features may, however, be part of the clinical presentation of an ASD during adult life. Most adults present with symptoms of breathlessness on exertion or palpitations usually in the third or fourth decade of life.

Examination reveals:

- right ventricular heave;
- pulmonary ejection systolic flow murmur;
- fixed splitting of the second heart sound (S_2) during all respiration phases;
- tricuspid diastolic flow murmur (with large defects).

Chest radiograph

This most frequently shows a normal or mildly increased cardiothoracic ratio with prominent pulmonary vascular markings and enlargement of the central pulmonary artery.

ECG

The most common findings include right axis deviation, right ventricular hypertrophy, and an RSR′ pattern in the right precordial leads with a QRS duration <120ms (incomplete right bundle branch block). Left axis deviation with right ventricular hypertrophy is found in ostium primum defects (see ➲Atrioventricular septal defect, p.334).

Cross-sectional echocardiography

The most important findings include right atrial and right ventricular dilatation, frequently occurring with pulmonary arterial dilatation and increased flow velocity across the pulmonary valve. Right heart volume loading may result in 'paradoxical' (anterior systolic) motion of the interventricular septum. The atrial defect should be visualized directly and is most obviously seen from a subcostal approach. Examination should include assessment of defect size, location within the septum, margin surrounding the defect, defect number, and associated anomalies (e.g. anomalous pulmonary venous drainage). A sinus venosus defect may be difficult to visualize, but should be suspected in all patients with unexplained right heart enlargement. A transoesophageal echocardiogram may be necessary to demonstrate this type of ASD. Diagnostic cardiac catheterization is almost never required, unless there is considerable doubt on the reversibility of pulmonary hypertension and increased pulmonary vascular resistance.

Natural history

Secundum ASDs rarely cause overt symptoms in childhood but these increase in frequency from early adulthood with the appearance of atrial arrhythmias (flutter or fibrillation) and exercise limitation due to right heart failure. Pulmonary vascular disease may also develop in adults. Pulmonary and paradoxical embolisms are occasional complications, but infective endocarditis is extremely rare in isolated secundum ASDs [84].

Management

Transcatheter occlusion usually with an Amplatzer device is currently the treatment of choice and is feasible in approximately 80% of cases [72] (➲Fig. 10.9; 10.7, and 10.8). Newer devices are currently being evaluated. In children, ASD closure is commonly undertaken electively at 3–5 years of age. Excellent results have been achieved, in both children and adults, with a very low incidence of embolization or perforation with damage to surrounding cardiac structures. Defects not suitable for transcatheter closure (including big defects, those with poorly developed margins, or some multiple defects) should be closed by surgery. Operative risks in children are very low, with occasional morbidity from pericardial effusion or transient postoperative arrhythmia. In adults, operative risks may be higher and depend on age and other risk factors. Closure should be undertaken during the preschool years or following later detection. Closure of an ASD at a young age, prevents right ventricular failure, pulmonary hypertension, and paradoxic embolism, and results in a normal life-expectancy. Closure of ASDs in adults may improve functional class and may prevent or improve signs and symptoms of right-sided heart failure and pulmonary hypertension, but survival remains reduced [85]. Atrial arrhythmias are likely to persist or develop following late ASD closure [82]. Closure of ASDs in adults is indicated in patients with signs of right ventricular overload. In 'asymptomatic' adults without any signs of right-sided pressure or volume overload, the long-term benefit of closure is doubtful and presently closure is not recommended in these patients with small ASDs. In patients with substantial pulmonary hypertension and pulmonary pressures above two-thirds of the systemic pressures, closure is still possible when the net left-to-right shunt exceeds 1.5 or when reversibility of the increased pulmonary vascular resistance is evident. In patients with atrial flutter, a right-sided Maze operation may be combined with surgical closure of the defect. It may also restore and maintain sinus rhythm [82].

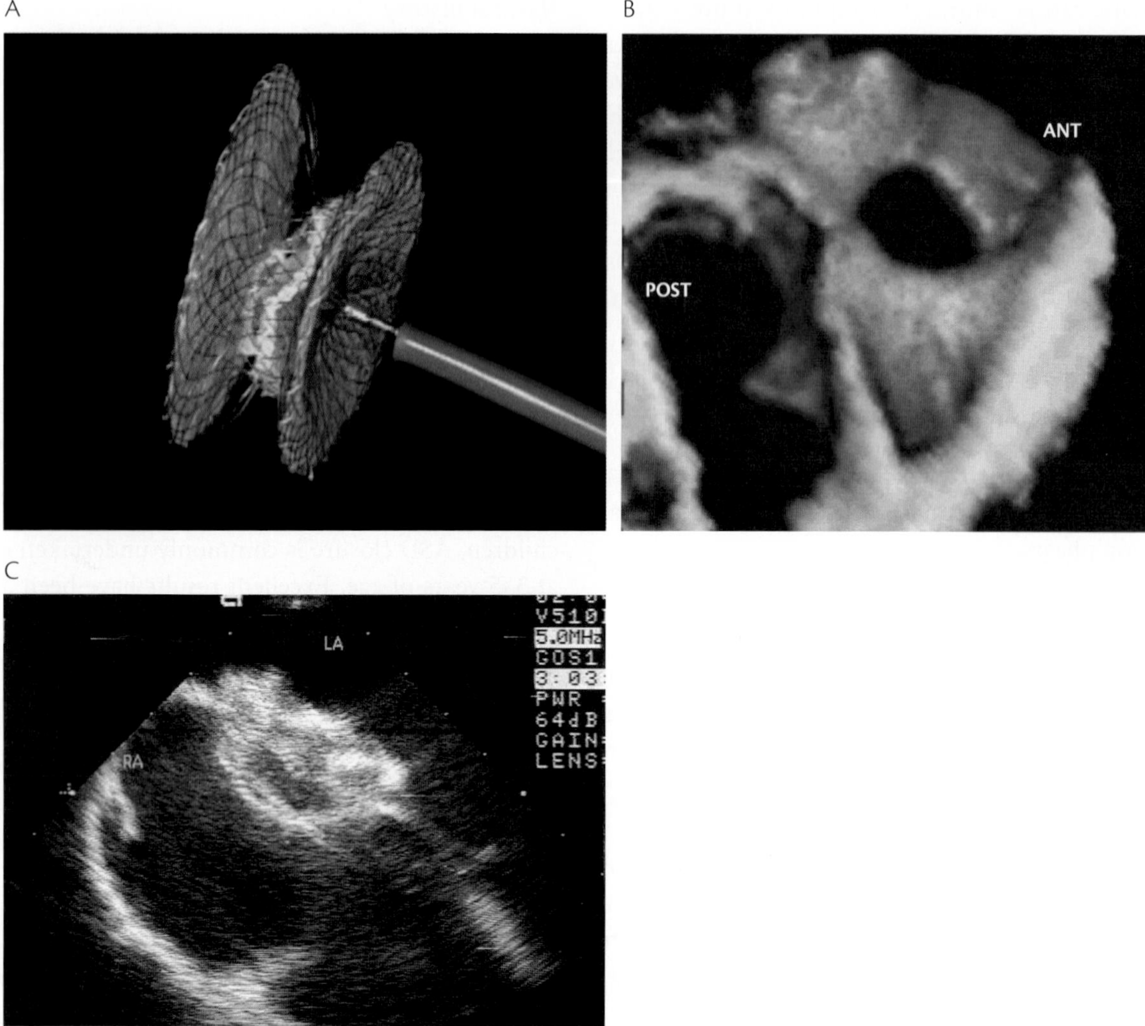

Figure 10.9 Transcatheter occlusion of atrial septal defect (ASD). (A) Amplatz ASD device attached to delivery wire and shown outside long delivery sheath. (B) Three-dimensional echocardiogram demonstrating ASD seen from right atrial aspect with clear superior and inferior margins. (C) Transoesophageal echocardiogram following delivery and release of Amplatz ASD device across defect. LA, left atrium; RA, right atrium.

Long-term outcome

After ASD closure at a young age, right ventricular size and function return rapidly to normal and patients do very well. Often in adults, the risk of atrial arrhythmia persists and long-term surveillance is indicated. This should also be undertaken if there was pulmonary hypertension or associated lesions were present. No restrictions in physical activities are required in patients after successful ASD closure. Pregnancy is well tolerated in patients after ASD closure unless there is pulmonary hypertension.

Atrioventricular septal defect

This group of abnormalities is characterized by a defect at the site of the atrioventricular septum. It accounts for approximately 4% of all congenital cardiovascular malformations and there is a strong association with trisomy 21 (Down syndrome). Well over half of children having surgery for an AVSD will have trisomy 21.

Morphology (➲ Fig. 10.10)

These defects are characterized by a lack of continuity between atrial and ventricular septal structures. The atrioventricular valve, which is common to both ventricles is fundamentally different from either a mitral or a tricuspid valve and is usually composed of five leaflets (🎥 10.9). The size of both the atrial communication above the leaflets of the valve and the ventricular defect below the leaflets can vary from non-existent to very large. When there is no ventricular defect, the common atrioventricular valve has separate orifices into each ventricle. It is more accurately described as a common atrioventricular valve with separate orifices but also referred to as a 'partial' AVSD or ostium primum ASD. Associated with the

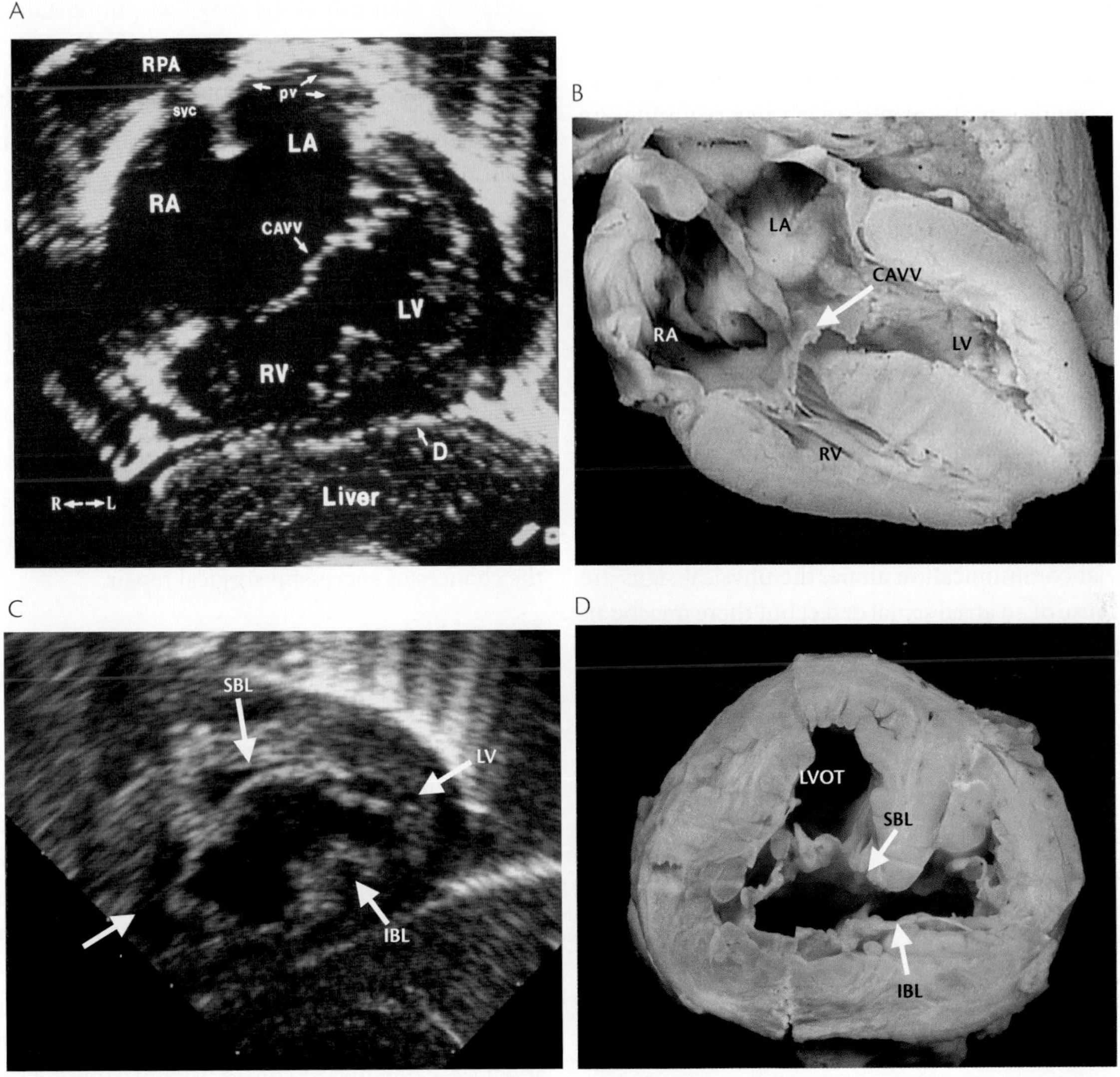

Figure 10.10 Echocardiographic and morphological correlates of atrioventricular septal defect (AVSD). (A) Subcostal four-chamber view of AVSD demonstrating large atrial and ventricular defects together with common atrioventricular valve. RPA, right pulmonary artery; SVC, superior caval vein; PV, pulmonary veins; LA, left atrium; RA, right atrium; CAVV, common atrioventricular valve; RV, right ventricle; LV, left ventricle; D, diaphragm. (B) Equivalent view of a morphological specimen (abbreviations as in A). (C) Subcostal short-axis view of AVSD demonstrating complete atrioventricular valve orifice. SBL, superior bridging leaflet; LV, left ventricle; IBL, inferior bridging leaflet. (D) Equivalent view of a morphological specimen demonstrating the same features (abbreviations as in C).

abnormal atrioventricular junction, there is displacement of the left ventricular outflow tract anterosuperiorly causing elongation and predisposing to anatomical obstruction. The morphology of the common atrioventricular valve leaflets is also variable and may affect valve function. The various types of valve abnormalities have been described according to the Rastelli classification, but an accurate description of the valvar leaflets has been shown to reflect more closely clinical outcomes [86]. Atrioventricular septal defects are commonly associated with other abnormalities both within the heart itself and in the great vessels. Some of these may influence prognosis and operability and include ventricular disproportion, abnormalities of the outflow tracts including left ventricular outflow tract obstruction, ToF, and double outlet right ventricle. It should also be noted that this cardiac malformation is frequently seen with isomerism of the atrial appendages and in this setting, is associated with abnormalities of cardiac position as well as abnormalities of systemic and pulmonary venous drainage.

Pathophysiology

The haemodynamic consequences of this lesion and therefore, the clinical presentation, depend on a number of different morphological features. Large atrial and ventricular components to the defect will cause clinical features similar to those of a large VSD. If the defect is limited to a communication at atrial level, the clinical findings are similar to those of a secundum atrial septal defect provided there is no significant atrioventricular valve regurgitation (🎥 10.10). This is a key determinant of presentation and outcome. Presentation also depends on the presence of additional abnormalities such as right or left ventricular outflow tract obstruction.

Diagnosis

Clinical

The diagnosis of an AVSD may be made as part of an early screening programme for babies with trisomy 21 in the absence of symptoms. Most children with a complete AVSD will become symptomatic in the first few months of life, with features of a large left-to-right shunt. In patients with an atrial communication alone, the physical signs are similar to those of an atrial septal defect but there may be an additional pansystolic murmur related to atrioventricular valve regurgitation. For those with a defect having both atrial and ventricular components, the signs are similar to those found in large VSDs, with additional murmurs related to atrioventricular valve regurgitation.

Chest radiograph

An isolated AVSD is associated with normal cardiac position and cardiomegaly. Pulmonary plethora is evident and is partly a reflection of the size of the ventricular component of the defect. In patients who have AVSD with atrial isomerism, there may be dextrocardia and/or pulmonary oligaemia, if there is right ventricular outflow tract obstruction/pulmonary atresia.

ECG

The ECG almost invariably demonstrates a leftward or a superior QRS axis and an AVSD is one of the few congenital cardiovascular malformations associated with a superior QRS axis in the neonatal period (others include a large VSD and tricuspid atresia). When present with left atrial isomerism, abnormalities of cardiac rhythm are frequent, including complete heart block.

Echocardiography

The echocardiographic diagnosis of an AVSD is usually straightforward and requires recognition of classic features which include:

- absence of normal atrioventricular valve offsetting;
- presence of a common atrioventricular valve with abnormal atrioventricular valve leaflets;
- abnormality in the normal inlet to outlet ratio of the ventricles.

Having established the diagnosis, important additional features include:

- atrioventricular function and the degree of regurgitation;
- ventricular and valvar disproportion which may preclude surgical repair;
- additional abnormalities involving the outflow tracts and great arteries;
- in the presence of atrial isomerism, detailed echocardiographic examination of the points of entry of both the systemic and pulmonary veins should be undertaken.

Cardiac catheterization and angiography

This investigation is not required unless there is concern about pulmonary vascular resistance which may influence the chances of successful surgical repair.

Natural history

Partial AVSDs have a similar natural history to that of secundum defects unless there is significant atrioventricular valve regurgitation, apart from the risk of infective endocarditis. Significant atrioventricular valve regurgitation results in cardiac failure and requires early surgical intervention. Patients with complete AVSD usually present with heart failure from early infancy, rapidly developing pulmonary vascular disease unless the defect is repaired early. Many have Down syndrome and for years surgical intervention was not performed. In these circumstances, pulmonary vascular obstructive disease results, with premature death and a slow downward course usually from the second decade of life. The high surgical mortality for repair at some centres justified this approach in the early era of treatment. As this has fallen substantially, a conservative strategy for children with Down syndrome cannot be justified on medical grounds.

Management

With rare exceptions, all patients with AVSD will require surgical correction. The precise approach to repair depends on the individual variation and anatomy, which is considerable. Key elements are closure of the atrial and ventricular communications and creation of a non-stenotic, competent left atrioventricular valve. Success of the left atrioventricular valve repair is the major determinant of long-term outcome and results have improved dramatically, with better understanding its trifoliate nature [87]. Morphological factors determining postoperative atrioventricular valve regurgitation include quality of atrioventricular valve tissue, deficiency of the mural leaflet, and important abnormalities of the subvalvar mechanisms. There has been a trend towards early repair for both complete and partial AVSD. Surgical results for complete AVSD repair are best with surgery undertaken at around 3 months of age [88]. Traditionally, partial AVSDs have been managed like secundum atrial septal defects, unless associated with significant atrioventricular valve regurgitation. Morphological evidence, however, suggests that early repair may be easier and a trial is awaited to assess this approach. Options for repair may also be affected by valvar or ventricular disproportion. Occasionally, a 'small ventricle' can be enlarged at repair by judicious dissection of intraventricular muscle bundles to release the interventricular septum. The ability to deal with valvar or disproportion depends largely on the chordal position and distribution. AVSDs can now be repaired successfully, even when associated with other cardiac malformations, including ToF.

Long-term outcome

Long-term results of repair are excellent, provided the left atrioventricular valve repair is adequate [89]. No restrictions to activity are necessary and infrequent follow-up visits suffice. Repeat surgery and valve replacement may be required in older patients. Early heart block is now rare and late arrhythmia is uncommon. If atrial arrhythmia develops, full haemodynamic assessment should be undertaken. Late survival in some patients will be complicated by the non-cardiac complications of Down syndrome. There are still many such patients with unoperated AVSDs in adult practice and an increasing number of patients immigrating from countries without advanced paediatric services may have unoperated AVSDs and pulmonary vascular disease. Substantial improvement in their life expectancy can be achieved by simple measures such as avoidance of unnecessary anaesthesia and other circumstances leading to systemic vasodilatation. New therapies for pulmonary vascular disease are under evaluation but as yet there are no data to support their use in patients with CHD and Eisenmenger syndrome.

Patent arterial duct

Persistent patency has been estimated to represent 7% of all congenital cardiac malformations, excluding those in premature infants.

Morphology

The arterial duct is derived from the sixth aortic arch and is almost always a unilateral left-sided structure, irrespective of the laterality of the aortic arch. Occasionally, when the arch is right sided, a right-sided arterial duct arises from the ventrolateral aspect of the aortic arch just distal to the right subclavian artery. Patency of the arterial duct is actively maintained in utero by local prostaglandin synthesis but at birth, the duct undergoes rapid constriction. A persistent arterial duct may therefore have a variable shape depending on whether constriction has occurred circumferentially or longitudinally or indeed if constriction has occurred at all. In cyanotic CHD with pulmonary atresia, the arterial duct tends to be smaller and more tortuous as it only carries the relatively small amount of blood required to supply the fetal lungs during pregnancy. In contrast, when there is aortic atresia, the arterial duct tends to be shorter and may be larger than normal.

Pathophysiology

Pathophysiological distinctions should be made between ductal patency in a pre-term infant whose mechanisms for ductal closure are immature and that of the term infant in whom patency is a true congenital malformation possibly related to an abnormality of the elastic tissue within the wall of the duct. In the former, providing the infant does not succumb to the complications of prematurity or the duct itself, ductal closure would be expected as the infants matures. The clinical findings and management of patent arterial duct in the premature infant is beyond the scope of this chapter.

In patients in whom continued ductal patency is required to maintain either the systemic or pulmonary circulation, spontaneous closure is associated with profound clinical deterioration. This can be reversed medically with the use of prostaglandin infusion within the first few days of life until either operative repair or a palliative procedure is undertaken.

Diagnosis

Clinical

Most term infants and children with continued ductal patency remain asymptomatic, with a cardiac murmur detected at routine medical examination being the most common presentation. Occasionally, continued patency of a large duct will cause heart failure in infancy. The combination of a patent arterial duct with a large atrial communication may result in a disproportionately symptomatic patient because of left-to-right shunts at multiple sites within the heart. With larger ducts, the left-to-right shunt causes an increased volume load, similar to that from a VSD. Physical signs in small ducts are minimal except for a soft continuous murmur beneath the left clavicle. In larger ducts, pulses may be brisk, the left ventricle may be hyperdynamic, and there is often a continuous machinery type murmur which obscures the S_2.

Chest radiograph

This may be unremarkable in small ducts. In large ducts, the cardiothoracic ratio is increased and there is evidence of pulmonary plethora.

ECG

Normal in cases with a small patent arterial duct but increased left ventricular forces are present when the duct is large.

Echocardiography

The arterial duct can almost always be adequately imaged. Important features to note are the size of the duct, the direction and velocity of blood flow through the arterial duct, as well as assessment of left atrial and left ventricular size. Echocardiography should exclude additional structural cardiac abnormalities of which, coarctation of the aorta is most important.

Cardiac catheterization and angiography

This has become a therapeutic rather than a diagnostic procedure.

Natural history

The natural history is no longer seen, as once the clinical diagnosis of persisting patency of the arterial duct is made, closure should be undertaken even if the shunt is small (10.11–10.15). A large duct may lead to heart failure and pulmonary vascular disease. Infective endocarditis may occur more commonly in large ducts and a persistent duct may calcify in adults. Closure of small ducts is more controversial, but is usually undertaken to reduce the risk of endocarditis [90]. In the era of high resolution echocardiography, it is not uncommon to demonstrate trivial patency of the duct in the absence of a murmur ('silent duct') [91]. The natural history is unknown. Most cardiologists would ignore this finding as endocarditis in these circumstances has not been described.

Management

In the premature baby, medical management includes fluid restriction and diuretics. Indomethacin should be given to encourage duct closure and success depends on dosage, timing and, importantly, on gestational and postnatal age. Protocols and dosing vary. Indomethacin treatment is not entirely benign and has been associated with increased bleeding, renal dysfunction, and necrotizing enterocolitis [92, 93].

In small symptomatic patients with a large duct, surgical closure is recommended, usually via a left thoracotomy. Complications are rare and complete closure is achieved in most [94]. A patent arterial duct can be closed by interventional cardiac catheterization and this is now the treatment of choice for almost all patients. Since Portsman's first procedures in 1971, a range of devices and delivery systems have been developed which can be applied to ducts of different morphologies and increasingly smaller infants. Success rate is >90% and late results are excellent. Occasional reports of device embolization, pulmonary artery and aortic narrowing, as well as device-related endocarditis have been reported [95].

Long-term outcome

If closure has been achieved, patients can be discharged and endocarditis prophylaxis is no longer required. Closure of a PDA in adults is rarely required and can usually be undertaken by interventional catheterization.

Common arterial trunk

Persistent CAT is a rare (1.6% of all congenital cardiovascular malformations) but serious abnormality in which a single vessel arises from the heart and supplies the systemic, pulmonary, and coronary circulations.

Morphology

CAT results from failure of normal septation of the developing arterial trunk. There is always a VSD, overridden by the solitary arterial trunk that gives rise to the coronary, pulmonary, and systemic arteries. Occasionally, CAT may arise predominantly or exclusively from one ventricle. The truncal valve frequently has an abnormal number of cusps and may be stenotic or regurgitant or both. In most cases, atrial situs is normal and there is laevocardia. The aortic arch may be right- or left-sided and on occasion there may be complete interruption of the aortic arch. A classification was devised by Collett and Edwards [96] according to the origin of the pulmonary arteries from the trunk, but description of the pulmonary artery pattern in each case is more important. Occasionally, CAT may be the solitary outlet from a heart with a functionally single ventricle.

Pathophysiology

Pulmonary blood flow is governed by the size of the pulmonary arteries, the presence of pulmonary artery obstruction, and the pulmonary vascular resistance. Once pulmonary vascular resistance has started to fall postnatally, patients with unobstructed pulmonary flow develop signs of early severe congestive cardiac failure. As this is a common mixing situation at great artery level, there is mild cyanosis. The clinical manifestations will be exacerbated if there is significant truncal regurgitation. Occasionally, there may be acute cardiovascular collapse in patients with CAT and aortic arch interruption.

Diagnosis

Clinical

The majority of patients present in the newborn period with mild cyanosis and increasing cardiac failure. Symptoms include poor feeding, poor weight gain, and tachypnoea with an overactive precordium. The first heart sound (S_1) is normal and there is a single S_2. There may be an associated ejection click. If there is significant truncal valve stenosis or regurgitation, there may be associated systolic ejection or early diastolic murmurs respectively. The association between this lesion and 22q11 deletion should be remembered and actively investigated.

Chest radiograph

There is usually normal cardiac position and almost always there is cardiomegaly with pulmonary plethora. High 'take-off' of the pulmonary artery may be present. Approximately 25% of patients will have a right aortic arch.

ECG

The findings are non-specific, but include evidence of right ventricular hypertrophy, often associated with ST-segment and T-wave changes.

Echocardiography

In the majority of cases, this provides all the necessary information to enable planning of neonatal surgical repair. Careful assessment of the VSD will normally confirm that this is a muscular defect. Occasionally there will be additional muscular VSDs. Detailed evaluation of the truncal valve function may be difficult in the face of the increased cardiac output passing through the single arterial valve. This may result in overestimation of the degree of stenosis. Regurgitation is usually easier to assess and is of great importance in relation to surgical repair. Careful evaluation of the aortic arch is important to ensure that there is continuity and no interruption.

Cardiac catheterization and angiography

Preoperative cardiac catheterization and angiography is now very rarely performed, but may occasionally be necessary in patients when there is suspicion that one of the pulmonary arteries arises from the descending aorta or from an arterial duct (🎥 10.16 and 10.17).

Natural history

The majority of children born with CAT would die during the first year without surgery, and many present as cardiac emergencies during the first weeks of life. The natural history is influenced by the associated malformations, especially abnormalities of the pulmonary arteries, aortic arch (including interruption), and function of the truncal valve. Survivors without pulmonary obstruction develop pulmonary obstructive disease. As a result, surgical intervention is indicated in all patients.

Management

Pulmonary artery banding no longer has a place in surgical management of CAT, and definitive neonatal repair is now performed. This consists of closure of the VSD to commit the CAT to the left ventricle, disconnection of the pulmonary arteries from the trunk, and insertion of a conduit (usually a homograft) between the right ventricle and the pulmonary artery.

Long-term outcome

Outcome depends considerably on the nature and function of the truncal valve and the survival of the right ventricle to pulmonary artery conduit. Malfunction of the truncal valve may require intervention. Surgical results have improved dramatically over the last 20 years. However, right ventricle to pulmonary artery conduit replacement will be required during childhood and adolescence, and long-term follow-up is mandatory for all. In the future, percutaneous pulmonary valve implantation may limit the lifetime number of reoperations required by such patients.

Aortic arch obstruction

Flow in the aorta can be compromised by coarctation (3% of congenital cardiac malformations) or interruption of the aortic arch.

Morphology

The most common site for aortic coarctation is between the left subclavian artery and the aortoductal junction. If the duct is open, there is infolding of the posterolateral wall of the aorta, causing a discrete ductal shelf. In neonates and small infants, there tends to be a variable degree of tubular hypoplasia. Frequently associated cardiac abnormalities include anomalous origin of the right subclavian artery, bicuspid aortic valve with or without aortic stenosis, VSD, and varying degrees of mitral valve stenosis. Coarctation occurring beyond the duct in the neonatal period is one of the few remaining surgical emergencies, as clinical improvement does not occur despite prostaglandin infusion.

Pathophysiology

The manifestations of aortic coarctation depend on the severity of obstruction. In neonates, severe obstruction may develop rapidly following closure of the arterial duct, causing cardiac failure, systemic hypoperfusion, and acidosis. In infants, aortic obstruction may develop more slowly if there is delayed ductal constriction. In the majority of cases, this occurs within the first few months of life and these infants present with cardiac failure including tachypnoea, poor feeding, excessive perspiration, and absent femoral pulses. In neonates and infants, cardiac murmurs are usually due to associated cardiac lesions rather than to the coarctation itself. Coarctation may not present until childhood or adult life if it is not severe or if there is rapid development of a collateral circulation. The diagnosis is usually made at a routine medical examination, which reveals upper limb hypertension with absent femoral pulses or a cardiac murmur. On direct questioning, patients may complain of symptoms of claudication, cold feet, and headaches. The typical continuous murmur of coarctation is audible, usually best heard over the back.

Diagnosis

Clinical

See ➲Table 10.9.

Chest radiograph

Cardiomegaly with pulmonary plethora is present in infants. In older children (>4 years), there is a normal cardiothoracic ratio with possible rib notching.

ECG

It is not widely appreciated that neonates and infants with coarctation have right ventricular dominance with extreme rightward axis, and that left ventricular hypertrophy only develops later.

Table 10.9 Clinical features of aortic coarctation at different ages

	Neonate	Infant	Older child
Presenting feature	Circulatory collapse	Cardiac failure	Hypertension
Femoral pulses	Absent	Absent	Reduced or absent
Apex beat	Normal	Hyperdynamic	Displaced → apex, LV heave
Heart sounds	S_1, normal S_2, single	S_1, S_2 normal, often with S_3	S_1, S_2 normal
Murmurs	Absent	Short ESM at LSE	Continuous murmur at back, ESM at LSE
Hypertension	Absent	Usually	Invariably
Chest X-ray	↑CTR, plethora	↑CTR	CTR normal Rib notching
ECG	Right axis	Biventricular hypertrophy	Left axis
	Right ventricular hypertrophy		Left ventricular hypertrophy

CTR, cardiothoracic ratio; ESM, ejection systolic murmur; LSE, left sternal edge; S_1, first heart sound; S_2, second heart sound.

Echocardiograph

This is the investigation of choice in neonates and infants. Views from the suprasternal notch allow assessment of the severity of arch obstruction, the size of the transverse aortic arch and associated abnormalities of the head and neck vessels (10.18). Additional information about left ventricular contractility and a search for associated abnormalities, including persistent left superior caval vein, aortic stenosis, VSD, and mitral stenosis, should be performed. In older children, assessment of left ventricular hypertrophy and the Doppler-derived coarctation gradient provide the most important information.

CMR and CT

Both these forms of non-invasive imaging provide very detailed anatomical information about aortic arch anatomy, with the added advantage of being able to demonstrate the relations of the area of coarctation to adjacent structures (10.1 and 10.19). CMR can also quantify the functional severity of the coarctation.

Cardiac catheterization and angiography

This is no longer required for preoperative assessment of aortic coarctation. However, there is increasing use of this technique as a therapeutic option (see ➲Management, p.340).

Natural history

Coarctation presenting in the neonatal period requires urgent surgical correction. In patients presenting in childhood or during adult life the natural history is poor, with systemic hypertension, as well as morbidity and premature death from coronary disease, heart failure, and cerebrovascular complications. Occasionally, the first presentation may be a catastrophic cardiovascular event such as aortic dissection or rupture. There is also a risk of endocarditis. The average age of death of patients with coarctation who have survived childhood without intervention is 34 years [97].

Management

Symptomatic neonates presenting with coarctation may have a duct-dependent systemic circulation requiring urgent medical management with prostaglandin infusion and inotropic support for impaired left ventricular function. Prompt surgical correction is required, usually via a left thoracotomy. This can be achieved by a number of surgical techniques, including resection and end-to-end anastomosis and subclavian flap angioplasty [98, 99]. Dacron patch angioplasty is no longer performed as the incidence of late aneurysm has been higher than with other techniques. A more extended arch reconstruction may be required if the aorta is hypoplastic, in addition to a discrete narrowing [100]. Operative results are excellent, although there is a small risk of paraplegia due to impairment of spinal cord blood supply [101]. The risk is higher in patients with anomalous origin of the right subclavian artery from the descending aorta. If additional cardiac lesions such as VSD are present, a 'complete repair' on cardiopulmonary bypass may be indicated [102]. Alternatively, coarctation repair and pulmonary artery banding may be performed, with later VSD closure and debanding. Recoarctation in neonates occurs in up to 20% of cases [103].

Elective repair of coarctation is the treatment of choice for children when the diagnosis is made beyond infancy. Surgery is usually favoured, although balloon dilatation of native coarctation has been advocated. For both approaches, restenosis rates are higher in younger patients and late aneurysms are recognized [104].

In patients presenting in childhood or adult life, intervention is required in cases when there is a significant resting gradient (≥30mmHg) together with rest- and/or exercise-induced hypertension. Balloon dilatation with stent implantation is an attractive option for native coarctation in the older patient and is increasingly the treatment of choice (10.20–10.22) [105].

Long-term outcome

The long-term outcomes of patients with coarctation have been disappointing even after successful repair [3]. Long-term follow-up in specialists units is important despite the apparent 'simplicity' of the malformation. Surveillance for local aortic arch abnormalities including recoarctation and aneurysm [106] is important and CMR/CT has been invaluable. The progressive nature of systemic hypertension (especially systolic hypertension on exercise) has been less well appreciated. This may develop even after successful arch repair and is the major determinant of late morbidity and mortality.

Understanding of the pathophysiology of late hypertension is incomplete, but it involves conduit artery, central aorta and resistance vessel abnormalities [107] Some of these changes may be acquired, as late hypertension is more common when coarctation repair is undertaken at an older age.

The successful use of stents for recoarctation has lowered the threshold for re-intervention after arch repair. Nevertheless, late outcome of stenting requires further research. Antihypertensive therapy is under-prescribed and the optimal regimems remain unknown.

Aortic arch interruption

Morphology

Interruption of the aortic arch occurs with equal frequency distal to the left subclavian (type A) or distal to the left common carotid (type B). Infrequently, there will be interruption distal to the innominate artery (type C). Almost all cases have associated anomalies, most frequently a posterior malalignment VSD causing subaortic obstruction and associated patency of the arterial duct. Other forms of VSD may exist but are less common. There may be abnormal ventriculoarterial connections including discordance, and double outlet right ventricle (Taussig–Bing anomaly). The presence of 22q11 deletion should be considered in all cases of aortic arch interruption.

Pathophysiology

Most commonly, when interruption is associated with patency of the arterial duct, the infant will remain well until constriction of the duct precipitates a critical reduction in lower body perfusion. In the majority of cases, infants are admitted to specialist units within the first 2 weeks of life with acute onset of heart failure, often complicated by shock and acidosis. Rarely, the arterial duct remains open and excess pulmonary blood flow develops as pulmonary vascular resistance falls.

Diagnosis

Clinical

The most specific sign is differential upper body pulses with weakness of one or both arm pulses or one carotid pulse (these findings may change with pharmacological manipulation of the duct). Auscultation is usually unhelpful, with murmurs due to the presence of associated cardiac abnormalities.

Chest radiograph

- The heart is usually left sided with evidence of cardiomegaly.
- Pulmonary vascular markings are usually increased.
- An absent thymic shadow may suggest 22q11 deletion.

ECG

There are no specific electrocardiographic features.

Echocardiography

Echocardiography should enable a complete description of the aorta, the site of interruption, as well as the origin of the head and neck vessels. Detailed evaluation of intracardiac anatomy for additional abnormalities is most important for planning of surgical strategy.

Cardiac catheterization

This is not normally required as a diagnostic investigation and has largely been superseded by echocardiography, sometimes with additional CMR or CT.

Management

Complete repair of the interrupted aortic arch together with closure of VSD is usually undertaken in the neonatal period. Operative results depend on the nature and severity of the aortic arch obstruction and the clinical condition of the child. Long-term surveillance of the arch is required because of the possibility of residual or recurrent arch obstruction, as in patients after coarctation repair.

Left ventricular outflow obstruction

Left ventricular outflow obstruction comprises 4% of all congenital cardiac malformations and may occur at subvalvar, valvar or supravalvar level (🎥 10.23–10.25). This excludes bicuspid aortic valve, which does not usually produce problems during childhood. Aortic valve stenosis may occur as an isolated lesion, but may also be associated with other left heart obstructive lesions at multiple levels (Shone's complex). In this condition, there is usually mitral valve stenosis with subaortic and/or aortic stenosis, as well as hypoplasia of the aortic arch and discrete coarctation.

Morphology

Valvar aortic stenosis is the commonest form of left ventricular outflow obstruction (75%). Valve morphology and severity are highly variable. In more severe cases, diagnosed in utero or presenting in the first hours or days after birth, there may be a small left ventricle precluding consideration for a biventricular circulation. Furthermore, there may be associated endocardial fibroelastosis affecting left ventricular function.

When the obstruction is subvalvar, three different morphological types are identifiable. The commonest form is a discrete fibromuscular shelf, which is usually circumferential and may be adherent to the aortic valve leaflets and to the anterior mitral valve leaflets. In the 'tunnel' type of subaortic stenosis, there is usually narrowing of the aortic valve in addition to a small left ventricular outflow, which is often lined with fibrous tissue. Muscular outflow tract obstruction forms part of the spectrum of hypertrophic obstructive cardiomyopathy. Supravalvar aortic stenosis accounts for only 1–2% of left ventricular outflow tract obstruction in childhood. It may be sporadic or more commonly part of Williams–Beuren syndrome. Different morphological entities have been described, including discrete and diffuse narrowing, as well as association with abnormalities of the aortic arch, including coarctation. In Williams–Beuren syndrome, there are often coexisting multiple systemic and pulmonary arterial stenosis associated with deletion of the elastin gene on chromosome 7 [108].

Pathophysiology

Severe left ventricular outflow obstruction during the neonatal period is a medical emergency and most have either critical aortic valve stenosis or outflow obstruction at multiple levels. The obstruction is so severe that the left ventricle cannot maintain systemic circulation which depends on the right-to-left flow through the ductus arteriosus. When critical aortic stenosis is diagnosed in fetal life, the outlook is poor [89]. A cardiac chamber that does not receive an adequate amount of blood flow antenatally does not grow normally. In case of a very severe aortic stenosis, almost the entire cardiac output will be taken care of by the right ventricle and both left atrium and left ventricle will hardly develop. With serial antenatal echocardiograms the evolution of worsening left heart hypoplasia can be documented in these patients. This has prompted the use of prenatal cardiac interventional catheterization in an attempt to encourage ventricular growth [109]. Postnatally, presentation of aortic valve stenosis depends on the severity of obstruction and left ventricular size and function. The degree of obstruction may be underestimated in the presence of poor left ventricular function and assessment requires evaluation of both the peak systolic pressure gradient (≥75mmHg is severe) as well as the aortic valve area (≤0.5cm^2/m^2 is severe).

The most common form of aortic valve abnormality is a bicuspid aortic valve. This can cause critical aortic stenosis, but the most common presentation is much more benign. It rarely gives rise to significant stenosis in childhood and in general there is a very small, but steady, increase in gradient across the valve throughout life. From a young adult age onwards, patients with a bicuspid aortic valve can present with sufficient stenosis as to warrant intervention. It should be appreciated that, in some cases, the ascending aorta is also abnormal with histology similar to those seen in Marfan syndrome, with cystic medial degeneration. This can lead to severe dilatation of the ascending aorta with increased risk of dissection.

Supravalvular aortic stenosis is often present from birth and can progress throughout life. The coronary arteries lie in the high pressure area, distal to the valve but proximal to the stenosis. Theoretically, this could lead to advanced atherosclerosis in the coronary circulation, but there are no data so far to support this.

Discrete subaortic stenosis is, as a rule, not present antenatally or at birth, develops throughout life. The exact denominators for the development of the subaortic stenosis are not known. The most accepted theory is that an altered shear stress in the left ventricular outflow tract as a result of a—sometimes minimal—anatomic abnormality in the left ventricle can stimulate development and growth of the subaortic stenosis. Sometimes this can occur very rapidly, within the first few months after birth and early surgical removal is indicated in these cases. There is a risk of recurrence in such cases. When subaortic stenosis develops more slowly, recurrence rates are lower.

Diagnosis

Clinical

Critical aortic stenosis in the neonate results in rapid development of cardiac failure, with a severe reduction in left ventricular function. Patients may be tachypnoeic with tachycardia and pallor and have decreased or absent peripheral pulses. The S_2 is often single and there may be a gallop rhythm. An ejection systolic murmur may be present. These findings in the neonate contrast with the majority of patients who present later in childhood, with a murmur, but are who are entirely asymptomatic. In the more severe cases, this may be associated with exercise intolerance and occasionally with chest pain. Physical signs in such patients include normal or decreased peripheral pulses, a diminished aortic component to the S_2 with a systolic ejection click and an ejection systolic murmur radiating to the neck. Supravalvar aortic stenosis is usually detected when Williams–Beuren syndrome is diagnosed and routine cardiac screening is undertaken. The findings of subaortic stenosis resemble those for aortic valve stenosis but patients do not have an ejection click.

Chest radiograph

Neonatal critical aortic valve stenosis is usually associated with laevocardia, cardiomegaly and pulmonary oedema. In older children, the chest radiograph findings are frequently normal. In case of a bicuspid aortic valve in an adult patient, dilatation of the ascending aorta can sometimes be seen.

ECG

There is usually left axis deviation and evidence of left ventricular hypertrophy. In more severe cases, there may be repolarization changes suggestive of ischaemia and strain in the lateral precordial leads.

Echocardiography

Aortic stenosis can be diagnosed by cross-sectional echocardiography. In the neonatal period, it is crucial to evaluate:

- left ventricular size/volume;
- size of the mitral valve;
- evidence of mitral regurgitation;
- size of aortic outflow and aortic valve;
- severity of aortic valve stenosis using Doppler;
- presence or absence of endocardial fibroelastosis;
- left ventricular systolic function.

This enables appropriate decision making regarding treatment. In all forms of aortic stenosis in all age groups, poor left ventricular function can lead to underestimation of the severity of the aortic stenosis.

In older children and adults, assessment of the severity of valve stenosis by Doppler-derived gradients is the most widely accepted method for assessment of severity. Evaluation of left ventricular hypertrophy and function is also important in deciding on timing of intervention. The degree of aortic regurgitation, which may coexist, will influence suitability for interventional catheter treatment (see ➲Management, p.343). Echocardiography can usually define the nature and estimate the severity of the left ventricular outflow tract obstruction in patients with subaortic stenosis. With Doppler echo, the maximal flow velocity over the left ventricular outflow tract can be measured It may, however, not be possible to derive a reliable pressure gradient from this velocity as in complex outflow obstruction, the simplified Bernouilli equation cannot be used. Severity of the stenosis in terms of pressure gradient can only be assessed with invasive measurements.

In supravalvar aortic stenosis, it is important to determine for the extent and severity of aortic arch abnormalities as well as to assess the degree of left ventricular hypertrophy, which may be out of proportion to the degree of supravalvar aortic stenosis. Recently, newer echocardiographic techniques using Doppler tissue imaging can be used to evaluate diastolic function and to relate this to the severity of the left ventricular outflow obstruction. This may help to define the optimal timing of intervention.

Cardiac catheterization and angiography

This is not required for diagnosis but is increasingly used as a treatment of valvar aortic stenosis, both in neonates and older children (see ➲Management, p.343). It is sometimes indicated in subaortic stenosis in order to measure the gradient. In supra-aortic stenosis it may be dangerous. CMR and CT have a role in the evaluation of all forms of left ventricular and aortic arch obstruction.

Management

In critical aortic valve stenosis in neonates, maintenance of patency of the arterial duct by prostaglandin may be lifesaving, before relief of the obstruction can be attempted by either balloon dilatation or surgery. Infants and children with mild aortic stenosis may remain stable for many years, with slow progression, and intervention can be delayed until adulthood. Those with moderate or severe aortic stenosis progress more rapidly, and those with a gradient >75mmHg and left ventricular hypertrophy have a risk of sudden death. Infective endocarditis is a serious complication at all ages.

Both balloon dilatation and surgery can be performed in the neonatal period. The results appear comparable in published series, although no randomized trial has been undertaken [110]. Outcome after both approaches is determined by the severity of the valve deformity as well as by the left ventricular changes, which may include endocardial fibroelastosis, and infarction of the papillary muscles of the mitral valve. If the left ventricular cavity is small or if multiple obstructive lesions are present, an alternative Norwood approach may be preferable (see ➲Hypoplastic left heart syndrome, p.345). Children who present beyond infancy should remain under careful cardiological follow-up, which should include regular ECG, echocardiography, and exercise testing. Although solid data are lacking, the common opinion is that intervention in childhood is indicated if there are symptoms, progressive gradient increase, left ventricular hypertrophy, repolarization changes on resting or exercise ECG, or an abnormal exercise blood pressure response. Valve area should be calculated as gradients can be misleading if cardiac output is reduced. Balloon dilatation is usually the procedure of choice in the older child, unless there is significant aortic regurgitation [111]. This can be undertaken by anterograde or retrograde approaches at all ages (📹 10.26), and use of balloons one size below the valve diameter reduces the risk of important new aortic regurgitation [112]. Similar principles apply to surgery in the child. Aortic valvotomy, leaving a small gradient and little or no aortic regurgitation, is the preferred result. Risk of surgery or catheter intervention is high in neonates, but significantly lower in older patients [113]. Both treatments are palliative, however, and gradual restenosis is the rule. A second valvotomy in childhood can be attempted, unless the valve is calcified or significantly regurgitant, but aortic valve replacement is almost always eventually required. However, in the US Natural History Study of Congenital Heart Disease, only 27% of children who underwent aortic valvotomy at age >2 years required a second intervention within 20 years.

In a small child, the Ross or 'autograft' operation is the approach of choice for valve replacement (implanting the pulmonary valve in the left ventricular outflow tract and a homograft in the right ventricular outflow tract) [114]. This permits growth of the neo-aortic valve and does not require anticoagulants. However, the homograft will require replacement and the long-term fate of the neo-aortic valve is still uncertain. In the older child, both bioprosthesis and the Ross operation can be considered. For adolescents and adults, the Ross operation is a less popular choice and most patients and physicians opt for a mechanical or biological prosthesis [115]. The most important reason not to choose for a Ross operation in adult patients is progressive dilatation of neo-aorta—the part of the original pulmonary trunk that is attached to the pulmonary valve and that forms the most proximal part of the aortic trunk after the Ross procedure—and of the native ascending aorta, with its abnormal vascular wall that is prone to aneurysmatic dilatation. This may lead to progressive aortic regurgitation. Reoperation after a first Ross operation may be required for pulmonary homograft failure, aortic autograft failure, or ascending aorta dilatation. These problems may occur simultaneously and a complete re-do is often performed with a new homograft in pulmonary position in combination with a Bentall procedure (prosthetic valve in combination with synthetic aortic root replacement). The choice of surgical approach depends on a number of factors including age, desirability, and safety of anticoagulation and future pregnancy plans, as well as patient preference and local expertise. Occasionally more extensive surgery, such as a Konno procedure, is required when left ventricular outflow tract obstruction occurs at multiple levels, or if the aortic valve is small [116].

The severity of supravalvar aortic stenosis characteristically increases with time and patients may be at risk from sudden death [3]. The systemic arterial stenosis in key vessels such as the carotid and renal arteries may also progress. Indications for intervention are similar to those for aortic stenosis. Interventional catheterization, however, is not an option and surgery is required. This involves insertion of patches to enlarge the supravalvar area extending into the sinuses of Valsalva [107]. Induction of anaesthesia and onset of cardiopulmonary bypass may jeopardize coronary perfusion, and surgery may be difficult because a diffuse aortopathy is present in many cases.

Because of the progressive nature of subaortic stenosis, intervention is usually indicated at lower levels of severity than for aortic valve stenosis. This is controversial, as in some cases the malformation may be mild or stable for many years [117]. Most would recommend intervention if aortic regurgitation develops, as it can progress rapidly [118].

Interventional catheterization is not appropriate and surgical resection is required. The immediate and early results are excellent, but recurrence is common [119]. Complete removal of the obstruction at surgery is essential and recurrence risk appears lower when a myotomy or myectomy is also performed [120].

Life-long outcome

Lifelong follow-up is required for all types of left ventricular outflow tract obstruction, whether treated or untreated. This should include assessment of the structure and function of the left ventricular outflow tract (including valve stenosis and regurgitation) as well as of left ventricular size, structure, and function. Ventricular arrhythmias are more common in patients with left ventricular hypertrophy and may cause clinical problems including rarely sudden death. Vigorous activities are probably contraindicated in the presence of left ventricular hypertrophy or residual obstruction (>30mmHg), but social exercise should be permitted in most cases [121].

Pregnancy counselling is indicated as there may be an important impact on cardiac haemodynamics. There is also a recognized recurrence risk.

Hypoplastic left heart syndrome

This term is used to describe a group of closely related abnormalities whose common morphological feature is severe hypoplasia of the left heart structures. It accounts for between 2–4% of all congenital cardiovascular malformations.

Morphology

The pathogenesis of this group of abnormalities is poorly understood. Hypoplasia of left heart structures can be achieved by restricting inflow to the left side of the heart in animal models, but the increased recurrence risk in siblings and relatives [122] would suggest that there is more likely to be a genetic basis for this condition. The heart is usually left sided and enlarged with the cardiac apex formed by the right ventricle. The left atrium is small with or without a narrowed or occluded atrial foramen. There is either severe mitral stenosis or mitral atresia. The left ventricle is usually small and frequently, there is a diminutive ascending aorta with aortic atresia. The tricuspid valve is usually normal and there is right ventricular hypertrophy. The main pulmonary arteries are dilated with enlargement of the arterial duct. The pulmonary venous return is usually to the left atrium, but in association with an intact atrial septum (in about 10% of cases), there may be anomalous pulmonary venous return. There is almost invariably associated aortic coarctation.

Pathophysiology (➲ Fig. 10.11)

HLHS is a good example of the remarkable adaptability of the fetal circulation, permitting survival in the fetus despite such a complex cardiac abnormality. Cerebral and coronary circulation is maintained retrogradely round the aortic arch via the arterial duct. There are reports of congenital structural abnormalities in the brain in about 30% of patients [123]. Postnatally, the systemic circulation remains dependent on continued patency of the arterial duct. The pulmonary venous return must enter the right ventricle (usually through the atrial septum), to maintain the systemic circulation. An imperforate or restrictive atrial septum results in early pulmonary congestion. The proportion of flow to the pulmonary and systemic circulations is dependent on the balance between the systemic and pulmonary vascular resistances. Assuming the duct remains patent, as pulmonary vascular resistance falls postnatally, there will be progressive pulmonary over circulation and decreased systemic perfusion with acidosis.

Diagnosis

Clinical

Many infants with this condition will have had the diagnosis made prenatally by fetal echocardiography (10.27). This provides the opportunity to optimize postnatal management and limit complications. The clinical presentation described below reflects the situation when the diagnosis has not been anticipated prenatally. Immediately postnatally, most babies with this condition are well and relatively asymptomatic unless there is an intact or very restrictive atrial septum. Symptoms start following closure of the arterial duct, when babies will develop signs of acute congestive cardiac failure rapidly with increasing cyanosis, acidaemia, and respiratory distress. Prompt respiratory support and use of prostaglandin is needed to re-establish the fetal circulation and maintain ductal patency on which such infants depend. Physical signs in the newborn infant include:

- tachypnoea with dyspnoea;
- cyanosis with absent lower limb pulses and pallor;
- hyperdynamic precordium;
- normal S_1, single S_2, and a gallop rhythm;
- ejection systolic murmur (usually soft);
- hepatomegaly.

Chest radiograph

- Laevocardia with cardiomegaly.
- Large right atrial shadow.
- Pulmonary venous congestion/pulmonary oedema.

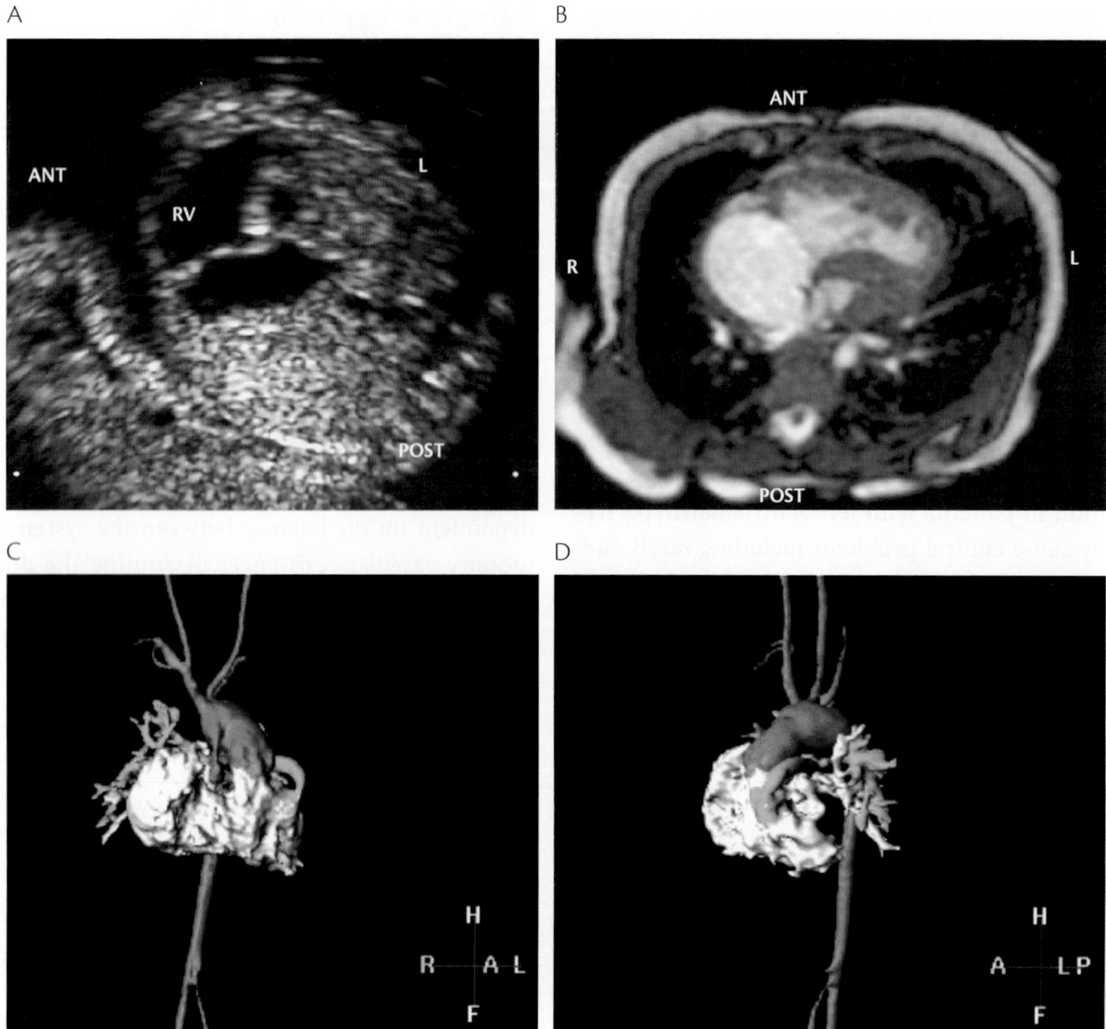

Figure 10.11 Images of hypoplastic left heart. (A) Four-chamber view through the fetal thorax demonstrating hypoplastic left heart. The left ventricle is seen as a small echogenic area adjacent to dilated right ventricle. ANT, anterior; RV, right ventricle; L, left; R, right; POST, posterior. (B) Axial MRI in postnatal scan of infant with hypoplastic left heart. The small hypertrophied left ventricle can be seen posterior to the dilated and apex-forming right ventricle (abbreviations as in A). (C, D) Three-dimensional MRI reconstructions of patient with hypoplastic left heart following Norwood stage I reconstruction with Sano modification. Images are colour coded, with white depicting the right ventricle, green the right ventricle to pulmonary artery conduit and branch pulmonary arteries, and red the aortic arch reconstruction and descending aorta. (C) View from the left side; note diminutive ascending aorta adjacent to much larger pulmonary valve incorporated into aortic arch reconstruction. (D) View from the left side; note anteriorly placed right ventricle to pulmonary artery conduit supplying branch pulmonary arteries. H, head; A, anterior; L, left; F, foot; P, posterior.

ECG

- This commonly shows rightward QRS axis with conspicuous right ventricular hypertrophy.
- Frequently, evidence of myocardial ischaemia.

Echocardiography

Having confirmed HLHS, the echocardiographic examination should be tailored towards identification of those features which will impact on the likelihood of surgical survival for such infants (10.28). This can be performed systematically in all patients with this condition:

- confirmation of normal pulmonary venous return;
- assessment of the size and flow characteristics of any atrial communication;
- evaluation of tricuspid valve function and incompetence;
- interrogation of the pulmonary valve excluding significant stenosis or incompetence;
- careful measurement of the dimensions of the ascending aorta and aortic arch;
- flow characteristics through the arterial duct;
- establishing whether aortic coarctation is present;
- assessment of ventricular function.

Cardiac catheterization and angiography

Diagnostic catheterization has little or no role in the initial management of such infants who are often critically unwell. Therapeutic catheterization has been used as part of the treatment for stage I palliation in this condition.

Natural history and management

The natural history of this condition without intervention is early postnatal demise following closure of the arterial duct, usually within the first week of life. The advent of prostaglandin infusions and the development of staged palliative procedures for surgical management have dramatically altered the outlook. Even with persistence of the arterial duct using prostaglandin infusion, appropriate and timely management of these infants is required to optimize survival and prevent progressive pulmonary over circulation with associated cardiac failure. Postnatal management of babies with HLHS can be divided into active surgical management (staged palliative surgery or rarely transplantation) and into compassionate care where no active postnatal intervention is undertaken.

A limited number of centres consider transplantation as first-line treatment for this condition: for most, the problem of donor availability limits this as a therapeutic option. Surgical palliation was pioneered in the 1980s and has resulted in steadily improving survival [124]. Initial surgery (the Norwood procedure) is performed in the neonatal period and requires trans-section of the pulmonary trunk, which is anastamosed to the hypoplastic aorta which in turn is augmented with a homograft patch. Supply to the detached pulmonary arteries is achieved through a modified right-sided Blalock–Taussig shunt or more recently by placement of a restrictive right ventricle to pulmonary artery conduit using a small GoreTex® tube (Sano modification; 10.29) [125]. The first stage is followed by a superior cavopulmonary anastamosis at 4–6 months and completion of the cavopulmonary connection with an inferior cavopulmonary connection at 2–3 years of age. Survival for stage I is now 80–90% in most centres and is usually higher for the second and third stages. Combined surgical and therapeutic catheterization (hybrid procedure) has been used with good effect in some centres achieving similar outcomes. Through a median sternotomy, bilateral pulmonary artery banding is performed surgically, followed by placement of a stent into the arterial duct through a purse-string suture in the main pulmonary artery to maintain ductal patency. An additional atrial septostomy is performed as required. Whilst this avoids the need for neonatal cardiopulmonary bypass surgery, the second stage becomes more difficult with aortic arch reconstruction, removal of the duct stent, and a superior cavopulmonary anastamosis.

In all series, there is continuing attrition of patients between stages and following the third stage. Furthermore, evidence would suggest that neurological outcome in the majority of patients treated along a Norwood protocol is not normal [40].

Long-term outcome

Few patients who have undergone a Norwood repair have yet reached adult life, but adult cardiologists need to be aware of the current enormous investment in the care of such patients during childhood and of the greatly improved early results. Survivors will all require follow-up in a specialist GUCH centre and problems can be anticipated. Their 'univentricular repair' leaves the morphologic right ventricle serving as the systemic ventricle. It is likely that there will be a gradual decline in ventricular function, with a significant number of patients developing features of the failing Fontan circulation.

Long-term management options for this group of patients include cardiac transplantation, but their previous surgery and the shortage of suitable donors reduces the likelihood of this as an exit strategy in all but a few patients.

Pulmonary valve stenosis

This is a common isolated cardiac abnormality representing almost 10% of all congenital cardiovascular malformations. However, it may also occur in association with a range of other complex defects.

Morphology

The most typical finding is fusion of the commissures of a trileaflet valve, associated with a small valve orifice, which may be central or eccentric. The degree of commissural fusion varies from severe, with presentation in the neonatal period or early infancy, to mild, which may result in minimal clinical sequelae other than an asymptomatic cardiac murmur. Right ventricular hypertrophy and frequently tricuspid incompetence are the consequences of severe obstruction. In Noonan syndrome, there is a characteristic pulmonary valve abnormality with little commissural fusion but thickened dysplastic valve cusps [126].

Isolated supravalvar pulmonary stenosis and branch pulmonary artery stenoses may occur (10.30). Frequently, this is associated with an identifiable genetic syndrome such as Noonan syndrome, Williams syndrome, Alagille syndrome, and 22q11 deletion.

Pathophysiology

The haemodynamic and clinical consequences of pulmonary stenosis depend mainly on the severity of the obstruction. When severe and presenting in the neonatal period, there is severe right ventricular hypertrophy with cavity obliteration. The oval foramen remains patent and decreased right ventricular compliance with increased right ventricular systolic pressures results in a significant right-to-left shunt at atrial level. In very severe stenosis, the pulmonary circulation may be duct dependent postnatally. When the valve is only moderately narrowed, there is usually continued valve growth through childhood and early infancy with the degree of narrowing remaining constant or even improving with age [127].

Diagnosis

Clinical

In its most severe form, cyanosis will be evident in the immediate postnatal period, with profound cyanosis developing following ductal closure. Such infants require urgent evaluation and treatment. Physical examination will confirm cyanosis and there may be associated respiratory distress. The S_1 is normal and there is a single S_2. Frequently, there is a pansystolic murmur due to associated tricuspid regurgitation.

In the older child with less severe stenosis, the predominant finding is a systolic ejection murmur loudest at the upper left sternal edge and which may radiate to the back. S_1 and S_2 are normal and there may be an associated ejection click. Occasionally, a thrill may be evident at the upper left sternal edge.

Chest radiograph

In severe neonatal pulmonary stenosis, there may be marked cardiac enlargement with a very prominent right atrial shadow. There is usually associated pulmonary oligaemia. In infants and children, the chest radiograph is usually normal but it may be possible to identify a prominent pulmonary artery shadow due to dilatation of the main pulmonary artery.

ECG

The right ventricular forces in the anterior precordial leads tend to correlate well with the degree of obstruction. In severe stenosis, there is associated right axis deviation and right atrial hypertrophy.

Echocardiography

Echo permits delineation of severity. Doppler studies can however, be misleading in the presence of very severe stenosis and continued ductal patency. Atrial septum should be assessed for presence of an atrial communication. In addition, the size of the tricuspid valve annulus, the presence of tricuspid valve regurgitation, and the size of the right ventricular cavity should be determined. In less severe cases, the Doppler-derived pulmonary valve gradient is used to monitor severity in those patients for whom medical surveillance rather than intervention is indicated.

Cardiac catheterization and angiography

This is no longer a diagnostic test but plays a major therapeutic role (see ➲Management, p.348).

Natural history

Neonates or infants may present with critical pulmonary stenosis and require urgent intervention. Outcome depends on the size and function of the right ventricle. The natural history of patients with mild and moderate pulmonary stenosis is much better and most are asymptomatic. Progression during childhood is rare and 25-year survival approached the normal population in the collaborative US study [127]. Obstruction may progress at valvar level and subvalvar narrowing with right ventricular hypertrophy may also develop.

There are few data for prognosis of pulmonary artery stenosis. Interestingly, in the Williams–Beuman syndrome, pulmonary artery narrowing tends to improve with time, in contrast to supravalvar aortic stenosis which may also be present [3].

Management

This has been revolutionized by balloon dilatation, which is now the treatment of choice and which obviates the need for surgery in the majority of patients. In neonates with critical stenosis, patency of the arterial duct should be maintained with prostaglandin infusion prior to intervention. There is some debate about levels of right ventricular outflow gradient that require intervention. In general, most cardiologists would undertake an interventional catheter if the gradient is >40mmHg. The results are excellent unless the valve is very dysplastic (as in some cases of Noonan syndrome). Subvalvar obstruction will often regress over months after valvar pulmonary stenosis has been relieved.

Surgery is limited to patients who have failed to respond adequately to interventional catheterization and consists of pulmonary valvotomy or valve excision. In adults, surgery is occasionally required if the valve is calcified or if multiple levels of obstruction are present. Infective endocarditis prophylaxis is necessary.

Peripheral pulmonary stenosis may also be amenable to balloon dilatation. Results may be disappointing due to recoil/restenosis and multiple sites of obstruction are often present. In the older patient, stent implantation can produce dramatic improvement even in arteries that would be inaccessible to the surgeon.

Long-term outcome

Long term results of relief or pulmonary stenosis are excellent, with a very low recurrence rate and a low need for repeat balloon valvotomy (approximately 5%), in the absence of a dysplastic pulmonary valve [128]. In comparison to surgery, the incidence and severity of pulmonary regurgitation is significantly lower. The adverse impact of late pulmonary regurgitation after surgery to the right ventricular outflow tract has been underestimated until recently. During long-term follow-up, significant right ventricular dilatation, triscupsid regurgitation and atrial arrhythmias may develop and contribute to functional decline. Pulmonary valve replacement (PVR) may be required and can produce significant clinical benefits, provided right ventricular dilatation and dysfunction are not too severe. In the future, new percutaneous catheter based approaches to pulmonary valve implantation may have a role and obviate the need for surgery.

Pregnancy is well tolerated and no specific limitation of exercise and sport is required, unless pulmonary stenosis is severe (in which case intervention would be indicated).

Pulmonary atresia with intact ventricular septum

This severe abnormality accounts for 2–3% of all cardiovascular malformations at birth. There is pulmonary atresia with a spectrum of abnormalities of the right ventricle.

Morphology

There is usually cardiac enlargement, which may vary from mild to massive, occasionally with huge enlargement of the right atrium, almost always with an atrial communication. The tricuspid valve is frequently small and may be dysplastic and regurgitant. The right ventricular cavity varies in size from being diminutive to almost normal, due to a variable degree of hypertrophy of its component parts. The extent of atresia of the pulmonary outflow tract varies from valvar alone to more severe forms where the atresia extends into the right ventricular infundibulum. Abnormalities of the coronary arteries involving fistulae between the right ventricular cavity and the coronary circulation are common and may influence management. These abnormal connections can result in cardiac ischaemia leading to the concept of 'a right ventricular coronary dependent circulation' [129] (🎥 10.31). The pulmonary arteries themselves are usually confluent and supply all the pulmonary segments (unlike those in ToF with pulmonary atresia). However, the branch pulmonary arteries are smaller than normal.

Pathophysiology

As the pulmonary valve is imperforate, systemic venous return will enter the left atrium through the oval foramen. The maintenance of any pulmonary blood flow postnatally relies on continued patency of the arterial duct. Duct closure postnatally results in acute hypoxia, cyanosis, acidosis, and rapid demise without early intervention.

Diagnosis

Clinical

Clinical cyanosis is evident in the immediate newborn period, becoming severe as the duct closes. Cardiac findings largely depend on tricuspid valve size and function. When there is severe tricuspid regurgitation with massive cardiomegaly, the precordium will be hyperactive. In contrast, with a minimally regurgitant tricuspid valve, the cardiovascular examination may be remarkably normal. Physical signs include:

- cyanosis;
- variable respiratory distress depending on severity of cardiac enlargement;
- normal S_1 and S_2;
- obvious pansystolic murmur when there is severe tricuspid regurgitation;
- hepatomegaly.

Chest radiograph

There is laevocardia with variable cardiac enlargement which can be correlated with the severity of the tricuspid regurgitation. With severe cardiomegaly, there may be pulmonary hypoplasia and pulmonary oligaemia.

ECG

There is a leftward QRS axis and decreased right ventricular forces. Evidence of right atrial enlargement with very large P-waves is common.

Echocardiography

Cross-sectional echocardiography is used to confirm a diagnosis of pulmonary atresia with an intact ventricular septum (🎥 10.32). A systematic approach should include assessment of:

- size of the atrial communication;
- size of the tricuspid valve annulus;
- severity of tricuspid regurgitation and right ventricle to right atrial pressure drop (by Doppler);
- individual components of the right ventricle including inlet, trabecular, and outlet portion;
- size of pulmonary valve annulus, main pulmonary artery, and branches;
- patency of the arterial duct;
- echocardiography may not demonstrate important right ventricular to coronary communications.

Cardiac catheterization and angiography

In many cases, initial palliation with placement of a systemic-to-pulmonary artery shunt is undertaken without the need for diagnostic angiography. Right ventricular decompression by interventional cardiac catheterization (see ➲Management, p.350) is often performed, providing it has been established that there are no major right ventricle to coronary artery communications.

Natural history

Without maintenance of ductal patency, the natural history of this condition would be early demise soon after ductal closure within the first few days to weeks of life.

Management

A prostaglandin infusion should be started following diagnosis, pending detailed echocardiographic assessment. The surgical approach will depend on right ventricular size, as well as the presence of right ventricle to coronary artery connections [130, 131]. In patients with tricuspid valve hypoplasia and muscular obliteration of the right ventricular apex and outflow tract, management will need to be planned along a single ventricle strategy, with surgical placement of a systemic to pulmonary artery shunt and therapeutic catheterization to perform a balloon atrial septostomy, if the atrial communication is restrictive. This patient would subsequently require a superior cavopulmonary anastamosis followed later by completion of the total cavopulmonary anastamosis.

In patients with an adequately-sized tricuspid valve, a reasonable right ventricular cavity and a patent outflow up to the level of the pulmonary valve, radiofrequency perforation and balloon dilatation of the pulmonary valve has become the treatment of choice (10.33–10.36). This has been shown to promote right ventricular growth, but it may be necessary to provide an additional source of pulmonary blood flow (systemic-to-pulmonary artery shunt or stenting the arterial duct) until right ventricular growth occurs.

Long-term outcome

The long term outcome for all approaches has been disappointing with late problems in those with a single ventricle circulation and difficulty in being able to predict adequate right ventricular growth and function in those managed along a biventricular track. Even with a good-sized right ventricle, there is frequently diastolic right ventricular dysfunction, predisposing to atrial dilatation and arrhythmias, and resulting in reduced exercise capacity. Furthermore, optimal management of the abnormal coronary circulation remains unclear [127].

Tetralogy of Fallot

Morphology

ToF constitutes 7% of all congenital cardiac malformations and consists of right ventricular outflow obstruction, a subaortic VSD with overriding aorta, and right ventricular hypertrophy. These morphological features arise from anterior and cephalad deviation of the infundibular septum, which results in muscular outflow tract obstruction. This may be aggravated by a small pulmonary valve ring and valvar pulmonary stenosis. Right ventricular hypertrophy reflects the myocardial response to right ventricular hypertension. The VSD is typically large and perimembranous but may be a muscular outlet defect. The degree of aortic override varies, and in some cases the majority of the aorta is committed to the right ventricle (double outlet right ventricle). Associated abnormalities of the origin and calibre of the pulmonary arteries are common, and the right or left pulmonary artery may originate from the arterial duct or from the aorta. Abnormal coronary artery distribution (such as origin of the left anterior artery from the right coronary system in approximately 5%) may influence the timing and approach of surgical repair. In its most severe form, ToF is associated with atresia of the right ventricular outflow tract, and these patients have marked variations in the arterial blood supply to the lungs. In the most favourable situation, the pulmonary arteries are central and confluent, and supply is derived from the arterial duct. At the other end of the spectrum, the pulmonary arterial supply is derived entirely from aortopulmonary collateral arteries, with no discernible central pulmonary arteries (10.37). In a significant proportion of cases, the pulmonary blood supply is mixed, with some lung segments being supplied by aortopulmonary collateral arteries whilst others are supplied by pulmonary arteries, which may or may not communicate with the aortopulmonary collateral arteries.

Pathophysiology

Right ventricular ejection in the presence of right ventricular outflow obstruction results in shunting of blood into the ascending aorta, causing systemic arterial desaturation. Right and left ventricular pressures are equal. The degree of arterial desaturation will depend on the severity of the outflow tract obstruction, which tends to increase with time. The pulmonary blood flow may be augmented by persistent patency of the arterial duct or by coexisting aortopulmonary collateral arteries.

Diagnosis

Clinical

This depends mainly on the severity of the right ventricular outflow obstruction. A haemodynamically 'well-balanced' situation may be present and these patients may merely have an asymptomatic murmur. However, cyanosis usually becomes detectable as the right ventricular outflow obstruction gradually increases. ToF, with cyanosis from birth or in early infancy, may require early intervention. Hypercyanotic spells, resulting from the dynamic nature of the infundibular obstruction, may be triggered by crying or feeding and may result in syncope, convulsions, and occasionally death. In contrast, some patients with minimal or mild right ventricular outflow obstruction may have a significant left-to-right shunt with no cyanosis and occasionally develop cardiac failure in infancy.

Physical signs include:

- cyanosis, polycythaemia, and clubbing;
- parasternal heave due to right ventricular hypertrophy;
- ejection systolic murmur at upper left sternal edge, due to right ventricular obstruction;
- single S_2.

Chest radiograph

This typically shows:

- left-sided heart (boot-shaped);
- concave pulmonary artery segment (hollow pulmonary bay);
- pulmonary oligaemia (with cyanosis);
- right-sided aortic arch (in 25% of cases).

ECG

This is not diagnostic but shows sinus rhythm, rightward QRS axis, and right ventricular hypertrophy.

Echocardiography

This is the most important single investigation. Patients are often referred for surgery, when primary repair is planned or following systemic to pulmonary shunt, without preoperative cardiac catheterization. The important features to establish include:

- size and position of the VSD (10.38);
- severity and nature of right ventricular outflow obstruction (10.39);
- size of the main pulmonary artery, pulmonary artery branches and their confluence;
- side of the aortic arch;
- coronary artery distribution;
- identification of additional abnormalities (including ASD, additional VSD, arterial duct, aortopulmonary collateral arteries, and persistence of the left superior caval vein).

Cardiac catheterization and angiography

This is rarely required for preoperative diagnosis. The use of CMR or CT, with contrast angiography and three-dimensional reconstruction, has further reduced the need for diagnostic cardiac catheterization, even after initial palliation by a systemic to pulmonary artery shunt. Haemodynamic evaluation may occasionally be required when there is concern about pulmonary hypertension, in cases with non-confluent branch pulmonary arteries, and also in patients in whom aortopulmonary collateral arteries have been detected (10.40 and 10.41). In such patients, the demonstration of central pulmonary arteries, even if small, has a major impact on management (10.42) and angiography, with pulmonary venous wedge injection should be considered early in infancy. A further indication for cardiac catheterization is the evaluation of the coronary artery distribution, when this cannot be adequately detected by echocardiography.

Natural history

Treatment for ToF is surgical and it is rare to encounter the natural history in developed countries. Right ventricular outflow obstruction is progressive and results in increasing cyanosis. There may also be increasingly frequent cyanotic spells, which may be fatal. Without surgery, only 10% of patients are alive by 25 years, although prolonged survival is possible. The natural history is further complicated by the risk of infective endocarditis and cerebral abscess as well as the systemic complications of cyanosis with polycythaemia (see ➲ Clinical, p.350).

Management

Hypercyanotic spells should be treated by placing the child in the knee–elbow position, establishing intravenous access, and administering oxygen. Morphine sulphate (0.1mg/kg) can be helpful but the main treatment is intravenous beta-blocker (propranolol 0.1mg/kg). Acidosis should be corrected with sodium bicarbonate. Propranolol may be given as prophylaxis against further spells, prior to surgery. Palliation, by creation of a surgical systemic to pulmonary shunt, ushered in the era of surgical treatment of congenital cardiac malformations [132]. ToF has been corrected since the 1950s (closure of VSD and relief of right ventricular outflow obstruction) [133]. The important decision for each case is whether a prior palliative shunt is required. As the results of neonatal and infant cardiac surgery have improved, the trend has been towards earlier primary repair, reserving palliation for cases with complicating features. These include hypoplastic pulmonary arteries, anomalous coronary arteries, and other associated lesions. Units differ in their approach [134]. Many routinely perform primary repair in infants presenting at >3 months of age. Operative mortality is now very low and long-term survival is excellent, approaching that of the general population in favourable subgroups [135].

Long-term outcome

The most important issue after surgical correction in long-term care is now recognized to be the impact of pulmonary regurgitation [136, 137]. This is very common and is well tolerated in most patients for decades. In others, however, it leads to progressive right ventricular dilatation, right heart failure, tricuspid regurgitation, and supraventricular arrhythmia [138]. PVR is required in these circumstances and produces significant clinical benefits in most patients [139]. However, right ventricular function does not appear to improve in all patients and hence optimal timing of pulmonary valve implantation to preserve cardiac function is a key issue for ongoing research [140]. Evidence is accumulating that earlier treatment may be more beneficial, but the beneficial effects of PVR have to be weighed against the risk for repeat surgery PVR [141]. The new option of percutaneous pulmonary valve implantation may influence management in the near future (Fig. 10.12) (10.43–10.47) [142]. Peripheral pulmonary branch stenosis is not uncommon in Fallot patients and can be treated by stent implantation during PVR.

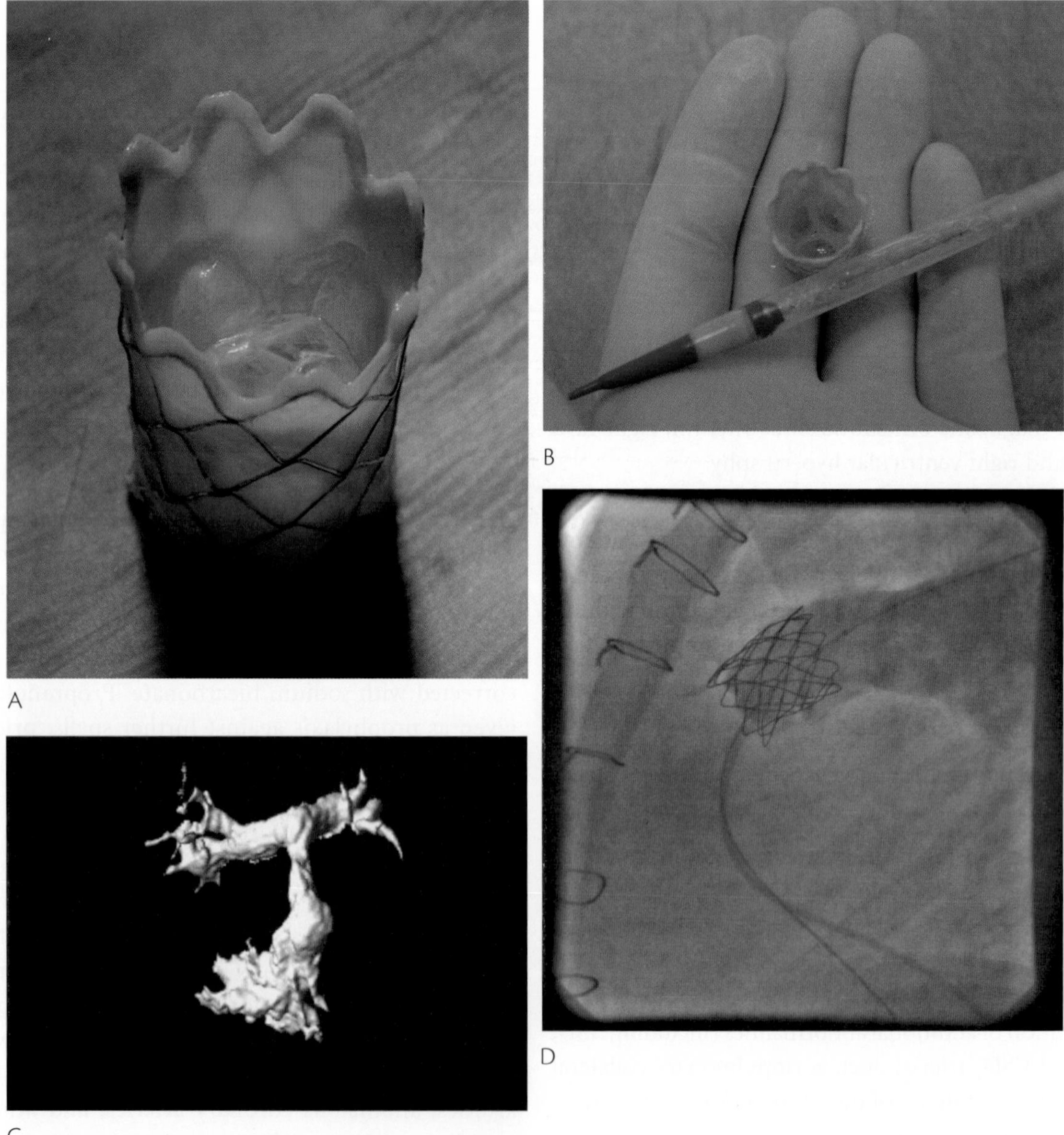

Figure 10.12 (A) Stent-mounted tissue valve used for percutaneous pulmonary valve insertion. (B) Delivery catheter with covered balloon developed for percutaneous pulmonary valve insertion. (C) Three-dimensional MRI reconstruction of right ventricular outflow tract and branch pulmonary arteries for improved visualization of ideal placement of stent-mounted valve. (D) Lateral angiogram following placement of stent-mounted valve confirming good relief of obstruction and valve competency.

Sudden death is not common and occurs in 0.5–0.6% over 30 years. It accounts for approximately one-third of late deaths [143]. Non-sustained ventricular arrhythmia is very common but not an indicator of risk, so that routine antiarrhythmic therapy is not indicated for asymptomatic patients [144]. The usual arrhythmia focus is the right ventricular outflow tract in the area of infundibulectomy or the VSD closure site. The combination of pulmonary regurgitation, right ventricular dilatation, and late ventricular arrhythmia with QRS duration >180ms on the ECG may identify increased risk [145, 146](➲Fig. 10.13). Reoperation of correctable lesions is often the best treatment for ventricular arrhythmias. Atrial tachyarrhythmias may contribute substantially to late morbidity and even mortality. Supraventricular arrhythmia (atrial flutter or fibrillation) is relatively common and occurs in up to one-third of adult patients with previous repair[147]. It may be the first sign of haemodynamic deterioration and a thorough cardiac examination of underlying causes is warranted. Improvement of haemodynamics by means of reoperation will lead to disappearance of arrhythmias in most patients.

If palpitation or syncope develops, patients should receive prompt attention and full haemodynamic and electrophysiological review are indicated. In most centres, this would include an electrophysiological study if no sustained arrhythmia is documented on non-invasive monitoring. Management of sustained ventricular tachycardia (which is rare) should include consideration of correction of underlying haemodynamic abnormalities, where feasible radiofrequency ablation, and an implantable cardiac defibrillator [148, 149].

Pregnancy is well tolerated in women with a good haemodynamic repair and functional status, even in the presence

A

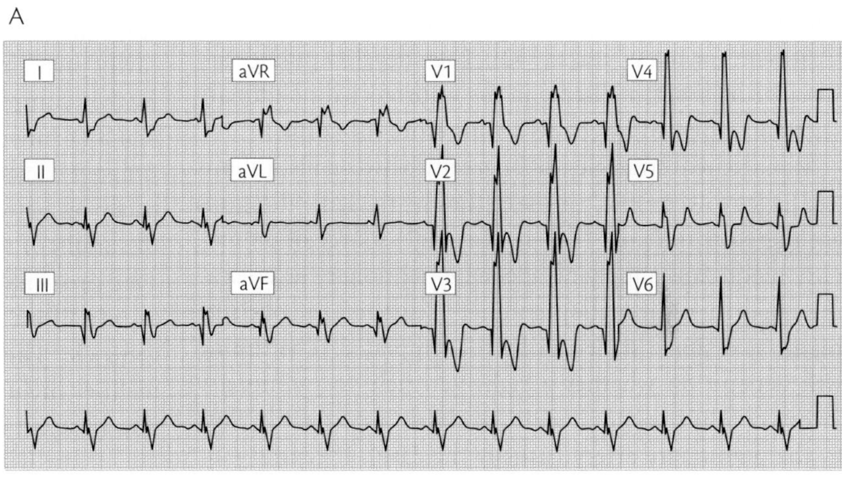

B

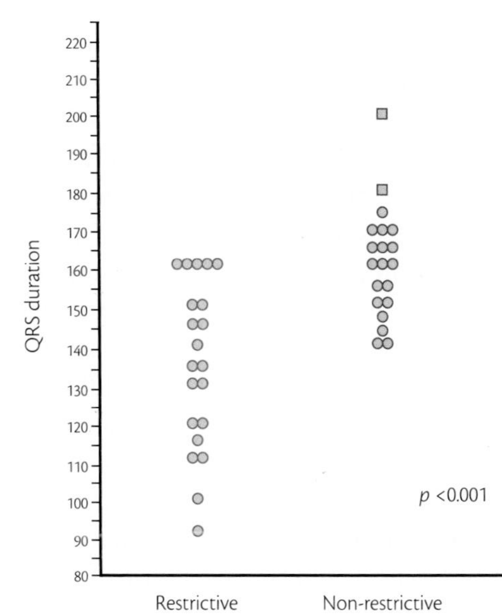

Figure 10.13 (A) 12-lead ECG in adult patient following surgical repair of tetralogy of Fallot demonstrating right bundle branch block pattern together with prolonged QRS duration measuring > 180 ms. (B) Comparison of QRS duration in patients in whom there was restrictive and non-restrictive physiology following surgical repair of tetralogy of Fallot. QRS duration > 180 ms predicted a greater risk of sudden-onset ventricular tachycardia. Reproduced with permission from Gatzoulis MA, Till JA, Somerville J, *et al.* Mechanoelectrical interaction in tetralogy of Fallot. QRS prolongation relates to right ventricular size and predicts malignant ventricular arrhythmias and sudden death. *Circulation* 1995; **92**: 231–7.

of pulmonary regurgitation. There is no need to restrict physical activities in the patient with a good repair of ToF and no documented arrhythmia.

Late aortic dilatation and aortic regurgitation is observed increasingly frequently [150, 151]. Signs of medial degeneration in the aortic wall, similar to those seen in patients with Marfan syndrome, have been demonstrated. When the diameter of the aortic root exceeds 55mm, aortic root replacement may be indicated.

Management of patients with ToF and pulmonary atresia is one of the biggest challenges in CHD. Their pulmonary blood supply is highly variable and this determines the presentation, natural history, management, and outcomes (see ➲Fig. 10.5). Neonates with pulmonary atresia and duct-dependent pulmonary blood supply require prostaglandin infusion, followed by urgent surgery to survive. Others may have increased pulmonary blood supply as a result of multiple major aortic pulmonary collateral arteries (MAPCAs) and present with heart failure. A third group with a 'balanced' pulmonary supply can remain well without any treatment for many years [152]. They develop pulmonary vascular obstructive disease in the unprotected pulmonary segments supplied by vessels arising from the aorta.

Management strategies differ greatly between institutions and have evolved rapidly in the last few years. Generalizations are therefore difficult. If there is a single source of pulmonary blood flow supplying adequate pulmonary arteries to the majority of bronchopulmonary segments, a complete repair as a single stage can be contemplated. The timing will depend on whether a right ventricle to pulmonary artery conduit is required to establish anterograde flow to the pulmonary artery (usually the case). If central pulmonary arteries are diminutive or absent, many consider such patients as uncorrectable and treatment concentrates on optimizing the pulmonary circulation by surgery or interventional catheterization as the clinical condition dictates. Other patients have a small central pulmonary artery, supplying a variable proportion of pulmonary segments, supplemented by an almost infinite variety of MAPCAs. Prospects for repair depend on establishing a single source of pulmonary blood flow ('unifocalization') which can then be connected to the right ventricle, together with closure of the VSD. Multiple-stage palliative procedures may be required to achieve this result and some patients may never become candidates for repair. Long-term results for these surgical protocols are only beginning to appear [153]. Although encouraging, patients may be left with right ventricular hypertension that is likely to limit life expectancy and quality of life. Right ventricle to pulmonary artery conduits will deteriorate with time and require further surgical replacement or percutaneous pulmonary valve insertion.

Ebstein's malformation

This is characterized by downward displacement of the tricuspid valve into the right ventricle. It is an uncommon disorder, accounting for 0.5% of all congenital cardiovascular malformations in live-born infants, but is disproportionately represented in adults. The reported association between Ebstein's malformation and maternal lithium ingestion is not borne out in most studies [12].

Morphology

Most hearts with typical Ebstein's malformation will have laevocardia and concordant atrioventricular and ventriculoarterial connections. Ebstein's malformation of the tricuspid valve has also been described in association with congenitally corrected TGA (ccTGA). The degree of displacement of the tricuspid valve into the right ventricular cavity varies from minimal to very severe. The findings are further complicated by dysplasia of the valve and abnormal attachments of the leaflets. Because of the abnormally situated tricuspid valve orifice, a portion of the right ventricle lies between the true atrioventricular valve ring and the origin of the valve, in continuity with the right atrium. This proximal portion of the right ventricle is described as 'atrialized' and leaves a small distal functional right ventricle. The most commonly associated cardiac abnormalities include varying degrees of right ventricular outflow obstruction, ASD, and, much less commonly, VSD.

Pathophysiology

Ebstein's malformation has an extremely variable course, depending on the degree of abnormality of the tricuspid valve apparatus and the associated cardiac abnormalities [154] (➲Fig. 10.14). If the deformity of the tricuspid valve is severe, intrauterine death may result or neonates may present with profound congestive cardiac failure and cyanosis. The cardiac malformation may be compounded by respiratory problems as a result of pulmonary hypoplasia due to massive cardiomegaly. Survival is particularly poor in the presence of pulmonary stenosis or atresia. Presentation in childhood with palpitation, a murmur, or cyanosis is associated with a better outcome, with an actuarial survival of 85% at 10 years. Patients presenting in adolescence or adult life generally have mild symptoms, are acyanotic, and have a good prognosis. Arrhythmia (atrial flutter or fibrillation) is the most common presenting feature and is

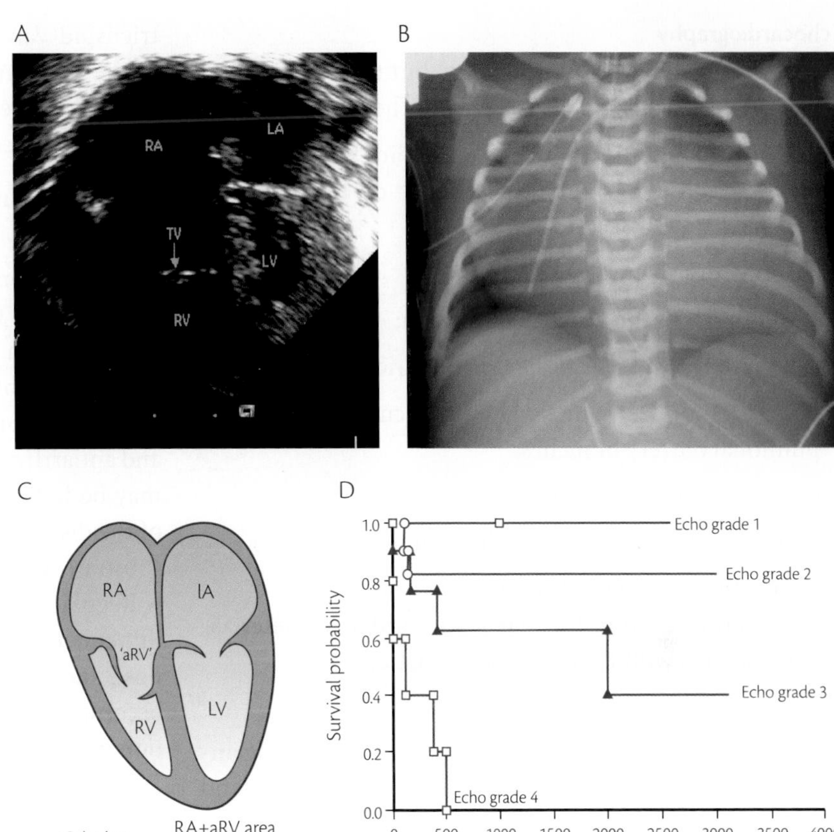

Figure 10.14 Features of Ebstein's malformation. (A) Apical view from transthoracic echocardiogram demonstrating apical displacement of tricuspid valve with large right atrium and atrialized component of right ventricle. Functional right ventricular size is small. There is moderate right heart dilatation. (B) Severe Ebstein's anomaly in the newborn period demonstrating massive cardiomegaly in a ventilated patient due to severe tricuspid regurgitation and massive right atrial enlargement. This is associated with severe pulmonary hypoplasia. (C) Grading of the severity of Ebstein's anomaly as a measure of prognosis using a ratio of right atrial size to the size of the other cardiac chambers at end diastole. Grading used to define increasing severity: grade I, < 0.5; grade II, 0.5–0.99; grade III, 1–1.49; grade IV, > 1.5. (D) Survival probability of patients with Ebstein's anomaly according to previous grading system. Reproduced with permission from Celemajer DS, Cullen S, Sullivan ID, *et al.* Outcomes in neonates with Ebstein's anomaly. *J Am Cardiol Coll* 1992; **19**: 104–6.

often, but not always, associated with pre-excitation. This may be difficult to treat medically or by ablation and may occasionally precipitate heart failure in a previously well patient. The true 'natural history' is difficult to assess because of selection bias in series collected before the introduction of echocardiography, which can now pick up the problem much earlier. It may also be difficult, sometimes, to separate Ebstein's malformation from other forms of tricuspid valve dysplasia.

Diagnosis

Clinical

In severe disease, neonatal heart failure, often with severe cyanosis, occurs. Physical signs include:

- cyanosis with tachycardia and tachypnoea;
- an overactive precordium;
- S_1 and S_2 are usually normal, but there is frequently an audible S_3 and S_4;
- pansystolic murmur loudest at the lower left sternal edge is present, due to tricuspid regurgitation;
- there may be an ejection murmur due to right ventricular outflow obstruction.

In milder cases, there may be few manifestations other than variable exertional dyspnoea, fatigue and cyanosis during childhood. In such cases, physical findings may include widely split S_1 and S_2 with prominent S_3 and S_4, so that auscultation has an almost rhythmical quality. There is frequently a pansystolic murmur at the lower left sternal edge.

Chest radiograph

- Babies presenting in the newborn period will almost always have cardiomegaly, which may be massive.
- Pulmonary hypoplasia with pulmonary oligaemia.
- In milder forms, the only finding may be mild to moderate cardiomegaly.

ECG

Most frequently, there is a low-voltage QRS complex pattern with a right bundle branch block morphology and prolonged PR interval. Right atrial enlargement is suggested by tall peaked T waves. Supraventricular arrhythmias may occur in the neonatal period but are more common in older patients. There may be evidence of ventricular pre-excitation.

Echocardiography

This clearly defines the abnormality, but there are specific features that need detailed assessment. These include:

- accurate evaluation of the tricuspid valve leaflets, their attachments and the severity of regurgitation (10.48 and 10.49);
- the integrity of the atrial septum;
- the integrity of the ventricular septum;
- estimation of the size of the right ventricle;
- patency and size of the right ventricular outflow and pulmonary artery branches;
- patency of the arterial duct;
- exclusion of associated left-sided lesions.

Cardiac catheterization and angiography

There is no indication for diagnostic cardiac catheterization in patients with Ebstein's malformation.

Management

Treatment of the critically ill neonate involves prostaglandin infusion to maintain patency of the arterial duct and the use of pulmonary vasodilators, including prostacyclin and nitric oxide. Many babies improve spontaneously as the pulmonary vascular resistance falls, but intensive support may be required for the first few days. Most older children, adolescents, and adults are asymptomatic and can be managed conservatively. Arrhythmias are notoriously difficult to manage by antiarrhythmic drugs or radiofrequency ablation, as patients have distorted tricuspid valve anatomy, a dilated right atrium and often multiple accessory pathways. Heart failure may be treated with diuretics or afterload reducers, if there is left ventricular dysfunction [155].

In the newborn period, a systemic-to-pulmonary shunt is indicated for cyanosis and right ventricular outflow obstruction and of more definitive surgery can be considered at a later date [156]. In the older child and adult, surgery should be undertaken if there is progressive functional decline, increasing cyanosis, right heart failure, or paradoxical emboli. Selection of cases remains difficult, however. Results are poor in 'end-stage' patients and there is no evidence that surgery reduces the risk of late sudden death. As a result, most units reserve surgery for symptomatic cases.

A superior cavopulmonary anastomosis and Fontan operation have been performed in cases where the right ventricle is not considered adequate to sustain the cardiac output. Occasionally, an ASD with left-to-right shunt can be closed as an isolated procedure. In most cases, surgery has been directed at reconstruction or replacement of the tricuspid valve apparatus, often with plication/resection of the right atrial wall. Tricuspid valve reconstruction has been performed by a variety of approaches and results have been good in selected patients at expert centres [157, 158].

Long-term outcome

The adult cardiologist may well encounter patients with Ebstein's anomaly who have not had surgery as patients may remain well for decades. There is no indication for restriction in physical exercise in the absence of heart failure or arrhythmia. Awareness of the high incidence of arrhythmia (predominantly supraventricular) is important and antiarrhythmic therapy and/or radiofrequency ablation may be indicated. The latter is often challenging because of the distorted anatomy and complex electrophysiological substrate which may include multiple accessory pathways.

Regular functional testing is helpful as symptoms are difficult to assess. Surgery should be considered if cyanosis increases, functional status declines, or arrhythmia becomes difficult to manage. In the future, earlier intervention is likely to practised as surgical results improve.

Most patients have improved functional status and tricuspid valve competence after surgery, although late tachyarrhythmias may remain a problem [159]. However, the long-term fate of survivors is still unknown and lifelong follow-up is required.

Total anomalous pulmonary venous connection

TAPVC accounts for approximately 2% of all congenital cardiac malformations in live births.

Morphology (Fig. 10.15)

Most commonly, the pulmonary vein joins a confluence or chamber behind the left atrium. Arising from this confluence, one or more primitive vessels persist and drain pulmonary venous blood into a systemic vein or directly into the atrium. Persistence of the left cardinal vein drains blood to the innominate vein. Drainage to the right cardinal vein is to the superior caval vein, azygos vein, or directly to the right atrium. This type of anomalous pulmonary venous drainage is described as 'supracardiac' and may not be obstructed. Flow may also be directed from the confluence into the coronary sinus, producing 'cardiac' TAPVC. Finally, there may be persistence of a descending channel that passes beneath the diaphragm and enters the portal system ('infradiaphragmatic' TAPVC), and this type is almost always obstructed. There is always an atrial communication present, which may rarely become restrictive

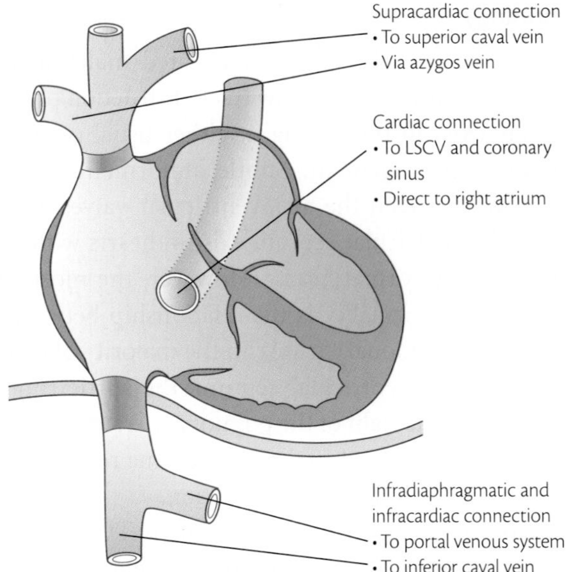

Figure 10.15 Schematic representation of the potential sites of anomalous pulmonary venous drainage in the heart.

postnatally. When pulmonary venous drainage may occur in association with right atrial isomerism, in the context of complex cardiac abnormalities, the pattern of pulmonary venous drainage is different (➲Fig. 10.1).

Pathophysiology

In TAPVC, both systemic and pulmonary venous returns enter the right atrium and some of the mixed blood passes across the atrial foramen into the left side of the heart. In obstructed TAPVC, the increased pulmonary blood flow postnatally causes marked pulmonary venous congestion and increased pulmonary vascular resistance. In the absence of ductal patency, right ventricular systolic pressure becomes suprasystemic and the right ventricle fails. If the duct remains patent, there is profound cyanosis with right-to-left flow across the arterial duct. If there is no obstruction to pulmonary venous return, there is a large left-to-right shunt with features similar to a large ASD associated with mild to moderate cyanosis.

Diagnosis

Clinical

Obstructed TAPVD presents in the neonatal period as a medical emergency with profound respiratory distress, associated with severe hypoxaemia. Cardiovascular findings are unimpressive, with a normal S_1, a single loud S_2, and there are frequently no murmurs.

When unobstructed, the features are suggestive of a large ASD associated with cyanosis. Patients are tachypnoeic with a normal S_1, a widely split S2, and a pulmonary systolic murmur loudest at the upper left sternal edge. There is usually an associated right ventricular heave.

Chest radiograph

In obstructed TAPVC, the heart is of normal size or small, with diffuse shadowing through both lung fields due to pulmonary venous congestion. This may be confused with lung disease.

In unobstructed TAPVC, there is cardiomegaly with pulmonary plethora. In supracardiac TAPVC, there may be a left-sided vertical vein shadow and a prominent superior caval vein, producing the 'snowman' appearance.

ECG

There are no specific findings but right ventricular hypertrophy with right axis deviation is almost universal.

Echocardiography

TAPVC as an isolated abnormality can be diagnosed on cross-sectional echocardiography and, with patience and multiple views, it is possible to confirm the site of drainage for all four pulmonary veins in almost all cases. A clinical index of suspicion needs to be maintained to ensure that this diagnosis is not overlooked in the critically ill neonate. Obstructed infracardiac TAPVC can be diagnosed by the presence of prominent and dilated veins within the hepatic system, as well as by a descending channel flowing from the heart and traversing the diaphragm to enter the portal system (often adjacent to the inferior caval vein). In the supracardiac type, demonstration of an ascending channel to join the innominate or superior caval vein is associated with dilatation of the superior caval vein and prominent venous return into the right atrium from the superior caval vein. Flow at atrial level is exclusively right to left. In most cases, it is also possible to identify the presence of a pulmonary venous confluence, into which the pulmonary veins drain, with clear separation from the left atrium. There is almost always marked right-to-left ventricular disproportion. However, the left ventricle is usually apex forming, and despite its appearance is able to support the systemic circulation. Obstructed types may be associated with features of severe pulmonary hypertension. Careful evaluation to exclude additional abnormalities is mandatory. The echo diagnosis can be extremely difficult in critically ill neonates who are on extra-corporal membrane oxygenation (ECMO), because the cardiac output—and with that the flow velocity of pulmonary venous return—is very low. Colour Doppler, with velocity settings as low as possible to detect very low-velocity flows, can be helpful in this situation.

Cardiac catheterization

Echocardiography has superseded cardiac catheterization as the diagnostic technique for this condition. Cardiac catheterization may occasionally be used for delineation of anomalous pulmonary venous drainage of mixed type, when some veins may drain to the superior caval vein and others to the innominate vein via an ascending vertical vein. The advent of CMR and CT is likely to eliminate the need for preoperative catheterization (see ➲Fig. 10.4).

Natural history

The natural history depends on the degree of obstruction to pulmonary venous return, which is influenced by the pattern of anomalous pulmonary venous connection. Obstructed TAPVC, presenting as a cardiac emergency in the neonate, is fatal without surgery. The clinical course is unfavourable, even without obstruction: without surgical treatment, 75–90% of the patients die in the first year of life. Very exceptionally, survival until older age has been reported.

Management

Patients with unobstructed TAPVC also require repair early. The only place for medical management is for resuscitation of the critically sick neonate and balloon atrial septostomy has no role. Surgery involves cardiopulmonary bypass and creation of a wide communication between the pulmonary veins and left atrium, closure of anomalous pulmonary vein connections to the systemic circulation, and usually closure of the atrial communication. Mixed forms of pulmonary venous return may be particularly challenging operations. Early results of surgery have improved dramatically, with a low incidence of recurrent pulmonary venous obstruction (unless there are intrinsic abnormalities extending into the pulmonary veins themselves [160]. Reoperation in these circumstances carries a high risk but interventional catheterization has also not been very successful.

Long-term outcome

The late results of TAPVC are excellent, with a very low incidence of pulmonary venous obstruction, arrhythmia, and essentially normal quality of life [161]. In the absence of haemodynamic problems, patients can be managed by primary care and regular cardiac clinics.

Complete transposition of the great arteries

In complete TGA (4.4% of congenital cardiac malformations), the aorta arises from the right ventricle and the pulmonary artery from the left ventricle (ventriculoarterial discordance) (🎥 10.50).

Morphology

TGA may be complicated by associated malformations (VSD or left ventricular outflow tract obstruction or both). TGA may exist in the setting of either usual or mirror-image atrial arrangement. Subtle abnormalities of the relationship between the atrioventricular valves and the shape of the ventricular septum exist in hearts with TGA, compared with normal hearts. However, the most obvious external abnormality is the relationship between the aorta and the pulmonary trunk. In the majority of cases of TGA with intact ventricular septum, the aortic root lies anterior and to the right of the pulmonary artery. However, uncommon variations do exist and become relevant when considering the arterial switch operation.

Defects in the ventricular septum in TGA have the same spectrum as those in the normal heart. Left ventricular outflow obstruction, seen most frequently in association with a VSD, is due to caudal displacement of the infundibular septum, causing subpulmonary and pulmonary stenosis. With an intact ventricular septum, left ventricular outflow obstruction may be caused by an abnormal pulmonary valve, dynamic subpulmonary outflow tract obstruction, or, occasionally, abnormal mitral valve attachments. The anatomy of the coronary arteries has assumed major importance since the introduction of the arterial switch operation. The coronary arteries usually originate from the facing or posterior sinuses of the aortic valve. The most noteworthy abnormality is the presence of an intramural segment of either right or left proximal coronary artery, making coronary artery transfer during the arterial switch operation significantly more difficult [162].

Pathophysiology

In TGA, the two circulations operate in parallel, with desaturated systemic blood flow routed back to the body and saturated pulmonary venous return routed back to the lungs. With closure of the normal fetal shunts, there is no mixing within the circulation, and without early intervention, profound hypoxaemia with acidosis develops rapidly. Providing the foramen remains open, mixing of blood at atrial level can achieve sufficient 'effective' pulmonary blood flow.

In patients with TGA and intact ventricular septum, cyanosis usually becomes evident soon after birth and may progress rapidly. Differential cyanosis may be evident, with lower extremities that are pinker than upper extremities due to flow from pulmonary artery to aorta through the arterial duct.

Diagnosis

Clinical

Physical signs include cyanosis, prominent right ventricular impulse, soft mid-systolic murmur, and single S_2. In those with an associated VSD or large patent arterial duct, the onset of cyanosis is usually slower and less severe.

Chest radiograph

The classical appearances are laevocardia (but dextrocardia is recognized) with a normal or slightly increased cardiothoracic ratio, but with an 'egg on side' appearance due to the anteroposterior relationship of great arteries. Pulmonary vascular markings are usually mildly increased.

ECG

This is not helpful in diagnosis but shows sinus rhythm, rightward QRS axis, and right ventricular hypertrophy.

Echocardiography

Cross-sectional echocardiography has made the identification of TGA straightforward. Multiple views and serial images have meant that there is now little or no role for angiography in the initial evaluation. The important echocardiographic features include:

- confirmation of atrioventricular concordance and ventriculoarterial discordance;
- assessment of adequacy of the interatrial communication;
- assessment of any VSDs;
- exclusion of left ventricular outflow obstruction;
- confirmation of morphologically normal semilunar valves;
- evaluation of the spatial relationships of the great arteries;
- assessment of the patency of the arterial duct;
- exclusion of coarctation of the aorta;
- detailed assessment of coronary artery anatomy.

Natural history

Unless treated promptly, TGA is a lethal condition and 90% of patients die within the first year of life. The associated malformations affect presentation and management.

Management and long-term outcome

Early treatment is directed towards improving mixing between the two parallel circulations to increase systemic arterial saturation. This can be achieved by maintaining patency of the arterial duct using prostaglandin infusion and/or by enlarging the intra-atrial communication by balloon atrial septostomy (10.51). This can be performed under echo guidance, which will also permit assessment of the adequacy of the resulting ASD.

Definitive surgery was performed for many years using either the Mustard or Senning operation. Both involve creation of an intra-atrial baffle to re-route the systemic and pulmonary systemic venous return to the pulmonary artery and aorta respectively [162]. Accordingly, the GUCH specialist should understand the intra-atrial repair and its consequences, even though this surgical approach has now been superseded by the arterial switch operation.

During long-term follow-up after the Mustard and Senning operations a number of complications have emerged, and the late results have been disappointing [73, 163]. Venous pathway problems (including stenosis and baffle leaks) may require intervention and these may be amenable to interventional catheterization (e.g. stenting and device closure). Progressive loss of stable sinus rhythm has proved inevitable and occurs with equal frequency after the Mustard and Senning procedures [164].

Junctional rhythm is common with bradycardia and tachycardias. Pacemaker insertion was often undertaken but no improvement in survival has been documented [165]. A pacemaker should be reserved for the rare patient with symptomatic bradycardia or those requiring antiarrhythmic therapy for tachycardia (in association with bradycardia). The most worrying issue is the fate of the right ventricle in the systemic circulation. In many subjects, right ventricular dysfunction develops together with tricuspid regurgitation [166]. The combination of atrial tachycardias, venous pathway restriction, and right ventricular dysfunction is the likely risk substrate for late sudden death which may often occur during or after physical exertion [167].

Risk stratification and treatment remains challenging. ACE inhibitors have been used with questionable rationale and beta-blockers may be preferable. Regular follow-up of such patients in specialized GUCH units is required [168].

Some patients are considered for transplantation or conversion to an arterial switch. However, this is not straightforward and the left ventricle needs to be 'retrained' by pulmonary artery banding to deal with the higher after load of the systemic circulation. The increasing evidence of late problems after atrial redirection operations has led to the widespread adoption of the neonatal arterial switch procedure (anatomical repair) [169].

In patients with an intact ventricular septum, this should be performed within the first few weeks (ideally <4 weeks) of life before left ventricular pressure falls and 'detraining' occurs. The early mortality is now very low and medium-term data suggest excellent survival with a much lower incidence of arrhythmia and preserved ventricular function [170].

The change in surgical approach from intra-atrial to arterial switch repair represents a powerful argument for life-long follow-up of CHD, with the close collaboration between paediatric and grown-up congenital cardiologists. Potential long-term problems after the arterial switch, especially related to 'neo-aortic' regurgitation and coronary artery patency, will need evaluation [171].

For infants with TGA and a large VSD or a large arterial duct, an arterial switch operation with closure of the VSD/patent arterial duct should be performed, ideally within the first 2 months of life. If there is a VSD and pulmonary stenosis, a palliative systemic-to-pulmonary shunt in infancy may be required followed by later repair, which often involves insertion of a right ventricle to pulmonary artery conduit (Rastelli operation) [171].

Congenitally corrected transposition of the great arteries

Congenitally corrected transposition of the great arteries (ccTGA) or atrioventricular and ventriculoarterial discordance is uncommon, accounting for <1% of all congenital cardiovascular malformations. There is a wide spectrum of morphological features and associated abnormalities and the nomenclatures that has been used has been confusing [172].

Morphology

The abnormal connections in 'double' discordance may be present in hearts with usual or mirror-image atrial arrangement. The heart itself may be left-sided, right-sided, or in the midline. The ventricles are inverted when compared with the normal situation, with the aorta arising anteriorly from the right ventricle and the pulmonary artery arising posteriorly from the left ventricle. The aorta arises from a free-standing infundibulum, which separates the aortic valve from the tricuspid valve. In contrast, the pulmonary valve is in fibrous continuity with the mitral valve. Associated lesions are common (80–90%). Usually a VSD is present (75% of cases), often in a perimembranous subpulmonary position, but VSDs may occur anywhere and are frequently multiple. The left-sided tricuspid valve may have features of Ebstein's malformation and straddling of either atrioventricular valve is well recognized. Pulmonary stenosis or atresia occurs in almost half of cases (usually with VSD).

Pathophysiology

Isolated ccTGA may have no haemodynamic consequences in childhood and early adulthood. The pathophysiology is determined by the associated lesions.

Diagnosis

Clinical

Fetal diagnosis may be triggered by detection of a prenatal arrhythmia. Patients with isolated ccTGA are often asymptomatic through childhood and into middle age. They may be detected because of an abnormal chest radiograph or ECG (often at routine medical examination). The physical signs depend on the nature of the associated malformations. In patients with a large VSD, congestive cardiac failure may develop in infancy. When there is a VSD and pulmonary stenosis, increasing cyanosis may develop or the patient may deteriorate acutely when the duct closes, if pulmonary atresia is present.

Chest radiograph

In isolated ccTGA with laevocardia, there is a normal cardiothoracic ratio with an abnormally straight left heart border due to the left and anterior position of the ascending aorta. The cardiothoracic ratio may be increased with pulmonary plethora when there is an associated VSD or atrioventricular valve regurgitation.

ECG

This shows variable degrees of atrioventricular block, abnormal P-wave axis, and abnormal QRS activation with reversal of the Q-wave pattern in the precordial leads.

Cross-sectional echocardiography

This is able to identify the morphological characteristics of ccTGA. The inverted position of the ventricles can be recognized by the fundamental differences between the two ventricles. The anatomic right ventricle has increased trabecularization, a moderator band, and a more apically inserted tricuspid valve. There is a discontinuity between the atrioventricular valve and the arterial valve. In the left ventricle, the mitral valve has a higher insertion, the muscular wall is smoother, and a continuity exists between the mitral valve and the arterial valve. It is particularly important to identify associated anomalies, particularly atrioventricular valve straddling, VSD, left ventricular outflow obstruction, and atrioventricular valve regurgitation. It is usually possible to plan appropriate management strategies without invasive testing.

Cardiac catheterization and angiography

This is rarely indicated as a diagnostic procedure.

Natural history

The natural history and management are usually determined by the associated cardiac malformations. Without associated lesions, a patient with congenitally corrected transposition is often asymptomatic until late adulthood [173, 174]. Dyspnoea and exercise intolerance from systemic right ventricular failure and significant left atrioventricular valve regurgitation (especially with an Ebstein-like tricuspid valve) will usually manifest itself by the fourth or fifth decade. Palpitations from supraventricular arrhythmias may arise in the fifth or sixth decade and there is a progressive tendency to develop atrioventricular conduction problems (reported as 2% per year incidence of complete heart block) [175]. Tachyarrhythmia associated with ventricular pre-excitation may also develop.

Management

In patients with VSD and/or left ventricular outflow obstruction, surgery is complicated because of the location of the conduction tissue and resultant operative risk of complete heart block [176]. Relief of pulmonary stenosis often requires insertion of a left ventricle to pulmonary artery conduit. A 'double-switch' approach (atrial redirection by Mustard or Senning operation with an arterial switch or connection of the left ventricle to aorta via a VSD if present) is a novel approach that restores the left ventricle to the systemic circulation [177]. However, the results remain uncertain. Intervention is not required for the asymptomatic patient with isolated ccTGA, apart from the insertion of a pacemaker if complete heart block develops.

Patients with significant tricuspid regurgitation require surgery as regurgitation is progressive and associated with 'right ventricular' failure Valve replacement has been the most common procedure and results have been better when undertaken before ventricular function is severely compromised [178]. Tricuspid regurgitation may be improved by a residual left ventricular outflow obstruction which can cause a shift in the interventricular septum towards the dilated systemic right ventricle.

Recently, banding of the pulmonary artery has been performed to obtain a similar beneficial effect on the dilated systemic right ventricle and tricuspid regurgitation (10.52 and 10.53). A double switch can be considered in patients after such 'left ventricular' retraining. Too few patients have reached adult life after the various surgical approaches for comparison of outcome.

Long-term outcome

Long-term surveillance of all operated and unoperated patients with ccTGA should be undertaken in specialist GUCH centres. This should focus on the function of the systemic ventricle, the systemic AV-valve, the development and progression of aortic regurgitation, as well as the cardiac rhythm [179].

Pregnancy counselling should be provided by experts as the volume load of pregnancy may compromise the systemic load of the right ventricle. Exercise recommendations should also be provided by experts in GUCH [180].

Univentricular atrioventricular connection (single ventricle)

Hearts with a univentricular atrioventricular connection (including tricuspid atresia, mitral atresia, and double-inlet ventricle) are characterized by the output from both atria being directed into a single ventricular chamber. This heterogeneous group of abnormalities accounts for 1.5–2% of all congenital cardiac malformations. The principle of management for all such hearts in whom a biventricular repair is not feasible has been to aim for a Fontan-type circulation. Even after a successful operation patients have considerable problems during long-term follow-up and are perhaps the most challenging cases in GUCH practice.

Morphology

Description of the morphological abnormalities in this group has long been an area of contention because of a lack of consensus about the definition of a ventricle. Most commonly, there is a dominant right or left ventricle and an additional second ventricular chamber, which is rudimentary. The 'mode' of connection (see Nomenclature, p.314) may include absent atrioventricular connection (right or left) or double-inlet ventricle with two separate or a common atrioventricular valve. The arterial connections can be concordant, discordant, double outlet, or solitary outlet with atresia of the pulmonary artery or of the aorta. In practice, there are usually two arterial trunks with stenosis of one or other artery. The sequential segmental approach, together with description of associated abnormalities, facilitates classification of these complex hearts.

Pathophysiology

Pathophysiology depends mainly on the pulmonary and systemic blood flows and the associated malformations. In all cases, there is a degree of cyanosis, as a result of mixing at ventricular level.

Diagnosis

Clinical

Most patients present in the neonatal period with a varied clinical picture, unless prenatal diagnosis has already been made. If they have pulmonary stenosis, there is cyanosis, a ventricular heave, a normal S_1 and a single S_2. There is usually an ejection systolic murmur caused by pulmonary outflow obstruction. In contrast, those with unobstructed pulmonary blood flow have much less severe cyanosis and may have features of cardiac failure. Physical signs include an overactive precordium with a normal S_1 and a variable S_2 with a loud pulmonary component. There is usually a soft systolic murmur. Other patients may present in critical condition with obstructed systemic flow (caused by subaortic stenosis, coarctation or interrupted aortic arch) or the consequences of coexisting abnormalities (e.g. TAPVC with atrial isomerism).

Chest radiograph

Abnormalities of cardiac position are common and there may be discordance between the side of the stomach and the heart, in association with atrial isomerism. There is almost always cardiomegaly. In cases with pulmonary outflow obstruction, there will be pulmonary oligaemia, whereas pulmonary plethora is usually seen in those with unobstructed pulmonary blood flow.

ECG

The ECG findings are diverse. Attention should be paid to rhythm abnormalities, particularly in patients with suspected atrial isomerism. A superior P-wave axis is a strong clue for the presence of left isomerism, with interruption of the inferior caval vein.

Echocardiography

Demonstration of the cardiac connections as well as the intracardiac and extracardiac malformations is usually possible, but is time-consuming. In particular, definition of the systemic and pulmonary venous connections of the heart has important immediate and long-term management implications. Atrioventricular valve function and obstruction of the pulmonary or aortic valve must also be assessed.

Cardiac catheterization and angiography

There may still be a role for diagnostic cardiac catheterization and angiography in the evaluation of some of these complex patients, who have abnormalities of systemic and pulmonary venous connection that may not be defined completely by echocardiography. However, CMR and CT are usually able to provide this important information less invasively.

Natural history

The natural history is highly variable and depends particularly on the degree of obstruction in the systemic and pulmonary outlets and, to a lesser extent, on the ventricular morphology and atrioventricular connection. Most patients who present as neonates require urgent or early palliative surgery to ensure survival. If the circulation is 'well balanced', survival into adult life with relatively few symptoms is possible. Predicted survival curves can be created for combinations of malformations (patients with double-inlet left ventricle, two atrioventricular valves with ventriculoarterial discordance and pulmonary stenosis do best). An adequate arterial saturation in these complete mixing situations requires a high pulmonary blood flow and consequently greatly increased load on the ventricle. As a result, progressive deterioration with ventricular failure usually begins from the second or third decade of life.

Management

In the neonate or infant, palliative surgery is often required, for example systemic-to-pulmonary shunt, pulmonary artery band, complex surgery for subaortic stenosis, together with treatment of any associated malformations such as TAPVC or coarctation. Since its introduction in 1971, the Fontan operation has become the definitive procedure of choice for suitable patients [181]. Surgery involves separation of the systemic and pulmonary venous returns without a subpulmonary ventricle. A number of modifications have been made since the original surgical description, aimed largely at streamlining the systemic venous return to the pulmonary arteries. The cardiopulmonary connection has been abandoned in favour of a total cavopulmonary connection (TCPC), either intracardiac or with an extra cardiac conduit between the inferior caval vein and the pulmonary artery, together with a superior caval vein to pulmonary artery connection (bidirectional Glenn) [182]. Frequently, this cavopulmonary circulation is established in two stages, with an initial bidirectional Glenn anastamosis. The TCPC completion is sometimes fenestrated, creating a small communication between the cavopulmonary connection and atrium to allow controlled right-to-left shunting [183].

It is now appreciated that both operative mortality and postoperative outcome after TCPC depend on suitability of the circulation and adherence to defined criteria dealing with pulmonary artery size and anatomy, pulmonary vascular resistance, atrioventricular valve and ventricular function. In the best cases, operative risk is now <5% [184, 185].

Long-term outcome

A number of important problems have emerged during long-term follow-up and premature decline in function, with reduced survival, is 'built in' to the Fontan circulation [186–188]. Key issues contributing to the 'failing Fontan' include the function of the systemic ventricle (which is 'preload deprived'), a rise in pulmonary vascular resistance, atrioventricular valve regurgitation, the development of pulmonary arteriovenous malformations, and the consequences of chronic venous hypertension [189]. These include massive right atrial dilatation, pulmonary venous obstruction, protein-losing enteropathy, and, particularly, supraventricular arrhythmia. Approximately 20% of patients have clinically important arrhythmia (including intra-atrial re-entry tachycardias and atrial flutter) by 10 years after Fontan and this incidence increases with longer follow-up [190]. Surgical modifications such as TCPC, which excludes the hypertensive right atrium from the subpulmonary circulation, may result in a lower incidence of long-term arrhythmia but this is not yet proven [190]. Protein-losing enteropathy results in peripheral oedema, pleural effusions, and ascites. It can be diagnosed by gastrointestinal clearance of alpha$_1$-antitrypsin and has an ominous prognostic significance, with a 5-year survival rate of <50% [191].

Comprehensive investigation is mandatory for patients with any of these manifestations of the failing Fontan complex. In particular, it is crucial to exclude obstruction to the systemic venous return, as even a minor degree may have major clinical consequences. Appropriate investigations include transoesophageal echocardiography, CMR, and/or cardiac catheterization. Intervention by stent implantation or surgery may be required. Right atrial blood stasis, coagulation abnormalities, development of right atrial thrombus, and, in particular, the potential for recurrent subclinical pulmonary emboli have led many to advise lifelong anticoagulant therapy, although this is not yet supported by rigorous long-term data. Arrhythmia must be treated actively, as loss of sinus rhythm itself leads to accelerated haemodynamic decline. Antiarrhythmic drugs, apart from amiodarone, have been disappointing. Results of radiofrequency ablation of the often multiple atrial re-entry circuits have improved, but these procedures remain challenging [192]. Treatment of protein-losing enteropathy includes sodium restriction, high protein diet, diuretics, ACE inhibitors, steroids, albumin infusions, chronic subcutaneous heparin, and creation of a fenestration (by interventional catheter) [193].

Patients with a failing Fontan should be considered for surgical conversion or for transplantation. Conversion of an atriopulmonary connection to a more energy-efficient TCPC, together with arrhythmia surgery, has produced good results in selected patients, but has a surgical mortality and ongoing postoperative morbidity [194]. Patients with the Fontan procedure have the most severe limitation of exercise capacity amongst patients with CHD. Twenty-five years after surgery, the percentage of patients without a serious complication (reoperation, arrhythmias, thromboembolic complications may be <10%). The long-term prognosis of patients even with an 'excellent' Fontan circulation is unknown, but life-expectancy can be anticipated to be substantially reduced. Adult cardiologists should therefore appreciate that the Fontan operation, in its various manifestations, should be considered the 'best' palliation for patients with these complex cardiac malformations and lifelong specialist follow-up is required for the many unresolved treatment issues.

Personal perspective

The management of congenital cardiac malformations has been one of the biggest success stories of modern medicine. As a result of improvements in medical and surgical management, the majority of children born with congenital cardiac malformations now survive to adulthood and adults presently outnumber children with congenital cardiac malformations. Increasingly, therefore, adult cardiologists need to become involved in the lifetime management of this new population of patients and are likely to encounter patients with a range of complex malformations in their practice. In order to manage such patients effectively, the adult practitioner must understand the paediatric presentation, natural history, and interventions undertaken in childhood. Similarly, paediatric practitioners need to be aware of the long-term outcome of their management strategies in order to refine early care. The management of TGA is a wonderful example of this 'feedback', with the change from atrial to arterial switch operation.

A number of important trends have emerged in the lifetime management of CHD. Investigation has shifted away from invasive cardiac catheterization towards non-invasive modalities as echocardiography, and more recently CMR and CT, have become able to define anatomy and physiology accurately. In parallel with the reduction of diagnostic cardiac catheterization, there has been a spectacular rise in the range and number of therapeutic cardiac catheterization procedures. These are now often integrated into a long-term management strategy together with surgery and will, in some cases, obviate the need for surgery completely. The outcome after such novel approaches will need rigorous testing in structured trials.

Improvements in diagnosis, neonatal intensive care, cardiopulmonary bypass, and surgical skill and confidence has resulted in a clear shift away from palliation towards primary definitive repair wherever possible. This has contributed to a dramatic reduction in surgical morbidity and mortality and improved haemodynamic results. With better outcome prospects, the goals of treatment have changed from merely early survival towards 'lifetime' management aimed at optimizing life expectancy and quality of life. Paediatric cardiology and adult cardiology will need to reintegrate in order to provide the best care for the increasing number of survivors of treatment for congenital cardiac malformations, and this will be a major challenge for the profession in the next few years.

Further reading

Chessa M, Arciprete P, Bossone E, *et al.* A multicentre approach for the management of adults with congenital heart disease. *J Cardiovasc Med* (Hagerstown) 2006; **7**: 701–5.

Deanfield J, Thaulow E, Warnes C, *et al.* Management of grown up congenital heart disease. *Eur Heart J* 2003; **24**: 1035–84.

Report of the British Cardiac Society Working Party. Grown-up congenital heart (GUCH) disease: current needs and provision of service for adolescents and adults with congenital heart disease in the UK. *Heart* 2002; **88**(Suppl.1):i1–i14.

Therrien J, Webb G. Clinical update on adults with congenital heart disease. *Lancet* 2003; **362**: 1305–13.

Therrien J, Dore A, Gersony W, *et al.* Canadian Cardiovascular Society. CCS Consensus Conference 2001 update: recommendations for the management of adults with congenital heart disease. Part I. *Can J Cardiol* 2001; **17**: 940–59.

Therrien J, Gatzoulis M, Graham T, *et al.* Canadian Cardiovascular Society Consensus Conference 2001 update: recommendations for the management of adults with congenital heart disease. Part II. *Can J Cardiol* 2001; **17**: 1029–50.

Therrien J, Warnes C, Daliento L, *et al.* Canadian Cardiovascular Society Consensus Conference 2001 update: recommendations for the management of adults with congenital heart disease. Part III. *Can J Cardiol* 2001; **17**: 1135–58.

Warnes CA, Williams RG, Bashore TM, *et al.* ACC/AHA 2008 Guidelines for the Management of Adults with Congenital Heart Disease: a report of the American College of Cardiology/American Heart Association Task Force on Practice Guidelines (writing committee to develop guidelines on the management of adults with congenital heart disease). *Circulation* 2008; **118**: e714–833.

Online resources

London Medical Database for Dysmorphology: http://www.lmdatabases.com/

Additional online material

10.1 Multislice three-dimensional CT scan reconstruction of complex cardiac lesion with dextrocardia, functional univentricular heart, total anomalous pulmonary venous drainage and anterior aorta with coarctation.

10.2 MRI white blood image showing subaortic ventricular septal defect in unrepaired tetralogy of Fallot.

10.3 Demonstration of Amplatz muscular septal occluder being deployed in a model heart across the ventricular septum through a muscular ventricular septal defect.

10.4 Transthoracic two-dimensional echocardiogram showing Amplatz muscular septal occluder after deployment in the muscular portion of the atrial septum to occlude muscular ventricular septal defect.

10.5 Transthoracic two-dimensional echocardiogram showing secundum type atrial septal defect.

10.6 Transthoracic two-dimensional echocardiogram showing sinus venosus type atrial septal defect with the superior caval vein sitting astride the defect and left-to-right flow across the defect seen on colour flow mapping.

10.7 Occlusion of a secundum type atrial septal defect being demonstrated in a model heart viewed from the left and right sides using an Amplatz septal occluder.

10.8 Transoesophageal two-dimensional echocardiogram showing Amplatz septal occluder across the atrial septum post release with colour flow mapping confirming the absence of any residual left-to-right shunt across the atrial septum.

10.9 Transthoracic three-dimensional echocardiogram demonstrating a complete atrioventricular septal defect with a common atrioventricular valve seen in an apical four-chamber view.

10.10 White blood axial MRI cut demonstrating a complete atrioventricular septal defect with common atrioventricular valve orifice and showing evidence of left-sided atrioventricular valve regurgitation.

10.11 Transthoracic two-dimensional echocardiogram in a parasternal short-axis view with colour flow mapping demonstrating a modest sized, restrictive patent arterial duct.

10.12 Angiogram in a lateral projection showing flow through a restrictive patent arterial duct into the main pulmonary artery after aortic injection.

10.13 Lateral image during fluoroscopic screening showing Amptatz duct occluder (type 2) in position across the arterial duct prior to release form delivery wire.

10.14 Aortogram in a lateral projection post deployment of Amplatz duct occluder (type 2) confirming appropriate positioning of the device and minimal residual shunt.

10.15 Post procedure two-dimensional transthoracic echocardiogram in a parasternal short-axis view showing the occlusion device across the arterial duct with no residual flow seen through the duct on colour flow mapping.

10.16 Angiogram in an anteroposterior projection with injection into the root of a common arterial trunk showing ascending aorta and dilated right pulmonary artery.

10.17 Pulmonary venous wedge angiogram in an anteroposterior projection with injection into the left upper pulmonary vein demonstrating delayed retrograde filling of a small left pulmonary artery disconnected from the common arterial trunk.

10.18 Two-dimensional transthoracic echocardiogram with colour flow mapping from a suprasternal view showing aortic coarctation.

10.19 Three-dimensional MRI angiographic reconstruction of discrete aortic coarctation with the development of multiple collateral arteries.

10.20 Aortogram in a lateral projection showing severe discrete aortic coarctation with collateral formation.

10.21 Aortogram in a lateral projection showing stent placement at the site of severe discrete aortic coarctation.

10.22 Repeat aortogram in a lateral projection showing result after stent placement at the site of severe discrete aortic coarctation.

10.23 Two-dimensional echocardiogram in a parasternal long-axis view showing subvalvar aortic stenosis due to a discrete fibomuscular ridge with colour flow mapping confirming that the flow disturbance occurs below the aortic valve at the site of the ridge.

10.24 Two-dimensional echocardiogram in a parasternal long-axis view showing valvar aortic stenosis with narrow left ventricular outflow tract, doming aortic valve with colour flow mapping confirming that the flow disturbance occurs at the level of the aortic valve.

10.25 Two-dimensional echocardiogram in a parasternal long-axis view showing supravalvar aortic stenosis with narrowing at the level of the aortic sinotubular junction and colour flow mapping confirming that the flow disturbance occurs above the level of the aortic valve.

10.26 Fluoroscopic screening in an anteroposterior view during balloon inflation in a patient with aortic valve stenosis.

10.27 Two-dimensional fetal echocardiogram showing a four-chamber view of the fetal heart in hypoplastic left heart syndrome.

10.28 Two-dimensional transthoracic echocardiogram in an apical view with colour flow mapping in a patient with hypoplastic left heart syndrome.

10.29 Three-dimensional MRI angiographic reconstruction of a heart with hypoplastic left heart syndrome after initial palliation with a Norwood stage 1 operation using the Sano modification.

10.30 Pulmonary arteriogram in a four-chamber projection in a patient with Alagille syndrome showing supravalvar pulmonary stenosis as well as diffuse peripheral branch pulmonary artery stenosis characteristic of this condition.

10.31 Right ventricular angiogram in an anteroposterior projection showing hypoplastic right ventricle with atretic right ventricular outflow tract.

10.32 Two-dimensional echocardiogram with colour flow mapping from an apical view showing features of pulmonary atresia with intact ventricular septum.

10.33 Right ventricular angiogram in an anteroposterior projection showing hypoplastic right ventricle with atretic right ventricular outflow tract up to the level of the pulmonary valve.

10.34 Fluoroscopic screening in a lateral projection following perforation of the pulmonary valve showing initial balloon dilatation of the pulmonary valve using a 'balloon on a wire' technique.

10.35 Fluoroscopic screening in a lateral projection following perforation of the pulmonary valve showing further balloon dilatation of the pulmonary valve.

10.36 Final right ventricular angiogram in an anteroposterior projection after dilatation of the pulmonary valve showing filling of the confluent pulmonary artery system from the right ventricular injection.

10.37 Three-dimensional angiographic CT reconstruction of distal aortic arch and descending aorta in a patient with pulmonary atresia and multifocal pulmonary blood supply.

10.38 Two-dimensional echocardiogram in a parasternal long-axis view showing subaortic ventricular septal defect and aortic override in unrepaired tetralogy of Fallot.

10.39 Two-dimensional echocardiogram in a parasternal short-axis view showing subaortic ventricular septal defect and pulmonary outflow tract obstruction with small main pulmonary artery in unrepaired tetralogy of Fallot.

10.40 Descending aortogram in an anteroposterior projection showing pulmonary blood flow derived from multiple aortopulmonary collateral arteries arising from the descending aorta.

10.41 Angiographic injection in an anteroposterior projection into aortopulmonary collateral artery arising from descending aorta.

10.42 Angiographic injection in an anteroposterior projection into aortopulmonary collateral artery arising from ascending aorta.

10.43 Angiogram in the main pulmonary artery in a lateral projection in a patient with severe tetralogy of Fallot repaired with a right ventricle to pulmonary artery conduit which has become stenosed with valvar regurgitation.

10.44 Angiogram in the main pulmonary artery in a lateral projection in a patient with severe tetralogy of Fallot repaired with a right ventricle to pulmonary artery conduit showing positioning of bare metal stent prior to implantation in right ventricular outflow.

10.45 Fluoroscopic screening in a lateral projection in a patient with severe tetralogy of Fallot repaired with a right ventricle to pulmonary artery conduit.

10.46 Fluoroscopic screening in a lateral projection in a patient with severe tetralogy of Fallot repaired with a right ventricle to pulmonary artery conduit.

10.47 Main pulmonary artery angiogram in a lateral projection in a patient with severe tetralogy of Fallot repaired with a right ventricle to pulmonary artery conduit.

10.48 Two-dimensional echocardiogram with colour flow mapping from an apical view showing dilatation of right heart structures with apical displacement of the septal leaflet of the tricuspid valve and severe tricuspid regurgitation.

10.49 Two-dimensional echocardiogram with colour flow mapping from an apical view showing dilatation of right heart structures with apical displacement and tethering of the leaflets of the tricuspid valve to the right ventricular apex and significant tricuspid regurgitation.

10.50 White blood MRI image in a lateral projection showing parallel arrangement of great arteries in simple transposition of the great arteries.

10.51 Two-dimensional echocardiogram from a subcostal view showing echo-guided balloon atrial septostomy in a patient with transposition of the great arteries.

10.52 Two-dimensional echocardiogram from an apical view with colour flow mapping showing significant left-sided tricuspid regurgitation in a patient with congenitally corrected transposition.

10.53 Two-dimensional echocardiogram from an apical view with colour flow mapping showing marked improvement in left-sided tricuspid regurgitation after pulmonary banding in a patient with congenitally corrected transposition.

For full references and multimedia materials please visit the online version of the book (http://esctextbook.oxfordonline.com).

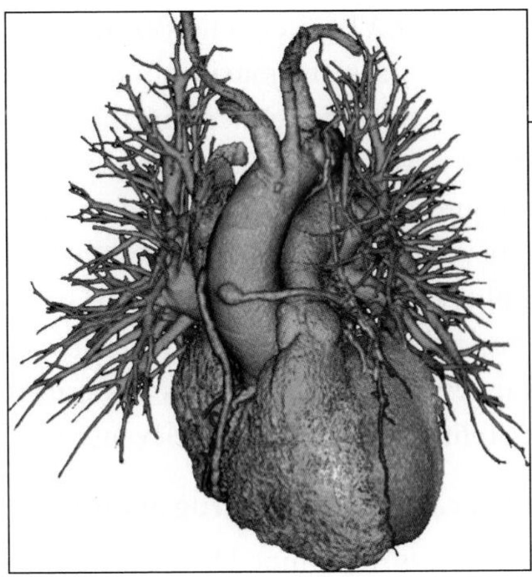

CHAPTER 11

Clinical Pharmacology of Cardiovascular Drugs

Faiez Zannad, Pascal Bousquet, and Laurent Monassier

Contents

Summary

Treatment of cardiovascular (CV) disease often requires the administration of numerous medications for long periods of time to patients likely to be old and suffering from a range of comorbid conditions. Rational prescribing informed by clinical pharmacology is essential if the right drug is to be administered to the right patient, at the right time, and for the right price. This requires an appreciation of the key principles of clinical pharmacology, and specific knowledge of individual therapies. Knowledge of polypharmacy and drug interactions is crucial, and the pharmacokinetic and pharmacodynamic challenges associated with advanced patient age, comorbidity, and sometimes frailty must be addressed and overcome. The environmental and genetic determinants of variability in response to treatment are increasingly well understood, and new biomarkers and pharmacogenetic techniques provide the foundations of the emerging discipline of personalized medicine. Long-term preventive medication raises issues concerning safety, adherence, and cost to healthcare providers. A basic familiarity with the principles of pharmaco-vigilance, pharmaco-epidemiology, and pharmaco-economics may therefore be of some value to practitioners.

No other medical discipline has progressed as fast as CV medicine. The high incidence and prevalence of CV disease has created a huge epidemiological challenge, and an enormous potential market for the pharmaceutical industry, which continues to play a very important role in research and development. The aim of CV therapy is as much to improve quality of life as to prolong survival. Its efficacy is often measured using hard morbidity and mortality endpoints requiring sophisticated long-term clinical trials. Consequently, therapeutic decisions in CV medicine are more evidence based than is possible in other specialties, and the results of major trials have shaped routine practice. It is therefore essential for those training in cardiology and CV medicine to be taught to assess the evidence provided by the literature and use it to make informed individual therapeutic decisions.

This chapter summarizes the principles of clinical pharmacology relevant to CV drug therapy and introduces fundamental concepts in the critical appraisal of trial data. It provides an overview of the critical characteristics of drugs commonly used to treat CV disease.

Basic concepts in clinical pharmacology

Pharmacodynamics

Pharmacodynamics is the study of the biochemical and physiological effects of drugs on the body, the mechanisms of drug action, and the relationship between drug concentration and effect.

The activity of most CV drugs mainly reflects interaction with enzyme, structural or carrier proteins, interaction with ion channels, and ligand binding to hormone, neuromodulator, and neurotransmitter receptors. Occasionally, they act via cellular membrane disruption (general anaesthetics) or a chemical reaction (cholestyramine, a cholesterol-binding agent that acts as a chelating agent). Enzyme-substrate binding is a means of altering the production or metabolism of key endogenous substances. For example, aspirin irreversibly inhibits the enzyme prostaglandin synthetase (cyclooxygenase, COX) thereby preventing inflammatory response. Angiotensin-converting enzyme (ACE) inhibitors prevent the production of angiotensin II and concomitantly suppress degradation of bradykinin, thereby raising its concentration and enhancing its vasodilating effects. Digitalis inhibits the activity of the carrier molecule, the Na–K–ATPase pump.

Agonist–antagonist mechanism of action

The majority of drugs act as ligands which bind to receptors responsible for cellular effects. Binding may elicit the receptor's normal action (agonist, partial agonist), block it (antagonist), or even reverse it (inverse agonist). The binding of a ligand (medication) to a receptor is governed by the law of mass action, and the rates of binding and dissociation can be used to determine the equilibrium concentration of bound receptors. Response to a drug relates to the proportion of bound receptors—known as occupancy. The relationship between occupancy and pharmacological response is usually non-linear.

The underlying principles of drug–receptor interaction are based on the assumption that an agonist interacts reversibly with its receptor and consequently induces an effect. Antagonists bind to the same receptors as the agonists, but usually have no effect other than to prevent agonist molecules from binding and thereby inhibiting their effect. Antagonists are considered competitive if they bind reversibly. When antagonists reduce the maximum agonist effect, the antagonism is considered non-competitive or insurmountable. Experimental pharmacology indicates that some angiotensin receptor AT1 antagonists exert insurmountable effects; in other words, the maximum potential agonistic effect of angiotensin II is reduced in the presence of the antagonist. However, the clinical significance of this property has been questioned, as agonist and antagonist levels in humans never reach the high concentrations used in experimental pharmacology, and the actions of all these antagonists are basically competitive and reversible in nature. In the dose ranges of AT1 antagonists prescribed clinically, insurmountability is of little or no relevance [1].

Specificity/selectivity of cardiovascular drug action

The specificity of a molecule is determined by its activity at a single receptor, enzyme, or receptor subtype. Depending on the therapeutic target, it is possible to achieve a degree of specificity of drug action within the CV system. For example, because voltage-gated calcium channels make only a small contribution to the control of venous smooth muscle tone, calcium-channel blockers are selective arterial dilators [2]. Similarly, vasopressin agonists produce a degree of preferential splanchnic vasoconstriction, and are used in the treatment of portal hypertension [3]. The selective dilator effects of sildenafil (a type V phosphodiesterase (PDE) inhibitor) on the penile and pulmonary vasculature may reflect expression of that enzyme in those particular vascular beds [4]. However, many such receptors are expressed in other cells and tissues, and when activated there result in the recognized adverse effects of 5HT1 and vasopressin agonists (coronary spasm), and PDE V inhibitors (systemic hypotension). Moreover, loss of specificity is commonly seen as the dose increases; ➲Fig. 11.1 shows the dose–response curves for a drug acting at two receptors

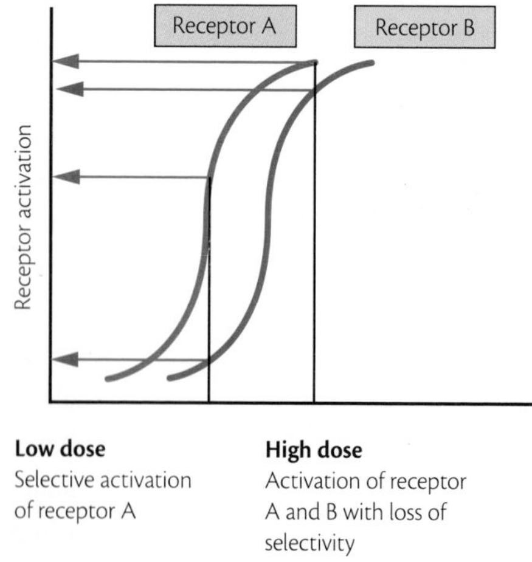

Figure 11.1 Dose–response curves for a drug acting at two receptors but with different potencies. At low doses, receptor A is specifically activated but at higher doses, where the curves converge, there is equivalent activation of receptors A and B.

but with different potencies. At low doses, receptor A is specifically activated but at higher doses, where the curves converge, there is equivalent activation of receptors A and B. Selectivity of drugs is relative, not absolute. Cardioselective beta-receptor antagonists (beta-blockers) are supposed to act only on cardiac beta-1 receptors. However, at higher doses they may also act on beta-2 receptors in bronchi and blood vessels, thereby inducing bronchoconstriction and vasoconstriction. Drug selectivity may be expressed as ratios of the relative potencies of individual antagonists. Highly selective drugs may be preferred for a targeted action.

Potency and efficacy of drugs

Though potentially highly non-linear, the intensity of effect of an agonist or antagonist relates to the number of receptors occupied. The theoretical maximum effect is achieved when all receptors are occupied. Observed dose- or concentration-effect relationships are conventionally plotted semi-logarithmically (linear effects on the ordinate versus log concentrations on the abscissa), and display a typical sigmoid shape. Potency refers to the concentration (or dose) of a drug required to achieve a given effect. By increasing the concentration of the agonist, antagonist molecules are displaced, inhibition overcome, and the same maximum effect obtained as in the absence of the antagonist, but with much higher agonist concentrations. In a graphic plot, the resulting agonist dose-effect curve will appear shifted to the right by the antagonist. The degree of this parallel shift in the semi-log plot depends on the antagonist dose and in turn allows for a quantification of the antagonist's activity. It is expressed as the ratio of the agonist concentrations (or doses) that elicit an identical response both in the presence and the absence of the antagonist, and is defined as 'dose ratio' and usually derived at agonist concentrations producing half the maximum effect (E50). E50s of drugs with similar mechanisms of action reflect their relative potencies. The IC50 is comparable to EC50, but for antagonist drugs. It represents the concentration required for 50% inhibition *in vitro*.

➲Fig. 11.2A shows the relative potencies of two drugs that inhibit the same hypothetical enzyme. Drug A is more potent than drug B, as lower concentrations are required to achieve a given response and the dose–response curve is shifted to the left on the x-axis. The effect increases as a function of concentration up to a maximum, beyond which higher concentrations produce no greater response. This plateau defines the efficacy of the agent concerned. Note that drugs A and B both achieve the same maximal effect, and are therefore of equivalent efficacy despite the difference in potency. Evidently, co-administration of A and B at their maximal doses will produce no greater effect than either A or B alone. That is why drugs with different mechanisms of action and different molecular targets tend to be used in combination therapy for CV, rather than combining drugs with the same mechanism. Drug C is both less potent and less efficacious than A or B.

Modest differences in potency between drugs with the same mechanism of action are rarely of clinical importance. First, most prescribers are unaware of the molecular weights of the drugs they are prescribing, without which it is impossible to accurately compare potency. For example, weight for weight, amlodipine is approximately six times more potent than nifedipine (60mg of nifedipine is needed to produce the same blood pressure lowering effect as 10mg of amlodipine), but mole for mole, amlodipine is closer to ten times more potent because of its greater molecular weight. Second, differences in potency are seldom of material interest to the prescriber or patient as long as the drugs concerned have the same vasodilator effect (efficacy). Atorvastatin is approximately fourfold more potent than simvastatin (weight for weight), but over most of the dose-range the effect of atorvastatin can be reproduced by administering a larger dose of simvastatin [5]. Occasionally, the issue of potency may become a problem if other effects of the drug molecule produce unwanted events that have a

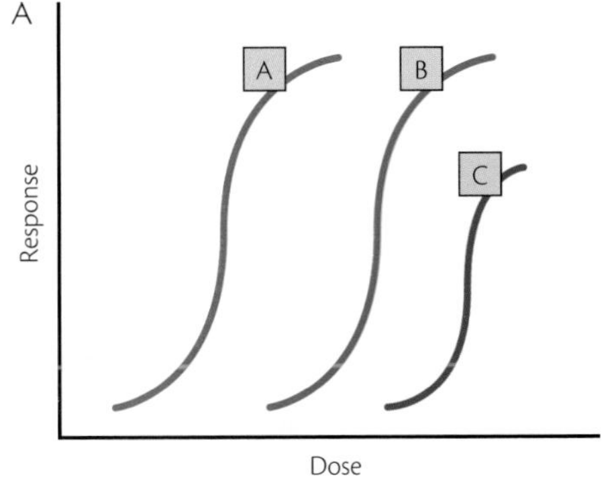

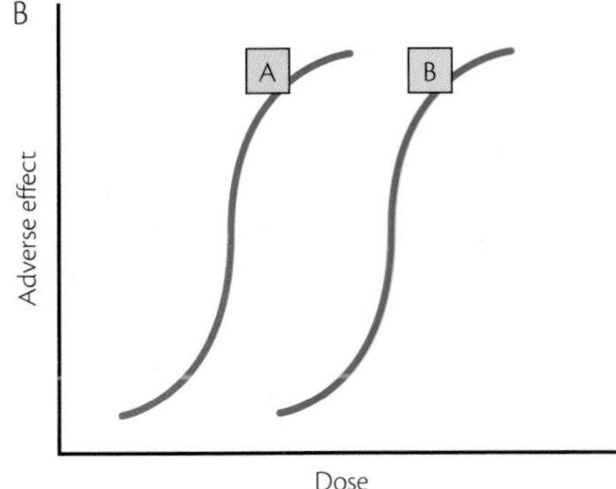

Figure 11.2 The relative potencies of two drugs that inhibit the same hypothetical enzyme. Drug A is more potent than drug B, as lower concentrations are required to achieve a given response and the dose–response curve is shifted to the left on the *x*-axis. Drug C is both less potent and less efficacious than A or B.

concentration-response relationship substantially different from that of the desired (therapeutic) effect. However, given that 90% of all adverse reactions to drugs are a consequence of their primary mechanism of action [6], the dose–response curve and the dose–adverse effect curve will usually both be shifted leftward for a more potent drug (➲Fig. 11.2B). There is evidence that this is the case with statins; the most potent statin, cerivastatin, had its marketing licence withdrawn because of toxicity [7], and dose for dose, the toxicity of atorvastatin is greater than that of simvastatin [8].

Adverse reactions to drugs are not always a consequence of their primary mechanism of action and may relate to secondary activity. When that is the case, care should be taken to select a dose that treats the disease effectively while remaining safe. The range between the minimum amount that is effective and the amount that results in more adverse events than desired effects is called the therapeutic window. Medication with a narrow therapeutic window, such as digoxin, must be administered and monitored with care, for example by frequently measuring blood concentrations in order to avoid adverse effects such as arrhythmias.

Dose–response relationships

Classical molecular pharmacology deals with the interaction of a drug with its receptor. At a molecular level, the relationship between drug concentration (on a log scale) and response is typically sigmoidal. Clinically, a similar relationship can be seen between the dose administered and the physiological response (➲Fig. 11.3), although the dose–response relationship *in vivo* will also depend on pharmacokinetic parameters that determine the concentration of a drug that actually reaches its receptor.

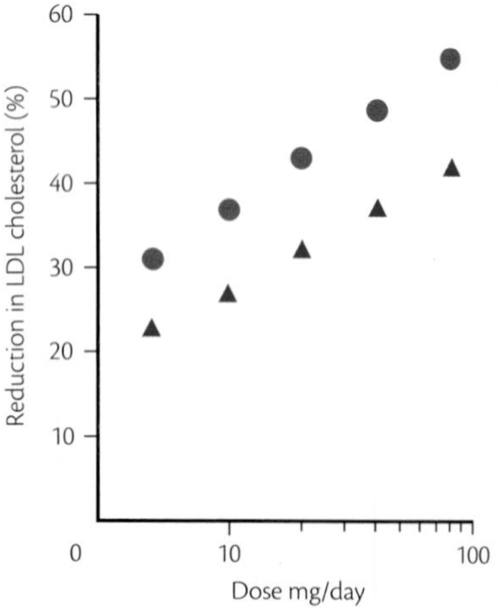

Figure 11.3 Dose–response curve of the effect of statins on low-density lipoprotein (LDL) cholesterol. Atorvastatin, red circles; simvastatin, blue triangles.

During the clinical development of a medication, its dose–response relationship must be established in order to determine the useful dose range and the 'optimal dose'—often defined as the lowest dose providing maximal efficacy. In turn, maximal efficacy is defined by the maximal effect achieved at the plateau of the dose–effect relationship. When a drug is introduced into clinical practice, the licensed dose range should fall on the steep part of the dose–response curve to facilitate titration (➲Fig. 11.3). However, more often than not, therapies are introduced into practice at a dose close to that producing a maximal response. That is the case with most antihypertensive agents, leaving little room for dose up-titration. Maximal effective doses of antihypertensive agents are close to the top of the dose–response range, beyond which little additional blood pressure effect can be obtained by further increasing the dose. Additional efficacy with further dose increments is usually minimal, leading to a plateau in the dose–effect relationship curve.

A real dose–effect relationship is not always documented over a wide range of doses. Dose finding in phase II clinical trials is one of the most challenging tasks in drug development. Captopril was introduced at initial doses above 600mg daily, resulting in significant first-dose hypotension [9]. Subsequently, it was found that 150mg a day achieved the maximal blood pressure lowering effect and was much safer. Similarly, thiazide diuretics were used at supramaximal hypotensive doses for many years before it was realized that five-to tenfold lower doses produced similar reductions in blood pressure while minimizing adverse effects [10]. It may be useful to plot on the same graph the placebo-corrected dose–effect relationship of drugs from the same class, so as to compare their relative efficacy (➲Fig 11.4) [11].

Pharmacokinetics

Pharmacokinetics refers to the fate of substances administered externally to a patient. In contrast to pharmacodynamics, which explores what a drug does to the body, pharmacokinetics explores what the body does to the drug. This includes the routes and mechanisms of absorption and excretion, the rate at which a drug's activity begins and its duration, biotransformation of the molecule in the body, and the effects and routes of excretion of its metabolites.

Absorption of drugs

The majority of CV drugs are administered orally, which suits patients being treated for the conditions outlined

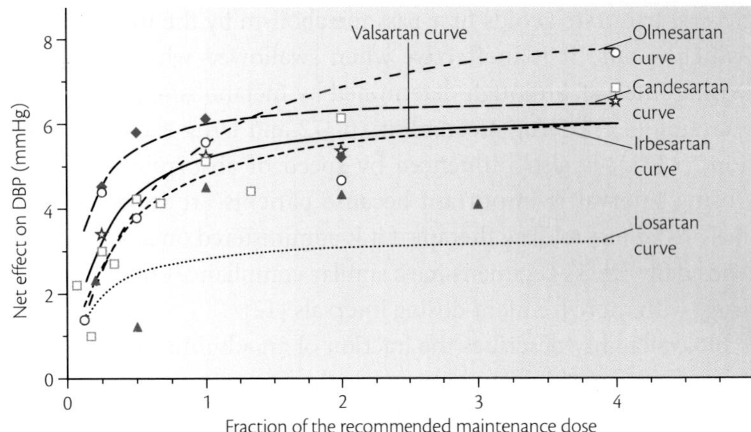

Figure 11.4 Examples of dose–effect relationships with antihypertensive angiotensin receptor blockers [11]. Candesartan, green diamonds; irbesartan, orange squares; losartan, red triangles; olmesartan, blue circles; valsartan, purple stars.

in ➲Fig. 11.5. The intravenous (IV) route is restricted to drugs that are not readily absorbed through the gastrointestinal tract (heparin) or are digested (for example, proteins such as thrombolytics, nesiritide). IV drugs may also be indicated when faster onset of action is required (IV nitrates, inotropes), when it is important to rapidly titrate drug dose against effect (IV heparin in patients at high risk of bleeding), and when the gut is unavailable (patient is unconscious) or non-functioning (diuretics in severe heart failure to avoid uncertain absorption due to gut oedema). The sublingual route is used for drugs that undergo extensive rapid hepatic metabolism; sublingual absorption of

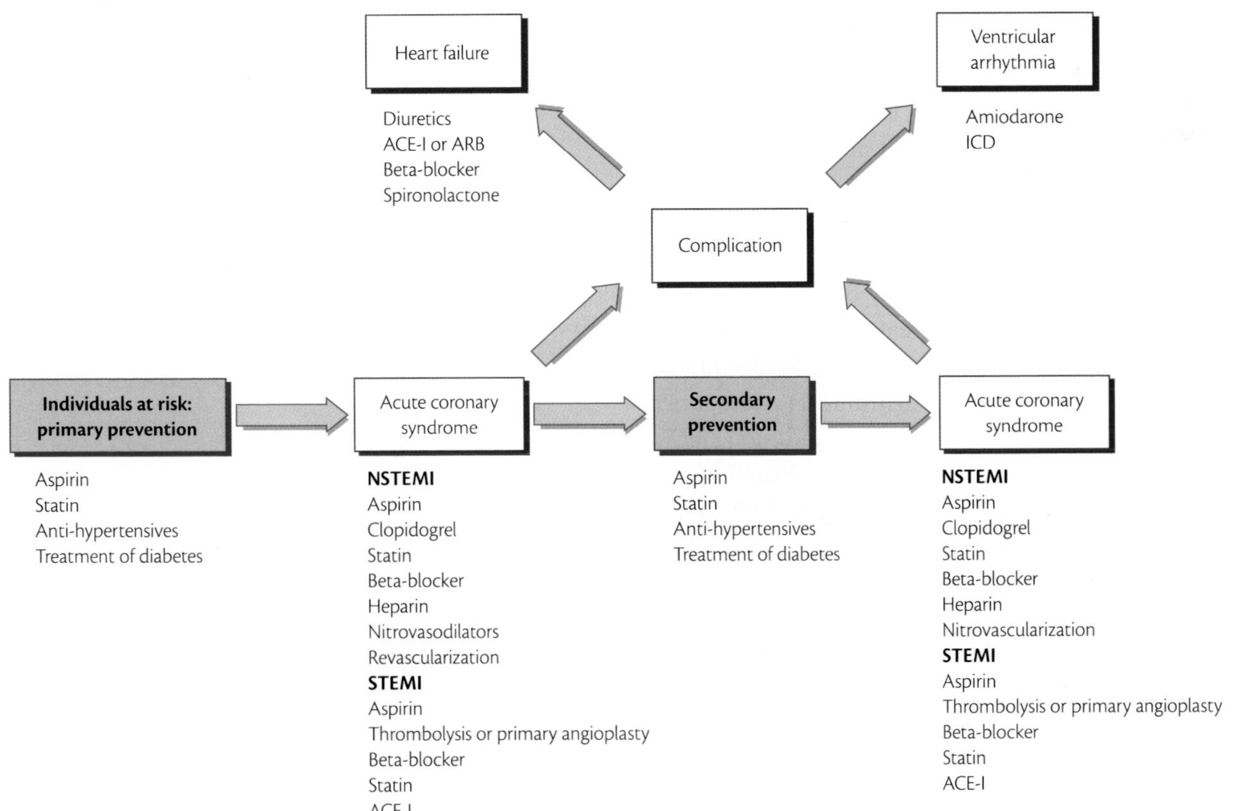

Figure 11.5 Place of drug therapies in treatment as defined by the natural history of atherothrombotic CV disease. ACE-1, angiotensin-converting enzyme inhibitor; ICD, automatic implantable cardioverter defibrillator; ARB, angiotensin receptor blocker; NSTEMI, non-ST segment elevation myocardial infarction; STEMI, ST segment elevation myocardial infarction.

glyceryl trinitrate avoids first-pass metabolism by the liver (which is why it is ineffective when swallowed whole). Dosing interval, although determined by metabolism and excretion (see ➲Drug metabolism, p.372 and Drug excretion, p.373), is also influenced by speed of absorption. Dosing interval is important because patients are more likely to adhere to drug therapy if it is administered once or twice daily (these regimens have similar compliance) than drugs with more frequent dosing intervals [12].

Bioavailability describes the fraction of an administered dose of unchanged drug that reaches the systemic circulation, one of the principal pharmacokinetic properties of any agent. By definition, a medication administered IV is 100% bioavailable. However, when administered via other routes (such as orally), its bioavailability decreases due to incomplete absorption and first-pass metabolism.

Drug distribution

Most CV drugs distribute freely throughout the CV system, and will have generalized effects in all vascular beds that contain target receptors and enzymes. Widespread distribution of drugs outside the CV system is also to be expected, though water- and lipid-soluble agents differ in this respect. Lipid-soluble molecules tend to have larger volumes of distribution. The volume of distribution (VD), also known as the apparent volume of distribution, is a pharmacological measure of the distribution of a medication between plasma and the rest of the body. It is defined as the volume in which the amount of drug would need to be uniformly distributed to produce the observed blood concentration. VD may be increased by renal failure (due to fluid retention) and liver failure (due to altered body fluid and plasma protein binding). Conversely, it may be decreased due to dehydration. Digitalis and, to a greater extent, amiodarone are sequestered in body fat due to very high lipid solubility. This results in a large volume of distribution and the need for loading doses when initiating therapy, and a long period of elution when treatment is discontinued. Penetration of the blood–brain barrier by the lipid-soluble beta-blocker propranolol may be responsible for some adverse effects (notably sleep disturbance and nightmares) that can be alleviated by switching to a water-soluble member of the same class, such as atenolol.

Drug metabolism

Many CV drugs require metabolism to become active. Such so-called prodrugs include nitrate vasodilators (an as yet unknown process yields the active moiety, nitric oxide), and many ACE inhibitors (for example, enalapril is metabolized to enalaprilat). Metabolism of most drugs leads to increased water solubility, allowing for excretion in the urine. Phase 1 reactions result in oxidation or reduction of drug molecules, leading to inactivity. Subsequent phase 2 reactions (conjugation with glucuronide, sulphate, or acetate) lead to water solubility and excretion in the urine. Phase 1 reactions are of most interest, as many involve CYP enzymes—a family of molecules responsible for the metabolism of a large number of antiarrhythmic drugs. Genetic variation in CYP affects 10% of Europeans, and can lead to poor metabolism of these drugs, accumulation, and toxicity [13]. One CYP inhibited by a constituent of grapefruit juice is associated with an increased effect of calcium-channel blockers [14].

CYP enzymes exhibit common and potentially important polymorphisms. Several variants influence the metabolism of CV drugs. Among the most important of these is variation in the CYP2C9 enzyme that metabolizes warfarin. Two common variants (*CYP2C9*2* and *CYP2C9*3*) have been identified, and about 20% of individuals carry at least one copy. Carriage of these variants is associated with reduced warfarin requirement, and a 1.5-to twofold increase in risk of haemorrhage. However, whether information on *CYP2C9* genotyping will impact on bleeding rates in clinical practice will require prospective evaluation in clinical trials [15].

The first-pass effect is a phenomenon of drug metabolism whereby the concentration of a drug is greatly reduced before it reaches the systemic circulation (➲Fig. 11.6). After a drug is

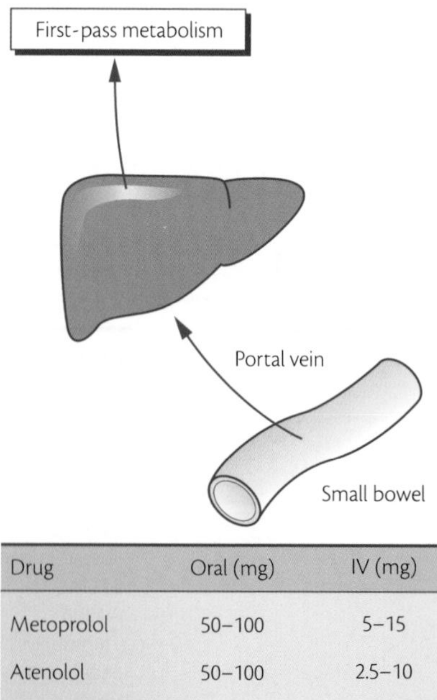

Drug	Oral (mg)	IV (mg)
Metoprolol	50–100	5–15
Atenolol	50–100	2.5–10

Figure 11.6 Metabolism by the liver reduces the oral bioavailability of beta-blockers and aspirin; consequently, when the first-pass metabolism is bypassed by intravenous administration of beta-blockers, the dose required is substantially smaller than for the oral dose.

swallowed, it is absorbed by the digestive system and enters the hepatic portal system. It is carried through the portal vein into the liver before it reaches the rest of the body. The liver metabolizes many agents, sometimes to such an extent that only a small amount of active drug emerges from the liver to reach the rest of the circulatory system. This first pass through the liver thus greatly reduces bioavailability. Alternative means of administration such as the IV and sublingual routes, avoid the first-pass effect for nitrates. Verapamil is extensively metabolized in the liver and exposed to first-pass metabolism. Beta-blockers also undergo extensive first-pass metabolism, which is why the IV dose of atenolol is tenfold lower than the oral dose.

Higher concentrations of aspirin in the portal circulation than the systemic circulation (because of first-pass metabolism) may be important in its effect on platelet function. In the time taken to absorb aspirin from the gut, most of the circulating platelets will have traversed the portal circulation and been exposed to concentrations of aspirin sufficient to maximally block COX, while systemic concentrations, being much lower, may have less effect on endothelial COX [16].

Drug excretion

The kidneys, which excrete water-soluble substances, are the principal organs of excretion. The biliary system contributes to excretion to the degree that a drug is not reabsorbed from the gastrointestinal tract. Generally, the contributions of the intestine, saliva, sweat, breast milk, and lungs to excretion is small, except for exhalation of volatile anaesthetics. Excretion via breast milk, although not important to the mother, may affect the breastfeeding infant. Hepatic metabolism often makes drugs more polar and thus more water soluble. The resulting metabolites are then more readily excreted.

Renal excretion

Renal filtration accounts for most drug excretion. With aging, renal drug excretion decreases, and at age 80 years, clearance is typically reduced to half of what it was at the age of 30. Drugs bound to plasma proteins remain in the circulation; only unbound drug is contained in the glomerular filtrate. Urine pH, which varies from 4.5–8.0, may markedly affect drug reabsorption. Acidification of urine increases reabsorption and decreases excretion of weak acids, and decreases reabsorption of weak bases. Alkalinization of urine has the opposite effect. Drugs compete with each other for secretion; for example, secretion of dofetilide by the renal tubules can be inhibited by cimetidine, trimethoprim, and ketoconazole.

Biliary excretion

Some drugs and their metabolites are extensively excreted in bile. Agents with a molecular weight above 300 and with both polar and lipophilic groups are more likely to be excreted in the bile; smaller molecules are generally excreted only in negligible amounts. Conjugation, particularly with glucuronic acid, facilitates biliary excretion. In the enterohepatic cycle, a drug secreted in bile is reabsorbed into the circulation from the intestine. Biliary excretion eliminates substances from the body only to the extent that enterohepatic cycling is incomplete—when some of the secreted drug is not reabsorbed from the intestine.

Duration of action and biological half-life

The duration of action of a drug is dependent on its half-life, defined as the time it takes to lose half of its pharmacological activity. Biological half-life is determined by elimination half-life, but for a number of drugs the two differ significantly. Elimination half life is mainly determined by drug metabolism, distribution, and excretion. However, even when measurable, the plasma concentrations of a given compound may not predict its duration of action. Indeed, many substances may leave the blood compartment and become undetectable but still remain bound in the tissues and more specifically to their selective receptors.

Knowledge of the equilibrium dissociation constant (Kd) is critical. Molecules that bind strongly to receptors (low Kd) and insurmountable antagonists tend to have durations of action longer than would be expected on the basis of elimination half-life. As estimation of biological half-life is sometimes difficult, assessment of time-effect profiles rather than time-concentration profile may be more informative.

Trough-to-peak ratio was introduced as a method of assessing the time-effect profile of antihypertensive drugs. The original recommendations for its proper application required repeated conventional blood pressure measurements to be performed in comparable standardized conditions, both at peak and at trough. The ratio between the average values of these multiple trough and peak measurements was suggested to provide a reliable and reproducible index of drug effect–time distribution.

Variation in response to drug therapy

In principle, one would aim for a target plasma concentration of the drug for a desired level of response. In reality, there are many factors affecting this goal. There appears to be substantial interindividual variation in the dose–response to drug therapy, which can arise because of differences in drug metabolism or elimination (pharmacokinetic), or because of physiological differences in the receptor or systems targeted (pharmacodynamic).

Pharmacokinetic factors determine peak and steady state concentrations, and concentrations cannot be maintained with absolute consistency because of interindividual variations in absorption, distribution, metabolic breakdown, and excretory clearance. Population pharmacokinetics is the study of the sources and correlates of variability in drug concentrations among individuals who are the target patient population receiving clinically relevant doses of a drug of interest. Certain patient demographic, pathophysiological, and therapeutic features, such as body weight, excretory and metabolic functions, and the presence of other therapies, can consistently alter dose–concentration relationships. For example, steady-state concentrations of drugs eliminated mostly by the kidney are usually greater in patients suffering from renal failure than they are in patients with normal renal function receiving the same dosage. Population pharmacokinetics seeks to identify the measurable pathophysiologic factors that cause changes in the dose–concentration relationship and the extent of these changes so that, if such changes are associated with clinically significant shifts in the therapeutic index, dosage can be appropriately modified. Because response to unfractionated heparin is variable due to unpredictable absorption and protein binding following subcutaneous administration, therapy needs to be monitored by measuring the activated partial thromboplastin time. Low-molecular-weight heparin has much more reliable absorption and interacts predictably with proteins. It can therefore be administered at a dose based solely on body weight rather than on clotting times.

An extreme example of pharmacodynamic sources of variability is low-renin hypertension. This is common in patients of Afro-Caribbean origin and is responsible for a poor hypotensive response to therapies that block the renin–angiotensin system (beta-blockers, ACE inhibitors, and angiotensin II receptor blockers) when used as monotherapy [17].

Genetic factors may alter metabolism or drug action itself, and a patient's immediate status may also affect indicated dosage. For example, a single gene defect can dramatically affect responses to drugs; individuals deficient in glucose-6-phosphatase dehydrogenase are prone to haemolytic anaemia in response to oxidizing drugs such as antimalarials [18]. A later section of this chapter deals specifically with the pharmacogenetics of CV drugs (see ➲Pharmacogenomics, pharmacogenetics, and cardiovascular drugs, p.377).

Lastly, variation in response may be factitious; a patient might not be adhering to medication, an occurrence that is not uncommon when (as in CV disorders) the preventative therapies being used have no apparent symptomatic benefit to the patient.

In the case of warfarin, variation may relate to all of the above mechanisms. Pharmacokinetics may be affected by environmental factors, such as food; variation in response may result from differential antagonism by endogenous vitamin K between individuals and/or differences in drug metabolism arising from common genetic variations; variation in the gene for the enzyme cytochrome CYP2C9, a determinant of warfarin metabolism, might account for a proportion of the variability in the effect of warfarin and susceptibility to bleeding [15]. Finally, non-adherence is one of the main reasons for lack of response (or excess response) to oral anticoagulant activity. Biochemical monitoring of drug action is one way to tailor response to a desired target. In the case of oral anti-vitamin K agents, INR has proven to be a reliable biomarker.

The mean dose–response of a drug is in effect the aggregate of individual curves from individual patients. To avoid over-treatment, it is common practice to perform some degree of dose-titration when initiating therapy; for example, elderly patients are often more sensitive than younger people to the effects of vasodilators and therefore start at lower doses.

Class effect

Major advances in therapy follow from the discovery of new molecular targets and new molecules to modulate their function, but it is much more common for a new chemical entity to mimic the action of an established one ('me-too' drugs). A prescriber can choose from several ACE inhibitors, angiotensin receptor blockers, beta-blockers, and calcium-channel blockers, and five statins. The main reason for the proliferation of similar drugs is the commercial imperative; pharmaceuticals companies need market share, especially when the market is large (as in CV disease).

An important premise behind the development of a new agent in an established class is that efficacy is the result of a 'class effect'. Marketing usually tends to highlight real, yet frequently marginal differences among agents belonging to the same class. Although there is little reason to expect drugs that target the same mechanism to have substantially different effects, the story of cerivastatin withdrawal shows that all statins are not alike. Importantly, class effect may be used by regulators and reimbursement bodies to mandate the use of the cheapest available drug within a class.

However, the choice of agent should be made on the basis of evidence from appropriate clinical trials. Only trials provide accurate evidence concerning the benefit:risk ratio and the size of the effect of a given dose of a given drug. Prescribers should adhere to using drugs within a class with the best available trial based evidence.

Pleiotropic effects of drugs

Additional mechanisms of action may be proposed for a particular class of CV drugs. Such multiplicity of effects/action is known as pleiotropic, and pleiotropic effects have been ascribed to ACE inhibitors (not only vasodilatory, but antiproliferative, antioxidant, etc.) and statins (anti-inflammatory effects as well as reducing low-density lipoprotein cholesterol). Often these adventitious effects are observed solely in *in vitro* or animal studies and of uncertain clinical relevance. The cardiovascular effects of ACE inhibitors are just as easily explained by their vasodilator and blood pressure lowering effects [19], and the protective effects of statins by their reduction in blood cholesterol [20]. However, recent trials provide evidence of possible dissociation between the clinical benefit of renin–angiotensin–aldosterone system antagonists and their blood pressure lowering effect—Heart Outcomes and Prevention Evaluation (HOPE), the Anglo-Scandinavian Cardiac Outcomes Trial (ASCOT), Ongoing Telmisartan Alone and in combination with Ramipril Global Endpoint Trial (ONTARGET), as well as between the clinical benefit of statins and LDL lowering, Justification for the Use of Statins in Prevention: an Intervention Trial Evaluating Rosuvastatin (JUPITER).

Drug interactions

Patients with CV disease will generally be taking several medications and such polypharmacy predisposes to drug interactions. Whole books have been written about them, so it is impractical to remember them all (especially when many are clinically unimportant). A few basic concepts will suffice, together with an awareness of the possibility that an interaction may occur in any patient. A number of websites offer the practitioner an updated and referenced guide to drug–drug interactions and may be searched online as needed.

Pharmacodynamic interactions

Interactions between vasodilator drugs result in augmented hypotensive responses, a desirable interaction when treating hypertension, undesirable when patients are taking organic nitrates and PDE V inhibitors (e.g. sildenafil) and when they increase symptomatic hypotension and risk of falls in the elderly (who are more prone to hypotension due to age-related physiological blunting of the baroreflexes). Conversely, drugs that cause sodium and water retention (non-steroidal anti-inflammatories, corticosteroids) commonly block the effects of diuretics. Antiplatelet drugs and anticoagulants mutually increase the risk of bleeding in patients taking both. All classes of antiarrhythmic drugs become more pro-arrhythmic when used together either as causes of ventricular arrhythmias (for example, amiodarone and flecainide) or bradycardia (concomitant use of beta-blockers, calcium-channel blockers, and digoxin). Co-administration of ACE inhibitors, angiotensin-receptor blockers, aldosterone antagonists, and potassium-sparing diuretics predisposes to hyperkalaemia.

Pharmacokinetic interactions

These occur when the metabolism or excretion of drugs is altered. Important examples include the induction (anti-epileptic drugs) or inhibition (certain antibiotics, amiodarone) of CYP enzymes to reduce or enhance respectively the anticoagulant effect of warfarin. Other clinically important interactions include the reduction of renal excretion of digoxin by amiodarone and calcium-channel blockers, or the range of drugs (fibrates, antifungal and antiviral drugs) that impair the metabolism of statins and increase the risk of myositis and rhabdomyolysis. Prescribers should be aware of such common and important problems.

Drugs with a narrow therapeutic index merit special consideration; for such a drug the effective therapeutic plasma concentration is close to the concentration range where adverse effects occur. Therefore, even minor changes in plasma concentration can have adverse effects. Good examples are warfarin, digoxin, anti-epileptic drugs, and cyclosporin; drug interactions should be anticipated when these therapies are co-prescribed with other cardiovascular medications.

Adverse effects of cardiovascular drugs

The high incidence and prevalence of CV disease mean that the drugs used to treat it are widely prescribed, often for many years, with the attendant risk of adverse effects. The major reason for the high absolute number of adverse events attributable to the use of CV medications is not that they are inherently unsafe, but rather that they include some of the most commonly prescribed medications in current use.

In the last 10 years xamoterol (a beta-agonist for heart failure), mibefradil (a calcium-channel blocker), flosequinan (a vasodilator for heart failure) cerivastatin (a statin lipid-lowering drug), ximelagatran (an oral anticoagulant), and rimonabant (a cannabinoid agonist for metabolic syndrome), have had their licences revoked or been withdrawn as a result of toxicity. Others, such as sibutramine (a 5HT receptor antagonist for weight loss), have had their labels significantly changed because of safety issues.

The most common adverse events are of type 1 (a consequence of the mechanism of action of the drug; for example, asthma precipitated by a beta-blocker). Type 2 adverse events are unrelated to the mechanism of action of the drug and are unpredictable and often serious, but rare. By the time any new agent comes to market, it has usually been administered to only about 5000 individuals. If serious adverse events occur at a rate of 1 in 5000 or less, it is unlikely that they will come to light until the drug becomes available. Type 2 adverse events can only be detected by post-marketing surveillance, which is an integral component of the assessment of the performance of any new drug. National Drug Regulatory Authorities in European countries have their own arrangements for reporting adverse drug reactions, with global coordination of reports through the World Health Organization (WHO) Collaborating Centre for International Drug Monitoring (http://www.who-umc.org). Within the CV field, examples of utility of spontaneous reporting include the withdrawal of encainide and flosequinan (excess mortality), mibefradil (multiple drug interactions), and terfenadine (fatal cardiac arrhythmias).

Note that serious but unpredictable adverse effects can occur in just one member of a particular class of drugs that target the same mechanism of action. A good example is practolol, a beta-blocker withdrawn because it increased the risk of retroperitoneal fibrosis, a complication that was not evident with other beta-blockers. More recently, cerivastatin was withdrawn because it had an unacceptably high risk of rhabdomyolysis compared to other statins. The limited safety information that is usually available when a drug is licensed remains a persuasive reason for avoiding newer members of a class until there is a compelling reason to use them.

Cardiovascular safety of non-cardiovascular drugs

Most recently, the CV toxicity of rofecoxib a non-steroidal anti-inflammatory drug (NSAID) led to its temporary withdrawal, and raised concerns about all other COX-2 inhibitors [21]. The NSAIDs are not the first drugs for non-cardiovascular targets to exhibit unexpected CV risk after market release. In 1997, fenfluramine and dexfenfluramine (anorexigens for obesity) were withdrawn when data suggested that they could cause cardiac valvular disease. The following year, terfenadine (an antihistamine for allergic conditions) was withdrawn because of association with fatal cardiac arrhythmias when it was administered with cytochrome p450 enzyme system inhibitors; 2 years later, cisapride (a serotonin 5-HT4 receptor agonist for gastro-oesophageal reflux) was withdrawn following reports of cardiac arrhythmia and death.

Beneficial effects on non-CV targets may be associated with unfavourable CV events. However, CV testing is not a major focus of the evaluation and development of non-CV drugs. Consequently, at approval, the relation between non-CV benefit and CV risk may not be adequately defined. Pre-approval deficiencies are difficult to remedy within current regulatory algorithms, which create barriers to detecting relatively uncommon adverse events before approval. Existing laws do not permit regulatory agencies to mandate post-approval safety studies. Thus, new approaches are needed to document the CV effects of new pharmacological agents not intended for CV targets. Surrogates may be used to predict CV risk. Both the US Food and Drug Administration (FDA) and the European Medicines Agency (EMEA) mandate measurement of the electrocardiographic QT interval during drug development on the basis that a substantial increase predicts potentially lethal arrhythmia. International Conference of Harmonisation (ICH) documents E14 and S7B emphasize the need for thorough assessment of the QT interval during preclinical and clinical testing, supported by *in vivo* CV safety studies and *in vitro* electrophysiological studies; assessment should also include a dedicated study specifically looking at effect on cardiac repolarization [22, 23]. However, inferences concerning adverse events from such data can be overcome only with trials that measure clinical events directly [24].

Uncertainty may be minimized only with pharmacogenomic and other novel initiatives. Nonetheless, in the present, we can and must improve our efficiency in defining the risk:benefit ratios of non-CV drugs. This will happen only if patient exposure is increased in number and duration in pre- and post-approval studies sufficiently large and long enough to enable exclusion, with reasonable certainty, of unacceptable CV risks. Strategies to achieve this goal are available [25].

Cardiotoxic drugs

The heart is a target of injury for many drugs. Potentially cardiotoxic agents are particularly prominent in cancer treatment. As survival of cancer patients continues to improve, cardiologists are increasingly faced with new cardiac disorders related to drug toxicities [26].

The most common CV complications of anthracyclines and related drugs (doxorubicin, daunorubicin, epirubicin, idarubicin, and mitoxantrone) are heart failure (HF) and left ventricular (LV) dysfunction, and, very rarely, potentially fatal myocarditis-pericarditis syndrome. The risk of HF is higher with greater cumulative dose and older age, after chest radiotherapy, or when the patient has a history of cardiac disease. Continuous (versus rapid) infusion or concurrent administration of dexrazoxane may decrease the risk of HF. Baseline assessment of LV function with echocardiography before starting any potentially cardiotoxic treatment is indicated. Pre-existing cardiac disease may preclude the use of anthracyclines. Echocardiography should be repeated beyond a cumulative dose of 360mg/m^2 until the completion of therapy and also subsequently. There is no consensus on the frequency of echocardiography or the optimal approach to long-term surveillance. Acute toxicity (non-specific electrocardiogram changes and arrhythmia) is rare and usually not clinically significant.

- **Alkylating agents** such as cyclophosphamide may cause myocarditis and HF. The risk increases with the cumulative dose and after chest radiotherapy or anthracycline administration. Acute toxicity generally occurs 1–10 days after treatment. Rare cases of haemorrhagic myocarditis have been reported.
- Among **monoclonal antibodies**, trastuzumab may cause HF and LV dysfunction, particularly when combined with anthracyclines, cyclophosphamide, or paclitaxel. Baseline and serial assessment of LV function are recommended until the completion of therapy and also subsequently. There is no consensus on the frequency of monitoring or optimal long-term surveillance. Rituximab may acutely cause hypotension, angio-oedema or arrhythmias.
- **Interleukins** may cause hypotension associated with vascular leak syndrome with transient LV dysfunction during infusion. Patients receiving rituximab or interleukins should be clinically monitored for evidence of haemodynamic instability.
- **Antimetabolites** capecitabine, and fluorouracil may cause ischaemia probably related to vasospasm or thrombosis, particularly among patients with a history of coronary artery disease. Clinical and telemetric monitoring are recommended during treatment. Cytarabine may cause pericarditis and, rarely, HF.
- **Vinca alkaloids** may also cause ischaemia and should be monitored in a similar way. Patients with pre-existing coronary artery disease may need additional anti-anginal treatment. Paclitaxel may cause hypotension as a hypersensitivity reaction or arrhythmia (supraventricular or ventricular tachyarrhythmias, atrioventricular block).
- **Tyrosine kinase inhibitors** sunitinib and imatinib also produce HF and LV dysfunction and the same monitoring recommended for the other anti-cancer agents also applies here. HF generally improves after cessation of treatment.

Pharmacogenomics, pharmacogenetics, and cardiovascular drugs

Pharmacogenomics is the branch of pharmacology that deals with the influence of genetic variation on drug response in patients by correlating gene expression or single nucleotide polymorphisms (SNPs) with a drug's efficacy or toxicity. The aim is to develop rational means of optimizing drug therapy with respect to a patient's genotype in order to ensure maximum efficacy with minimal adverse effects. Such approaches promise the advent of 'personalized medicine', in which drugs and drug combinations are optimized for each individual's unique genetic makeup [27, 28].

Pharmacogenomics is the whole-genome application of pharmacogenetics, which examines single gene interactions with drugs. Data on pharmacogenomics are available on a website for the Pharmacogenetics and Pharmacogenomics Knowledge Base (http://www.pharmgkb.org)

Whether and how to use genetic information in the clinical setting is still debated. One of the challenges regarding the use of pharmacogenetic information clinically is the lack of readily available genetic testing and of a dosing algorithm/equation. To date, no polymorphic variant has been identified that exerts an effect sufficiently profound to mandate altering prescribing patterns for CV drugs.

Genetic variation in pharmacokinetics

There are about 60 distinct CYP genes in humans. An up-to-date list of CYP gene polymorphisms is available on the Internet (http://www.imm.ki.se/CYPalleles/). Most CYP-mediated drug metabolism in humans is catalyzed by the CYP enzyme subfamilies CYP2D6, CYP3A, and CYP2C. Individuals with genetically determined low or no CYP2D6 enzyme activity are referred to as poor metabolizers, whereas individuals with fully functional enzyme activity are known as extensive metabolizers. Poor metabolizers are at increased risk of excessive or prolonged therapeutic effect or toxicity, whereas ultra-rapid metabolizers may not achieve sufficient levels of the drug to be therapeutic. For example, clearance of the beta-blocker metoprolol is decreased in poor metabolizers, leading to a risk of hypotension or bradycardia. Calcium-channel blockers and statins are metabolized by the CYP3A family. Antivitamin K anticoagulants are metabolized by the CYP2C family.

Enzymatic metabolism is not the sole determinant of drug pharmacokinetics. Drug transporters, which can be subdivided into uptake and efflux systems, have received increased attention for their role in determining drug disposition, intestinal absorption, and renal elimination. Polymorphisms of ABCB1, also known as P-glycoprotein, have been associated with a higher risk of toxicity of digoxin.

Genetic variation in pharmacodynamics

There are several pharmacological targets including receptors, enzymes, ion channels, lipoproteins, coagulation factors, and signal transduction pathways. These targets may present variations within their gene sequence that can alter the effect of the administered drug. A few examples of such polymorphisms are: α-adducin (Gly460Trp), angiotensinogen (Met235Thr), angiotensin-II receptor type 1 (A1166C), ACE (insertion/deletion (I/D), cholesteryl ester transfer protein (CETP) (B1/B2), apolipoprotein E (APOE) (E2/E4), factor V Leiden (Arg506Gln), and the glycoprotein IIIa (GPIIIa) (PlA1/A2polymorphism) gene. A number of common variants in candidate genes that might influence statin responsiveness have been evaluated. Of these, small effects of polymorphisms in the 3-hydroxy-3-methylglutaryl-coenzyme A (HMG-CoA) reductase and APOE genes have been reported but, given the inconsistency of genetic association studies of common variants, these findings require validation in very large studies. Even if confirmed, the effects are likely to be small and unlikely to alter prescribing decisions for this group of drugs.

Warfarin

Warfarin has the strongest pharmacogenetics data of all CV drugs. Genetic variability helps explain differences in dose requirements. Between 30–60% variability in warfarin dose can be explained by genetic, demographic, and clinical factors. Genetic factors may explain two-thirds of that variability. Two genes have been clearly associated with a variable warfarin dose: those encoding the major enzyme responsible for the metabolism of warfarin (cytochrome P450 2C9, *CYP2C9*) and the protein on which warfarin exerts its pharmacological effect (vitamin K epoxide reductase, *VKORC1*). There are two polymorphisms, CYP2C9*2 and CYP2C9*3, both of which reduce the normal metabolic activity of the enzyme. The *3 polymorphism does so to a greater extent than the *2 polymorphism. Carriers of at least one variant copy of the *2 allele require less warfarin daily and those carrying at least one copy of the *3 allele require even less. Individuals with *CYP2C9* variant alleles require a longer period of time to achieve a stable dose and are at increased risk of bleeding, particularly during the period of therapy initiation. The CYP2C9 genotype is associated with bleeding [29]. Warfarin creates an anticoagulant effect by inhibiting the enzyme vitamin K epoxide reductase (VKOR), leading to decreased regeneration of vitamin K. The influence on warfarin kinetics and metabolism has been demonstrated to be significant, with carriers of the VKORC1 AA genotype requiring a significantly higher daily dose of warfarin than those carrying the GA or GG genotypes. Together, CYP2C9 and VKORC1 account for nearly 55% of the variability in warfarin daily dose requirements. Patients with VKORC1 polymorphisms and GA and GG genotypes were found to need approximately 75% of the mean daily requirement of patients with the AA genotype. The average dose needed by GG homozygotes is higher than in GA genotype patients, with AA homozygotes requiring the lowest dose. The distribution of CYP genoptypes is influenced by ethnicity. As many as 10% of Caucasians and African Americans have decreased activity of CYP2D6.

Whether and how to use genetic information about warfarin in the clinical setting is still debated. One of the challenges is the lack of availability of a dosing algorithm/equation.

Antiplatelet agents

Resistance to aspirin has been suggested as a possible explanation for failure to respond to its anticipated antiplatelet effect, and as a potential contributor to stent thrombosis, and increased risk of myocardial infarction, stroke, and CV death. Platelet response to aspirin is a complex phenotype involving multiple genes and molecular pathways. Aspirin response phenotypes can be categorized as directly or indirectly related to COX-1 activity, with phenotypic variation indirectly related to COX-1 being much more prominent. Pharmacogenomic differences have been proposed to explain part of the variability in platelet response to aspirin, but the specific gene variants that contribute to phenotypic variation are not known [30].

Clopidogrel is a prodrug that requires oxidation to its active metabolite, 2-oxoclopidogrel, by CYP3A4 and other CYP enzymes. This active thiol metabolite inhibits adenosine diphosphate (ADP)-induced platelet aggregation by blocking the platelet P2Y12 receptor, resulting in reduction in ADP-mediated platelet aggregation. Response to clopidogrel is reported to vary widely, with non-response rates ranging from 4–30% at 24 hours. Suggested mechanisms for this variability have included under-dosing, drug interactions with CYP3A4 substrates and inhibitors, and intrinsic interindividual differences resulting from genetic polymorphisms in the pathways of clopidogrel pharmacokinetics and pharmacodynamics [31].

Beta-blockers

Multiple polymorphisms have been identified for beta-adrenoreceptor (AR)-blocking drugs and may account for the differences in and predictability of response to these agents in hypertension and HF. However, genomic characterization of every patient who is a candidate for beta-blockers is unlikely to be a clinically useful tool.

Both beta(1)- and beta(2)-AR subtypes are polymorphic. There are two major SNPs in the beta(1)-AR gene: the Ser49Gly and Arg389Gly beta(1)-AR polymorphisms; and three major SNPs in the beta(2)-AR gene: Arg16Gly, Gln27Glu, and Thr164Ile beta(2)-AR. Beta-AR polymorphisms do not play a role in CV diseases such as hypertension, coronary artery disease, and chronic HF. However, patients homozygous for the Arg389 beta(1)-AR polymorphism should be good responders, and those homozygous for the Gly389 beta(1)-AR polymorphism should be poor responders or non-responders. Finally, the Arg16Gln27 beta(2)-AR haplotype appears to be susceptible to agonist-induced desensitization and has been associated with poor outcome of HF. However, large prospective studies are needed to replicate these results and determine their clinical relevance [32].

Certain patients with increased gene expression for the beta-adrenergic receptor may have an increased basal heart rate and blood pressure and show increased response to beta-adrenergic-blocking drugs.

The pharmacokinetics of certain beta-adrenergic-blocking drugs (e.g. metoprolol, carvedilol, timolol, and propranolol) may be influenced by polymorphisms in the CYP2D6 isozyme. Poor metabolizers of carvedilol (5–10% of Caucasians) may achieve higher concentrations than rapid metabolizers. Pharmacodynamic rather than pharmacokinetic factors are important predictors of interindividual variation in the efficacy of beta-blocker treatment. Even so, there are big differences between patients in the optimal dosages of each beta-blocker [33].

Drugs influencing the renin–angiotensin–aldosterone system

Polymorphisms in the ACE I/D gene, the angiotensinogen gene, and the angiotensin II type 1 receptor (AT1R) gene have been identified and research is ongoing to explain some of the genetic differences. The distribution and frequency of these polymorphisms may explain the differences in response observed among black and white patients. Different alleles may be associated with toxicity related to ACE inhibitors, in particular reductions in renal function and the occurrence of cough [34]. At the start of treatment, clinical characteristics are not sufficient to distinguish between patients who will and will not benefit from ACE inhibition. Although pharmacogenetic research is still at an early stage, it may be expected to provide useful tools with which to optimize and individualize ACE inhibitor therapy.

Risks and benefits of prescribing for special groups

Elderly people

Elderly people make up the largest group of patients in whom special considerations apply. They have a particularly high burden of concurrent CV and non-CV disease and are usually taking many different medications. Drug excretion via the kidneys declines with age; the elderly should therefore be considered renally insufficient. Reduced metabolic clearance is most marked for drugs with high levels of hepatic elimination, and reduction of metabolic drug clearance is more pronounced in malnourished or frail subjects. The water content of the body decreases with age, and the fat content rises; hence, the distribution volume of hydrophilic compounds is reduced in the elderly, and that of lipophilic compounds is increased. These age-related pharmacokinetic changes underpin the widely held view that drugs should be used at low doses when initiating therapy [35]. The increased risk of digoxin toxicity in elderly patients can be primarily attributed to reduced renal excretion and a decrease in the volume of distribution. Changes in diuretic and natriuretic effects with age are associated with pharmacokinetic changes and are not pharmacodynamic in nature. Because of a decrease in total body water with advancing age, an equal volume of fluid loss in young and older patients represents more severe dehydration in the elderly. Combined with the decrease in thirst, fluid intake, and CV reflexes, hypovolaemia may contribute to deficits in haemoperfusion of vital organs. Reduced renal clearance of loop and thiazide diuretics in the elderly results in higher plasma levels and systemic toxicity, whereas the diuretic and natriuretic effect is decreased.

The pharmacodynamic response to CV drugs may be diminished in the elderly. The most important pharmacodynamic difference with age as far as CV agents are concerned is the decreased effect of beta-blockers due to a decline in response in vascular, cardiac, and pulmonary tissue. This is thought to be attributable to a decrease in

Gs protein interactions. Most studies indicate that there is no decrease in alpha-receptor sensitivity with age. ACE inhibitors do not show age-related differences in elderly patients. With regard to calcium-channel blockers, a slight increase in the effect of dihydropyridines has been reported among older adults, but no change in non-dihydropyridines has been observed, other than a decrease in PR interval prolongation. One of the characteristics of old age is a progressive decline in counter-regulatory homeostatic mechanisms. Therefore the rate of adverse effects is higher and their intensity greater. Such events include postural hypotension with agents that lower blood pressure, dehydration, hypovolaemia, and electrolyte disturbances in response to diuretics, bleeding complications with oral anticoagulants, hypoglycaemia with anti-diabetics, and gastrointestinal irritation with NSAIDs. Drug-induced orthostatic reactions, that are estimated to occur at a frequency of 5–33% in geriatric patients, contribute to the risk of syncope and falls. The greater incidence of adverse effects of drugs in the elderly is related not only to the specific effect of aging but also to the high rates of polypharmacy and comorbidity [36, 37].

There are no simple rules for prescribing that can be applied to the entire elderly population; rather the dose has to be determined individually, paying particular attention to reductions in body weight and renal elimination. Monitoring of digoxin serum concentrations may be useful. However, it is generally recommended to start with a smaller initial dose than is given to younger adults (for example, 50%), and the dose should be titrated to a clearly defined therapeutic response. Therapeutic drug monitoring as a guide to dosage is not very helpful in older patients because of the lack of established target concentrations. Older adults are underrepresented in clinical trials, thus clinical judgment is required to determine how intensively to implement adult guidelines.

Children

Particular problems arise when treating children because many drugs are unlicensed for use in young people, necessitating extrapolation from data in adults. The most obvious problem is that the dose range will not have been established during drug development. The laws and regulatory processes that govern the pharmaceutical industry have historically led to exclusion of children from the drug development process. Many of the medicines prescribed to children are unlicensed or off-label forms (i.e. forms outside of the terms of the licence, such as unapproved doses or agents licensed for use in a different disease or age group). New European Union legislation provides the pharmaceutical industry with incentives to consider children in the drug development process, and industry practice is expected to improve in several areas related to paediatrics. Meanwhile, the use of CV drugs in children remains empirical, at best with dose adjustment according to body weight or body surface area.

Young women of childbearing potential

Prescribing in young women of childbearing potential poses problems related to the real risk of unplanned pregnancy while receiving a teratogenic drug. Because organogenesis takes place during the first 8 weeks of pregnancy, the fetus is at most risk when the woman may not even realize that she is pregnant. It is therefore best to treat this patient population only with drugs for which there is evidence of safety. These are typically older agents that have been safely used to treat hypertension in early pregnancy (e.g. thiazides and beta-blockers). The teratogenic potential of a drug that has recently been licensed is bound to be unknown (because no studies will have been performed in pregnant women). Its use in this context therefore poses an unknown risk that can be avoided by choosing a safe alternative.

If a potentially teratogenic drug is being used, such as an ACE inhibitor, angiotensin-receptor blocker (responsible for ear and kidney malformation), or statin, the prescriber must warn the patient of the risks and provide advice on effective contraception. If pregnancy is planned, all medications must be reviewed for teratogenic potential and safe alternatives substituted as necessary. A particular problem is warfarin, which is teratogenic in early pregnancy (facial abnormalities) and poses a high risk of fetal bleeding and peri-partum haemorrhage in the third trimester. Heparin would be the alternative of choice because it does not cross the placenta [38].

Patients with liver disease

In patients with liver disease, accumulation of calcium-channel blockers, and angiotensin-receptor blockers requires dose reduction because of impaired metabolism. Special care is needed with anticoagulants, as many patients will have prolonged clotting times. Liver disease may reduce activation of prodrugs (for example, many ACE inhibitors including enalapril and ramipril); lisinopril is not a prodrug and may be preferred. Statins are a recognized cause of raised transaminases and it is usual to monitor hepatic function more frequently when the patient has established liver disease.

Patients with impaired kidney function

Patients with impaired kidney function, as defined by a serum creatinine >133μmol/L in men, >124μmol/L in women, or proteinuria >300mg/24 hours, display a very high added CV risk [39]. Of note, impaired kidney function may be more accurately defined using an estimated (using the modification of diet in renal disease (MDRD) or the Gault–Cockcroft formulas) creatinine clearance <60mL/min/1.73m2 for 3 months or more; intensive blood pressure lowering targeted to a blood pressure <130/80mm Hg [40], preferentially using ACE-I or ARB [41], has been shown to slower the progression of the renal insufficiency and of proteinuria, and may improve CV outcomes [42]. A worsening of renal function is expected after the introduction of ACE-I or ARB and is not considered clinically important unless substantial and/or associated with a life-threatening hyperkalaemia. A concomitant use of mineralocorticoid receptor antagonists should be reduced in order to minimize the risk of hyperkalaemia. In the setting of HF, the latest European Society of Cardiology (ESC) guidelines state that an increase of serum creatinine of up to 50% from baseline or to an absolute concentration of 265μmol/L, whichever is lower, is acceptable. If the creatinine rises above 265μmol/L but below 310μmol/L, halve dose of ACE-I and monitor blood chemistry closely (i.e. mainly K+). If creatinine rises to 310μmo/L or above, stop ACE-I immediately and monitor blood chemistry closely. In a setting of hyperkalaemia, check for use of other agents causing hyperkalemia such as potassium supplements and potassium-sparing diuretics (spironolactone, eplerenone, amiloride), and stop them. If potassium rises above 5.5mmol/L, halve dose of ACE-I and monitor blood chemistry closely. If potassium rises above 6mmol/L, halve dose of ACE-I and monitor blood chemistry and ECG closely.

The use of diuretics or other agents is often necessary to reach the blood pressure target in chronic kidney disease patients. Such patients are indeed prone to develop resistant hypertension; Loop diuretics should be preferentially used in patients with severe kidney dysfunction (creatinine clearance <30mL/min/1.73m^2 i.e. stage 5 according to the Kidney Disease Outcome Quality Initiative (K/DOKI) classification), because thiazide diuretics lose most of their efficiency at this stage.

A recent metanalysis showed that the risk of CV events and CV mortality is reduced by statin treatment in people at different stages of chronic kidney disease (pre-dialysis, dialysis, and transplant), and the magnitude of CV benefit achieved seems broadly similar in these groups and approximates that of statin treatment in other populations. Statins were associated with lipid lowering, CV, and antiproteinuric benefits in chronic kidney disease. They seem to be safe in chronic kidney disease, with respect to the risk of rhabdomyolysis and hepatotoxicity and because limited withdrawals occurred in the treatment group [43].

Clinical trials and assessment of evidence

Evidence-based medicine as the basis for pharmacotherapy

Evidence-based medicine (EBM) involves administering only those agents for which there is established evidence of a positive benefit:risk ratio. EBM has led to an impressive improvement in the health status and outcome of patients with CV disease, and is the basis for drug approval.

Evidence may stem from the results of a variety of clinical investigations, including observational and case–control studies as well as randomized controlled clinical trials (RCTs). Data from the latter are strongest because only RCT results can establish causality (that the intervention actually causes a response). RCTs are designed to test a pharmacological hypothesis. All pharmacological mechanism-based hypotheses should be subjected to clinical trial.

A number of promising pharmacological mechanisms have failed the clinical trial test, and many pharmacological agents never become licensed medications. Occasionally, the results of RCTs conducted on apparently very sound pharmacological foundations are negative and reveal excess risk, including, in a number of trials, excess mortality. Mechanism-based medicine (MBM) does not allow for the estimation of risk related to pharmacotherapy. Not all adverse effects are attributable to the main pharmacological mechanism of the drug concerned. Some are unexpected. The frequency and consequences of expected and unexpected adverse effects can be addressed only with prospective studies, including RCTs and case–control pharmaco-epidemiological investigations. Beyond benefit and risk, adoption of new treatments by physicians practising EBM is also influenced by cost—more specifically the benefit:cost ratio. Again, this requires RCTs and cannot be established using MBM. EBM is the safest and most efficient way to treat patients. Pharmacological mechanisms underpin the hypotheses tested in RCT.

Equipoise is an ethical concept in the design and conduct of clinical trials that states that we can only conduct clinical trials in areas of uncertainty. However, investigators and institutional review boards do not always agree about what constitutes uncertainty, which may vary according to individual, local, national, or international concepts.

Statistical aspects of clinical trials

The usual approach to testing the potentially superior efficacy of a new treatment over placebo (or the existing best therapy) is to develop the null hypothesis that the experimental treatment offers no therapeutic advantage.

When a well designed trial (a randomized study with no bias) compares two treatments, any variation observed is likely to be attributable to a difference between the drugs. Significance tests are applied to answer the following questions: how strong is the evidence that the difference is real? Could it be due to chance? Significance tests yield p (probability)-values; the smaller the p-value, the stronger the evidence. As an arbitrary guideline, p is set at <0.05, defining statistical significance at the 5% level. However, this does not prove that there is or is not a treatment difference. A real difference may not be identified because the study is too small to prove it beyond doubt. The estimate of the treatment effect obtained (sometimes called the point estimate) is surrounded by a degree of uncertainty. One way of expressing uncertainty is to estimate the 95% confidence interval (95% CI). For example, an observed relative risk of 0.33 with a 95% CI of 0.15–0.53 means that we may be 95% sure that the true relative risk is in this interval (and there is 5% chance that the true relative risk does not lie in the CI). The size of this confidence limit depends on the number of subjects studied, the rate of outcome measures used to define efficacy (for example, death, myocardial infarction, or stroke), and the size of the treatment effect. Therefore, estimation of the difference between treatments is more accurate in large studies and the bigger the study the smaller the CI. Increasing the sample size fourfold may halve the width of the CI. $P < 0.05$ means that the 95% CI for relative risk does not include the value of 1 and $p > 0.05$ means 95% CI includes 1.

The size of the population (number of patients) enrolled in a trial needs to be set during the planning phase, based on initial assumptions. This is called the power calculation and is based on setting the α value (risk of type I error, false-positive result) that is, the risk of claiming a difference when none exists. It is usually set at $\alpha = 0.05$, that is $p < 0.05$. The risk of type II error (β = a false negative result, the risk of not claiming a difference when there is one) is usually set at $\beta = 0.1$ or 0.2, that is power $= 100\ (1 - \beta) = 90\%$ or 80%. Power calculation also requires estimation of the rate of occurrence of the primary endpoint in the control group and the size of the effect of the study drug. Both estimates must be realistic and clinically significant, and are usually derived from available databases from previous trials and/or observational studies.

Standards of reporting of clinical trials

The aim of EBM is to change clinical practice. Because it stems mainly from clinical trial findings, great care is necessary when interpreting their results. For several reasons, there is a general tendency to 'put a positive spin' on results. This is true even of major investigations published in well-respected journals. Therefore, the reader is advised to remain vigilant in order to spot biased trial design, poor quality conduct, distorted reporting of results, and unreliable conclusions. The CONSORT Guidelines, for authors, journals, and readers [44] have been adopted by most major journals and provide checklists of criteria (➲Table 11.1). The main and most common biases are: post hoc emphasis of positive results, reliance on multiple outcomes, credit given to subgroup analyses, obsession with the p-value <0.05, confusion between relative and absolute benefit, misinterpretation of estimates of the treatment effect size and their precision, misinterpretation of graphics, and distorted graphics.

What is a positive result?

Difference (superiority) trials, by far the most frequent type, aim to determine whether there is sufficient evidence that one treatment arm is different from another. A difference is considered to have been demonstrated if a p-value <0.05 is obtained.

Equivalence (non-inferiority) trials aim to determine whether two treatment arms are equivalent (or nearly so). This is most often done to show that a less expensive or a better tolerated new treatment has clinical benefit very similar to that of the standard therapy [45]. Equivalence trials can never establish identical equivalency, which would require an infinitely large study. The aim is to demonstrate that the observed treatment difference(s) is close to zero with a tight CI. Showing lack of statistically significant difference is not enough, particularly if the trial is small. In fact, true equivalence trials are rare. More commonly, non-inferiority trials aim to assess whether one treatment is at least as good as an alternative. The statistical approach is to declare the smallest treatment difference Δ (non-inferiority margin) which, if true, would be of sufficient magnitude to declare non-equivalence. Δ is expressed as a percentage or odds ratio for binary responses, and as the mean difference for quantitative responses. Non-inferiority is confirmed if the 95% CI for difference excludes Δ. Non-inferiority trials are increasingly common; because they need to be large, it is tempting to choose too large a non-inferiority margin.

Table 11.1 Consolidated Standards of Reporting Trials (CONSORT)

	Item number	Descriptor	Reported on page number
Title and abstract	1	How participants were allocated to interventions (e.g. 'random allocation', or 'randomly assigned').	
Introduction			
Background	2	Scientified background and explanation of rationale.	
Methods			
Participants	3	Eligibility criteria for participants and the settings and locations where the data were collected.	
Interventions	4	Precise details of the interventons intended for each group and how and when they were actually administered.	
Objectives	5	Specific objectives and hypotheses.	
Outcomes	6	Clearly defined primary and secondary outcome measures and, when applicable, any methods used to enhance the quality of measurements (e.g. multiple observations, training of assessors, etc.).	
Sample size	7	How sample size was determined and, when applicable, explanation of any interim analyses and stopping rules.	
Randomization			
Sequence generation	8	Method used to generate the random allocation sequence, including details of any restriction (e.g. blocking, stratification).	
Allocation concealment	9	Method used to implement the random allocation sequence (e.g. numbered containers or central telephone), clarifying whether the sequence was concealed until interventions were assigned.	
Implementation	10	Who generated the allocation sequence, who enrolled participants, and who assigned participants to their groups.	
Blinding (masking)	11	Whether or not participants, those administering the interventions, and those assessing the outcomes were aware of group assignment. If not, how the success of masking was assessed.	
Statistical methods	12	Statistical methods used to compare groups for primary outcome(s); methods for additional analyses, such as subgroup analyses and adjusted analyses.	
Results			
Participant flow	13	Flow of participants through each stage (a diagram is strongly recommended). Specifically, for each group, report the numbers of participants randomly assigned, receiving intended treatment, completing the study protocol, and analysed for the primary outcome. Describe protocol deviations from study as planned, together with reasons.	
Recruitment	14	Dates defining the periods of recruitment and follow-up.	
Baseline data	15	Baseline demographic and clinical characteristics of each group.	
Numbers analysed	16	Number of participants (denominator) in each group included in each analysis and whether the analysis was by 'intention to treat'. State the results in absolute numbers when feasible (e.g. 10/20, not 50%).	
Outcomes and estimation	17	For each primary and secondary outcome, a summary of results for each group, and the estimated effect size and its precision (e.g. 95% CI).	
Ancillary analyses	18	Address multiplicity by reporting any other analyses performed, including subgroup analyses and adjusted analyses, indicating those prespecified and those exploratory.	
Adverse events	19	All important adverse events or side effects in each intervention group.	
Discussion			
Interpretation	20	Interpretation of the results, taking into account study hypotheses, sources of potential bias or imprecision and the dangers associated with multiplicity of analyses and outcomes.	
Generalizability	21	Generalizability (external validity) of the trial findings.	
Overall evidence	22	General interpretation of the results in the context of current evidence.	

Checklist of items to include when reporting a randomized trial. Reproduced with permission from Moher D, Schulz KF, Altman DG. The CONSORT statement: revised recommendations for improving the quality of reports of parallel-group randomised trials. *Lancet* 2001; **357**:1191–4.

Endpoints in clinical trials

The main result of a trial should be relative to the primary endpoint. Bad practice when the primary endpoint is not reached includes post hoc emphasis of positive results with regard to other outcomes, and highlighting possible positive results on a secondary endpoint, in a subgroup of patients or on a composite endpoint or one component of a primary composite endpoint. The selection of a primary endpoint is an important step in a clinical trial. Along with the treatments and the definition of the target population, it defines the research question. The trial is designed and powered to answer the primary endpoint. Any other result can only be supportive of the main result regarding the primary endpoint (internal validity) or raise new hypotheses to be tested in another trial. In the ELITE I trial, losartan was compared to captopril in patients with HF and the primary endpoint was the tolerability measure of a persisting increase in serum creatinine of 26.5μmol/L or more (≥0.3mg/dL) on therapy [46]. The 'interpretation' section of the abstract of the main section was as follows: 'In this study of elderly heart-failure patients, treatment with losartan was associated with an unexpected lower mortality than that found with captopril. Although there was no difference in renal dysfunction, losartan was generally better tolerated than captopril and fewer patients discontinued losartan therapy'. Therefore, the mortality result as a post hoc endpoint was emphasized, although, the authors conceded that 'A further trial, evaluating the effects of losartan and captopril on mortality and morbidity in a larger number of patients with HF, is in progress'. ELITE II, a trial specifically designed and powered with mortality as the primary endpoint was negative [47]. This example highlights that post hoc non-primary endpoint findings may be the result of chance and should not be relied on.

Many trials use a composite endpoint as a primary or secondary outcome. This may be defined as 'an event that is considered to have occurred if any one of several different events or outcomes is observed'. [48]. Use of composites is a common way to deal with multiple outcomes that increases event rates and consequently requires a smaller sample than using one of the components as the primary end point. It assumes that the treatment effect is similar for each component of the composite outcome, which is not always the case. Therefore, composite endpoints are difficult to interpret if effects are not similar for all components, or if the effect of treatment is primarily on a more common, less serious component of the composite. The conclusion of the report of the ValHeFT trial, which compared valsartan to placebo in patients with HF, correctly referred to the primary endpoint: 'Valsartan significantly reduces the combined end point of mortality and morbidity.' However, in this trial, mortality was not affected by valsartan and the main driver of the benefit was the effect on HF hospitalization; 'Overall mortality was similar in the two groups. The incidence of the combined end point, however, was 13.2% lower with valsartan than with placebo (relative risk, 0.87; 97.5% CI, 0.77 to 0.97; p = 0.009), predominantly because of a lower number of patients hospitalized for HF; 455 (18.2%) in the placebo group and 346 (13.8%) in the valsartan group (p <0.001)' [49].

Another inadequate way to report composite outcomes is to imply that the results apply to the individual components rather than only to the overall composite. A good example is the CURE study of clopidogrel in acute coronary syndromes, where the primary endpoint was non-fatal myocardial infarction (detected solely by a rise in troponin T in many cases), stroke, or CV death [50]. It demonstrated that clopidogrel caused an 18% relative risk reduction (RRR) in the rate of non-fatal myocardial infarction, stroke, or death. However, it turns out that clopidogrel reduced the incidence of non-fatal myocardial infarction alone (absolute risk reduction (ARR) 1.5; number needed to treat (NNT) 67 per year), with no significant effect on death or stroke. Combining these endpoints contributes to the common misconception that clopidogrel reduces the risk of myocardial infarction, cardiovascular death *and* stroke rather than myocardial infarction, CV death *or* stroke [51]. Clopidogrel might reduce these other endpoints but we do not have the data to show that it does. Finally, it is usually not wise to combine safety and efficacy outcomes into a composite, such as thrombotic events and bleeding for an antithrombotic trial. Such outcomes need to be examined separately to balance risks and benefits.

In the examples considered so far, most of the endpoints have been the so-called 'real' endpoints of death or major CV events. However, not all trials consider such responses. A surrogate endpoint is a result that is easy to measure and believed to predict an outcome of direct clinical relevance. Examples would be blood pressure, serum cholesterol, carotid artery intima-media thickness, or the number of ectopic beats or periods of ST-segment depression on a 24-hour ECG recording. Because the relationship between the surrogate measure and the real endpoint is often uncertain, trials that evaluate surrogate endpoints alone must be interpreted with a high degree of caution. In the CAST trial [52], the effects of class 1 antiarrhythmic drugs (including flecainide and encainide) on cardiovascular mortality were examined in patients with myocardial infarction.

Although previous studies had shown that these drugs reduced ventricular ectopy following MI, and other studies had shown an association between ventricular ectopy and adverse outcome, there were no firm data prior to the CAST trial on the effect of these agents on mortality. The CAST study showed that arrhythmia suppression notwithstanding, mortality rates over 10 months were higher at 8.3% among the patients receiving antiarrhythmic drugs compared to 3.5% among those receiving placebo, in direct contrast to the expectation from earlier trials that had used surrogate outcome measures. For instance, and until further knowledge, neither drug licensing nor changes in clinical practice should be based on surrogate endpoints. Blood pressure and blood cholesterol levels are the only two exceptions to this rule.

Subgroup analyses

Practitioners and regulatory agencies are keen to know whether there are subgroups of patients who are more (or less) likely to benefit (or to be harmed) by the study drug. The vast majority of published trial reports include subgroup analyses. Regulatory guidance encourages appropriate subgroup analyses, particularly to derive information on subgroups of patients who may be harmed. For instance, a clinical alert was published following the unexpected finding in the BARI (Bypass Angioplasty Revascularisation Investigation) trial that mortality after angioplasty in patients with diabetes was nearly double that after bypass-graft surgery (p = 0.003) [53].

Subgroup analysis may identify heterogeneity in responses to trial interventions across clinically important patient categories. However, interpretation of subgroup analyses is restricted by multiplicity of testing and low statistical power. Reporting of subgroup analysis is often characterized by poor practice. This includes emphasis on 'positive'findings in specific subgroups when the result in the main population is negative [54], seen in the case of the BEAUTIFUL trial published in *The Lancet*. This looked at whether ivabradine (a heart-rate slowing agent) reduces CV death and morbidity in patients with coronary artery disease and LV systolic dysfunction. The 'interpretation' section of the publication stated the following: 'Reduction in heart rate with ivabradine does not improve cardiac outcomes in all patients with stable coronary artery disease and LV systolic dysfunction, but could be used to reduce the incidence of coronary artery disease outcomes in a subgroup of patients who have heart rates of 70bpm or greater.' Although the use of the conditional 'could be used' is cautious, the reader may misinterpret this subgroup finding as reliable enough to consider using ivabradine in patients with heart rates >70bpm [55].

One cautious rule is to keep the emphasis on the overall result. Because a finding in a subgroup may be chance, as the result of multiple testing, its only value is in generating hypotheses for future trials and is in no way a final answer. A well-publicized example comes from the ISIS-2 trial. A subgroup analysis of data from the aspirin arm, conducted to illustrate the dangers of a subgroup analysis even in a very large RCT, indicated an apparent difference in the effect of aspirin on mortality after myocardial infarction by astrological birth sign, aspirin being apparently ineffective for those born under Libra or Gemini.

Measuring the size of treatment effects: absolute risk reduction and relative risk reduction

If a trial is considered positive, that is the therapy under evaluation offers a therapeutic advantage, the next important question is 'how large is the treatment benefit?' The degree of statistical significance (the p-value) provides no information about the size of the treatment effect. A very small treatment benefit could be detected very precisely by a very large trial and, conversely, a substantial treatment effect might be detected with only marginal levels of significance in a small trial. What then is the best measure of the effect of treatment—an important issue in assessing if the new treatment warrants a change in clinical practice?

Consider a hypothetical clinical trial of an antiplatelet treatment being evaluated among 2000 men and women at high risk of coronary heart disease (CHD). Let us assume that 1000 subjects were allocated to the treatment and 1000 to placebo, and that follow-up was complete at 5 years when the trial closed. The results are presented as Trial A in ➲Table 11.2. Among the group allocated placebo, 200/1000 suffered a CHD event, but among those allocated the treatment only 100/1000 suffered an event. This difference is statistically significant ($p < 0.0001$), but is this an important treatment benefit?

If we first consider the participants allocated to placebo, 200/1000 suffered a CHD event. In other words, the 5-year event rate, or 5-year absolute risk, of CHD was 20%, confirming the high risk of the participants. In the intervention arm of the trial, the treatment lowered the absolute risk to 10% over 5 years. Two measures of the treatment effect can now be derived, the ARR and the RRR. The formulae for deriving these values are simple and are shown in the footnote to ➲Table 11.2. The ARR is simply the difference in risks (or event rates) between the two groups, while

Table 11.2 Calculation of treatment benefits in three hypothetical clinical trials (see text for explanation)

Profile of trial participants	No. of events in placebo group (n = 1000)	No.of events in treatment group (n = 1000)	Percentage absolute risk reduction (ARR) (95% CI)	Percentage relative risk reduction (RRR) (95% CI)	X^2-statistic, P-value	Number-needed-to- treat (95% CI)
Trial A High risk	200	100	10 (6.9, 13.1)	50 (37.5, 60)	$X^2 = 38.5$, $p < 0.0001$	10 (8, 14)
Trial B Intermediate-risk	100	50	5 (2.7, 7.3)	50 (30.6, 64)	$X^2 = 17.3$ $p < 0.0001$	20 (14, 37)
Trial C Low-risk	20	10	1 (−0.1, 2.1)	50 (−6.3, 76.5)	$X^2 = 2.74$ $p = 0.098$	100 (48, 1000)

ARR, event rate in control group minus event rate in treatment group; RRR = ARR/control group event rate; NNT = 100/ARR.

the RRR is this difference expressed as a proportion of the control group event rate. It is clear that in our hypothetical trial the ARR is 10% (20 – 10%), and the RRR is 50% (ARR/control group event rate (i.e. 10/20) × 100%). For completeness, the 95% confidence limits around these values are also shown.

By analogy with the previous aspirin example, a 10% ARR equates to ten fewer events for every 100 patients treated in this trial for 5 years. The RRR tells us that this treatment halves the event rate. Which of these, the ARR or RRR, provides the best single indication of the treatment benefit? To answer this, consider a second clinical trial of the same drug in a different group of 2000 individuals at lower risk of CHD (➲Table 11.2, Trial B). In this study, the event rate among the control group over 5 years is lower (10%), but this is still halved by the treatment to 5%. Thus the RRR remains the same (50%) but the ARR is smaller (5%). In a third trial (Trial C, ➲Table 11.2), an even lower risk population has been studied. The corresponding event rates in the placebo and treatment groups are 2% and 1% respectively, the RRR is again unchanged at 50% but the ARR is smaller still at 1%. Some important points emerge from these examples.

First, because the same RRR can be observed in trials with very different ARRs, the RRR does not distinguish trivial from substantial treatment effects. This helps us answer which is the best single measure of the treatment effect—it is the ARR. Second, for a given proportionate reduction in risk, the ARR is highly dependent on the event rate among the participants being studied. Indeed the ARR can be described by the equation ARR = RRR × control group event rate. The higher the event rate, the higher the ARR. Two things follow from this. First, it may make sense to target treatment to those with the highest likely event rate (or risk). This is the strategy currently used to guide statin or antiplatelet therapy in the primary prevention of CHD events. Second, it illustrates why the control group event rate is such an important determinant of sample size and of the confidence limits surrounding the treatment effect. Scrutiny of the χ^2-statistics and p-values in ➲Table 11.2 shows that as the control group event rate falls (from Trial A to Trial C), a study of 2000 participants becomes progressively underpowered to detect a 50% RRR.

Number needed to treat

Although it is a good indicator of treatment benefit, the ARR can be difficult to conceptualize. In Trial A the ARR of 10% indicates that ten CHD events are prevented for every 100 subjects treated for 5 years. By extrapolation, one event would be prevented for every ten subjects treated. The number of subjects that need to receive treatment to prevent one adverse event is defined as the NNT. In this trial, the NNT is therefore 10. The NNT is related to the ARR by the formula NNT = 100/ARR (when this is expressed as a percentage, as in this case) or 1/ARR (if the ARR is expressed as a decimal).

Despite the value of the ARR and NNT, scrutiny of the abstract or promotional material of many clinical trials will reveal a recurring pattern. Treatment benefit will usually be expressed as the RRR (a larger number, with greater immediate impact than the ARR), whereas rates of adverse events will usually be expressed as absolute rather than relative risks, perhaps to minimize the impact of information on drug toxicity.

The ideal NNT would be one—that is every patient who receives treatment, benefits. NNTs of one are rare. Insulin treatment to prevent ketoacidosis in type I diabetes mellitus, and thyroxine treatment to prevent symptoms in patients with hypothyroidism, might be two examples. NNTs of fewer than ten are seen with antimicrobial treatments for certain infections. In CV disease, however, NNTs to prevent major clinical endpoints are substantially higher (➲Fig. 11.7). Though estimates of treatment benefits are rarely presented to patients in this way in clinical practice (though many

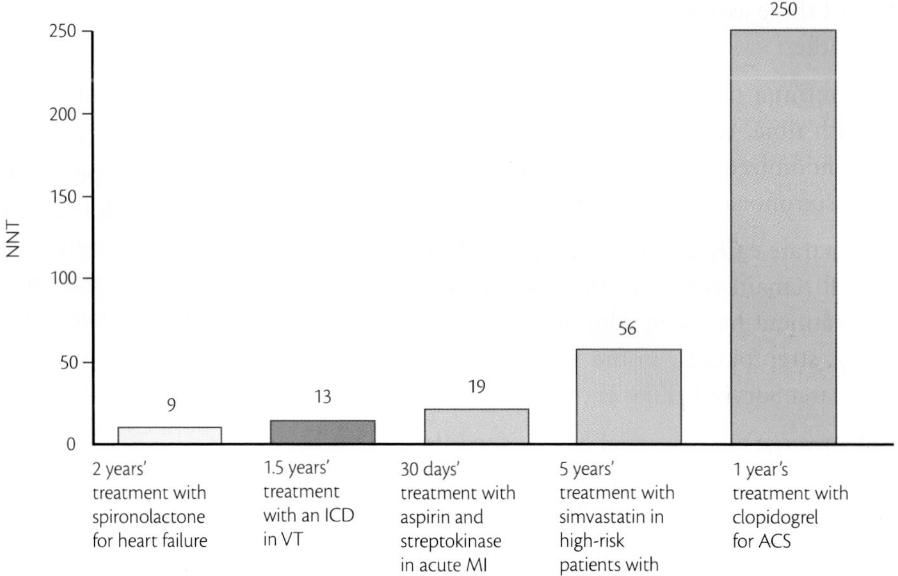

Figure 11.7 Number needed to treat (NNT) of common cardiovascular interventions for mortality reduction. The lower the NNT the more effective the therapy is in preventing death. Note that some interventions are effective in relatively short periods of time [thrombolysis and aspirin in acute myocardial infraction (MI)], some require lengthy treatment (statins) and some are relatively ineffective (clopidogrel; for mortality the absolute risk reduction is not significant (NS) and the confidence intervals for the NNT span infinity). VT, ventricular tachycardia; ACS, acute coronary syndrome.

argue they should be), studies have shown that when such information is provided patients are reluctant to take medications with NNTs greater than 30 [56].

A related concept is the number needed to harm (NNH), which is a measure of the risks of drug treatment. The Cardiac Arrhythmia Suppression (CAST) trial provides a good example; in patients post myocardial infarction, class I antiarrhythmic drugs increased the relative risk of death by 60%, and the absolute risk by 4.8% [45]. The NNH was therefore 100/4.8 = 21. For every 21 patients treated an additional one patient died who would not otherwise have done so. All drugs carry risks and benefits and a comparison of NNT and NNH is a useful quantitative way of expressing this. A good recent example is the use of COX-2 inhibitors to reduce the incidence of peptic ulceration and its complications (NNT = 100) at the cost of increased CV events (NNH = 100).

The RRR observed across a wide range of baseline event rates or risks is relatively constant for a number of preventive treatments in CV disease (➲Table 11.3). Thus the proportional reduction in risk is fairly similar for antihypertensive agents in the primary prevention of stroke or coronary events, for warfarin in the primary prevention of stroke in atrial fibrillation, and for statins or aspirin in the primary and secondary prevention of coronary events [57], whichever patient group is studied, though, as we have seen, the absolute benefits depend on the risk profile of the group being treated.

Survival curve interpretation

Because figures are so effective in creating an enduring impression of results, their construction—and interpretation by readers—must be handled with care. Pocock *et al.* have published an excellent guide on what constitutes good practice in reporting trials and using figures to aid the presentation of trial results [63]. Effective CV drugs reduce the rate of events but do not abolish them. Whether patients take a placebo or an active drug, survival curves inexorably slope downward (➲Fig. 11.8), and if the trial is long enough (or the death rate is high enough as it is in cancer trials) survival curves will converge when all participants have died. The vertical difference between the curves is a measure of the ARR at any given time point (➲Fig. 11.8A) Note that the ARR (and hence the NNT) will vary depending on the time point chosen. The ARR reported at the end of the trial will therefore be specific to that particular time point.

If the study has a low event rate (as is the case for many CV trials), the survival curves will be shallow and the trial will only provide data about the early part of the survival curve. Extrapolating beyond the available data will require

Table 11.3 Relative risk reduction in some common trials

Intervention	Outcome	Relative risk reduction	Reference
Thiazide diuretics for primary prevention in hypertension	Myocardial infarction Stroke	22% 31%	61
Statins in secondary prevention	CHD mortality or non-fatal myocardial infarction	25%	62
Aspirin in long-term secondary prevention	Any serious vascular event	25%	63
ACE inhibitors in HF	Death	20%	48
Beta-blockers in HF	Death	37%	64

one of three assumptions to be made. The survival curves will either:

1) Continue to diverge (treatment benefit will increase with time, e.g. the Heart Protection Study (HPS), the Randomized Aldactone Evaluation Study (RALES) study of spironolactone in HF [64]).
2) Separate early and then run parallel (treatment benefit will remain constant; this pattern is expected when a treatment has been administered on a single occasion, e.g. streptokinase in the Second International Study of Infarct Survival (ISIS-2) cohort [65]).
3) Converge after the trial has finished (treatment benefit will wane with time; the Protein C Worldwide Evaluation in Severe Sepsis (PROWESS) study of activated protein C in bacterial sepsis [66]).

The second point to make about survival curves is that the horizontal separation is a measure of the event-free time gained (➲Fig. 11.8B). In ISIS-2, the combination of aspirin and streptokinase separated the curves (prolonged life) by approximately 1 year; a similar estimate describes the treatment effect of ACE inhibitors in HF [67]. As for estimates of risk reduction, event-free time will depend on the time point chosen and cannot be extrapolated with certainty beyond the trial closure.

Interpreting a trial report

When interpreting a trial report, one should keep in mind four areas of concern:

1) Was the trial a fair comparison?—internal validity;
2) Were enough patients studied?—appropriate sample size;
3) Are the results consistent with other available knowledge?;
4) Is the trial directly relevant to daily clinical practice?—external validity.

Internal validity

A scientifically valid comparison between two treatment groups depends on the groups being as much alike as possible, with the only exception being the specific treatments under investigation. The best way to achieve such a balance is randomization, whereby chance determines the treatment administered. Randomization ensures that assignment to a specific treatment is not known in advance by either the clinician or the patient. The primary benefit is elimination of both conscious and unconscious bias. Randomization also helps ensure identical ancillary care and patient evaluation. Although it does not guarantee balanced treatment groups, it will tend to produce groups that are alike on average. Because imbalances may still occur by chance, baseline characteristics should be reviewed and adjustments made if necessary. Stratified randomization offers some protection against imbalance: patients are formed into risk groups (strata) based on one or more prognostic factors, and a separate randomization is conducted for each.

When reading the report of a clinical trial one should check whether randomization was adequately reported and whether it was done properly. There are several methods of randomization, not all of which are foolproof. Central randomization using specific software to generate random numbers for allocation is standard, and the only acceptable method in open (unblinded) trials. All randomized patients in pragmatic trials, whatever their fate during the study (and, notably, disregarding whether they have taken the drug, been discontinued from the trial, have crossed to the comparator treatment, are poor compliers, etc.) should be included in the main analysis in their allocated groups.

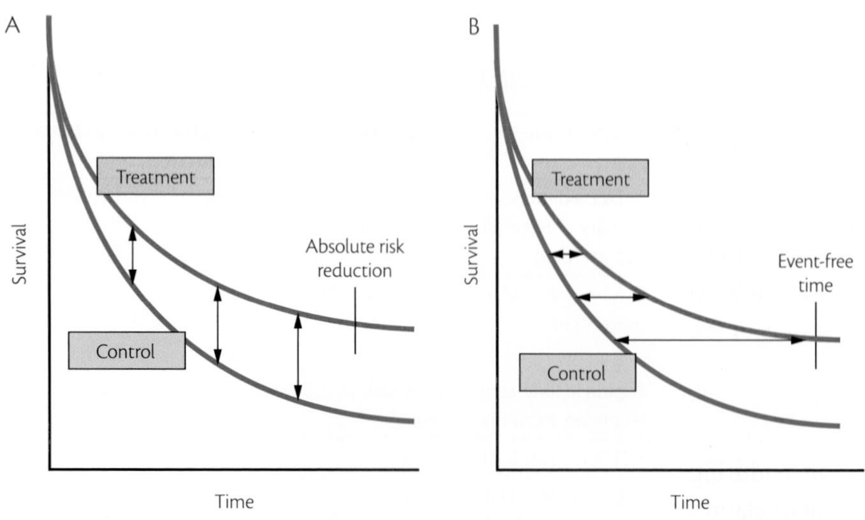

Figure 11.8 Survival curves showing the treatment effect of a cardiovascular drug compared to the placebo group. At the start of the trial survival is 100% in both groups but with time more patients in the placebo group reach the endpoint (e.g. death) and the curves diverge. (A) shows that the absolute reduction in death (vertical difference between the two curves) depends on the time point chosen. Similarly, (B) shows how the event-free time (horizontal difference between the two curves) also depends on the time point evaluated.

This is called analysis by intention to treat (ITT) providing for an unbiased comparison of strategies.

Other tests of internal validity involve assessing the quality of blinding, for example, double-blinding of patient, caregiver, assessor, and those responsible for data processing and analysis. Other factors to assess include: the quality and comprehensiveness of patient follow-up; proper handling of problems related to drop-outs and non-compliance; concordance between conclusions and pre-defined aims and results; optimal reporting of benefit versus risk; and a statement of the trial's limitations.

External validity

The external validity of the results of a trial refers to their generalizability—whether they can reasonably be applied to a definable group of patients in a particular clinical setting in routine practice [68]. Some trials such as GISSI-1 [69] and HPS [70] have very good external validity. The GISSI-1 trial of thrombolysis for acute myocardial infarction avoided selective recruitment, enrolling 90% of patients admitted within 12 hours of the event with a definite diagnosis and no contraindications. As a consequence, it has excellent external validity and is one of very few RCTs in acute myocardial infarction with a control group mortality (13%) remotely consistent with routine clinical practice at the time.

The setting is important, particularly in global trials performed in countries with different healthcare systems. Patient selection with strict eligibility criteria, usually set to reduce heterogeneity, enrich risk levels, and reduce sample size may create a study population with characteristics remote from those of a real-life patient group. One way to assess external validity is to evaluate the ratio of randomized patients to eligible non-randomized patients in participating centres, and the proportion of patients who declined randomization. The practitioner may also compare the baseline clinical characteristics of randomized patients with those seen in daily practice.

Treatment should be compared to standard of care with regard to the appropriateness/relevance and adequacy of the control intervention, and prohibition of certain non-trial treatments. The clinical relevance of outcome measures is usually left to the practitioner's own judgement. Whether management of patients (frequency of follow-up, adequacy of its length) in the trial is relevant to common practice needs to be assessed. External validity of safety results requires complete reporting of relevant adverse effects. It is seriously compromised when patients at risk of complications and/or those who experienced adverse effects during a run-in period are excluded. The HOPE [71] and ONTARGET [72] trials excluded patients who did not tolerate ramipril during the run-in. As a consequence, the rate of adverse effects cannot be estimated from the trial data, and the unusually low reported rate of ramipril-related cough sheds no light on its real incidence.

Meta-analysis

Meta-analysis is an objective quantitative approach to combining evidence from separate (but similar) studies in order to derive a single summary measure of treatment effect. The rationale is that any one trial is too small, and the results of individual trials are insufficiently generalizable. Objective combining of trial evidence is desirable. Therefore, the purpose of meta-analysis is to combine information from all available trials, display consistent objective data, test an overall null hypothesis, estimate an average treatment effect, and investigate consistency among trial results (non-heterogeneity).

Importantly, only randomized trials should be included in a meta-analysis. Trials should involve similar treatments, patients, and endpoints, with unbiased and comparable study designs, ITT analysis, and complete follow-up. All such trials should be included, which is not an easy task, because some will not have been published and data may be unavailable. Because all published meta-analyses are not of good quality, some may be perceived as statistical tricks which make unjustified assumptions to produce oversimplified generalizations out of a complex of disparate studies. Another inherent limitation is that meta-analysis is a 'semi-quantitative' descriptive tool rather than an exact estimation method.

Good examples of useful meta-analyses are the individual participant data meta-analysis of trials of thrombolysis in acute myocardial infarction [73], ACE inhibitors in HF [67], and carotid endarterectomy in patients with transient ischaemic attacks or minor stroke and a carotid stenosis [74]. As a result of these analyses, it is accepted that the benefits of thrombolysis are greatest in patients presenting with ST-segment elevation on the ECG, or new left bundle branch block, that ACE inhibitors are effective in HF at all clinical grades of disease, and that endarterectomy should be confined to patients with a >70% stenosis of the carotid artery.

There are several examples of misleading meta-analyses, in which the combined results of smaller trials have subsequently been refuted or modified by the publication of a very large RCT. The most notable example is that of intravenous magnesium in the treatment of acute myocardial infarction, where the results of a meta-analysis published in 1993 [75] were subsequently overturned by the publication of the very large ISIS-4 trial in 1995 [76]. Other examples include studies of aspirin in the prevention of pre-eclampsia [77].

Table 11.4 Inotropic drugs [78, 79]

Indications	Mechanism(s)	Pharmacokinetics [80, 81]	Adverse effects	Major non-recommended combinations (contraindications)
Digoxin (digitalislike compounds) [82]				
Heart failure [83–86].	Na^+/K^+ pump inhibitor (periphery). Vagal stimulation (central).	Oral bioavailability: 75%. Plasma protein binding: 20%. Clearance: kidney 90%. Plasma half-life: 36 hours.	Low therapeutic index: drug monitoring recommended. Cardiac: ventricular arrhythmias, ECG changes. Non-cardiac: nausea, colour vision troubles, psychiatric [87].	Numerous interactions. Loop diuretics. Antiarrhythmics. Beta-blockers (atrioventricular block 2 and 3 if no pacemaker, premature ventricular beats, atrial tachycardia with WPW syndrome, ventricular tachycardia, non-corrected hypokalaemia)
Enoximone [88] Milrinone [89]				
Acute heart failure.	PDE 3 inhibitors: increase cardiac contractility. Vasodilatation.	Intravenous routes only. Rapid increase in contractility (5–15min), stable during infusion, rapid washout.	Cardiac arrhythmias. Headache.	No major (obstructive cardiomyopathy, severe aortic stenosis, atrial fibrillation, hypovolaemia, LV aneurysm).
Sympathomimetics [90]				
Epinephrine Acute heart failure. Anaphylactic shock.	Alpha and beta adrenergic agonist: vasoconstriction, positive inotropic and chronotropic.	Intravenous. Subcutaneous.	Allergy to sodium disulfite (if present).	Alpha- and beta-blockers (ventricular arrhythmia, obstructive cardiomyopathy, angina pectoris).
Isoprenaline/isoproterenol Atrioventricular blocks. Cardiac arrest. Low cardiac output after cardiac surgery.	Non selective beta adrenergic agonist: increase cardiac output, vasodilatation, bronchodilatation.	Plasma half-life: 3–7 hours. Urinary clearance.	Tachycardia, arrhythmias, angina pectoris, headache. Allergy to sodium disulfite.	Halogen gas anaesthetics (increase cardiac arrhythmias). Beta-blockers (reduction of efficacy) (tachycardia >130bpm, digoxin intoxication, myocardial infarction).
Dopamine [91, 92] Low cardiac output after cardiac surgery. Cardiogenic shock.	Dopaminergic agonist (low dose): diuretic, positive inotropic. Beta adrenergic agonist (medium dose): positive inotropic, vasodilatation. Alpha adrenergic agonist (high dose): vasoconstriction.	Intravenous only. Plasma half-life: 2min.	Cardiac arrhythmias, nausea, angina pectoris. Allergy to sodium disulfite.	Not to be diluted with alkaline solutions. Halogen gas anaesthetics. MAO inhibitors (obstructive cardiomyopathy, severe aortic stenosis).
Dobutamine [93, 94] Acute heart failure.	Beta1 adrenergic agonist: increase cardiac contractility and output.	Intravenous only. Plasma half-life: 2min.	Tachycardia. Increase blood pressure. Arrhythmias. Cardiac ischaemia.	Beta blockers (reduction of efficacy) (obstructive cardiomyopathy, severe aortic stenosis).
Dopexamine Acute heart failure.	Beta-2 (norepinephrine reuptake inhibitor) and dopaminergic agonist: increase cardiac output, vasodilatation.	Intravenous only. Plasma half-life: 6–7min.	Tachycardia, cardiac arrhythmias, nausea, angina pectoris.	Beta-blockers (reduction of efficacy). MAO inhibitors (obstructive cardiomyopathy, severe aortic stenosis, pheochromocytoma).
Levosimendan [95, 96]	Calcium sensitizer. Inotrope and vasodilator.	Intravenous only. half-life 1 hour. Active metabolite half-life of 70–80 hours.	Cardiac arrhythmias, headache, nausea, palpitation, and dizziness, hypotension.	

The most likely explanation in each case is that the meta-analyses of smaller RCTs that predated the very large and definitive mega-trial were biased by the preferential publication of positive results. Publication bias remains one of the greatest obstacles to reliable meta-analysis, but can be minimized by actively seeking out unpublished data.

Individual drug classes

Major pharmacological characteristics and information on therapeutic use of cardiovascular drugs are summarized in ➲Table 11.4–11.13. Drugs are ordered according to their pharmacological classes.

Table 11.5 Antiarrhythmic drugs [97]

Indications	Mechanism(s)	Pharmacokinetics	Adverse effects	Major non-recommended combinations (contraindications)
Class I [98]				
Cibenzoline [99, 100] Prevention of reoccurrence of ventricular tachycardia, without pump failure.	Negative inotropic. Increase conduction time. Blockade of accessory conduction.	Oral bioavailability: 90%. No relevant plasma protein fixation. Plasma half-life: 7 hours (increased in elderly). Urinary clearance (60% unchanged).	Heart failure, cardiac blocks, arrhythmias, tremor, dizziness, nausea.	Beta-blockers, class I antiarrhythmics, arrhythmogenic drugs (myocardial infarction, cardiac failure, atrioventricular blocks without pacemaker).
Disopyramide [101] Ventricular arrhythmias, supraventricular tachycardia, prevention of electric shocks for patients with automatic cardiovertors.	Reduction of action potential amplitude, reduction of automaticity, increase of refractory periods, slowing of conduction. Negative inotropic.	Oral and intravenous. Oral bioavailability: 90–100%. Great variability for plasma half-life. Metabolite with anticholinergic properties.	Heart failure, cardiac blocks, arrhythmias. Associated with atropinic effects: acute urinary retention, mouth dryness, visual troubles.	Beta-blockers, class I antiarrhythmics, arrhythmogenic drugs, erythromycin (myocardial infarction, cardiac failure, atrioventricular blocks without pacemaker, long QT, glaucoma, myasthenia).
Flecainide [102] Ventricular arrhythmias, supraventricular tachycardia, prevention of electric shocks for patients with automatic cardiovertors.	Increase of refractory periods, slowing of conduction. Negative inotropic.	Oral bioavailability: 90–100%. Plasma half-life: 14 hours. Urinary clearance.	Heart failure, atrioventricular block, arrhythmias, neurologic troubles.	Beta-blockers, class I antiarrhythmics, acetylcholine esterase inhibitors, bupropion (myocardial infarction, cardiac failure, atrioventricular blocks without pacemaker).
Lidocaine Prevention of ventricular arrhythmias in acute myocardial infarction.	Action at the ventricular level. Reduction of excitability. No effect on conduction, no negative inotropic effects.	Intravenous only. Liver metabolism (CYP1A2, 3A4). Urinary clearance.	Central nervous system ++. Respiratory. Reduction of blood pressure, arrhythmias, cardiac arrest.	Class I antiarrhythmics, Cimetidine, amiodarone, beta blockers (atrioventricular blocks, epilepsy).
Phenytoine Cardiac arrhythmias due to digitalis.	Antiepileptic drug.	Intravenous only.	Ventricular fibrillation, troubles of cardiac conduction, hypotension. Central nervous system.	(Allergy.)
Propafenone [103]	Atria: increase conduction time and refractory periods. Atrioventricular: slows conduction. Ventricular: increases conduction time and refractory periods. Beta blocker and negative inotropic.	Oral bioavailability: 100%. Plasma half-life: 4 hours. Excretion: liver.	Heart failure, arrhythmias, atrioventricular block. Nausea, taste troubles, tremor, headache. Rare hepatitis.	Beta blockers, class I anti-arrhythmics (myocardial infarction, cardiac failure, atrioventricular blocks, cirrhosis of the liver).
Hydroquinidine [104] Ventricular arrhythmias, supraventricular tachycardia, prevention of electric shocks for patients with automatic cardiovertors.	Reduction of automaticity, reduction of speed of conduction, reduction of excitability, negative inotropic effect, anticholinergic, vasodilatation.	Oral bioavailability: 80%. High tissue uptake. Plasma half-life: 7–9 hours. Urinary excretion.	Arrhythmias, conduction troubles, photosensitization, anaemia, gut problems.	Other antiarrhythmics, beta-blockers, some antipsychotics (atrioventricular blocks without pacemaker, digoxin intoxication, 'torsades de pointes', long QT, cardiac failure).

(Continued)

Table 11.5 *(Continued)* Antiarrhythmic drugs [97]

Indications	Mechanism(s)	Pharmacokinetics	Adverse effects	Major non-recommended combinations (contraindications)
Class II: beta blockers: see Table 11.9.				
Class III				
Amiodarone [105] Prevention of LV and supraventricular tachycardia and fibrillation. Slowing and reduction of atrial fibrillation and flutter [106].	Mainly acting on phase 3 of the action potential. Bradycardia. Reduction of adrenergic responses. Increase in refractory periods. Slowing of conduction in accessory pathways. Increase in coronary blood flow. No negative inotropic property.	Oral bioavailability: 30–80%. Slowly acting via oral route. Loading dose recommended. Long and variable plasma half-life: 20–100 days. Mainly eliminated by the liver. Still acting 10–30 days after stopping the treatment [107]. Intravenous [108].	Cornea deposits. Optic neuropathy. Photosensitization. Hypothyroidism, hyperthyroidism. Interstitial pneumopathy. Tremor, hepatitis, bradycardia, nausea.	All drugs that slow repolarization (risk of torsades de pointes). Antipsychotics. Antiarrhythmics inducing bradycardia. Cyclosporin (reduction of its metabolism by amiodarone). Control of plasma potassium. (bradycardia, sinus disease, atrioventricular blocks without pacemaker, hyperthyroidism, iodine allergy, pregnancy, breastfeeding).
Dronedarone [109, 110] Prevention of LV and supraventricular tachycardia and fibrillation. Slowing and reduction of atrial fibrillation and flutter.	Same as amiodarone.	Well-absorbed after oral administration (70–94%) in fed conditions Bioavailability due to presystemic first-pass metabolism is under fed conditions only 15%. Food increases absorption. plasma protein binding (>98%), Large volume of distribution. extensively metabolized (>84%) into N-debutyl metabolite, 3–10× less potent. 84% of dose excreted as metabolites in faeces. Steady state terminal half-lives 30 hours.	No iodine related adverse effects.	Same as amiodarone.
Ibutilide [111, 112] Reduction of atrial fibrillation and flutter.	Increase action potential duration.	Intravenous only. Low plasma protein fixation. Plasma half-life: 6 hours. Liver metabolism. Urinary excretion.	Torsade de pointes. LV tachycardia (mainly for patients with LV dysfunction). Intracardiac blocks.	All drugs that slow repolarization (risk of torsade de pointes). Control of plasma potassium (LV tachycardia, heart failure, long QT, atrioventricular blocks, sinus disease, myocardial infarction, hypokalaemia, hypomagnesemia)
Class IV: calcium blockers (verapamil, diltiazem): see Table 11.10.				
Adenosine–adenosine trisphosphate Reduction of junction tachycardia.	Purinergic agonists. Slowing of atrioventricular node conduction.	Intravenous only. Very short plasma half-life.	Headache, vertigo, anxiety, nausea.	Dipiridamole (inhibition of adenosine reuptake). Theophyllin, caffeine (adenosine antagonists) (atrioventricular blocks without pacemaker, long QT, hypotension, unstable angina pectoris, heart failure, asthma)

Table 11.6 Lipid-lowering drugs

Indications	Mechanism(s)	Pharmacokinetics	Adverse effects	Major non-recommended combinations (contraindications)
Nicotinic acid [113, 114] Hypercholesterolaemia (high LDL and low HDL) in combination with a statin.	Reduction of free fatty acids release by adipocytes. Stimulation of lipoprotein lipase. Reduce LDL (8–16%), triglycerides (14–35%). Increase HDL (16–26%).	Resorption: 60-76%. Hepatic first-pass: high and variable. Liver metabolism. Urinary clearance.	Cutaneous flush. Allergy. Increase in plasma ASAT and ALAT.	Nicotinic acid can increase liver and muscle toxicities due to HMG-CoA reductase inhibitors (statins) (allergy, liver insufficiency, stomach ulcer, arterial bleeding).
Fibrates [115, 116]				
Bezafibrate, ciprofibrate, fenofibrate Hypercholesterolaemia (type IIa). Hypertriglyceridaemia (type IIb, III and IV).	PPAR alpha agonists Inhibition of cholesterol and triglycerides synthesis. Reduce LDL (15–25%), triglycerides (30–50%). Increase HDL (10–15%)	Good oral bioavailability. Highly transported by plasma albumin. Plasma half-life variable from one drug to the other. Urinary excretion.	Transient increase in ALAT and ASAT (stop if >3× normal values) Rhabdomyolysis (stop if CPK >5× normal values).	HMG-CoA reductase inhibitors (potentiation of muscle toxicity). Drugs that affect kidney function. Vitamin K antagonists. Cyclosporin (liver insufficiency, kidney insufficiency, photosensitivity to fibrates).
Gemfibrozil [117] Hypercholesterolaemia if contraindication to a statin. Hypertriglyceridaemia.	Increase peripheral lipolysis. Increase liver cholesterol turnover. Reduction of VLDL synthesis.	Oral bioavailability: 100%. Highly transported by plasma albumin. Liver metabolism. Inhibition of a lot of liver enzymes: CYP2C8, CYP2C9, CYP2C19, CYP1A2, UGTA1, and UGTA3. Urinary excretion.	Rhabdomyolysis (stop if >5× normal values).	HMG-CoA reductase inhibitors (potentiation of muscle toxicity). Numerous interactions: repaglinide, rosiglitazone, vitamin K antagonists (allergy, liver insufficiency, kidney insufficiency, photosensitivity to fibrates, biliary lithiasis).
Ezetimibe [118] Hypercholesterolaemia in combination with a statin.	Inhibition of Niemann–Pick C1-like 1 (NPC1L1) in the small intestine (reduction of cholesterol and phytosterols resorption).	High liver metabolism. Highly transported by plasma albumin. Biliary excretion [119].	Rare: headache, abdominal pain, diarrhoea.	Colestyramine, vitamin K antagonists (allergy, pregnancy, breastfeeding, liver insufficiency).
Statins				
Atorvastatin, fluvastatin, pravastatin, rosuvastatin, simvastatin [120] Hypercholesterolaemia (type IIa). Hypertriglyceridaemia (type IIb, III). Primary (hypertension, type 2 diabetes) and secondary prevention of coronary events.	Inhibition of HMG-CoA reductase. Reduce LDL (40–60%), triglycerides (20–40%). Increase HDL (5–10%) [121, 122].	High first-pass effect. Clearance: depending on the drug.	Muscle pain, rhabdomyolysis. [123, 124]. Transient increase in ALAT and ASAT (stop if >3× normal values). Rhabdomyolysis (stop if CPK >5× normal values).	Fibrates (potentiation of muscle toxicity). Itraconazole, ketoconazole, stiripentol, delavirdine, telithromycine. (allergy, liver insufficiency, pregnancy, breastfeeding) [125].
Colestyramine Hypercholesterolaemia.	Blocks enterohepatic biliary acids cycle and increases rate of cholesterol incorporation into these acids.	No resorption.	Reduction of lipophilic vitamins resorption (A, D, E, K). Constipation, diarrhoea, abdominal pain.	Biliary acids, vitamin K antagonists, digitalis like compounds, thyroid hormones (allergy, liver insufficiency, biliary lithiasis).

ALAT, alanine amino transferase; ASAT, aspartate amino transferase; CPK, creatine phosphokinase; HDL, high-density lipoprotein, HMG-CoA, 5-hydroxy-3-methylglutaryl-coenzyme A; LDL, low-density lipoprotein.

Table 11.7 Diuretic drugs

Indications	Mechanism(s)	Pharmacokinetics	Adverse effects (contraindications)	Major non-recommended associations
Potassium-sparing diuretics				
*Spironolactone (see also ➲ Table 11.8) Hypertension [126]. Congestive heart failure with low ejection fraction and stages III-IV NYHA [64]. Diuretic-induced hypokalaemia. Primary aldosteronism. Secondary aldosteronism associated with cirrhotic, nephrotic syndrome, congestive heart failure oedema [127].	High doses: potassium-sparing diuretics (Na^+K^+ATPase inhibitors).	Prodrug, activated into potassium canreonate Delayed action (48 hours). Long duration of action. Liver metabolism.	Hyperkalaemia, gynaecomastia, dysmenorrhoea, impotence. Hypotension, dehydration (severe/acute renal failure; liver insufficiency).	Potassium salts/other potassium-sparing diuretics
Amiloride, triamterene Hypertension. Diuretic-induced hypokalaemia. Cirrhotic, congestive heart failure oedema.	Block the sodium/potassium exchanger in the distal tubule	Oral bioavailability: ? Plasma protein binding: ? Clearance: kidney ? Plasma half-life: ?	Hyperkalaemia, hypotension, dehydration (severe renal failure).	Severe renal failure; potassium salts/other potassium-sparing diuretics
Loop diuretics				
Furosemide, bumetanide Congestive heart failure [128, 129]. Hypertension (when thiazide diuretics are contra-indicated i.e. creatinine clearance <30mL/min/1.73m^2). Heart failure or renal insufficiency oedema. Hypercalcaemia	Natriuresis by blocking the Na/K/2CL exchanger in the medullary thick ascending limb of the loop of Henle. Intravenous administration causes pulmonary vasodilatation in acute heart failure.	Oral bioavailability: 65%. Plasma protein binding: 96–98%. Clearance: kidney. Plasma half-life: 50min.	Metabolic adverse effects: increased glycaemia, diabetes. Hypokalaemia. Hypomagnesemia. Hypotension, dehydration. Deafness. Hyperuricaemia, gout. Cutaneous allergies.	Functional acute renal failure; liver encephalopathy, severe hypokalaemia, hyponatraemia, dehydration, urinary obstruction
Thiazide diuretics				
Benflumethiazide, hydrochlorothiazide, indapamide Hypertension [130–132].	Natriuresis by blocking sodium/chloride co-transporter in the distal tubule, open potassium channels.	(Hydrochlorothiazide) Oral bioavailability: 60–80%. Plasma protein binding: 40%. Clearance: kidney 90% Plasma half-life: 6–25 hours.	Metabolic adverse effects: increased glycaemia, diabetes. Hypokalaemia. Hyponatraemia. Hypotension, dehydratation. Hyperuricaemia, gout. Hypercalcaemia. Cutaneous allergies.	Sulfamid allergy; severe kidney insufficiency; liver encephalopathy.
Arginine-vasopressin antagonist				
Tolvaptan Acute decompensated heart failure for relief of symptoms (not licensed) [133, 134]. Hyponatraemia.	Vasopressin receptor antagonist. Aquaresis.	Plasma half-life 6–8 hours.	Thirst. Dry mouth. Hypernatraemia.	

Table 11.8 Drugs acting on the renin–angiotensin–aldosterone system

Indications	Mechanism(s)	Pharmacokinetics	Adverse effects	Adverse effects (contraindications)
Angiotensin-converting enzyme inhibitors (ACEI)				
Benazepril, captopril, cilazapril, enalapril, fosinopril, imidapril, lisinopril, moexipril, perindopril, quinapril, ramipril, trandolapril, zofenopril Hypertension (all) [135, 136]. All grades of heart failure with low ejection fraction (captopril, enalapril, lisinopril, ramipril, trandolapril) [137, 138]. Secondary prevention following myocardial infarction (captopril, enalapril, perindopril, quinapril, ramipril, trandolapril) [139], stroke (perindopril) [140], kidney disease (benazepril, captopril, enalapril, lisinopril, perindopril, trandolapril) [41], and in high cardiovascular risk patients (ramipril) [50].	Inhibition of ACE leading to reduced formation of angiotensin II and impaired breakdown of bradykinin, vasodilatation, antiproliferative.	Depending on the drug prodrugs activated in the liver: benazeprilate, cilazaprilate, enalaprilate, fosinoprilate, moexiprilate, perindoprilate, quinaprilate, ramiprilate, trandolaprilate, zofenoprilate. Liver elimination and likely to accumulate with liver insufficiency: cilazapril, lisinopril, ramipril, zofenopril. Kidney elimination and likely to accumulate with renal failure: all.	Hypotension. Cough (5–10%). Hyperkalaemia. Renal impairment (especially in presence of bilateral artery stenosis). Angio-oedema.	Angio-oedema, Pregnancy 2nd, 3rd quarter.
Angiotensin receptor blockers (ARBs)				
Candesartan cilexitil, eprosartan, irbesartan, losartan, olmesartan, medoxomil telmisartan, valsartan Hypertension (all) [135] Heart failure with low ejection fraction, as an altenative to ACE inhibitors (candesartan, valsartan) or in addition to ACE inhibitors (candesartan). Heart failure with preserved ejection fraction (candesartan). Secondary prevention following myocardial infarction (valsartan), kidney disease (candesartan, losartan, irbesartan, telmisartan, valsartan) [141], and in high cardiovascular risk patients (telmisartan) and in hypertensive patients with LVH (losartan) [142].	Block angiotensin II receptor, vasodilatation, antiproliferative.	Depending on the on the drug prodrugs activated in the liver: candesartan, glucuronid irbesartan, carboxylic losartan, olmesartan. Liver elimination and likely to accumulate with liver insufficiency:losartan, olmesartan, telmisartan, valsartan. Kidney elimination and likely to accumulate with renal failure: all but valsartan (although its use is not recommended in patients with creatinine clairance below 20mL/min).	Same ACE inhibitors (except cough).	Pregnancy 2nd, 3rd quarter.
Renin inhibitor				
Aliskiren Hypertension [143–145].	Direct inhibition of renin leading to reduced formation of angiotensin II, vasodilatation, antiproliferative.	Oral bioavailability: low. Plasma protein binding: 50%. Clearance:biliary excretion Plasma half-life 30 hours. Pharmacokinetics unaffected by hepatic or renal impairment.	Hyperkalaemia Renal impairment. Diarrhoea.	?
Aldosterone antagonists				
Spironolactone Hypertension [126]. Congestive heart failure with low ejection fraction and stages III-IV NYHA [64]. Diuretic-induced hypokalaemia. Primary aldosteronism. Secondary aldosteronism associated with cirrhotic, nephrotic syndrome, congestive heart failure oedema.	Mineralocorticoid receptor antagonist.Low doses: anti-inflammatory, anti-fibrosis, and anti-remodelling. High doses: potassium sparing diurerics (Na^+K^+ATPase inhibitors).		Hyperkalaemia, gynecomastia, dysmenorrhea, impotence. Hypotension, dehydration.	Severe/acute renal failure; liver insufficiency; potassium salts/other potassium sparing diuretics.
Eplerenone Congestive heart failure and LV systolic dysfunction post-myocardial infarction [146–149].	Mineralocorticoid receptor (MR) antagonist: same as spironolactone, but more specificity toward MR vs. sexual steroid receptors.	Plasma protein binding: 50%. Clearance: kidney 67%. Plasma half-life: 3–5 hours.	Hyperkalaemia. Hypotension. Dehydration.	Severe/moderate renal failure; liver insufficiency; hyperkalaemia; potassium salts/other potassium-sparing diuretics CYP3A4 inhibitors.

Table 11.9 Beta-blockers [150–152]

Indications	Mechanism(s) per indication	Pharmacokinetics	Adverse effects (contraindications)	Major non-recommended combinations
Angina pectoris	Blockade of cardiac beta-adrenoceptors, negative inotropic and chronotropic effets, reduction of myocardial O_2 consumption.	Lipophilic drugs such as propranolol are rapidely metobolized in the liver; some active metabolites; large volume of distribution, including brain; short half life. Carvedilol, propranolol: poor bioavailability.	Bronchospasm (asthmatic disease).	Bradycardic agents. Verapamil. Diltiazem. Pilocarpine. Centrally acting antihypertensives.
Hypertension	Negative inotropic and chronotropic effects, reduction of cardiac output. Reduction of renin release.	Hydrophilic drugs such as atenolol and sotalol: opposite properties.	Bradycardia (atrio-ventricular blocks).	Hypotensive agents. Floctafenine.
Supraventricular arrhythmias (atrial fibrillation)	Blockade of cardiac beta-adrenoceptors, negative chronotropic effects.		Lipophilic drugs: nightmares, sleep disturbances.	Drugs causing ventricular arrhythmias, torsades de pointe. Sultopirine. Bepridil. Amiodarone.
Chronic heart failure	Bradycardic effect increases diastolic filling time.		Fatigue.	Antidiabetics: masking of the early signs of hypoglycaemia. Insulin. Sulfamids.
Obstructive cardiomyopathy	Negative inotropic effect.		Impotence.	
Secondary prevention of myocardial infarction	Reduction of myocardial O_2 consumption and antiarrhythmic effects.		Cold extremities (Raynaud's syndrome).	

Notes:

There are 2 different subtypes of beta-adrenergic receptors: $beta_1$ and $beta_2$; $beta_1$-adrenergic receptors are mainly located in the heart; $beta_1$-selective antagonists have less non-cardiac adverse effects.

Non- selective beta antagonists propranolol, partially $beta_1$-selective: acebutolol.

Third generation beta-blockers: i.e. with vasodilating properties:
labetalol: additional alpha-adrenergic properties. Specific indication: acrosyndromes;
celiprolol: additional $beta_2$ agonistic activity;
carvedilol: additional antioxidant and alpha-adrenergic blocking properties;
nebivolol: additional property, NO donor. Specific indication: congestive heart failure.

Some drugs have a quinidine-like antiarrhythmic effect (ex. propranolol)
sotalol: additional antiarrhythmic effects due to action potential prolongation (amiodarone-like action);
pindolol: partial agonist (agonist/antagonist) less bradycardic side effects.

Table 11.10 Vasodilators (except drugs of the renin–angiotensin–aldosterone system)

Indications	Mechanism(s)	Pharmacokinetics	Adverse effects	Major non recommended combinations
Calcium-channel blockers				
Dihydropyridines [153–155] Amlodipine besylate; felodipine; isradipine; lacidipine; lercanidipine; manidipine; nicardipine chlorhydrate; nifedipine; nimodipine; nisoldipine; nitrendipine.				

Table 11.10 *(Continued)* Vasodilators (except drugs of the renin–angiotensin–aldosterone system)

Indications	Mechanism(s)	Pharmacokinetics	Adverse effects	Major non-recommended combinations
Angina pectoris Hypertension	Blockade of L-type calcium channels; Selectivity for vascular channels.	Amolodipine: half life: about 40 hours.	Flushes; headaches; ankle oedema; tachycardia, palpitations.	Dantrolene (arrhythmias).
Bradycardic drugs (verapamil, diltiazem) [156, 157]				
Angina pectoris. Hypertension. Supraventricular arrhythmias. Verapamil: post MI protection in patients intolerant to beta-blockers.	Blockade of cardiac and vascular calcium channels. Inhibition of atrioventricular nodal conduction, slowing of heart rate, decreased myocardial oxygen consumption.	Verapamil: plasma protein binding about 90%; diltiazem: almost completely metabolized.	Bradycardia; sino-atrial block, AV block.	Other bradycardic agents (beta-blockers).
Alpha-adrenergic receptor blockers [158]				
Prazosin Urapidil				
Hypertension (not first-line agents, only in combination in non-controlled hypertension).	Antagonism of alpha-adrenergic receptors.	Prazosin: plasma protein binding 97%.	Orthostatic hypotension Flushes Headaches.	
NO donors [159]. Glyceryl trinitrate, isosorbide mononitrate, isosorbide dinitrate.				
Angina pectoris. Heart failure.	NO release. Vascular smooth muscle cell relaxation.	Metabolized to release NO; Variable duration of action; Important hepatic metabolism.	Headaches Flushes Syncopes	PDE inhibitors (severe hypotension)

Table 11.11 Antiplatelet drugs

Indications	Mechanism(s)	Pharmacokinetics	Adverse effects	Major non-recommended combinations
Aspirin [160]				
Acute coronary syndrome.	Irreversible inhibition of platelet COX-1.	Oral administration, once daily.	Gastric ulceration Gastro-intestinal haemorrhage.	Other non steroidal anti-inflammatory drugs.
Stable and unstable angina.	Resulting inhibition of thromboxane synthesis.	Because of irreversible COX inhibition, platelet function normalizes 7 days after withdrawal.	Allergy.	Anticoagulants.
Stroke.			Exacerbation of bronchospasms.	
Transient ischaemic attack.				
Primary and secondary prevention of vascular events.				
Coronary stent implantation.				
Clopidogrel and derivatives.				
Same acute interventions as aspirin (usually in addition to aspirin).	Antagonism of ADP receptors	Oral administration, once daily.	Gastro-intestinal haemorrhage.	Anticoagulants.
Secondary prevention in patients intolerant to aspirin.	Resulting prevention of GPIIb/IIIa receptor complex activation by ADP. Inhibition of platelet aggregation	Prodrug. Important hepatic metabolism.	Rash.	Non-steroidal anti-inflammatory drugs.

(Continued)

Table 11.11 *(Continued)* Antiplatelet drugs

Indications	Mechanism(s)	Pharmacokinetics	Adverse effects	Major non-recommended combinations
GP IIb/IIIa receptor blockers [161]				
Tirofiban Eptifibatide Abciximab				
Acute coronary syndrome.	Blockade of interaction between GPIIb/IIIa receptor complex and fibrinogen.	Abciximab: IV administration.	Haemorrhage.	Anticoagulants.
Percutaneous coronary intervention.	Resulting prevention of platelet bridging.	Platelet function restored after 48h.	Thrombocytopenia.	

Table 11.12 Anticoagulant and fibrinolytic drugs [162]

Indications	Mechanism(s)	Pharmacokinetics	Adverse effects	Non-recommended combinations
Heparins				
Unfractionated				
Venous thromboembolism.	Common to unfractionated and fractionated: activation of antithrombin III.	Subcutaneous administration: variable absorption.	Haemorrhages.	
Pulmonary and deep vein embolism.	Resulting inhibition of thrombin (IIa) and Xa.	IV administration adjusted to activated partial thromboplastin time.	Thrombocytopenia.	
Coronary artery disease (acute phase of myocardial infarction).	Specfic to unfractionated: Direct inhibition IIa.		Osteoporosis.	
Valvular diseases.	Anti-Xa action = anti-IIa action.			
Prevention of arterial thromboembolism.				
Coagulopathies.				
Low-molecular-weight heparins				
Deep venous thrombosis.	Fractionated: Anti-Xa action > anti-IIa.	Subcutaneous administration.	Same as unfractionated.	
Prevention of postsurgery venous thromboembolism.		Weight adjustment.	Plus cutaneous necrosis at the injection site.	
Unstable angina and myocardial infarction.		If necessary, monitoring by Xa assay.		
Oral anticoagulants [163]				
Warfarin Acenocoumarol Fluindione				
Venous thromboembolic disease.	Antagonism of vitamin K.	Adjustment according INR.	Haemorrhage.	Non-steroidal anti-inflammatory drugs, including aspirin.
Atrial fibrillation.	Resulting inhibition of synthesis of the active forms of factors II, VII, IX, X.	Hepatic metabolism (CYP2C9): many drug interactions.	Low therapeutic index.	
Prevention of thromboembolism in patients with mechanical valves.			Hepatitis.	
Complicated myocardial infarction.				

Table 11.12 *(Continued)* Anticoagulant and fibrinolytic drugs [162]

Indications	Mechanism(s)	Pharmacokinetics	Adverse effects	Non-recommended combinations
Fibrinolytics [164]				
Alteplase Reteplase Streptokinase Tenecteplase Urokinase				
Acute myocardial infarction with ST elevation.	Promotion of conversion of plasminogen to plasmin.		Haemorrhages+++	Other anticoagulants.
	Direct mechanism for alteplase (tPA).	IV bolus followed by infusion.		
	Indirect mechanism for streptokinase by forming a complex with plasminogen.	IV infusion 30–60min.	Hypotension. Allergy.	

Table 11.13 Ivabradine [165]

Indications	Mechanism(s)	Pharmacokinetics	Adverse effects (contraindication)	Non-recommended combinations
Angina (when beta-blockers are contraindicated are not tolerated).	Channel if inhibition; slowing of sinus rhythm.		Visual disturbances, bradycardia (sick sinus, III AV block, HR <60bpm).	Other bradycardic agents, cytochrome P450 3A4 inhibitors; macrolides; anti-proteases.

Personal perspective

Future advances will bring incremental benefits to those already achieved, but new treatments are likely to be expensive, and balancing clinical benefits and costs will present a challenge to all healthcare systems. Moreover, not all new developments represent a substantial therapeutic advance. In the future, it will become more important than ever to quantify both the treatment effect and the cost, as choices will have to be made that will have an impact on public health as much as on the individual patient.

Therapeutics used to be as much a science as an art. Now, incremental regulatory requirements, concerns with safety, and cost constraints make managing CV disorders increasingly challenging as manifested in the requirements of mechanism-based drug discovery and evidence-based drug therapy. Basic mechanistic hypothesis-driven drug discovery has delivered few novel agents. New pharmacogenomic tools and high throughput techniques promise to identify a large number of therapeutic targets for testing in clinical trials. Translational research in CV medicine is lagging behind that in oncology. Cancer genomics may be useful as a template for CV medicine. This also applies to the low uptake of the use of biomarkers in CV drug discovery and clinical trials as compared to oncology.

In their efforts to maximize return on investment and develop 'blockbuster' drugs, pharmaceutical companies have ignored important unmet needs, such as acute HF, CV protection in chronic kidney disease, and other conditions where outcome is still dismal. Companies have also paid considerable attention to safe 'me-too' drugs, which offer little advantage over other members of their class. Furthermore, the 'one size fits all' policy, with drugs developed to be prescribed to the largest possible population may no longer be applicable. Pharmacogenetics, and more generally personalized medicine, have not delivered significant advances so far. Research on predictors of response is still very marginal and needs to be overhauled. Dose-finding and proof of concept studies are areas where progress may be made and may be improved by using biomarkers more appropriately.

The design and conduct of clinical trials is another challenging area. Because of safety concerns and regulatory requirements, companies have grown wary of ambitious and costly programmes. Models where new drugs may be approved conditionally with re-assessment of drug label and/or licence after completion of ambitious post-marketing surveillance programmes and genuine phase IV safety trials should be encouraged. Within this context, obsession with morbidity/mortality endpoints should be abandoned. Alternative endpoints, such as slowing disease progression, are worth considering. Unconventional well designed endpoints, mixing in composite morbidity/mortality endpoints with validated measures of quality of life, are a challenging area for future research. Well accepted safety requirements for drugs used in primary prevention in large populations over long periods of time should not be applied to drugs destined for shorter use in very severe patients. This is true in acute HF syndromes, common conditions that are associated with higher event rates than acute coronary syndromes and yet receive far less attention, with very few new drug candidates or positive trials.

Polypharamcy has become the rule, partly because the current model of drug development is based on testing new entities on top of 'conventional' therapy. In certain circumstances, such as in HF, head-to-head comparisons between new and 'conventional' treatments will become necessary. In HF, it is uncertain whether high doses of few combined medications or low doses of multiple medications are to be preferred. Polypharmacy is also needed for primary prevention in high-risk populations as well as in secondary prevention. This is related to the multifactorial determinants of CV risk. Pleiotropic effects of some single agents will not be sufficient to address the multiple mechanisms of atherosclerosis. Therefore, multiple drug combinations will become more popular and the need for a polypill has already been highlighted. Methodological and regulatory challenges are still to be overcome before polypills become standard practice.

Finally, implementation of the results of clinical trials is a new and emerging science that requires as good an understanding of the external validity of trial results as of barriers in real life therapy. This includes better understanding of adherence, referral models, cost models, and reimbursement systems as well as generic drug use and self-medication—all areas where more pharmaco-epidemiological research is needed.

Even so, CV medicine is way ahead of other disciplines in terms of evidence-based practice; but it is a daily observation that evidence-based guidelines are not being implemented appropriately. Knowledge, specifically in the area of clinical pharmacology, and understanding of the methodology and interpretation of trials need to be disseminated through educational and training initiatives. Testing and incorporation of guideline-based algorithms into disease management programmes may also help. More research is needed in order to develop and assess specific implementation strategies. The science of guideline and trial result implementation is nascent and will probably develop much as the science of clinical trials has done over the last 30 years.

Further reading

Antman EM. *Cardiovascular Therapeutics: A Companion to Braunwald's Heart Disease*, 3rd edn., 2006. Philadelphia, PA: WB Saunders.

Douglas SA, Ohlstein EH, Johns DG. Techniques: Cardiovascular pharmacology and drug discovery in the 21st century. *Trends Pharmacol Sci* 2004; **25**:225–33.

Johnson GD. *Fundamentals of Cardiovascular Pharmacology*, 1999. Chichester: John Wiley & Sons, Ltd.

Kipshidze NN, Fareed J, Moses JW, *et al.* (eds.). *Textbook of Interventional Cardiovascular Pharmacology*, 2007. London: Informa Healthcare.

Machin D, Day S, Green S (eds.). *Textbook of Clinical Trials*, 2nd edn., 2006. Chichester: John Wiley & Sons, Ltd.

Pocock SJ. *Clinical Trials: A Practical Approach*, 1984. Chichester: John Wiley & Sons, Ltd.

Online resources

- American College of Cardiology—Cardiosource: http://www.cardiosource.com/clinicaltrials/index.asp

- ClinicalTrials.gov, a registry of federally and privately supported clinical trials conducted in the US and around the world: http://www.clinicaltrials.gov/
- Home Page of the Human Cytochrome P450 (CYP) Allele Nomenclature Committee: http://www.imm.ki.se/CYPalleles/
- Pharmacogenetics and Pharmacogenomics Knowledge Base: http://www.pharmgkb.org
- WHO Collaborating Centre for International Drug Monitoring: http://www.who-umc.org

For full references and multimedia materials please visit the online version of the book (http://esctextbook.oxfordonline.com).

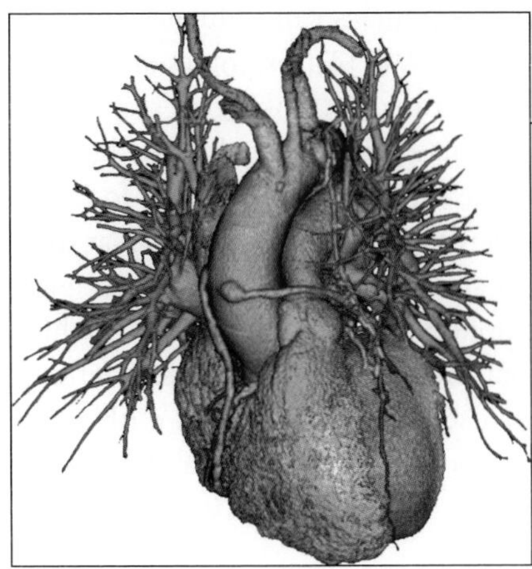

CHAPTER 12

Prevention of Cardiovascular Disease

Annika Rosengren, Joep Perk, and Jean Dallongeville

Contents

Summary

The global increase in cardiovascular disease (CVD) during the 20th century is partially explained by an increasing proportion of older adults in the population, but also by changes in work conditions, transport, diet, and social networks, all of which have a direct impact on risk factors for CVD. Although the mortality rate is falling markedly in some European countries, it is increasing in others and CVD is expected to remain the leading cause of premature death in Europe in the coming decades.

CVD is strongly related to individual lifestyle characteristics and associated risk factors. In seeking to prevent CVD in the population, the objectives are to reduce mortality and morbidity and improve the chances of a longer life expectancy with preserved quality of life. Risk behaviour can be modified successfully through lifestyle management. Single risk factors such as hyperlipidaemia and hypertension can be controlled by adding pharmacotherapy. Thus, there are effective tools both for the detection and for the modification of CVD risk.

In this chapter, prevention strategies and priorities are presented in agreement with the recent guidelines of the Fourth Joint European Societies Task Force on CVD prevention in clinical practice. The detection and modification of risk factors is described in the sections on smoking, physical activity, blood pressure, nutrition, obesity, and lipids. The chapter includes specific methods for lifestyle counselling; drug therapy has been recommended, whenever deemed appropriate. Finally, new evidence on the importance of psychosocial risk factors and the influence of gender will also be discussed.

Introduction

Societal causes of CVD

In order to understand cardiovascular prevention, cardiologists need to understand that CVD reflects not only individual choices and genetic susceptibility, but also conditions in society. Before World War I, death from CVD was, if not unusual, at least was vastly outnumbered by deaths in early childhood, and deaths from infectious diseases and malnutrition. The increase in CVD during the 20th century is partially explained by an increasing proportion of older adults in the population, but also by economic and human development such as urbanization and industrialization, with concomitant changes in work conditions, transportation, diet, and social networks, all of which have a direct impact on risk factors for CVD. In the year 1970, 37% of the world's population were living in cities. Currently, about 50% are living in cities, and this proportion is expected to increase to 61% by 2020 [1]. In high-income countries, urbanization is already widespread, with the most rapid urbanization now taking place in low- and middle-income countries.

Economic growth and changes in food production has lead to changes in diet and, coupled with less physical activity, caloric imbalance with a worldwide epidemic of obesity. Adverse changes include an increased consumption of foods of high caloric density, high in fats, meats, refined carbohydrates, and low in fibre. Diet, in turn, is a major determinant for the development of dyslipidaemia, hypertension, and other conditions which lead to the development of CVD.

Low levels of physical activity are connected to the development of obesity, particularly abdominal obesity, insulin resistance, and diabetes, all of which are linked to increased risk for CVD. Increases in mechanization at work, and in the home, more sedentary leisure time activities, such as TV watching and computer activities, and changes in transportation all contribute to decreasing energy expenditure. Even moderate physical activity protects against CVD but societal factors can influence opportunities for walking or riding bicycles as a mode of transportation [2], such as mixed residential and commercial tenants, street connectivity, the presence or absence of sidewalks, bicycle lanes, and the perception of a safe environment, both from crime and the dangers of heavy traffic.

Tobacco use is another factor, where societal factors are important. In many high-income countries, tobacco consumption is decreasing, whereas tobacco companies are increasing their marketing efforts in low- and middle-income countries. Legislation and policies can influence smoking habits, and thereby risk of CVD [3]. Examples are regulation of advertising, restriction of smoking in restaurants and other public places, dissemination of knowledge, and attitudes. In Scotland, the number of admissions for acute coronary syndrome decreased markedly in the year after the implementation of smoke-free legislation, with fewer admissions in both smokers and non-smokers [4], which illustrates the potential impact of legislative restrictions. Additionally, tobacco use is often clustered with other adverse factors, such as poor diet, sedentary habits, and low socio-economic factors.

Facts and figures about CVD in Europe

Diseases of the heart and circulatory system (CVD) cause >4.3 million deaths in the European Region (ER) each year and 2.0 million deaths in the 27 states of the European Union (EU). It accounts for 42% of all deaths in the EU, and 48% in the ER [5]. Currently, >800,000 persons aged <65 years die from CVD each year in the ER and >230,000 in the EU.

Coronary heart disease (CHD) is the single most common cause of death in Europe, and alone accounts for one in five deaths in men and women in the ER. In the EU, 16% of men and 15% of women die from CHD (➲Figs. 12.1 and 12.2). Stroke is the second most common cause of death in the ER, more so for women than for men, with 17% of women and 11% of men dying from stroke each year. Corresponding figures for the EU are 12% and 9% for women and men, respectively.

Within Europe, there is a considerable variation in CVD between nations and regions. There is a clear north–east to south–west gradient in age-standardized mortality within Europe [6, 7] (➲Figs. 12.3 and 12.4). In particular, countries from Central and Eastern Europe have high mortality rates compared with other European countries. The lowest mortality rates are found in France, Portugal, Italy, Spain, Switzerland, and the Netherlands. There is a considerable within-country variation in CHD in Germany, the UK, and Poland.

The highest age-adjusted mortality rate for CHD in men <65 years of age is currently reported from the Russian Federation at 242 per 100,000, and the lowest from France at 17 per 100,000 (➲Fig. 12.5). Corresponding figures for women <65 years of age are 74 (Ukraine) and 3 (France) per 100,000 (➲Fig. 12.6). The rate ratio of dying from CHD between the EU countries with the highest mortality compared with

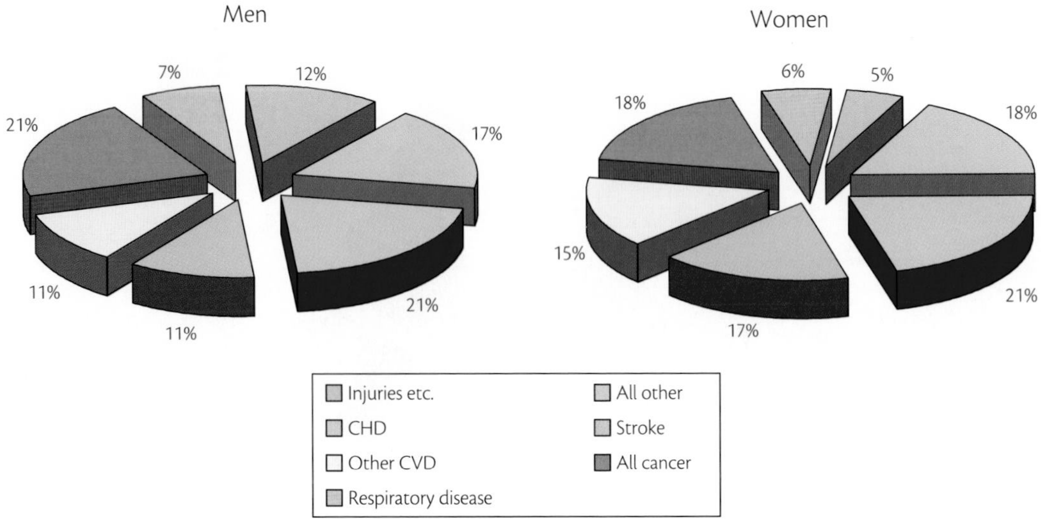

Figure 12.1 Proportion of deaths by cause in European men and women, all ages, latest available year. Adapted with permission from British Heart Foundation. *European Cardiovascular Disease Statistics 2008*, 2008. London: British Heart Foundation.

the lowest mortality is 7.1 (95% confidence interval (CI), 6.6–7.6) for men (Latvia vs. France) and 9.9 (95% CI, 8.5–11.5) for women (Estonia vs. France) [7].

Apart from the marked regional variations, there are also very rapid and pronounced variations over time. Traditionally, countries around the Mediterranean Sea had markedly lower risk than European countries in the north and west. However, as a result of the decreasing coronary mortality in these countries, differences within the EU are now much smaller (➲Figs. 12.7 and 12.8). Among persons aged <65 years, there is little difference between a former high-risk country such as the UK and a Mediterranean country like Greece. The Scandinavian countries Denmark, Norway, and Sweden currently have lower rates than Greece and are approaching the exceptionally low rates for France.

In order to attempt to explain the observed decline in CHD mortality, researchers have used models of various degrees of complexity [8–13]. Major advancements in the treatment of acute coronary syndromes, hypertension, and heart failure have been made, as well as improvements in secondary prevention. Combining data on major risk factors in the population (cholesterol, blood pressure, smoking, diabetes, obesity, and physical inactivity) with data on medical treatment and interventions has been used in epidemiological models to simplify and help explain a complex reality. The majority of the models consistently suggest that risk factor improvements explain more of the mortality decline than treatments, ranging from 44% in the USA to 72% in Finland (➲Fig. 12.9). However, unmeasured factors such as cohort effects related to nutrition in childhood

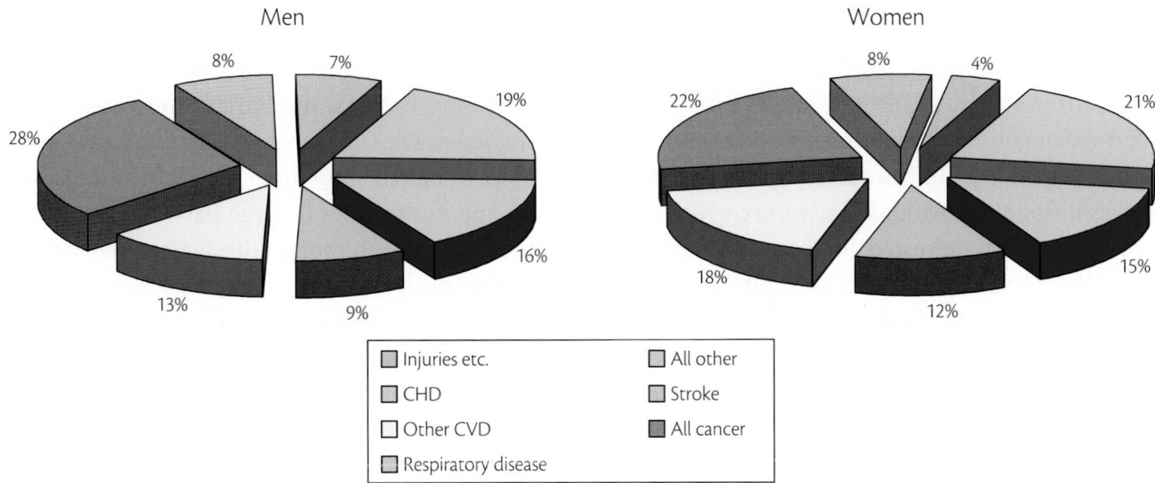

Figure 12.2 Proportion of deaths by cause in EU men and women, all ages, latest available year. Adapted with permission from British Heart Foundation. *European Cardiovascular Disease Statistics 2008*, 2008. London: British Heart Foundation.

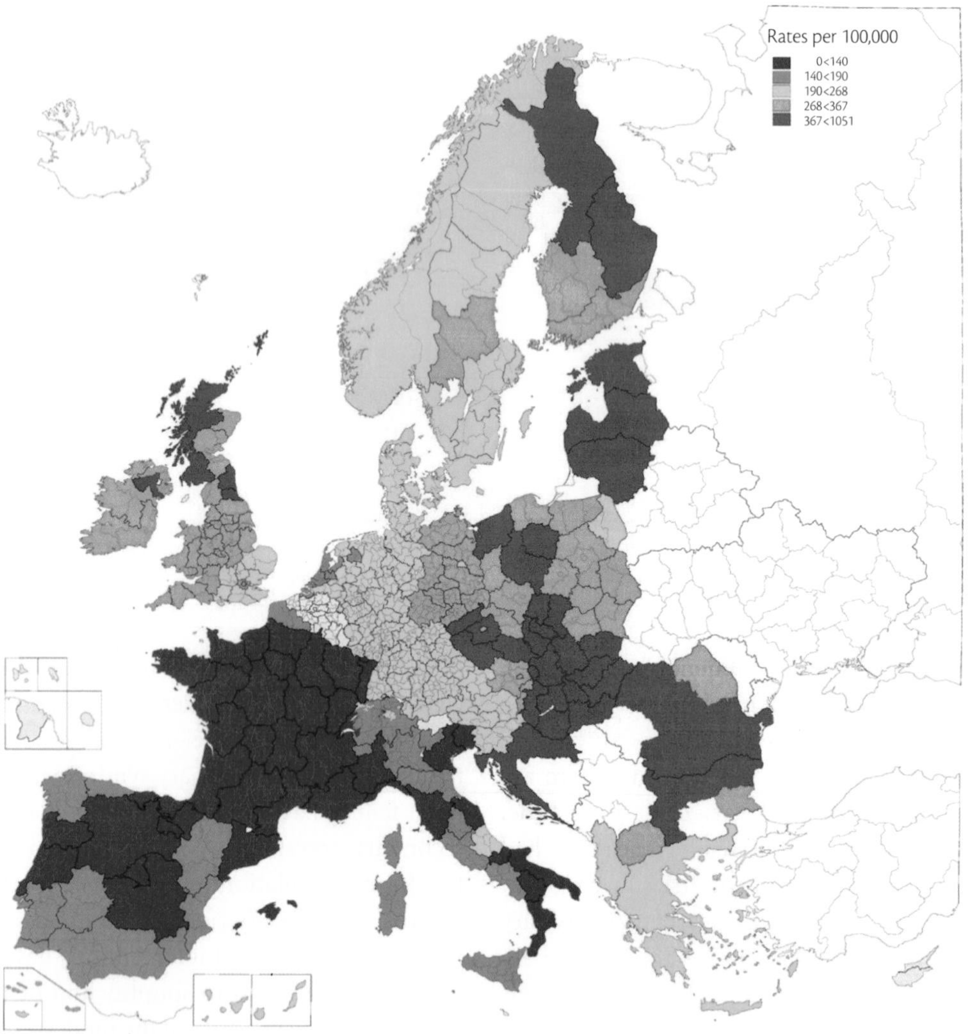

Figure 12.3 Age-standardized mortality from ischaemic heart disease in European regions (men; age group 45–74 years; year 2000). Reproduced with permission from Müller-Nordhorn J, Binting S, Roll S, *et al.* An update on regional variation in cardiovascular mortality within Europe. *Eur Heart J* 2008; **29**: 1316–26.

or adolescence, or changes in psychosocial factors related to the workplace and to the social environment may also contribute.

Even though CVD mortality, particularly with respect to CHD, but also from stroke, has decreased very substantially in many European countries, the same is not entirely true for morbidity. Morbidity can be measured in several ways, for instance as hospital admissions (or, more correctly, discharges) or as disability-adjusted life years (DALY)—an aggregate of life lost and years of healthy life lost due to disability. The DALY is the measure which is used in the WHO Burden of Disease project [14]. The proportion of DALYs lost due to CVD in Europe in 2002 was 23%, compared to 11% for cancer and 20% for neuropsychiatric disorders. The proportions of DALYs lost due to CVD in the EU was lower, or 19%, compared to 16% for cancer, and 25% for neuropsychiatric disorders. Hospital discharge rate as a measure of morbidity is not a reliable tool for measuring morbidity because it is influenced by administrative routines, and thresholds for admission, but even so, it is notable that in many countries where mortality is decreasing rapidly, hospital discharge rates for CVD have not decreased to the same extent.

CVD results in substantial disability and loss of productivity and contributes in large part to the escalating costs of healthcare. Even though the age-standardized mortality rates have declined over the past decades in many European countries, the prevalence of CVD is increasing because of improved treatment and higher survival rates and because of the increasing elderly population. The prevalence of patients who are at risk of recurrent disease (re-infarction, recurrent stroke, heart failure, sudden death) is likewise on the increase. Furthermore, with the current pandemic of obesity in childhood and adolescence, CVD may extend into

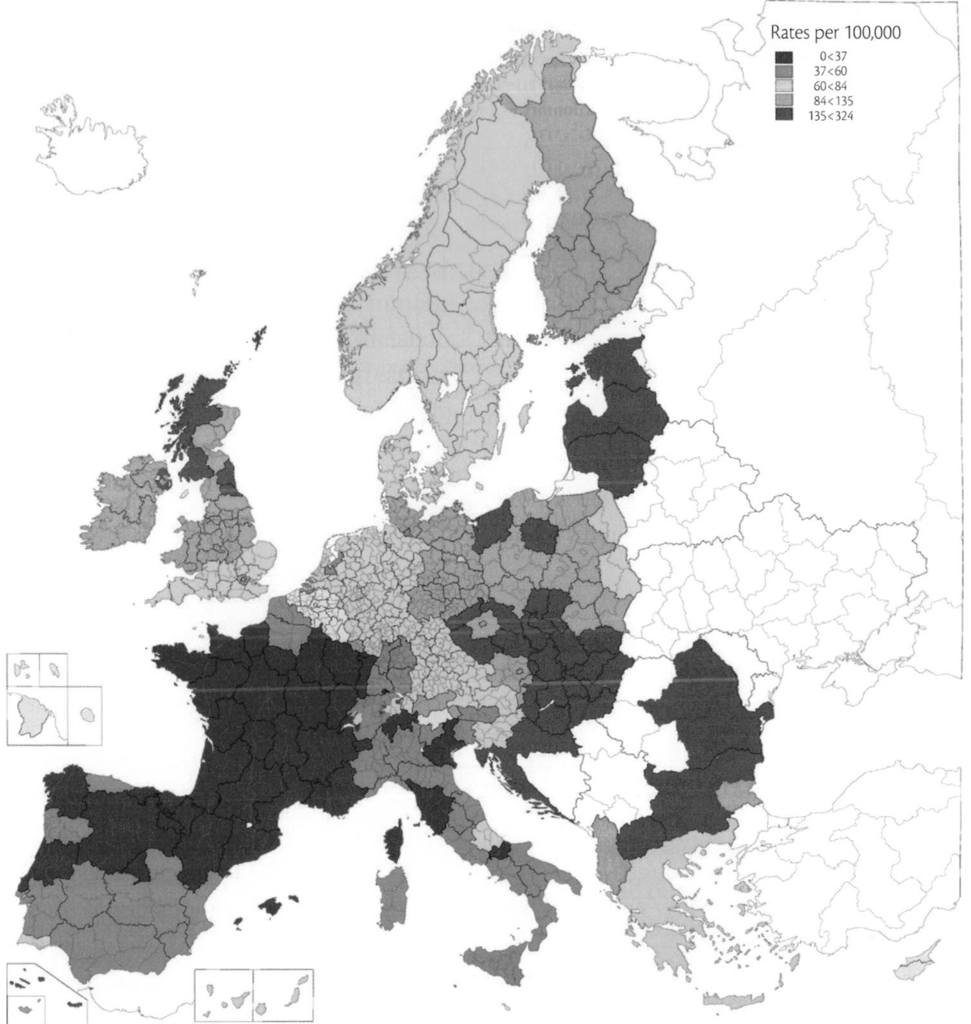

Figure 12.4 Age-standardized mortality from ischaemic heart disease in European regions (women; age group 45–74 years; year 2000). Reproduced with permission from Müller-Nordhorn J, Binting S, Roll S, *et al.* An update on regional variation in cardiovascular mortality within Europe. *Eur Heart J* 2008; **29**: 1316–26.

younger age groups in the future. Thus, CVD is expected to remain the largest burden on healthcare in Europe in the coming decades.

Prevention strategies

In seeking to prevent CVD in European populations the objectives are to reduce mortality and morbidity and improve the chances of a longer life expectancy with preserved quality of life [15]. CVD is strongly related to lifestyle characteristics and associated risk factors. There is clear scientific evidence that lifestyle modification and risk factor reduction can influence the development and progression of the disease both before and after the occurrence of a clinical event.

Traditionally, preventive cardiology has been concerned with unifactorial risk assessment, as in the management of hypertension, hyperlipidaemia, or diabetes. This has resulted in emphasis being placed on single high-risk factors rather than on the overall level of risk based on a combination of factors. In contrast, the concept of total risk, which has been a cornerstone of the European guidelines since the first (1994) edition [16] acknowledges that CVD has a multifactorial aetiology and that risk factors can have a multiplicative effect, enhancing the effect of one another. Accordingly, treatment of risk factors is directed at reducing total risk, more than at the treatment of the individual factors. As an example, the most effective treatment in a smoker with moderate hypercholesterolaemia can be to quit smoking, rather than to prescribe a statin.

The importance of comprehensive risk factor intervention in patients with established CVD and in high-risk

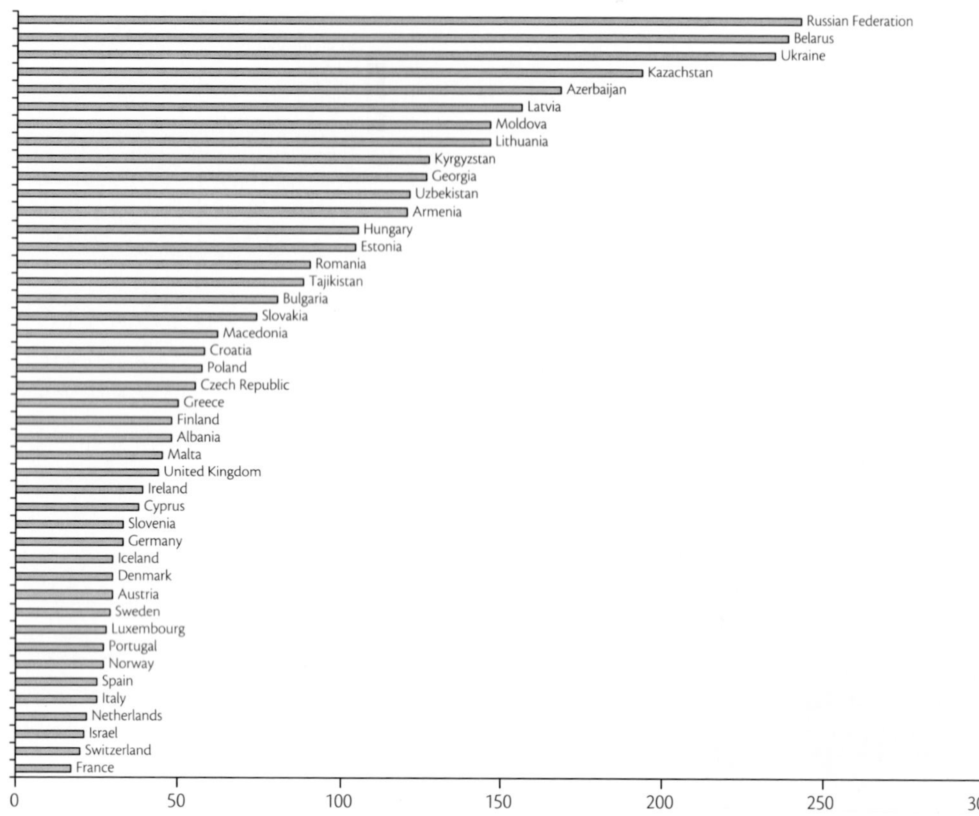

Figure 12.5 Age-standardized death rates for CHD in European countries in men <65 years. Adapted with permission from British Heart Foundation. *European Cardiovascular Disease Statistics 2008*, 2008. London: British Heart Foundation.

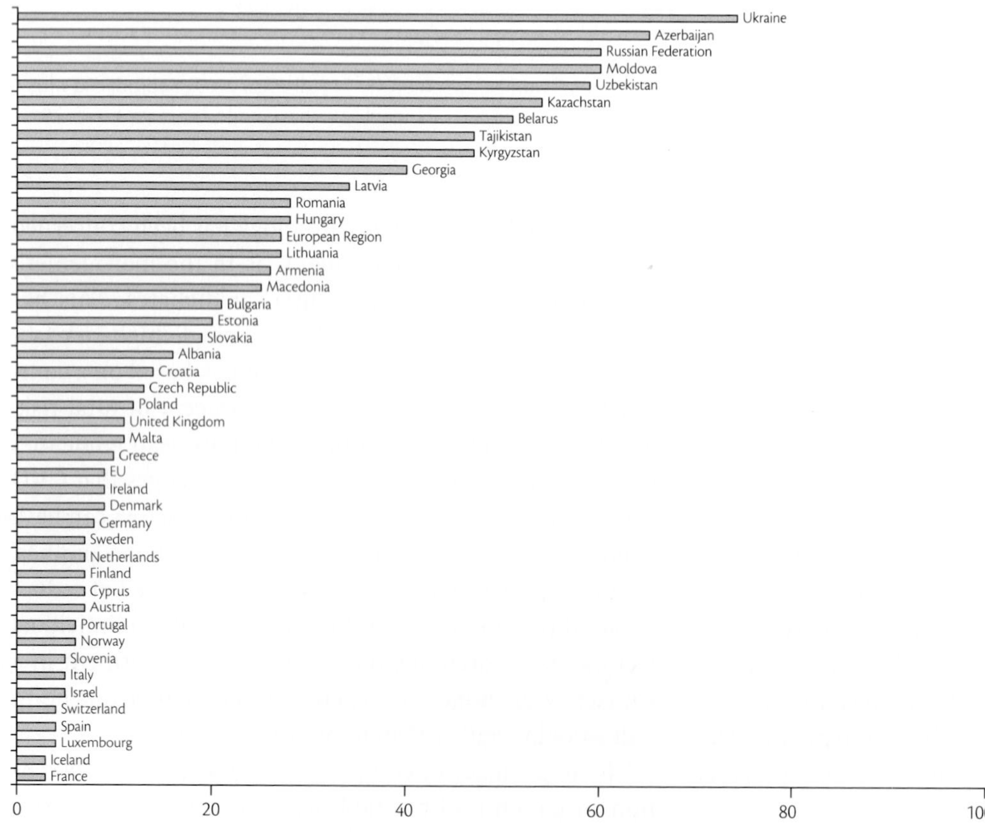

Figure 12.6 Age-standardized death rates for CHD in European countries in women <65 years. Adapted with permission from British Heart Foundation. *European Cardiovascular Disease Statistics 2008*, 2008. London: British Heart Foundation.

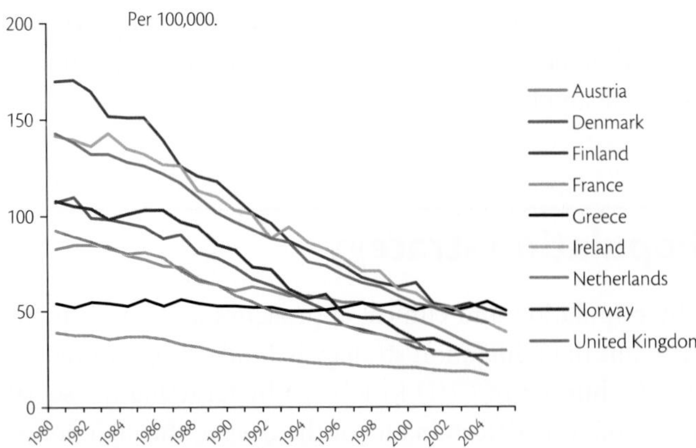

Figure 12.7 Death rates from CHD in selected European countries for men aged <65 years. Adapted with permission from British Heart Foundation. *European Cardiovascular Disease Statistics 2008*, 2008. London: British Heart Foundation.

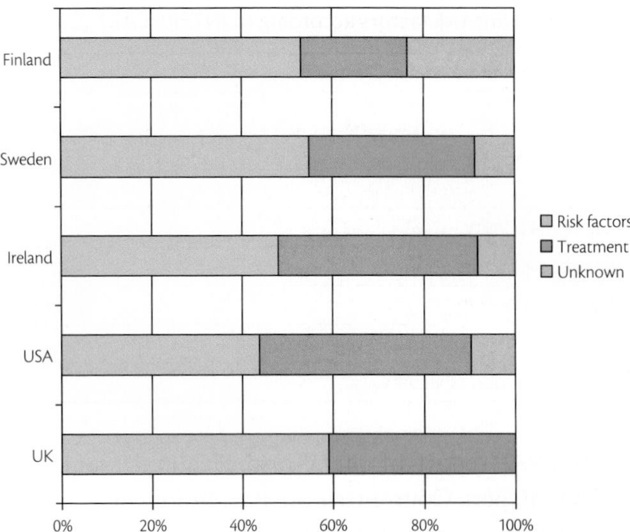

Figure 12.9 Relative contributions from changes in treatment and risk factors to the decrease in CHD death rates in IMPACT models from selected countries [9–13].

subjects has been emphasized by several expert groups. Previous recommendations were based on reports from the Framingham Study [17]. Because this risk score was based on a limited North American sample its applicability to European populations has been questioned. Accordingly, the development of a risk estimation system based on a large pool of representative European data was instigated: the SCORE (Systematic COronary Risk Evaluation) for total CVD risk [18]. The design of this project allows the development of methods for creating national or regional risk charts based on published mortality data. Thus, there is unanimity on the clinical priorities for coronary prevention and the need to target those at highest risk on the basis of a comprehensive multifactorial risk assessment. Yet, surveys have revealed that there is considerable potential to improve risk factor management [19–22].

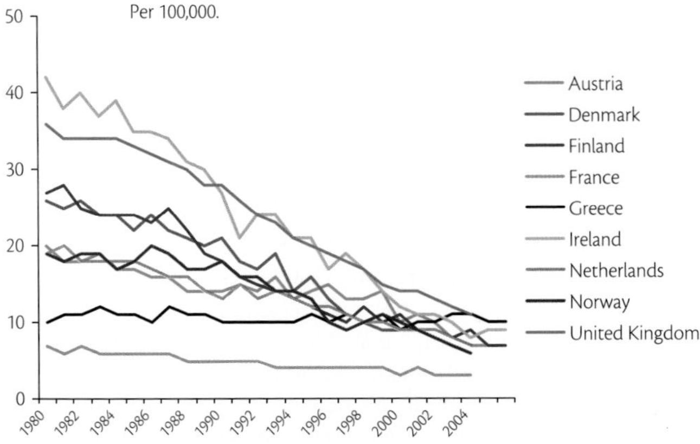

Figure 12.8 Death rates from CHD in selected European countries, women aged <65 years. Adapted with permission from British Heart Foundation. *European Cardiovascular Disease Statistics 2008*, 2008. London: British Heart Foundation.

A genetic predisposition does play a role in the development of CVD and a detailed family history of CHD or other atherosclerotic disease should be part of the assessment of all patients with CVD and in the identification of high-risk individuals. However, except in rare cases, as for example in familial hypercholesterolaemia, the influence of a positive family history is not among the strongest risk factors. Moreover, it is not amenable to intervention and serves alongside other risk factors to identify individuals who are at increased risk. Even with a positive family history, CVD only rarely occurs in the absence of other risk factors.

There is a wealth of evidence that tobacco smoking, lack of physical activity, nutritional habits, and psychosocial factors play important roles both as causes of the mass occurrence of CVD in populations and as contributing factors to the risk of CVD in individuals within populations. In the INTERHEART study, almost 70% of all cases with a first myocardial infarction could be related to smoking and lipids, and up to 90% could be related to nine easily identifiable and modifiable risk factors, demonstrating the importance of continuing efforts to prevent CVD [23] (➲Table 12.1). The cumulative effect of these risk factors on the odds ratio for myocardial infarction is shown in ➲Fig. 12.10.

For a proper assessment of the total cardiovascular risk, each individual risk factor has to be considered and the impact of modifying risk has to be assessed against the background set by the non-modifiable risk characteristics. Therefore, the concept of total CVD risk estimation is an important principle in the development of preventive strategies.

Table 12.1 Nine risk factors according to INTERHEART [23]

ApoB/ApoA1-ratio
Smoking
Hypertension
Diabetes
Abdominal obesity
Psychosocial factors
Low physical activity
Low consumption of fruit and vegetables
Low consumption of alcohol

The 1982 report of the World Health Organization (WHO) Expert Committee on Prevention of Coronary Heart Disease considered that a comprehensive action for prevention has to include three components:

- **Population strategy**—for altering at the population level lifestyle and environmental factors and their socioeconomic determinants, which are the underlying causes of CHD.
- **High-risk strategy**—identification of high-risk individuals and action to reduce their risk factor levels.
- **Secondary prevention**—prevention of recurrent events and progression of the disease in patients with clinically established CHD.

The last two correspond to prevention activities targeted at individuals and should be an integral part of clinical practice. They are the focus of this chapter. The population strategy, targeted at entire communities, should be an integral part of food and nutrition, transport, employment, education, health, and other policies at European, national, regional, and local levels.

Population strategy

The population and clinical approaches are complementary, but the population strategy is fundamental to reducing the burden of CVD in Europe by targeting the social and economic determinants of the disease through political action. The population strategy must lead eventually to changes in lifestyle: a reduction in the number of people who smoke, enhancement of physical activity, and the promotion of adequate and balanced food habits. These goals can be reached in different ways, but political will and development of ad hoc policies and investments at all levels are a condition without which they cannot be achieved.

Social inequalities affect cardiovascular health. A population strategy should ensure actions against the determinants of these inequalities. The strategy has to ensure equity of access to preventive advice and to diagnostic and therapeutic interventions, to reduce the social differences in health. A preventive population strategy can be successful, as demonstrated in Finland [24], but is critically dependent on the participating parties such as government, insurance companies, and the food industry, among others. Physicians, nurses, and other members of the medical profession, however, should not underestimate the impact that they can have in the public domain.

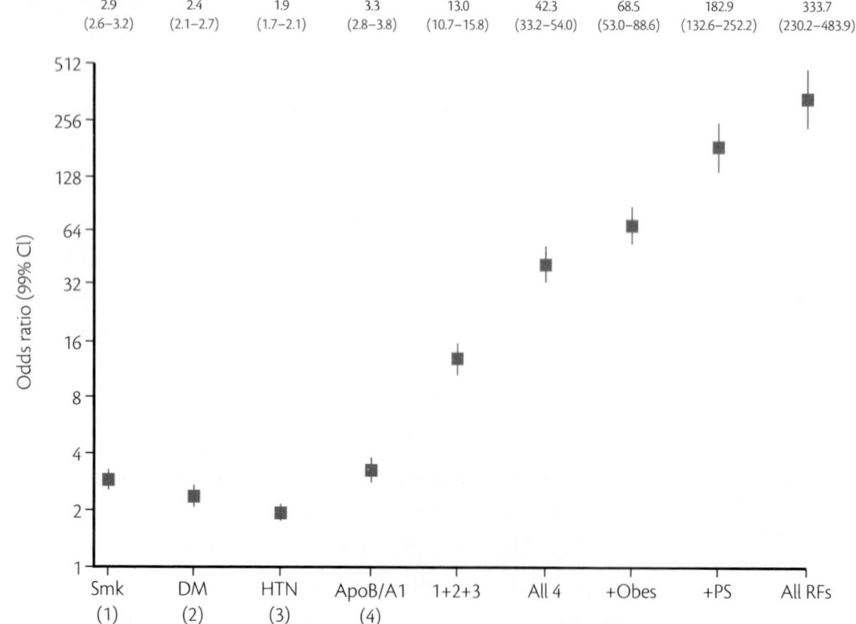

Figure 12.10 Risk of AMI associated with exposure to multiple risk factors. Smk, smoking; DM, diabetes mellitus; HTN, hypertension; Obes, abdominal obesity; PS, psychosocial; RF, risk factors. The odds ratios are based on current never smoking, top lowest tertile for abdominal obesity, and top lowest quintile for ApoB/ApoA1. Adapted with permission from Yusuf S, Hawken S, Ôunpuu S, *et al.* Effect of potentially modifiable risk factors associated with myocardial infarction in 52 countries (the INTERHEART study): case-control study. *Lancet* 2004; **364**: 937–52.

Modifying CVD risk at the individual level

Even though marked differences exist between the prevalence of cardiovascular disease between countries, there is within every society a great variation in absolute risk between individuals. The absolute lifetime risk of CHD (angina and myocardial infarction) has been estimated at almost 50% in white American men, and one-third in women [25]. By way of systematically comparing persons with and without manifest CVD a number of risk factors have been identified. Risk factors can be defined as easily identified and measurable factors, which are associated with increased risk. The most important risk factors are dyslipidaemia, hypertension, smoking, poor nutrition, low physical activity, obesity, diabetes, and mental stress. Most risk factors reflect complex aetiologies, comprising individual choices, societal factors, and genetic factors. Risk factors are important, first, because they provide information on aetiology. A second advantage of the risk factor concept is the potential to quantify these complex factors and determine the individual risk by the use of statistical models and algorithms.

It is important to recognize that, by the time, risk factors are identified and treated, atherosclerosis may already be advanced. Interventions towards risk factors in middle age are efficient in reducing risk but will only achieve a partial reduction. Although reductions in CVD death rates in some European countries have been impressive, the burden of disease is still substantial. It has been held that as much as 90% of heart attacks could be prevented, but only if control of the major risk factors starts in youth [26].

Priorities in clinical practice

The number of patients with established CVD and of otherwise healthy individuals who are at high risk is large. This presents a considerable challenge to the medical community for which the tasks of CVD prevention are difficult to accomplish in the context of the daily workload. Therefore, it is useful to define priorities for CVD prevention. The Fourth Joint European Societies Task Force on CVD prevention in clinical practice [15] has developed guidelines proposing the order in which preventive action should be taken, because with limited resources full-scale action directed to all groups potentially needing preventive advice may not be feasible in the national healthcare structure. As soon as progress has been made in the top priority groups, action may be directed to groups with a lower rank order in the list. The highest priority is given to patients with established CVD, the lowest to the general population met in clinical practice.

Furthermore, cardiologists and other physicians should act as opinion leaders and influence public health decisions, aiming at facilitating healthy lifestyles at a broad population level (➲ Table 12.2)

Proposed list of priorities

1) Patients with established CHD, peripheral artery disease, and cerebrovascular atherosclerotic disease.
2) Asymptomatic individuals who are at high risk of developing atherosclerotic CVD.
3) First-degree relatives of patients with early-onset CVD (defined as males <55 years, females <65 years).
4) First-degree relatives of asymptomatic individuals at high risk.
5) Other individuals met in connection with ordinary clinical practice.

Effects of age and gender

The most important individual predictor for CVD is increasing age. However, age in itself does not cause CVD but rather reflects the risk factor burden, accumulated over the years. Young people with a high risk factor burden have, despite this, a low risk of developing clinical disease in a short-term perspective. In contrast, among the elderly the absolute risk is high even with a very moderate risk factor burden.

Women and men differ in risk throughout life. This is most evident for coronary disease, where younger men

Table 12.2 Characteristics of people who tend to stay healthy

No smoking
Healthy food choices
Physical activity: 30min of moderate activity a day
BMI <25 kg/m^2 and avoidance of central obesity
BP <140/90mmHg
Total cholesterol <5mmol/L (~190mg/dL)
LDL cholesterol <3mmol/L (~115mg/dL)
Blood glucose <6mmo/L (~110mg/dL)

Adapted with permission from Graham I, Atar D, Borch-Johnsen K, *et al.* European guidelines on cardiovascular disease prevention in clinical practice: full text. Fourth Joint Task Force of the European Society of Cardiology and other societies on cardiovascular disease prevention in clinical practice (constituted by representatives of nine societies and by invited experts). *Eur J Cardiovasc Prev Rehabil* 2007; **14**(Suppl.2): S1–S113.

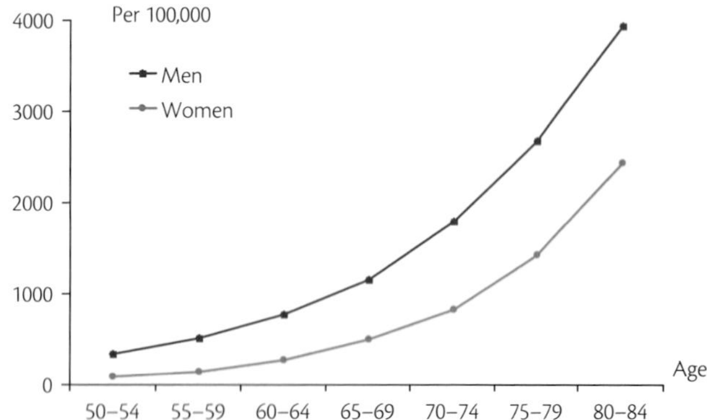

Figure 12.11 Incidence of AMI per 100,000 population in Swedish men and women aged 50–84 years, by age, in the year 2005. Swedish AMI register.

have an about four- to fivefold higher risk than women (➲Fig. 12.11). The difference in mortality and morbidity diminishes with age, but even at ages between 75 and 85, the incidence is almost twofold in men compared to women. Eventually, however, almost as many women as men die from coronary disease and in large parts of the world, CHD is the most important single cause of death in both men and women. The sex difference with respect to stroke is less marked, but at least in the age span <65, stroke is twice as common in men as in women (➲Fig. 12.12). Even so, because women live longer, the absolute numbers who die from stroke and the proportion dying from stroke is higher in women than men. Currently, just over 200,000 male deaths from stroke occur yearly in the EU, corresponding to a total of 9% of all deaths [5]. Among EU women, almost 300,000 deaths from stroke occur annually, or 12% of all deaths in women.

The reason for the lower risk of CVD in women is generally assumed to be due to the protective effect of oestrogen. Evidence for a heart-protective effect of oestrogen include observational studies on rates of CVD in men and women

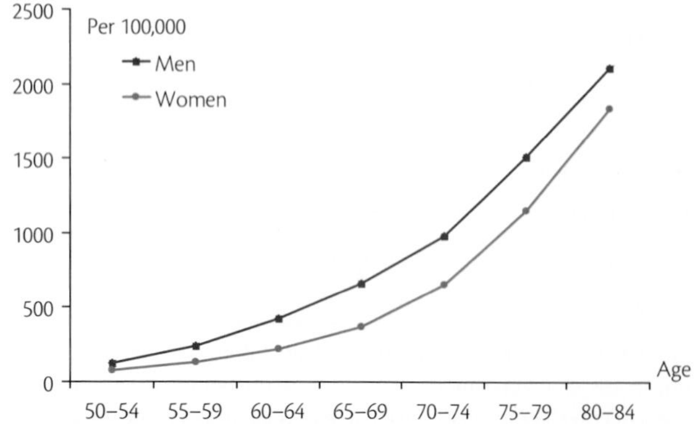

Figure 12.12 Incidence of stroke per 100,000 population in Swedish men and women aged 50–84 years, by age, in the year 2004. Swedish linked hospital discharge and death registries.

[27], effects of early menopause/oophorectomy on risk of CVD, observational studies on risk factors [28], and observational studies of women taking oestrogen [29]. Women who take oestrogen are 35–50% less likely to develop CHD than women who do not take oestrogen. Large randomized trials testing the effect of hormone therapy on clinical coronary outcomes, however, have not confirmed a cardioprotective effect [30, 31]. This is probably due to the fact that oestrogen has several and opposing effects, on the one hand slowing the earlier stages of atherosclerosis through beneficial effects on lipid profile and endothelial function but on the other potentially triggering acute coronary events through prothrombotic and inflammatory mechanisms in advanced disease [32]. However, the male-to-female ratio in CVD, varies considerably between countries and over time, indicating that other factors are probably also important. Alternative explanations may include changes in the prevalence of risk factors, e.g. smoking, but potentially also sex-related vulnerability to other risk factors [33].

Estimation of total risk

It is well established that risk factor management decisions should not be based on consideration of a single risk factor. Total risk means the likelihood of a person developing a fatal cardiovascular event over a defined period of time. ➲Table 12.3 illustrates how a 60-year-old woman with a cholesterol level of 8mmol/L can have a nine times lower CVD mortality risk than a man with a cholesterol level of 5mmol/L if the man smokes and is hypertensive. Estimating the combined effect on CVD mortality of several major risk factors is more complex than assessing single risk factors. It is essential for the clinician to be able to assess risk rapidly and with sufficient accuracy to allow evidence-based management decisions. To this end, risk charts have been published [17, 18]. These charts use age, sex, smoking status, total cholesterol, and systolic blood pressure to estimate the risk of coronary or cardiovascular events over the next 10 years. In the widely used Framingham risk charts a 10-year

Table 12.3 Examples of how other risk factors may negate the advantages of having a desirable cholesterol level. Risk figures refer to the 10-year risk of CVD death

Sex	Age	Serum cholesterol (mmol/L)	Blood pressure (mm Hg)	Smoking	Risk (%)
Female	60	8	120	–	2
Female	60	7	140	+	5
Male	60	6	160	–	8
Male	60	5	180	+	19

risk of 20% or more was used arbitrarily as a threshold for risk factor intervention. However, the charts had several weaknesses: they were derived from North American data and the applicability of the risk chart to European populations was uncertain. In addition, the dataset used for the chart was small and the definition of non-fatal endpoints differed from that used in other studies.

The risk chart currently used in the Task Force recommendations was developed as part of an EU Concerted Action Project: the SCORE (➲ Figs. 12.13 and 12.14) [18]. The SCORE risk prediction system is derived from 12 European cohort studies and comprises >200,000 persons, 3 million person-years of observation, and >7000 fatal cardiovascular events. The main differences from the Framingham charts are:

- CVD mortality, rather than total events, is used as a primary endpoint because this allows risk to be calculated for countries or regions where only mortality data are available.
- All atherosclerotic deaths (not only CHD) are included in the risk model by using a calculation method that allows stroke deaths to be considered separately from CHD deaths if required. Stroke deaths may be proportionately more important in low-risk populations.
- The risk chart has been modified to provide more detail for middle-aged subjects in whom risk changes more rapidly with age.
- Separate charts have been prepared for higher- and lower-risk areas of Europe. In the future it will be possible to produce individualized risk charts for individual countries, provided reliable mortality information is available.

It should be stressed that the SCORE charts are only for use in subjects without known vascular disease, and only in those aged 65, or less. Subjects with manifest atherosclerotic vascular disease are already at high risk of vascular events and should be treated accordingly.

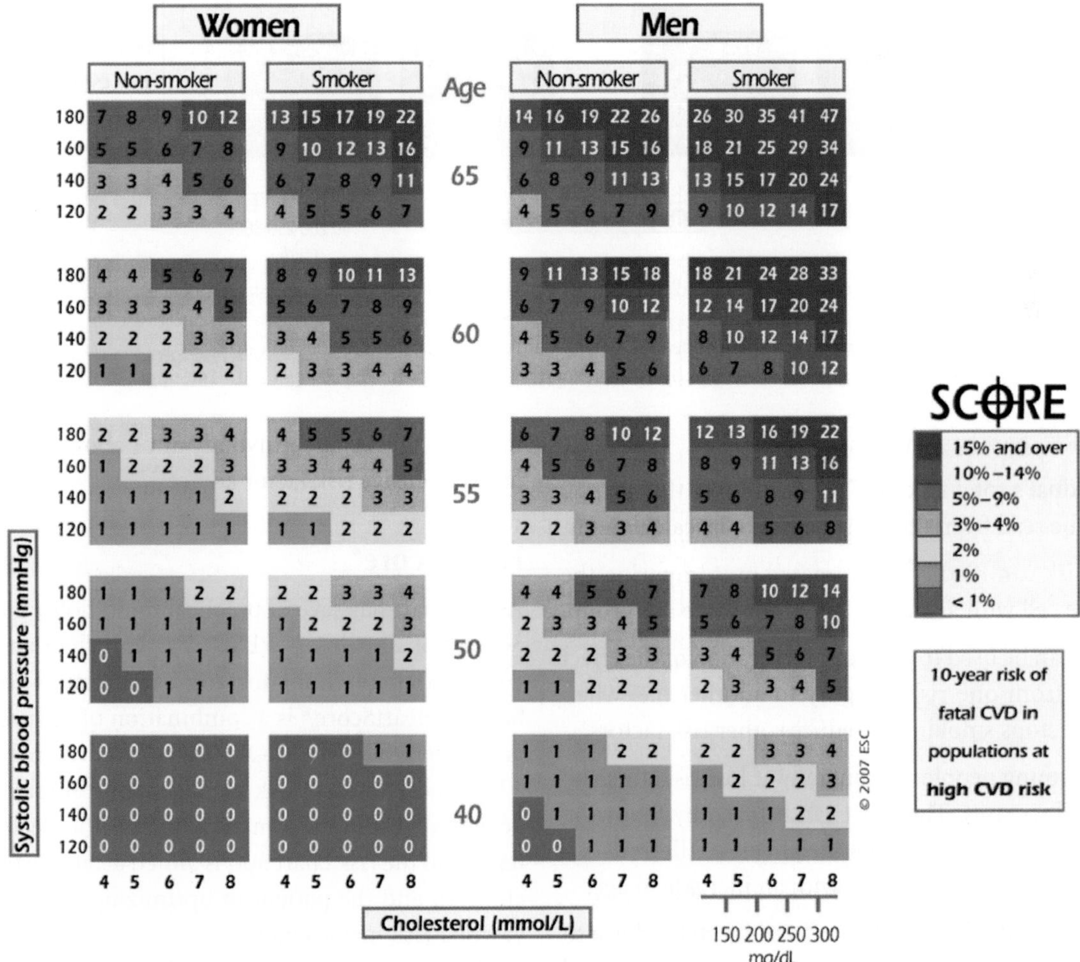

Figure 12.13 SCORE chart: 10-year risk of fatal CVD in populations at high CVD risk based on the following risk factors: age, gender, smoking, SBP and total cholesterol. Reproduced with permission from Graham I, Atar D, Borch-Johnsen K, *et al.* European guidelines on cardiovascular disease prevention in clinical practice: full text. Fourth Joint Task Force of the European Society of Cardiology and other societies on cardiovascular disease prevention in clinical practice (constituted by representatives of nine societies and by invited experts). *Eur J Cardiovasc Prev Rehabil* 2007; **14**(Suppl.2): S1–S113.

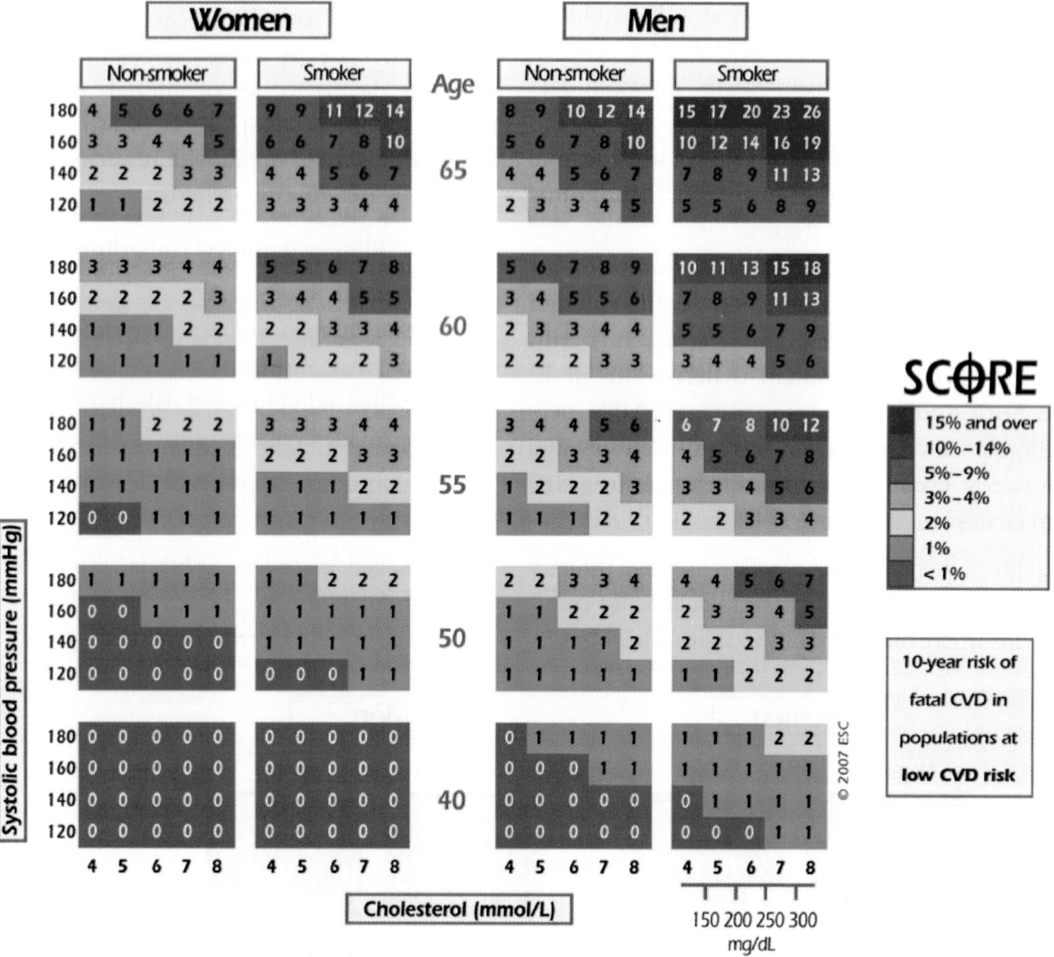

Figure 12.14 SCORE chart: 10-year risk of fatal CVD in populations at low CVD risk based on the following risk factors: age, gender, smoking, SBP, and total cholesterol. Reproduced with permission from Graham I, Atar D, Borch-Johnsen K, *et al.* European guidelines on cardiovascular disease prevention in clinical practice: full text. Fourth Joint Task Force of the European Society of Cardiology and other societies on cardiovascular disease prevention in clinical practice (constituted by representatives of nine societies and by invited experts). *Eur J Cardiovasc Prev Rehabil* 2007; **14**(Suppl.2): S1–S113.

The SCORE chart has several functions:

- An individual's total risk of CVD death over the next 10 years can be read from the chart without any calculations.
- Relative risk can readily be estimated by comparing the risk in one cell with any other cell in the same age group.
- The chart can be used to give some indication of the effect of change from one risk category to another, i.e. when the subject stops smoking or reduces other risk factors.
- Although young people are generally at low risk, this will rise as age increases. The chart can be used by following the tables upward to illustrate the effects of lifetime risk by observing the increased risk with an increase in age.

Low-risk individuals should be offered lifestyle advice to maintain their low-risk status. In the previous chart, based on the Framingham study results, high risk for CHD mortality and morbidity was defined as a level of 20% or more. This equates to a risk of approximately 5% CVD mortality in the SCORE chart. Anybody at or above this level would merit intensive risk factor advice.

HeartScore®

As the chart has several practical limitations, the European Society of Cardiology (ESC) has launched an interactive computer-based tool for total risk estimation—HeartScore®. HeartScore® is a combination of the precard® program operating with SCORE data. The precard® program is a health educational risk management program which has been developed in Denmark [34]. It is the electronic counterpart to the risk chart and is aimed at supporting both the clinician and the patient in optimizing individual cardiovascular risk management.

The program operates with the same risk factors, endpoints, colours, etc. as the risk chart. The expected effect of intervention is calculated from large randomized clinical trials in hypertension and hypercholesterolaemia and is also shown in a bar chart. At the end of the consultation an individual sheet of health advice based on the actual risk profile can be printed.

The program is flexible and interactive. It can be updated as new cohort studies become available, and can incorporate new languages, new risk factors, and new endpoints as knowledge evolves. Several countries have adapted the program using updated mortality data, which allow clinicians to have immediate and interactive access to appropriate local preventive advice.

HeartScore® is available for downloading in a version for low-risk and high-risk regions via the ESC website (see ➲Online resources, p.435) National versions will be gradually made available from this website. However, given the rapidly evolving changes, where several former high-risk countries now have CHD mortality levels approaching or even lower than some low-risk countries, some caution is warranted when using the charts. Although not formally tested, physicians in former high-risk countries which have had a steep decline may consider using the low-risk charts instead.

How to use the charts

- To estimate a person's total 10-year risk of CVD death, find the table for their gender, smoking status, and age. Within the table find the cell nearest to the person's systolic blood pressure (mmHg) and total cholesterol (mmol/L or mg/dL).
- The effect of lifetime exposure to risk factors can be seen by following the table upwards. This can be used when advising younger people.
- Low-risk individuals should be offered advice to maintain their low-risk status. Those who are at 5% risk or higher, or who will reach this level in middle age, should be given maximal attention.
- To define a person's relative risk, compare their risk category with that of other people of the same age and gender.
- The effect of changing cholesterol, smoking status, or systolic blood pressure can be estimated from the chart.

Qualifiers

Total CVD risk may be higher than indicated in the chart:

- as the person approaches the next age category;
- in asymptomatic people with paraclinical evidence of atherosclerosis (e.g. computed tomography scan, ultrasonography);
- in people with a strong family history of premature CVD;
- in people with low high-density lipoprotein (HDL) cholesterol levels, with raised triglyceride levels, with impaired glucose tolerance, with raised C-reactive protein, fibrinogen, homocysteine, apolipoprotein B, or lipoprotein(a) levels;
- in obese and sedentary people.

High-risk strategy

Prevention targeted at individuals who are at high risk but otherwise healthy should be an integral part of clinical practice. The usefulness of screening has been debated; it has been held that screening for high-risk individuals represents a costly and relatively ineffective strategy that distracts from cheaper and more effective policy interventions which benefit entire populations [15]. Even so, a substantial number are identified in daily practice without having to resort to cardiovascular screening of the entire population and they will have to be managed through the best available and evidence-based clinical strategies, including lifestyle changes for all, and medication, when appropriate. Some patients will come to the attention of the medical profession by their lifestyle, e.g. smoking cigarettes or obesity, others through the presence of a family history of early CVD. Others will be identified by the detection of hypertension, hyperlipidaemia, diabetes, or by a combination of risk factors, as in the metabolic syndrome. The cost-effectiveness of primary prevention using medication to treat hypertension or dyslipidaemia in patients at high risk appears to be good, but will obviously depend on the cost of medication, as well as the absolute risk and estimated duration of treatment [35].

In the 2003 European guidelines, a 10-year risk of CVD death of 5% or more was arbitrarily considered high risk. As a 95% chance of survival may be considered as relatively good by many, the new nomenclature used in the 2007 guideline is that everyone with a 10-year risk of cardiovascular death of 5% or more are at *increased risk.*

The SCORE diagram only uses fatal events, because non-fatal event rates are critically dependent upon definitions and the methods used in their ascertainment. Considerable changes in diagnostic tests and definitions, particularly with respect to myocardial infarction, have occurred since the SCORE cohorts were assembled. In addition, survival rates, particularly for hospitalized patients but also for out-of hospital deaths, have improved. Clinicians naturally wish for the total risk of non-fatal plus fatal events but because many fatal events occur out-of-hospital, figures for total events are not easily available. Still, recent analyses from the Swedish linked hospital discharge and death registries suggest that, in first CHD events, for each fatal case, the total risk of a first non-fatal or fatal CHD event can currently be calculated to be five times higher in people <55 years of age, four times higher among those aged 55–64 years and three times higher among those aged 65–74 years [36].

Individuals at increased risk can be defined as those with:

- multiple risk factors resulting in a 10-year fatal CVD risk of ≥5% at present according to SCORE;
- markedly raised levels of single risk factors, i.e. blood pressure ≥180/110mmHg, or persistent blood pressure of ≥160/110mmHg. These levels should be treated with antihypertensive drugs, irrespective of other risk factors;
- total cholesterol ≥8mmol/L (320mg/dL);
- low-density lipoprotein (LDL)-cholesterol ≥6mmol/L (≥240mg/dL);
- diabetes mellitus.

Secondary prevention

The most cost-effective strategy for preventing cardiovascular events starts by targeting patients who have had a CVD event. They are at the highest risk, there are relatively few of them, they are easy to identify, and they are likely to be more motivated than patients without symptoms [37]. Long-term prognosis in patients with past acute myocardial infarction (AMI) has improved substantially, probably due both to the availability of effective secondary prevention strategies and also to changes in clinical presentation [38] and lowering of the threshold for diagnosis. Even so, 10-year risk can vary substantially, from <10% in young patients with previous myocardial infarction to >40% among patients aged 65–74 years. Patients who present with CVD have already declared themselves to be at high risk and therefore their modifiable risk factors need to be reduced. These include the basic elements of lifestyle counselling (stopping smoking, modifying food and physical activity habits, taking action against psychosocial stress and depression) and pharmacological treatment, and are an integral part of post-event cardiological or stroke care.

The treatment goals of prevention in patients with established CVD, or with increased risk, are:

- stopping smoking;
- healthy food choices;
- physical activity: at least 30min of moderate activity each day;
- body mass index (BMI) <25kg/m^2 and avoidance of central obesity;
- total cholesterol <4.5mmol/L (175mg/dL) with an option of <4mmol/L (155mg/dL) if feasible;
- LDL cholesterol <2.5mmol/L (100mg/dL) with an option of <2mmol/L (80mg/dL) if feasible;
- blood pressure <130/80mmHg, if feasible.

Smoking

Smoking as a risk factor for CVD

Tobacco use is one of the most important causes of AMI and CVD globally. All forms of tobacco use, including different types of smoking and chewing tobacco and second-hand smoke, increase risk [39]. Over 1 million men and 200,000 women in Europe die from smoking each year; of which 375,000 men and 78,000 women die from CVD [5]. Smoking remains the single most important preventable cause of disease and early death, with an estimated 30% of all CHD cases due to smoking [23].

Smoking behaviours are contagious. In a densely interconnected social network of >12,000 people in the Framingham Heart Study it was found that smoking behaviour spread through close and distant social ties, and that groups of interconnected people stopped smoking in concert [40]. This finding suggests that decisions to quit smoking reflect choices made by groups of people connected to each other.

The adverse effect of smoking is related to the amount of tobacco smoked daily [39] (➲Fig. 12.15) and the risk of future CVD is particularly high if smoking starts before the age of 15 years [41]. Both active and passive smoking are associated with progression of atherosclerosis [42]. In the presence of other risk factors (diabetes, hypertension, dyslipidaemia, overweight), smoking-related risk increases even further.

Quitting smoking is the most effective of all preventive measures. The effect is more pronounced in patients with CHD: a recent review [43] has shown that quitting smoking is associated with a substantial reduction in risk of all-cause mortality: pooled crude relative risk (RR) 0.64 (95% CI 0.58–0.71). There was also a reduction in non-fatal myocardial infarctions—RR 0.68 (95% CI 0.57–0.82).

Assessment of smoking

A full assessment of the smoking status of the patient is mandatory. This includes: motivation to quit smoking,

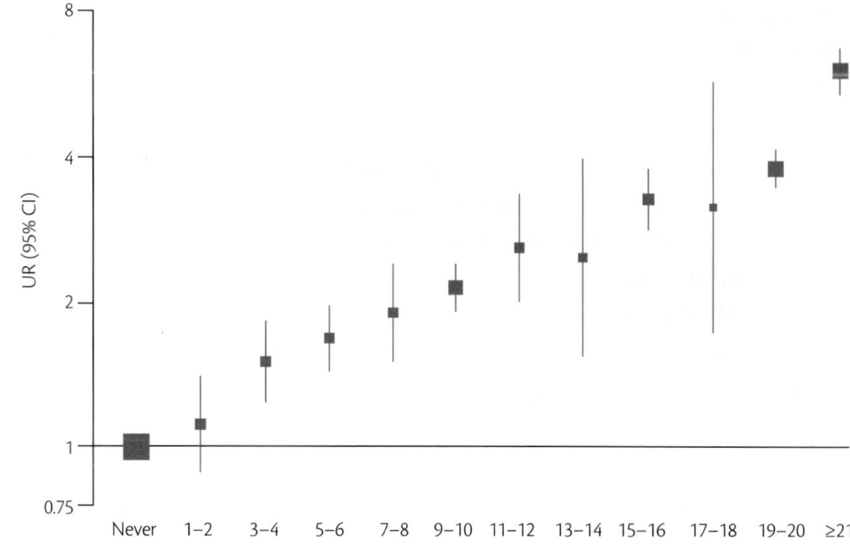

Figure 12.15 Risk of AMI with increasing numbers of cigarettes smoked, compared with never smoked; ≥21 cigarettes smoked per day represents about 1.5 pack of cigarettes per day, associated with OR 6.00–7.00. Reproduced with permission from Teo KK, Ôunpuu S, Hawken S, *et al.* Tobacco use and risk of myocardial infarction in 52 countries in the INTERHEART study: a case-control study. *Lancet* 2006; **368**: 647–58.

amount and type smoked, social and family environment, knowledge of nicotine's role in health, signs of nicotine dependence, earlier cessation experience and existing relevant comorbidity, especially chronic obstructive lung disease. A simple lung function test may be valuable. In addition, the degree of addiction and the state of changing smoking habits are highly relevant. Here, the Fagerström test for nicotine dependence can be used (➲Table 12.4) [44, 45].

Management of smoking, quitting smoking programmes

Clear and strict advice that a cardiac patient should quit smoking is of decisive importance in the smoking cessation process. At the time of an acute cardiac event or coronary intervention patients may be highly motivated to change lifestyle, and this is an opportunity to initiate or reinforce anti-smoking advice that should not be missed. Continued reinforcement and encouragement are also important.

There is a broad variety of options in smoking cessation therapy varying from simple self-help interventions to drug therapy:

- **Self-help interventions**: smokers may give up smoking on their own but leaflets with advice and information may help. Standard self-help materials may increase quitting rates compared to no intervention but the effect is limited. Materials that are tailored for individual smokers may be more effective [46].
- **Individual behavioural counselling**: when compared to control or minimal intervention, individual counselling is more effective and may lead to a quitting smoking rate of up to 40% 6 months after starting the programme [47].
- **Group therapy programmes**: these provide smokers with an opportunity to learn behavioural techniques combined with mutual support within the group, although not all smokers accept this option. Groups are better than self-help and other less intensive interventions. However, there is not enough evidence on their effectiveness, or cost-effectiveness, compared to individual counselling with similar intensity. Addition of group

Tablel 12.4 The Fagerström test for nocotine dependence

Question	Answer	Points
1 How soon after you wake up do you smoke your first cigarette?	Within 5min	3
	6–30min	2
	31–60min	1
	After 60min	0
2 Do you find it difficult to refrain from smoking in places where it is forbidden?	Yes	1
	No	0
3 Which cigarette would hate most to give up?	The first in the morning	1
	Any other	0
4 How many cigarettes per day do you smoke?	≤10	0
	11–20	1
	21–30	2
	≥31	3
5 Do you smoke more frequently during the first hours after waking than during the rest of the day?	Yes	1
	No	0
6 Do you smoke if you are so ill that you are in bed most of the day?	Yes	1
	No	0

Average score in representative samples of smokers: 3–4 points.
Questions 1 and 4 have the highest informative value.

therapy to treatment, such as advice from a health professional or nicotine replacement, has limited additional benefit [48].

- **Nicotine replacement therapy (NRT)**: the aim is to replace nicotine from cigarettes, thus reducing withdrawal symptoms associated with smoking. Different forms of nicotine replacement are available: chewing gum, transdermal patches, nasal spray, inhalers, and tablets. All of the commercially available forms of NRT (gum, transdermal patch, nasal spray, inhaler, and sublingual tablets/lozenges) can help people who make a quit attempt to increase their chances of successfully stopping smoking. NRTs increase the rate of quitting by 50–70%, regardless of setting [49]. Provision of more intense levels of support is not essential to the success of NRT. The use of nicotine patches is well tolerated by CVD patients. Nicotine patches have been demonstrated to be safe even in patients with acute coronary syndromes [50].
- **Antidepressants**: smoking cessation and nicotine withdrawal may precipitate depression. The antidepressants bupropion and nortriptyline aid long-term smoking cessation but selective serotonin reuptake inhibitors (e.g. fluoxetine) do not [51]. Evidence suggests that the mode of action of bupropion and nortriptyline is independent of their antidepressant effect and that they are of similar efficacy to nicotine replacement. Adverse events with both medications are rarely serious or lead to stopping medication.

Despite these options, many patients who succeed in quitting manage to do this without any special programmes or treatment. Support by the spouse and family is important in smoking cessation.

A community approach will remain an important part of health promotion activities. In several European countries smoke-free environments have been created, with restrictions of smoking at work sites, in public places, restaurants, etc. These changes are important public-health developments that may support individual smoking cessation efforts.

Physical activity

Physical inactivity as a risk factor for CVD

Physical inactivity is a major and growing component in the burden of chronic disease. At least 60% of the global population fails to achieve the minimum recommendation of 30min' moderate intensity physical activity daily and the proportion of people doing no physical activity in a week can reach up to 25%.

The risk of CVD increases by at least 1.5 times in people who are inactive. Decreasing physical activity in the younger generation will likely have a major impact on CVD rates in the future. In the younger age groups, activity patterns decline consistently from ages 12 through 21 years. In young adulthood (18–29 years) deterioration continues, whereas in middle age (30–64 years) the activity pattern stabilizes, with a tendency to improve in older age [52]. The combination of excessive caloric intake and insufficient exercise are lifestyle factors contributing to the development of the metabolic syndrome, which has reached an almost epidemic level in Europe and elsewhere.

Regular physical activity is protective through a wide variety of beneficial effects, all of which converge to reduce incidence and mortality from CVD. Physical activity helps maintain body weight, has a beneficial effect on lipid profile, mainly through raising HDL and decreasing triglyceride levels, increases insulin sensitivity, and reduces blood pressure. Physical inactivity, a state not natural to man, will have the opposite effect. Thus, the promotion of regular physical activity and maintenance of fitness at school, at work and during commuting, at home, during leisure time, and after old-age retirement is an important task for preventive cardiology. However, although counselling may result in a greater amount of physical activity, a review of interventions for promoting physical activity revealed only a moderate effect on achieving the predetermined levels of physical activity and cardiorespiratory fitness [53].

Children and adolescents

The risk of a premature onset of atherosclerosis is increasing as children are becoming less active. Today children expend 600kcal/day less than their counterparts 50 years ago [54]. School children rarely exercise the recommended daily 60–90min daily. More than half of adolescents become physically inactive after leaving school.

Atherosclerosis begins in childhood: the first stage, a reversible fatty streak, is seen in most children. The harmful later stage, the atheromatous plaque, does not appear until after puberty in boys and much later in girls [55]. Traditional risk factors, such as hypertension, dyslipidaemia, and smoking, act in the early stages of this process. At present, blood pressure levels in children are rising, the prevalence and the degree of obesity increases, insulin resistance and type 2 diabetes mellitus (non-insulin dependent diabetes mellitus) are more often found in young individuals [56].

Healthy adults

Changes in society and the individual adaptations to these contribute to a sedentary lifestyle. The exertional demands at the work place have decreased; only a minority of labourers will experience breathlessness in their daily work. Commuting has become less physically demanding. There is lower energy expenditure at home and during leisure time.

Since the landmark studies by the groups of Morris and Paffenbarger [57, 58] the relation between physical activity and CVD has become well established. Maintaining physical fitness has a direct protective effect independent of other risk factors and exercise capacity, as well as physical activity, are powerful predictors of mortality [59–61]. Regular exercise diminishes the risk of a myocardial infarction under strenuous exertion [62].

Adults with CVD

CVD patients tend to restrict physical activity for fear or because of symptoms. Overprotection by the family may contribute. Restoration and maintenance of physical fitness are both needed and beneficial.

Many of the effects of an active lifestyle observed in the healthy population apply to the CVD patient. Physical activity reduces the progression of atherosclerosis by improving endothelial dysfunction. It affects the production of free radicals, protecting patients from oxidative stress; it improves insulin sensitivity and reduces plasma homocysteine levels. Protection against malignant arrhythmias and less myocardial wall stress is obtained through modifying the sympatho-vagal balance [63–65]. In a meta-analysis including 8440 patients, a 27% reduction of total mortality as a result of exercise training was estimated, and cardiac mortality was reduced by 31% [66]. In spite of these benefits only a minority of patients are referred to exercise training programmes. Physical inactivity, additionally, is common in patients with congestive heart failure. The benefit of improving physical fitness in these patients has been clearly demonstrated [67].

The elderly

Age-related physiological changes may result in physical inactivity: a decrease in maximum heart rate, stroke volume, cardiac output, and down-grading of beta-adrenergic receptors. Peripheral changes contribute with decreases in muscular strength and coordination, peripheral O_2 uptake, bone mineral content, and lung function. With increasing age, the activities of daily life put a greater demand on work capacity. Regular physical activity will counteract or effectively slow down age-related changes, improving quality of life, and extending disease-free survival. As the elderly account for most myocardial infarctions and coronary interventions, cardiologists need to use the therapeutic potential of physical activity. This might even ameliorate the decline caused by concomitant diseases often seen among the elderly.

Assessment of physical activity

In youth, assessment of physical activity remains a challenge for research: differing stages of growth, discrepancies between physical strength and fitness, and difficulties with the validity of questionnaires confound assessment. Formal exercise testing including measuring oxygen consumption or direct observation are resource-consuming methods. Yet, assessment is needed to evaluate physical activity programmes. Heart rate monitors, pedometers, and accelerometers are used, although they do not register all forms of physical activity in children. Accelerometers may be the preferred choice [68]. In high-risk children, as in hereditary dyslipidaemia, a heavy family CVD burden or diabetes mellitus, standard exercise testing can provide a ground for lifestyle advice and follow-up.

In healthy adults a brief interview concerning physical activity at work and in leisure time if needed, together with a recall questionnaire, diary, or pedometer may act as a base for the physician's advice. For research purposes the IPAQ (international physical activity questionnaire) is recommended [69]. This may be used in conjunction with an exercise test using a bicycle ergometer or treadmill to obtain an objective assessment of exercise capacity.

In adults with CVD the patient's history usually needs objective assessment by exercise testing to detect myocardial ischaemia, to stratify for risk of a new event, to select for coronary intervention, or to assess the effect of revascularization or the response to medication. We refer to guidelines issued by the ESC [70] and the American Heart Association [71].

In the elderly the patient interview remains the cornerstone in assessing physical activity. The specific problems of deteriorating physical capacity should be addressed, especially regarding the activities of daily living and the need for support. Concomitant diseases must be taken into account. Exercise testing on a bicycle ergometer or treadmill may be indicated in persons with symptoms of CVD. However, less demanding methods, such as the 6-min walk test or the shuttle walk test, may also provide valuable information on the physical capacity of the elderly.

Management of physical activity

Children and adolescents

Every child should be encouraged to spend a minimum of 60–90min every day in physical activities that increase heart rate to a significant degree, be it in school or during leisure time. Special efforts should be made to maintain activity levels during and after adolescence.

Healthy adults

In high-risk individuals the family doctor should specifically promote regular physical exercise. For all healthy adults, regardless of risk, an active lifestyle should include work, commuting, domestic life, and leisure time. According to recent recommendations [72], healthy adults aged 18–65 years need moderate-intensity aerobic (endurance) physical activity for a minimum of 30min on 5 days each week or vigorous-intensity aerobic physical activity for a minimum of 20min on 3 days each week. Combinations of moderate- and vigorous-intensity activity can be performed to meet this demand.

Recommended intensity may be defined as heart rate during exercise at 60–75% of the maximum. As a simple method for estimating maximum heart frequency the formula of '220 – age = maximal heart rate' can be used. Alternatively, the Borg scale of perceived exertion may be applied, using the level of 'moderate exertion' as the target [73].

A practical method for calculating energy expenditure is the use of metabolic equivalents: MET. One MET represents an individual's resting energy expenditure. Walking at 5km/hour on a flat surface will expend about 3.3METs, jogging and running on a similar surface results in approximately 8METs. For example, a person walking at 5km/hour (moderate intensity) for 30min would accumulate 99METs/30min of activity (3.3METs × 30min). If jogging at 8km/hour for 20min one would expend 160MET/20min (8METs × 20min). Accordingly, the minimum recommendation for moderate-intensity activity (walking for 30min on 5 days of the week) would amount up to 495METs per week (99 × 5), or not very different from the vigorous-intensity recommendation (jogging for 20min on 3 days), which would result in 480METs weekly (160 × 3). Notably, these recommendations still result in much lower calorie expenditure than that registered for some indigenous, nomadic populations [74].

By using the MET method different combinations of activity can be calculated to ascertain the recommended minimum. When combining moderate- and vigorous-intensity activity to meet the recommendation, the minimum goal should be in the range of 450–750METs weekly. Non-trained individuals should start at the lower end of this range when beginning an activity programme and progress towards the higher end as they become fitter. Listed in ➲Table 12.5 are the MET values for a variety of common physical activities.

Although aerobic endurance training remains the cornerstone of physical activity, anaerobic resistance training has become increasingly popular and can at present be considered as a valuable addition to conventional endurance training. Resistance training enhances muscular strength and endurance, functional capacity and independence, and quality of life while reducing disability both in persons without and with CVD [75].

Short bouts of vigorous physical activity can increase the risk of sudden cardiac death and AMI in susceptible persons. Maintaining physical fitness may help to reduce this risk. The use of screening healthy individuals before participation in strenuous exercise has not been systematically evaluated [76].

Adults with CVD

Recommendations for CVD patients should be based on a clinical examination including exercise testing. Patients with stable angina pectoris or recovering from a myocardial infarction or coronary intervention should be referred to a rehabilitation programme provided by a multidisciplinary team on an ambulatory basis or for selected cases to a specialized in-patient institute. Individual home training programmes and other aids (books, CD-Rom, Internet, etc.) are available and effective although regular follow-up and encouragement are needed. Heart-rate monitors or pedometers may be helpful in home-based programmes. We refer to ➲Chapter 25 (Cardiac Rehabilitation) for detailed information. The prescription of physical training programmes in congenital heart disease should remain in the hands of paediatric cardiologists and specially trained physiotherapists.

The elderly

The recommendations for the healthy elderly are similar to those for adults. Daily physical activity should be maintained at a moderate and agreeable level. Brisk walking at a pace at which a conversation still can be held ('walk-and-talk model') is a good example. Activities that improve flexibility are recommended and balance exercises are indicated for older adults at risk of falls. Senior citizens should have an activity plan for achieving recommended physical activity that integrates both preventive and therapeutic recommendations. This includes moderate-intensity aerobic activity, muscle-strengthening activity, reducing sedentary behaviour, and risk management [77].

Senior CVD patients will benefit equally from rehabilitation programmes: training is safe, improves strength, aerobic fitness, endurance, and physical function. It will improve risk factors, mental state, and quality of life [78]. Resistance

Table 12.5 MET equivalents of common physical activities (also see Table 25.11, p.946 and Table 32.1, p.1216)

Light <3.0METs	Moderate 3.0–6.0METs	Vigorous >6.0METs
Walking Walking slowly around home, store or office = 2.0*	**Walking** Walking 5km/hour = 3.3* Walking at very brisk pace (7km/hour) = 5.0*	**Walking** Walking at very very brisk pace (8km/hour) = 6.3* Walking/hiking at moderate pace and grade with no or light pack (>5kg) = 7.0
Household and occupation Sitting: using computer work at desk using light hand tools = 1.5 Standing performing light work such as making bed, washing dishes, ironing, preparing food, or store clerk = 2.0–2.5	**Household and occupation** Carpentry: general = 3.6 Carrying and stacking wood = 5.5 Cleaning: heavy: washing windows, car, clean garage = 3.0 Mowing lawn: walk power mower = 5.5 Sweeping floors or carpet, vacuuming, mopping = 3.0–3.5	**Household and occupation** Carrying heavy loads such as bricks = 7.5 Heavy farming such as bailing hay = 8.0 Shovelling, digging ditches = 8.5 Shovelling sand, coal, etc. = 7.0
Leisure time and sports Arts and crafts, playing cards = 1.5 Billiards = 2.5 Boating (power) = 2.5 Croquet = 2.5 Darts = 2.5 Fishing (sitting) = 2.5 Playing most musical instruments = 2.0–2.5	**Leisure time and sports** Badminton: recreational = 4.5 Basketball: shooting around = 4.5 Bicycling: on flat: light effort (12–15km/hour) = 6.0 Dancing — ballroom slow = 3.0; fast = 4.5 Fishing from river bank and walking = 4.0 Golf: walking pulling clubs = 4.3 Sailing boat, wind surfing = 3.0 Swimming leisurely = 6.0† Table tennis = 4.0 Tennis doubles = 5.0 Volleyball: noncompetitive = 3.0–4.0	**Leisure time and sports** Basketball game = 8.0 Bicycling: on flat: moderate effort (16–20km/hour) = 8.0; fast (> 20km/hour) = 10 Hiking at steep grades and pack 5–20 kg = 7.5–9.0 Jogging at 9km/hour = 8.0* Jogging at 11km/hour = 10.0* Running at 13km/hour = 11.5* Skiing cross country: slow (4km/hour = 7.0; fast (8–12km/hour) = 9.0 Soccer: casual = 7.0; competitive = 10.0 Swimming: moderate/hard = 8–11† Tennis singles = 8.0 Volleyball: competitive at gym or beach = 8.0

* On flat, hard surface.

† MET values can vary substantially from person to person during swimming as a result of different strokes and skill levels.

training may be an attractive alternative as it can be used in training at home (thera-band, weight lifting, etc.). The goal should be the prevention of physical inactivity with the efforts of an active lifestyle rewarded by cardiovascular and other health benefits.

Blood pressure

Hypertension as a risk factor for CVD

Hypertension, defined as a systolic blood pressure (SBP) ≥140mmHg and/or a diastolic blood pressure (DBP) ≥90mmHg, is one of the most important preventable causes of premature death worldwide, contributing to approximately half of all global CVD (see Chapter 13, Hypertension). In many countries, up to 30% of adults have hypertension; a further 50–60% would be in better health if they reduced their blood pressure by increasing physical activity, maintaining an ideal body weight and eating more fruits and vegetables. CVD doubles for every 10mmHg increase in DBP or every 20mmHg increase in SBP [79].

Blood pressure usually rises with age, except where salt intake is low, physical activity high, and obesity largely absent. Most natural foods contain salt; processed food may be high in salt; and individuals may add salt for taste. Dietary salt increases blood pressure in most people with hypertension, and in about a quarter of normotensives, especially with increasing age. In addition to effective lifestyle changes medication may be needed for control of hypertension.

Lifestyle management

Blood pressure can be reduced either by lifestyle interventions or by pharmacotherapy. Lifestyle interventions have been evaluated in mild blood pressure elevation [80]. Blood pressure was moderately reduced in individuals exposed to dietary sodium reduction, increased potassium intake, decreased alcohol consumption, body weight reduction, dietary regimens based on fish oils, increased physical activity, and cessation of smoking [80, 81]. In compliant individuals lifestyle changes reduce the total CVD risk, prevent a restart of medication after drug treatment has been stopped, and may decrease the number and doses of drugs needed. Treatment based on these interventions alone may be sufficient for patients with mild hypertension and should always be advised even for patients on antihypertensive drugs. Frequent reinforcement is needed because long-term compliance in lifestyle changes may be lacking.

Lifestyle recommendations include:

- weight reduction in overweight individuals;
- reduction of salt intake to <6g daily;
- restriction of alcohol consumption to <10–30g/day (men) and <10–20g/day (women);
- regular physical activity in sedentary individuals;
- quitting smoking;
- dietary changes in cases of hyperlipidaemia.

Drug treatment (also see Chapter 13)

The decision to start treatment depends both on the level of blood pressure and on the assessment of total CVD risk. Because risk factors may interact, the total cardiovascular risk of hypertensive patients may be high even if blood pressure is only mildly elevated [82]. In patients with established CVD or if target organ damage, such as left ventricular hypertrophy, or microalbuminuria, is present the choice of drugs depends on the underlying disease.

Large-scale randomized controlled trials have conclusively demonstrated that pharmacological blood pressure reduction substantially reduces CVD mortality and morbidity [15]. Drug therapy is needed in case of a sustained SBP ≥160mmHg and/or DBP ≥100mmHg, or if target damage is present. Patients with SBP 140–159mmHg and/or DBP 90–99mmHg are managed according to their total risk, which usually means medications, unless risk is very low (<1%) [15]. Individuals with SBP <140mmHg and DBP <90mmHg and no other risk factors do not require drug therapy as a rule.

Nutrition

Nutritional treatment for the prevention of CVDs

The relation between nutritional habits and cardiovascular risk is well established. Several clinical and epidemiological studies have shown strong associations between nutritional factors and CVD risk factors, such as hypertension, cholesterol, and diabetes, as well as with the occurrence of fatal and non-fatal cardiovascular events. Furthermore, multifactorial or targeted nutritional interventions have clearly demonstrated the beneficial effects of preventive or therapeutic nutritional approaches. In view of this strong evidence nutrition therapy is a full component of cardiovascular risk prevention.

Diet and CVDs

The principal properties of foods and nutrients are summarized in Table 12.6.

Total fat, saturated, monounsaturated, and trans fatty acids

Dietary lipids play a major role in the formation of the atheromatous plaque and thrombotic complications. In Western countries, dietary intake of fat is often >100g/day. Dietary fatty acids affect cholesterol and lipoprotein levels [83], arterial blood pressure, and haemostasis. In cohort studies, the positive relationship between fat intake and CVDs was linked to their saturated fatty acid content

Tablel 12.6 General recommendations for high cardiovascular risk subjects, to be adapted according to local and cultural circumstances

Nutrient and food	Goal	Affect cardiovascular risk factors	Affect cardiovascular events
Energy	Keep BMI <25kg/m^2 and waist girth <102cm in men and <88cm in women	Triglycerides, HDL-cholesterol, insulin, glycaemia, blood pressure	Effect of BMI reduction Unknown
Total fat	30% of total energy	LDL-cholesterol and body fat	Little evidence
Saturated fat	10% of total energy	LDL-cholesterol, HDL-cholesterol, body fat, glycaemia	Yes
Trans fatty acids	<2% of total energy	LDL-cholesterol, HDL-cholesterol	Yes
Polyunsaturated	≥10% of total energy	LDL-cholesterol, HDL-cholesterol	Yes
Monounsaturated	≥10% of total energy		Yes
n-3 fatty acid	1g/day;	Triglycerides, blood pressure, haemostasis, heart rate	Decrease fatal cardiovascular events
Dietary cholesterol	<300mg/day	LDL-cholesterol	Little evidence
Fruit and vegetable	≥ five portions a day	Blood pressure	Yes
Salt	<6 g/day	Blood pressure	Little evidence

BMI, body mass index.

[84, 85]. Animal products, industrially manufactured meals, and certain cooking fats are the principal sources of saturated fats. These fatty acids increase LDL-cholesterol concentrations. Epidemiological data for monounsaturated fatty acids are scarcer. However, intake of monounsaturated fatty acids have been associated with reduced coronary risk compared to saturated fatty acids [84].

Trans fatty acids are produced during industrial hydrogenation of vegetable fats and oils and during the natural digestion process in ruminant animals. Metabolic studies and meta-analyses show a clear and consistent association between increasing trans fatty acid intakes and an adverse lipid profile [86]. Epidemiological studies have shown positive associations between trans fatty acids and cardiovascular morbidity and mortality. As a consequence of these and other potential deleterious effects (➲Fig. 12.16) [87], trans fatty acids have been banned from foods in a number of European countries.

N-6 and n-3 polyunsaturated fatty acids

Linoleic acid is the main representative of the n-6 group. These fatty acids are mainly derived from vegetal oils. Clinical studies have shown that the consumption of n-6 polyunsaturated fatty acids decreases LDL-cholesterol. In cohort studies, the intake of polyunsaturated fatty acids is associated with a reduced coronary risk compared to saturated fatty acids or trans fatty acids. Intervention studies combining a reduction in risk factors and an increase in polyunsaturated fatty acid intake have shown reduced CVD incidence and mortality [88].

Alpha-linolenic acid is the precursor of the n-3 fatty acid group. Primary food sources are soy beans, rapeseed, safflower, and linseed oil. In cohort studies, the intake of-alpha-linolenic acid is inversely correlated to cardiovascular events and in secondary prevention trials coronary deaths were less frequent in patients randomly assigned to a Mediterranean diet with a high alpha-linolenic acid content [88].

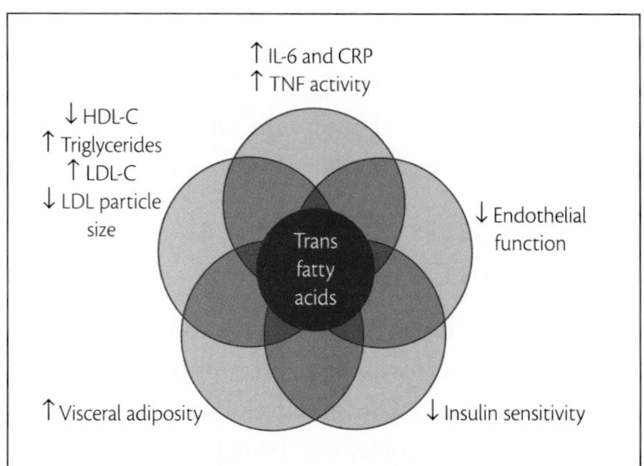

Figure 12.16 Effects of trans fatty acids on biological and metabolic variables. Adapted from with permission from Mozaffarian D, Willett WC Trans fatty acids and cardiovascular risk: a unique cardiometabolic imprint? *Curr Atheroscler Rep* 2007; **9**: 486–93.

Eicosapentaenoic acids and docosahexaenoic acids are two important members of the n-3 group that are mainly derived from oily fish. The intake of eicosapentaenoic acids and docosahexaenoic acids reduces plasma triglycerides, arterial blood pressure, and improves haemostasis. Prospective studies show a reduced risk of fatal cardiovascular events in people who regularly eat fish [89]. In patients with CVD, the intake of fish and of eicosapentaenoic acids and docosahexaenoic acids supplements reduces coronary mortality [88].

The cardioprotective effects of fish oil have been attributed to antiarrhythmic effects of eicosapentaenoic acids and docosahexaenoic acids. Preclinical data indicate that altering ion-channel function and preventing cytosolic free calcium levels from reaching toxic levels in cardiac myocytes. Three recent clinical trials have examined whether omega-3 fatty-acid supplementation suppresses arrhythmias in patients with implantable cardioverter defibrillators. The results of these studies are controversial and do not permit to conclude definitely on the properties of fish oil towards major events [90].

In conclusion, the dose response of eicosapentaenoic acids and docosahexaenoic acids seems to vary depending on the different endpoints (➲Fig. 12.17) [91]. It increases rapidly to reach a plateau corresponding to 750mg/day for sudden death, whereas the triglyceride-lowering properties depend directly on the dosage.

Fruits, vegetables, vitamins, and vitamin supplements

Fruits and vegetables are important sources of vitamins and fibre. Intervention trials have demonstrated that regular intake of a diet with a high fruit and vegetable content and reduced dairy product content lowers SBP and DBP [92]. In observational cohort studies, the risks of coronary events (➲Fig. 12.18) and strokes are reduced by 7% and 5%, respectively, for one additional portion of fruit and vegetable per day [93, 94].

Antioxidant vitamins have beneficial effects on cardiovascular risk factors in laboratory experiments. Most epidemiological observation studies have shown negative associations between the intake of vitamin E or carotenoids and CVD [95]. Similarly, leaf vegetable vitamins have a clear impact on homocysteine levels, another vascular risk factor. However, when intervention therapeutic trials were conducted, results were disappointing, showing at best no protective effect of vitamin supplements.

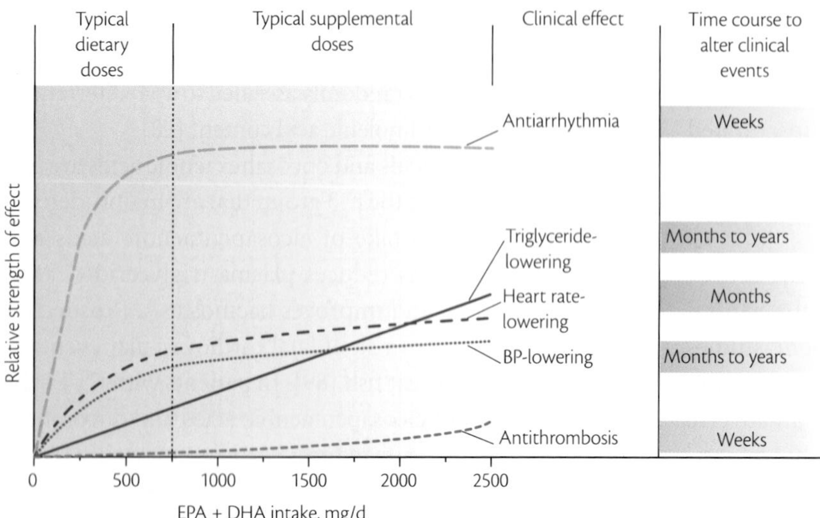

Figure 12.17 Potential dose responses and time courses for clinical events and control of cardiovascular risk factors of DHA and EPA intake. Adapted with permission from Mozaffarian D, Rimm EB Fish intake, contaminants, and human health: evaluating the risks and the benefits. *JAMA* 2007; **296**: 1885–99.

Alcohol

In the population, the connection between alcohol use and mortality follows a U- or J-shaped curve. Optimum consumption ranges between 10–30g of alcohol per day for men, and is lower for women [96]. Reduced coronary mortality is the major cause for the reduction in mortality, with no evidence of higher benefit with any specific type of drink [97]. Conversely, 'binge drinking' is associated with a higher risk of sudden death and cerebrovascular stroke. Despite the protective association of low to moderate alcohol consumption, alcohol cannot be recommended in the prevention of CVD. In contrast to cardioprotective pharmacological agents, there exists no randomized study to prove the benefit of alcohol in the prevention of CVD. However, low to moderate consumption can probably be continued.

Salt

Sodium intake affects arterial pressure levels. Community-based intervention studies and meta-analyses of randomized trials have shown that a reduction in salt intake resulted in reduced arterial blood pressure in normo- and hypertensive subjects [98].

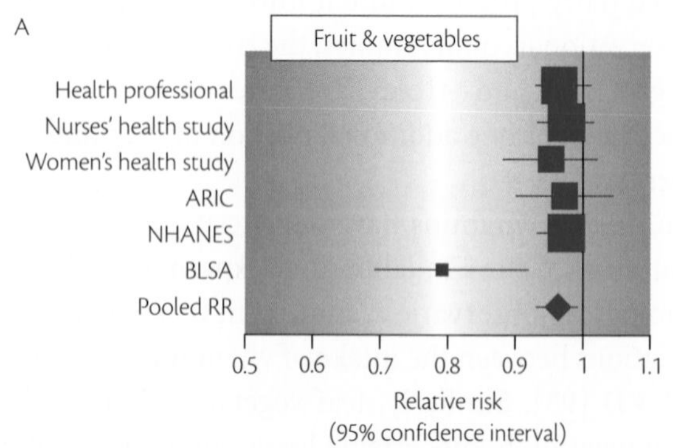

Figure 12.18 Pooled relative risk (95% CI) of coronary events for one daily portion of fruit and vegetable intake per day. Adapted with permission from Dauchet L, Amouyel P, Hercberg S, *et al.* Fruit and vegetable consumption and risk of coronary heart disease: a meta-analysis of cohort studies. *J Nutr* 2007; **136**: 2588–93.

Mediterranean diet

The traditional Mediterranean diet is characterized by moderate energy intake, low animal fat, high olive oil, high cereals, high legumes, nuts, and vegetables, and regular and moderate wine. The potential benefits of a Mediterranean-type diet are supported by clinical dietary interventions which demonstrated that adherence to such diet reduces several cardiovascular risk factors in high-risk subjects. A recent trial comparing Mediterranean, low-carbohydrate and low-fat diets has shown similar reduction in body weight with the low-carbohydrate and Mediterranean diets. However the effects on lipids were more favourable with the low-carbohydrate diet and those on glycaemic control with the Mediterranean diet [99]. Numerous epidemiological studies suggest that adherence to the traditional Mediterranean diet is beneficial for health and particularly protects against CVD [100] (➲Fig. 12.19). In contrast, there are a limited number of intervention studies to confirm these observations in patients with coronary disease.

Practical aspects of nutritional prevention of CVDs

The principal objective of dietary intervention is to control risk factors to prevent the formation and rupture of the atheromatous plaque. Dietary recommendations should be individually adapted taking into account the patient's risk profile and eating habits as well as the cultural characteristics.

General issues: recommendations

- A varied and balanced diet is important to preserve good cardiovascular health.

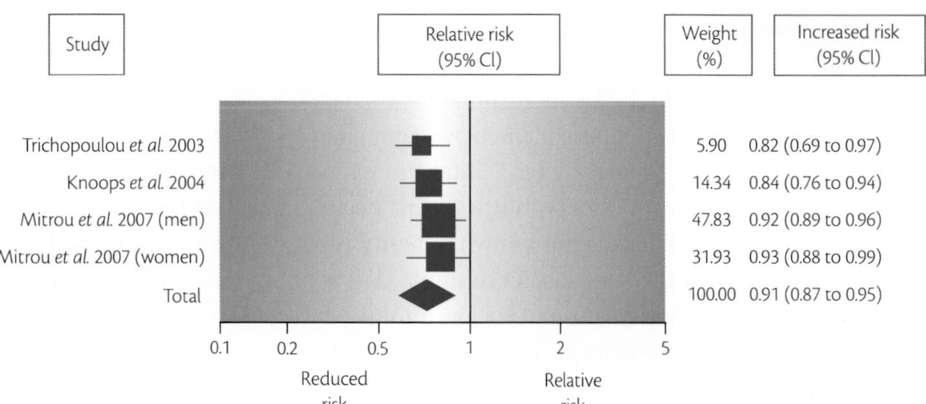

Figure 12.19 Pooled relative risk of CVD associated with increase in adherence of Mediterranean diet. Adapted with permission from Sofi F, Cesari F, Rosanna A, *et al.* Adherence to Mediterranean diet and health status: meta-analysis. *BMJ* 2008; **337**: a1344.

- Regular fish intake because the n-3 fatty acids which they contain protect against fatal cardiovascular events.
- Fruits and vegetables, 3–5 portions per day, cereals and grain products, skimmed dairy products, and low-fat meat.
- To maintain the ideal weight the intake of calories should be adjusted to energy expenditure by restricting fatty products and products with a high caloric density.
- The total fat intake should not exceed 30% of calorie intake. The saturated fatty acid intake should not exceed 30% of total lipids and the rest monounsaturated or polyunsaturated fats.
- The cholesterol intake should be <300mg/day.

Nutritional treatment of dyslipidaemias

- Reduction of LDL-cholesterol is the main objective of dietary treatment of subjects at high cardiovascular risk, aiming at less saturated and trans fatty acid intake, and, to a smaller degree, food cholesterol intake. The primary sources of trans and saturated fatty acids are hard margarines and products of animal origin, such as meat and dairy products.
- Increasing intake of omega-3 fatty acids from fish oils and certain vegetal oils to decrease plasma concentrations of triglycerides and prevent sudden death.
- Increasing intake of polyunsaturated fatty acids, soluble fibres, and phytosterols to reduce plasma concentrations of LDL-cholesterol.
- Exercise, body weight reduction in the obese, and normalization of glycaemia in diabetic patients to increase blood HDL-cholesterol levels.
- Reduction in the intake of refined sugars, which is associated with reduced concentrations of HDL-cholesterol and increased triglycerides in sensitive subjects. They may be replaced by complex sugars from fruits, vegetables, and grain products.

Weight control

A reduction in the weight of obese subjects is associated with improvement of the main risk factors:

- Weight loss is obtained by reducing calorie intake and increasing exercise.
- The calorie intake is obtained by decreasing high energy density food such as dietary lipids (9kcal/g) and alcohol (7kcal/g). The reduction of saturated fats of animal origin is the favoured target because of their effects on the lipoprotein profile.
- The lipid intake should be <30% of the energy intake.
- Aim at a weight loss from 0.5–1kg/week until target weight has been achieved. Upon weight loss completion, the objective becomes to maintain a stable weight and block weight recovery. Exercise should be adjusted to the physiological condition of the patient.

In conclusion, nutritional strategies have proven to be an efficient means of reducing events in subjects at high cardiovascular risk. Therefore, all patients with manifest CVD and subjects with high cardiovascular risk should receive professional advice on food and dietary choices to lower their risk.

Obesity and problems related to obesity

The obesity epidemic

Obesity and conditions related to obesity are major determinants of cardiovascular morbidity in Europe and worldwide. Whereas obesity has primarily been considered to result from individual choices against a background of genetics, it is becoming increasingly clear that the current obesity epidemic is driven by an environment that promotes obesity, by affecting individual lifestyle in the context of society. The rapid increase in obesity over the past few decades, during which the environment has changed markedly, will obviously not be explained by major changes in genetic make-up. Ultimately, energy intake in excess of caloric expenditure causes obesity, but why this occurs in some but not all individuals is not known. Obesity is usually more prevalent in the lower socioeconomic classes but even so, there is a varying relation of socioeconomic status with obesity between countries at different stages of development and, even in the Western world, socioeconomic gradients with respect to obesity are both heterogeneous and in transition.

Smoking rates are declining in many countries in Europe, whereas obesity is a growing problem worldwide; for this reason an increasing number of future cardiovascular events will be attributable to obesity. Figures from the latest pan-European study conducted in the mid-1990s indicated that obesity (defined as BMI ≥30kg/m^2) affects more than one in five in several European middle-aged populations, and that less than half have normal BMI (<25kg/m^2) [5]. Recent WHO estimates, based on national survey data, show that the prevalence of obesity in men aged 15 years and above ranges from 5% in Uzbekistan to 26% in Greece, and in women from 6% in Norway to 30% in Turkey [5]. Still, while all states, with one single exception (Colorado), in the USA currently have obesity rates of 20% in the adult population, or more (see ➲Online resources, p.435), with a prevalence of obesity ≥30% in three states, rates in the European region are much lower. Only a small proportion of the 34 ER countries with available recent data on obesity have rates comparable to the US. By and large, the situation in Europe today with respect to obesity rates is similar to the US in the early 1990s. Because, in a social context, obesity appears to spread through social ties [101], the same is probably true for maintaining normal weight. The future developments of the obesity epidemic in Europe will therefore rest not only with political decisions but also with social and cultural contexts. Some hope is offered by recent findings on the levelling off of obesity trends in children [102–104].

The current rapid increase in the prevalence of obesity is determined by environmental factors but it is equally clear that genetic factors predispose some individuals to develop overweight and obesity in the presence of abundant food. Twin, adoption, and family studies have shown that genetic factors play a significant role in the pathogenesis of obesity. However, in the absence of environmental factors, obesity will not develop.

Despite the fact that overweight and obesity are linked to hypertension, dyslipidaemia, diabetes, and thrombotic and fibrinolytic processes, as well as inflammatory reactions, findings with respect to CHD and stroke have not been consistent. Whereas serum cholesterol, smoking, and high blood pressure have established roles as predictors of CVD, studies with respect to obesity are more heterogeneous, with many of the early studies showing no, or only a weak, relation with cardiovascular outcomes [105]. In later years, however, several sufficiently large studies have, in fact, demonstrated significant associations between BMI, the most widely used measure of fatness, and CVD [106, 107], although usually at a relatively high BMI, and thus identifying limited subsets of the population at increased risk.

The inconsistent findings with respect to BMI are, to some extent, the result of methodological problems, because BMI does not discriminate between muscle and fat, which may be why moderately elevated levels have generally not been significantly associated with CVD. In addition, BMI does not take the distribution of excess fat into account. Several studies indicate that abdominal fat, as measured by the waist to hip ratio, is a more important predictor than BMI. In the INTERHEART study, waist-to-hip ratio showed a graded and highly significant association with myocardial infarction risk worldwide (➲Fig. 12.20). Redefinition of obesity based on waist-to-hip ratio instead of BMI increased the estimate of myocardial infarction attributable to obesity in most ethnic groups [108]. Another methodological problem is that many studies have used multivariate techniques to investigate whether the effect of obesity is independent of hypertension and dyslipidaemia, conditions that are a result of excess body fat. Even though obesity alone may not be sufficient to produce cardiovascular complications, this is an approach that will lead to an underestimation of the effects of obesity.

In later years there is more than sufficient documentation to support the role of obesity in the pathogenesis of CVD, either directly or via intervening factors. Several studies show increasing risk of myocardial infarction, coronary deaths, and stroke with increasing BMI, or abdominal obesity. Recent autopsy studies in young men and women have demonstrated that obesity is associated with more extensive and severe early atherosclerotic lesions [109, 110]. Some studies have indicated that the optimal BMI with respect to coronary disease and stroke is probably in the lower reference range [111, 112]. Even so, measures of obesity are still not included in cardiovascular risk prediction, probably mostly as a result of the methodological problems and inconsistencies in prior research.

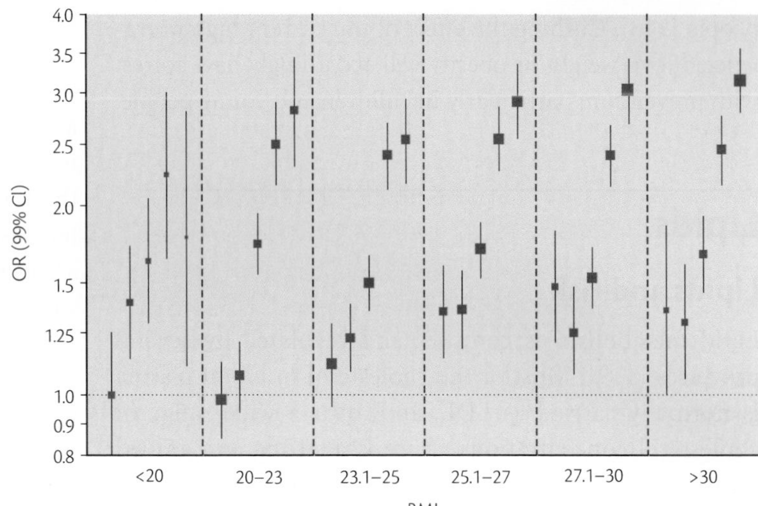

Figure 12.20 Association of waist-to-hip ratio within BMI categories with myocardial infarction risk in the INTERHEART study [108]. Within each BMI category risk increases with increasing waist-to-hip ratio. Reproduced with permission from Yusuf S, Hawken S, Ôunpuu S, *et al.* Obesity and the risk of myocardial infarction in 27,000 participants from 52 countries: a case-control study. *Lancet* 2005; **366**: 1640–9.

Consequences of obesity

Overweight and abdominal obesity are associated with several adverse factors, such as low HDL-cholesterol, high serum triglycerides, small and dense atherogenic LDL, hypertension, glucose intolerance, insulin resistance, and diabetes. The clustering of these factors has been termed the metabolic syndrome [113]. According to one definition [114], a diagnosis of metabolic syndrome can be made if a person has three or more of the following five features:

- increased waist circumference (>102cm in men and >88cm in women);
- elevated triglycerides (≥1.7mmol/L, ≥150mg/dL);
- reduced HDL-cholesterol (<1mmol/L, <40mg/dL in men and <1.3mmol/L, <50mg/dL in women);
- elevated blood pressure (≥130mmHg SBP and/or ≥85mmHg DBP or on treatment for hypertension);
- elevated glucose (≥6.1mmol/L, ≥110mg/dL), or previously recognized diabetes.

A recent, even more stringent definition, was introduced by the International Diabetes Federation [115].

- Central obesity defined by ethnic-specific waist circumference criteria (≥94cm in Europid men and ≥80cm in Europid women) and any two of the following four components:
    - elevated triglycerides (≥1.7mmol/L, ≥150mg/dL), or specific treatment for this lipid abnormality;
    - reduced HDL-cholesterol (<1mmol/L, <40mg/dL in men and <1.3mmol/L, <50mg/dL in women), or specific treatment;
    - elevated blood pressure (≥130mmHg SBP and/or ≥85mmHg DBP or on treatment for hypertension);
    - elevated glucose (≥5.6mmol/L, ≥100mg/dL), or previously recognized diabetes.

There is a strong association between multiple metabolic risk factors and insulin resistance, and the metabolic syndrome has alternatively been termed the insulin resistance syndrome. The interactions between the various components of the metabolic syndrome and insulin resistance are complex and partly determined by genetic factors. However, the increasing prevalence of the metabolic syndrome worldwide is predominantly the result of increasing rates of overweight and obesity. In the US population, who have high obesity rates, the prevalence of the metabolic syndrome, using the first of the definitions above, was stated to be >40% in the early 1990s in people aged 60 years or more [116].

Treatment of obesity

Treatment of obesity, once established, is notoriously difficult. Although there is evidence for short-term effects with medical treatment (orlistat, sibutramine) the relapse rate remains high. New potential anti-obesity drugs such as rimonabant, a selective cannabinoid receptor type 1 (CB_1 receptor) antagonist has been shown to reduce body weight consistently in obese and overweight individuals, but at the price of side effects, mainly depressed mood disorders and anxiety [117], eventually causing the drug to be withdrawn from the market. Surgical intervention has been demonstrated to be associated with sustained weight loss in patients with a BMI between 35–40kg/m^2 but is an option only in a small proportion of all overweight and obese people [118]. Curbing the effect of the current high prevalence of overweight or obesity will accordingly have to rest with prevention, particularly in children and young people.

Lipids

Lipids and risk

Lipid metabolism is complex and regulated by several processes [119]. Most of the cholesterol in blood plasma is normally carried as LDL, and, over a wide range of cholesterol concentrations, there is a strong and graded positive association in men and women between total as well as LDL-cholesterol and the risk of CVD [120]. In a recent meta-analysis of individual data from 61 prospective studies with 55,000 vascular deaths, total cholesterol was positively associated with IHD mortality in both middle and old age and at all blood pressure levels (➲ Fig. 12.21). A 25-year follow-up of the populations of the Seven Countries Study [121] showed that the relative risk associated with high as opposed to low serum cholesterol was virtually identical in men from Finland, Italy, Greece, the Netherlands, and the former Yugoslavia, with Japan, which had only very few cases, as the only exception. However, the absolute risk associated with any particular level of serum cholesterol varied markedly between different countries. Coronary artery disease is rare in populations with total cholesterol <3–4mmol/L, even in the presence of other risk factors, but even in a very-low-risk population with low cholesterol levels, such as the Chinese, an association has been found between serum cholesterol and coronary mortality [122].

By itself, hypercholesterolaemia produces no symptoms; it is only an indicator of elevated risk. Except in rare cases with inherited lipid disorders, such as familial hypercholesterolaemia, an elevated serum cholesterol can be associated

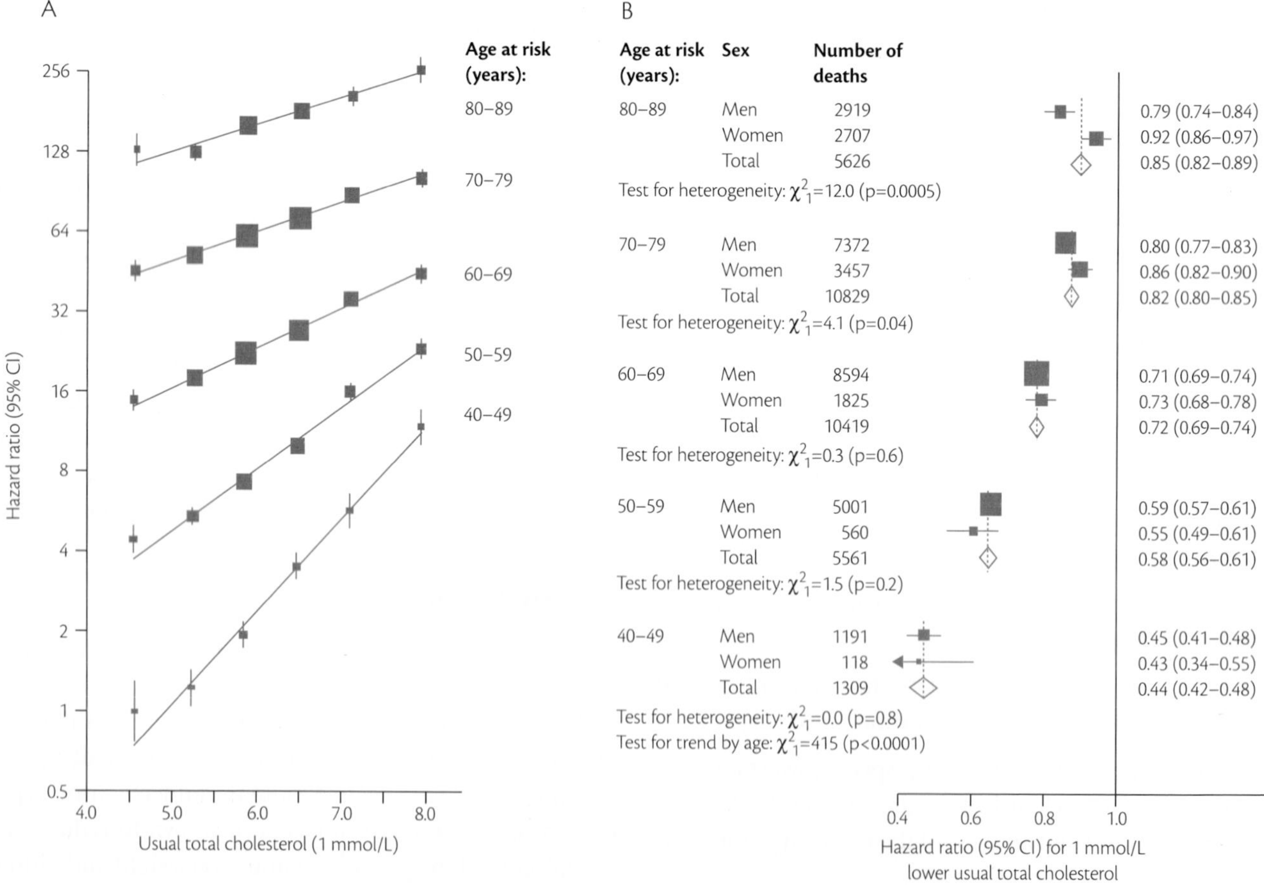

Figure 12.21 (A) IHD mortality (33,744 deaths) versus usual total cholesterol. Age-specific associations. (B) Age-specific and sex-specific hazard ratios for 1mmol/L lower usual total cholesterol. Hazard ratios on the left are plotted on a floating absolute scale of risk (so each log hazard ratio has an appropriate variance assigned to it). The slopes of the age-specific lines on the left are given on the right, subdivided by sex. Each square (left or right) has an area inversely proportional to the variance of the log of the hazard ratio that it represents. Reproduced with permission from Lewington S, Whitlock G, Clarke R, *et al.* Blood cholesterol and vascular mortality by age, sex, and blood pressure: a meta-analysis of individual data from 61 prospective studies with 55,000 vascular deaths. *Lancet* 2007; **370**: 1829–39.

with almost any risk of developing coronary disease. In an otherwise healthy non-smoking woman the risk may be next to negligible, but the risk increases with the number of other risk factors and can be up to ten times higher in a man of the same age who is also a smoker [123]. The highest absolute risk associated with high serum cholesterol is run by people who already have manifest coronary disease or who have diabetes.

In contrast to LDL-cholesterol, increased concentrations of HDL-cholesterol protect against atherosclerotic disease in populations at high risk. The cardioprotective effects of HDL-cholesterol have been attributed to reverse cholesterol transport, positive effects on endothelial cells, and to antioxidant activity [124]. Elevated serum triglycerides are associated with increased risk of CVD but the association is not as strong, nor as consistent, as it is for serum cholesterol. Low HDL levels and increased triglycerides are both components of the metabolic syndrome, and are also associated with a number of other adverse factors, for example type 2 diabetes, hypertension, low physical activity, obesity, and low consumption of fruits and vegetables. Statistically, lipid fractions in the blood are highly intercorrelated; in particular, there is an inverse correlation between serum triglycerides and HDL-cholesterol. Accordingly, an independent role for serum triglycerides has been difficult to establish. However, given the complex pathophysiology concerning lipids and atherosclerotic disease, the concept of statistical independence does little to enhance our understanding of the role of triglycerides in risk estimation. Even so, a meta-analysis of 17 population-based studies, comprising >46,000 men and >10,000 women, showed that risk of CVD in fact does increase with increasing degrees of hypertriglyceridaemia, independently of serum cholesterol [125]. The effect of serum triglycerides seems to be stronger for women than for men [120].

In recent years, apolipoproteins, such as apolipoprotein B (apoB) which is the major protein component of LDL, apolipoprotein A1, the major apoprotein of HDL, and particularly the ratio between these two apoproteins have received much attention. However, even though the apoB/apoA1 ratio promises to be a very useful and accurate tool in prediction of CHD [126], its role as a treatment goal is not yet firmly established.

Drug treatment of dyslipidaemia

Pharmacological agents that reduce serum cholesterol have long been available. However, the WHO clofibrate trial published in the early 1980s [127], which showed that patients on active treatment, although they had significantly fewer coronary events, had higher all-cause mortality, led to a therapeutic nihilism that lasted for more than a decade. In 1994, the 4S study was published [128]. This was the first large study that unequivocally demonstrated a survival advantage in coronary patients on active treatment with a statin. This study, and several more large placebo-controlled trials, have clearly demonstrated that patients with coronary disease benefit from cholesterol-lowering treatment, with an estimated 20–40% reduction in coronary events, almost regardless of initial serum cholesterol level [129]. In addition, primary prevention trials have demonstrated significant reductions in coronary events [130].

A recent prospective meta-analysis of data from 90,056 individuals in 14 randomized trials of statins found that for about one-fifth per mmol/L LDL-cholesterol reduction there were almost 50 fewer people per 1000 randomized in the trials who had major vascular events over the next 5 years among those with pre-existing CHD at baseline, compared with 25 per 1000 among participants with no such history [131]. There was no evidence that statins increased the incidence of cancer overall or at any particular site.

Data derived from several sources show a log-linear relation between LDL-cholesterol and risk of coronary disease. As the absolute reduction in LDL-cholesterol induced by cholesterol-lowering drugs will be larger with higher initial levels and, as the relation between LDL-cholesterol is curvilinear, this larger reduction will result in a proportionately greater net reduction in coronary events. In terms of reduction in absolute risk in a particular individual, the reduction will be determined as much by his or her overall coronary risk, as by the initial cholesterol level. The presence of coronary disease, diabetes, or an accumulation of other risk factors means a higher absolute risk and the same net benefit in terms of reduced coronary events can therefore be expected at lower lipid levels in patients with any of these conditions.

A recent study, the JUPITER (Justification for the Use of Statins in Prevention: an Intervention Trial Evaluating Rosuvastatin) trial, compared rosuvastatin with placebo in a group characterized by low LDL and high-sensitivity C-reactive protein levels, as a marker of inflammation[132]. Rosuvastatin was found to significantly reduce the incidence of major cardiovascular events. The implications of this trial remain uncertain, first, because only a small proportion of those screened were randomized; second, because the absolute event rate, even among those treated with placebo, was low; and third, the long-term safety of rosuvastatin has not been as clearly established as for other statins.

However, together with other evidence for the benefits of statin treatment in a broad range of patients, the JUPITER trial will probably contribute to lower the threshold for statin treatment of dyslipidaemia in healthy people.

In contrast to findings for CHD, plasma cholesterol is not associated with overall mortality from stroke [133]. However, stroke aetiology is rather more complicated than coronary heart disease, and stroke mortality is probably not an ideal proxy for overall stroke risk. Notwithstanding, treatment with a statin is still associated with a reduction in stroke risk [131].

Several Western countries have, in fact, experienced important decreases in mortality from CHD during the last decades, largely resulting from lifestyle changes. One example is Finland, which has experienced a very large decrease in CHD mortality since 1970. During the same period, intake per day of saturated fat from liquid dairy products and spreadable fat decreased from 45g to 16g in men [134]. Both in Finland and in Sweden a sizable reduction in serum cholesterol was found to explain 30–50% of the decline in coronary mortality [8, 12].

In terms of life-years saved or coronary events avoided, a population strategy makes more sense as the reduction in risk factors and attack rate will also involve those with moderately increased levels and the intervention will be targeted at more than one risk factor. Optimal serum cholesterol, as defined by the European guidelines as being a serum cholesterol <5mmol/L, is found in a minority of European middle-aged populations. If normotension, normal weight, and non-smoking are added, only a tiny fraction have truly optimal risk factor status [135]. Most cases of coronary disease occur in the large group in the population with combinations of moderately elevated levels of risk factors. From a population perspective, intervention only in persons with high cholesterol will achieve comparatively little with respect to reduction in coronary disease incidence and mortality.

When changing perspective from the population to the individual patient with high serum cholesterol, however, the aim must be to attempt to minimize risk in that individual patient. In accordance with the recommendations on prevention of coronary disease from the Joint European Societies and other national recommendations, this will mean not only treatment with a statin in an important number of patients, but also aiming for reducing overall risk. This will involve anti-smoking advice, treatment of hypertension, weight-reducing regimens, and advice on physical activity, whenever appropriate. Although the reduction in risk achieved by treatment is more or less the same regardless of initial risk, the gain in terms of absolute risk is greater the higher the risk in the individual.

Current European recommendations hold that, for healthy people, total plasma cholesterol should be <5mmol/L (<190mg/dL), and LDL-cholesterol should be <3mmol/L (<115mg/dL). Concentrations of HDL-cholesterol and triglycerides are not used as goals of therapy, but as markers of increased risk: HDL-cholesterol <1.0mmol/L (<40mg/dL) in men and <1.2mmol/L (>46mg/dL) in women; fasting triglycerides >1.7mmol/L (>150mg/dL). Both low HDL and raised triglycerides reflect abdominal obesity and low physical activity, stressing the importance of lifestyle in patients with these aberrations.

In asymptomatic subjects (➲Fig. 12.22), the first step is to assess total cardiovascular risk. If the 10-year risk of cardiovascular death is <5%, advice concerning diet, physical activity, and smoking should be given to keep the cardiovascular risk low. If the 10-year risk of cardiovascular death is ≥5%, serum LDL-cholesterol, HDL-cholesterol, and triglyceride should be analysed and intensive lifestyle advice should be given. If total and LDL-cholesterol levels <5mmol/L and <3mmol/L, respectively, are achieved, and the total CVD death risk estimate has become <5%, yearly follow-up is warranted to ensure that cardiovascular risk remains low. If total CVD risk remains elevated or progresses to ≥5%, lipid-lowering drug therapy should be considered to lower total and LDL-cholesterol.

Several trials have unequivocally demonstrated the benefits of long-term use of statins in the prevention of new ischaemic events and mortality in patients with coronary heart disease. The targets established by the Fourth Joint Task Force of the ESC and other societies in patients after infarction are: for total cholesterol: 175mg/dL (4.5mmol/L) with an option of 155mg/dL (4.0mmol/L) if feasible and for LDL-cholesterol 100mg/dL (2.5mmol/L) with an option of 80mg/dL (2.0mmol/L) if feasible. Although pharmacological treatment is highly efficient in treating dyslipidaemia, diet remains a basic requirement for all patients. Even with maximal therapy, targets will not be achieved in some patients, but they will still benefit from treatment.

The most recent controversy on lipid-lowering treatment has been focused on intensive versus standard lipid-lowering therapy. A recent meta-analysis of randomized controlled trials that compared different intensities of statin therapy identified a total of seven trials, with a total of 29,395 patients with coronary artery disease [136]. Compared with less intensive statin regimens, the more intensive regimens further reduced LDL-cholesterol levels and reduced the risk of myocardial infarction and stroke. Although there was no effect on mortality among patients with chronic coronary artery disease, all-cause mortality was reduced among

Managing total CVD risk: lipids

Treatment goals are not defined for HDL cholesterol and triglycerides, but HDL cholesterol <1.0mmol/L (~40mg/dL) for men and <1.2mmol/L (~45mg/dL) for women and fasting triglycerides of >1.7mmol/L (~150mg/dL) are markers of increased cardiovascular risk

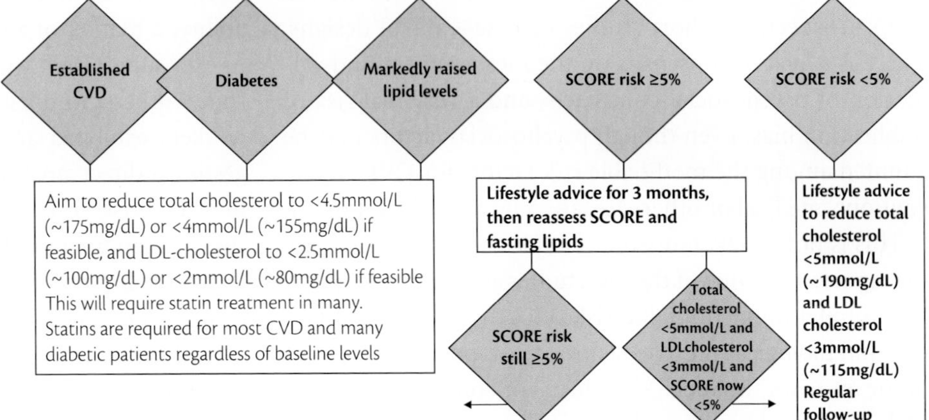

Figure 12.22 Managing total CVD risk: Lipids. Adapted with permission from Graham I, Atar D, Borch-Johnsen K, *et al.* European guidelines on cardiovascular disease prevention in clinical practice: full text. Fourth Joint Task Force of the European Society of Cardiology and other societies on cardiovascular disease prevention in clinical practice (constituted by representatives of nine societies and by invited experts). *Eur J Cardiovasc Prev Rehabil* 2007; **14**(Suppl.2): S1–S113.

patients with acute coronary syndromes treated with more intensive statin regimens. About half of the patients treated with more intensive statin therapy did not achieve an LDL-cholesterol level of <80mg/dL (2.0mmol/L), and none of the trials tested combination therapies. The analysis supports the use of more intensive statin regimens in patients with established coronary artery disease, but no strong evidence was found to advocate treating to particular LDL targets, using combination lipid-lowering therapy to achieve these targets. Still, there is, additionally, no lower threshold beyond which LDL reduction has been shown to have no effect. There is also evidence to suggest that a number of patients are not adequately treated, and existing targets may serve to emphasize the importance of using statins in sufficient dosages.

In acute coronary syndromes, treatment with statins should be initiated while patients are still in hospital. An additional reason for this is to ensure patient adherence. In patients with AMI, plasma lipids should be evaluated at 4–6 weeks after initiation of therapy, and after 3 months. The second control after 3 months is important, because the acute phase reaction associated with AMI can lead to lowered serum cholesterol concentrations over the first 2 to 3 months, particularly in large infarctions.

In patients who do not tolerate statins, or who have contraindications, other lipid-lowering therapy may be warranted. In a study with gemfibrozil (a fibrate) [137] patients with HDL-cholesterol levels ≤40mg/dL (1.04mmol/L) but LDL-cholesterol levels ≤140mg/dL (3.6mmol/L) and triglycerides ≤300mg/dL (7.7mmol/L) and with a previous infarction benefited from gemfibrozil with a 24% reduction in the combined endpoint of death from coronary artery disease, non-fatal infarction, and stroke. In the Bezafibrate Infarction Prevention (BIP study) [138], bezafibrate given to patients with a previous infarction or stable angina and with low (≤45mg/dL (1.2mmol/L) HDL-cholesterol levels) was associated with a non-significant 7.3% reduction in the incidence of fatal or non-fatal (re)infarction or sudden death. A larger benefit was seen for this endpoint in patients with high triglycerides at baseline. Ezetimibe, a compound which reduces cholesterol uptake from the intestine, decreases LDL-cholesterol (and C-reactive protein) but there are no clinical data to support its current use.

Psychosocial factors

During the last two decades, considerable evidence has accumulated with respect to the association of markers of stress and other psychosocial factors with coronary disease [139–141]. However, compared to other major risk factors, psychosocial variables are more difficult to define objectively because several different dimensions are involved. Despite this, several separate constructs within the broad conceptual framework of psychosocial factors are increasingly considered as being causally related to CHD. Stress at work and in family life, life events, low perceived control, lack of social support, socioeconomic status, and depression are some of the dimensions that have been shown to either influence the risk of CHD or affect prognosis in CHD patients.

In the world of evidence-based medicine, psychosocial factors hold a precarious position. With few exceptions, there are overall not many meta-analyses, systematic reviews, and randomized controlled trials of interventions. Most data are purely descriptive and observational, derived from prospective cohort studies or case–control designs. There is a lack of consensus on the measurement and validation of psychosocial constructs, and a very real risk of publication bias. Even though psychosocial factors may be counted among the modifiable risk factors for CVD, interventions, medical or otherwise, are only rarely investigated.

This is not to say, however, that psychosocial factors are unimportant. In one of the few studies attempting to quantify population attributable risk of both psychosocial factors and biological/lifestyle factors, a composite of stress (at home, at work, financial) low locus of control, life events, and depression was found to have a population attributable risk of 32%, comparable to the effect of smoking [142]. Even so, the importance of psychosocial factors is still controversial and it has been argued, based on prospective data, that factors such as vital exhaustion, psychological stress, and social class add little to the overall prediction of CHD [143].

There are several methodological problems in the study of psychosocial factors and health outcomes. First, compared to other biological and lifestyle risk factors, psychosocial factors represent a more problematic construct in that there is little uniformity with respect to either definition or measurement of these factors. Second, most of the dimensions involved are subjective, and hence potentially open to biases and confounding. Third, even though some persons may be more vulnerable than others with respect to adverse circumstances, exposure probably varies considerably over a lifetime, and hence, prospective follow-up studies with extended follow-up may not adequately capture short-term influences.

According to popular opinion, stress is one of the most important risk factors for CHD but this view has not so far been altogether accepted by the medical profession. However, accumulating evidence does, in fact, demonstrate that it is likely that stress is causally related to CHD, and possibly even to stroke. To date, most studies have dealt with stress at work, with stress outside the workplace receiving less attention. Both cross-sectional and prospective studies have demonstrated a positive association between level of work stress and disease [142, 144–148]. Even so, not all studies have found an association between indices of job stress and CVD [149], arguing that associations between stress and coronary disease are mainly the result of confounding by low socioeconomic status [149] or that associations may be spurious, because people with stress tend to report more symptoms [150].

Shift work has been described as increasing future risk of CHD, both in women and men. Decreased heart-rate variability, a marker of autonomic imbalance, has been related to exposure to shift work [151]. In the Helsinki Heart Study shift workers, who had a 50% excess risk of CHD over day workers, exhibited large increases in perceived job stress, suggesting a direct stress-related mechanism explaining part of the CHD risk [152]. In addition to perceived stress at work, stressful conditions in family life have been shown to increase CHD risk. In women in Stockholm, marital discord was found to worsen prognosis in acute coronary syndrome and reduce event-free survival over and above the effects of standard clinical prognostic factors [153]. Although most of the women were employed outside the home, the hazards of marital stress were stronger than those of stress at work in these women.

Clinical depression, depressive symptoms, and other negative emotions have been associated with an increased risk of CHD incidence in both men and women [154]. In established CHD, clinical depression is associated with an increased risk for recurrent major cardiac events [155], particularly if there was also a lack of social support [156].

Men and women with low socioeconomic status have an increased risk of coronary disease. There is a large body of literature concerning socio-economic status and coronary heart disease. A much-cited review published in 1993 [157] indicated that there is a substantial body of evidence for a consistent relation between socio-economic status and the incidence and prevalence of CVD, secular trends in cardiovascular mortality, survival with CVD, and the prevalence of cardiovascular risk factors. By and large, more recent findings have not challenged these conclusions, at least not for Western populations.

There are several ways of measuring socio-economic status, with education, income, and occupational position most often used, but there is an increasing awareness that these variables cannot be used interchangeably [158]. Because there are differences in the distribution of risk factors, there has been a debate whether the effect of socio-economic status merely reflects these differences, or whether there is an independent effect [159, 160]. In addition, a relation between low socio-economic status and occupation has not been consistently observed in all populations. In one study in Europe a north–south gradient was observed with CHD mortality strongly related to occupational class in England and Wales, Ireland, Finland, Sweden, Norway, and Denmark, but not in France, Switzerland, and

Mediterranean countries [161]. Ignoring socio-economic status in risk factor estimation has been suggested to underestimate CVD risk in deprived people [162].

The mechanism by which psychosocial factors increase the risk of CVD is complex. In experimental studies, worsened coronary atherosclerosis [163] and endothelial dysfunction [164] occur in response to social disruption. Several studies have demonstrated links between psychosocial variables and vascular function [165, 166], inflammation [167], increased blood clotting, and decreased fibrinolysis [168]. The exact pathophysiological nature of the influence of psychosocial factors remains to be determined, as does the temporal sequence of events.

Taken together, these studies suggest a role for psychosocial factors as causes and prognostic factors in CVD. However, there is, so far, no or little evidence that any interventions targeting these factors improves prognosis in patients with CVD. Stress management training, with the aim to reduce stress and other psychological interventions can form part of cardiac rehabilitation programmes. A recent Cochrane review aimed to determine the effectiveness of psychological interventions, in particular stress management interventions, on mortality and morbidity, psychological measures, quality of life, and modifiable cardiac risk factors, in patients with coronary heart disease [169]. Small reductions in anxiety and depression in patients were found. The authors considered that the poor quality of trials, heterogeneity observed between trials, and significant publication bias made the pooled finding of a reduction in non-fatal myocardial infarction uncertain. Findings from studies including psychological treatment, usually as a component of comprehensive cardiac rehabilitation and with highly heterogeneous designs have not been conclusive [170–172]. Even though depression has been shown to be a negative prognostic factor in patients with CHD, it is at present not proven that treatment of depression helps improve survival [173, 174].

Gender aspects in prevention

Smoking may be a stronger risk factor for AMI in middle-aged women than in men, but relative risks associated with serum total cholesterol and blood pressure are similar [123]. However, serum triglycerides, which are strongly related to obesity, have been demonstrated to be a better predictor of future coronary events in women, compared to men [120].

The INTERHEART case–control study demonstrated similar odds ratios for AMI in women and men for several risk factors, including abnormal lipids, current smoking, abdominal obesity, high-risk diet, and psychosocial stress factors, but the increased risk associated with hypertension, diabetes, and low physical activity seemed to be greater in women than in men [175]. The population attributable risk of all nine risk factors exceeded 94%, and was similar among women and men. Men were significantly more likely to suffer a myocardial infarction prior to 60 years of age than were women; however, after adjusting for levels of risk factors, the sex difference in the probability of myocardial infarction cases occurring before the age of 60 years was reduced by more than 80%, implying that the difference in age is largely explained by the higher risk factor levels at younger ages in men compared to women.

Because smoking is more prevalent among men than in women in most nations of the world, more cases of AMI are attributable to this factor among men, compared to women, whereas hypertension and diabetes cause proportionately more AMIs among women than among men.

In primary prevention, the higher absolute risk among men in a 10-year perspective should be taken into account, for example when pharmacological treatment of hypertension or hypercholesterolaemia is being considered. In a lifetime perspective, however, the absolute risk among women is not much different from that among men. Hence, lifestyle modifications with respect to anti-smoking advice, diet, physical activity, and avoidance of obesity should be the same, irrespective of gender. Women with manifest CVD or diabetes lose all female protection, and have essentially the same risks as men with the same conditions. Accordingly, in secondary prevention, treatment should be the same for men and women.

Conclusion

CVD is preventable. As many as nine out of ten fatal CHD attacks in younger people need probably never occur. The large variations over time and over location bear witness to this. The marked decline in CHD mortality in several European countries is the result of better treatment in the acute phase, but also more importantly of lifestyle changes in the population and better identification and treatment of risk factors. However, despite the expanding knowledge in this area, many men and women still die prematurely from CHD and stroke.

Personal perspective

What does the physician dealing with cardiovascular disorders need to know about prevention? First, he or she needs to have an understanding that these diseases, by and large, are produced by societal factors, and that they are preventable. Second, within each society, cardiovascular risk can be influenced by individual behaviour. Tobacco smoking, inactivity, the consumption of food rich in calories, sugar and the wrong kind of fats, and the resulting development of hypertension, dyslipidaemia, and abdominal obesity are all amenable to change. Genetic disposition plays a part in determining our response to environmental factors. Third, patients at increased risk can be identified by detecting and assessing risk factors: either as total risk as a result of multiple risk factors, the presence of clinically manifest CVD or diabetes mellitus, or as marked raised levels of single risk factors (dyslipidaemia, hypertension, smoking).

Modification of risk should be tailored to the needs of the individual patient. Treatment includes lifestyle management and the use of pharmacotherapy, when needed. The main targets of risk modification are a cessation of smoking, an active lifestyle with 30–60min daily of physical activity on at least a moderate level, healthy food choices, and reducing excess weight, which, in turn, help preserve normal levels of blood pressure and lipids. The cardiologist has a decisive initial role in motivating the patient to commit to a healthy lifestyle once significantly raised risk and/or the presence of CVD has been confirmed. Yet, special attention should be paid to a lasting maintenance of risk reduction, for which long-term follow-up in cooperation with the family doctor is mandatory.

The burden of disease is now shifting towards low- and middle-income countries, in Europe and elsewhere. Some European countries have had an exceptional decline in CHD death rates, with some former high-risk countries now with CHD rates approaching those of some Mediterranean countries. However, these favourable trends may now be turning, with rates in younger people shown to be levelling out. The worldwide epidemic of obesity is rampant, in Europe as elsewhere, but the prevalence is still much lower in many European countries than in the US. To curb the rise in obesity is one of the next great challenges. Atherosclerotic changes start early in life, symptoms occur decades later. Control of major risk factors in the young and middle aged will substantially reduce CHD and CVD in middle age and later. If caloric excess and sedentary behaviours continue we will be facing increasing obesity rates, and more premature CHD, stroke, and diabetes throughout Europe. Increasing CVD rates may, however, not yet be apparent in the next decade, because rates of heart disease and stroke are low among the young. It is likely that the medical profession will be better at identifying and treating risk factors in the middle-aged and older, because of the dissemination of knowledge and availability of effective treatments. This will substantially reduce risk in those who are treated, but to what extent better treatment will reduce population CVD rates is not known. In order to substantially improve CVD rates in the future, behaviours in young people need to be targeted, not through medical interventions, but through attitudes, knowledge, policies, and legislation.

Further reading

Graham I, Atar D, Borch-Johnsen K, *et al.* European guidelines on cardiovascular disease prevention in clinical practice: full text. Fourth Joint Task Force of the European Society of Cardiology and other societies on cardiovascular disease prevention in clinical practice (constituted by representatives of nine societies and by invited experts). *Eur J Cardiovasc Prev Rehabil* 2007; **14**(Suppl.2): S1–113.

Hu FB, Willett WC. Optimal diets for prevention of coronary heart disease. *JAMA* 2002; **288**: 2569–78.

Kuper H, Marmot M, Hemingway H. Systematic review of prospective cohort studies of psychosocial factors in the etiology and prognosis of coronary heart disease. *Semin Vasc Med* 2002; **2**: 267–314.

Lewington S, Clarke R, Qizilbash N, *et al.* Age-specific relevance of usual blood pressure to vascular mortality: a meta-analysis of individual data for one million adults in 61 prospective studies. *Lancet* 2002; **360**: 1903–13.

Lewington S, Whitlock G, Clarke R, *et al.* Blood cholesterol and vascular mortality by age, sex, and blood pressure: a meta-analysis of individual data from 61 prospective studies with 55,000 vascular deaths. *Lancet* 2007; **370**: 1829–39.

Unal B, Critchley JA, Capewell S. Explaining the decline in coronary heart disease mortality in England and Wales between 1981 and 2000. *Circulation* 2004; **109**: 1101–7.

Yusuf S, Hawken S, Ôunpuu S, *et al.* Effect of potentially modifiable risk factors associated with myocardial infarction in 52 countries (the INTERHEART study): case-control study. *Lancet* 2004; **364**: 937–52.

Yusuf S, Reddy S, Ôunpuu S, *et al.* Global burden of cardiovascular diseases: part I: general considerations, the epidemiologic transition, risk factors, and impact of urbanization. *Circulation* 2001; **104**: 2746–53.

Online resources

- HeartScore®, an interactive computer-based tool for total risk estimation available from the ESC: http://www.heartscore.org
- Maps of US obesity trends (1985–2007) from the US Centers for Disease Control and Prevention: http://www.cdc.gov/nccdphp/dnpa/obesity/trend/maps/

For full references and multimedia materials please visit the online version of the book (http://esctextbook.oxfordonline.com).

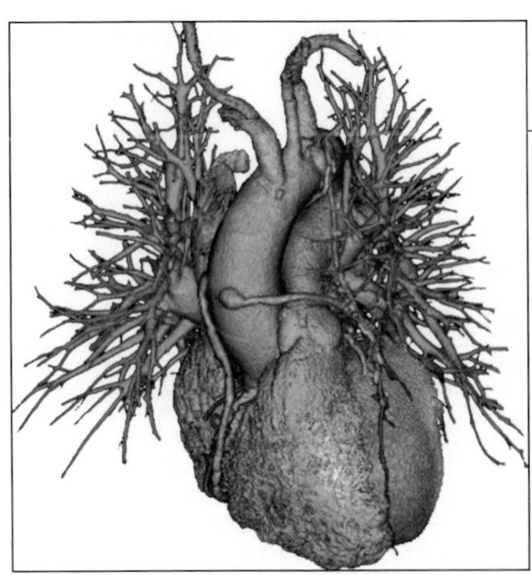

CHAPTER 13

Hypertension

Sverre E. Kjeldsen, Tonje A. Aksnes, Robert H. Fagard, and Giuseppe Mancia

Contents

Summary

Hypertension, usually defined as persistent blood pressure at 140/90mmHg or higher, affects about a quarter of the adult population in many countries and particularly in Western societies. Hypertension is a risk factor for most, if not all, cardiovascular diseases and renal failure. While blood pressure should be measured repeatedly for the diagnosis, new techniques such as 24-hour ambulatory blood pressure and self-measured, home blood pressure taking are increasingly being used for diagnosis and assessment during treatment. Modern work-up of hypertensive patients focuses on the detection of target organ damage, i.e. left ventricular hypertrophy and renal effects including microalbuminuria.

While diagnosis of secondary causes of hypertension should be kept in mind, the detection of concomitant diseases or risk factors should be clearly identified for the purpose of assessing total cardiovascular risk and choosing the optimal treatment. While lifestyle changes may be appropriate, i.e. increase physical exercise, reduce body weight if needed, and eat healthily, these kinds of interventions should not unnecessarily delay initiation of drug treatment for hypertension when clearly indicated. Drug treatment has repeatedly proven effective in outcome studies in preventing stroke, heart failure, deteriorated renal function, new-onset diabetes and, to some extent, coronary heart disease and other complications. Modern drug treatment of hypertension usually contains a combination of well-tolerated doses of two or more drugs aiming at blood pressure below 140/90mmHg and below 130/80mmHg in patients with diabetes and already established cardiovascular disease. Acetylsalicylic acid and statins are recommended as add-on treatment if total 10-year cardiovascular risk is above 20%.

Introduction

This chapter is based on the 2003 and 2007 *Guidelines for the Management of Arterial Hypertension* jointly issued by the European Society of Hypertension (ESH) and the European Society of Cardiology (ESC) [1, 2]. For in-depth reading of the pathophysiology and aetiology of essential hypertension, the most common form of hypertension, extensive reviews have been published [3–5].

Definition and classification of hypertension

Systolic, diastolic, and pulse pressures as predictors

Both systolic and diastolic blood pressures show a continuous graded independent relationship with risk of stroke and coronary events [6]. The relationship between systolic blood pressure and relative risk of stroke is steeper than that for coronary events, reflecting a closer aetiological relationship with stroke, but the attributable risk—excess deaths due to raised blood pressure—is greater for coronary events than stroke. However, with population ageing the relative incidence of stroke is increasing, as shown in randomized controlled trials [7].

The apparently simple direct relationship between increasing systolic and diastolic blood pressure levels and increasing cardiovascular risk is complicated by the relationship that normally prevails between blood pressure and age, namely systolic blood pressure rises throughout the adult age range, whereas diastolic blood pressure peaks at about age 60 years in men and 70 years in women, and falls gradually thereafter [8]. Although both the continuous rise in systolic blood pressure and the rise and fall in diastolic blood pressure with age are usual, they represent the results of some of the pathological processes that underlie 'hypertension' and cardiovascular diseases [9].

These observations help to explain why, at least in elderly populations, a wide pulse pressure (systolic blood pressure minus diastolic blood pressure) has been shown in some observational studies to be a better predictor of adverse cardiovascular outcomes than either systolic or diastolic pressures individually [10, 11]. However, in the largest compilation of observational data in almost 1 million patients from 61 studies [12], both systolic and diastolic blood pressures were independently predictive of stroke and coronary mortality, and more so than pulse pressure.

Table 13.1 Definitions and classification of blood pressure levels (mmHg)

Category	Systolic		Diastolic
Optimal	<120	and	<80
Normal	120–129	and/or	80–84
High normal	130–139	and/or	85–89
Grade 1 hypertension	140–159	and/or	90–99
Grade 2 hypertension	160–179	and/or	100–109
Grade 3 hypertension	≥180	and/or	≥110
Isolated systolic hypertension	≥140	and	<90

Isolated systolic hypertension should be graded (1, 2, 3) according to systolic blood pressure values in the ranges indicated, provided that diastolic values are <90mmHg.

In practice, given that there are randomized controlled trial data supporting the treatment of isolated systolic hypertension [13, 14] and treatment based purely on diastolic entry criteria [15], one should continue to use both systolic and diastolic blood pressures as part of guidance for treatment thresholds.

Classification of hypertension

The continuous relationship between the level of blood pressure and cardiovascular risk makes any numerical definition and classification of hypertension arbitrary.

The real threshold of hypertension should therefore be considered to be mobile, being higher or lower on the basis of the total cardiovascular risk of each individual. Accordingly, the definition of high normal blood pressure in ➲Table 13.1 includes blood pressure values that may be considered as 'high' (i.e. hypertension) in high-risk subjects or fully normal in low-risk individuals.

Total cardiovascular risk

Because of the clustering of risk factors in individuals and the graded nature of the association between each risk factor and cardiovascular risk [16] (➲Chapter 12), a contemporary approach is to determine the threshold for therapeutic intervention at least for cholesterol and blood pressure lowering, on the basis of estimated global coronary or cardiovascular (coronary plus stroke) [17] risk over a defined relatively short-term (e.g. 5- or 10-year) period. It should be noted that although several methods may be used, most risk estimation systems are based on the Framingham study [18]. Although this database has been shown to be reasonably applicable to some European populations [19], estimates require recalibration in other populations [20] owing to important differences in the prevailing incidence of coronary and stroke events. The main disadvantage associated with intervention threshold based on relatively short-term absolute risk is

Table 13.2 Stratification of cardiovascular risk

	Blood pressure (mmHg)				
Other risk factors, OD, or disease	**Normal** SBP 120–129 or DBP 80–84	**High normal** SBP 130–139 or DBP 85–89	**Grade 1 HT** SBP 140–159 or DBP 90–99	**Grade 2 HT** SBP 160–179 or DBP 100–109	**Grade 3 HT** SBP ≥180 or DBP ≥110
No other risk factors	Average risk	Average risk	Low added risk	Moderate added risk	High added risk
1–2 risk factors	Low added risk	Low added risk	Moderate added risk	Moderate added risk	Very high added risk
3 or more risk factors, MS, OD, or diabetes	Moderate added risk	High added risk	High added risk	High added risk	Very high added risk
Established CV or renal disease	Very high added risk	Very high added risk	Very high added risk	Very high added risk	Very high added risk

SBP: systolic blood pressure; DBP: diastolic blood pressure; CV: cardiovascular; HT: hypertension; MS: metabolic syndrome; OD: subclinical organ damage; Low, moderate, high, very high risk refer to 10-year risk of a CV fatal or non-fatal event. The term 'added' indicates that in all categories risk is greater than average.

that younger adults (particularly women), despite having more than one major risk factor, are unlikely to reach treatment thresholds despite being at high risk relative to their peers. By contrast, most elderly men (e.g. >70 years) will often reach treatment thresholds although being at very little increased risk relative to their peers. This situation results in most resources being concentrated on the oldest subjects, whose potential lifespan, despite intervention, is relatively limited, and young subjects at high relative risk remain untreated despite, in the absence of intervention, a predicted significant shortening of their otherwise much longer potential lifespan [21, 22].

On the basis of these considerations, total cardiovascular risk classification may be stratified as suggested in ➲Table 13.2. The terms *low*, *moderate*, *high*, and *very high added risk* are calibrated to indicate, approximately, an absolute 10-year risk of cardiovascular disease of <15%, 15–20%, 20–30% and >30%, respectively, according to Framingham criteria [17] or an approximate absolute risk of fatal cardiovascular disease <4%, 4–5%, 5–8%, and >8% according to the SCORE chart [23] (➲Chapter 12). The term'added' indicates that in all categories risk is greater than average.

➲Table 13.3 indicates the most common risk factors, subclinical organ damage, diabetes mellitus, and established cardiovascular and renal diseases to be used to stratify risk and prognosis.

- Obesity is indicated as 'abdominal obesity' in order to give specific attention to an important sign of the metabolic syndrome [24].
- Diabetes is listed as a separate criterion in order to underline its importance as risk, at least twice as large as in absence of diabetes [25] (➲Chapter 14).
- Microalbuminuria is indicated as a sign of organ damage, but proteinuria as a sign of established renal disease (➲Chapter 15).
- Slight elevation of serum creatinine as sign of subclinical organ damage is indicated as a serum creatinine concentration of 115–133μmol/L (1.3–1.5mg/dL) in men and 107–124μmol/L (1.2–1.4mg/dL) in women, and concentrations >133μmol/L (>1.5mg/dL) in men and >124μmol/L (>1.4mg/dL) in women as renal disease [26, 27].

Diagnostic evaluation

In hypertension, diagnostic procedures are aimed at:

- establishing the blood pressure levels;
- excluding or identifying secondary causes of hypertension;
- evaluating the overall cardiovascular risk of the subject by searching for other risk factors, subclinical organ damage and concomitant diseases or accompanying clinical conditions.

The diagnostic procedures consist of:

- repeated blood pressure measurements;
- medical history;
- physical examination;
- laboratory and instrumental investigations: some of which should be considered essential in all subjects with high blood pressure; some are recommended and may be used extensively; some are useful only when suggested by some of the more widely recommended examinations or the clinical course of the patient.

Blood pressure measurement

Blood pressure is characterized by large spontaneous variations both within 24 hours and between days. The diagnosis of hypertension should thus be based on multiple blood

Table 13.3 Factors influencing prognosis

Risk factors	Subclinical organ damage	Diabetes mellitus	Established cardiovascular or renal disease
◆ Systolic and diastolic BP levels ◆ Levels of pulse pressure (in the elderly) ◆ Age (men >55 years; women >65 years) ◆ Smoking ◆ Dyslipidaemia ◆ TC >5.0mmol/L (190mg/dL) or LDL-C >3.0 mmol/L (115mg/dL) or HDL-C: men <1.0mmol/L (40mg/dL) women <1.2mmol/L (46mg/dL) or TG >1.7mmol/L (150mg/dL) ◆ Fasting plasma glucose 5.6–6.9mmol/L (102–125 mg/dL) ◆ Abnormal glucose tolerance test ◆ Abdominal obesity (waist circumference: men >102cm; women >88cm) ◆ Family history of premature CV disease (men at age <55 years; women at age <65 years)	◆ Electrocardiographic LVH (Sokolow–Lyon >38mm; Cornell >2440mm × ms) or echocardiographic LVH (LVMI: men ≥125g/m^2; women ≥110 g/m^2) ◆ Carotid wall thickening (IMT >0.9 mm) or plaque ◆ Carotid-femoral pulse wave velocity >12m/s ◆ Slight increase in plasma creatinine: men 115–133μmol/L (1.3–1.5mg/dL); women 107–124μmol/L (1.2–1.4mg/dL) ◆ Low estimated glomerular filtration rate (<60mL/min/1.73m^2) or creatinine clearance (<60mL/min) ◆ Ankle–brachial BP index <0.9 ◆ Microalbuminuria 30–300mg/24 hours or albumin–creatinine ratio: men ≥22mg/g creatinine; women ≥31mg/g creatinine	◆ Fasting plasma glucose ≥7.0mmol/L (126 mg/dL) on repeated measurement ◆ Postload plasma glucose >11.0mmol/L (198mg/dL)	◆ Cerebrovascular disease: ischaemic stroke, cerebral haemorrhage, transient ischaemic attack ◆ Heart disease: myocardial infarction, angina pectoris, coronary revascularization, heart failure ◆ Renal disease: diabetic nephropathy, renal impairment (serum creatinine men >133; women >124mmol/L), proteinuria (>300mg/24 hours) ◆ Peripheral artery disease ◆ Advanced retinopathy: haemorrhages or exudates, papilloedema

TC, total cholesterol; LDL-C, low-density lipoprotein cholesterol; HDL-C, high-density lipoprotein cholesterol; IMT, intima media thickness; LVH, left ventricular hypertrophy; LVMI, left ventricular mass index.

pressure measurements, taken on separate occasions. The correct method for measurement of blood pressure is summarized in ➲Table 13.4. If blood pressure is only slightly elevated, repeated measurements should be obtained over a period of several months to define as accurately as possible the patient's 'usual' blood pressure. If, on the other hand, the patient has a more marked blood pressure elevation, evidence of hypertension-related organ damage, or a high or very high cardiovascular risk profile, repeated measurements should be obtained over shorter periods of time, i.e. weeks or days. Blood pressures can be measured by the doctor or the nurse in the office or in the clinic (office or clinic blood pressure), by the patient at home, or automatically over 24 hours. These procedures are summarized in the following sections [28].

Office or clinic blood pressure measurement

Blood pressure can be measured by a mercury sphygmomanometer, whose various parts (rubber tubes, valves, quantity of mercury, etc.) should be kept in proper condition. Other non-invasive devices (aneroid and auscultatory or oscillometric semi-automatic devices) can also be used and will indeed become increasingly important because of the progressive banning of medical use of mercury. These devices, however, should be validated according to standardized protocols (http://www.dableducational.org) [29] and their accuracy should be periodically checked by comparison with mercury sphygmomanometric values.

Table 13.4 Assessment of blood pressure using the correct method for diagnosis [1, 2]

When measuring blood pressure, care should be taken to:
◆ Allow the patients to sit for several minutes in a quiet room before beginning blood pressure measurements
◆ Take at least two measurements spaced by 1–2min, and additional measurements if the first two are quite different
◆ Use a standard bladder (12–13cm long and 35cm wide) but have a larger and a smaller bladder available for fat and thin arms, respectively. Use the smaller bladder in children
◆ Have the cuff at the heart level, whatever the position of the patient
◆ Use phase I and V (disappearance) Korotkoff sounds to identify systolic and diastolic blood pressure, respectively
◆ Measure blood pressure in both arms at first visit to detect possible differences due to peripheral vascular disease. In this instance, take the higher value as the reference one
◆ Measure blood pressure 1 and 5min after assumption of the standing position in elderly subjects, diabetic patients, and in other conditions in which postural hypotension may be frequent or suspected
◆ Measure heart rate by pulse palpation (at least 30s) after the second measurement in the sitting position

Ambulatory blood pressure measurement

Several devices (mostly oscillometric) are available for automatic blood pressure measurements in patients who are allowed to conduct a near-normal life. This allows information to be obtained on 24-hour average blood pressure, as well as on average blood pressure values on more restricted portions of the 24 hours, such as the day, the night, and the morning (➲Fig. 13.1) [28]. This information should not be regarded as a substitute for information derived from conventional blood pressure measurements. It may be considered, however, of additional clinical value because cross-sectional and longitudinal studies have shown that office blood pressure has a limited relationship with 24-hour, and thus daily life, blood pressure [30]. These studies have also shown that ambulatory blood pressure:

- correlates with the subclinical organ damage of hypertension more closely than office blood pressure [31–34];
- predicts, both in populations and in hypertensive patients, the cardiovascular risk more and above the prediction provided by office blood pressure values [35–38];
- improves, when added to clinic blood pressure measurements, the accuracy of the prediction of the patients' risk; and
- measures more accurately than office blood pressure the extent of blood pressure reduction induced by treatment, because of the absence of a 'white coat' [39], a placebo [40] effect, and a higher reproducibility over time [41].

Although some of these advantages can be obtained by increasing the number of office blood pressure measurements [42], 24-hour ambulatory blood pressure monitoring before and during treatment can be recommended at the time of diagnosis and, occasionally, during treatment, whenever the facilities make it possible.

When measuring 24-hour blood pressure [28] care should be taken to:

- Use only devices validated by international standardized protocols.
- Use cuffs of appropriate size and compare the initial values with those from a sphygmomanometer to check that the differences are not > ±5mmHg.
- Set the automatic readings at no more than 30-min intervals to obtain an adequate number of values and have most hours represented if some readings are rejected because of artefacts.
- Instruct the patients to engage in normal activities but to refrain from strenuous exercise, and to keep the arm extended and still at the time of cuff inflations.
- Ask the patient to provide information in a diary on unusual events, and on duration and quality of night sleep; although in the population and the hypertensive patients at large, day and night blood pressures normally show a close correlation, there is evidence that subjects in whom nocturnal hypotension is blunted and thus exhibit a relatively high night blood pressure may have an unfavourable prognosis [43].
- Obtain another ambulatory blood pressure monitoring if the first examination has <70% of the expected values because of a high number of artefacts.
- Remember that ambulatory blood pressure is usually several mmHg lower than office blood pressure [44–46].

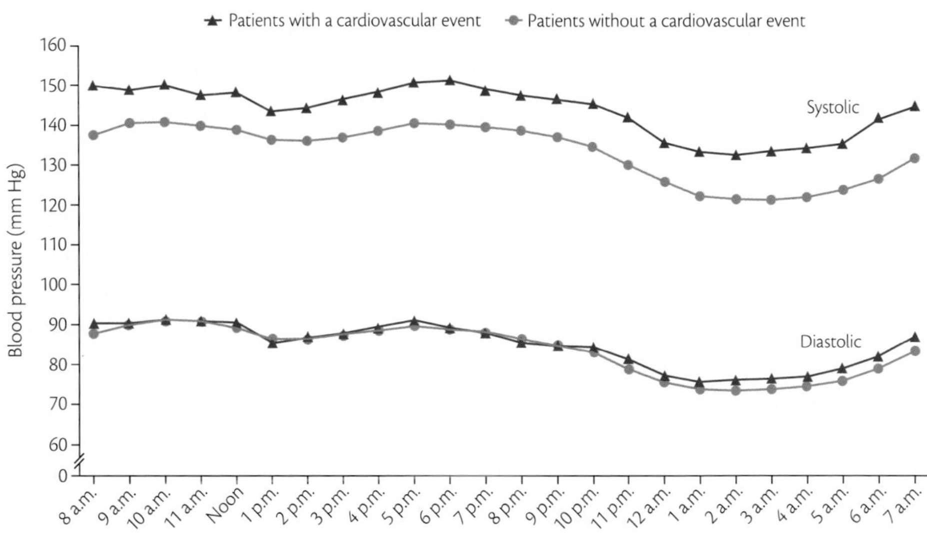

Figure 13.1 Graph shows 24-hour ambulatory blood pressure in two patients with hypertension in order to illustrate that a patient who has suffered a cardiovascular event typically has higher systolic blood pressure indicating more severe hypertension than a patient without a cardiovascular event.

Table 13.5 Blood pressure thresholds (mmHg) for definition of hypertension with different types of measurement

	Systolic blood pressure	Diastolic blood pressure
Office or clinic	140	90
24-hour	125–130	80
Day	130–135	85
Night	120	70
Home	130–135	85

As shown in ➲Table 13.5, in the population office values of 140/90mmHg correspond to about 125–130/80mmHg 24-hour systolic and diastolic blood pressure average values, and to about 130–135/85mmHg daytime average values. These values may be approximately taken as the threshold values for diagnosing hypertension by ambulatory blood pressure.

- Base clinical judgement on average 24-hour, day or night values only; other information derivable from ambulatory blood pressure (e.g. blood pressure standard deviations, trough–peak ratio, smoothness index) is clinically promising but is still in the research phase.

Home blood pressure

Self-measurements of blood pressure at home cannot provide the extensive information on 24-hour blood pressure values provided by ambulatory blood pressure monitoring. It can provide, however, values on different days in a setting close to daily life conditions. When averaged over a period of a few days these values have been shown to share some of the important advantages of ambulatory blood pressure, i.e. to have no white coat effect and to be more reproducible and predictive of the presence and progression of organ damage than office values [31, 47]. Evidence is also available that home blood pressure may predict the cardiovascular risk better than clinic blood pressure. Home blood pressure measurements for suitable periods (e.g. a few weeks) before and during treatment can therefore be recommended also because this relatively cheap procedure may improve the patient's adherence to treatment regimens [48].

When advising self-measurement of blood pressure at home, care [28] should be taken to:

- Advise only use of validated devices; few of the currently available wrist devices for measurement of blood pressure are satisfactorily validated—should any of these wrist devices be used, the subject should receive recommendation to keep the arm at heart level during measurement.
- Use semi-automatic devices rather than mercury sphygmomanometer to avoid the difficulty posed by patient's instruction and the error originated from hearing problems in elderly individuals.
- Instruct the patient to perform measurement in the sitting position after several minutes' rest—inform them that values may differ between measurements because of spontaneous blood pressure variability.
- Avoid asking for an excessive number of values to be measured and ensure that measurements include the period prior to drug intake to have information on duration of the treatment effect.
- Remember that, as for ambulatory blood pressure, normality values are lower for home than office blood pressure—take 130–135/85mmHg as the values of home blood pressure corresponding to 140/90mmHg measured in the office or clinic (➲Table 13.5).
- Give the patient clear instructions on the need to provide the doctor with proper documentation of the measured values and to avoid self-alterations of the treatment regimens.

Isolated office or white coat hypertension

In some patients, office blood pressure is persistently elevated, whereas daytime or 24-hour blood pressure falls within their normality range. This condition is widely known as *white coat hypertension* [49], although the more descriptive and less mechanistic term *isolated office (or clinic) hypertension* is preferable because the office ambulatory blood pressure difference shows only a limited correlation with the office blood pressure elevation induced by the alerting response to the doctor or the nurse, i.e. the true *white coat effect* [50]. Regardless of the terminology, evidence is now available that isolated office hypertension is not infrequent (about 15% in the general population) [51] and that it accounts for a noticeable fraction of individuals in whom hypertension is diagnosed. There is also evidence that in individuals with isolated office hypertension, cardiovascular risk is less than in individuals with both office and ambulatory blood pressure elevations [51, 52]. In a meta-analysis of outcome studies [52] the risk for cardiovascular events was on average 12% higher in white coat hypertension than in true normotension, the 95% confidence limits being compatible with a 50% higher to a 16% lower risk in white coat hypertension. Therefore more studies are needed to clarify whether or not white coat hypertension carries a greater risk than true normotension. In addition, several, although not all, studies, have reported this condition to be associated with a prevalence of organ damage and metabolic abnormalities greater than those of normal subjects, which suggests that it may not be an entirely innocent phenomenon [53].

Physicians should diagnose isolated office hypertension whenever office blood pressure is >140/90mmHg at several visits, whereas 24-hour and daytime ambulatory blood pressure are <125–130/80 and <130–135/85mmHg, respectively. Diagnosis can also be based on home blood pressure values (average of several day readings <130–135/85mmHg). Identification should be followed by a search for metabolic risk factors and subclinical organ damage. Drug treatment should be instituted when there is evidence of organ damage or a high cardiovascular risk profile. However, lifestyle changes and a close follow-up should be implemented in all patients with isolated office hypertension in whom the doctor elects not to start pharmacological treatment.

Isolated ambulatory or masked hypertension

The reverse phenomenon of white coat hypertension has also been described, namely individuals with normal office blood pressure (<140/90mmHg) may have elevated ambulatory or home blood pressure values [53–56]. The prevalence in the population is about the same as that of isolated office hypertension [55, 57]. These individuals have been shown to display a greater than normal prevalence of organ damage [53, 57], with an increased prevalence of metabolic risk factors than truly normotensive individuals [55–57]. In addition, meta-analyses of outcome studies have indicated that masked hypertension increases cardiovascular risk, which appears to be close to that of in- and out-of-office hypertension [52, 58].

Family and clinical history

A comprehensive family history should be obtained, with particular attention to hypertension, diabetes mellitus, dyslipidaemia, premature coronary heart disease, stroke, or renal disease.

Clinical history should include:

- duration and previous levels of high blood pressure;
- symptoms suggestive of secondary causes of hypertension and intake of drugs or substances that can raise blood pressure, such as liquorice, cocaine, amphetamines, oral contraceptives, steroids, non-steroidal anti-inflammatory drugs, erythropoietin, and cyclosporins;
- lifestyle factors, such as dietary intake of fat (animal fat in particular), salt, and alcohol, quantification of smoking and physical activity, weight gain since early adult life;
- past history or current symptoms of coronary disease, heart failure, cerebrovascular or peripheral vascular disease, renal disease, diabetes mellitus, gout, dyslipidaemia, bronchospasm or any other significant illnesses, and drugs used to treat those conditions;
- previous antihypertensive therapy, its results and adverse effects;
- personal, family and environmental factors that may influence blood pressure and cardiovascular risk, as well as the course and outcome of therapy.

Physical examination

In addition to blood pressure measurement, physical examination should search for evidence of additional risk factors (in particular abdominal obesity), for signs suggesting secondary hypertension, and for evidence of organ damage.

Laboratory investigations

Laboratory investigations are also aimed at providing evidence of additional risk factors, at searching for hints of secondary hypertension, and at assessing absence or presence of subclinical organ damage. The younger the patient, the higher the blood pressure and the faster the development of hypertension, the more detailed the diagnostic work-up will be.

Essential laboratory investigations should include: blood chemistry for fasting glucose, total cholesterol, low- (LDL) and high-density lipoprotein (HDL) cholesterol, triglycerides, uric acid, creatinine, estimated creatinine clearance (Cockroft–Gault formula), or glomerular filtration rate (Modification of Diet in Renal Disease (MDRD) formula) (➲Chapter 15), sodium, potassium, haemoglobin, and haematocrit; urinalysis (complemented by microalbuminuria dipstick test and microscopic examination); and an electrocardiogram. Whenever fasting glucose is >5.6mmol/L (100mg/dL), post-prandial blood glucose should also be measured or a glucose tolerance test performed [60]. A fasting glucose of 7.0mmol/L (126mg/dL) or a 2-hour post-prandial glucose of 11mmol/L (198mg/dL) is now considered threshold value for diabetes mellitus in repeated findings [60] (➲Chapter 14).

Searching for subclinical organ damage

Owing to the importance of subclinical organ damage in determining the overall cardiovascular risk of the hypertensive patient, evidence of organ involvement should be sought carefully. Recent studies have shown that without ultrasound cardiovascular investigations for left-ventricular hypertrophy and vascular (carotid) wall thickening or plaque, up to 50% of hypertensive subjects may be mistakenly classified as at low or moderate added risk, whereas presence of cardiac or vascular damage stratifies them within a higher risk group. Likewise, searching for microalbuminuria can be strongly recommended because of the mounting evidence that it may be a sensitive marker of organ damage, not only in diabetes, but also in hypertension.

Heart

Electrocardiography (➲Chapter 2) should be part of all routine assessment of subjects with high blood pressure. Its sensitivity to detect left-ventricular hypertrophy is low but, nonetheless, hypertrophy detected by the Sokolow–Lyon index or of the Cornell voltage QRS duration product is an independent predictor of cardiovascular events [61]. Electrocardiography can also be used to detect patterns of ventricular overload ('strain'), known to indicate more severe risk [61], ischaemia, conduction defects, and arrhythmias. Echocardiography is undoubtedly much more sensitive than electrocardiography in diagnosing left-ventricular hypertrophy [62] and predicting cardiovascular risk [63]. An echocardiographic examination (➲Chapter 4) may help in more precisely classifying the overall risk of the hypertensive patient and in directing therapy. The best evaluation includes measurements of interventricular septum and posterior wall thickness and of end-diastolic left-ventricular diameter, with calculation of left-ventricular mass according to available formulae [64]. Classifications in concentric or eccentric hypertrophy, and concentric remodelling by also using the wall–radius ratio have been shown to have risk predicting value [65]. Echocardiography also provides means of assessing left-ventricular diastolic distensibility (diastolic function) by Doppler measurement of the ratio between the E and A waves of transmitral blood flow (and, more precisely, by adding measurement of early diastolic relaxation time and evaluating patterns of pulmonary vein outflow into the left atrium) [66].

There is current interest to investigate whether patterns of 'diastolic dysfunction' can predict onset of dyspnoea and impaired effort tolerance without evidence of systolic dysfunction, frequently occurring in hypertension and in the elderly ('diastolic heart failure') [67]. Finally, echocardiography can provide evidence of left-ventricular wall contraction defects due to ischaemia or previous infarction and, more broadly, of systolic dysfunction. Other diagnostic cardiac procedures, such as cardiac magnetic resonance (➲Chapter 5), cardiac scintigraphy (➲Chapter 7), exercise test (➲Chapter 2 and 25), and coronary angiography (➲Chapter 8), are obviously reserved for specific indications (diagnosis of coronary artery disease, cardiomyopathy, etc.). On the other hand, a radiograph of the thorax may often represent a useful additional diagnostic procedure, when information on large intrathoracic arteries or the pulmonary circulation is sought.

Blood vessels

Ultrasound examination of the carotid arteries with measurement of the intima media complex thickness and detection of plaques [68] has repeatedly been shown to predict occurrence of both stroke and myocardial infarction. A survey indicates that it can usefully complement echocardiography in making risk stratification of hypertensive patients more precise.

Evidence of arterial damage may also be suggested by a low ankle–brachial blood pressure index (<0.9), using a continuous wave Doppler unit and a blood pressure manometer. A low ankle–brachial blood pressure index signals advanced peripheral artery disease and in general advanced atherosclerosis [69] (➲Chapter 36).

The increasing interest in systolic blood pressure and pulse pressure as predictors of cardiovascular events [70] has stimulated the development of techniques for measuring large artery distensibility or compliance [71, 72]. This has been further supported by the observation that a reduction of arterial distensibility per se may have a prognostic significance [73]. One of these techniques, the pulse wave velocity measurement [73], may be suitable because of its simplicity for diagnostic use. Another technique, the augmentation index measurement device [74], has also raised wide interest as a possible tool to obtain an assessment of aortic blood pressure from peripheral artery measurement in view of the evidence that aortic blood pressure (and therefore the pressure exerted on the heart, brain and the kidney) may be different from that which is usually measured at the arm, and may be differently affected by different antihypertensive drugs.

Finally, there has been widespread interest in investigating endothelial dysfunction or damage as an early marker of cardiovascular damage [75, 76]. The techniques used so far for investigating endothelial responsiveness to various stimuli are either invasive or too laborious and time consuming to envisage their use in the clinical evaluation of the hypertensive patient. However, current studies on circulating markers of endothelial activity, dysfunction, or damage may soon provide simpler tests of endothelial dysfunction and damage to be investigated prospectively.

Kidney

The diagnosis of hypertension-induced renal damage is based on the finding of an elevated value of serum creatinine, of a decreased (measured or estimated) creatinine clearance, or the detection of an elevated urinary excretion of albumin below (microalbuminuria) or above (macroalbuminuria) the usual laboratory methods to detect proteinuria. The presence of mild renal insufficiency has been defined as serum creatinine values equal or above 133μmol/L (1.5mg/dL) in men and 124μmol/L (1.4mg/dL) in women [77, 78] or by the finding of estimated creatinine clearance values below 60mL/min [27]. Estimation from serum creatinine of glomerular filtration rate (MDRD formula requiring age, gender, and race) or creatinine clearance (Cockroft–Gault formula requiring also body size) should be routine procedures [74, 78, 79]. A slight increase in serum creatinine and urate may sometimes occur when antihypertensive therapy is instituted or potentiated, but this should not be taken as a sign of progressive renal deterioration. Hyperuricaemia, defined as a serum uric acid level in excess of 416μmol/L (7mg/dL), is frequently seen in untreated hypertensives and has also been shown to correlate with the existence of nephrosclerosis [80] (➲Chapter 15).

Although an elevated serum creatinine concentration points to a reduced rate of glomerular filtration, an increased rate of albumin or protein excretion points to a derangement in the glomerular filtration barrier [81]. Microalbuminuria has been shown to predict the development of overt diabetic nephropathy in both type 1 and type 2 diabetics [82] (➲Chapter 14), whereas the presence of proteinuria generally indicates the existence of established renal parenchymatous damage [81]. In non-diabetic hypertensive patients, microalbuminuria, even below the threshold values currently considered [83], has been shown to predict cardiovascular events, and a continuous relation between urinary albumin excretion and cardiovascular, as well as non-cardiovascular, mortality has been found in a general population study [84].

The finding of deranged renal function in a hypertensive patient, expressed as any of the earlier mentioned alterations, is frequent and constitutes a very potent predictor of future cardiovascular events and death [26, 27]. It is therefore recommended that serum creatinine (possibly with estimated creatinine clearance calculated) and serum urate levels are measured, and urinary protein (by dipstick) searched in all hypertensive patients. In dipstick negative patients low grade albuminuria (microalbuminuria) should be determined in spot urine by a validated commercial method (24-hour or night urine samples are discouraged due to the inaccuracy of urinary sampling) and related to urinary creatinine excretion [85].

Fundoscopy

In contrast with the 1930s, when the Keith Wagener and Barker classification of hypertensive eye ground changes in four grades [86] was formulated, nowadays most hypertensive patients present early in the process of their illness, and haemorrhages and exudates (grade 3), or papilloedema (grade 4), are very rarely observed. In an evaluation of 800 hypertensive patients attending a hypertension outpatient clinic [87] the prevalence of grades 1 and 2 retinal changes was as high as 78% (in contrast with 43% for carotid plaques, 22% for left-ventricular hypertrophy, and 14% for microalbuminuria). It is therefore doubtful whether grades 1 and 2 retinal changes can be used as a sign of subclinical organ damage to stratify total cardiovascular risk, whereas grades 3 and 4 are certainly markers of severe hypertensive complications.

Brain

In patients who have suffered a stroke, imaging techniques allow improved diagnosis of the existence, nature and location of a lesion [88, 89]. Cranial computerized tomography (CT) is the standard procedure for diagnosis of a stroke but, with the exception of prompt recognition of an intracranial haemorrhage, CT is progressively being replaced by magnetic resonance imaging (MRI) techniques. Diffusion-weighted MRI can identify ischaemic injury within minutes after arterial occlusion. Furthermore, MRI, particularly in fluid attenuated inversion recovery (FLAIR) sequences, is much superior to CT in discovering silent brain infarctions, the large majority of which are small and deep (lacunar infarction). As cognition disturbances in the elderly are, at least in part, hypertension related [90, 91], suitable cognition evaluation tests, such as the Mini Mental State Evaluation, should probably be used more often in assessment of the elderly hypertensives.

Screening for secondary forms of hypertension

A specific cause of blood pressure elevation can be identified in a minority (<5–10%) of adult patients with hypertension. Therefore, screening for secondary forms of hypertension is indicated, if possible before initiation of antihypertensive therapy. Findings suggesting a secondary form of blood pressure elevation are severe hypertension, sudden onset of hypertension, and blood pressure responding poorly to drug therapy.

Hypertension induced by hormonal contraceptives, conjugated oestrogens and by pregnancy is briefly summarized and commented upon in ➲Table 13.6.

Renal parenchymal hypertension

Renal parenchymal disease is the most common cause of secondary hypertension, detected in about 5% of all cases

Table 13.6 Hypertension induced by hormonal contraceptives, conjugated oestrogens, and by pregnancy [1, 2]

Oral contraceptives
Even low-dose oral contraceptives are associated with an increased risk of hypertension, stroke, and myocardial infarction. The progestogen-only pill is a contraceptive option for women with high blood pressure, but its influence on cardiovascular outcomes has been insufficiently investigated
Hormone replacement therapy
There is evidence that the only benefit of this therapy is a decreased incidence of bone fractures and colon cancer, accompanied, however, by increased risk of coronary events, stroke, thromboembolism, breast cancer, gallbladder disease, and dementia. This therapy is not recommended for cardioprotection in postmenopausal women
Hypertension in pregnancy
Hypertensive disorders in pregnancy, particularly pregnancy-induced hypertension with proteinuria (also known as pre-eclampsia), may adversely affect neonatal and maternal outcomes
Non-pharmacological management (including close supervision and restriction of activities) should be considered for pregnant women with systolic blood pressure 140–149mmHg or diastolic blood pressure 90–95mmHg. In the presence of gestational hypertension (with or without proteinuria) drug treatment is indicated at blood pressure levels ≥140/90 mmHg, but in the case of pre-existing hypertension without organ damage, threshold for drug treatment may be 150/95mmHg. Systolic blood pressure levels ≥170 or diastolic blood pressure ≥110mmHg should be considered an emergency requiring hospitalization
In non-severe hypertension, oral methyldopa, labetalol, calcium antagonists, and (less frequently) beta-blockers are drugs of choice
In pre-eclampsia with pulmonary oedema, nitroglycerine is the drug of choice. Diuretic therapy is inappropriate because plasma volume is reduced
As emergency, intravenous labetalol, oral methyldopa, and oral nifedipine are indicated. Intravenous hydralazine is no longer the drug of choice because of an excess of perinatal adverse effects
Intravenous infusion of sodium nitroprusside is useful in hypertensive crises, but prolonged administration should be avoided
Calcium supplementation, fish oil, and low-dose aspirin are not recommended. However, low-dose aspirin may be used prophylactically in women with a history of early onset pre-eclampsia

of hypertension (➲Chapter 10). The finding of bilateral upper abdominal masses at physical examination is consistent with polycystic kidney disease and should lead to an abdominal ultrasound examination. Renal ultrasound has now almost completely replaced intravenous urography in the anatomical exploration of the kidney. While the latter requires the injection of nephrotoxic contrast media, ultrasound is non-invasive and provides all necessary anatomic data about kidney size and shape, cortical thickness, urinary tract obstruction, and renal masses, in addition to evidence of polycystic kidneys. Assessment of the presence of protein, erythrocytes and leucocytes in the urine and measurement of serum creatinine concentration are the proper functional screening tests for renal parenchymal disease [92, 93], and should be performed in all patients with hypertension. Renal parenchymal disease may be excluded if urinalysis and serum creatinine concentration are normal at repeated determinations. The presence of erythrocytes and leucocytes should be confirmed by microscopic examination of the urine. If the screening tests for renal parenchymal hypertension are positive, a detailed work-up for kidney disease should ensue.

Renovascular hypertension

Renovascular hypertension is caused by one or several stenoses of the extrarenal arteries and is found in about 2% of adult patients with blood pressure elevation. In about 75% of these patients, the renal artery stenosis is caused by atherosclerosis (particularly in the elderly population). Fibromuscular dysplasia accounts for up to 25% of total cases (and is the most common variety in young adults). Hypertension of abrupt onset or worsening as well as high blood pressures increasingly difficult to treat suggest the presence of this condition. Signs of renal artery stenosis are an abdominal bruit with lateralization, hypokalaemia, and progressive decline in renal function. However, these signs are not present in many patients with renovascular hypertension. Determination of the longitudinal diameter of the kidney using ultrasound can be used as a screening procedure. However, a difference of >1.5cm in length between the two kidneys—which is usually considered as being diagnostic for renal stenosis—is only found in about 60–70% of the patients with renovascular hypertension. Colour Doppler sonography is able to detect stenosis of the renal artery, particularly stenosis that is localized close to the origin of the vessel [94], but the procedure is highly observer dependent. There is evidence that investigation of the renal vasculature by breath-hold, three-dimensional, gadolinium-enhanced magnetic resonance angiography is the diagnostic procedure of choice for renovascular hypertension [95]. Another imaging procedure with similar sensitivity is spiral CT, which, however, requires the application of contrast media and relatively high X-ray doses. Once there is a strong suspicion of renal artery stenosis, intra-arterial digital subtraction angiography should be performed for confirmation. This invasive procedure is still the gold standard for the detection of renal artery stenosis (➲Fig. 13.2).

Phaeochromocytoma

Phaeochromocytoma is a very rare secondary hypertensive state (0.2–0.4% of all cases of elevated blood pressure) with an estimated annual incidence of 2–8 per million population [96]. The diagnosis is based on establishing an increase in plasma or urinary catecholamines or their metabolites (noradrenaline, adrenaline, metanephrines). In most

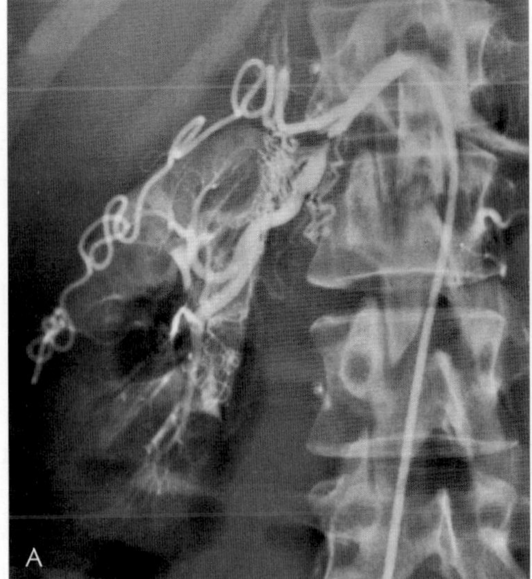

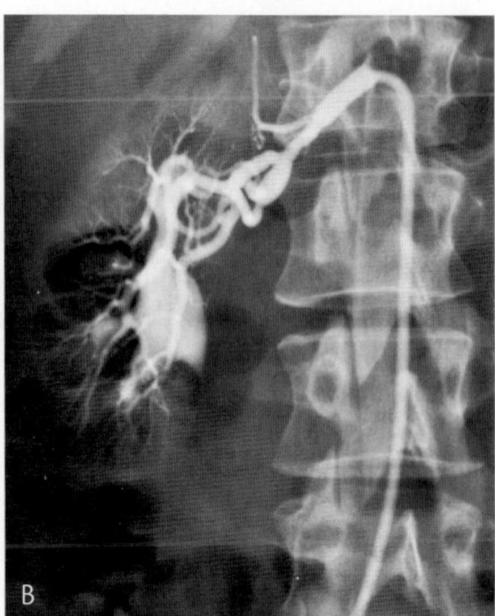

Figure 13.2 Renal arteriograms in a patient with renal artery stenosis, before (A) and after (B) percutanous transluminal arterioplasty.

patients with phaeochromocytoma, no further confirmation is required [97]. If the urinary excretion of catecholamines and their metabolites is only marginally increased or normal despite a strong clinical suspicion of phaeochromocytoma, the glucagon stimulation test can be applied. This test requires the measurement of catecholamines in plasma and should be performed after the patient has been effectively treated with an alpha-blocker. This pre-treatment prevents marked blood pressure rises after injection of glucagon. The clonidine suppression test is used to identify patients with essential hypertension, who have slight elevations of the excretion of catecholamines and their metabolites in urine [98]. Once the diagnosis of phaeochromocytoma has been established, localization of the tumour is necessary. As phaeochromocytomas are often big tumours localized in, or in the close vicinity of, the adrenal glands, they often are detected by ultrasound. A more sensitive imaging procedure is CT (➲Fig. 13.3). The meta-iodobenzylguanidine scan is useful in localizing extra-adrenal phaeochromocytomas and metastases of the 10% of phaeochromocytomas that are malignant.

Primary aldosteronism

Primary aldosteronism accounts for about 1% of all patients with hypertension. The determination of serum potassium levels is considered to be a screening test for the disease. However, only about 80% of the patients have hypokalaemia in an early phase [99], and some authorities maintain that hypokalaemia may even be absent in severe cases. Particularly in patients with bilateral adrenal hyperplasia, serum potassium levels may be normal or only slightly decreased [100]. The diagnosis is confirmed by a low plasma renin activity (<1ng/mL/hour) and elevated plasma aldosterone levels (after withdrawal of drugs influencing renin, such as beta-blockers, angiotensin-converting enzyme (ACE) inhibitors, angiotensin receptor antagonists, and diuretics) and in recent years there has been a move to measure the aldosterone-to-renin ratio [101]. A plasma

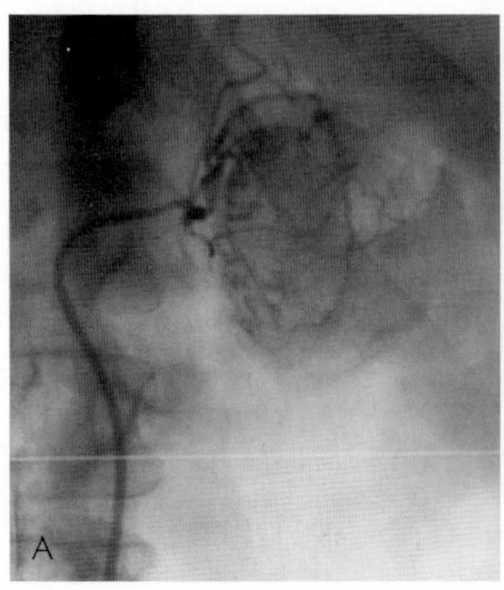

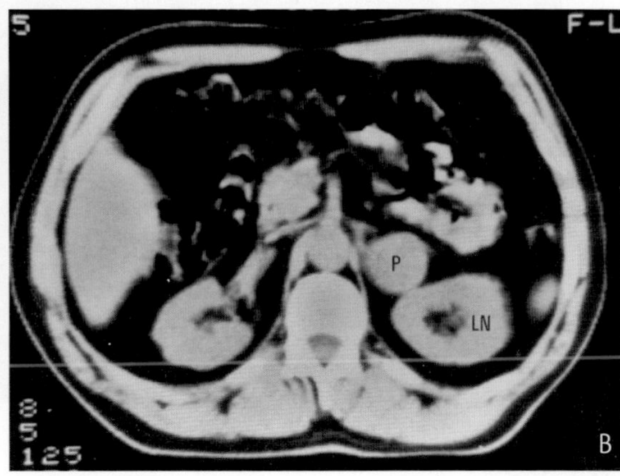

Figure 13.3 Hormone producing tumor shown on arteriogram (A) and on CT (B). LN, left kidney; P, pheochromocytoma.

aldosterone (pg/mL)–plasma renin activity (ng/mL/hour) ratio of >50 is highly suggestive of primary aldosteronism [100]. The diagnosis of primary aldosteronism is confirmed by the fludrocortisone suppression test [102]. Imaging procedures such as CT and MRI are used to localize an aldosterone-producing tumour, but adrenal morphology correlates poorly with function, and adrenal venous sampling, although invasive and difficult to perform, is considered by some investigators to be a more reliable procedure [103].

Cushing's syndrome

Cushing's syndrome affects <0.1% of the total population. On the other hand, hypertension is a very common finding in Cushing's syndrome, affecting about 80% of such patients. The syndrome is suggested by the typical habitus of the patient. The determination of 24-hour urinary cortisol excretion is the most practical and reliable index of cortisol secretion and a value exceeding 110nmol (40mcg) is highly suggestive of Cushing's syndrome. The diagnosis is confirmed by the 2-day, low-dose dexamethasone suppression test or the overnight dexamethasone suppression test. A normal result of either of the two suppression tests excludes the possibility of Cushing's syndrome [104]. Further tests and imaging procedures have to be used to differentiate the various forms of the syndrome [105].

Coarctation of the aorta

Coarctation of the aorta is a rare form of hypertension in children and young adults (➲Fig. 13.4). The diagnosis is usually evident from physical examination. A mid-systolic murmur, which may become continuous with time, is heard over the anterior part of the chest and also over the back. Hypertension is found in the upper extremities concomitantly with low or not measurable blood pressure in the legs.

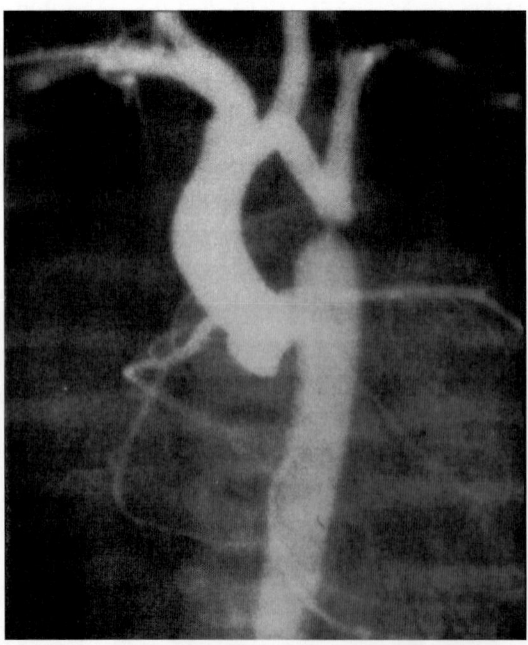

Figure 13.4 Arteriogram showing coarctation of the decending part of the thoracic aorta after left subclavian artery.

Genetic analysis

There is often a family history of high blood pressure in hypertensive patients, suggesting that inheritance contributes to the pathogenesis of this disorder. Essential hypertension has a highly heterogeneous character, which points to a multifactorial aetiology and polygenic abnormalities [106, 107] (➲Chapter 9). Variants in some genes might render an individual sensitive to a given factor in the environment. A number of mutations in the genes encoding for major blood pressure controlling systems has been recognized in humans, but their exact role in the pathogenesis of essential hypertension is still unclear. The search for candidate gene mutations in the individual hypertensive is therefore not useful at present. However, the patient's genetic disposition might influence drug-metabolizing enzymes, which might translate into differences in drug effects or tolerability, and several extremely rare monogenic forms of inherited hypertension have been described.

Therapeutic approach

When to initiate antihypertensive treatment

Guidelines for initiating antihypertensive treatment are based on two criteria: (1) the level of total cardiovascular risk, as indicated in ➲Table 13.2, and (2) the level of systolic and diastolic blood pressure, as classified in ➲Table 13.1. Consideration of subjects with systolic blood pressure of 120–139mmHg and diastolic blood pressure of 80–89mmHg for possible initiation of antihypertensive treatment is so far limited to subjects with established diabetes mellitus, renal and cardiovascular disease [108–110]. Antihypertensive treatment is recommended within this blood pressure range only for patients at least at high total risk. Close monitoring of blood pressure and no blood pressure intervention is only recommended for patients at moderate or low total risk, who are considered to mostly benefit from lifestyle measures and correction of other risk factors (e.g. smoking).

In patients with grade 1 and 2 hypertension, antihypertensive drug treatment should be initiated promptly in subjects who are classified as at high or very high risk, whereas in subjects at moderate or low added risk, blood pressure, as well as other cardiovascular risk factors, should be monitored for several weeks or months under non-pharmacological treatment only (➲Table 13.7). However, even in these patients lack of blood pressure control after a suitable period of non-pharmacological intervention should lead to the institution of drug treatment in addition to life-style changes.

➲Table 13.7 also includes recommendations about initiation of treatment in patients with grade 3 hypertension. In these subjects confirmation of elevated blood pressure values should be obtained within a few days, and treatment instituted immediately, without the preliminary need of establishing the absolute risk (high even in absence of other risk factors). Complete assessment of other risk factors, subclinical organ damage, or associated disease can be carried out after institution of treatment, and lifestyle measures can be recommended at the same time as initiation of drug therapy.

Several studies have shown that in high or very high-risk patients, treatment of hypertension is very cost-effective, i.e. the reduction in the incidence of cardiovascular disease and death largely offsets the cost of treatment despite its lifetime duration. Some pharmacoeconomical studies suggest that treatment may be less cost-effective in grade 1 or 2 hypertensives who are at low or moderate added risk. This may be more apparent than real, however, because in these patients the purpose of treatment is not to prevent an unlikely morbid or fatal event in the subsequent few years but rather to oppose appearance and/or progression of organ damage that will make the patient a high risk in the long term. Several trials of antihypertensive therapy, foremost the HDFP (Hypertension Detection and Follow-up Program) [111] and HOT (Hypertension Optimal Treatment) [112, 113] studies, have shown that under these circumstances and despite intensive blood pressure lowering, residual cardiovascular risk remains higher than in patients with initial moderate risk. This suggests that some of the major cardiovascular risk changes may be difficult to reverse and that restricting antihypertensive therapy to patients at high or very high risk may be far from an optimal strategy.

Goals of treatment

The primary goal of treatment of the patient with high blood pressure is to achieve the maximum reduction in the long-term total risk of cardiovascular morbidity and mortality. This requires treatment of all the reversible risk factors identified, including smoking, dyslipidaemia, or obesity and the appropriate management of associated clinical conditions like diabetes mellitus, as well as treatment of the raised blood pressure per se (➲Chapter 12).

As to the blood pressure goal to be achieved, evidence from old and recent randomized prospective trials [2, 114] justifies the recommendation to always try to reach values below 140mmHg systolic and 90mmHg diastolic. This is also supported by the results of retrospective analysis of the trials which have shown that regardless of which drugs were employed, patients in whom treatment reduced blood pressure below these values had fewer cardiovascular events than patients in whom blood pressure control had not been

Table 13.7 Initiation of antihypertensive treatment

Other risk factors, OD, or disease	Normal SBP 120–129 or DBP 80–84	High normal SBP 130–139 or DBP 85–89	Grade 1 HT SBP 140–159 or DBP 90–99	Grade 2 HT SBP 160–179 or DBP 100–109	Grade 3 HT SBP ≥180 or DBP ≥110
No other risk factors	No BP intervention	No BP intervention	Lifestyle changes for several months then drug treatment if BP uncontrolled	Lifestyle changes for several weeks then drug treatment if BP uncontrolled	Lifestyle changes + immediate drug treatment
1–2 risk factors	Lifestyle changes	Lifestyle changes	Lifestyle changes for several weeks then drug treatment if BP uncontrolled	Lifestyle changes for several weeks then drug treatment if BP uncontrolled	Lifestyle changes + immediate drug treatment
3 or more risk factors, MS, or OD	Lifestyle changes	Lifestyle changes and consider drug treatment	Lifestyle changes + drug treatment	Lifestyle changes + drug treatment	Lifestyle changes + immediate drug treatment
Diabetes	Lifestyle changes	Lifestyle changes + drug treatment			
Established CV or renal disease	Lifestyle changes + immediate drug treatment	Lifestyle changes + immediate drug treatment	Lifestyle changes + immediate drug treatment	Lifestyle changes + immediate drug treatment	Lifestyle changes + immediate drug treatment

CV: cardiovascular; MS: metabolic syndrome; OD: subclinical organ damage.

reached [115, 116]. There is also evidence, however, that in diabetic subjects as well as in non-diabetic subjects characterized by a high cardiovascular risk, further benefit can be obtained by more intensive blood pressure lowering interventions. In the diabetic hypertensive patients of the HOT study [112, 113, 117], the incidence of cardiovascular events was lower in the group randomized to a target diastolic blood pressure of 80mmHg or less than in the group randomized to a target diastolic blood pressure of 90mmHg or less [112, 113, 117]. In the diabetic patients recruited for the ABCD study, the group in which a more intensive treatment reduced blood pressure below 130/80mmHg had fewer strokes than the group in which a less intensive treatment was adopted [118]. In patients with a history of coronary or cerebrovascular disease, a reduction in the incidence of cardiovascular events was seen both in initially hypertensive and in initially normotensive (blood pressure <140/90mmHg) patients, the latter group achieving on-treatment blood pressure values <130/80mmHg [108, 109, 119–122]. Although in some of these studies the role played by the blood pressure reduction (versus that due to the specific protective properties of the drugs employed) is not entirely clear, these studies suggest that it is appropriate to try to lower blood pressure well below 140/90mmHg when patients present with diabetes (➲Chapter 14) or with a history of cardiovascular disease.

Whether this is the case in non-diabetic patients as well as in patients at lower degrees of risk has not yet been established. However, observational data provide evidence that in lower-risk individuals the relationship between blood pressure and cardiovascular risk is linear down to systolic and diastolic values of about 110mmHg and 70mmHg, respectively [12]. Furthermore, although in the non-diabetic patients of the HOT study reducing diastolic blood pressure more intensively was not associated with a reduced incidence of cardiovascular morbidity and mortality (except for a significant reduction in myocardial infarction), randomization to the lowest target blood pressure was not accompanied by an increased cardiovascular risk either [112, 113, 117]. This is relevant to the clinical practice because setting lower blood pressure goals allows a greater number of subjects to at least meet the traditional ones. The problem lays in that reaching blood pressures well below 140/90mmHg is not easy, as shown by the fact that so far trials have never been able to obtain in diabetic patients on treatment average systolic values below 130mmHg [123]. In the recent ACCOMPLISH (Avoiding Cardiovascular events through COMbination therapy in Patients Living with Systolic Hypertension) trial, however, the combination treatments employed have reduced systolic blood pressure to an average value of 130mmHg, which raises hopes for a more effective blood pressure control in the future [124]. Evidence is available that rigorous blood pressure control is also necessary to delay progression of renal disease in diabetic patients with nephropathy, and that target blood pressures <130/80mmHg maximize nephroprotection, particularly in the presence of proteinuria, in which case even lower blood pressure values may be desirable [125]. Data are less consistent for non-diabetic nephropathy [126] but overall the protective role of rigorous blood pressure control per se for the kidney cannot be disputed. Indirectly, this means cardiovascular protection as well because of the association between advanced renal damage and cardiovascular risk [127].

An important problem that physicians face when dealing with the achievement of blood pressure goals lower than the traditional ones, is whether this could eventually incur in the J-curve phenomenon, i.e. an increase in cardiovascular risk due to an excessive blood pressure reduction and thus an impaired perfusion of vital organs. No J-curve phenomenon down to blood pressure values of about 110/70mmHg has been reported on healthy subjects (discussed earlier) [12], but this does not exclude its occurrence at higher blood pressure values in subjects in whom hypertension, organ damage, or cardiovascular disease may impair the ability to preserve, via autoregulation, blood flow in the face of a blood pressure reduction. Retrospective analysis of prospective trials have suggested that in hypertension a J-curve may be seen when blood pressure falls below 70mmHg diastolic and 120mmHg systolic [80, 128]. However, whether and to what extent this is caused by an excessive blood pressure reduction versus a high initial risk condition that leads to a greater blood pressure fall is not clear.

As to the blood pressure goal to be achieved, randomized trials comparing less with more intensive treatment [110, 113, 116, 129] have shown that in diabetic patients more intensive blood pressure lowering is more protective [110, 112, 116, 130]. This is not yet conclusively established in non-diabetic subjects, because the only trial not exclusively involving diabetics is the HOT study [112, 116], which presently, because of the small diastolic blood pressure differences achieved (2mmHg) among the groups randomized to ≤90, ≤85, or ≤80mmHg, was unable to detect significant differences in the risk of cardiovascular events (except for myocardial infarction, p-value = 0.05) between adjacent target groups. However, the results of the HOT study have confirmed that there is no increase in cardiovascular risk in the patients randomized to the lowest target group, which is relevant to clinical practice because, as already mentioned, setting lower blood pressure goals allows a greater number of subjects to at least meet the traditional ones. Observational studies in healthy subjects show a direct linear relationship with cardiovascular events of systolic and diastolic blood pressure values as low as 115–110 and 75–70mmHg, respectively, without evidence within this range of a J-curve phenomenon [12]. Furthermore, a subgroup analysis of the HOT study [117] suggests that, except for smokers, a reduction of diastolic blood pressure to an average of 82mmHg rather than 85mmHg significantly reduces major cardiovascular events in non-diabetic patients at high or very high risk (50% of HOT study patients), as well as in patients with previous ischaemic heart disease, in patients >65 years, and in women. Finally, in patients with a history of stroke or transient ischaemic attack, the PROGRESS trial [108] showed less cardiovascular mortality and morbidity by reducing diastolic blood pressure to 79mmHg (active treatment group) rather than 83mmHg (placebo group). Similar observations have been made in patients with coronary disease, although the role of blood pressure reduction in these trials has been debated [123]. As far as systolic blood pressure is concerned, evidence of a greater benefit by a more aggressive reduction is limited to the UKPDS study, which has shown, through retrospective analysis of the data, fewer cardiovascular morbid events at values below 130–120 compared with 140mmHg. Most trials, however, have been unable to reduce systolic blood pressure below 140mmHg, and in no trials on diabetic and non-diabetic patients have values below 130mmHg been achieved [123].

As for patients with non-diabetic renal disease, data about the effects of more or less intensive blood pressure lowering on cardiovascular events are scanty: the HOT study was unable to find any significant reduction in cardiovascular events in the subset of patients with plasma creatinine >115μmol/L (>1.3mg/dL) [117] or >133μmol/L (>1.5mg/dL) [27] when subjected to more versus less intensive blood pressure lowering (139/82 versus 143/85mmHg). However, evidence, suggests that values lower than 130/80mmHg may help preserve renal function, especially in the presence of proteinuria, and none of these trials suggests an increased cardiovascular risk at the lowest blood pressure achieved.

In conclusion, on the basis of current evidence from trials, it can be recommended that blood pressure can be intensively lowered at least below 140/90mmHg and to definitely lower values if tolerated, in all hypertensive patients, and below 130/80mmHg in diabetics and in high or very high risk patients, such as those with associated clinical conditions (stroke, myocardial infarction, renal dysfunction, proteinuria). The achievable goal may depend on the pre-existing blood pressure level, and systolic values below 140mmHg may be difficult to achieve, particularly in the elderly.

When home or ambulatory blood pressure measurement are used to evaluate the efficacy of treatment, it must be remembered that daytime values provided by these methods (compared with office measurement) are on average at least 5–10mmHg lower for systolic and 5mmHg lower for diastolic blood pressure, although these differences tend to become smaller at lower office blood pressure values, such as those recommended as treatment goals [45].

Lifestyle changes

Lifestyle measures should be instituted whenever appropriate in all patients, including subjects with high normal blood pressure and patients who require drug treatment. The purpose is to lower blood pressure and to control other risk factors and clinical conditions present (➲Chapter 12). However, lifestyle measures are undocumented in preventing cardiovascular complications in hypertensive patients and should never delay the initiation of drug treatment unnecessarily, especially in patients at higher levels of risk, or detract from compliance to drug treatment.

Smoking cessation

Smoking cessation is probably the single most powerful lifestyle measure for the prevention of a large number of non-cardiovascular and cardiovascular diseases, including stroke and coronary heart disease [131]. Those who quit before middle age typically have a life expectancy that is not different to that of lifelong non-smokers. Although smoking cessation does not lower blood pressure [132], smoking may predict a future rise in systolic blood pressure [133], and global cardiovascular risk is greatly increased by smoking [131]. For several reasons, therefore, hypertensive smokers should be counselled on smoking cessation. In addition, some other data suggest that smoking may interfere with the beneficial effects of some antihypertensive agents, such as beta-blockers, or may prevent the benefits of more intensive blood pressure lowering [117]. Where necessary, nicotine replacement, or buspirone or varenicline therapy should be considered, as they appear to facilitate smoking cessation [134].

Moderation of alcohol consumption

There is a linear relationship between alcohol consumption, blood pressure levels, and the prevalence of hypertension in populations [135]. Beyond that, high levels of alcohol consumption are associated with high risk of stroke [136]; this is particularly so for binge drinking. Alcohol attenuates the effects of antihypertensive drug therapy, but this effect is at least partially reversible within 1–2 weeks by moderation of drinking by around 80% [137]. Heavier drinkers (five or more standard drinks per day) may experience a rise in blood pressure after acute alcohol withdrawal and are more likely to be diagnosed as hypertensive at the beginning of the week if they have a weekend drinking pattern. Accordingly, hypertensive patients who drink alcohol should be advised to limit their consumption to no more than 20–30g of ethanol per day for men, and no more than 10–20g per day for women. They should be warned against the heightened risks of stroke that are associated with binge drinking.

Weight reduction and physical exercise

Excess body fat predisposes to raised blood pressure and hypertension [138]. Weight reduction reduces blood pressure in overweight patients and has beneficial effects on associated risk factors, such as insulin resistance, diabetes mellitus, hyperlipidaemia, and left-ventricular hypertrophy. In a meta-analysis of available studies, the mean systolic and diastolic blood pressure reductions associated with an average weight loss of 5.1kg were 4.4 and 3.6mmHg, respectively [139]. The blood pressure lowering effect of weight reduction may be enhanced by simultaneous increase in physical exercise [140], by alcohol moderation in overweight drinkers [141], and by reduction in sodium intake [142]. Physical fitness is a rather strong predictor of cardiovascular mortality, independent of blood pressure and other risk factors [143]. Thus, sedentary patients should be advised to take up moderate levels of aerobic exercise on a regular basis, such as walking, jogging, or swimming, for 30–45min on most, preferably all days of the week [144, 145]. The extent of the pre-training evaluation will depend on the extent of the envisaged exercise and on the patient's symptoms, signs, overall cardiovascular risk, and associated clinical conditions. Even mild exercise may lower systolic blood pressure by about 4–8mmHg [146, 147]. Whereas dynamic resistance training may decrease blood pressure by about 3mmHg [148], purely isometric exercise such as heavy weightlifting can have a pressor effect and should be avoided. If hypertension is poorly controlled, and always in severe hypertension, heavy physical exercise should be discouraged or postponed until appropriate drug treatment has been instituted and found to work.

Reduction of high salt intake and other dietary changes

Epidemiological studies suggest that dietary salt intake is a contributor to blood pressure elevation and to the prevalence of hypertension [149]. The effect appears to be enhanced by a low dietary intake of potassium-containing foods. Randomized controlled trials in hypertensive patients indicate that reducing sodium intake by 80–100mmol (4.7–5.8g) per day from an initial intake of around 180mmol (10.5g) per day will reduce blood pressure by an average of 4–6mmHg [150] or even more if combined with other dietary counselling [151]. Patients should be advised to avoid added salt, to avoid obviously salted food, particularly processed foods, and to eat more meals cooked directly from natural ingredients containing more potassium. Counselling by trained nutritionists may be useful. Hypertensive patients should also be advised to eat more fruit, vegetables [152], and fish [153], and to reduce their intake of saturated fat and cholesterol.

Pharmacological therapy

Introduction

Recommendations about pharmacological therapy (➲Chapter 11) are here preceded by analysis of the available evidence (as provided by large randomized trials based on fatal and non-fatal events) of the benefits obtained by antihypertensive therapy and of the comparative benefits obtained by the various classes of agents. This is the strongest type of evidence available. It is commonly recognized, however, that event-based randomized therapeutic trials have some limitations; among these, the special selection criteria of the subjects included: the frequent selection of high-risk patients in order to increase the power of the trial, so that the vast majority of uncomplicated and lower risk hypertensives are rarely represented; the therapeutic programmes that often diverge from usual therapeutic practice; and the stringent follow-up procedures enforcing patients' compliance well beyond that obtained in common medical practice. The most important limitation is perhaps the necessarily short duration of a controlled trial, in most cases 4–5 years, whereas additional life expectancy and hence expectancy of therapeutic duration for a middle-aged hypertensive is of 20–30 years [21, 154].

Long-term therapeutic benefits and long-term differences between benefits of various drug classes may also be evaluated by using intermediate end-points (i.e. subclinical organ damage changes), as some of these changes have predictive value of subsequent fatal and non-fatal events. Several of the recent event-based trials have also used 'softer' end-points, such as congestive heart failure (certainly clinically relevant, but often based on subjective diagnosis), hospitalization, angina pectoris and coronary revascularization (highly subjected to local clinical habits and facilities), etc. Treatment-induced alterations in metabolic parameters, such as serum LDL- or HDL-cholesterol, serum potassium, glucose tolerance, induction or worsening of the metabolic syndrome, or diabetes, although they can hardly be expected to affect cardiovascular event incidence during the short term of a trial, may have some impact during the longer course of the patient's life.

Trials based on mortality and morbidity end-points comparing active treatment with placebo

The results of trials performed in mostly systolic–diastolic hypertension and in elderly with isolated systolic hypertension have been included in meta-analyses [6, 154–157]. Antihypertensive treatment resulted in significant and similar reductions of cardiovascular and all-cause mortality in both types of hypertension. With regard to cause-specific mortality, Collins and colleagues [15] observed a significant reduction in fatal stroke (–45%, *p*-value <0.001), but not in fatal coronary heart disease (–11%, NS). This could be related to age because coronary mortality was significantly reduced by 26% (*p*-value <0.01) in a meta-analysis on elderly with systolic–diastolic hypertension [158]. Fatal and non-fatal strokes combined and all coronary events were significantly reduced in the two types of hypertension. The Blood Pressure Lowering Treatment Trialists Collaboration (BPLTTC) [130] performed separate meta-analyses of placebo-controlled trials in which active treatment was initiated by a calcium antagonist or by an ACE inhibitor and showed the reductions in cardiovascular end-points were similar to those found in the trials in which active treatment was based on diuretics or beta-blockers. The proportional reduction of the cardiovascular risk appears to be similar in women and in men [159].

Additional information has more recently been provided by other trials, not yet included in the previously mentioned meta-analysis. Placebo-controlled trials addressed the effect of the angiotensin receptor antagonists losartan [160] and irbesartan [161, 162] in patients with type 2 diabetes and nephropathy. All studies concluded that the drug treatment was renoprotective but that there was no evidence of benefit in secondary cardiovascular end-points (for the evaluation of which, however, these trials had insufficient power). It can be concluded from these recent placebo-controlled trials that blood pressure lowering by angiotensin antagonists can also be beneficial, particularly in stroke prevention, and, in patients with diabetic nephropathy, in slowing down progression of renal disease.

Trials based on mortality and morbidity end-points comparing treatments initiated by different drug classes

During the last decade, a large number of controlled randomized trials has compared antihypertensive regimens initiated with different classes of antihypertensive agents, most often comparing older (diuretics and beta-blockers) with newer ones (calcium antagonists, ACE inhibitors, angiotensin receptor antagonists, alpha-blockers), and occasionally comparing newer drug classes. Several trials [163–171] with >67,000 randomized patients, comparing calcium antagonists with older drugs, have been reviewed [172]. For none of the outcomes considered in this analysis, including all-cause and cardiovascular mortality, all cardiovascular events, stroke, myocardial infarction and heart failure, did the *p*-values for heterogeneity reach statistical significance (0.12 ≤ *p*-value ≤ 0.95). The pooled odds ratios expressing the possible benefit of calcium antagonists over old drugs were close to unity and non-significant for total mortality, cardiovascular mortality, all cardiovascular events and myocardial infarction (➲ Fig. 13.5). Calcium antagonists provided slightly better protection against fatal and non-fatal stroke than old drugs (➲ Fig. 13.6). For the trials combined, the odds ratio for stroke reached formal significance (0.90, 95% confidence interval 0.82–0.98, *p*-value = 0.02) after CONVINCE (Controlled ONset Verapamil INvestigation of Cardiovascular Endpoints) [171], the only large trial based on verapamil, was excluded. For heart failure, calcium antagonists appeared to provide less protection than conventional therapy, regardless of whether or not the CONVINCE trial was incorporated in the pooled estimates.

Six trials with about 47,000 randomized patients compared ACE inhibitors with older drugs [164, 167, 173, 174]. The pooled odds ratios expressing the possible benefit of ACE inhibitors over conventional therapy were close to unity, and non-significant for total mortality, cardiovascular mortality, all cardiovascular event and myocardial infarction (➲ Fig. 13.5). Compared with old drugs, ACE inhibitors provided slightly less protection against stroke (➲ Fig. 13.6), heart failure, and all cardiovascular events. For all-cause and cardiovascular mortality, stroke, and myocardial infarction, *p*-values for heterogeneity among the trials of ACE inhibitors were non-significant (0.16 ≤ *p*-value ≤ 0.90). In contrast, for all cardiovascular events and heart failure, heterogeneity was significant owing to the ALLHAT (Lipid-Lowering Treatment to Prevent Heart Attack Trial) [164] findings. Compared with chlorthalidone, ALLHAT patients allocated to lisinopril had a greater risk of stroke, heart failure and hence combined cardiovascular disease [164]. Similar findings were previously reported for the comparison of the alpha-blocker doxazosin with chlorthalidone, an ALLHAT arm that was interrupted prematurely [163]. Although ALLHAT [164] stands out as the largest double-blind trial undertaken in hypertensive patients, interpretation of its results is difficult in several aspects, which may account for the

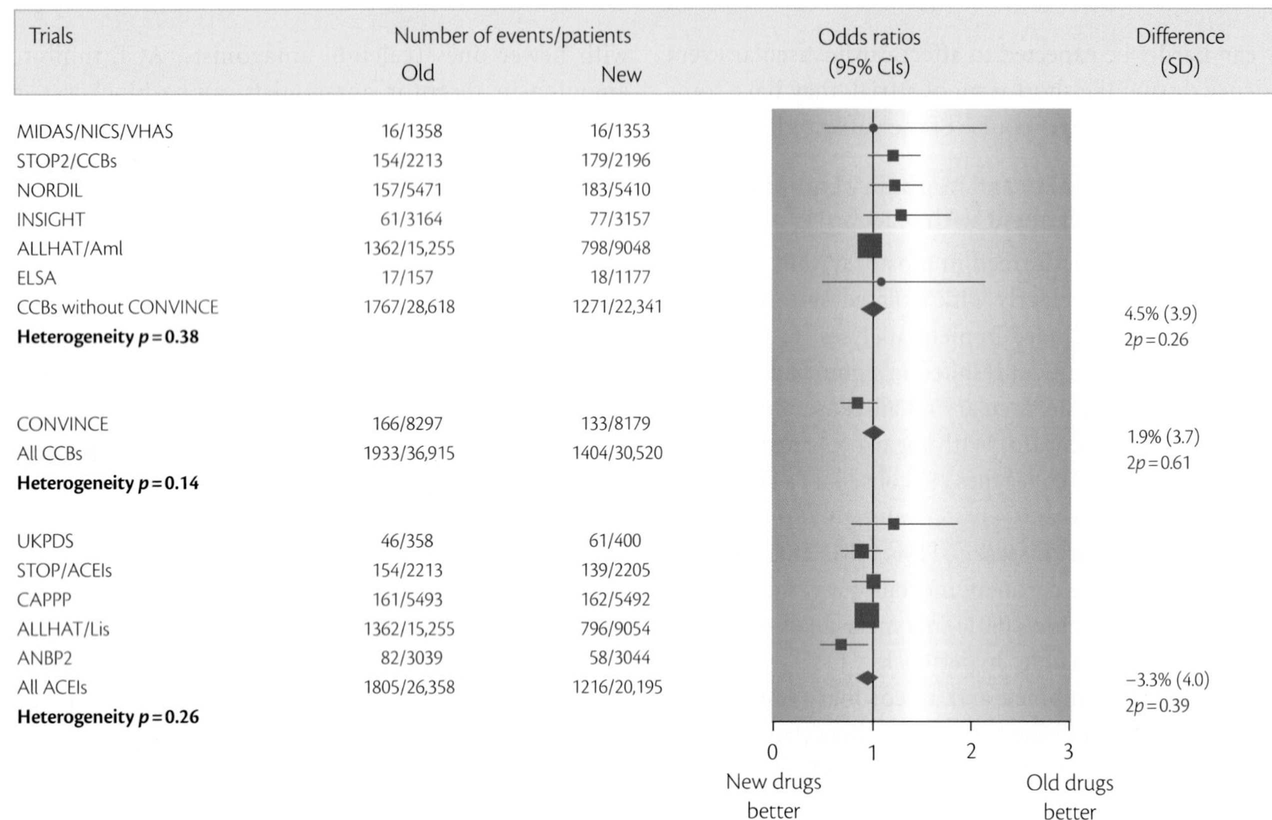

Figure 13.5 Fatal and non-fatal myocardial infarction. Modified after Staessen JA, Wang JG, Thijs L. Cardiovascular prevention and blood pressure reduction: a quantitative overview updated until 1 March 2003. *J Hypertens* 2003; **21**:1055–76.

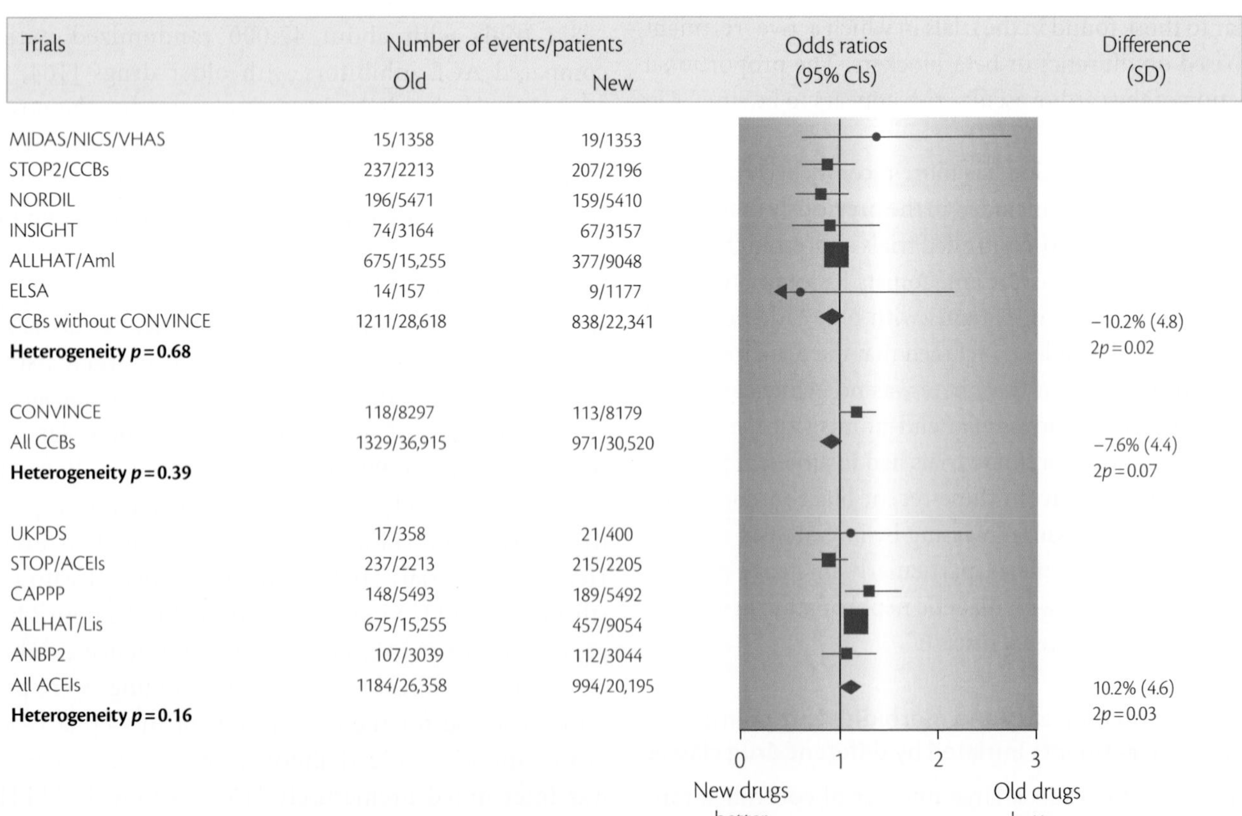

Figure 13.6 Fatal and non-fatal stroke. Modified after Staessen JA, Wang JG, Thijs L. Cardiovascular prevention and blood pressure reduction: a quantitative overview updated until 1 March 2003. *J Hypertens* 2003; **21**:1055–76.

heterogeneity of ALLHAT results with respect to those of the other trials.

- In ALLHAT, 90% of the patients at randomization were already on antihypertensive treatment, most often diuretics, thus ALLHAT tested 'continuing a diuretic' versus 'switching drug classes'. Patients on diuretics with latent or compensated heart failure were deprived of their therapy when they were not randomized to chlorthalidone.
- The achieved systolic pressure was higher on doxazosin, amlodipine, and lisinopril than on chlorthalidone. Presumably, these factors explain why the Kaplan–Meier curves started to diverge immediately after randomization for heart failure and approximately 6 months later also for stroke.
- The sympatholytic agents used for step-up treatment (atenolol, clonidine, and/or reserpine at the physician's discretion) led to a somewhat artificial treatment regimen, which does not reflect modern clinical practice, is not usually recommended, and is known to potentiate the blood pressure response to diuretics much more than to ACE inhibitors or alpha-blockers.
- ALLHAT did not include systematic end-point evaluation, which may have particularly affected evaluation of 'softer' end-points, such as congestive heart failure.

These limitations notwithstanding, ALLHAT [163, 164], either alone or in combination with the other trials, supports the conclusion that the benefits of antihypertensive therapy largely depend on blood pressure lowering, thus being in line with the findings of the meta-analysis of the BPLTTC (Blood Pressure Lowering Treatment Trialists' Collaboration) [130, 175]. The conclusion that a substitution of portion of the benefit of antihypertensive treatment depends on blood pressure reduction per se is also supported by the findings of the INVEST (INternational VErapamil SR-trandolapril Study) [176], in which cardiovascular disease was similarly frequent in patients treated with verapamil compared with those treated with atenolol (± hydrochlorotiazide). It is not entirely supported by the data of the Second Australian Blood Pressure study [177], in which ACE inhibitor-based treatment was found to be more protective against cardiovascular disease than diuretic-based treatment. The difference was modest, however, and significant only when the second morbid event in the same patient was included in the analysis. The conclusion of the paramount importance of blood pressure control for prevention of cardiovascular complications is supported by the results of the VALUE (Valsartan Antihypertensive Long-Term Use Evaluation) trial [178, 179], in which cardiac disease (the primary endpoint) was similarly frequent in high-risk hypertensive patients who were treated with valsartan or amlodipine. Amlodipine reduced blood pressure to a greater degree in the months that followed randomization than using the other drug regimens, and this was accompanied by a lower risk of events [179].

The LIFE (Losartan Intervention For End point reduction in hypertension) study [180] compared the angiotensin receptor antagonist losartan with the beta-blocker atenolol in hypertensive patients with left-ventricular hypertrophy for an average of 4.8 years, and found a significant 13% reduction in major cardiovascular events, mostly due to a significant 25% reduction in stroke incidence. There were no blood pressure differences between the treatment groups. The SCOPE (Study on COgnition and Prognosis in the Elderly) study [181] was initiated as a comparison of elderly patients receiving candesartan or placebo but, because for ethical reasons 85% of the placebo-initiated patients received antihypertensive therapy (mostly diuretics, beta-blockers, or calcium antagonists), the study is a comparison of antihypertensive treatment with or without candesartan. After 3.7 years of treatment there was a non-significant 11% reduction in major cardiovascular events, and a significant 28% reduction in non-fatal strokes among candesartan-treated patients, with an achieved blood pressure slightly lower (3.2/1.6mmHg) in the candesartan group.

In a meta-analysis of the BPLTTC that included angiotensin receptor antagonist treatment [175], it was concluded that angiotensin receptor antagonist based regimens showed a greater effect than other control regimens on the risk of stroke, heart failure, and major cardiovascular events, but not on coronary heart disease, cardiovascular death, and total mortality. However, angiotensin receptor antagonist treatment compared to calcium channel blocker treatment with amlodipine is balanced when assessing the VALUE Trial [178] and the CASE-J (Candesartan Antihypertensive Survival Evaluation in Japan) study [182].

Randomized trials based on intermediate end-points

Left-ventricular hypertrophy

The studies that have tested the effects of various antihypertensive agents on hypertension-associated left-ventricular hypertrophy, mostly evaluated as left-ventricular mass at the echocardiogram (➲Chapter 4), are almost innumerable, but only a few of them have followed strict enough criteria to provide reliable information. The very few studies adhering to these strict criteria do not yet provide incontrovertible answers, although meta-analyses suggest that, for a similar blood pressure reduction, newer agents (ACE inhibitors, calcium antagonists, and angiotensin receptor antagonists) may be more effective than conventional drugs [183, 184]. The large and long-term (4.8 years) LIFE Study is particularly relevant, as the greater regression of electrocardiographically determined left-ventricular hypertrophy with losartan was accompanied by a reduced incidence of cardiovascular events [180]. The same findings were obtained in a LIFE substudy in which left-ventricular hypertrophy was determined by echocardiography. Future studies should investigate treatment-induced effects on indices of collagen content of the ventricular wall rather than on its mass only.

Arterial wall and atherosclerosis

A number of randomized trials have compared the long-term (2–4 years) effects of different antihypertensive regimens on carotid artery wall intima media thickness. The most convincing evidence has been obtained for calcium antagonists, which comes from trials with different agents, concluding with a long-term study on more than 2000 patients [185, 186]. The data show [185–188] that for a similar reduction in blood pressure these drugs slow down carotid artery wall thickening and plaque formations more than conventional drugs. Evidence of a greater benefit is also available for ACE inhibitors [189], although less consistently.

Renal function

The most abundant evidence concerns renal function in diabetic patients [190] (➲Chapter 14). Progression of renal dysfunction (➲Chapter 15) can be retarded by adding an angiotensin receptor antagonist [160, 161] (compared with placebo) in diabetic patients with advanced nephropathy. Consistent effects of more intensive blood pressure lowering were found on urinary protein, both overt proteinuria and microalbuminuria. Of several studies in diabetic patients comparing treatments initiated by different agents, some did not show a difference in the renal protective effect of the drugs that were being compared [110, 170, 173], whereas one indicated the angiotensin receptor antagonist irbesartan to be superior to the calcium antagonist amlodipine in retarding development of renal failure [161], and the other indicated the angiotensin receptor antagonist losartan to reduce incidence of new overt proteinuria better than the beta-blocker atenolol [191].

As to patients with non-diabetic renal disease, a meta-analysis of 11 randomized trials comparing antihypertensive regimens including or excluding an ACE inhibitor [192] indicates a significantly slower progression in patients achieving blood pressure of 139/85mmHg rather than 144/87mmHg. It is not clear, however, whether the benefit should be ascribed to ACE inhibition or to the lower blood pressure achieved. Some light on the matter is shed by the AASK (African American Study of Kidney Disease and Hypertension) study [193]. ACE inhibitors were shown to be somewhat more effective than beta-blockers [193] or calcium antagonists [194] in slowing glomerular filtration rate decline. It appears, therefore, that in patients with non-diabetic renal disease the use of an ACE inhibitor may be more important than an aggressive blood pressure reduction, whereas in diabetic patients aggressive lowering of blood pressure may be equally important as blockade of the renin–angiotensin system.

Several studies have also investigated the combination of an angiotensin receptor antagonist with an ACE inhibitor (compared with monotherapies). The COOPERATE (Combination treatment of angiotensin-II receptor blocker and angiotensin-converting-enzyme inhibitor in non-diabetic renal disease) study has reported a reduced progression of non-diabetic nephropathy by the combination versus the combination components in monotherapy without a blood pressure difference between treatment groups [195]. A recent meta-analysis concluded that the combination in patients with chronic proteinuric renal disease was safe and confirmed greater antiproteinuric action, at least in short term, but additional trials with longer follow-up are needed to determine whether the decrease in proteinuria will result in significant preservation of renal function [196].

New-onset diabetes

Diabetes (➲Chapter 14) and hypertension are often associated and awareness that several antihypertensive agents may exert undesirable metabolic effects has prompted investigation (often post-hoc) of the incidence of new diabetes in antihypertensive treatment trials [197]. Almost all trials of antihypertensive therapy using new-onset diabetes as an endpoint have shown a significantly greater incidence in patients treated with diuretics and/or beta-blockers compared with ACE inhibitors, angiotensin receptor antagonists or calcium antagonists [109, 164, 170, 174, 176, 181, 198], with a few exceptions [167, 168] (➲Fig. 13.7). Administration of the angiotensin receptor antagonist valsartan and candesartan have been more beneficial on this end-point than administration of amlodipine [178, 182]. There are thus differences between different antihypertensive drugs on this end-point. This is likely to be clinically relevant because, in the long term, treatment-induced diabetes is accompanied by an increased incidence of cardiovascular disease as much as native diabetes [199–201].

Atrial fibrillation

Two large hypertension trials (VALUE [202] and LIFE [203]) have shown that the angiotensin receptor blockers are associated with a relative risk reduction of new atrial

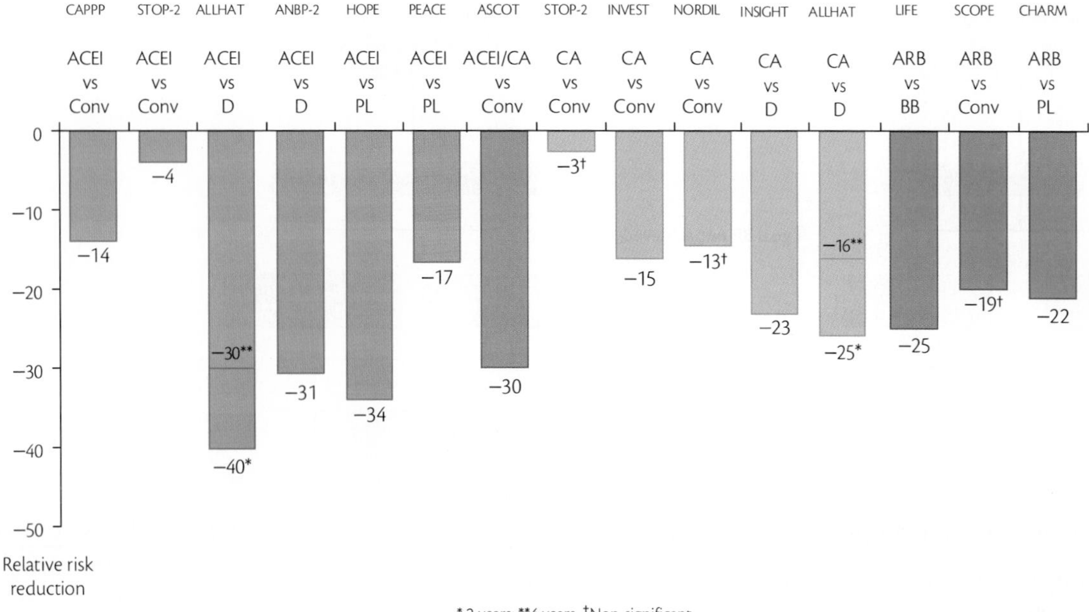

* 2 years; **4 years, †Non-significant

ACEI; ACE inhibitor, ARB; angiotensin receptor antagonist, BB; beta-blockers Conv; conventional treatment (BB/D), D; diuretics, PL; placebo

Figure 13.7 Prevention of new-onset diabetes: new versus placebo or conventional antihypertensive treatment.

fibrillation of 33% compared with beta-blocker in LIFE and 23% compared with calcium antagonist in VALUE, respectively (➲ Chapter 29). A lower incidence of new atrial fibrillation has also been observed in heart failure trials using ACE inhibitors and angiotensin receptor antagonist and some smaller studies have shown effects of angiotensin receptor antagonists on recurrent atrial fibrillation in patients with previous episodes of arrhythmia when used in addition to amiodarone [204]. No significant difference was seen between the ACE inhibitor ramipril, the angiotensin receptor antagonist telmisartan or the combination of both (ACE inhibitor + angiotensin receptor antagonist) in case of new-onset atrial fibrillation in the ONTARGET™ (Ongoing Telmisartan Alone and in Combination with Ramipril Global Endpoint Trial) [205]. Possible mechanisms for the reduction of atrial fibrillation seen after treatment with blockers of the renin-angiotensin system may in addition to the blood pressure reduction per se be prevention of left atrial dilatation, cardiac fibrosis and dysfunction, as well as a possible direct anti-arrhythmic effect [204].

Therapeutic strategies

Principles of drug treatment: monotherapy versus combination therapy (➲ Chapter 11)

In most, if not all, hypertensive patients, therapy should be started gently, and target blood pressure values achieved progressively through several weeks. To reach target blood pressure, it is likely that a large proportion of patients will require combination therapy with more than one agent. The proportion of patients requiring combination therapy will also depend on baseline blood pressure values. In grade 1 hypertensives, monotherapy is likely to be successful more frequently [113, 163, 164]. In trials on diabetic patients, the vast majority of patients were on at least two drugs, and in two trials on diabetic nephropathy [160, 161] an average of 2.5 and 3.0 non-study drugs were required in addition to the angiotensin receptor antagonist used as study drug.

According to the baseline blood pressure and the presence or absence of complications, it appears reasonable to initiate therapy either with a low dose of a single agent or with a low-dose combination of two agents (➲ Fig. 13.8). If low-dose monotherapy is chosen and blood pressure control is not achieved, the next step is to switch to a low dose of a different agent or to increase the dose of the first compound chosen (with a greater possibility of eliciting adverse disturbances) or to make recourse to combination therapy. If therapy has been initiated by a low-dose combination, a higher dose combination can subsequently be used or a low dose of a third compound added.

The following two-drug combinations have been found to be effective and well tolerated, but other combinations are possible (➲ Fig. 13.9):

- diuretic and ACE inhibitor;
- diuretic and angiotensin receptor antagonist;

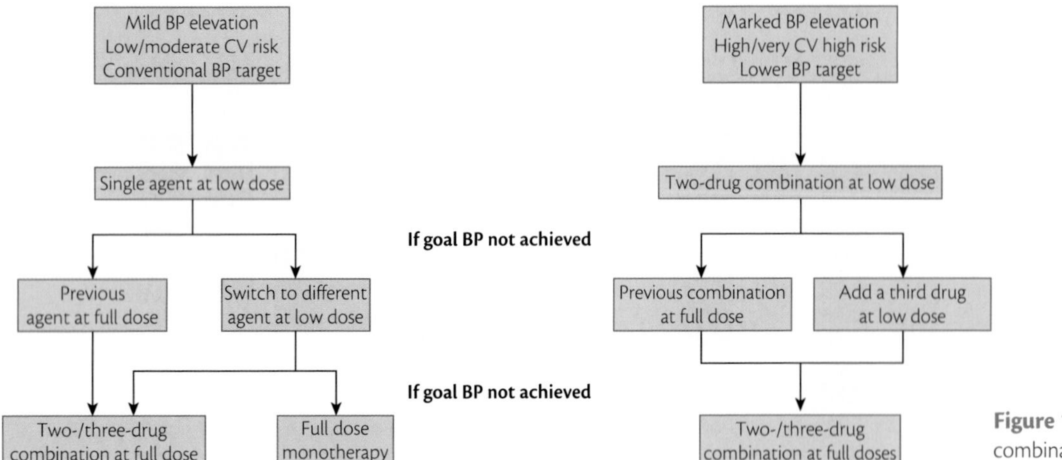

Figure 13.8 Monotherapy versus combination strategies.

- calcium antagonist (dihydropyridine) and beta-blocker;
- calcium antagonist and ACE inhibitor;
- calcium antagonist and angiotensin receptor antagonist;
- calcium antagonist and diuretic;
- other combinations can be used if necessary, and three or four drugs may be required in special cases.

The use of long-acting drugs or preparations providing 24-hour efficacy on a once-daily basis is recommended. The advantages of such medications include improvement in adherence to therapy and minimization of blood pressure variability, thus possibly providing greater protection against the risk of major cardiovascular events and the development of organ damage [206, 207].

Particular attention should be given to adverse events, even purely subjective disturbances, because they may be an important cause of non-compliance. Patients should always be asked about adverse effects, and dose or drug changes made accordingly. Even within the same drug class, there may be compounds less prone to induce a specific adverse effect (e.g. among beta-blockers, less fatigue or Raynaud's phenomenon with vasodilating compounds; among calcium antagonists, no constipation with dihydropyridines, no tachycardia with verapamil and diltiazem, variable degree of dependent oedema with different compounds).

Choice of antihypertensive drugs

A large number of randomized trials confirm that the main benefits of antihypertensive therapy are due to lowering of blood pressure per se, largely independently of the drugs used to lower blood pressure. There is also evidence, however, that specific drug classes may differ in some effect or in special groups of patients. Finally, drugs are not equal in terms of adverse disturbances, particularly in individual patients, and patients' preference is a prerequisite for compliance and therapy success.

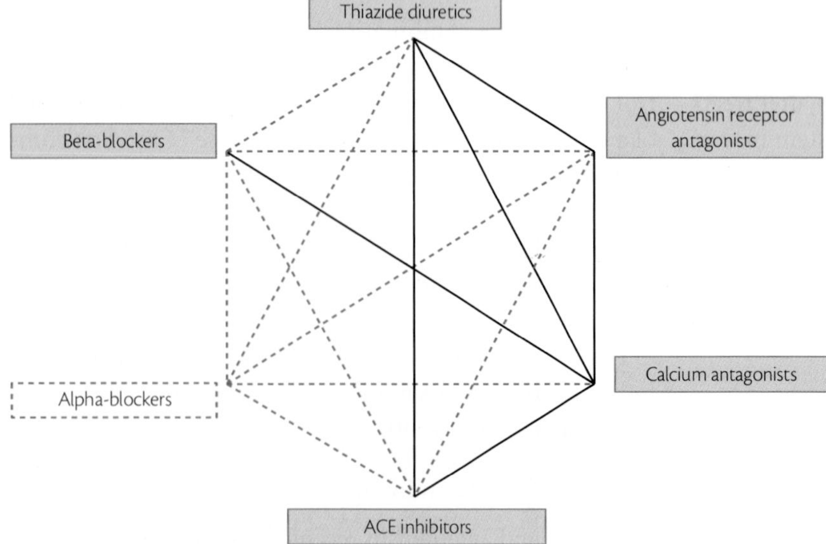

Figure 13.9 Possible combinations between some classes of antihypertensive drugs. The preferred combinations in the general hypertensive population are represented as black lines. The frames indicate classes of agents proven to be beneficial in controlled intervention trials.

It can therefore be concluded that the major classes of antihypertensive agents—diuretics, beta-blockers, calcium antagonists, ACE inhibitors, and angiotensin receptor antagonists—are suitable for the initiation and maintenance of antihypertensive therapy. Evidence favouring the use of alpha-blockers is less than evidence of the benefits of other antihypertensive agents, and it appears prudent to use alpha-blockers mostly for combination therapy. Emphasis on identifying the first class of drugs to be used is probably outdated by the awareness that two or more drugs in combination are necessary in the majority of patients, particularly those with higher initial blood pressures, or subclinical organ damage, or associated diseases, in order to achieve target blood pressure. Not withstanding, the two-drug combination that has been proven most effective in preventing endpoint is calcium-channel blocker plus ACE inhibitor. In the ASCOT (Anglo-Scandinavian Cardiac Outcomes Trial) [208], the combination of amlodipine plus perindopril was superior to atenolol plus bendroflumethiazide (second drug in about 60% in both arms) in preventing most CV endpoint and new-onset diabetes, and in ACCOMPLISH the combination of benazepril plus amlodipine was superior to benazepril plus hydrochlorothiazide (HCTZ) [209].

Because of the diabetogenic effects and inferiority in at least one major trial (ASCOT), the combination diuretic and beta-blocker is no longer recommended as first-line treatment in uncomplicated hypertensives with high metabolic risk.

Within the array of available agents, the choice of drugs will be influenced by many factors including:

- the previous favourable or unfavourable experience of the individual patient with a given class of compounds;
- the effect of drugs on cardiovascular risk factors in relation to the cardiovascular risk profile of the individual patient;
- the presence of subclinical organ damage, clinical cardiovascular disease, renal disease, and diabetes, which may be more favourably treated by some drugs than others;
- the presence of other coexisting disorders that may either favour or limit the use of particular classes of antihypertensive drugs;
- the possibility of interactions with drugs used for other conditions present;
- the cost of drugs, either to the individual patient or to the health provider, although cost considerations should not predominate over efficacy and tolerability in any individual patient;

The physician should tailor the choice of drugs to the individual patient, after taking all these factors, together with patient preference, into account. Indications and contraindications of specific drug classes are listed in ➲Tables 13.8 and 13.9, and therapeutic approaches to be preferred in special conditions are discussed in the next section.

Therapeutic approaches in special conditions

Elderly

There is little doubt from randomized controlled trials that older patients benefit from antihypertensive treatment in terms of reduced cardiovascular morbidity and mortality, whether they have systolic–diastolic hypertension [158] or isolated systolic hypertension [157]. Whereas trials in the elderly usually include patients who are at least 60 years old, a meta-analysis concluded that fatal and non-fatal cardiovascular events combined were significantly reduced in participants in randomized, controlled trials of antihypertensive drug treatment, who were aged 80 years and over, but all-cause mortality was not reduced [210]. However, with the recent publication of HYVET [211], treatment of hypertension also in the very old is proven to reduce mortality. In HYVET (Hypertension in the Very Elderly Trial) [211], the diuretic indapamide plus the ACE inhibitor perindopril was given; a reduction in systolic BP from about 173 to about 140mmHg largely reduced stroke, heart failure, and mortality.

The larger randomized controlled trials of antihypertensive treatment versus placebo or no treatment in elderly patients with systolic–diastolic hypertension used a diuretic or a beta-blocker as first-line therapy [158]. In trials on isolated systolic hypertension, first-line drugs consisted of a diuretic [13] or a dihydropyridine calcium antagonist [12, 212, 213]. In all of these trials, active therapy was superior to placebo or no treatment. Other drug classes have only been used in trials in which 'newer' drugs were compared with 'older' drugs [164, 167, 180, 181, 214]. It appears that benefit has been shown in older patients for at least one representative agent of several drug classes, i.e. diuretics, beta-blockers, calcium antagonist, ACE inhibitors, and angiotensin receptor antagonists. A recent meta-analysis of the BPLTTC concluded that reduction of blood pressure produces benefit in younger (<65 years) and older (≥65 years) adults, with no strong evidence that protection against major cardiovascular events afforded by different drug classes varies substantially with age [215].

Initiation of antihypertensive treatment in elderly patients should follow the general guidelines. Many patients will have other risk factors, subclinical organ damage, and associated cardiovascular conditions, to which the choice of the first

Table 13.8 Preferred drugs and conditions favouring use of some antihypertensive drugs

Subclinical organ damage	**Drug**
Left ventricular hypertrophy	ACE inhibitors, calcium antagonists, angiotensin receptor antagonists
Asymptomatic atherosclerosis	Calcium antagonists, ACE inhibitors
Microalbuminuria	ACE inhibitors, angiotensin receptor antagonists
Renal dysfunction	ACE inhibitors, angiotensin receptor antagonists
Clinical event	
Previous stroke	Any BP lowering agent
Previous myocardial infarction	Beta-blockers, ACE inhibitors, angiotensin receptor antagonists
Angina pectoris	Beta-blockers, calcium antagonists
Heart failure	Diuretics, beta-blockers, ACE inhibitors, angiotensin receptor antagonists, antialdosterone agents
Atrial fibrillation:	
recurrent	ACE inhibitors, angiotensin receptor antagonists
continuous	Beta-blockers, non-dihydropiridine calcium antagonists
Renal failure/proteinuria	ACE inhibitors, angiotensin receptor antagonists, loop diuretics
Peripheral artery disease	Calcium antagonists
Condition	
Isolated systolic hypertension (elderly)	Diuretics, calcium antagonists
Metabolic syndrome	ACE inhibitors, angiotensin receptor antagonists, calcium antagonists
Diabetes mellitus	ACE inhibitors, angiotensin receptor antagonists
Pregnancy	Calcium antagonists, methyldopa, beta-blockers
Hypertension in blacks	Diuretics, calcium antagonists

Thiazide diuretics	**Beta-blockers**	**Calcium antagonists (dihydropyridines)**	**Calcium antagonists (verapamil/ diltiazem)**
◆ Isolated systolic hypertension (elderly) ◆ Heart failure ◆ Hypertension in blacks	◆ Angina pectoris ◆ Post-myocardial infarction ◆ Heart failure ◆ Tachyarrhythmias ◆ Glaucoma ◆ Pregnancy	◆ Isolated systolic hypertension (elderly) ◆ Angina pectoris ◆ LV hypertrophy ◆ Carotid/coronary atherosclerosis ◆ Pregnancy ◆ Hypertension in blacks	◆ Angina pectoris ◆ Carotid atherosclerosis ◆ Supraventricular tachycardia
ACE Inhibitors	**Angiotensin receptor antagonists**	**Diuretics (antialdosterone)**	**Loop diuretics**
◆ Heart failure ◆ LV dysfunction ◆ Post-myocardial infarction ◆ Diabetic nephropathy ◆ Non-diabetic nephropathy ◆ LV hypertrophy ◆ Carotid atherosclerosis ◆ Proteinuria/ microalbuminuria ◆ Atrial fibrillation ◆ Metabolic syndrome	◆ Heart failure ◆ Post-myocardial infarction ◆ Diabetic nephropathy ◆ Proteinuria/microalbuminuria ◆ LV hypertrophy ◆ Atrial fibrillation ◆ Metabolic syndrome ◆ ACEI-induced cough	◆ Heart failure ◆ Post-myocardial infarction	◆ End stage renal disease ◆ Heart failure

drug should be tailored. Furthermore, many patients will need two or more drugs to control blood pressure, particularly due to the fact that it is often difficult to lower systolic pressure to below 140mmHg [123, 216]. A post hoc analysis of the Syst-Eur (Systolic Hypertension in Europe) trial suggests that antihypertensive treatment can be intensified to prevent cardiovascular events when systolic blood pressure is not under control in older patients with systolic hypertension, at least until diastolic blood pressure reaches about 55mmHg. However, a prudent approach is warranted

Table 13.9 Compelling and possible contraindications to use of antihypertensive drugs

	Compelling	Possible
Thiazide diuretics	Gout	Metabolic syndrome Glucose intolerance Pregnancy
Beta-blockers	Asthma A–V block (grade 2 or 3)	Peripheral artery disease Metabolic syndrome Glucose intolerance Athletes and physically active patients Chronic obstructive pulmonary disease
Calcium antagonists (dihydropyridines)		Tachyarrhythmias Heart failure
Calcium antagonists (verapamil, diltiazem)	A–V block (grade 2 or 3) Heart failure	
ACE inhibitors	Pregnancy Angioneurotic oedema Hyperkalaemia Bilateral renal artery stenosis	
Angiotensin receptor antagonists	Pregnancy Hyperkalaemia Bilateral renal artery stenosis	
Diuretics (anti-aldosterone)	Renal failure Hyperkalaemia	

in patients with concomitant coronary heart disease, in whom diastolic blood pressure should probably not be lowered to less than 70mmHg [217].

Diabetes mellitus

The prevalence of hypertension is increased in patients with diabetes mellitus [218] (➲Chapter 14). Type 2 diabetes is by far the most common form, occurring about 10–20 times as often as type 1. Hypertensive patients frequently exhibit a condition known as 'metabolic syndrome', i.e. a syndrome associating insulin resistance (with the concomitant hyperinsulinaemia), central obesity, and characteristic dyslipidaemia (high plasma triglyceride and low HDL- cholesterol) [24, 219]. These patients are prone to develop type 2 diabetes.

In type 1 diabetes, hypertension often reflects the onset of diabetic nephropathy [220], whereas a large fraction of hypertensive patients have still normoalbuminuria at the time of diagnosis of type 2 diabetes [221]. The prevalence of hypertension (defined as a blood pressure ≥140/90mmHg) in patients with type 2 diabetes and normoalbuminuria is very high up to about 70%, and increases even further to 90% in the presence of microalbuminuria [222].

The coexistence of hypertension and diabetes mellitus (either of type 1 or 2) substantially increases the risk of macrovascular complications, including stroke, coronary heart disease, congestive heart failure, and peripheral vascular disease, and is responsible for an excessive cardiovascular mortality [220, 223]. The presence of microalbuminuria is both an early marker of renal damage and an indicator of increased cardiovascular risk [224, 225]. There is also evidence that hypertension accelerates the development of diabetic retinopathy [226]. The level of blood pressure achieved during treatment greatly influences the outcome of diabetic patients. In patients with diabetic nephropathy, the rate of progression of renal disease is in a continuous relationship with blood pressure until a level of 130mmHg systolic and 70mmHg diastolic is reached. Aggressive treatment of hypertension protects patients with type 2 diabetes against cardiovascular events. The primary goal of antihypertensive treatment in diabetics should be to lower blood pressure below 130/80mmHg whenever possible, the best blood pressure being the lowest one that remains tolerated. This concept was further supported by the recently published ADVANCE (Action in Diabetes and Vascular Disease: Preterax and Diamicron MR Controlled Evaluation) trial [227].

Weight gain is a critical factor in the progression to type 2 diabetes and intensive lifestyle measures should be implemented with particular emphasis on interventions (caloric restriction and increased physical activity) favouring weight reduction to decrease blood pressure and improve glucose tolerance [228]. To fight against overweight by calorie restriction and a decrease in sodium intake is essential, as a strong relationship exists between obesity, hypertension, sodium sensitivity and insulin resistance [229].

No major trial has been performed to assess the effect of pharmacological blood pressure lowering on cardiovascular morbidity and mortality in hypertensive patients with type 1 diabetes. There is, however, good evidence that beta-blocker and diuretic-based antihypertensive therapy delays the progression of nephropathy in these patients [230]. In albuminuric patients with type 1 diabetes the best protection against renal function deterioration is obtained by ACE inhibition [231]. It remains unknown whether angiotensin receptor antagonists are equally effective in this indication.

As to antihypertensive treatment in type 2 diabetes [190, 232], evidence of the superiority or inferiority of different drug classes is still vague and contradictory. Superiority of ACE inhibitors in preventing the aggregate of major cardiovascular events is limited to two trials, one against diuretics/beta-blockers [174] and the other against a calcium antagonist [129], or on analyses of cause-specific events for which the trial power was even less. The ALLHAT trial [164] has also failed to find differences in cardiovascular outcomes in the larger number of type 2 diabetes patients included in the trial, randomized to a diuretic, a calcium antagonist or an ACE inhibitor. Evidence concerning angiotensin receptor antagonists has shown a significant reduction of cardiovascular events, cardiovascular death, and total mortality in diabetics when losartan was compared with atenolol [191], but not when irbesartan was compared with amlodipine [161]. If renal end-points are also considered, the benefits of angiotensin receptor antagonists become more evident, as the IDNT (Irbesartan in Diabetic Nephropathy Trial) [161] showed a reduction in renal dysfunction and failure by the use of irbesartan rather than amlodipine, and LIFE [191] indicated losartan reduced proteinuria better than atenolol. In conclusion, in view of the consensus that blood pressure in type 2 diabetic patients must be lowered, whenever possible, to <130/80mmHg, it appears reasonable to recommend that all effective and well-tolerated antihypertensive agents can be used, frequently combinations of two or more drugs are needed. Available evidence indicates that lowering blood pressure also exerts a protective effect on appearance and progression of renal damage and some additional protection can be obtained by the use of a blocker of the renin–angiotensin system (either an angiotensin receptor antagonist or an ACE inhibitor). Antihypertensive drugs should also be considered when blood pressure is in the high normal range and in the presence of microalbuminuria. In the presence of microalbuminuria or diabetic nephropathy, treatment should start with or include a drug acting against the renin–angiotensin system. Lipid lowering agents should also be considered because of the result of the CARDS (Collaborative Atorvastatin Diabetes Study) trial [233], which indicated that diabetic patients benefit from having their lipids tightly controlled.

Concomitant cerebrovascular disease

Evidence of the benefits of antihypertensive therapy in patients who had already suffered a stroke or a transient ischaemic attack (TIA) (secondary prevention) was equivocal [234], and no definite recommendation could be given until the PROGRESS (Perindopril Protection Against Recurrent Stroke Study) clearly showed the benefits of lowering blood pressure in patients with previous episodes of cardiovascular disease, even when their initial blood pressure was in the normal range [108]. The benefit was proven for the combination of indapamide and perindopril [108]. The recent PRoFESS (Prevention Regimen For Effectively Avoiding Second Strokes) study of telmisartan versus placebo on top of other antihypertensive medication showed a trend for less recurrent stroke but did not reach significance likely because of loss of statistical power [235].

The other issue, whether elevated blood pressure during an acute stroke should be lowered at all, or to what extent and how, is still a disputed one, for which there are more questions than answers, but trials are in progress. A statement by a special International Society of Hypertension (ISH) panel has been published [236].

Concomitant coronary heart disease and congestive heart failure

The risk of a recurrent event in patients with coronary heart disease is significantly affected by the blood pressure level [237], and hypertension is frequently a past or present clinical problem in patients with congestive heart failure [238] (➲Chapter 23). However, few trials have tested the effects of blood pressure lowering in patients with coronary heart disease or congestive heart failure. The HOT Study showed a significant reduction of strokes when the target blood pressure in hypertensives with previous signs of ischaemic heart disease was lowered, and found no evidence of a J-shaped curve [113, 117].

Apart from the INVEST study [176], many of the more common blood pressure lowering agents have been assessed in patients with coronary heart disease or heart failure with objectives other than reduction of blood pressure. Beta-blockers, ACE inhibitors, and anti-aldosterone compounds are well established in the treatment regimens for preventing cardiovascular events and prolonging life in patients after an acute myocardial infarction and with heart failure, but how much of the benefit is due to concomitant blood pressure lowering and how much to specific drug actions has never been clarified. There are also data in support of the use of angiotensin receptor antagonists in congestive heart failure as alternatives to ACE inhibitors, especially in ACE inhibitor intolerance or in combination with ACE inhibitors [239, 240]. The role of calcium antagonists in prevention of coronary events has been vindicated by the ALLHAT trial, which showed a long-acting dihydropyridine to be equally effective as the other antihypertensive compounds [164]. Calcium antagonists are possibly less effective in prevention of congestive heart failure, but a long-acting compound such as amlodipine may be used, if hypertension is resistant to other compounds [241].

Hypertensive patients with deranged renal function

Renal vasoconstriction is found in the initial stages of essential hypertension and this is reversed by the administration of calcium antagonists and ACE inhibitors. In more advanced stages of the disease, renal vascular resistance is permanently elevated as a consequence of structural lesions of the renal vessels (nephrosclerosis). Before antihypertensive treatment became available, renal involvement was frequent in patients with primary hypertension. Renal protection in diabetes requires two main accomplishments: first, to attain a very strict blood pressure control (<130/80mmHg and even lower, <125/75mmHg, when proteinuria >1g per day is present) and, second, to lower proteinuria or albuminuria (micro- or macro-) to values as near to normalcy as possible. In order to attain the latter goal, blockade of the effects of angiotensin II (either with an ACE inhibitor or with an angiotensin receptor antagonist) is required. In order to achieve the blood pressure goal, combination therapy is usually required, even in patients with high normal blood pressure [190]. The addition of a diuretic as second-step therapy is usually recommended (a loop diuretic if serum creatinine >2mg/dL), but other combinations, in particular with calcium antagonists, can also be considered. To prevent or retard development of nephrosclerosis, blockade of the renin–angiotensin system has been reported to be more important than attaining very low blood pressure [193]. On the whole, it seems prudent to start antihypertensive therapy in patients (diabetic or non-diabetic) with reduced renal function, especially if accompanied by proteinuria, by an ACE inhibitor, or an angiotensin receptor antagonist, and then add other antihypertensive agents in order to further lower blood pressure (➲Chapter 15).

Resistant hypertension

Hypertension may be termed resistant to treatment, or refractory, when a therapeutic plan that has included attention to lifestyle measures and the prescription of at least three drugs (including a diuretic) in adequate doses has failed to lower systolic and diastolic blood pressure sufficiently. In these situations, referral to a specialist should be considered because resistant hypertension may be due to secondary hypertension and is often associated with subclinical organ damage and a high added cardiovascular risk. More specific causes of resistant hypertension are listed in ➲Table 13.10.

Table 13.10 Causes of resistant hypertension [1, 2]

Poor adherence to therapeutic plan
Failure to modify lifestyle including:
weight gain
heavy alcohol intake (NB: binge drinking)
Continued intake of drugs that raise blood pressure (liquorice, cocaine, glucocorticoids, non-steroidal anti-inflammatory drugs, etc.)
Obstructive sleep apnoea
Unsuspected secondary cause
Irreversible or scarcely reversible organ damage
Volume overload due to:
inadequate diuretic therapy
progressive renal insufficiency
high sodium intake
hyperaldosteronism
Causes of spurious resistant hypertension:
isolated office (white coat) hypertension
failure to use large cuff on large arm
pseudohypertension

Hypertensive emergencies

Hypertensive emergencies are observed when severe forms of high blood pressure are associated with acute damage to target organs. The most important emergencies are listed in ➲Table 13.11. Such emergencies are rare but can be life threatening and the management of hypertension must be rapid. Care should be taken, however, that extremely rapid falls in blood pressure may not be associated with complications such as underperfusion of the brain and cerebral infarction or damage to the myocardium and kidneys.

Malignant hypertension embraces a syndrome of severe elevation of arterial blood pressure (diastolic blood pressure usually but not always >140mmHg) with vascular damage that can be particularly manifest as retinal haemorrhages, exudates, and/or papilloedema. Malignant hypertension may be seen in a variety of conditions and must be regarded as a hypertension emergency. Oral medication can be used if blood pressure is responsive, with the goal to bring diastolic blood pressure down to 100–110mmHg over 24 hours.

Table 13.11 Hypertensive emergencies

Hypertensive encephalopathy
Hypertensive left ventricular failure
Hypertension with myocardial infarction
Hypertension with unstable angina pectoris
Hypertension and dissection of the aorta
Severe hypertension associated with subarachnoid haemorrhage or cerebrovascular accident
Crisis associated with phaeochromocytoma
Use of recreational drugs such as amphetamines, LSD, cocaine, or ecstasy
Hypertension perioperatively
Severe pre-eclampsia or eclampsia

Personal perspective

In hypertensive patients, the primary goal of treatment is to achieve maximum reduction in the long-term total risk of cardiovascular disease. Modern antihypertensive treatment should usually be given as a combination of well-tolerated drugs, not withholding lifestyle changes when appropriate. There is solid documentation of cardiovascular protection; although most benefit is related to the blood pressure reduction per se, there is evidence in certain patient groups, such as diabetics and patients with left-ventricular hypertrophy, that benefits may be better with certain drugs. However, blood pressure control among patients is still on average suboptimal or even poor, and this applies even more so to patients with complicated hypertension and particular high risk. The challenge for the future is to implement the knowledge from the research and provide equal levels of care for all hypertensive patients. Newer drugs seem better tolerated than the old ones, but they have not been studied in the vast majority of patients—namely those with mild blood pressure elevation only. It is a challenge for all to document more solid prognostic improvements among these patients, including examining the cost–benefit of treating these patients. Treatment of associated risk factors with lipid lowering agents, antiplatelet therapy, and glycaemic control in diabetics should also be considered. Full implementation of ambulatory and home blood pressure assessments in clinical practice still needs better documentation. Isolated office or white coat hypertension, and also the reversed phenomenon in patients with high ambulatory but low office blood pressure, need better understanding. Prevention of certain not so 'hard' but still important end-points, such as new-onset diabetes, atrial fibrillation, and vascular dementia, needs extensive investigations. The breakthrough of genetic stratification in the field of hypertension research is also still to come.

Further reading

Mancia G, De Backer G, Dominiczak A, *et al.* 2007 Guidelines for the management of arterial hypertension: The Task Force for the Management of Arterial Hypertension of the European Society of Hypertension (ESH) and of the European Society of Cardiology (ESC). *Eur Heart J* 2007; **28**: 1462–536.

Parati G, Stergiou GS, Asmar R, *et al.* European Society of Hypertension guidelines for blood pressure monitoring at home: a summary report of the Second International Consensus Conference on Home Blood Pressure Monitoring. *J Hypertens.* 2008; **26**: 1505–26.

Ruilope L, Kjeldsen SE, Sierra A, et al. The kidney and cardiovascular risk – implications for management: A Consensus Statement from the European Society of Hypertension. *Blood Pressure* 2007; **16**: 72–9.

Zanchetti A, Mancia G, Black H, *et al.* Facts and fallacies of blood pressure control in recent trials: Implications in the management of patients with hypertension. *J Hypertens* 2009; **27**: 673–9.

Online resources

dabl® Educational Trust: blood pressure monitors-validations, papers, and reviews: http://www.dableducational.org/welcome.html

For full references and multimedia materials please visit the online version of the book (http://esctextbook.oxfordonline.com).

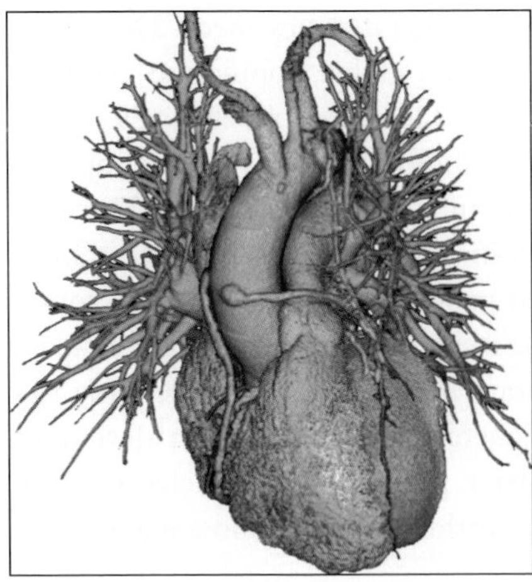

CHAPTER 14

Diabetes Mellitus and Metabolic Syndrome

Francesco Cosentino, Lars Rydén, Pietro Francia, and Linda G. Mellbin

Contents

Summary

This chapter reviews an evidence-based approach to diagnosis and treatment of diabetes mellitus and metabolic syndrome according to recent scientific evidence and recommendations of major international guidelines. The pathophysiology and clinical management of atherosclerotic complications are considered as a continuum rather than separate issues, merging basic and clinical sciences into a 'bench-to-bedside' approach.

It is estimated that diabetes affects about 246 million people world-wide, with an expected 55% increase to 380 million in 2025. Approximately 50% of persons above the age of 60 years will meet current diagnostic criteria for metabolic syndrome in the near future. Hyperglycaemia, insulin resistance, and the consequent cellular shift to an increased oxidative stress carry a high risk for development of comorbidities and cardiovascular risk factors, mainly hypertension, lipid disorders, a proinflammatory state, and activation of coagulation and thrombosis. As a consequence, the incidence of and mortality from all forms of cardiovascular disease are two- to eightfold higher in persons with diabetes, and coronary artery disease accounts for 75% of all deaths in such individuals. The impressive burden of the disease supports the employment of comprehensive risk stratification systems to identify patients who, besides glycaemic control, will benefit from a multifactorial management with statins, aspirin, renin–angiotensin system antagonists, and coronary interventions supplemented by drug-eluting stents and antithrombotic agents to prevent cardiovascular events.

Introduction

Diabetes mellitus is characterized by a state of long-standing hyperglycaemia, hyperinsulinaemia, and excess circulating free fatty acids resulting from environmental and genetic factors. The prevalence of diabetes is increasing rapidly, and individuals with diabetes are at high risk for cardiovascular disorders that affect the heart, brain, and peripheral vessels. Although cardiovascular disease (CVD) accompanying diabetes is on the rise, many open issues remain concerning the temporal relations between diabetes and CVD, the contribution of conventional risk factors, and the role of diabetes-specific risk factors. The major CVD risk factors, including elevated low-density lipoprotein (LDL)-cholesterol, hypertension, and smoking, remain important determinants of CVD in diabetic patients (➲Chapter 12). In addition, emerging risk factors such as hyperglycaemia, insulin resistance, albuminuria, fibrinogen and enhanced inflammatory activation, further affect the risk. Hence the significant clustering of atherogenic risk factors links the current epidemic of diabetes and CVD. Indeed, diabetes mellitus magnifies the risk of cardiovascular morbidity and mortality [1]. Besides the well-recognized microvascular complications of diabetes, such as nephropathy and retinopathy, macrovascular complications, including diseases of coronary, peripheral, and carotid vessels, cause common problems.

This chapter will consider the pathophysiology and management of atherosclerotic complications of diabetes as a continuum and not as separate sections. Nowadays, physicians caring for patients with CVD must understand the effects of diabetes mellitus and the detrimental accumulation of risk factors on the heart and blood vessels. Early detection and intervention of the atherogenic metabolic abnormalities and glucose intolerance that precede development of diabetes is mandatory. A high priority is given to the modification of the major risk factors for CVD. Increasing evidence indicates that controlling CVD risk factors will reduce onset of CVD and its complications in patients with diabetes [2].

Epidemiology of diabetes and impaired glucose tolerance

In 1997, Amos and colleagues [3] estimated the global burden of diabetes to be 124 million people, and projected an increase to 221 million by the year 2010. The most recent predictions made by the International Federation of Diabetes supercedes these numbers, estimating that diabetes affects 246 million people in 2007 (6% of the global population) with an expected 55% increase to 380 million in 2025 (7% of the global population). In addition, 308 million have impaired glucose tolerance (IGT) in 2007 with an expected increase of 36% to 418 million in 2025 (➲Fig. 14.1). A substantial proportion of affected people are unaware of their condition and do not receive treatment. The increasing frequency of obesity and sedentary lifestyles, major underlying risk factors for type 2 diabetes, and IGT in both developed and developing countries, portends that diabetes will continue to be a growing worldwide entity and a major cause of CVD.

Diagnostic criteria

The diagnosis of type 1 diabetes is often prompted by symptoms such as increased thirst and urinary volume, recurrent infections, unexplained weight loss, and glycosuria. A glucose value above the diagnostic targets presented in ➲Table 14.1 establishes the diagnosis while type 2 diabetes not infrequently remains without symptoms until a cardiovascular event leads to the measurement of plasma glucose levels. A fasting plasma glucose (FPG) of <6.1mmol/L (<110mg/dl) is considered normal. Impaired fasting glucose encompasses FPGs >6.1mmol/L but <7mmol/L (<126mg/dL). An FPG >7.0mmol/L establishes the diagnosis of diabetes mellitus.

Among routine tests of glucose metabolism, the 2-hour oral glucose tolerance test (OGTT) most closely reflects postprandial glucose disposal. Patients fast overnight, then have blood drawn for plasma glucose before and 2 hours after the ingestion of an oral load of 75g of dextrose. IGT corresponds to a 2-hour glucose concentration between 7.8mmol/L (140mg/dL) and 11.1mmol/L (199mg/dL), while diabetes is defined as a value >11.1mmol/L (>200mg/dL) [4].

For clinical purposes, an OGTT should be considered if causal blood glucose values lie in the uncertain range (i.e. between the levels that establish or exclude diabetes) and FPG levels are below those which establish the diagnosis of diabetes. In this regard, despite the recent lowering by the American Diabetes Association (ADA) [5] of the value of normal FPG concentration to 5.5mmol/L and impaired fasting glucose (IFG) (from >5.5mmol/L to <7.0mmol/L), many individuals with abnormal glucose metabolism remain unidentified if not challenged with a 2-hour post-glucose value. In particular, lower fasting glucose levels may be seen in persons who have 2-hour post-load glucose values that are diagnostic for diabetes in less obese subjects and the elderly. On the other hand, middle-aged,

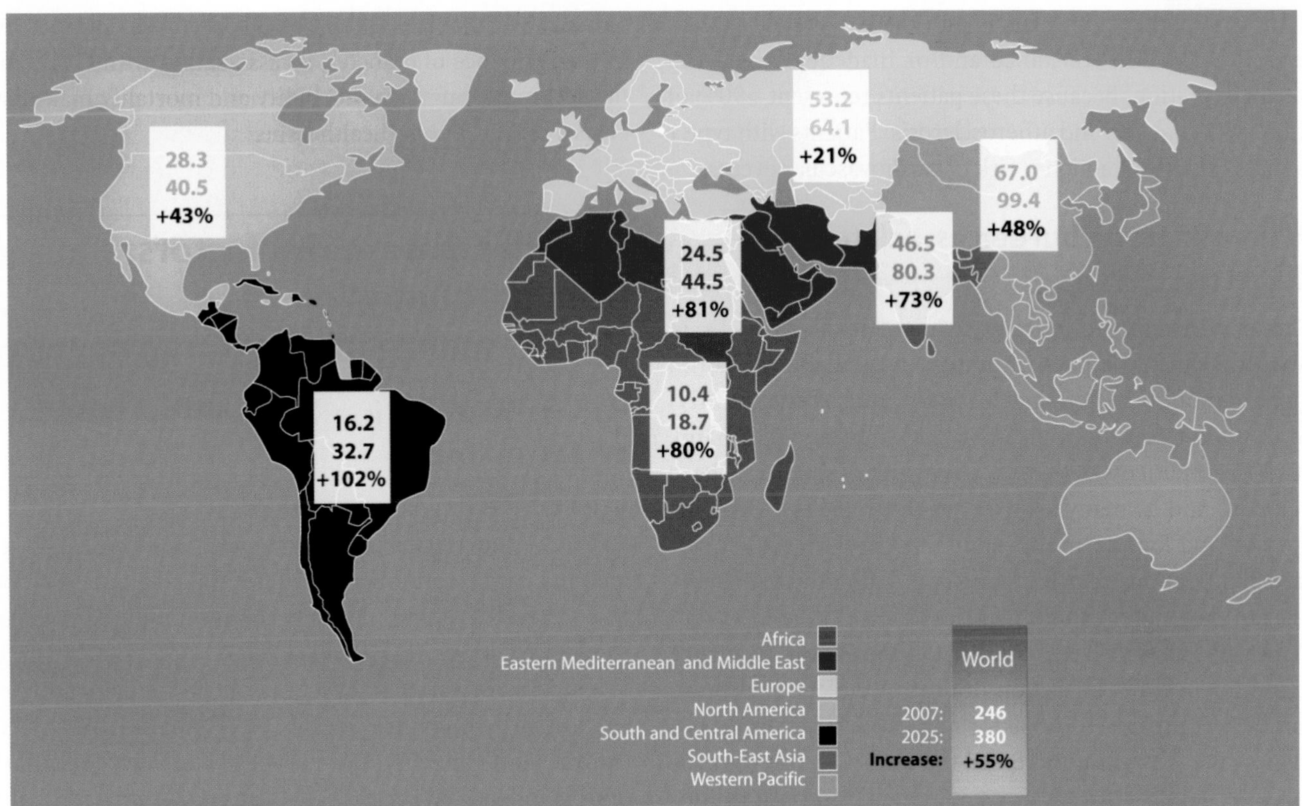

Figure 14.1 Global projections for the number of people with diabetes (20–79 years age group), 2007 and 2025 (millions). Reproduced with permission from *IDF Atlas*, 3rd edn., ©International Diabetes Federation 2006. http://www.eatlas.idf.org/prevalence

more obese patients are more likely to have diagnostic fasting values. Diagnosis requires the identification of individuals at risk for development of complications in whom early preventive strategies are indicated. Ideally both the 2-hour and the fasting value should be used [6]. IGT or IFG are not clinical entities, but rather risk categories for future diabetes and/or CVD. IGT is often associated with the metabolic syndrome (insulin-resistance syndrome). Thus, IGT may not be directly involved in the pathogenesis of CVD, but rather act as a marker of enhanced risk.

Table 14.1 Values for diagnosis of diabetes mellitus and other categories of hyperglycaemia

	Venous glucose concentration, mmol/L (mg/dL)	
	Whole blood	**Plasma**
Diabetes mellitus		
Fasting	≥6.1 (≥110)	≥7.0 (≥126)
or		
2-hour post glucose load	≥10.0 (≥180)	≥11.1 (≥200)
or both		
Impaired glucose tolerance (IGT)		
Fasting (if measured)	<6.1 (< 110)	<7.0 (<126)
and		
2-hour post glucose load	≥6.7 (≥120) and <10.0 (<180)	≥7.8 (≥140) and <11.1 (<200)
Impaired fasting glycaemia (IFG)		
Fasting	≥5.6 (≥100) and <6.1 (<110)	≥6.1 (≥110) and <7.0 (<126)
and (if measured)		
2-hour post glucose load	<6.7 (<120)	<7.8 (<140)

Modified with permission from WHO. *Definition, diagnosis and classification of diabetes mellitus and its complications. Part 1: Diagnosis and classification of diabetes mellitus. Report of a WHO consultation*. Geneva: WHO.

In this chapter, the focus is on type 2 diabetes, characterized by insulin resistance and/or inadequate beta-cell insulin secretion, because these patients represent >90% of those with diabetes and atherosclerosis. Patients with type 1 diabetes also have a higher risk of cardiovascular events.

Atherosclerotic burden associated with diabetes

The incidence of and mortality from all forms of CVD are two- to eightfold higher in persons with diabetes than in those without diabetes, and coronary artery disease (CAD) accounts for 75% of all deaths [7, 8]. On the other hand, 20–30% of patients with an acute coronary syndrome have diabetes, and as many as 40% have IGT [9–11]. Both in-hospital and long-term mortality rates after an acute myocardial infarction are twice as high for patients with diabetes than among those without diabetes (➲Fig. 14.2).

In a population-based study [12] the 7-year incidence of first myocardial infarction or death for diabetic patients was 20% compared to 3.5% for non-diabetics. A history of myocardial infarction increased the rate of recurrent myocardial infarction or cardiovascular death in both groups (18.8% in non-diabetic persons and 45% in those with diabetes). Thus patients with diabetes, but without previous myocardial infarction, carry the same level of risk for subsequent acute coronary events as non-diabetic patients with previous myocardial infarction. This led the Adult Treatment Panel III of the National Cholesterol Education Program to establish diabetes as a CAD risk equivalent, mandating aggressive antiatherosclerotic treatment [13]. Comorbidities—including renal insufficiency, peripheral and cerebral vascular disease—that are more prevalent in patients with diabetes, often worsen outcomes. The increase in the incidence of diabetes, its association with CVD, and the accompanying high morbidity and mortality make diabetes a serious public-health issue.

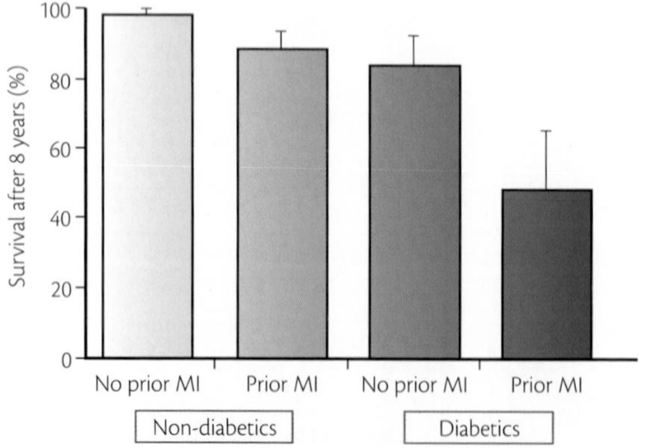

Figure 14.2 Mortality in diabetics after myocardial infarction. Modified with permission from Haffner SM, Lehto S, Ronnemaa T, *et al.* Mortality from coronary heart disease in subjects with type 2 diabetes and in nondiabetic subjects with and without prior myocardial infarction. *N Engl J Med* 1998; **339**: 229–34.

Vascular disease risk factors: from pathophysiology to clinical management

Hyperglycaemia, insulin resistance, and oxidative stress

Hyperglycaemia

Hyperglycaemia characterizes both type 1 and type 2 diabetes mellitus. Since a number of studies linked elevated blood glucose levels to excess mortality and morbidity from vascular disease [14], growing efforts focus on clarifying the effects of glucose on vascular function, in particular endothelial function and nitric oxide (NO) bioavailability. The endothelium contributes to the control of vascular smooth muscle tone by NO release that causes vasodilatation and platelet inhibition, thereby preventing vasoconstriction and thrombus formation. NO is generated from a terminal guanidino nitrogen of l-arginine and is catalysed by a family of enzymes called NO synthases (NOSs). One of these enzymes, endothelial NOS (eNOS), is Ca^{2+}-dependent and is constitutively present in various cell types, including endothelial cells.

The activity of the l-arginine/NO pathway is a balance between synthesis and breakdown of NO by its reaction with the superoxide anion (O_2^-). Under physiological conditions the production of this molecule is not markedly affected by O_2^-. Hence, NO may exert its vascular protective effects favouring an anti-atherosclerotic environment. However, in the presence of cardiovascular risk factors, an excessive production of O_2^- occurs rapidly, inactivating NO and leading to the formation of high concentrations of peroxynitrite ($ONOO^-$), a very powerful oxidant (➲Fig. 14.3).

Endothelial dysfunction, an early feature of diabetic vascular disease, is characterized by a decrease in NO bioavailability and a concomitant increase in vascular O_2^- production [15–17] (➲Fig. 14.4). Loss of NO bioavailability precedes the development of overt atherosclerosis and is an independent predictor of adverse cardiovascular events [18].

Mitochondrial O_2^- production has been recognized as an important mediator of hyperglycaemic vascular damage [16]. A further increase in O_2^- is driven by a vicious circle involving

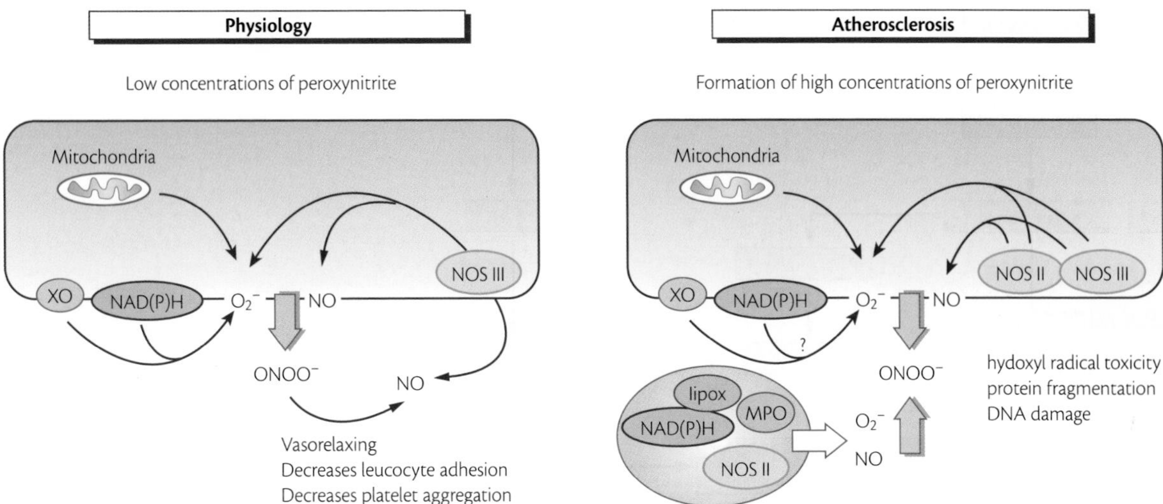

Figure 14.3 In the atherosclerotic setting, an excessive production of O_2^- occurs. O_2^- rapidly inactivates NO leading to the formation of high concentrations of peroxynitrite ($ONOO^-$), a condition associated with cellular toxicity. Please note the putative sources of O_2^- in the left panel. Reproduced with permission from Wever RM, Lüscher TF, Cosentino F, *et al.* Atherosclerosis and the two faces of endothelial nitric oxide synthase. *Circulation* 1998; **97**: 108–12.

ROS-induced activation of protein kinase C (PKC) [15] and vice versa PKC-mediated ROS production. Indeed, activation of PKC by glucose has been implicated in the regulation and activation of NAD(P)H-dependent oxidase, a major vascular source of O_2^- production [16, 19]. NAD(P)H activity and subunit protein expression are enhanced in the internal mammary arteries and saphenous veins of diabetic patients [20]. Although a high glucose-dependent PKC activation leads to an upregulation of eNOS expression, this is outbalanced by the increased NO breakdown causing a net reduction of its bioavailability. Thus, activation of the PKC pathway represents a proximal node in the intracellular signalling leading to hyperglycaemia-induced oxidative stress and endothelial dysfunction [21] (➲Fig. 14.5).

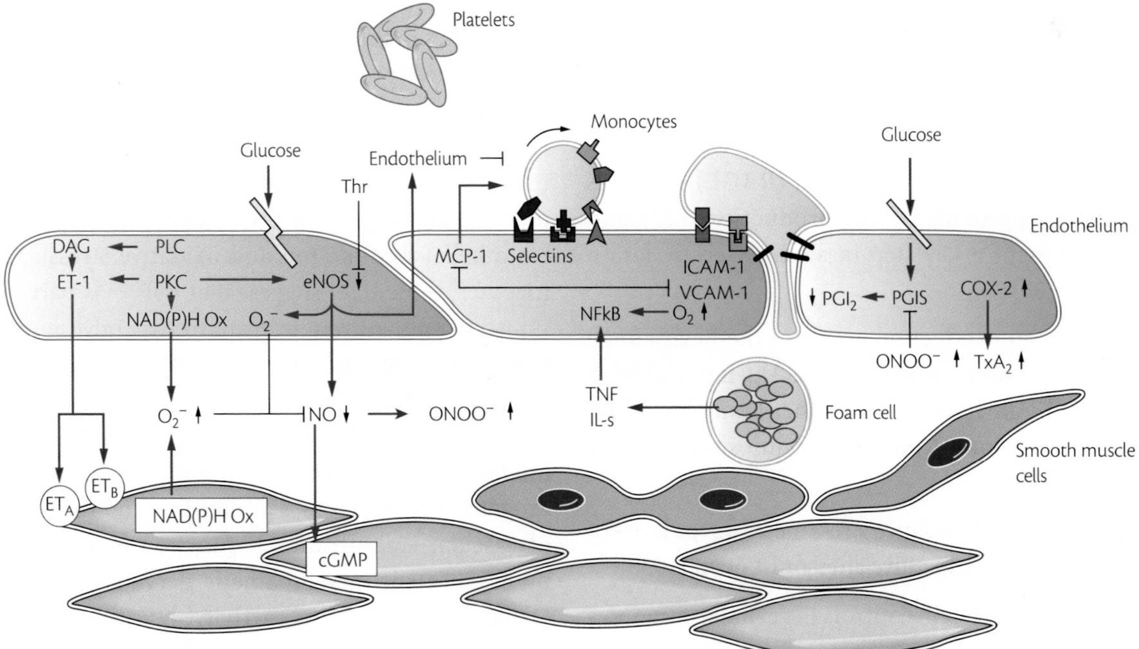

Figure 14.4 Hyperglycaemia and endothelium-derived vasoactive substances. COX-2 cyclooxygenase-2; DAG, diacylglycerol; eNOS, endothelial nitric oxide synthase; ILs interleukins; MCP-1, monocyte chemoattractant factor-1; NADPH Ox, nicotinamide adenine dinucleotide phosphate oxidase; NF-kB, nuclear factor kappa B; O_2^-, superoxide anion; $ONOO^-$, peroxynitrite; PKC, protein kinase C; PLC, phospholipase C; Thr, thrombin; TNF, tumor necrosis factor. Reproduced with permission from Creager MA, Lüscher TF, Cosentino F, *et al.* Diabetes and vascular disease: pathophysiology, clinical consequences and medical therapy: Part I. *Circulation* 2003; **108**: 1527–32.

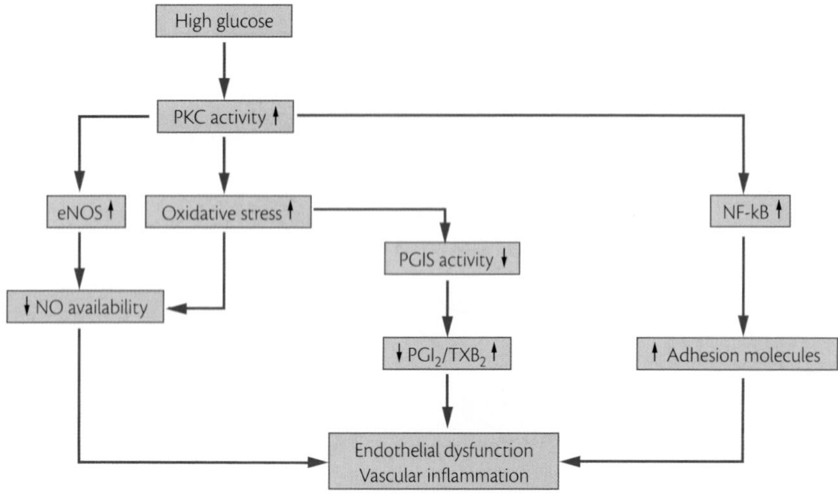

Figure 14.5 A single unifying PKC-dependent mechanism is the triggering step by which hyperglycaemia induces endothelial dysfunction and vascular inflammation. PGI_2/TXB_2, prostacyclin/thromboxane; PGIS, prostacyclin synthase; PKC, protein kinase C.

Oxygen-derived free radical excess affects endothelial function via a number of different pathways:

- Superoxide anion rapidly inactivates NO to peroxynitrite [22], a powerful oxidant which easily penetrates across phospholipid membranes and produces substrate nitration, thereby inactivating regulatory receptors and enzymes, such as free radical scavengers [23, 24] and key NOS co-factors, for instance tetrahydrobiopterin [25].
- Mitochondrial production of superoxide increases intracellular formation of advanced glycation end-products (AGEs) which adversely affect endothelial function by increasing ROS production and inflammatory cytokines from vascular cells, thereby enhancing endothelial expression of various adhesion molecules implicated in atherogenesis [26].
- Activation of the receptor for AGEs (RAGE) increases intracellular superoxide anion production [27] and seems to represent a key step in atherosclerotic lesion development [28].
- Superoxide anion production activates the hexosamine pathway, which lowers protein kinase Akt-induced NOS activation [29]. Akt activation is further limited by PKC-dependent inhibition of phosphatidylinositol-3 kinase (PI-3K) pathway.
- High glucose-induced oxidative stress increases the levels of dimethylarginine, a competitive antagonist of NOS [30].

The $p66^{Shc}$adaptor protein controls the cellular responses to oxidative stress. Mice lacking $p66^{Shc}$($p66^{Shc-/-}$) have an increased resistance to ROS, prolonged life span, and exhibit less atherosclerosis during a high-fat diet, suggesting that $p66^{Shc}$ is involved in aging and aging-associated disease [31, 32]. Accordingly, it was demonstrated that old $p66^{Shc-/-}$ mice maintain endothelium-dependent relaxations compared with age-matched wild-type littermates [33]. In addition, $p66^{Shc-/-}$ cells exhibit reduced levels of intracellular ROS and decreased mitochondrial DNA alterations, indicating that $p66^{Shc}$ is a critical component of the intracellular redox state [34]. Although the exact biochemical role of $p66^{Shc}$ remains to be determined, it participates in mitochondrial ROS production by serving as a redox-sensitive enzyme that oxidizes cytochrome c, thus generating proapoptotic ROS in response to specific stress signals (➲Fig. 14.6). These data support the concept that $p66^{Shc}$ plays a pivotal role in controlling oxidative stress and participates in the pathogenesis of vascular disease [35]. The $p66^{Shc}$ gene expession is significantly increased in monocytes in blood obtained from patients with diabetes mellitus and is correlated with plasma isoprostanes, an *in vivo* marker of oxidative stress [36]. Furthermore, genetic deletion of $p66^{Shc}$ adaptor protein prevents hyperglycaemia-induced endothelial dysfunction and oxidative stress [37]. Taken together, these data suggest that $p66^{Shc}$ is part of a signal transduction pathway relevant to hyperglycaemia-induced vascular damage and may represent a potential therapeutic target against diabetic vascular complications.

The impact of diabetes on vascular function is not limited to the endothelium. Thus the vasodilator response to exogenous NO donors is diminished and the dysregulation of vascular smooth muscle function is further enhanced by impairment in sympathetic nervous system function. Diabetes increases PKC activity, NF-κB production, and generation of oxygen-derived free radicals in vascular smooth muscle as well. Moreover, diabetes heightens migration of vascular smooth muscle cells into nascent atherosclerotic lesions, where they replicate and produce extracellular matrix, important steps in mature lesion formation [38].

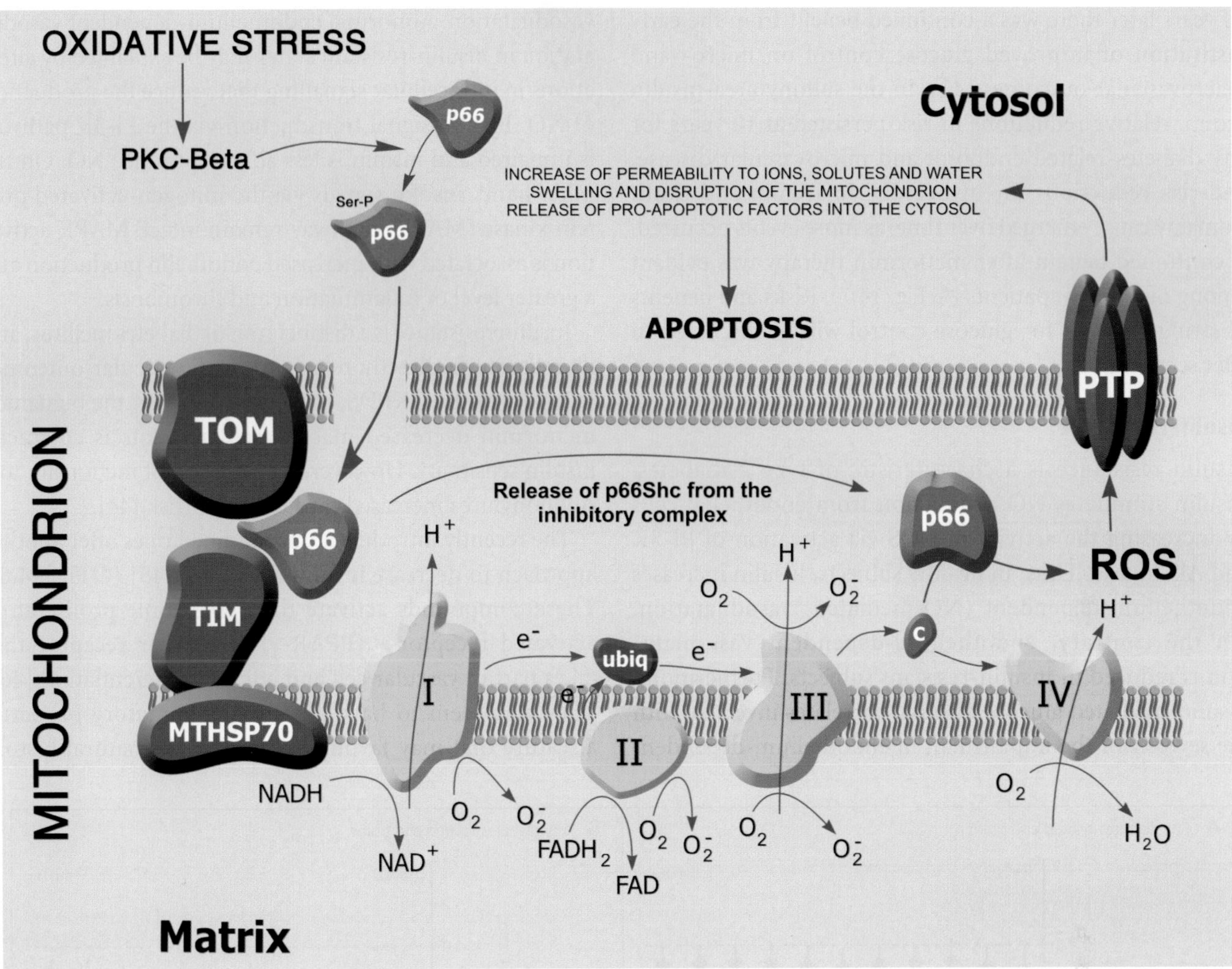

Figure 14.6 Biochemistry from the p66Shc pathway in the mitochondrial electron transport chain. Free radicals activate protein kinase C-β isoform to induce Ser^{36} phosphorylation of the $p66^{Shc}$, allowing transfer of the protein from the cytosol to the mitochondrion. In the mitochondrion, $p66^{Shc}$ binds to a complex which includes members of the TIM-TOM import complex. Proapoptotic stimuli destabilizes the $p66^{Shc}$-mtHsp70 complex and lead to the release of $p66^{Shc}$ in its monomeric form [8, 10]. Once activated, $p66^{Shc}$ oxidizes cytochrome c and catalyzes the reduction of O_2 to H_2O_2. This latter induces opening of the mitochondrial permeability transition pore (PTP), with subsequent increase of mitochondrial membrane permeability to ions, solutes and water, swelling and disruption of the organelle, and consequent release of proapoptotic factors into the cytosol. Reproduced with permission from Cosentino F, Francia P, Camici GG, *et al.* Final common molecular pathways of aging and cardiovascular disease: role of the p66Shc protein. *Arterioscler Thromb Vasc Biol* 2008; **28**: 622–8.

Vascular smooth muscle cell apoptosis in atherosclerotic lesions is also increased, such that patients with diabetes tend to have fewer smooth muscle cells in the lesions, which increases the propensity for plaque rupture [39]. Elaboration of cytokines diminishes the vascular smooth muscle synthesis of collagen and increases production of matrix metalloproteinases, yielding an increased tendency for plaque destabilization.

Given the above-mentioned effects of hyperglycaemia on vascular function, one might speculate that tight glycaemic control would protect from micro- and macrovascular damage and improve the prognosis. Epidemiological studies support the notion that increasing blood glucose levels relate to cardiovascular events. Less is, however, known on the effect of strict glycaemic control. Few clinical trials with sufficient periods of follow-up have focused on the effect of different glucose-lowering agents on mortality and cardiovascular events in diabetic patients. The United Kingdom Prospective Diabetes Study (UKPDS), a randomized, prospective, multicentre trial, showed that intensive glucose therapy in patients with newly diagnosed type 2 diabetes mellitus was associated with a reduced risk of microvascular complications and a non-significant reduction in the risk of myocardial infarction ($p = 0.052$). In the overweight patients, who primarily received metformin, reductions in the risk of myocardial infarction of 39% ($p = 0.01$), and of death from any cause of 36% ($p = 0.01$) were observed [40]. In a post-interventional follow-up of the UKPDS survivor performed

10 years later there was a continued benefit from the early institution of improved glucose control on micro- and macrovascular outcomes [41]. In the sulfonylurea-insulin group, relative reductions in risk persisted at 10 years for any diabetes-related endpoint and microvascular disease, and risk reductions for myocardial infarction and death from any cause emerged over time, as more events occurred. A continued benefit after metformin therapy was evident among overweight patients (➲Fig. 14.7). Risks and benefits of stringent goals for glucose control will be discussed in later sections.

Insulin resistance

Insulin resistance is a characteristic of type 2 diabetes. Insulin stimulates NO production from endothelial cells by increasing the activity of NOS via activation of PI-3K and Akt kinase. Thus, in healthy subjects, insulin increases endothelium-dependent (NO-mediated) vasodilatation. On the contrary, endothelium-dependent vasodilatation is reduced in insulin-resistant subjects. Furthermore, insulin-mediated glucose disposal correlates inversely with the severity of the impairment in endothelium-dependent vasodilatation. Abnormal endothelium-dependent vasodilatation in insulin-resistant states may be explained by alterations in intracellular signalling that reduce the production of NO. Insulin signal transduction via the PI-3K pathway is impaired and insulin is less able to produce NO. On the other hand, insulin signals via the mitogen-activated protein kinase (MAPK) pathway remain intact. MAPK activation is associated with increased endothelin production and a greater level of inflammation and thrombosis.

Insulin resistance is a distinct trait of diabetes mellitus, and its magnitude directly relates to cardiovascular outcomes [42, 43]. In the UKPDS, a likely reason that the biguanide metformin decreased macrovascular events is enhanced insulin sensitivity. However, the addition of metformin to a sulphonylurea increased cardiovascular risk [44].

The recently introduced thiazolidinediones offer another approach to decrease insulin resistance [45] (➲Fig. 14.8). These compounds activate the peroxisome proliferator-activated receptor-γ (PPAR-γ), a nuclear receptor that takes part in vascular cell and adipose differentiation [46]. They also seem to have an anti-inflammatory property, a feature that may favourably impact the natural history

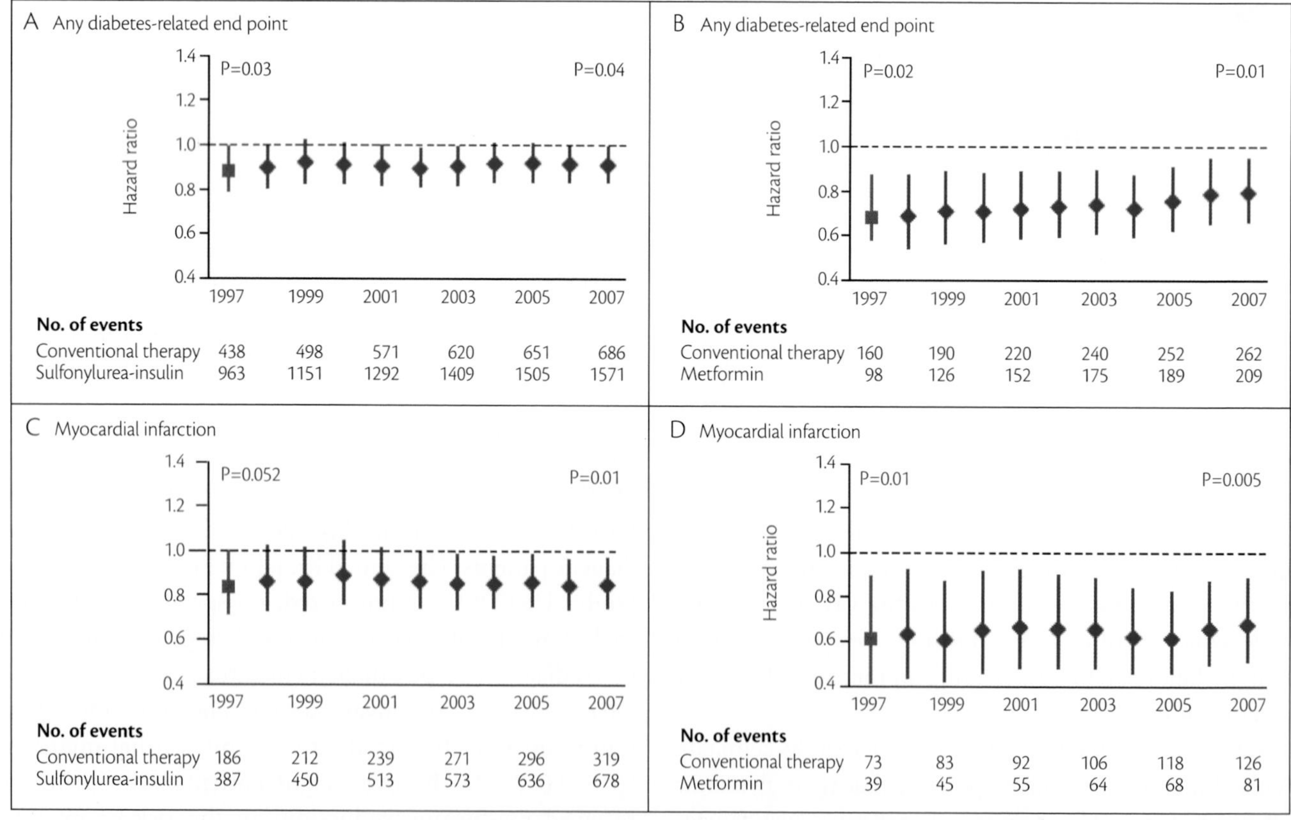

Figure 14.7 Hazard ratios for any diabetes related endpoint (upper part) and for myocardial infarction (lower part) in patients with type 2 diabetes in the UKPDS study. (A) and (C) intensive glucose control by means of sulfonylurea-insulin is compared to conventional therapy while the similar comparisons for metformin are presented in (B) and (D). Intensive therapy improves the prognosis in particular when based on metformin. The overall values at the end of the study in 1997, are shown (red squares), along with the annual values during the 10-year post-trial monitoring period (blue diamonds). Adapted with permission from Holman RR, Paul SK, Bethel MA, *et al.* 10-year follow-up of intensive glucose control in type 2 diabetes. *N Engl J Med* 2008; **359**: 1577–89.

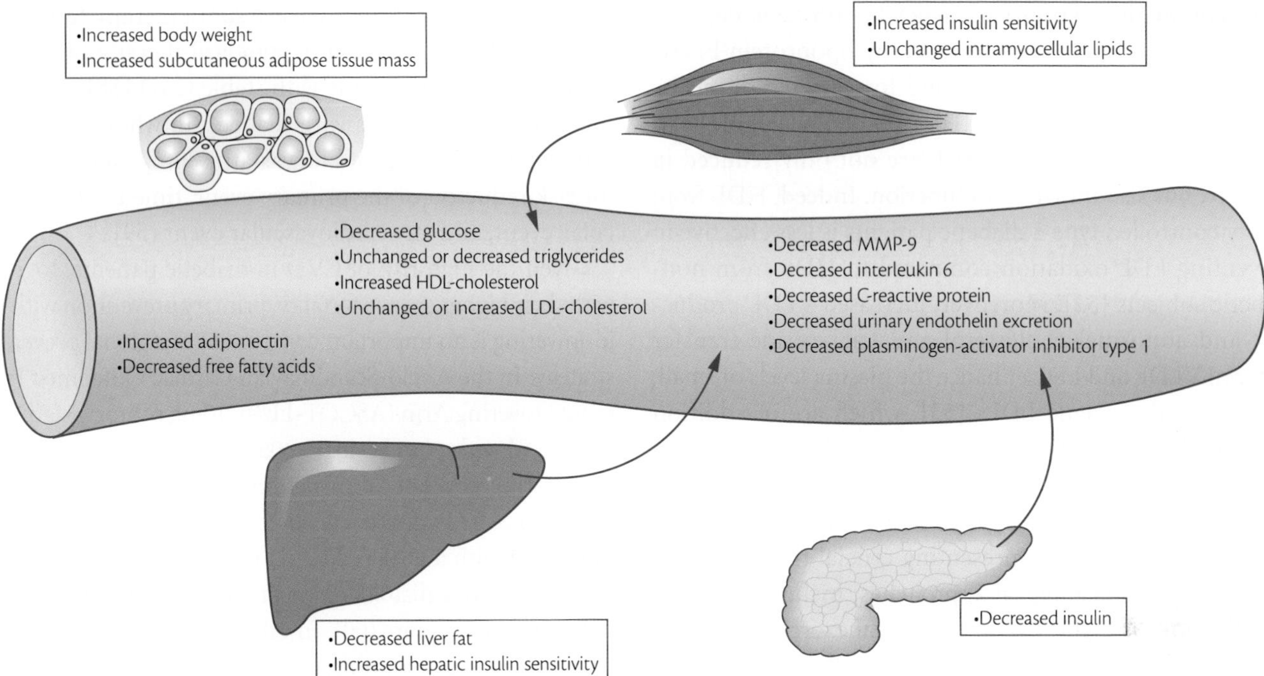

Figure 14.8 Mechanism of action of thiazolidinediones *in vivo* in humans. HDL, high-density lipoprotein; LDL, low-density lipoprotein; MMP-9, matrix metalloproteinase-9. Reproduced with permission from Yki-Jarvinen H. Thiazolidinediones. *N Engl J Med* 2004; **351**: 1106–18.

of the atherosclerotic process. Drug therapies that increase insulin sensitivity, such as metformin and the thiazolidinediones, improve endothelium-dependent vasodilatation. At present, and after elimination of troglitazone because of hepatotoxic effects, rosiglitazone and pioglitazone are approved in most countries for the treatment of hyperglycaemia in patients with type 2 diabetes (➲ for further information see ➲ Glycaemic control, p.480).

Oxidative stress

Given the pivotal role of oxidative stress in endothelial function and atherosclerotic processes in diabetes, growing efforts focus on the putative effects of antioxidant therapy. Despite evidence indicating the reversal of endothelial dysfunction by different antioxidant agents [47], data from clinical trials do not support antioxidant therapy in diabetes mellitus [48, 49]. These data would seem to refute a role of oxidative stress in the pathogenesis of atherosclerosis.

There are several reasons to believe that this conclusion is not justified but rather that treatment with antioxidative is perhaps not the best approach for reducing oxidative stress. The rate of reaction between vitamin E and superoxide is several orders of magnitude less than the rate of reaction between superoxide with NO. Moreover, many of the oxidative events occur in the cytoplasm and in the extracellular space, and would not be affected by lipid-soluble antioxidants, which are concentrated in lipid membranes and lipoproteins. Finally, antioxidants may become pro-oxidants after scavenging a radical, vitamins E and C become tocopheroxyl and ascorbyl radicals, respectively. The tocopheroxyl radical can be regenerated by other antioxidants such as vitamin C or co-enzyme Q10. For this reason, the use of cocktails of antioxidants rather than high doses of a selected one may be more effective. Given the above considerations, it is possible that antioxidant vitamins will never prove suited to limit vascular oxidant stress. To prevent the development of the earliest stages of diabetic vascular disease, future research should focus on identifying substances which have antioxidant effects not because they scavenge radicals but because they block their production.

Lipid disorders

Classically, diabetes induces elevation of triglycerides and LDL-cholesterol and a decline of high-density lipoprotein (HDL) plasma levels. These changes affect the natural history of the atherosclerotic disease, and render the patients more prone to develop CAD, stroke, and peripheral vascular disease. Diabetes-related enhanced free fatty acid liberation is crucial for the well-described changes in lipid profile. Excess circulating levels of free fatty acids result from both enhanced release from adipose tissue and reduced uptake from skeletal muscle [50]. The liver responds to free fatty acid excess by increasing very-low-density lipoprotein (VLDL) production and cholesteryl ester synthesis [51].

The accumulation of triglyceride-rich lipoproteins, depending also on their reduced clearance by lipoprotein lipase, triggers hypertriglyceridaemia and lowers HDL levels by promoting exchanges from HDL to VLDL via cholesteryl ester transfer protein [51]. HDL are not only reduced in quantity, but also impaired in function. Indeed, HDL from poorly controlled type 2 diabetic patients is less effective in preventing LDL oxidation compared to HDL from non-diabetic subjects [52]. Moreover, increased VLDL production and abnormal cholesterol and triglyceride transfer between VLDL and LDL enhance the plasma levels of small, dense, proatherogenic LDLs [53], which are in addition more prone to oxidation because of impaired antioxidant defence mechanisms in the plasma of diabetics.

These changes in lipid profile have important clinical consequences, thereby representing crucial treatment targets. Non-pharmacological approaches, including dietary modifications, weight loss, and physical exercise [54] represent first-line therapy although are often insufficient. The 3-hydroxy-3-methylglutaryl coenzyme A reductase inhibitors (or statins), by increasing LDL clearance and decreasing VLDL secretion, represent the cornerstone of lipid-lowering therapy.

In the landmark Scandinavian Simvastatin Survival Study (4S) [55], simvastatin reduced the risk of total mortality and myocardial infarction by 43% and 55%, respectively, in diabetic patients, compared to 29% and 32% in non-diabetic patients. Accordingly, the Cholesterol and Recurrent Events (CARE) trial [56] demonstrated a 24% reduction in cardiovascular events in diabetic patients with CAD and elevated or average LDL-cholesterol with statins. In the Heart Protection Study (HPS) [49], which enrolled 3000 diabetic subjects without evidence of atherosclerosis at entry, simvastatin reduced the combined endpoint of acute coronary syndrome, stroke, or revascularization by 34% over a 5-year follow-up period in the diabetic subgroup.

More recently the added benefit of achieving LDL cholesterol concentrations lower than levels previously advocated has been tested. In the Pravastatin or Atorvastatin Evaluation and Infection Therapy (PROVE-IT) Trial, standard statin therapy (pravastatin 40mg/day) was compared to intensive therapy (atorvastatin 80mg/day) in 4162 patients within 10 days of an acute coronary syndrome [57]. More intensive therapy (achieved mean LDL 1.6mmol/L (62mg/dL)) was associated with a significant 16% risk reduction in cardiovascular events, compared to standard therapy (mean LDL 2.5mmol/L (97mg/dL)). PROVE-IT included diabetic patients (18%) and there was no heterogeneity of effect in this subgroup. Treat to New Target Trial (TNT) compared the effects of intensive statin therapy (atorvastatin 80mg/day), compared to standard therapy (atorvastatin 10mg/day), in patients with stable CAD [58]. The TNT recruited 1501 patients with diabetes in whom significant differences in favour of atorvastatin 80mg were observed for risk reducton of the primary event, time to cerebrovascular event, and any cardiovascular event [59].

Given the high risk of CVD in diabetic patients, together with their higher event mortality, primary prevention with lipid-lowering is an important component of a global preventive strategy. In the Anglo-Scandinavian Cardiac Outcomes Trial-Lipid Lowering Arm (ASCOT-LLA), 10mg of atorvastatin was compared with placebo in 10,305 hypertensive patients with non-fasting cholesterol of 6.5mmol/L (251mg/dL) or less, of whom 2532 had type 2 diabetes. Atorvastatin therapy was associated with a 36% reduction in the primary endpoint of non-fatal myocardial infarction and fatal CAD after a median follow-up of 3.3 years [60]. In HPS, there were 2912 diabetic patients without symptomatic vascular disease [43]. In this cohort, the risk reduction was 33% with simvastatin.

The primary preventive Collaborative Atorvastatin Diabetes Study (CARDS) [61] assessed atorvastatin for primary prevention of major cardiovascular events in patients with type 2 diabetes and without high cholesterol [LDL-cholesterol below 4.14mmol/L. In this study, 2838 patients without a history of CVD were randomized to placebo or 10mg of atorvastatin daily if they had at least one further risk factor (retinopathy, albuminuria, current smoking, or hypertension). The trial was terminated after a median duration of follow-up of 3.9 years because of the beneficial effects of atorvastatin. Acute coronary heart disease events were reduced by 36%, coronary revascularizations by 31%, and stroke by 48%. Moreover, atorvastatin reduced the death rate by 27%, which was borderline significant.

As a result of its ability to increase HDL and decrease triglyceride levels without affecting glucose control, niacin would be an ideal drug in dyslipidaemic diabetic patients [62]. However, the effect on cardiovascular outcomes is still unproven in diabetics. This and well-known side effects [63] still make niacin a second-line agent.

Fibric acid derivatives, such as PPAR-α agonists, also raise HDL and lower triglyceride levels. The Veterans Affairs High-Density Lipoprotein Cholesterol Intervention Trial (VA-HIT) [64] showed a 24% risk reduction in death from CAD, non-fatal myocardial infarction, and stroke in diabetic patients with normal LDL and low HDL levels treated with gemfibrozil. The FIELD study (Fenofibrate Intervention and Event Lowering in Diabetes) which assessed the effect of fenofibrate compared to placebo in type 2 diabetes, with and without previous CVD presented conflicting results [65]. After a mean duration of 5 years, fenofibrate therapy was associated with a relative risk reduction of 11% in the primary endpoint of CHD death and non-fatal MI, which did not reach statistical significance. Total cardiovascular events (cardiac death, MI, stroke, coronary and carotid revascularization) were significantly reduced. Total mortality was 6.6% in the placebo and 7.35 in the fenofibrate group (p = 0.18). The major conclusion following these results is that statins remain the major treatment choice in a majority of patients with diabetes.

As a result of the potential risk of myositis [66], the joint use of fibric acid derivatives and statins requires careful monitoring and should be considered only in selected patients.

Hypertension

Hypertension is a common comorbidity of diabetes. Indeed, high blood pressure is more common in patients with type 2 diabetes than in matched controls [67]. Hypertension is often the result of underlying nephropathy in type 1 diabetes while the association of type 2 diabetes and high blood pressure is a typical feature of the metabolic syndrome. In 1998, UKPDS first documented the benefits of tight blood pressure control in diabetic patients, underlining the need for two or three drugs in combination to control blood pressure in a majority of enrolled subjects.

According to the European Society of Cardiology (ESC) and European Association for the Study of Diabetes (EASD) guidelines on diabetes, pre-diabetes, and CVD, as well as the European Society of Hypertension (ESH)/ESC guidelines for the management of hypertension, a target blood pressure <130/80mmHg is the goal in diabetic hypertensive patients [2, 68]. Although diuretics, beta-blockers, angiotensin-converting enzyme (ACE) inhibitors, angiotensin receptor blockers (ARBs), and calcium-channel blockers are all effective in lowering blood pressure in diabetics (➲Table 14.2), the modern approach starts with modulation of the renin–angiotensin system (➲Fig. 14.9) by ACE inhibitors, or ARBs, which exert vascular protective effects beyond blood pressure control [69–72]. In the HOPE trial, ramipril significantly reduced death, myocardial infarction, and stroke in more than 3000 high-risk non-hypertensive diabetic patients [73]. Losartan was superior to atenolol in reducing the combined endpoint of cardiovascular death, stroke, or myocardial infarction and total mortality in a large subgroup of hypertensive diabetic patients in the LIFE trial [74, 75]. Since both drugs had the same blood pressure-lowering capacity the difference in effect seems to be independent of blood pressure lowering. Such benefits support the front-line use of ACE inhibitors and ARBs in high-risk diabetic patients, probably regardless of whether they are hypertensive. A further reason to stress the key role of renin–angiotensin system modulation in diabetic hypertensive patients is the well-demonstrated ability of ACE inhibitors and ARBs to slow the deterioration of renal function and rate of progression to end-stage renal disease [69, 71].

The recent guidelines [2, 68, 76] emphasize that diabetic patients are exposed to a high cardiovascular risk at blood pressure levels in the high-normal range, supporting the early initiation of pharmacological antihypertensive treatment in addition to lifestyle measures. In this regard, the Action in Diabetes and Vascular disease: preterAx and diamicroN modified release Controlled Evaluation; (ADVANCE) trial was carried out with the purpose of evaluating a fixed combination of perindopril and indapamide-based strategy in 11,140 patients with type 2 diabetes, regardless of their blood pressure levels [51]. The perindopril/indapamide group experienced statistically significant relative risk reductions compared with the placebo group in total and cardiovascular mortality, total coronary events, and new microalbuminuria.

The putative added value of combining an ACE inhibitor (ACEI) with an ARB in diabetic patients is still under evaluation. The recently published results of the the ONgoing Telmisartan Alone and in combination with Ramipril Global Endpoint Trial (ONTARGET) trial shed a new light on the cardiovascular protection of patients at high risk of a cardiovascular events [77]. The question of the equivalence of ACEIs and ARBs remained unanswered until the ONTARGET trial showed that an ARB, telmisartan 80mg is equally effective as an ACEI, ramipril 10mg, when prescribed to patients at high risk in terms of the composite outcome of cardiovascular death, myocardial infarction, and stroke. Telmisartan was, as could be expected, slightly better tolerated. The comparator ramipril was chosen as the current gold standard ACE-inhibitor following the HOPE trial. Moreover, ONTARGET is the first trial to test the hypothesis of superiority of adding an ARB to an ACEI over the ACEiIor ARB monotherapy. Surprisingly, the combination of the two agents, telmisartan and ramipril, did not further reduce the event rate. It did, however, cause significantly more side effects compared to monotherapy. A parallel study investigated the efficacy of telmisartan in patients who are intolerant to an ACEI. This trial, Telmisartan Randomised AssessmeNt Study in aCE-inhibitor iNtolerant subjects with cardiovascular Disease (TRANSCEND), surprisingly did not show a significant reduction of cardiovascular death, myocardial infarction, or stroke [78].

Table 14.2 Relationship between blood pressure lowering and risk of cardiovascular disease in patients with diabetes

Trial	No. of patients	Duration (years)	Blood pressure control		Initial therapy	Outcome	Risk reduction (%)
			Less tight	Tight			
SHEP, 1996	583	5	155/72*	143/68*	Chlorthalidone	Stroke	NS
						CVD events	34
						CHD	56
Syst-Eur, 1999	492	2	162/82	153/78	Nitrendipine	Stroke	69
						CV events	62
HOT, 1998	1501	3	144/85*	140/81*	Felodipine	CV events	51
						MI	50
						Stroke	NS
						CV mortality	67
UKPDS, 1999	1148	8.4	154/87	144/82	Captopril or atenolol	Diabetes-related endpoints	34
						Death	37
						Stroke	44
						Microvascular endpoints	37
HOPE, Micro-HOPE, 2000	3577	4.5	Changes in systolic (2.4mmHg) and diastolic (1.0mmHg)	–	Ramipril vs. placebo	CV events	25
						CV mortality	37
						MI	22
						Stroke	33
						Total mortality	24
						New-onset diabetes	34
CAPP, 2001	572	7	155/89 vs. 153/88	–	Captopril vs. diuretics or ß-blockers	Fatal + NFMI + stroke + CV deaths	41
IDNT, 2001	1715	2.6	≤135/85	–	Irbesartan vs. amlodipine or placebo	Doubling of serum creatinine + end-stage renal disease + death from any cause	23 (vs. amlodipine) 20 (vs. placebo)
IRMA, 2001	590	2	144/83	–	Irbesartan 150mg or 300mg vs. placebo	Onset of diabetic nephropathy	35 (150mg)
			143/83				
			141/83				65 (300mg)
RENAAL, 2001	1513	3.4	152/82 vs. 153/82	–	Losartan vs. placebo in addition to conventional therapy	Doubling of serum creatinine	25
						End-stage renal disease	28
						Death	NS
LIFE, 2002	1195	4.8	146/79 vs. 148/79	–	Losartan vs. atenolol	CV events	22
						Total mortality in diabetics	39
						New-onset diabetes	25
INSIGHT, 2003	6321	4	145/82 vs. 144/82		Nifedipine 30mg or hydrochlorothiazide 25mg + amiloride 2.5mg	CV death + MI + heart failure + stroke	NS
						Composite of primary e.p., including all-cause mortality and death from vascular and non-vascular causes	24 (Nifedipine)
VALUE, 2004	15245	4	139/79 vs 137/78	–	Valsartan vs. amlodipine	Cardiac mortality + morbidity	NS
ASCOT-BPLA, 2005	19237 (13% diabetics)	5.5	130/80 in 32% of both treatment groups	–	Amlodipine ± perindopril vs. atenolol ± thiazide diuretic	NFMI and fatal CHD	NS

Table 14.2 *(Continued)* Relationship between blood pressure lowering and risk of cardiovascular disease in patients with diabetes

Trial	No. of patients	Duration (years)	Blood pressure control		Initial therapy	Outcome	Risk reduction (%)
			Less tight	Tight			
UKPDS, 2008	884	10 (partial monitoring)	No difference	–	No attempt to maintain previously assigned therapies	Diabetes-related endpoints	NS
						Death	NS
						Stroke	NS
						Microvascular endpoints	NS
ADVANCE, 2008	11140	4.3	136/73 vs. 140/73	–	Perindopril + indapamide vs. placebo	Total mortality	14
						Total coronary events	14
						Major vascular events	9
						New microalbuminuria	21
ONTARGET, 2008	25620 (37% with diabetes)	4.8	Changes in BP 0.9/0.6mmHg and 2.4/1.4mmHg in the telmisartan and combination therapy group, respectively	–	Ramipril vs. telmisartan vs. combination	Composite primary endpoint including death from CV causes, MI, stroke or hospitalization for heart failure	NS
TRANSCEND, 2008	5926 (35% with diabetes)	4.8	Changes in BP 3.2/1.8mmHg	–	Telmisartan vs. placebo (in addition to usual therapy)	Composite primary endpoint including CV death, MI, stroke, hospitalization for heart failure	NS

ADVANCE, Action in Diabetes and Vascular disease: preterAx and diamicroN modified release Controlled Evaluation; ASCOT, Anglo-Scandinavian Cardiac Outcomes Trial; CAPP, CAptopril Prevention Project; CHD, coronary heart disease; CV, cardiovascular; CVD, cardiovascular disease; HOT, Hypertension Optimal Treatment; IDNT, Irbesartan Diabetic Nephropathy Trial; IRMA, IRbesartan MicroAlbuminuria in type 2 diabetes; MI, myocardial infarction; NFMI, non-fatal myocardial infarction; NS, not significant; ONTARGET, ONgoing Telmisartan Alone and in combination with Ramipril Global Endpoint Trial; RENAAL, Reduction in End points in NIDDM with Angiotensin II Antagonist Losartan; SHEP, Systolic Hypertension in the Elderly Program; Syst-Eur, Systolic hypertension in Europe; TRANSCEND, Telmisartan Randomized AssessmeNt Study in ACE iNtolerant subjects with cardiovascular Disease; UKPDS, United Kingdom Prospective Diabetes Study.

*Blood pressure in diabetic + non-diabetic population because blood pressure not reported for diabetic patients alone.

Data derived from Sowers JR, Haffner S. Treatment of cardiovascular and renal risk factors in the diabetic hypertensive. *Hypertension* 2002; **40**: 781–8. Modified from Lüscher TF, Creager MA, Beckman JA, et al. Diabetes and vascular disease pathophysiology, clinical consequences, and medical therapy: Part II. *Circulation* 2003; **108**: 1655–61.

In summary, patients with type 2 diabetes and hypertension are at increased cardiovascular and renal risk over the whole range of blood pressure. Effort should be directed to block their renin–angiotensin system regardless of the blood pressure levels. The use of combination therapy, starting at early stages of blood pressure elevation, can be expected to facilitate the objective to prevent micro- and macrovascular complications.

Thrombosis and coagulation

Platelet function is crucial in determining the natural history of atherosclerosis and the consequences of plaque rupture. It is therefore not surprising that cardiovascular risk is closely linked to platelet function abnormalities and coagulation disorders that are common in the diabetic patient. The intracellular platelet glucose concentration mirrors the extracellular environment and is associated with increased superoxide anion formation, PKC activity, and decreased platelet-derived NO [79, 80]. Moreover, diabetic patients show increased expression of glycoprotein Ib and IIb/IIIa, which enhances both platelet–von Willebrand factor and platelet–fibrin interactions [79] (➲Fig. 14.10). Hyperglycaemia further affects platelet function by impairing calcium homeostasis [81] and thereby altering platelet conformation, secretion and aggregation, and thromboxane formation. Other abnormalities affecting platelet function include impaired endothelial production of NO and prostacyclin, and increased production of fibrinogen, thrombin, and von Willebrand factor [79].

Moreover, blood coagulability is enhanced in diabetic patients. Indeed, plasma coagulation factors (e.g. factor VII and thrombin), lesion-based coagulants (e.g. tissue factor), and atherosclerotic lesion content of plasminogen

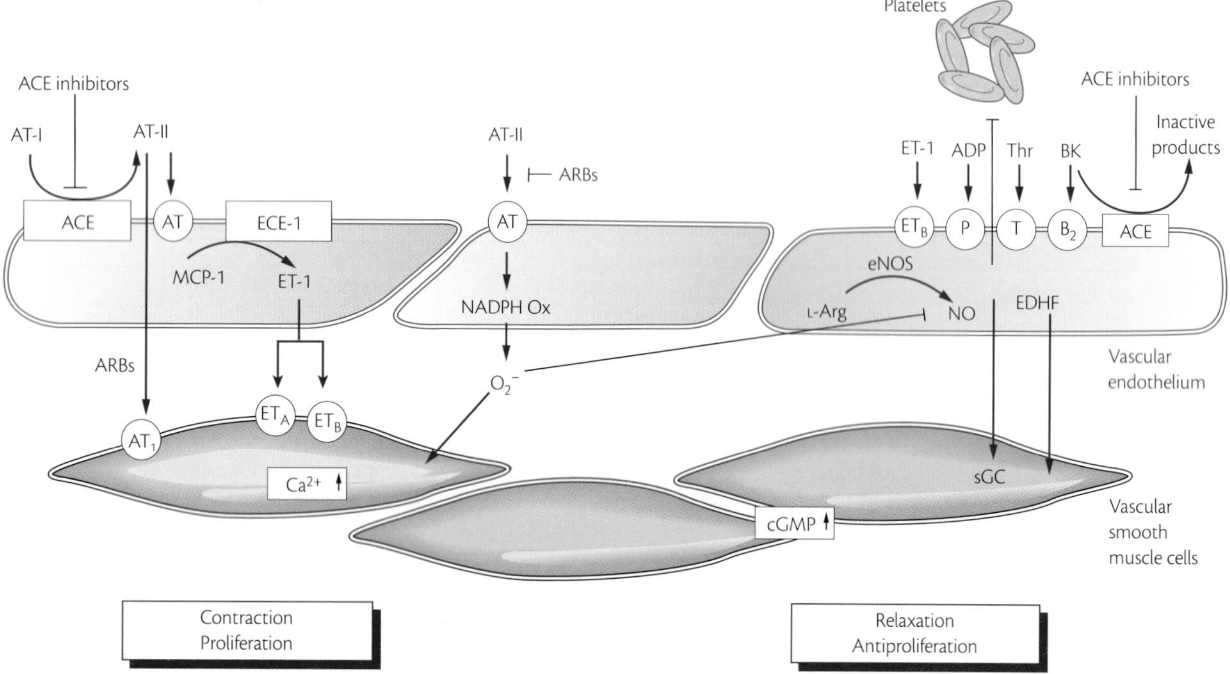

Figure 14.9 Effects of ACE inhibitors and angiotensin receptor blockers (ARBs) on endothelium-derived vasoactive substances. ACE, angiotensin converting enzyme; AT1, angiotensin receptor-1; AT-I, angiotensin-I; AT-II, angiotensin-II; bET-1, big endothelin-1; BK, bradykinin; cGMP, cyclic guanosine monophosphate; ECE-1, endothelin converting enzyme-1; EDHF, endothelium-derived hyperpolarizing factor; eNOS, endothelial nitric oxide synthase; ET-1, endothelin-1; ET_A & ET_B, endothelin receptor subtypes; L-Arg, L-arginine; sGc, soluble guanylate cyclase; Thr, thrombin.

activator inhibitor-1 (a fibrinolysis inhibitor) are increased, and endogenous anticoagulants (e.g. thrombomodulin and protein C) are decreased [81, 82–85]. Thus, a propensity for platelet activation and aggregation, coupled with a tendency for coagulation, amplify the risk that plaque rupture results in thrombotic occlusion of arteries (➲Fig. 14.10).

Results from several trials have consistently demonstrated that increased propensity for platelet aggregation in diabetics strongly relates to cardiovascular outcomes. The Antiplatelet Trialists' Collaboration analysed the results of 195 trials of >135,000 patients at high risk of arterial disease and found that platelet antagonists lowered the risk of stroke, myocardial infarction, and vascular death [86] (➲Fig. 14.11). In the Early Treatment of Diabetic Retinopathy Study (ETDRS), aspirin reduced the risk of myocardial infarction in patients with type 1 or type 2 diabetes without increasing the risk of vitreous or retinal bleeding, even in patients with retinopathy [87].

In acute coronary syndromes, platelet antagonists seem to be particularly effective in diabetics. The PRISM-PLUS study showed that addition of tirofiban (a platelet glycoprotein IIb/IIIa antagonist) to heparin decreased the risk of death and myocardial infarction particularly in diabetics [88]. A meta-analysis of six large-scale trials of intravenous glycoprotein IIb/IIIa inhibitors in the management of acute coronary syndromes in diabetics showed that these agents reduce mortality by 25% at 30 days in diabetic patients [89]. In the Clopidogrel in Unstable Angina to Prevent Recurrent Ischaemic Events (CURE) study the addition of clopidogrel to aspirin led to a reduction in death, myocardial infarction, or stroke in patients with unstable angina/non-ST-segment-elevation myocardial infarction (NSTEMI), irrespective of their diabetes status [90]. In addition, specific and amplified benefits of clopidogrel treatment have been reported in diabetics [91].

It is therefore appropriate to recommend the use of aspirin both as a secondary prevention strategy in diabetics already affected by myocardial infarction, cerebrovascular disease, or peripheral artery disease, and as a primary prevention strategy in diabetics who have additional risk factors for CVD.

Clinical presentation and management of cardiovascular disease

Coronary artery disease and glucose metabolism

Prevalence

Abnormal glucose metabolism is common in patients with CVD. When OGTTs are performed before hospital

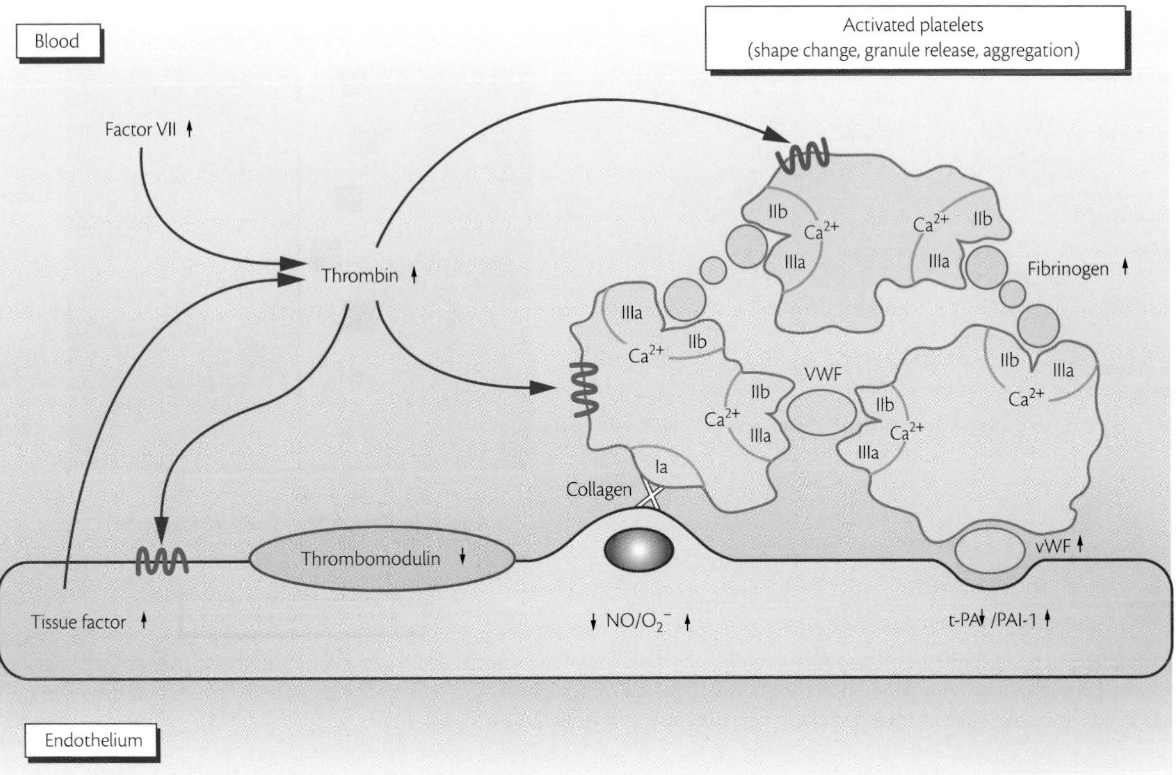

Figure 14.10 Platelet function and plasma coagulation factors are altered in diabetes, favouring platelet aggregation and a propensity for thrombosis. There is increased expression of glycoprotein Ib and IIb/IIIa, augmenting both platelet–von Willebrand (vWF) factor and platelet–fibrin interaction. The bioavailability of NO is decreased. Coagulation factors, such as tissue factor, factor VII, and thrombin, are increased; plasminogen activator inhibitor (PAI-1) is increased; and endogenous anticoagulants such as thrombomodulin are decreased. t-PA, tissue plasminogen activator. Reproduced with permission from Creager MA, Lüscher TF, Cosentino F, *et al.* Diabetes and vascular disease: pathophysiology, clinical consequences and medical therapy: Part I. *Circulation* 2003; **108**: 1527–32.

discharge in patients with myocardial infarction but without previously known diabetes, 35% have IGT and 31% newly detected diabetes [84]. This prevalence persists 3 and 12 months later, suggesting that increased sympathetic drive induced by the acute illness was not the main reason for the metabolic imbalance, and that an OGTT performed before hospital discharge provides a reasonable estimate of the glucometabolic status [92]. Similar findings were reported in two larger studies, i.e. the Euro Heart Survey [83] and China Heart Survey [93]. The Euro Heart Survey involved 110 centres in 25 countries recruiting 4196 patients with CAD. Thirty-one percent had known type 2 diabetes at the time for recruitment. An OGTT was used for the characterization of glucose metabolism in patients without known glucose perturbations. In patients with acute CAD, 36% had impaired glucose regulation and 22% newly detected diabetes, and in patients with stable CAD, 37% and 14% respectively.

The China Heart Survey, mimicking the design of the Euro Heart Survey, enrolled 3513 Chinese patients with CAD. Type 2 diabetes was known in approximately one-third of those recruited for the study. Among the remaining patients OGTT diagnosed type 2 diabetes in 27% and IGT or IFG in another 37%. Even patients with peripheral or cerebrovascular disease presumed free from glucometabolic disturbances have high proportions of glucose abnormalities when investigated with an OGTT [94]. Taken together these studies provide strong and universal evidence that normal glucose regulation is indeed less common than abnormal glucose regulation in patients with CVD, highlighting the need for strategies for glucometabolic screening.

Prognostic implications

Due to better management the overall prognosis has improved following acute coronary events but patients with diabetes continue to have a considerably more dismal prognosis than their non-diabetic counterparts [95, 96]. The prognosis in patients with diabetes presenting with acute coronary syndrome has been evaluated in several randomized clinical trials. The first Global Utilization of Streptokinase and Tissue Plasminogen Activator for Occluded Coronary Arteries trial (GUSTO I) enrolled 41,021 patients presenting

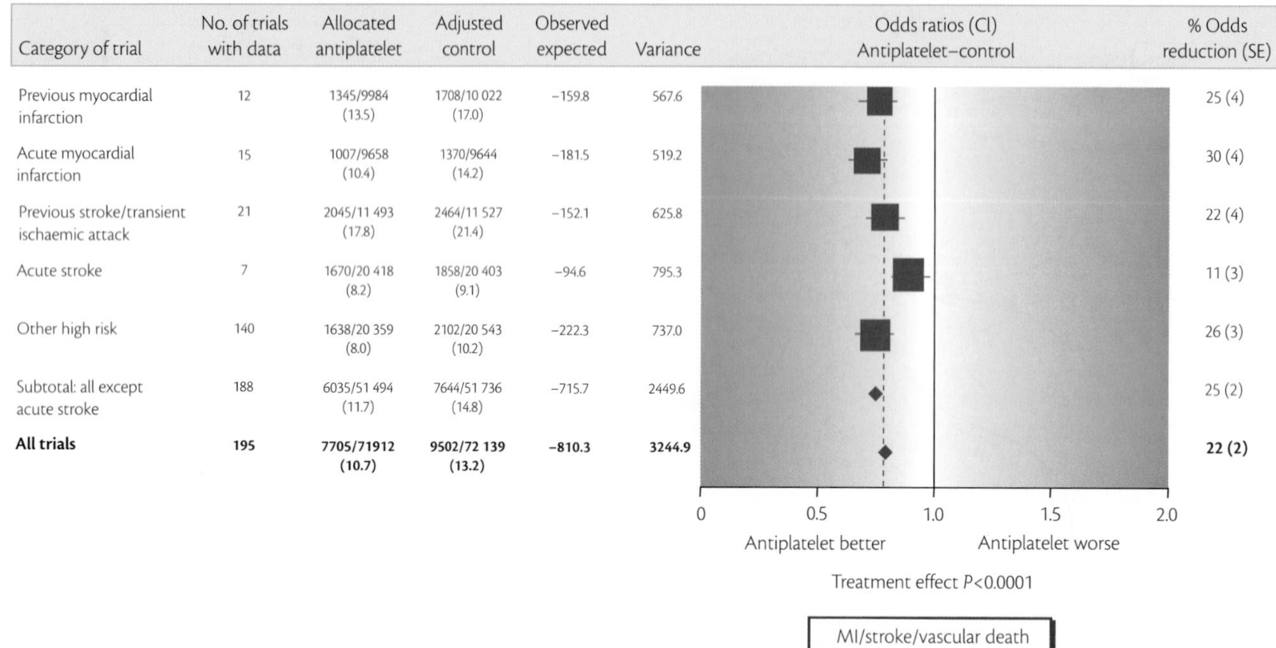

Category of trial
No. of trials with data
Allocated antiplatelet
Adjusted control
Observed expected
Variance
Odds ratios (CI) Antiplatelet–control
% Odds reduction (SE)
Previous myocardial infarction | 12 | 1345/9984 (13.5) | 1708/10 022 (17.0) | −159.8 | 567.6 | 25 (4)
Acute myocardial infarction | 15 | 1007/9658 (10.4) | 1370/9644 (14.2) | −181.5 | 519.2 | 30 (4)
Previous stroke/transient ischaemic attack | 21 | 2045/11 493 (17.8) | 2464/11 527 (21.4) | −152.1 | 625.8 | 22 (4)
Acute stroke | 7 | 1670/20 418 (8.2) | 1858/20 403 (9.1) | −94.6 | 795.3 | 11 (3)
Other high risk | 140 | 1638/20 359 (8.0) | 2102/20 543 (10.2) | −222.3 | 737.0 | 26 (3)
Subtotal: all except acute stroke | 188 | 6035/51 494 (11.7) | 7644/51 736 (14.8) | −715.7 | 2449.6 | 25 (2)
All trials | 195 | 7705/71912 (10.7) | 9502/72 139 (13.2) | −810.3 | 3244.9 | 22 (2)
0
0.5
1.0
1.5
2.0
Antiplatelet better
Antiplatelet worse
Treatment effect P<0.0001
MI/stroke/vascular death

Figure 14.11 Effects of antithrombotic therapy in myocardial infarction, stroke and vascular death in the Antithrombotic Trialists' Collaboration. Reproduced with permission from Antithrombotic Trialists' Collaboration. Collaborative meta-analysis of randomised trials of antiplatelet therapy for prevention of death, myocardial infarction, and stroke in high risk patients. *BMJ* 2002; **324**: 71–86.

with STEMI, including insulin-treated and non-insulin-treated patients with diabetes [7]. The 30-day mortality rate was significantly higher for diabetic than non-diabetic patients. A meta-analysis was also performed with data from six large-scale trials enrolling patients without and with diabetes hospitalized for NSTEMI and/or unstable angina [89]. The 30-day mortality rate was found to be significantly higher in the diabetic subgroup. In the Organization to Assess Strategies for Ischaemic Syndromes (OASIS) registry, a six-nation NSTEMI/acute coronary syndrome outcome study, diabetes increased mortality by 57% [8].

Notably all stages of glucose abnormalities are associated with an increased risk of cardiovascular morbidity and mortality. Indeed dysglycaemic individuals often develop vascular damage during the pre-diabetic stage, although glucometabolic perturbations often remain undetected until the first cardiovascular event. Follow-up of the GAMI patients demonstrated that abnormal glucose regulation detected a few days after an acute myocardial infarction is an independent predictor of a dismal prognosis [10]. One-year mortality in the Euro Heart Survey was 2.2% in patients with CAD and normal glucose metabolism, 5.5% in those with newly diagnosed type 2 diabetes, and 7.7% in patients with known type 2 diabetes [97]. Based on these studies, an aggressive treatment strategy with maximization of life-saving therapies is crucial for patients with diabetes and CAD.

Glycaemic control

Acute management

The concept of improving metabolic support to the ischaemic myocardium has been tested. The CREATE-ECLA trial randomized over 20,000 patients with STEMI, out of whom 18% had type 2 diabetes, to high dose glucose–insulin–potassium (GIK) or usual care. There was no positive effect of GIK on mortality, cardiac arrest, or cardiogenic shock [98]. This and similar trials did not aim for glucose control as a primary target. On the contrary, glucose levels increased during the infusion, which may have contributed to the lack of effect. The results from CREATE-ECLA suggest that acute metabolic intervention by means of GIK has no place in contemporary treatment of patients with acute myocardial infarction as recently debated [99].

Since hyperglycaemia is associated with an impaired prognosis in patients with CAD, it is reasonable to assume that tight glycaemic control would improve the outcome. This hypothesis was verified in the Diabetes and Insulin–Glucose Infusion in Acute Myocardial Infarction (DIGAMI) study [100]. Of 620 diabetic patients with acute myocardial infarction, 306 were randomly assigned to an insulin–glucose infusion of at least 24 hours followed by multidose subcutaneous insulin with the intention to rapidly and consistently lower glucose to preset targets, while 314 patients were randomized to routine glucose-lowering therapy. During an average follow-up of 3.4 years, 33% of the patients in the intensive insulin group and 44% in the control group died ($p = 0.011$). Metabolic control, mirrored by blood glucose and HbA1c, improved significantly more in patients on intensive insulin treatment than in the control group, but it was unclear whether the benefit was the result of the initial insulin–glucose infusion or the chronic insulin therapy.

The second DIGAMI trial, recruiting 1253 patients with type 2 diabetes and acute myocardial infarction [101], was designed to further study this aspect. DIGAMI 2 did not verify that an acutely introduced, long-term intensive insulin treatment strategy improved survival. The different outcome between these two trials may have several explanations. The overall mortality in DIGAMI 2 was lower than expected, most likely due to an aggressive use of evidence-based treatment including revascularization, and glucose control was better in DIGAMI 2 already at the study start. Moreover, the targeted glucose levels were not reached in the intensive insulin group resulting in similar glycaemic control between the different treatment arms. The DIGAMI 2 trial clearly confirmed that the glucose level is a strong and independent predictor of long-term mortality following myocardial infarction in patients with type 2 diabetes. That glucose control rather than insulin treatment per se is of prognostic importance in patients with acute myocardial infarction or under intensive care is also indicated by other trials [102, 103]. The current guideline recommendation is that diabetic patients with myocardial infarction benefit from tight glycaemic control which may be accomplished by different treatment strategies, and insulin is usually the drug of choice in an acute setting [2, 104].

Chronic treatment

Long-term glucose control with a HbA1c level of <6.5% and a fasting glucose <6.0mmol/L (108mg/dL) has been recommended to reduce macrovascular complications in patients with CAD and diabetes [2]. Following the recently published ADVANCE [105] and ACCORD [106] trials it has, however, been questioned if intensive glucose lowering is truly beneficial. In the ADVANCE trial, microvascular, but not macrovascular, complications were improved during a follow-up of 5 years, while ACCORD was prematurely stopped after 3.4 years due to an increased mortality in the intensively treated group, although the rate of non-fatal myocardial infarction and stroke were lower in the intensively treated group at that time. There are several possible explanations for these negative results, for example, too short follow-up to demonstrate an effect on macrovascular complications, too rapidly and aggressively instituted glucose-lowering treatment with an increased incidence of severe hypoglycaemia, and potentially harmful drug combinations including an extensive use of thiazolidinediones and insulin in ACCORD.

Few clinical trials with sufficient periods of follow-up have focused on the effect of different glucose-lowering agents on mortality and cardiovascular events in diabetic patients. This may explain the lack of generally accepted evidence-based treatment strategies for patients with type 2 diabetes. An exception is the UKPDS experiences with the use of metformin in overweight patients with type 2 diabetes, in whom this drug had a favourable effect on cardiovascular events and mortality after an average follow-up of 11 years, as further consolidated in a recent post-trial follow-up [41].

An opinion, shared by all major guidelines is that lifestyle intervention and metformin should be the platform in all patients without contraindications to this drug [107], but many patients need combinations of medications to reach the recommended glucose targets. The treatment has to be individualized with the risk–benefit balance in mind, and there is a need for studies on this subject since emerging evidence suggests that glucose-lowering drugs may not only be of benefit. Thiazolidinediones are known to increase fluid accumulation which may induce heart failure and recent meta-analyses relate rosiglitazone to an increased risk for myocardial infarction [108]. Pioglitazone, on the contrary, decreased the risk of a composite of MI, stroke, and death in the PROACTIVE trial [109]. Another group of glucose-lowering agents, sulphonylureas, has been associated with untoward cardiac effects in the experimental setting, essentially interference with ischaemic preconditioning, but this does not appear to have clinical implications, especially not with the use of newer sulphonylureas [110, 111].

The safety of insulin, mandatory for the treatment of many patients, has also been questioned [112]. As revealed by the Euro Heart Survey and a post-hoc analysis of the DIGAMI 2 study, chronic insulin treatment in patients with CAD may increase the risk of cardiovascular events compared with oral glucose-lowering agents at a similar level of glucose control [110, 113]. These findings underline the importance to reach adequate glucose control if insulin is used in order to balance benefits of lowering glucose against possible untoward effects.

Until further information is available, patients with type 2 diabetes should be managed according to a multifactorial treatment strategy in which glucose lowering is one of several interventions. Glucose targets as outlined in available guidelines are still valid but the glucose-lowering agents should be chosen and used with caution.

Revascularization strategies

Patients with diabetes have a higher complication rate and a higher long-term mortality and morbidity following revascularization (➲Chapter 17) than their non-diabetic counterparts both after bypass surgery [114, 115] and percutaneous coronary interventions [65], even in the era of drug eluting stents [116]. In the National Heart, Lung, and Blood Institute (NHLBI) percutaneous coronary intervention (PCI) registry, patients with diabetes had a greater incidence of three-vessel disease and more diffuse disease in both proximal and distal coronary artery segments when compared with patients without diabetes. In the Fast Revascularization during Instability in Coronary Artery Disease (FRISC-II) trial it was the presence of diabetes itself, rather than a diffuse or multivessel disease, that related to an unfavourable prognosis [117]. Unfortunately most outcome information is derived from registry studies or sub-group analyses from clinical trials recruiting patients with and without diabetes. These diabetic cohorts may be subjected to selection bias and their disease state is inadequately characterized, as is their glucose-lowering therapy. The influence of glycaemic control on both short- and long-term outcome seems to be of importance but prospective clinical trials testing this in well-defined patient cohorts are not available [118, 119].

Bypass surgery versus percutaneous coronary intervention

Mak and Faxon [115] summarized five randomized trials of patients, which included 627 patients with diabetes, comparing coronary artery bypass graft surgery (CABG) with PCI in patients with multivessel disease. During a period of follow-up between 1–8 years the overall mortality was 34% among diabetic patients treated with PCI and 19% among those randomized to CABG (95% CI 28–39%) with an increasing mortality difference with long periods of follow-up. The Bypass Angioplasty Revascularization Investigation (BARI) [120, 121] is the largest of these randomized trials. BARI enrolled 1829 patients with multivessel disease of whom 353 (19%) had diabetes. In patients without diabetes the cumulative 10-year survival was virtually identical for CABG and PCI (73% and 71% respectively). Patients with diabetes had significant survival advantage after CABG (58%) compared with PCI (45%; p = 0.025). Moreover, there was a significantly higher need for repeated revascularization among diabetic PCI-treated patients than in the group without diabetes (➲Fig. 14.12). Following CABG the survival rate was better in diabetic patients who received at least one arterial graft (64%) than those given vein grafts only (45%).

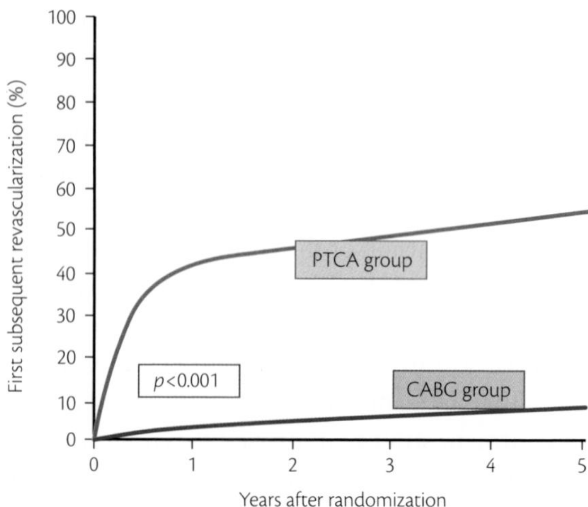

Figure 14.12 In the BARI trial, the subgroup of diabetic PTCA patients had significantly higher need for repeated revascularization than did PTCA patients without diabetes. Reproduced with permission from The Bypass Angioplasty Revascularization Investigation (BARI) Investigators. Comparison of coronary bypass surgery with angioplasty in patients with multivessel disease. *N Engl J Med* 1996; **335**: 217–25.

Revascularization in acute coronary syndromes

Revascularization of diabetic patients in the setting of acute coronary syndromes was evaluated in a subgroup of the FRISC-II trial. This revealed that early revascularization, either by CABG or PCI, was at least as effective among diabetic as in non-diabetic patients, with an almost 40% reduction of the combined endpoint re-infarction and mortality during the first year of follow-up. Since the risk for events was higher in the diabetic subgroup, fewer diabetic than non-diabetic patients needed to be treated to save one event (11 vs. 32). A management strategy based on early coronary angiography and, if possible, an early coronary intervention is therefore recommended for diabetic patients [117]. Primary PCI has been compared to fibrinolytic therapy for treatment of STEMI in a pooled analysis of 6315 patients among whom 877 (14%) with diabetes. Thirty-day mortality was higher in patients with diabetes (9.4% vs. 5.9%; p <0.001) and the use of primary PCI improved 30-day survival in both patient groups (diabetes-adjusted odds ratio (OR) 0.50; 95% CI, 0.31–0.80; p = 0.003) as well as recurrent infarction and stroke [122].

Coronary restenosis and stenting

Short-term angiographic success rates of stenting in diabetics (92–100%) are about the same as in non-diabetic patients [123]. The composite endpoint of mortality, non-fatal myocardial infarction, and urgent CABG is usually similar in diabetic and non-diabetic patients although a trend toward higher rates of subacute stent thrombosis has been found in diabetics. The main reason for the less favourable long-term results of PCI in patients with compared to those without diabetes is the substantially higher rate of restenosis. Van Belle and colleagues [124] found a lower angiographic restenosis rate in diabetic patients treated with coronary stents compared with those treated with balloon angioplasty. Still, diabetics have a less favourable clinical outcome and a lower event-free survival than non-diabetic patients. The incidence of both restenosis and stent-vessel occlusion is significantly higher in the former group of patients [125]. A subgroup analysis of the Arterial Revascularization Therapy Study (ARTS) trial [126], including 112 diabetic patients, revealed that surgical revascularization with routine use of arterial bypass conduits provides a superior 1-year clinical outcome compared with PCI in patients with diabetes and multivessel CAD, even following a strategy of stented angioplasty. The PCI group had the lowest event-free survival rate (63%) because of a higher demand of repeated revascularization compared with those treated with CABG (84%; $p < 0.001$) and non-diabetic patients treated with stents (76%, $p < 0.04$) (➲Fig. 14.13).

Several studies reveal that diabetes is an independent risk factor for in-stent restenosis after balloon angioplasty, ranging from 35% to 71% [127]. Coronary stenting with bare metal stents (BMSs) reduces this risk, but restenosis still remains more frequent in diabetics with a restenosis rate of at least 30% compared to 20% or less in patients without diabetes [128]. Tight glycaemic control, aggressive risk factor modification, and the use of glycoprotein IIb/IIIa inhibitors have been attempted to improve the outcome of coronary stenting in diabetics, with some success.

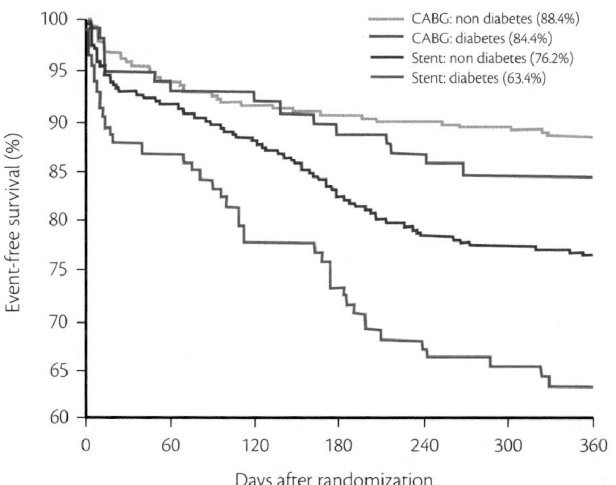

Figure 14.13 In the ARTS trial, diabetic patients treated with stenting had the lowest event-free survival rate (63.4%) because of a higher incidence of repeat revascularization compared with both diabetic patients treated with CABG (84.4%, $p < 0.001$) and non-diabetic patients treated with stents (76.2%, $p = 0.04$). Reproduced with permission from Abizaid A, Costa MA, Centemero M, *et al.* Clinical and economic impact of diabetes mellitus on percutaneous and surgical treatment of multivessel coronary disease patients: insights from the Arterial Revascularization Therapy Study (ARTS) trial. *Circulation* 2001; **104**: 533–8.

The high demand for repeat revascularization procedures exposes the diabetic patients to an increased risk for periprocedural complications. The introduction of drug-eluting stents (DESs) coated with sirolimus (rapamycin), which has anti-inflammatory and antiproliferative properties, reduced restenosis significantly in several prospective, multicentre, randomized trials [129, 130]. A meta-analysis comparing DESs to BMSs in diabetic subpopulations in several clinical trials revealed that DESs were associated with an 80% relative risk reduction for restenosis during the first year of follow-up, but the restenosis rate remained higher in diabetic compared to non-diabetic patient [131].

In DIABETES, one of very few prospective trials specifically performed on a population of diabetic patients, 160 patients with one or more significant coronary stenoses in one, two, or three vessels were randomized to PCI with either a DES (sirolimus) or a BMS. After 2 years the rate of target lesion revascularization was significantly lower in the DES than in the BMS group (8 vs. 35%; $p < 0.001$). However, the total demand for revascularization was similar in both groups and related to progression of atherosclerosis in coronary segments remote from the target lesion (8% in DES group vs. 10% in BMS group) [132].

Adjunctive therapy

Potent platelet inhibition by glycoprotein IIb/IIIa inhibitors improves the outcome after PCI. Glycoprotein IIb/IIIa receptor blockade seems to have an even greater effect in diabetics, decreasing the need for repeat interventions among stented patients [133]. Abciximab, tirofiban, and eptifibatide achieved similar levels of inhibition of platelet aggregation and similar reduction in the platelet–monocyte interaction in patients undergoing coronary stenting. Pooled data from the EPIC, EPILOG, and EPISTENT trials [134], including 1462 diabetic patients, showed that, compared to placebo, abciximab decreased the 1-year mortality among patients with diabetes to the same order as that in patients without diabetes, while the impact of abciximab on patients without diabetes was much more limited (➲Fig. 14.14). In the PRISM-PLUS Study, a comparison of treatment outcomes in the diabetic subgroup revealed that the combination therapy (tirofiban and heparin) compared with heparin alone was associated with reductions in the incidence of cardiac adverse events, but these results did not reach statistical significance [135]. Furthermore, there is increasing evidence that glycoprotein IIb/IIIa inhibitors

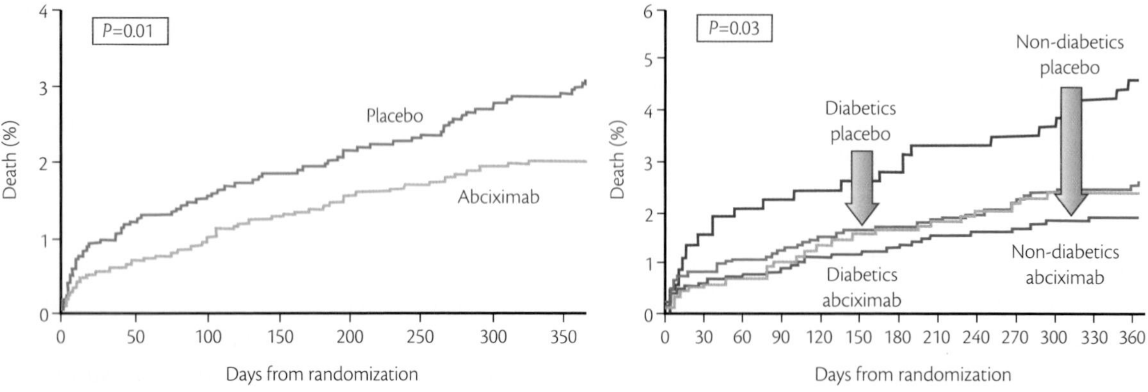

Figure 14.14 Pooled data from the EPIC, EPILOG, and EPISTENT trials showed that abciximab decreases the 1-year mortality of diabetic patients to that of placebo-treated non-diabetic patients. Reproduced with permission from Bhatt DL, Marso SP, Lincoff AM, *et al.* Abciximab reduces mortality in diabetics following percutaneous coronary intervention. *J Am Coll Cardiol* 2000; **35**: 922–8.

are of particular value in the diabetic patients with non-ST-elevation acute coronary syndromes during PCI [89].

Cerebrovascular disease

Diabetes increases the risk of stroke [136] (➲Chapter 20). As an example, the risk of stroke among patients on glucose-lowering drugs was increased threefold among the nearly 350,000 men in the Multiple Risk Factor Intervention Trial [137]. In the Baltimore–Washington Cooperative Young Stroke Study, stroke risk increased more than tenfold in diabetic patients younger than 44 years, ranging as high as 23-fold in young Caucasian men [138]. Diabetes also increases stroke-related mortality and doubles the rate of recurrent stroke [139, 140].

Measures to prevent stroke should include a multifactorial strategy [141, 142] aimed at treatment of hypertension, hyperlipidaemia, microalbuminuria, hyperglycaemia, and the use of antiplatelet medications. Results from the HOPE study and the Perindopril Protection Against Recurrent Stroke Study (PROGRESS) suggest that the reduction of stroke incidence in diabetic subjects during treatment based on ACEIs was greater than would be anticipated from blood pressure-lowering effect alone and the effect was also evident in normotensive individuals [73, 143]. In the LIFE trial the same trend was found with an ARB [75]. However, in several other trials, including Anti-hypertensive and Lipid Lowering Treatment to Prevent Heart Attack Trial (ALLHAT), there was no apparent benefit of one class of antihypertensive drug over another in this respect [144, 145]. Treatment with statins also reduces the incidence of stroke in high-risk patients [49] as well as antiplatelet therapy, which is indicated for both primary and secondary prevention of stroke. Aspirin in a low dose (75–250mg daily) should be the initial choice. Clopidogrel 75mg once daily may be given in case of intolerance [91, 146]. The combination with aspirin and clopidogrel seems less safe since it was associated with an increased risk of bleeding without any benefit in term of cardiovascular outcome in the MATCH-Trial, performed in 7599 patients of whom 68% had diabetes [147]. Nor did the CHARISMA-Study, combining aspirin and clopidogrel, show any benefit [148].

Diabetic patients with cerebrovascular atherosclerosis should receive platelet antagonists, statins, and ACEIs. A strategy of surgical revascularization combined with medical therapy for asymptomatic and symptomatic patients with haemodynamically significant internal carotid artery atherosclerosis resulted in fewer strokes than medical therapy alone [149, 150]. Diabetic subjects represented 23% of the total population in the Asymptomatic Carotid Atherosclerosis Study (ACAS) [149] and 19% in the North American Symptomatic Carotid Endarterectomy Trial (NASCET)[150]. Consequently, they should be managed as non-diabetic patients with carotid artery disease. Cardiovascular mortality following carotid endarterectomy is increased in diabetic patients after 30 days and 1 year because of an increased rate of coronary events [151, 152]. The rates of perioperative major and minor stroke, however, do not differ between diabetic and non-diabetic patients [153], even if the need for hospitalization was somewhat longer. Thus, despite a lack of direct outcome data in diabetic patients, evidence suggests that the use of stenting for the treatment of carotid artery atherosclerosis is as rational in patients with diabetes as in those without diabetes [154].

Peripheral arterial disease

Diabetes increases the incidence and severity of limb ischaemia approximately two- to fourfold [155] (➲Chapter 36). Data from the Framingham cohort and Rotterdam studies show increased rates of absent pedal pulses, femoral bruits, and diminished ankle–brachial indices [156]. Diabetic peripheral arterial disease (PAD) often affects the distal limb vessels, such as the tibial and peroneal arteries, limiting the potential for collateral vessel development and reducing options for revascularization [157]. As such, patients with diabetes are at a particularly high risk to develop symptomatic forms of PAD, such as intermittent claudication and critical limb ischaemia, and to undergo amputation. In the Framingham cohort, the presence of diabetes increased intermittent claudication more than threefold in men and more than eightfold in women.

Diabetic persons have a particular propensity to develop foot ulcers with male sex, hyperglycaemia, and diabetes duration as important risk factors. Foot ulcers often result from severe macrovascular disease, and diabetic neuropathy exacerbates the risk [158, 159]. Once ulceration occurs, patients with diabetes have a much higher risk of amputation, highlighting the importance of prevention.

An objective measure of PAD is the ankle–brachial blood pressure index, defined as the ratio between the arterial pressure at the ankle level and in the brachial artery with the highest pressure (➲Chapter 36). A Doppler device is used to record the pulse in the dorsal pedal artery or the posterior tibial artery, while decreasing pressure in a cuff placed at the ankle level. Measurement is made in a supine position after 5min of rest. The reproducibility of this method is good and the ankle–brachial blood pressure index should normally be >0.9. This measurement is valuable for early detection of PAD and also for a better stratification of overall cardiovascular risk. An ankle–brachial blood pressure index <0.5 or an ankle pressure <50mmHg is indicative of severely impaired circulation of the foot.

For diabetic patients with PAD, general measures to reduce overall cardiovascular risk should be intensive [141, 142]. Smoking cessation is mandatory and regular exercise is also important. All patients with type 2 diabetes and PAD are recommended treatment with low-dose aspirin; treatment with clopidogrel or low-molecular weight heparin may be considered in certain cases [2].

Two non-invasive therapies have demonstrated benefit in improving walking distance in patients with PAD: exercise and cilostazol [160, 161]. Supervised exercise increases walking distance impressively. Patients with progressively disabling claudication and those with critical limb ischaemia should be considered for revascularization. Decisions regarding endovascular or open surgical procedures depend in large part on the severity and distribution of the arterial lesions. Outcomes of iliac artery percutaneous transluminal angioplasty (PTA) and stenting in patients with diabetes have been reported as being similar to or sometimes worse than those in non-diabetic patients [162], and the long-term patency after femoral–popliteal PTA is less in diabetic than non-diabetic patients [163]. The long-term patency of tibio–peroneal artery PTA is low in both diabetic and non-diabetic patients, but may be sufficient in the short term to facilitate healing of foot ulcers. Graft patency rates are similar in diabetic and non-diabetic patients following surgical revascularization. Still there is a greater rate of limb loss in diabetic patients with critical limb ischaemia as a result of persistent foot infection and necrosis [164]. Moreover, the risk of perioperative cardiovascular events is increased in patients with diabetes [165].

Selected issues

Cardiac autonomic neuropathy and silent myocardial ischaemia

Autonomic neuropathy is a serious and common complication of diabetes. It has been estimated that about 20% of asymptomatic diabetic patients have abnormal cardiovascular autonomic function [166, 167]. The risk for cardiovascular autonomic neuropathy depends on the duration of diabetes and the degree of glycaemic control. It is caused by injury to the autonomic nerve fibres that innervate the heart and blood vessels. The hypotheses concerning its aetiology include metabolic insult to nerve fibres, neurovascular insufficiency, neurohormonal growth factor deficiency, and autoimmune damage [168]. The main consequences are dysfunctional heart rate control, abnormal vascular dynamics and cardiac denervation, which become clinically overt as exercise intolerance, orthostatic hypotension, intraoperative cardiovascular morbidity [169], and silent myocardial ischaemia.

The earliest sign is often a vagal deficiency leaving sympathetic innervation unopposed. A manifestation of this is that diabetic patients tend to have a higher resting heart rate and less heart rate variability during the day than their non-diabetic counterparts. A clinical setting where this may be particularly unfavourable is at the onset of a myocardial infarction, causing unnecessary myocardial oxygen consumption in a situation with decreased nutritional blood supply. The autonomic nervous system influences coronary blood flow regulation independently of endothelial cell function. Diabetic patients with sympathetic nervous system dysfunction have impaired dilatation of coronary resistance vessels in response to cold pressure testing when compared with diabetics without defects in cardiac adrenergic nerve density. Global myocardial blood flow and coronary flow reserve, studied by positron emission tomography in response to adenosine provocation, were subnormal in diabetics with cardiovascular autonomic neuropathy. It is obvious that cardiovascular autonomic neuropathy may provoke ischaemic episodes by upsetting the balance between myocardial supply and demand. As a result of autonomic neuropathy, silent myocardial ischaemia is common in diabetic patients and is often symptomatically apparent only in advanced stages of disease. Instead of typical angina, patients frequently complain of shortness of breath, diaphoresis, or profound fatigue.

Knowledge on the actual prevalence of cardiovascular autonomic neuropathy and its related mortality rates is conflicting. However, different studies and meta-analyses reveal that mortality rates among diabetic subjects with cardiovascular autonomic neuropathy are many times higher than among those without. Subjects with diabetes and low levels of autonomic function parameters (baroreflex sensitivity, heart rate variability, and classical Ewing tests) had an approximately doubled risk of mortality in the Hoorn Study [170].

In the Detection of Ischaemia in Asymptomatic Diabetics (DIAD) study [171], cardiac autonomic dysfunction, assessed by the Valsalva manoeuvre, was a strong predictor of ischaemia, whereas traditional and emerging risk factors were not. Impaired angina perception largely accounts for such an increased mortality. Indeed, silent myocardial ischaemia delays treatment of acute coronary events and makes it more difficult to monitor anti-ischaemic treatment or determine whether restenosis has occurred after a coronary intervention. Although silent myocardial ischaemia has a reported prevalence of 10–20% in diabetic populations compared with only 1–4% in non-diabetic populations, routine screening for silent myocardial ischaemia in diabetics remains debatable.

In the DIAD study [171], 22% of 522 type 2 diabetic patients randomized to adenosine stress testing with myocardial perfusion imaging by means of single photon emission computerized tomography (SPECT) had silent ischaemia. This would indicate that asymptomatic diabetic patients have at least an intermediate probability of CAD, a prevalence that may justify routine screening for CAD by non-invasive testing. In a series of 203 diabetic patients [172], the prevalence of functional silent myocardial ischaemia, assessed by stress electrocardiogram (ECG) and thallium myocardial scintigraphy, was 15.7%. In this study, the positive predictive value of exercise ECG was 90%, compared with 63% of thallium myocardial scintigraphy. Thus, available evidence highlights the need for non-invasive screening by means of stress-testing in diabetic subjects, especially considering the high sensitivity, feasibility and low costs of exercise ECG.

Based on cardiovascular autonomic neuropathy-associated coronary blood flow impairment, misdiagnosed CAD, and the consequently higher risk of mortality, it is presently recommended that a baseline determination of cardiovascular autonomic function is performed upon diagnosis in type 2 diabetes and within 5 years of diagnosis for type 1 diabetes, followed by yearly repeated tests [173].

Diabetes and cardiac arrhythmias

Atrial fibrillation

With a prevalence of 0.4% in the general population, and roughly 10% in subjects older than 80 years, atrial fibrillation (AF) is the most common cardiac rhythm disorder and the major risk factor for stroke [174] (➲Chapter 29). On an epidemiological basis, diabetes is associated with AF and seems to favour the occurrence of the arrhythmia. Indeed, in the Framingham Heart Study [175], diabetes was shown to favour new-onset AF in a large cohort of men and women followed-up for 38 years (OR, 1.4 for men and 1.6 for women).

In a recent community-based observational study revealing that diabetes and/or hypertension are associated with the development of AF, the association of combined diabetes and hypertension with AF was significant when adjusted for cardiovascular risk factors, while it lost its significance when adjusted for Homeostasis Model Assessment (HOMA)-index, a marker of insulin resistance [176]. This would suggest that insulin resistance rather than hyperglycaemia per se may account for the increased risk for new-onset AF in patients with diabetes and hypertension. These observations suggest that insulin resistance may account for the increased risk of AF in patients with diabetes and/or hypertension, and set the rational for a role of RAAS blockade in preventing AF.

Diabetes is among the main risk factors for stroke in AF patients. Data from the pooled control groups of five primary prevention trials with aspirin or warfarin in AF patients (AF Investigators group, AFI) [181] reveal that risk factors predicting the occurrence of stroke in AF are age, hypertension, previous stroke or TIA, and diabetes (➲Chapter 29). In particular, patients with AF not receiving anticoagulants had a relative risk of stroke of 1.7. Although antithrombotic therapy prevents stroke in patients with AF, the choice of the anti-thrombotic agent is determined by the risk:benefit ratio between initial risk of stroke and absolute risk of bleeding. Indeed, the greater the initial risk of cerebrovascular events, the larger the benefit of oral anticoagulation as compared to aspirin [182]. Diabetes is a moderate risk factor for stroke according to the 2006 guidelines on AF from the ACC/AHA/ESC task force [183], and is included in most risk stratification algorithms for stroke. In CHADS2 [184], one of the most recent score-based risk stratification schemes, two points are given for prior stroke or TIA, and one point for each of the following: congestive heart failure, hypertension, age >75 years, and diabetes. The presence of a single moderate risk factor (e.g. diabetes) carries an annual risk of stroke of 1.5% without warfarin, while a score of 2 or 3 (e.g., diabetes and hypertension or diabetes and prior TIA) carries an annual risk of 2.5% and 5.2%, respectively. Current guidelines [2] recommend (➲ Chapter 29):

- oral anticoagulation (INR 2–3) for all patients with prior stroke or TIA (class I, level of evidence A);
- oral anticoagulation (INR 2–3) for patients with more than one risk factor among: age 75 years or greater, hypertension, congestive heart failure, impaired left ventricular systolic function, diabetes (class I, level of evidence A);
- either oral anticoagulation (INR 2–3) or aspirin (81–325mg daily), according to the individual risk of bleeding and patient preference, in subjects with a single risk factor (e.g., diabetes) (class IIa, level of evidence A);
- oral anticoagulation (INR 2–3) for patients aged 65–74 years and diabetes mellitus (class I).

As far as therapeutic strategies for rhythm control in AF are concerned, anti-arrhythmic drugs failed to show any consistent advantages over a rate control approach in large clinical trials [185, 186]. Among different treatments for AF, catheter ablation was recently shown to be a safe and effective option [187] when 70 patients with type 2 diabetes were randomized to catheter ablation or antiarrhythmic drug therapy for symptomatic drug-refractory AF (29 with paroxysmal and 41 with persistent). At 1 year, 80% of patients treated with pulmonary vein isolation were free from AF as compared with 43% of patients treated with anti-arrhythmic drugs only. Moreover, patients treated with anti-arrhythmic drugs developed drug-related adverse effects (17%) and were more likely to be hospitalized during follow-up (➲ Chapter 29).

Sudden cardiac death

In Western countries, ischaemic heart disease is the main substrate for the development of life-threatening cardiac arrhythmias and sudden cardiac death (SCD) [188] (➲ Chapter 30). As diabetes considerably increases the risk of CAD and worsens prognosis after acute myocardial infarction, it is not surprising that in many analyses diabetes is regarded as predictor of SCD. However, proving this concept was far more complex than anticipated. Indeed, mode of death in large cardiovascular trials may be difficult to determine (especially when death is unwitnessed and/or autopsy is unavailable), and the definition of diabetes or glucose intolerance among different studies may vary significantly.

The Framingham Study [189] was one of the first long-term follow-up studies revealing that diabetes was associated with an almost fourfold increased risk of SCD. This has been confirmed in the Nurses' Health Study [190], which included >120,000 women aged 30–55 years and followed for 22 years. Diabetes was associated with an almost threefold increase in the risk of SCD. The link between diabetes and SCD was assessed in the Honolulu Heart Program [191], Paris Prospective Study [192], and by the Group Health Cooperative [193], all of which confirmed that diabetes is a strong risk factor. Still it remains unclear whether CAD, left ventricular dysfunction, or arrhythmias perhaps triggered by hypoglycaemia account for this association.

Cardiovascular autonomic neuropathy is frequent among diabetics, occurring in 22% of patients with type 2 diabetes [194]. In patients with diabetes mellitus, cardiac autonomic neuropathy has been reported to be a poor prognostic factor associated with an increased incidence of SCD [195]. Indeed, reduction in heart rate variability (➲ Chapter 2) and impaired parasympathetic–sympathetic balance play a role in the genesis of ventricular arrhythmia [196]. In particular, patients with severe distal left ventricular sympathetic denervation display proximal areas of myocardial hyperinnervation, which constitute a pattern of autonomic and electrical instability predisposing to life-threatening arrhythmias [197]. Moreover, corrected QT (QTc) interval prolongation and dispersion, which have been reported in 26% and 33% of patients with type 2 diabetes, increase the risk for ventricular arrhythmias and sudden death [198].

In line with the view that cardiovascular risk is a *continuum* that increases well below the present thresholds for diabetes, the focus has recently shifted from the traditional dichotomous risk stratification (i.e. diabetics versus non-diabetics) to the identification of the risk of SCD according to blood glucose levels. Hence, Jouven *et al.* [199] showed that the risk increases with glycaemia, and that even patients with non-fasting glycaemia between 7.8–11.1mmol/L (140 and 200mg/dL) have an increased risk of sudden death.

Hyper- or hypokalaemia induced by hypoglycaemia has been associated with repolarization abnormalities and prolongation of QT-intervals which may lead to ventricular arrhythmias. However, these assumptions are mainly based on mechanistic studies, case reports, and registry- and trial-based retrospective subgroup analyses, and the clinical importance is not proven [200, 201]. Beta-blockers corrected, at least in part, these abnormalities in experimental models [202] and, despite the risk of masking symptoms of hypoglycaemia, the general consensus is to recommend their use as they improve survival in diabetic subjects [203].

Diabetes and heart failure

Epidemiology

The prevalence of heart failure has been estimated to be 0.6–6.2% in Swedish men and to increase by age (➲Chapter 23). Similar proportions were reported among both genders in the Rotterdam population and the Reykjavík Study [204, 205]. Regarding the prevalence of the combination of diabetes and heart failure, the most recent and extensive data are from the Reykjavík Study showing that it is 0.5% in men and 0.4% in women, increasing by age. Heart failure was found in 12% of people with diabetes compared to only 3% in those without this disease [206]. Regarding incidence data from the Framingham study revealed that the likelihood of developing heart failure was doubled among males and five times higher in females with diabetes during 18 years of follow-up compared to patients free from diabetes.

In a general population of elderly Italians the incidence of diabetes was significantly higher among heart failure patients (OR = 3.2 (2.6–4.0) during 3 years of follow-up and diabetes predicted the subsequent development of heart failure [207]. In the Reykjavik study there was a linear and independent relationship between increasing fasting glucose and the development of heart failure. Following standardization for age and gender the incidence of heart failure was 5.3/1000/year, of diabetes 4.6/1000/year, and abnormal glucose regulation 12.6/1000/year respectively. Increasing fasting glucose by 1mmol/L increased the risk for heart failure by 14% ($p = 0.04$) after adjusting for ischaemic heart disease, body mass index, and other risk factors for CVD. The association between diabetes (OR 3.0; 95% CI 2.3–4.0) and abnormal glucose regulation (OR 1.8; 95% CI 1.5–2.3) and heart failure was strong [208].

Pathophysiology

Analysis of the Framingham Cohort showed that diabetic individuals, particularly women, had greater left ventricular wall thickness and cardiac mass than control subjects. More recent studies reported a link between diabetes and some forms of 'idiopathic' dilated cardiomyopathy [209, 210], and claimed that diabetes-related cardiomyopathy is independent from CAD 211. An early manifestation of myocardial engagement in a diabetic patient is diastolic dysfunction, which is seen in animal models [212] and in humans [213, 214]. The reduction of left ventricular compliance is associated with the severity and duration of diabetes but is detectable already early in the course of diabetes [215]. The frequent coexistence of hypertension and diabetes does, however, cloud the actual contribution of the diabetic state to the diastolic dysfunction. After the onset of diastolic dysfunction, progressive myocardial dysfunction occurs in a time-dependent fashion subsequently leading systolic dysfunction and the classical features of heart failure. Because of the common coexistence of diabetes, hypertension, and CAD, it has been debated whether the myocardial dysfunction is primarily triggered by the glucometabolic disorder itself rather than by the synergistic action of these factors. From a clinical perspective, prevention of the development of left ventricular systolic dysfunction and subsequent heart failure is currently focused on pharmacological treatment of the comorbidities. It may also explain why meticulous antihypertensive treatment seems to be particularly effective in the diabetic subject.

Further evidence for the existence of a distinct diabetes-specific cardiomyopathy emerges from basic reports of changes in cardiac structure and cardiomyocyte ultra structure plausibly attributable to the diabetic milieu. In diabetic patients, as well as in animal models, the heart displays a reduction in cardiac mass, myocardial hypertrophy, interstitial fibrosis, and cell loss over time [216]. Although similar pathoanatomical changes may be seen even in the hypertensive heart, cardiac cell death is still believed to be a direct consequence of hyperglycaemia-induced metabolic abnormalities, sub cellular defects, and abnormal gene expression [217].

A prominent role is currently conferred to enhanced intramyocardial deposition of collagen [218], abnormalities in calcium handling [219], changes in troponin T [220], and PKC-mediated cardiac hypertrophy and failure [221]. Moreover, recent evidence in diabetic patients [222] and in streptozotocin-induced diabetic mice [223] suggests that increased incidence of cell apoptosis occurs in the diabetic heart, mainly as a consequence of oxidative stress-triggered receptor-independent cell death pathway activation [224].

Thus, oxidative stress rather than hyperglycaemia per se may account for subcellular remodelling, cardiomyocyte apoptosis, and the subsequent onset of cardiomyopathy. Accordingly, a significant increase in 3-nitrotyrosine-containing proteins, typical end-products of the reaction of peroxynitrite with biological compounds [225], has been reported in cardiomyocytes from diabetic patients and streptozotocin-induced diabetic animals. This evidence suggests a causative link between hyperglycaemia, oxidative/nitrosative stress, cardiomyocyte apoptosis, and diabetic cardiomyopathy. Still attempts to improve early signs of myocardial dysfunction by means of glucose normalization have so far not been successful although previous uncontrolled observations in more severe diabetes seemed promising [226].

Prognostic implications

The combination of diabetes and heart failure has a serious prognosis including patients with left ventricular dysfunction due to ischaemic heart disease [227, 228]. In a general population in Reykjavík there was a significant increase in mortality with the concomitant presence of heart failure and glucose abnormalities even after adjustment for cardiovascular risk factors and ischaemic heart disease (OR; 95%CI for men = 2.1 (1.5–2.9) and for women = 1.9; 1.2–2.8) [229]. This may be seen as an indicator of the serious implication of the combination of diabetes and heart failure.

Therapy

Few clinical trials have specifically addressed treatment of heart failure in a well-defined diabetic population. Thus available information on treatment efficacy has to be based on diabetic subgroups, often in the magnitude of 20–35%, from various heart failure trials. Although the characterization of these subgroups lacks in completeness and information on glucose-lowering therapy, available data favour a proportionately similar efficacy of diuretics, ACEIs, and beta-blockers in patients with and without diabetes. Since the absolute risk for morbidity and mortality is substantially higher in patients with diabetes the absolute treatment efficacy is higher in patients with than among those without diabetes. Drugs, like trimetazidine, etomoxir, and dichloroacetate, aimed to shift myocardial metabolism from oxidation of free fatty acids towards glycolysis, have been tested in patients with myocardial dysfunction and diabetes. The usefulness must still be considered controversial despite some recent promising results [230–232].

The metabolic syndrome

Insights from pathophysiology for better clinical management

In 1988, Reaven [233] noted that several risk factors (e.g. dyslipidaemia, hypertension, hyperglycaemia) commonly cluster together. He defined this clustering as syndrome X, and identified it as a risk factor for CVD.

Nowadays, extended panels of metabolic risk factors have been identified to better understand pathogenesis, predict outcomes, and improve clinical management of the so-called metabolic syndrome (MS). Two independent efforts to identify definition criteria have been carried out by the National Cholesterol Education Program's Adult Treatment Panel III (ATP III) [13] and the World Health Organization (WHO) [234].

ATP III identified six components of the MS that relate to CVD:

- abdominal obesity;
- atherogenic dyslipidaemia;
- raised blood pressure;
- insulin resistance and/or glucose intolerance;
- proinflammatory state;
- prothrombotic state.

All of these components are part of a larger body of risk factors for CVD that ATP III identifies as underlying (obesity, physical inactivity, atherogenic diet), major (cigarette smoking, hypertension, elevated LDL-cholesterol, low HDL-cholesterol, family history of premature coronary heart disease, aging) and emerging (elevated triglycerides, small LDL particles, insulin resistance, glucose intolerance, proinflammatory state, and prothrombotic state).

To facilitate diagnosis and preventive interventions, ATP III proposed a clinical definition based on having at least three of five criteria (➲Table 14.3) [235]. Using ATP III definition, the estimated prevalence of the MS among men and women in NHANES III [236] ranges from 5% (normal weight) to 60% (obese) in men, and from 6% (normal weight) to 50% (obese) in women. Currently it exceeds 20% of individuals who are at least 20 years of age, and 40% of the population >40 years [237].

The WHO criteria (➲Table 14.4) require insulin resistance for diagnosis, by demonstrating the presence of type 2 diabetes, IFG, or IGT by OGTT in patients without IFG. In addition to insulin resistance, two other risk factors are sufficient for a diagnosis of MS.

On the contrary, ATP III claims that information obtained from an OGTT does not outweigh the inconveniences and costs of applying this test in the clinical routine.

Notably, both ATP III and WHO recognize CVD as the primary outcome of the MS. In the Framingham Study the MS alone predicted 25% of all new-onset CVD. In the absence of diabetes the MS generally did not raise the 10-year risk for CAD to >20% (the threshold for the CAD risk equivalent in ATP III). Notably, the 10-year cardiovascular risk in men with MS ranged from 10–20%, whereas it did not exceed 10% in most women, who also displayed a lower rate of CAD events during the 8-year follow-up.

Table 14.3 ATP III clinical identification of the metabolic syndrome

Risk factor	Defining level
Abdominal obesity, given as waist circumference*†	
Men	>102cm (>40 inches)
Women	>88cm (>35 inches)
Triglycerides	≥150mg/dL
HDL cholesterol	
Men	<40mg/dL
Women	<50mg/dL
Blood pressure	≥130/≥85mmHg
Fasting glucose	≥110mg/dL‡

* Overweight and obesity are associated with insulin resistance and the metabolic syndrome. However, the presence of abdominal obesity is more highly correlated with the metabolic risk factors than is an elevated BMI. Therefore, the simple measure of waist circumference is recommended to identify the body weight component of the metabolic syndrome.

† Some male patients can develop multiple metabolic risk factors when the waist circumference is only marginally increased, e.g. 94–102cm (37–39 inches). Such patients may have a strong genetic contribution to insulin resistance. They should benefit from changes in life habits, similarly to men with categorical increases in waist circumference.

‡ The ADA has recently established a cutpoint of ≤100mg/dL, above which persons have either prediabetes (impaired fasting glucose) or diabetes. This new cutpoint should be applicable for identifying the lower boundary to define an elevated glucose as one criterion for the metabolic syndrome.

Reproduced from Grundy SM, Brewer HB, Jr., Cleeman JI, *et al.* Definition of metabolic syndrome: Report of the National Heart, Lung, and Blood Institute/American Heart Association conference on scientific issues related to definition. *Circulation* 2004; **109**: 433–8. Reprinted with permission ©2004 American Heart Association, Inc.

A new definition of MS has been recently proposed by the International Diabetes Federation [238]. To be defined as having MS, one must have:

- central obesity (defined as waist circumference ≥94cm (≥37 inches) for European men and ≥80cm (≥31.5 inches) for European women, **with ethnicity specific values for other groups);**

Table 14.4 WHO clinical criteria for metabolic syndrome

Insulin resistance, identified by 1 of the following:
Type 2 diabetes
Impaired fasting glucose
Impaired glucose tolerance
Or for those with normal fasting glucose levels (<110mg/dL), glucose uptake below the lowest quartile for background population under investigation under hyperinsulinemic, euglycaemic conditions.
Plus any 2 of the following:
Antihypertensive medication and/or high blood pressure (≥140mmHg systolic or ≥90mmHg diastolic)
Plasma triglycerides ≥150mg/dL (≥1.7mmol/L)
HDL cholesterol <35mg/dL (<0.9mmol/L) in men or <39mg/dL (1.0mmol/L) in women
Body mass index >30kg/m^2 and/or waist:hip ratio >0.9 in men, >0.85 in women
Urinary albumin excretion rate ≥20mcg/min or albumin:creatinine ratio ≥30mg/g

Reproduced from Grundy SM, Brewer HB, Jr., Cleeman JI, *et al.* Definition of metabolic syndrome: Report of the National Heart, Lung, and Blood Institute/American Heart Association conference on scientific issues related to definition. *Circulation* 2004; **109**: 433–8. Reprinted with permission ©2004 American Heart Association, Inc.

plus any two of the following four factors:

- **raised TG level:** ≥150mg/dL (1.7mmol/L), or specific treatment for this lipid abnormality;
- **reduced HDL cholesterol:** <40mg/dL (1.03mmol/L) in males and <50mg/dL (1.29mmol/L) in females, or specific treatment for this lipid abnormality;
- **raised blood pressure:** systolic blood pressure ≥130mmHg or diastolic blood pressure ≥85mmHg, or treatment of previously diagnosed hypertension;
- **raised fasting plasma glucose** (FPG) ≥ 100mg/dL (5.6mmol/L), **or previously diagnosed type 2 diabetes.** If above 5.6mmol/L or 100mg/dL, OGTT is strongly recommended but is not necessary to define presence of the syndrome.

This new definition is easy to use in clinical practice as it avoids the need for measurements that may only be available in research settings.

In this section, specific risk factors and new emerging and contributing conditions will be analysed in the attempt to identify a continuum between pathogenesis, clinical management, and treatment of MS risk factors.

Obesity

In ATP III, abdominal obesity, recognized by increased waist circumference, is the first criterion listed. Its inclusion reflects the pivotal role assigned to abdominal obesity as a contributor to the MS: obesity contributes to hypertension, high serum cholesterol, low HDL-cholesterol, and hyperglycaemia, and it associates with higher CVD risk. Excess visceral adipose tissue releases several products that apparently exacerbate these risk factors, including:

- non-esterified fatty acids, which overload muscle and liver with lipid, thus enhancing insulin resistance;
- plasminogen activator inhibitor type 1 (PAI-1), which contributes to a prothrombotic state;
- C-reactive protein (CRP), which may signify cytokine excess and a proinflammatory state.

The strong connection between abdominal obesity and risk factors led ATP III to define the MS essentially as a cluster of metabolic complications of obesity.

As stated by the NHLBI and the National Institute of Diabetes and Digestive and Kidney Diseases (NIDDK) [239], overweight and obesity are defined by a body mass index (BMI) of 25–29.9kg/m^2 and ≥30kg/m^2, respectively. Abdominal obesity, defined as a waist circumference ≥102cm (≥40 inches) in men and ≥88cm (≥35 inches) in women, is associated with several of the components of the MS. In ATP III, the rationale for using waist criteria rather than BMI arises from data showing that measures of overall obesity are relatively insensitive indicators of the risk for metabolic and cardiovascular complications of obesity, as compared with measures of central or abdominal adiposity [240]. Waist circumference reflects both abdominal subcutaneous adipose tissue and abdominal visceral adipose tissue. The visceral adipose tissue is presumed to be the major determinant of metabolic and cardiovascular complications of obesity [241]. It is presently unclear whether more accurate measures of specific abdominal subcutaneous and visceral adipose tissue using computerized tomography or magnetic resonance imaging may provide superior information regarding obesity complications [242].

It is generally accepted that obesity should be the primary target of intervention in MS. First-line therapy should be weight reduction obtained by lowering caloric intake and reinforcing physical activity. Weight loss lowers serum cholesterol and triglycerides, raises HDL-cholesterol, lowers blood pressure and glucose, and reduces insulin resistance. Recent data further show that weight reduction can decrease serum levels of CRP and PAI-1.

Extreme diets are often ineffective in producing long-term results. More effective and healthful for long-term weight loss are reduced-energy diets, consisting of a modest calories/day reduction. General recommendations for diet composition include low intake of saturated fats, trans fats and cholesterol; reduced consumption of simple sugars; increased intake of fruits, vegetables, and whole grains. Regular physical activity is highly recommended, with a daily minimum of 30min of moderate–intensity activity [243]. More exercise (i.e. 1 hour daily) is even more efficacious for weight control. A realistic goal is to reduce body weight by 7–10% over 6–12 months. Long-term maintenance of weight loss is best achieved when regular exercise is included in the weight-reduction regimen and professional support (such as nutrition counselling) and group training is often helpful.

Insulin resistance

Insulin resistance per se is believed to play a significant role in the pathogenesis of MS, and many investigators claim that this is the pathophysiological process behind the clustering of cardiovascular risk factors in the MS. Insulin resistance predicts atherosclerosis and cardiovascular events independently from other risk factors, including fasting glucose and lipid levels [244]. Recent data from the STOP-NIDDM trial [245] have convincingly demonstrated that acute cardiovascular events in subjects with IGT may be prevented by treatment that reduces postprandial glucose levels. Moreover, the impressive results of the Finnish Diabetes Prevention Study and the Diabetes Prevention Programme led the ADA and the NIDDK to recommend that people aged over 45 years with a BMI ≥25 should be screened for high blood glucose and given appropriate counselling on the importance of weight loss if found to have evidence of a pre-diabetic state.

Mechanisms by which insulin resistance impacts other MS risk factors are:

- diversion of excess non-esterified fatty acids from lipid-overloaded insulin-resistant muscles to the liver, thus promoting fatty liver and atherogenic dyslipidaemia;
- enhanced output of VLDL;
- predisposition to glucose intolerance, which can be worsened by increased hepatic gluconeogenesis in the insulin-resistant liver;
- blood pressure raising, by a variety of mechanisms (see following section for details).

Insulin resistance generally rises with increasing body fat and most people with a BMI ≥30kg/m^2 have postprandial hyperinsulinaemia/reduced insulin sensitivity [246] while persons with a BMI between 25–29.9kg/m^2 exhibit a spectrum of insulin sensitivities as well. In some populations (such as South Asians), insulin resistance is common even with BMI <25kg/m^2, a condition termed primary insulin resistance.

Various measures have been used to define insulin sensitivity [247]. While hyperinsulinaemic clamp and glucose tolerance testing-based approaches accurately define insulin resistance, prolonged insulin infusion and/or repeated blood sampling are required, which may be undesirable in routine clinical practice. Surrogate measures of insulin sensitivity including the Homeostasis Model Assessment (HOMA) and Quantitative Insulin Sensitivity Check Index (QUICKI) have been developed, showing a good correlation with direct gold-standard measures [248] and predicting the development of CVD and type 2 diabetes mellitus [249].

The reduction of insulin resistance is an attractive pharmacological target to prevent CVD in MS patients and there are currently two classes of drugs available: metformin and insulin sensitizers, such as thiazolidinediones. Both drugs reduce insulin resistance and favourably impact different metabolic risk factors. Metformin has been used in overweight patients with type 2 diabetes in the UKPDS and was shown to reduce cardiovascular events and mortality after 11 years of follow-up. [41]. Among thiazolinideniones, rosiglitazone has been related to an excess of risk for myocardial infarction [108] whereas pioglitazone decreased the risk of a composite endpoint of MI, stroke, and death in the PROACTIVE trial [109].

Atherogenic dyslipidaemia

Atherogenic dyslipidaemia is often recognized in MS and manifests itself by raised triglycerides, low HDL-cholesterol, increased remnant lipoproteins, elevated apolipoprotein B, and small LDL and HDL particles. It is commonly believed that hypertriglyceridaemia is the result of enhanced triglyceride hepatic synthesis driven by an increased flux of free fatty acids from the periphery to the liver in an insulin-resistant setting [250]. The causes of hypertriglyceridaemia in the MS are, however, most likely multifactorial and the increased free fatty acid flux hypothesis is one side of this issue. In the same view, low HDL-cholesterol, often ascribed to elevated triglycerides because of increased transfer of triglycerides to HDL and cholesterol from HDL [251], are likely to have a more complex origin, because HDL-cholesterol levels are often reduced in patients with insulin resistance even when fasting triglyceride levels are normal.

More recently, activation of innate immunity and immunity-related inflammation have been proposed as potential links between insulin resistance and dyslipidaemia. In animal models activation of innate immunity leads to changes in lipoproteins, enzymes, transfer proteins and receptors [252] commonly seen also in human MS. Inflammation-driven increase in lipase production has been proposed as a mechanism promoting reduction of lipid content of HDLs [253].

While lipid-lowering therapy is mandatory in dyslipidaemic MS patients, most of them do not display elevated LDL-cholesterol levels, and there is no consensus on the appropriate LDL target in the MS. It is conceivable that in the presence of additional traditional (smoking, family history of CAD) or new (high CRP levels, evidence of a prothrombotic state) risk factors, the MS should be considered a CVD equivalent rather than a 'sum' of risk factors. Statin therapy with a target LDL-cholesterol <100mg/dL (or even lower, based on evidence in 'very-high-risk patients') would then be the appropriate target.

Several drugs are available for patients with atherogenic dyslipidaemia. Statins reduce all apolipoprotein B-containing lipoproteins, often achieving ATP III goals for LDL/non-HDL-cholesterol. Their impact on CV events is well documented [254]. Fibrates improve all components of atherogenic dyslipidaemia, and post hoc analysis of recent trials strongly suggests that they reduce CVD endpoints in patients with atherogenic dyslipidaemia and MS [255]. Since clinical studies demonstrate that abnormal lipoprotein patterns are better controlled by statin–fibrate therapy, a combined therapeutic strategy would seem attractive. However, both fibrates and statins have the potential to produce myopathy, and their combined use enhances this risk [64]. Nicotinic acid shares some features with fibrates, and is considered especially efficacious for raising HDL-cholesterol levels. Its combined use with statins is promising. Still awaiting proven efficacy confirmation from randomized clinical trials is the category of dual PPAR agonists. They are promising agents targeting both PPAR-α and PPAR-γ, thereby simultaneously treating insulin resistance, glucose intolerance, elevated triglycerides, and low HDL-cholesterol levels.

High blood pressure

In obese patients, blood pressure is sensitive to sodium intake, and this sensitivity is related to fasting insulin levels [256]. The antinatriuretic effect of insulin, together with its ability to activate the sympathetic nervous system [257] and to drive abnormal vascular function, contributes to the development of hypertension. Moreover, both hyperglycaemia and insulin activate the renin–angiotensin system by enhancing the expression of angiotensin II, which contributes to raising the blood pressure of patients with insulin resistance (➲Fig. 14.15) (➲Chapter 13).

The majority of MS patients fall into the categories of normal and high-normal blood pressure levels (systolic: 120–139mmHg or diastolic: 80–89mmHg) or stage 1 hypertension (systolic blood pressure: 140–159mmHg or diastolic blood pressure: 90–99mmHg). Lifestyle modification is

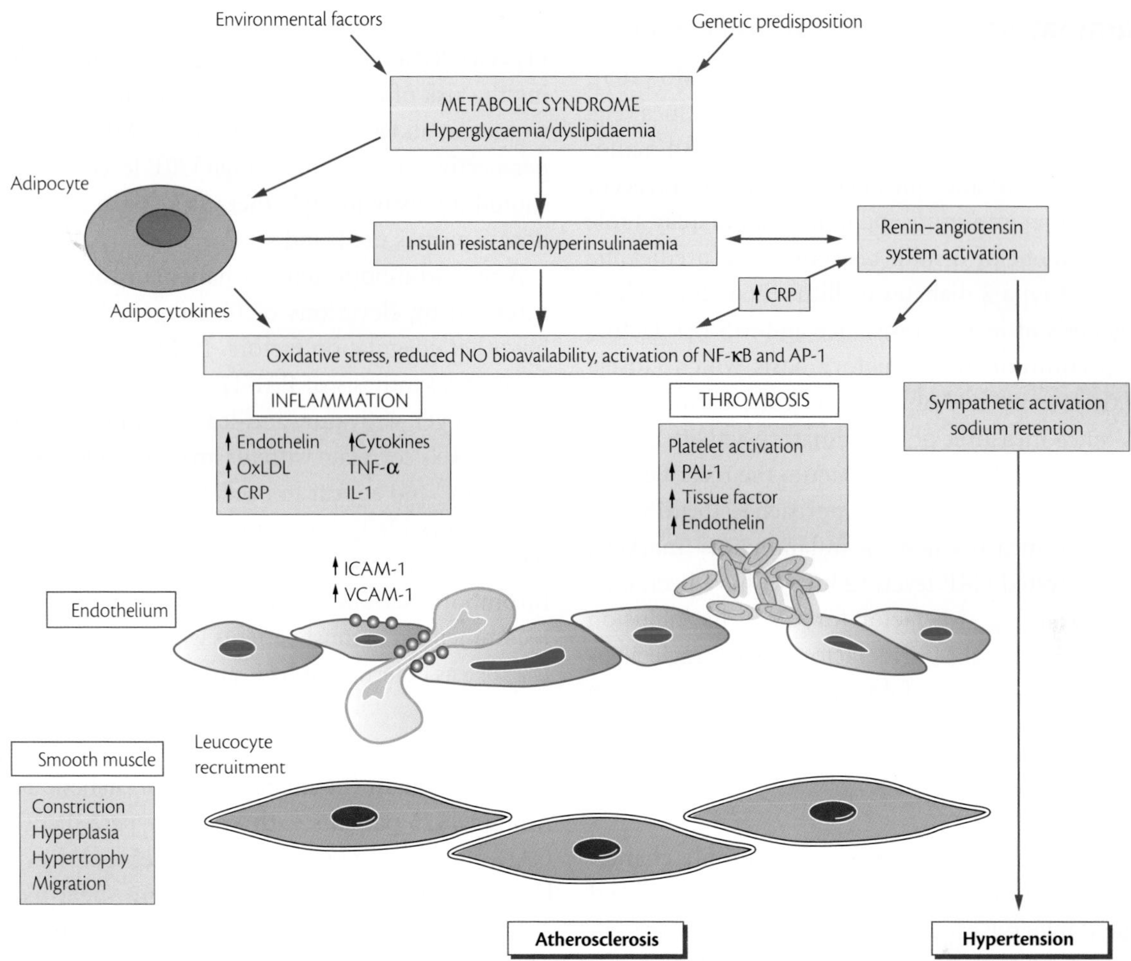

Figure 14.15 Pathophysiology of cardiovascular disease in metabolic syndrome. AP-1, activator protein-1; CRP, C-reactive protein; ICAM-1, intercellular adhesion molecule; IL-1, interleukin-1; oxLDL, oxidized low density lipoprotein; PAI-1, plasminogen activator inhibitor-1; TNF-α, tumor necrosis factor-α; VCAM-1, vascular cell adhesion molecule. Reproduced with permission from Prasad A, Quyyumi AA. Renin-angiotensin system and angiotensin receptor blockers in the metabolic syndrome. *Circulation* 2004; **110**: 1507–12.

the cornerstone of management in all patients with high-normal blood pressure levels or with the MS. If blood pressure exceeds 140/90mmHg, pharmacological therapy is indicated according to both JNC7 [258] and ESH-ESC [259] recommendations. In patients with established diabetes, antihypertensive drugs should be introduced at even lower blood pressures (>130/80mmHg) (see ➲Chapter 13). No class of antihypertensive drugs has been identified as being uniquely efficacious in patients with MS. Diuretics and beta-blockers in high doses can worsen insulin resistance and atherogenic dyslipidaemia. However, beta-blockers are cardioprotective in patients with established CAD and are no longer contraindicated in patients with type 2 diabetes.

As mentioned, a rationale for antagonizing the renin–angiotensin system in MS has been proposed [260]. ACE inhibition improves insulin sensitivity and glycaemic control in diabetic patients [261] and was shown to induce a 14% relative reduction in the incidence of new-onset type 2 diabetes in the Captopril Prevention Project (CAPP) [262]. This was confirmed by the Heart Outcomes Prevention Evaluation (HOPE) trial, in which ramipril significantly reduced by 34% the incidence of new-onset diabetes [263]. Moreover, in the Losartan Intervention for Endpoint Reduction (LIFE), conducted on patients with hypertension and left ventricular hypertrophy, losartan reduced the composite cardiovascular event rate by 13% and the incidence of new-onset diabetes by 25% compared with atenolol [74, 75]. Similarly, treatment with valsartan, compared with amlodipine, was associated with a reduction in the incidence of diabetes in high-risk hypertensive patients in the Valsartan Antihypertensive Long-term Use Evaluation (VALUE) [264]. ACE inhibitors and angiotensin receptor antagonists also have a reno-protective capacity, not least in the diabetic patient.

In summary, ACEIs and ARBs are useful, first-line antihypertensives. Some evidence exists that they carry advantages over other drugs in patients with MS.

Proinflammatory and prothrombotic state

Chronic subclinical inflammation is part of the MS [265]. This condition is characterized by elevated cytokines (e.g. tumour necrosis factor-α and interleukin-6) and acute-phase reactants (CRP and fibrinogen). Of interest, recent studies suggest that immunity and inflammation play a role in the development of insulin resistance and predict the development of type 2 diabetes mellitus [266, 267]. Thus, the pathogenesis of insulin resistance and MS risk factors may have a common inflammatory basis which closely relates to the occurrence of atherosclerotic cardiovascular events. Since measures of inflammatory activity do not presently provide additional insights into the risk of events in MS patients, the current clinical approach to the MS does not incorporate measurement of inflammatory markers. However, as elevated CRP levels (≥3mg/L) have been outlined as an emerging risk factor for CVD, its inclusion together with traditional MS risk factors into a single algorithm is likely to provide a useful approach to risk prediction in MS patients. Indeed, in a recently published study [268], plasma CRP levels provided prognostic information regarding the risk of cardiovascular events in apparently healthy women at all levels of severity of the MS. From a practical perspective, the finding of high CRP levels in a MS patient should intensify lifestyle therapies, make certain that low-dose aspirin is used, and set lower LDL goals.

A prothrombotic state in patients with the MS is characterized by elevations of fibrinogen, PAI-1, and possibly other coagulation factors. In MS, activation of NF-kB promotes synthesis of PAI-1, a natural inhibitor of tissue plasminogen activator, and leads to impaired fibrinolysis. PAI-1 levels correlate with plasma insulin levels and insulin resistance, and appear to predict the likelihood of developing diabetes [269]. Since no drugs are available that target PAI-1 and fibrinogen, the alternative approach to the prothrombotic state is antiplatelet therapy. Use of aspirin is recommended in most patients whose 10-year risk for CHD is ≥10% as determined by Framingham risk scoring.

Personal perspective

Type 2 diabetes is a complex disease not only characterized by insulin resistance, beta-cell dysfunction, and subsequent hyperglycaemia, but also comorbidities such as hypertension, hyperlipidaemia, and a prothrombotic state. These factors interact synergistically thereby contributing to the total risk of cardiovascular complications and to the more dismal prognosis in these patients. A comprehensive approach, aiming at correction of all modifiable risk factors, is a prerequisite for a successful prevention of CVD manifestations and it is mandatory to initiate the needed measures without any delay [2].

The value of a multifactorial intervention was clearly demonstrated by the STENO 2 study recruiting 160 diabetic patients with microalbuminuria. In this trial early instituted, intensive, and target-driven multifactorial therapy resulted in a reduction of micro- and macrovascular events by about 50% during a mean follow-up of 7.8 years [141]. At that time all patients were given target-driven therapy. An extended follow-up until 13 years after study start still demonstrated a lasting effect of the initial intervention with an absolute mortality and cardiovascular mortality reduction of 20% and 29% respectively, underlining the importance of early treatment initiation [142].

Data from the Euro Heart Survey on Diabetes and the Heart support that a multifactorial approach should be a cornerstone in the management of diabetic patients. Among 1425 patients with known type 2 diabetes and CAD, 44% received a complete package of evidence-based medications including aspirin, beta-blockade, renin–angiotensin–aldosteron inhibitors, and statins. The diabetic patients on this combination had a significantly lower all-cause mortality (3.5 vs. 7.7%; $p = 0.001$) and fewer combined cardiovascular events (11.6 vs. 14.7%; $p = 0.050$) compared to those not receiving a full combination of evidence based medications [270].

Important information in this chapter is also that macrovascular complications are already common at the time when diabetes is diagnosed. Thus it is essential to identify people at high risk for developing diabetes, such as those with IGT and other components of MS, to allow the institution of preventive measures to stop or retard the development of diabetes and its complications. Lifestyle-oriented advice, when needed supplemented with drugs, such as acarbose or metformin, is effective in this respect [271–274].

Multifactorial treatment is mandatory and rewarding when it comes to improving cardiovascular prognosis for patients with type 2 diabetes. The increasing epidemic of diabetes and the metabolic syndrome is, however, not an isolated medical problem. To handle it at a population basis necessitates societal reforms including agricultural and food-processing political considerations [275].

Further reading

Alberti KG, Zimmet P, Shaw J. The metabolic syndrome—a new worldwide definition. *Lancet* 2005; **366**: 1059–62.

Camici GG, Schiavoni M, Francia P, *et al.* Genetic deletion of p66(Shc) adaptor protein prevents hyperglycemia-induced endothelial dysfunction and oxidative stress. *Proc Natl Acad Sci USA* 2007; **104**: 5217–22.

Dandona P, Thusu K, Cook S, *et al.* Oxidative damage to DNA in diabetes mellitus. *Lancet* 1996; **347**: 444–5.

Gaede P, Lund-Andersen H, Parving HH, *et al.* Effect of a multifactorial intervention on mortality in type 2 diabetes. *N Engl J Med* 2008; **358**: 580–91.

Gerstein HC, Miller ME, Byington RP, et al. Effects of intensive glucose lowering in type 2 diabetes. *N Engl J Med* 2008; **358**: 2545–559.

Holman RR, Paul SK, Bethel MA, *et al.* 10-year follow-up of intensive glucose control in type 2 diabetes. *N Engl J Med* 2008; **359**: 1577–89.

Lindstrom J, Ilanne-Parikka P, Peltonen M, *et al.* Sustained reduction in the incidence of type 2 diabetes by lifestyle intervention: follow-up of the Finnish Diabetes Prevention Study. *Lancet* 2006; **368**: 1673–9.

Ryden L, Standl E, Bartnik M, *et al.* Guidelines on diabetes, pre-diabetes, and cardiovascular diseases: executive summary. The Task Force on Diabetes and Cardiovascular Diseases of the European Society of Cardiology (ESC) and of the European Association for the Study of Diabetes (EASD). *Eur Heart J* 2007; **28**: 88–136.

➲ **For full references and multimedia materials please visit the online version of the book (http://esctextbook.oxfordonline.com).**

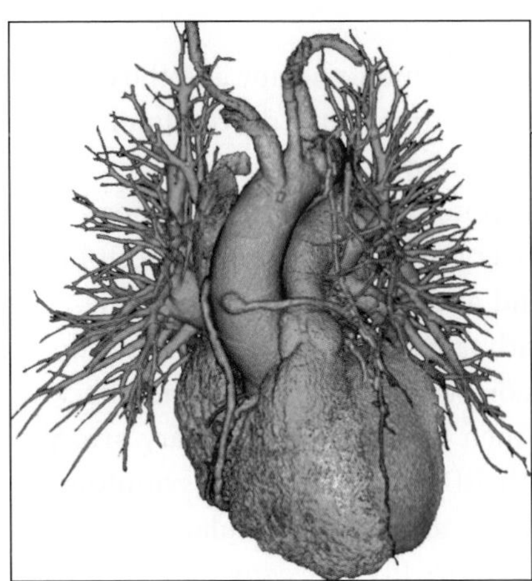

CHAPTER 15

Heart and Other Organs

Frank Ruschitzka

Contents

Introduction

Innovation in medicine emerges at the crossroads of different specialities.

Paul Hugenholtz

While the development of novel imaging techniques, interventions, and devices has transformed our specialty, cardiologists will have to continue to look beyond the borders of their discipline. Reaching out to our colleagues from different disciplines will not only further optimize the care of our patients, particularly the elderly presenting with comorbidities, but will also impact scientific exchange in a way that is best described as 'cross-fertilization'. As such, this chapter was introduced to this edition of the textbook to give those who already know 'everything about something' a chance to learn 'something about everything'. In particular, chapters on stroke, kidney disease, and erectile dysfunction (ED) have been added.

ED, kidney disease, or stroke are all highly prevalent in patients with cardiovascular disease. They particularly benefit from increased cardiovascular disease risk-factor surveillance and intervention and heightened awareness of the associated risk factors that need to be vigorously screened and treated accordingly.

Kidney disease is both a cause and a consequence of cardiovascular disease. Cardiovascular disease critically determines life expectancy of patients with chronic kidney disease. While death from cardiovascular disease is ten times more likely in dialysis patients than in the general population, even mild impairment of kidney function already substantially increases the risk of developing cardiovascular disease. Therefore, screening for cardiovascular disease is of high yield among patients with renal disease, even in those who do not report any history of cardiovascular symptoms.

Conversely, the presence of even mild renal impairment is an established risk factor for the development of heart disease. As such, in cardiac patients appropriate assessment of renal function (serum creatinine, estimated glomerular filtration rate, and proteinuria) is now obligatory.

Stroke ranks third after coronary heart disease as a cause of death worldwide. Eighty per cent of strokes are caused by focal cerebral ischaemia due to arterial occlusion, and the remaining 20% are caused by haemorrhages. Atherosclerosis (leading to thromboembolism or local occlusion) and cardioembolism are the leading causes. Striking similarities exist with regard to non-modifiable risk (age >55 years, African American race, male gender, prior transient ischaemic attack (TIA) or stroke and family history) and modifiable risk factors (hypertension, dyslipidaemia, cigarette smoking) of heart disease and stroke.

While blood pressure control is the mainstay in the primary prevention of stroke, only very high blood pressure values exceeding 220/110mmHg should be treated in acute stroke.

Secondary prevention of stroke following a cardiogenic TIA or stroke should mostly be performed with oral anticoagulation which is clearly superior to acetylsalicylic acid (ASA). Antiplatelet therapy is indicated in patients with ischaemic stroke and no cardiac source of embolism. Both clopidogrel monotherapy and the combination of ASA plus extended-release dipyridamole are superior to ASA monotherapy.

In patients with a symptomatic high degree stenosis of the internal carotid artery, stenting and endarterectomy are well established and offer similar clinical outcome.

ED is predominantly a vascular disease sharing the same risk factors as coronary artery disease and affects up to two-thirds of men with known coronary artery disease. All men with ED and no cardiac symptoms should be considered as cardiac (or vascular) patients until proven otherwise. Since ED is an early warning sign for silent coronary and vascular disease, men presenting with ED and no cardiac symptoms should undergo a full medical assessment with cardiovascular risk as high, medium, or low and have their cardiovascular risk factors treated accordingly.

While phosphodiesterase type 5 (PDE-5) inhibitors have transformed the management of ED, they remain contraindicated in patients with concomitant nitrates.

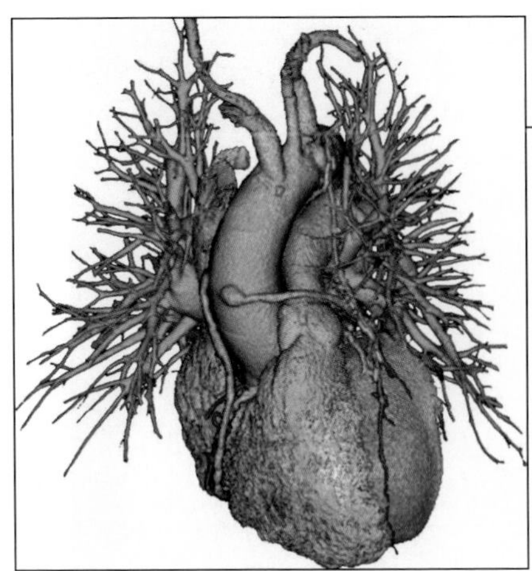

CHAPTER 15a

The Heart and the Brain

Hans-Christoph Diener, Heinrich Mattle, Michael Böhm, and Frank Ruschitzka

Contents

Summary

Stroke is the third most common reason for death, the second for dementia, and the most common cause for permanent disability. About 25% of all strokes are caused by a cardiac source of embolism, most frequently atrial. Acute stroke should be treated in dedicated stroke units. Systemic thrombolysis with recombinant tissue plasminogen activator in a time window up to 4.5 hours or endovascular recanalization up to 6 hours is effective in decreasing permanent disability after ischaemic stroke. Secondary prevention of stroke following a cardiogenic transient ischaemic attack or stroke should mostly be performed with oral anticoagulation which is clearly superior to acetylsalicylic acid (aspirin). Antiplatelet therapy is indicated in patients with ischaemic stroke and no cardiac source of embolism. Both clopidogrel monotherapy and the combination of aspirin plus extended-release dipyridamole are superior to aspirin monotherapy. In patients with a symptomatic high-degree stenosis of the internal carotid artery, endarterectomy has a slightly lower complication rate compared to stenting and balloon angioplasty with a similar long-term outcome.

Pathophysiology of acute ischaemic stroke and diagnostic procedures

Patients with ischaemic stroke experience sudden focal neurological deficits lasting >24 hours. Mortality following ischaemic stroke is 20–30% due to brain oedema and secondary complications such as aspiration pneumonia, deep vein thrombosis, and pulmonary embolism, sepsis or heart failure. Predictors for poor outcome are: initial loss of consciousness, age >70 years, hemiplegia with forced eye deviation, prior stroke, and concomitant coronary heart disease [1].

The reduced blood flow leads to neural and glial death in the core of the infarct. The core of the stroke area is surrounded by the so-called penumbra with diminished cerebral blood flow and functional loss of neurons and glia with the potential to survive. The best strategy to rescue this tissue is recanalization. Ischaemia triggers a complex cascade of release of excitatory amino acids, Ca^{2+} influx, and release of intracellular calcium and production of free radicals. Neuroprotective therapy aiming at interrupting these processes has failed so far for treatment of human stroke [2].

The first diagnostic procedure after physical and neurological examination is computer tomography (CT) or magnetic resonance imaging (MRI) of the brain to exclude cerebral haemorrhage. Indirect signs of cerebral ischaemia can be seen in CT within 2–3 hours. Diffusion-weighted MRI shows ischaemia immediately (➲ Fig. 15a.1) also in areas in which CT visualizes tissue poorly e.g. the posterior fossa. CT or MR angiography or duplexsonography will identify significant stenosis or occlusion of brain-supplying arteries. Diffusion- and perfusion-weighted MRI allows identification of the penumbra and can identify patients who qualify for either systemic or local thrombolysis beyond the 4.5-hour window.

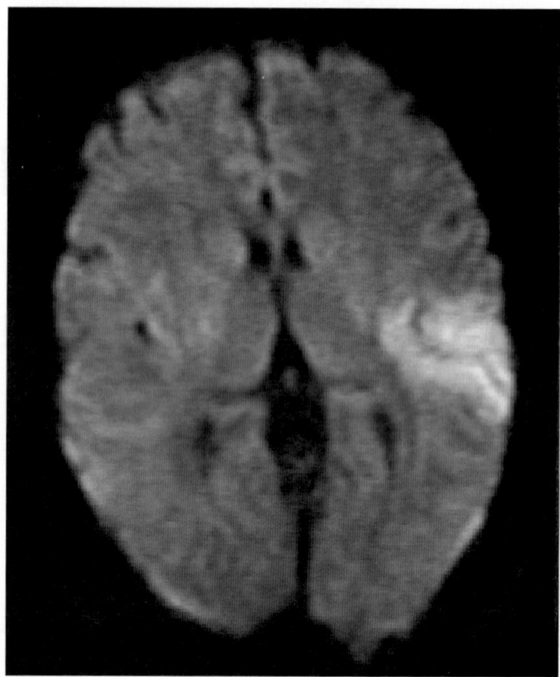

Figure 15a.1 Diffusion weighted magnetic resonance imaging of an acute infarct in the left middle cerebral artery 1.5 hours after the onset of symptoms. The underperfused brain area is shown in white.

Characteristics of cardioembolic stroke

Typically, stroke due to cardiac emboli appears suddenly, mostly without further progression of deficits [3]. The clinical symptoms and signs depend on the part of the brain involved. They include motor and sensory hemiparesis, visual field deficits, dysphasia, disorientation, vertigo, ataxia, and loss of consciousness, and may be accompanied initially by palpitations or retrosternal pain. Emboli preferentially lodge in the main trunks of the cerebral arteries or are scattered in the pial branches, much more often than in the small deep penetrating arteries. The resulting infarct is mostly a wedge–shaped, cortico-subcortical territorial infarct and rarely a deep lacune. Sometimes, multiple infarcts in one or multiple vascular territories are seen, and haemorrhagic transformation is more common than in atherothrombotic stroke. When emboli lyse, rapid recovery from a major hemispheral deficit ('spectacular shrinking deficit') can occur. Emboli arising from infectious endocarditis or atrial myxoma may lead to the formation of cerebrovascular aneurysm, which are usually fusiform.

Neither clinical presentation nor findings of brain imaging are specific. Therefore, cardioembolic stroke should always be suspected, when a cardiac disease or arrhythmia is found to be present and other causes of stroke have been excluded. As to the diagnosis of cardioembolic stroke, considerable disagreement exists among experts. If history and physical examination, electrocardiography, telemetry, chest X-ray, CT, or MRI of the brain show primary haemorrhage or cerebral micro- or macroangiopathy, further cardiac workup might not be needed. If clinical signs or ancillary findings indicate heart disease, a rational approach might be to perform transthoracic echocardiography (TTE), but if clinical signs or ancillary findings are normal it might be more appropriate to proceed directly to transoesophageal echocardiography (TOE) and extended monitoring for arrhythmias. Also in young patients in whom TTE has a low detection rate it might be more cost-effective to skip TTE and move directly to TOE [4].

Treatment of acute ischaemic stroke

Patients with acute stroke should be admitted to a dedicated stroke unit (➲Table 15a.1). Stroke unit care decreases mortality and permanent severe disability by 20% [5, 6]. In the initial phase after a stroke, treatment aims at keeping or bringing physiological parameters into the normal range. Prospective studies showed a negative effect on outcome of too low or high blood pressure, sudden drops of blood pressure, increased blood glucose, increased temperature, fluid loss, or hypoxia. Blood pressure increases in the acute phase of stroke and returns to normal or prior levels after a few days. Therefore only very high blood pressure values exceeding 200/110mmHg should be treated [7]. The following approach is recommended although not proven by randomized trials:

- Systolic blood pressure should be maintained between 120–200mmHg.
- If systemic thrombolysis is considered blood pressure should be lowered below 180 mmHg.
- Increased blood glucose should be lowered with insulin.
- Increased temperature is lowered by paracetamol or cooling blankets.
- Infections leading to fever are treated with antibiotics.
- Monitoring of pO_2 and O_2 is necessary as well as monitoring of heart rhythm.
- Prophylaxis of deep vein thrombosis in patients with paretic leg or immobilization by low-molecular-weight heparin, heparin, stockings, and physical therapy.
- Early mobilization, physical therapy, speech therapy, occupational therapy and neuropsychological therapy as needed depending on the neurological deficits.

The only specific therapy in acute ischaemic stroke is systemic thrombolysis with recombinant tissue plasminogen activator (rtPA) [8] (➲Fig. 15a.2). Efficacy was originally demonstrated in a 3-hour time window, but recently efficacy in a 4.5-hour window has been observed [9]. The most important contraindications are cerebral bleeds, severe stroke, age >80 years, recent surgery, coagulation disorders, and blood pressure >180mmHg. Thrombolysis is effective in anterior and posterior circulation strokes. The most dangerous complication is cerebral haemorrhage which occurs in about 5% of all patients. Based on the results of diffusion-weighted and perfusion-weighted MRI some centres use thrombolysis off-label in the time window beyond

Table 15a.1 Recommended requirements for centres managing acute stroke patients

Primary stroke centre	**Comprehensive stroke centre**
Availability of 24-hour CT scanning	MRI /MRA /CTA
Established stroke treatment guidelines and operational procedures, including intravenous rtPA protocols 24/7	TOE
Close cooperation of neurologists, internists, and rehabilitation experts	Cerebral angiography
Specially trained nursing personnel	Transcranial Doppler sonography
Early multidisciplinary stroke unit rehabilitation including speech therapy, occupational therapy, and physical therapy	Extracranial and intracranial colour-coded duplex sonography
Neurosonological investigations within 24 hours (extracranial Doppler sonography)	Specialized neuroradiological, neurosurgical, and vascular surgical consultation (including telemedicine networks)
TTE	Carotid surgery
Laboratory examinations (including coagulation parameters)	Angioplasty and stenting
Monitoring of blood pressure, ECG, oxygen saturation, blood glucose, body temperature	Automated monitoring of pulse oximetry, blood pressure
Automated ECG monitoring at bedside	Established network of rehabilitation facilities to provide a continuous process of care, including collaboration with outside rehabilitation centre

CT, computed tomography; CTA, computed tomography angiography; ECG, electrocardiogram; MRA, magnetic resonance angiography; MRI, magnetic resonance imaging; rtPA, recombinant tissue plasminogen activator; TOE, transoesophageal echocardiography; TTE, transthoracic echocardiography.

Adapted with permission from European Stroke Organisation (ESO) Executive Committee and ESO Writing Committee. Guidelines for management of ischaemic stroke and transient ischaemic attack 2008. *Cerebrovasc Dis* 2008; **25**: 457–507.

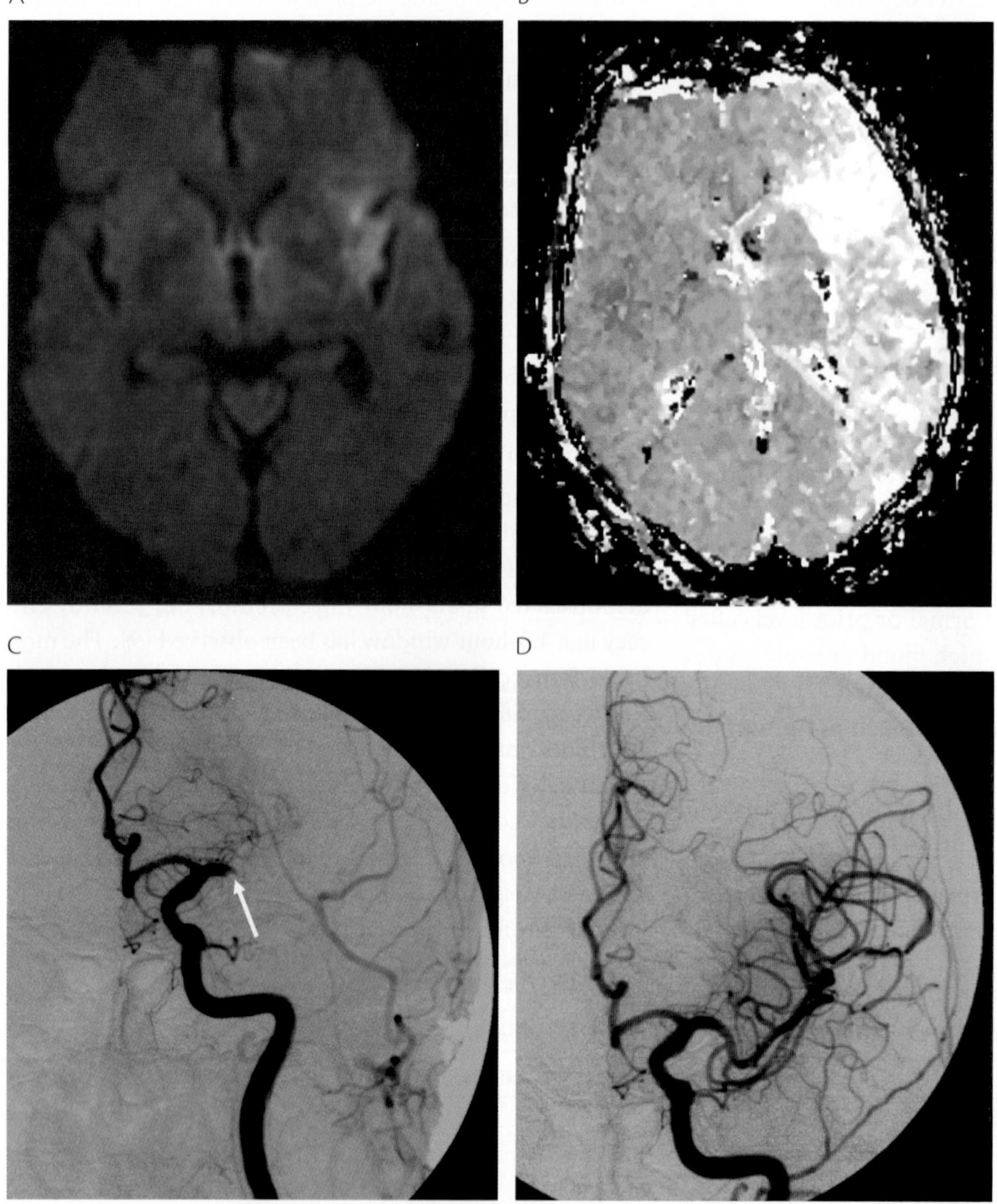

Figure 15a.2 74-year-old woman with acute sensorimotor hemiplegia on the right and aphasia. There is a small lesion on diffusion-weighted images (A) and a large reduction of perfusion (B) indicating a 'mismatch' and salvageable tissue in the territory of the left middle cerebral artery. Angiography showed an occlusion of the left middle cerebral artery main stem which was recanalized with intra-arterial thrombolysis (C, D).

4.5 hours, when penumbra is still present. Specialized centres may alternatively perform local thrombolysis via microcatheter with urokinase or rtPA, use thrombus extraction devices, e.g. the MERCI retriever, or suction devices, e.g. PENUMBRA.

Stroke in the posterior fossa can lead to occlusive hydrocephalus requiring the insertion of a shunt by a neurosurgeon. In space-occupying cerebellar infarctions, craniectomy of the posterior fossa and resection of the ischaemic brain tissue is necessary. Malignant middle cerebral artery infarction in patients <60 years can be treated by hemicraniectomy. This procedure dramatically reduces mortality (from 80% to 30%) and shows a trend for reduced morbidity in surviving patients [10, 11]. The use of corticosteroids, haemodilution, or the systemic use of streptokinase is ineffective or even damaging.

Cryptogenic stroke and patent foramen ovale

The prevalence of a patent foramen ovale (PFO) is up to 25% in the general population. To date, epidemiologic studies have not shown thromboembolic events to occur more frequently in subjects with PFO, and therefore no special primary intervention is needed [12]. In patients with stroke of unknown cause (cryptogenic stroke), however, the prevalence of PFO is substantially higher and approximates 40% [13]. Case reports and case–control studies of cryptogenic strokes compared to strokes with known aetiology or non-stroke controls confirmed an association of PFO and stroke. Therefore, the presence of a PFO after stroke or emboli to other organs raises important questions on the management of such patients. Prospective cohort studies have shown that treatment with aspirin or anticoagulation with a vitamin K antagonist such as warfarin reduces the risk of recurrent stroke in the average patient with PFO to levels similar to those without PFO. As aspirin was as effective as anticoagulation, aspirin should be considered the treatment of choice [14]. Among patients with PFO, those with spontaneous or large right-to-left shunts, with a coinciding atrial septal aneurysm or multiple ischaemic events prior to the PFO diagnosis are at higher risk of recurrent stroke than the average PFO patient. Percutaneous device closure (PDC) becomes therefore an attractive alternative to medical treatment in such patients, but data from randomized controlled trials comparing the effect of percutaneous device closure with medical therapy are still lacking [15]. At present, general use of PDC cannot be recommended.

Secondary stroke prevention in patients with atrial fibrillation

The evidence that oral anticoagulation prevents recurrent stroke in patients with atrial fibrillation results from the European Atrial Fibrillation Trial [16]. This randomized placebo-controlled trial showed a 68% relative risk reduction (RRR) for a recurrent stroke in patients with atrial fibrillation treated with warfarin compared to only 19% for patients receiving 300mg of aspirin per day. Numbers needed to treat are 12 per year. Therefore, oral anticoagulation in patients with atrial fibrillation is by far the most effective treatment for secondary stroke prevention. Similarly, a Cochrane analysis concluded that oral anticoagulation is more effective than aspirin for the prevention of vascular events (odds ratio (OR), 0.67; 95% confidence interval (CI), 0.50– 0.91) or recurrent stroke (OR, 0.49; 95% CI, 0.33– 0.72) [17]. As expected, the risk of major bleeding complications is increased with anticoagulation, but not the risk of intracranial bleeds. Patients with intermittent atrial fibrillation have a similar stroke risk as patients with permanent atrial fibrillation [18, 19]. The optimal international normalized ratio (INR) range for oral anticoagulation is between 2–3 [20]. INR values >4.0 lead to an increased risk of major bleeding complications particularly in the elderly [21]. The bleeding risk with anticoagulants is also increased when high blood pressure is not well controlled.

The ACTIVEW study compared the combination of aspirin and clopidogrel vs. oral anticoagulation with warfarin in patients with atrial fibrillation [22]. The study was terminated prematurely due to a significant reduction of stroke and systemic embolism in favour of warfarin. The rate of major bleeding complications was not different between the two regimens.

In conclusion, stroke patients with a cardiac source of embolism, in particular atrial fibrillation, should be treated with oral anticoagulation (INR 2–3). Patients with mechanical heart valves should be anticoagulated with an INR between 2–3.5. In patients with transient ischaemic attacks (TIAs) or minor stroke, oral anticoagulation can be initiated immediately after the exclusion of cerebral haemorrhage. Patients with contraindications or unwilling to use oral anticoagulation should receive aspirin 300mg per day.

Secondary stroke prevention with antiplatelet drugs

Antiplatelet drugs are effective in secondary stroke prevention after TIAs or ischaemic stroke. This has been shown in many placebo-controlled trials and in several meta-analyses [23–25]. The RRR for non-fatal stroke achieved by antiplatelet therapy in patients with TIA or stroke is 23% (reduced from 10.8% to 8.3% in 3 years). The combined endpoint of stroke, MI, and vascular death is reduced by 17% (from 21.4% to 17.7 over 29 months).

A meta-analysis of the eleven randomized and placebo-controlled trials investigating aspirin monotherapy in secondary stroke prevention found a RRR of 13% (95% CI, 6–19%) for the combined endpoint of stroke, MI, and vascular death [26]. There is no relationship between the dose of aspirin and its efficacy in secondary stroke prevention [26, 27]. Gastrointestinal side effects and bleeding complications are, however, dose dependent and bleeding rates increase significantly beyond a daily dose of aspirin of 150mg per day [28, 29]. Therefore, the recommended dose of aspirin is 75–150mg per day.

In CAPRIE (Clopidogrel vs. Aspirin in Patients at Risk of Ischaemic Events), clopidogrel monotherapy (75mg/day) was compared to ASA (325mg/day) in almost 20,000 patients with stroke, myocardial infarction, or peripheral arterial disease (PAD) [30]. The combined endpoint of stroke, myocardial infarction, and vascular death was reduced by 8.7% under clopidogrel with an ARR of 0.51% per year. The largest benefit of clopidogrel was seen in patients with PADs. The risks of gastrointestinal bleeds (1.99% vs. 2.66%) and gastrointestinal side effects (15% vs. 17.6%) were smaller with clopidogrel than with aspirin.

The MATCH (Management of ATherothrombosis with Clopidogrel in High-risk patients with recent transient ischaemic atteck or ischaemic stroke) study compared the combination of clopidogrel 75mg and aspirin 75mg per day with clopidogrel monotherapy in high-risk patients with TIA or ischaemic stroke [31]. It failed to show superiority of combination antiplatelet therapy for the combined endpoint of stroke, myocardial infarction, vascular death, and hospitalization due to a vascular event. Instead, the combination resulted in an increase of bleeding complications, and therefore is not recommended.

The CHARISMA trial (Clopidogrel for High Atherothrombotic Risk and Ischaemic Stabilization, Management, and Avoidance) was a combined primary and secondary prevention study in 15,603 patients and compared the combination of clopidogrel and aspirin with aspirin monotherapy [32]. Similar to MATCH, the study failed to show a benefit for combination therapy and displayed a higher bleeding rate under the combination. Symptomatic patients, however, appeared to derive significant benefit from dual antiplatelet therapy [33].

The combination of low-dose aspirin and extended-release dipyridamole (ER-dipyridamole) was investigated in the second European stroke prevention study (ESPS2) with 6602 patients with TIAs or stroke [34]. Patients were randomized to aspirin (25mg BID), ER-dipyridamole (200mg BID), the combination of aspirin and ER-dipyridamole, or placebo. For the primary endpoint stroke, the combination was superior to aspirin monotherapy (RRR, 23%; absolute risk reduction (ARR 3%) and placebo (RRR, 37%; ARR, 5.8%). Aspirin monotherapy lowered the risk of stroke by 18% (ARR 2.9%) and dipyridamole monotherapy by 16% (ARR 2.6%) compared to placebo. Major bleeding complications were seen more frequently with aspirin and the aspirin plus ER-dipyridamole combination, whereas dipyridamole monotherapy had a similar bleeding rate as placebo. Cardiac events occurred in similar frequency in the groups treated with dipyridamole compared to aspirin. Patients with coronary heart diseased had no increased risk of angina or MI when treated with extended-release dipyridamole [35]. The investigator-initiated, open European/Australasian Stroke Prevention in Reversible Ischaemia Trial (ESPRIT) randomized 2739 patients with presumed atherothrombotic TIA or minor stroke to aspirin (30–325mg per day) or the combination of aspirin with dipyridamole and followed them for a mean period of 3.5 years. The primary endpoint was the combination of vascular death, stroke, myocardial infarction, and major bleeding complications. The event rate for the primary endpoint was 16% with aspirin monotherapy and 13% with aspirin plus dipyridamole resulting in a RRR of 20% (ARR, 1%) [36]. In the combination arm, 34% of patients terminated the trial prematurely mostly because of adverse events like headache (13% in the aspirin arm of the study). A meta-analysis of all stroke prevention trials testing aspirin monotherapy vs. aspirin plus dipyridamole showed a RRR in favour of the combination for the combined vascular endpoint by 18% (95% CI, 9–26%).

A direct comparison of clopidogrel and aspirin plus ER-dipyridamole was performed in the PRoFESS study [37]. There was no difference in efficacy across all endpoints and various subgroups of patients. Aspirin plus ER-dipyridamole resulted in more intracranial bleeds and a higher drop out rate due to headache compared with clopidogrel (5.9% vs. 0.9%). ➲Table 15a.2 summarizes the recommendations for antithrombotic therapy from the Stroke Council of the American Heart Association [38].

Secondary stroke prevention and hypertension

Hypertension is the most important risk factor for stroke (➲Table 15a.3; see also ➲Chapter 13) [39]. Stroke mortality is strongly related to the level of blood pressure (➲Fig. 15a.3) [40]. There are only few studies investigating the efficacy of classes of antihypertensive drugs in secondary stroke prevention. A meta-analysis comprised seven studies in 15,527 patients with TIA, ischaemic, or haemorrhagic stroke who were followed for 2–5 years [41]. Treatment with antihypertensives reduced the risk of stroke (OR, 0.76), of non-fatal stroke (OR, 0.79), of MI (OR 0.79), and the risk of all vascular events (OR 0.79). For prevention of stroke, the combination of an angiotensin-converting enzyme (ACE)-inhibitor with a diuretic seemed most effective. ACE-inhibitors and angiotensin receptor blockers are supposed to exhibit pleiotropic and protective vascular effects beyond lowering high blood pressure. Under this assumption, the Heart Outcomes Prevention Evaluation

Table 15a.2 Recommendations for antithrombotic therapy from the Stroke Council of the American Heart Association

Antiplatelet agent	Recommendation	Class, level of evidence
Aspirin	50–325 mg/day is an acceptable initial therapy	IIa, A
	Addition of aspirin to clopidogrel increases the risk of haemorrhage and is not recommended for ischaemic stroke or TIA	III, A
	For patients who have an ischaemic cerebrovascular event while on aspirin, there is no evidence that increasing the dose of aspirin provides additional benefit	IIa, B
Clopidogrel	Clopidogrel is an acceptable initial therapy	IIa, A
	Clopidogrel may be considered over aspirin alone on the basis of direct comparison trials	IIb, B
	Clopidogrel may be used for patients who are allergic to aspirin	IIa, B
Dipyridamole	In combination with aspirin, dipyridamole is an acceptable initial therapy	IIa, A
	The combination of aspirin plus dipyridamole is suggested over aspirin alone	IIa, A
	Compared with aspirin alone, the combination of aspirin plus dipyridamole is safe	IIa, A
General	For patients with noncardioembolic ischaemic stroke or TIA, antiplatelet therapy rather than oral anticoagulants is recommended to reduce the risk of recurrent stroke and other cardiovascular events	I, A
	Insufficient data are available to make evidence-based recommendations with regard to choices between antiplatelet options other than aspirin. Selection of an antiplatelet agent should be individualized based on patient risk factor profiles, tolerance, and other clinical characteristics	IIb, B
	Although alternative antiplatelet agents are often considered for noncardioembolic patients, no single agent or combination has been well studied in patients who have had a cerebrovascular ischaemic event while on aspirin	IIa, B

(HOPE) study compared ramipril with placebo [42]. In the subgroup of patients with TIAs or stroke as the qualifying event, ramipril resulted in a relative reduction of the combined endpoint of stroke, MI, or vascular death by 24% or an ARR of 6.3% over 5 years.

PROGRESS (Perindopril Protection Against Recurrent Stroke Study) was the first large-scale trial on secondary stroke prevention in 6105 patients who were randomized to either perindopril with or without indapamide or placebo [43]. Across the 4-year observation period, blood pressure in the treatment group was lowered on average by 9/4mmHg. The ARR for recurrent stroke was 4% and the RRR was 28%. For the combination of perindopril and indapamide, the RRR was 43% whereas the ACE inhibitor alone did not achieve the same level of blood pressure lowering and was not significantly superior to placebo.

MOSES (Morbidity and Mortality After Stroke – Eprosartan vs Nitrendipine for Secondary Prevention) included 1352 hypertensive patients who had suffered a stroke in the previous 24 months [44]. Patients were randomized to either eprosartan (600mg per day) or nitrendipin (10mg per day) on top of additional antihypertensive therapy when appropriate. Despite an identical blood pressure reduction, eprosartan was superior to nitrendipin to prevent recurrent vascular events (21% RRR). Optimal systolic blood pressure in the MOSES trial was 120–140mm Hg.

PRoFESS (Prevention Regimen For Effectively avoiding Second Strokes) randomized 20,332 patients with a recent ischaemic stroke to telmisartan 80mg/day or placebo in

Table 15a.3 Prevalence and relative risk of modifiable risk factors for ischaemic stroke in the general population

Risk factor	Prevalence (%)	Relative risk
Hypertension	25–40	3–5
Elevated total cholesterol (> 240mg/dL [6.21 mmol/L])	6–40	1.8–2.6
Smoking	25	1.5
Physical inactivity	25	2.7
Obesity	18	1.8–2.4
Asymptomatic carotid stenosis (> 50%)	2–8	2
Alcohol consumption (> 5 drinks/day)	2–5	1.6
Atrial fibrillation	1	5 (nonvalvular) 17 (valvular)

Reproduced with permission from Straus SE, Majumdar SR, McAlister FA. New evidence for stroke prevention: scientific review. *JAMA* 2002; **288**: 1388–95.

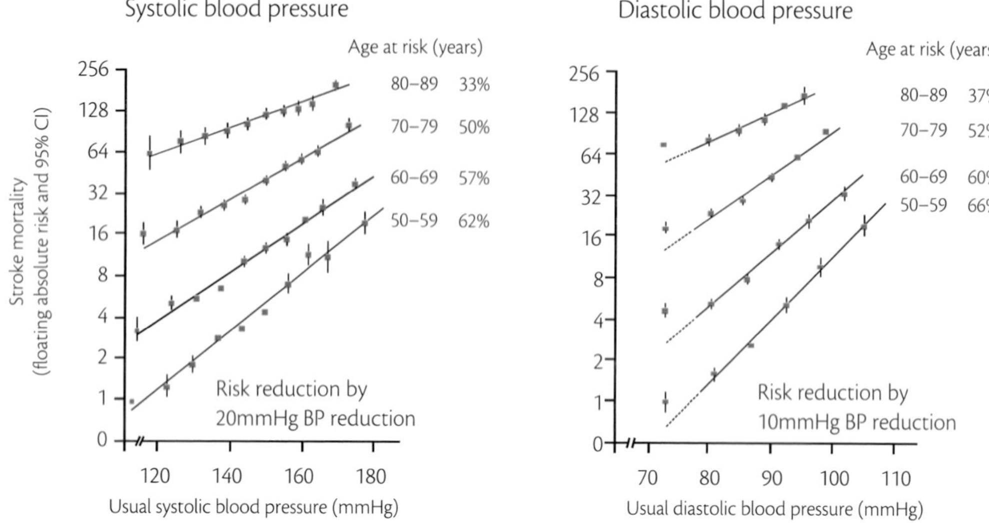

Figure 15a.3 Stroke mortality and blood pressure. Reproduced with permission from Lewington S, Clarke R, Qizilbash N, *et al*. Age-specific relevance of usual blood pressure to vascular mortality: a meta-analysis of individual data for one million adults in 61 prospective studies. *Lancet* 2002; **360:** 1903–13.

addition to other antihypertensive therapies, for a median follow-up of 2.4 years [45]. Mean blood pressure in the telmisartan group was lower by 3.8/2.0mmHg over the trial period. Recurrent strokes occurred in 8.7% in the telmisartan group compared to 9.2% in the placebo group, which was not significant. Initiation of telmisartan early after a stroke, and continued for a median of 2.4 years, did neither significantly lower the rate of recurrent strokes, major vascular events or new-onset diabetes.

In conclusion, all antihypertensive drugs are most likely effective in secondary stroke prevention. Beta-blockers (atenolol) show the lowest efficacy. More important than the choice of antihypertensive is the degree of blood pressure-lowering achieved. Currently recommended targets for systolic and diastolic blood pressure are 140/90mmHg in non-diabetics and 130/80mmHg in diabetics; however, even lower pressures may provide additional benefit. Achieving target blood pressure frequently requires combination therapy. Concomitant diseases (kidney failure, congestive heart failure) have to be considered. Lifestyle modification will lower blood pressure and should be recommended in addition to drug treatment.

Secondary stroke prevention in patients with coronary heart disease

Cardiologists and neurologists are faced in their clinical routine with patients with manifest disease of the coronary arteries and stroke or TIA. In this section we will give recommendations for the treatment of stroke patients with acute coronary syndrome and patients with coronary heart disease and an acute stroke. All these recommendations are not evidence based.

Patients with a history of ischaemic stroke who present with an acute coronary syndrome may receive thrombolysis, heparin, and/or stenting. In contrast, in patients with disabling strokes or cerebral haemorrhage, thrombolysis and standard dose heparin should be avoided. The use of clopidogrel plus aspirin after an acute coronary syndrome and/or a stent implantation carries a higher bleeding risk than monotherapy. However, the benefit of dual platelet inhibition in terms of preventing vascular events and stent thrombosis is clearly higher than with monotherapy. Patients with a cardioembolic stroke in the past who are anticoagulated and need a coronary stent might be treated for a limited time with triple therapy (aspirin, clopidogrel, and oral anticoagulation). The optimal time period when the increased rate of bleeding complications might offset the prevention of stent thrombosis is, however, not known.

In patients with atrial fibrillation receiving oral anticoagulation who suffer a cerebral haemorrhage anticoagulation should be stopped. Oral anticoagulation might be reintroduced if the expected risk of a cardioembolic stroke is higher than the risk of recurrent brain haemorrhage.

In patients with atrial fibrillation and stable coronary heart disease, cardiologists tend to combine oral anticoagulation with low-dose aspirin. The results from the two SPORTIF trials, however indicate that the combination of oral anticoagulation with ASA does not reduce the risk of vascular events but results in a significant increase in bleeding complications [46].

Secondary stroke prevention in patients with significant stenosis of brain-supplying arteries

Two large randomized trials (North American Symptomatic Carotid Endarterectomy Trial, NASCET and European Carotid Surgery Trial, ECST) found a clear benefit for carotid endarterectomy compared to medical treatment in patients with high degree symptomatic stenosis of the internal carotid artery (ICA) [47, 48]. Taken together, the trials found an ARR of 13.5% over 5 years for the combined endpoint of stroke and death in favour of carotid endarterectomy [49]. The risk reduction was even higher in patients with an ICA stenosis >90%. In patients with an ICA stenosis of 50–69%, the 5-year ARR for the endpoint ipsilateral stroke was 4.6%. This benefit was mainly apparent in men. Patients with an ICA stenosis <50% do not benefit from carotid endarterectomy. The short-term complication rates (stroke and death) were 6.2% with an ICA stenosis >70% and 8.4% for an ICA stenosis of 50–69%. Aspirin should be given prior to, during and after carotid surgery [50]. Several studies randomized patients with significant ICA stenosis to carotid endarterectomy or balloon angioplasty with stenting (➲Fig. 15a.4). Surgeons and interventional neuroradiologists had to meet defined quality standards. SPACE (Stent-protected Percutaneous Angioplasty of the Carotid vs. Endarterectomy) randomized 1200 symptomatic patients with a >50% stenosis (according to the NASCET criteria) or >70% (according to ESC criteria) within 6 months after a transient ischaemic attack or minor stroke to carotid endarterectomy or stenting [51]. The primary endpoint, ipsilateral stroke or death within 30 days, occurred in 6.84% of patients undergoing stenting and 6.34% of patients undergoing carotid endarterectomy. A post hoc subgroup analysis identified age <68 years as a factor being associated with a lower complication rate in patients treated with stenting. The complication rate of surgery was not age dependent [52]. In this study, the use of protection system did not influence the complication rate. In the SAPPHIRE study, enrolling high risk patients, complication rates were even slightly lower with carotid stenting than with carotid endarterectomy (➲Table 15a.4) [53]. In contrast, the EVA-3S (Endarterectomy Versus Angioplasty in Patients with Severe Symptomatic Carotid Stenosis) was terminated prematurely after 527 patients were randomized due to a significant difference in the 30-day complication rate favouring carotid surgery (9.6% vs. 3.9%; OR, 2.5; 95% CI, 1.25–4.93) [54]. Of note, however, EVA-3S involved a considerable number of centres with very limited experience in carotid stenting which makes the interpretation of this study difficult. In addition the complication rate of surgery was much lower than

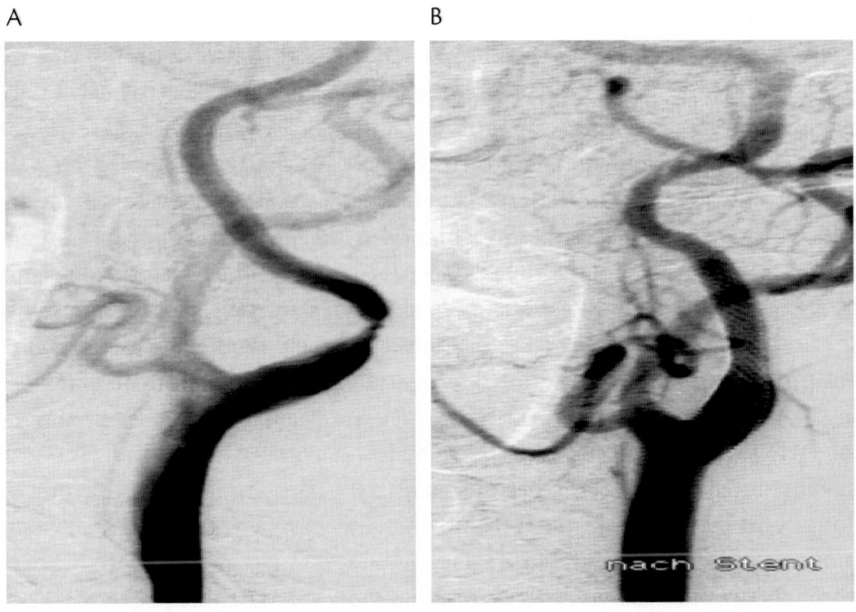

Figure 15a.4 Severe stenosis of the internal carotid artery prior to (A) and after (B) stenting.

Table 15a.4 Risk of stroke or death from large-scale randomized trials comparing endovascular (CAS) and surgical (CEA) treatment in patients with severe carotid artery stenosis

Outcome	Any stroke or death at 30 days		Disabling stroke or death at 30 days		Ipsilateral stroke after 30 days	
	CAS n (%)	CEA n (%)	CAS n (%)	CEA n (%)	CAS n (%)	CEA n (%)
CAVATAS	25 (10.0)	25 (9.9)	16 (6.4)	15 (5.9)	6†	10†
SAPPHIRE	8 (4.8)	9 (5.4)	unk	unk	unk	unk
SPACE	46 (7.7)	38 (6.5)	29 (4.8)	23 (3.9)	4 (0.7)*	1 (0.2)*
EVA3S	25 (9.6)	10 (3.9)	9 (3.4)	4 (1.5)	2 (0.6)*	1 (0.3)*

CAS, carotid artery stenting; CEA, carotid endarterectomy; Intention-to-treat data; unk, unknown. † follow-up duration 1.95 years in mean; * up to 6 months. CAVATAS [58]; SAPPHIRE [53]; SPACE [51]; EVA3S [54].

Adapted with permission from European Stroke Organisation (ESO) Executive Committee and ESO Writing Committee. Guidelines for management of ischaemic stroke and transient ischaemic attack 2008. *Cerebrovasc Dis* 2008; **25**: 457–507.

observed in the SPACE study. Taken together, the results of the studies published to date show a similar and in some instances lower complication rate for endarterectomy compared to carotid stenting [55].The reported medium-time outcomes in a 2-4-year follow-up were comparable but the restenosis rate was higher after carotid stenting [56, 57]. It is likely that the success of carotid stenting (and for that matter also of carotid endarterectomy) depend heavily on the experience of a given centre.

In conclusion, symptomatic patients with significant stenosis of the ICA should preferably undergo carotid endarterectomy. In experienced centres, carotid stenting may be a valuable alternative to carotid endarterectomy. The benefit of surgery (and most likely also that of stenting) increases with the degree of stenosis between 70–95%. The benefit of surgery is highest in the first 2–4 weeks after the initial transient ischaemic attacks or minor stroke. The benefit of surgery is lower in patients with a stenosis between 50–70%, in high degree stenosis (pseudo-occlusion), in women or when surgery is performed 12 weeks or later after the initial event. The benefit of surgery is no longer present when the complication rate exceeds 6%. Patients should receive aspirin prior to, during, and after endarterectomy. Clopidogrel should be replaced by aspirin 5 days before surgery. At present, carotid stenting has a slightly higher short-term complication rate (particularly in less experienced centres) and similar medium time outcomes. The use of protection systems did not decrease the complication rate in some trials, but the favourable outcomes in SAPPHIRE suggest that the use of such devices should be preferred. The restenosis rate is higher after stenting. Whether this translates into higher long-term event rates is not yet known. The complication rate of carotid stenting is age dependent and increases beyond an age of 65–68 years. The combination of clopidogrel (75mg) plus aspirin (75–100mg) is recommended in patients after stenting for 1–3 months.

Secondary stroke prevention in heart failure

The SAVE trial in patients after MI and impaired left ventricular function as well as the SOLVD trial in stable heart failure have shown that the risk of stroke increases in parallel to the impairment of ventricular function as judged from ejection fraction [59, 60]. Most likely, left ventricular dilatation and impaired ejection fraction increases the likelihood to develop left ventricular thrombi in cardiomyopathy [61]. Impairment of left ventricular function produces atrial dilatation and stretch and therefore, produces an increased rate of atrial fibrillation depending on the severity of heart failure, which can amount to a prevalence of 49.8% in severe heart failure. In some trials the incidence of thromboembolic strokes was even higher in patients, in which atrial fibrillation was not detected. Therefore, it was subject of debate whether in patients with highly impaired left ventricular function and heart failure anticoagulation should be performed even in the presence of sinus rhythm. However, all cause mortality as well as cardiovascular endpoints are increased when patients receive warfarin therapy [62]. Therefore, in patients with sinus rhythms oral anticoagulation is not recommended unless atrial fibrillation or other striking indications are present. Even though there are arguments in favour of using platelet inhibitors like aspirin [63], there is evidence that in heart failure aspirin might interfere with the beneficial effects of ACE-inhibitors on outcome [64].

Personal perspective

Prevention and therapy of stroke based on randomized controlled trials has made major progress in the last 20 years. The implementation of the new therapy, however, has been too slow. Many countries still do not provide stroke unit care for patients with acute stroke and as a consequence the rate of systemic thrombolysis is low. Secondary prevention of patients with atrial fibrillation or PFO is a good example of the need of cardiologists and neurologists to cooperate for the benefit of the optimal treatment. At present many treatments are available for secondary stroke prevention. Long-term compliance and adherence is low. One possibility to improve this situation would be integrated stroke care with risk factor control and medical or surgical (interventional) therapy provided and organized by stroke centres. At a later time, when the risk of recurrent stroke has declined, care can be handed over to the internist or general practitioner in private practice.

Further reading

Adams RJ, Albers G, Alberts MJ, *et al.* Update to the AHA/ASA recommendations for the prevention of stroke in patients with stroke and transient ischemic attack. *Stroke* 2008; **39**: 1647–52.

Doufekias E, Segal AZ, Kizer JR. Cardiogenic and aortogenic brain embolism. *J Am Coll Cardiol* 2008; **51**: 1049–59.

European Stroke Organisation (ESO) Executive Committee and ESO Writing Committee. Guidelines for management of ischaemic stroke and transient ischaemic attack 2008. *Cerebrovasc Dis* 2008; **25**: 457–507.

O'Donnell MJ, Hankey GJ, Eikelboom JW. Antiplatelet therapy for secondary prevention of noncardioembolic ischemic stroke: a critical review. *Stroke* 2008; **39**: 1638–46.

Singer DE, Albers GW, Dalen JE, *et al.* Antithrombotic therapy in atrial fibrillation: American College of Chest Physicians Evidence-Based Clinical Practice Guidelines (8th Edition). *Chest* 2008; **133**: 546S–592S.

➲ **For full references and multimedia materials please visit the online version of the book (http://esctextbook.oxfordonline.com).**

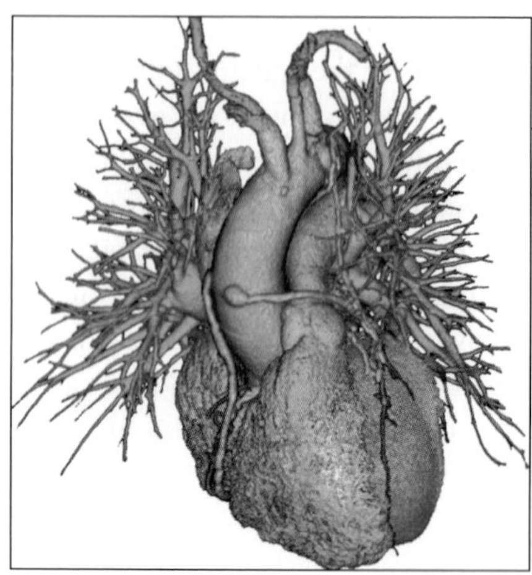

CHAPTER 15b

Cardiovascular Problems in Chronic Kidney Disease

Eberhard Ritz and Andrew Remppis

Contents

Summary

Until recently, impaired kidney function was an orphan in the cardiological assessment of patients with heart disease, while in patients with chronic kidney disease (CKD) cardiological assessment was not considered a high priority. However, impressive evidence has now been provided that cardiovascular problems critically determine life expectancy of patients with CKD.

Cardiological examination of patients with advanced CKD should be obligatory. Importantly, invasive diagnostic workup and revascularization procedures should not be withheld in CKD patients presenting with myocardial ischaemia.

Conversely, in cardiac patients appropriate assessment of renal function employing modern methodology (estimated glomerular filtration rate, albuminuria) is obligatory as well, since kidney function critically determines systemic neurohumoral activation.

In the management of renal patients the most important aspect is appropriate control of blood pressure, but cardiovascular prevention in these patients comprises the full spectrum of beta blockade, blockade of the renin–angiotensin–aldosterone system, aspirin, and statins.

Chronic kidney disease as a cardiovascular risk factor

It has been recognized only recently that minor CKD is a powerful cardiovascular risk factor [1]. The recent Consensus Group therefore stated that renal evaluation should be part and parcel of the evaluation of patients with cardiac problems [2].

The assessment of renal function is based primarily on two parameters, the *glomerular filtration rate* (GFR) on the one hand and *urinary excretion of albumin* (or in more advanced stages of CKD unselective proteinuria) on the other hand.

For the clinical assessment of GFR, one has to be aware of the fact that in early stages of CKD a major reduction of GFR may still be compatible with serum creatinine concentrations within the normal range, because the serum creatinine concentration depends apart from the GFR also on non-renal factors, particularly on muscle mass. This frequently causes underestimation of the severity of CKD in the elderly and cachectic patient. This dilemma has led to efforts to provide more accurate estimates of GFR (*eGFR*) by standardizing the measurement of serum creatinine (Cleveland clinic protocol) and by using an algorithm correcting for age, gender, and ethnicity:

$$\text{eGFR} = 175 \times (\text{standardized S-creatinine})^{-1.154} \times (\text{age})^{-0.203} \times 0.742 \text{ (for females)} \times 1.212 \text{ (for blacks)} \ [3].$$

For eGFR values >60mL/min/1.73m^2, the estimate is imprecise and the laboratory should state only that the value is >60mL/min/1.73m^2. It is known, however, from studies in large cohorts that already minor reductions of eGFR in the range of values above 60mL/min increase the cardiovascular risk [4]. One of the reasons for the insensitivity of GFR to detect incipient kidney damage is the fact that the remaining nephrons respond to nephron loss with compensatory hyperfiltration, thus masking the extent of renal damage by initially still maintaining the whole kidney GFR within the normal range. Importantly, in the normal and near-normal range of GFR cystatin C is more precise than creatinine based eGFR. The measurement, however, is costly and currently not (yet) used for routine measurements.

Currently the severity of chronic kidney disease is graded from CKD1–CKD5 (➲Fig. 15b.1).

Apart from GFR, *urinary excretion of albumin* is a powerful independent predictor of cardiovascular risk: the risk increases progressively with rising urinary albumin concentrations. For historic reasons, one still distinguishes between normoalbuminuria and microalbuminuria (definition of microalbuminuria: excretion of 30–300mg albumin/day), but the cardiovascular risk steadily increases

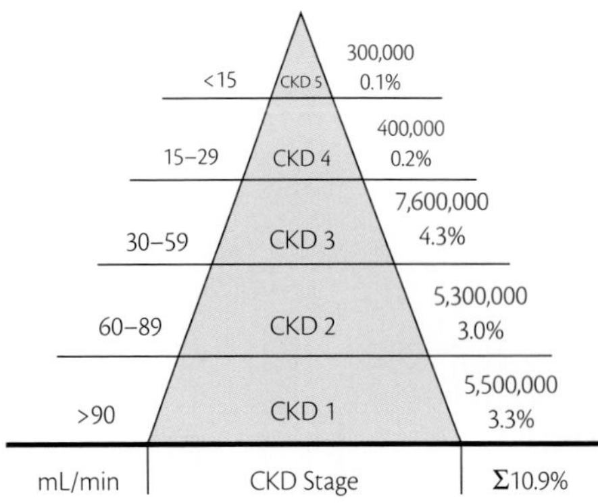

Figure 15b.1 Stages of chronic kidney disease (CKD) and their frequency in the general population. Adapted with permission from K/DOQI clinical practice guidelines for chronic kidney disease: evaluation, classification, and stratification. *Am J Kidney Dis* 2002; **39**(Suppl.1): S1–S266.

even in the range of normoalbuminuria. The most convenient and adequately sensitive procedure is to measure albumin in the morning urine without correction for urinary creatinine concentration.

It is important to note that *both GFR* and *albuminuria* independently contribute to the cardiovascular risk [5]. In the absence of albuminuria, the cardiovascular risk of reduced renal function is markedly less than if a combination of low GFR plus albuminuria is present (➲Fig. 15b.2).

The impact of *impaired renal function on the cardiovascular risk* is not only relevant in patients with *primary kidney disease*, but is also pronounced in patients with *primary cardiac disease*, particularly in patients with the acute coronary syndrome (ACS). ➲Fig. 15b.3 shows that in patients with ACS the entire spectrum of complications is progressively

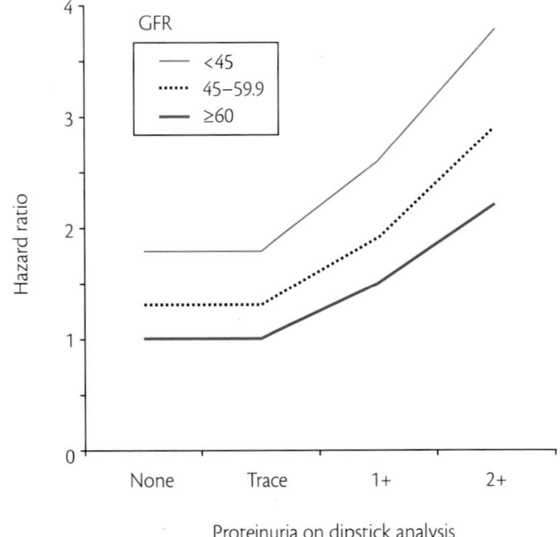

Figure 15b.2 Adjusted all-cause mortality according to proteinuria and kidney function. Adapted with permission from Tonelli M, Jose P, Curhan G, *et al*. Proteinuria, impaired kidney function, and adverse outcomes in people with coronary disease: analysis of a previously conducted randomised trial. *BMJ* 2006; **332**: 1426.

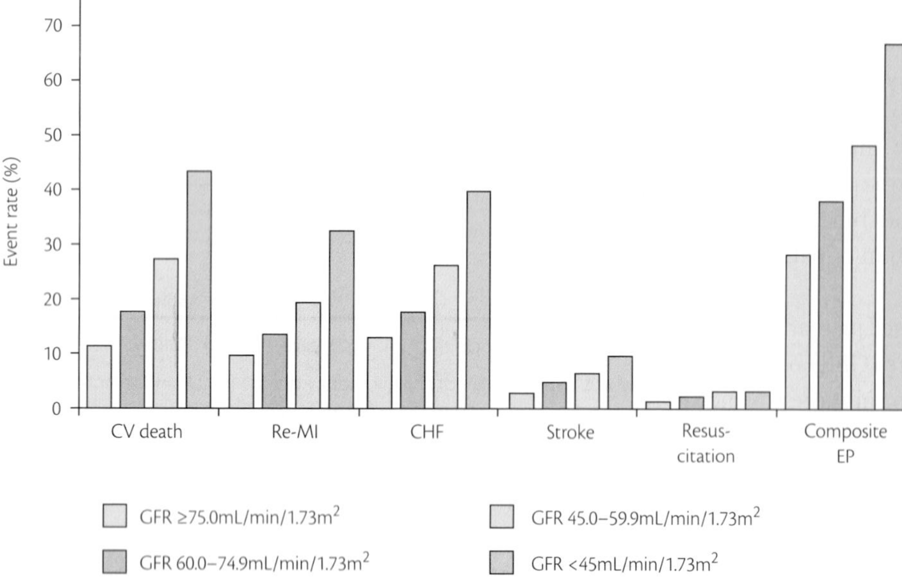

Figure 15b.3 Impact of CKD on different types of cardiac events in patients with MI. Adapted with permission from Anavekar NS, McMurray JJ, Velazquez EJ, *et al.* Relation between renal dysfunction and cardiovascular outcomes after myocardial infarction. *New Engl J Med* 2004; **351**: 1285–95.

more frequent the more advanced the CKD [6] is. CKD is also a powerful predictor of risk in patients with congestive heart failure.

A most important part of the assessment in renal malfunction is the evaluation of *blood pressure*. In renal patients this apparently simple problem becomes problematic. ➲Table 15b.1 makes this point: office blood pressure is notoriously unreliable. Many studies showed that self-measured blood pressure is a much more reliable parameter. Renal patients, particularly diabetic patients with nephropathy, are characterized in early stages of CKD by nocturnal non-dipping which makes ambulatory blood pressure measurement a very valuable tool.

Vascular stiffening is a main consequence of impaired renal function. This changes vascular impedance and contributes to large blood pressure amplitudes. In renal patients, central blood pressure (in the aorta) is usually considerably higher than brachial blood pressure, thus complicating the issue of target blood pressures on treatment. Because coronary perfusion occurs only during diastole, it appears wise not to lower diastolic blood pressure to values <70mmHg [7], at least in patients with known coronary heart disease. To halt progression of CKD, current guidelines recommend a *target blood pressure* of 130/80mmHg (or lower values if proteinuria exceeds 1g/day) in patients with diabetic and non-diabetic CKD [8]. Renin–angiotensin system (RAS) blockade further intensifies reduction of proteinuria independent of blood pressure [8]. Since reducing albuminuria has a significant impact on cardiovascular events [9], one should consider intensifying RAS blockade to reduce proteinuria even to values <1g/day, if necessary by using doses of RAS blockers beyond those licensed for blood pressure-lowering.

Table 15b.1 Blood pressure in chronic kidney disease

Office blood pressure: risk of white coat hypertension and masked hypertension
Home blood pressure, i.e. self-measurement: superior to office blood pressure
Ambulatory blood pressure measurement: useful because of frequency of inappropriately high night-time blood pressure in CKD; non-dipping!
Systolic blood pressure: highest predictive value for cardiovascular events
Pulse pressure: additional predictive value
Diastolic blood pressure: low values <70mmHg—higher mortality in coronary heart disease patients

Chronic kidney disease and cardiovascular mortality

It has been recognized that in patients with primary kidney disease the risk to ultimately require haemodialysis is much lower than to die mainly from cardiovascular causes—by a factor of 20 (CKD2) in early, and a factor of three in late stages of CKD (CKD4) [10]. This clearly highlights the importance of diagnosing renal dysfunction in early stages of CKD in order to obtain a complete assessment of the cardiovascular risk in patients with primary kidney disease. Due to the systemic impact of kidney failure on, amongst others, neurohumoral activation, detection of CKD is especially relevant in patients with primary heart disease.

The mechanisms by which renal impairment affects cardiac function are not entirely clear, but the most important aspects for the management of patients are the early appearance of:

- sympathetic overactivity and the reduced breakdown of catecholamines (renalase);
- lipid abnormalities, e.g. Lp(a), small dense low-density lipoprotein, remnants, modified apolipoproteins;
- increased oxidative stress and microinflammation;
- increased serum-phosphate (which has been identified as a cardiovascular risk factor in cardiac patients even when renal function is normal) [11];
- early increase in asymmetric dimethylarginine (ADMA), an important risk factor which is not susceptible to current therapies [12].

Causes of death and underlying pathology in end-stage renal disease

The prospective 4D study [13] in haemodialysed type 2 diabetic patients showed that cardiac arrest (26% of deaths), heart failure (6%), and death from other cardiac causes (3%) are more frequent causes than myocardial infarction (9%), although myocardial infarction is much more frequent than in the background population. This finding has been confirmed by the US Renal Data System Registry in non-diabetic patients as well.

Left ventricular systolic dysfunction with a low ejection fraction at echocardiography is well known as a strong predictor of cardiovascular survival [14]. The importance of diastolic malfunction, however, a typical finding early on in kidney failure, has been vastly underestimated in the past.

Accelerated large vessel disease with increased arterial stiffening and calcification leads to an increased afterload to the heart inducing left ventricular hypertrophy, which in turn is greatly amplified independent of blood pressure, since kidney malfunction affects the heart by (currently poorly characterized) factors other than volume and pressure. The resulting *uremic cardiomyopathy* is mainly characterized by cardiomyocyte drop-out with interstitial fibrosis (demonstrable with magnetic resonance imaging, MRI), by right and left ventricular hypertrophy, and by microvessel disease with wall thickening of post-coronary arteries and capillary deficit leading to a marked decrease of ischaemia tolerance. In addition, our experimental studies documented diminished insulin-dependent glucose uptake. Importantly, the *pro-arrhythmic mechanisms* triggered in this molecular concert of hypertrophy encompass changes on various levels of the organ ranging from autonomic failure down to dysfunctional subcellular Ca^{2+} handling, all these components paving the way for triggered activity and re-entry mechanisms as the basis of ventricular tachycardias.

The loss of the 'Windkessel' effect causes an increase of *wave propagation velocity* imposing an increased pulsatile pressure and flow to the peripheral vasculatures, which again induces small vessel damage and end organ dysfunction. Furthermore the resulting greater blood pressure amplitude with low diastolic pressures jeopardizes coronary perfusion.

To assess large vessel disease, an important contributor to the cardiovascular risk, it is useful to have pelvic and abdominal X-rays to assess calcification of iliac arteries and the aorta (both of which are powerful predictors of cardiovascular risk).

What clinical examinations are useful or necessary in the patient with end-stage renal disease?

Cardiological workup of the renal patient initially includes electrocardiogram and echocardiographic evaluation to detect inappropriate left ventricular hypertrophy and pericardial effusion. Because in end-stage renal disease metabolic myopathy often precludes a meaningful evaluation by treadmill testing, pharmacologic stress testing has become the gold standard in non-invasive detection of cardiac ischaemia. MRI technology has recently allowed the differentiation of two major types of uremic cardiomyopathy, one with a more subendocardial late enhancement possibly reflecting silent ischaemia, and another one with a diffuse pattern of late enhancement characteristically found in patients with more pronounced left ventricular hypertrophy. Moreover, MRI is a powerful tool to detect cardiac amyloidosis. Unfortunately gadolinium application is critical in end-stage renal disease due to its toxicity (see ➲Acute reactions and nephrogenic skin fibrosis after gadolinium, p.514).

The *coronary angiogram represents the gold standard* for the diagnosis of coronary artery disease (CAD) allowing direct treatment. It is still underused in renal patients because of concern about radiocontrast nephropathy, but should definitely not be omitted in patients with an ACS because cardiac mortality significantly outweighs the potential further reduction of GFR. Observational data (USRDS) show that in dialysed patients percutaneous intervention

(PCI) with stenting results in superior short-term outcome, while bypass surgery, using internal mammary grafts, provides superior 1-year survival [15, 16]. In the future, hybrid approaches employing a combination of minimally invasive direct coronary artery bypass grafting (MIDCAB) and PCI might prove beneficial especially in elderly multimorbid renal patients.

Radiocontrast nephropathy

Acute renal failure (or according to recent nomenclature: acute kidney injury (AKI)) after radiocontrast administration is a complication in CKD patients, particularly diabetic CKD patients.

Patients with pre-existing CKD account for 30–35% of patients with acute renal failure in general and in such patients dialysis independence at day 90 is less than in patients without CKD. The long-term outcome is also worse in patients with acute renal failure who had pre-existing CKD: 28.2% after 3 years vs. 7.6% of patients without pre-existing CKD. These long-term consequences add to the problem of increased hospitalization and cost due to radiocontrast nephropathy. Several studies show a significantly increased mortality with odds ratios up to 5–10, while an increased rate of delayed death was also shown after radiocontrast-induced acute renal failure during percutaneous coronary intervention [17].

Recent studies show that measurement of indicators of renal damage (kidney injury molecule-1 (KIM-1), neutrophil gelatinase-associated lipocalin (NGAL) and others) [18] allow the recognition of high renal risk within hours of exposure to an intervention, e.g. cardiac surgery; they promise to become clinically useful tools. Whether they also predict radiocontrast nephropathy is unknown.

The first step to prevent contrast nephropathy is to identify patients at higher risk: the elderly and the patients with diabetes, with elevated serum creatinine, and with hypertension. Drugs which should best be avoided in patients scheduled for radiocontrast investigation are non-steroidal anti-inflammatory agents (both COX-1 and COX-2), aminoglycosides, cyclosporine, tacrolimus, amphothericin, etc. There is some recent information that intensive blockade of the RAS may aggravate the risk of acute renal failure.

A long list of interventions has been proposed for the prevention of radiocontrast nephropathy. The only intervention for which uncontroversial evidence is available is the administration of saline, half normal saline [19] or better, normal saline [20]. There have been proposals to administer N-acetyl cysteine [21] or to use sodium bicarbonate [22] instead of saline, but the efficacy of these interventions has not been consistently confirmed. Prophylactic haemodialysis is also not useful.

A bone of contention is the type of radiocontrast agent administered: it has been reported that the iso-osmolar, dimeric, non-ionic radiocontrast agent iodixanol is superior to the low osmolar, monomeric, non-ionic agent iohexol [23], but again this has not been confirmed by subsequent studies. The roles of radiocontrast ionicity, osmolality, and viscosity in the genesis of radiocontrast nephropathy remain currently unresolved. Therefore, the best advice remains to hydrate the patient with normal saline and to administer the lowest possible dose of radiocontrast agents in high risk patients.

Acute reactions and nephrogenic skin fibrosis after gadolinium

MRI has become a powerful diagnostic tool in cardiology as gadolinium-containing contrast agents (Gd-contrast) allow the sensitive detection of myocardial scarring in various specific cardiac diseases such as ischaemic heart disease, myocarditis, cardiomyopathies, amyloidosis etc. Although Gd-contrast has initially been embraced as a non-toxic contrast material in renal patients, both acute and chronic toxicity have been observed especially in end-stage renal patients on haemodialysis and chronic ambulatory peritoneal dialysis.

Nephrogenic systemic fibrosis (NFS) is a rare but potentially fatal condition first described as a scleromyxoedema-like fibrosing syndrome in association with renal insufficiency [24]. It is initially characterized by red and painful plaques that coincide with oedema. Subsequently thickening, induration, and hardening of the skin in the distal extremities and the trunk occurs, while the face is usually spared. Notably, other organs including the lungs, liver, muscles, and the heart may also be involved causing considerable morbidity and mortality. The underlying mechanism is thought to be transmetallation whereby in exchange for endogenous metals free gadolinium is released from the chelate with subsequent binding to tissue. Circulating cells are then recruited causing fibrosis by cytokine production and T-cell activation. Since no effective therapeutic intervention is available, it is of paramount importance to identify the patients at highest risk for NFS. As the majority of patients with NFS were preterminal or on renal replacement therapy (GFR $<30 \mathrm{mL/min/1.73m^2}$), it is expert opinion that

Gd-contrast should only be administered to patients with CKD1–CKD3. Moreover, in observational studies inflammatory state, metabolic acidosis, high calcium and phosphate levels as well as high erythropoietin (EPO) dosages were aggravating factors. Importantly, the vast majority of NFS cases appeared in patients who received gadodiamide (Omniscan®), a contrast agent with a linear and uncharged molecular configuration. It is thus wise to not only to minimize the dose of contrast agent, but also to use Gd-contrast with cyclic and charged configuration posing the least risk of transmetallation.

Recently in dialysis patients a gadolinium-exposure induced systemic inflammatory response was observed in 13 out of 136 patients receiving Gd-DTPA (Magnevist®) [25]. A peracute septicaemia-like clinical picture evolved with fever, malaise, hypotension, vomiting, and dyspnoea. While steroids did not improve symptoms, significant improvement was seen within the first 5 hours of dialysis. Interestingly, C-reactive protein levels remained markedly elevated up to 14 days. Lymphopenia was seen in all patients, PMN remained normal, and none of these patients developed nephrogenic systemic fibrosis.

Interventions to reduce the cardiovascular risk

A major dilemma is the fact that in the past renal patients were deliberately excluded from major intervention studies. As a result, current therapeutic recommendations are mainly based on observational data or based on post hoc analyses in patients with early stages of CKD who had been included in large cardiological intervention studies. Controlled prospective information is available only for few interventions (➲Table 15b.2).

Table 15b.2 Summary of interventions

Statins #
Renin–angiotensin system blockade #
EPO §§
Beta-blockers §§
Vitamin D §§
Phosphate binders §; §§
Salt restriction§
Folate†

#Evidence from *controlled trials* in CKD patients;

§Suggested by *observational data* in CKD patients; §§in dialysis patients.

†No evidence.

Blood pressure control

The most important component of treatment is blood pressure control (➲target values listed in 'Chronic kidney disease as a cardiovascular risk factor', p.511). There is a caveat, however, in patients on haemodialysis. They often develop hypotensive episodes during fluid removal by ultrafiltration. Not only high, but even more potently low blood pressure predicts death in this high-risk population, particularly in the elderly with high comorbidity and low diastolic blood pressure values. The advice is to gradually lower blood pressure close to or within the normal range, but not to tolerate hypotensive episodes.

Statins

Statins, if anything, were equally effective or even more effective, in patients with reduced kidney function who had been included in intervention trials. Statins are safe and no excessive frequency of rhabdomylosis is seen in CKD patients. One interventional study, the 4D study in haemodialysed type 2 diabetics, however, failed to document a significant effect on the primary composite endpoint. But adjudicated coronary death was lowered to the same extent as in studies on non-renal patients. Therefore it is widespread opinion that all renal patients should be on statins. Most fibrates are metabolized by the kidney. Because of the risk of rhabdomyolysis they require monitoring and dose adjustment: they are therefore little used.

Correction of anaemia by erythropoietin

Observational studies showed that in dialysed patients with baseline haemoglobin (Hb) <10g/dL cardiac function was improved and left ventricular hypertrophy partially reversed when Hb was raised by the administration of EPO. Recent controlled studies showed no significant benefit when Hb concentrations were raised by EPO treatment above the recommended target of 11–12g/dL [26]. There is recent concern about adverse effects when Hb is increased further. Therefore Hb values >13g/dL should be avoided.

Beta-blockers

Even when GFR is not yet decreased, sympathetic activity is increased in patients with primary kidney disease and hypertension as documented by microneurography. In addition, breakdown of circulating catecholamines is reduced in advanced CKD because catecholamine breakdown by the amino-oxidase renalase from the kidney is diminished. Excessive sympathetic activation provides a good a priori rationale for the use of beta-blockers. The modern beta-blockers (carvedilol, nevibolol) with less metabolic and renal circulatory side effects are advisable [27]. The only prospective evidence of cardiovascular benefit available is one single study [28] in haemodialysed patients with cardiomyopathy and reduced EF. It documented significant reduction of total mortality and cardiovascular death. Nevertheless, not to the least because of the high frequency of sudden death, many experts believe that administration of beta-blockers is indicated unless there are specific contraindications.

Renin–angiotensin system blockade

Inappropriate activation of the RAS is a hallmark of CKD. The PEACE study [29] documented significantly reduced all-cause mortality in patients with stable coronary heart disease and eGFR <60mL/min/1.73m^2 who had received 4mg trandolapril, but not in patients with eGFR >60mL/min/1.73m^2, suggesting increased RAS activity or increased responsiveness to RAS blockade in CKD. Intervention studies in renal patients, usually to prevent progression of CKD, are underpowered to show a significant benefit on CV endpoints and this is true also for one intervention study [30] in haemodialysed patients.

In CKD patients RAS blockade by ACE inhibitors or ARB is also indicated because of the well-documented effect of RAS blockade to reduce progression of CKD. Their administration is safe, specifically also with respect to hyperkalaemia [31].

In dialysis patients, maintenance of residual renal function is associated with better survival. Both ACE inhibitors and ARB prolong the persistence of residual renal function. Therefore their administration is rational even in the absence of controlled evidence.

The safety of additional aldosterone blockade for patients with impaired renal function is currently not well documented and hyperkalaemia is a major concern.

Vitamin D

Recently, a large number of observational studies in patients with coronary heart disease and in CKD patients (predialysis and on dialysis) suggest improved survival and less cardiovascular events with administration of the precursor 25(OH)vitamin D_3 and of active vitamin D compounds which obviously have actions beyond bones and mineral metabolism. This area is currently in flux and large studies are ongoing. It is wise to measure 25(OH)D concentrations in CKD patients (measurement of 1,25$(OH)_2D_3$ is not necessary except in unusual hypercalcaemic cases). Cholecalciferol should be administered if the 25(OH)D level is <30ng/mL. Administration of active vitamin D should currently be based on the guidelines is restricted to lowering elevated PTH, but cardiovascular protection by active vitamin D may become a topic in the future.

Phosphataemia

Even in non-renal patients, serum-phosphate predicts cardiovascular events [11]. The impact of phosphataemia on survival and coronary heart disease has been grossly underestimated in the past. According to current guidelines in CKD patients, serum-phosphate should be kept within the normal range by restriction of dietary phosphate intake and, if necessary oral phosphate binders (for details see guidelines to be published soon). In dialysed patients serum-phosphate should be <6mg/dL.

Salt restriction and volume control

Sodium retention and hypervolaemia are common in renal patients. Dietary salt restriction (recommendation: 6g/day) and use of diuretics is therefore an integral part of patient management. The plausibility of this recommendation is heightened by experimental and observational evidence that salt—apart from increasing blood pressure—causes also blood pressure-independent CV target organ damage.

In dialysed patients, the issue of salt restriction is controversial.

One important predictor of death is loss of residual renal function, i.e. diuresis. Diuretics increase the amount of urine excreted, but do not extend the duration of residual diuresis. In contrast, RAS blockade maintains residual diuresis for longer periods of time.

With respect to volume control, continuous ambulatory peritoneal dialysis (CAPD) has the advantage of slow low-intensity fluid removal, thus avoiding the large volume swings seen with haemodialysis. An alternative currently under investigation is daily dialysis.

Homocysteine

Observational studies showed a strong correlation between serum-homocysteine concentrations and survival on dialysis. One interventional study to lower homocysteine by folate showed no benefit.

Sleep apnoea and depression

These two factors are impressively strong predictors of mortality and adverse cardiovascular events, both in CKD and haemodialysis patients. Unfortunately procedures with proven benefit are currently not available.

Diuretic therapy

The use of diuretics for the treatment of kidney and heart failure is an essential component of the therapeutic regimen both in CKD patients and in patients with heart failure. Diuretics are beneficial by potentiating the pressure lowering effect of inhibitors of the RAS and relieving symptomatic episodes of decompensated heart failure. On the other hand, however, diuretics trigger counterbalancing antinatriuretic mechanisms, e.g. ACE II, aldosterone, decreased systemic blood pressure. Such systemic *neurohumoral counterregulation* has adverse effects on heart and kidneys. Therefore it is expert opinion that the lowest effective dose should be administered. Even relatively low doses of diuretics allow to uptitrate blood pressure lowering medication, e.g. inhibitors of the RAS and beta-blockers—medications with proven benefit in both heart and kidney failure.

In combination with RAS inhibitors low dose *thiazide diuretics* augment the reduction of albuminuria—a powerful cardiovascular and renal risk factor. RAS inhibitors diminish the thiazide-induced reduction in GFR. As a result, the filtered sodium load is increased, permitting more effective natriuresis.

In patients with a GFR less than approximately 30mL/min, thiazides cause only a minor increase of natriuresis. At this level of GFR they should be exchanged for, or combined with, *loop diuretics* which are effective even in advanced kidney failure. The combination makes sense because frequently resistance to loop diuretic monotherapy develops because of a compensatory increase of distal tubular Na^+ reabsorption; this can be overcome by the addition of a thiazide. It is important that in proteinuric patients the efficacy of diuretics is decreased because in the tubulus lumen diuretics are up to 90% protein bound while only the concentration of the free diuretic inhibits tubular Na^+ reabsorption. In this situation higher doses of diuretics are required. It is important to pay attention to the half-life of the diuretic; e.g. furosemide is fully effective only with three times daily administration.

Na^+ reabsorption is also increased by aldosterone. The plasma aldosterone concentration usually decreases initially after administration of ACE-inhibitors and ACE receptor blockers, but in the long term a secondary increase in plasma aldosterone frequently occurs ('escape').

Table 15b.3 How to deal with insufficient response to diuretic treatment in patients with renal failure and patients with heart failure

Reduction of salt intake—diet, restriction of Na^+-containing infusions
Selection of appropriate diuretic and diuretic dose—half-life, pharmacokinetics frequently influenced by GFR and proteinuria
Interaction by medications affecting renal function—non-steroidals, thiazolidinedione ...
Potentiation of efficacy of diuretics by combining loop diuretics and distally acting diuretics—sequential nephron blockade
Haemodialysis/ultrafiltration, positive inotropic interventions, intra-aortic ballon pump, assist devices

In proteinuric CKD this is usually associated with an increase in proteinuria. In this situation *spironolactone* is helpful, particularly in patients with low K^+ serum levels. Unfortunately at low GFR the risk of hyperkalaemia is significantly increased.

A frequent cause of insufficient efficacy of diuretic treatment is an excessive dietary *sodium intake* or administration of Na^+ by infusions. In such patients even though an adequate diuresis may be achieved the sodium balance may not become negative.

In oedematous patients with advanced heart failure, *delayed intestinal absorption of diuretics* may occur as a result of mucosal oedema in the gut so that less diuretic is delivered to the tubule accounting for an inadequate natriuretic response. If in such cases the intravenous application of diuretics fails to establish diuresis, more invasive measures e.g. ultrafiltration, haemodialysis, inotropic support, or left assist devices may be needed depending on the prevailing pathophysiology of either renal or cardiac failure (➲Table 15b.3).

Particularly in elderly patients, mostly women, thiazides and particularly the combination of thiazides with loop diuretics ('sequential nephron blockade') may cause *hypovolaemic hyponatraemia*. This is usually associated with an excess of antidiuretic hormone (ADH). Discontinuation of thiazide diuretics may be sufficient. Hypovolaemic hyponatraemia predicts poor outcome particularly in end-stage heart failure. The treatment is largely empirical: fluid (water) restriction (<1.5L) and discontinuation of diuretics. Small studies found an increased efficacy from concomitant hypertonic saline infusions. Since the primary problem is water retention from ADH excess, this procedure is not recommended: it may contribute to further volume expansion if diuresis is not adequate [32]. The water retention underlying hyponatraemia in heart failure is the result of unopposed baroreceptor activity causing inappropriate non-osmotic release of arginine vasopressin leading to water retention. The administration of vasopressin V_2 receptor blockers represents a novel therapeutic option in hypovolaemic hyponatraemia, but long-term benefit on survival has not been demonstrated.

Loop diuretics, and to a lesser degree, thiazides increase the renal production of *prostaglandins*. They act as vasodilators and regulate renal blood flow. *Non-steroidal anti-inflammatory drugs* impair prostaglandin synthesis and thus cause renal ischaemia by unopposed actions of angiotensin II. They also reduce natriuresis. Therefore it is risky to administer them in patients with CKD and advanced cardiac disease.

Personal perspective

The major challenge in the future will be to improve the interaction between cardiologists and nephrologists and to make renal evaluation an integral part of cardiological assessment. In view of the shocking excess mortality in ESRD patients it is necessary to start treatment aimed at reduction of cardiovascular risk in the earliest possible stage of CKD; yet currently the majority of patients with end-stage renal disease is first seen and adequately treated immediately prior to or at the time of start of renal replacement therapy.

The pathogenesis of the unique acceleration of atherogenesis and of the development of a specific form of cardiomyopathy even in the earliest stages of renal disease is currently poorly understood. Exciting new data argue for an important role of salt and cardiotonic steroids. Serum phosphate and vitamin D are unexpected newcomers in the orchestra of cardiovascular risk factors and pathophysiology. We shall certainly be confronted with many more surprises in the future.

Further reading

Mancia G, De Backer G, Dominiczak A, *et al.* 2007 Guidelines for the Management of Arterial Hypertension: The Task Force for the Management of Arterial Hypertension of the European Society of Hypertension (ESH) and of the European Society of Cardiology (ESC). *J Hypertens* 2007; **25**: 1105–87.

Sarnak MJ, Levey AS, Schoolwerth AC, *et al.* Kidney disease as a risk factor for development of cardiovascular disease: a statement from the American Heart Association Councils on Kidney in Cardiovascular Disease, High Blood Pressure Research, Clinical Cardiology, and Epidemiology and Prevention. *Circulation* 2003; **108**: 2154–69.

Stevens LA, Coresh J, Greene T, *et al.* Assessing kidney function—measured and estimated glomerular filtration rate. *N Engl J Med* 2006; **354**: 2473–83.

Tonelli M, Jose P, Curhan G, *et al* . Proteinuria, impaired kidney function, and adverse outcomes in people with coronary disease: analysis of a previously conducted randomised trial. *BMJ* 2006; **332**: 1426.

de Zeeuw D, Remuzzi G, Parving HH, *et al.* Albuminuria, a therapeutic target for cardiovascular protection in type 2 diabetic patients with nephropathy. *Circulation* 2004; **110**: 921–7.

➲ **For full references and multimedia materials please visit the online version of the book (http://esctextbook.oxfordonline.com).**

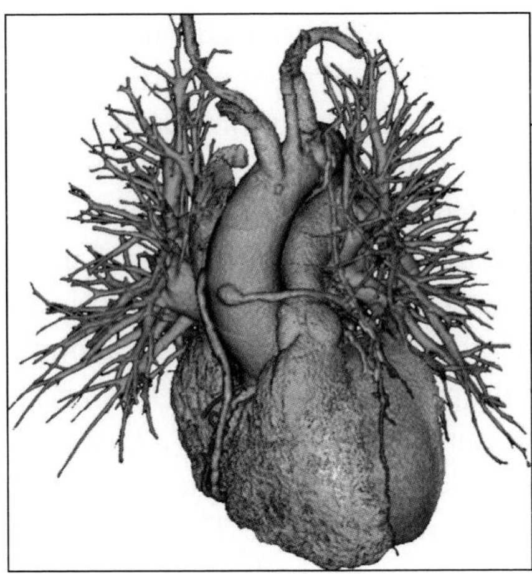

CHAPTER 15c

Erectile Dysfunction

Graham Jackson

Contents

Summary

Erectile dysfunction (ED) is common, affecting up to two-thirds of men with known coronary artery disease (CAD) and endothelial dysfunction is now considered the common denominator, explaining the link between ED and CAD in men over 40 years of age with organic ED. Due to the smaller size of the penile arteries (1–2mm), the same degree of endothelial dysfunction may present with ED ahead of CAD (vessel size 3–4mm). It is now established that ED may be a marker of and potentially an independent risk factor for silent CAD with a time window of 2–5 years from the onset of ED to the coronary event. This provides an opportunity for reducing cardiovascular risk in men with ED and no cardiac symptoms, with ED being considered a cardiac or vascular disease equivalent unless and until proved otherwise. ED may present before chronic coronary disease as well as acute coronary syndromes. Exercise testing will not identify subclinical lipid-rich plaque of <50% stenosis which is vulnerable to rupture but recent studies using 64-channel multi-detector computer tomography (MDCT) have identified plaque disease in the presence of normal maximal treadmill exercise electrocardiograms (ECGs) in men with ED and no cardiac symptoms.

Men (and women) with cardiac disease should be routinely advised on sexual activity as part of a comprehensive approach to rehabilitation. Several therapies are available for the treatment of ED with encouraging significant success rates. There is no evidence that any therapy for ED increases cardiac risk provided the men (and their partners) are properly assessed. Sexual activity is a normal part of life for all age groups and there is no reason why patients with cardiac disease cannot experience a satisfying relationship.

Introduction

Erectile dysfunction (ED) is common and currently affects >150 million men worldwide [1]. In the Massachusetts Male Aging Study (MMAS) the prevalence of ED was 52% in American men aged 40–70 years [2]. ED increases in incidence with age with men aged >70 years being three times more likely to have ED than men in their 40s. As we are an aging population and as age is not a barrier to sexual activity, the challenge of identifying and managing ED can only increase. The predicted prevalence of ED is expected to be >300 million men by the year 2025.

There is now a large body of evidence supporting the concept that ED is predominantly a vascular disease sharing the same risk factors as CAD and often presenting 2–5 years before cardiac symptoms occur [3]. The common pathophysiology is endothelial dysfunction and the possibility of using ED as a marker or independent risk factor for asymptomatic CAD has excited a great deal of interest with regard to reducing cardiovascular risk factors in men with ED in order to prevent a subsequent cardiac event [4].

Whilst the commonest cause of ED in men >40 years of age is organic (vascular), it is important not to compartmentalize ED. The organic cause invariably has psychological consequences, especially depression, with the man losing self-esteem, feeling inadequate and a failure. ED is an important cause of relationships breaking down and the partner must not be overlooked, so management needs to embrace more than just trying to establish an erect penis as a lot of psychosocial support is needed. Similarly a man with predominantly psychological ED may have cardiovascular risk factors which need to be addressed.

When advising cardiac patients about sexual activity it is important to individualize the advice. We have a statistical framework to support our recommendations but each person being advised will have, as well as a general cardiac condition (e.g. post-myocardial infarction), varying degrees of effort restriction, determined by, for example, the size of the infarction. In addition, each person will have personal issues regarding safety of sex, treatment of ED, and their confidence in returning to normal activities including sex. As we advise on sex we need to remember that the problems may have preceded the cardiac event with important relationship issues as a consequence.

Cardiovascular response to sex

The cardiovascular response to sexual activity including intercourse is similar to mild to moderate daily non-sexual effort. Several studies have been performed using ambulatory electrocardiography and blood pressure monitoring comparing heart rate, electrocardiographic, and blood pressure responses during sexual activity and other normal daily activities. Nemec and colleagues evaluated ten healthy males comparing heart and blood pressure responses during sexual intercourse with their wives in their homes [5]. They recorded only modest changes whether the male was on top or underneath. In the on top position the peak heart rate was 114 ± 14 beats per minute (bpm) returning to 69 ± 12bpm by 120s post-orgasm, and when the male was underneath a similar peak heart rate of 117 ± 4bpm was recorded. The peak blood pressure responses were similar for both positions with a systolic reading at orgasm of 160mgHg. Bohlen and colleagues, again evaluating ten healthy males, looked at man on top, woman on top, self-stimulation and partner stimulation, and found no significant difference in heart rates or blood pressure response [6]. Though there is less information available in women in a post-myocardial infarction study, cardiovascular responses were similar with a peak heart rate in men of 111bpm and women 104bpm with a similar time to recovery of 3.1min and 2.6min respectively [7]. In a study of stable angina patients using 24-hour ECG monitoring, the heart rate response averaged 122bpm with a range of 102–137 (30 men and 5 women) during intercourse compared to a maximum of 124bpm during the rest of the day [8].

Expressed as a multiple of the metabolic equivalent of the task or MET (one MET is the energy expenditure at rest which is approximately 3.5mL of oxygen per kg body weight per minute) sexual activity between couples in a long standing relationship is associated with a peak workload of 3–4 METs at orgasm, though younger couples, who may be more vigorous in their activity, may expend 5–6 METs. The average duration of intercourse is 5–15min so sexual intercourse is not an extreme or sustained cardiovascular stress. Casual sex may involve a greater cardiac workload due to lack of familiarity and age mismatch, most often an older man with a younger woman [9].

Using our knowledge of METs we can advise patients on sexual activity using a simple comparison with other activities such as walking 1 mile (1.6km) on the level in 20min (➲Table 15c.1).

Cardiac risk

There is only a small risk of myocardial infarction associated with sexual activity [10]. The relative risk of a myocardial infarct during the 2 hours after sexual intercourse is shown in ➲Table 15c.2.

Table 15c.1 Metabolic equivalent of task units (METs) as a guide to relating daily activity to sexual activity

Daily activity	METs
Sexual intercourse with established partner	
Lower range (normal)	2–3
Lower range orgasm	3–4
Upper range (vigorous activity)	5–6
Lifting and carrying objects (9–20kg)	4–5
Walking 1.6 km (1 mile) on the level in 20min	3–4
Golf	4–5
Gardening (digging)	3–5
'Do-it-yourself', wallpapering, etc.	4–5
Light housework; e.g. ironing, polishing	2–4
Heavy housework; e.g. making beds, scrubbing floors, cleaning windows	3–6

The baseline absolute risk of a myocardial infarction during normal daily life is low—1 chance in a million per hour for a healthy adult, and 10 chances in a million per hour for a patient with documented cardiac disease. Therefore, during the 2 hours after sexual intercourse, the risk increases to 2.5 in a million for a healthy adult and 25 in a million for a patient with documented cardiac disease; importantly, there is no increased risk in those who are physically active [11].

A similar study from Sweden has reported identical findings [12]. If we take a baseline annual rate of 1% for a 50-year-old man, as a result of weekly sexual activity the risk of a myocardial infarction increases to 1.01% in those without a history of a previous myocardial infarction and to 1.1% in those with a previous history.

Coital sudden death is very rare. In three large studies death related to sexual activity was 0.6% in Japan, 0.18% in Frankfurt, and 1.7% in Berlin [13]. Extramarital sex was responsible for 75%, 75%, and 77% respectively, and the victims were men in 82%, 94%, and 93% of cases respectively.

Table 15c.2 Relative risk of myocardial infarction during the 2 hours after sexual activity: physically fit equals sexually fit

Patient type	Relative risk (95% confidence interval)
All patients	2.5 (1.7–3.7)
Men	2.7 (1.8–4.0)
Women	1.3 (0.3–5.2)
Previous myocardial infarction	2.9 (1.3–6.5)
Sedentary life	3.0 (2.0–4.5)
Physically active	1.2 (0.4–3.7)

The partnership of an older man with a younger woman was the most common setting. Excessive drinking and sex too close to a large meal were frequently associated.

Assessing the risk of sex activity

In spite of taking a careful clinical history and using the MET equivalents in ➲Table 15c.1 there will be occasions when the physical ability of the individual is unclear. In this setting exercise testing can be used to help resolve any doubts. Using METs, sexual intercourse is equivalent to 3–4min of the standard Bruce treadmill protocol. If a person can manage at least 4min on the treadmill without significant symptoms, ECG evidence of ischaemia, a decrease in systolic blood pressure, or dangerous arrhythmias, it will be safe to advise on sexual activity. Using ambulatory ECGs and bicycle exercise tests, Drory and colleagues studied 88 men with CAD who were not receiving medication [14]. On ambulatory ECGs one-third of the men had ischaemia during sexual intercourse and all had ischaemia on the bicycle exercise ECG. All those who did not exhibit ischaemia on exercise test (n = 34) also had no ECG changes during sexual intercourse. All ischaemic episodes during sexual intercourse were associated with an increasing heart rate, identifying a potentially important therapeutic role for drugs that decrease the heart rate (β-adrenoreceptor antagonists, Ivabradine, verapamil, diltiazem).

If a patient is unable to perform an exercise test because of mobility problems, a pharmacological stress test should be utilized (e.g. dobutamine stress echocardiography).

A man who cannot achieve 3–4 METs should be further evaluated by angiography if appropriate.

Advice on METs in the clinical setting and relating this advice to sexual intercourse should also include advice on the avoidance of stress, a heavy meal, or excess alcohol consumption before sexual intercourse.

Though advocated as a means of evaluating cardiac risk in men with ED and no cardiac symptoms, exercise electrocardiography will not identify sub 50% lesions which may be lipid rich and vulnerable to rupture [15].

Erectile dysfunction and the cardiac patient

ED and CAD commonly co-exist with endothelial dysfunction the common denominator. ED and CAD share the same risk factors which explains the endothelial link [16].

The clinical consequences of endothelial dysfunction include the development of atherosclerosis, acute coronary syndromes, cardiac failure, and ED. It is now recognized that a defect in the NO-cyclic guanosine 3′5′-monophosphate system in smooth-muscle cells is an early marker of systemic vascular abnormalities before the development of overt cardiovascular disease in men with ED.

Measures of endothelial dysfunction have been shown to be improved by drugs that benefit cardiovascular morbidity and mortality (e.g. angiotensin-converting enzyme (ACE) inhibitors in cardiac failure; statin and ACE inhibitors in ischaemic heart disease) and by drugs used in the treatment of erectile dysfunction, heart failure, and diabetes (e.g. phosphodiesterase type 5 (PDE-5) inhibitors). Over the past decade, as the direct relationship of ED and endothelial dysfunction has become elucidated, it has become similarly apparent that ED may be treated with PDE-5 inhibitors which improve endothelial dysfunction by acting within the smooth-muscle cell [17].

Cardiovascular risk factors

The shared risk factors between ED and vascular disease include smoking, hyperlipidaemia, diabetes, hypertension, obesity, and a sedentary lifestyle (➲Table 15c.2).

In the MMAS involving a large population-based random sample of 1290 healthy men aged 40–70 years, the age-adjusted probability of complete ED was 15% in treated hypertensives compared to 9.6% of the whole population [2]. In another study, ED was reported in 17% of men with untreated hypertension in comparison with 25% of men who were receiving current antihypertensive treatment.

However, more recent analyses of hypertensive patients suggest that the prevalence of ED in hypertensive populations is even higher. Burchardt and colleagues mailed the International Index of Erectile Function (IIEF) questionnaire to 476 male patients with hypertension [18]. One hundred and four patients (mean age 62.2 years) completed the questionnaire. Of these, 68.3% had some degree of ED. ED was mild in 7.7%, moderate in 15.4%, and severe in 45.2%. Compared to the general population of ED cases, patients with hypertension had more severe ED (45.2% in hypertensives vs. ~10% in a general population as reported by the MMAS). The authors concluded that ED was more prevalent in patients with hypertension than in age-matched controls and that the degree of ED was more severe in patients with hypertension than the general male population. Another study has also confirmed a very high rate of ED among hypertensive patients [19]. In a survey of 7689 patients (mean age 59 years) using the Sexual Health Inventory in Men (SHIM) questionnaire, in 3906 men with hypertension alone (no diabetes) ED was present in 67%, similar to the 68% figure mentioned earlier. In 2377 men with diabetes, ED was present in 71% and of 1186 men with both hypertension and diabetes ED was present in 77%. Of concern, ED was untreated in 65% even though the majority of men said that they wanted treatment. It is clear that a significant number of hypertension patients are likely to have ED.

In the MMAS, smoking doubled the chance of ED developing over an 8-year follow-up period and increased the rate of occurrence in hypertensives. Smoking is well known as a risk factor for endothelial damage and vascular disease. Although cessation of smoking later in life may still be of some benefit to the 3–4mm coronary arteries, it may be too late to reverse damage to the small (1–2mm) penile arteries [20].

Hyperlipidaemia increases the risk of ED by 1.8 times, with a raised high-density lipoprotein (HDL) cholesterol level being protective. For every 1mmol/L increase in cholesterol, there is an increase by a factor of 1.32 in the risk of developing ED. For every 1mmol/L increase in HDL there is a 0.38 risk factor decrease of ED. In contrast to what might be expected, lipid-lowering therapy does not benefit ED and in some cases can actually cause or exacerbate ED, possibly due to a central action secondary to blood–brain barrier penetration, though additional multiple risk factors may also be causative [21].

Diabetics suffer from both endothelial and neurological ED, with ED prevalence recorded as high as 80% in those >60 years of age. It is possible that early and vigorous glucose control might be preventative. In addition, the early use of statins and perhaps prophylactic PDE-5 inhibitors as daily therapy theoretically could preserve endothelial function [22].

Erectile dysfunction as a predictor of occult coronary artery disease

The question 'Is erectile dysfunction a marker for cardiovascular disease' has now been answered in the affirmative as a result of several studies [23]. The artery size hypothesis has been used to explain how ED acts as a silent marker of vascular disease elsewhere in the body, and more significantly as a marker of CAD [24]. Artery size varies considerably according to location within the vascular system (➲Table 15c.3).

Table 15c.3 Artery size and atherothrombosis. A significant restriction to flow in the penile arteries may be subclinical in larger vessels

Artery	Diameter (mm)	Clinical event
Penile	1–2	ED
Coronary	3–4	Ischaemic heart disease
Carotid	5–7	TIA/stroke
Femoral	6–8	Claudication

TIA, transient ischaemic attack.

For example, the lumen of the penile arteries is considerably smaller (1–2mm) compared with that of the coronary (3–4mm), carotid (5–6mm), and femoral (6–8mm) arteries. Because of their smaller size, the same level of plaque burden and/or endothelial dysfunction has a greater effect on blood flow through the penile arteries than through the coronary, carotid, and femoral arteries. Therefore the clinical manifestations of penile endothelial dysfunction may become evident before the consequences of coronary or peripheral vascular disease. By the time the lumen of the larger arteries become significantly obstructed (>50%), the penile blood flow may have already decreased considerably, which explains why so many men with CAD have ED.

Thus on the basis of artery size hypothesis and the fact that the endothelium is the same throughout the arterial tree, a malfunction in the penile arteries causing ED may be a predictor of silent subclinical cardiovascular disease (CVD). Furthermore, because an acute coronary syndrome often arises as the result of the rupture of a subclinical plaque, the presence of ED may also be an early warning sign of an acute event as well as being a manifestation of advanced obstructive CAD [25].

In 1999 Pritzker presented a preliminary report entitled 'The Penile Stress Test: A window to the hearts of man' [26]. He reviewed the results of exercise stress testing, risk factor profiles, and, in selected cases, angiography in 50 men with ED, who had no cardiac symptoms or past history. Multiple cardiovascular risk factors were present in 80%. Exercise tests positive for ischaemia were found in 28 of the 50 men. Coronary angiography was performed in 20 men and revealed left main stem or severe three-vessel disease in six men, moderate two-vessel disease in seven men, and significant single-vessel disease in seven men. This study identified the significant incidence of occult coronary disease in cardiologically asymptomatic men presenting with ED to a urological service. Others have reported similar findings and noted the occurrence of ED before cardiac symptoms developed [3]. In a study comparing the velocity of cavernosal artery blood flow with the presence of ischaemic heart disease in men with ED, a low peak systolic velocity (PSV) predicted the presence of CAD [27]. A PSV <35cm/s was associated with CAD in 41.9% of men and above 35cm/s in only 3.7% of men.

In support of this concept, a series of 300 patients with acute chest pain and angiographically proven CAD were evaluated with a semi-structured interview to assess their medical and sexual histories prior to presentation [25]. The prevalence of ED among these patients was 49% (n = 147). In these 147 men with both ED and CAD, ED was experienced before CAD symptoms in 99 patients (67%). The mean time interval between the occurrence of ED and the occurrence of CAD was 38.8 months (range: 1–168 months). Interestingly, all men with ED and type 1 diabetes developed sexual dysfunction before the onset of CAD symptoms. The authors do point out the absence of a control group with CAD and normal erections, but their findings clearly identify the need to assess cardiovascular risk in all males presenting with ED without obvious psychosexual aetiology, especially in patients with diabetes.

Speel and colleagues evaluated 158 men aged 40–69 years with penile pharmacoduplex ultrasonography in order to determine whether there was cavernous arterial insufficiency and related these findings to the Framingham risk with the results extrapolated to the Dutch aging male population [28]. Cavernous insufficiency identified a significantly increased risk of CAD in the group aged 50–59 years but not in the age groups 40–49 years and 60–69 years. Overall, it was predicted that one in four men with ED aged 40–69 years and without known CAD would developed CAD over the next 12 years.

Roumeguére and colleagues compared 215 patients with ED and 100 patients without ED in order to evaluate undiagnosed hyperlipidaemia and coronary risk [29]. The prevalence of hypercholesterolaemia was 79.6% vs. 52% in the ED and non-ED groups (p = 0.06). Increased 10-year CAD risk was 56.6% vs. 32.6% (ED vs. no ED; p <0.05). Low HDL cholesterol and high total cholesterol to HDL ratio, both established important risk markers for CAD, were identified as predictors of ED. This study suggested that ED might serve as a 'sentinel event' for coronary heart disease.

ED is also more frequent in diabetic patients with silent CAD than in those without. In a study of men with type II diabetes (n = 260) the incidence of ED (IIEF questionnaire) was significantly higher in the population with asymptomatic CAD than in the population without CAD (33.8 vs. 4.7%; p <0001) [30]. ED not only predicted CAD independently of other risk factors but also was the strongest predictor of silent CAD in this study.

The large Prostate Cancer Prevention Trial provided the first evidence of a strong association between ED and the subsequent development of clinical cardiovascular events [31]. ED at entry or that developed during follow up was found to significantly predict any cardiac event with a hazard ratio of 1.45 ($p < 0.001$; 95% confidence interval (CI): 1.25–1.69). The data also showed that the cardiovascular risk associated with incident ED (that is, developed during follow up) was at least as great as the risk associated with a family history of myocardial infarction, current smoking or hypercholesterolaemia.

A similar strong correlation between ED and increased cardiovascular risk was also reported in a health screening project using the IIEF-5 questionnaires [32]. In this analysis of 2561 patients, the presence of moderate to severe ED (IIEF-5 score 5–16) was calculated to increase the 10 year relative risk of developing CAD by 65% ($p<0.001$) and of stroke by 43% ($p = 0.04$). Although mild ED (IIEF-5 score 17–21) was associated with increased risk (18–24%), this observation was not statistically significant.

In a recently reported population-based study (the Krimpen study) a single question on erectile rigidity (from the International Continence Society male sex questionnaire) was shown to be a predictor for the combined outcome of acute myocardial infarction, stroke and sudden death, independently of risk factors in the Framingham risk profile [33]. Men (aged 50–75; free of prostate and bladder disease) were followed up for an average of 6.3 years. Of those men who did not have CVD at baseline (n = 1248), 258 (22.8%) had severely reduced erectile rigidity. Fifty-eight cardiovascular events occurred in the 7945 person-year follow-up. After adjusting for age and CVD risk score, the hazard ratios (95% CI) were 1.6 (1.2–2.3) and 2.6 (1.3–5.2) for reduced and severely reduced erectile rigidity, respectively.

Recent findings suggest that there is a strong temporal relationship between ED and CAD, with ED preceding a cardiovascular event by at least 2–5 years. This temporal relationship was investigated in a questionnaire-base study that included 207 patients with CVD attending cardiovascular rehabilitation programmes and 165 age-matched controls from general practice in the UK [34]. Patients completed up to four questionnaires including the IIEF. Of the individuals with CVD 56% were experiencing symptoms of ED at the time of the study and had done so for a mean of 5 ± 5.3 years. In contrast, 37% of individuals in the control group had ED symptoms for a mean of 6.6 ± 6.8 years. Of particular concern, the study highlighted that only 53% of the CVD group and 43% of the control group had actually discussed their ED symptoms with a health professional.

In a study of 147 men presenting with acute coronary syndrome (plaque rupture), documented ED and CAD, Montorsi and colleagues reported the presence of clinically evident ED symptoms in 99 patients (67%) developed approximately 3 years (mean 38.8 month, range 1–168 months) prior to the acute event [25].

In the subsequent AssoCiation Between eRectile dysfunction and coronary Artery disease (COBRA) trial 93% of patients with a chronic coronary syndrome reported ED symptoms before the onset of angina pectoris, with a mean interval of 24 (range 12–36) months [35]. This finding further reinforces the concept of a lead time of at least 2–5 years between the development of ED and symptomatic CAD. The time intervals (range) for patients with one-, two- and three-vessel disease were 12 (9.5–24), 24 (16.5–36), and 33 (21–47) months respectively. There was a significant relationship between the length of time from ED to CAD onset and the number of vessels involved ($p = 0.016$). Importantly, given that men with ED may be at cardiovascular risk, this 'long' lead time provides an early opportunity for cardiovascular risk reduction [4].

Treating erectile dysfunction in men with cardiovascular disease

Recognizing the need for advice on management of erectile dysfunction, two consensus panels (in the UK and the USA) have produced similar guidelines dividing cardiovascular risk into three practical categories, with recommendations for management [36,37]. The Princeton consensus guidelines have recently been updated. It is recommended that all men with ED should undergo a full medical assessment. Baseline physical activity needs to be established and cardiovascular risk graded as low, intermediate, or high (➲Table 15c.4). Most patients with low or intermediate cardiac risk can have their ED managed in the outpatient or primary care setting.

There is no evidence that treating ED in patients with cardiovascular disease increases cardiac risk; however, this is with the provisos that the patient is correctly assessed and that the couple or individual (self-stimulation may be the only form of sexual activity) is appropriately counselled. Oral drug treatment is the most widely used, because of its acceptability and effectiveness, but all treatments have a place in management. The philosophy is to be always positive during what, for many men and their partners, is an uncertain time.

Table 15c.4 Risk from sexual activity in cardiovascular diseases: Second Princeton Consensus Conference

Low risk: typically implied by the ability to perform exercise of modest intensity without symptoms
Asymptomatic and <3 major risk factors (excluding sex)
Major CVD risk factors include age, male sex, hypertension, diabetes mellitus, cigarette smoking, dyslipidemia, sedentary lifestyle, and family history of premature CAD
Controlled hypertension
Beta-blockers and thiazide diuretics may predispose to erectile dysfunction
Mild, stable angina pectoris
Non-invasive evaluation recommended
Antianginal drug regimen may require modification*
Post revascularization and without significant residual ischaemic
ETT may be benefical to assess risk
Post myocardial infarction (>6–8 weeks), but asymptomatic and without ETT-induced ischaemia, or post revascularization
If post revascularization or no ETT-induced ischaemia, intercourse may be resumed 3–4 weeks after myocardial infarction
Mild valvular disease
May include selected patients with mild aortic stenosis
LVD (NYHA class I)
Most patients are low risk
Intermediate or indeterminate risk: evaluate to reclassify as high or low risk
Asymptomatic and ≥3 CAD risk factors (excluding sex)
Increased risk for acute myocardial infarction and death
ETT may be appropriate, particularly in sedentary patients
Moderate, stable angina pectoris
ETT may clarify risk
Myocardial infarction with previous 2–6 weeks
Increased risk of ischaemia, reinfarction, and malignant arrhythmias
ETT may clarify risk
LVD/CHF (NYHA class II)
Moderate risk of increased symptoms
Cardiovascular evaluation and rehabilitation may permit reclassification as low risk
Non-cardiac atherosclerotic sequelae (peripheral arterial disease, history of stroke, or transient ischaemic attacks)
Increased risk of myocardial infarction
Cardiological evaluation should be considered
High risk: defer resumption of sexual activity until after cardiological assessment and treatment
Unstable or refractory angina
Increased risk of myocardial infarction
Uncontrolled hypertension
Increased risk of acute cardiac and vascular events (i.e. stroke)
CHF (NYHA class III, IV)
Increased risk of cardiac decompensation
Recent myocardial infarction (within 2 weeks)
Increased risk of reinfarction, cardiac rupture, or arrhythmias, but impact of complete revascularization on risk is unknown
High-risk arrhythmias
Rarely, malignant arrhythmias during sexual activity may cause sudden death
Risk is decreased by an implanted defibrillator or pacemaker

(Continued)

Table 15c.4 *(Continued)* Risk from sexual activity in cardiovascular diseases: Second Princeton Consensus Conference

High risk: defer resumption of sexual activity until after cardiological assessment and treatment
Obstructive hypertrophic cardiomyopathies
Cardiovascular risks of sexual activity are poorly defined
Cardiovascular evaluation (i.e. ETT and echocardiography) may guide patient management
Moderate to severe valve disease
Use vasoactive drugs with caution

CAD, coronary artery disease; CHF, congestive heart failure, CVD, cardiovascular disease; ETT, exercise tolerance test; LVD, left ventricular dysfunction; NYHA, New York Heart Association.

*Avoid nitrates with PDE-5 inhibitors.

Adapted with permission from Jackson G. Safety and efficacy of the medical treatment of erectile dysfunction. *Heart Metab* 2005; **28**: 14–21.

Lifestyle changes

The commonest modifiable lifestyle factors associated with ED are obesity, cigarette smoking, hyperlipidaemia, and a sedentary lifestyle. In the Second Princeton Consensus on Sexual Dysfunction and Cardiac Risk the role of lifestyle factors was emphasized regarding associated risk and evidence of benefit from intervention [3, 37].

Obesity

Obesity has been confirmed as a risk factor for ED in large-scale cross-sectional and longitudinal studies. In the Health Professionals Follow-up Study the impact of obesity, physical activity, alcohol use, and smoking on ED was assessed in 22,086 men aged 40–75 years over 14 years [38]. Of men who were healthy with no ED in 1986, 17.7% developed ED during follow-up. Obesity nearly doubled the risk of ED (multivariate relative risk 1.9 compared with risk in men of ideal weight in 1986). In a study of 1700 Dutch men aged between 5–75 years, increased body mass index (BMI) was found to be a significant predictor of ED and, similarly, obesity was found to be a significant independent risk factor for ED in the Men in Australia Telephone Survey (MATeS) study [39,40].

Obesity is an independent risk factor for CAD and is associated with elevated levels of inflammatory markers, which in turn are associated with endothelial dysfunction. This low-grade inflammation may be an important pathophysiologic link between obesity, ED, CAD, and the 'metabolic syndrome' [17].

A study of 110 obese men aged 35–55 years with a BMI of 30kg/m^2 or greater (normal ≤25kg/m^2; pre-obese, 25–30kg/m^2) assessed the degree to which weight loss combined with increased physical activity affected erectile function [41]. None of the patients had diabetes, hypertension, or hyperlipidaemia. In a single-blind fashion half were randomly assigned to active intervention and half were given general information about healthy eating and exercise. The intervention group was given detailed advice about how to lose 10% or more of body weight, attended monthly group sessions, were set targets, were taught how to reduce calories, and were allocated food diaries. In addition to being given detailed advice about food types, they also had personal activity training, including advice on walking and activities such as soccer and swimming. After 1 year of monthly meeting with their nutritionalists and exercise trainers, they met twice monthly for a further year.

When assessed at 2 years, the BMI had decreased from 36.9 to 31.2kg/m^2 in the intervention group, and from 36.4 to 35.7kg/m^2 in the control group ($p <0.001$). Of interest, the inflammatory markers interleukin-6 ($p = 0.03$) and C-reactive protein (CRP) also decreased ($p = 0.02$). Physical activity increased more in the intervention group from 48 to 195min/week, compared with 51 to 84min/week in the controls ($p < 0.001$). ED improved significantly more in the intervention group; their International Index of Erectile Function (IIEF) scores increased from a mean of 13.9 to 17 ($p <0.001$), and in 17 men the score was >22 (normal). The mean score in the control group was stable (13.5–13.6) though three achieved a score >22. The authors showed, using multivariate analysis, that improvements in BMI and physical activity as well as CRP were independently and significantly associated with improved IIEF score. They concluded that one-third of obese men with ED can improve their erectile functions as a result of intensive lifestyle changes. They also identified a reduction in inflammatory markers that may well have had a significant impact on endothelial function, emphasizing again the link between obesity, ED, and CAD.

Physical activity

A sedentary, inactive lifestyle has been linked to ED. In the Health Professionals' Follow-up Study ED was associated with the level of physical activity as well as with BMI [38]. When the men were categorized according to their level of physical fitness, the least active levels (higher levels of sedentary behaviour) were independently linked to ED. All types of exercise reduced the incidence of ED. Running at least 2.5 hours a week was associated with a 30% RRR for ED when compared with no regular activity, and 1.5 hours of running or 3 hours of rigorous outdoor work reduced the relative risk by 20%.

In the Global Study of Sexual Attitudes and Behaviour (GSSAB), 31.8% of men who had less than average levels of physical activity had ED, compared with 13.9% of men who exercised more than average [42].

With obesity increasing the incidence of ED by 30%, and weight loss combined with physical activity decreasing ED by 30%, the Princeton Consensus emphasized the importance of lifestyle intervention particularly in men with ED and CAD because of the benefit throughout the vascular tree.

Smoking

In the Health Professionals' Study, smoking increased the risk of developing ED by 50% [38]. In the MMAS men who smoked at baseline increased their risk of developing moderate or total ED to 24%, compared with non-smokers at 14% ($p = 0.01$) [2]. Smoking has been shown to significantly adversely interfere with the cavernous venoocclusive mechanism and to reduce the erectile response to intracavernous injections. When considering overall vascular health, advice and support to enable individuals to stop smoking are an essential lifestyle intervention.

The metabolic syndrome

The metabolic syndrome consists of a cluster of risk factors that increase the risk of cardiovascular disease and type 2 diabetes [17, 44]. It is characterized by abdominal obesity, hyperlipidaemia, glucose intolerance, hypertension, and insulin resistance. It is associated with proinflammatory markers and endothelial dysfunction and an increased incidence of moderate to severe ED in men >50 years of age. Furthermore, ED may predict the metabolic syndrome in men with a BMI of <25kg/m^2 who otherwise would be considered at low cardiovascular risk [45].

As the components of the metabolic syndrome increase, so does the presence of organic ED. In addition, a threefold increase in the prevalence of hypogonadism has been reported, and as the number of criteria for the metabolic syndrome increased, so did the incidence of hypogonadism [46]. The strong association between the metabolic syndrome and hypogonadism has led to the speculation that testosterone replacement might be a therapeutic option. To date, however, the evidence supports primarily a lifestyle approach.

The Mediterranean-style diet (rich in whole grain, fruits, vegetables, legumes, walnuts, and olive oil) was evaluated in 35 men, with 30 acting as control subjects [47]. All had the metabolic syndrome and ED. The intervention group was given detailed dietary advice, targets were set, and monthly small-group sessions were held to offer support. Men in the control group were given general oral and written information about healthy foods but no individualized support. After 2 years, markers of endothelial function and inflammation significantly improved in the intervention group but not in the control group. In the intervention group, 13 men achieved an IIEF of 22 or higher, compared with only two in the control group. The intervention group had a significant decrease in glucose, insulin, LDL cholesterol, triglycerides, and blood pressure, with a significant increased in HDL cholesterol. Fourteen men in the intervention group had glucose intolerance and six had diabetes at baseline, but by 2 years the numbers had reduced to eight and three respectively.

We see here the evidence that multiple risk factor reduction benefits a multiple risk factor state in terms of both ED and CAD risk. A potentially important link is also emerging between inflammatory markers and their modification in the ED/CAD context and its therapy.

Alcohol

Excessive alcohol intake per se increases cardiovascular risk but there is little evidence of ED risk other than the acute effect of binge drinking. In addition, men with a very high alcohol intake are unlikely to participate in studies of risk association and reduction, so data are at present inconclusive [3].

Drug therapy

Phosphodiesterase type 5 inhibitors

PDE-5 inhibitors have transformed the management of ED [48]. The mechanism of action by blocking the degradation of cyclic guanosine 3′5′-monophosphate (cGMP) by PDE-5 promotes blood flow into the penis and the restoration of erectile function. They do not initiate an erection and sexual stimulation is needed to obtain an erection (➲Fig. 15c.1). They are not aphrodisiacs.

Haemodynamically, PDE-5 inhibitors have mild nitrate-like actions (sildenafil was originally intended to be a drug

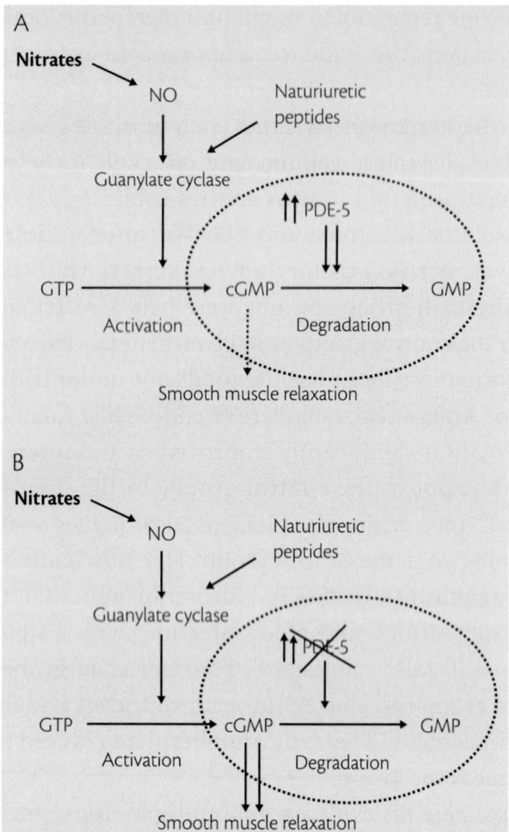

Figure 15c.1 (A) By degrading cyclic guanosine monophosphate (cGMP), phosphodiesterase type-5 (PDE-5) reduces smooth muscle relaxation, and the resulting effect on penile blood flow may cause erectile dysfunction. (B) A PDE-5 inhibitor reduces the degradation of cGMP, promotes smooth muscle relaxation, and improves penile blood flow. In the presence of nitrates, there may be an exaggerated vasodilatory response throughout the vasculature, leading to profound hypotension.

for the treatment of stable angina). As PDE-5 is present in smooth muscle cells throughout the vasculature and the nitric oxide/cGMP pathway is involved in the regulation of blood pressure, PDE-5 inhibitors have a modest hypotensive action. In healthy men, a single dose of sildenafil 100mg transiently decreased blood pressure by an average of 10/7mmHg with a return to baseline at 6 hours after the drug was given [49]. There was no effect on heart rate. As nitric oxide is an important neurotransmitter throughout the vasculature and is involved in the regulation of vascular smooth muscle relaxation, a synergistic and clinically important interaction with oral or sublingual nitrates can occur, and a profound decrease in blood pressure can result [50]. The mechanism involves a combination of increased formation of cGMP when nitrates activate guanylate cyclase, and decreased breakdown of cGMP as a result of the action of PDE-5 inhibitors. The concomitant administration of PDE-5 inhibitors and nitrates is thus contraindicated, and this recommendation also extends to other nitric oxide donors such as nicorandil. Clinical guidelines recommend that sublingual nitrate should be taken 12 hours after the PDE-5 inhibitors sildenafil or vardenafil; tadalafil, which has a longer half-life, ceases to react with nitrates only after 48 hours [3]. Oral nitrates are not prognostically important drugs, and they can therefore be discontinued and, if necessary, alternative agents substituted [51]. After cessation of oral nitrate, and provided there has been no clinical deterioration, PDE-5 inhibitors can be used safely. It is recommended that the time interval before the use of a PDE-5 inhibitor be five half-lives, which equates to 5 days in the case of most popular once-daily oral nitrate agents.

Sildenafil (Viagra®)

Sildenafil was the first oral treatment for ED and is the most extensively evaluated [52]. Overall success rates of 80% or more in patients with cardiovascular disease have been recorded with no evidence of tolerance. Patients with diabetes, with or without risk factors, in whom the pathophysiology is more complex and extensive, have an average success rate of 60%. To date, randomized trials, open-label studies, and outpatient monitoring studies have not found the use of sildenafil to be associates with any excess risk of myocardial infarction, stroke, or mortality.

In patients with stable angina pectoris, there is no evidence of an ischaemic effect caused by coronary steal, and in one large, double-blind, placebo-controlled exercise study, sildenafil 100mg increased exercise time and diminished ischaemia [53]. A study of the haemodynamic effects of sildenafil in men with severe CAD identified no adverse cardiovascular effects, and a potentially beneficial effect on coronary blood flow reserve [54]. Studies in patients with and without diabetes have demonstrated improved endothelial function acutely and after long-term oral administration, which may have implications beyond the treatment of erectile dysfunction. Sildenafil has also been shown to attenuate the activation of platelet IIb/IIIa receptor activity [48]. Hypertensive patients receiving monotherapy or being treated with several drugs have experienced no increased in adverse events, with the exception of those receiving doxazosin, a non-selective α-adrenoceptor antagonist. Occasional postural effects have occurred with sildenafil when it was taken within 4 hours of doxazosin 4mg; advice to avoid this time interval is now in place [55]. Sildenafil has also been proved to be effective in patients with heart failure who were deemed suitable for treatment of erectile dysfunction; the incidence of erectile dysfunction inpatients with heart failure is 80%, making this finding of major clinical importance [56].

On average, the dose of sildenafil is 50mg; 25mg is advised initially for those older than 80 years because of delayed excretion. Onset of action is 30–60min with a peak effect from 1–12 hours. A dose of 100mg is invariably needed in patients with diabetes. An empty stomach and the avoidance of alcohol or cigarette smoking facilitate the effect of the drug. Sildenafil 100mg has no adverse cardiac effects additional to those associated with the 50mg dose and should be routinely prescribed if, after four attempts, the 50mg dose is not effective.

Adverse effects are generally mild in nature (➲Table 15c.3) with drop out rates similar to placebo in the randomized studies.

The short half-life of sildenafil makes it the drug of choice in patients with more severe cardiovascular disease, allowing early use of supportive treatment if an adverse clinical event occurs.

Tadalafil (Cialis®)

Tadalafil also has been extensively evaluated in patients with cardiovascular disease, and has a safety and efficacy profile similar to that of sildenafil [57]. Studies have shown no adverse effects on cardiac contraction, ventricular repolarization or ischaemic threshold. A similar hypotensive effect has been recorded with a dose of doxazosin 8mg so caution is needed: as hypotension does not occur when the patient is in the supine position, and as tadalafil has a long half-life, it is suggested that tadalafil is taken in the morning and doxazosin in the evening. There is no interaction of tadalafil with the selective α-adrenoceptor antagonist, tamsulosin, which can therefore be prescribed as an alternative to doxazosin for benign prostate hypertrophy [58]. Tadalafil is effective from 30min after administration, but its peak efficacy occurs at 2 hours. Efficacy is maintained for up to 36 hours and is not influenced by food. It is administered in 10–20mg doses. The recommended starting dose is 10mg and should be adjusted according to the patient's response and side effects. Adverse events (➲Table 15c.3) are generally mild in nature and the drop-out rate due to adverse events is similar to placebo.

Tadalafil improved erections by 67% and 81% in men taking 10mg and 20mg of tadalafil compared with 35% of men in the control placebo group [59]. Tadalafil also improved erections in difficult-to-treat subgroups. In diabetic patients 64% reported improved erections compared to 25% of patients in the control group.

Because of its long half-life, tadalafil may not be the drug of first choice for patients with a more complex cardiovascular disease. However, as 80% of patients with cardiovascular disease stratify as low risk it does represent an alternative for the majority.

Tadalafil is now approved as a daily therapy (2.5 and 5mg) which may improve spontaneity and effectiveness [60].

Vardenafil (Levitra®)

Because vardenafil has a chemical structure very similar to that of sildenafil, it is not surprising that it has a similar clinical profile. One study has reported no impairment of exercise ability in patients with stable CAD receiving vardenafil 20mg [61]. Daily therapy provides no advantage probably due to the short half-life [62].

Vardenafil is effective after 30min from administration. Its effect is reduced by a heavy fatty meal. It is administered in 5, 10, and 20mg doses. The recommended starting dose is 10mg and should be adjusted according to the patient's response and side effects. Adverse events (➲Table 15c.5) are generally mild in nature with a drop-out rate similar to placebo.

After 12 weeks of treatment in a dose-response study, improved erections were reported by 66%, 76%, and 80% of men taking 5mg, 10mg, and 20mg of vardenafil respectively, compared with 30% of men taking placebo [63]. Vardenafil has also improved erections in difficult to treat subgroups. In diabetic patients 72% reported improved erections compared to 13% of patients taking placebo.

Cardiovascular safety

Clinical trial results and post-marketing data of sildenafil, tadalafil, and vardenafil have demonstrated no increase in myocardial infarction rates in patients that received these agents compared to expected rates in age-matched populations of men [64]. None of the PDE-5 inhibitors were found to adversely affect total exercise time or time to ischaemia

Table 15c.5 Common adverse events of all three PDE-5 inhibitors (from EMEA statements on product characteristics)

Adverse event	Sildenafil	Tadalafil	Vardenafil
Headache	12.8 %	14.5 %	16 %
Flushing	10.4 %	4.1 %	12 %
Dyspepsia	4.6 %	12.3 %	4 %
Nasal congestion	1.1 %	4.3 %	10 %
Dizziness	1.2 %	2.3 %	2 %
Abnormal vision	1.9 %		<2 %
Back pain		6.5 %	
Myalgia		5.6 %	

during exercise testing in men with stable angina. In addition to established benefit in treating pulmonary hypertension, these are encouraging results in cardiac failure [65].

Organic nitrates (e.g. nitroglycerine, isosorbide mononitrate, isosorbide dinitrate) and other nitrate preparations used to treat angina, as well as amyl nitrite or amyl nitrate ('poppers' used for recreation) are absolute contraindications to the use of PDE-5 inhibitors. They result in cGMP accumulation and unpredictable falls in blood pressure and symptoms of hypotension. The duration of interaction between organic nitrates and PDE-5 inhibitors is dependent upon the PDE-5 inhibitor and nitrate under study.

If a PDE-5 inhibitor is taken and the patient develops chest pain, nitroglycerine must be withheld for at least 12 hours if sildenafil (and likely vardenafil) was used (half-life 4 hours) and for at least 48 hours if tadalafil was used (half-life 17.5 hours). If a patient develops angina while taking a PDE-5 inhibitor he should be told to discontinue sexual activity and stand up, as the venous pooling will imitate a nitrate [3]. If pain continues under hospital supervision alternate agents should be prescribed, though intravenous nitrates can be used under careful medical observation.

Co-administration of PDE-5 inhibitors with antihypertensive agents (ACE inhibitors, ACE receptor blockers, calcium blockers, beta-blockers, diuretics) may result in small additive drops in blood pressure, which are usually minor. In general, the adverse event profile of the PDE-5 inhibitor [5] is not worsened by a background of antihypertensive medicines, even when the patient is on multiple antihypertensive agents.

Injection therapy

Direct intracavernosal injection of vasodilating agents began in the 1980s. Prostaglandin E1 is a natural substance that relaxes smooth muscle cells and dilates the arterioles, increasing blood flow into the penis. Alprostadil is a commercially available form of prostaglandin E1 that is effective in 5–15min, with an erection that usually lasts 30min but occasionally may persist for several hours [66]. The starting dose is 1.25mcg and can be increased to 40mcg, depending on effect. It is important that patients be taught the correct technique for injection; men with poor dexterity (e.g. arthritic hands or tremor) will need their partner's help with the injection. In fact, partners may often perform the injection as part of the sexual activity. On removal of the needle, firm pressure is applied and the drug should be gently massaged into the penis for approximately 30s. Men on anticoagulants, however, should compress the injection site for 5–10min.

The resulting erection occurs without stimulation, although stimulation may enhance its effects. The erections are occasionally painful, but usually feel natural. It is recommended that this treatment not be used more frequently than every 4 days.

Alprostadil is effective in up to 80% of the cases and is associated with a return to spontaneous erections in 35%. It is safe and effective in diabetic patients who are used to self-injection of insulin. Although its efficacy rates are impressive, the discontinuation rate for alprostadil is high, with local pain and loss of spontaneity being the most commonly cited reasons.

Transurethral therapy

Intraurethral therapy of alprostadil presents an alternative to injections [67]. Medicated urethral system for erection (MUSE) is a single-use transurethral system that involves the insertion of a 1.4mm pellet into the urethra using a hand-held applicator just after micturition and about 15min prior to sexual activity. As with injection therapy, the patient must be taught the correct technique of insertion. Patients should receive an initial dose of 250mcg with dosage titration between 125–1000g under medical supervision until the patient achieves a satisfactory response. These numbers are much higher than with injection therapy due to drug loss in the general circulation. A maximum of two doses are allowed per 24-hour period. Once the correct dose has been identified, success rates of up to 60% have been recorded, although in a comparative study with injections this fell to 43% (injections 70%).

Non-drug therapy

Psychosexual therapy

If psychogenic ED is present, appropriate counselling should be arranged. Even organic cases of ED may have a psychological component secondary to the dysfunction itself. Cooperative teamwork between the physician and the therapist is valuable when the organic and psychological causes of ED overlap.

Vacuum constriction devices

The vacuum constriction device is a long-established means of treating ED [68]. It is a non-invasive method that produces an erection by creating a pressure vacuum of up to 250mmHg, causing blood flow into the penis. The erection is then maintained with the placement of a rubber constriction ring at the base of the penis. The constriction ring must not be left in place longer than 30min, since ischaemic damage could occur.

It should be recognized that a significant haematoma (minor in 10% of cases) may occur in men on anticoagulants; so, this is a relative contraindication. Specific training and advice before commencing the use of a vacuum device are needed. Vacuum devices are also not recommended for men with penile curvature.

Surgical treatment

When all else fails or when there is a history of trauma, penile surgery offers another therapeutic route. Cardiac patients should not be denied this option. Clearly, specialist referral and advice is needed and referral to the urologist is advised, with the cardiologist outlining the risk from a cardiac perspective.

Testosterone

In men there is increasing evidence that a low testosterone is associated with all-cause death and especially cardiovascular death [69]. This begs the question as to whether replacement may be beneficial which in an ageing population could be particularly important considering the age-related decline in androgens that frequently occurs.

A low testosterone is associated with several cardiovascular risk factors including visceral fat accumulation [70, 71]. As testosterone replacement in hypogonadal men decreases adiposity, and obesity is an independent risk factor for cardiovascular disease, the concept of replacement therapy reducing cardiac risk is of considerable interest [72]. In addition, low testosterone levels are associated with glucose intolerance and type II diabetes (independent of adiposity) and the metabolic syndrome [46]. This has raised the possibility that replacement of testosterone in men with low levels could help prevent the development of type II diabetes, and progression of the metabolic syndrome to type II diabetes and the cardiovascular risk associated with both clinical entities [73].

With regard to coagulation, there is some evidence that testosterone replacement decreases fibrinogen levels and augments the fibrinolytic system as well as decreasing platelet aggregation [70]. A low testosterone is associated with increased inflammatory markers (interleukin 6 and C-reactive protein) which are established cardiovascular risk factors. The data with hyperlipidaemia is conflicting with replacement resulting in a 10% fall in the LDL cholesterol (beneficial) being offset by a 10% fall in the HDL cholesterol (adverse potential) [74].

Vascular effects of testosterone are also potentially beneficial with a direct action on smooth muscle via an action on calcium or potassium channels [75]. Experimental studies have demonstrated coronary artery dilatation after acute administration of testosterone [76]. In men with stable angina, 3 months of transdermal testosterone improved exercise-induced ischaemia and the angina threshold [77].

Recently, the European Prospective Investigation into Cancer in Norfolk (EPIC-Norfolk) Study has been published [78]. This 6–10-year nested case–control study looked at testosterone levels and all-cause, cancer, and cardiovascular deaths. Endogenous testosterone levels at baseline were found to be inversely related to all-cause mortality, cardiac and cancer deaths. Whilst the authors concluded that a low testosterone may be a marker for those at high risk of cardiovascular events, they emphasized the need for randomized placebo controlled trials. The Rancho-Bernardo study reported similar findings over a 20-year follow up period with men in the lowest testosterone quartile having a 40% greater chance of dying mainly from cardiac and respiratory disease. Interestingly this excess was independent of age, lifestyle, hyperlipidaemia, and obesity [79].

Whilst at present we have no definitive evidence that testosterone replacement will reduce cardiovascular risk, there is clearly a need to formally evaluate its role in a large placebo controlled trial. Reassuringly, replacement is not associated with increased cardiac risk and can be safely initiated for those who are hypogonadal and symptomatic.

Quick guide to specific cardiac conditions and sex

Hypertension

- This is not a contraindication to sex when controlled.
- Controlled patient: antihypertensives (single or multiple) are not a contraindication, but use caution with doxazosin (and other nonselective α-blockers) and PDE-5 inhibitors.
- All ED therapies can be utilized.
- Antihypertensives least likely to cause ED are the angiotensin II receptor antagonists and doxazosin.

Angina

- For stable patients, there is minimal risk for sex or ED therapy.
- Nitrates and nicorandil are contraindications to the PDE-5 inhibitors. On most occasions these can safely be discontinued.
- Heart rate-slowing drugs are the most effective antianginal agents: β-blockers, verapamil, diltiazem.
- Use an exercise ECG to stratify risk if unsure.

Post-myocardial infarction

- Use pre- or post-discharge exercise ECG to guide advice; no need to delay sex resumption if satisfactory.
- Advise gentle return to allow for loss of confidence by both patient and partner.
- Rehabilitation programmes are a positive advantage.
- Avoid sex in the first 2 weeks (period of maximum risk).

Post surgery or percutaneous intervention

- If successful, risk is low
- Sternal scar may be painful; advise side-to-side position or patient on top position. Use a soft cushion over the sternal scar.
- Use exercise ECG if unsure of ability.

Cardiac failure

- The risk is low if ability is good.
- If symptomatic, adjust medication accordingly; patient may need to be the more passive partner.
- If severely symptomatic, sex many not be possible owing to physical limitation and can occasionally trigger decompensation.
- An exercise programme can facilitate the return to sex; physically fit equals sexually fit.

Valve disease

- For mild cases, there is no increased risk.
- Significant aortic stenosis may lead to sudden death and can be worsened by the vasodilatory effects of PDE-5 inhibitors.

Arrhythmias

- Controlled atrial fibrillation is not an increased risk depending on cause and exercise ability.
- Warfarin does not contraindicate the vacuum device but care is needed and caution is required with injections.
- Complex arrhythmias: arrange for 24–48-hour ambulatory ECG monitoring and exercise testing. Treat and retest.
- Pacemakers are not a contraindication.
- With implanted defibrillators, use exercise test for safety before advising. This is usually not a problem.

Other conditions

- For pericarditis, await full recovery; there is no specific increased risk thereafter.
- With peripheral vascular disease, stroke, or TIAs there is increased risk of myocardial infarction, therefore screen.
- With hypertrophic obstructive cardiomyopathy, there is increased risk of syncope and sudden death on exercise. Exercise ECG is advised. PDE-5 inhibitors and alprostadil may increase the degree of obstruction owing to vasodilatory effects. Test dose under hospital supervision is recommended.

Conclusion

Cardiac patients may have anxieties about sexual activity because of their false belief of substantially increased risk. ED is common in cardiac patients because of the shared risk factors that adversely impact endothelial function. Signs of ED often present before overt cardiac symptoms develop; therefore a cardiac workup may be warranted for these patients, even without relevant cardiovascular histories. There is now increasing awareness of therapy for ED, but many patients remain reluctant to come forward for advice. The question of sexual activity and ED therapy should be raised by healthcare professionals as a routine part of the management of cardiac patients. Treatment is available. With reassurance, support, and careful explanation, sexual relationships can be enjoyed by cardiac patients who receive appropriate advice.

Personal perspective

With the recognition that ED is an early warning sign for silent coronary and vascular disease, screening for men presenting with ED and no cardiac symptoms is widely advocated. According to the second Princeton Consensus Guidelines, all men with ED and no cardiac symptoms should be considered as cardiac (or vascular) patients until proven otherwise. Such patients should undergo a full medical assessment with stratification of cardiovascular risk as high, medium, or low. Those patients at low risk should receive lifestyle advice regarding physical activity and weight control and undergo regular monitoring by their general practitioner. Patients at increased risk for cardiovascular events should ideally undergo stress testing and referral for risk reduction therapy.

Although an exercise ECG is advocated to identify patients at increased cardiovascular risk, this method will identify only those people with obstructive flow-limiting CAD. Wherever possible, intermediate and high-risk patients should be considered for elective computed tomography coronary angiography to identify the presence of non-flow limiting lipid plaques that are potentially vulnerable to rupture. By implementing these measures, it should be possible to initiate early aggressive cardiovascular risk reduction in 'at-risk' patients, thereby taking advantage of the 2–5-year window of opportunity between the development of symptomatic ED and CAD. However, for the full potential of this approach to be realised, comprehensive education programmes are required to encourage men with ED to present to their general practitioner as soon as possible. In addition, a multidisciplinary approach is required, involving teamwork between the family doctor, nurse, pharmacist, urologist, diabetologist, and cardiologist.

Further reading

Jackson G. *Sex, The Heart and Erectile Dysfunction*, 2004. London: Taylor and Francis.

Jackson G, Hutter A. Cardiovascular issues in male and female sexual dysfunction. In Porst H, Buvat J (eds.) *Standard Practice in Sexual Medicine*, 2006. Oxford: Blackwell Publishing, pp. 376–86.

Kloner RA (ed.). *Heart Disease and Erectile Dysfunction*, 2004. Totoma, NJ: Humane Press.

Lue TF, Basson R, Rosen R, *et al.* (eds.). *Sexual Medicine, Sexual Dysfunction in Men and Women*, 21st edn., 2004. Paris: Health Publications.

➲ **For full references and multimedia materials please visit the online version of the book (http://esctextbook.oxfordonline.com).**

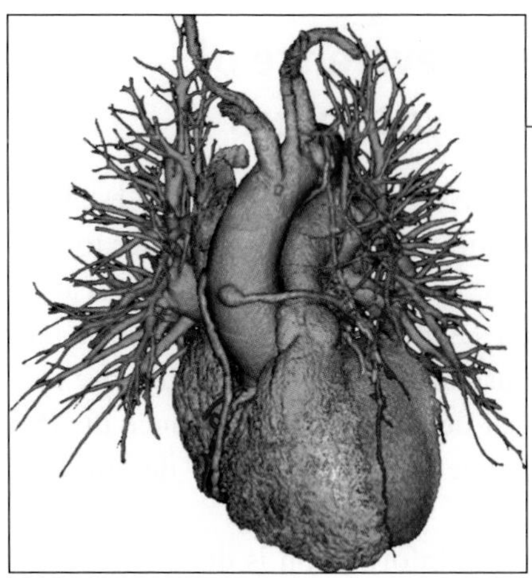

CHAPTER 16

Acute Coronary Syndromes

Christian W. Hamm, Helge Möllmann, Jean-Pierre Bassand, and Frans Van de Werf

Contents

Summary

Acute coronary syndrome (ACS) is the clinical manifestation of the critical phase of coronary artery disease (CAD). Based on electrocardiogram (ECG) and biochemical markers it is distinguished from ST-elevation myocardial infarction (STEMI), non-ST-elevation myocardial infarction (NSTEMI), and unstable angina. The common underlying pathophysiology is related to plaque rupture or erosion with subsequent thrombus formation. Despite the decreasing age-adjusted mortality for myocardial infarction, the disease prevalence for non-fatal components of ACS remains high and the economic costs are immense. Treatment of patients presenting with an ACS aims at immediate relief of ischaemia and the prevention of serious adverse events, including death, myocardial (re)infarction, and life-threatening arrhythmias. The general management is predominately guided by the ECG and biomarkers. All patients should be admitted to an inpatient unit with careful observation for recurrent ischaemia, ECG monitoring, and frequent assessment of vital signs. The implementation of chest pain units and treatment networks with standardized care improve delivery of best management. In general, treatment options include antiplatelet therapy, antithrombins, fibrinolytics, percutaneous coronary interventions (PCI), and cardiac surgery. In patients with persistent ST-segment elevation rapid (within 6 hours after onset of pain) and sustained reperfusion of the infarct related artery by primary PCI or fibrinolysis improves early and long-term outcome. In patients presenting without ST-segment elevation (NSTE-ACS) the further management is guided by risk stratification (troponin, ECG, risk scores etc.). High-risk patients benefit from an early (<72 hours) invasive strategy. It is well established that adherence to guidelines recommended therapy reduces mortality and morbidity in this high risk population.

Introduction

As early as 2600 BC, Egyptian papyrus scrolls recorded that patients with acute chest pain were at high risk of death. Today, the term acute coronary syndrome (ACS) is used to denote the acute phases of ischaemic coronary artery disease with or without myocardial cell necrosis. This term is preferred to earlier symptom-related terminology because it encompasses the common underlying pathophysiology.

ACS describes the spectrum of clinical manifestations which follow disruption of a coronary arterial plaque, complicated by thrombosis, embolization, and varying degrees of obstruction to myocardial perfusion. The clinical features depend upon extent and severity of myocardial ischaemia. Complete coronary occlusion in the absence of collateral perfusion results in STEMI or NSTEMI. Transient or partial coronary occlusion may also result in myocyte necrosis as a result of embolization of thrombus and plaque fragments into the distal coronary circulation and changes in vascular tone. The release of sensitive markers of myocardial necrosis (troponins) is regarded as indicative of myocardial cell necrosis and fulfils the definition of myocardial infarction [1]. If no rise in markers is detected, the term unstable angina is used and non-cardiac differential diagnoses must be considered [2].

In the clinical setting the term 'acute coronary syndrome' is used as an initial working diagnosis which initiates a diagnostic cascade (➲Fig 16.1). According to the ECG and biomarker results the diagnosis is later refined. The first therapeutic steps are based on the ST-segment in the initial ECG.

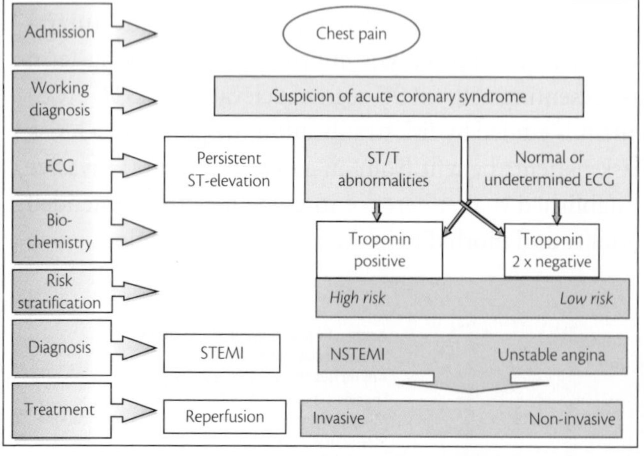

Figure 16.1 The spectrum of acute coronary syndromes.

Incidence and prevalence of acute coronary syndromes

The diagnosis of NSTE-ACS is more difficult to establish than STEMI and therefore its prevalence is harder to estimate. In addition, in recent years, a new definition of acute myocardial infarction (AMI) has been introduced taking into account the use of more sensitive and more specific biomarkers of cell death [3]. The incidence of AMI increased by approximately 10%, if the new definition is applied [4].

Internationally, robust information is documented for coronary heart disease deaths and for AMI with specific ECG and enzyme/marker characteristics. The American Heart Association estimates that 1.1 million myocardial infarctions occur in the USA alone and that 40% of these patients will die. Approximately half of the deaths occur prior to the patient receiving medical attention [5]. Taken together with corresponding figures for myocardial infarction in the UK [6], these data suggest that the incidence of AMI is in the range of 1 per 250 to 1 per 500 of the population per year. To date, there are no reliable estimates for Europe as a whole, because of the absence of a common centre for centralised health statistics.

The prevalence of NSTE-ACS, relative to STEMI, has been determined from multiple surveys and registries [7–16]. Overall, data suggest that the annual incidence of NSTE-ACS is higher than that of STEMI. Based on registry data, the incidence for all ACS is approximately threefold the incidence of STEMI [9]. Thus, the annual incidence of ACS in Europe is estimated at between 1 per 80 to 1 per 170 of the population per year. The incidence of chest pain leading to hospital assessment for suspected ACS may, however, be substantially higher and varies regionally, depending on the threshold for referral or presentation to an emergency department.

The ratio between NSTE-ACS and STEMI has changed over time, as the rate of NSTE-ACS increased relative to STEMI, without any clear explanation for the reasons behind this evolution [17]. This change in the pattern of NSTE-ACS could actually be linked to changes in the management of disease, and greater efforts in prevention of CAD over the last 20 years [18–21].

An apparent paradox exists with respect to the prevalence of ACS. Although age-adjusted death rates from CAD are falling in many economically developed communities, the prevalence appears to be rising. This apparent contradiction is explained by increased awareness in both the public and primary care physicians of ACS, especially suspected myocardial infarction, together with lowered thresholds for presentation and evaluation of suspected ACS. This now includes patients of advanced age and those with significant comorbidity. Previously, many of these patients may not have presented for evaluation of suspected ACS. Thus, although the true incidence of ACS may follow the declining trends for myocardial infarction, the higher prevalence is accounted for by more patients being evaluated for the condition.

Time trends

Analysis of data from the MONICA centres over a 10-year trend indicates an average 4% annual reduction in CAD mortality for men and women. However, this varies from a 7–8% annual reduction in some countries, for example Australia, Finland, and Sweden, to annual increases in some geographic regions [22]. The decline in death rates from coronary heart disease amongst developed economies in Europe, North America, Australia, and New Zealand (between 39 and 52% fall in age-adjusted death rates in men and women from 1989–1999) is contrasted with an increase in mortality in several countries of Eastern and Central Europe, most notably countries of the former USSR. For example, in Ukraine between 1989–1999 age-adjusted death rates rose by 60% in both men and women.

In the UK a 36% fall in age-adjusted death rates has occurred over the past decade; for men aged 35–74 years the death rate from coronary heart disease per 100,000 of the population fell from 364 to 199 [6]. The most rapid fall in death rates has occurred amongst men aged 55–64 years and women aged 55–64 years with lesser falls demonstrated in older and younger age groups. Recent large-scale multinational surveys and registries have used predefined case definitions and methods to minimize the influence of bias on patient inclusion and have provided robust information for the full spectrum of ACS [9, 11].

Longitudinal studies within specific regions can provide important insights into changes over the course of time. In south-western France, for example, the 28-day case fatality rate has fallen between 1985–1993 by about 3% a year for first myocardial infarction [23]. It was concluded that this mainly reflects improvements in acute management rather than in prevention. Similarly, longitudinal studies in Sweden between 1984–1991 demonstrated that 2-year mortality after AMI fell from 36% to 25%. Most of the reduction in mortality occurred during the in-hospital phase [24]. In considering the decline in coronary heart disease mortality in Scotland, it was estimated that 40% of the decline was attributed to improved therapeutic treatments and 51%

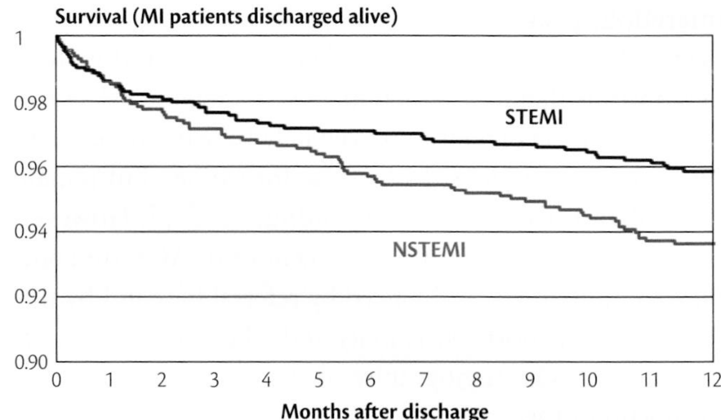

Figure 16.2 Longterm survival of patients discharged alive after ST elevation myocardial infarction or non-ST elevation myocardial infarction according to EuroHeart Survey.

to measurable risk factor reductions [25]. Whereas the in-hospital mortality is significantly higher in STEMI-patients, the long-term mortality is higher in NSTEMI-patients (➲Fig. 16.2).

Health economic implications

Despite the falling age-adjusted mortality for myocardial infarction, the disease prevalence for non-fatal components of ACS remains high and the economic costs are immense. The annual cost of coronary heart disease ranks highest of all diseases for which comparable analyses have been performed [26].

The economic cost of coronary heart disease relates not only to the direct cost to the healthcare system but also to loss of productivity and to the provision of formal and informal care of patients. For example, in the UK, the economic burden of coronary heart disease has been estimated at €2.6 billion for direct healthcare costs in 1999 and a further €3.6 billion for the provision of care for CAD subjects, and €4.4 billion for loss of productivity.

General risk factors for acute coronary syndromes

A series of modifiable risk factors (e.g. hyperlipidaemia, hypertension, diabetes, and metabolic syndrome) and non-modifiable risk factors (e.g. gender and age) relate to the development of atherosclerosis and the risk of presenting with ACS. Also see ➲Chapter 17.

Age and gender

The most powerful independent predictor for the development of ACS, including presentation with myocardial infarction, is age. Among men, risk increases with each decile of age and comparisons between men and women demonstrate that for premenopausal women the risk corresponds with that of men approximately 10 years younger [6]. Post menopause, the risks increase for women but remain lower than for men of corresponding age [27]. However, interpretations of the impact of gender in ACS are complex and potentially influenced by referral bias and by differences in diagnostic sensitivity of the ECG and stress tests with gender. On angiography of suspected ACS a higher proportion of women do not have significant obstructive coronary heart disease. For example, in the RITA 3 study, 37% of women who fulfilled symptomatic and ECG criteria for NSTE-ACS did not have a stenosis >50%, whereas the corresponding figure for men was 12%. Similarly, 26% of men, but only 16% of women had significant disease in three or more vessels [28]. Adjusted for age, women have higher rates of diabetes and hypertension but are less frequently smokers [29].

Family history

Having accounted for all known risk factors, family history remains a significant independent risk factor for the development of coronary heart disease. In addition, genetic traits contribute to the specific risk phenotypes, including those related to hyperlipidaemia. Twin studies reveal higher concordance among identical than non-identical twins.

Metabolic syndrome

The term metabolic syndrome describes the combination of several factors often clustering together, which increase the risk of diabetes mellitus and cardiovascular disease (➲ Table 16.1).

The dramatic increase in the prevalence of obesity among children and adolescents has been demonstrated across many economically developed and developing communities. In the year 2000, >20% of the US adult population from 22 states had a body mass index >30kg/m^2. In contrast, none of the states had >20% of the population with this level of obesity in 1990 [30]. This rise has serious implications for future coronary events, including ACS. Among obese children and adolescents, the prevalence of metabolic syndrome approaches 50% (38.7% in moderately obese subjects and 49.7% in severely obese subjects) [31]. C-reactive protein (CRP) and interleukin-6 are markers of inflammation and their levels can be used as predictors for future cardiovascular events; the concentrations of these markers rise with the extent of obesity. In addition, adiponectin, a biomarker of insulin sensitivity which also has a role in preventing atherosclerosis development, is decreased in obesity [31]. The findings provide a link between obesity, metabolic syndrome and future risk of acute coronary events.

In the Third National Health Nutrition Examination Survey (TNHNES) of more than 10,000 subjects, the presence of the metabolic syndrome independently increased the risk of myocardial infarction twofold [odds ratio (OR) 2.01] [32]. Other independent predictors of cardiac events were low levels of high-density lipoprotein (HDL)-cholesterol (OR 1.35), hypertension (OR 1.44) and hypertriglyceridaemia (OR 1.66).

The strongest influence on all components of the metabolic syndrome can be accounted to lifestyle and, therefore, the main emphasis in the management of these patients should be in professionally supervised lifestyle changes with particular efforts to reduce body weight and increase physical activity. Both interventions have been shown to radically reduce the risk of developing diabetes and to beneficially influence other risk factors like hypertension and hyperlipidaemia [33].

Table 16.1 Original NCEP-ATP III definitions of the metabolic syndrome

At least three of the following five components:
Central obesity: waist circumference >102cm in men, >88cm in women
Elevated triglycerides: >1.7mmol/L (>150mg/dL)
Low HDL cholesterol: <1.03mmol/L (<40mg/dL) in men, <1.29mmol/L (<50mg/dL) in women
Raised blood pressure (BP): systolic BP>130mmHg and/or diastolic BP>85mmHg, or treatment of previously diagnosed hypertension
Impaired fasting glycaemia: fasting plasma glucose >6.1mmol/L (>110mg/dL) or previously diagnosed type 2 diabetes
The revised version uses lower cut-off values for impaired fasting glycaemia (>5.6mmol/L (>100mg/dL)).

Diabetes mellitus (➲ Chapter 14)

Clinical and animal studies demonstrate the importance of diabetes as a risk factor for the development of atherosclerosis as well as for ACS, and the increasing prevalence of obesity in specific populations is implicated in the increased frequency of metabolic syndrome and type 2 diabetes. Patients with type 2 diabetes mellitus have a risk of death from cardiovascular causes that is two- to sixfold elevated compared to those without diabetes. ACSs and cardiovascular deaths account for more than one-quarter of all new cardiovascular events among diabetic patients. Intensive intervention involving multiple risk factor reduction among patients with type 2 diabetes and microalbuminuria demonstrates that five patients need to be treated to prevent one cardiovascular event over the course of 8 years [34].

A target-driven long-term intensified intervention aimed at modifying several risk factors in patients with type 2 diabetes and microalbuminuria reduces the risk of cardiovascular and microvascular events by approximately 50% [34].

The treatment regimen of diabetic patients should not only concentrate on dietary advice and adequate glucose control. In these patients it is of paramount importance to orchestrate therapeutical interventions for all risk factors including stringent antihypertensive and lipid-lowering treatment. Treatment targets for patients with type 2 diabetes are given in ➲Table 16.2 [33].

Hypertension (➲Chapter 13)

Elevated blood pressure is not only a risk factor for CAD [35], but also heart failure, peripheral vascular disease, and renal failure in both men and women [36]. Furthermore, there is a particularly strong influence of elevated blood pressure on stroke. Approximately two-thirds of cerebrovascular disease burden and half of ischaemic heart disease burden are attributable, at least in part, to elevated blood pressure [27]. The stroke and CAD-related mortality increase progressively and linearly from blood pressure levels as low as 115mmHg systolic and 75mmHg diastolic upward [37]. The Blood Pressure Lowering Treatment Trialists' Collaboration has examined the influence of blood pressure lowering on mortality and the development of major cardiovascular events [38]. The overview examined data from 29 randomized trials (n = 162 341 patients) revealing that the reduction in blood pressure (irrespective of the regimen used) is directly related to the reduction in risk of cardiovascular events. Thus, blood pressure lowering is critically important not only in secondary prevention but in the primary prevention of major cardiovascular events including the development of ACS. The goal of blood pressure lowering should be values lower 140/90mmHg in all hypertensive patients qualifying for drug treatment and even lower if lack of side effects permits. Patients with established cardiovascular disease and diabetic patients are at especially high risk. Therefore, antihypertensive treatment should be more intense with a goal lower than 130/80mmHg [33].

Table 16.2 Treatment targets in patients with type 2 diabetes mellitus

HbA_{1c}	<6.5% if feasible
Fasting plasma glucose	<6.0mmol/L (<110mg/dL)
Blood pressure	<130/80mmHg
Total cholesterol	<4.5mmol/L (<175mg/dL)
	<4.0mmol/L (<155mg/dL) if feasible
Low-density lipoprotein-cholesterol	<2.5mmol/L (<100mg/dL)
	<2.0mmol/ L (>80mmg/dL) if feasible

Lipid abnormalities (➲Chapters 9 and 17)

Extensive studies have demonstrated that elevated plasma total cholesterol, low-density lipoprotein (LDL) cholesterol and very-low-density lipoprotein (VLDL) cholesterol are associated with atherogenesis and that lowering total cholesterol and LDL cholesterol is associated with reduced atherogenesis. A 10% reduction of plasma total cholesterol is associated with a 25% reduction in the incidence of CAD after 5 years. Likewise, a reduction of LDL cholesterol of 1mmol/L (~40mg/dL) is followed by a 20% reduction in cardiovascular events [39]. Elevated levels of HDL-cholesterol are protective whereas reduced levels of HDL confer increased risk.

Multiple large-scale cholesterol-lowering trials have demonstrated a reduced number of cardiovascular events among treated individuals without manifest CAD at the time of inclusion (West of Scotland Coronary Prevention Study, WOSCOPS; The Air Force/Texas Coronary Atherosclerosis Prevention Study AFCAPS/TexCAPS). Among those patients with hypertension at baseline, a 3-year treatment with a statin (atorvastatin) reduced the risk of major cardiovascular events by approximately one-third (hazard ratios for myocardial infarction or fatal coronary heart disease 0.64, $p < 0.01$) [40].

The first therapeutic principle should be to assess the individual cardiovascular risk and to advise patients with regard to smoking, exercise, nutrition, and blood pressure control. In general, total plasma cholesterol should be below 5mmol/L (190mg/L), and the LDL-fraction below 3mmol/L (115mg/dL). Similar to the treatment of hypertension, high-risk-patients with established cardiovascular disease or diabetes should be treated more aggressive with a total plasma cholesterol lower than 4.5mmol/L (<175mg/dL) or—if feasible—<4mmol/L (<155mg/dL) and a LDL-fraction <2.5mmol/L (<100mg/dL) with an option of <2mmol/L (<80mg/dL) [33].

Other modifiable and potentially modifiable risk factors

Up-regulation of systemic inflammation provides a plausible mechanism for accelerating atherogenesis and its acute complications. A series of risk factors may be directly or indirectly related to increased coronary and vascular risk (for example, elevated homocysteine, CRP, fibrinogen, plasminogen activator inhibitor type 1, and altered platelet reactivity).

A series of additional 'environmental factors' are influenced by lifestyle but may also interact with the genetically influenced factors listed earlier. These include high-fat, low-antioxidant diets (experimentally and clinically), smoking, a lack of exercise, and obesity. Infectious agents may also contribute to the up-regulation of the inflammatory response and acceleration of atherogenesis.

Individuals born with low birth weight exhibit a two- to threefold increased risk in later life of non-fatal coronary heart disease compared with normal birth weight infants [41]. Low birth weight is also associated with several coronary risk factors including the subsequent development of hypertension, type 2 diabetes, and elevated cholesterol and fibrinogen concentrations. The risk factors are related not only to birth weight but to other indicators of restriction of fetal growth including small head circumference and altered placental development. The associations between size at birth and coronary heart disease are not explained by premature birth. They are also independent of the risks of subsequent obesity, smoking, and socioeconomic classification. The findings have led to the hypothesis that coronary heart disease is programmed in fetal life ('the Barker hypothesis') [42]. *In utero* programming of steroid metabolism may explain, at least in part, the re-setting of vascular tone in the arterial system and insulin sensitivity [43, 44].

Based upon the INTERHEART case–control study in 52 countries, nine potentially modifiable risk factors account for >90% of the risk of AMI, consistently across geographic regions and ethnic groups [45] (➲Chapter 12). Identified risk factors include abnormal lipids reflected by the apolipoprotein B:apolipoprotein A1 ratio, smoking, hypertension, diabetes, abdominal obesity, psychosocial factors, consumption of fruits and vegetables, alcohol, and regular physical activity. The findings suggest that these phenotypes are potentially amenable to modification across countries and diverse ethnic populations. This has major implications for primary and secondary prevention strategies.

Genetic influences in atherothrombosis and the initiation of acute coronary syndromes

Common forms of atherosclerosis are multifactorial and relate principally to polygenic disorders rather than to single gene defects. Nevertheless, rare Mendelian disorders have provided insights into disease mechanisms. These include familial hypercholesterolaemia with abnormalities of the LDL receptor and familial disorders of apolipoprotein B-100. Similarly, there are single gene defects associated with low HDL, including apolipoprotein A-1 deficiency and ABC transporter defects (Tangier disease). Specific genetic traits relate to disorders of haemostasis and elevated homocysteine is linked to a defect of cystathionine β-synthase (a regressive metabolic disorder with severe occlusive vascular disease). Type 2 diabetes is associated with altered expression of hepatocyte nuclear factor 4α, hepatocyte nuclear factor 1α, and glucokinase. Hypertension is linked with 11β-hydroxylase abnormalities and mineralocorticoid receptor defects (see ➲Chapter 9).

In contrast, a series of relatively common genetic variations contribute to coronary heart disease and to coronary heart disease risk factors. These include the apolipoprotein E defects which explain about 5% of the variance in cholesterol levels (LDL and VLDL). Various polymorphisms influence HDL through hepatic lipase, lipoprotein lipase, and defects in transfer proteins. A series of alleles explain >90% of the variance in lipoprotein (a). Polymorphisms influence tetrahydrofolate reductase and hence homocysteine levels. Specific polymorphisms influence fibrinogen, plasminogen activator inhibitor type 1, and coagulation factor VIII and hence defects in coagulation and endogenous fibrinolysis. Similarly, polymorphisms of angiotensinogen, the beta-2 receptor, and α-adducin affect blood pressure. Specific defects influence angiotensin-converting enzyme and endothelial nitric oxide synthase, contributing to vascular tone [46]. A series of polymorphisms influence the risk of plaque rupture, including those regulating matrix metalloproteinases. As further data emerge, unravelling the contribution of groups of polymorphisms may allow a more accurate genetic basis of risk for atherogenesis and its acute complications to be established. Genetic and environmental factors interact to produce specific clinical phenotypes where underlying genetic risk is amplified or modified by environmental and therapeutic interventions.

A new approach addressing the complex interplay between environmental and genetic factors in cardiovascular disease are genome-wide association studies. These studies using chip-based genotyping technologies are capable to identify hundreds of thousands of single nucleotide polymorphisms within a short time frame thereby facilitating genetic studies in large cohorts. Particular interest gained the publication of the Wellcome Trust Case Control Consortium (WTCCC) that analyzed data from approximately 2000 people and a shared set of 3000 controls for each of seven complex diseases including CAD. Whereas no candidate genes for essential hypertension could be discovered, several genetic loci were identified, which substantially affect the risk of development of CAD [47, 48].

Pathophysiology of acute coronary syndromes

Atherosclerosis

Atherosclerosis is by far the most frequent cause of CAD, carotid artery disease, and peripheral artery disease, but atherosclerosis alone is rarely fatal [49]. ACSs as a life-threatening manifestation of atherosclerosis are usually induced by acute thrombosis. These thromboses occur on a ruptured or eroded atherosclerotic plaque, with or without concomitant vasoconstriction, and cause a sudden and critical reduction in blood flow [49–51]. In rare cases, ACS may have a non-atherosclerotic aetiology such as arteritis, trauma, spontaneous dissection, thromboembolism, congenital anomaly, cocaine abuse, or complications of cardiac catheterization.

Atherosclerosis is a chronic and multifocal immunoinflammatory, fibroproliferative disease of medium-sized and large arteries mainly driven by lipid accumulation [51]. Atherosclerosis begins to develop naturally early in life and progresses with time. The speed of progression is unpredictable and differs markedly among different subjects. Likewise, there is substantial variation in the amount of evolved atherosclerosis as a response to risk factor exposure, probably because the individual vulnerability to atherosclerosis and its risk factors varies greatly. However, even in vulnerable individuals, it usually takes several decades to develop obstructive or thrombosis-prone plaques, so in principle there should be ample time to inhibit, or at least delay plaque development and its complications by timely screening and, where necessary, risk-reducing interventions (➲Figs. 16.3 and 16.4) [52, 53].

Serial angiographic and pathoanatomical observations indicate that the natural progression of CAD involves two distinct processes: a fixed and generally reversible process causing gradual luminal narrowing slowly over years or decades caused mainly by atherosclerosis, and a dynamic and potentially reversible process that punctuates the slow progression in a sudden and unpredictable way leading to rapid coronary occlusion caused by thrombosis or vasospasm, or both. Thus, symptomatic coronary lesions contain a variable mix of chronic atherosclerosis and acute thrombosis but, because the exact nature of the mix is unknown in the individual patient, the term atherothrombosis is frequently used. Generally, atherosclerosis predominates

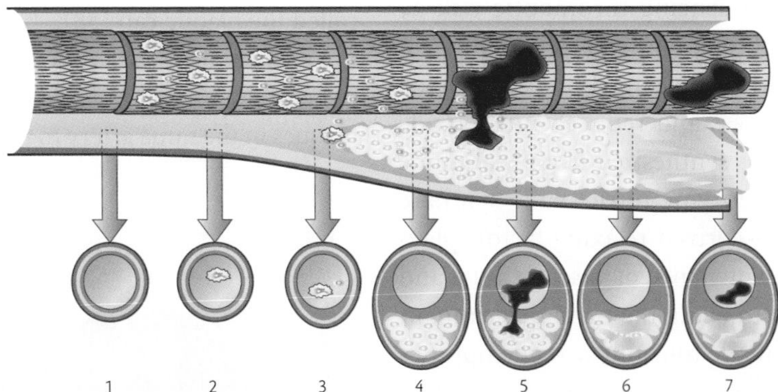

Figure 16.3 Development of the vulnerable plaque. Top, Longitudinal section of artery depicting 'timeline' of human atherogenesis from normal artery (1) to atheroma that causes clinical manifestations by thrombosis or stenosis (5, 6, 7). Bottom, Cross-sections of artery during various stages of atheroma evolution. 1, Normal artery. 2, Lesion initiation occurs when endothelial cells, activated by risk factors such as hyperlipoproteinaemia, express adhesion and chemoattractant molecules that recruit inflammatory leucocytes such as monocytes and T lymphocytes. Extracellular lipid begins to accumulate in intima at this stage. 3, Evolution to fibrofatty stage. Monocytes recruited to artery wall become macrophages and express scavenger receptors that bind modified lipoproteins. Macrophages become lipid-laden foam cells by engulfing modified lipoproteins. Leucocytes and resident vascular wall cells can secrete inflammatory cytokines and growth factors that amplify leucocyte recruitment and cause smooth muscle cell migration and proliferation. 4, As lesion progresses, inflammatory mediators cause expression of tissue factor, a potent pro-coagulant, and of matrix-degrading proteinases that weaken fibrous cap of plaque. 5, If fibrous cap ruptures at point of weakening, coagulation factors in blood can gain access to thrombogenic, tissue factor-containing lipid core, causing thrombosis on non-occlusive atherosclerotic plaque. If balance between prothrombotic and fibrinolytic mechanisms prevailing at that particular region and at that particular time is unfavourable, occlusive thrombus causing ACS may result. 6, When thrombus resorbs, products associated with thrombosis such as thrombin and mediators released from degranulating platelets, can cause healing response, leading to increased collagen accumulation and smooth muscle cell growth. In this manner, the fibrofatty lesion can evolve into an advanced fibrous and often calcified plaque, one that may cause significant stenosis, and produce symptoms of stable angina pectoris. 7, In some cases, occlusive thrombi arise not from fracture of fibrous cap but from superficial erosion of endothelial layer. Resulting mural thrombus, again dependent on local prothrombotic and fibrinolytic balance, can cause acute myocardial infarction. Superficial erosions often complicate advanced and stenotic lesions, as shown here. Superficial erosions do not necessarily occur after fibrous cap rupture. Adapted from Libby P. Current concepts in of the pathogenesis of the acute coronary syndromes. *Circulation* 2001; **104**: 365–72.

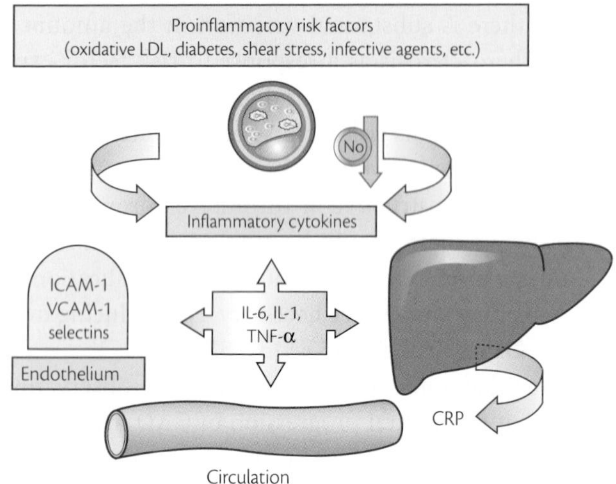

Figure 16.4 The pathophysiology of atherosclerosis with respect to lesion development, progression and destabilization. Biomarkers with distinct pathophysiological profile can be used to assess disease activity.

in lesions responsible for chronic stable angina, whereas thrombosis constitutes the critical component of culprit lesions responsible for the ACS [49, 51].

Endothelial dysfunction and pathological thrombogenicity

The endothelium plays a critical role in both regulating the vasomotor tone and influencing thrombotic risk by release of prostacyclin, endothelin-1, hyperpolarizing factor, and nitric oxide. Endothelial dysfunction is associated with enhanced oxidative stress and reduced nitric oxide bioavailability. Nitric oxide is synthesized from L-arginine under the influence of the enzyme nitric oxide synthase and is the key endothelium-derived relaxing factor, playing a pivotal role in the maintenance of vascular tone and reactivity [54]. In addition to being the main determinant of basal vascular smooth muscle tone, nitric oxide opposes the actions of potent endothelium-derived contracting factors such as angiotensin-II and endothelin-1. Furthermore, nitric oxide inhibits platelet and leucocyte activation and maintains the vascular smooth muscle in a non-proliferative state. This pivotal role of nitric oxide is reflected in diabetic patients, who are known to be at especially high risk for cardiovascular events. Endothelial dysfunction in patients with diabetes mellitus may additionally result from a decreased bioavailability of nitric oxide (secondary to insulin resistance) coupled with an exaggerated production of endothelin-1 (stimulated by hyperinsulinaemia or hyperglycaemia) [55].

Endothelial dysfunction has been implicated in the pathogenesis and clinical course of all known cardiovascular diseases and is associated with future risk of adverse cardiovascular events [56]. Systemic endothelial dysfunction is a major predictor of recurrence of instability in patients with ACSs [57].

The plaque

The typical fibrolipid plaque consists of a lipid core surrounded by a dense capsule of connective tissue. The core contains both, an acellular mass of lipid and numerous macrophages containing abundant intracytoplasmic droplets of cholesterol. Likewise, the extracellular lipids are mainly cholesterol or its esters, some of which in a crystalline form. The macrophages derive from moncytes having left the arterial lumen and invaded the plaque by crossing the endothelium. These macrophages are refered to as 'foam cells' given their intracellular lipid accumulation. They are highly activated and produce several procoagulant and inflammatory mediators, such as tissue factor, tumor necrosis factor α (TNFα), interleukins, and metalloproteinases. This lipid mass and the inflammatory cells are surrounded by a connective tissue capsule composed mainly from collagen synthesised from fibroblasts, myofibroblasts, and smooth muscle cells. The part of the fibrous capsule that is located between the arterial lumen and the plaque is called the plaque cap [58].

Coronary atherosclerotic plaques are very heterogeneous structurally as well as biologically, and even neighbouring plaques in the same artery may differ markedly (➲Fig. 16.5).

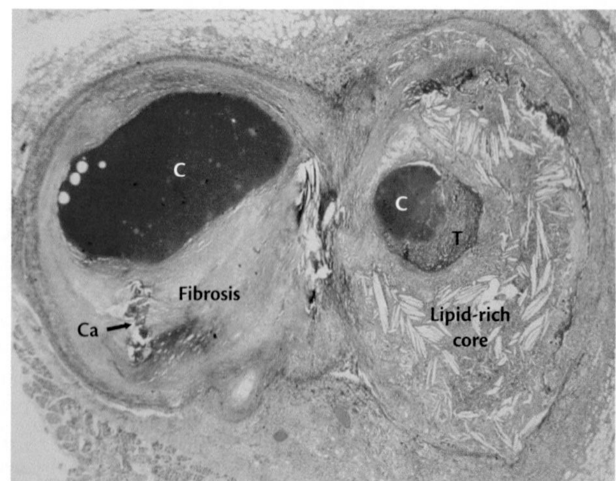

Figure 16.5 Atherothrombosis: a variable mix of chronic atherosclerosis and acute thrombosis. Cross-sectioned arterial bifurcation illustrating a collagen-rich (blue-stained) plaque in the circumflex branch (left), and a lipid-rich and ruptured plaque with a non-occlusive thrombus superimposed in the obtuse branch (right). Ca, calcification; T, thrombus; C, contrast in the lumen. (Courtesy of E. Falk.)

The great majority of coronary plaques are, and will remain, quiescent, at least from a clinical point of view. In fact, during a lifetime, none or only few coronary plaques become complicated by clinically significant thrombosis, and these rare but dangerous thrombosis-prone plaques are called vulnerable. Thus, a vulnerable plaque is a plaque assumed to be at high short-term risk of thrombosis, i.e. causing an ACS [59]. The challenge is to identify the presence of the thrombosis-prone plaques, treat them (or rather the patients harbouring them), and thus avoid ACS [60, 61].

Arterial remodelling is bidirectional. Plaques responsible for ACS are usually relatively large and associated with compensatory enlargement called positive or outward remodelling that tends to preserve a normal lumen despite the presence of significant, and potentially dangerous, vessel wall disease [62, 63]. Such lesions, hidden in the arterial wall, may not be seen by angiography. As many as three-quarters of all infarct-related thrombi appear to evolve over plaques causing only mild-to-moderate stenosis prior to infarction, partly because their propensity for outward remodelling, partly because of their much greater prevalence compared to stenotic plaques. Thus, the great majority of myocardial infarction originate from atherosclerotic lesions that, prior to the acute events, were haemodynamically insignificant and probably asymptomatic. In contrast, plaques responsible for stable angina are usually smaller but, nevertheless, may cause more severe luminal narrowing because of concomitant local shrinkage of the artery (negative or inward remodelling) [63].

The vulnerable plaque

Approximately 75% of all coronary thrombi responsible for ACS are precipitated by plaque rupture [49]. Plaque ruptures are caused by a structural defect (a gap) in the fibrous cap that normally separates the lipid-rich core of an inflamed plaque from the lumen of the artery (➲Fig. 16.6). Based on the morphological appearance of ruptured plaques, it is assumed that a rupture-prone plaque will possess the features illustrated in ➲Figs. 16.7 and 16.8. Lipid accumulation [64], thinning of the plaque's fibrous cap with local loss of smooth muscle cells [48], and inflammation with many activated macrophages and few mast cells and neutrophils [51, 65, 66], and intraplaque haemorrhage [67] destabilize plaques, making them vulnerable to rupture. In contrast, smooth muscle cell-mediated healing and repair processes stabilize plaques, protecting them against rupture [68]. Plaque size or stenosis severity reveals nothing, or only a little, about a plaque's vulnerability [62].

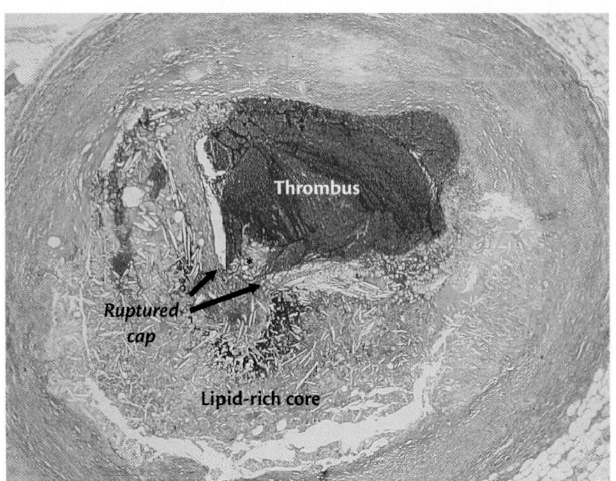

Figure 16.6 Plaque rupture. Cross-sectioned coronary artery containing a lipid-rich atherosclerotic plaque with occlusive thrombosis superimposed. The fibrous cap covering the lipid-rich core is ruptured (between arrows) exposing the thrombogenic core to the blood in the lumen. Atheromatous plaque content is displaced through the gap in the cap into the lumen (cholesterol crystals at asterisk), clearly indicating the sequence of events: plaque rupture preceded thrombus formation. Trichrome stain, rendering luminal thrombus and intraplaque haemorrhage red and collagen blue. (Courtesy of E. Falk.)

Clinical observations suggest that culprit lesions responsible for ACSs generally are less calcified than plaques responsible for stable angina, indicating that calcium confers stability to plaques rather than the opposite [69]. The total amount of calcification (the calcium score) is a marker of plaque burden (and thus a marker of cardiovascular risk) rather than a marker of risk conferred by the individual calcified plaque [70].

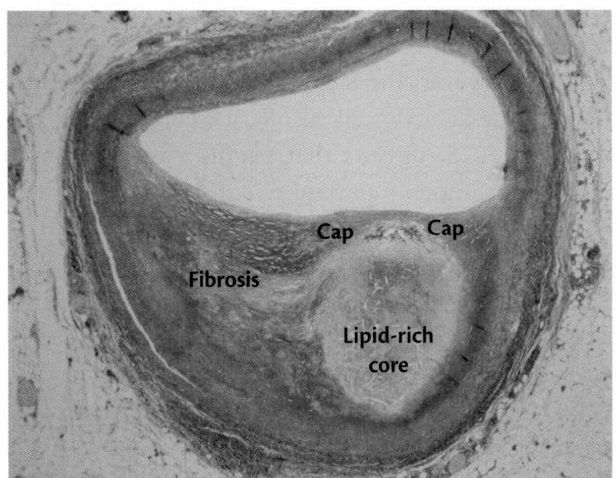

Figure 16.7 Vulnerable plaque. Cross-section of a coronary artery containing a plaque assumed to be rupture-prone, consisting of a relatively large lipid-rich core covered by a thin and fragile fibrous cap. Trichrome stain, rendering collagen blue and lipid colourless. (Courtesy of E. Falk.)

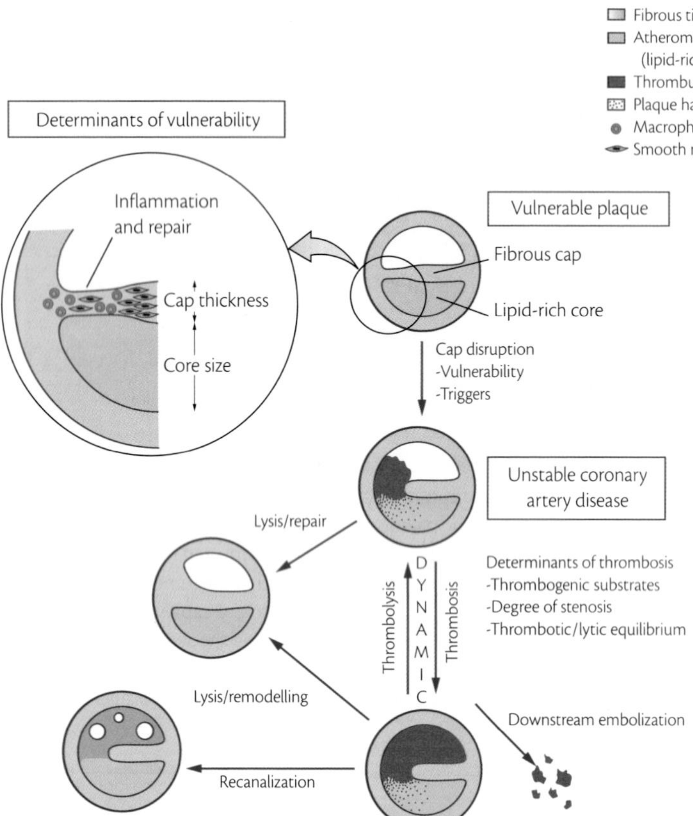

Figure 16.8 Plaque vulnerability, rupture and thrombosis. Lipid accumulation, cap thinning, macrophage infiltration, and local loss of smooth muscle cells destabilize plaques, making them vulnerable to rupture. It is unknown whether rupture of a vulnerable plaque is a random (spontaneous) or triggered event. The thrombotic response to plaque rupture is dynamic and depends on local (e.g. exposed substrate and shear forces) as well as systemic factors (e.g. platelets, coagulation and fibrinolysis).

Plaque rupture

Sudden rupture of a thin and inflamed fibrous cap may occur spontaneously but triggering could also play a role and thus help explain the non-random onset of ACS [71]. Potential triggers may include extreme physical activity, especially in someone unaccustomed to regular physical activity, severe emotional trauma, sexual activity, exposure to illicit drugs such as cocaine or amphetamines, cold exposure, and acute infections—or simply normal daily activities [71]. However, the fact that exercise stress testing in individuals with advanced coronary atherosclerosis rarely triggers an ACS suggests that plaque vulnerability ultimately plays a more important role in plaque rupture than physiological stresses or other potential triggers. Rupture of the plaque surface occurs frequently during plaque growth [72]. Most frequently, a small 'resealing' mural thrombus forms at the rupture site, and only occasionally does a major and life-threatening luminal thrombosis evolve.

After an ACS, the risk of a recurrent ischaemic event is high during the following 3–6 months. Many of these 'new' events are probably caused by reactivation of the original culprit lesion (rethrombosis), but both postmortem and clinical observations indicate that patients with ACSs often have many ruptured and/or 'active' plaques in their coronary arteries, indicating widespread disease activity [73]. The role of active non-culprit lesion (vulnerable plaques) for subsequent ischaemic events is unknown.

Plaque erosion

The term plaque erosion is generally used for intact plaques with superimposed thrombosis, i.e. there is no underlying plaque rupture but the endothelium is missing at the plaque-thrombus interface (➲Fig. 16.9) [74]. These plaques have identified themselves as being relatively thrombogenic, but the precipitating factor or condition may, in fact, be found outside rather than inside the plaque (e.g. a hyperthrombotic tendency or so-called vulnerable blood).

The term plaque erosion is an attractive model for the minority of thrombi not preceded by plaque rupture (~20% in males and ~40% in females) [29, 74]. It refers to a heterogeneous group of atherothrombotic plaques where no deep injury is present explaining the overlying thrombus but the endothelium is missing at the plaque–thrombus interface.

The precise mechanisms of thrombosis over eroded plaques are not fully understood but probably reflect the heterogeneity of these plaques. It is conceivable that systemic thrombogenic factors such as platelet hyperaggregability, hypercoagulability, circulating tissue factor, and/or

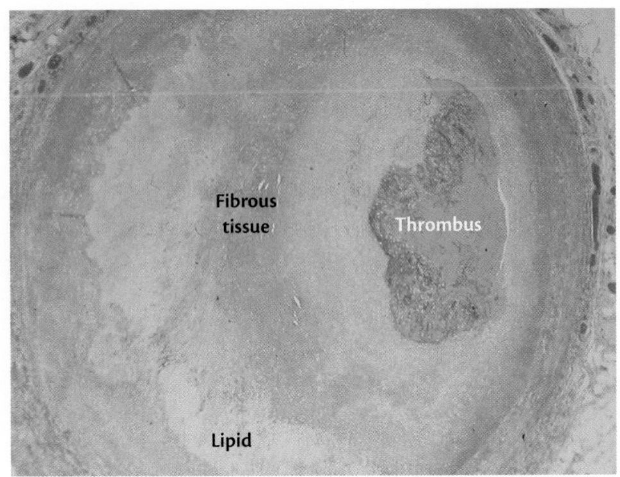

Figure 16.9 Plaque erosion. Cross-section of a coronary artery containing a severely stenotic atherosclerotic plaque with occlusive thrombosis superimposed. The lipid located deeply in the plaque is covered by a thick and intact fibrous cap. The endothelium is missing at the plaque–thrombus interface but the plaque surface is otherwise intact. Thus, there is no obvious local cause (no ruptured plaque) of thrombosis. Trichrome stain, rendering thrombus red, collagen blue, and lipid colourless. (Courtesy of E. Falk.)

depressed fibrinolysis play a major role in thrombosis over plaques that are only eroded (vs. ruptured). Recent studies have suggested that activated circulating leucocytes may transfer active tissue factor by shedding microparticles and conferring them onto adherent platelets [75, 76]. Accordingly, such circulating sources of tissue factor rather than plaque-derived tissue factor can contribute to thrombosis at sites of endothelial denudation as seen in plaque erosion.

Thrombotic response

There are three major determinants of the thrombotic response to plaque rupture or the amount of thrombosis formed on top of an eroded plaque: the local thrombogenic substrate, local flow disturbances, and the systemic thrombotic propensity.

Local thrombogenic substrate

Ongoing inflammation in terms of further macrophage infiltration and activation bears further risk after plaque rupture since these plaque components are highly thrombogenic when exposed to the flowing blood [77]. Activated macrophages express tissue factor, and the lipid-rich atheromatous core contains high amounts of active tissue factor, probably originating from dead macrophages [75, 78]. Culprit lesions responsible for the ACSs contain more tissue factor than plaques responsible for stable angina [79]. Oxidized lipids in the lipid-rich core may also directly stimulate platelet aggregation.

Local flow disturbances

In contrast to venous thrombosis, rapid flow and high shear forces promote arterial thrombosis, probably via shear-induced platelet activation [80]. A platelet-rich thrombus may indeed form and grow within a severe stenosis, where the blood velocity and shear forces are highest. Irregularities of the exposed surface further increase the platelet-mediated thrombus formation.

Systemic thrombotic propensity

The activation status of platelets, coagulation, and fibrinolysis is critical for the outcome of plaque rupture, documented by the protective effect of antiplatelet agents and anticoagulants in patients at risk of coronary thrombosis. Tissue factor probably plays an important prothrombotic role both locally (expressed by macrophages in the culprit lesion) and systemically (expressed by activated leucocytes in the peripheral blood) [75, 76, 79].

Platelets, fibrin, and thrombotic burden

In coronary thrombosis, the initial flow obstruction is usually caused by platelet aggregation, but subsequently fibrin is important for the further stabilization of the early and fragile platelet thrombus. Thus, both platelets and fibrin are equally involved in the evolution of a stable and persisting coronary thrombus.

If the platelet-rich thrombus (macroscopically white) at the site of plaque disruption occludes the lumen totally—as is usually the case in STEMI—the blood proximal and distal to the occlusion will stagnate and may coagulate, giving rise to a secondarily formed venous-type stagnation thrombosis (macroscopically red, ➲Fig. 16.10). Stagnation thromboses may contribute significantly to the overall thrombotic burden, particularly in occluded vein grafts (no side branches), and thus hamper recanalization. Clinical observations indicate that it is indeed very difficult to recanalize an occluded vein graft rapidly by intravenous thrombolytic therapy alone.

Dynamic thrombosis and microembolization

The thrombotic response to plaque rupture is dynamic: thrombosis and thrombolysis, often associated with vasospasm, tend to occur simultaneously, causing intermittent flow obstruction and distal embolization (➲Fig. 16.11) [29].

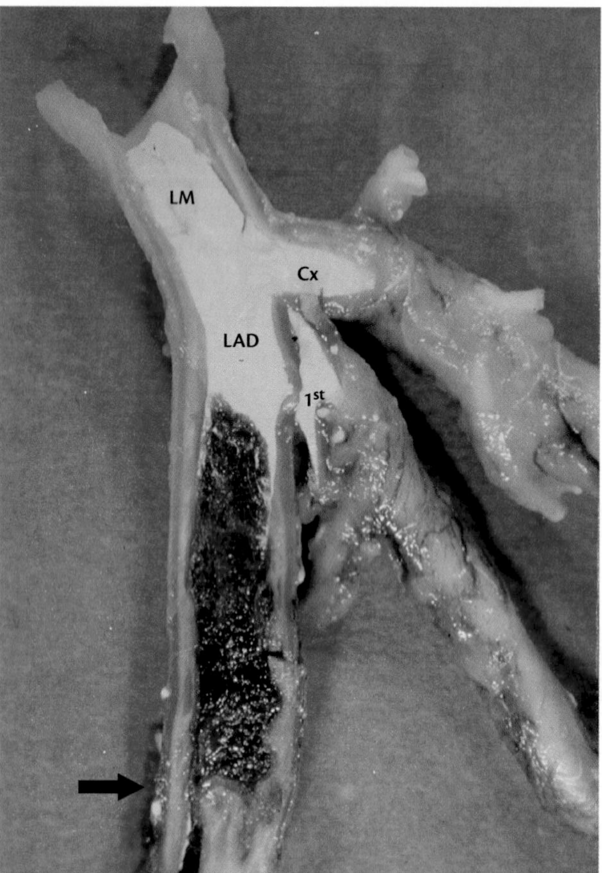

Figure 16.10 Thrombotic burden. Thrombosed coronary artery cut open longitudinally, illustrating a voluminous erythrocyte-rich stagnation thrombosis (dark black on screen) that has developed secondarily to blood stagnation caused by an occlusive platelet-rich thrombus (white) formed on top of a severely stenotic and ruptured plaque (arrow). The white material in the lumen is contrast medium injected post-mortem. LM, left main stem; LAD, left anterior descending coronary artery; Cx, circumflex branch; 1st; first diagonal branch. (Courtesy of E. Falk.)

The latter leads to microvascular obstruction, which may prevent myocardial reperfusion despite a 'successfully' recanalized infarct-related artery [81].

The purpose of coronary recanalization is, of course, to provide oxygenated blood to the ischaemic myocardium, and 'successful' recanalization (a patent culprit artery with brisk flow angiographically) is assumed to improve the perfusion at the tissue level. However, mechanical crushing and fragmentation of atherothrombotic lesion during percutaneous coronary intervention has emerged as a major cause of intracoronary (micro) embolization leading to downstream microvascular occlusion and thus preventing optimal reperfusion of the ischaemic myocardium despite 'successful' recanalization of the infarct-related artery [81]. Both spontaneous as well as iatrogenic coronary microembolization appear to be associated with an unfavourable long-term prognosis.

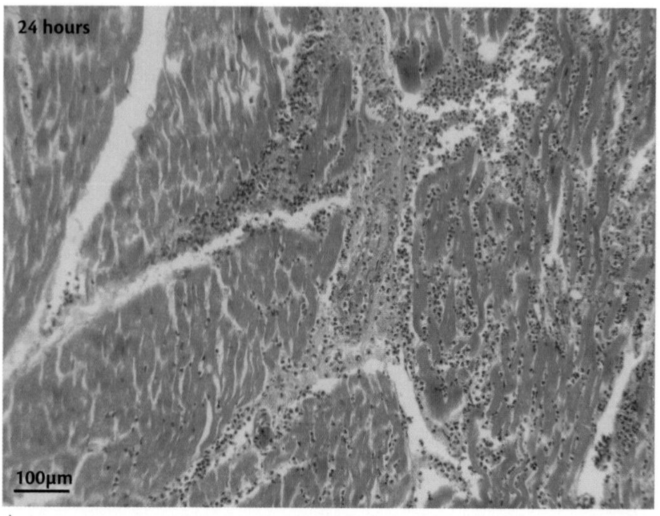

A

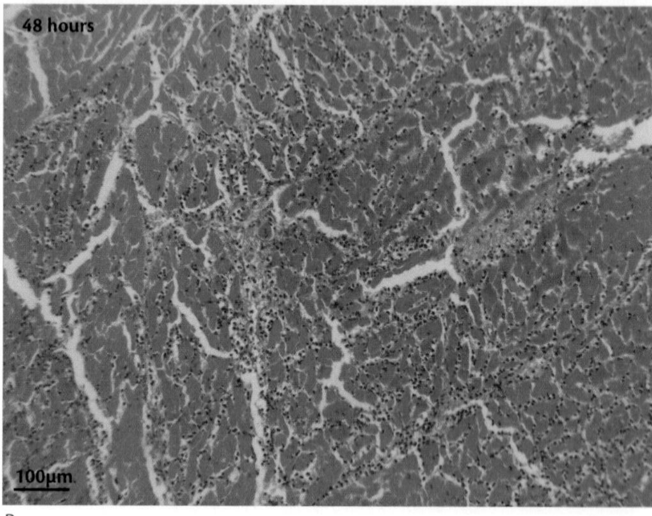

B

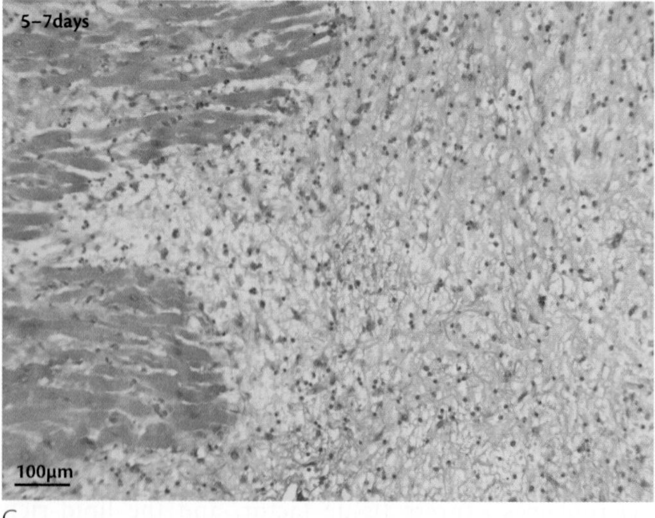

C

Figure 16.11 Typical histological alterations after myocardial infarction. (A) Invasion of neutrophil granulocytes during the first 24 hours. (B) Myocytolysis with loss of nuclei. (C) Beginning replacement fibrosis. (Courtesy of E. Falk.)

Development of myocardial infarction

Myocardial infarction (i.e. irreversible injury) caused by complete coronary artery occlusion begins to develop as soon as 15–20min of severe ischaemia (lack of forward or collateral flow). Within the perfusion area of the occluded artery, flow deprivation and myocardial ischaemia are usually most severe subendocardially (apart from the innermost 10 or so cell layers nourished from the cavity) and, at least in dogs, cell death progresses from the subendocardium to the subepicardium in a time-dependent fashion, called the 'wavefront phenomenon' (➲Figs. 16.12 and 16.13) [82]. Although the susceptibility to ischaemic necrosis differs significantly among patients (related to, for example, variability in preconditioning and oxygen demand/consumption), there are two well-characterized major determinants of the ultimate extent of infarction: First, the location of the occlusion, defining the 'area at risk' (amount of jeopardized myocardium) and second, the severity and duration of myocardial ischaemia (residual flow and rapidity of recanalization).

The speed and completeness of infarct development and, consequently, the potential for myocardial salvage by reperfusion therapy is difficult to assess in the individual patient presenting with an evolving AMI. The amounts of residual or spontaneously restored forward flow and collateral flow differ substantially among AMI patients. Rapid recruitment of collateral flow at the time of coronary occlusion (via preexisting collaterals) does not exist in some patients with myocardial infarction because they do not have such protective collaterals. They rapidly develop a transmural AMI, (like rabbits and pigs, which functionally lack collaterals), whereas other myocardial infarction patients have collaterals, probably because of the presence of severe collateral-promoting atherosclerotic stenoses prior to the acute occlusion. Patients in this second set slowly develop a relatively small myocardial infarction, or possibly none at all, in the same way as cats and guinea-pigs, which possess native collaterals.

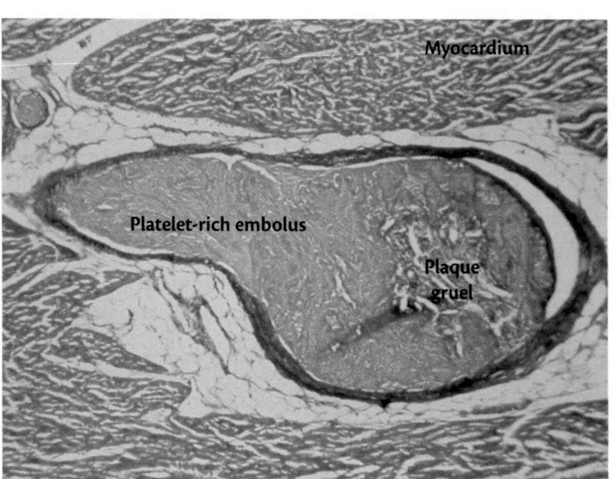

Figure 16.12 Distal embolization. Microvascular occlusion, caused by embolized platelet-rich thrombus and atheromatous 'gruel', in the myocardium downstream of a thrombosed epicardial coronary artery. If extensive, microvascular obstruction may prevent myocardial reperfusion despite 'successful' recanalization of the infarct-related artery. (Courtesy of E. Falk.)

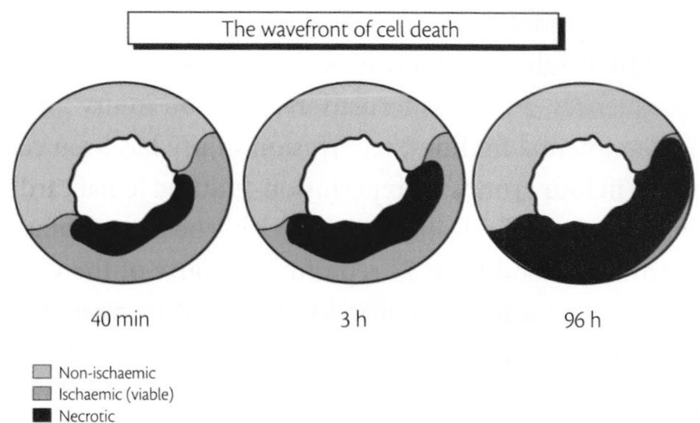

Figure 16.13 The wavefront phenomenon. Following coronary occlusion in dogs, ischaemic cell death progresses from the subendocardium to the subepicardium in a time-dependent fashion—the wavefront phenomenon. Adapted with permission from Reimer KA, Jennings RB. The 'wavefront phenomenon' of myocardial ischemic cell death. II. Transmural progression of necrosis within the framework of ischemic bed size(myocardium at risk) and collateral flow. *Lab Invest* 1979; **40**: 633–44.

The available collateral flow, at the time of occlusion, may limit or even avert the development of myocardial infarction. In unstable angina with pain at rest, about 10% of patients have an occluded culprit artery at the time of presentation, but no definite infarction evolves because of well-developed collateral circulation [32]. In infarction without Q-wave development, about 25% of patients have an occluded culprit artery at early angiographic examination, increasing to 40% in the subsequent few days, but a significant amount of myocardium is salvaged because of parallel development of collateral vessels [32]. Conversely, in STEMI, nearly all patients initially have an occluded culprit artery. Unless recanalization occurs rapidly, these patients usually develop extensive transmural infarction with Q-waves on the ECG because of poor collateral circulation. Thus, collaterals may save myocardium at risk, and improve clinical outcome.

Reperfusion and reperfusion injury

Timely, complete, and sustained reperfusion may save myocardium at risk of undergoing necrosis in patients with evolving STEMI. Such infarcts nearly always remain anaemic and pale if not reperfused. In contrast, therapeutic reperfusion is often associated with extravasation of erythrocytes in the ischaemic tissues that have already passed the point of no return, giving rise acutely to a haemorrhagic red infarct.

However, besides beneficial effects of reperfusion in term of myocardial salvage, reperfusion itself may cause harmful consequences, a process termed 'reperfusion injury'. Based on experimental findings, reperfusion injury has been categorized in four groups: 1) reperfusion-induced lethal cardiomyocyte injury of cells that are still viable before restoration of coronary blood flow; 2) reperfusion injury of the vasculature causing a loss of coronary vasodilatory reserve and contributing to the phenomenon of no-reflow; 3) stunned myocardium, e.g. prolonged contractile dysfunction of cardiomyocytes due to severely disturbed intracellular metabolism or depleted energy supply; 4) malignant arrhythmias in terms of ventricular tachycardia or fibrillation occurring after successful coronary reperfusion [83]. However, it is difficult to attribute these points solely to reperfusion and not to the preceding ischaemia. Therefore, the potential for reperfusion injury should not diminish efforts to achieve timely reperfusion in the setting of acute myocardial infarction.

No-reflow phenomenon

No-reflow describes the absence of distal myocardial reperfusion despite successful recanalization of an occluded infarct related artery. The classical—experimental—no-reflow model claims mechanical and functional factors to be responsible for the disturbed coronary flow. Mechanical factors include luminal obstruction through neutrophil plugging, atherothrombotic emboli (➲Fig. 16.11), platelets, or vascular endothelial cell swelling and external compression of the coronary arteries caused by oedema or haemorrhage [84].

No-reflow in human AMI is more complex than that seen after ligation of a normal coronary artery in animals (classical no-reflow model), because the clinical setting involves an atherothrombotic dynamic occlusion with both an innate risk of distal embolization and an embolization risk when crushed or fragmented mechanically during percutaneous coronary intervention [81]. Thus, coronary no-reflow and myocardial hypoperfusion after otherwise successful recanalization of infarct-related arteries do not simply represent non-reperfusion confined to myocardium that is already dead. No-reflow may also result from PCI-induced (micro)vascular obstruction caused by distal (micro)embolization and/or microvascular spasm [81].

Diagnosis and risk stratification of acute coronary syndromes

Diagnosis and risk stratification in patients with ACS are closely linked. During the process of establishing the diagnosis and excluding differential diagnoses the risk is repeatedly assessed and serves as a guide for the therapeutic management. Risk must not be understood in a binary way, but rather as a continuum from patients with very high risk to patients with low risk.

The prognosis of patients with ACS can be derived from surveys carried out around the world that have included >100,000 patients. Data consistently show that the mortality rate at 1 and 6 months is higher in survey populations than in randomized clinical trials. Hospital mortality is higher in patients with STEMI than among those with NSTE-ACS (7% vs. 5% respectively), but at 6 months, the mortality rates are very similar in both conditions (12% vs. 13% respectively) [85, 86] (➲Fig. 16.2). Long-term follow-up of those that survive to reach hospital showed that death rates were higher among those with NSTE-ACS than STE-ACS, with a twofold difference at 4 years [87]. This difference in mid- and long-term evolution may be due to different patient profiles, since NSTE-ACS patients tend to be older, and have more comorbidities, especially diabetes and renal failure. The difference could also be due to the greater extent of coronary artery and vascular disease, or persistent triggering factors such as inflammation [44, 88].

History and clinical presentation

An accurate history is essential in distinguishing the onset of ACS from alternative diagnoses. When faced with a symptomatic patient, there are several clinical findings that increase the probability of a diagnosis of CAD and therefore ACS. These include older age, male gender, and known atherosclerosis in non-coronary territories, like peripheral or carotid artery disease. The presence of risk factors, in particular diabetes mellitus and renal insufficiency, as well as prior manifestation of CAD, i.e. previous AMI, percutaneous intervention (PCI), or coronary bypass graft surgery (CABG), also raises the likelihood of NSTE-ACS. However, all of these factors are not specific, so that their diagnostic value should not be overestimated.

The prodrome is characterized by chest discomfort, usually at rest or on minimal exertion. Of patients with STEMI, two-thirds have prodromal symptoms in the preceding week and one-third have symptoms for up to 4 weeks. Overall, only 20% have symptoms for <24 hours. Accordingly, increased awareness of prodromes and correct interpretation of these signals during history taking can prevent the progress to myocardial infarction and sudden death.

The clinical presentation of patients with ACS encompasses a large variety of symptoms. The typical clinical presentation is retro-sternal pressure or heaviness ('angina') radiating to the left arm, neck, or jaw, which may be intermittent (usually lasting several minutes) or persistent. These complaints may be accompanied by other symptoms such as diaphoresis, nausea, abdominal pain, dyspnoea, or a syncope.

Chest pain can be graded according to the Canadian Cardiovascular Society Classification (CCS). Chest pain characteristic of an ACS has the following characteristics:

- prolonged (>20mim) anginal pain at rest;
- new onset (*de novo*) severe (CCS class III) angina; or
- destabilization of previously stable angina with at least CCS III angina characteristics (crescendo angina).

In patients with NSTE-ACS prolonged pain is observed in 80%, while *de novo* or accelerated angina is observed in only 20% of patients [89]. In contrast to patients with myocardial infarction, the pain waxes and wanes, is dependent on the level of exercise, and usually lasts no more than 20min. Patients with STEMI usually have most severe chest pain with fear of dying. Although the pain is typically located in the centre or the left lateral chest and radiates to the left shoulder, arm, neck, or jaw, pain may also be epigastric, particularly in inferior myocardial infarction. Perception of pain in the right side of the chest does not exclude myocardial ischaemia. If the pain is related to inspiration (pleuritic pain), or radiates to the back, other differential diagnoses including aortic dissection must be considered (➲Table 16.3). Pain that persists over many days or pain that can be provoked mechanically is less likely to be ischaemic. It is important to note that a reliable distinction between ACS with or without ST elevation cannot be solely based on symptoms.

Atypical presentations are not uncommon in ACS [90]. These include epigastric pain, recent-onset indigestion, stabbing chest pain, chest pain with some pleuritic features, or increasing dyspnoea. Atypical complaints are often observed in younger (25–40 years) and older (>75 years) patients, in women, and in patients with diabetes, chronic renal failure, or dementia [90, 91]. Absence of chest pain leads to under-recognition of the disease and under-treatment [92]. In the Multicenter Chest Pain Study, acute myocardial ischaemia was diagnosed in 22% of patients presenting to emergency departments with sharp or stabbing chest pain, 13% of those with chest pain that had some pleuritic features, and in a small proportion (7%) of those whose pain was fully reproduced by palpation [93]. In addition, variant angina, as a result of coronary spasm, forms part of the spectrum of ACS and may not be recognized at initial presentation. The diagnostic and therapeutic challenges arise especially when the ECG is normal or nearly normal, or conversely when the ECG is abnormal at baseline due to underlying conditions such as intraventricular conduction defects or LV hypertrophy [14].

There are certain features regarding the symptoms that may support the diagnosis of CAD and guide the management. The exacerbation of symptoms by physical exertion and their relief at rest or after nitrates support a diagnosis of ischaemia. Symptoms at rest carry a worse prognosis than symptoms elicited only during physical exertion. In patients with intermittent symptoms, an increasing number of episodes preceding the index event may also have an impact on outcome. The presence of tachycardia, hypotension, or heart failure upon presentation indicates a poor prognosis and needs rapid diagnosis and management. It is important to identify clinical circumstances that may exacerbate or precipitate NSTE-ACS, such as anaemia, infection, inflammation, fever, and metabolic or endocrine (in particular thyroid) disorders.

In up to one-half of patients with STEMI, physical and/or emotional factors are identified in the prodrome and may have influenced plaque rupture. A circadian pattern of presentation with STEMI is well documented. The peak incidence of events coincides with the early waking hours, possibly associated with rises in catecholamines and cortisol and increases in platelet aggregability. Population studies reveal that approximately 30% of myocardial infarctions occur silently or with less severe symptoms.

Table 16.3 Differential diagnosis in ACS

Cardiac	Pulmonary	Haematological	Vascular	Gastrointestinal	Orthopaedic
Myocarditis Pericarditis Myopericarditis Cardiomyopathy Valvular disease Apical ballooning (Tako-Tsubo syndrome)	Pulmonary embolism Pulmonary infarction Pneumonia Pleuritis Pneumothorax	Sickle cell anaemia	Aortic dissection Aortic aneurysm Aortic coarctation Cerebrovascular disease	Oesophageal spasm Oesophagitis Peptic ulcer Pancreatitis Cholescystitis	Cervical discopathy Rib fracture Muscle injury/inflammation Costochondritis

They are detected only by chance on subsequent ECG recordings [94].

To recognize subgroups of patients with unstable angina who are at different levels of cardiac risk, the Braunwald classification was introduced [92]. This empirically developed classification is based on symptoms with respect to pain severity and duration as well as the pathogenesis of myocardial ischaemia and was validated in prospective studies [95, 96]. Patients with unstable angina at rest within the last 48 hours (class IIIB) have been shown to be at highest risk of an adverse cardiac event (11% in-hospital event rate). The Braunwald classification has become an accepted standard for grading patients, designing study protocols, and improving the comparability of study results. For further risk assessment, troponins have been introduced to this classification (➲Table 16.4) [97].

Physical examination

Physical examination of patients with chest pain includes chest examination, auscultation, and measurement of heart rate and blood pressure. There are no individual physical signs diagnostic of STEMI, but many patients have evidence of autonomic nervous system activation (pallor, sweating) and either hypotension or a narrow pulse pressure. Features may also include irregularities of the pulse, bradycardia or tachycardia, a third heart sound, and basal rales. Signs of heart failure or haemodynamic instability must prompt the physician to expedite the diagnosis and treatment of patients. An important goal of the physical examination is to exclude non-cardiac causes of chest pain, and non-ischaemic cardiovascular disorders (e.g., pulmonary embolism, aortic dissection, pericarditis, valvular heart disease), or potentially extra-cardiac causes, such as acute pulmonary diseases (e.g. pneumothorax, pneumonia, pleural effusion). In this regard, differences in blood pressure between the upper and lower limbs, an irregular pulse, heart murmurs, a friction rub, pain on palpation, and abdominal masses are physical findings that may suggest a diagnosis other than NSTE-ACS. Other physical findings such as pallor, increased sweating, or tremor may orientate towards precipitating conditions, such as anaemia and thyrotoxicosis. Also see ➲Chapter 1.

The electrocardiogram

The resting ECG plays a central role in the early assessment of patients with suspected ACS. In all patients admitted with acute chest pain, a resting 12-lead ECG should be recorded and interpreted by an experienced physician within 10min [95]. Dynamic changes, particularly during episodes of chest pain, have a very high diagnostic value. Continuous ST-segment monitoring was shown to provide better ECG prediction, but should not delay invasive management in symptomatic patients [98]. Ideally, a tracing should be obtained when the patient is symptomatic and compared with a tracing obtained when symptoms have resolved. Comparison with a previous ECG, if available, is extremely valuable, particularly in patients with coexisting cardiac pathology such as left ventricular hypertrophy or a previous myocardial infarction [93, 98]. Exercise testing is contraindicated in symptomatic patients and in patients with elevated biomarkers like troponins. After stabilization and in absence of other high-risk features, treadmill testing is useful for risk assessment (➲Chapters 1 and 25).

ST-segment shifts and T wave changes are the paramount ECG signs of unstable CAD [85, 99]. The number of leads showing ST depression and the magnitude of ST depression are indicative of extent and severity of ischaemia and correlate with prognosis [100]. ST-segment depression ≥0.5mm (0.05mV) in two or more contiguous leads, in the appropriate clinical context, is suggestive of NSTE-ACS and linked

Table 16.4 Braunwald classification of unstable angina

Severity	Clinical circumstances		
	A—develops in presence of extracardiac condition that intensifies myocardial ischaemia (secondary UA)	**B—develops in absence of extracardiac condition (primary UA)**	**C—develops within 2 weeks of acute myocardial infarction (post-infarction UA)**
I—new onset of severe angina or accelerated angina, no rest pain	IA	IB	IC
II—angina at rest within past month but not within preceding 48 h (angina at rest, subacute)	IIA	IIB	IIC
III—Angina at rest within 48 h (angina at rest, acute)	IIIA	IIIB-T_{neg} IIIB-T_{pos}	

Reproduced with permission from Hamm CW, Braunwald E. A classification of unstable angina revisited. *Circulation* 2000; **102**: 118–22.

to prognosis [101]. Minor (0.5mm) ST depression may be difficult to measure in clinical practice. More relevant is ST depression of ≥1mm (0.1mV) which is associated with an 11% rate of death and myocardial infarction at 1 year [99]. ST depression of ≥2mm carries about a sixfold increased mortality risk [102]. ST depression combined with transient ST elevation also identifies a high-risk subgroup [103].

Patients with ST depression have a higher risk for subsequent cardiac events compared to those with isolated T-wave inversion (>1mm) in leads with predominant R-waves, who in turn have a higher risk than those with a normal ECG on admission. Some studies have cast doubt on the prognostic value of isolated T-wave inversion. However, deep symmetrical inversion of the T-waves in the anterior chest leads is often related to a significant stenosis of the proximal left anterior descending coronary artery or main stem [104].

New ST-segment elevations in the presence of appropriate symptoms indicate transmural ischaemia as a result of acute coronary occlusion. In the very early phase of AMI giant T-waves are a rare finding. Persistent ST-segment elevation at the J-point (in absence of left bundle branch block) with the cut-off points ≥0.2mV in men or ≥0.15mV in women in leads V2 through V3 and/ or ≥0.1mV in other leads characterizes evolving myocardial infarction (STEMI). The ST-segment vector points to the region of injury, which allows the infarct-related artery to be identified in many cases (➲Table 16.5). Right precordial leads (V3r to V6r) may be useful in identifying right ventricular involvement and V7 to V9 in detecting true posterior infarction.

Transient ST-segment elevation may be observed in ACS and particularly in Prinzmetal's angina. To detect or to rule out transient ST-segment changes during recurrent episodes of chest pain or in silent ischaemia, continuous multi-lead ST-segment monitoring can be useful.

ST-segment depression may occur in reciprocal leads (➲Figs. 16.14 and 16.15) as an electrical mirror or as the result of true ischaemia in another territory ('ischaemia at a distance'). In the absence of ST-segment elevation, depression of the ST-segment is indicative of subendocardial ischaemia. Only biochemical markers of myocardial cell injury (e.g. troponins) will determine whether this patient is having a NSTEMI in the absence of typical ST-segment elevations. Isolated ST-segment depression in the right precordial leads may occur in strictly posterior myocardial infarction. Borderline ST-segment elevations confined to leads V1 and V2 may be the result of early repolarization and should critically be interpreted when typical clinical symptoms are lacking.

During the evolution of cell necrosis the amplitude of the R-wave is reduced, T-waves become negative, and Q-waves develop. Clinically established myocardial infarction is defined by any Q-wave in leads V_2 through V_3 ≥0.02s, or Q-wave ≥0.03s and ≥0.1mV or QS complex in leads I, II, aVL, aVF, or V4 to V6 in any of a continguous lead grouping (I, aVL,V6; V4–V6; II, III, aVF). However, the absence or presence of Q-waves is not a reliable sign of a transmural or non-transmural infarct expansion. In addition, creatine kinase (CK) levels do not always correlate with the development of Q-waves. Accordingly, the terms Q-wave and non-Q-wave myocardial infarction have fallen out of use [105].

It is important to note that even a completely normal ECG in patients presenting with suspicious symptoms does not exclude the possibility of an ACS. In several studies about 5% of patients with normal ECG who were discharged from the emergency department were ultimately

Table 16.5 Acute myocardial infarction based on electrocardiographic entry criteria with angiographic correlation

Location	Anatomy of occlusion	ECG	1-year mortality (%)*
Proximal left anterior descending	Proximal to first septal perforator	ST↑ V1–6, I, aVL and fascicular bundle or bundle branch block	25.6
Mid left anterior descending	Proximal to large diagonal but distal to first septal perforator	ST↑ V1–6, I, aVL	12.4
Distal left anterior descending or diagonal	Distal to large diagonal or to diagonal itself	ST↑ V1–V4 or ST↑ I,V5,6 aVL, V5–V6	10.2
Moderate to large inferior (posterior, lateral, right ventricular)	Proximal right coronary artery or left circumflex	ST↑ II, III, aVF and any or all of the following: 1) V1, V3R, V4R 2) V5V6 3) R > S in V1, V2	8.4
Small inferior sdsds	Distal righ coronary artery or left circumflex branch occlusion	ST↑ II, III, aVF only	6.7

*Based on GUSTO-I cohort population in each of the 5-year categories, all receiving reperfusion therapy.

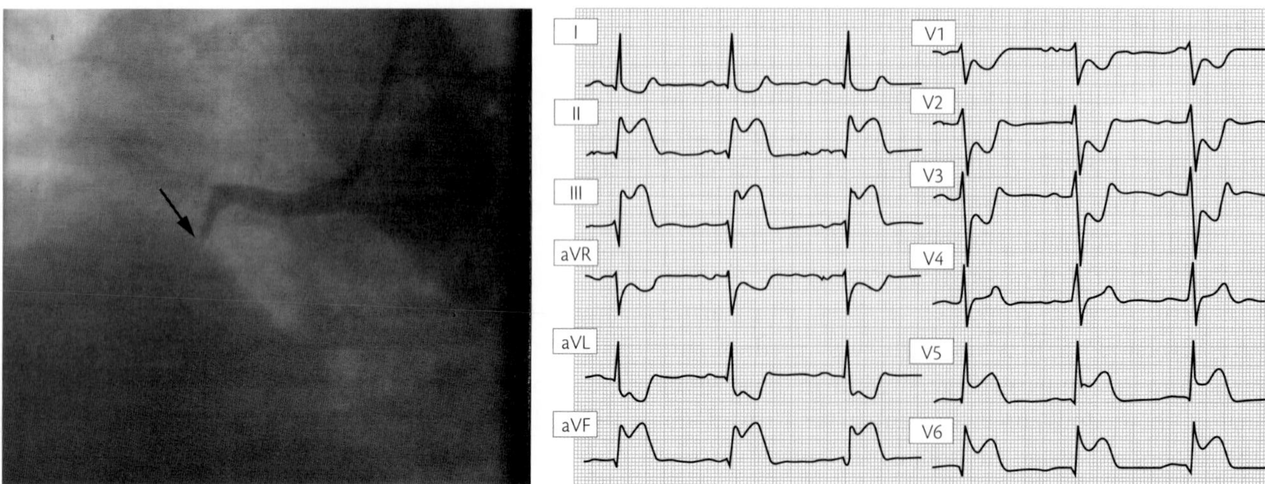

Figure 16.14 Inferior AMI: occluded right coronary artery, ST-segment elevation in leads II, III and aVF; ST depression in V1 to V4.

found to have either an AMI or unstable angina [104, 106, 107]. This false diagnosis especially occurs in cases, where the left circumflex artery represents the culprit lesion. However, a completely normal ECG recording during an episode of significant chest pain should direct attention to other possible causes for the patient's complaints.

Biochemical markers

Biochemical markers play a central role in evaluating patients with chest pain. Besides routine laboratory measurements (haemoglobin, white blood cell count, thyroid hormones, etc.) special markers reflecting distinct pathophysiological processes play today a central role in evaluating this high-risk group of patients. Many of the novel biomarkers have been useful in elucidating the underlying mechanisms of ACS, but only some of these have entered routine application [108].

Markers of myocardial necrosis

Pathohistological studies in patients with unstable angina have disclosed focal cell necroses in the myocardium distal to the culprit artery. These were attributed to repetitive thrombus embolization [109, 110]. Focal cell necroses, are only very infrequently detectable by routine CK and CK-MB measurements. Even improved test systems for the quantitative determination of CK-MB based on immunological determination, which are superior to enzyme activity measurements, did not substantially increase the sensitivity for the detection of minor myocardial injury. Myoglobin is

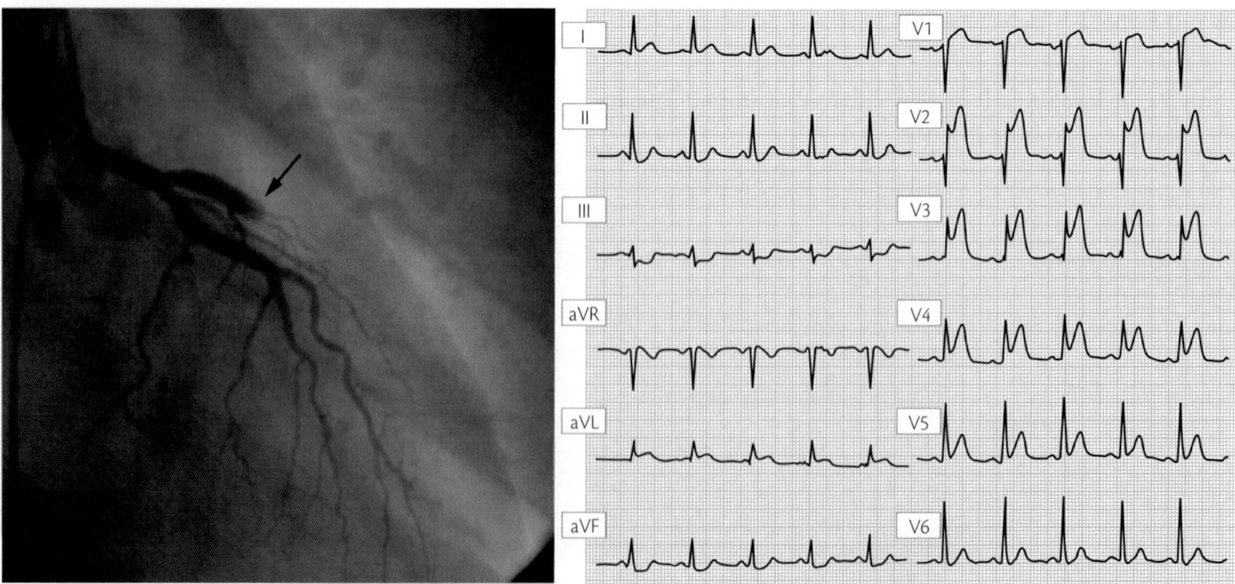

Figure 16.15 Anterior AMI: occluded left anterior descending coronary artery, ST-segment elevation.

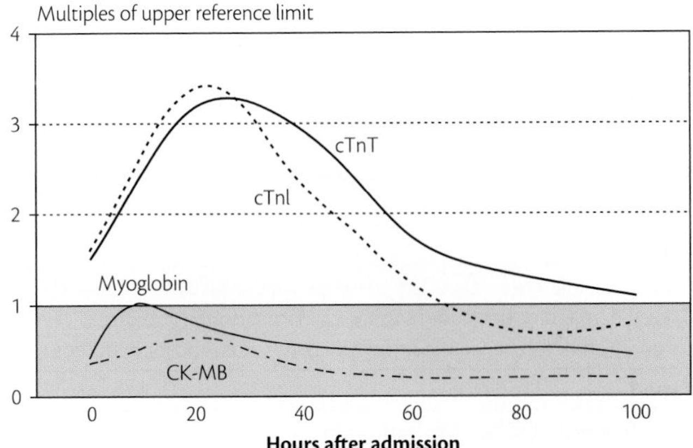

Figure 16.16 Typical time course of cardiac enzymes in patients with non-ST-elevation myocardial infarction.

a marker, which rises earlier than CK-MB in AMI but has similar limitations with respect to specificity (➲Fig. 16.16; Table 16.6).

These biochemical limitations of CK-MB and myoglobin measurements for the detection of minor myocardial injury have been overcome by the introduction of cardiac troponin T and troponin I measurements in the early 1990s. The troponin complex is formed by three distinct structural proteins (troponins I, C, and T) and is located on the thin filament of the contractile apparatus in both skeletal and cardiac muscle tissue regulating the calcium-dependent interaction of myosin and actin. Cardiac isoforms for all three troponins, however, are encoded each by different genes and can be distinguished by monoclonal antibodies recognizing the amino acid sequence distinct for the cardiac isoform [111]. However, only the cardiac isoforms of troponin T and troponin I are exclusively expressed in cardiac myocytes. Accordingly, the detection of cardiac troponin T and troponin I are highly specific for myocardial damage, attributing these markers the role of a new gold standard. In conditions of 'false-positive' elevated CK-MB, such as skeletal muscle trauma, troponins will clarify any cardiac involvement. Accordingly, the definition of myocardial infarction was based on biomarkers of necrosis, i.e. troponins.

In patients with a myocardial infarction, an elevation of troponin in peripheral blood can first be observed as early as 3–4 hours because of its release from a cytosolic pool (➲Fig. 16.16), followed by a prolonged appearance of up to 2 weeks related to continuous proteolysis of the contractile apparatus in the necrotic myocardium. The high proportional rise of troponins, relative to the low plasma troponin concentrations in healthy controls, allows the detection of myocardial damage in about one-third of patients presenting with unstable angina even without elevated CK-MB [112–120].

Definition of acute myocardial infarction

The traditional clinical definition of myocardial infarction by the WHO did not require elevations of biochemical markers, and hence was revised by the Joint European Society of Cardiology/American College of Cardiology Committee. The new AMI definition was based on biomarker criteria, namely troponin elevation as a result of irreversible cell damage, combined with clinical features [121]. This concept has been reinforced by the 'Universal definition of myocardial infarction' in 2007 [1]. According to this document, a myocardial infarction is defined by a typical rise or fall of cardiac troponins together with one of the following clinical signs of myocardial ischaemia: typical symptoms, ECG changes, loss of viable myocardium, or regional wall motion abnormalities detected by imaging techniques (➲Table 16.7). Furthermore, a classification of five types of myocardial infarction was introduced reflecting the mechanism of cell injury (➲Table 16.8). The changed definition increased the frequency of the diagnosis of myocardial infarction and has important implications for the interpretation of epidemiological research and clinical trials as well as for clinical care. Although many physicians had conceptual difficulties with the translation of this change in paradigm into clinical practice, the increased risk in patients with elevated troponin levels justifies the revised criteria.

Troponins for risk stratification

It has been demonstrated in numerous clinical trials that troponin T and troponin I are strongly associated with increased risk both in the acute phase of hospitalization and during long-term follow-up. In the first report on troponin T in a small cohort of patients with unstable angina, it was

Table 16.6 Biochemical markers for the detection of myocardial necrosis

	MW (kDa)	Specificity	Sensitivity	First rise after AMI	Peak after AMI	Return to normal
CK-MB mass	85.0	++	+	4 hours	24 hours	72 hours
Myoglobin	17.8	+	+	2 hours	6–8 hours	24 hours
Troponin T	33.0	+++	+++	4 hours	24–48 hours	5–21 days
Troponin I	22.5	+++	+++	3–4 hours	24–36 hours	5–14 days

Table 16.7 Definition of myocardial infarction

Criteria for acute myocardial infarction
The term myocardial infarction should be used when there is evidence of myocardial necrosis in a clinical setting consistent with myocardial ischaemia. Under these conditions any one of the following criteria meets the diagnosis for myocardial infarction: ◆ Detection of rise and/or fall of cardiac biomarkers (preferably troponin) with at least one value above the 99th percentile of the upper reference limit (URL) together with evidence of myocardial ischaemia with at least one of the following: • Symptoms of ischaemia; • ECG changes indicative of new ischaemia [new ST-T changes or new left bundle branch block (LBBB)]; • Development of pathological Q waves in the ECG; • Imaging evidence of new loss of viable myocardium or new regional wall motion abnormality. ◆ Sudden, unexpected cardiac death, involving cardiac arrest, often with symptoms suggestive of myocardial ischaemia: and accompanied by presumably new ST elevation, or new LBBB, and/or evidence of fresh thrombus by coronary angiography and/or at autopsy, but death occurring before blood samples could be obtained, or at a time before the appearance of cardiac biomarkers in the blood ◆ For percutaneous coronary interventions (PCI) in patients with normal baseline troponin values, elevations of cardiac biomarkers above the 99th percentile URL are indicative of peri-procedural myocardial necrosis. By convention, increases of biomarkers greater than 3 x99th percentile URL have been designated as defining PCI-related myocardial infarction. A subtype related to a documented stent thrombosis is recognized ◆ For coronary artery bypass grafting (CABG) in patients with normal baseline troponin values, elevations of cardiac biomarkers above the 99th percentile URL are indicative of peri-procedural myocardial necrosis. By convention, increases of biomarkers greater than 5 x 99th percentile URL plus either new pathological Q waves or new LBBB, or argiographically documented new graft or native coronary artery occlusion, or imaging evidence of new loss of viable myocardium have been designated as defining CABG-related myocardial infarction ◆ Pathological findings of an acute myocardial infarction
Criteria for prior myocardial infarction
Any one of the following criteria meets the diagnosis for prior myocardial infarction
◆ Development of new pathological Q waves with or without symptoms ◆ Imaging evidence of a region of loss of viable myocardium that is thinned and fails to contract, in the absence of a non-ischaemic cause. ◆ Pathological findings of a healed or healing myocardial infarction

Table 16.8 Clinical classification of different types of myocardial infarction

Type 1
Spontaneous myocardial infarction related to ischaemia due to a primary coronary event such as plaque erosion and/or rupture, fissuring, or dissection
Type 2
Myocardial infarction secondary to ischaemia due to either increased oxygen demand or decreased supply, e.g. coronary artery spasm, coronary embolism, anaemia, arrhythmias, hypertension, or hypotension
Type 3
Sudden unexpected cardiac death, including cardiac arrest, often with symptoms suggestive of myocardial ischaemia, accompanied by presumably new STelevation, or new LBBB, or evidence of fresh thrombus in a coronary artery by angiography and/or at autopsy, but death occurring before blood samples could be obtained, or at a time before the appearance of cardiac biornarkers in the blood
Type 4a
Myocardial infarction associated with PCI
Type 4b
Myocardial infarction associated with stent thrombosis as documented by angiography or at autopsy
Type 5
Myocardial infarction associated with CABG

demonstrated that the risk of death and myocardial infarction during hospitalization was increased even in the presence of antithrombotic therapy with aspirin and heparin [113]. In a later trial the prognostic value was shown to correlate with the absolute concentrations of troponin T over a 5-month period [116]. The peak value during the first 24 hours provided the best independent prognostic information and the absence of troponin T was superior to CK-MB for identification of the low-risk group [122]. Furthermore, the combination of the troponin T test with a predischarge exercise test represents an excellent risk assessment for unstable coronary disease [123]. During the 5-month follow-up, death and myocardial infarction occurred at a rate of only 1%, if both the troponin test and the predischarge exercise test were normal, whereas the event rate was as high as 50% when both tests were abnormal. Moreover, the prognostic potential of troponin T in the entire spectrum of patients with ACS, including myocardial infarction, was evaluated in a substudy of the GUSTO (Global Use of Strategies To Open occluded coronary arteries) IIA trial [124]. A single measurement within 2 hours after admission was highly predictive of 30-day mortality and other major complications. The prognostic value was independent of ECG findings and was superior to CK-MB measurements.

For elevations of cardiac troponin I, a similar prognostic impact was evidenced as for troponin T elevations. In the TIMI IIIB trial including patients with unstable angina and non-Q-wave myocardial infarction, the mortality rate was closely related to troponin I levels reaching 7.5% after 42 days' follow-up in patients with the highest troponin I values [115].

Troponin is a particularly appealing marker, because in addition to its prognostic value it has important therapeutic implications. The increased risk in patients with elevated troponin levels is reduced by glycoprotein IIb/IIIa inhibitors and early invasive management [125].

Analytical aspects of troponin measurements

Since measurement of troponins plays a central role for the diagnosis of myocardial infarction and the therapeutic decision making in patients with ACSs, clearly defined decision limits are mandatory. The difficulty with defining the appropriate diagnostic threshold for troponins is compounded by the availability of multiple assays for troponin I with different reference ranges [126]. The recommended threshold for an abnormal troponin level is the concentration above the 99th percentile of a healthy reference population [1, 125]. In addition, the analytical quality depends on sufficient analytical precision, which is defined as a coefficient of variation (CV) below 10%. In the past, commercially available troponin assays were not able to measure a troponin concentration at the 99th percentile with the required precision. In fact the lowest concentration that could be determined with a CV <10% was about 1.4–4.4-fold higher then the concentration at the 99th percentile [127]. With the introduction of newly developed high- or ultrasensitive troponin assays it is possible to measure troponin concentrations at the 99th percentile with the required precision. Some of these new assays have already been launched to the market and are commercially available; others will be introduced for routine clinical application in the near future.

Since the decision limits of these new high sensitive troponin assays will be lower than those of the currently available assays, the number of detectable myocardial infarction will increase, and in addition the diagnosis of a myocardial infarction will be possible at an earlier time point. On the other side, with these high sensitive assays, troponin elevations will be detectable in chronic cardiovascular diseases other than ischaemic heart disease and may also occur after extreme exercise or from other causes of severe cardiac stress without coronary disease. Thus it will be important to consider the differential diagnosis of troponin elevation and to carefully look at dynamic troponin changes with a rise and fall, to correctly classify patients as having myocardial infarction and to assign the patients to the appropriate therapeutic strategy.

The difficulty with defining the appropriate diagnostic threshold for troponins is compounded by the availability of multiple assays for troponin I for with different reference ranges. Many manufacturers report two decision limits: a 'diagnostic' limit for the definitive diagnosis of myocardial infarction based on prior comparisons to CK-MB and a lower limit 'suggestive' of myocardial injury that is important for the patients' prognosis. Though the challenge of developing terminology and diagnostic thresholds around low-level troponin elevation is still debated, the clinical importance of increased troponin levels in suspected ACS is firmly established.

There is no clinical difference between troponin T and troponin I. Differences between study results are predominantly explained by varying inclusion criteria, differences in sampling patterns and use of assays with different diagnostic cut-offs. The decision limits must be based on carefully conducted clinical studies for individual troponin I assays and should not be generalized between different troponin I assays.

Suspected ACS represents a possibly life-threatening condition in which savings in time for therapeutic decision-making and further patient management may be decisive. It was shown prospectively that risk stratification based on a protocol scheduling rapid testing of troponin on the patient's arrival in the emergency room, and again 6–12 hours later, provides, in general, reliable risk stratification [117, 125]. A single test result obtained on admission of the patient is inappropriate for risk stratification, because up to 10% of high-risk patients will be missed.

Non-cardiac causes of elevated cardiac troponins

One initial barrier to the universal acceptance of troponins as the gold standard for the detection of myocardial injury has been the observation that troponin concentrations are increased rarely in non-cardiac conditions, but are more commonly elevated in patients with renal failure. Although measurements of cardiac troponins are generally assessed as highly specific for myocardial injury, elevated cardiac troponin, unrelated to myocardial damage, has been reported in a number of conditions including cerebrovascular accidents, subarachnoid haemorrhage, endocrine disease, polymyositis, dermatomyositis, and haematological malignancies [127, 128] (➲Table 16.9). Studies in intensive-care units have demonstrated increased troponin levels in septic patients. Importantly, troponin concentrations in these patients correlated with left ventricular dysfunction and the presence of multiorgan failure. However, it remains unclear whether troponin elevation affected either hospital length of stay or survival [129].

Elevated levels of cardiac troponins are frequently found in patients with end-stage renal disease in the absence of unstable heart disease. Even using more specific second-generation troponin T assays, up to 53% of asymptomatic patients with end-stage renal disease remain positive for cardiac troponin T [130–132]. An elevated concentration identifies patients at greater risk of all-cause mortality [130–133]. Given the

Table 16.9 Causes of elevated troponin

Cardiac contusion, or other trauma including surgery, ablation, pacing, etc.
Congestive heart failure–acute and chronic
Aortic dissection
Aortic valve disease
Hypertrophic cardiomyopathy
Tachy- or bradyarrhythmias, or heart block
Apical ballooning syndrome
Rhabdomyolysis with cardiac injury
Pulmonary embolism, severe pulmonary hypertension
Renal failure
Acute neurological disease, including stroke or subarachnoid haemorrhage
Infiltrative diseases, e.g. amyloidosis, haemochromatosis, sarcoidosis, and scleroderma
Inflammatory diseases, e.g. myocarditis or myocardial extension of endo-/pericarditis
Drug toxicity or toxins
Critically ill patients, especially with respiratory failure or sepsis
Burns, especially if affecting >30% of body surface area
Extreme exertion

lower frequency of abnormal troponin I in asymptomatic patients with end-stage renal disease, it has been suggested that this may be a more specific marker of cardiac ischaemia than troponin T for this group of patients [133, 134]. Several factors are likely to explain the discrepancy between troponins I and T. Free cytosolic proteins are released earlier when cells are damaged, estimated to be 7% for troponin T as compared to 3.5% for troponin I [135]. There is roughly twice as much troponin T as troponin I per gram of myocardium [136]. Moreover, uraemia increases the free serum concentration and the clearance of protein-bound factors. As troponin I is released from the myocardium only as a complex and troponin T is released as a complex as well as free troponin T, it is possible that uraemia may affect the detection, release, or clearance of different troponin subunits. Since free and bound troponin T are large molecules (37 and 77kDa, respectively), it is unlikely that the kidney is responsible for clearance. Indeed, the half-life and clearance of troponin I after an AMI appear similar between patients with normal renal function and end-stage renal disease [137].

A number of studies investigated the prognostic role of serum troponins in patients with renal failure using newer cardiac troponin assays. In the largest of these trials [138] troponin T was more commonly elevated than troponin I, but both were predictive of increased mortality. In the setting of an ACS, an analysis of >7000 patients disclosed that troponin T is an important predictor for adverse outcome in both patients with and without renal failure [139]. In conclusion, serum cardiac troponin concentrations are frequently increased in asymptomatic patients with renal failure. This is likely representing multifactorial pathology, potentially including cardiac dysfunction, left ventricular hypertrophy, as well as subclinical myocardial infarction, and is associated with an increased risk of morbidity and mortality.

Markers of myocardial stress (natriuretic peptides)

Myocardial stress leading to neurohormonal activation of the heart can be monitored by measuring systemic levels of natriuretic peptides secreted from the heart. Atrial natriuretic peptides (ANP) are primarily produced in the cardiac atria, whereas B-type natriuretic peptides (BNP) are mainly synthesized in the ventricular myocardium. Both peptides are generated as pro-hormones (proANP and proBNP) that upon secretion are cleaved into the biologically active peptides (ANP and BNP) and the N-terminal pro-hormone fragments (NT-proANP and NT-proBNP). Natriuretic peptides are released mainly in response to increased stretch or wall tension and are involved in the regulation of blood pressure, blood volume, and sodium balance via modulation of natriuresis, vasodilatation, and inhibition of the renin–angiotensin–aldosterone system as well as the sympathetic nervous system. In disease states, BNP and NT-proBNP have a greater proportional rise than ANP and NT-proANP, and have received most of the interest for a clinical application [140].

Even though, there are differences between BNP and NT-proBNP in their physiological functions as well as in clearance and half-life time, there seems to be no clinically meaningful difference between the two markers for the application as diagnostic and prognostic markers.

Both natriuretic peptides are highly sensitive and fairly specific markers for the detection of left ventricular dysfunction. Therefore, investigators originally focused on the predictive value of natriuretic peptides in patients with congestive heart failure. However, there is also good evidence from animal studies and experimental data, that myocardial ischaemia itself, independently form demonstrable haemodynamic changes, is a stimulus for BNP and NT-proBNP release [141, 142]. Thus, the focus has expanded and the diagnostic and prognostic value of natriuretic peptides in patients with ischaemic heart disease, stable coronary heart disease, as well as ACSs, has been evaluated.

In patients with stable coronary heart disease, levels of B-type natriuretic peptides are elevated with an association to the extent of inducible myocardial ischaemia and to the severity of coronary artery involvement [143]. However, BNP and NT-proBNP as indicators for myocardial ischaemia lack sufficient sensitivity and specificity. Therefore, they are not useful as diagnostic markers in clinical routine in this setting. B-type natriuretic peptides have been demonstrated to provide strong prognostic information for mortality independent of left ventricular function, clinical signs of heart failure, and conventional risk factors [144, 145]. Similarly, it has been reported from numerous studies, that patients presenting with ACS and elevated levels of B-type natriuretic peptides, have a three- to fivefold increase in mortality as compared to those with lower levels of NT-proBNP or BNP [146–151]. In fact this association of elevated B-type natriuretic peptides with mortality remained strong even after adjusting for age, Killip class, left ventricular ejection fraction determined by echocardiography, and established clinical risk scores such as the TIMI risk score [152]. But even more importantly, B-type natriuretic peptides are able to discriminate high-risk patients among troponin-negative patients presenting with suspected ACS or chest pain, who are generally considered to be at low risk [153]. Consequently, assessment of B-type natriuretic peptides has entered current guidelines [125]. Noteworthy, even though B-type natriuretic peptides are able to predict mortality and heart failure, they failed to predict recurrent ischaemic events [147].

According to currently available data, a threshold of BNP above 80pg/mL and for NT-proBNP above 500pg/mL as an indicator for high-risk patients can be recommended.

Despite their strong prognostic value, it remains undetermined whether specific therapeutical implications can be derived from the assessment of B-type natriuretic peptides in patients with ischaemic heart disease. From retrospective analyses of clinical trials including patients with ACS, data has been reported suggesting a benefit from an early invasive treatment of patients with elevated NT-proBNP. However, at present no general recommendation can be given [148, 154–156]. The potential of B-type natriuretic peptides to predict a benefit from an ACE inhibitor treatment in patients with stable ischaemic heart disease has been investigated in retrospective analyses of two large trials. Conclusively, it was found in both trials that ACE inhibitor treatment was equally effective independently of B-type natriuretic peptide levels [157].

In summary, assessment of B-type natriuretic peptides in patients with clinical symptoms of ACS adds prognostic information beyond that derived from traditional risk assessment. However, with the currently available data no clear recommendations regarding management for patients with increased BNP or NT-proBNP can be ascertained.

Markers of inflammation

Of the numerous inflammatory markers that have been investigated over the past decade, high sensitive C-reactive protein (hsCRP) is the most widely studied in populations covering the entire range from apparently healthy individuals to patients with cardiovascular risk factors, with stable coronary heart disease, and with ACS. The physiological role of CRP is not fully elucidated; however, its properties are consistent with non-specific defence mechanisms. In response to tissue injury or local inflammation, CRP synthesis occurs in hepatocytes in response to stimulation by various cytokines [158, 159]. In addition, there are some data suggesting a local release of CRP from atherosclerotic plaques. In patients with myocardial infarction, an acute inflammatory process induced by myocardial damage also contributes to CRP increase [119, 147].

Several epidemiologic studies have shown that increases in hsCRP concentrations, within the reference interval, are associated with an increased risk for future myocardial infarction, stroke, peripheral arterial disease, and sudden cardiac death in apparently healthy men and women [160–163]. These findings are consistent with findings form basic research studies demonstrating that inflammation plays an important role for the initiation and progression of atherosclerosis. In primary prevention studies, however, hsCRP added little to the predictive value provided by the assessment of traditional risk factors, including LDL-cholesterol [164–167].

In ACS a large number of studies including thousands of patients, have demonstrated that hsCRP was able to predict short-term as well as long-term cardiovascular complications. The association of hsCRP and the risk of death in patients with ACS was independent from the therapeutic strategy and the predictive information was incremental to TIMI risk score and other biomarkers. There is also robust evidence that, even among patients with troponin-negative ACS, elevated levels of CRP are predictive of future risk [119, 168, 169]. The FRISC study confirmed that mortality is associated with elevated CRP levels at the time of the index event and continues to increase for several years [119, 168–174].

Since CRP is not only a passive bystander but plays an active role in the promotion of atherosclerosis, hsCRP levels might be useful to target therapy. And in fact, several studies demonstrated that the effect of aggressive lipid lowering with statins was most effective in patients in whom LDL was lowered below 70mg/L and hsCRP below 2mg/L

[175–177]. Even plaque regression could be observed by IVUS under high dose statin treatment with the largest reduction in those patients in whom both, LDL and hsCRP, were lowered below the median [178]. Therefore, there is substantial evidence in favour of the application of hsCRP to identify those patients who might benefit most from the use of HMG CoA reductase inhibitors.

As decision limits for risk classification of patients with stable ischaemic disease or in primary prevention a concentration of hsCRP below 1mg/dL identifies patients at low risk, between 1–3mg/dL patients at intermediate risk, and above 3mg/dL patients at high risk. For risk assessment in the acute phase of an ACS a higher decision limit of 10mg/L should be used for the assessment of prognosis [179].

Point-of-care testing

Point-of-care tests are characterized as assays to be performed either directly at the bedside or at 'near-patient' locations such as the emergency department, chest pain evaluation centre, or intensive care unit. Therefore, the rationale behind point-of-care testing is the improvement in analytical turnaround time.

Point-of-care assays are available for the determination troponins, CK-MB, myoglobin, and B-type natriuretic peptides [180–182]. These hand-held, disposable assays use small quantities of anticoagulated blood to determine the presence or absence of abnormal concentrations of cardiac proteins within 15–20min. Based on immunochromatic methods these assays allow qualitative determination of myocardial proteins by utilization of mono- or polyclonal antibodies directed against the target protein. Application of a defined amount of whole blood or plasma onto the test strip initiates the assay process. From whole blood samples cellular blood components are separated by a permeable membrane. If abnormal concentrations of cardiac markers are present, colour-labelled antibodies will bind to the proteins. By means of solid-phase technology the antibody-protein complex adheres to an immobilized ligand as part of the test kit and the process of antibody binding and migration finally results in an identifiable colour development at a specified region of the test kit.

The National Academy of Clinical Biochemistry as well as the ESC Task Force Report advise implementation of point-of-care testing systems if the hospital logistics cannot consistently deliver cardiac marker results within 1 hour [79, 183, 184]. Point-of-care techniques must be analytically accurate and equivalent to centralized laboratory methods. In large series, bedside tests results were validated against quantitative measurements and could be reliably performed by paramedical staff [117, 118, 185–187].

Reading of point-of-care tests is performed visually and therefore is observer dependent. A further major limitation is that visual assessment only allows a yes or no statement without definitive information regarding the concentration of the marker in the blood. In general, a darker or earlier developing signal line indicates a higher concentration of the marker in the sample but remains subjective. Careful reading exactly at the assay-specific indicated time under good illumination is essential to avoid observer misinterpretation especially in cases of marginal antibody binding. Even the faintest colouring should be read as a positive test result. No special skill or prolonged training is required to read the result of these assays. Accordingly, these tests can be performed by a variety of members of the health-care team [188]. Numerous studies have shown that point-of-care test systems are reliable, provided the above precautions were taken into consideration [117, 189]. Time to signal appearance (<10min) has been shown to identify a subgroup of patients that is at particular risk [190]. Nowadays, an optical reading system for most point of care tests is offered which also provides a printout of the quantitative result [187, 191].

Multimarker approach in clinical practice

Since ACS is a complex event, several markers reflecting the respective pathophysiological pathways may be advantageous for risk stratification (➲Fig. 16.17). Markers for the acute risk of myocardial infarction and for long-term mortality can be distinguished. The combined use of markers for myocardial necrosis, inflammation, and neurohumoral activation may significantly add to our ability to correctly identify patients who are at high risk for future cardiovascular events. Several studies have demonstrated that a multimarker approach improves risk stratification [27, 192]. Currently, it is advised to use troponins for the acute risk stratification on arrival of the patient in the hospital. During the subsequent days, BNP or NTproBNP allows estimation of the area that was at risk during the acute event and the impact on long-term outcome. For the detection of

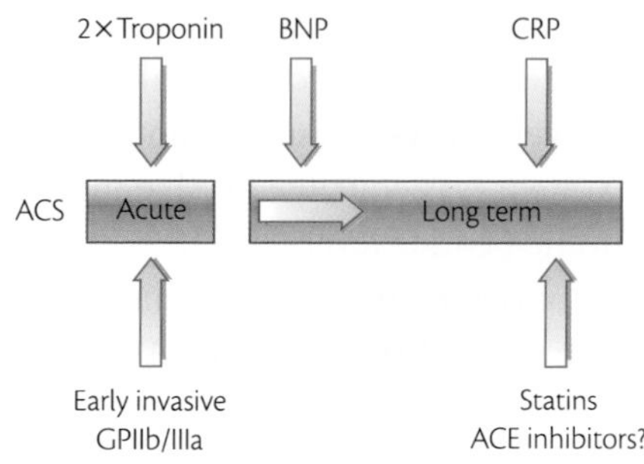

Figure 16.17 Multimarker testing in ACS during hospitalization.

the underlying inflammatory activity being responsible for the long-term mortality of the patients, currently only CRP is available on a routine basis and may be measured at the time before discharge.

Novel biomarkers

There are still a considerable number of patients who are at increased risk undetectable by established biomarkers currently available for routine use, i.e. troponins, BNP, and hsCRP. Since the pathophysiology of ACS is complex, not a single marker but a combination of markers will likely be used in the future, resembling different mechanisms. Accordingly, the search goes on for a combination of ideal markers with the aim to further improve diagnosis and risk assessment.

In the last decade an inflationary number of novel biomarkers have been identified and investigated. This has become possible for several reasons. The advanced understanding of the underlying pathophysiology of atherosclerosis and atherothrombosis allowed the examination of numerous enzymes, cytokines, adhesion molecules, and soluble receptors as potentially useful biomarkers. In addition, new technologies enabling a proteomic and genomic approach were capable of identifying new proteins or genes associated with different disease states. Furthermore, existing serum and plasma banks from large clinical trials were available to perform retrospective studies on the prognostic and diagnostic value of these novel biomarkers.

From an academic perspective, it can be distinguished between markers reflecting platelet activation, coagulation, endothelial dysfunction, inflammation, plaque destabilization and rupture, ischaemia and necrosis, as well as myocardial stress (➲Fig. 16.18). Many have yielded promising results but are still far from introduction into clinical routine and must undergo different phases of evaluation. This roadmap includes various steps from first experimental studies, studies on analytical and preanalytic conditions, followed by clinical studies as a proof of concept, confirmatory and comparative analyses, as well as interventional trials. A new marker can only be recommended for broad clinical application, if it is validated comprehensively and demonstrated that it provides incremental information which can be transferred in an improvement in patient care [193, 194].

Imaging modalities in acute coronary syndromes

Imaging modalities are secondary tools in the diagnosis of ACS. They usually only confirm or exclude the working diagnosis based on biochemical markers and the ECG.

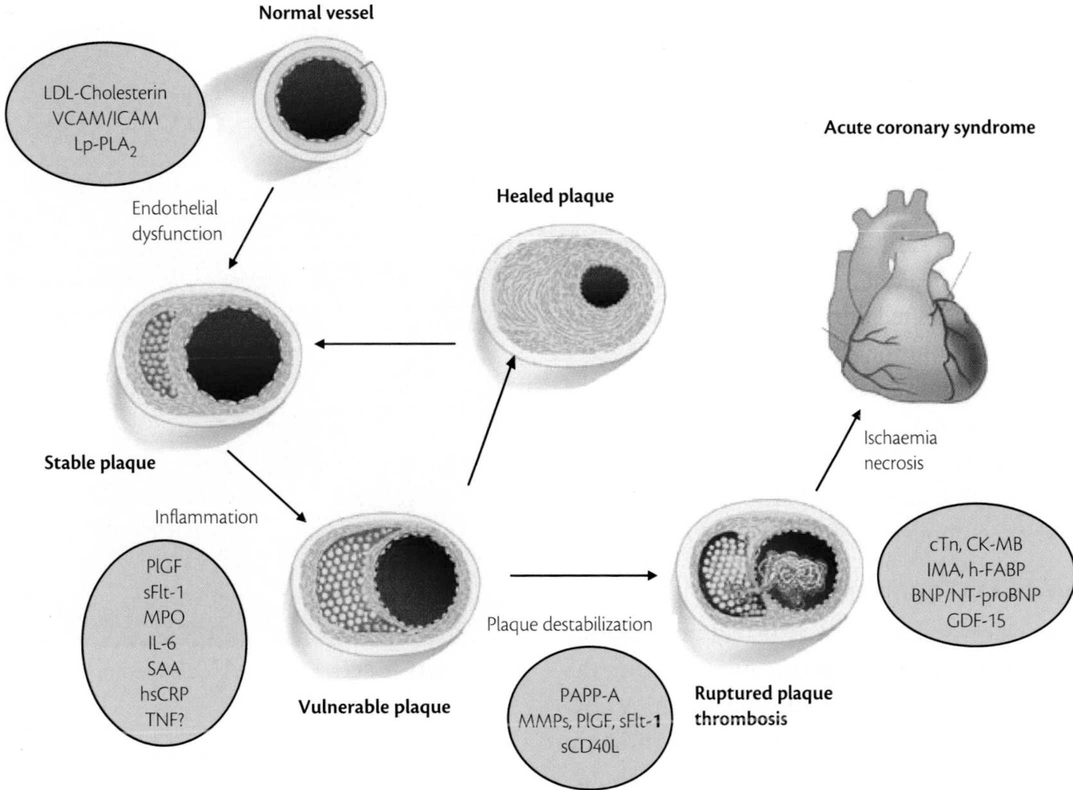

Figure 16.18 Biomarkers in acute coronary syndromes.

Coronary angiography

Coronary angiography is the gold standard to prove or exclude CAD. Patients with multiple vessel disease as well as those with left main stenosis are at highest risk of serious cardiac events [195]. Angiographic assessment of the characteristics and location of the culprit lesion as well as other lesions is essential if revascularization is being considered. Complex, long, heavily calcified lesions, angulations, and extreme tortuosity of the vessel are indicators of risk. Highest risk is associated with the occurrence of filling defects indicating intra coronary thrombus formation. In approximately 10–15% of patients presenting with chest pain no high-grade lesion can be identified, or CAD is excluded. Also see ➲Chapter 8.

Cardiac computed tomography

Currently, cardiac computed tomography (CT) cannot replace coronary angiography in ACS, because of its still suboptimal diagnostic accuracy. Furthermore, because of the high likelihood of a percutaneous intervention, time is lost and the patient is exposed to unnecessary radiation and contrast medium utilization, if CT is used as the first diagnostic option. Also see ➲Chapter 6.

Two-dimensional echocardiography

Two-dimensional echocardiography in experienced hands is a useful bedside technique in the triage of patients with acute chest pain. Left ventricular systolic function is an important prognostic variable in patients with ischaemic heart disease which can easily and accurately be assessed by echocardiography. Regional wall-motion abnormalities occur within seconds after coronary occlusion well before necrosis. However, these are not specific for acute events and may be the result of old infarction. Transient localized hypokinesia or akinesia in segments of the left ventricle wall may be detected during ischaemia, with normal wall motion on resolution of ischaemia. The absence of wall-motion abnormalities excludes major myocardial infarction. Echocardiography is of additional value for the diagnosis of other causes of chest pain such as acute aortic dissection, hypertrophic cardiomyopathy, pericarditis, or massive pulmonary embolism [196]. Also see ➲Chapter 4.

Myocardial perfusion scintigraphy

Myocardial perfusion scintigraphy is usually not readily available and is therefore only infrequently used for the triage of patients presenting with acute chest pain. A normal resting technetium-99 myocardial perfusion scintigram effectively excludes major myocardial infarction. An abnormal acute scintigram is not diagnostic of acute infarction unless it is known previously to have been normal, but it does indicate the presence of CAD and the need for further evaluation.

Magnetic resonance imaging

Cardiac magnetic resonance (CMR) imaging is a new technology, which is available in an increasing number of centres. CMR is not yet capable of imaging coronary arteries in routine settings. However, the multimodality characteristic of CMR provides a comprehensive examination, combining regional contractile function, myocardial perfusion, and viability. This allows identification of patients with ACS and differentiation of patients with myocardial infarction. More importantly, CMR can rule out other potential causes for acute chest pain, such as myocarditis, pericarditis, aortic dissection, and pulmonary embolism (➲Fig. 16.19) [105, 197]. Also see ➲Chapter 5.

Risk scores

Risk scores summarize various parameters to improve risk assessment. Several scores have been developed and validated in large patient populations. Although the contributions of individual risk factors are difficult to estimate at the bedside for each individual patient, established risk-score

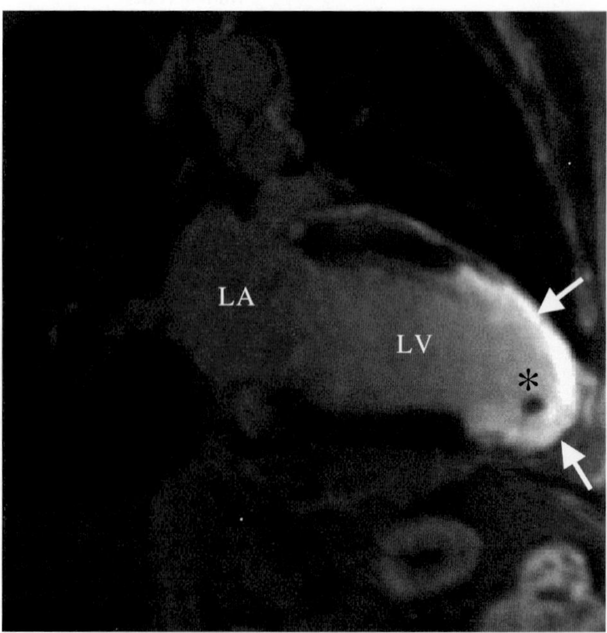

Figure 16.19 Vertical long axis of the left ventricle (LV) using an inversion recovery T1-weighted gradient echo sequence 10 min after injection of gadolinium DTPA showing a large region of hyperenhancement in the anterior wall and the apex (i.e. late enhancement) representing a transmural infarction (arrow). An apical thrombus shows no contrast uptake (*). LA, left atrium.

tools like GRACE or TIMI provide simple methods to estimate the risk of death and MI, and hence guide in-hospital and postdischarge management.

The GRACE risk scores [198, 199] are based upon a large unselected population of an international registry of full spectrum of ACS patients. The risk factors were derived with independent predictive power for in-hospital deaths [200] and post-discharge deaths at 6 months [9]. Easy to assess variables such as age, heart rate, systolic blood pressure, serum creatinine level, Killip class at admission, presence of ST deviation, and elevated cardiac biomarkers as well as cardiac arrest are included in the simplified calculation. The models were validated in various study populations and registries exhibiting good discriminative power. Their complexity, however, requires special tools (graphs, tables, or computer programs) to estimate risk at the bedside. Computer or PDA software of a simplified nomogram are freely available at http://www.outcomes.org/grace (➲Fig. 16.20). According to the GRACE risk score result three risk categories have been developed for NSTE-ACS (➲Table 16.10). Based on direct comparisons [200], the GRACE risk score is recommended as preferred classification in NSTE-ACS to apply on admission and at discharge in daily clinical routine practice. Similar predictive value was evidenced for patients presenting with ST-elevations [198].

The TIMI risk score for unstable angina/non-ST elevation MI is derived from the TIMI-11B trial population and was validated in various patient cohorts as well as applied in analyzing treatment efficacy in various risk groups [201]. It is less accurate in predicting events, but its simplicity makes it useful. For STEMI, the TIMI risk score is a weighted integer score that can be easily assed on admission based

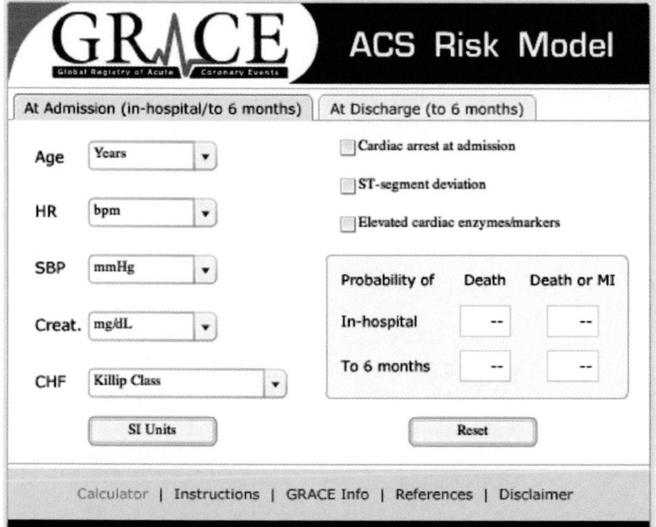

Figure 16.20 GRACE ACS risk model.

Table 16.10 Risk assessment according to the GRACE risk score [198, 199]

Risk category (in hospital) (tertiles)	GRACE risk score	In-hospital deaths (%)
Low	≤108	<1
Intermediate	109–140	1–3
High	>140	>3
Risk category (6 months) (tertiles)	**GRACE risk score**	**Post-discharge to 6 months deaths (%)**
Low	≤88	<3
Intermediate	89–118	3–8
High	>118	>8

upon data from clinical trials and tested in STEMI populations [202, 203]. This score allocates points on the basis of historical and clinical findings in addition to ST-segment elevation or left bundle branch block on the ECG and time to reperfusion of >4 hours. Application of the data to registry patients demonstrated a higher risk of death than in the overall trial populations [204]. Among patients not receiving reperfusion therapy the risk score underestimated death rates and offered lower discriminatory capacity. Nevertheless, this score provides a simple and valid bedside tool for the triage of patients into different risk categories.

Risk stratification in NSTE-ACS

The treatment of the individual patient with NSTE-ACS is tailored according to the risk for subsequent events and should be assessed immediately at the initial presentation as well as repeatedly thereafter in the light of continuing or repetitive symptoms and additional information from clinical chemistry or imaging modalities. It has to be distinguished between short-term and long-term risk. The short-term risk is related to the acute thrombotic event, whereas the long-term risk is determined by the progression of the underlying disease.

The algorithm for the work-up of patients presenting with chest pain to the emergency room is depicted in ➲Fig. 16.21. Based on the ECG the patient will be assigned to ST or NSTE-ACS. In NSTE-ACS troponin elevations play the central role for the acute risk assessment. Patients with persistent or recurrent angina associated with dynamic ST-segment depression or deep negative T waves, critical arrhythmias (ventricular tachycardia, ventricular fibrillation), or haemodynamic instability (symptoms of shock) can be assigned to high risk before the troponin result is available prompting immediate invasive evaluation. Increased risk is also associated with features like diabetes, renal dysfunction or reduced left ventricular function.

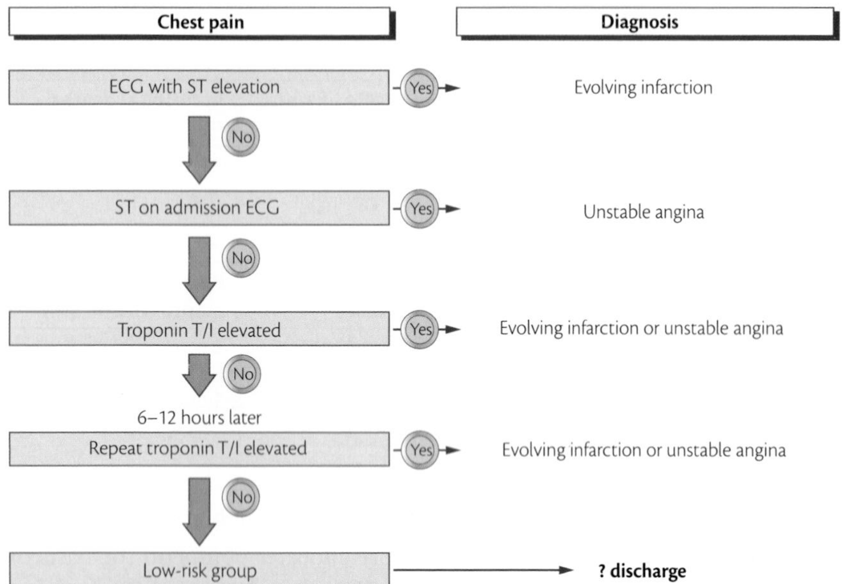

Figure 16.21 Algorithm of work-up of patients with chest pain.

The long-term risk of mortality is related to well-established parameters. These include age and the established risk factors. From imaging modalities the extent of CAD (main stem lesion) and reduced left ventricular function are predictors of future outcome. Biochemical markers of inflammation (CRP), myocardial stress (BNP, NT-proBNP), and of renal insufficiency (creatinine clearance) are further strongly associated with increased mortality.

Risk stratification in STEMI

Analysis of the risk for adverse outcome after presentation with STEMI is most important in guiding management and therapeutic decisions in the acute phase and after discharge. However, the use of any risk assessment tool should not lead to delays in providing the time-sensitive assessment and treatment strategies that patients with STEMI require.

Five rather simple baseline parameters can be used to independently predict >90% of the 30-day mortality: older age, lower systolic blood pressure, Killip class, elevated heart rate, and anterior infarct location [205]. Other independent predictors are previous infarction, height, time to treatment, diabetes, weight, and smoking status (➲Fig. 16.22).

The prognosis of myocardial infarction is related to the extent of myocardium at risk and thereby related to the site of coronary occlusion. Patients with main stem occlusions only rarely reach the hospital for reperfusion therapy. Occlusion of the proximal left anterior descending coronary artery proximal to the first septal branch is associated

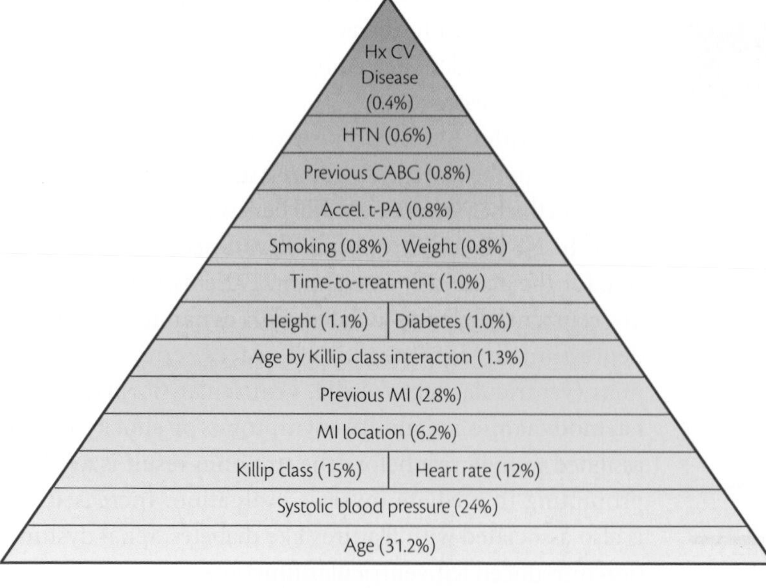

Figure 16.22 Multivariate model of 30-day mortality according to GUSTO I trial. Adapted with permission from Lee KL, Woodlief LH, Topol EJ, *et al.* Predictors of 30-day mortality in the era of reperfusion for acute myocardial infarction. Results from an international trial of 41,021 patients. GUSTO-I Investigators. *Circulation* 1995; **91**: 1659–68. Hx, history.

with high early and late mortality ('widow-maker'). Large inferior myocardial infarction as a result of occlusion of a dominant right coronary artery is also a high risk, particularly when the right ventricle is involved. Other locations, such as apical (distal left anterior descending), lateral (diagonal branch), or small inferior infarction (distal right or circumflex), show ST-segment elevations in only a few leads and have a better outcome. Strictly posterior myocardial infarction (marginal branch of left circumflex) may escape routine ECG leads or only be evident through ST depression in V1 to V4, but usually have a good outcome.

The ECG allows the rough location of the infarct artery and identification of the extent of the territory at risk. The development of a bundle branch block or atrioventricular block in anterior myocardial infarction suggests involvement of a proximal septal artery and is associated with increased mortality. Atrioventricular blocks in inferior myocardial infarction are frequent and mostly transient.

The haemodynamic impact of the evolving myocardial infarction is clinically most evident by the symptoms of shock. The Killip classification is widely used and linked to outcome. Killip class IV ('cardiogenic shock') is found in about 5% of AMI patients and is associated with extremely high mortality of up to 80%, particularly if associated with mechanical complications (septal rupture) [206, 207].

Blood sampling for serum markers must be routinely performed in the acute phase, but one should not wait for the results to initiate reperfusion treatment. The finding of elevated markers of necrosis may sometimes be helpful (e.g. in patients with left bundle branch block), but should not retard decision making. Elevation of markers of necrosis (troponin) on arrival in hospital is associated with adverse outcome [208]. Natriuretic peptides measured 2–4 days after admission have shown to represent potent predictors of long-term mortality [209].

Outcome of patients with STEMI is related to reperfusion success. However, epicardial flow proved to be inadequate to completely reflect myocardial perfusion. Abnormal microvascular perfusion appears the better indicator with prognostic implications. Useful techniques to assess microperfusion are the blush grade on angiography and myocardial contrast echocardiography. A relatively simple and readily available tool is the ECG ST-segment resolution in the lead showing the worst initial deviation that exceeds 50% at 60–90min after reperfusion [210]. This surrogate marker for mortality is also associated with enhanced recovery of LV function, reduced infarct size. More than 70% ST-segment resolution has more predictive value than infarct artery patency [211].

Differential diagnoses

There are several cardiac and non-cardiac conditions that may mimic ACS (see ➲Table 16.3). Underlying chronic heart conditions such as hypertrophic cardiomyopathy and valvular heart disease (i.e. aortic stenosis, aortic regurgitation) may be associated with typical clinical symptoms, elevated cardiac biomarkers, and ECG changes [212]. Since some patients with these underlying conditions also have CAD, the diagnostic process can be difficult.

Myocarditis, pericarditis, or myopericarditis of different aetiologies may be associated with chest pain that resembles the typical angina of ACS and be associated with a rise in cardiac biomarker levels, ECG changes, and wall motion abnormalities. A flu-like, febrile condition, with symptoms attributed to the upper respiratory tract often precedes or accompanies these conditions. However, infections, especially of the upper respiratory tract, also often precede or accompany ACS [212, 213]. The definitive diagnosis of myocarditis or myopericarditis may frequently only be established during the course of hospitalization.

Some non-cardiac, life-threatening conditions may mimic ACS and must be diagnosed. Among these, pulmonary embolism may be associated with dyspnoea, chest pain, ECG changes, as well as elevated levels of cardiac biomarkers similar to that of ACS [214]. Aortic dissection is another condition to be considered as an important differential diagnosis. ACS may be a complication of aortic dissection when the dissection involves the coronary arteries. In a patient with undiagnosed aortic dissection, the current antithrombotic therapies for ACS may exacerbate the patient's condition and result in detrimental outcomes. Stroke may be accompanied by ECG changes, wall motion abnormalities, and a rise in cardiac biomarker levels [198]. Conversely, atypical symptoms such as headache and vertigo may in rare cases be the sole presentation of myocardial ischaemia.

Treatment of non-ST-elevation acute coronary syndromes

The treatment options in patients with NSTEMI-ACS are based on evidence from numerous clinical trials or meta-analyses. Four categories of acute treatment are discussed: anti-ischaemic agents, anticoagulants, antiplatelet agents, and coronary revascularization. In general, the therapeutic approach is based on whether the patient is to be only medically treated, or in addition referred to angiography and revascularization.

Anti-ischaemic agents

These drugs decrease myocardial oxygen consumption (decreasing heart rate, lowering blood pressure or depressing LV contractility) and/or induce vasodilatation. Thereby they reduce ischaemia and relieve angina.

Nitrates

Nitrates are the oldest drugs used in treatment of angina. Their use in patients with ACS is largely based on pathophysiological considerations and clinical experience. The therapeutic benefits of nitrates and similar drug classes such as sydnonimines are related to their effects on the peripheral and coronary circulation. The major therapeutic benefit is probably related to the venodilator effects that lead to a decrease in myocardial preload and LV end-diastolic volume resulting in a decrease in myocardial oxygen consumption. In addition, nitrates dilate normal as well as atherosclerotic coronary arteries and increase coronary collateral flow (➲Chapter 11).

Studies of nitrates in unstable angina have been small and observational [215–217]. There are no randomized placebo controlled trials to confirm the benefits of this class of drugs either in relieving symptoms or in reducing major adverse cardiac events. Only very scarce data exist about the best route for administrating nitrates (intravenous, oral or sublingual or topical), and about the optimal dose and duration of therapy [218, 219].

In patients with NSTE-ACS who require hospital admission, intravenous nitrates may be considered in the absence of contraindications. The dose should be titrated upwards until symptoms (angina and/or dyspnoea) are relieved unless side effects (notably headache or hypotension) occur. A limitation of continuous nitrate therapy is the phenomenon of tolerance, which is related both to the dose administered and to the duration of treatment. When symptoms are controlled, intravenous nitrates may be replaced by nonparenteral alternatives with appropriate nitrate-free intervals. An alternative is to use nitrate-like drugs, such as sydnonimines or potassium channel activators.

Beta-blockers

Evidence for the beneficial effects of beta-blockers in unstable angina is based on limited randomized trial data, along with pathophysiological considerations and extrapolation from experience in stable angina and STEMI. Beta-blockers competitively inhibit the myocardial effects of circulating catecholamines. In NSTE-ACS, the primary benefits of beta-blockers are related to their effects on beta-1 receptors that result in a decrease in myocardial oxygen consumption.

Only two trials have compared beta-blockers to placebo in unstable angina [220, 221]. A meta-analysis suggested that beta-blocker treatment was associated with a 13% relative reduction in risk of progression to STEMI [222]. Although no significant effect on mortality in NSTE-ACS has been demonstrated in these relatively small trials, the results may be extrapolated from larger randomized trials of beta-blockers in patients with unselected MI [223].

Beta-blockers are recommended in NSTE-ACS in the absence of contraindications and are usually well tolerated. In most cases oral treatment is sufficient. The target heart rate for a good treatment effect should be between 50–60 bpm. Patients with significantly impaired atrioventricular conduction, a history of asthma or of acute LV dysfunction should not receive beta-blockers (see ➲Chapter 11).

Calcium-channel blockers

There are three subclasses of calcium blockers which are chemically distinct and have different pharmacological effects: the dihydropyridines (such as nifedipine), the benzothiazepines (such as diltiazem), and the phenylalkylamines (such as verapamil). The agents in each subclass vary in the degree to which they cause vasodilatation, decrease myocardial contractility and delay atrioventricular (AV) conduction. AV block may be induced by non-dihydropyridines. Nifedipine and amlodipine produce the most marked peripheral arterial vasodilatation, whereas diltiazem has the least vasodilatory effect. All subclasses cause similar coronary vasodilatation (see ➲Chapter 11).

There are only small trials testing calcium-channel blockers in NSTE-ACS. Generally, they show efficacy in relieving symptoms that appears equivalent to beta-blockers [224, 225]. A larger randomized trial tested nifedipine and metoprolol [221]. Although no statistically significant differences were observed, there was a trend towards an increased risk of MI or recurrent angina with nifedipine (compared to placebo), whereas treatment with metoprolol, or with a combination of both drugs, was associated with a reduction in these events.

The beneficial effect after discharge is somewhat controversial [226, 227]. A meta-analysis of the effects of calcium-channel blockers on death or non-fatal MI in unstable angina suggests that this class of drugs does not prevent the development of acute MI or reduce mortality [228]. In particular, several analyses of pooled data from observational studies suggest that short-acting nifedipine might be associated with a dose-dependent detrimental effect on mortality in patients with coronary heart disease [229, 230]. On the other hand, there is evidence for a protective role of diltiazem in NSTEMI in one trial [231]. Nevertheless, calcium-channel blockers, particularly dihydropyridines are the drugs of choice in vaso-spastic angina.

Newer drugs

New antianginal drugs with different modes of action have been investigated in recent years. Ranolazine exerts antianginal effects by inhibiting the late sodium current [232], but failed to an impact on outcome in NSTEMI-ACS [233]. Ivabradine selectively inhibits the primary pacemaker current in the sinus node and could be used in patients with beta-blocker contraindications [234]. Trimetazidine exerts metabolic effects without haemodynamic changes [235]. Nicorandil has nitrate-like properties and significantly reduced the rate of occurrence of the composite endpoint of coronary death, non-fatal MI or unplanned hospital admission for cardiac pain in chronic stable angina patients [236]. However, none of these drugs have been shown to improve outcome in the setting of NSTE-ACS (see ➲Chapter 17).

Anticoagulants

Anticoagulants are used in the treatment of NSTE-ACS to inhibit thrombin generation and/or activity, thereby reducing thrombus-related events. Anticoagulation is effective in addition to platelet inhibition and the combination of the two is more effective than either treatment alone [237, 238]. With all anticoagulants, there is an increased risk of bleeding. Several anticoagulants have been investigated in NSTE-ACS, namely, unfractionated heparin (UFH), low-molecular-weight heparin (LMWH), fondaparinux, direct thrombin inhibitors (DTI), and vitamin-K antagonists (VKA).

Unfractionated heparin

UFH is a heterogenous mixture of polysaccharide molecules, with a molecular weight ranging from 2000–30,000 (mostly 15,000–18,000) Daltons. One-third of the molecules only contain the pentasaccharide sequence, which binds to antithrombin and accelerates the rate at which antithrombin inhibits factor-Xa. Inhibition of factor-IIa is achieved only if the chains containing the pentasaccharide sequence comprise at least 18 saccharide units. Intravenous infusion is the preferred route of administration. The therapeutic window is narrow, requiring frequent monitoring of activated partial thromboplastin time (aPTT), with an optimal target level of 50–75s, corresponding to 1.5–2.5 times the upper limit of normal. The weight adjusted regimen, most likely to achieve target aPTT values is an initial bolus of 60–70IU/kg (maximum of 5000IU), followed by an infusion of 12–15IU/kg/hour, to a maximum of 1000IU/hour [237]. Heparin-induced thrombocytopenia is not infrequent with UFH, and may be associated with severe thrombotic complications.

The meta-analysis of six trials testing short-term UFH vs. placebo or untreated controls showed a significant risk reduction for death and MI of 33% [239]. In trials testing UFH in aspirin-treated patients, a trend towards a benefit was observed in favour of the UFH-aspirin combination, but at the cost of an increase in the risk of bleeding [239] (➲Fig. 16.23).

Low-molecular-weight heparins

LMWH represent a class of heparin-derived compounds with molecular weights ranging from 2000–10,000 Daltons. Anti-Xa activity is achieved thanks to linkage of the pentasaccharide sequence to antithrombin. The anti-IIa

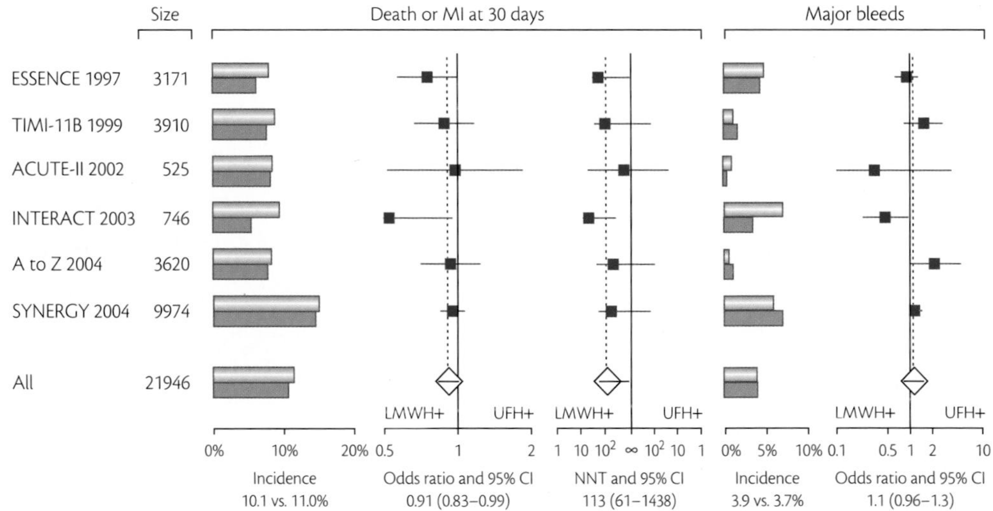

Figure 16.23 Death, myocardial infarction, and major bleeds at 30 days in randomized trials of Enoxaparin (dark blue bars) vs. UFH (light blue bars). NNT = number of patients who needed to be treated to avoid one event.

activity is lower than with UFH and depends on the molecular weight of the molecule. LMWHs are almost completely absorbed after subcutaneous administration. Protein binding and platelet activation are lower with LMWH than with UFH so that the dose-effect relationship is more predictable. The risk of heparin-induced thrombocytopenia is lower with LMWH as compared to UFH. As LMWH are partially eliminated by the renal route, in patients with a CrCl <30mL/min a replacement by other substances should be considered or their dose has to be carefully adjusted. LMWH are injected subcutaneously every 12 hours in NSTE-ACS at body-weight adjusted doses. An initial intravenous bolus in high risk patients has also been advocated. Monitoring of anti-Xa activity is not necessary, except in special populations of patients, such as those with renal failure and obesity [236].

Dalteparin in aspirin-treated patients led to a significant risk reduction for death and MI, with a modest increase in bleeding risk. Dalteparin and nadroparin were shown to be equally as efficacious and safe as UFH in aspirin-treated patients. Enoxaparin is the most widely investigated LMWH. In a meta-analysis of all enoxaparin trials, a significant 9% reduction in the combined endpoint of death or MI was observed at 30 days in favour of enoxaparin vs. UFH [240]. LMWH have been used in combination with aspirin, thienopyridines and GP IIb/IIIa inhibitors in many recent trials or observational studies. No significant increase in the risk of bleeding was observed as compared to UFH in the same situation (➲Fig. 16.24).

Selective factor Xa Inhibitor (fondaparinux)

Fondaparinux is a synthetic pentasaccharide that exerts a selective, indirect, anti-thrombin mediated inhibition of factor Xa. It has a 100% bio-availability after subcutaneous injection and a long half life, and can therefore be given once daily. It is eliminated mainly by the renal route, and is contraindicated if CrCl is <20mL/min. No formally-documented case of heparin-induced thrombocytopenia has been reported with this drug. Monitoring of platelet count is therefore not necessary. In NSTE-ACS, a 2.5-mg fixed dose is recommended. No monitoring of anti-Xa activity is required [237, 238].

Fondaparinux was tested versus enoxaparin in the Oasis-5 study [241]. Similar efficacy was observed with both drugs at 9 days in terms of death, MI and refratory ischaemia. At the same timepoint, major bleeds were halved with fondaparinux (2.2% versus 4.1%). At 30 days and 6 months, there was a significant risk reduction for death. The composite outcome of death, MI or stroke was significantly lower (−11%) with fondaparinux as compared to enoxaparin at 30 days, and at 6 months. In patients submitted to PCI, thrombus formation on the angioplasty material during PCI was observed in both groups, though at a significantly higher rate with fondaparinux than with enoxaparin.

Direct thrombin inhibitors

DTI bind directly to thrombin (factor-IIa) and thereby inhibit the thrombin-induced conversion of fibrinogen to fibrin. They inactivate fibrin-bound and fluid-phase thrombin. As they do not bind to plasma proteins, the anticoagulant effect is more predictable. Currently several DTI (hirudin, argatroban, bivalirudin) are available. Monitoring of the anticoagulant activity of hirudin and bivalirudin can be achieved with aPTT. There is no risk of heparin-induced thrombocytopenia. Hirudin and its derivatives are eliminated by the renal route, therefore, dose adaptation is needed in case of sever renal failure. No striking advantages have been observed in initial trials with hirudin versus UFH in the setting of NSTE-ACS [237, 241].

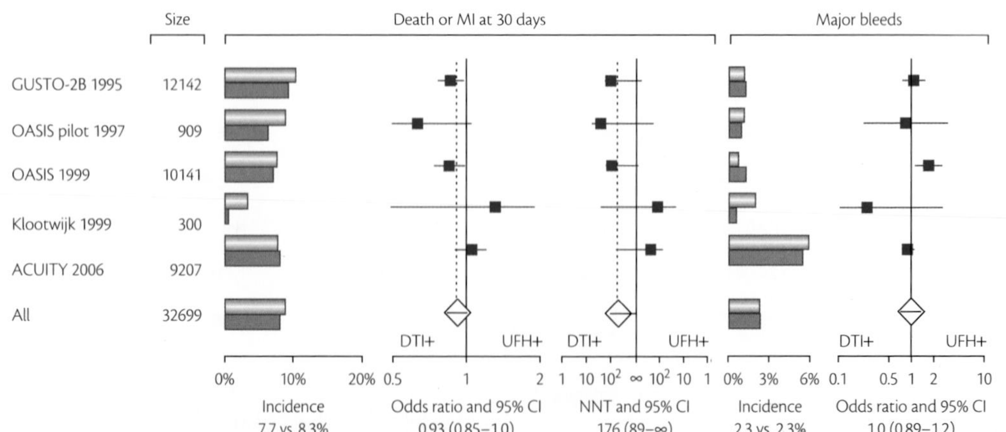

Figure 16.24 Death, myocardial infarction, and major bleeds at 30 days in randomized trials of direct thrombin inhibitors (dark blue bars) vs. unfractionated heparin/low-molecular-weight heparin (light blue bars). NNT = number of patients who needed to be treated to avoid one event. (For ACUITY, the arms unfractionated heparin/low-molecular-weight heparin and bivalirudin both with glycoprotein IIb/IIIa inhibitors as background therapy are presented. In addition, the composite ischaemic endpoint includes unplanned revascularization.)

Bivalirudin was tested in the ACUITY (Acute Catheterization and Urgent Intervention Triage Strategy) trial, in which patients with moderate to high risk NSTE-ACS planned for invasive strategy were included [240]. Bivalirudin alone as compared to a combination of anticoagulants plus systematic GP IIb/IIIa inhibitors was shown to be non-inferior in preventing ischaemic events (7.3% vs. 7.7%, respectively) in the whole population. However, in patients not pretreated with clopidogrel a significant 29% excess of composite ischaemic endpoints was observed for bivalirudin alone vs. UFH/LMWH plus GP IIb/IIIa inhibitors. A significant risk reduction for bleeding (3.0% vs. 5.7%, −47%) was also observed with bivalirudin alone, but without impact on the rate of death or further ischaemic events as observed in other trials [241].

Vitamin-K-antagonists

VKA have been tested as long-term treatment following ACS with INR ranging from 2–3. VKA treatment and especially VKA in combination with aspirin were shown to be more effective than aspirin alone in the long-term prevention against death, re-MI and stroke, but at the cost of a higher risk of major bleeding [242]. VKA are mostly used in the presence of other indications for anticoagulation, such as atrial fibrillation, or after implantation of a mechanical heart valve. Treatment decisions must be made on an individualized basis and should include information on key factors, including bleeding and thromboembolic risks. The triple combination of VKA, aspirin and clopidogrel should be avoided because of a significant excess of bleeding was reported with this regimen [243].

Anticoagulants during PCI procedures

Aspirin and systemic anticoagulation with UFH is currently the standard of care in PCI [244]. UFH is administered as an intravenous bolus of 100IU/kg or 50–60IU/kg if GP IIb/IIIa inhibitors are given [244]. The efficacy of UFH can be monitored by activated clotting time (ACT), but the real utility of ACT monitoring remains controversial.

Bivalirudin was tested during PCI procedures in comparison to UFH/LMWH or bivalirudin plus GP IIb/IIIa inhibitors in ACUITY trial [245]. As already mentioned, a significant risk reduction for bleeding was observed with bivalirudin alone as compared to UFH/LMWH or bivalirudin with GP IIb/IIIa inhibitors, but with a significantly higher rate of ischaemic events in patients not pre-treated with clopidogrel.

Enoxaparin (1mg/kg twice daily) was compared to UFH as antithrombotic agent in a PCI setting in 4687 NSTE-ACS in the SYNERGY (Superior Yield of the New strategy of Enoxaparin, Revascularisation, and Glycoprotein IIb/IIIa inhibitors) trial. There was no difference in outcome during or after PCI, whatever the drug used in the catheterization laboratory. However, there was a strong trend towards an excess of bleeding (non-CABG-related TIMI major bleeds) with enoxaparin, as compared to UFH, possibly augmented by post-randomization crossover antithrombotic therapy [246]. Lower doses of enoxaparin may be favourable with respect to bleeding [247]. An additional 0.3mg/kg intravenous bolus of enoxaparin is recommended if the last subcutaneous injection was given >8 hours before PCI [237].

Enoxaparin and fondaparinux were used in the setting of PCI in 6239 patients in OASIS-5 (Fifth Organization to Assess Strategies in Acute Ischemic Syndromes). There was a significantly higher risk of vascular access site complications (+ 59%) with enoxaparin than with fondaparinux. However, catheter thrombi were significantly more common with fondaparinux as compared to enoxaparin (0.4% vs. 0.9%). Accordingly, a bolus dose of UFH (50IU/kg bodyweight) at the time of PCI is mandatory in case of PCI in patients initially treated with fondaparinux [241].

Summary

Fondaparinux has demonstrated a better efficacy-safety profile than enoxaparin, but it cannot be used as stand-alone anticoagulant in the setting of PCI, where an additional bolus of UFH has to be given. Enoxaparin can be used as initial anticoagulant and during PCI, and the indication for this drug has to be weighed against the bleeding risk. Bivalirudin was shown to be as efficacious as a combination of conventional anticoagulants plus GP IIb/IIIa inhibitors in the setting of PCI in NSTE-ACS, but safer as regards bleeding complications. Fondaparinux, enoxaparin and bivalirudin are either contraindicated, or require dose adaptation in case of severe renal failure. UFH can be used in all indications, but it is somewhat more cumbersome to use.

Antiplatelet therapy

Effective antiplatelet therapy is a cornerstone of treatment in ACS, since platelet activation and aggregation plays a key pathophysiological role. Platelets need to be seen not only in the frame of the acute plaque rupture, but also as a contributor to subsequent atherothrombotic events. Three complementary strategies provide effective platelet inhibition: cyclooxygenase-1 inhibition (acetylsalicylic acid, aspirin), inhibition of ADP mediated platelet activation with thienopyridines (clopidogrel, ticlopidine), and glycoprotein IIb/IIIa receptor inhibition (tirofiban, eptifibatide, abciximab).

Acetylsalicylic acid (aspirin)

Acetylsalicylic acid, commonly named aspirin, inhibits platelet activation by irreversible inhibition of platelet derived cyclooxygenase-1, thereby reducing the formation of thromboxane A2. In three trials conducted 20 years ago it was consistently shown that aspirin decreases death or myocardial infarction in patients with unstable angina [248–250]. The meta-analysis by the Antithrombotic Trialists Collaboration confirmed a 46% reduction in the rate of vascular events [251]. This meta-analysis also elucidated that 75–150mg aspirin is as effective as higher doses for chronic therapy. An initial dose of non-enteric (chewed or intravenously administered) aspirin from 160–325mg is recommended to minimize delay before platelet inhibition occurs [251]. In another meta-analysis, including four studies, the reduction in the rate of vascular events was 53%, with a number-needed-to-treat of 17 [238].

The most common side effect of aspirin is gastrointestinal intolerance, which occurs in 5–40% of aspirin-treated patients. Gastro-intestinal bleeding increases with higher doses [252]. Proven hypersensitivity ('allergy') to aspirin is rare, as its prevalence depends on the clinical manifestation. More serious reactions such as anaphylactic shock are extremely rare [253, 254]. Rarely aspirin-exacerbated asthma is observed. Aspirin-induced rash or skin manifestations occur in 0.2–0.7% of the general population.

Aspirin resistance refers to the variability in the magnitude of platelet aggregation inhibition measured *ex vivo* achieved in a treated population. Up to 50% of individuals exhibit a relative aspirin resistance in *ex vivo* tests. Some patients may develop treatment failure over time, even with increasing doses resulting in different degrees of thromboxane A2 inhibition and a difference in event rates [255]. However, until now an unequivocally accepted standard method for testing for aspirin resistance is missing.

Thienopyridines

Adenosine diphosphate (ADP) receptor antagonists block the ADP-induced pathway of platelet activation by specific inhibition of the P2Y12 receptor. The first compound used in ACS was ticlopidine [256] which today is replaced by clopidogrel because of potentially serious side effects, like the risk of neutropenia or thrombocytopenia. New antiplatelet agents that block the P2Y12 receptor with more potent receptor affinity and more rapid onset of action are currently introduced to the market or still under evaluation (e.g. prasugrel, AZD6240, cangrelor).

The value of clopidogrel on top of aspirin (75–325mg) vs. aspirin alone was demonstrated in the large CURE (Clopidogrel in Unstable Angina to Prevent Recurrent Ischemic Events) trial. Patients received placebo or a loading dose of 300mg clopidogrel followed by 75mg daily in addition to conventional therapy. A 20% risk reduction at 12 months for death from cardiovascular causes, non fatal MI, or stroke was observed in the treatment arm. The risk reduction was significant for myocardial infarction, and there was a trend towards reduction of death and stroke. The risk reduction was consistent across all risk groups as well as various subsets of patients (elderly, ST deviation, with or without elevated cardiac biomarkers, diabetic patients) [257]. The benefit was obtained early, with a significant 34% risk reduction of cardiovascular death, myocardial infarction, stroke or severe ischaemia at 24 hours in the clopidogrel group (1.4% vs. 2.1%, OR, 0.66; 95% CI, 0.51–0.86, p <0.01) and was maintained throughout the 12 months of the study period (➲Fig. 16.25).

In the TRITON–TIMI (Trial to Assess Improvement in Therapeutic Outcomes by Optimizing Platelet Inhibition with Prasugrel Thrombolysis in Myocardial Infarction) 38 trial the third generation thienopyridine prasugrel was compared with clopidogrel in patients with ACS undergoing PCI [258]. Prasugrel is more rapid in onset, more consistent and more potent in action. In the population of patients with UA/NSTEMI followed for 6–15 months, a 18% reduction in the primary endpoint of cardiovascular death, non-fatal MI or non-fatal stroke was observed with prasugrel (12.1% vs. 9.9%).

Bleeding risk

A major concern is the risk of bleeding of dual antiplatelet treatment, because there is no known antidote to clopidogrel or other ADP receptor antagonists (➲Fig. 16.26). In CURE, an increased rate of major bleedings was observed in clopidogrel plus aspirin treated patients (3.7% vs. 2.7%, RR, 1.38; 95% CI, 1.13–1.67, p =0.001), but with a non-significant increase in life-threatening and fatal bleeds.

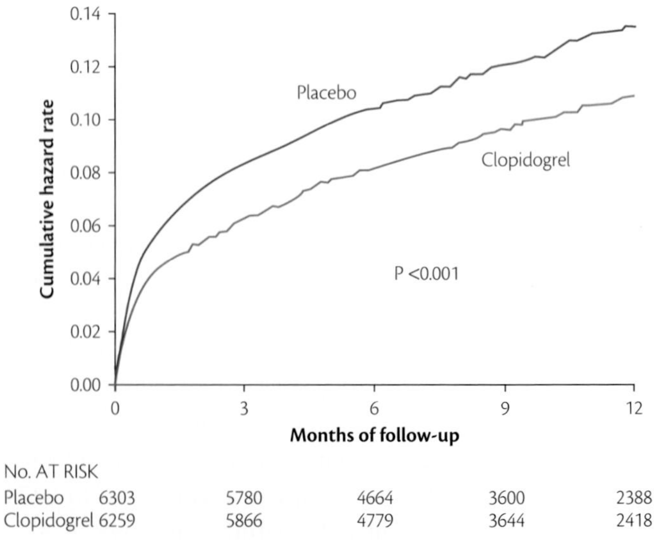

Figure 16.25 Cumulative hazard rates for the first primary outcome (death from cardiovascular causes, nonfatal myocardial, or stroke) during the 12 Months of the study.

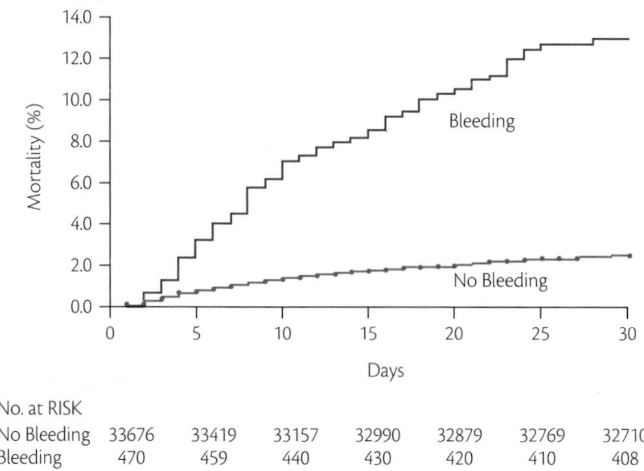

No. at RISK							
No Bleeding	33676	33419	33157	32990	32879	32769	32710
Bleeding	470	459	440	430	420	410	408

Figure 16.26 Kaplan-Meier estimates of mortality during the first 30 days among patients who developed and those who did not develop major bleeding. According to Eikelboom JW, Mehta SR, Anand SS, *et al.* Adverse impact of bleeding on prognosis in patients with acute coronary syndromes. *Circulation* 2006; **114**: 774–82.

Bleeding rates were higher in patients who underwent CABG, but this reached only borderline significance in 912 patients submitted to surgery <5 days after cessation of clopidogrel treatment (9.6% vs. 6.3%, RR, 1.53; 95% CI, 0.97–2.40, p =0.06). For those treated >5 days after interruption of clopidogrel there was no significant increase in bleeding [259]. However, in the entire cohort, the benefit of clopidogrel treatment, including among patients submitted to revascularization by both PCI and CABG, outweighed the risk of bleeding. In total, treating 1000 patients resulted in 21 fewer cardiovascular deaths, MI or stroke, at the cost of an excess of 7 patients requiring transfusions, and a trend for 4 patients to experience life-threatening bleeds [259]. The excess bleeding risk in patients submitted to surgery can be attenuated or eliminated by stopping clopidogrel 5 days before surgery. However, it is not known whether this results in increased complication rates during wash-out.

In the TRITON – TIMI 38 study, treatment with prasugrel also resulted in more bleeding than with standard dose clopidogrel. The key safety endpoint of TIMI major bleeding was increased from 1.8 to 2.4% over 15 months (HR 1.32 [1.03–1.68], p =0.03). This increase in bleeding was also observed for life-threatening and fatal bleeding.

Dose and timing of clopidogrel

In patients with ACS it is recommended that clopidogrel be given at first contact both to prevent events prior to PCI and to allow adequate time for drug effect prior to PCI. It was shown in several trials that pretreatment of unselected patients with clopidogrel before angiography results in better outcome of PCI [260–262]. Accordingly, postponing clopidogrel administration until coronary anatomy is known by angiography is discouraged, as the highest rates of events are observed in the early phase of ACS. The only potential advantage of this approach is to reduce higher bleeding risk in patients requiring immediate surgery. However, this situation is rare and frequently surgery can be deferred safely by 5 days. In patients who cannot be given clopidogrel before PCI, GP IIb/IIIa inhibitors may be chosen alternatively.

Multiple smaller studies have tested higher loading doses of clopidogrel (600 or 900mg) demonstrating a more rapid inhibition of platelet aggregation than achieved with 300mg. However, no large-scale outcome clinical trials are yet available in the setting of ACS. Nevertheless, first clinical experience suggests that faster platelet inhibition with higher loading doses (600mg, ~2 hours) may be more effective in reducing clinical endpoints [263–266]. The definitive answer to the risk vs. benefit will be provided by ongoing large-scale clinical trials.

Clopidogrel resistance

Clopidogrel is an inactive compound, which needs oxidation by hepatic cytochrome P450 to generate an active metabolite. CYP3A4 and CYP3A5 are the P450 isoforms responsible for the oxidation of clopidogrel, which produce the active form of the drug. The standard dose of clopidogrel achieves approximately 30–50% inhibition of ADP induced platelet aggregation through antagonism to the P2Y12 platelet ADP receptor [267].

Clopidogrel resistance or more aptly termed variability in response is not clearly defined and depends on the in vitro test system used. With these limitations, clopidogrel resistance has been reported to occur in 4–30% of patients [267]; the incidence of dual nonresponiveness to clopidogrel and aspirin is 6%. The mechanism of clopidogrel resistance is still under investigation. Despite small studies that have shown higher rate of events associated with low inhibition of platelet aggregation [268–270] the clinical importance of this phenomenon remains uncertain.

Drug interaction

Reduced bio-availability through drug interactions has recently been discussed, particularly with particular statins which are metabolised by CYP3A4 and CYP3A5 and which have been shown in *in vitro* studies to limit by 90% the degradation of clopidogrel into its active metabolite form [267]. However, this has not been translated into any demonstrable negative clinical effect [271]. Indeed, in the GRACE registry, the combination of clopidogrel and statins is suggestive of an additive beneficial effect [272].

The combination of clopidogrel with oral vitamin K antagonists (warfarin, phencoumon) is recommended only after careful benefit risk assessment, since it may potentially increase the risk of bleeding. This combination can be necessary in the context of mechanical heart valves or in the case of high risk of thromboembolic events. Under these circumstances the lowest efficacious INR and shortest duration of clopidogrel treatment should be targeted.

Withdrawal of oral antiplatelet agents

Some reports have shown that in patients with CAD, withdrawal of antiplatelet agents may result in an increased rate of recurrence of events [273]. Similar as after coronary stenting, interruption of dual antiplatelet treatment soon after the acute phase of ACS may expose patients to a high risk of recurrence of events, even though only few data are available to support this notion. However, the interruption of dual antiplatelet therapy in case of necessary surgical procedures >1 month after ACS in patients without drug-eluting stents may be reasonable. If during the early phase interruption of dual antiplatelet therapy becomes mandatory, such as need for urgent surgery or major bleeding that cannot be controlled by local treatment, no proven effective alternative therapy can currently be recommended as a substitute. LMWHs have been advocated but without tangible proof of efficacy and safety.

Summary

A 300-mg loading dose of clopidogrel is recommended, followed by 75mg clopidogrel daily for patients with ACS. Clopidogrel should be maintained for at least 12 months unless there is an excessive risk of bleeding. Prolonged or permanent withdrawal of aspirin, clopidogrel or both is discouraged unless strongly clinically indicated. For all patients with aspirin contraindication clopidogrel should be given as substitute. In patients considered for an invasive procedure/PCI, a loading dose of 600mg of clopidogrel may be used to achieve more rapid inhibition of platelet function, although randomized evidence is not yet available. In patients pretreated with clopidogrel who need to undergo CABG, surgery should be postponed for 5 days for clopidogrel withdrawal if clinically feasible. The triple combination of aspirin, clopidogrel, and vitamin K antagonists (warfarin) should be restricted to compelling indications, in which case, the lowest efficacious INR and shortest duration of triple treatment should be anticipated.

Glycoprotein IIb/IIIa receptor inhibitors

Three GP IIb/IIIa inhibitors are approved for clinical use, the antibody fragment abciximab, as well as the small molecules eptifibatide and tirofiban. They block the final common pathway of platelet activation by binding to the fibrinogen and, under high shear conditions, to the von Willebrand factor, and thereby inhibiting the bridging between activated platelets. Abciximab is a monoclonal antibody fragment, eptifibatide is a cyclic peptide, and tirofiban a peptido-mimetic inhibitor. The results in randomized trials obtained with GP IIb/IIIa inhibitors differ according to their use in a conservative or an invasive strategy of ACS.

Conservative strategy

GP IIb/IIIa inhibitors have only a modest benefit on outcome in a conservative strategy. A meta-analysis including 31,402 ACS patients treated in clinical trials using GP IIb/IIIa inhibitors showed only a 9% risk reduction for death and MI at 30 days with GP IIb/IIIa inhibitors [274]. This risk reduction was consistent across multiple sub-groups, and was evident particularly in high risk patients, (diabetic patients, ST segment depression, troponin-positive patients) and in patients submitted to PCI during initial hospitalization. GP IIb/IIIa inhibitors had no effects in troponin-negative patients and in women. However, women with troponin release derived the same benefit as men. The use of GP IIb/IIIa inhibitors was associated with an increase in major bleeding complications, but intra-cranial bleeding was not significantly increased [274].

In a further meta-analysis the outcome as a function of the utilisation of GP IIb/IIIa inhibitors in patients initially medically managed and submitted to PCI was explored [275]. A 9% risk reduction overall was confirmed, but the benefit was non-significant in purely medically managed patients receiving GP IIb/IIIa inhibitors vs. placebo, with a rate of death and MI at 30 days of 9.3% vs. 9.7%. The only significant beneficial effect was observed when GP IIb/IIIa inhibitors were maintained during PCI (10.5% vs. 13.6%). These data confirm previous reports showing a risk reduction for ischaemic events in patients pre-treated with GP IIb/IIIa inhibitors before PCI [276, 277]. In diabetic patients, a meta-analysis showed a highly significant risk reduction for death at 30 days with the use of GP IIb/IIIa inhibitors [278], particularly pronounced when submitted to PCI.

Abciximab in a conservative management exhibited no benefit, but was associated with increased bleeding risk [279]. In contrast, for eptifibatide a significant reduction of the 30-day composite endpoint of death or non-fatal MI was observed (14.2 vs. 15.7%, eptifibatide vs. placebo, $p = 0.04$). The benefit was maintained over 6 months. There was an excess risk of TIMI major bleeding (10.6 vs. 9.1%, $p = 0.02$), but no excess of intracranial bleedings. The rate of mild or severe thrombocytopenia was not statistically different in both treatment arms. Tirofiban has been tested in two separate randomized trials against combination with or without UFH [280, 281]. The tirofiban-alone approach was associated with an excess of adverse events. However, a 32% reduction of the risk of death, MI, and refractory ischaemia was obtained at 7 days and maintained at 30 days and 6 months in the tirofiban plus UFH group, as compared to UFH alone in patients at high risk. Major bleeding complications were statistically not more frequent in the tirofiban group. In patients with less risk a 33% reduction in the composite endpoint of death, MI or refractory ischaemia was observed at 48 hours and maintained at 30 days, but not thereafter. However, the benefit was highly significant throughout follow-up in troponin positive patients [282]. The rate of thrombocytopenia (defined as platelet count <90,000/mm^3) was significantly more frequent with tirofiban than with UFH (1.1% vs. 0.4%, p = 0.04).

Invasive strategy

GP IIb/IIIa inhibitors exert their beneficial potential best in patients with ACS and planned invasive management. Consistent results have been obtained in three different meta-analyses exploring the impact of the use of GP IIb/IIIa inhibitors in the setting of PCI. Two meta-analyses showed that a significant risk reduction for death and MI at 30 days could be achieved when GP IIb/IIIa inhibitors were administered before taking patients to the catheterization laboratory, and maintained during PCI [275, 276]. Another meta-analysis demonstrated a 27% risk reduction in 30-day mortality among a total of 20,186 patients [283]. However, thienopyridines and stents were not routinely used in these trials.

Abciximab

Abciximab was the first drug to be tested in three trials as an adjunct to PCI in the setting of ACS [284–286]. In total 7290;patients were included revealing a significant reduction of the combination of death and MI or need for urgent revascularization at 30 days. Pooled data from these three trials showed also a significant late mortality benefit (HR 0.71; 95% CI, 0.57–0.89, p = 0.003) [287].

In CAPTURE (c7E3 Antiplatelet Therapy in Unstable Refractory Angina) trial, abciximab has been tested in patients with NSTE-ACS with planned single vessel PCI without routine use of stents and clopidogrel. Treatment with abciximab for 24 hours before and 12 hours after the intervention significantly reduced the rate of death, MI and need for urgent intervention for recurrent ischaemia as compared to placebo at 30 days (11.3% vs. 15.9%, p = 0.012) [288]. The benefit as in other trial was restricted to patient with elevated troponin levels [289].

In the more recent ISAR-REACT-2 (Intracoronary Stenting and Antithrombotic Regimen: Rapid Early Action for Coronary Treatment 2) study high-risk NSTE-ACS patients were randomized following pre-treatment with aspirin and 600mg of clopidogrel to either abciximab or placebo [290]. There was a similar rate of diabetic patients in each group (average 26.5%); 52% of patients had elevated troponins, and 24.1% had previous MI. The 30-day composite endpoint of death, MI or urgent target vessel revascularization was significantly reduced in abciximab treated patients vs. placebo (8.9% vs. 11.9%; RR, 0.75; 95% CI, 0.58–0.97, p = 0.03). Most of the risk reduction generated by abciximab resulted from a reduction in the occurrence of death and MI. The effect was more pronounced in certain pre-specified subgroups, particularly troponin-positive patients (13.1% vs. 18.3%; RR, 0.71; 95% CI, 0.54–0.95, p = 0.02). The duration of pre-treatment with clopidogrel had no influence on outcome, and there was no beneficial effect in troponin-negative patients or among diabetic patients.

The TARGET trial (Do Tirofiban and ReoPro Give Similar Efficacy Outcome Trial) is the only larger head-to-head comparison of abciximab vs. tirofiban, in which two-thirds of the patients had recent or ongoing NSTE-ACS. Abciximab was shown to be superior to tirofiban in standard doses in reducing the risk of death, MI and urgent revascularization at 30 days, but the difference was not significant at 6 months and 1 year [291].

Eptifibatide

Eptifibatide was first tested in patients undergoing PCI including 38% with unstable angina (IMPACT-2) and exhibited no significant benefit as compared to placebo [292]. Subsequently, eptifibatide was tested in the ESPRIT (European/Australasian Stroke Prevention in Reversible Ischaemia Trial) trial with an increased dose of eptifibatide and including 46% of patients with ACS [293]. Compared to placebo a significant reduction in the risk of death, MI, urgent target vessel revascularization and bail-out use of GP IIb/IIIa inhibitors was revealed at 48 hours, maintained at 30 days, and at 6 months (6.6% vs. 10.5%; RR, 0.63; 95% CI, 0.47–0.84, p = 0.0015 at 48 hours). The secondary composite endpoint of death, MI or urgent target vessel revascularization was also significantly reduced at this time point (6.0% vs. 9.3%; RR, 0.65; 95% CI, 0.47-0.87, p = 0.0045).

Tirofiban

Tirofiban was tested in the RESTORE (Randomized Efficacy Study of Tirofiban for Outcomes and Restenosis) trial, in 2139 patients with recent ACS. A significant 38% relative-risk reduction in the primary composite endpoint of death, MI, repeat revascularization or recurrent ischaemia at 48 hours was observed at 7 days but not at 30 days [294]. Tirofiban was used at the same dose in the TARGET and RESTORE trials. In retrospect the dose may have been too low.

Recent, smaller trials explored higher doses of tirofiban (bolus 25mcg/kg and infusion 0.15mcg/kg/min for 24–48 hours) in various clinical settings. In a trial of 202 patients, the high dose was shown to reduce the incidence of ischaemic thrombotic complications vs. placebo during high-risk PCI [295]. TENACITY, designed as a large scale study testing high dose tirofiban against abciximab was stopped for non-scientific reasons after inclusion of 383 patients.

Upstream use of GP IIb/IIIa inhibitors prior to revascularization

It has been discussed whether so-called upstream use of glycoprotein IIb/IIIa inhibitors could be of benefit with the intention to reduce thrombus burden before PCI and to avoid complications in the waiting phase. This strategy has been shown in meta-analyses to further reduce the risk of death and MI at 30 days, if GP IIb/IIIa inhibitors are started upstream of and maintained during the PCI procedure [275, 276]. This question will be further explored prospectively in upcoming trials (EARLY-ACS) [296].

In ACUITY-TIMING study deferred selective vs. routine upstream administration of GP IIb/IIIa inhibitors was tested in a 2 × 2 factorial open-label design [297]. GP IIb/IIIa inhibitors were used in 55.7% of patients for 13.1 hours in the deferred selective and in 98.3% of patients for 18.3 hours in the routine upstream strategy. The deferred selective strategy resulted in a reduced 30day major bleeding rate (4.9% vs. 6.1%; RR, 0.80; 95% CI, 0.67–0.95). The rate of ischaemic events did not meet the set criteria for non-inferiority, although a trend towards a higher rate was noted (7.9% vs. 7.1%; RR, 1.12; 95% CI, 0.97–1.29, $p = 0.13$). TIMI minor bleeding rate was significantly lower (5.4% vs. 7.1%, $p < 0.001$; deferred selective vs. routine upstream), whereas TIMI major bleeding rate was not significantly different (1.6% vs. 1.9%, $p = 0.20$). The ischaemic composite endpoint was achieved more frequently in patients submitted to PCI with deferred selective vs. routine upstream GP IIb/IIIa inhibitors (9.5% vs. 8.0%; RR, 1.19; 95% CI, 1.00–1.42, $p = 0.05$). From these results it can be concluded that more frequent and more prolonged use of GP IIb/IIIa inhibitors in an upstream strategy leads to an excess risk of bleedings, however, there is a potentially higher protection against ischaemic events.

GP IIb/IIIa inhibitors and CABG

Inhibition of platelet aggregation increases bleeding complications associated with cardiac surgery. However, surgery in patients receiving GP IIb/IIIa inhibitors can safely be performed when appropriate measures are taken to ensure adequate haemostasis and the pharmacokinetics of the different compounds are understood. GP IIb/IIIa inhibitors should be discontinued at the time cardiac surgery starts. Eptifibatide and tirofiban have a short half-life (4–6 hours) allowing platelet function to recover by the end of CABG. Abciximab has a longer effective half-life (~6–12 hours) and earlier discontinuation is warranted. If excessive bleeding occurs, fresh platelet transfusions may be considered. Fibrinogen supplementation with fresh frozen plasma or cryoprecipitate either alone or in combination with platelet transfusion can also be used for restoring the haemostatic potential after the administration of small-molecule GP IIb/IIIa inhibitors [298].

Adjunctive therapy

GP IIb/IIIa inhibitors must be used in combination with an anticoagulant. Unfractionated heparin is safe, if the dose is adjusted. Several trials and observational studies in PCI have shown that LMWH, predominantly enoxaparin, can be safely used with GP IIb/IIIa inhibitors without compromising efficacy [240, 299–301]. The combination with fondaparinux was shown to be safe in the OASIS-5 study. Bivalirudin and UFH/LMWH were shown to have equivalent safety and efficacy when used with triple antiplatelet therapy, including GP IIb/IIIa inhibitors in the ACUITY trial [245].

Bivalirudin alone was associated with a lower bleeding risk as compared to any combination with GP IIb/IIIa inhibitors and may therefore be used as alternative in patients with high bleeding risk [245].

Summary

Patients at intermediate to high risk, namely patients with elevated troponins, ST-depression, or diabetes, either eptifibatide or tirofiban for initial early treatment are recommended in addition to dual oral antiplatelet treatment. The initial treatment with these drugs prior to angiography should be maintained during and after PCI. For high risk patients not pretreated with tirofiban or eptifibatide proceeding to PCI, abciximab is the drug with best evidence. The use of eptifibatide or tirofiban in this setting is less well established. Bivalirudin may be used as an alternative to GP IIb/IIIa inhibitors plus UFH/LMWH in patients with high risk of bleeding.

Special populations and conditions

Several groups of patients are at substantial risk of adverse cardiac events and merit alternative therapeutic strategies. There is great overlap between these subgroups, i.e. many elderly patients are women and/or have renal dysfunction, diabetes, or anaemia. As a rule, these subgroups are usually at higher risk of death and further ischaemic events, as well as at higher risk of bleeding than the general population. In addition, registries have consistently shown that these subgroups are treated less optimally than the general population.

The elderly

Depending on how 'elderly' is defined (>65 or >75 years of age), the rate of elderly patients hospitalized for ACS ranges from 27–34% in Europe. In ACS, the risk of death increases in a continuous curvilinear manner with each decade after age 50. In patients >75 years, the death rate is at least twice as high as in patients aged <75 years. Older age is also a strong predictor of bleeding complications. Elderly patients are poorly represented in clinical trials, with the result that trials findings cannot always be generalised to this subset of patients. As a general rule, elderly patients should be managed on a case by case basis, taking into account the risk of further ischaemic events and bleeding complications. Attention must be paid to the combination and to the dosage of drugs, as excess dosing is frequent in elderly patients. Invasive strategy leads to better outcome in elderly patients but at the cost of a higher risk of bleeding [302, 303].

Gender

Women suffering from NSTE-ACS tend to be older, and to have more,illnesses, including renal impairment, diabetes and heart failure. In registries in Europe, the average age of women with NSTE-ACS was 6 years higher than in men (71 vs. 65 years). After long debate, data have confirmed that there is no significant difference in terms of efficacy in pharmacological approach and revascularization procedures between women and men. Differences in outcomes reported between women and men disappeared after adjustment for baseline characteristics and comorbidities [304].

Diabetes mellitus (➲Chapter 14)

Diabetes mellitus is an independent predictor of higher mortality among patients with NSTE-ACS, and is associated with a twofold higher risk of death as compared to non-diabetic patients, placing diabetic patients in a high-risk category. The rate of diabetes mellitus, mainly type 2, is increasing among patients with NSTE-ACS, and ranges between 29–35% in Europe. Diabetic patients are more frequently women (41.6% vs. 30.7% in men), more often hypertensive (81% vs. 66% in non-diabetic patients), or obese (BMI >30, 28.5% vs. 18.6% in diabetic vs. non-diabetic patients) and more frequently suffer from renal failure (7.2% vs. 2.4% among non-diabetic patients). When impaired glucose tolerance or impaired fasting glycaemia are considered, in addition to established diabetes type 2, two-thirds of all patients suffering from either acute or chronic CAD have established glucose regulation abnormalities [305].

Tight glycaemic control at the acute phase of ACS has not been consistently shown to improve prognosis. However, glucose level at admission is a strong, independent predictor of long-term mortality in patients with type 2 diabetes. Insulin infusion may be needed in diabetic patients with high blood glucose levels at admission in order to reach normoglycaemia as soon as possible.

Invasive strategy improves outcome in diabetic patients. However, debate continues surrounding the best type of revascularization strategy (PCI vs. CABG). In the BARI trial, an advantage was shown in favour of CABG, but PCI was carried out with old technology. Drug-eluting stents have shown similar efficacy in diabetic vs. non-diabetic patients when compared to bare metal stents [306]. Ongoing trials comparing revascularization with drug-eluting stents or surgery may help to define the best revascularization strategy in diabetic patients.

As diabetic patients constitute a high risk population, optimal pharmacological approach and invasive strategy should be offered in the setting of ACS.

Chronic kidney disease (➲Chapter 15)

Chronic kidney disease (CKD) is a marker of risk of CAD. Among the general population, CKD is associated with a higher risk of cardiovascular and all-cause mortality, which increases exponentially with progressive decrease of GFR, with swift increase in events for GFR<60mL/min/1.73m^2 [307]. The high prevalence of CAD in CKD patients is due to a high incidence of traditional and also non-traditional risk factors such a intense pro-inflammatory state, hyperhomocysteinaemia, and pro-thrombotic state [308]. Diabetes which accounts for about 50% of all cases of end-stage renal dysfunction is an aggravating factor.

Moderate to severe renal dysfunction can be present in up to 40–50% of patients hospitalized for ACS. Renal dysfunction is a potent independent predictor of bleeding risk. Great caution should be paid to dosage of anticoagulants and GP IIb/IIIa inhibitors, since most are eliminated at least partially by the renal route. The dose of LMWH has to be carefully adjusted in patients with a CrCl <30mL/min. Fondaparinux is contraindicated if CrCl <20mL/min. Dose adaptation is required with bivalirudin. In case of severe renal dysfunction, UFH must be used, since anticoagulant activity can be monitored with aPTT.

Renal dysfunction can be worsened by the use of contrast medium at the time of angiography/angioplasty. CIN has an impact on prognosis, and can be kept under control with appropriate preventive measures, including hydration, use of small amounts of preferably iso-osmolar contrast medium, and staged procedures if multi-vessel disease submitted to PCI.

Patients with CKD form a high risk group, and should be treated as any other NSTE-ACS patients, particularly as regards revascularization and use of aspirin, clopidogrel, statins, and ACE inhibitors [309].

Troponin elevations are sometimes found in asymptomatic patients with renal dysfunction, particularly those under haemodialysis, without clear evidence of ongoing NSTE-ACS. These troponin elevations may render the diagnosis of NSTE-ACS difficult in this setting. However, the prognosis of patients with CKD is impaired in case of any troponin elevation independent of the anginal status.

Anaemia

According to the World Health Organization (WHO) criteria (haematocrit <39% or haemoglobin levels <13g/dL in men, and <12g/dL in women), anaemia may be present in 5–10% of patients with NSTE-ACS [256]. Anaemia is associated with higher mortality across the whole spectrum of CAD, including STEMI, NSTE-ACS, PCI, and CABG [310].

Anaemia is associated with more comorbidities, such as older age, presence of diabetes, and renal failure but also non-cardiovascular conditions (haemorrhagic diathesis or malignancy), which may account partly for the adverse prognosis. However, there seems to be a causal link between anaemia and risk of cardiovascular death [247]. Low baseline haemoglobin was also shown to be an independent predictor of the risk of bleeding.

Normal coronary arteries

About 15% of patients with proven NSTE-ACS actually have normal, or nearly normal coronary arteries. The pathophysiology of NSTE-ACS in patients with patent coronary arteries is not homogeneous and possible mechanisms include: 1) a coronary artery spasm (Prinzmetal's angina); 2) an intramural plaque complicated by acute thrombosis with subsequent recanalization; 3) coronary emboli; and 4) syndrome X. Important atherosclerotic burden may be present even in the absence of angiographically significant stenoses, because it may occur in a diffuse manner and lead to arterial wall remodelling in which the wall thickens and expands outwards without encroaching on the lumen.

The prognosis of patients with patent coronary arteries depends on the causative factors. Prinzmetal's angina can frequently be controlled with appropriate medical treatment. Syndrome X has a very good prognosis. In all other situations, the prognosis depends on the extent of myocardial damage, propensity for recurrence of events, and presence of comorbidities. In all circumstances where documented NSTE-ACS patients present with patent coronary arteries, optimal antithrombotic therapy and secondary prevention is necessary with antiplatelet agents and statins.

Apical ballooning, also referred to as Tako-Tsubo cardiomyopathy or stress cardiomyopathy, may present clinically as NSTE-ACS and is characterized by normal coronary arteries at angiography accompanied by apical and sometimes medioventricular akinesis unrelated to the distribution of a coronary artery. It typically occurs in postmenopausal women after an episode of severe emotional or physical stress. The pathogenesis is not entirely elucidated yet, however, there exists robust data that a catecholamine excess may play an important role. Apical ballooning may be accompanied by severe complications, such as cardiogenic shock or malignant arrhythmias. The regional wall motion abnormalities typically normalize within weeks [311, 312].

Complications

Bleeding complications

Bleeding complications are the most frequent non-ischaemic complications observed in the management of NSTE-ACS. The frequency of major bleeding ranges from 2–8% across the spectrum of NSTE-ACS and depends greatly on the type of treatment used, particularly type and dose of antithrombotic and antiplatelet therapy, invasive procedures, and on the baseline characteristics of patients, as well as on the definition used to define bleeding.

The strongest independent predictors of major bleedings were shown to be advanced age, female sex, history of bleeding, use of PCI, history of renal insufficiency, and use of IIb/IIIa inhibitors [313]. Excessive dosage of drugs, especially in case of renal dysfunction, plays a critical role, as bleeding risk exponentially increases with decreasing creatinine clearance (CrCl) (➲Table 16.11).

Major bleeding was shown to be associated with a fourfold increase in the risk of death, a fivefold increase in risk of recurrent MI, and a threefold increase in risk of stroke at 30 days [314, 315]. Several factors contributing to worse outcome have been discussed. Withdrawal of antiplatelet and antithrombotic drugs may play a major role, as well as the prothrombotic and pro-inflammatory consequences of bleeding.

Management of bleeding complications

Reduction in bleeding was shown to improve outcome, and thus, prevention of bleeding has become an important target in the management of ACS. Prevention of bleeding encompasses the choice of safer drugs, appropriate dosage

Table 16.11 Multivariate model for major bleeding in patients with non-ST elevation MI

Variable	Adjusted OR	95%CI	P-value
Age (per 10-year increase)	1.22	1.10–1.35	0.0002
Female sex	1.36	1.07–1.73	0.0116
History of renal insufficiency	1.53	1.13–2.08	0.0062
History of bleeding	2.18	1.14–4.08	0.014
Mean arterial pressure (per 20mmHg decrease)	1.14	1.02–1.27	0.019
Diuretics	1.91	1.46–2.49	<0.0001
LMWH only	0.68	0.50–0.92	0.012
LMWH and UFH*	0.72	0.52–0.98	0.035
GP IIb/IIIa inhibitors only	1.86	1.43–2.43	<0.0001
Thrombolytics and GP IIb/IIIa inhibitors	4.19	1.68–10.4	0.002
IV inotropic agents	1.88	1.35–2.62	0.0002
Right-heart catheterization	2.01	1.38–2.91	0.0003

Reference groups: male gender; UFH for LMWH only, both LMWH and UFH, and neither LMWH nor UFH; neither thrombolytics nor GP IIb/IIIa inhibitors for thrombolytics only, GP IIb/IIIa inhibitors only, and both thrombolytics and GP IIb/IIIa inhibitors; no for other variables. Hosmer–Lemeshow goodness of fit test P-value = 0.70; C-statistic = 0.73.

(taking into account age, gender, and CrCl), reduced duration of antithrombotic treatment, use of combination of antithrombotic and antiplatelet agents according to proven indications, as well as the choice of radial over femoral approach if angiography or PCI is being considered.

Interruption and neutralization of both antiplatelet and antithrombotic treatments are required if major bleeding cannot be controlled. This of course induces a risk of acute thrombotic events, which is maximum after 4–5 days, but persists for up to 30 days [315].

Protamine sulphate fully neutralizes factor-IIa activity, with the result that its impact is major with UFH, but only partial with LMWH. Recombinant factor VII has been recommended in case of major bleeding occurring with fondaparinux [237, 238].

Platelet transfusion can only reverse the effects of irreversible antiplatelet agents like aspirin and clopidogrel. Platelet transfusion is also recommended in case of bleeding with abciximab, but with tirofiban or eptifibatide, fibrinogen-containing plasma supplementation may also be needed in addition platelet transfusion because of the large amount of freely circulating molecules with these compounds [316].

Impact of blood transfusion

Blood transfusion can be required to control anaemia and haemodynamic compromise. However, there is ongoing controversy about its real efficacy and safety, because it has been shown that blood transfusion was associated with poorer outcome, even after adjustment for baseline characteristics, and in-hospital procedures [317].

It is not clearly understood why transfusion may be associated with adverse outcome. Alterations in erythrocyte, nitric oxide biology in stored blood cells, and impaired oxygen transport capabilities have been put forward. Many other factors have also been suggested, but as yet, the exact mechanisms remain to be elucidated.

A restrictive blood transfusion policy was shown to lead to better results than a liberal strategy in terms of mortality and organ failure at 30 days in critically ill patients. Therefore, it is now increasingly advocated that blood transfusion be avoided in patients with haemoglobin >7g/dL in the absence of haemodynamic compromise. In patients with haemoglobin <7g/dL, blood transfusion should be administered. Appropriate post-transfusion target haematocrit or haemoglobin levels remain poorly defined, but a target of 8–9g/dL appears to be adequate [238].

Thrombocytopenia

Thrombocytopenia can occur as a result of heparin-induced thrombocytopenia (HIT) or as a complication of the use of GP IIb/IIIa inhibitors. HIT must be suspected when there is a drop of >50% in platelet count, or a decrease in platelet count to <100,000/μL. Immediate interruption of UFH or LMWH is mandatory, as soon as HIT is suspected. Alternative antithrombotic therapy must be introduced. Direct thrombin-inhibitors, such as argatroban, or hirudin or derivatives, which do not carry any risk of thrombocytopenia, represent the optimal treatment [318].

Severe and profound thrombocytopenia due to GP IIb/IIIa inhibitors was observed in 0.5–5.6% of patients in clinical trials with GP IIb/IIIa inhibitors. Discontinuation of GP IIb/IIIa inhibitors, UFH and/or LMWH is required in case of severe thrombocytopenia. In case of bleeding, platelet transfusion, fresh frozen plasma, or cryoprecipitate, either alone or in combination, has been advocated [316].

Invasive versus conservative strategy

Choice of strategy

Coronary angiography should be planned as soon as possible (urgent invasive strategy) in patients with severe ongoing angina, profound or dynamic ECG changes, major arrhythmias or haemodynamic instability upon admission or thereafter. These patients represent 2–15% of the patients admitted with NSTE-ACS [319–321]. In patients with intermediate to high risk features, but without the aforementioned life-threatening features, early coronary angiography (within 72 hours) followed by revascularization when possible and indicated, or initial medical stabilization and selective performance of coronary angiography based on the clinical course have been tested as alternative strategies. In low-risk patients, a non-invasive assessment of inducible ischaemia should be performed prior to discharge. If this is positive, coronary angiography should be performed [322].

A meta-analysis of seven randomized trials (including early studies prior to the widespread use of stents and multidrug adjunctive therapy) comparing routine angiography followed by revascularization with a more conservative strategy (invasive care only in patients with recurrent or inducible ischaemia) showed reduced rate of death and MI at end of follow-up (12.2% vs. 14.4%) routine invasive vs. selective invasive [323]. At the same timepoint, there was a non-significant trend towards fewer deaths (5.5% vs. 6.0%), while a significant reduction in MI alone was observed (7.3% vs. 9.4%, p <0.001). These results were obtained despite an early hazard observed during initial hospitalization in the routine invasive group, where a significantly higher risk of death and MI was noted. The beneficial effect was actually achieved from hospital discharge to end of follow-up. Over a mean follow-up of 17 months, recurrent angina was reduced by 33% and re-hospitalization by 34% in the routine invasive group. Many of the trials analysed in this meta-analysis were not contemporary [323]. In four of the trials, namely TIMI (Thrombolysis in Myocardial Infarction)-3B, VANQWISH (Veterans Affairs Non–Q-Wave Infarction Strategies in-Hospital), MATE (Medicine versus Angiography in Throm-bolytic Exclusion), and FRISC (Framingham and Fast Revascularization During Instability in Coronary Artery Disease)-2, the use of stents and GP IIb/IIIa inhibitors was low or non existent [324–326]. In another meta-analysis including six contemporary trials, the OR was 0.84 for early invasive vs. conservative strategy (➲Fig. 16.27). The benefit of the routine invasive strategy was present in patients with elevated troponins at baseline, but not in troponin-negative patients (from the analysis of the 3 most recently performed trials with available troponin data) [327–329]. A more recent meta-analysis including 7 trials with 8,375 patients available for analysis showed after a mean follow-up of 2 years a significant risk reduction for all-cause mortality and the incidence of non-fatal MI [330]. Long-term mortality reduction has been confirmed in the follow-up of RITA-3 (Third Randomized Intervention Treatment of Angina) at 5 years [331][325] and FRISC-2 at 2 and 5 years [327, 329]. More recently, a review of the most contemporary trials by the Cochrane collaboration confirmed the existence of a trend towards an

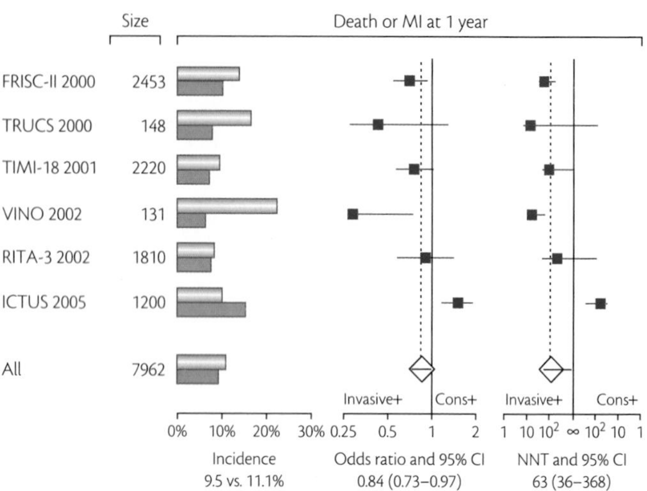

Figure 16.27 Death or myocardial infarction in six contemporary randomized trials comparing early invasive (dark blue bars) vs. conservative strategy (light blue bars). NNT, number of patients who needed to be treated to avoid one event.

early excess of mortality with invasive strategy (RR 1.59), but with a significant long-term benefit in terms of death (RR 0.75) or MI (RR 0.75) with invasive vs. conservative at 2–5 year' follow-up [332]. In contrast, in the more recent ICTUS (Invasive vs. Conservative Treatment in Unstable Coronary Syndromes) trial no difference could be found between early vs. selective invasive strategy in the incidence of the primary composite endpoint of death, MI or re-hospitalization for angina at 1- and 3-year follow-up [333, 334]. In keeping with prior studies, routine intervention was associated with a significant early hazard. However, the discrepancy between this and prior trials could be attributed in part to the small difference in revascularization rates between the two study groups and the high overall rate of revascularization before discharge (76% in the routine invasive and 40% in the selective group).

In all randomized trials, a large proportion of patients in the conservative arm eventually underwent revascularization ('cross-over') such that the true benefit of revascularization is underestimated [335]. When comparing the relative mortality benefit between routine and selective revascularization strategies with the actual difference in the revascularization rates between arms, a linear relationship emerges, the greater the difference in the rate of revascularization, the greater the benefit on mortality (➲Fig. 16.28).

Timing of invasiveness

With the exception of indications for emergency angiography and revascularization, controversy remains as to the optimal timing between hospital admission, initiation of medical therapy, and invasive evaluation. In the ISAR-COOL (Intracoronary Stenting with Antithrombotic

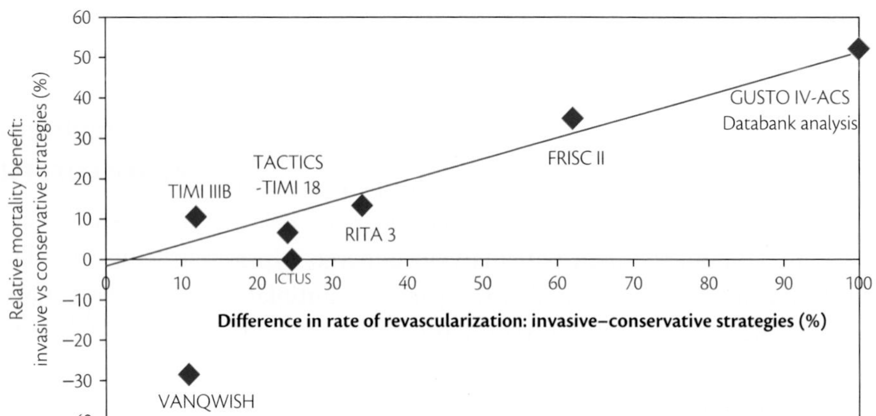

Figure 16.28 The ability to demonstrate relative mortality benefit with the revascularization strategy depends on the gradient in rates of revascularization between both randomization arms.

Regimen Cooling-Off Trial) trial, deferral of intervention did not improve outcome [336]. Patients randomized to immediate PCI (on average 2.4 hours after admission) had a lower incidence of death or MI at 30 days than patients randomized to deferred PCI (86 hours after admission and medical therapy). Likewise, no early hazard was observed in TACTICS-TIMI (Treat Angina with Aggrastat and Determine Cost of Therapy with an Invasive or Conservative Strategy-Thrombolysis in Myocardial Infarction)-18 (mean delay for PCI was 22 hours) with upstream treatment with GP IIb/IIIa inhibitors [289].

At variance with these findings, expedite catheterization was associated with worse outcome in the GRACE (Global Registry of Acute Coronary Events) and CRUSADE (Can Rapid risk stratification of Unstable angina patients Suppress ADverse outcomes with Early implementation of the ACC/AHA guidelines) registry [337, 338]. A current study (Timing of Intervention in Acute Coronary Syndrome, TIMACS) indicates, however, that patients with high risk according to the GRACE risk score benefit from early (<24 hours after presentation) invasive strategy. Accordingly, currently available evidence does not mandate a systematic approach of immediate angiography in NSTE-ACS patients stabilized with a contemporary pharmacological approach, but favours this in high risk patients.

Percutaneous coronary intervention

Outcome after PCI in NSTE-ACS has been markedly improved with the use of intracoronary stenting and contemporary antithrombotic and antiplatelet therapy. The risk of bleeding complications should be balanced against the severity of ischaemia and the patient's risk profile. The choice of access site depends on operator expertise and local preference. Non pharmacological strategies to reduce access site bleeding complications include the use of closure devices and the radial approach. The femoral approach is preferred in haemodynamically compromised patients to permit the use of intra-aortic balloon counterpulsation. As for all patients undergoing PCI, stent implantation in this setting helps to reduce the threat of abrupt closure and restenosis. The safety and efficacy of drug-eluting stents has not been prospectively tested in this specific population, although registry data suggest a benefit in terms of long-term mortality [339]. The approved DES appear to be equally effective in reducing restenosis in this setting as shown from subgroup analyses of randomized trials and real world data [340]. While the incidence of (sub)acute stent thrombosis is higher in NSTE-ACS patients, as compared to stable patients undergoing PCI, the use of DES does not seem to portend a higher risk of (sub) acute stent thrombosis in this specific setting [341]. In view of the potentially severe consequences of acute or sub-acute stent thrombosis, it is advisable to use a bare metal stent (BMS) in patients scheduled to undergo extra-cardiac interventions or surgery that will require interruption of clopidogrel within the first year after stent implantation [342, 343]. This strategy should be also considered in patients requiring long-term VKA treatment. Accordingly, the choice between use of BMS or DES should be based on an individual assessment of benefit versus potential risk [344, 345].

The main issue with PCI for NSTE-ACS remains the relatively high incidence of periprocedural MI, up to 10% [333]. The use of antiplatelet therapy has significantly reduced the incidence of periprocedural MI [346]. However, embolization of debris or plaque fragments cannot entirely be prevented by state-of-the-art antithrombotic and antiplatelet adjunctive therapy [347]. A wide variety of filter and/or distal protection devices have been tested but failed to improve clinical outcome, with the exception of the subset of saphenous vein graft interventions [348].

Currently there is no outcome data supporting routine PCI in non-significant culprit or non-culprit coronary obstructions, as perceived by angiography, even with the use of DES ('plaque sealing') [349]. Only exceptionally, non-significant culprit lesions presenting features of plaque rupture (e.g. haziness, irregular borders, dissections) may justify a mechanical intervention.

Coronary artery bypass graft

The proportion of patients with NSTE-ACS undergoing bypass surgery during the initial hospitalization is about 10% [333]. It is important to consider the risk of bleeding complications in patients who undergo bypass surgery while initially treated with aggressive antiplatelet treatment [350, 351]. Overall, pre-treatment with triple or even dual antiplatelet regimen should be considered as only a relative contraindication to early bypass surgery but does require specific surgical measures to minimize bleeding and platelet transfusions.

Respective indications for PCI or CABG

With the exception of an urgent procedure, the choice of revascularization technique in NSTE-ACS is the same as for elective revascularization procedures. From the randomized controlled trials comparing multivessel stented PCI with bypass surgery, there was no interaction between the presence of NSTE-ACS, treatment strategy and outcome [351, 352]. In patients with multivessel disease, all significant stenoses can be treated at once. A staged procedure may be considered, with immediate PCI of the culprit lesion and subsequent reassessment of the need for treatment of other lesions.

Management concept of non-ST-elevation acute coronary syndrome (➲Fig. 16.29)

NSTE-ACS encompasses a heterogeneous spectrum of patients with different levels of risk in terms of death, MI or recurrence of MI. A stepwise standardized strategy based on the available scientific data may be applicable to most patients admitted with suspected NSTE-ACS. It must be appreciated, however, that specific findings in individual patients may result in appropriate deviations from the proposed strategy. For every patient, the physician must make an individual decision taking into account the patient's history (comorbid illnesses, age etc.), his/her clinical condition, findings during the initial assessment on first contact, and the available pharmacological and non-pharmacological treatment options.

Initial evaluation

Chest pain or discomfort will be the symptom that leads to the patient seeking medical attention or hospitalization. A patient with suspected NSTE-ACS must be evaluated in a hospital and immediately seen by a qualified physician.

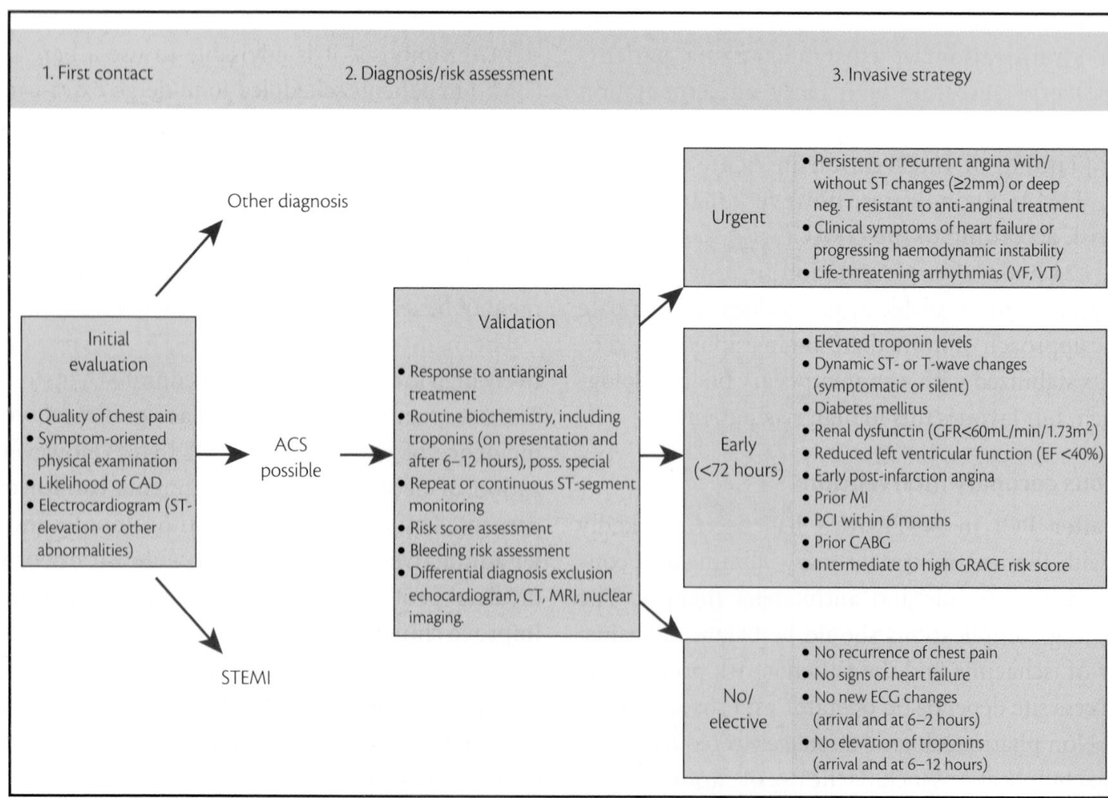

Figure 16.29 Decision-making algorithm for the management of patients with non ST-elevation acute coronary syndrome.

Specialized chest pain units provide the best and expeditious care [353].

The initial step is to assign the patient without delay to a working diagnosis on which the treatment strategy will be based. The criteria are:

- Quality of chest pain and a symptom-oriented physical examination;
- Assessment of the likelihood of CAD (e.g. age, risk factors, previous MI, CABG, PCI);
- ECG (ST deviation or other ECG abnormalities).

Based on these findings which should be available within 10min after first medical contact the patient can be assigned to one of the 3 major working diagnoses:

- STEMI requiring immediate reperfusion;
- NSTE-ACS;
- ACS (highly) unlikely.

The assignment to the category 'unlikely' must be done with caution and only when another explanation is obvious (e.g. trauma). Additional ECG leads (V3R and V4R, V7–V9) should be recorded, especially in patients with persisting chest pain.

Blood is drawn on arrival of the patient in hospital and the result should be available within 60min to be used in the second strategy step. Initial blood tests must at least include: troponin T or troponin I, creatine kinase (-MB), creatinine, haemoglobin, and leucocyte count.

Table 16.12 Initial treatment regimen for patients with acute coronary syndromes

Oxygen	Insufflation (4–8L/min) if oxygen saturation is <90%
Nitrates	Sublingually or intravenously (caution if systolic blood pressure <90mmHg)
Aspirin	Initial dose of 160–325mg non-enteric formulation followed by 75–100mg/day (intravenous administration is acceptable)
Clopidogrel	Loading dose of 300mg (or 600mg for rapid onset of action) followed by 75mg daily
Anticoagulation	Choice between different options depends on strategy: ◆ UFH intravenous bolus 60–70IU/kg (maximum 5000IU) followed by infusion of 12–15IU/kgh (maximum 1000IU/h) titrated to aPTT 1.5–2.5 times control ◆ Fondaparinux 2.5mg/daily subcutaneously ◆ Enoxaparin 1mg/kg twice daily subcutaneously ◆ Dalteparin 120IU/kg twice daily subcutaneously ◆ Nadroparin 86IU/kg twice daily subcutaneously ◆ Bivalirudin 0.1mg/kg bolus followed by 0.25mg/kg/h
Morphine	3–5mg intravenously or subcutaneously, depending on pain severity
Oral beta-blocker	Particularly if tachycardia or hypertension without sign of heart failure
Atropine	0.5–1mg intravenously if bradycardia or vagal reaction

Diagnosis validation

After the patient is assigned to the group NSTE-ACS, intravenous and oral treatments will be started according to ➲Table 16.12. The first-line treatment includes nitrates, beta-blockers, aspirin, clopidogrel, and anticoagulation. The further management will be based on additional information/data as listed in ➲Table 16.13.

The treatment of the individual patient is tailored according to the risk for subsequent events and should be assessed early at the initial presentation as well as repeatedly thereafter in the light of continuing or repetitive symptoms and additional information from clinical chemistry or imaging modalities. Risk assessment is an important component of the decision-making process and is subject to constant re-evaluation. It encompasses assessment of both ischaemic and bleeding risk. The risk factors for bleeding and ischaemic events overlap considerably, with the result that those patients at high risk of ischaemic events are also at high risk of bleeding complications. Therefore, the choice of the pharmacological environment (dual or triple antiplatelet therapy, anticoagulants) has become critical, as has the dosage of the drugs. In addition, in case invasive strategy is needed, the choice of the vascular approach is very important, since the radial approach has been shown to reduce the risk of bleeding as compared to the femoral approach. In this context, particular attention has to be paid to renal dysfunction, shown to be particularly frequent in elderly patients and among diabetics.

During this step other diagnoses may be confirmed or excluded, like acute anaemia, pulmonary embolism, aortic aneurysm (➲Table 16.13).

Table 16.13 Diagnosis validation

- Routine clinical chemistry, particularly troponins (on presentation and after 6–12 h) and other markers according to working diagnoses (e.g. D-dimers, BNP, NT-proBNP);
- Repeat, preferably continuous, ST-segment monitoring (when available);
- Echocardiogram, MRI, CT, or nuclear imaging for differential diagnoses (e.g. aortic dissection, pulmonary embolism);
- Responsiveness to antianginal treatment;
- Risk score assessment;
- Bleeding risk assessment.

During this step the decision has to be made whether the patient should go on to cardiac catheterization or not.

Invasive strategy

Cardiac catheterization is advised to prevent early complications and/or to improve long-term outcome. Accordingly, the need for and timing of invasive strategy has to be tailored according to the acuteness of risk into three categories: conservative, early invasive or urgent invasive.

Patients that fulfil all below criteria may be regarded as low risk and should not be submitted to early invasive evaluation:

- no recurrence of chest pain;
- no signs of heart failure;
- no abnormalities in the initial ECG or a second ECG (6–12 hours);
- no elevation of troponins (arrival and at 6–12 hours).

Low risk as assessed by a risk score (see ➲ Risk stratification, p.1269) can support the decision-making process for a conservative strategy. The further management in these patients is according to the evaluation of stable CAD [354]. Before discharge a stress test for inducible ischaemia is useful for further decision making.

Patients that cannot be excluded by the above criteria should go on to cardiac catheterization.

Urgent invasive strategy

Urgent invasive strategy should be undertaken for patients who are without ECG evidence of transmural infarction (e.g. occlusion of the circumflex artery) or are estimated to be at high risk of rapid progression to vessel occlusion. These patients are characterized by:

- refractory angina (e.g. evolving MI without ST abnormalties);
- recurrent angina despite intense antianginal treatment associated with ST depression (>2mm) or deep negative T waves;
- clinical symptoms of heart failure or haemodynamic instability ('shock');
- life-threatening arrhythmias (ventricular fibrillation or ventricular tachycardia).

In addition to the medication of ➲ Table 16.12, a GP IIb/IIIa inhibitor (tirofiban, eptifibatide) or bivalirudin should be added in symptomatic patients bridging the time to catheterization.

Early invasive strategy

Some patients initially respond to the antianginal treatment, but are at increased risk and need early angiography.

Table 16.14 Indications for routine early angiography

- elevated troponin levels;
- dynamic ST or T-wave changes (symptomatic or silent) (≥0.5mm);
- diabetes mellitus;
- reduced renal function (GFR<60mL/min/1.73m^2);
- depressed LVEF<40%;
- early post-MI angina;
- PCI within 6 months;
- previous CABG;
- intermediate to high risk according to a risk score (Table 5).

The timing depends on the local circumstances, but it should be performed within 72 hours.

The features in ➲ Table 16.14 indicate patients that should undergo routine early angiography.

The decision about the timing of catheterization must continuously be re-evaluated and modified according to clinical evolution and occurrence of new clinical findings.

Revascularization modalities

If the angiogram shows no critical coronary lesions, patients will be referred for medical therapy. The diagnosis of NSTE-ACS may be reconsidered and particular attention should be given to other possible reasons for symptoms at presentation before the patient is discharged. However the absence of critical coronary lesions does not rule out the diagnosis if clinical presentation was suggestive of ischaemic chest pain and if biomarkers were positive. In the setting of significant left main disease a PCI should be considered instead of CABG if treatment is deemed urgent.

Recommendations for the choice of a revascularization modality in NSTE-ACS are similar to those for elective revascularization procedures. In patients with single vessel disease, PCI with stenting of the culprit lesion is the first choice. In patients with multivessel disease the decision for PCI or CABG must be made individually. A sequential approach with treating the culprit lesion by PCI followed by elective CABG may in some patients be advantageous.

If angiography shows no options for revascularization, owing to the extent of the lesions and/or poor distal run-off, freedom from angina at rest should be achieved by intensified medical therapy and secondary preventive measures should be instituted.

Discharge and postdischarge management

Although in NSTE-ACS most adverse events occur in the early phase, the risk for MI or death remains elevated over several months. Patients treated with early revascularization are at low (~2.5%) risk for developing life-threatening arrhythmias, with 80% occurring during the first 12 hours after onset of symptoms [355]. Accordingly, monitoring of the patients beyond 24 – 48 hours is not warranted. Discharge from hospital depends on clinical and angiographic findings. Patients with NSTE-ACS should be hospitalized for at least 24 hours after successful stenting of the culprit lesion.

Treatment of ST-elevation acute coronary syndromes

Management of ST-elevation acute coronary syndromes (➲ Fig. 16.30)

Over the last 50 years, the treatment of acute STEMI has considerably changed the outcome of this life-threatening condition. The introduction of defibrillators and coronary care units in the 1960s reduced hospital mortality from about 30% to 15%. In the late 1970s and early 1980s the introduction of reperfusion with fibrinolytic therapy was associated with hospital mortality rates raging from 7–10%. A further reduction to around 5% occurred with the use of mechanical reperfusion and optimal adjunctive therapies (at least in randomized studies). In the 'real world' mortality rates are much higher due to, among others, the absence of reperfusion therapy in around 30% of STEMI patients.

For patients with the clinical presentation of STEMI within 12 hours after onset of symptoms and with persistent ST-segment elevation or new or presumed new left bundle-branch block, early mechanical (PCI) or pharmacological reperfusion should be performed unless clear contraindications are present.

There is general agreement that reperfusion, i.e. primary PCI, should also be considered after 12 hours, if there is clinical and/or electrocardiographic evidence of ongoing ischaemia, since occlusion is a dynamic process and the patients' information is often unclear. This paradigm change is supported by a meta-analysis of ten studies in which patients presenting later than 12 hours after onset of symptoms were randomized between medical treatment or PCI. Patients who underwent PCI benefited with a significantly better left ventricular function and improved clinical outcome [356].

Fibrinolytic treatment

The benefit of fibrinolytic therapy is well established [357]: approximately 30 early deaths are prevented per 1000 patients treated within 6 hours of symptom onset. Overall, the largest absolute benefit is seen among patients with the highest risk. Several factors like the fibrinolytic agent, adjunctive medication, and timing of treatment have an impact on the result.

Fibrinolytic agents

Streptokinase was the first fibrinolytic agent and it is still used in many countries. GISSI (Gruppo Italiano per lo Studio della Sopravvivenza nell'Infarto Miocardico)-1 (11,806 patients; published in 1986) and ISIS (Second International Study of Infarct Survival)-2 (17,187 patients; published in 1988) are the major landmark studies of fibrinolytic therapy, demonstrating a 23% reduction in 30-day mortality among patients randomized to streptokinase compared to control therapy [358, 359]. Fibrinolysis with this agent was also associated with a small, but significant, excess risk of intracranial haemorrhage

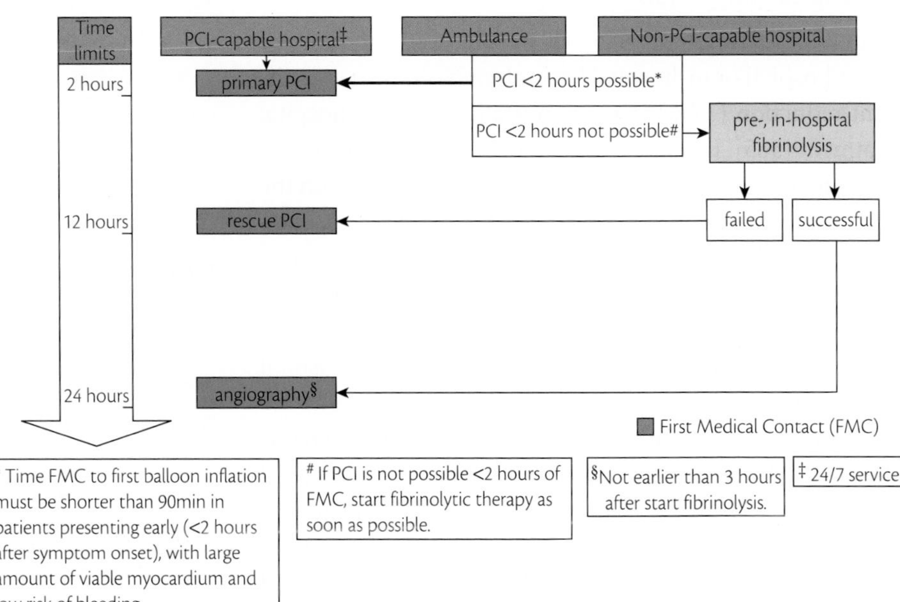

Figure 16.30 Reperfusion strategies. Thick arrow indicates preferred strategy.

(0.4% vs. 0.1%) events. In the GUSTO (Global Use of Strategies To Open occluded coronary arteries in acute coronary syndromes) trial [360] an accelerated infusion of the fibrin-specific agent t-PA (alteplase) with concomitant aPTT (activated partial thromboplastin time) adjusted intravenous heparin resulted in 10 fewer deaths per 1000 patients treated when compared to streptokinase at the cost of 3 additional strokes. In assessing the net clinical benefit of t-PA (survival without a neurological deficit) one must take into account that only one of these additional strokes survived with a residual neurological deficit. Several mutants of t-PA were developed with a longer half-life, so that these agents could be administered via bolus injection. Double-bolus r-PA (reteplase) does not offer any advantage over accelerated t-PA except for its ease of administration [361]. Single-bolus weight-adjusted TNK-tPA (tenecteplase) is equivalent to accelerated t-PA with respect to 30-day mortality and is associated with a significantly lower rate of non-cerebral bleedings and less need for blood transfusion [362]. Thus, the bolus fibrinolytic agents have a similar effectiveness, and have a slightly more favourable (tenecteplase) safety profile than alteplase. Their use should facilitate pre-hospital administration.

If there is evidence of persistent occlusion, re-occlusion or reinfarction with recurrence of ST-segment elevations after fibrinolysis, the patient should be immediately transferred to a centre with PCI capabilities. If rescue PCI is not available, a second administration of a non-immunogenic fibrinolytic agent (not streptokinase) may be considered only in case of a large infarct and provided the risk of bleeding is not high [363]. However, this approach has not yet proven to be efficient [364].

Prehospital fibrinolysis

Analysis of studies in which >6000 patients were randomized to pre-hospital or in-hospital fibrinolysis has shown a significant reduction (17%) in early mortality with pre-hospital treatment [365]. In a meta-analysis of 22 trials a much larger mortality reduction was found in patients treated within the first 2 hours than in those treated later [366]. These data support pre-hospital initiation of fibrinolytic treatment if this reperfusion strategy is indicated. More recent post hoc analyses of several randomized trials and data from registries have confirmed the clinical usefulness of pre-hospital fibrinolysis [367]. Most of these studies reported outcome data similar to that of primary PCI, provided early angiography and PCI were performed in those patients who needed intervention. However, whether pre-hospital fibrinolysis is associated with a similar or better clinical outcome than primary PCI in early presenting patients has not been studied prospectively in an adequately sized randomized fashion.

Provided that fibrinolytic therapy is the most appropriate reperfusion strategy, pre-hospital fibrinolysis should be the treatment of choice, when appropriate logistics are existing, including trained medical or paramedical staff able to analyse on-site or to transmit the ECG to the hospital. In this case, the aim is to start fibrinolytic therapy within 30min after first contact with the patient.

Hazards of fibrinolysis

Fibrinolytic therapy is associated with a small but significant excess of strokes [357] with all of the excess hazard appearing on the first days after treatment. The early strokes are largely attributable to cerebral haemorrhage; later strokes are more frequently thrombotic or embolic. Advanced age, lower weight, female gender, prior cerebrovascular disease, systolic and diastolic hypertension on admission have been identified to be significant predictors of intracranial haemorrhage [368]. In the latest trials, intracranial bleeding occurred in 0.9 to 1.0% of the total population studied [361, 362]. Major non-cerebral bleeds (bleeding complications requiring blood transfusion or that are life-threatening), can occur in 4 up to 13% of the patients treated [362, 369].

Contraindications to fibrinolytic therapy

Absolute and relative contraindications to fibrinolytic therapy are shown in ➲Table 16.15. Diabetes (more particularly

Table 16.15 Absolute and relative contraindications for fibrinolytic therapy

Absolute contraindications
Haemorrhagic stroke or stroke of unknown origin at any time
Ischaemic stroke in preceding 6 months
Central nervous system trauma or neoplasms
Recent major trauma/surgery/head injury (within preceding 3 weeks)
Gastrointestinal bleeding within the last month
Known bleeding disorder
Aortic dissection
Non-compressible punctures (e.g. liver biopsy, lumbar puncture)
Relative contraindications
Transient ischaemic attack in preceding 6 months
Oral anticoagulant therapy
Pregnancy or within 1 week post-partum
Refractory hypertension (systolic blood pressure > 180mmHg and/or diastolic blood pressure >110mmHg)
Advanced liver disease
Infective endocarditis
Active peptic ulcer
Refractory resuscitation

diabetic retinopathy) and successful resuscitation are no contraindication to fibrinolytic therapy. Fibrinolytic therapy should not be given to patients refractory to resuscitation.

Angiography after fibrinolytic therapy

If it is likely that fibrinolysis was successful (ST-segment resolution of >50% at 60–90min, occurrence of typical reperfusion arrhythmias, disappearance of chest pain) angiography should be arranged. This is supported by data from the CARESS (Combined Abciximab Reteplase Stent Study) and TRANSFER-MI trials in which patients referred to angiography only in case of failed fibrinolysis had a significantly worse clinical outcome compared to a strategy of referring all patients for angiography and (if indicated) PCI [358]. In order to avoid an early PCI during the prothrombotic period following fibrinolysis on the one hand, and to minimize the risk of reocclusion on the other hand, a time window of 3–24 hours following successful fibrinolysis is most appropriate [359, 370].

Adjunctive anticoagulant and antiplatelet therapy

Convincing evidence of the effectiveness of aspirin was demonstrated by the ISIS-2 trial [371], in which the benefits of aspirin and streptokinase were additive. The first dose of 150–325mg should be chewed (no enteric-coated aspirin because of slow onset of action) and a lower dose (75–100mg) given orally daily thereafter. If oral ingestion is not possible, aspirin can be given intravenously (250–500mg). The benefit of dual antiplatelet treatment with aspirin and clopidogrel was demonstated in the CLARITY (Clopidogrel as Adjunctive Reperfusion Therapy) and COMMIT (Clopidogrel and Metoprolol in Myocardial Infarction Trial) trials [372, 373]. Adjunctive therapy with clopidogrel reduced the composite endpoint of death from cardiovascular causes, recurrent myocardial infarction, or need for urgent revascularization at 30 days by 20% in CLARITY [372]. In COMMIT clopidogrel administration resulted in 9 fewer events (death, reinfarction or stroke) per 1000 patients treated for about 2 weeks [365]. Thus, clopidogrel should be routinely used in the acute phase of myocardial infarction in patients who are treated with fibrinolytic therapy.

Heparin has been extensively used during and after fibrinolysis, especially with alteplase. Heparin does not improve immediate clot lysis but coronary patency evaluated in the hours or days following fibrinolytic therapy with alteplase appears to be higher with intravenous heparin [374]. No difference in patency was apparent in patients treated with either subcutaneous or intravenous heparin and streptokinase [375]. Intravenous heparin administration until discharge has not been shown to prevent reocclusion after angiographically proven successful coronary fibrinolysis [376]. Heparin infusion after fibrinolytic therapy may be discontinued after 24–48 hours. Close monitoring of heparin therapy is mandatory; aPTT values over 70s are associated with higher likelihood of mortality, bleeding and reinfarction [377].

The low-molecular-weight enoxaparin treatment is associated with a significant reduction in the risk of death and reinfarction at 30 days compared to a weight-adjusted heparin dose [378]. This is, however, achieved at the cost of a significant increase in non-cerebral bleeding complications. The net clinical benefit (absence of death, non-fatal infarction or intracranial haemorrhage) favours enoxaparin. When the dose is adjusted for age and renal function, this benefit was observed regardless of the type of fibrinolytic agent and the age of the patient.

Fondaparinux was superior to placebo or heparin in preventing death and reinfarction in patients who received fibrinolytic therapy [379]. This was not the case, when heparin was deemed to be indicated. The data for bivalirudin in combination with streptokinase are not sufficiently convincing to recommend this anticoagulant [380].

Percutaneous coronary interventions

The role of percutaneous coronary interventions (PCI) during the early hours of STEMI can be divided into primary PCI, PCI combined with pharmacological reperfusion therapy (facilitated PCI), and 'rescue PCI' after failed pharmacological reperfusion.

Primary percutaneous coronary interventions

Primary PCI is defined as angioplasty and/or stenting without prior or concomitant fibrinolytic therapy, and is the preferred therapeutic option when it can be performed expeditiously by an experienced team including interventional cardiologists and a skilled supporting staff. This means that only hospitals with an established interventional cardiology programme (24 hours/7 days) should use primary PCI as a routine treatment option for patients with STEMI. Lower mortality rates among patients undergoing primary PCI are observed in centres with a high volume of PCI procedures [381, 382].

Primary PCI is effective in securing and maintaining coronary artery patency and avoids some of the bleeding risks of fibrinolysis. In randomized clinical trials comparing timely performed primary PCI with in-hospital fibrinolytic therapy in high-volume, experienced centres have

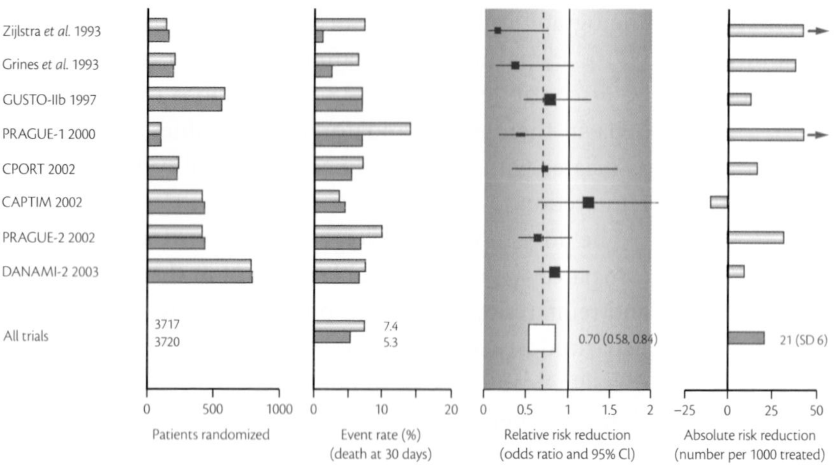

Fig 16.31 Death at 30-day follow-up in randomized trials of primary PCI (dark blue bars) vs. fibrinolytic therapy (light blue bars) in patients with ST-elevation acute coronary syndrome. Results are shown from selected trials that randomized at least 200 patients. Overall results are based on all 22 trials that were conducted between 1990 and 2003 (see text).

shown more effective restoration of patency, less reocclusion, improved residual LV function and, most important, a better clinical outcome with primary PCI (➲Fig. 16.31) [383]. Routine coronary stent implantation in patients with STEMI decreases the need for target-vessel revascularization but is not associated with significant reductions in death or reinfarction rates [384] compared to primary angioplasty. In addition, several randomized clinical trials with medium-term follow-up, including patients with STEMI, have shown that drug-eluting stents reduce the risk of reintervention compared to bare metal stents, without having a significant impact on the risk of stent thrombosis, recurrent myocardial infarction and death [385–387]. These findings have recently been challenged by a large-scale registry, which demonstrated a significantly reduced mortality in patients who were treated for acute myocardial infarction with drug-eluting stents in comparison to bare metal stents [339].

Long delay before primary PCI has been shown to be associated with a worse clinical outcome (➲Fig. 16.32) [388, 389]. Several delay times can be defined: time from symptom onset to first medical contact (FMC), time from FMC to arrival in cath lab, time from FMC to balloon inflation. The 'PCI-related delay time' is the difference between the times of FMC to balloon inflation minus the theoretical time from FMC to start of fibrinolytic therapy. The extent to which the PCI-related time delay diminishes the advantages of PCI over fibrinolysis has been the subject of many analyses and debates. Because no specifically designed study has addressed this issue, caution is needed when interpreting the results of these post-hoc analyses. A number of randomized trials have calculated that the PCI-related time delay potentially mitigating the benefit of the mechanical intervention varies between 60min [390] and 110min [391]. Another analysis of these trials calculated a benefit of primary PCI over fibrinolytic therapy up to a PCI-related delay of 120min [392]. In 192,509 patients included in the NRMI 2-4 registry [393] the mean PCI-related time delay where mortality rates of the two reperfusion strategies were equal was calculated at 114min. This study also indicated that this time delay varied considerably according to age, symptom duration and infarct location: from <1 hour for an anterior infarction in a patient <65 years presenting <2 hours of symptom onset to almost 3 hours for a non-anterior infarction in a patient >65 years presenting >2 hours after symptom onset. Although these results were derived from a post-hoc analysis of a registry and reported delay times are sometimes inaccurate, this study suggests that an individualized rather than a uniform approach for selecting the

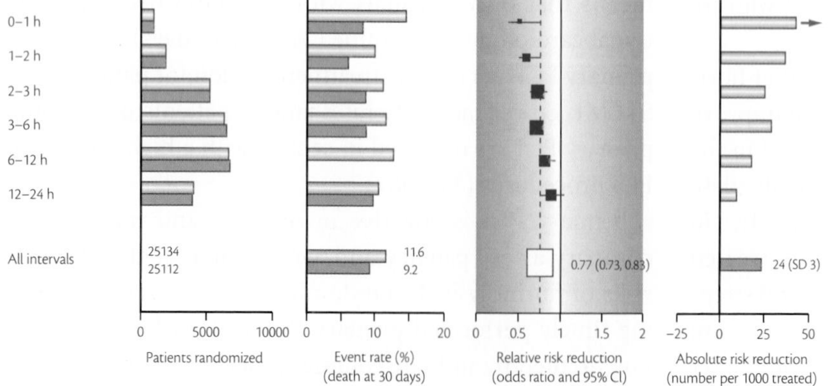

Fig 16.32 Death at 30-day follow-up in randomized trials of fibrinolytic therapy (dark blue bars) vs. control (light blue bars) in patients with ST-elevation acute coronary syndrome, in subgroups according to time from symptom onset to treatment.

optimal reperfusion modality could be more appropriate when PCI cannot be performed within a short timeframe.

Taken all available data together, primary PCI (balloon inflation) should be performed within 2 hours after first medical contact in all cases and within 90min in patients presenting early with a large amount of viable myocardial at risk.

Patients with contraindications to fibrinolytic therapy have a higher morbidity and mortality than those eligible for this therapy. Primary PCI can be performed with success in these patients [394]. Primary PCI is also the preferred treatment for patients with cardiogenic shock [395]. Only the culprit lesion should be dilated in the acute setting, except for patients in shock. Complete revascularization of the non-culprit lesions may be performed at a later time point depending on the remaining ischaemia.

Facilitated percutaneous coronary interventions

Facilitated PCI is defined as a pharmacologic reperfusion treatment delivered prior to a planned PCI, in order to bridge the PCI-related time delay. Full-dose lytic therapy, half-dose lytic therapy with a GPIIb/IIIa inhibitor and GPIIb/IIIa inhibitor alone have been tested for this indication. Despite the fact that pre-PCI patency rates were higher with lytic-based therapies there was no evidence of as clinical benefit with lytic-based treatments no mortality benefit but more bleeding complications were observed. The pre-PCI patency rates with upfront abciximab and tirofiban were not higher than with placebo. Also with this strategy no significant benefit was observed. Therefore, facilitated PCI as it has been tested in these trials cannot generally be recommended.

Rescue percutaneous coronary interventions

Rescue PCI is defined as PCI performed on a coronary artery, which remains occluded despite prior fibrinolytic therapy. The non-invasive identification of failed fibrinolysis remains a challenging issue, but <50% ST-segment resolution in the lead(s) with the highest ST-segment elevations 60–90min after start of fibrinolytic therapy has increasingly been used as a surrogate. Rescue PCI has been shown to be feasible and relatively safe. A recent meta-analysis showed that rescue PCI is associated with a significant reduction in heart failure and reinfarction and a trend towards lower all-cause mortality compared to a conservative strategy, at the cost, however, of an increased risk of stroke and bleeding complications [396]. Rescue PCI should be considered when there is evidence of failed fibrinolysis based on clinical signs and insufficient ST–segment resolution (<50%), when there is clinical or ECG evidence of a large infarct and when the procedure can be performed within a reasonable time delay (up to 12 hours after onset of symptoms).

Adjunctive antithrombotic treatments and devices

Aspirin, NSAID, COX-2 inhibitors: aspirin should be given to all patients with STEMI as soon as possible after the diagnosis is deemed probable. There are few, if any, absolute contraindications to the use of aspirin, but it should not be given to those with a known hypersensitivity, active gastrointestinal bleeding, known clotting disorders or severe hepatic disease. Aspirin may occasionally trigger bronchospasm in asthmatic patients. Aspirin should be started at a dose of 150–325mg in a chewable form (enteric-coated aspirin should not be given because of slow onset of action). An alternative approach, especially if oral ingestion is not possible, is intravenous administration of aspirin at a dose of 250–500mg, although no specific data are available on the relative merits of this strategy. A lower dose (75–100mg) is given orally daily thereafter for life. Non-steroidal anti-inflammatory drugs (NSAIDs) apart from aspirin and selective COX-2 inhibitors have been demonstrated to increase the risk of death, reinfarction, cardiac rupture and other complications in STEMI patients and should therefore be discontinued at the time of STEMI [397].

Clopidogrel

Although clopidogrel is less studied in patients with STEMI treated with primary PCI, there is abundant evidence on its usefulness as an adjunctive antiplatelet therapy on top of aspirin in patients undergoing PCI [259, 372, 398]. Based on these data, clopidogrel should be given as soon as possible to all patients with STEMI undergoing PCI. It is started with a loading dose of at least 300mg, but a 600mg loading dose achieves a more rapid and stronger inhibition of platelet aggregation [266]. This should be followed by a daily dose of 75mg for 1 year.

GPIIb/IIIa inhibitors

Platelet glycoprotein IIb/IIIa inhibitors block the final pathway of platelet aggregation. Most of the studies on the role of GPIIb/IIIa antagonists in STEMI have focused on abciximab rather than on the other two compounds, tirofiban and eptifibatide. Several randomized trials have assessed the value of periprocedural administration of intravenous abciximab in addition to aspirin and heparin in this setting. A systematic review of these trials showed that abciximab reduced 30-day mortality by 32% without affecting the risk of haemorrhagic stroke and major bleeding [399]. Abciximab did not have a significant impact on the patency of infarct-related vessels and its administration upstream of a planned PCI procedure did not offer advantages compared to the administration in the catheterization lab [400]. Abciximab is given intravenously as a bolus of 0.25mg/kg, 0.125mcg/kg per min infusion (maximum 10mcg/min for 12 hours). However, it remains to be elucidated whether abciximab provides an additional benefit to STEMI patients who receive an optimal clopidogrel treatment prior to PCI. The pre-hospital initiation of high-bolus dose tirofiban in association with aspirin, clopidogrel (600mg), and heparin improved ST-segment resolution and showed a trend towards an improved clinical outcome but was not associated with more patency of the infarct vessel when compared to placebo [401].

Heparins

Unfractionated heparin is the standard anticoagulant during PCI in STEMI. The lack of randomized clinical trials of heparin vs. placebo during PCI in STEMI is due to the common belief that anticoagulation therapy is essential. Heparin is given as an intravenous bolus at a starting dose of 100U/kg weight (60U/kg if GPIIb/IIIa antagonists are used). It is recommended to perform the procedure under activated clotting time (ACT) guidance: heparin should be given at a dose able to maintain an ACT of 250–350s (200–250s if GPIIb/IIIa antagonists are used). LMWHs have been studied in a limited number of STEMI patients undergoing primary PCI. Thus, there is little evidence to support their use instead of heparin in this setting.

Bivalirudin

The direct thrombin inhibitor bivalirudin, has also been investigated as an adjunct antithrombotic therapy in patients undergoing PCI. In a recent trial (HORIZONS-AMI) 3602 patients undergoing PCI were randomly assigned in an unblinded fashion to receive either bivalirudin with provisional use of GPIIb/IIIa inhibitor or heparin (or enoxaparin) plus a GPIIb/IIIa inhibitor [402]. The primary endpoint, the composite of 30-day incidence of major adverse cardiac events or major bleeding, was significantly reduced by bivalirudin due to a 40% reduction in major bleeding. All-cause mortality at 30 days was lowered by an absolute 1%. However, acute stent thrombosis occurred more frequently. Bivalirudin is usually given as an intravenous bolus followed by an infusion during PCI and does not have to be titrated to ACT.

Fondaparinux

Fondaparinux, a selective factor Xa inhibitor, has been compared with heparin or placebo in 12,092 STEMI patients treated with fibrinolytic agents or PCI or no reperfusion therapy [379]. In the PCI subset, fondaparinux was associated with a non-significant 1% higher incidence of death or recurrent infarction at 30 days. These findings together with the increased rate of catheter thrombosis do not lend support to the use of fondaparinux as the sole anticoagulant in patients undergoing primary PCI.

Adjunctive device

Adjunctive devices aiming at the prevention of distal embolization have been investigated intensively and have shown heterogeneous results in subsequent meta-analyses with no overall clinical benefit despite a lower rate of distal embolization angiographically [403]. However, in a recent randomized study in 1071 patients aspiration of thrombus prior to PCI was associated with improved tissue reperfusion measured as myocardial blush grades and with improved survival at 1 year compared to conventional PCI [404, 405].

'No reflow'

The 'no-reflow' phenomenon in STEMI patients is characterized by inadequate myocardial reperfusion after successful re-opening of the epicardial infarct-related artery. Depending on the technique used, 10–40% of patients undergoing reperfusion therapy for STEMI may show evidence of no-reflow [406–409].

No-reflow may occur as a consequence of downstream microvascular embolization of thrombotic or atheromatous (lipid-rich) debris, reperfusion injury, microvascular disruption, endothelial dysfunction, inflammation and myocardial oedema [410, 411]. No-reflow can cause prolonged myocardial ischaemia, may result in severe arrhythmias and critical haemodynamic deterioration, and is associated with a significantly increased risk of clinical complications [407, 412]. Consequently, reversing no-reflow is associated with a favourable effect on LV remodelling even in the absence of significant improvement in regional contractile function [413]. Therapeutic options for no-reflow include intracoronary administration of vasodilators like adenosine, verapamil, nicorandil, papaverine and nitroprusside [414, 415]. High-dose intravenous infusion of adenosine was also associated with a reduction in infarct size but clinical outcomes were not significantly improved [416]. The glycoprotein IIb/IIIa receptor antagonist abciximab was found to improve tissue perfusion [417, 418] and is recommended as antithrombotic co-therapy with primary PCI.

Coronary bypass surgery

The number of patients who need CABG in the acute phase is limited but CABG may be indicated after failed PCI, coronary occlusion not amenable for PCI, presence of refractory symptoms after PCI, cardiogenic shock, or mechanical complications such as ventricular rupture, acute mitral regurgitation, or ventricular septal defect [419, 420]. In patients with an indication for CABG, e.g. multivessel disease, it is recommended to treat the infarct-related lesion by PCI and to perform CABG later in more stable conditions.

Antithrombotic therapy without reperfusion therapy

In patients presenting within 12 hours after onset of symptoms not receiving reperfusion therapy for any reason and in patients presenting later than 12 hours after onset of symptoms aspirin, clopidogrel and an anticoagulant (heparin, enoxaparin, or fondaparinux) should be given [373, 421–423]. Fondaparinux was superior to heparin in this special subgroup and might therefore be the preferred agent in this setting [422]. Angiography before hospital discharge is recommended, if no contraindications are present.

Acute complications of ST-elevation myocardial infarction

Pump failure

Pump failure is usually due to myocardial damage but may also be the consequence of arrhythmias or mechanical complications such as mitral regurgitation or ventricular septal defect. Heart failure during the acute phase of STEMI is associated with a poor short- and long-term prognosis [424]. The clinical features are those of breathlessness, sinus tachycardia, a third heart sound, and pulmonary rales which are basal but may extend throughout both lung fields. The degree of failure may be categorized according to the Killip classification (➲Table 16.16). General measures include monitoring for arrhythmias, checking for electrolyte abnormalities, and the presence of concomitant conditions such as valvular dysfunction or pulmonary disease. Pulmonary congestion can be assessed by chest X-rays. Echocardiography is the key diagnostic tool and should be performed to assess the extent of myocardial dysfunction and possible complications, such as mitral regurgitation and ventricular septal defect.

Oxygen should be administered early by mask or intranasally, but caution is necessary in the presence of chronic pulmonary disease. Monitoring blood oxygen saturation is indicated. Minor degrees of failure often respond quickly to nitrates and low doses of diuretics. The dose of nitrates should be titrated while monitoring blood pressure to avoid hypotension. In the absence of hypotension, hypovolaemia or significant renal failure, ACE inhibitors (or an angiotensin receptor blocker if ACE inhibitors are not tolerated) should be initiated within 24 hours. In severe heart failure and shock (Killip class III and IV) continuous positive airway pressure or endotracheal intubation with ventilatory support may be required. Unless the patient is hypotensive, intravenous nitroglycerine should be given until a fall in systolic blood pressure of 30mmHg or more is observed or until the systolic blood pressure falls to <90mmHg. Inotropic agents may be of value in severely hypotensive patients. Pulmonary artery catheterization may be considered for treatment monitoring.

Table 16.16 Killip classification

Killip class I:	includes individuals with no clinical signs of heart failure
Killip class II:	includes individuals with rales or crackles in the lungs, S_3 gallop, and elevated jugular venous pressure
Killip class III:	describes individuals with frank acute pulmonary oedema
Killip class IV:	describes individuals in cardiogenic shock or hypotension (blood pressure <90mmHg), and evidence of peripheral vasoconstriction (oliguria, cyanosis or sweating)

Patients with acute heart failure may have stunned (reperfused but with delayed contractile recovery) or hypoperfused, viable myocardium. Identification of viable myocardium followed by revascularization can lead to improved LV function.

Cardiogenic shock

Cardiogenic shock is a clinical state of hypoperfusion characterized by a systolic pressure <90mmHg and a central filling pressure (wedge pressure) >20mmHg, or a cardiac index <1.8L/min/m^2 often caused by extensive loss of viable myocardial tissue (➲Fig. 16.33). Shock is also considered present, if intravenous inotropes and/or intra-aortic balloon pump are needed to maintain a systolic blood pressure >90mmHg and a cardiac index of >1.8L/min/m^2. The diagnosis of cardiogenic shock should be made when other causes of hypotension have been excluded such as hypovolaemia, vasovagal reactions, electrolyte disturbances, pharmacological side effects, tamponade or arrhythmias. It is usually associated with extensive LV damage, but may occur in right ventricular infarction. LV function and associated mechanical complications should be evaluated urgently by two-dimensional Doppler echocardiography. Haemodynamic assessment with a pulmonary artery (Swan–Ganz) catheter is useful in managing patients. The pulmonary wedge (= filling) pressure should be at least 15mmHg and cardiac index >2L/min/m^2. In some cases of cardiogenic shock, inotropic agents (dopamine, dobutamine) may stabilize patients at risk of progressive haemodynamic collapse or serve as a life-sustaining bridge to a more definitive therapy.

Supportive treatment with a balloon pump is strongly recommended as a bridge to haemodynamic recovery or

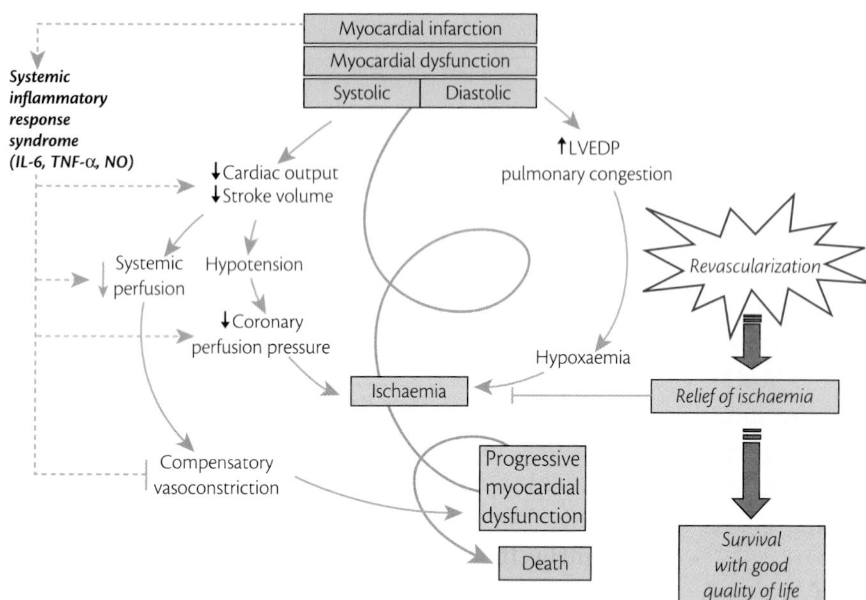

Figure 16.33 Myocardial injury causes contractile dysfunction. A decrease in cardiac output leads to a decrease in systemic and coronary perfusion. This exacerbates ischaemia. Inadequate systemic perfusion triggers compensatory vasoconstriction. Systemic inflammation may play a role in limiting the peripheral vascular compensatory response and may contribute to myocardial dysfunction. Revascularization leads to relief of ischaemia and significantly increases the likelihood of survival with good quality of life. IL-6 indicates interleukin-6; TNF-{alpha}, tumor necrosis factor-{alpha}; LVEDP, LV end-diastolic pressure. Adapted with permission from Reynolds HR, Hochman JS. Cardiogenic shock: current concepts and improving outcomes. *Circulation* 2008; **117**: 686–97.

bridge to further mechanical interventions. The intra-aortic balloon pump IABP improves diastolic coronary blood flow and reduces myocardial work. Both effects of the IABP are especially helpful in patients with STEMI with ongoing or recurrent ischaemic discomfort, hypotension from ischaemia-mediated LV dysfunction, and cardiogenic shock.

Selected patients with cardiogenic shock, especially in whom revascularization is technically not possible, a short- or long-term mechanical support device may be considered for either a bridge to recovery or to subsequent cardiac transplantation. Some of these support devices include extracorporeal membrane oxygenation (ECMO) via a cardiopulmonary bypass system placed through either the femoral or intrathoracic vessels and may especially serve patients with heart failure and concomitant respiratory failure. These systems are limited by their short-term usefulness [425, 426].

Cardiac rupture

Acute free wall rupture is characterized by cardiovascular collapse with electromechanical dissociation, i.e. continuing electrical activity with a loss of cardiac output and pulse. It is usually fatal within a few minutes, and does not respond to standard cardiopulmonary resuscitation. Only very rarely is there time to bring the patient to surgery.

In about 25% of patients with cardiac rupture the presentation is subacute because of thrombus or adhesions sealing the defect. The clinical picture may simulate reinfarction because of the recurrence of pain and re-elevation of ST-segments. More frequently there is sudden haemodynamic deterioration with transient or sustained hypotension due to cardiac tamponade. Echocardiography is not always able to show the site of rupture, but it can demonstrate pericardial fluid with or without signs of tamponade. However, the presence of pericardial fluid alone is not sufficient to diagnose a subacute free wall rupture, because effusion is relatively common after STEMI. The typical finding is an echo-dense mass in the pericardial space consistent with clot (haemopericardium). Immediate surgery is the treatment of choice.

Ventricular septal rupture must be considered in case of sudden severe clinical deterioration. The diagnosis is confirmed by a new, loud systolic murmur, by echocardiography and/or by detecting an oxygen step-up in the right ventricle. Echocardiography reveals the location and size of the ventricular septal defect. The left-to-right shunt can be depicted by colour Doppler and further quantified by pulsed Doppler technique. Pharmacological treatment with vasodilators, such as intravenous nitroglycerine, may produce some improvement, if there is no cardiogenic shock. Intra-aortic balloon counter pulsation is the most effective method of providing circulatory support while preparing for further therapy. Even if there is no haemodynamic instability early surgery is usually indicated, because the defect may increase [427]. However, there is still no consensus on the optimal timing of surgery because early surgical repair is difficult due to friable necrotic tissue. Therefore, percutaneous closure of the defect using an occluder-device may be an option, either as bridge to subsequent surgery or as definite therapy [428].

Mitral regurgitation

Mitral regurgitation is common and occurs usually after 2–7 days. There are three mechanisms of acute mitral regurgitation in this setting: 1) mitral valve annulus dilatation due to LV dilatation and dysfunction; 2) papillary muscle dysfunction usually due to inferior myocardial infarction; and 3) rupture of the trunk or tip of the papillary muscle. In most patients acute mitral regurgitation is secondary to papillary muscle dysfunction rather than rupture. The most frequent cause of partial or total papillary muscle rupture is a small infarct of the posteromedial papillary muscle in the right or circumflex coronary artery distribution [429]. Papillary muscle rupture typically presents itself as a sudden haemodynamic deterioration. Due to the abrupt and severe elevation of left atrial pressure, the murmur is often of low intensity. Chest radiography shows pulmonary congestion (this may be unilateral). The presence and severity of mitral regurgitation is best assessed by colour Doppler-echocardiography. Initially, a hyperdynamic left ventricle can be found. The left atrium is usually of normal size or slightly enlarged. In some patients transoesophageal echocardiography may be necessary to clearly establish the diagnosis. A pulmonary artery catheter can be used to guide patient management; the pulmonary capillary wedge pressure tracing may show large V-waves. Most patients with acute mitral regurgitation should be operated early because they may deteriorate suddenly. Cardiogenic shock and pulmonary oedema with severe mitral regurgitation require emergency surgery. Most patients need intra-aortic balloon pump placement during preparation for coronary angiography and surgery. Valve replacement is the procedure of choice for rupture of the papillary muscle, although repair can be attempted in selected cases [430].

Arrhythmias and conduction disturbances

Life-threatening arrhythmias, such as ventricular tachycardia (VT), ventricular fibrillation (VF), and total atrioventricular (AV) block, may be the first manifestation of ischaemia and require immediate correction. These arrhythmias cause many of the reported sudden cardiac deaths in patients with acute ischaemic syndromes. VF or sustained VT has been reported in up to 20% of patients who present themselves with STEMI [431].

The mechanisms of arrhythmias during acute ischaemia may be different from those seen in chronic stable ischaemic heart disease. Often, arrhythmias are a manifestation of a serious underlying disorder, such as continuing ischaemia, pump failure, or endogenous factors such as abnormal potassium levels, autonomic imbalances, hypoxia, and acid-base disturbances that should be corrected immediately. The necessity for arrhythmia treatment and its urgency depend mainly upon the haemodynamic consequences of the rhythm disorder.

Ventricular ectopic beats are common during the initial phase, but do not have—irrespective of their complexity (multiform QRS complex beats, short runs of ventricular beats, or the R-on-T phenomenon)—value as predictors of VF and do not require specific therapy.

Neither non-sustained VT (lasting <30s) nor accelerated idioventricular rhythms (usually a harmless consequence of reperfusion with a ventricular rate <120 bpm) occurring in the setting of STEMI serve as reliably predictive markers of early VF. As such, these arrhythmias do not require prophylactic antiarrhythmic therapy. Sustained and/or haemodynamically compromising VT, occurs in approximately 3% of all myocardial infarctions [432].

The incidence of VF occurring within 48h after the onset of STEMI may be decreasing due to increased use of reperfusion treatment and beta-blockers [433]. VF occurring early after STEMI has only been associated with an increase in hospital mortality but does not influence long-term mortality. Use of prophylactic beta-blockers in the setting of STEMI reduces the incidence of VF [434]. Similarly, correction of hypomagnesaemia and hypokalaemia is encouraged because of the potential contribution of electrolyte disturbances to VF. Prophylaxis with lidocaine may reduce the incidence of VF but appears to be associated with increased mortality likely owing to bradycardia and asystole and has therefore been abandoned. There is no reason to treat asymptomatic ventricular arrhythmias in the absence of established benefit. Pulseless VT and VF should be managed according to the resuscitation guidelines [435–443]. Prophylactic drug infusion with amiodarone plus a beta-blocker may be continued after resuscitation.

Atrial fibrillation (AF), which complicates 10–20% of STEMIs, is more prevalent in older patients and in those with severe LV damage and heart failure. AF in combination with STEMI is associated with higher stroke rates and with an increased in-hospital mortality [444]. In many cases—especially if present already before myocardial infarction—the arrhythmia is well tolerated and no specific treatment is required. In other instances, if fast conductance contributes to heart failure, AF should be treated (cardioversion, beta-blockers, or amiodarone). Administration of an intravenous anticoagulant is indicated if the patient is not already on such therapy. Other supraventricular tachycardias are rare and usually self-limiting. They may respond to carotid sinus pressure, beta-blockers or intravenous adenosine.

Sinus bradycardia is common (9–25%) in the first hour, especially in inferior infarctions [445]. Specific treatment is only necessary if the arrhythmias are haemodynamically compromising. A new left bundle-branch block usually indicates extensive anterior infarction with a high likelihood for developing complete AV block and pump failure. AV blocks occur in almost 7% [446] and a persistent bundle-branch block is seen in up to 5.3% of cases of STEMI [447]. In contrast to early ventricular arrhythmias, patients with peri-infarction AV block have a higher in-hospital and late mortality than those with preserved AV conduction [448]. The increased mortality is related to the extensive myocardial damage required to develop heart block rather than to the heart block itself. While pacing has not been shown to increase long-term survival, it is indicated in symptomatic bradyarrhythmias associated with STEMI [449]. AV block associated with inferior wall infarction is usually transient, with a narrow QRS escape rhythm above 40 bpm. and low mortality, whereas AV block related to anterior wall infarction is more often located below the AV node and associated with an unstable, wide QRS escape rhythm due to the extensive myocardial necrosis. Recommendations for permanent cardiac pacing for persistent conduction disturbances (≥14 days) due to STEMI are outlined in the ESC guidelines for cardiac pacing [450].

Adjunctive therapy in the acute phase

Beta-blockers

The benefit of long-term beta-blockers after STEMI is well established; the role of routine early intravenous administration is less conclusive. Two randomized trials of intravenous beta-blockade in patients receiving fibrinolysis [451, 452] were too small to draw conclusions. A post-hoc analysis of the use of atenolol in the GUSTO-I trial and a systematic review did not support the routine early intravenous use of beta-blockers [453, 454].

In the large-scale COMMIT CCS 2 trial intravenous metoprolol followed by oral administration until discharge or up to 4 weeks in patients with suspected infarction [455] did not improve survival when compared to placebo. Fewer patients had reinfarction or VF with metoprolol but this was counterbalanced by a significant increase in cardiogenic shock. Early intravenous use of beta-blockers is clearly contraindicated in patients with clinical signs of hypotension or congestive heart failure. Early use may be associated with a modest benefit in low-risk, haemodynamically stable, patients. In most patients, however, it is prudent to wait for the patient to stabilize before starting an oral beta-blocker.

Nitrates

The routine use of nitrates in the initial phase of a STEMI has not convincingly been shown to be of value and is therefore not recommended.

Calcium antagonists

A meta-analysis of trials involving calcium antagonists early in the course of STEMI showed a non-significant adverse trend [229]. There is no case for using calcium antagonists for prophylactic purposes in the acute phase.

Angiotensin-converting enzyme inhibitors and angiotensin receptor blockers

It is well established that ACE inhibitors should be given to patients with impaired EF (≤40%) or who have experienced heart failure in an early phase. The GISSI-3 [456], ISIS-4 [457] and the Chinese Study [458] have shown that ACE inhibitors started on the first day reduce mortality in the succeeding 4-6 weeks by a small but significant degree. A systematic overview of trials of ACE inhibition early in STEMI indicated that this therapy is safe, well tolerated and associated with a small but significant reduction in 30-day mortality with most of the benefit observed in the first week [457]. Therefore, ACE inhibitors should be started in the first 24h if no contraindications are present [459]. Patients who do not tolerate an ACE inhibitor should be given an ARB.

Magnesium

The large ISIS-4 trial [457] does not support the use of magnesium, although it has been argued that the magnesium regimen was not optimal. The large MAGIC (Magnesium in Coronaries) trial confirmed that there is no indication for the routine administration of intravenous magnesium in patients with STEMI.

Glucose-insulin-potassium

Although smaller studies have shown a favourable effect on the metabolism of the ischaemic myocardium, the CREATE-ECLA (Clinical Trial of Reviparin and Metabolic Modulation in Acute Myocardial Infarction Treatment and Evaluation-Estudios Clinicos Latino America) trial [423] has shown that a high-dose glucose-insulin-potassium infusion had a neutral effect on mortality, cardiac arrest and cardiogenic shock in the >20,000 patients studied. Therefore, there is no indication for this therapy in STEMI.

Specific types of infarction and subgroups

Right ventricular infarction

The recognition of right ventricular infarction is important because it may manifest itself as cardiogenic shock, but the appropriate treatment strategy is quite different from that of shock due to severe LV dysfunction. Right ventricular infarction may be suspected by the specific, but insensitive,

Table 16.17 Right ventricular infarction. Sensitivity and specificity of different diagnostic tools.

	Sensitivity	Specificity
Physical examination	88	69
ECG (ST-elevation V4R)	83	77
Echocardiography (right ventricular dilatation and akinesia)	92	82
Haemodynamics (RAP>10mmHg; RAP/PCWP >0.8)	82	97
Radionuclide ventriculography	92	82

Modified from O'Rourke RA, Dell'Italia LJ. Diagnosis and management of right ventricular myocardial infarction. *Curr Probl Cardiol* 2004; **29**: 6–47.

clinical triad of hypotension, clear lung fields, and raised jugular venous pressure in a patient with inferior STEMI. ST-segment elevation in V4R is very suggestive of the diagnosis; this lead should certainly be recorded in all cases of inferior STEMI and shock, if not done routinely. Q-waves and ST-segment elevation in V1–V3 also suggest right ventricular infarction. Echocardiography may confirm the diagnosis. Various degrees of right ventricular involvement in inferior STEMI can be found. See ➲Table 16.17.

When right ventricular infarction can be implicated in hypotension or shock, it is important to maintain right ventricular preload. It is desirable to avoid (if possible) vasodilator drugs such as opioids, nitrates, diuretics and ACE inhibitors/ARBs. Intravenous fluid loading is effective in many cases: initially, it should be administered rapidly. Careful haemodynamic monitoring is required during fluid loading. Atrial fibrillation often complicates right ventricular infarction. This should be corrected promptly as the atrial contribution to right ventricular filling is important in this context. Likewise, if heart block develops, dual chamber pacing should be installed. Revascularization by PCI should be performed as soon as possible as it may result in rapid haemodynamic improvement [460]. There has been some question of the effectiveness of fibrinolytic therapy in right ventricular infarction, [300] but it certainly seems appropriate in the hypotensive patient if PCI is not available.

Diabetic patients

Up to 20% of all patients with infarction have diabetes and this figure is expected to increase [461]. Patients with diabetes mellitus may present themselves with atypical or even without symptoms, and early development of heart failure is a common complication. Diabetic patients who sustain STEMI still have doubled mortality compared to non-diabetic patients [462, 463]. Despite this, patients with diabetes often do not receive the same extensive treatment as do non-diabetic patients. This has been shown to be associated with poorer outcome, and is presumably triggered by fear for treatment-related complications [464]. Fibrinolysis should not be withheld in patients with diabetes when indicated, even in the presence of retinopathy [465]. Furthermore, treatment with statins, beta-blockers and ACE inhibitors seems to be at least as effective and safe in diabetic as in non-diabetic patients [466–469].

Deterioration of the glucometabolic state of diabetic patients at the time of admission reflecting an acute stress response to sudden impairment of LV function, appears to have an effect on outcome. Higher glucose levels on admission are indeed associated with increased mortality rates in diabetic patients presenting with STEMI [470, 471]. Strict attention to the glycaemic control by use of insulin infusion followed by multiple-dose insulin treatment has been shown to reduce long-term mortality as compared to routine oral antidiabetic therapy in diabetic patients [472–474]. In the more recent DIGAMI (Diabetes and Insulin-Glucose Infusion in Acute Myocardial Infarction)-2 study, however, mortality did not significantly differ between diabetic patients randomized to either acute insulin infusion followed by insulin-based long-term glucose control, insulin infusion followed by standard glucose control or standard glucometabolic management, probably reflecting a lack of difference in glucose control in the three groups [475]. Because hyperglycaemia remained one of the most important predictors of outcome in this study, however, it appears to be reasonable to keep glucose levels within normal ranges in diabetic patients. Target glucose levels between 90 and 140mg/dL (5mmol/L and 7.8mmol/L) have been suggested [476]. Blood glucose levels below 80–90mg/dL (4.4–5mmol/L) should be avoided, as hypoglycaemia-induced ischaemia might also affect outcome [477]. Also see ➲Chapter 14.

Patients with renal dysfunction

The two-year mortality rate among STEMI patients with end-stage renal disease (creatinine clearance <30mL/min) is considerably higher than in the general population [478]. This may be explained by a higher proportion of cardiovascular risk factors as well as the fact that acute reperfusion strategies are offered to these patients less frequently because of fear of higher bleeding rates and contrast medium-induced renal failure [479, 480]. Although recommendations for STEMI patients with renal dysfunction are essentially the same as for patients without renal disease the risk of a further deterioration of renal function must be taken into account when administering contrast medium during primary PCI and when giving drugs such as ACE inhibitors, ARBs, and diuretics. Also see ➲Chapter 15.

Management of the later in-hospital complications

Pericarditis

Pericarditis associated with acute myocardial infarction may cause chest pain that can easily be misinterpreted as recurrent infarction or post-infarction angina. However, contrary to these entities, pericarditis-induced pain is usually of a sharp nature and related to posture and respiration. It is often accompanied by a pericardial rub. The pain may be relieved by high-dose intravenous aspirin (1000mg/24 hours) or non-steroidal inflammatory agents. Echocardiography should be regularly performed in order to early diagnose complicating pericardial effusions.

Late ventricular arrhythmias

VT and VF occurring during the first 24–48 hours have a low predictive value for recurring arrhythmias risk over time. Arrhythmias developing later are liable to recur and are associated with an increased risk of sudden death [481].

Aggressive attempts should be made to treat heart failure and to search for and to correct myocardial ischaemia in patients with ventricular tachyarrhythmias. Myocardial revascularization should be performed, when appropriate, to reduce the risk of sudden death in patients experiencing VF or polymorphic VT [482]. No controlled trials, however, have evaluated the effects of myocardial revascularization on VT or VF after STEMI. Observational studies suggest that revascularization is unlikely to prevent recurrent cardiac arrest in patients with a markedly abnormal LV function or sustained monomorphic VT, even if the original arrhythmia appeared to result from transient ischaemia [483].

Several prospective multicentre clinical trials in high-risk patients with LV dysfunction (EF <40%) due to prior infarction have documented improved survival with ICD therapy [484–486]. Compared to conventional antiarrhythmic drug therapy, ICD therapy was associated with a reduction in mortality from 23% to 55%, depending on the risk group studied. The ICD is therefore the primary therapy to reduce mortality in patients with significant LV dysfunction, who present with haemodynamically unstable sustained VT or who are resuscitated from VF occurring later than in the first 24–48 hours [482]. Electrophysiological testing with catheter ablation may occasionally be of benefit if a curable arrhythmia, such as bundle-branch reentry, is revealed. Also see ➲Chapter 30.

Patients with sustained monomorphic VT without haemodynamic instability are usually, but not always, at relatively low risk for sudden death (2% yearly) [487]. If episodes are relatively infrequent, the ICD alone may be the most appropriate initial therapy in order to avoid the relative ineffectiveness and adverse complications of drug therapy. ICD implantation is in this context also reasonable for treatment of recurrent sustained VT in patients with normal or near normal LV function. Alternatively, catheter ablation is, in experienced hands, a good therapeutic option for monomorphic VT.

With the exception of beta-blockers, randomized clinical trials have not shown antiarrhythmic drugs to be effective in the primary management of patients with life-threatening ventricular arrhythmias or in the prevention of sudden death and should not be used as primary therapy for this indication. Only amiodarone therapy may be considered in special situations. No benefit of amiodarone was shown in patients with NYHA functional class II heart failure and even showed potential harm in patients with NYHA functional class III heart failure and EF ≤35% [484].

Left ventricular thrombus

The development of mural left ventricular thrombi is a common complication of myocardial infarction typically developing within the first two weeks. They are the most common source of stroke. The likelihood of developing a left ventricular thrombus after an acute myocardial infarction depends on infarct location and size. Left ventricular thrombus is most often seen in patients with large anterior infarctions with aneurysm formation and akinesis or dyskinesis. In patients treated with fibrinolysis or primary PCI the rate of mural thrombus formation is around 4 to 5% [488–490].

Post-infarction angina and ischaemia

Angina, recurrent ischaemia or reinfarction in the early post-infarction phase following successful primary PCI or fibrinolysis should prompt urgent (repeated) coronary angiography and if indicated (repeated) PCI or CABG.

Although analyses from several trials have identified a patent infarct-related vessel as a marker for good long-term outcome, it has yet not been convincingly shown that late PCI with the sole aim of restoring patency is beneficial. In the OAT trial, successful PCI of the occluded infarct-related artery 3–28 days after the acute event did not reduce death, reinfarction, or heart failure in stable patients without chest pain or signs of ongoing ischaemia, but was associated with an excess reinfarction during 4 years of follow-up [491].

Coronary artery bypass surgery may be indicated if symptoms are not controlled by other means or if coronary angiography demonstrates lesions, such as left main stenosis or three-vessel disease with poor LV function.

Secondary prevention

Coronary heart disease is a chronic condition and patients who have recovered from a STEMI are at high risk for new events and premature death. Eight to ten per cent of post-infarction patients have a recurrent infarction within a year after discharge [492], clearly demonstrating the necessity of an effective secondary prevention (see Chapter 12).

Several evidence-based interventions can improve prognosis. Even though long-term management of this large group of patients will be the responsibility of the general practitioner, these interventions will have a higher chance to be implemented if initiated during hospital stay. In addition, lifestyle changes should be explained and proposed to the patient before discharge. However, habits of a lifetime are not easily changed and the implementation and follow-up of these changes are a long-term undertaking. In this regard a close collaboration between the cardiologist and the general practitioner is critically important.

Smoking cessation

Unselected ACS patients who are smokers, are twice as likely to present as STEMI, compared to non-smokers [493], indicating a strong prothrombotic effect of smoking. Evidence from observational studies shows that those who stop smoking reduce their mortality in the succeeding years by at least one-third compared to those who continue to smoke [494]. Stop smoking is potentially the most effective of all secondary prevention measures and much effort should be devoted to this end. Patients do not smoke during the acute phase of a STEMI and the convalescent period is ideal for health professionals to help smokers to quit. However, resumption of smoking is common after returning home and continued support and advice is needed during rehabilitation. Nicotine replacement, buproprione and antidepressants may be useful [495]. Nicotine patches have been demonstrated to be safe in ACS patients [496]. Also see Chapter 25.

Diet, dietary supplements, and weight control

Evidence from systematic reviews of randomized controlled trials on food and nutrition in secondary prevention has recently been published [497]. Current guidelines on prevention [495] recommend: 1) to eat a wide variety of foods; 2) adjustment of calories intake to avoid overweight; 3) increased consumption of fruit, vegetables, along with wholegrain cereals and bread, fish (especially oily), lean meat, and low-fat dairy products; 4) to replace saturated fats with monounsaturated and polyunsaturated fats from vegetable and marine sources and to reduce total fats to <30% of calories intake, of which less than 1/3 should be saturated; 5) to reduce salt intake if blood pressure is raised. Many processed and prepared foods are high in salt, and in fat of doubtful quality.

There is no evidence for the use of antioxidant supplements, low glycaemic index diets, or homocysteine-lowering therapies post STEMI. The role of omega-3 fatty acid supplements for secondary prevention after STEMI is unclear [495]. In an unselected heart failure population including 50% patients with ischaemic cardiomyopathy, polyunsaturated fatty acids provided a small beneficial advantage in terms of mortality and admission to hospital for cardiovascular reasons [498]. In the only (open-label) randomized study in patients post myocardial infarction, the GISSI prevenzione trial, 1g of fish oil daily on top of a Mediterranean diet significantly reduced total and cardiovascular mortality [456]. However, a meta-analysis, including GISSI prevenzione, showed no significant effect on mortality or cardiovascular events [412] and no evidence that the source or dose affected outcome.

Obesity is an increasing problem in patients with STEMI. At least one third of the European women and one in four men with ACSs below the age of 65 have a BMI of 30kg/m^2 or more [499]. Current ESC guidelines [495] define a BMI <25kg/m^2 as optimal and recommend weight reduction when BMI is 30kg/m^2, or more, and when waist circumference is more than 102/88cm (men/women) because weight loss can improve many obesity-related risk factors. However, it has not been established that weight reduction per se reduces mortality (see Chapter 25).

Physical activity

Exercise therapy has long been used for rehabilitation purposes following STEMI and the benefit of regular physical exercise in stable CAD patients is also well established. Four mechanisms are considered to be important mediators of a reduced cardiac event rate: 1) improvement of endothelial function, 2) reduced progression of coronary lesions, 3) reduced thrombogenic risk and 4) improved collateralization. In a large meta-analysis exercise training as part of coronary rehabilitation programs was associated with a 26% reduction in cardiac mortality [500]. It should be appreciated that apart from its influence on mortality, exercise rehabilitation can have other beneficial effects. Exercise capacity, cardio-respiratory fitness, and perception of well-being have also been reported to improve, at least during the actual training period, and even in elderly patients. Thirty minutes of moderate intensity aerobic exercise at least five times per week is recommended [495]. Each single-stage increase in physical work capacity is associated with a reduction in all-cause mortality risk in the range of 8–14%. Also see ➲Chapter 25.

Antiplatelet and anticoagulant treatment

The Antiplatelet Trialists Collaboration [251] meta-analysis demonstrated a 25% reduction in reinfarction and death for post-infarction patients treated with aspirin in a dose range from 75–325mg daily. There is evidence that the lower dosages (75–100mg) are effective with fewer bleeding complications [251]. Clinical trials undertaken before the widespread use of aspirin have shown that oral anticoagulants (vitamin K antagonists) are effective in preventing reinfarction and death in infarct survivors [501, 502]. Aspirin can be replaced by oral anticoagulants at recommended INR if there is an indication for oral anticoagulation (e.g. atrial fibrillation, LV thrombus, mechanical valves). In a large meta-analysis of patients with ACSs followed for up to 5 years (including >10,000 patients with infarction), the combination of aspirin and oral anticoagulation at INR 2–3 prevented three major adverse events and caused one major bleed per 100 patients treated compared to aspirin alone [503]. This combination therefore seems to be a reasonable treatment in STEMI survivors who have a high risk of thromboembolic events. In some patients, there is an indication for dual antiplatelet therapy and oral anticoagulation (e.g. stent placement and AF). In the absence of prospective randomized studies, no firm recommendations can be given [243, 504, 505]. Triple therapy seems to have an acceptable risk: benefit ratio provided clopidogrel cotherapy is kept short and the bleeding risk is low [504, 505]. Oral anticoagulants plus a short course of clopidogrel might be an alternative in patients with a higher risk of bleeding [504]. Most importantly, drug-eluting stents should be avoided in patients who need oral anticoagulation. Oral anticoagulants may also be considered in patients who do not tolerate aspirin or clopidogrel.

Clopidogrel given on top of aspirin for a median of 9–12 months has been studied for secondary prevention after an ACS without persistent ST-segment elevation [252]. The use of clopidogrel for primary PCI and in conjunction with fibrinolytic therapy has been described earlier (see ➲Reperfusion therapy, p.587). The optimal duration of clopidogrel treatment after STEMI has not been determined. Extrapolating the long-term effect of clopidogrel in patients after NSTE-ACS with a treatment duration of 12 months is recommended whether or not a stent has been placed [252, 259].

Beta-blockers

Several trials and meta-analyses have demonstrated that beta-blockers reduce mortality and reinfarction by 20–25% in those who have recovered from an infarction. Most of these trials have been performed in the pre-reperfusion era. A meta-analysis of 82 randomized trials provides strong evidence for long-term use of beta-blockers to reduce morbidity and mortality after STEMI, even if ACE inhibitors are co-administered [454]. The significant mortality reductions observed with beta-blockers in heart failure in general further support the use of these agents after STEMI. Evidence from all available studies suggests that beta-blockers should be used indefinitely in all patients who recovered from a STEMI and do not have a contraindication [454].

Calcium antagonists

Trials with verapamil [506] and diltiazem [507] have suggested that these agents may prevent reinfarction and death. In a small trial with STEMI patients treated with fibrinolytic agents, but without heart failure, the 6-month use of diltiazem (300mg daily) reduced the rate of coronary interventions [230]. However, the use of verapamil and diltiazem is only appropriate when beta-blockers are contraindicated or not tolerated. Caution must be exercised in the presence of impaired LV function. Trials with dihydropyridines (nifedipine) have failed to show a benefit in terms of improved prognosis. They should, therefore, only be prescribed for clear clinical indications such as hypertension or angina [229].

Nitrates

There is no evidence that oral or transdermal nitrates improve prognosis. The ISIS-4 [457] and GISSI-3 [456] trials failed to show a benefit at 4–6 weeks after the event. Nonetheless, nitrates continue to be first-line therapy for symptomatic angina pectoris.

Angiotensin-converting enzyme inhibitors and angiotensin receptor blockers

Several trials have established that ACE inhibitors reduce mortality after STEMI with reduced residual LV function (<40%) [508–511]. There exists strong evidence for administering ACE inhibitors to patients having experienced symptoms of heart failure in the acute phase, even after full recovery, or to patients who have an EF of ≤40%, provided there are no contraindications. There is a case for giving ACE inhibitors to all patients with STEMI from admission [456, 512]. Against such a policy is the increased incidence of hypotension and renal failure in those receiving ACE inhibitors in the acute phase, and the small benefit in those at relatively low risk, such as patients with small inferior infarctions. In favour are observations from studies in populations with stable cardiovascular disease but without LV dysfunction showing a 1.1% absolute risk reduction of the combined endpoint of cardiovascular death, non-fatal myocardial infarction and stroke. Use of ACE inhibitors should be considered in all patients with atherosclerosis, but given the relatively modest effect, their long-term use is not mandated in post-STEMI patients who are normotensive, without heart failure or compromised systolic left ventricular function.

Two trials have evaluated ARBs in the context of STEMI as alternatives to ACE inhibitors: the OPTIMAAL (Optimal Trial in Myocardial Infarction with Angiotensin II Antagonist Losartan) trial with losartan failed to show superiority or non-inferiority over captopril [513]. Conversely, the VALIANT (VALsartan in acute myocardial iNfarcTion trial) trial compared high-dose valsartan alone, full-dose captopril or both. Mortality was similar in the three groups, but discontinuations were more frequent in the groups receiving captopril [514]. Therefore, valsartan in dosages as used in the trial represents an alternative to ACE-inhibitors in patients who do not tolerate ACE-inhibitors and have clinical signs of heart failure and/or an EF ≤40%.

Aldosterone blockade

The EPHESUS (Eplerenone Post-Acute Myocardial Infarction Heart Failure Efficacy and Survival Study) trial randomized post-STEMI patients with LV dysfunction (EF ≤40%) and heart failure or diabetes to eplerenone, a selective aldosterone blocker, or placebo. After a mean follow-up of 16 months, there was a 15% relative reduction in total mortality and a 13% reduction in the composite of death and hospitalization for cardiovascular events [515]. However, serious hyperkalaemia was more frequent in the group receiving eplerenone. The results suggest that aldosterone blockade may be considered for post-STEMI patients with an EF ≤40% and/or heart failure provided that creatinine is <2.5mg/dL in men and 2.0mg/dL in women, and potassium is ≤5.0mEq/L. Routine monitoring of serum potassium is warranted and should be particularly careful when other potential potassium-sparing agents are used.

Management of diabetes

Glucometabolic disturbances are common in patients with coronary disease and should be actively searched for. Since an abnormal glucose tolerance test is a significant risk factor for future cardiovascular events after myocardial infarction [516], it seems meaningful to perform such a test before, or shortly after, discharge [305]. In patients with established diabetes the aim is to achieve HbA1c levels ≤6.5%. This calls for intensive modification of lifestyle (diet, physical activity, weight reduction), usually in addition to pharmacotherapy. Coordination with a physician specialized in diabetes is advisable. In patients with impaired fasting glucose level or impaired glucose tolerance only lifestyle changes are currently recommended [305].

Interventions on lipid profile

Several trials have unequivocally demonstrated the benefits of long-term use of statins in the prevention of new ischaemic events and of mortality in patients with coronary heart disease. The targets established by the Fourth Joint Task Force of the ESC and other societies in patients after infarction are: for total cholesterol: 175mg/dL (4.5mmol/L) with an option of 155mg/dL (4.0mmol/L) if feasible and for lower LDLc 100mg/dL (2.5mmol/L) with an option of 80mg/dL (2.0mmol/L) if feasible [495]. Although pharmacological treatment is highly efficient in treating dyslipidaemia in heart disease, diet remains a basic requirement for all patients with coronary heart disease. The most recent controversy on lipid-lowering treatment has been focused on intensive, versus standard lipid-lowering therapy. A recent meta-analysis of randomized controlled trials that compared different intensities of statin therapy identified seven trials with nearly 30,000 patients suffering from CAD [517]. Compared with less intensive statin regimens, more intensive regimens further reduced LDLc-levels and reduced the risk of myocardial infarction and stroke. Although there was no effect on mortality among patients with chronic CAD, all-cause mortality was reduced among ACS patients with more intensive statin regimens. All seven trials reported events by randomization arm rather than by LDLc-level achieved. About half of the patients treated with more intensive statin therapy did not achieve an LDLc-level of <80mg/dL (2.0mmol/L), and none of the trials tested combination therapies. The analysis supports the use of more intensive statin regimens in patients with established CAD.

Prophylactic implantation of an implantable cardioverter defibrillator

The ICD is the only specific antiarrhythmic treatment proved consistently effective to reduce risk of both sudden death and total mortality. Primary preventive ICD therapy has been shown to reduce the risk of sudden death in two patient groups: 1) patients whose EF is ≤40% and who have spontaneous non-sustained VT and sustained monomorphic VT inducible by electrophysiological testing [518], and 2) patients whose EF is ≤30% as a result of an infarction that occurred at least 40 days earlier when heart failure (NYHA functional class II or III symptoms) is present [484, 519–521]. In view of this, ICD therapy after STEMI is reasonable in patients with an EF ≤30–35%, and who are in NYHA functional class I on chronic optimal medical therapy. In general, ICD implantation should be deferred until at least 40 days after the acute event. Evaluation of the need for an ICD and implantation should be deferred until at least 3 months after revascularization procedures to allow adequate time for recovery of LV function. Prophylactic antiarrhythmic drug therapy is not indicated to reduce mortality (see Chapter 30).

Personal perspective

The prevalence of CAD and consecutively the prevalence of ACS are continuously increasing as a result of growing life expectancy and increasing rates of obesity and diabetes. A further increase is expected not only in highly industrialized countries but also, and most pronounced, in the rapidly developing, densely populated regions of the world. It is already conceivable that diagnosis and risk assessment of individual patients in the near future will be guided by sophisticated biochemical markers that capture earlier stages of pathophysiology long before fatal events have occurred. Further contributions to the early detection of patients at risk are expected from improved non-invasive imaging techniques. Several promising drugs developments are under evaluation which may further increase efficacy and safety. However, the treatment has already reached a very high level of success and more attention needs to be directed in implementing the current achievements. Particularly health-education programmes directed towards better early identification may contribute most effectively to reducing fatal outcomes.

Further reading

Bassand JP, Hamm CW, Ardissino D, *et al.* Guidelines for the diagnosis and treatment of non-ST-segment elevation acute coronary syndromes. *Eur Heart J* 2007; **28**: 1598–660.

Bassand JP. Bleeding and transfusion in acute coronary syndromes: a shift in the paradigm. *Heart* 2008; **94**: 661–6.

Clappers N, Brouwer MA, Verheugt FW. Antiplatelet treatment for coronary heart disease. *Heart* 2007; **93**: 258–65.

Graham I, Atar D, Borch-Johnsen K, *et al.* European guidelines on cardiovascular disease prevention in clinical practice: executive summary. *Eur Heart J* 2007; **28**: 2375–414.

Hillis LD, Lange RA. Optimal management of acute coronary syndromes. *N Engl J Med* 2009; **360**: 2237–40.

Korff S, Katus HA, Giannitsis E. Differential diagnosis of elevated troponins. *Heart* 2006; **92**: 987–93.

Mollmann H, Nef H, Elsasser A, *et al.* Stem cells in myocardial infarction: from bench to bedside. *Heart* 2009; **95**: 508–14.

Thygesen K, Alpert JS, White HD. Universal definition of myocardial infarction. *Eur Heart J* 2007; **28**: 2525–38.

Van de Werf F, Bax J, Betriu A, *et al.* Management of acute myocardial infarction in patients presenting with persistent ST-segment elevation: the Task Force on the Management of ST-Segment Elevation Acute Myocardial Infarction of the European Society of Cardiology. *Eur Heart J* 2008; **29**: 2909–45.

White HD, Chew DP. Acute myocardial infarction. *Lancet* 2008; **372**: 570–84.

Wiviott S. *Antiplatelet therapy in ischemic heart disease*, 2009. Chichester: Wiley-Blackwell.

Online resources

- The Global Registry of Acute Coronary Events: http://www.outcomes.org/grace

For full references and multimedia materials please visit the online version of the book (http://esctextbook.oxfordonline.com).

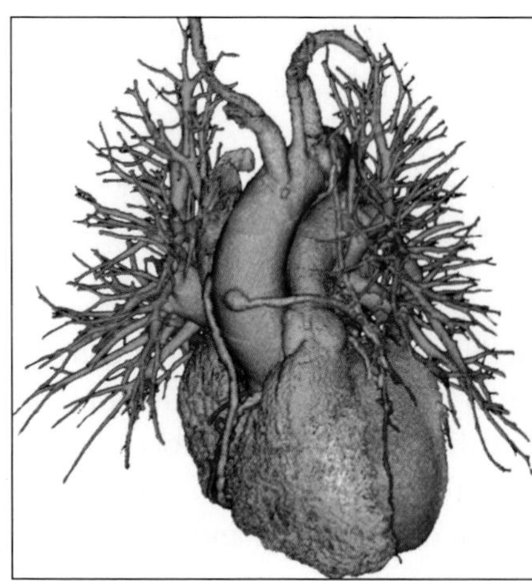

CHAPTER 17

Chronic Ischaemic Heart Disease

Filippo Crea, Paolo G. Camici, Raffaele De Caterina, and Gaetano A. Lanza

Contents

Summary

The coronary circulation serves the purpose of matching myocardial oxygen supply and consumption. A transient mismatch causing reversible myocardial ischaemia is the dominant feature of chronic ischaemic heart disease (IHD), which is also characterized by stable symptoms over a period of months, years, or even decades. Stable angina is the most frequent presentation of chronic IHD; other clinical presentations are microvascular angina, vasospastic angina, and ischaemic cardiomyopathy. Stable angina is mainly caused by obstructive coronary atherosclerosis. ECG exercise stress test is the first-line test for diagnosis and risk stratification; when it cannot be performed or is not interpretable imaging stress tests are indicated. The aims of treatment are to improve prognosis and to reduce symptoms. Prognosis is improved by the reduction of coronary risk factor burden, by the administration of antiplatelet agents, and, in high risk patients, by myocardial revascularization. Symptoms are improved by anti-anginal drugs which act through different mechanisms, including reduction of myocardial oxygen consumption and improvement of myocardial perfusion, and by myocardial revascularization in patients who do not satisfactorily respond to drugs. Microvascular angina is caused by coronary microvascular dysfunction; its prognosis is good, but symptoms can be invalidating and frequently do not fully respond to conventional anti-anginal drugs. Vasospastic angina is caused by coronary artery spasm; prognosis is good if spasm is prevented by treatment with coronary vasodilators. Ischaemic cardiomyopathy is dominated by symptoms and signs of left ventricular dysfunction; prognosis is mainly determined by the degree of left ventricular dysfunction and seems improved by myocardial revascularization in patients with large areas of myocardial viability.

Introduction

Chronic IHD is characterized by stable symptoms over a period of months, years, or even decades. It may represent the first clinical presentation of IHD, more frequently in women than in men, or it may follow an acute coronary syndrome. Angina, caused by episodes of transient myocardial ischaemia, is the dominant symptom of chronic IHD, which includes three different clinical presentations: stable angina, microvascular angina, and vasospastic angina. Myocardial ischaemia, however, may be silent in all anginal syndromes. A fourth clinical presentation of IHD is ischaemic cardiomyopathy, which is characterized by signs and symptoms of heart failure.

In chronic stable angina transient myocardial ischaemia is mainly caused by obstructive coronary stenoses which reduce coronary flow reserve, thus preventing the matching between myocardial oxygen supply and myocardial oxygen demand when subendocardial coronary flow reserve is exhausted. Symptom severity can be modulated by dynamic vasomotion at the site of pliable stenoses and/or by coronary microvascular dysfunction [1].

In microvascular angina transient myocardial ischaemia is caused by coronary microvascular dysfunction in patients with angiographically normal epicardial coronary arteries, in the absence of any other specific cardiac disease.

In vasospastic angina transient myocardial ischaemia is caused by coronary spasm. Angina attacks typically occur at rest, usually with a stable, predictive pattern, but sometimes with phases of worsening symptoms which can mimic an acute coronary syndrome.

Finally, ischaemic cardiomyopathy (➲Chapter 18) can result from a large myocardial infarction (MI) or from multiple smaller infarctions followed by left ventricular dilatation and dysfunction.

Knowledge of anatomy and function of coronary arterial system and of pathophysiology of myocardial ischaemia are needed for a full comprehension of the different clinical presentations of chronic IHD.

Notably, angina and transient myocardial ischaemia may also occur in patients with non atherosclerotic obstructive coronary artery disease, including those with congenital abnormalities of coronary arteries, myocardial bridging, coronary arteritis in association with systemic vasculitis, and radiation-induced coronary disease [2]. These forms of angina are not discussed in this chapter. Angina can also occur in heart diseases not primarily involving epicardial coronary arteries, including myocardial (see ➲Chapter 18) and valvular (see ➲Chapter 21) diseases, in which coronary microvascular dysfunction, however, plays an important contributory pathogenetic role [3].

The coronary circulation

The coronary circulation is composed of three vascular systems arranged in series: 1) the arterial system conveys blood from the aorta to the site of metabolite and gas exchanges with myocardial cells, and controls most of the resistance to flow; 2) the capillary system controls the regional microdistribution of blood flow and blood-tissue exchanges; and 3) the venous system controls intramyocardial blood volume at the end of diastole, thus influencing end-diastolic myocardial fibre length.

Although all the components of the coronary circulation are essential for its correct functioning, evidence accrued over the past few decades has proved that a number of different abnormalities in the arterial system are involved in the pathogenesis of many cardiac diseases.

Coronary arterial system

The coronary arterial system is composed of three compartments with different functions, although their precise borders cannot be clearly defined anatomically or histologically (➲Fig. 17.1) [1].

The proximal compartment is represented by the large epicardial coronary arteries which have a capacitance function and offer little resistance to coronary blood flow. During systole, epicardial coronary arteries accumulate elastic energy as they increase their blood content by about 25%. This elastic energy is transformed into blood kinetic energy at the beginning of diastole and contributes to the prompt reopening of intramyocardial vessels that are squeezed closed by systole.

The intermediate compartment is represented by pre-arterioles. They are characterized by a measurable pressure drop along their length. They are not under direct vasomotor control by diffusible myocardial metabolites because of their extramyocardial position and arterial wall thickness. Proximal pre-arterioles are more responsive to changes in flow, while distal pre-arterioles are more responsive to changes in pressure. Their specific function is to maintain pressure at the origin of the arterioles within a narrow range when coronary perfusion pressure and/or flow change.

The distal compartment is represented by arterioles. They are characterized by a considerable pressure drop along their length and represent the site of the metabolic regulation of myocardial blood flow, as their tone is influenced

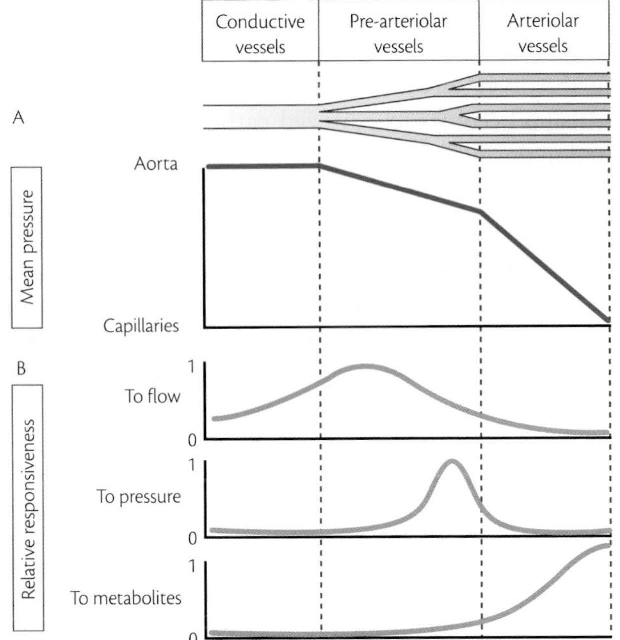

Figure 17.1 (A) Schematic representation of the functional subdivision of the coronary arterial system in conductive vessels, pre-arterioles and arterioles. The pressure drop along conductive vessels is negligible, that through pre-arterioles is appreciable and that through the arterioles is the largest. Pre-arterioles, by definition, are not exposed to myocardial dilator metabolites because of their extramyocardial position or their wall thickness. (B) Conductance vessels and, to an even greater extent, proximal pre-arterioles are more responsive to flow-dependent dilatation. Distal pre-arterioles are more responsive to changes in intravascular pressure and are mainly responsible for autoregulation of coronary blood flow. Arterioles are more responsive to changes in the intramyocardial concentration of metabolites and are mainly responsible for the metabolic regulation of coronary blood flow. Reproduced from Maseri A. *Ischemic Heart Disease*, 1995. New York: Churchill Livingstone Inc, with permission from Elsevier.

by substances produced during myocardial metabolism. Their specific function is the matching of myocardial blood supply and myocardial oxygen demand.

Large epicardial arteries have a diameter ranging from a few millimetres to ~500μm and are visible at coronary angiography. Pre-arterioles (diameter from ~500 to ~100μm) and arterioles (diameter <100μm) are below the resolution of current angiographic systems and hence are not visible at angiography. Notably, each compartment is governed by distinct regulatory mechanisms.

Distribution of coronary vascular resistance in series

The vascular resistance is distributed in series along the coronary vascular bed, but it also varies in parallel vascular segments in different layers of the ventricular wall.

The individual contribution of successive coronary vascular segments to total resistance can be inferred from the progressive drop in mean pressure from the aorta to the coronary sinus. About 10% of the pressure drop occurs in epicardial coronary arteries, 30% in pre-arterioles, 40% in arterioles, and 20% from capillaries to large veins (➲Fig. 17.2) [4]. Notably, such an inference is an approximation as the vascular cross-section varies considerably during the cardiac cycle. Indeed, because the left ventricular wall compresses intramyocardial vessels during systole, most of the coronary blood flow to the left ventricle occurs during diastole. Thus, the contracting heart obstructs its own blood supply. At peak systole there is even backflow in the coronary

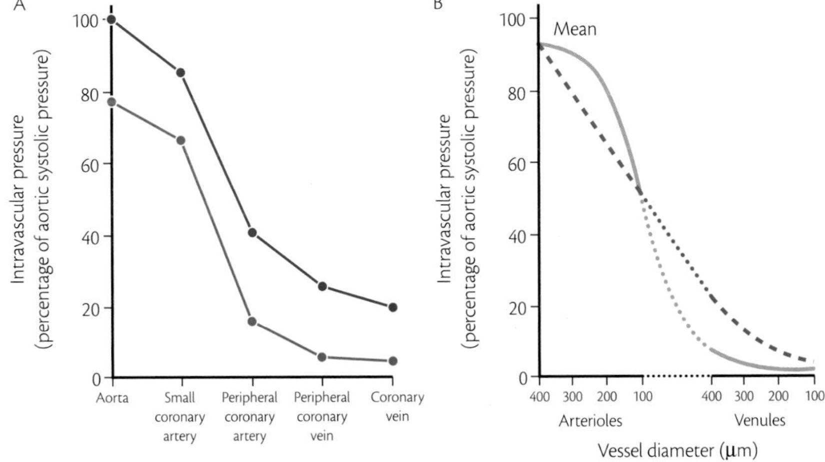

Figure 17.2 (A) Systolic (blue line) and diastolic (red line) pressures in a distal epicardial coronary artery, in a coronary arteriole, in a small coronary vein and in a large coronary vein of anaesthetized dogs, expressed as percentages of aortic pressure. The greatest pressure drop occurs through small coronary arteries. (B) Mean coronary pressure drop from the aorta to small coronary arteries and veins in a rabbit heart, measured on the surface of the epicardium (orange line). The greatest pressure drop occurs at the level of arterioles less than 100μm in diameter. During intravenous dipyridamole infusion (green line) the pressure drop across pre-arteriolar vessels increases, indicating insufficient flow-mediated dilatation. Adapted with permission from Klassen GA, Armour JA, Garner JB. Coronary circulatory pressure gradient. *Can J Physiol Pharmacol* 1987; **65**: 520–31; and Chilian WM, Layne SM, Klausner EC, *et al.* Redistribution of coronary microvascular resistance produced by dypiridamole. *Am J Physiol* 1989; **256**: 383–92.

arteries, particularly in the intramural and small epicardial vessels. During diastole the driving pressure is the pressure gradient between the coronary arteries and either the right atrium or the left ventricle (for veins that drain directly into the ventricle). If perfusion pressure is progressively lowered, diastolic blood flow ceases when the coronary driving pressure reaches 40–50mmHg, the so-called *pressure at zero flow*, which is largely determined by diastolic compressive forces.

Distribution of coronary vascular resistance in parallel

The distribution of coronary resistance in parallel vascular segments in different layers of the ventricular wall can be studied by pressure/flow curves which provide information on the differences in vascular resistance between subendocardial and subepicardial layers of the ventricular wall. In non-beating hearts, maximal conductance is higher in the subendocardial than the subepicardial layers (➲Chapter 8). Conversely, in beating hearts, maximal conductance is lower in the subendocardial layers because of greater extravascular compressive forces during both systole and diastole. The extravascular systolic compressive forces have two components. The first is the intracavitary left ventricular pressure, which is transmitted fully to the subendocardium, but falls off to almost zero at the epicardial surface. The second is the vascular narrowing caused by compression and bending of vessels coursing through the ventricular wall from subepicardium to subendocardium (intramyocardial pressure). Hence, during ventricular contraction, subendocardial arterioles become more narrowed relative to those in the subepicardium and, at the onset of diastole, they present a higher resistance to flow, needing a longer time to resume their full diastolic calibre.

Tachycardia impairs the subendocardial blood flow, particularly in the presence of myocardial hypertrophy. In fact, the time constant of diastolic filling of intramyocardial vessels does not shorten with heart rate and becomes a limiting factor for the perfusion of subendocardial layers. Nevertheless, in conscious dogs, under normal resting conditions, the subendocardial flow is higher than the subepicardial flow (with a ratio of about 1.25:1), because of a greater conductance in the subendocardial arterioles. The latter finding is consistent with the higher subendocardial oxygen demand which is secondary to the greater wall stress in the subendocardial than in the subepicardial layers [5]. Thus, given a sufficiently high perfusion pressure, a sufficiently long diastole and an adequate systolic expansion of conductive arteries, the subendocardium is adequately perfused. However, when perfusion pressure at the origin of arteriolar vessels is reduced compared to that of the aorta (e.g. due to epicardial coronary stenosis or aortic stenosis) perfusion becomes jeopardized earlier in the inner compared to the outer layers of the left ventricle. The inner layers then become even more susceptible to underperfusion if diastolic time is short and in the presence of myocardial hypertrophy. Of note, selective constriction of subepicardial vessels can influence perfusion pressure in subendocardial vessels and hence subendocardial flow. Overperfusion of the subepicardial layers, in particular during exercise, when subendocardial perfusion is hampered by the shortening of diastolic time, might be prevented by sympathetic-system-mediated selective constriction of the subepicardial vessels, as proposed by Feigl [6]. Accordingly, potent constrictors, such as endothelin and alpha-adrenergic agonists, or adenosine antagonists, such as theophylline [7], cause selective subepicardial constriction which secondarily improves subendocardial perfusion.

Response to changes in flow

The shear stress, the tractive force that acts on the vascular wall, is proportional to the shear rate or velocity and to viscosity. Arteries exhibit an intrinsic tendency to maintain a constant shear stress, despite changes in shear rate or in viscosity. Indeed, very high or very low shear stress may jeopardize the interaction between blood elements and the endothelium. In the absence of changes in distending pressure, variations of flow in epicardial coronary arteries can be achieved by intracoronary injection of arteriolar vasodilators such as adenosine. Angiographic studies in man have shown that epicardial coronary arteries dilate in response to an increase in coronary blood flow and that the increase in coronary diameter is proportional to the increase in flow, thus maintaining shear stress constant [8].

Flow-mediated dilatation occurs also in proximal pre-arterioles during the dilatation of distal pre-arterioles in response to a reduction in perfusion pressure and during arteriolar dilatation in response to increased myocardial oxygen consumption or following myocardial ischaemia. In this setting, flow-mediated dilatation serves mainly to minimize any fall in pressure along the course of proximal pre-arterioles during dilatation of more distal vessels [9].

Mechanisms of flow-mediated dilatation

Flow-mediated dilatation is determined by vasodilators released by endothelial cells in response to an increase in shear stress, in particular nitric oxide (NO), endothelium-derived hyperpolarizing factor (EDHF), and prostacyclin.

EDHF causes hyperpolarization and relaxation of smooth muscle cells by opening K^+ channels, whereas prostacyclin causes relaxation by activating adenylate cyclase, which leads to the formation of cyclic adenosine monophosphate. (➲Fig. 17.3).

NO is synthesized from the amino acid L-arginine by NO synthases (NOSs). The endothelial isoform, eNOS (or NOS III), is constitutive and is predominantly, although not exclusively, found in endothelial cells. eNOS is a highly regulated protein at both transcription and functional levels.

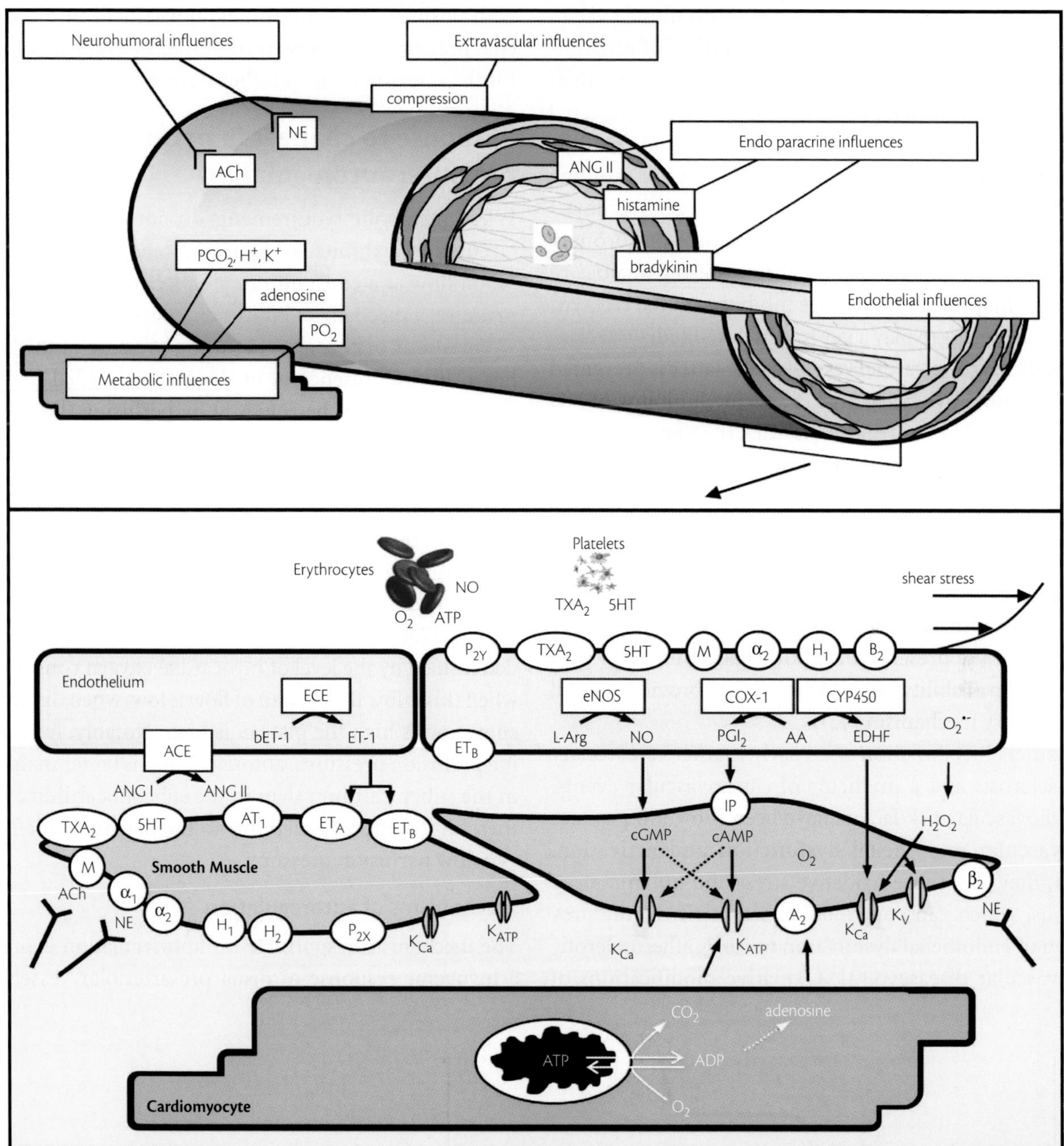

Figure 17.3 Schematic drawing of a coronary arteriole and the various influences that determine coronary vasomotor tone and diameter. PO_2, oxygen tension; TxA_2, thromboxane A_2 (receptor); 5HT, serotonin or 5-hydroxytryptamine (receptor); P2X and P2Y, purinergic receptor subtypes 2X and 2Y that mediate ATP-induced vasoconstriction and vasodilation, respectively; ACh, acetylcholine; M, muscarinic receptor; H1 and H2, histamine receptors type 1 and 2; B2, bradykinin receptor subtype 2; ANG I and ANG II, angiotensin I and II; AT1, angiotensin II receptor subtype 1; ET, endothelin; ETA and ETB, endothelin receptor subtypes A and B; A2, adenosine receptor subtype 2; β2, β2-adrenergic receptor; β1 and α2, α-adrenergic receptors; NO, nitric oxide; eNOS, endothelial NO synthase; PGI2, prostacyclin; IP, prostacyclin receptor; COX-1, cyclooxygenase-1; EDHF, endothelium derived hyperpolarizing factor; CYP450, cytochrome P450 2C9; K_{Ca}, calcium-sensitive K channel; K_{ATP}, ATP-sensitive K channel; K_V, voltage-sensitive K channel; AA, arachidonic acid; L-Arg, L-arginine; O_2^{-}, superoxide. Receptors, enzymes, and channels are indicated by an oval or rectangle, respectively. Adapted with permission from Duncker DJ, Bache RJ. Regulation of coronary blood flow during exercise. *Physiol Rev* 2008; **88:** 1009–86.

Full function of the enzyme is dependent on its existence as a dimer, disassociation from the membrane protein caveolin, activation through calcium-calmodulin, and sufficient supply of substrate (L-arginine) and cofactors, most notably tetrahydrobiopterin. The normal coronary endothelium can cause vasodilatation as constitutive NOS produces NO, which causes relaxation of vascular smooth muscle via an increase in cGMP and consequent activation of calcium-activated potassium channels, possibly ATP-dependent K-channels. Endothelial production of NO can be triggered by specific receptors (e.g. muscarinic, bradykinin, and histamine receptors) or by mechanical deformation resulting from shear forces or pulsatile strain caused by blood flow.

The contribution of NO to maintenance of coronary blood flow has been studied by administering analogs of L-arginine that act as competitive inhibitors of the NO synthesis. NO appears to play a key role in flow-mediated relaxation of the large epicardial vessels, as the latter is prevented by N^g-monomethyl-L-arginine, a specific inhibitor of NO synthesis [10]. The contribution of EDHF to endothelium-dependent relaxation varies as a function of the size of the artery; indeed, it is more pronounced in resistance vessels and might play an important role in pre-arteriolar flow-mediated dilatation [11]. In contrast, the contribution of prostacyclin to flow-mediated relaxation appears to be modest. Yet, prostacyclin-mediated relaxation might be important in the presence of endothelial dysfunction with reduced bioavailability of NO, when it may provide a useful compensatory mechanism [12].

Endothelial dysfunction is an early marker of coronary atherosclerosis and a predictor of cardiovascular events. All cardiovascular risk factors have been shown to produce early vascular endothelial dysfunction and activation. Indeed, they also cause oxidative stress and inflammatory reactions, which can contribute substantially to the progression of endothelial dysfunction towards atherosclerotic cardiovascular diseases [13]. Oxidative modifications of lipids, in particular, play a central role in propagating the inflammatory response.

The techniques generally used to test endothelial function are invasive and involve intracoronary administration of drugs such as acetylcholine during coronary angiography. More recently, measurement of myocardial blood flow with positron emission tomography (PET) in response to cold pressure test has been employed as a non-invasive tool for the assessment of endothelial function.

Response to changes in perfusion pressure: autoregulation

When metabolic requirements do not vary, the coronary circulation exhibits an intrinsic tendency to maintain blood flow at a constant rate despite changes in perfusion pressure, a mechanism known as autoregulation.

Variations of coronary perfusion pressure in the beating heart, in the presence of unaltered myocardial metabolic requirements, can be achieved by perfusing the coronary circulation independently from the aorta, so that aortic pressure (a determinant of myocardial oxygen consumption) remains constant when coronary arterial pressure is varied. In this setting, pressure/flow curves show that when perfusion pressure is varied, flow remains almost constant over a wide range of pressures, i.e. from 60–120mmHg (➲Fig. 17.4). The level at which flow remains constant is determined by the level of myocardial oxygen consumption; when this is low the plateau of flow is low, when oxygen consumption is high the plateau is high. Notably, for decreasing perfusion pressures, autoregulation is better maintained in the subepicardium than in the subendocardium, which, therefore, is more susceptible to the detrimental effects of very low perfusion pressures.

Mechanisms of autoregulation

The mechanism responsible for autoregulation is probably a myogenic response of distal pre-arteriolar vessels: they

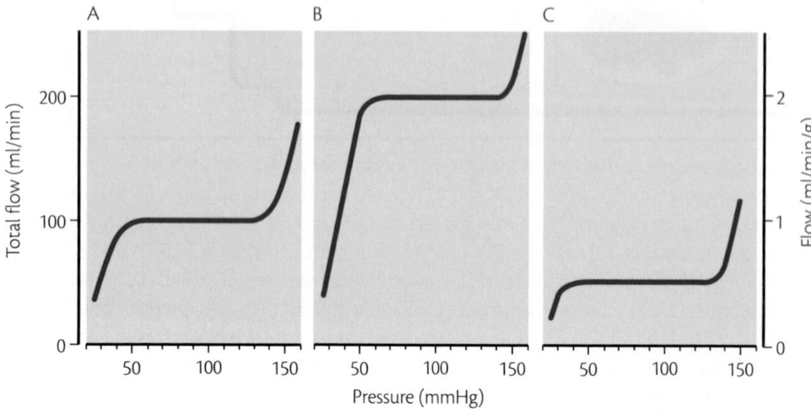

Figure 17.4 Autoregulation of coronary blood flow in anaesthetized dogs in the presence of normal (A), high (B), or low (C) oxygen consumption. In the presence of autoregulation, coronary flow is determined by the level of myocardial oxygen consumption, by the oxygen saturation of arterial blood and by neurohumoral modulation of coronary vasomotor tone. Autoregulation fails when perfusion pressure either decreases or increases beyond the range of pressures within which autoregulation acts.

dilate in response to a reduction of perfusion pressure and constrict in response to an increase of perfusion pressure (➲Fig. 17.5) [14]. Myogenic responsiveness in the coronary microcirculation, independent of the endothelium, has been directly demonstrated *in vivo* in vessels that contribute to coronary microvascular resistance, and it is more pronounced in subepicardial than in subendocardial pre-arterioles. The mechanisms of the myogenic constriction in response to an increase in distending pressure are not well understood. They probably involve activation of a non-selective cation channel and subsequent influx of Na^+, K^+ and Ca^{2+} ions. The consequent membrane depolarization enables the recruitment of voltage-dependent calcium channels, which contributes to the increased calcium inflow. Furthermore, stretch initiates hydrolysis of membrane phospholipids, a process which contributes to increased intracellular calcium release. Myogenic contraction is ultimately caused by activation of myosin light chain kinase [15].

Response to changes in myocardial oxygen consumption: metabolic regulation

Energy production in the normally functioning heart is primarily dependent on oxidative phopshorylation. Because of this dependence on oxidative energy production, increases of cardiac activity require almost instantaneous parallel increases of oxygen availability. In contrast to skeletal muscle, which is quiescent with very low metabolic requirements during resting conditions, the heart has high oxygen consumption already at rest (20-fold higher than that of skeletal muscle). As an adaptation to the high oxygen demands, the heart maintains a very high level of oxygen extraction already under resting conditions so that 70–80% of the arterially delivered oxygen is extracted, compared with only 30-40% in skeletal muscle. Therefore, any further increase in oxygen demand can only be met by augmenting myocardial perfusion. The coronary circulation supplies the myocardium with blood for its widely and rapidly changing needs. It can supply oxygen in amounts up to five times the baseline consumption, and carries substrates and removes metabolic waste products, all to ensure optimal working conditions for myocardial cells. This demanding function takes place in an organ that generates its own perfusion pressure.

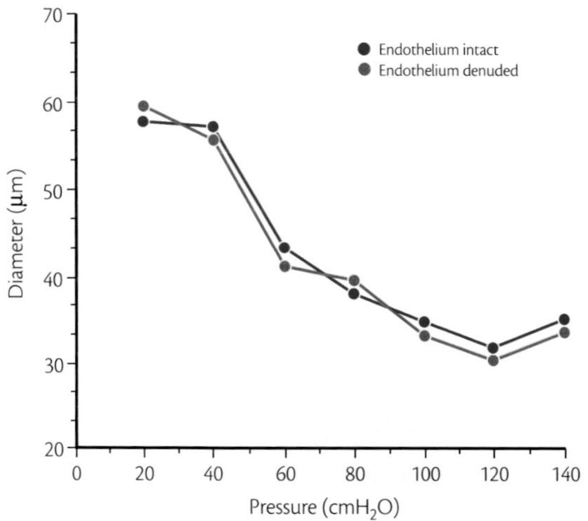

Figure 17.5 Effects of increasing pressures in a dog arteriole. Arteriolar dilatation and constriction were observed at lower and higher pressures, respectively. After mechanical denudation of the endothelium, spontaneous tone and myogenic responses were preserved. Thus, endothelium-independent pressure-induced myogenic constriction in arterioles is the main determinant of coronary autoregulation. Adapted with permission from Kuo L, Chilian WM, Davis MJ. Coronary arteriolar myogenic response is independent of endothelium. *Circ Res* 1990; **66**: 860–6.

Under basal resting conditions the tone of coronary resistive vessels is high and coronary blood flow is at its lowest level. This intrinsically high resting tone provides the coronary circulation with the ability to increase flow by reducing vasomotor tone when myocardial oxygen consumption increases, a mechanism known as functional hyperaemia. This metabolic control of coronary blood flow is very precise and is fundamental for adequate myocardial oxygen supply. Indeed, in normal humans myocardial oxygen extraction is already considerably raised under resting conditions and does not change appreciably during increased cardiac work up to submaximal levels [16].

For any level of myocardial oxygen consumption, average coronary vascular resistance, and hence flow, can be modulated by a wide variety of neurotransmitters, by autacoids produced by the vessel wall, blood-borne substances, and drugs acting on different segments of resistive vessels. Neurotransmitters are released at nerve endings. Autacoids are generated locally by endothelial cells (NO, prostaglandins, EDHF, endothelin) or by adventitial cells (histamine, kinins, leukotrienes) while others are released by circulating platelets (thromboxane A_2, serotonin) or carried in the bloodstream (adrenaline). Notably, when myocardial oxygen consumption remains constant, any change in flow caused by neurohumoral modulation is mirrored by a change in oxygen extraction, so that vasodilatation or constriction are associated, respectively, with a proportional increase or decrease in coronary sinus PO_2 and oxygen saturation [17].

Determinants of myocardial oxygen consumption

The most important determinant of oxygen consumption is cardiac work, as in the non-beating heart oxygen consumption is only 15-20% of that under normal resting conditions.

Oxygen consumption, as for other tissues, is also influenced by the type of substrate used; indeed, it is higher when using predominantly fatty acids (which have a respiratory quotient of 0.7) than when using carbohydrates (which have a respiratory quotient of 1.0). Furthermore, myocardial oxygen consumption is about 15–20% higher in the subendocardium than the subepicardium.

Most of the time the factors that influence myocardial metabolic activity vary concurrently. However, when they are artificially separated under experimental conditions in a canine model, they rank in the following order [18].

- *Heart rate.* Myocardial oxygen consumption approximately doubles during atrial pacing when heart rate is doubled. However, this is probably an underestimate, as during pacing (but not during exercise) the stroke volume decreases, also causing a decrease in ventricular volume and wall tension.
- *Aortic pressure.* Myocardial oxygen uptake approximately doubles as mean aortic pressure is increased from 75 to 175mmHg at constant heart rate and stroke volume.
- *Myocardial inotropic state.* Myocardial oxygen consumption increases by about 30% when d*P*/dt (the first derivative of systolic left ventricular pressure over time) is doubled by extrasystolic potentiation or by noradrenaline administration at constant heart rate, aortic pressure and cardiac output.
- *Stroke volume.* Myocardial oxygen consumption increases by about 20% when stroke volume is increased by 60% at constant rate-pressure product (i.e. heart rate times systolic blood pressure).
- An accurate measurement of myocardial oxygen consumption requires the determination of coronary blood flow and of arterial-venous difference in blood oxygen content (which is generally achieved by sampling blood simultaneously from the aorta and the coronary sinus). As coronary sinus sampling is required, and as the measurement of coronary flow presents considerable methodological problems, a number of indirect indices have been proposed. Of these, the rate-pressure product is the simplest and yet it correlates closely in a wide range of values with measured changes in myocardial oxygen consumption [16].

Mechanisms of metabolic regulation of myocardial blood flow

By acting on coronary arterioles, adenosine is probably the key mediator of metabolic blood flow regulation. Adenosine is formed by degradation of adenine nucleotides under conditions in which adenosine triphosphate (ATP) utilization exceeds the capacity of myocardial cells to re-synthesize high energy compounds (a process dependent on oxidative phosphorylation in mitochondria). This results in the production of adenosine monophosphate, which is converted to adenosine by the enzyme 5'-nucleotidase. Adenosine then diffuses from the myocytes into the interstitial fluid, where it exerts powerful arteriolar dilator effects through the stimulation of A_2 adenosine receptors on smooth muscle cells. Several findings support the critical role of adenosine in the metabolic regulation of myocardial flow. Indeed, its production increases in cases of imbalance in the supply/demand ratio of myocardial oxygen, and the rise in interstitial concentration of adenosine parallels the increase in coronary blood flow. Inhibition of adenosine, however, does not reduce the magnitude of functional hyperaemia entirely, thus suggesting that other substances can play a critical role [19].

It is worth emphasizing that the response of the coronary circulation to changes in myocardial oxygen consumption triggers a complex and integrated microvascular response. The arterioles dilate in response to the release of myocardial metabolites and this dilatation decreases both resistance in the overall network and pressure in distal pre-arterioles, which in turn induces myogenically sensitive vessels to dilate. Furthermore, dilatation of distal pre-arterioles and arterioles results in an increase in shear stress and triggers flow-dependent dilatation in larger pre-arterioles and in conductance arteries.

Thus, as proposed by Chilian [20], the coronary circulation matches blood flow with oxygen requirements by coordinating the resistances within different microvascular domains, each governed by distinct regulatory mechanisms. Such integration appears advantageous because the system does not rely on a single mechanism of control. Accordingly, if a pathological process renders a mechanism dysfunctional, other mechanisms, at least to some extent, can compensate for it, although the price to pay is a reduction of regulatory mechanism reserve.

Response to a brief coronary occlusion: reactive hyperaemia

When a major epicardial coronary artery is occluded for a short period of time, occlusion release is followed by a significant increase in coronary blood flow, a phenomenon known as reactive hyperaemia. The maximum increase in blood flow occurs within a few seconds after the release of the occlusion and the peak flow, which has been shown to reach four or five times the value of pre-ischaemic flow, is dependent on the duration of the ischaemic period for occlusion times up to 15–20s. Although occlusions of longer duration do not modify further the peak of the hyperaemic response, they do affect the duration of the entire hyperaemic process, which increases with the length of the occlusion [21]. Generally, the excess flow that follows the occlusion, known as flow repayment, is larger than the flow debt incurred during the ischaemic period (➲Fig. 17.6) [22].

From the previous observations it is generally accepted that myocardial ischaemia, even of brief duration, is the most effective stimulus for vasodilatation of coronary resistive vessels and that, under normal circumstances, reactive hyperaemic peak flow represents the maximum flow available at a given coronary perfusion pressure. Values of coronary blood flow comparable to the peak flow of reactive hyperaemia can be achieved using coronary vasodilators such as adenosine or dipyridamole, which induce a 'near maximal' vasodilatation of the coronary microcirculation. This concept, however, has been challenged by studies in experimental animals, as well as in human subjects, that have demonstrated that reactive hyperaemic peak flow may not represent the true ceiling of blood flow achievable at a given perfusion pressure [23, 24]. Reactive hyperaemia occurs also in denervated isolated hearts, thus suggesting that flow-mediated, myogenic and metabolic mechanisms (see previous sections) are the main determinants of this phenomenon [25].

Coronary flow reserve

The concept of coronary flow reserve was first introduced by Gould and colleagues in 1974 [26] as an indirect parameter to evaluate the global function of the coronary circulation (➲Chapter 9). Coronary flow reserve is the ratio of coronary blood flow during near maximal coronary vasodilatation to resting flow and is an integrated measure of flow through both the large epicardial coronary arteries and the microcirculation (➲Fig. 17.7) [27].

Coronary flow reserve must be considered a relative, rather than absolute, value that depends on four main variables:

- resting blood flow;
- cross-sectional area of arteriolar vessels per unit volume of myocardium;
- extravascular coronary resistance;
- arteriolar perfusion pressure.

Since resting blood flow is the denominator in the formula used to compute coronary flow reserve, any increase in resting blood flow (e.g. the increase in resting perfusion seen in patients with arterial hypertension) will lead to a net decrease in the available coronary flow reserve.

The total cross-sectional area of resistive vessels per unit volume of myocardium influences coronary flow conductance and hence the slope of the pressure/flow curve in inner and outer layers of the ventricular wall. The greater the vascular cross-sectional area, the steeper the slope of

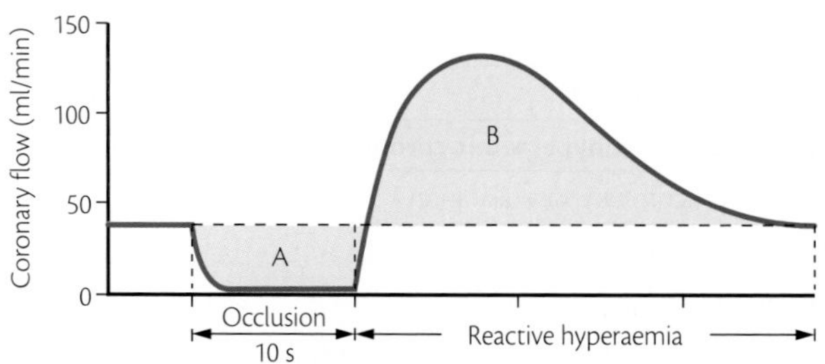

Figure 17.6 Mean coronary blood flow before, during and after coronary occlusion. Area A is the flow debt acquired during occlusion, whereas area B is its repayment following restoration of blood flow (see text for definitions). Typically, the repayment is larger than the flow debt incurred during the ischaemic period. Adapted with permission from Meredith IT, Currie KE, Anderson TJ, *et al.* Postischemic vasodilation in human forearm is dependent on endothelium-derived nitric oxide. *Am J Physiol* 1996; **270**: 1435–40.

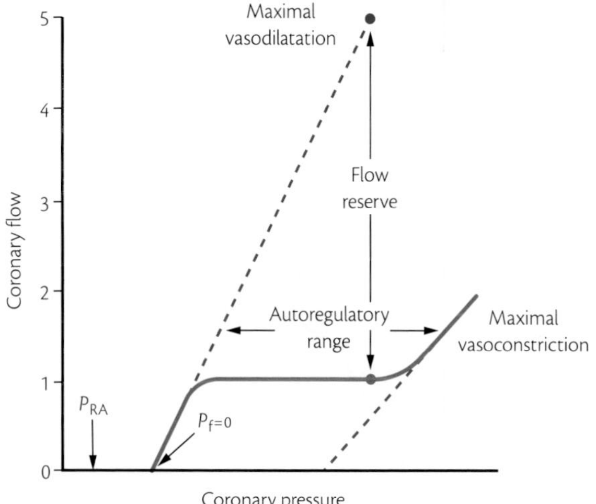

Figure 17.7 Relationship between coronary blood flow and coronary arterial pressure in the left ventricle. At a constant level of myocardial oxygen consumption, coronary blood flow is maintained constant over a wide range of coronary perfusion pressures (red line), included within the boundaries of maximal resistive coronary vessel dilatation or constriction (dashed lines). In the presence of maximal resistive vessel dilatation coronary blood flow and coronary arterial pressure are proportional (dashed line on the left). The red and blue circles represent the basal state and the maximal coronary blood flow, respectively, under normal conditions, giving a coronary flow reserve of 5.0. P_{RA} = right atrial pressure, $P_{f=0}$ = pressure at zero flow. Reproduced from Maseri A. *Ischemic Heart Disease*, 1995. New York: Churchill Livingstone Inc, with permission from Elsevier.

the pressure/flow curve (the greater the increase in flow per unit increase in pressure). In the presence of maximal vasodilatation the vascular conductance per unit volume of myocardium can be reduced because the total number of resistive vessels per unit volume is decreased or because the lumen of individual vessels is reduced.

Extravascular compressive forces reduce coronary flow reserve mainly in subendocardial layers, in particular during tachycardia and in the presence of elevated diastolic ventricular pressures (➲Fig. 17.8) [28].

The perfusion pressure that determines flow for any given level of vascular resistance is the pressure at the origin of arteriolar vessels. During maximal coronary dilatation, the slope of the pressure/flow curve is very steep; thus the increase of coronary flow reserve with increasing pressure is substantial. Under physiological conditions the coronary perfusion pressure that determines myocardial blood flow corresponds closely to aortic pressure.

In patients, a reduced coronary flow reserve can be the result of a narrowing of epicardial coronary arteries or may reflect a dysfunction of the coronary microcirculation. The latter can be caused by structural (e.g. vascular remodelling with a reduced lumen to wall ratio) or functional (e.g. vasomotor abnormalities) changes, which may involve neurohumoral factors and/or endothelial dysfunction. An abnormal coronary flow reserve may also reflect changes in systemic haemodynamics (e.g. hypotension) as well as changes in extravascular coronary resistance (e.g. increased intramyocardial pressure).

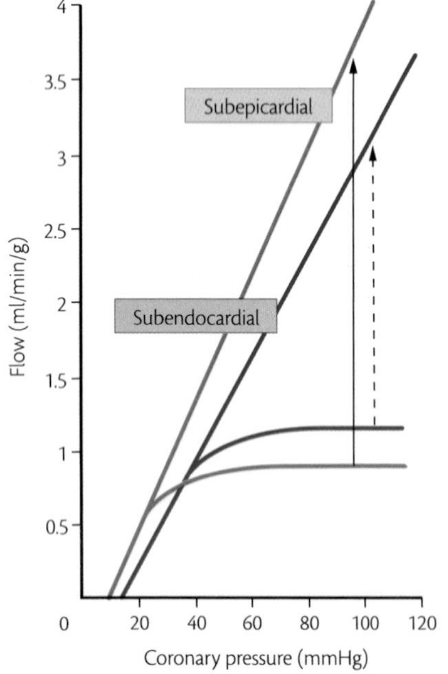

Figure 17.8 Coronary blood flow reserve in subendocardial and subepicardial layers. Under physiological conditions the coronary flow reserve is lower in the subendocardial layers, where there is a higher resting blood flow as a result of a higher oxygen consumption and a lower pressure/flow curve because of higher extravascular compressive forces. This difference between subepicardial and subendocardial layers increases progressively with tachycardia and with elevation of diastolic pressure. Adapted from Bache RJ, Vrobel TR, Arentzen CE, *et al.* Effect of maximal coronary vasodilation on transmural myocardial perfusion during tachycardia in dogs with left ventricular hypertrophy. *Circ Res* 1981; **49**: 742–9.

Resting and hyperaemic myocardial blood flows are heterogeneous both between and within individuals and exhibit a similar degree of spatial heterogeneity, which appears to be temporally stable [29]. Since resting coronary/myocardial blood flow parallels myocardial oxygen consumption, care must be taken to normalize coronary flow reserve measurements obtained on different occasions by using a 'corrected' resting flow. This is generally obtained by correcting resting flow for the relative rate-pressure product. Furthermore, several factors may influence resting coronary blood flow, including gender (women tend to have higher resting coronary/myocardial blood flow) and drugs, which, therefore, must also be taken into account. The value of hyperaemic coronary/myocardial blood flow can be influenced by a number of factors which may 'artificially' limit the maximum flow response (➲Table 17.1). These include sub-maximal coronary vasodilatation caused by the consumption of substances, such as caffeine, that antagonize the effect of some vasodilator drugs (adenosine and dipyridamole). Of note, there is a direct linear relation between age and resting myocardial blood flow, partly related to changes in external cardiac workload with age, whereas hyperaemic myocardial blood flow declines in

Table 17.1 Factors affecting coronary flow reserve

Factors that affect resting coronary/myocardial blood flow
Oxygen consumption (heart rate and blood pressure)
Gender
Drugs
Endothelial dysfunction
Presence of scar/fibrosis
Factors that affect hyperaemic coronary/myocardial blood flow
Sub-maximal coronary vasodilatation
Perfusion pressure
Caffeine and caffeine derivatives*
Anatomical remodelling of the microcirculation
Increased microvascular tone
Increased extravascular resistance
Endothelial dysfunction
Presence of scar/fibrosis
Cardiac denervation

* When adenosine or dipyridamole are used to assess coronary flow reserve.

people over 65 years of age [30]. The type of vasodilator stimulus used can also influence the assessment of coronary flow reserve. Indeed, hyperaemic myocardial blood flow, for example, was found to reach higher values in subjects in whom the standard dose of adenosine (140mcg/kg/min) was used compared to those in whom dipyridamole (0.56mg/kg infused over 4min) was used [29]. On the whole, the inter-individual variability of hyperaemic myocardial blood flow is greater than that observed for resting myocardial blood flow.

Assessment of coronary flow reserve in man

The assessment of coronary flow reserve in humans implies the measurement of coronary or myocardial blood flow (➲Chapter 8). Several techniques, including Doppler wires and coronary sinus thermodilution, are available for measuring coronary blood flow. These techniques are invasive and affected by serious limitations [31]. While coronary blood flow has units of volume per time (i.e. mL/min), Doppler measurements usually allow assessment of flow velocity (cm/s) and only a few techniques provide volumetric flow [32]. Measurement of inert tracer clearance, the assessment of which can be invasive (based on arterial-venous sampling) or non-invasive (based on external detection of radionuclide wash-out, e.g. ^{133}Xe), provides estimates of regional perfusion, although the mass of tissue subtended by the artery under study is unknown. Single-photon emission computed tomography (SPECT) allows the non-invasive assessment of directional changes in regional tissue perfusion, but its physical limitations do not permit quantification of myocardial blood flow [33]. More recently, non invasive assessment of coronary blood flow velocity in the left anterior descending coronary artery (LAD) by Doppler echocardiography and of myocardial perfusion by echocontrastography has also become possible. Notably, PET has been shown to allow non-invasive and accurate quantification of regional myocardial blood flow per gram of tissue, if suitable tracers are used and appropriate mathematical models are applied [34].

In normal humans, the range of regional coronary flow reserve is wide, with important clinical implications. A regional coronary flow reserve of <2.5 is often interpreted as abnormal. Yet, many normal left ventricular regions have a coronary flow reserve of <2.5 [30].

Myocardial ischaemia

Ischaemia is caused by an imbalance between myocardial oxygen supply and consumption (➲Fig. 17.9). The imbalance can be caused by a primary reduction of myocardial oxygen supply which, in turn, can be caused by a reduction of coronary blood flow (for instance in presence of occlusive coronary thrombosis or spasm or of severe hypotension) or by a reduction of O_2-carrying capacity (for instance caused by anaemia or carbon monoxide poisoning). The imbalance also occurs when coronary flow reserve is reduced by an increase of coronary vascular resistance caused by critical coronary stenoses, coronary microvascular dysfunction or extracoronary conditions (for instance aortic stenosis). Under these circumstances ischaemia occurs when an increase of myocardial oxygen consumption exhausts coronary flow reserve. As subendocardial coronary flow reserve is more limited than subepicardial reserve, ischaemia caused by an increase of myocardial oxygen consumption is typically subendocardial and is made even more severe by the 'steal phenomenon'. Indeed, after exhaustion of subendocardial coronary flow reserve, any further dilation of subepicardial

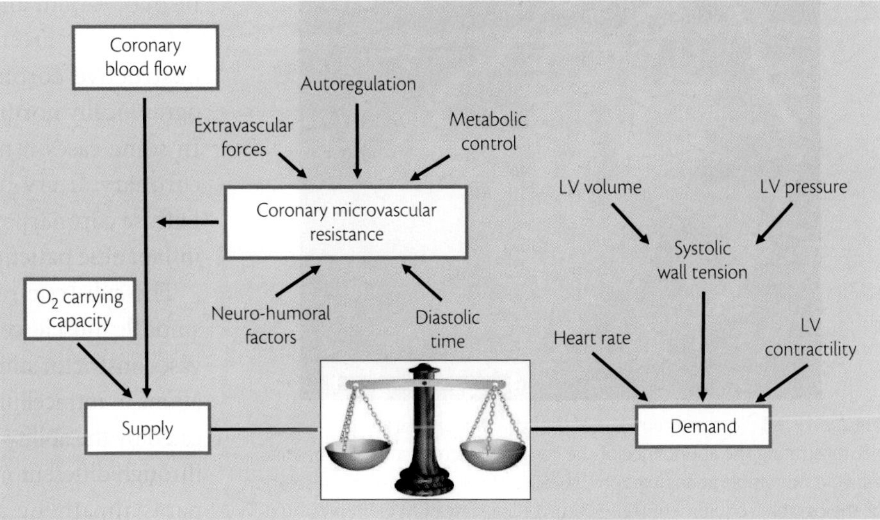

Figure 17.9 Synopsis of determinants of myocardial blood supply (on the left) and of myocardial oxygen consumption (on the right). Mismatch between supply and consumption causes myocardial ischaemia.

arterioles causes a further drop of post-stenotic pressure and subendocardial perfusion [6].

Causes of myocardial ischaemia

Macro and microvascular disease

Atherosclerotic disease of the vascular system is a continuum. Disease may begin early in life, but it does not become clinically overt until atherosclerotic plaques reach a critical stage. The clinical manifestations of the disease are related to the progressive impairment of tissue perfusion due to the growth of the plaque inside the lumen of the vessel causing impairment of blood flow and ischaemia which may lead to symptoms such as angina pectoris. Its diagnosis is based on the use of a number of diagnostic techniques based either on identification of the anatomical changes (stenoses) in the large epicardial coronary arteries or on the functional consequences of these stenotic lesions on coronary flow reserve and/or on the electrical activity of the heart and/or on regional left ventricular function.

The development and refinement of non-invasive cardiac imaging over the past two decades, in particular, has provided new tools for the identification of pre-clinical disease. A bulk of studies, mainly using PET for the non-invasive quantification of regional myocardial blood flow (mL/min/g of tissue), have demonstrated that dysfunction of the coronary microcirculation, which represents about 95% of coronary circulation (➲Fig. 17.10), occurs in many clinical conditions in the absence of demonstrable stenoses on the large epicardial arteries. Studies in asymptomatic subjects, but with risk factors for coronary artery disease such as hypercholesterolemia, essential hypertension, diabetes mellitus, and smoking, have provided evidence of how these risk factors translate into measurable damage to the coronary microcirculation in the absence of demonstrable stenoses of the epicardial coronary arteries. In some cases these abnormalities represent mere epiphenomena, whilst in others they contribute to the pathogenesis of myocardial ischaemia and even represent important markers of risk, thus becoming possible therapeutic targets [3].

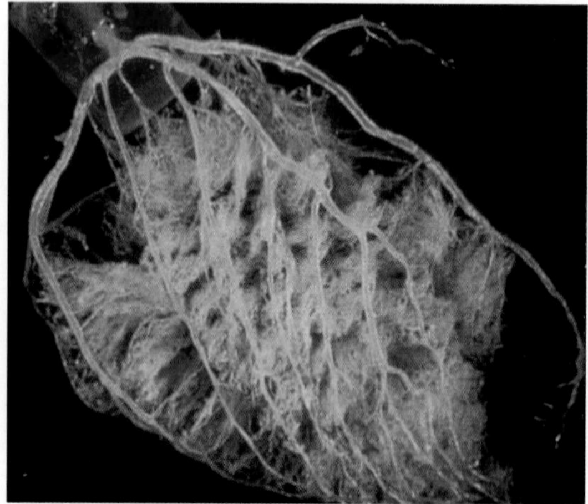

Figure 17.10 Post-mortem cast of the coronary circulation demonstrating the abundance of the coronary microcirculatory network which is not visible at angiography, because of the limited spatial resolution of angiographic equipment (i.e.~500μm). (Courtesy of M Gibson.)

Flow limiting stenosis

Under normal circumstances, large epicardial coronary arteries (conduit arteries) offer very little resistance to flow whilst the pre-arterioles and arterioles, below 500μm in diameter, are the principal determinants of coronary vascular resistance [35]. Atherosclerotic plaques which determine a reduction of luminal diameter add an extra resistance 'in series', that results in a post-stenotic pressure drop. The latter is compensated for by vasodilatation of resistive vessels and does not have any appreciable effect on coronary flow reserve for reductions of internal luminal diameter up to 50%. Thereafter, however, this compensatory mechanism is progressively exhausted for increasing values of stenosis severity and coronary flow reserve becomes close to unity (i.e. hyperaemic flow = resting flow) for reduction of luminal diameter >80% (➲Fig. 17.11) [36]. Functionally, this process progressively limits the ability of the coronary circulation to increase blood flow to meet an increased metabolic demand and is the basis for exercise-induced myocardial ischaemia and angina pectoris in patients with obstructive coronary atherosclerosis.

Occlusive spasm and dynamic stenoses

Coronary artery spasm, consisting of a paroxysmal, intense occlusive vasoconstriction usually involving a segment of an epicardial coronary artery, which results in transmural myocardial ischaemia, is the unique pathogenetic mechanism of variant angina [37].

Coronary artery spasm may occur at the site of an obstructive coronary atherosclerotic plaque or in angiographically normal or near normal coronary arteries [38]. In some cases it may involve more segments in the same coronary artery branch or even more than one branch. Diffuse coronary spasm may also be observed, in particular in Japanese patients.

The substrate of coronary spasm is a hyperreactivity of smooth muscle cells of the involved coronary segment to vasoconstrictor stimuli [39]. This is likely to be related to alterations in intracellular transduction mechanisms [38], as indicated by the ability of different vasoconstrictor stimuli, acting through different membrane receptors (e.g. sympathetic and parasympathetic activation [40], ergonovine, histamine,

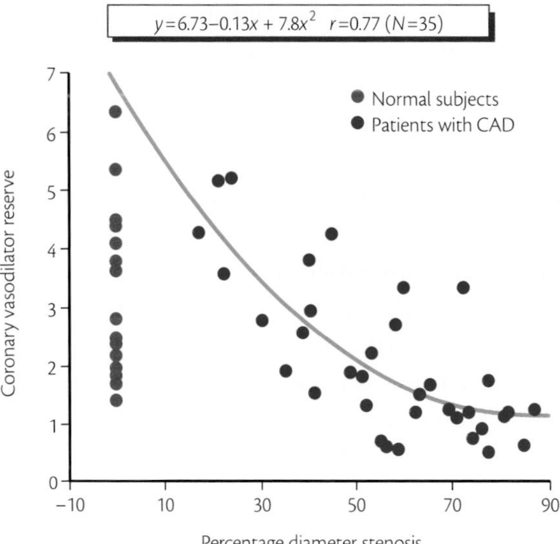

Figure 17.11 Relationship between severity of coronary stenosis (measured by quantitative coronary angiography) and coronary flow reserve (measured non-invasively by positron emission tomography and oxygen-15 labelled water) in patients with coronary artery disease (CAD, blue circles). There is a progressive decline in flow reserve for stenoses with a severity ≥50% and the flow reserve approaches unity for stenoses ≥80% (i.e. maximum flow, after adenosine, is not different from resting flow). When flow reserve is close to unity, any increase in cardiac workload cannot be met by an adequate increase in blood flow leading to myocardial ischaemia in the region subtended by the stenotic coronary artery. A massive interindividual variability of coronary flow reserve is noted, however, among apparently normal subjects (red circles), thus making the interpretation of coronary flow reserve in the presence of obstructive coronary atherosclerosis rather difficult. Adapted from Uren NG, Melin JA, Bruyne B, *et al.* Relation between myocardial blood flow and the severity of coronary-artery stenosis. *N Engl J Med* 1994; **330**: 1782–8. Copyright ©1994 Massachusetts Medical Society. All rights reserved.

dopamine, acetylcholine, serotonin, alkalosis) to precipitate coronary spasm, even in the same patient [39].

The causes of smooth muscle cell hyperreactivity are unknown, but several possible contributing factors have been suggested, including increased cellular rho-kinase activity [41], abnormalities in ATP-sensitive potassium channels [42] and membrane Na^+-H^+ countertransport [43].

Coronary spasm must be distinguished from dynamic stenoses observed in patients with stable angina. Coronary spasm is caused by hyperreactivity of smooth muscle cells of a localized coronary segment and is occlusive or subocclusive. Dynamic stenoses, instead, are mainly caused by endothelial dysfunction, which facilitates vasoconstriction at the site of pliable critical or subcritical coronary stenoses in response to sympathetic stimuli (such as exercise and mental stress), resulting in a transient worsening of stenosis severity. This may facilitate the occurrence of transient myocardial ischaemia in the presence of an increased myocardial oxygen consumption or even at rest [44].

It is worth noting that, although the main pathogenetic component of acute coronary syndromes is coronary thrombosis [45], abnormal coronary vasomotion of variable severity often plays a contributory role.

Thrombosis

Local thrombosis that occurs at the site of eroded or fissured plaques is central to the initiation of myocardial ischaemia in acute coronary syndromes. Notably, in about two-thirds of patients thrombus formation occurs at the site of atherosclerotic plaques which reduce lumen diameter by <50%, and in 97% of patients at the site of plaques which reduce lumen diameter by <70%. In this setting a crucial role is played by local tissue factor expression, and probably also by tissue factor transported by circulating leucocyte-derived microparticles, which interacts with factor VIIa to initiate a cascade of enzymatic reactions resulting in the local generation of thrombin and fibrin deposition. Furthermore, thrombin and collagen exposed by endothelial cell disruption, trigger platelet aggregation, followed by the release of powerful vasoconstrictors.

Microvascular dysfunction

Until quite recently, causes of transient myocardial ischaemia were investigated in conduit coronary arteries. However, recent advances have highlighted the crucial involvement of microcirculation in several clinical manifestations of ischaemic heart disease (IHD). Microvascular dysfunction can be the result of either functional (e.g. endothelial and/or smooth muscle cell dysfunction) or structural (e.g. remodelling of intramural coronary arteries with a reduced lumen to wall ratio) alterations.

A new concept is emerging where 'coronary microvascular disease' is a well-defined condition that often precedes the development of full-blown IHD and may have an independent prognostic value [46]. Indeed, coronary microvascular dysfunction has been documented in asymptomatic subjects with risk factors for IHD, including not only hypertension and diabetes [47], but also hypercholesterolaemia, obesity, and smoking [48-50], and can be severe enough to cause angina even in patients with minimal to moderate disease of the epicardial coronary arteries.

Coronary microvascular dysfunction can be observed following percutaneous coronary interventions (PCI) in patients with stable angina [51] and appears to play an important role also in patients with unstable angina [52]. The 'no reflow phenomenon' is an extreme form of microvascular dysfunction which can occur in the territory of an acute MI despite restoration of epicardial blood flow by successful thrombolysis or primary PCI, thus negating the potential prognostic advantages of the treatment [53].

A dysfunction of the coronary microcirculation has also been demonstrated in some cardiac diseases unrelated to coronary artery disease, in particular dilated and hypertrophic cardiomyopathies (➲Table 17.2) [54, 55]. It is worth noting that microvascular dysfunction has been suggested to be a strong predictor of major cardiac events at follow-up in these groups of patients [54, 55], whereas it remains unclear whether it may have any prognostic value in other clinical conditions characterized by left ventricular hypertrophy.

Finally, microvascular dysfunction has been suggested to be involved in the pathogenesis of microvascular angina. The hypothesis that angina is of ischaemic origin was based on the presence of ST-segment depression during spontaneous chest pain episodes and on ECG stress tests, as well as on the evidence of reversible stress-induced myocardial perfusion defects [56], reduced endothelium-dependent and independent coronary vasodilation [57], and metabolic evidence of myocardial ischaemia in some studies [58]. Other studies, however, failed to find evidence of abnormal myocardial blood flow or coronary flow reserve [59], or metabolic evidence of ischaemia during stress tests [60]. An ischaemic origin of angina is contradicted also by the lack of transient wall motion abnormalities in the presence of angina and typical transient ST-segment [61]. Maseri and colleagues however, proposed that focal ischaemia in small myocardial regions scattered throughout the myocardium caused by pre-arteriolar dysfunction might explain the paradox of angina and ST-segment depression in the absence of wall motion changes [62].

Table 17.2 Clinical conditions associated with evidence of coronary microvascular dysfunction

Spontaneous
Risk factors for ischaemic heart disease
Smoking
Hyperlipidaemia
Hypertension
Obesity
Diabetes
Secondary left ventricular hypertrophy
Primary cardiomyopathies
Acute coronary syndromes (no-reflow)
Syndrome X
Iatrogenic
Percutaneous coronary interventions
Bypass surgery

Extracoronary cardiac and non-cardiac causes of ischaemia

About 90% of myocardial blood flow occurs in diastole because of the high extravascular compressive forces during systole. An increase of diastolic ventricular pressure causes an elevation of extravascular compressive force, which can limit myocardial perfusion, thus facilitating effort-induced myocardial ischaemia. An increase of diastolic ventricular pressure is typically observed in hypertrophic cardiomyopathy, in restrictive cardiomyopathy and in hypertensive heart disease. In aortic stenosis both an increase of diastolic left ventricular pressure and a reduction of coronary perfusion pressure contribute to the pathogenesis of effort-induced myocardial ischaemia.

Finally effort-induced myocardial ischaemia can be favoured by a reduction of oxygen content in arterial blood, as observed in anaemia or in patients with severe pulmonary diseases, or by increased metabolic requests, as in hyperthyroidism.

Consequences of myocardial ischaemia

Structural and ultrastructural alterations

Most of our understanding of the early cellular consequences of myocardial ischaemia is derived from experimental studies in animals. It is generally accepted that ischaemia for up to 15–20min is associated with reversible injury, whereas ischaemia of longer duration leads to a progressively more extensive area of irreversible injury. Most of the ultrastructural alterations seen early in ischaemic myocardium, such as cell swelling, glycogen depletion, margination of nuclear chromatin and elongation of myofibrils, become progressively more severe in the irreversible phase. There are, however, two distinctive signs of irreversible damage: amorphous matrix densities in the mitochondria and breaks in the sarcolemma [63].

In the dog, irreversible damage is initially detectable (15–20min after coronary occlusion) in subendocardial layers, which are more susceptible to ischaemia because of the higher myocardial oxygen consumption, and then propagates towards the subepicardial layers (the wavefront of necrosis). Apoptosis appears to be a significant complicating factor of acute MI, increasing the magnitude of myocyte cell death associated with coronary artery occlusion, and might play an important role in cardiac remodelling [64].

Metabolic alterations

Under conditions of myocardial ischaemia, oxygen shortage leads to a reduced rate of substrate oxidation (both free fatty acids and glucose) resulting in ATP depletion and accumulation of reduced coenzymes, that are re-oxidized to some extent in the mitochondria by way of the maleate–aspartate cycle. Thus, despite greater glucose availability through both an increased uptake of exogenous glucose and activation of glycogen breakdown, glucose oxidation during ischaemia is negligible. Pyruvate formed through glycolysis cannot be oxidized and, in the presence of increased amounts of reduced nicotinamide adenine dinucleotide (NADH), is converted to lactate by lactate dehydrogenase, thus contributing to tissue acidosis. In addition, a greater amount of alanine, produced via transamination of pyruvate, is released from myocardial fibres. Finally, major changes involve K^+ and Ca^{2+} ions. Loss of intracellular K^+ begins within seconds of the onset of ischaemia and extracellular concentration markedly increases during the first few minutes. The mechanisms of this loss, which begins before substantial ATP depletion, are still largely unknown. The decrease of transmembrane K^+ gradient is a major cause of abnormalities detectable on surface ECG. The early increase in cytosolic Ca^{2+} results from increased influx and decreased sequestration in the sarcoplasmic reticulum and is thought to be one of the mechanisms of irreversible cell death [65].

After an ischaemic episode, myocardial glucose utilization is higher than in resting conditions despite normalization of the haemodynamic conditions (➲Fig. 17.12) [66]. This extra glucose is probably used for rebuilding of the glycogen stores that had been depleted during ischaemia.

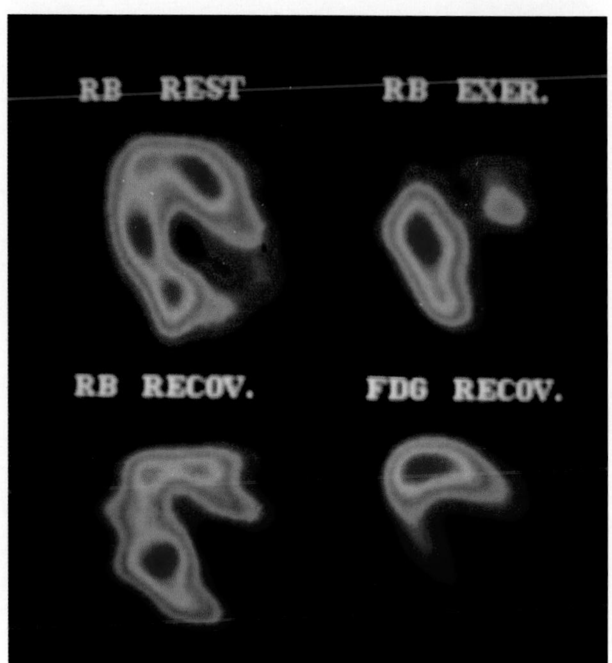

Figure 17.12 Positron emission tomography scans of rubidium-82 (^{82}Rb)- and ^{18}F-labelled deoxyglucose (FDG) uptake in the left ventricle of a patient with left anterior descending coronary artery disease. In each image, the left ventricular free wall is in the 6 o'clock to 10 o'clock position, the anterior wall and septum are in the 10 o'clock to 3 o'clock position, and the remaining open area is in the plane of the mitral valve. The scan at rest (top left) shows a homogeneous cation uptake in all myocardial walls. The ^{82}Rb scan recorded during exercise (top right) shows a severely reduced cation uptake in the anterior left ventricular wall, while the ^{82}Rb scan recorded in the recovery phase (when the patient had neither pain nor ECG changes) shows that perfusion is similar to baseline (bottom left). FDG was injected in the recovery phase after the last ^{82}Rb scan. The FDG scan, recorded 60 minutes after tracer injection, shows a greater FDG uptake in the previously ischaemic area (bottom right). FDG uptake in the anterior wall is 1.55 times higher than that in the non-ischaemic muscle. Adapted with permission from Camici PG, Araujo L, Spinks T, *et al.* Increased uptake of 18F-fluorodeoxyglucose in postischemic myocardium of patients with exercise-induced angina. *Circulation* 1986; **74:** 81–8.

Cardiac function alterations

Over 70 years ago Tennant and Wiggers [67] demonstrated that acute ischaemia rapidly impairs myocardial contractile function. For many years it was believed that relief of ischaemia led to an almost immediate normalization of function, provided that necrosis had not occurred. In 1975, Heyndrickx *et al.* [68] demonstrated, in a conscious dog model, that a 15-min coronary occlusion (a time period generally not associated with cell death), followed by reperfusion, produced a marked depression in regional contractile function that persisted for at least 6 hours after reperfusion. The term 'myocardial stunning' was coined to describe this viable tissue that exhibited prolonged post-ischaemic ventricular dysfunction. More recently, stunning has been demonstrated to occur in patients with IHD both after exercise-induced and dobutamine-induced ischaemia (➲Fig. 17.13) [69, 70]. Another more persistent form of post-ischaemic left ventricular dysfunction has been demonstrated in patients with chronic IHD: 'hibernated myocardium'. This can be defined as chronically dysfunctional myocardium, subtended by a stenotic coronary artery (with severe limitation of coronary flow reserve), that improves function upon coronary revascularization. The pathophysiology of myocardial hibernation in humans is more complex than initially postulated. The recent evidence that repetitive ischaemia in patients with IHD can be cumulative and leads to more severe and prolonged stunning, further supports the hypothesis that, at least initially, stunning and hibernation are two facets of the same coin [71].

Finally, a consequence of myocardial ischaemia is 'myocardial preconditioning', where a short episode of ischaemia can reduce the morphofunctional effects of a subsequent episode of ischaemia. The term was introduced by Murry *et al.* [72], who found a reduction in myocardial infarct size in dogs, when persistent coronary occlusion was preceded by one or more brief episodes of ischaemia. Preconditioning was subsequently demonstrated in other animal species,

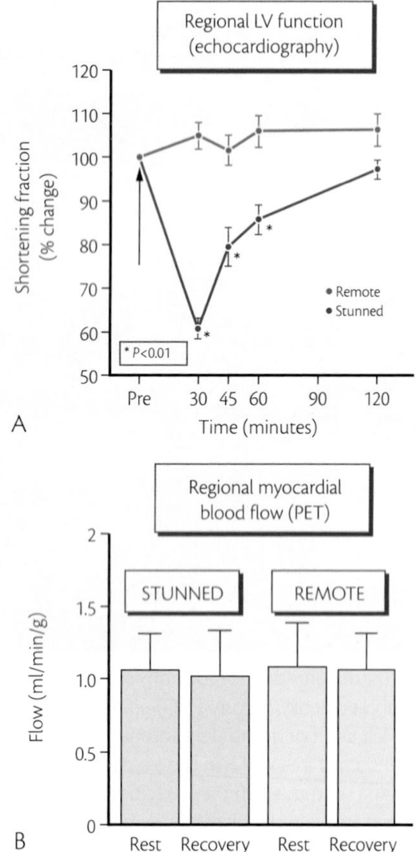

Figure 17.13 Demonstration of stunning in patients with single vessel coronary artery disease and exercise-induced ischaemia. (A) Regional left ventricular wall motion assessed by echocardiography at baseline and at different time points during dobutamine stress test. Shortening fraction in the recovery phase was unchanged in the control territory subtended by a non-diseased coronary artery (red line). By contrast, the shortening fraction was severely reduced in the ischaemic territory (blue line) and returned towards baseline only after 120 minutes from the cessation of dobutamine stress test. (B) In the ischaemic region, myocardial blood flow, as measured by positron emission tomography (PET) and 15 oxygen-labelled water, was comparable to blood flow in the non-ischaemic territory, both at baseline and also 30 minutes after dobutamine stress test, when shortening fraction was still severely depressed, thus demonstrating the occurrence of stunning in man. Adapted from Barnes E, Hall RJ, Dutka DP, *et al.* Absolute blood flow and oxygen consumption in stunned myocardium in patients with coronary artery disease. *J Am Coll Cardiol* 2002; **39**: 420–7, ©2002, with permission from Elsevier.

and further studies have also shown that a second window of protection can be demonstrated approximately 24 hours after the ischaemic stimulus, lasting for 48–72 hours [73]. In humans, ischaemic preconditioning has also been found to occur as a reduced myocardial suffering during repeated spontaneous or provoked (e.g. by balloon inflation during coronary angioplasty) transient ischaemic episodes [74].

Arrhythmias

Myocardial ischaemia can trigger electrophysiological changes that favour the development of arrhythmias. These are rare during transient episodes of subendocardial ischaemia, whereas they are more common when myocardial ischaemia is transmural and in the setting of acute MI. The most common forms of arrhythmia during ischaemia and infarction are ventricular tachyarrhythmias and fibrillation whilst atrioventricular block and asystole occur less frequently. In the canine model, but not in man, life-threatening ventricular arrhythmias are frequently found at the time of post-ischaemic reperfusion.

Reflex sympathetic activation

Ischaemia stimulates the terminal endings of both vagal and sympathetic fibres that innervate the myocardium. Sympathetic activation can further exacerbate myocardial ischaemia by increasing contractility and triggering vasoconstriction and ventricular arrhythmias. Following acute MI continued sympathetic activation contributes to ventricular remodelling and hypertrophy and to myocardial beta-adrenoceptor down-regulation [75].

Cardiac ischaemic pain

Cardiac ischaemic pain is a late consequence of myocardial ischaemia. Notably, transient myocardial ischaemia and even necrosis can occur in the absence of pain. More than 200 years after the original description of angina pectoris by Heberden [76], the mechanisms that lead to the genesis of cardiac ischaemic pain are still not fully elucidated. However, it now appears that substances released during myocardial ischaemia, that are able to stimulate afferent nerves, trigger the pain signal [77].

An important chemical stimulus is adenosine release by cardiomyocytes during ischaemia [78]. Adenosine plays a major role in the metabolic regulation of myocardial blood flow, because of its powerful vasodilator effect on arterioles. Interestingly, adenosine is also a powerful algogenic substance. Indeed, its intracoronary injection causes angina-like chest pain in the absence of signs of ischaemia. The algogenic effect of adenosine is mediated by A_1 receptors located on the membranes of afferent cardiac nerve fibres, whereas its vasodilator effect is mediated by A_2 receptors on vascular smooth muscle cells. Cardiac ischaemic pain, however, can still be induced after administration of adenosine inhibitors, suggesting that mechanisms other than adenosine are involved in its origin. In particular, bradykinin and substance P have been found to induce or modulate angina pain in man.

Cardiac pain signals are transmitted throughout sympathetic and, in part, vagal nerves to neurons in the dorsal horns of the spinal cord, from here to the thalamus, and from the thalamus to the cortex, where they are processed and decoded as pain [79] (➲Fig. 17.14).

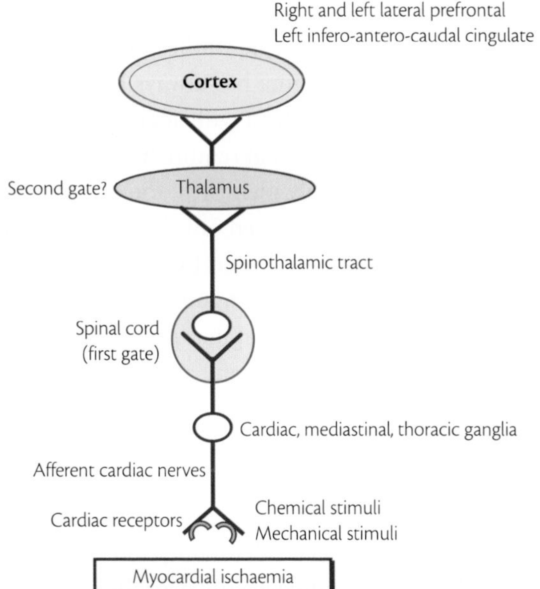

Figure 17.14 Transmission of cardiac ischaemic pain signals to cortical centres. Cardiac ischaemic pain signals generated by chemical (e.g. adenosine) or mechanical stimuli (e.g. stretching of intramyocardial or periarterial nerve fibres) travel throughout sympathetic and, in part, vagal nerves to neurons in the dorsal horns of the spinal cord. From there pain signals are transmitted to the thalamus and to the cortex where they are processed and decoded as pain. Profound modulation of pain signals occurs at spinal and, probably, at supraspinal level.

The central transmission of pain signals generated from the heart is modulated in the central nervous system by both ascending and descending signals. An important modulation is believed to occur in the dorsal horns of the spinal cord, where, according to the gate theory, a group of intermediate neurons may inhibit the transmission of the pain signal [80].

The somatic location of cardiac ischaemic pain does not allow us to predict the site of myocardial ischaemia. Indeed, about 70% of patients who suffer from both anterior and inferior MI at different times of their life experience pain in the same body region during the infarctions [81]. Accordingly, separate infusions of adenosine into the right or left coronary artery result in a similar distribution of pain in about 75% of the patients [82]. On the other hand, different locations of angina in the same patient at different times suggest ischaemia originating from different myocardial regions [83].

The ischaemic cascade

The clinical consequences of transmural myocardial ischaemia occur in a rather predictable sequence known as the 'ischaemic cascade' and are characterized by the following events (➲Fig. 17.15):

- reduction in pH and increase in the concentration of K^+ ions in venous blood draining the ischaemic region;

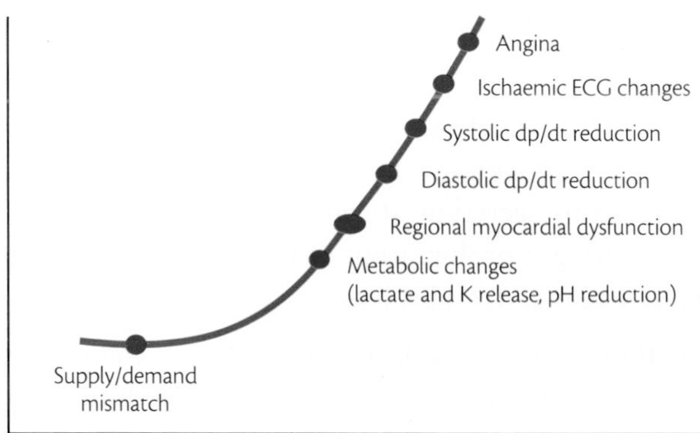

Figure 17.15 The 'ischaemic cascade'. Sequence of events following mismatch between oxygen supply and oxygen demand.

- regional wall motion abnormalities and signs of global diastolic and systolic left ventricular dysfunction;
- development of ST-segment changes;
- cardiac ischaemic pain.

This sequence of events helps to explain why imaging techniques based on the assessment of regional wall motion are more sensitive than ECG in the detection of myocardial ischaemia.

It has been proposed that severe microvascular dysfunction might be followed by a different 'ischaemic cascade' characterized by the early onset of ECG changes and chest pain in the absence of regional wall motion abnormalities [62].

Coronary collateral circulation

Collaterals develop from pre-existing anastomotic channels (thin-walled structures ranging in diameter from 20–200μm), as a result both of the establishment of a pressure gradient between their origin and termination and of chemical mediators released during tissue hypoxia, a process called arteriogenesis. A pressure gradient of about 10mmHg has been shown to be sufficient to elicit the development of collateral flow. Intercoronary arterial anastomoses are present in variable numbers in different species: they are so numerous in guinea-pigs that they can prevent infarction following sudden coronary occlusion, whereas, at the other extreme, they are virtually absent in rabbits. In dogs the density of anastomotic channels can deliver 5–10% of preocclusional resting flow. Humans have a slightly worse collateral circulation than dogs, but with a marked interindividual variability [84].

Arteriogenesis occurs in three stages [85]:

- the first stage (first 24 hours) is characterized by passive widening of pre-existing channels and endothelial activation, followed by secretion of proteolytic enzymes which dissolve extracellular matrix;

- the second stage (from 1 day to about 3 weeks) is characterized by migration of monocytes into the vascular wall, followed by secretion of cytokines and growth factors, which trigger proliferation of endothelial and smooth muscle cells and of fibroblasts;
- the third phase (3 weeks to ~3 months) is characterized by thickening of the vascular wall as a result of deposition of extracellular matrix.

In its final stage the mature collateral vessels may reach ~1mm in luminal diameter. Tissue hypoxia can favour collateral development by acting on the promoter gene of vascular endothelial growth factor (VEGF), but it is not an essential requirement for collateral development. There is no consistent evidence that exercise can favour collateral development. Among risk factors diabetes might impair the ability to develop collateral vessels [86].

Well-developed collateral circulation can be sufficient to prevent myocardial ischaemia in man in the presence of a sudden collateral occlusion, but it rarely provides blood flow adequate to meet myocardial oxygen consumption during maximal physical exercise.

Collateral vessels may also form through angiogenesis, which involves sprouting of new vessels from pre-existing vessels and usually results in the formation of capillary-like structures. This was clearly demonstrated following mammary artery implants in the myocardium of dogs with gradual total occlusion of a major coronary artery. The collateral blood supply provided by such newly formed vessels is rather small compared with that provided by arteriogenesis [87].

Epidemiology of chronic ischaemic heart disease

Cardiovascular diseases remain a major cause of mortality and morbidity in Western countries, although, after peaking in the 1960s of the previous Century, a decreasing trend of their incidence has been shown in the last decades, mainly explained by the dramatic improvement in the control of cardiovascular risk factors and preventive medical therapies [88]. The decreased burden of cardiovascular diseases has been paralleled by a reduction of the incidence of angina. However, the prevalence of angina seems to remain stable, likely due to the longer mean life [89, 90].

The exact prevalence and incidence of chronic stable angina in Europe as well as in other countries, however, is poorly known in the contemporary era, due to the lack of recent large-scale epidemiologic studies. In fact, the prevalence and incidence of angina has always been difficult to assess adequately, as, in contrast with acute coronary events (acute MI, unstable angina) that require hospitalization and therefore can be more easily identified, the extent of angina in the population can be assessed only by means of surveys or questionnaires. The largest used tool in this scope is the Rose questionnaire, which distinguishes between definite and possible (type 1 and 2) angina, mainly based on the presence of effort related chest pain, and has been shown to correlate significantly with clinical outcome [91]. Although these tools allow an estimate of the prevalence of subjects with anginal symptoms in the population, a correct diagnosis of true angina (i.e. chest pain caused by coronary artery abnormalities) would need documentation of myocardial ischaemia, due to the limited accuracy of the symptom as a predictor of coronary artery disease.

Several previous old studies from different cohorts of patients, however, suggested an annual incidence of uncomplicated angina of about 0.5% in Western people with age >40, although geographic variations are evident. For instance, in a study the incidence of angina was 0.54% in Belfast (Northern Ireland), but only 0.26% in France [92]. These geographical variations have also been confirmed in recent studies showing that angina incidence paralleled that of mortality for IHD. Overall, it can be estimated that between 20,000 and 40,000 new patients are affected by angina pectoris every year in most European countries.

The prevalence of angina increases with age in both genders. At the age of 45–54 years, indeed, it is around 2–5%, whereas it is 10–20% at the age of 65–74. The prevalence of chronic IHD, however, is certainly much higher given the frequent absence of anginal symptoms in stable or stabilized IHD patients [93].

Interestingly, the prevalence of angina seems to be slightly higher in women than in men through several age decades and countries in the world, with an average ratio of 1.2 [94] (➲Fig. 17.16). These figures, however, refer to the assessment of symptoms only, whereas in anginal patients a definite diagnosis of obstructive coronary atherosclerosis can be demonstrated more frequently in men than in women. Indeed, among patients with chest pain suggestive of myocardial ischaemia who undergo coronary angiography, 10–30% are found to have normal or near normal coronary arteries at angiography and 70–80% of these patients are women. Although some of these patients may have vasospastic angina and others may have a non cardiac cause of chest pain, most of them present typical features of cardiac microvascular angina, i.e. a clinical picture compatible

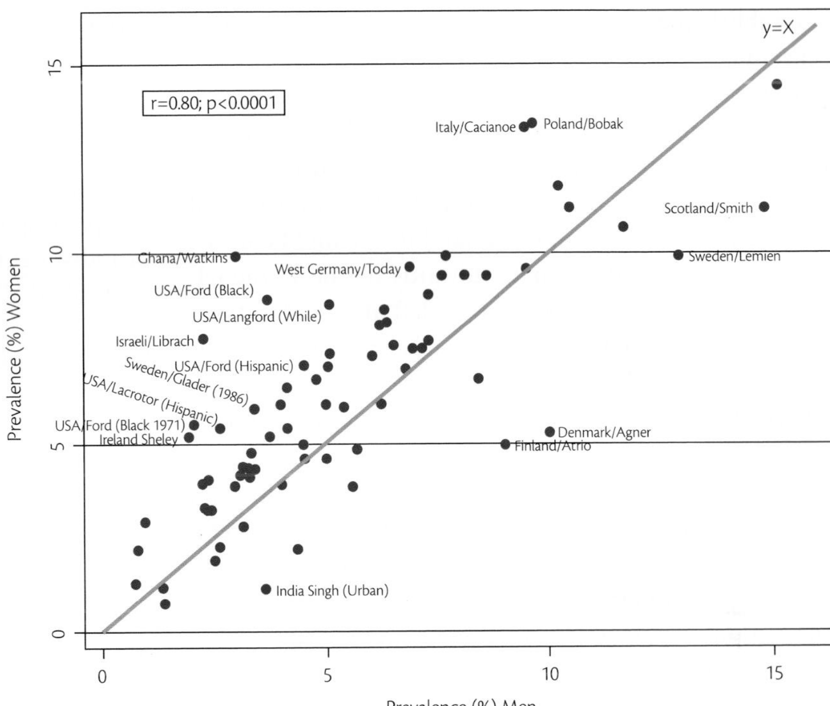

Figure 17.16 Angina prevalence in women and in men in several countries in the World. Angina prevalence is higher in women than in men. References are given for populations showing the largest differences between the two genders. Adapted from Hemingway H, Langenberg C, Damant J, *et al.* Prevalence of angina in women versus men: a systematic review and meta-analysis of international variations across 31 countries. *Circulation* 2008; **117**: 1526–36.

with angina caused by coronary microvascular dysfunction [95]. Several recent findings suggest, in fact, that coronary microvascular mechanisms may play a pathophysiological role in angina symptoms more frequently in women than in men [96].

Some studies have suggested that angina is associated with similar odds ratios for cardiovascular events in men and women, but data from the WISE study show that the risk of major coronary events (i.e. coronary death, acute MI) is low in women with angina but without obstructive coronary artery disease [96], thus underscoring the importance to clarify the pathophysiolgic mechanism of anginal symptoms. Why women who develop microvascular angina have a low risk of obstructive coronary atherosclerosis and of acute coronary complications is a challenging unresolved issue, but some protective mechanism must play a role [97].

The first clinical manifestation of IHD also presents some differences between men and women, further suggesting the existence of some differences between the two sexes in the development of IHD. In the Framingham study [98], among 5127 initially asymptomatic subjects (aged from 30 to 62 years) followed up for 14 years, the mode of first presentation of IHD was predominantly an acute coronary syndrome in man (68%) and predominantly a stable angina in women (56%).

The frequent occurrence of acute coronary syndromes as first manifestation of IHD, particularly among men, has been confirmed in the GISSI-2 study [99]. Indeed, among 12,381 patients admitted with a first acute MI, about 65% had no previous history of IHD, whereas about one half of the remaining patients had pre-infarction unstable angina (<1 month) and about one half had history of chronic stable angina. Among patients who present with an acute MI, 45% of men, but only 15% of women, developed a syndrome of stable angina in the Framingham study [98].

Assessment of angina pectoris

> There is a disorder of the breast, marked with strong and peculiar symptoms, considerable for the kind of danger belonging to it, and not extremely rare, of which I do not recollect any mention among medical authors. The seat of it, and sense of strangling and anxiety with which it is attended, may make it not improperly be called Angina Pectoris.
>
> William Heberden, 1768

Characteristics of angina pectoris

Independent of its causes, the most typical clinical manifestation of myocardial ischaemia is represented by angina pectoris (*angina*, from the Latin for anguish) [100] (➲Chapter 1). The features of chest pain that should be investigated to diagnose and characterize angina pectoris include type, location, irradiation and duration of pain, modalities of pain onset and offset, and response to cessation of effort and nitrate administration. Importantly, a careful assessment of characteristics of chest pain may help to establish the mechanisms responsible for myocardial ischaemia.

In its typical presentation, angina is referred as a constrictive, aching sensation, or pressure or tightness discomfort in the retrosternal area or in the anterior portion of the chest. Typically, the area of pain is indicated by the patient with a clenched fist or an open hand in the middle of the chest. Pain frequently radiates towards the neck, the left shoulder and the medial side of the left arm, and lasts no more than 10–15min. Angina responds promptly to cessation of effort and short-acting nitrates.

Several variants, however, exist to this typical presentation. Thus, pain can be represented by a heavy or burning sensation and can radiate towards the epigastrium, the right shoulder or arm, the interscapular area, the jaw and teeth, and, exceptionally, it can also be referred to the upper right abdominal quadrant or to the head [101]. Angina in atypical locations, although rare, may represent the main or only symptom of IHD.

Since the correct diagnosis of chest pain is extremely important to orient further therapeutic efforts, algorithms to improve the reliability of the diagnosis of myocardial ischaemia based on symptoms have been devised (➲Table 17.3) [102].

In most cases it is possible to identify conditions which trigger angina. These are more often represented by physical efforts, but they may consist of stressful or emotional states, exposure to cold, abundant meals or hypertensive episodes. Angina usually subsides by removing the triggering cause, but short-acting nitrates may be necessary to shorten angina duration. Finally, angina can also occur at rest without any apparent triggering cause.

Table 17.3 Clinical classification of chest pain

Typical angina (definite)	Meets three of the following characteristics: ◆ substernal chest discomfort of typical quality ◆ provoked by exertion or emotional stress ◆ relieved by rest or GTN
Atypical angina (probable)	Meets two of the previous characteristics
Non cardiac chest pain	Meets one or none of the previous characteristics

GTN, glyceryl trinitrate.

Adapted from Fox K, Garcia MA, Ardissino D, *et al.* Guidelines on the management of stable angina pectoris: executive summary: The Task Force on the Management of Stable Angina Pectoris of the European Society of Cardiology. *Eur Heart J* **27**: 1341–81.

Differential diagnosis of chest pain

Angina pectoris can be simulated by several non-ischaemic cardiac diseases or by extracardiac diseases. Indeed, somatic or visceral pain signals may converge on the same neurons in the spinal dorsal horns which also receive cardiac ischaemic pain signals, thus resulting in a pain sensation similar or indistinguishable, as to type and location, from angina (➲Table 17.4).

Cardiovascular causes of chest pain

In the absence of obstructive coronary stenoses, spasm or thrombosis, chest pain, usually related to effort or to other conditions of increased myocardial oxygen demand, may occur in patients with severe left ventricular hypertrophy, caused by aortic stenosis, hypertrophic cardiomyopathy, arterial hypertension, or, less frequently, by aortic regurgitation or dilated cardiomyopathy. In these conditions, the increased left ventricular mass is often not matched by a parallel growth of coronary microcirculation; thus, increased oxygen demand cannot be satisfied. Diastolic dysfunction, with increased diastolic pressure, is also present and facilitates subendocardial ischaemia. Finally, coronary microvascular dysfunction can contribute to myocardial ischaemia [3]. Distinction from angina caused by obstructive coronary artery disease may be difficult even after full non-invasive diagnostic investigation and may eventually require coronary angiography.

Notably, angina in the absence of signs of myocardial ischaemia is sometimes experienced by patients who have recently undergone coronary stent implantation [103]. Stretching of the coronary arterial wall at the site of stenting is the likely mechanism in these cases. In very rare cases, angina is triggered by the intermittent appearance of heart rate-dependent left bundle branch block, in the absence of any evidence of myocardial ischaemia [104]. Stretching of afferent nerve fibres caused by dyssynergic myocardial contraction at the appearance of left bundle branch block is the likely mechanism of pain in these cases.

Aortic dissection must be carefully excluded in patients presenting with chest pain. In this condition chest pain is usually of sudden onset and severe, but in some cases it is subacute and atypical. It often radiates to the back, lasts for hours, is not influenced by breathing or turning and may tend to migrate. A history of hypertension or a marfanoid habitus in young patients should raise suspicions. Differences in peripheral pulses and an enlarged aorta on chest X-ray should also suggest the diagnosis of aortic dissection, which is then confirmed by transoesophageal

Table 17.4 Differential diagnosis of chest pain

Cardiovascular causes
Ischaemic
Flow-limiting coronary stenosis
Coronary vasospasm
Coronary thrombosis
Microvascular dysfunction*
Non-ischaemic
Coronary arterial wall distension
Dyssinergic myocardial contraction
Aortic dissection
Pericarditis
Pulmonary embolism or hypertension
Non-cardiovascular causes
Gastrointestinal
Oesophageal spasm
Gastro-oesophageal reflux
Gastritis/duodenitis
Peptic ulcer
Cholecystitis
Respiratory
Pleuritis
Mediastinitis
Pneumothorax
Neuromuscular/skeletal
Chest wall pain syndrome
Nevritis/radiculitis
Herpes zoster
Tietze's syndrome
Psychogenetic
Anxiety
Depression

echocardiography, computed tomography (CT) or cardiac magnetic resonance (CMR).

Chest pain caused by pericarditis is usually easily recognized because of typical changes in breathing and exacerbation by assuming the supine position; pericardial rubs can be present and the ECG usually shows typical diffuse ST-segment elevation.

Chest pain caused by pulmonary embolism (➲Chapter 37) is frequently associated with dyspnoea and tachypnoea; the presence of typical predisposing conditions (e.g. recent surgery, prolonged bed rest) should raise suspicions. The ECG, laboratory investigation and imaging techniques usually allow the correct diagnosis.

Finally, pulmonary hypertension (➲Chapter 24), either primary or secondary, may also be associated with chest pain, caused by increased stress on the pulmonary arterial wall or by right ventricular ischaemia. A careful physical examination and appropriate diagnostic tests (e.g. ECG, chest X-ray, echocardiography) usually allow the correct diagnosis of pulmonary hypertension.

Non-cardiovascular causes of chest pain

These include four major groups of clinical syndromes.

Gastro-intestinal disorders are among the most frequent disorders mimicking angina. Oesophageal spasm and reflux, in particular, may cause typical retrosternal or epigastric pain, which can radiate towards the neck, jaw and arms, and can occasionally be relieved by short-acting nitrates. Chest pain caused by gastro-oesophageal reflux usually appears immediately after a meal or at night. Yet, angina can occur under the same circumstances. Furthermore, both reflux and angina can be triggered by exercise. Of note, reflux and oesophageal spasm may coexist with angina, as the latter may be facilitated by autonomic reflexes and pain related to gastro-enteric disorders. The response to anti-acid treatment and endoscopy may help in the differential diagnosis.

Peptic ulcer and gastritis (and/or duodenitis) may sometimes mimic angina. However, the link to meals, the absence of a relation to effort and the response to anti-acid treatment suggest the diagnosis, which can be confirmed by endoscopy.

Acute or chronic cholecystitis can also sometimes simulate atypical angina, but the pain is not relieved by nitrates. Abdominal ultrasound examination is usually sufficient to document the presence of cholecystitis.

Respiratory diseases (pneumothorax, pleuritis, mediastinitis) may cause chest pain, but symptom features and an accurate physical examination usually establish the correct diagnosis, which can subsequently be confirmed by imaging techniques.

Neuromuscular disorders, including chest wall pain syndrome and neuritis, are among the most common causes of chest pain. Neuromuscular chest pain is usually modified by breathing and/or chest movement, and can be induced by pressure on specific points of the chest. Pain is usually long-lasting (hours, days), does not have any relation with effort and is not relieved by nitrates, whereas it is relieved by anti-inflammatory drugs. Tietze's syndrome (swelling and pain of left chondro-sternal joints) is a rare condition that can be easily recognized.

Psychogenic causes should, finally, be taken into account after organic causes of chest pain have all been excluded. Indeed, anxiety and depression are possible causes of chest pain simulating angina pectoris.

Angina equivalents

In some patients myocardial ischaemia is expressed by transient symptoms that are different from angina pectoris, including dyspnoea, arrhythmias and presyncope or syncope.

Dyspnoea may occur when transient ischaemia involves a large myocardial mass, thus resulting in severe left ventricular dysfunction and pulmonary congestion/oedema. In this case cardiac auscultation may reveal a third heart sound and basal pulmonary rales might be heard on thorax auscultation. Dyspnoea may also occur when myocardial ischaemia causes left ventricular papillary muscle dysfunction, resulting in severe mitral valve regurgitation. In this case, a new, or worsening of a previous, apical systolic murmur is appreciated on cardiac auscultation during ischaemia.

Arrhythmias induced by myocardial ischaemia can be appreciated by the patient as palpitation (e.g. correlated to effort). Severe tachyarrhythmias (e.g. ventricular tachycardia), but also bradyarrhythmias (e.g. atrioventricular or sinoatrial block) may result in presyncope or syncope, as a result of a fall in left ventricular output.

Silent ischaemia

A large number of studies using Holter monitoring have consistently shown that most spontaneous episodes of myocardial ischaemia (i.e. 70–80%), regardless of their causes, are silent, as they are not associated with angina, or angina equivalents [105]. Furthermore, silent ischaemia can also be frequently documented during diagnostic stress tests. The proportion of silent ischaemic episodes is similar in the different coronary ischaemic syndromes, being unrelated to the causes of ischaemia. Of note, from a clinical point of view, prognosis of painful and silent myocardial ischaemia is similar, being dictated in both cases by the underlying causes of myocardial ischaemia.

The causes of silent ischaemia are not completely clear, but several mechanisms are likely to contribute to this phenomenon. A relation between extent and severity of myocardial ischaemia and the occurrence of angina has been suggested by some reports. Most studies, however, failed to find differences between patients with painful or painless ischaemia with regard to severity of ST-segment changes, wall motion abnormalities or haemodynamic changes during ischaemic episodes [105]. Thus, on the whole, the association between severity and extent of myocardial ischaemia and occurrence of pain is poor, even in the same patient.

The causes of painless ischaemia can be different in patients who present both painless and painful myocardial ischaemia during the same day, or even in a short period of time, despite similar duration and severity of ischaemia, and in those who predominantly or exclusively present silent ischaemia.

In the former group silent ischaemic episodes are probably the result of a dynamic peripheral and/or central modulation of cardiac pain signals [79, 106]. Instead, in patients with predominant, or even only, silent myocardial ischaemia, the failure to develop pain could be because of a generalized defective perception of painful stimuli. Indeed, these patients, compared with those with predominantly painful ischaemia, have a higher threshold and tolerance for pain stimuli, including forearm ischaemia, cold pressor, skin electrical stimulation, intravenous adenosine infusion, and dental pulp stimulation [100]. Increased central release of endogenous opioids, which inhibit nociceptive dorsal horn-convergent neurons, has been proposed as a possible mechanism, but studies comparing plasma levels of endogenous endorphins in patients with predominantly painful or painless ischaemia have given controversial results [100]. Finally, psychological factors may play an important role, as patients exhibiting predominantly silent ischaemia have been found to present lower scores for nervousness, 'excitability' and tendency to complain.

In contrast with current beliefs, there is no definite evidence that silent ischaemia is more prevalent among diabetic patients [107,108] than in the general population. In diabetic patients, however, both silent myocardial ischaemia and microalbuminuria independently affect prognosis [109].

Stable angina: diagnosis

Symptoms and physical examination

Stable angina is characterized by a pattern of angina which has remained stable for at least 2 months. It can be the first manifestation of IHD or can appear in patients who had suffered a previous acute coronary event. Typically, angina is induced by efforts or conditions that increase myocardial oxygen demand (e.g. emotional and psychological stresses, hypertensive episodes). Angina is promptly relieved by interrupting the precipitating event, although short-acting nitrates can accelerate pain relief.

The pathologic substrate of stable angina is the presence of coronary flow-limiting stenoses, which do not allow an adequate increase in coronary blood flow during increased myocardial oxygen demand. Typically, myocardial ischaemia is limited to the subendocardial layers, which is most frequently manifested by ST-segment depression in one or more ECG leads (more often V4–V6).

In stable angina, myocardial ischaemia can occur reproducibly for a given level of exercise or in specific conditions, suggesting fixed stenoses. In most patients, however, the ischaemic threshold is variable, and angina can occasionally occur at rest (mixed angina). This variability can be the result of vasomotion at the site of pliable stenoses, modulating their severity (dynamic stenoses) and/or of vasomotor changes in the coronary microcirculation or collateral vessels [110, 111].

The Canadian Cardiovascular Society (CCS) classification of stable angina is the most widely used to assess the severity of angina pectoris (➲Table 17.5) [112].

Alternative classification systems have also been proposed, such as the Duke specific activity index [113] and the Seattle angina questionnaire [114], which may offer better prognostic capability [115].

In patients with stable angina general physical examination is often unremarkable, but findings suggesting lipid disorders (i.e. cutaneous xanthomata, xanthelasma, corneal arcus) (➲Chapter 1) can be observed on visual inspection. Peripheral pulse examination may reveal bruits and murmurs suggesting arterial stenoses, in particular in the carotid and femoral arteries.

Cardiac physical examination is usually uninformative. However, a rapid pulse may be a clue to thyrotoxicosis or anaemia, which can exacerbate angina pectoris. A third and/or fourth heart sound may be heard during angina because of transient cardiac failure. A transient paradoxical splitting of the second heart sound appears in cases of ischaemia-induced left bundle branch block, whereas a transient systolic murmur may indicate mitral regurgitation following papillary muscle dysfunction, in particular in patients with a dilated left ventricle. Finally, a systolic murmur may suggest that aortic stenosis or hypertrophic cardiomyopathy is a possible cause of angina.

A flow chart summarizing the diagnostic work-up in patients with stable angina symptoms is shown in ➲Fig. 17.17.

Table 17.5 Canadian Cardiovascular Society classification of angina pectoris

I. Ordinary physical activity, such as walking and climbing stairs, does not cause angina. Angina results from strenuous or rapid or prolonged exercise at work or recreatio
II. Slight limitation of ordinary activity: walking or climbing stairs rapidly, walking uphill, walking or climbing stairs after meals, in cold in wind, or when under emotional stress, or only during the few hours after awakening. Walking more than two blocks on the level and climbing more than one flight of ordinary stairs at a normal pace and under normal conditions
III. Marked limitations of ordinary physical activity: walking one or two blocks on the level and climbing the more than one flight under normal conditions
IV. Inability to carry on any physical activity without discomfort. Anginal syndrome may be present at rest

Data from Campeau L. Grading of angina pectoris. *Circulation* 1976; **54**: 522.

Non-invasive tests

Laboratory tests

They can provide information related to possible causes of ischaemia. Haemoglobin and, where there is a clinical suspicion of a thyroid disorder, thyroid hormone levels provide information related to possible causes of ischaemia. If there is a clinical suspicion of instability, biochemical markers of myocardial damage such as troponin or creatinine kinase myocardial band (measured by the mass assay) should be employed to exclude myocardial injury. If these markers are elevated, management should continue as for an acute coronary syndrome rather than stable angina. After initial assessment, these tests are not recommended as routine investigations during each subsequent evaluation. Routine laboratory chemical tests are recommended in the initial assessment of patients with suspected angina to well characterize the cardiovascular risk profile (glucose, lipids) and to identify possible comorbidities, including hepatic and renal function.

Resting ECG

In patients with suspected angina pectoris a resting 12-lead ECG should be recorded, although only occasionally it is of diagnostic value (➲Chapter 2). Indeed, resting ECG is normal in about 50% of cases and, when abnormal, will show abnormalities (e.g. minor ST-segment/T wave changes, atrioventricular or intraventricular conduction disorders, supraventricular or ventricular arrhythmias) that are not sufficiently specific for the diagnosis of IHD because they can be frequently found in several other conditions. However, the detection of pathologic Q/QS waves, even in the absence of any history of previous MI, or of typical negative symmetric T waves and/or ST-segment depression, strongly suggests an ischaemic origin of symptoms.

Chest X-ray

Although routinely performed in most patients, chest X-ray has poor diagnostic value in suspected stable angina.

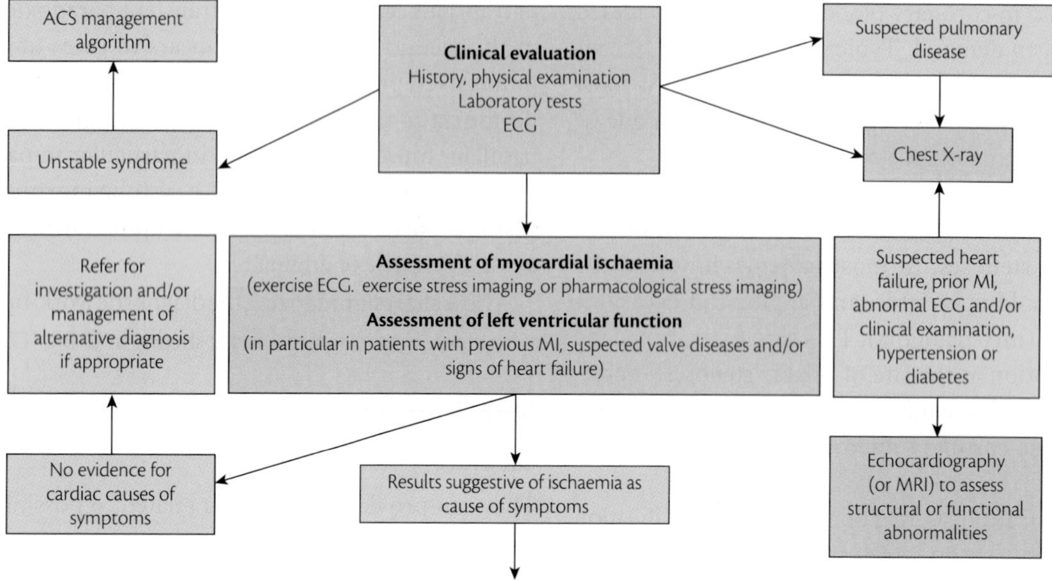

Figure 17.17 Flow chart showing the diagnostic work up in patients with suspected stable angina. Adapted from Fox K, Garcia MA, Ardissino D, *et al.* Guidelines on the management of stable angina pectoris: executive summary: The Task Force on the Management of Stable Angina Pectoris of the European Society of Cardiology. *Eur Heart J* **27**: 1341–81.

The detection of coronary calcifications, however, is associated with a high probability of obstructive IHD [116].

Echocardiography at rest

Resting two-dimensional and Doppler echocardiography is useful to detect or rule out the possibility of other disorders such as valvular heart disease or hypertrophic cardiomyopathy as a cause of symptoms and to evaluate ventricular function (➲Chapter 4). For purely diagnostic purposes, echo is useful in patients with clinically detected murmurs, history and ECG changes compatible with hypertrophic cardiomyopathy or previous MI and symptoms or signs of heart failure. Recent developments in tissue Doppler imaging and strain rate measurement have greatly improved the ability to study diastolic function, but the clinical implications of isolated diastolic dysfunction in terms of treatment or prognosis are less well defined.

Ambulatory ECG Holter monitoring

Holter monitoring (➲Chapter 2) rarely adds additional diagnostic information on top of what is achievable by an ECG exercise stress test (ECG-EST), but it may reveal myocardial ischaemia during normal daily activities [117] in up to 10–15% of patients with stable angina who do not develop diagnostic ST-segment depression during ECG-EST [118]. This can occur in patients in whom coronary vasoconstriction plays an important role in the pathogenesis of myocardial ischaemia. Accordingly, ECG monitoring is more helpful for diagnostic purposes in patients with symptoms suggestive of dynamic stenosis or coronary vasospasm.

ECG exercise stress test

Treadmill or bicycle ECG-EST during 12-lead ECG monitoring is the test of choice to diagnose myocardial ischaemia in the majority of patients with suspected stable angina, because of its simplicity and the excellent cost: benefit ratio (➲Table 17.6) [102] (➲Chapters 8 and 25).

The main diagnostic ECG abnormality during EST consists of a rectilinear or downsloping ST-segment depression ≥0.1mV, persisting for at least 0.06–0.08s after the J-point, in one or more ECG leads (➲Fig. 17.18) [119].

It is worth noting that in about 15% of patients diagnostic ST-segment changes appear during the recovery phase, rather than during the active phase, of exercise [120].

To obtain maximal diagnostic information from ECG-EST, the latter should be symptom/sign limited and performed without the influence of anti-ischaemic drugs. There are numerous reviews and meta-analyses of the performance of exercise ECG for the diagnosis of coronary disease [121–123], showing variable diagnostic yield according to the threshold selected for the diagnosis. Using exercise ST-depression ≥0.1mV or 1mm to define a positive test, the reported sensitivity and specificity for the detection of significant coronary artery disease range between 23–100% (mean 68%) and 17–100% (mean 77%), respectively. Restricting the analysis to those studies designed

Table 17.6 Non-invasive tests for diagnosis and prognostic stratification of stable angina

Test	Recommended use	Comments
Exercise ECG	First choice in most patients	Difficult to interpret in presence of abnormal basal ECG
Exercise myocardial perfusion scintigraphy or echocardiography	Patients with non-interpretable ECG Non-conclusive exercise ECG results For accurate location of ischaemia	Imaging techniques more predictive than ECG Exercise more physiologic than pharmacologic stressors Echocardiography more informative than nuclear techniques and radiation free, but interpretation more operator-dependent and poor image quality in some patients
Myocardial perfusion scintigraphy or echocardiography during infusion of pharmacologic stressors	Patients unable to exercise Preferable if assessment of viable myocardium is also needed	Echocardiography more informative than nuclear techniques and radiation free, but interpretation more operator-dependent and poor image quality in some patients

ECG, electrocardiogram.

to avoid work-up bias, sensitivity was 50% and specificity 90% [124].

The positive predictive value for coronary artery disease of exercise-induced ST-segment depression increases up to 90% if it is accompanied by typical angina pain, if it occurs in the early stages of exercise or persists for >5min in the recovery phase, and if it is >0.2mV [125]. Early appearance, extensive lead involvement and slow normalization after exercise are also clues to the presence of multivessel IHD.

When assessing the accuracy of ECG-EST, as well as of other non-invasive techniques, for the diagnosis of obstructive IHD, intrinsic bias should be considered, which may account for a proportion of erroneous results. This bias consists of considering the presence or absence of obstructive coronary stenoses at angiography as the gold standard for diagnostic accuracy. Indeed, on the one hand non-invasive stress tests detect myocardial ischaemia, which may be caused by coronary spasm or microvascular dysfunction. On the other hand, obstructive atherosclerosis does not always cause myocardial ischaemia during stress (e.g. for the presence of well-developed collateral circulation).

Several other variables have been suggested to improve the diagnostic accuracy of ECG-EST, including QRS and U wave changes, ST/HR slope or ST/HR index and the ST/HR recovery loop, but, despite their potential, they have not been yet fully implemented in clinical practice [126, 127].

The interpretation of ST-segment changes during ECG-EST should be individualized, particularly considering the pre-test probability for the patient to have obstructive coronary artery disease, which mainly depends on the characteristics of symptoms, but is also influenced by risk factors, in particular age (➲Table 17.7) [102]. Indeed, owing to the

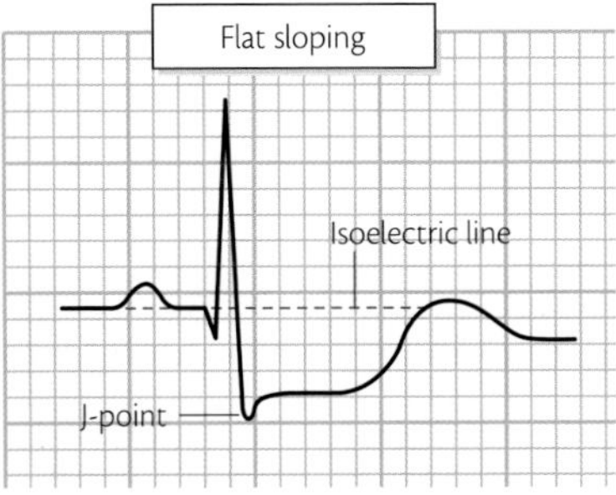

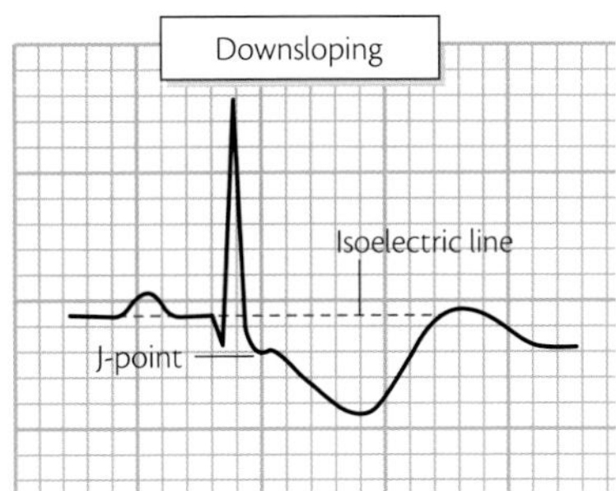

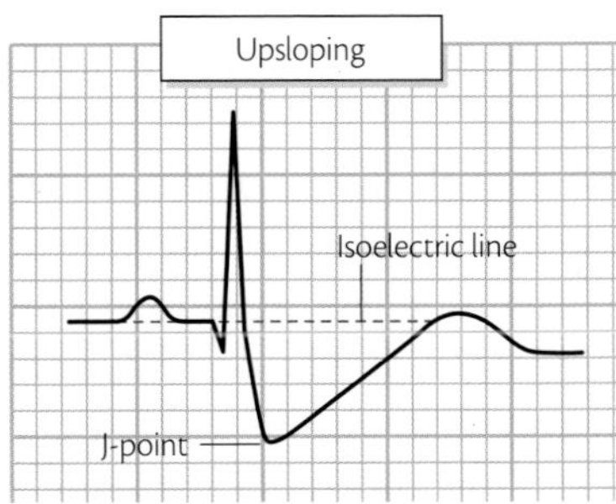

Figure 17.18 Three different types of ST-segment depression that can be seen during exercise-stress test: horizontal (flat sloping), upsloping, and downsloping. Horizontal or downsloping ST-segment depression ≥1.0mm is usually taken as cut off for the diagnosis of obstructive coronary artery disease. with downsloping ST segment depression having higher specificity. Upsloping ST-segment depression is less specific for coronary artery disease, but an upsloping ST segment depression ≥2.0 or ≥1.5mm at 0.08s from the J-point has sufficient specificity to suggest coronary artery disease. Adapted with permission from Barnabei L, Marazia S, De Caterina R. Receiver operating characteristic (ROC) curves and the definition of threshold levels to diagnose coronary artery disease on electrocardiographic stress testing. Part I: The use of ROC curves in diagnostic medicine and electrocardiographic markers of ischaemia. *J Cardiovasc Med* (Hagerstown) 2007; **8**: 873–81.

Table 17.7 Pre-test (top table) and post-test ECG exercise stress test (bottom table) likelihood of ischaemic heart disease, according to chest pain features, sex, and age. Values represent the percentage of patients found to have significant obstructive coronary atherosclerosis at angiography

Age (years)	Typical angina		Atypical angina		Non-anginal chest pain	
	Male	**Female**	**Male**	**Female**	**Male**	**Female**
30–39	69.7	25.8	21.8	4.2	5.2	0.8
40–49	87.3	55.2	46.1	13.3	14.1	2.8
50–59	92.0	79.4	58.9	32.4	21.5	8.4
60–69	94.3	90.1	67.1	54.4	28.1	18.6

Age (years)	ST depression (mV)	Typical angina		Atypical angina		Non-anginal chest-pain	
		Male	**Female**	**Male**	**Female**	**Male**	**Female**
30–39	0.00–0.04	25	7	6	1	1	<1
	0.05–0.09	68	24	2	4	5	1
	0.10–0.14	83	42	38	9	10	2
	0.15–0.19	91	59	55	15	19	3
	0.20–0.24	96	79	76	33	39	8
	>0.25	99	93	92	63	68	24
40–49	0.00–0.04	61	22	16	3	4	1
	0.05–0.09	86	53	44	12	13	3
	0.10–0.14	94	72	64	25	26	6
	0.15–0.19	97	84	78	39	41	11
	0.20–0.24	99	93	91	63	65	24
	>0.25	>99	98	97	86	87	53
50–59	0.00–0.04	73	47	25	10	6	2
	0.05–0.09	91	78	57	31	20	8
	0.10–0.14	96	89	75	50	37	16
	0.15–0.19	98	94	86	67	53	28
	0.20–0.24	99	98	94	84	75	50
	>0.25	>99	99	98	95	91	78
60–69	0.00–0.04	79	69	32	21	8	5
	0.05–0.09	94	90	65	52	26	17
	0.10–0.14	97	95	81	72	45	33
	0.15–0.19	99	98	89	83	62	49
	0.20–0.24	99	99	96	93	81	72
	>0.25	>99	99	99	98	94	90

Adapted with permission from Management of stable angina pectoris. Recommendations of the Task Force of the European Society of Cardiology. *Eur Heart J* 1997; **18:** 394–413.

suboptimal sensitivity and specificity of ECG-EST, pre-test probability influences the predictive value for IHD, according to Bayes theorem.

Bayes theorem allows the calculation of the probability of a subject to be affected by a disease in the presence of a positive or negative diagnostic test. According to Bayes theorem, the probability of the disease depends not only on the sensitivity and specificity of the test but also on the pre-test probability of the disease in the population of individuals to which the subject belongs (➲Fig. 17.19) [128]. Accordingly, diagnostic tests are particularly useful and maximally informative in patients with an intermediate probability of disease. Indeed, in patients with estimated low pretest probability of IHD (e.g. a 30-year-old woman with atypical angina), ST-segment depression has low predictive value for IHD, because of a high proportion of false-positive results. As a consequence, the test is not usually recommended for diagnostic purposes in

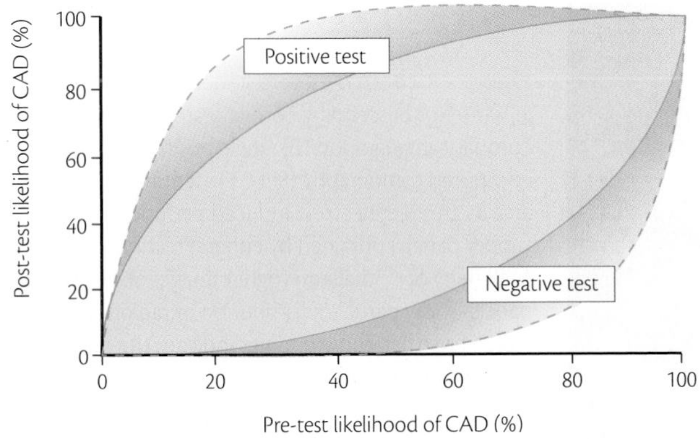

Figure 17.19 The relationship between pre-test probability of obstructive coronary artery disease and the post-test probability of the disease according to the result of a diagnostic non-invasive test with a sensitivity and specificity of 75% (solid lines) and a test with a sensitivity and specificity of 90% (dashed lines). In the former condition, it can be seen that, in the case of a positive test (upper solid line), the probability of disease becomes sufficiently high (50%) only when pre-test probability is at least 20%, and progressively increases with the increase of the pre-test probability. On the other hand, if pre-test probability is elevated, the probability of disease remains high, even in the case of a negative test (bottom solid line). Diagnostic accuracy improves significantly with a test with a very high sensitivity and specificity; indeed, in the case of a pre-test probability of 20%, such a test is associated with a positive predictive value of disease of 85%. However, it can be observed that, in this case also, when pre-test probability is very low (e.g. 5%) a positive test is associated with a presence of disease of only 45% (upper dashed line). At the other extreme, if the pre-test probability is high, post-test probability remains high even in the presence of a negative test (bottom dashed line). Adapted from Epstein SE. Implications of probability analysis on the strategy used for noninvasive detection of coronary artery disease. Role of single or combined use of exercise electrocardiographic testing, radionuclide cineangiography and myocardial perfusion imaging. *Am J Cardiol* 1980; **46**: 491–9, ©1980 with permission from Elsevier.

asymptomatic individuals with a good risk factor profile. At the other extreme, in patients with estimated high pre-test probability of IHD (e.g. a 60-year-old diabetic man with typical angina) ECG-EST is only confirmatory, whereas a negative test does not allow obstructive coronary artery disease to be excluded. Nevertheless, ECG-EST is useful in these patients, providing additional information on the severity of ischaemia, the degree of functional limitation and prognosis [129]. The exact definition of the upper and lower boundaries of intermediate probability is a matter of physician judgement in individual patients, but values of 10% and 90%, respectively, have been suggested [124].

The ECG-EST has limited value in patients with basal ECG abnormalities, including left bundle branch block, paced rhythm or Wolff–Parkinson–White syndrome, which preclude a correct interpretation of ST-segment changes. False-positive results are also more frequent in patients with resting ST-segment/T wave abnormalities, because of left ventricular hypertrophy, electrolyte imbalance, or drug effects (e.g. digitalis).

An important issue with ECG-EST is the diagnosis of obstructive IHD in women, in whom ST-segment depression has been found to have lower specificity (i.e. it is more often a false-positive result) than in men. However, when pre-test probability is accurately determined, and patients with a normal ECG at rest are selected, ECG-EST has the same reliability in women as in men [130].

Stress tests in combination with imaging

The best established stress imaging techniques are perfusion scintigraphy and echocardiography. Both may be used in combination with either exercise stress or pharmacological stress. Novel stress imaging techniques now also include stress MRI, usually performed with pharmacological stress.

Stress imaging techniques have several advantages over conventional ECG-EST, including superior diagnostic performance (➲Table 17.6) for the detection of obstructive coronary artery disease, the ability to quantify and localize areas of ischaemia, and the ability to provide diagnostic information in the presence of resting ECG abnormalities or inability of the patient to exercise. Such techniques are often preferred in patients with previous percutaneous PCI or coronary artery bypass grafting (CABG) because of their ability to localize ischaemia. Furthermore, in patients with intermediate coronary lesions at angiography, evidence on imaging stress tests of myocardial ischaemia in the corresponding myocardial territory predicts future events, whereas a negative test identifies patients at low cardiac risk, who can be reassured.

Stress imaging techniques, therefore, might be considered as an alternative to standard ECG-EST to detect ischaemia; however, they are more expensive and time-consuming, and less cost-effective. Thus, for diagnostic purposes they are only indicated in patients with non-conclusive results of ECG-EST or when ECG is not interpretable [102].

Scintigraphic stress tests

Exercise myocardial perfusion scintigraphy is a robust, non-invasive method of assessing regional myocardial perfusion and allows the diagnosis of myocardial ischaemia by showing a reversible reduction of isotope myocardial uptake at peak exercise, as compared to rest, in myocardial regions supplied by stenotic coronary artery branches (➲Fig. 17.20).

The three commercially available flow perfusion tracers, ^{201}thallium, and ^{99m}technetium-labelled sestamibi or tetrofosmin, have similar accuracies for the detection of IHD.

Published figures of sensitivity and specificity for the diagnosis of coronary disease vary widely and depend upon

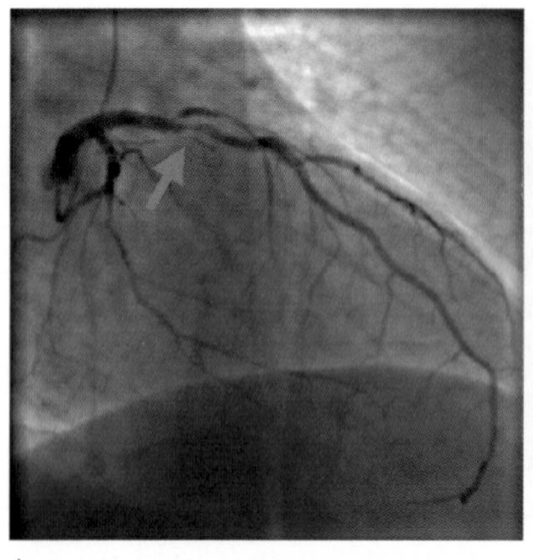
A

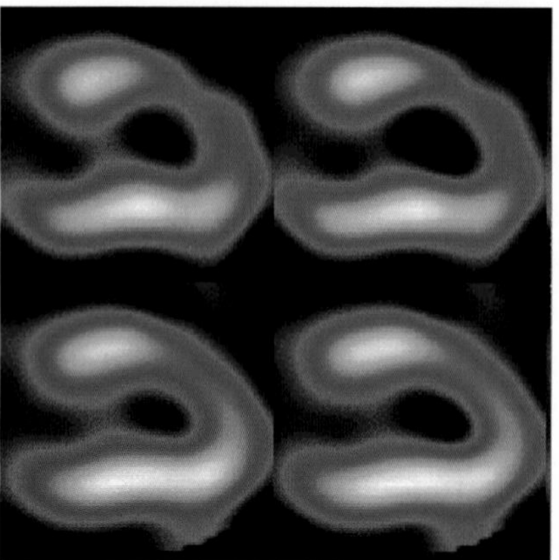
B

Figure 17.20 (A) A severe stenosis is present in the left anterior descending coronary artery (arrow) at coronary angiography. (B) Single positron emission computed tomography (SPECT) identifies the ischaemic area as an exercise stress-induced perfusion defect (upper panels) obtained by either ^{99}technetium-labelled MIBI (left) or ^{201}thallium (right). Images at rest (bottom panels) show partial redistribution of radioisotopes. Taken together, these findings indicate the presence of a previous antero-apical myocardial infarction with inducible myocardial ischaemia in the peri-infarct region. (By courtesy of Dr. Paolo Marzullo, Laboratory of Nuclear Cardiology, CNR Institute of Clinical Physiology, Pisa, Italy).

the characteristics of the studied population (e.g. gender, presenting symptoms, medication, presence of previous infarction, etc.), the imaging technique (planar or SPECT, qualitative or semi-quantitative analysis) and the experience of the centre. Overall, exercise myocardial scintigraphy is more sensitive than ECG-EST for IHD detection, Using SPECT imaging, and without correction for referral bias, sensitivity has been found to range between 70–98%, and specificity 40–90% [102].

Scintigraphic studies are more accurate than ECG-EST in predicting the presence of multivessel IHD and in detecting the location and extent of myocardial ischaemia [102]. Thus, they can be indicated when this information is important.

Pharmacological stressors can be used as an alternative to exercise in patients who are unable to exercise adequately (e.g. elderly patients or patients with peripheral vascular disease or those limited by dyspnoea) [131]. They include the sympathetic agonist dobutamine, which causes an increase of myocardial oxygen consumption simulating physical exercise, and the arteriolar vasodilators dipyridamole and adenosine, which cause subendocardial underperfusion in myocardial regions supplied by stenotic coronary artery branches, because of the coronary blood flow steal phenomenon.

The diagnostic accuracy with pharmacological stressors has been reported to be similar to that with exercise [132]. The latter, however, is preferable because of the more obvious relation of exercise levels with real-life activities and of the additional diagnostic and prognostic information provided by the results of exercise stress per se.

Radionuclide angiography has been used in previous years to diagnose obstructive coronary artery disease, but it has now fallen out of favour because it adds no relevant diagnostic information to that provided by other non-invasive tests.

Echocardiographic stress tests

Exercise echocardiography is an alternative to exercise myocardial perfusion scintigraphy as a second-tier test to standard ECG-EST, presenting similar indications and advantages, including a more reliable diagnosis of multivessel disease and location of myocardial ischaemia [133]. Its indications as a real first-step alternative to ECG-EST are similarly doubtful (➲Table 17.6).

Diagnosis of IHD on echocardiography is based on the detection of stress test-induced reversible regional left ventricular wall motion abnormalities. Compared with scintigraphy, inconveniences include poor image quality in about 15% of patients, higher operator-dependent interpretation, lower sensitivity (in particular for single-vessel disease of the left circumflex coronary artery), the need for special training for a correct performance and interpretation, and more difficult assessment of ischaemia in the presence of basal left ventricular wall motion abnormalities. The inability to image at peak exercise is only a minor disadvantage because contractile abnormalities do not usually normalize immediately after peak exercise.

Exercise echocardiography, however, also has some advantages over exercise perfusion scintigraphy, including a slightly higher specificity, the possibility of a more extensive evaluation of cardiac anatomy and function, greater availability, lower cost, and a greater safety (being free of radiation exposure).

Pharmacological stressors are used more frequently than exercise in echocardiography. Indications and stressors for echocardiography are the same as those for pharmacological scintigraphic stress tests. In patients with negative tests, however, atropine is often added, either to dobutamine (especially in patients on beta-blockers) or to dipyridamole, to increase heart rate and the sensitivity of the test.

In a direct comparison of the different stress tests, sensitivity of exercise and dobutamine echocardiography for the diagnosis of obstructive coronary artery disease was similar, whereas sensitivity of dipyridamole echocardiography was lower and specificity did not differ among tests [134].

Stress cardiovascular magnetic resonance

CMR stress testing in conjunction with dobutamine infusion can detect wall motion abnormalities induced by ischaemia, and compares favourably to dobutamine stress echo because of higher quality imaging [135] (➲Chapter 5). A low event rate when dobutamine CMR is normal has been reported [136]. Myocardial perfusion CMR now achieves comprehensive ventricular coverage using multislice imaging. Although still in development, the results are already good in comparison with other imaging techniques [137]. The restricted availability, the higher costs, and also some difficulties in continuous monitoring of the patient during the stress test, limit at present the utilization of this technique for diagnostic purposes in clinical practice.

Non-invasive techniques to assess coronary anatomy

Computed tomography

Recent considerable advances in technology have largely overcome problems of spatial resolution and movement artefact, which have long been limiting factors for this type of imaging. Two imaging techniques of this kind include ultra-fast or electron beam CT (EBCT) and multi-detector or multi-slice CT (MDCT). Both techniques have been validated for quantification of the extent of coronary calcifications, which correlates more closely with the overall burden of plaque than with the location or severity of stenoses [138, 139]. Assessment of coronary calcification is not however recommended routinely for the diagnostic evaluation of patients with stable angina [102].

The improvement in image acquisition times and resolution can now allow coronary arteriography be performed by injection of intravenous contrast agents, with MDCT being the most promising technique for the non-invasive imaging of the coronary arteries. MDCT angiography accurately identifies the presence and severity of obstructive coronary artery disease and subsequent revascularization in symptomatic patients. However the negative and positive predictive values in the most recent comparative studies indicate that MDCT angiography cannot replace invasive coronary angiography for diagnostic purposes, and additionally involves a higher radiation exposure [140].

Magnetic resonance arteriography

CMR contrast coronary arteriography also permits the non-invasive assessment of the coronary lumen [141], and, in addition, also holds the potential for plaque characterization [142] (➲Chapter 5). Additional advantages of the technique are that it has a considerable potential for evaluation of the overall cardiac anatomy and function. However at present it is still an investigational tool not recommended in clinical practice.

Invasive tests

Coronary angiography

By definition, obstructive coronary artery disease, as the cause of stable angina, is ultimately diagnosed by documenting flow-limiting coronary artery stenoses at angiography. Yet, because of the small, but definite, risk of complications and its cost, coronary angiography cannot be recommended as a routine diagnostic procedure to assess chest pain. The composite rate of major complications associated with routine diagnostic catheterization in patients is 1–2%. The composite rate of death, MI, or stroke of the order of 0.1–0.2%.

Coronary angiography (➲Chapter 8) for diagnostic purposed is indicated in specific subsets of patients including: 1) patients who have a high probability of needing myocardial revascularization; 2) patients at high risk because of resuscitated sudden death or life-threatening ventricular arrhythmias in whom a definitive diagnosis regarding the presence or absence of coronary disease is important in clinical decision making; 3) patients with a non conclusive diagnosis of IHD on noninvasive testing. In contrast, coronary angiography for diagnostic purposes should not be performed in: 1) anginal patients who refuse myocardial revascularization; 2) anginal patients in whom the diagnosis of IHD is clearly confirmed by the results of non invasive testing. Recommendations for diagnostic coronary angiography are summarized in ➲Table 17.8.

Intracoronary diagnostic techniques

Intravascular ultrasound

Intravascular ultrasound allows the production of images from within the coronary arteries by passing an ultrasound catheter into the coronary artery lumen (➲Chapter 8). It allows for accurate measurement of coronary luminal diameter, assessment of eccentric lesions and of vessel remodelling, and also for quantification of atheroma and calcium deposition. It also allows a detailed assessment of interventional target lesions, of placement, apposition and expansion of coronary stents, and of transplant vasculopathy [143]. The technique has achieved an important role in specialized clinical settings, particularly as an adjunct to PCI. However it is more appropriately used in such specific settings and for research purposes than for widespread applications as first-line investigation for coronary artery disease (see ➲Chapter 8) [102].

Table 17.8 Recommendations for diagnostic coronary angiography

Evidence and/or general agreement that diagnostic coronary angiography is indicated
Patients with severe stable angina (Class 3 or greater of Canadian Cardiovascular Society Classification) in spite of optimal medical treatment
Survivors of cardiac arrest
Patients with life-threatening ventricular arrhythmias
Patients previously treated by myocardial revascularization who develop early recurrence of moderate or severe angina
Conflicting evidence and/or a divergence of opinion that diagnostic coronary angiography is indicated, but weight of evidence/opinion is in favour
Patients with moderate to high pre-test probability of ischaemic heart disease after clinical assessment and an inconclusive diagnosis on non-invasive testing or conflicting results from different non-invasive modalities
Patients with a high risk of restenosis on non invasive testing, after a percutaneous coronary intervention, performed in a prognostically important site.
Evidence or general agreement that diagnostic coronary angiography is not indicated
Patients in whom the diagnosis of ischaemic heart disease is clearly confirmed by non invasive testing
Patients who refuse myocardial revascularization

Invasive assessment of functional severity of coronary lesions

The functional severity of coronary lesions after angiography can be assessed invasively by measuring either coronary flow reserve, by an intracoronary Doppler wire [144], or intracoronary artery pressure fractional flow reserve (FFR) [145.146]. Both techniques involve the induction of hyperaemia through the intracoronary injection of vasodilating agents. Such physiological measurements may facilitate diagnosis in cases of intermediate angiographic stenoses (visual estimates 30–70% in diameter), and may allow better decisions on the suitability of revascularization. They should not however be used routinely [102].

Stable angina: risk stratification

Prognostic information in stable IHD patients can be derived mainly from clinical evaluation and from non-invasive laboratory tests, which allow careful assessment of two major prognostic risk factors, i.e. left ventricular function and presence and severity of myocardial ischaemia. In specific cases the invasive assessment of coronary anatomy by angiography also provides important clues to the risk of the patient.

Based on clinical evaluation

The severity and frequency of chest pain, as expressed by the CCS classification, have prognostic implications. Indeed, a low anginal threshold is usually associated with severe coronary flow reserve reduction [147]. Symptoms of acute left ventricular dysfunction during angina, possibly indicating extensive myocardial ischaemia, also predict a worse outcome. However, the relationship between symptoms and IHD severity is less than optimal, thus limiting the value of symptoms for predicting clinical outcome. Physical examination may also help in determining risk. The presence of peripheral vascular disease (either lower limb or carotid) identifies patients at increased risk of subsequent cardiovascular events in stable angina. In addition, signs related to heart failure (which reflect left ventricular function) convey an adverse prognosis.

Fasting plasma glucose and fasting lipid profile including total cholesterol, high density lipoprotein (HDL) and low density lipoprotein (LDL) cholesterol, and triglycerides should be evaluated in all patients with suspected ischaemic disease, including stable angina, to establish the patient's risk profile and ascertain the need for treatment. Obesity and, in particular, evidence of the metabolic syndrome are predictive of adverse cardiovascular outcome in patients with established disease as well as in asymptomatic populations. The presence of the metabolic syndrome can be determined from the assessment of waist circumference, blood pressure, HDL, triglycerides, and fasting glucose levels and offers additional prognostic information to that obtained from the conventional Framingham risk scores without major additional cost in terms of laboratory investigation. Further laboratory testing, including measures of apolipoproteins, homocysteine, lipoprotein (a), haemostatic abnormalities, and markers of inflammation, such as C-reactive protein, has been the subject of much interest as methods to improve current risk prediction. More recently, NT-BNP has been shown to be an important predictor of long-term mortality independent of age, left ventricular ejection fraction, and conventional risk factors. As yet, the additional prognostic information of these biochemical indices in stable IHD patients seems limited and there is no adequate information regarding how modification can significantly improve on current treatment strategies to recommend their use in all patients, particularly given the constraints of cost and availability.

The presence of abnormalities on standard 12-lead ECG (i.e. Q waves, persistent ST-T wave abnormalities) and left ventricular enlargement or pulmonary venous congestion on chest X-ray are also associated with a poorer outcome [148].

Several widely available equations based on multiple risk factors exist to calculate the absolute risk of developing coronary or cardiovascular disease in patients without established disease. However, such risk scores do not apply to a population with symptoms. Although several scores have been developed to predict the presence of coronary disease by using clinical or exercise variables or their combination prognostic scores are comparatively few and applicability is limited by restriction of the population studied to those who can exercise. A modified version of the Framingham risk equation exists, which has been adapted for use in patients with pre-existing cardiovascular disease, but this does not allow discrimination between initial manifestations of coronary artery disease or presenting symptoms. Data from institutional databases, such as the Duke database, have also been used to synthesize nomograms to assign absolute probabilities of coronary disease and mortality given various combinations of data from clinical assessment, non-invasive testing, and coronary angiography. However, these tools were developed in populations assessed up to 30 years ago, are not specific to a stable angina population, and may not be widely applicable [149]. Recently, the Euro heart angina score has been developed, which is a simple and objective score that allows an estimate of the probability of death or non-fatal MI among patients with a clinical diagnosis of stable angina, using six simple predictors: comorbidities, diabetes, angina score, symptom duration, left ventricular function, and repolarization abnormalities on resting ECG [150]. The predictive accuracy of this score is comparable to that of older predictive models but is more relevant to a contemporary population (➲Fig. 17.21).

Based on the assessment of left ventricular function

The strongest single predictor of long-term survival in patients with stable IHD is left ventricular ejection fraction (LVEF). In patients with stable angina mortality increases as LVEF declines. In the Coronary Artery Surgery Study (CASS) study the 12-year survival rate of patients with LVEF >50%, 35–49%, and <35% were 73%, 54%, and 21%, respectively [151]. Clinical evaluation, as outlined earlier may indicate which patients have heart failure, and thus at substantially increased risk for future cardiovascular events. However, the prevalence of asymptomatic ventricular dysfunction is not inconsiderable and has been reported to be as high as twice that of overt heart failure. Thus, an estimation of left ventricular function is desirable for risk

Risk factor	Score contribution	Individual's score
Comorbidity*		
No	0	
Yes	86	
Diabetes		
No	0	
Yes	57	
Angina score		
Class I	0	
Class II	54	
Class III	91	
Duration of symptoms		
≥6 months	0	
<6 months	80	
Abnormal ventricular function		
No	0	
Yes	114	
ST depression or T wave inversion on resting electrocardiogram		
No	0	
Yes	34	
		Total=

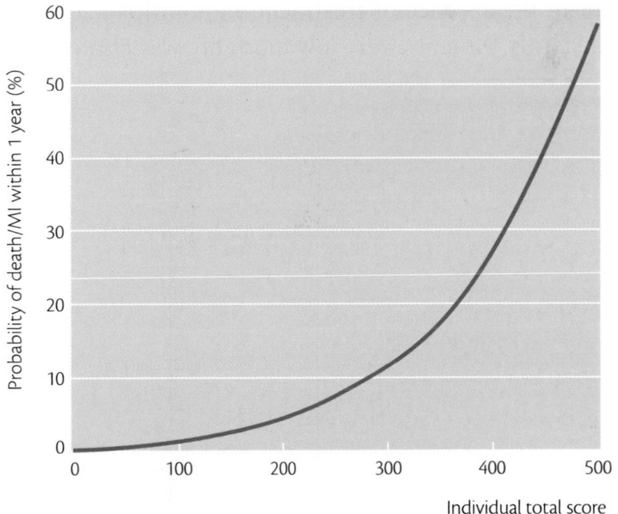

Figure 17.21 Left: score sheet to calculate risk score for patients presenting with stable angina based on the findings of the Euro heart survey of stable angina, a pan-European survey in 156 outpatient cardiology clinics. Right: plot to assign estimated probability of death or non-fatal myocardial infarction within one year of presentation according to combination of clinical and investigative features in patients with stable angina. MI, myocardial infarction. *One or more of previous cerebrovascular event; hepatic disease defined as chronic hepatitis or cirrhosis, or other hepatic disease causing elevation of transaminases more than three times upper limit of normal; peripheral vascular disease defined as claudication either at rest or on exertion, amputation for arterial vascular insufficiency, vascular surgery (reconstruction or bypass) or angioplasty to the extremities, documented aortic aneurysm, or non-invasive evidence of impaired arterial flow; chronic renal failure defined as chronic dialysis or renal transplantation or serum creatinine greater than 200μmol/L; chronic respiratory disease defined as a diagnosis previously made by physician or patient receiving bronchodilators or FEV_1 <75%, arterial pO_2 <60%, or arterial pCO_2 >50% predicted in previous studies; chronic inflammatory conditions defined as a diagnosis of rheumatoid arthritis, systemic lupus erythematosis or other connective tissue diseases, polymyalgia rheumatica, and so on; malignancy defined as a diagnosis of malignancy within a year or active malignancy. Adapted with permission from Daly CA, De Stavola B, Lopez Sendon JL, *et al.* Predicting prognosis in stable angina results from the Euro heart survey of stable angina: prospective observational study. *BMJ* 2006; **332**: 262–7.

stratification of patients with stable angina. Left ventricular function can be easily assessed by two-dimensional echocardiography. Due to technical issues (inadequate echo window), however, echocardiography may fail to allow valid assessment of left ventricular function in about 10% of cases. In these cases utilization of other imaging methods (e.g. scintigraphy, CMR) are therefore required. In other cases also it can be more convenient to assess left ventricular function by other methods. For example, in patients undergoing a stress imaging test with myocardial scintigraphy or CMR, left ventricular function can be assessed during the test using these imaging modalities. Similarly, in patients scheduled for coronary angiography left ventricular systolic function can be assessed by left ventricular angiography during the invasive procedure.

Based on the assessment of myocardial ischaemia

ECG-EST is the key test for the assessment of the amount of myocardium at risk of ischaemia. A good effort tolerance in the absence of ischaemia is associated with a good outcome [152]. Indeed, in the CASS registry, completing stage 2 of the Bruce protocol on treadmill EST, in the absence of ischaemia, was associated with a yearly mortality < 1%, even in the absence of treatment with antiplatelet agents and statins. Notably, very low mortality was also observed in patients who went beyond stage 4 of the Bruce protocol, despite three-vessel disease [153].

Table 17.9 High risk findings of major non-invasive stress tests

Exercise ECG	ST segment depression ≥1mm at Bruce stage 1 Slow ST depression recovery (>5min) after exercise Achievement of workload < 4 METs Abnormal blood pressure response Duke treadmill score ≤−11
Stress myocardial scintigraphy	Multiple and/or large and/or severe reversible perfusion defects Stress-induced left ventricular dilation Stress-induced lung thallium-201 uptake
Stress echocardiography	Multiple and/or large and/or severe regional wall motion abnormalities Stress-induced left ventricular dilatation

The occurrence of myocardial ischaemia during exercise, in particular if it appears at low workload and is associated with a low ejection fraction, portends an ominous prognosis [129]. High-risk features of ECG-EST are summarized in ➲Table 17.9.

Composite scores, which take into account symptoms, ECG signs of ischaemia and other exercise parameters, have been proposed to improve prognostic stratification of stable angina patients. The Duke treadmill score [154] (➲Fig. 17.22), which has been prospectively validated in large cohorts of patients, is based on exercise capacity (as exercise duration), severity of myocardial ischaemia

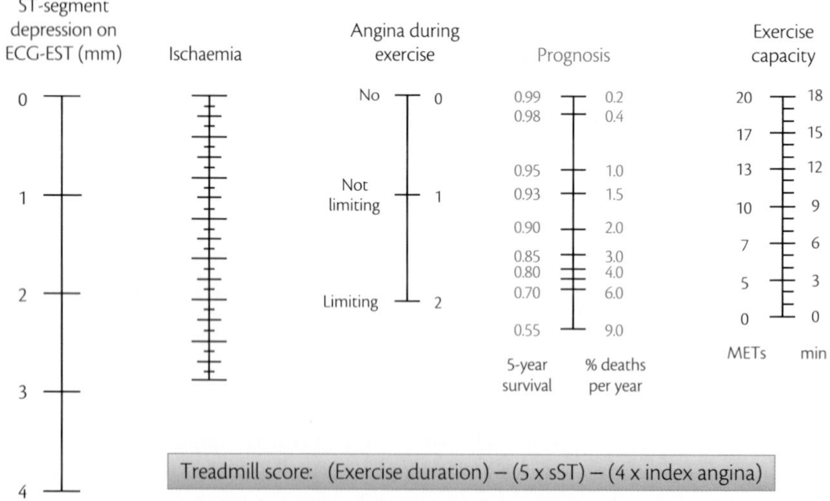

Figure 17.22 Diagram to derive an estimate of prognosis in patients with ischaemic heart disease undergoing treadmill ECG exercise stress test (ECG-EST) by Bruce protocol. To obtain an estimate of 5-year survival or yearly death rate ('prognosis' line) a line from the maximal ST-segment depression recorded during ECG-EST ('ST-segment' line) to the line of exercise induced 'angina' must be drawn, which will cross the 'ischaemia' line in a point; a second line, from this point to the point on the 'exercise capacity' line expressing the METs or exercise duration achieved during the test, must therefore be drawn. The latter line will cross the 'prognosis' line in a point that will indicate the estimate of prognosis. The formula to calculate the Duke treadmill index score for risk stratification of patients in low, intermediate and high risk, is also shown (see text for details). Adapted from Mark DB, Shaw L, Harrell FE, Jr., *et al.* Prognostic value of a treadmill exercise score in outpatients with suspected coronary artery disease. *N Engl J Med* 1991; **325**: 849–53.

(as maximal ST-segment depression) and appearance of angina, and is calculated from the following formula:

Exercise duration (Bruce protocol, in min) –
(5 × ST-segment depression during exercise test, in mm) –
(4 × angina index),

where the angina index assumes a value of '0' if there is no angina induced by exercise, '1' if non-limiting angina occurs during exercise, and '2' if angina is the reason for stopping the test. Among patients with suspected IHD, the two-thirds of patients with a Duke score >5 had a 4-year survival rate of 99% (average annual mortality rate 0.25%), whereas, at the other extreme, the 4% of patients, with a score of −11 or less, had a 4-year survival rate of 79% (average annual mortality rate 5%) [154].

In patients who can undergo exercise and exhibit an interpretable ECG, the additional prognostic value of imaging stress tests compared to that of ECG-EST is clinically limited [155]. The extent of perfusion defects and/or signs of left ventricular dysfunction on radionuclide scintigraphic tests and the extent of left ventricular wall motion abnormalities on echocardiography, induced by either exercise or pharmacological stressors, have been found to be associated with an adverse clinical outcome in stable IHD patients (➲Table 17.9) [156, 157].

Frequent transient ischaemic episodes during daily life, detected by ECG Holter monitoring, are also associated with a worse prognosis [158], although the information that this finding adds to full assessment of ECG-EST remains uncertain. Ambulatory ECG Holter monitoring, however, might be prognostically helpful in patients unable to undergo exercise stress test.

Based on coronary angiography

It is important to recognize that diagnostic techniques able to identify vulnerable plaques responsible for future acute coronary events are still lacking [159] (➲Chapter 8). Thus, the major current focus for risk stratification is on non-invasive techniques, the rationale being the identification of patients in whom revascularization might decrease mortality.

Several prognostic indices have been proposed to relate disease severity to the risk of subsequent cardiac events. The simplest and most widely used is the classification into one, two, three, and left main (LM) vessel disease. Recently, the extent of coronary atherosclerosis assessed at angiography has been found to be a better predictor of outcome than its severity (i.e. number of coronary artery branches presenting critical stenoses) [160]. Thus the higher mortality rates in patients with multivessel disease, as compared with those with one-vessel disease, are probably the consequence of a higher number of mildly stenotic, or even non-stenotic, plaques that are potential sites for acute coronary events. However, the clinical applicability of scores based on the extent of coronary atherosclerosis is still limited.

In the CASS registry of medically treated patients, the 12-year survival rate of patients with normal coronary arteries was 91% compared with 74% for those with single vessel disease, 59% for those with two vessel disease, and 50% for those with three-vessel disease [151]. Patients with severe LM stenosis have a poor prognosis when treated medically. The presence of severe proximal LAD disease also significantly reduces the survival rate. The 5-year survival rate with three-vessel disease plus ≥95% proximal LAD stenosis was reported to be 54% compared with a rate of 79% with three-vessel disease without proximal LAD stenosis [161].

When appropriately used, clinical assessment and non-invasive tests have an acceptable predictive value for adverse events. This is most true when the pre-test probability of severe coronary artery disease is low. When the estimated annual cardiovascular mortality rate is less than or equal to 1%, the use of coronary arteriography to identify patients whose prognosis can be improved is low. In contrast, it is appropriate for patients whose cardiovascular mortality risk is >2% per annum. Decisions regarding the need to proceed to arteriography in the intermediate risk group, those with an annual cardiovascular mortality of 1–2% should be guided by a variety of factors including the patient's symptoms, functional status, lifestyle, and occupation [162], as well as comorbidity, and response to initial therapy [102]. Coronary angiography should not be performed in patients who refuse invasive procedures, prefer to avoid revascularization, or who are not candidates for myocardial revascularization [162]. ➲Table 17.10 summarizes the recommendations for the use of coronary angiography for risk stratification.

Table 17.10 Recommendations for risk stratification by coronary angiography

Patients undergoing diagnostic coronary angiography (see ➲Table 17.8)
Patients determined to be at high risk for adverse outcome on the basis of non-invasive testing including clinical evaluation, assessment of the amount of myocardium at risk of ischaemia, and assessment of left ventricular function.
Patients who are being considered for major non-cardiac surgery, especially vascular surgery (repair of aortic aneurysm, femoral bypass, carotid endoarterectomy) determined to be at moderate to high risk for adverse outcome on the basis of non-invasive testing including assessment of the amount of myocardium at risk of ischaemia and of left ventricular function

Chronic stable angina: medical treatment

Clinical management of patients with stable angina has two main objectives. The first objective is to improve prognosis by preventing MI and death. Efforts to prevent MI and death in stable angina focus primarily on reducing the incidence of acute coronary events and the development of left ventricular dysfunction. Lifestyle changes and drug treatment play vital role in modifying the atherosclerotic disease process and 'stabilizing' coronary plaques, as well as in reducing platelet activation and fibrinolytic and inflammatory abnormalities which predispose to acute coronary events. Such interventions may also slow progression or even induce regression of coronary atherosclerosis. In high risk patients myocardial revascularization offers additional opportunities to further improve prognosis by improving existing perfusion.

The second objective is to minimize or abolish symptoms using anti-anginal drugs, reverting to myocardial revascularization in patients who do not respond to medical treatment.

Interventions to improve outcome: lifestyle changes

The major lifestyle changes which improve clinical outcome in IHD are summarized in ➲Table 17.11.

Smoking

There is overwhelming evidence of an adverse effect of smoking on health. Smoking already kills 1 in 10 adults and is expected to cause 10 million deaths annually world-wide by 2030 [163]. The adverse effect of smoking is related to the amount of tobacco smoked daily and to the duration of smoking [164]. The effects of smoking on cardiovascular disease interact synergistically with other risk factors such as age, gender, arterial hypertension, and diabetes. Passive smoking has also been shown to increase the risk of IHD. Long-term smoking is associated with impaired endothelium-dependent coronary vasodilatation [165]. Smoking-enhanced platelet aggregation and platelet thrombus formation may be important mechanisms for the increased risk of acute coronary events in smokers [166]. The assessment of smoking status should be done at every opportunity and stopping smoking should be actively encouraged in all smokers [167]. The benefits of smoking cessation have been extensively reported and apply to all ages. Some of the advantages are almost immediate, others take more time.

Quitting smoking, however, is a complex and difficult process, because the habit is strongly addictive both pharmacologically and psychologically. Quitting can be facilitated by professional assistance. The physician's firm and explicit advice that a person should stop smoking completely is the most important factor in getting the smoking cessation process started. The momentum for smoking cessation is particularly strong at the time of diagnosing an acute vascular event and in connection with an invasive treatment, such as coronary artery bypass grafting, percutaneous transluminal coronary angioplasty, or vascular surgery. The physician's advice is equally important in helping healthy high risk individuals to attempt to quit smoking. Assessing whether the person is willing to try to quit, brief reiteration of the cardiovascular and other health hazards of smoking, and agreeing on a specific plan with a follow-up arrangement are decisive steps and essential features of the brief initial advice of smoking cessation in clinical practice. Both individual and group behavioural interventions are effective in helping smokers to quit. However, the quality of physician–patient communication seems to be more relevant than the quantity of counselling sessions or the intervention format. Support by the partner and family is very important in smoking cessation. Involvement of the family in the smoking cessation process and getting other smoking family members to quit smoking together with the patient is also of great help.

Nicotine chewing gum and transdermal nicotine patches, bupropion, and varenicline, a partial nicotine acetylcholine receptor agonist, all appear superior to placebo at promoting smoking abstinence [168, 169].

Table 17.11 Recommendations for lifestyle changes

Smoking cessation
Assess smoking status and advise to quit and to avoid passive smoking
Bupropione, varenicline, or nicotine treatment in patients who keep smoking
Physical activity
Exercise test-guided moderate intensity aerobic exercise at least five times per week
Medically supervised rehabilitation programmes for high-risk patients
Diet and weight reduction
Weight reduction is aimed at BMI <25 kg/m^2 and waist circumference <102/88cm (men/women)
Diet based on low intake of salt and saturated fats, and regular intake of fruit, vegetables, and fish
Moderate alcohol consumption should not be discouraged

Diet, dietary supplements, and weight control

Dietetics is an integral part of cardiovascular patient risk management. A varied and energy-balanced regimen together with regular exercise is critical to the preservation of a good cardiovascular health. Notably, fatty acids regulate cholesterol homeostasis and concentrations of blood lipoproteins, and affect the levels of other cardiovascular risk factors, such as blood pressure, haemostasis, and body weight, through various mechanisms. There are strong, consistent and graded relationships between saturated fat intake, blood cholesterol levels, and the occurrence of cardiovascular diseases. The relationships are accepted as causal. Sodium intake, especially in the form of sodium chloride, influences arterial blood pressure and therefore the risk of arterial hypertension, stroke, IHD, and heart failure. In contrast dietary patterns including fruit and vegetables, monounsaturated fatty acid-rich oil (such as olive oil), and low fat dairy products, have been associated with decreased incidence of cardiovascular events. Evidence from randomized controlled trials on food and nutrition in secondary prevention has recently been reviewed [170, 171]. Dietetic recommendations should be defined individually, taking into account the subject's risk factors, in particular dyslipidaemia, hypertension, diabetes, and obesity. Current guidelines on prevention recommend: (i) to eat a wide variety of foods; (ii) adjustment of calorie intake to avoid overweight; (iii) increased consumption of fruit and vegetables, along with wholegrain cereals and bread, fish (especially oily), lean meat, and low-fat dairy products; (iv) to replace saturated and trans fats with monounsaturated and polyunsaturated fats from vegetable and marine sources and to reduce total fats to <30% of total calorie intake, less than one-third of which should be saturated; and (v) to reduce salt intake if blood pressure is raised. Furthermore, alcohol in moderation (one-two glasses per day) may be beneficial, but excessive consumption is harmful [172]. Many processed and prepared foods are high in salt, and in fat of doubtful quality and, therefore, should be avoided. There is no evidence for the use of antioxidant supplements, low glycaemic index diets, or homocysteine lowering therapies. The role of poly-unsatured (omega-3) fatty acid supplements for secondary prevention is unclear. In the only (open-label) randomized study in patients with a recent MI, 1g daily of fish oil on top of a Mediterranean diet significantly reduced total and cardiovascular mortality [173]. However a recent meta-analysis showed no effect on mortality or cardiovascular events and no evidence that the source or dose may affect the outcome [174].

Obesity

Obesity is becoming a panepidemics in both children and adults. Currently it is estimated that, worldwide, over 1 billion people are overweight, and >300 million are obese. Over one-third of children are overweight or obese. It is now clear that fat, and in particular intra-abdominal visceral fat, is a metabolically active endocrine organ that is capable of synthesizing and releasing into the bloodstream an important variety of peptides and non-peptide compounds that may play a role in cardiovascular homeostasis. Fat is associated with increased secretion of free fatty acids, hyperinsulinaemia, insulin resistance, hypertension, and dyslipidaemia which impact on risk factors and hence on risk. Interestingly, the effects of multivariate adjustment on the association between lipid levels and risk and between body weight and risk are different. Raised blood cholesterol levels, indeed, remain independently associated with risk after adjustment for other major risk factors, whereas the association between weight and risk tends to lose significance [172]. This should not be interpreted as indicating that body weight is not important, but, rather, that it determines an increase of cardiovascular risk when resulting in the appearance of one or more classical cardiovascular risk factors.

The achievement of an optimal body weight is based on an appropriate diet and on regular physical exercise. There is sufficient evidence available from intervention studies supporting the role of physical activity and moderate to vigorous exercise in promoting weight loss. Recent research has indicated that exercise may have beneficial effects before a training effect is apparent and may impact on abdominal fat metabolism before weight loss occurs [175]. This information may be valuable in motivating patients to initiate exercise. In contrast, the contribution of drug treatments aimed at reducing body weight through a variety of mechanisms, such as orlistat, an inhibitor of intestinal lipases, sibutramine and rimonabant, an endocannabinoid receptor inhibitor, is modest and, in the past, some products have had serious side effects.

Current guidelines define a BMI <25kg/m^2 and waist circumference <102/88cm (men/women) as the optimal target to reach [172].

Physical activity

Physical training has a wide variety of beneficial effects on the course of atherosclerosis, resulting in a 20–25% reduction in overall mortality [176]. Yet, only a minority of patients participate in exercise training programmes.

Several mechanisms are considered to be important mediators of a reduced cardiac event rate, including:

- improvement of endothelial function;
- reduced progression of coronary lesions;
- reduced thrombogenic risk;

- improvement of collateral coronary circulation; and
- improvement of autonomic sympathovagal balance.

In a large meta-analysis, exercise training as part of coronary rehabilitation programmes was associated with a 26% reduction in cardiac mortality rate in patients with coronary artery disease [177]. In addition to supervised physical exercise in patient groups, rehabilitation includes lifestyle advice and support as well as measures aimed at risk reduction. If patients prefer to perform the programme at home, they will need clear prescriptions, encouragement, and regular follow-up by their physician. In general, 30min of moderate intensity aerobic exercise at least five times per week is recommended. Each single-stage increase in physical work capacity is associated with a reduction in all-cause mortality risk in the range of 8–14%. It should also be appreciated that apart from its influence on mortality, exercise rehabilitation can have other beneficial effects. Exercise capacity, cardio-respiratory fitness, and perception of well-being have also been reported to improve, at least during the actual training period, even in elderly patients.

Behaviour change and management of behavioural risk factors

A number of specialized psychosocial intervention strategies have been demonstrated to have positive effects on risk factors, but the specific content and approaches taken by these interventions vary. Even if they intend to target only one behavioural risk factor, group-based behavioural interventions often contain elements which affect multiple risk factors. Interventions adding psychosocial and psychoeducational components to standard cardiological care can significantly improve quality of life and diminish cardiovascular risk factors [178, 179].

More importantly, a friendly and positive physician–patient interaction is a powerful tool to enhance patients' coping with stress and illness and adherence to recommended lifestyle change and medication. Social support provided by caregivers, including physicians, and shared decision making can help patients maintain healthy habits and adhere to medical advice.

Sexual activity and erectile dysfunction

Sexual intercourse may provoke anxiety, particularly for patients recovering after an acute MI. Studies have shown, however, that stable, optimally treated angina patients are not at greater cardiovascular risk during coitus [180] (see also ➲Chapter 15) Men with cardiovascular disease are more likely to have erectile dysfunction than the general population and may be prescribed agents such as sildenafil or tadalafil [181]. Interestingly, sildenafil appears to increase exercise duration and time to angina on treadmill testing [180]. As dramatic decreases in blood pressure may occur with administration of nitrates within 24 hours of taking sildenafil, their combination is contraindicated.

Interventions to improve outcome: pharmacological therapy

Pharmacological treatments to improve outcome in patients with stable IHD are summarized in ➲Fig. 17.23 and in ➲Table 17.12 (➲Chapter 11).

Managment of dyslipidemia

The relationship between a raised plasma cholesterol and cardiovascular diseases fulfils all of the criteria for causality. Indeed, the evidence that reducing plasma cholesterol reduces the risk of cardiovascular events is unequivocal. The higher the baseline risk, the greater the absolute benefit. A 10% reduction in plasma total cholesterol or a reduction of LDL cholesterol of 1mmol/L (40mg/dL) are associated with a 20–25% reduction in the rate of major coronary events [182]. Thus, reduction of serum cholesterol levels is increasingly recognized as essential for the prevention of cardiovascular events in patients with IHD. Dietary intervention is an important initial treatment in patients with elevated lipids, but only modest reductions (3–5%) in total cholesterol have been achieved in general population studies and they are insufficient to translate in a significant reduction of cardiovascular event rate. In contrast, treatment with 3-hydroxy-3-methylglutaryl coenzyme A (HMG-CoA) reductase inhibitors (statins) results in a robust reduction of LDL cholesterol levels which translates in a reduction of major cardiovascular events, like fatal and non-fatal MI, fatal and non-fatal stroke, and need for revascularization procedures, by about 30% [183]. Such findings support the view that statins stabilize lipid-rich atherosclerotic plaques of mild to moderate severity, and therefore make them less vulnerable to become unstable [184]. No trial has been performed specifically in patients with stable angina pectoris; nevertheless, patients with stable ischaemic disease represent a sizeable proportion in some of the major statin trials carried out in patients with known cardiovascular diseases. Key trials of statins in secondary prevention are summarized in ➲Table 17.13.

The most recent controversy on lipid-lowering treatment has been focused on intensive, versus standard lipid-lowering therapy. A recent meta-analysis of trials that compared different intensities of statin therapy identified a total of seven randomized controlled trials, with a total of 29,395 patients with coronary artery disease. Compared with less intensive

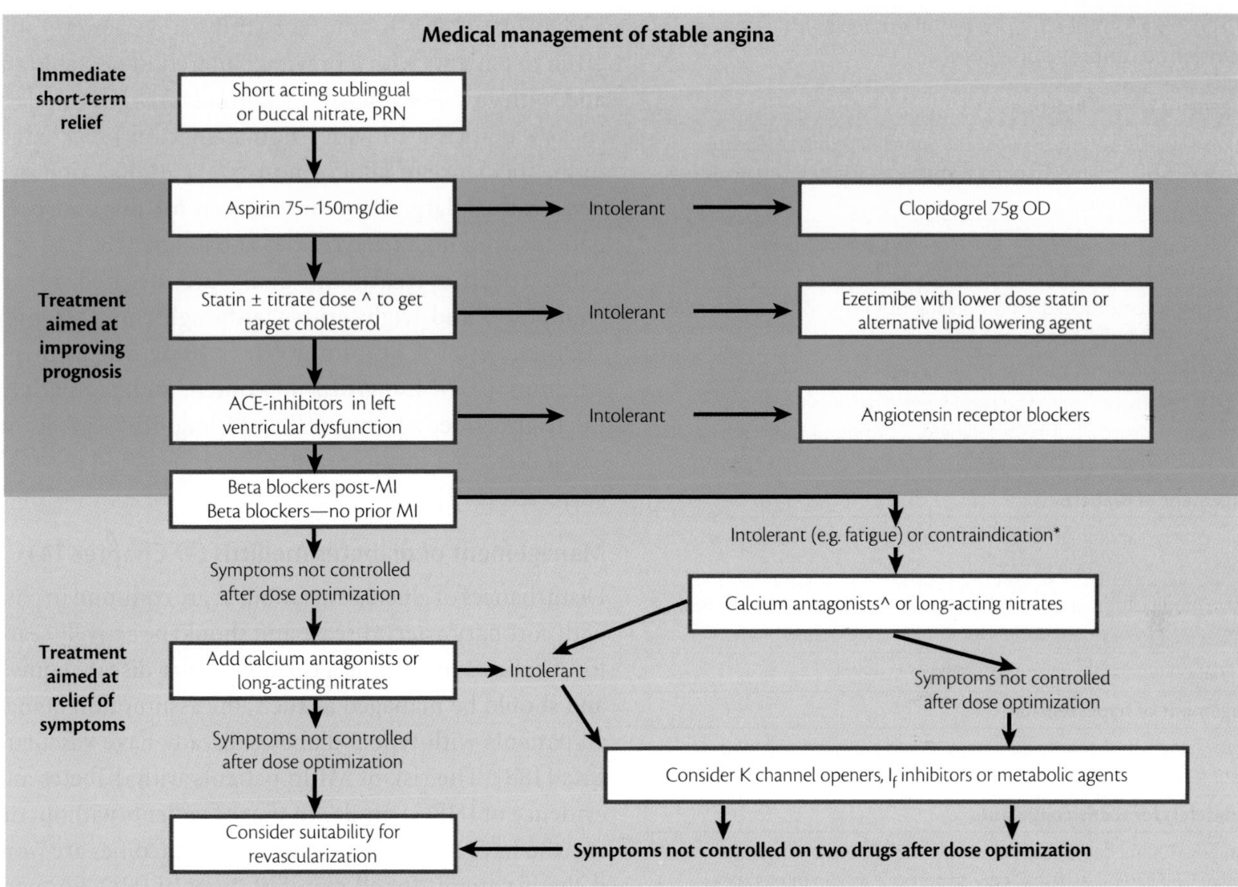

Figure 17.23 Algorithm for pharmacological treatment of stable angina. Treatment needed to improve prognosis are different of those needed to improve symptoms. *Relative contraindications to beta-blockade include asthma, symptomatic peripheral vascular disease and first-degree heart block. ^Avoid short-acting dihydropyridine formulations when not combined with a beta-blocker.

statin regimens, more intensive regimens further reduced the risk of MI (OR 0.85, 95% CI 0.77–0.93), stroke (OR 0.82, 95% CI 0.71–0.95), and coronary mortality (OR 0.84, 95% CI 0.71–0.98), although they failed to reduce total mortality (➲Fig. 17.24) [185].

Thus, statin therapy should always be given to patients with stable angina with the aim to achieve the following targets: for total cholesterol, 175mg/dL (4.5mmol/L) or even les [155mg/dL (4.0mmol/L)] if feasible; for LDL cholesterol, 100mg/dL (2.5mmol/L) or even less [80mg/dL (2.0mmol/L)] if feasible [172]. Therapy should utilize statin dosages documented to reduce morbidity/mortality in clinical trials. Because statins are prescribed on a long-term basis, possible interactions with other drugs (e.g. cyclosporin, macrolides, azole antifungals, calcium antagonists, protease inhibitors, sildenafil, warfarin, digoxin, nicotinic acid, and, in particular, fibrate) deserve particular attention.

Statin treatment is associated with few side-effects, but skeletal muscle damage (symptoms, CK elevations and, rarely, rhabdomyolysis) may occur, and liver enzymes should also be monitored after initiation of therapy. The increased efficacy of high-dose atorvastatin treatment is associated with a higher risk of enzymatic signs of liver damage, but no discernible increase in myalgia or rhabdomyolyisis.

If statins are poorly tolerated at high doses, or lipid control is not achieved with the highest statin dose, reduction of the statin dose and the addition of the cholesterol absorption inhibitor, ezetimibe, may afford adequate reduction of cholesterol levels. Effects on morbidity and mortality of such combination treatment, however, have not been documented yet. Other lipid lowering drugs, like fibrates, extended release nicotinic acid and their combinations with statins may be indicated to control the lipid levels among patients with severe dyslipidaemia. This is especially true for those with low HDL-cholesterol levels and high triglyceride levels. Adjunctive therapy to statins may be considered on an individualised basis in patients who have severe dyslipidaemia and remain at high risk after conventional measures.

Other lipid-lowering therapy may be warranted also in patients who do not tolerate or have contraindications to statins. In a study patients with HDL cholesterol

Table 17.12 Recommendations for pharmacological interventions to improve prognosis

Management of dyslipidemia
Statins in all patients, in the absence of contraindications, irrespective of cholesterol levels, initiated as soon as possible to achieve LDL cholesterol <100mg/dL (2.5mmol/L)
Further reduction of LDL cholesterol to achieve <80mg/dL (2.0mmol/L) should be considered in high-risk patients
Lifestyle change emphasized if TG > 150mg/dL (1.7mmol/L) and/or HDL cholesterol <40mg/dL (1.0mmol/L)
Selective inhibitors of cholesterol absorption, fibrates, nicotinic acid, or omega-3 supplements should be considered in patients who do not tolerate statins, especially if TG > 150mg/dL (1.7mmol/L) and/or HDL cholesterol <40mg/ dL (1.0mmol/L)
Management of diabetes
Lifestyle changes and pharmacotherapy to achieve HbA1c <6.5%, if possible
Intensive modification of other risk factors (dyslipidaemia, hypertension, obesity)
Coordination with a physician specialized in diabetes
Management of hypertension
Lifestyle changes and pharmacotherapy to achieve systemic blood pressure <130/80 mmHg
Antiplatelets/oral anticoagulants
Aspirin (75–100mg daily) in all patients without contraindications (i.e. active GI bleeding, aspirin allergy or previous aspirin intolerance)
Clopidogrel (75mg daily) in all patients with contraindications to aspirin
Oral anticoagulant at INR 2–3 in patients who do not tolerate aspirin and clopidogrel
Oral anticoagulant at recommended INR when clinically indicated (e.g. atrial fibrillation, LV thrombus, mechanical valve) in addition to low-dose aspirin and/or clopidogrel*
Beta-blockers and calcium-channel blockers
Oral beta-blockers in all patients without contraindications with left ventricular dysfunction or prior myocardial infarction
Rate lowering calcium-channel blockers in patients with a previous myocardial infarction and without heart failure who do not tolerate beta-blockers
Angiotensin converting enzyme-inhibitors (ACE-I) and angiotensin receptor blockers (ARBs)
ACE-inhibitor therapy in all patients with coincident indications for ACE-inhibition, such as hypertension, LV dysfunction, prior MI, or diabetes
ARBs in patients who do not tolerate ACE-inhibitors

* If long-term oral anticoagulation is required, use of a bare metal stent rather than a drug-eluting stent will expose the patient to a shorter duration of triple therapy and hence a lower bleeding risk.

levels <40mg/dL (1.04mmol/L) but LDL cholesterol levels >140mg/dL (3.6mmol/L) and triglycerides >300mg/dL (7.7mmol/L), and with a previous infarction benefited from gemfibrozil, with a 24% reduction in the combined end-point of death from coronary artery disease, non-fatal MI, and stroke [186]. In another study, however, bezafibrate given to patients with a previous infarction or stable angina and with low [<45mg/dL (1.2mmol/L)] HDL cholesterol levels was associated with a non-significant 7.3% reduction in the incidence of fatal or non-fatal (re)infarction or sudden death. A larger benefit was seen for this end-point in patients with high triglycerides at baseline [187].

No specific treatment goals are defined for HDL cholesterol and triglycerides, although concentrations of HDL cholesterol (<1.0mmol/L (<40mg/dL) in men and <1.2mmol/L (<45mg/dL) in women, and, similarly, fasting triglycerides >1.7mmol/L (>150mg/dL), serve as markers of increased cardiovascular risk and should probably be corrected [172].

Management of diabetes mellitus (➲ Chapter 14)

Disturbances of glucose metabolism are common in patients with coronary artery disease and should be actively searched for. Diabetes mellitus is a cardiovascular disease equivalent and should be managed as such, the assumption being that all patients with type 2 diabetes already have vascular disease [188]. The risk of MI in patients with diabetes and no evidence of IHD is similar to that of patients without diabetes who have had a MI. Furthermore, outcomes are worse in diabetic patients for all manifestations of IHD. For patients with known coronary disease and diabetes, rates of death approach 75% over 10 years [189]. Risk of cardiovascular events is further amplified in patients with the metabolic syndrome, in whom insulin resistance is present as a key characteristic. Aggressive medical management directed at optimizing glucose and blood pressure control, correcting dyslipidaemia and inhibiting platelet function reduces the likelihood of adverse cardiovascular events.

In patients with established diabetes, the aim is to achieve HbA1c levels <6.5%, if feasible [172]. This usually calls for intensive modification of lifestyle (diet, physical activity, weight reduction) in addition to pharmacotherapy. Coordination with a physician specialized in diabetes is advisable. In patients with impaired glucose tolerance, only lifestyle changes are currently recommended.

Management of hypertension (➲ Chapter 13)

Hypertension contributes to all of the major cardiovascular disease outcomes, increasing risk, on average, two- to three-fold. IHD is the most lethal and common consequence. Hypertension is also the most consistently powerful predictor of stroke. The risk of a recurrent event in patients with IHD is significantly affected by blood pressure level. Meta-analysis of 61 prospective observational studies has shown that even a 2-mmHg decrease in systolic blood pressure can

Table 17.13 Major statin clinical event trials in secondary prevention

Trial and agent	Follow-up (years)	Baseline LDL-C, mg/dL (mmol/L)	Changes in lipids	Primary end-point	Statin	Placebo	RRR	ARR*	NNT	Other clinical effects
4S Simvastatin 20–40mg/day	5.4	188 (4.9)	LDL-C ↓35% HDL-C ↑8% TG ↓10%	All-cause mortality	182/2221 (8.2%)	256/2223 (11.5%)	30% (*P* <0.001)	3.3%	30	CABG or PTCA ↓37% (*P* <0.001)
				Non-fatal MI, CHD death or resuscitated cardiac arrest (secondary)	431/2221 (19.4%)	622/2223 (28%)	34% (*P* <0.001)	8.6%	12	Post hoc: stroke or TIA ↓ 30% (*P* = 0.024)
CARE Pravastatin 40mg/day	5	139 (3.6)	LDL-C ↓32% HDL-C (5%† TG (14%	Non-fatal MI or CHD Death		274/2078 (13.2%)	24% (*P* = 0.003)	3.0%	33	No-excess non-CVD death CABG or PTCA ↓ 27% (*P* <0.001) Stroke ↓ 31% (*P* = 0.03)
LIPID Pravastatin 40mg/day	6.1	150 (3.9) median	LDL-C ↓ 25%† HDL-C ↑ 5%† TG ↓ 11%†	Non-fatal MI or CHD Death	557/4512 (12.3%)	715/4502 (15.9%)	24% (*P* <0.001)	3.6%	28	Total mortality ↓ 22% (*P* <0.001) CABG or PTCA ↓ 20% (*P* = 0.001) Stroke ↓ 19% (*P* = 0.048)
HPS‡ Simvastatin 40mg/day	5	131 (3.4)	LDL-C ↓ 29%† HDL-C ↑ 3%† TG ↓ 14%†	All-cause mortality	1328/ 10 269 (12.9%)	1507/ 10 267 (14.7%)	13% (*P* <0.001)	1.8%	56	Revascularization procedures ↓ 24% (*P* <0.001)
				Fatal or non-fatal vascular events	2033/ 10 269 (19.8%)	2585/ 10 267 (25.2%)	24% (*P* = 0.001)	5.4%	19	Stroke ↓ 25% (*P* <0.001)

* ARR was calculated as the placebo event rate minus the statin event rate. † Percentage average difference between statin and placebo. ‡ The HPS enrolled many types of high-risk patient, 35% of whom had not experienced a prior coronary event.

ARR, absolute risk reduction; CABG, coronary artery bypass graft; CARE, Cholesterol and Recurrent Events; CHD, coronary heart disease; CVD, cardiovascular disease; HDL-C, high-density lipoprotein cholesterol; HPS, Heart Protection Study; LDL-C, low-density lipoprotein cholesterol; LIPID, Long-Term Intervention with Pravastatin in Ischaemic Disease; MI, myocardial infarction; NNT, number needed to treat; PTCA, percutaneous transluminal coronary angioplasty; RRR, relative risk reduction; TG, triglycerides; TIA, transient ischaemic attack.

Data from Gotto AM, Amarenco P, Assman G, *et al. Dyslipedemia and Coronary Heart Disease*, 3rd edn, 2003. New York: International Lipid Information Bureau.

produce a 7% reduction in the risk of IHD mortality and a 10% reduction in risk of stroke mortality [190].

Treatment with any commonly used blood pressure-lowering regimen (beta-blockers, calcium-channel blockers, angiotensin converting enzyme (ACE)-inhibitors, angiotensin receptor blockers (ARBs) alpha blockers and diuretics) reduces the risk of total cardiovascular events, larger reductions in blood pressure producing larger reductions in risk. Choice of blood pressure-lowering agents, alone and in combination, is reviewed in recent guidelines. The goal is to achieve a blood pressure <130/80mmHg. Lifestyle modifications, in particular with respect to physical activity and weight loss will help pharmacological therapy to achieve these goals [172].

Antiplatelet agents

Low-dose aspirin

Aspirin is the prototypical platelet antagonist and has been available since the end of the nineteenth century. Aspirin was the first drug recognized to have important platelet-inhibitory effects. Its major antithrombotic effect is to irreversibly inhibit platelet thromboxane A2 synthesis, which has pro-aggregatory and vasoconstrictive properties. The inhibition is normally complete with chronic dosing

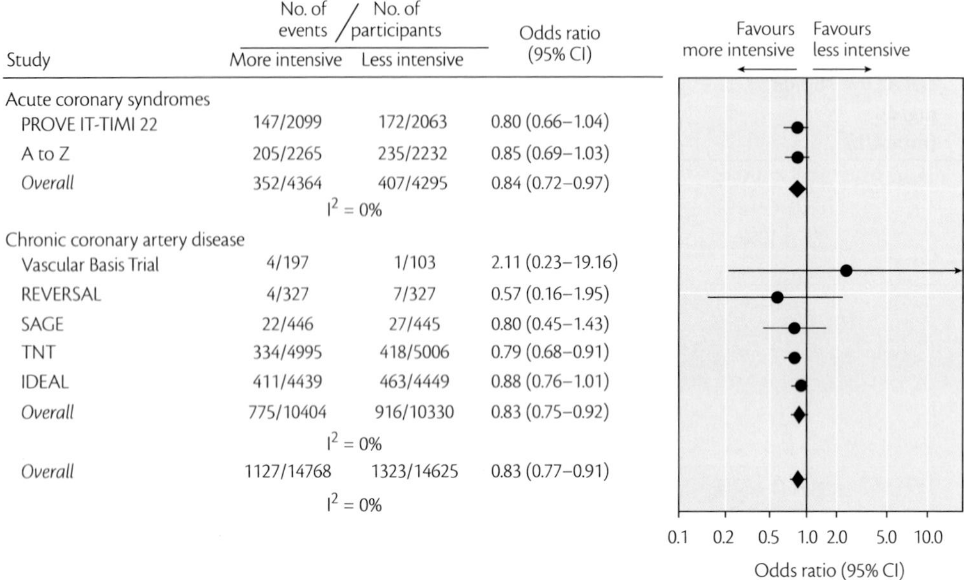

Study
No. of events / No. of participants
More intensive
Less intensive
Odds ratio (95% CI)
Favours more intensive
Favours less intensive
Acute coronary syndromes
PROVE IT-TIMI 22 147/2099 172/2063 0.80 (0.66–1.04)
A to Z 205/2265 235/2232 0.85 (0.69–1.03)
Overall 352/4364 407/4295 0.84 (0.72–0.97)
I2 = 0%
Chronic coronary artery disease
Vascular Basis Trial 4/197 1/103 2.11 (0.23–19.16)
REVERSAL 4/327 7/327 0.57 (0.16–1.95)
SAGE 22/446 27/445 0.80 (0.45–1.43)
TNT 334/4995 418/5006 0.79 (0.68–0.91)
IDEAL 411/4439 463/4449 0.88 (0.76–1.01)
Overall 775/10404 916/10330 0.83 (0.75–0.92)
I2 = 0%
Overall 1127/14768 1323/14625 0.83 (0.77–0.91)
I2 = 0%
0.1 0.2 0.5 1.0 2.0 5.0 10.0
Odds ratio (95% CI)

Figure 17.24 Meta-analysis of randomized trials that compared statin regimens of different intensities in adults with coronary artery disease. Risk of myocardial infarction or coronary death was significantly lower in patients randomized to more intensive statin treatment. Adapted with permission from Josan K, Majumdar SR, McAlister FA. The efficacy and safety of intensive statin therapy: a meta-analysis of randomized trials. *CMAJ* 2008; **178**: 576–84.

>75mg/day [191]. Aspirin's antiplatelet effects last for the life of the platelet (9–10 days). Aspirin is a mainstay in the treatment and prevention of vascular events.

The efficacy of aspirin has been clearly demonstrated in the Antithrombotic Trialists' Collaboration meta-analysis [192]. Thus, aspirin should always be given to patients with stable angina [193]. The ability to prevent platelet aggregation is the fundamental mode of action of aspirin, but additional favourable effects may reside in its ability to reduce haemostatic and inflammatory markers. High-risk patients derive the most benefit from aspirin, with a proportional risk reduction in serious vascular events of 46% in those with unstable angina and 33% among those with stable angina [192]. The benefits were clearly demonstrated in the SAPAT (The Swedish Angina Pectoris Aspirin Trial) trial. This randomized double-blind trial compared aspirin 75mg/day and placebo with concomitant treatment of sotalol (mean 160mg/day) in >2000 patients with stable angina over a mean period of 50 months. Compared with sotalol and placebo, the aspirin plus sotalol group had a 34% reduction in MI and sudden death. There was also a significant 22–32% reduction in vascular events, vascular death, stroke and total mortality in the aspirin group [194].

The optimal antithrombotic dosage of aspirin appears to be 75–150mg/day, as the relative risk reduction afforded by aspirin might decrease below this dose range. The relative risk of suffering an intracranial haemorrhage with aspirin treatment at doses >75mg/day increases by 30%, but the absolute risk of such complications is less than 1 per 1000 patient years [195]. Furthermore, in patients with atherosclerotic vascular disease, where the main aetiology of stroke is ischaemic, the net effect of aspirin treatment on stroke incidence is clearly beneficial. There is no evidence for a dose dependence of the risk of intracranial bleeding with aspirin in the therapeutically effective dose range. In contrast, gastrointestinal side-effects of aspirin increase at higher doses [196].

Thus, the dosage of aspirin should be the lowest effective one in order to optimize the balance between therapeutic gains and gastrointestinal side-effects during chronic therapy. In cases of mucosal erosions due to aspirin therapy, these may be alleviated by inhibiting gastric acid secretion. Eradication of *Helicobacter pylori* infection, if present, also reduces the risk of aspirin related gastrointestinal bleeding. A recent study showed that the addition of esomeprazole to aspirin (80mg/day) was better than switching to clopidogrel for the prevention of recurrent ulcer bleeding in patients with ulcers and vascular disease [197].

Possible problems related to 'aspirin resistance' are of considerable interest but in the absence of clear conclusions from this area of research and of a 'gold standard' test for assessment of aspirin resistance, further information is needed before management schemes can be implemented [198].

Clopidogrel

Clopidogrel and ticlopidine are thienopyridines that act as non-competitive ADP receptor antagonists and have antithrombotic effects similar to aspirin. Ticlopidine has been replaced by clopidogrel due to its risk of neutropenia and thrombocytpenia and the occurrence of more symptomatic side-effects. The main study documenting clopidogrel use in stable IHD is the CAPRIE (Clopidogrel vs. Aspirin in Patients at Risk of Ischaemic Events) trial, which included three equally large groups of patients with previous MI, previous stroke or peripheral arterial disease. Compared with aspirin 325mg/day, clopidogrel 75mg/day was slightly more effective (absolute risk reduction 0.51% per year; P <0.043) in preventing cardiovascular complications in high risk patients. When comparing outcomes in the three subgroups of patients enrolled in the CAPRIE trial the benefit with clopidogrel appeared in the subgroup with peripheral vascular disease only. Gastrointestinal haemorrhage was only slightly less common with clopidogrel when compared with aspirin treatment (1.99 versus 2.66% during 1.9 years of treatment), despite the relatively high dose of aspirin [199]. Clopidogrel is much more expensive than aspirin and should be given in patients intolerant to aspirin [193]. After coronary stenting or an acute coronary syndrome clopidogrel may be combined with aspirin during a finite period of time, but combination therapy is currently not warranted in stable angina pectoris not undergoing stent implantation [193].

One much discussed reason for variability of antiplatelet response to clopidogrel is pharmacological interaction with some statins, as clopidogrel forms its active metabolite(s) via CYP3A4 mediated metabolism, the activity of which can be influenced by statins; however, data are inconsistent. Notably, observational post-hoc analyses of outcomes among patients receiving maintenance treatment doses of clopidogrel and a potentially interacting statin have not shown differences in clinical outcome. On the other hand, there are no properly designed prospective studies aimed at addressing this issue [200].

Oral anticoagulants

Oral anticoagulants are not indicated in stable angina patients. They can be added to aspirin when needed for other reasons (for instance in patients with atrial fibrillation, cardiac prosthetic valves or pulmonary thromboembolism). In a large meta-analysis of patients with acute coronary syndromes followed for up to 5 years, the combination of aspirin and oral anticoagulation (with INR target of 2–3) caused one major bleed only per 100 patients treated compared with aspirin alone [201]. In some patients (e.g. stent placement in presence of atrial fibrillation) there is an indication for dual antiplatelet therapy and oral anticoagulation. However, there are no prospective trials assessing the risk/benefit ratio of triple antithrombotic therapy in such stable patients. Thus, in the absence of prospective randomized studies, no firm recommendation can be given. Triple therapy, however, seems to have an acceptable risk/benefit ratio provided that clopidogrel co-therapy is kept short and the bleeding risk is low [202].

Beta-blockers

Pharmacological properties of beta-blockers are summarized in ➲Table 17.14. Studies carried out in post-MI patients in the thrombolytic era established that the risk of suffering cardiovascular death or MI was reduced by beta-blockers [203]. A meta-regression analysis of the effects of different beta-blockers on mortality found non-significant benefits of acute treatment, but a significant 24% relative reduction of mortality with long-term secondary preventive treatment [204]. Most evidence is available for propranolol, timolol, and metoprolol, and it cannot be assumed that prognostic benefit will be achieved with other agents.

Beta-blockers are also an important treatment for several supraventricular and ventricular tachyarrhythmias and, in particular, for heart failure where their use is associated to a remarkable reduction in mortality. Yet, there are no large long-term studies assessing their effect on mortality in patients with stable angina. It can be extrapolated from the post-MI trials that beta-blockers may be cardioprotective also in patients with stable IHD. However, this has not been proven in a placebo-controlled trial. Furthermore, post-MI beta-blocker trials were performed before the implementation of other secondary preventive therapy, such as treatment with statins and ACE-inhibitors, thus leaving some uncertainty regarding their prognostic efficacy on top of a 'modern' treatment strategy. Notably, large beta-blocker trials in patients with stable angina did not show a significant difference in outcome between patients treated with beta-blockers or calcium-channel blockers, either nifedipine or verapamil [205,206]. A smaller study compared atenolol and placebo treatment and showed a lower rate of a combined endpoint, which included symptoms requiring treatment, in the atenolol group [207]. This study confirmed the anti-anginal effects of beta-blockers, but it failed to show beneficial effect on prognosis of patients with stable angina pectoris. Beta-1 blockade by metoprolol and bisoprolol, and the nonselective beta-blocker carvedilol, that also blocks alpha-1 receptors, have been shown to effectively reduce cardiac events in patients with congestive heart failure [208].

Thus, there is evidence of prognostic benefit from the use of beta-blockers in patients with stable angina who have suffered prior MI or have heart failure.

Table 17.14 Properties of beta-blockers

Drug	ISA	Cardioselective	Lipophilia	Plasma half-life (hours)	Dosage
Acebutolol	+	Yes	++	3–4	200–600mg BID
Atenolol	–	Yes	–	6–9	50–100mg OD
Betaxolol	–	Yes	++	14–22	5–20mg OD
Bisoprolol	–	Yes	+	13–14	5–20mg OD
Carvedilol*	–	No	++	6–7	3.125–50mg BID
Labetalol*	–	No	+++	3–4	100–400mg BID
Metoprolol	–	Yes	++	3–7	50–100mg BID–QID/ 50–400mg OD
Nadolol	–	No	+	20–24	40–80mg OD
Nebivolol	–	Yes	++	21	5mg OD
Oxprenolol	+	No	++	1–3	80mg BID
Pindolol	++	No	++	3–4	10–40mg/die (BID–TID)
Propranolol	–	No	+++	3–5	80–320mg/die (BID–TID) 80–160mg OD
Sotalol	–	No	–	9–10	80–160mg BID
Timolol	–	No	++	4	10–30mg BID

* Labetalol and carvedilol have additional α_2-blocking p-roperties.

ISA, intrinsic sympathomimetic activity

Calcium-channel blockers

Cardiovascular effects of calcium-channel blockers are summarized in Table 17.15. Heart rate lowering calcium-channel blockers may improve the prognosis of post-MI patients, as shown in the DAVIT (The Danish Verapamil Infarction Trial) II study for verapamil [209]. Similarly, diltiazem was found to improve prognosis in a subgroup analysis of post-MI patients without signs of heart failure in the MDPIT (The Multicenter Diltiazem Postinfarction Trial) study [210]. Furthermore, the INTERCEPT (Incomplete Infarction Trial of European Research Collaborators Evaluating Prognosis post-Thrombolysis) trial showed the safety, and to some degree the benefit, of diltiazem in patients with acute MI but without heart failure, who had received thrombolysis. Diltiazem was associated with a decrease in the combined event rate of non-fatal MI and refractory ischaemia [211]. The INVEST (International Verapamil SR-Trandolapril) trial examined mortality and morbidity outcomes in hypertensive patients with IHD by comparing a combined calcium channel inhibitor and ACE inhibitor strategy (verapamil–trandolapil) with a non-calcium antagonist treatment strategy (atenolol-hydrochlorothiazide) and showed both strategies to be equally effective [212]. Although verapamil and diltiazem have not been studied in an outcome trial in chronic stable angina, the above trials and other supplementary findings suggest that both drugs have a useful role, in this population, in the absence of heart failure.

Table 17.15 Properties of calcium-antagonists

	Diltiazem	Verapamil	Nifedipine	Amlodipine	Nicardipina	Felodipina
Heart rate	↓	↓	↔	↔	↔	↔
AV node conduction	↓	↓	↔	↔	↔	↔
Myocardial contractility	↓↓	↓↓↓	↔	↔	↔	↔
Peripheral vasodilatation	↑	↑	↑↑	↑↑	↑↑	↑↑
Myocardial oxygen demand	↓↓	↓↓	↓	↓	↓	↓
Dosage	60–120mg TID	80–120 TID	20–30mg BID*	5–10mg OD	20mg TID	5–10mg OD

AV, atrioventricular; ↑, increase; ↓, decrease; ↔, unchanged.

* Slow release forms.

In contrast, older trials of short-acting nifedipine showed no benefit on hard endpoints among patients with IHD, and even an increased risk of dying with high doses of the drug. The latter findings sparked an intense 'calcium antagonist debate' which pointed out the inappropriateness of treatment with short-acting vasodilator drugs such as dihydropyridine calcium-channel blockers in IHD patients. A meta-analysis of the safety of nifedipine in stable angina pectoris suggested, however, that the drug is safe. The recently published ACTION (A Coronary disease Trial Investigating Outcome with Nifedipine) trial, which compared treatment with long-acting nifedipine and placebo in patients with stable angina pectoris showed no benefit from treatment with regard to composite endpoints including death, MI, refractory angina, debilitating stroke and heart failure. Nifedipine treatment tended to increase the need for peripheral revascularization, but it reduced the need for coronary bypass surgery [213]. The authors concluded that nifedipine treatment is safe and reduces the need for coronary interventions. However, nifedipine did not affect hard endpoints. The CAMELOT (Comparison of Amlodipine versus Enalapril to Limit Occurrences of Thrombosis) study compared treatment with amlodipine, enalapril or placebo in patients with stable IHD and normal blood pressure during 2 years of follow-up. Amlodipine and enalapril treatment lowered blood pressure equally and tended to reduce the incidence of 'hard' endpoints similarly as compared with placebo, but these differences were not significant [214].

Thus, there is no evidence to support the use of calcium-channel blockers for prognostic reasons in uncomplicated stable angina, although heart rate lowering calcium-channel blockers may be used as an alternative to beta-blockers in post MI patients without heart failure who do not tolerate beta-blockers.

Angiotensin-converting enzyme-inhibitors

ACE-inhibitors have been available for over 20 years, initially for hypertension and then for treatment of heart failure. ACE-inhibitors prevent vasoconstriction by inhibiting the production of the vasoactive octapeptide angiotensin II from the decapeptide angiotensin I. This inhibition results in vasodilatation due to lowering of systemic vascular resistance and natriuresis from inhibition of aldosterone secretion. Inhibition of angiotensin II may also reduce sympathetic tone. Finally, ACE-inhibitors cause the inhibition of bradykinin degradation, which can contribute to their vasodilator effects. ACE-inhibitors are well established for the treatment of hypertension and heart failure (also in the absence of symptoms). These drugs are generally well tolerated. The most frequent adverse effect is a dry cough, in up to 20% of individuals. Angio-oedema is a comparatively rare but more serious adverse effect.

The clinical evidence of reductions in MI and cardiac mortality in trials of ACE-inhibitors for heart failure and the experimental evidence that inhibition of the renin-angiotensin system has important effects on improving endothelial dysfunction [215], prompted trials assessing the potential beneficial effects of ACE-inhibitors on cardiovascular events in patients with IHD without heart failure. This working hypothesis was confirmed in the HOPE (Heart Outcomes Prevention Evaluation) trial [216], which was conducted in patients aged 55 years or more, at high risk of cardiovascular complications, as indicated by a high prevalence of diabetes, hypertension, stroke and peripheral vascular disease. The HOPE trial showed a significant 22% reduction in the composite end-point of MI, stroke or death from cardiovascular disease among the patients assigned to ramipril. The EUROPA (European trial On reduction of cardiac events with Perindopril in stable coronary Artery disease) trial, conducted in a 'broad-risk' population with documented stable IHD without left ventricular dysfunction [217], treated with aspirin, statins and beta-blockers, showed that perindopril treatment was associated with a 20% relative risk reduction in cardiovascular death, MI or cardiac arrest. The results of the HOPE and EUROPE trails, however, are in contrast with those of the PEACE (Prevention of Events with Angiotensin Converting Enzyme inhibition) trial, which compared the effects of the ACE-inhibitor trandolapril and placebo, added to current standard therapy, in patients with stable coronary artery disease and preserved left ventricular function [218]. The incidence of the primary end-point (cardiovascular death, MI or coronary revascularization) was almost identical for trandolapril and placebo.

Thus, it is appropriate to consider ACE-inhibitors for the treatment of patients with stable angina pectoris and co-existing hypertension, diabetes, heart failure, asymptomatic left ventricular dysfunction or previous MI. In angina patients without co-existing indications for ACE-inhibitor treatment the anticipated benefit of treatment (possible absolute risk reduction) should be weighed against costs and risks for side-effects, and the dose and agent used should be of proven efficacy for this indication. Patients who do not tolerate an ACE-inhibitor might be given an ARB, based on the recent results of the ONTARGET (Ongoing Telmisartan Alone and in Combination With Ramipril Global Endpoint Trial) trial [219].

Interventions to improve symptoms and myocardial ischaemia

Symptoms of angina pectoris and signs of myocardial ischaemia (including silent ischaemia) may be reduced by drugs that reduce myocardial oxygen demand and/or increase blood flow to the ischaemic area. Commonly used anti-anginal drugs are beta-blockers, calcium-channel blockers, and organic nitrates.

Anti-anginal drug treatment should be tailored to the needs of the individual patient, and should be monitored individually. Short acting nitrate therapy should be prescribed for immediate angina relief. Although different types of drugs have been shown to have additive anti-anginal effects in clinical trials, this may not necessarily be so in the individual patient. More intense anti-anginal treatment is also likely to cause more side effects. Thus, the dosing of one drug should be optimized before adding a second drug, and it is advisable to switch drug combinations before attempting a three drug regimen. Poor adherence is always a factor to consider when drug therapy is unsuccessful.

The sequence of use of anti-anginal drugs is outlined in the treatment algorithm shown in ➲Fig. 17.23.

Short-acting nitrates

Rapidly acting formulations of nitroglycerin provide effective symptom relief in connection with attacks of angina pectoris, and may be used for 'situational prophylaxis'. The pain relieving and anti-ischaemic effects are mainly related to venodilatation and reduced diastolic filling of the heart (reduced intracardiac pressure), which also favours subendocardial perfusion. Coronary vasodilatation may contribute. Nitroglycerin causes dose-dependent vasodilator side-effects, such as headache and flushing. Overdosing may cause postural hypotension and reflexogenic cardiac sympathetic activation with tachycardia, leading to 'paradoxical' angina. Thus, patients should be carefully instructed about how to use short-acting nitroglycerin. Short-acting nitrate consumption is a simple and good measure of treatment effects with other anti-anginal drugs. Angina that does not respond to short-acting nitroglycerin should be regarded as a possible MI or non cardiac pain. About a half of patients with microvascular angina are unresponsive to or have incomplete benefit from sublingual nitrates.

Long-acting nitrates

Long-acting nitrates are only for symptomatic relief of angina. There are no data showing that long-term treatment with nitrates reduces mortality or the incidence of MI in patients with stable angina [102]. Tolerance to continuous oral or transdermal nitrates develops rapidly and, in order to overcome this inconvenient, nitrate-free intervals or a modified delivery system designed to provide a period of low blood nitrate concentration have been recommended [220]. The worry about intermittent nitrate therapy is that rebound exacerbation of symptoms may occur. Nevertheless, the safety of long-term use of nitrates has been established. Adverse effects include headache and occasionally postural hypotension. Only about 10% of patients are non-responders to nitrate therapy and a further 10% experience adverse effects requiring withdrawal of therapy [221].

Also available in certain countries is molsidomine, a vasodilator with an action similar to organic nitrates (i.e. increases levels of nitric oxide) and which has antianginal activity similar to long-acting nitrates without causing tolerance.

Beta-blockers

Beta-blockers are effective in reducing anginal symptoms and myocardial ischaemia and should be considered first-line treatment for the relief of angina [193].

Beta-blockers reduce oxygen demand by reducing heart rate and contractility, and by reducing blood pressure. Perfusion of ischaemic areas may be improved by prolonging diastole (i.e. the perfusion time), and by 'reverse coronary steal' due to increased vascular resistance in non-ischaemic areas. Beta-1 selective agents are preferred due to advantages concerning side-effects and precautions, when compared with non-selective beta-blockers. Commonly used beta-1 blockers with good documentation as anti-anginal drugs are metoprolol, atenolol, and bisoprolol [222]. To achieve 24-hour efficacy a beta-1 blocker with a long half-life (e.g. bisoprolol) or a formulation providing an extended plasma concentration profile (e.g. metoprolol CR) may be used. The degree of beta blockade may be assessed by exercise testing. Clinical parameters for an adequate beta-blocking effect are heart rate at rest <60bpm and heart at peak exercise <110bpm.

Some beta-blockers (like acebutolol and pindolol) exhibit intrinsic sympathomimetic activity and have less effect on resting heart rate, as they not only block β-receptors but also stimulate them, depending on the prevailing level of sympathetic activity. These agents cause less bradycardia at rest but exert adequate effect on exercise heart rate, and may offer advantages to patients who also have peripheral arterial disease. However, they seem less effective in angina prophylaxis. Different beta-blockers may also have a different rate of unwanted metabolic effects. In the recently reported GEMINI (Glycemic Effects in Diabetes Mellitus: Carvedilol-Metoprolol Comparison in Hypertensives) trial [223], for example, carvedilol improved cardiovascular risk factors and stabilized glycaemic control, while worsening of glycaemic control was observed with metoprolol. Such findings highlight potentially important metabolic effects that exist between beta-blockers and which may have important consequences in patients with diabetes.

About 15–20% of patients will not tolerate long-term use of beta-blockers. Side-effects of beta-blockade include cold extremities and symptomatic bradycardia, both of which are related to cardiac inhibition, and increased respiratory symptoms in asthma and chronic obstructive pulmonary disease (less common with beta-1 selective agents). Beta-blockers may cause fatigue, but only 0.4% of patients in trials discontinued treatment for this reason. Similarly, depression was not increased among beta-blocker treated patients, and sexual dysfunction was only found in 5 per 1000 patient years of treatment (leading to discontinuation in 2/1000) [224]. Quality-of-life, which has been extensively studied in the treatment of hypertension, is well preserved with beta-blocker treatment of hypertensive patients but this has not been systematically studied in patients with stable angina [225].

Thus, all anginal patients who require regular symptomatic treatment should be treated, unless contraindicated, with a beta-blocker. It should be noted that sudden withdrawal of beta-blockers may occasionally result in rebound angina and an increase in cardiac events.

Calcium-channel blockers

Calcium-channel blockers are structurally and pharmacologically heterogeneous compounds that share a common property: they inhibit entry of calcium into cells resulting in smooth muscle relaxation associated with peripheral and coronary vasodilatation. All these agents are effective in improving angina [214, 226, 227]. There are two main classes of calcium-channel blockers: non-dihydropyridines (e.g. verapamil and diltiazem) and dihydropyridines (e.g. nifedipine, amlodipine). Non dihydropyridines or heart rate lowering calcium-channel blockers reduce myocardial contractility, heart rate and A-V nodal conduction. Dihydropyridine also may cause some cardiodepression, but this is counteracted by reflexogenic cardiac sympathetic activation with slight increases in heart rate which usually, but not always, subside over time. Long-acting calcium-channel blockers (e.g. amlodipine) or sustained release formulations of short-acting compounds (e.g. nifedipine, felodipine, verapamil and diltiazem) are preferred, to minimize fluctuations of plasma concentrations and cardiovascular effects. Side-effects are also concentration-dependent, and mainly related to the arterial vasodilator responses (headache, flushing and ankle oedema); these effects are more pronounced with dihydropyridines. Verapamil and diltiazem may cause constipation.

The anti-anginal and anti-ischaemic effects of calcium-channel blockers may be additive to those of beta-blockers. Dihydropyridines are more suitable for combination with beta-blockers, which counteract the reflexogenic cardiac sympathetic activation. Non dihydropiridine calcium-channel blockers may cause conduction disturbances in susceptible patients treated with beta-blockers. All calcium-channel blockers may worsen heart failure. Attempts to use dihydropyridines for vasodilator treatment of heart failure have not been successful.

The principal adverse effect is ankle oedema, which is observed more frequently with dihydropiridines. Diltiazem may cause bradycardia, while constipation and flushing are sometimes seen with verapamil, which can also cause significant depression of myocardial contractility, requiring caution when used with beta-blockade.

In conclusion, calcium-channel blockers are effective anti-anginal drugs and can be used in addition to beta-blockers in patients who do not have good symptomatic control with beta-blockers only [102]. Combination of non dihydropyridine calcium-channel blockers and beta-blockers needs careful monitoring because can result in excessive bradycardia, which is not observed instead with dihydropyridines.

Comparison of beta-blockers and calcium-channel blockers treatment

Several studies compared the anti-anginal and anti-ischaemic effects of beta-blockers and calcium-channel blockers with variable results. The IMAGE (International Multicenter Angina Exercise) trial compared patients with stable angina treated with metoprolol or nifedipine [228]. Both drugs prolonged exercise tolerance over baseline levels, with greater improvement in patients receiving metoprolol. Responses to the two drugs, however, were variable and difficult to predict. In the APSIS (the Angina Prognosis Study In Stockholm) trial, verapamil was slightly more effective than metoprolol in increasing exercise tolerance [229]. The TIBBS (Total Ischemic Burden Bisoprolol Study) trial showed anti-ischaemic and anti-anginal effects of both bisoprolol and nifedipine, but bisoprolol was more effective [230]. The TIBET (Total Ischaemic Burden European Trial) trial compared the effects of atenolol, nifedipine or their combination on exercise-induced ischaemia and on total ischaemic burden [231]. Both medications, alone and in combination, caused significant improvements in exercise parameters and significant reductions in ischaemic activity during daily activities when compared with placebo but there were no significant differences between groups for any of the measured ischaemic parameters. There were significantly more withdrawals due to side effects in the nifedipine group when compared with the atenolol and the combination groups. Finally, a comprehensive meta-analysis showed that in stable angina beta-blockers are more effective than calcium-channel blockers in reducing anginal episodes, although the effects on exercise tolerance and ischaemia of the two drug classes are similar [232].

Thus, in the absence of prior MI, the available data suggest that the choice between a beta-blocker and calcium-channel blockers for anti-anginal treatment may be guided by individual tolerance and by the presence of other diseases and co-treatment. If these factors are equally weighted a beta-blocker is preferable as the first choice.

Comparison of nitrates with beta-blockers or calcium-channel blockers

There are relatively few studies comparing anti-anginal and anti-ischaemic effects of long-acting nitrates with beta-blockers or calcium-channel blockers, and there is no documentation concerning possible effects of nitrates on morbidity in stable angina pectoris. A meta-analysis found a non-significant trend towards less nitroglycerin use with beta-blockers, and fewer angina episodes per week with calcium-channel blockers compared with long-acting nitrates [232].

Thus, long-acting nitrates have no overall therapeutic advantages over beta-blockers or calcium-channel blockers.

Other antianginal drugs

New anti-anginal drugs include nicorandil, ivabradine, trimetazidine, and ranolazine. They can be used in symptomatic patients who do not tolerate beta-blockers or calcium-antagonists. They can also be used in patients who need combination treatment, but are intolerant to the combination of traditional anti-anginal drugs (beta-blockers, calcium-channel blocker, and long-acting nitrates).

Nicorandil

Adenosine triphosphate-sensitive potassium channels are ubiquitous in the heart and blood vessels and are important modulators of cardiovascular function. Nicorandil is a hybrid compound that comprises a potassium channel opener and a nitrate moiety [233]. Nicorandil has a dual mechanism of action on both preload and afterload, producing a dose-related improvement in haemodynamics. Angiographic studies have shown that the drug dilates both stenotic and non-stenotic coronary arteries and it is indicated for prophylaxis and treatment of angina, normally at a dose of 20mg twice daily. Nicorandil may mimic ischaemic preconditioning, which is a powerful protection mechanism against myocardial necrosis. Unlike classical nitrates there appears to be no haemodynamic tolerance to nicorandil. The IONA (Impact Of Nicorandil in Angina) trial has shown a significant early reduction of major coronary events in stable anginal patients treated with nicorandil when compared with placebo as add-on to conventional therapy. The result was driven by effects of nicorandil on 'hospital admission for cardiac chest pain', thus suggesting that it may be used in addition to conventional anti-anginal drugs [234], while the prognostic advantage was lost at follow-up. Headache is the most common side effect, usually occurring early on commencement of treatment and disappearing with chronic dosing.

Ivabradine

A high resting heart rate is associated with an increased risk of mortality and major cardiovascular events [235]. Drugs that lower heart rate, such as beta-blockers, have been shown to reduce the risk of sudden death and re-infarction in patients with IHD. Beta-blockers also play an important role in prevention of anginal attacks as described above. Because beta-blockers have haemodynamic effects other than lowering of heart rate and blood pressure (e.g. they are negatively inotropic), they are not well tolerated by all patients. The question remains whether agents, like ivabradine, which have a pure bradycardic action without other haemodynamic effects might also have clinical benefits in angina [236]. Ivabradine specifically inhibits I_f, a primary pacemaker current, and does not induce significant prolongation of repolarization over the dose range of 2.5–10mg twice daily. A recent randomized controlled trial over a 4-month period showed that ivabradine produces dose-dependent improvements in exercise tolerance and time to ischaemia during exercise [237]. Furthermore, in the ASSOCIATE trial this drug, compared to placebo, was found to significantly increase all exercise test end-points at 4-month follow-up in patients taking atenolol (50mg/day) [238]. Interestingly, the association of atenolol and ivabradine was well tolerated. In particular, only 1.1% of patients had to withdraw treatment because of bradyarrhythmia. The main side effect is represented by mild visual disturbances, mainly with the highest dose of ivabradine, which resolve spontaneously or with drug cessation. These may be linked to the presence of retinal ion channels similar to those mediating I_f [237].

Trimetazidine

Trimetazidine, which is available in some European countries, is a metabolic agent that has no haemodynamic effects. It has been shown to preserve energy balance and prevent disturbance of ion haemostasis during ischaemia. Its specific mechanism of action is unknown but its anti-anginal effects are attributed to modulatory effects on intracellular calcium. Trimetazidine also stimulates glucose oxidation and acts as a partial fatty acid oxidation inhibitor. Antianginal efficacy has been established with immediate-release formulations of trimetazidine three times daily [239] and, more recently, with a modified-release formulation of trimetazidine 35mg daily. The most commonly reported adverse effects with clinical doses are fatigue/drowsiness.

Ranolazine

Ranolazine, a new anti-ischaemic drug, is a selective inhibitor of the late sodium current that has the potential to reduce intracellular sodium-dependent calcium overload and its detrimental effects on cardiomyocyte function. Benefits have been shown in the clinical trials CARISA (Combination Assessment of Ranolazine In Stable Angina) and ERICA (Efficacy of Ranolazine in Chronic Angina) [240, 241]. Ranolazine in the dose range of 500–1500mg twice daily or ranolazine sustained release in doses of 750–1000mg twice daily, increased exercise tolerance and reduced angina attacks and myocardial ischaemia, providing also symptomatic relief in addition to atenolol, amlodipine or diltiazem at standard doses, without any effect, however, on long-term survival. More recently, ranolazine, compared to placebo, significantly reduced recurrent ischaemia and improved exercise performance in the subgroup of patients with acute coronary syndrome who reported prior chronic angina enrolled in the MERLIN-TIMI (Metabolic Efficiency With Ranolazine for Less Ischemia in Non-ST Elevation Acute Coronary Syndromes) 36 trial, [243]. The most commonly reported adverse effects with ranolazine are constipation, dizziness, nausea and asthenia.

Drugs potentially dangerous in stable angina patients

Cyclooxygenase-2 inhibitors and non-steroid anti-inflammatory drugs

Cyclooxygenase (COX)-2 inhibition reduces endothelial production of prostacyclin, which exhibits vasodilatory and platelet inhibiting effects. Attenuation of prostacyclin formation may predispose to elevated blood pressure, accelerated atherogenesis, and thrombosis upon plaque rupture. The recent withdrawal of rofecoxib, a highly selective COX-2 inhibitor, was caused by findings of an increased risk of serious coronary events in a placebo-controlled trial of cancer prevention. An increased risk of suffering fatal or non-fatal MI was also found in a meta-analysis of other randomized trials with rofecoxib [244]. In addition, COX-2 inhibition increases the risk of suffering stroke, heart failure and hypertension. It is worth noting that a recent meta-analysis of randomized trials has shown that both COX-2 inhibitors and traditional non-steroidal anti-inflammatory drugs (NSAIDs) similarly increase the risk of thrombotic cardiovascular events [245] (➲Fig. 17.25). Thus, the use of COX-2 inhibitors and NSAIDs should be avoided in patients with stable angina pectoris. When their administration is strongly indicated for clinical reasons, treatment duration should be as short as possible and always combined with low-dose aspirin to assure effective platelet inhibition. In such circumstances diclofenac should be preferred because it does not interfere with the antiplatelet effects of aspirin.

Hormone replacement therapy

Epidemiological evidence suggested substantial cardiovascular benefits of postmenopausal use of hormone replacement therapy (HRT). More recently, however, properly designed prospective, double blind, placebo-controlled trials have shown that HRT is not associated with cardiovascular benefit or may even increase the risk of stroke [246]. New guidelines therefore do not encourage routine use of HRT for chronic conditions and current users have been advised to taper doses downwards towards discontinuation [193].

Chronic stable angina: myocardial revascularization

There are two well-established approaches to revascularization for treatment of chronic stable angina caused by coronary atherosclerosis: PCI and CABG surgery. As in the case of pharmacological therapy the potential objectives of revascularization are twofold, to improve survival or survival free of infarction, or to diminish or eradicate symptoms. Individual risk as well as symptomatic status of patients represent key factors in the decision-making process.

Coronary revascularization procedures should be considered when the annual cardiovascular mortality rate, based on clinical evaluation and non-invasive testing, is >2% (for instance in patients with low Duke score at treadmill exercise test or with large regions of ischaemia at stress imaging

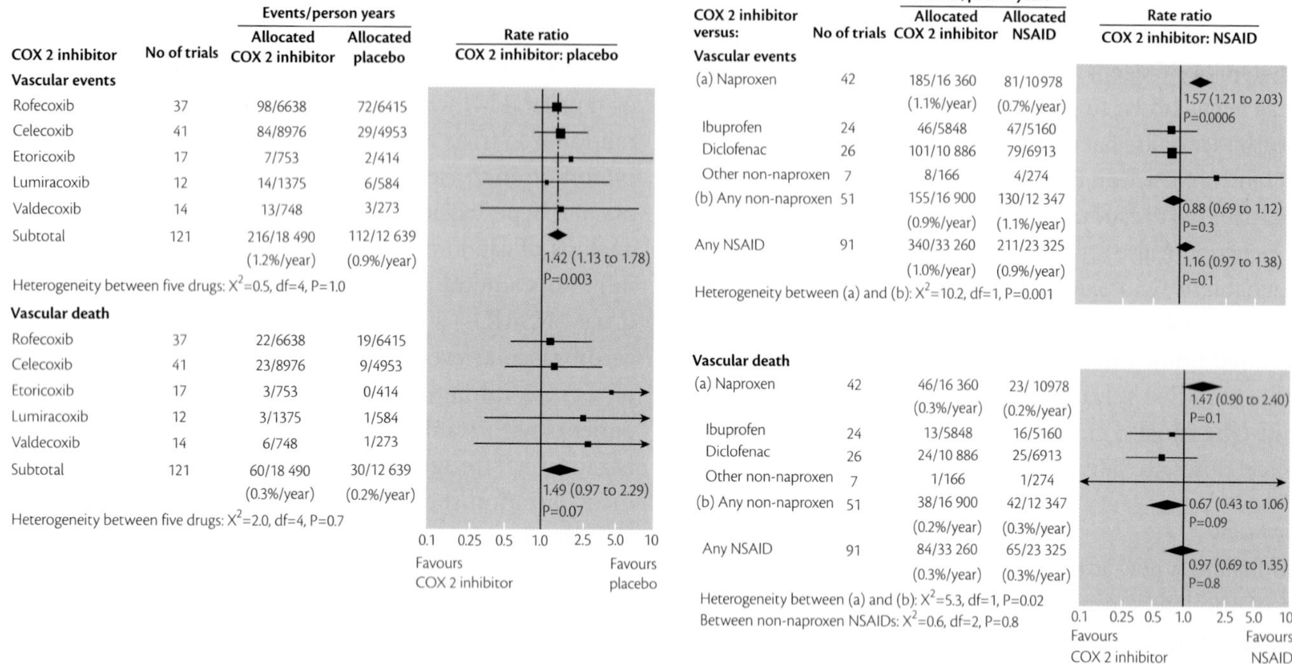

Figure 17.25 Meta-analysis of randomized trials that included a comparison of a selective COX 2 inhibitor versus placebo or a selective COX 2 inhibitor versus a traditional non-steroidal anti-inflammatory drugs (NSAIDs). Left: comparison of effects of different selective COX 2 inhibitors versus placebo on vascular events and vascular death. Event numbers and person years of exposure, with corresponding mean annual event rates in parenthesis, are presented for patients allocated to selective COX 2 inhibitor and placebo; COX 2 inhibitors significantly increase the risk of vascular events and vascular death compared to placebo by about 50%. Right: comparison of effects of selective COX 2 inhibitors versus NSAIDs on vascular events and vascular death; no difference is detectable between these two class with the exception of naproxen which is associated to a 57% lower risk of vascular events compared to COX 2 inhibitors Adapted with permission from Kearney PM, Baigent C, Godwin J, *et al.* Do selective cyclo-oxygenase-2 inhibitors and traditional non-steroidal anti-inflammatory drugs increase the risk of atherothrombosis? Meta-analysis of randomised trials. *BMJ* 2006; **332**: 1302–8.

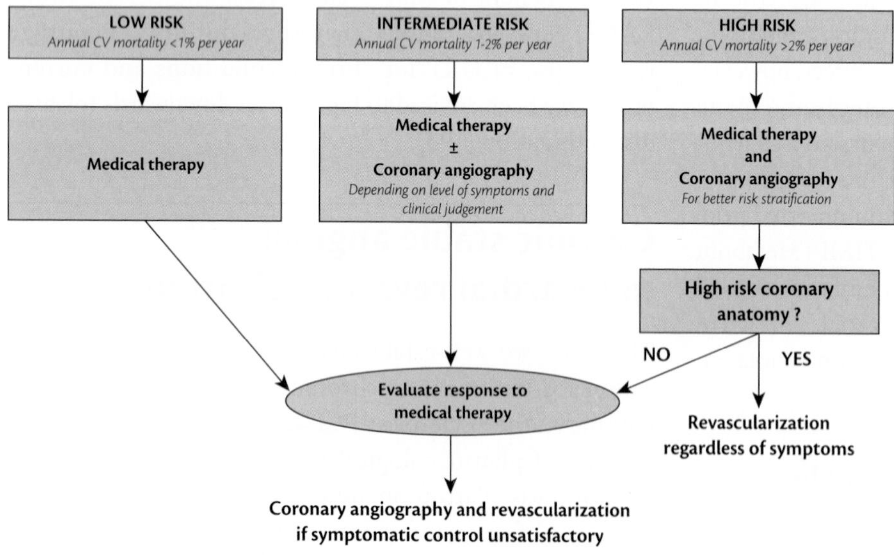

Figure 17.26 Flow chart summarizing the indications for myocardial revascularization based on clinical and no-invasive risk assessment. Risk of major cardiovascular events is mainly based on the measurement of left ventricular function and of amount of myocardium at risk of myocardial ischaemia as assessed in non-invasive testing. Adapted with permission from Fox K, Garcia MA, Ardissino D, *et al.* Guidelines on the management of stable angina pectoris: executive summary: The Task Force on the Management of Stable Angina Pectoris of the European Society of Cardiology. *Eur Heart J* **27**: 1341–81.

or with impaired left ventricular function, in particular if diabetics). In contrast, myocardial revascularization cannot be expected to improve the outcome, and therefore should not be considered for prognostic purposes, in patients at low risk with annual cardiovascular mortality <1%. In the presence of an intermediate risk the choice is difficult and should be carefully discussed with each individual patient, although in this setting diagnostic coronary angiography can add important prognostic information [102]. The algorithm in ➲Fig. 17.26 and ➲Table 17.16 outline recommendations for myocardial revascularization to improve prognosis in chronic stable angina.

Table 17.16 Recommendations for myocardial revascularization to improve prognosis

Evidence and/or general agreement that revascularization is beneficial
Significant left main stem disease or its equivalent (i.e. severe stenosis of ostial/proximal segment of left descending and circumflex coronary arteries)
Three-vessel disease with significant proximal stenoses: the survival benefit is greater in patients with abnormal left ventricular function or with extensive reversible ischaemia on non-invasive testing
Two-vessel disease with significant proximal LAD disease in patients with reversible ischaemia on non-invasive testing
Significant stenoses in patients with left ventricular dysfunction and a large area of viable myocardium
Conflicting evidence and/or a divergence of opinion that revascularization is beneficial, but weight of evidence/opinion is in favour
One- or two-vessel disease without significant proximal LAD coronary artery stenosis in patients who have survived sudden cardiac death or sustained ventricular tachycardia
Significant stenoses in patients with reversible ischaemia on non-invasive testing and evidence of frequent episodes of ischaemia during daily activities
Evidence or general agreement that revascularization is not useful/ effective and in some cases may be harmful
One or two vessel-disease without significant proximal LAD coronary artery stenosis in patients who have mild or no symptoms and have not received an adequate trial of medical therapy or have no demonstrable ischaemia or a limited area of ischaemia/viability only on non-invasive testing
Borderline (50–70%) coronary stenoses in locations other than left main stem and no demonstrable ischaemia on non-invasive testing
Non-significant (<50%) coronary stenoses
High risk of procedure-related morbidity or mortality unless the risk of the procedure is balanced by an expected significant improvement in survival or the patient's quality-of-life

LAD, left anterior descending.

Myocardial revascularization, however, is indicated, regardless of its effect on the outcome, in patients who remain symptomatic in spite of optimal medical treatment, if the operative risk is acceptable [102]. Both PCI and CABG are facing rapid development; thus the choice between these two approaches in the individual patient who needs myocardial revascularization may be difficult.

Percutaneous coronary interventions

Balloon angioplasty is aimed at restoring blood flow through stenotic coronary arteries by mechanical dilatation, i.e. inflation of a balloon catheter steered percutaneously to the narrowed site under fluoroscopic guidance. The procedure was introduced in 1977 by Grüntzig and has gained increasing clinical application since then [247]. In Europe, PCI is presently preferred over CABG in a ratio of 3:1 [248]. Following the availability of miniature and highly steerable guidewires, which have permitted access to virtually any branch of the epicardial coronary tree, the next decisive improvement resulted from the development and successful application of endovascular metallic scaffolds, called stents [249]. Stents are presently used in more than 80% of all PCI procedures. The stent implantation technique itself has been optimized by proper stent expansion and apposition against the wall, as learned from intravascular ultrasound imaging [250]. Stented angioplasty is superior to balloon angioplasty in technical success for the following reasons.

- Plaque fracture and dissection caused by balloon inflation often result in a pseudo-successful procedure while limited luminal enlargement is actually obtained.
- The dilated lesion shows greater stability after stenting, while abrupt closure within 48h following balloon treatment is not uncommon (up to 15% in the presence of severe residual dissection).
- The angiographic result obtainable after stenting is predictable irrespective of stenosis complexity.
- Follow-up studies show a lower restenosis rate with stent implantation.

Several randomized clinical trials support the above-mentioned statements, particularly the BENESTENT (BElgian NEtherlands Stent studies) family trials, which represent the foundations of the practice of PCI, at least in Europe. Other randomized clinical trials have shown that the benefits deriving from stent implantation are maintained up to 5 years after the initial procedure. In a meta-analysis of 29 trials involving 9918 patients, there was no evidence for a difference between routine coronary stenting and standard balloon angioplasty in terms of death or MI or the need for CABG surgery. However, coronary stenting reduced the rate of restenosis and the need for repeat PCI, findings confirmed in a further more recent meta-analysis [251, 252]. The risk of death associated with the procedure in routine angioplasty is 0.3–1%.

Despite the great improvement in technical success with stent implantation until fairly recently restenosis had remained the Achilles heel of PCI, still occurring in about 20–25% of cases.

Advances in the treatment and prevention of restenosis after percutaneous coronary interventions

Prior to the stent era, numerous mechanical and pharmacological approaches to the prevention of restenosis were tested and shown to be failures. Although a variety of devices have been developed to crack, break, stretch, scrape, shave or burn the atherosclerotic plaque, the durability of an initially successful procedure has been hindered by an incidence of angiographic restenosis within 6 months as high as 50%. This is because restenosis after balloon angioplasty or any other mechanical intervention, except stenting, is a complex wound healing process that results in exuberant neo-intimal proliferation as much as in constrictive remodelling of the vessel. Implantation of a metallic stent cage virtually eliminates vessel shrinkage and thereby significantly reduces clinical restenosis, i.e. the need for repeat intervention due to recurrent symptoms. At the same time, however, implantation of metallic stents exacerbates neo-intimal proliferation. Thus, particularly in small vessels, long lesions, saphenous vein graft disease and ostial lesions, stent implantation is followed by an angiographic restenosis rate above 30% [253]. Furthermore, restenosis inside a previously deployed metallic stent is difficult to treat; recurrence rates, indeed, range from 19–83% after any new intervention, albeit plain balloon angioplasty or a combined procedure involving plaque debulking [254]. This is particularly the case when diffuse or proliferative in-stent restenosis is present. Because in-stent restenosis has been shown to be almost exclusively due to neo-intimal proliferation, intracoronary irradiation was successfully applied, with either gamma or beta radiation. However, long-term results of brachytherapy have been plagued with exceedingly high rates of stent thrombosis and late vessel occlusion, presumably due to delayed re-endothelialization [255]. Vascular brachytherapy applied at the time of the initial stented angioplasty, in an attempt to prevent later proliferation of in-stent neointima, has been abandoned as well, due to a number of unexpected problems: subacute and late stent thrombosis, edge failure and geographical miss, acquired stent malapposition against the vessel wall due to vessel expansion and late recurrence of restenosis.

Presently, drug-eluting stents (DES) are replacing bare metal stents (BMS). These metallic scaffolds are covered with polymers from which less than 0.1mg of cytotoxic and anti-inflammatory compounds (e.g. paclitaxel, sirolimus, everolimus) are progressively eluted over the first weeks after stent implantation. Three drugs have shown significantly positive effects in prospective randomized trials of DES (paclitaxel, sirolimus, and its derivative everolimus).

Both angiographic restenosis rates and the need for repeat intervention due to symptom recurrence have been reduced by over 60%, at least with the use of the currently approved devices [256]. Reported incidence of major adverse cardiac events, including re-interventions, over 9 months ranges between 7.1–0.3% with DES stents compared with a range between 13.3–18.9 with BMS. More specific guidelines on the use of DES are available in the ESC guidelines on PCI [257]. Another development is the increasingly frequent use of direct stenting, i.e. stent implantation without balloon pre-dilatation. Animal experiments have suggested that direct stenting reduces endothelial and vessel wall damage and produces less neo-intimal proliferation [258]. When direct stenting is applicable with DES, restenosis rates as low as 2% have been observed [259]. Clinical follow-up for up to 4 years after DES seems to indicate durability of these results and additional long-term data are accumulating. Registries and surveillance data suggest that results obtainable in 'real life' are indeed comparable to those reported in randomized clinical trials, even in patient and lesion subsets considered at higher risk for poor outcome and which are usually excluded from such trials [260].

A drawback of stent implantation is the risk of stent thrombosis which is associated to a considerably high in hospital mortality. Stent thrombosis rate is about 2% during the first year and about 0.5% per year thereafter. The risk of stent thrombosis seems higher for DES than for BMS. The higher risk of stent thrombosis associated with DES implantation does not translate, however, in a higher rate of MI or mortality (➲Fig. 17.27). Thus, by markedly reducing the high rates of restenosis that would have occurred after BMS implantation, DES may directly reduce the subsequent occurrence of death and nonfatal MI, offsetting the incremental risk of stent thrombosis [261]. Taken together, meta-analyses and observational studies indicate that DES implantation does not significantly reduce the rate of major cardiac events, i.e. mortality and acute myocardial infarction, as compared to BMS implantation [262].

Thus, DES should be utilized in the treatment of coronary lesions at higher risk of restenosis and their implantation should be followed by a prolonged period of dual antiplatelet therapy.

Adjunctive pharmacological treatment

The mechanical trauma induced by PCI to the endothelium and deeper layers of the vessel wall and the

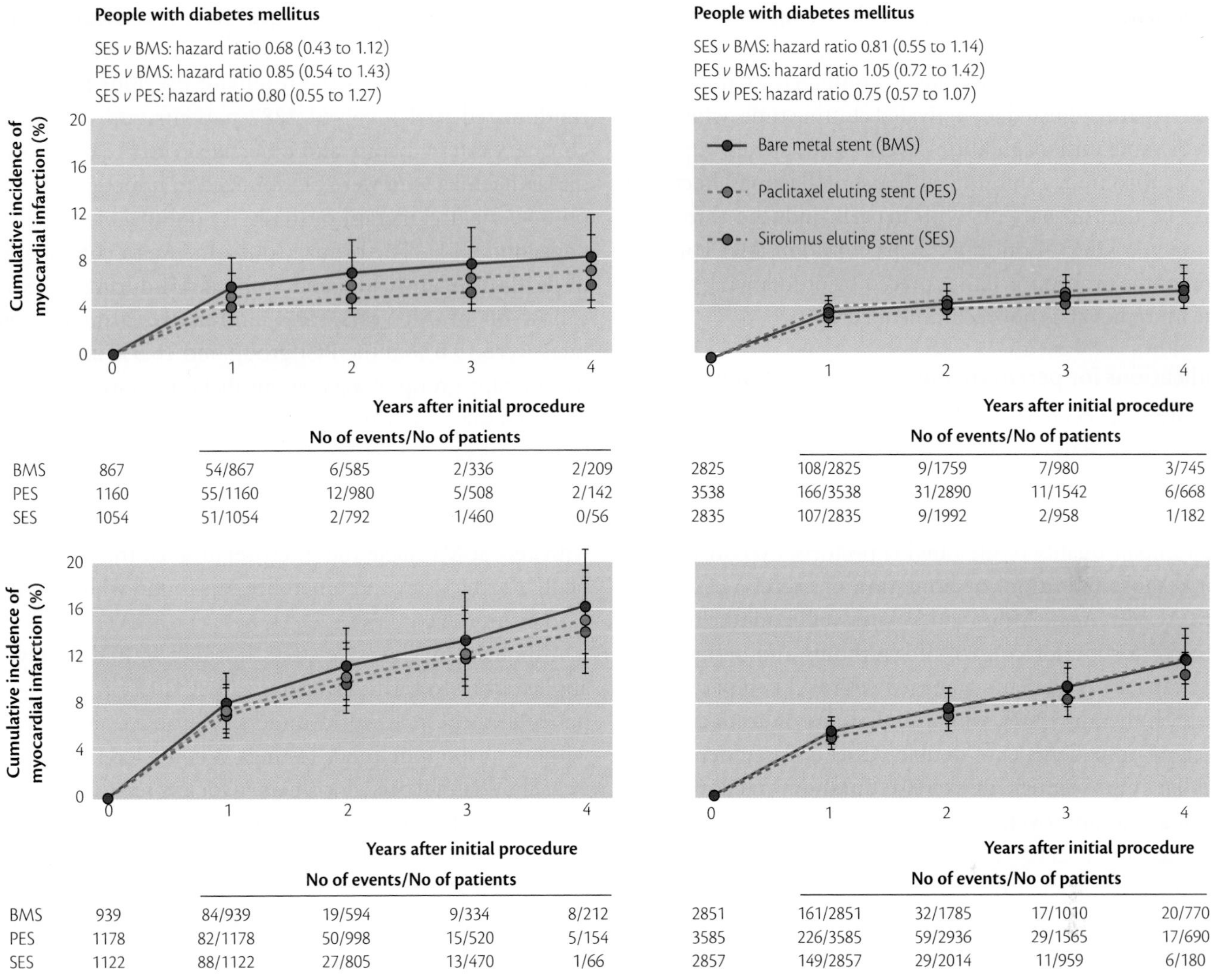

BMS	867	54/867	6/585	2/336	2/209	2825	108/2825	9/1759	7/980	3/745
PES	1160	55/1160	12/980	5/508	2/142	3538	166/3538	31/2890	11/1542	6/668
SES	1054	51/1054	2/792	1/460	0/56	2835	107/2835	9/1992	2/958	1/182

BMS	939	84/939	19/594	9/334	8/212	2851	161/2851	32/1785	17/1010	20/770
PES	1178	82/1178	50/998	15/520	5/154	3585	226/3585	59/2936	29/1565	17/690
SES	1122	88/1122	27/805	13/470	1/66	2857	149/2857	29/2014	11/959	6/180

Figure 17.27 Network meta-analysis with a mixed treatment comparison method to combine direct within trial comparisons between stents with indirect evidence from other trials while maintaining randomisation. The risk of myocardial infarction and of death or myocardial infarction was similar for sirolimus eluting stents (SES), paclitaxel eluting stents (PES) and bare metal stents (BMS) both in diabetic and non diabetic patients. Adapted from Stettler C, Alleman S, Wandel S, *et al.* Drug eluting and bare metal stents in people with and without diabetes: collaborative network meta-analysis. *BMJ* 2008; **337:** 1331.

presence of stents are a strong stimulus for platelet activation and clotting, which necessitates antithrombotic treatment.

All patients should receive aspirin and thienopyridine treatment [260]. To ensure full antiplatelet activity, clopidogrel should be initiated at least 6 hours prior to the procedure with a loading dose of 300mg, ideally administered the day before a planned PCI [263]. There is presently no consensus on the optimal duration of dual antiplatelet therapy after DES but many physicians empirically recommend prolonged treatment up to 1 year, particularly after stenting of complex or multiple lesions. The impact of possible resistance to antiplatelet agents requires further investigation.

Glycoprotein IIb/IIIa inhibitors, the most potent antiplatelet drugs available, that act by blocking the fibrinogen receptor, were proven beneficial in high-risk PCI, particularly during acute coronary syndromes. Given the overall low risk of PCI in stable IHD patients, the potential of glycoprotein IIb/IIIa receptor inhibitors of increasing the risk of bleeding complications and the considerable cost of their systematic use, these drugs are not a part of standard periprocedural medication but should be considered in complex or high-risk procedures [264].

Unfractionated heparin is given as an intravenous bolus either under activated clotting time guidance or in a weight-adjusted manner (usually 100IU/kg or 50IU/kg if glycoprotein IIb/IIIa receptor inhibitor is given). In a recent trial in patients undergoing elective PCI, a single intravenous bolus of 0.5mg of enoxaparin per kilogram was associated with reduced rates of bleeding as compared to unfractionated heparin adjusted for activated clotting time, with more predictable anticoagulation levels [265]. Bivalirudin is a direct thrombin inhibitor with a short-lasting effect that may be used in patients with heparin-induced thrombocytopenia [266]. Continued heparinization after completion of the procedure, either preceding or following arterial sheath removal, is not recommended.

Indications for percutaneous coronary interventions

On available evidence, PCI compared with medical therapy does not seem to provide substantial survival benefit in stable angina. Trial-based evidence indicates that PCI is more often effective than medical treatment in reducing events that impair quality of life (angina pectoris, dyspnoea, need for re-hospitalization, or limitation of exercise capacity). The ACME (Acute Mountain Sickness and Endothelin) trial showed a superior control of symptoms and better exercise capacity in patients managed with PCI compared with medical therapy [267], with a similar rate of death and MI. Of note, in patients with double-vessel disease, there was a similar improvement in exercise duration, freedom from angina, and improvement in quality-of-life at 6-month follow-up. In the RITA (Randomized Intervention Treatment of Angina)-2 trial, 1018 patients with stable angina (62% with multivessel CAD and 34% with significant disease in the proximal segment of the LAD coronary artery) were randomized to PCI or medical therapy and followed for a mean of 2.7 years [268]. Patients who had inadequate control of their symptoms with optimal medical therapy were allowed to cross-over to myocardial revascularization. This trial showed that PCI resulted in a better control of symptoms of ischaemia and improved exercise capacity compared with medical therapy, but it was associated with a higher combined endpoint of death and periprocedural MI. The AVERT (A Very Early Rehabilitation Trial) trial randomly assigned 341 patients with stable IHD, normal LV function, and Class I and/or II angina to PCI or medical therapy with 80mg daily atorvastatin [269]. At 18 months follow-up, 13% of the medically treated group had ischaemic events when compared with 21% of the PCI group. Angina relief, however, was greater in those treated with PCI. Accordingly, a recent comprehensive meta-analysis of PCI versus conservative therapy in non acute coronary artery disease including 2950 patients failed to find significant differences between the two treatment strategies with regard to total mortality, cardiac death or MI, nonfatal MI, CABG, or PCI during follow-up [270] (➲Fig. 17.28). The COURAGE (Clinical Outcomes Utilizing Revascularization and Aggressive Drug Evaluation trial nuclear substudy) trial has recently confirmed the results of previous trials. This randomized trial involved 2287 patients with significant coronary artery disease and objective evidence of myocardial ischaemia, who were randomized to undergo PCI with optimal medical therapy or to receive optimal medical therapy alone [271]. The primary outcome was a combination of death from any cause and nonfatal MI during a median follow-up of 4.6 years. The cumulative primary-event rates were 19.0% in the PCI group and 18.5% in the medical-therapy group. A very recent meta-analysis, which also included the COURAGE trial, found a lower total mortality in patients randomized to PCI as compared to those randomized to medical treatment [272]. However, several limitations, including the inclusion of trials enrolling patients with recent MI make the interpretation of the results difficult. Furthermore, no difference was found with regard to cardiac mortality.

Although non-invasive stress imaging should ideally be applied prior to cardiac catheterization [193], a majority of patients in the real world undergo coronary angiography without prior functional testing. When exercise-induced ischaemia has not been documented for any reason, the measurement of FFR can be applied during the invasive examination. This test is simple, easily obtained and lesion specific, and an FFR below 0.75 is a sufficiently reliable surrogate for inducible ischaemia. In the DEFER (Deferral of percutaneous coronary intervention) trial, PCI was either performed or deferred based on the FFR value. Event-free survival was similar between the deferral and PCI groups (92% versus 89% at 12 months and 89% versus 83% at 24 months), indicating that PCI does not improve outcome when performed on stenoses that are non-flow-limiting [273] (see ➲Chapter 8).

Taken together, currently available data suggest that in low- medium-risk patients with stable IHD, medical treatment including aggressive lipid-lowering therapy may be as effective as PCI in reducing major adverse cardiac events, while PCI is associated with a greater improvement in anginal symptoms and is therefore a viable option in patients who are symptomatic for angina in spite of optimal anti-anginal treatment.

Coronary artery bypass grafting

Introduction

CABG is the most documented, evaluated, and audited operation in the history of medicine. This surgical technique was initially introduced by Favaloro and colleagues in 1969 using saphenous vein grafts (SVG) interposed between

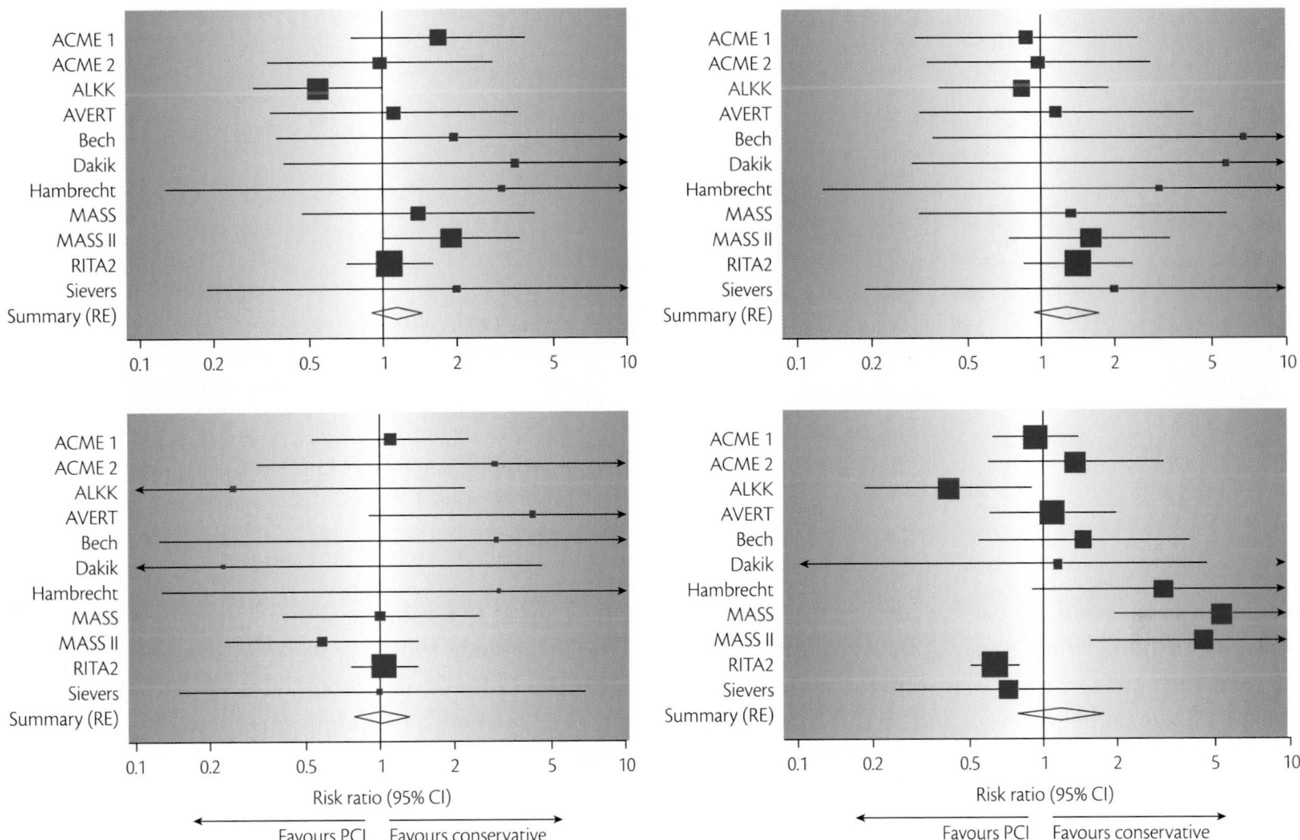

Figure 17.28 Meta-analysis of randomized trials comparing percutaneous coronary intervention (PCI) vs conservative medical treatment. The risk of cardiac death or any myocardial infarction (top left panel), nonfatal myocardial infarction (top right panel), coronary bypass grafting (bottom left panel), and repeat PCI during follow-up (bottom right panel) was similar for the two forms of treatment. Each study is shown by name along with point estimate of risk ratio and respective 95% CIs. In each panel, size of box denoting point estimate in each study is proportional to weight of study. Also shown are summary risk ratio and 95% CIs according to Der Simonian and Laird random effects model. Adapted with permission from Katritsis DG, Ioannidis JP. Percutaneous coronary intervention versus conservative therapy in nonacute coronary artery disease: a meta-analysis. *Circulation* 2005; **111**: 2906–12.

the aorta and epicardial coronary artery branches distal to critical stenoses [274]. Bypass surgery quickly became a cornerstone in the treatment of patients with IHD resulting in a striking improvement of anginal symptoms and of outcome in specific patient subsets.

Choice of conduit

By 10 years after CABG, 60% of SVG are stenosed or occluded. Since at least 70% of patients are alive 10 years after surgery, the recurrence of symptoms from vein graft disease remains a clinical problem. Large observational studies have shown that the use of the left internal mammary artery (LIMA) graft improves survival and reduces the incidence of late MI, recurrent angina, and the need for further cardiac interventions as compared to SVG [275, 276]. Accordingly, independent predictors of recurrence of angina after CABG are female gender, obesity, preoperative hypertension and lack of use of LIMA as a conduit to the LAD [277]. Over the last 20 years the standard procedure has been to graft the LAD with the LIMA and use SVG for the other epicardial coronary branches. There appears to be significant survival benefit, however, when using bilateral internal mammary artery (BIMA) grafts irrespective of age, ventricular function and the presence of diabetes [278, 279] (➲Fig. 17.29). Furthermore, the benefit of using BIMA increased with the duration of follow-up, particularly in terms of the need for repeat surgery. With the use of skeletonized IMA pedicles, the risk of sternal devascularization and subsequent dehiscence is much reduced, even in diabetics.

Other arterial grafts include the radial artery and the right gastroepiploic artery. The greatest experience has been with the radial artery, where reports have indicated patency rates greater than 90% at 3 years. There is a learning curve with radial artery grafts, however, and it is now clear that they should only be used for coronary vessels with high-grade stenosis or occlusion. In a prospective, randomized, single-centre trial, that compared angiographic patency of the radial artery with that of the free right internal mammary artery (RIMA) or SVG, no evidence emerged of a greater freedom from untoward events with radial artery use [280].

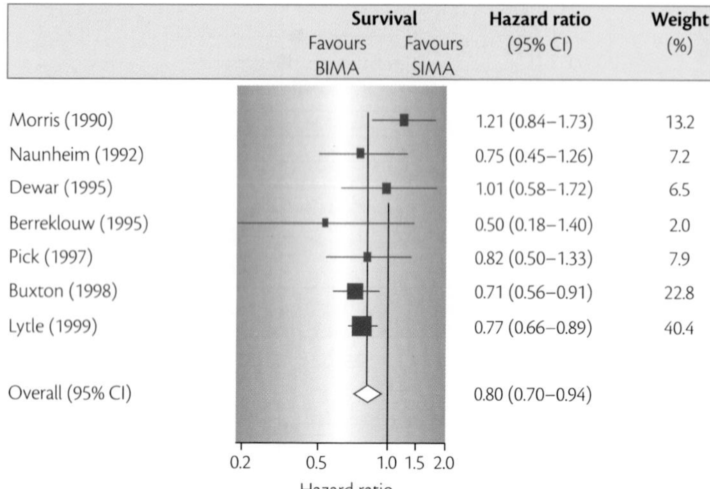

Survival
Favours BIMA
Favours SIMA
Hazard ratio (95% CI)
Weight (%)
Morris (1990) 1.21 (0.84–1.73) 13.2
Naunheim (1992) 0.75 (0.45–1.26) 7.2
Dewar (1995) 1.01 (0.58–1.72) 6.5
Berreklouw (1995) 0.50 (0.18–1.40) 2.0
Pick (1997) 0.82 (0.50–1.33) 7.9
Buxton (1998) 0.71 (0.56–0.91) 22.8
Lytle (1999) 0.77 (0.66–0.89) 40.4
Overall (95% CI) 0.80 (0.70–0.94)
0.2
0.5
1.0 1.5 2.0
Hazard ratio

Figure 17.29 Systematic review of trials comparing single internal mammary artery (SIMA) and bilateral internal mammary artery (BIMA) grafts. Survival was higher in patients treated with BIMA. Adapted with permission from Taggart DP, D'Amico R, Altman DG. Effect of arterial revascularisation on survival: a systematic review of studies comparing bilateral and single internal mammary arteries. *Lancet* 2003; **361**: 615–16.

Furthermore, a recent report has shown disappointing results for medium-term patency of the radial artery [281]. At 5 years the patency results were 92% for LIMA, 85% for RIMA, 64% for saphenous vein and 53% for radial artery grafts. There was a gender difference for the radial graft patency, with elderly females faring worse.

Beating heart surgery ('off-pump')

The use of extracorporeal circulation (cardiopulmonary bypass) for performing coronary artery surgery remains the most commonly used approach. However, there are risks, including a whole-body inflammatory response and the production of microemboli. The need for aortic cannulation and manipulation of the ascending aorta may lead to release of emboli, especially in elderly atheromatous patients, who constitute an increasing proportion of the patient pool accepted for coronary surgery. So-called 'off-pump' surgery may lead to a reduction in perioperative mortality and morbidity. The recent introduction of stabilization devices has enabled surgeons to treat patients with three-vessel disease in this way. Randomized trials comparing off-pump with the standard procedure are now available. Although the use of blood products was reduced in the off-pump group (3% vs. 13%) and the release of creatine kinase (CK)-MB isoenzyme was 41% less in the off-pump group, there were no differences in perioperative complication rates. There was also no difference in outcome in the first 1–3 years after surgery between off-pump and standard groups [282, 283]. A meta-analysis of six studies including 558 patients randomized to on-pump and 532 to off-pump CABG found no significant difference in the combined end-point of death, stroke, or MI [284]. A further randomized trial with angiographic follow-up at 3–6 months showed a significant reduction in graft patency (90% vs. 98%) in the off-pump group [285]. Accordingly, in a recent observational study including 49,830 patients, off-pump surgery was associated with lower in-hospital mortality and complication rates than on-pump CABG, but long-term outcomes were comparable, except for freedom from revascularization, which favoured on-pump CABG [286]. These studies suggest that the use of off-pump surgery should be applied cautiously and selectively to patients with good target vessels and significant comorbidity.

In the debates about on-pump and off-pump surgery, on-pump is usually treated as a single commodity. However, cardiopulmonary bypass can be conducted in several distinct ways. Cardioplegic arrest may be employed using a variety of solutions at different temperatures and by different routes, antegrade or retrograde or a combination of the two. Non-cardioplegic methods have a long pedigree and can be very effective. With the use of stabilizers, cardiopulmonary bypass can be employed without the insult of global ischaemia caused by aortic cross-clamping, and used to empty the heart while local stabilization of the target vessel is secured. When the vessel is opened a shunt may be placed, thus minimizing any regional ischaemia. This approach has proved effective in patients with myocardial hibernation and dilated hearts, and in repeat coronary surgery.

Repeat coronary artery surgery

The incidence of repeat coronary artery surgery, as a proportion of all coronary artery surgery, is less in Europe (5–10%) than in North America (10–15%). There is a higher morbidity and a two to three times higher mortality, compared to the first intervention [287]. Although the relief of angina is less predictable and less complete than after first-time surgery, the long-term outcome is encouraging, with 73% of patients being free of angina at 5 years. The indications for reoperation have not been defined by randomized trials, but the same principles apply as for first-time surgery. For instance, stenosis in a vein graft to the LAD is associated with a reduction in survival. A major improvement in survival after reoperation was especially evident for patients in this category. Among these patients, survival rates were 84% and 74% for the reoperation group at 2 and 4 years compared with 76% and 53% for the medically treated group [288].

Indications for coronary bypass surgery

There are two main indications for CABG: prognostic and symptomatic. Prognostic benefit of CABG is mainly because of a reduction in cardiac mortality, as there is less evidence for reduction in MI [289, 290]. In a meta-analysis of surgical trials comparing CABG with medical therapy prognostic benefit of CABG compared with medical therapy has not been found in low-risk patients (annual mortality < 1%), while CABG was shown to improve prognosis in those at medium to high-risk [290]. Further observational data from the Duke registry confirmed that long-term mortality benefit associated with surgery was limited to high-risk groups [291]. Analyses of observational and randomized controlled trial data revealed that the presence of specific coronary artery anatomy is associated with a better prognosis with surgery than with medical treatment. Such disease includes [292–294] (➲Table 17.17).

- Significant LM stenosis;
- Significant proximal stenosis of the three major coronary arteries;
- Significant stenosis of two major coronary arteries, including high-grade stenosis of the proximal LAD.

Significant stenosis was defined in these studies as >70% of major coronary arteries or >50% of the LM stem. The presence of impaired left ventricular function increases the absolute prognostic advantage of surgery over medical treatment in all categories. This information mainly comes from three major randomized studies, the European Coronary Artery study [295] the Coronary Artery Surgery study [296], and the Veterans Administration study [289].

Aside from studies dealing exclusively with the effects of either PCI vs. medical therapy or CABG vs. medical therapy, several hybrid studies have investigated the effects of revascularization (either PCI or surgery) compared with medical therapy. The ACIP (Asymptomatic Cardiac Ischemia Pilot) study provides additional information comparing medical therapy with PCI or CABG revascularization in patients with documented IHD and evidence of myocardial ischaemia by both exercise stress-testing and

Table 17.17 Mortality rates in a number of subgroups of patients with chronic ischaemic heart disease treated with medical therapy and statistical comparisons with mortality rates obtained in the same subgroups of patients treated with coronary artery by-pass surgery

Subgroup	Medical treatment	*p* value for CABG surgery vs. medical therapy
Vessel disease		
One vessel	9.9	0.18
Two vessels	11.7	0.45
Three vessels	17.6	<0.001
Left main artery	36.5	0.004
No LAD disease		
One or two vessels	8.3	0.88
Three vessels	14.5	0.02
Left main artery	45.8	0.03
Overall	12.3	0.05
LAD disease present		
One or two vessels	14.6	0.05
Three vessels	19.1	0.009
Left main artery	32.7	0.02
Overall	18.3	0.001
LV function		
Normal	13.3	<0.001
Abnormal	25.2	0.02
Exercise test status		
Missing	17.4	0.10
Normal	11.6	0.38
Abnormal	16.8	<0.001
Severity of angina		
Class 0, I, II	12.5	0.005
Class III, IV	22.4	0.001

* Systematic overview of the effect of coronary artery bypass graft (CABG) surgery versus medical therapy on survival based on data from the seven randomized trials comparing a strategy of initial CABG surgery with one of initial medical therapy. Subgroup results at 5 years are shown.

LAD, left anterior descending artery; LV, left ventricular.
Adapted with permission from Yusuf S, Zucker D, Peduzzi P, *et al.* Effect of coronary artery bypass graft surgery on survival: overview of 10-year results from randomised trials by the Coronary Artery Bypass Graft Surgery Trialists Collaboration. *Lancet* 1994; **344**: 563–70.

ambulatory ECG monitoring [297]. This small study randomized 558 such patients with or without anginal symptoms to one of three treatment strategies: angina-guided drug therapy, angina plus ischaemia-guided drug therapy, and revascularization by PCI or CABG surgery. At 2 years of follow-up, death or MI had occurred in 4.7% of the revascularization patients when compared with 8.8% of the ischaemia-guided group and 12.1% of the angina-guided group. Thus the results of the ACIP trial suggest that higher-risk patients who have demonstrable ischaemia during daily life and significant coronary artery disease may have a better outcome with revascularization with either CABG or PCI compared with those managed medically; this was a pilot study, however, underpowered to reach firm conclusions; indeed, no statistically significant difference in clinical outcome could be demonstrated between revascularization and ischaemia-guided medical therapy. Notably, other trials (TIME and Medicine, Angioplasty or Surgery Study, MASS) failed to show a reduction of major cardiac events in patients randomized to myocardial revascularization, as compared to those randomized to medical treatment [298, 299].

Surgery has been convincingly shown to reduce symptoms and ischaemia, and to improve quality-of-life in patients with chronic angina. These effects are evident in a much wider range of subgroups compared to those showing improvement of survival. In patients with three-vessel disease, the completeness of revascularization is a significant determinant of the relief of symptoms over a 5-year period. Approximately 80% of patients are angina-free 5 years after surgery and 63% at 10 years, but by 15 years only 15% are free of a coronary event [300].

The overall operative mortality for elective first-time CABG is 2–4% [301]. There are well-developed risk stratification models available for the assessment of risk in individual patients. Typically, the higher the risk of operation, the greater the benefit of surgical over medical treatment. Thus, individual risks and benefits should be discussed as thoroughly in low-risk patients in whom surgery is undertaken on symptomatic grounds alone, as in high-risk patients.

In conclusion, coronary artery bypass surgery remains the gold standard for the alleviation of symptoms in patients with coronary artery disease. In addition there are patient subsets in whom surgery will improve prognosis, notably those with LM stem or proximal anterior LAD disease, as well as those with impaired left ventricular function and three-vessel coronary disease. In addition, it is an important form of treatment for patients with ischaemic cardiomyopathy and large areas of myocardial viability, including those for whom angina is a minor component of their symptoms.

Percutaneous interventions versus coronary bypass surgery

A large number of clinical trials have compared PCI with CABG in order to establish the choice of revascularization technique, both before and after the introduction of stenting. Meta-analysis of trials conducted before 1995, when coronary stenting was rare, revealed no significant differences in the treatment strategy for either death or the combined endpoint of death or MI [302]. Mortality during the initial hospitalization for the procedure occurred in 1.3% of the CABG group and 1% of the PCI group. The need for subsequent revascularization was significantly higher in the PCI group, and although patients were significantly less likely to have angina 1 year after bypass surgery than after PCI, by 3 years this difference was no longer statistically significant. Results from the BARI (Bypass Angioplasty Revascularization Investigation) study, the largest single randomized trial of PCI vs. surgery, not included in this meta-analysis, were nonetheless consistent with these findings, although a survival advantage with bypass surgery was observed in the diabetic subgroup [303]. Compared with the balloon era, angioplasty using BMS has halved the risk difference for repeat revascularization at 1 year, which however remains at 18% after PCI vs. 4.4% after CABG [304, 305].

A meta-analysis including trials of stents suggests a mortality benefit with CABG compared with PCI at 5 years which continued to 8 years in patients with multivessel disease. Furthermore, a significantly lower incidence of angina and need for repeat revascularization was shown [306]. Subgroup analysis of trials with and without stents indicated significant heterogeneity between the two groups, with trials performed in the pre-stent era showing a trend towards reduced mortality favouring CABG which was not evident in the trials with stents. Accordingly, a more recent meta-analysis of four randomized controlled trials of PCI with stents compared with bypass surgery showed no significant difference between the treatment strategies in the primary endpoint of death, MI, or stroke at 1 year [307]. However, observational data on >60,000 patients from the New York Cardiac Registry indicated that for patients with two or more diseased coronary arteries, CABG was associated with higher adjusted rates of long-term survival compared to stenting [308]. Similar findings were confirmed, more recently, with observational data from the same Registry in the comparison between CABG and DES [309].

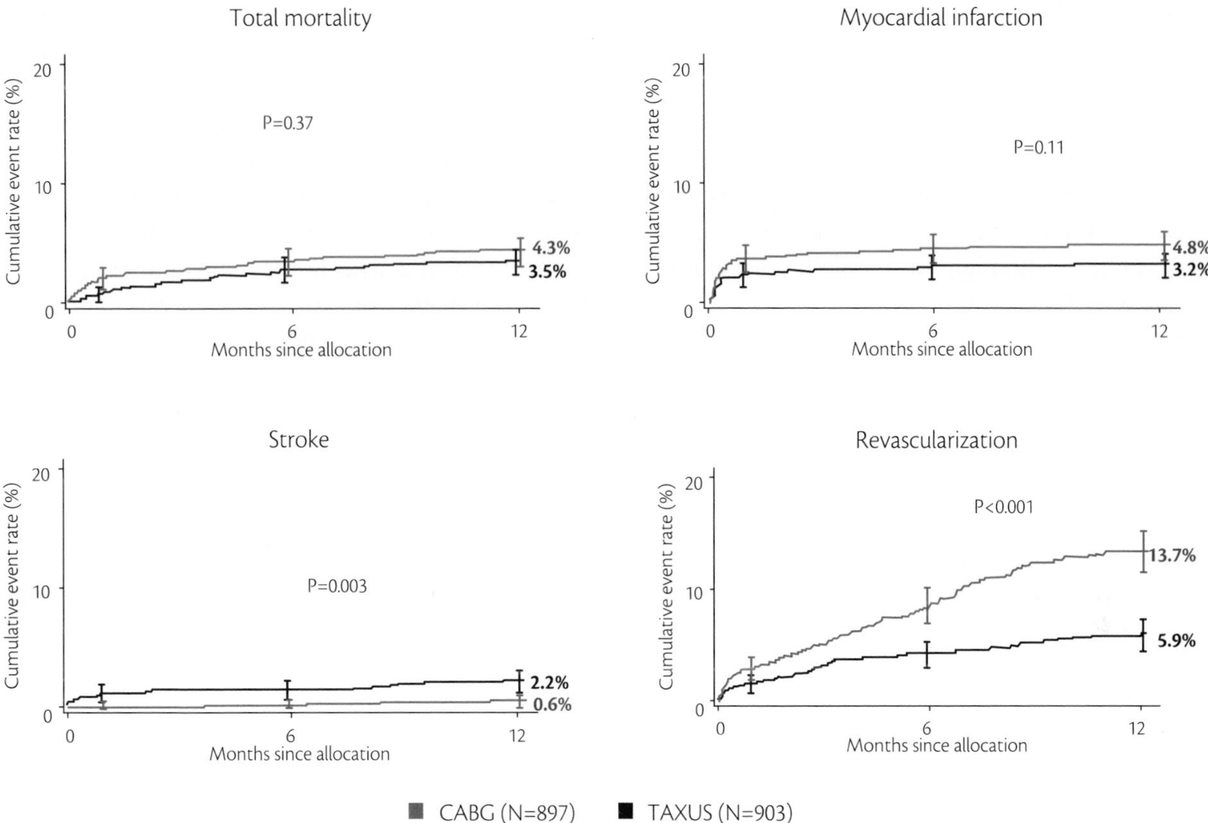

Figure 17.30 Comparison of percutaneous coronary intervention (PCI) by drug eluting stents vs. coronary bypass surgery for cardiac total mortality, myocardial infarction, stroke and repeat revascularization during one year follow-up in the SYNTAX trial. (Courtesy of P. Serruys.)

Above mentioned trials comparing PCI versus CABG have one or more of three important limitations: 1) they were limited to highly selected patient subpopulations (typically representing no more than 5% of screened patients); 2) they lacked an active control represented by patients screened but not randomized; 3) they did not utilize current, standard techniques for CABG and PCI. The SYNTAX (SYNergy between PCI with TAXus and cardiac surgery) trial has overcome these important limitations. This trial enrolled 3075 patients with 3-vessel and/or left main stem disease; 1800 patients, amenable to similar myocardial revascularization by PCI or CABG, were randomized; 1077 patients who underwent CABG because of contraindications to PCI and 198 who underwent PCI because of contraindications to CABG were followed in registries. The primary end-point was a composite of all cause death, cerebrovascular accident, documented MI or any repeat revascularization at 12 month follow up. The trial failed to demonstrate non inferiority of PCI vs. CABG for the primary end-point which occurred in 13.7% of the PCI group and 5.9% of the CABG group. This difference was mainly driven by a higher repeat revascularization rate (14.7% vs. 5.4%), while the rate of death, cerebrovascular accidents or MI was similar (7.7% vs. 7.6%, respectively). Interestingly, cerebrovascular accident rate was higher in the CABG group than in PCI group (2.2% vs. 0.6%), whereas acute MI rate was higher in the PCI group than in the CABG group (4.8% vs. 3.2%) (➲Fig. 17.30). Among patients in the CABG registry the primary end-point rate was 8.8%, thus indicating that about one third of patients with 3-vessel and/or left main stem disease were amenable to CABG only, and in these patients CABG was associated with an excellent outcome. Among patients in the PCI registry the primary end-point rate was 20.5%; in these patients, however, pre-procedural risk was considerably higher than that of randomized patients. Thus, PCI is a viable option for patients not eligible for CABG, although with a significant increase in the risk of major coronary events. Interestingly, the authors developed a new score to describe the complexity of coronary lesions which was predictive of the primary outcome. Among patients with a low score (about one third of randomized patients) the rate of the primary end-point was similar in the CABG and PCI groups [316].

Finally, some groups of patients warrant particular considerations when selecting revascularization options. They include: 1) patients with severely depressed LV function and/or high surgical risk; 2) patients with diabetes and multivessel disease; 3) patients with chronic total coronary occlusions; 4) patients with previous bypass surgery occlusions.

It is reasonable to assume that patients in whom surgical risk is prohibitively high may benefit from revascularization by PCI, particularly when residual viability can be demonstrated in dysfunctioning myocardium perfused by the target vessel(s), although this possibility has not been demonstrated in clinical trials.

As far as diabetic patients are concerned, although a direct comparison of PCI with CABG in diabetics is not yet available, subgroup or post hoc analyses of clinical trials have invariably shown a worse outcome with PCI than with CABG [310]. The BARI trial was the largest of these trials, and the only one in which a statistical difference in mortality was detected between the treatment groups in the diabetics [303]. In the ARTS (Arterial Revascularization Therapies Study) I trial, outcome for diabetics was poor in both treatment arms, but even more so following PCI. After 3 years, mortality was 7.1% in the PCI and 4.2% in the CABG group, with a still significant difference in event-free survival of 52.7% in the PCI group and 81.3% in the CABG group [311]. Preliminary data from the ARTS II, a prospective registry [312], suggest that the use of DES in patients with multivessel disease and/or diabetes mellitus might change this situation, although appropriate trials are expected to clarify this point.

Chronic total occlusions represent an anatomical condition where PCI is associated with low technical success and high complication rate, including extensive dissection, side-branch occlusion, distal embolization and coronary perforation [313]. When the occlusion can be crossed with a guidewire and the distal lumen has been reached, satisfactory results are obtainable with stent implantation albeit at the expense of a high restenosis rate (32–55%) [314]. In this case, the use of DES has been shown to improve these results in a significant way [315].

There are no randomized controlled trials comparing treatment options in patients with previous bypass surgery. Redo surgery may be undertaken on symptomatic grounds where the anatomy is suitable. However, the operative risk of re-do bypass surgery is as high as three-fold greater than initial surgery, and for those with a patent LIMA graft, there is the additional risk of damage to this graft during surgery. On the other hand PCI can be performed following previous surgical revascularization, either in the vein graft or arterial graft, or the native coronary tree, and may provide a useful alternative to redo surgery for symptomatic relief.

To summarize, after an initial pharmacological approach, revascularization may be recommended for patients with suitable anatomy who do not respond adequately to medical therapy. In asymptomatic patients, revascularization cannot improve symptoms and the only appropriate indication for revascularization would be to reduce the likelihood of future ischaemic complications. Evidence to support this strategy is limited only to those patients with objective evidence of extensive ischaemia and/or left ventricular dysfunction in whom revascularization (either PCI or CABG) may reduce the likelihood of mortality. In non-diabetic patients with one or two vessel disease without high grade stenosis of the proximal LAD in whom angioplasty of one or more lesions has a high likelihood of initial success, PCI is generally the preferred initial approach, influenced by factors such as the less invasive nature and the absence of survival advantage with CABG. For patients with more severe coronary artery disease each individual case should be carefully discussed between interventional cardiologists and cardiac surgeons. Some patients are eligible for PCI or CABG only. If both interventions can provide a similar myocardial revascularization, the choice should take into account the individual circumstances and the preferences of the patient with lesions of increasing complexity progressively favouring CABG. The following factors should always be taken into consideration for an optimal choise of the modality of myocardial revascularization: 1) risk of periprocedural morbidity and morbidity; 2) likelihood of success, including factors such as technical suitability of lesions for angioplasty or surgical bypass; 3) risk of restenosis or graft occlusion; 4) completeness of revascularization; 5) diabetic status; 6) local hospital experience in cardiac surgery and interventional cardiology; 7) patient's preference.

Management of refractory angina

Refractory angina pectoris is defined as the occurrence of frequent episodes of angina, significantly limiting daily activities of the patient (usually CCS class III–IV), which cannot be sufficiently controlled by optimal drug therapy and, at the same time, coronary anatomy is judged to be unsuitable for both percutaneous and surgical coronary intervention [317].

The exact prevalence of refractory angina has not been assessed adequately, but it will probably constitute a challenging issue in the next years, due to the progressively longer life expectancy of patients with complex or diffuse coronary artery disease. Of note, mortality is relatively higher in these patients, being around 4–8% per year.

Table 17.18 Proposed treatment options for refractory angina pectoris

Spinal cord stimulation (SCS)
Enhanced external counterpulsation
Surgical/percutaneous myocardial laser revascularization
Angiogenic therapy
Neuromodulatory therapies other than SCS (TENS, left stellate gangliectomy)
Epidural anaesthesia
Intermittent urokinase therapy
Chelation therapy
Shock wave therapy
Coronary sinus stenting
Heart transplantation

TENS, transcutaneous electrical nerve stimulation.

Several forms of therapy have been proposed for this condition (➲Table 17.18), but sufficient data and/or appropriate trials have been collected only for some of them [318].

Spinal cord stimulation (SCS)

While there is no evidence that clinical prognosis can be improved by any therapy, the body of evidence suggests that SCS may have beneficial effects in refractory angina. SCS has been used for about 20 years in these kind of patients and several studies have reported improvement in angina symptoms and quality of life, as well as a reduction in hospital re-admissions for angina [319, 320]. In a prospective multicentre Italian registry a significant improvement in symptoms at 13-month follow-up was observed in 73% of 104 patients [320]. Interestingly, in a small randomized study involving 103 chronic anginal patients with severe coronary artery disease, SCS was found to have similar effects as CABG on symptoms and quality of life, both at 6-month and at 5-year follow-up, with similar long-term survival [321]. Of note, no life-threatening complications related to SCS have been reported, while local infectious complications or catheter dislodgment requiring re-implant occur in a minority of patients.

Enhanced external counterpulsation

Comparable beneficial effects on angina symptoms have also been reported for EECP, which is increasingly used, in particular, in the USA [322, 323]. However, some conditions need caution or represent contraindications to EECP, including severe impairment of left ventricular function, uncontrolled hypertension, aortic disease, significant aortic regurgitation, peripheral venous disease and anticoagulant therapy, and the treatment can be associated with some troublesome side effects (e.g. leg or back pain, skin abrasion or oedema, headache, dizziness, epistaxis, and respiratory discomfort). In patients with depressed ventricular function EECP has also been associated with an appreciable occurrence of serious adverse events, including death and MI [324].

Myocardial laser revascularization

Myocardial laser revascularization has been investigated in several randomized trials using the epicardial surgical approach or the endocardial percutaneous approah. Although the early studies reported beneficial effects on symptoms [325], randomized 'sham-controlled' studies failed to show improvement of angina symptoms [326]. Furthermore, the risk of perioperative complications, including death (4–5%), MI (10%), and lung infections (5–30%) is rather high.

Angiogenic therapy

This latter form of therapy has been assessed in clinical trials by intracoronary or intramyocardial administration of growth factors or by gene therapy. The few controlled randomized trials, however, have given disappointing results, showing no or marginal effects on anginal symptoms and myocardial ischaemia [327, 328]. Furthermore, a small but significant number of serious adverse events occur during the treatment procedure. Unresolved issues relate to the risks from the stimulation of angiogenesis in the body which can potentially favour proliferative diseases, and the risk from the use of external genetic material, potentially favouring immunological reactions.

Other clinical manifestations of chronic ischaemic heart disease

Although chronic stable angina is the most frequent clinical syndrome in patients with recurrent, stable episodes of myocardial ischaemia, there are other relevant, distinct, although less frequent, clinical presentations than can be related to recurrent myocardial ischaemic episodes.

Microvascular angina

Microvascular angina is typically characterized by: 1) angina predominantly occurring on effort and typical enough to suggest IHD; 2) 'ischaemic like' ST segment depression during angina or provocative tests, mainly ECG-EST (➲Fig. 17.31); 3) normal coronary arteries at angiography; 4) absence of epicardial coronary artery spasm and of cardiac or systemic diseases known to cause microvascular dysfunction. This clinical presentation is also usually defined as cardiac syndrome X both in medical literature and clinical

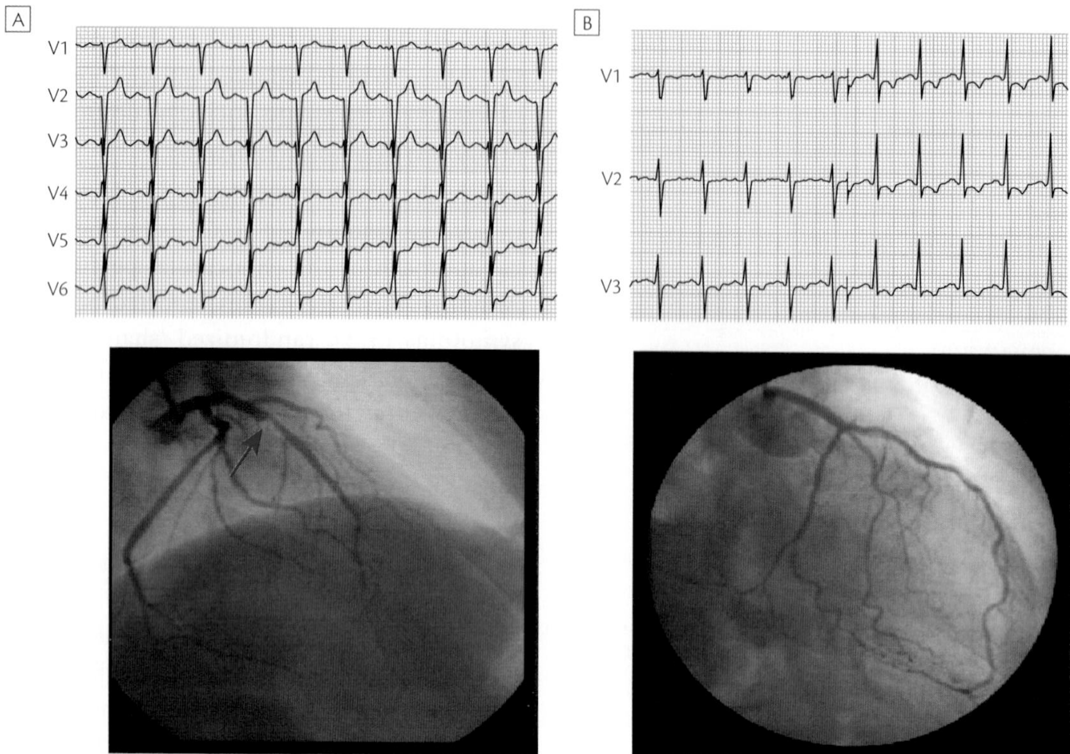

Figure 17.31 'Ischaemic' ST segment depression (~1.5mm) in anterior-lateral leads induced by treadmill exercise stress test (Bruce protocol) in two patients with stable effort angina *(upper panels)*. The morphology and severity of ST segment depression and the achieved workload (Bruce stage 2) is similar in the two patients. Yet, in patient A *(bottom left panel)* coronary angiography shows a tight stenosis of proximal left anterior descending coronary artery *(arrow)*, whereas in patient B *(bottom right panel)* angiography shows angiographically normal coronary arteries (microvascular angina).

practice, but the term microvascular angina will be used in this text as there is growing evidence of microvascular dysfunction and of an ischaemic origin of angina in this kind of patients [329].

The prevalence and incidence of microvascular angina is poorly known. However, among patients with chest pain suggestive of transient myocardial ischaemia who undergo coronary angiography, 10–30% are found to have normal or near normal coronary arteries and no evidence of coronary vasospasm. Although a number of these patients may not present a cardiac ischaemic syndrome, most of them present features compatible with microvascular angina, but their proportion remains uncertain.

Pathogenesis

There is still debate about whether microvascular dysfunction is the cause of myocardial ischaemia and chest pain in patients presenting with angina and normal coronary arteries. A reduced coronary flow reserve, however, has been consistently reported by several studies using different methods and techniques [330–332]. Both an impaired endothelium-dependent and endothelium-independent vasodilator function and an increased vasoconstrictor activity of coronary resistance arteries may be involved. The mechanisms are still incompletely known, but may include abnormal adrenergic activity, insulin resistance, inflammation, and, in women, oestrogen deficiency [329].

On the other hand, there is consensus that enhanced pain perception is present in a group of these patients, which could facilitate chest pain even for mild degrees of myocardial ischaemia. It remains controversial, however, whether increased cardiac pain perception is caused by a general nociceptive abnormality related to a cortical defect or rather by a specific peripheral cardiac neural alteration [333, 334].

Clinical presentation

In most cases the chest pain, which is induced by effort and relieved by rest, can not be distinguished between those with microvascular angina and those with obstructive coronary atherosclerosis. Some features of angina, however, strongly suggest microvascular angina, including a prolonged duration of chest pain after interruption of effort and a slow or inconstant response to sublingual nitrates.

Diagnosis

Physical examination is typically unremarkable, whereas ECG-EST shows results largely similar to those observed in patients with obstructive IHD (➲Fig. 17.31) and exercise myocardial perfusion scintigraphy is positive in about half of the patients [335]. The absence of left ventricular contractile abnormalities during echocardiographic stress test (dipyridamole, dobutamine or exercise), despite the induction of chest pain and ST-segment depression [336], strongly suggests microvascular angina, as does the lack of improvement of exercise induced angina and ST segment changes by short-acting nitrates [337].

Notably, while assessment of coronary microcirculation can be difficult to be done in each patient with angina and normal coronary arteries by invasive or sophisticated non invasive methods (e.g. CMR or PET imaging) due to time consumption and/or excessive costs, it has recently been suggested that coronary blood flow assessment in response to vasodilator stimuli might be done routinely by transthoracic Doppler recording of LAD [338] (➲Fig. 17.32) or by contrast stress echocardiography [339].

Prognosis

Prognosis of microvascular angina has consistently been shown to be excellent, as no increase in the risk of major cardiac events has usually been reported [340]. A significant impairment of left ventricular function at follow-up has been found in the small subset of patients who present with resting or stress induced LBBB [341], but these patients may have latent forms of dilated cardiomyopathy. Notably, recent data suggest that evidence of endothelial dysfunction in women with microvascular angina may be associated with the development of clinically silent, but angiographically detectable coronary artery disease at long-term follow-up [342].

In a recent long-term follow-up study (mean 11.6 years) no major cardiac events (death, acute MI) could be recorded in a population of 155 typical microvascular angina patients [343].

Despite the excellent prognosis, several patients with microvascular angina show persistence and even worsening of symptoms over time, with angina attacks becoming more frequent, severe, prolonged, and poorly responsive to drug therapy. Symptoms may considerably restrict patient's daily activities and lead to frequent non invasive, and even invasive, diagnostic investigation, as well as emergency room and hospital admissions. Thus, quality of life in these patients can be severely impaired, making microvascular angina a socially and economically relevant cardiac disease [340, 343].

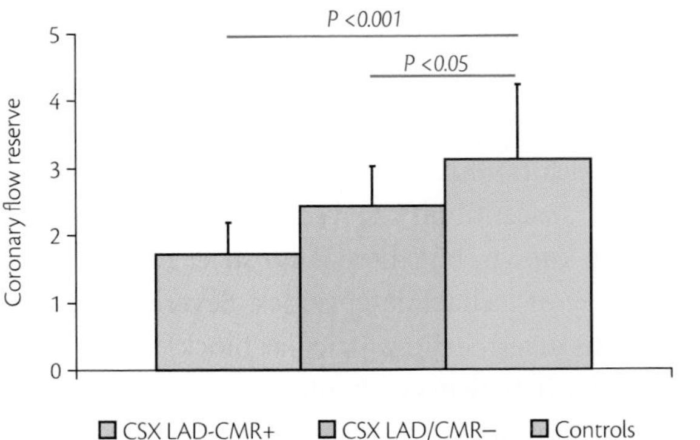

Figure 17.32 Increase in coronary blood flow velocity in the left anterior descending coronary artery (LAD) in response to infusion of adenosine (140μg/kg/min), assessed by transthoracic Doppler recording, in a group of patients with microvascular angina and with or without evidence of reversible perfusion defects in the LAD coronary artery territory at cardiovascular magnetic resonance during dobutamine stress test (LAD-CMR+ and LAD-CMR-, respectively). Patients showed lower vasodilator response to adenosine, compared to a control group of age and sex-matched healthy subjects, with the response being even lower in those with evidence of stress inducible perfusion defects on CMR. See [335].

Treatment

Treatment of microvascular angina is initially based on traditional anti-ischaemic drugs (beta-blockers, calcium antagonists and nitrates) in variable combination. In patients with persistent symptoms, benefits have been reported in small studies with the addition of ACE-inhibitors (which may counteract the vasoconstrictive and pro-oxidant effects of angiotensin II), xanthine derivatives (which can favour redistribution of myocardial blood flow towards ischaemic areas), statins (which may improve endothelial function), and (in pre-menopausal or menopausal women) estrogens (which may also improve endothelial function). In patients with angina refractory to medical treatment and with evidence of increased pain perception imipramine (which inhibits visceral pain transmission) can be added. Electrical neuromodulatory stimulation was found to reduce the number of angina episodes and might be therefore considered in this condition [95].

Vasospastic angina

Variant angina was first described by Prinzmetal and colleagues in 1959 [344]. It derives its name from the fact that, at variance with the most common effort angina, it occurs at rest and is associated with ST segment elevation on the ECG.

At its onset variant angina may present typical features of an acute coronary syndrome, due to recurrence of chest pain

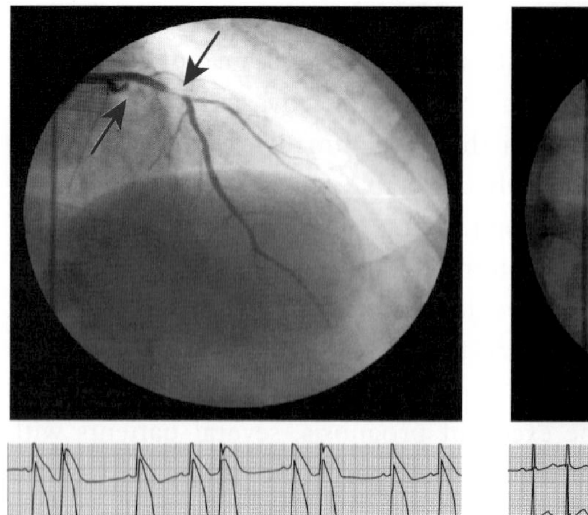

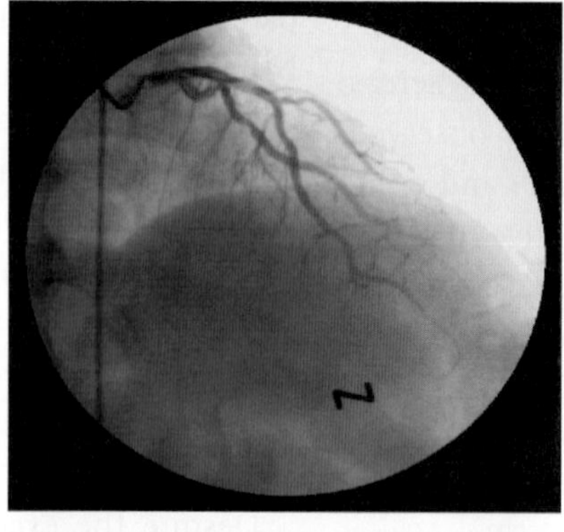

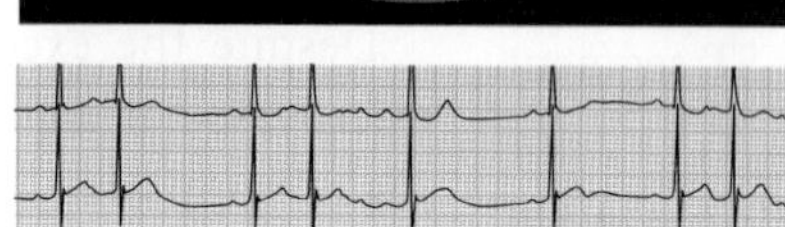

Figure 17.33 Documentation of occlusive coronary artery spasm of both left anterior descending coronary artery and circumflex coronary artery (arrows) following intracoronary administration of 16mcg of ergonovine in a patient with typical variant angina (top left). Coronary spasm promptly resolves after intracoronary administration of 2mg of isosorbide dinitrate (top right). The electrocardiogram shows marked ST segment elevation up to 20mm (bottom left) which resolves after nitrates (bottom right).

episodes at rest, although the usual typical short duration suggests the vasospastic nature of angina attacks. However, several patients seek medical attention or the correct diagnosis by physicians is achieved late, after weeks or months from symptom onset, when patients have a clear stable, most often predictive pattern of their anginal attacks. In particular, in Japan this condition is considered a chronic disease because of the frequent persistence of stable symptoms over months and years.

There have been no systematic studies assessing the epidemiology of variant angina, but in a recent study, variant angina was the final diagnosis in about 1.5% of patients admitted because of transient angina attacks, a figure similar to that reported in a previous older study [345]. The incidence, however, might be higher in Japanese than in Caucasian people [346].

Pathogenesis

Angiographic studies in the 1960s have demonstrated that variant angina has its unique mechanism in occlusive/subocclusive epicardial artery spasm, resulting in transient transmural ischaemia (➲Fig. 17.33) [347, 348]. As discussed earlier the pathogenetic mechanisms of coronary artery spasm are unknown, but an aspecific post-receptorial hyperreactivity to multiple vasoconstrictor stimuli of smooth muscle cells in one or more segments of epicardial coronary arteries has been shown to be responsible for the clinical syndrome [349].

Coronary angiography has shown that coronary artery spasm occurs at the site of significant (>50%) stenoses in about half of variant angina patients, whereas it occurs at the site of normal coronary arteries or non significant stenosis in the other patients [350].

Clinical presentation

Variant angina should be suspected in patients with angina occurring exclusively or predominantly at rest, without any apparent triggering cause. Angina is usually of short duration (2–5min), sometimes recurs in clusters, frequently shows a typical circadian pattern, with a more frequent occurrence in the early morning or in the night hours, and it promptly responds to short-acting nitrates. Several patients present ‘hot’ and ‘cold’ symptomatic phases, with periods of waxing and waning of symptoms lasting weeks or months. In some cases, however, symptoms can persist for years, reappearing when therapy is withdrawn. Effort tolerance is often well preserved, but exercise is a trigger of coronary artery spasm in about 25% of patients.

In some patients severe ventricular tachyarrhythmias may develop during myocardial ischaemic episodes caused by coronary artery spasm. These patients may present syncope or pre-syncope associated with angina and are at risk of sudden death [351, 352] (➲Fig. 17.34). The causes of the individual susceptibility to ventricular tachyarrhythmias are poorly known, but there is no strict relationship with the severity of ischaemic episodes. Severe bradyarrhythmias (sinus arrest, atrioventricular block) may also occur, in particular in patients with inferior transmural ischaemia. Prolonged, unrelieved occlusive spasm, on the other hand, may result in acute MI.

Despite the usual typical angina picture, variant angina is often underdiagnosed, with and consequent potential risks associated with transmural ischaemia. In a recent study, indeed, a definite clinical diagnosis of variant angina was achieved within 1 month of symptom onset only in less than a half of 202 consecutive patients, whereas more than 3 months was required in 32% [350].

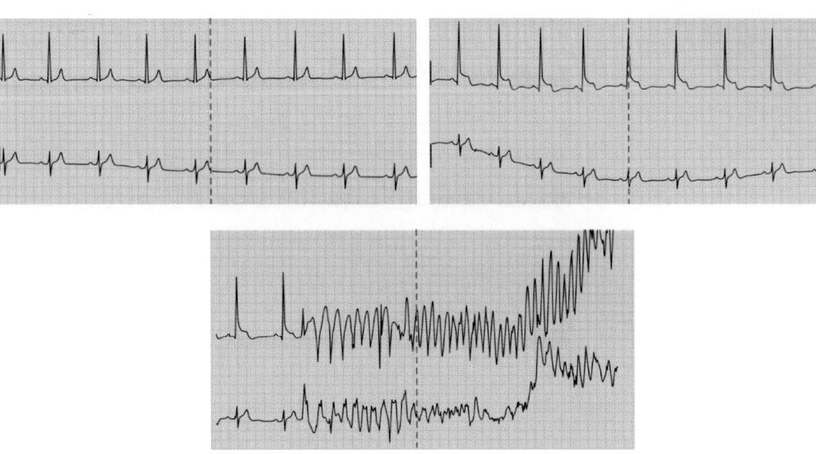

Figure 17.34 Episode of polymorphic ventricular tachycardia degenerated into ventricular fibrillation and cardiac arrest during an episode of transmural ischaemia started 3min before the arrhythmic event (non-continuous strips). This episode was recorded during long-term ECG monitoring by an external event loop-recorder in a patient with a history of undiagnosed pre-syncopal episodes. Prompt BLS by bystanders allowed saving life to the patient who underwent ventricular defibrillation after about 20min from the event. Coronary angiography showed normal coronary arteries with coronary spasm induced by intracoronary ergonovine administration.

Diagnosis

The clinical diagnosis of variant angina can be confirmed by the documentation of transient ST-segment elevation (≥1mm and up to 20–30mm) on the standard ECG during an anginal attack (➲Figs. 17.33 and 17.34). When it is difficult to record standard ECG during a chest pain episode, variant angina can be usually diagnosed by 24–48-hour ambulatory ECG monitoring, which allows also to assess the total ischaemic burden and the daily distribution of ischaemic episodes, most of which are silent [353]. ECG-EST can allow the diagnosis of vasospastic angina in a minority of patients by inducing reversible ST-segment elevation during or in the recovery phase of exercise.

Of note, the pre-test assumption of short-acting nitrates typically prevents exercise induced angina and ST-segment changes, in particular in patients without significant obstructive CAD lesions, whereas it hardly totally abolishes ischaemic changes when they are related to severe proximal stenosis of a coronary artery.

In about 10% of patients a provocative test of coronary artery spasm is necessary to confirm the diagnosis. Provocative tests of spasm can be performed either non invasively or during coronary angiography and are diagnostic when they induce anginal symptoms with typical ST-segment elevation. Non invasive tests are done mainly by administration of intravenous ergonovine, under careful clinical and ECG monitoring. As an alternative, hyperventilation test can be used, although it has a lower sensitivity.

Invasive provocative tests of spasm are usually performed by intracoronary infusion of ergonovine or acetylcholine during angiography. Advantages of invasive tests include the direct documention of coronary artery spasm and assessment of coronary anatomy. The invasive procedure is warranted in patients in whom use of systemic provocative tests of coronary spasm are associated with increased risk of refractory spasm (e.g. prolonged angina, delayed response to short-acting nitrates), as it allows direct intracoronary injection of vasodilator drugs (nitrates, calcium-channel blockers). Non invasive tests, on the other hand, can be repeated more easily to assess the effects of medication and changes in susceptibility to spasm during follow-up.

Prognosis

In early studies prognosis of variant angina was found to mainly depend on the presence of multivessel IHD [354]. Subsequent studies, however, showed that sudden death and cardiac arrest, as well as acute MI, may occur also in patients with normal or near-normal epicardial arteries [355, 356]. High risk includes multivessel spasm, severe ischaemia-related brady- or tachyarrhythmias, prolonged spasm, in particular when not promptly responding to nitrates, and, finally, spasm refractory to high doses of calcium-antagonists.

Importantly, prognosis of variant angina is strictly dependent on the time of diagnosis. Indeed, most events occur within days or months of symptom onset. Thus a prompt diagnosis is mandatory, even because initiation of medical vasodilator therapy is able to effectively prevent recurrence of spasm, thus reducing major coronary events and, therefore, significantly improving long-term prognosis in these patients [355].

Treatment

Chronic preventive treatment of variant angina is based mainly on the use of calcium-channel blockers. Usual average doses (e.g. 240–360mg/day of verapamil or diltiazem, 60–80mg/day of nifedipine) prevent spasm in about 90% of patients (➲Fig. 17.35). Long-acting nitrates (isosorbide dinitrate 20–40mg, or isosorbide mononitrate 10-20mg, both twice a day) can be added in some patients to improve the efficacy of treatment, and should be scheduled to cover

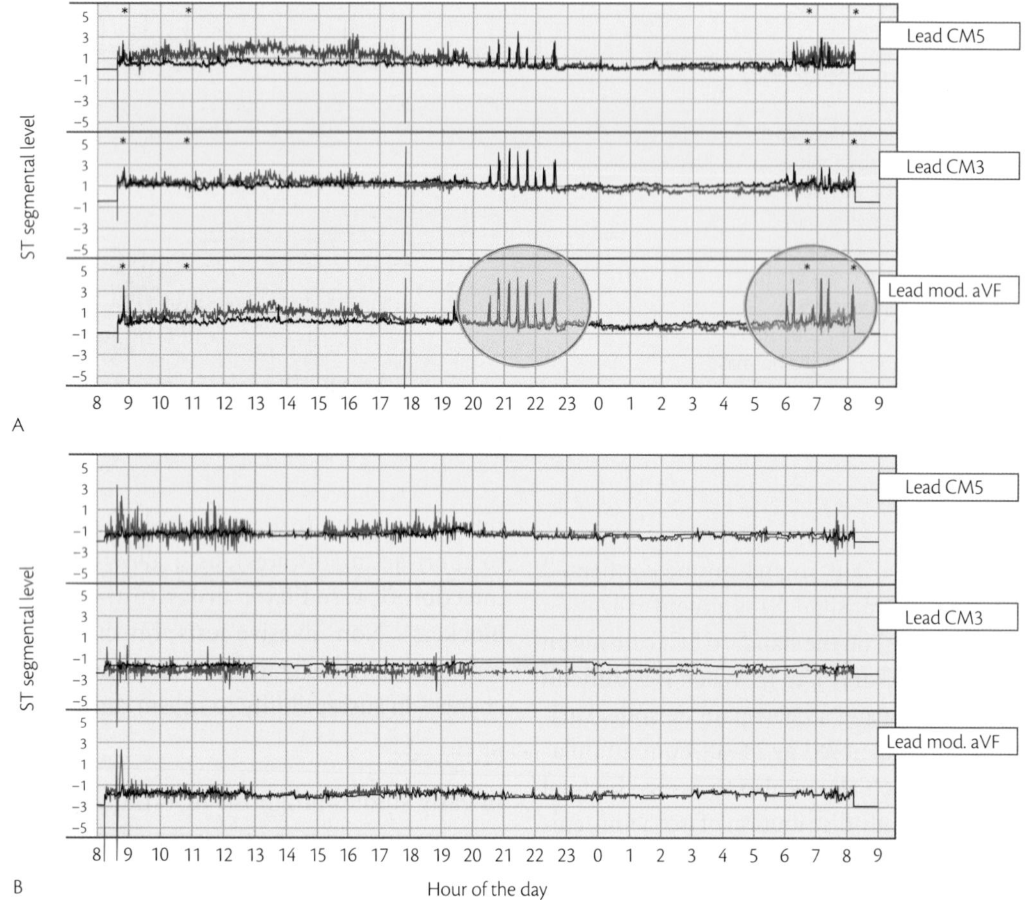

Figure 17.35 ST-segment trends of 24-hour 3-channel ambulatory ECG recordings (leads CM5-CM3-modified aVF) in a patient with a history of chest pain at rest lasting for 3 months. The blue lines indicate the ST-segment level, whereas the green lines indicate the ST segment slope. (A) Several short lasting episodes (n = 16) of ST-segment elevation can be observed, most typically grouped in clusters in the evening hours and in the early morning hours (red circles). (B) No episodes of ST-segment elevation are observed in the same patient 3 days after starting drug treatment with diltiazem 120mg TID.

the period of the day in which ischaemic episodes occur most frequently, in order to prevent nitrate tolerance. Beta-blockers are not indicated and should rather be avoided as they might favour spasm by leaving alpha-mediated vasoconstriction unopposed by beta-mediated vasodilation.

In about 10% of cases coronary artery spasm may be refractory to standard vasodilator therapy, although refractoriness is usually limited to brief periods in most patients. Use of very high doses of calcium-antagonists and nitrates (i.e. diltiazem 960mg/day, or verapamil 800mg/day, each associated with nifedipine 100mg and ISDN 80mg) usually control angina attacks in these periods. In the very rare cases in which this treatment is insufficient, the addition of the anti-adrenergic drugs guanethidine or clonidine might be helpful. Possible benefits have also been suggested from the use of anti-oxidant agents and of statins [356]. PCI with stent implantation at the site of spasm (even in the absence of significant stenosis) has also been reported to facilitate control of symptoms and efficacy of drug therapy in these patients [357]. Finally, implantation of an automatic cardioverter defibrillator or a pacemaker is indicated in patients with spasm-related life-threatening tachyarrhythmias or bradyarrhythmias, respectively, when coronary spasm presents a poor or uncertain response to medical therapy.

Ischaemic cardiomyopathy

In a number of cases the clinical picture of chronic stable IHD is dominated by symptoms and signs of left ventricular dysfunction, a condition defined as ischaemic cardiomyopathy [358]. Ischaemic cardiomyopathy constitutes the most common form of heart failure in developed countries accounting for two-thirds to three-quarters of cases of dilated cardiomyopathy.

Pathogenesis

Ischaemic cardiomyopathy can result from a single large infarction (usually >20% of myocardial mass) or from multiple smaller infarctions [359], followed by progressive ventricular dilatation and dysfunction, which may develop in a number of years. The reasons why for a similar extent of MI some patients, but not others, develop severe myocardial dysfunction are still largely debated [360].

Notably, in some cases ischaemic cardiomyopathy is the initial manifestation of IHD. The mechanisms responsible for ischaemic cardiomyopathy in these cases are not always clear. Some of these patients may have suffered from one or more silent MI, revealed by pathologic Q waves on a routine ECG. In other patients, however, there is no evidence of previous MI in clinical history as well as on the ECG and on imaging tests. Chronic ischaemic damage with progressive slow loss of cardiomyocyte, possibly involving multiple mechanisms, including focal necrosis, apoptosis [64], or even superimposed inflammation [361], is a plausible explanation.

In the GISSI-2 study, signs of cardiac failure at 6 months after a first MI were present in 9% of 9860 patients who received thrombolysis [362]. However, the growing survival rate after a first MI in the modern era of early coronary reperfusion and intensive effective medical therapy exposes patients to a progressive worsening of the underlying IHD thus increasing the risk of evolution towards left ventricular failure. Concomitant stable angina can be present in some of these patients.

Clinical presentation and diagnosis

Symptoms of left ventricular dysfunction typically include dyspnoea on effort, paroxysmal nocturnal dyspnoea, fatigue, weight gain, and reduced urinary output. Physical examination may reveal signs of heart failure, including a reduced first heart sound, presence of a third sound, ankle oedema, and pulmonary rales. A systolic murmur can be present when mitral regurgitation occurs as a consequence of left ventricular dilation or papillary muscle dysfunction.

Echocardiography shows left ventricular dilatation and reduced ejection fraction, with frequent diastolic dysfunction. Coronary angiography usually exhibits multivessel coronary artery disease. In some patients the extent and severity of coronary atherosclerosis is much less than predicted by left ventricular dysfunction, thus suggesting that the latter could mainly be caused, in fact, by a primary myocardial disease, such as myocarditis [361].

In patients with ischaemic cardiomyopathy it is important to establish the presence and extent of hibernated myocardium. Noninvasive imaging methods to assess myocardial metabolic activity, membrane integrity, and inotropic reserve are ideally suited for this assessment. Indeed, nuclear techniques allow to identify viable but dysfunctional myocardial regions, as viable myocardial fibres have intact cell membranes which take up specific labelled tracers like thallium (used with SPECT) or fluorodeoxyglucose (used with PET), while dobutamine echocardiography identifies regional inotropic reserve and contrast echocardiography allows to assess microvascular integrity. Contrast-enhanced cardiac CMR, on the other hand, is emerging as an important method for viability assessment. The relative merits of nuclear techniques, echocardiography and CMR for myocardial viability assessment are summarized in ➲Table 17.19. Cost, availability, and local expertise will always affect, however, the choice of a given diagnostic approach [363].

The assessment of myocardial viability has relevant therapeutic and prognostic implications, as myocardial revascularization seems to improve symptoms and perhaps prognosis in patients exhibiting viability of several hibernated myocardial regions, but not in patients without evidence of myocardial hibernation [364].

Prognosis

Ischaemic cardiomyopathy is associated with a poor outcome, compared to that of stable IHD without severe impairment of left ventricular function, and is also associated with a worse outcome compared with non ischaemic forms of dilated cardiomyopathy [365]. The reasons for the worse clinical outcome include higher risks of: 1) life-threatening ventricular arrhythmias; 2) severe left ventricular dysfunction during recurrence of ischaemia or a new MI; 3) potentially fatal systemic complications; and 4) iatrogenic complications due to use of multidrug therapy and of implantable devices.

Treatment

Management of heart failure is treated in detail in Chapter 23. If tolerated and in the absence of contraindications, typical drug therapy includes beta-blockers (mainly carvedilol), ACE-inhibitors (or ARBs). Spironolactone should also be considered in patients with creatinine levels <2.5mg/dL and serum potassium levels <5.5mmol/L. Furosemide or thiazide diuretics are indicated in patients with symptoms and/or signs of congestion, whereas digoxin can be considered in case of atrial fibrillation associated with high heart rate and/or symptoms. When antiarrhythmic treatment is needed for symptomatic supraventricular or ventricular tachyarrhythmias, amiodarone should be the drug of choice, whereas oral anticoagulant therapy should be added in patients with atrial fibrillation/flutter or documentation of intracardiac thrombus formation.

In IHD patients with dilated cardiomyopathy and significant impairment of systolic left ventricular function, clinical outcome can be improved by implantation of an automated cardiac defibrillator [366]; however, efforts to identify patients with higher risk of sudden death is

Table 17.19 Non-invasive techniques for the assessment of myocardial viability

Test	Advantages	Limitations
SPECT imaging	◆ High sensitivity ◆ Possibility of FDG imaging ◆ Quantitation of LV function ◆ Predictive of clinical outcome	◆ Areas of attenuation as non-viability ◆ Impossibility to differentiate endocardial and epicardial viability ◆ No absolute measure of blood flow ◆ Less specific than dobutamine echocardiography and less sensitive than PET
PET imaging	◆ Absolute quantification of myocardial blood flow and glucose utilization ◆ In conjunction with euglycaemic clamp allows inter-individuals and inter-centres comparison of glucose uptake ◆ More sensitive than other techniques ◆ No attenuation problem ◆ Predictive of outcome	◆ Less specific than dobutamine echocardiography and CMR ◆ Not ideal to differentiate endocardial and epicardial viability ◆ High cost and limited availability
Dobutamine echocardiography	◆ Higher specificity than nuclear techniques ◆ Assessment of both viability and ischaemia ◆ Assessment of LV function ◆ Predictive of outcome ◆ Low cost, wide availability	◆ Poor acoustic window in some patients ◆ Lower sensitivity than nuclear tests ◆ More operator-dependent
Contrast echocardiography	◆ Simultaneous assessment of microvascular integrity and systolic thickening ◆ Better examination of extent of viability than echocardiography ◆ Possibility to discriminate subendocardial from subepicardial perfusion	◆ Poor acoustic window in some patients ◆ Attenuation problems
Contrast CMR	◆ Accurate measurement of wall thickness ◆ Assessment of microvascular integrity ◆ Assessment of transmural extent of myocardial necrosis ◆ Good sensitivity and specificity for viability detection	◆ Need for faster automated techniques ◆ Information not in real time ◆ Patients with pace-maker or defibrillator* or claustrophobic cannot be studied ◆ High cost, limited availability

[18] FDG, fluorodeoxyglucose;CMR, cardiac magnetic resonance; LV left ventricular; PET, positron emission tomography; SPECT, single-photon emission computed tomography.

* Recent data, however, suggest that patients with electronic devices, including pacemakers, defibrillators and neurostimulators, can be studied by CMR without any significant increase in adverse events.

warranted, due to the high cost of the device and the non infrequent side effects (including inappropriate discharge) that can worsen patients' quality of life [367]. Predictors of sudden death include ventricular arrhythmias, late potentials on signal-averaged ECG, and, finally, depressed heart rate variability [368], heart rate turbulence [369] and baroreflex sensitivity [370], all expressions of an impairment of cardiac sympatho-vagal imbalance. However, the clinical relevance of predictors of sudden death different of ejection fraction is still uncertain.

In patients who remain symptomatic despite optimal medical therapy and have LVEF ≤30–40% and wide QRS (>130ms) due to left bundle branch block, biventricular pacing can improve both symptoms and survival [371], although about one third of patients do not respond to treatment [372].

The possibility that myocardial regeneration by stem cell therapy may improve left ventricular function and prognosis in these patients is a great hope for both patients and physicians, but these forms of treatment have until now given disappointing results and, therefore, need further

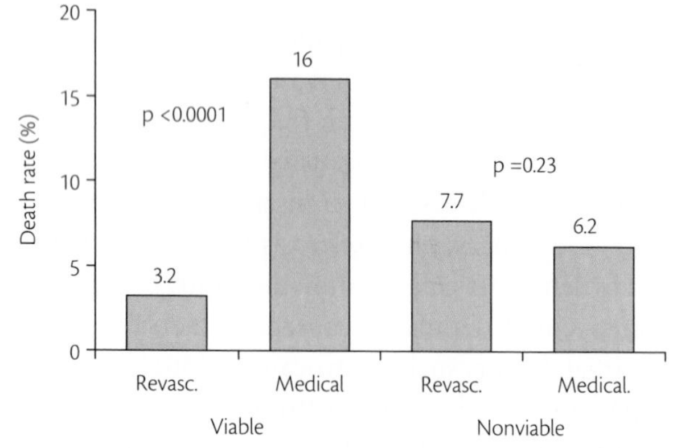

Figure 17.36 Systematic review of trials comparing coronary bypass surgery and medical treatment in patients with ischaemic cardiomyopathy. Bypass surgery was associated with a significant reduction in mortality in patients with myocardial variability, but not in those without evidence of myocardial viability, compared to medical therapy. Adapted with permission from Allman KC, Shaw LJ, Hachamovitch R, *et al.* Myocardial viability testing and impact of revascularization on prognosis in patients with coronary artery disease and left ventricular dysfunction: a meta-analysis. *J Am Coll Cardiol* 2002; **39**: 1151–8.

refinement and assessment before they can appear on the routine clinical scene.

Retrospective or registry studies suggest that coronary revascularization by CABG may improve long-term survival of patients with ischaemic cardiomyopathy who present evidence of large areas of viable myocardium, whereas it does not seem to improve clinical outcome when performed in the absence of evidence of significant areas of myocardial variability (➲ Fig. 17.36) [373]. Myocardial viability can be assessed by echocardiography, scintigraphy, PET or CMR, as recently extensively reviewed [374]. Caution, however, is required in accepting these findings as they do not derive from randomized controlled studies [364]. Whether coronary revascularization by PCI may achieve results similar to those suggested for CABG is also not well established.

Personal perspective

Chronic IHD is mainly characterized by four clinical presentations, i.e. stable angina, microvascular angina, vasospastic angina, and ischaemic cardiomyopathy. Although the improvements in our management of patients with chronic IHD over the past few decades have been impressive, the challenges we still face are enormous and different for these different presentations. In stable angina risk stratification is still imperfect; it is mainly based on the measurement of left ventricular function and of myocardium at risk of ischaemia. Although this is an acceptable initial approximation, it would be more cost-effective to identify those patients who harbour unstable coronary plaques, before the latter cause an acute coronary syndrome. In order to achieve this ambitious goal, it is necessary to improve our limited knowledge of the mechanisms responsible for the transition from coronary stability to instability. With regard to treatment aimed at improving prognosis, every endeavour should be made to ensure that measures and treatments known to reduce the burden of coronary risk factors are put into clinical practice. Unfortunately, the most recent surveys indicate that such preventive measures are still widely underutilized leaving considerable room for improvement. In particular, our ability to modify lifestyle is still remarkably limited, as witnessed by the pandemics of 'diabesity' (diabetes and obesity). Important technological advances in percutaneous and surgical myocardial revascularization will probably be obtained. In particular, efforts will be needed to further reduce the risk of restenosis which remains elevated even after the introduction of drug eluting stents. Efforts will also be needed to increase the utilization of arterial conduits in patients undergoing coronary bypass surgery. Such improvements will probably be more important for improving symptoms and quality of life, rather than for reducing the risk of major cardiovascular events. The increasing number of patients with refractory angina in whom myocardial revascularization is not feasible, however, remains a reason of concern also because their life expectancy is progressively increasing. It would be desirable to develop new forms of treatment for refractory angina, including new drugs, new interventions able to modulate the central processing of painful stimuli, and the utilization of stem cells. These considerations also apply to patients with microvascular angina who frequently present disabling symptoms, unresponsive to conventional anti-anginal drugs. In patients with vasospastic angina it would be desirable to improve our limited knowledge of the causes of smooth muscle cell hyper-reactivity responsible for coronary artery spasm, in order to develop more efficient forms of treatment in those refractory to standard medical vasodilator treatment. In patients with ischaemic cardiomyopathy it would be desirable to better identify patients in whom outcome is improved by myocardial revascularization. Indeed, current information is based on uncontrolled studies carried out before the implementation of drugs and devices currently utilized in the management of patients with heart failure. Finally, it will be extremely important to implement effective preventive measures before coronary atherosclerotic plaques and microvascular dysfunction become severe enough to cause symptoms.

Further reading

Babapulle MN, Joseph L, Belisle P, *et al.* A hierarchical Bayesian meta-analysis of randomised clinical trials of drug-eluting stents. *Lancet* 2004; **364**: 583–91.

Camici PG, Crea F. Coronary microvascular dysfunction. *N Engl J Med* 2007; **356**: 830–40.

Fox K, Garcia MA, Ardissino D, *et al.* Guidelines on the management of stable angina pectoris: executive summary: The Task Force on the Management of Stable Angina Pectoris of the European Society of Cardiology. *Eur Heart J* 2006; **27**: 1341–81.

Fourth Joint Task Force of the European Society of Cardiology and Other Societies on Cardiovascular Disease Prevention in Clinical Practice (Constituted by representatives of nine societies and by invited experts) European guidelines on cardiovascular disease prevention in clinical practice: executive summary. *Eur Heart J* 2007; **28**: 2375–414.

Freemantle N, Cleland J, Young P, *et al.* Beta-blockade after myocardial infarction: systematic review and meta regression analysis. *BMJ* 1999; **318**: 1730–7.

Lanza GA. Cardiac syndrome X: a critical overview and future perspectives. *Heart* 2007; **93**: 159–66.

Marazia S, Barnabei L, De Caterina R. Receiver operating characteristic (ROC) curves and the definition of threshold levels to diagnose coronary artery disease on electrocardiographic stress testing. Part II: the use of ROC curves in the choice of electrocardiographic stress test markers of ischaemia. *J Cardiovasc Med (Hagerstown)* 2008; **9**: 22–31.

Yusuf S, Zucker D, Peduzzi P, *et al.* Effect of coronary artery bypass graft surgery on survival: overview of 10-year results from randomised trials by the Coronary Artery Bypass Graft Surgery Trialists Collaboration. *Lancet* 1994; **344**: 563–70.

Additional online material

17.1 Reflow. Myocardial contrast echocardiography study. A) An example of a complete and homogeneous intramyocardial reflow.

17.2 No Reflow. Myocardial contrast echocardiography study. B) The transmural myocardial black apical zone is a no-reflow area appearing in this patient with acute myocardial infarction treated by primary PCI.

For full references and multimedia materials please visit the online version of the book (http://esctextbook.oxfordonline.com).

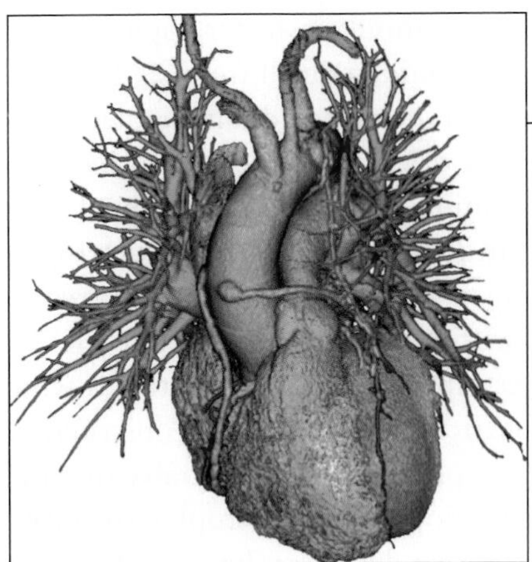

CHAPTER 18

Myocardial Disease

Otto M. Hess, William McKenna, and Heinz-Peter Schultheiss

Contents

Summary

Diseases of the myocardium are common and extend from primary forms (cardiomyopathies) to the secondary forms such as hypertensive heart disease, alcoholic cardiomyopathy, Takotsubo cardiomyopathy, and more rare forms of secondary myocardial disease such as muscular dystrophy cardiomyopathy or peripartum cardiomyopathy. The primary forms are typically genetically transmitted, whereas secondary myocardial diseases are mostly acquired. Secondary forms may also have a genetic background, which favours the development of secondary myocardial disease. A special form of myocardial disease represents inflammatory diseases of the myocardium such as myocarditis or viral cardiomyopathy.

A variant of the whole spectrum represents hypertrophic cardiomyopathy, which is—in contrast to other cardiomyopathies—associated with normal or supranormal myocardial function. The haemodynamic characteristics of this form of cardiomyopathy are: 1) the presence of systolic obstruction of the outflow tract; and 2) the existence of diastolic dysfunction. Most other forms show a reduction in systolic ejection performance (= systolic dysfunction).

Management of primary myocardial disease includes heart failure therapy in dilated cardiomyopathy, alcohol ablation of the septum in hypertrophic cardiomyopathy, defibrillator therapy in arrhythmogenic cardiomyopathy, immunomodulatory treatment in myocarditis or viral cardiomyopathy, and ultimately heart transplantation in end-stage myocardial disease.

Management of secondary myocardial disease is mainly linked to an identifiable source of myocardial dysfunction such as hypertension, diabetes, or excess alcohol consumption. A new form of secondary myocardial disease is Takotsubo cardiomyopathy, which shows a good prognosis over the short and mid-term follow-up and is thought to be due to excessive catecholamine exposure with coronary artery vasospasms.

Definition and classification

Primary myocardial diseases are described as cardiomyopathies. These are defined as disease of the myocardium associated with cardiac dysfunction. They are divided into five different groups (➲Fig. 18.1).

Inflammatory myocardial disease is defined as inflammation of the myocardium and its structures caused by infectious and non-infectious agents. The inflammation may involve the myocytes, interstitium, vessels, and/or pericardium. However, inflammation of the endocardium (endocarditis) is a disease on its own and is described in ➲Chapter 22.

Secondary myocardial diseases are defined as disease of the myocardium of known origin. There are nine subgroups:

- ischaemic cardiomyopathy;
- hypertensive cardiomyopathy;
- valvular cardiomyopathy;
- alcoholic cardiomyopathy;
- metabolic cardiomyopathy;
- Takotsubo cardiomyopathy;
- tachycardiomyopathy;
- muscular dystrophy cardiomyopathy;
- peripartum cardiomyopathy.

Primary myocardial disease (cardiomyopathies)

Hypertrophic cardiomyopathy

Definition, aetiology, and prevalence

The first account of hypertrophic cardiomyopathy (HCM) dates back to Donald Teare in 1958 who reported a common finding of asymmetric hypertrophy in the hearts of nine victims of sudden death from six families. Histological assessment of the myocardium revealed muscle bundles in different orientations separated by connective tissue. This seminal case series highlighted four cardinal features of the disease: unexplained hypertrophy of the left ventricle, myocyte disarray, familial occurrence, and an association with sudden cardiac death (SCD). The pathological description coincided with growing awareness of left ventricular outflow tract obstruction (LVOTO) in young people without aortic valve disease, an entity then termed 'idiopathic hypertrophic subaortic stenosis'. Over the next two decades it became clear that neither the asymmetric distribution nor the presence of obstruction was necessary for a diagnosis of HCM; concentric, apical, and eccentric patterns of hypertrophy are well recognized, while LVOTO has both clinical and prognostic importance but is present in less than one-quarter of these patients.

Genetics

A milestone in the understanding of HCM came with the identification of mutations in the cardiac β-myosin heavy chain gene [1] (see ➲Chapter 9). Later, other sarcomeric proteins were implicated in HCM, including α-tropomyosin, cardiac troponin T, troponin I, myosin-binding protein C, regulatory myosin light chain, essential myosin light chain, cardiac actin, titin, cardiac α-myosin heavy chain, and troponin C. This led to the concept that HCM is a disease of the sarcomere, the contractile apparatus of the cell. Analysis of genotype–phenotype correlations demonstrated that hypertrophy is not essential for diagnosis, e.g. mutations in troponin T may be associated with subtle or no hypertrophy but a high incidence of SCD [2]. This established the view of HCM as an inherited heart muscle disorder caused by mutations in sarcomeric proteins, resulting in myocyte disarray, with or without fibrosis, myocardial hypertrophy and small-vessel disease (narrowing of intramural coronary arteries by

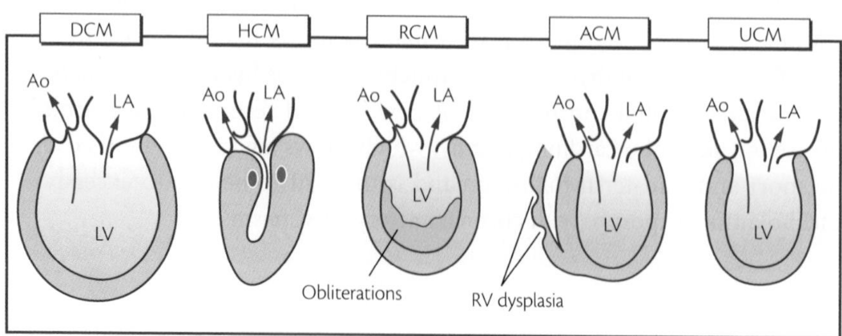

Figure 18.1 Classification of cardiomyopathies based on a report of the World Health Organization and International Society and Federation of Cardiology [38]. DCM, dilated cardiomyopathy; HCM, hypertrophic cardiomyopathy; RCM, restrictive cardiomyopathy; ACM, arrhythmic cardiomyopathy; UCM, unclassified cardiomyopathy.

medial thickening). The most common pattern of inheritance is autosomal dominant. Penetrance is incomplete and age-related: 55% for those aged 10–29 years, 75% for those aged 30–49, and 95% in gene carriers over the age of 50 [3].

Phenocopies

Recently, attention has focused on non-sarcomeric variants of HCM, termed 'phenocopies'. The prevalence of HCM in the adult population is estimated at 1 in 500. However, only about 60% of adults with HCM have mutations in sarcomeric genes. A small proportion of the remainder may have unknown defects in components of the sarcomere, but this is unlikely to fully account for the discrepancy. Indeed, the majority of young children with left ventricular hypertrophy (LVH) do not have sarcomeric disease but rather metabolic disorders, mitochondrial cytopathies, and syndromes with characteristic extracardiac features, disease states that may exist in adults with apparent HCM. Routine measurement of plasma α-galactosidase A levels among adult male HCM patients demonstrated a 4% prevalence of previously undiagnosed Anderson–Fabry disease [4]. Similarly, Danon disease, another X-linked lysosomal defect, was identified in 1% of HCM index cases by DNA testing [5].

Timely detection of cardiac phenocopies of HCM is important. First, the cardiac profile is frequently distinct from that of sarcomeric HCM, with an increased incidence of conduction disease and progression to cavity dilation and heart failure. Management of these disorders also requires vigilance for extracardiac complications, such as skeletal myopathy, renal impairment and neurological involvement. Furthermore, specific therapies such as enzyme replacement in Fabry disease may alter the natural history of the disease. Finally, recognition of recessive, X-linked and mitochondrial patterns of inheritance has major implications for familial assessment.

Towards a unifying hypothesis for the pathogenesis of HCM

The clinical, pathological and genetic diversity of HCM therefore precludes a comprehensive definition. LVH may be subclinical; myocyte disarray is present in Noonan syndrome and Friedreich's ataxia but otherwise rare among the phenocopies; and a broad spectrum of genetic defects can give rise to HCM (➲Table 18.1).

That a single unifying mechanism may underlie sarcomeric HCM and the cardiac phenocopies is an attractive concept. One of the first attempts to define the primary dysfunction in HCM was the contractile deficit hypothesis [6]. It was suggested that the various sarcomeric mutations result in diminished contractility of cardiac myocytes. This in turn leads to increased cell stress, which induces production of trophic and mitotic factors that ultimately cause hypertrophy, myocyte disarray, and fibrosis. Cytoskeletal function is impaired in dilated cardiomyopathy and after myocardial infarction, but preserved in HCM, accounting for the absence of cavity dilation in the latter. Early supporting evidence came primarily from *in vitro* studies demonstrating reduced contractility of cells expressing β-myosin heavy chain and troponin T mutations [7, 8]. Conversely, several mutations in β-myosin heavy chain are associated with enhanced enzymatic and mechanical properties [9], troponin T mutants show enhanced thin filament motility [10, 11], and mutant α-tropomyosin may allow increased force output at submaximal calcium concentrations [12]. Non-sarcomeric HCM is also less easily explained on the basis of diminished contractile performance.

More recently, Ashrafian *et al.* [13] have postulated a central role for compromised cellular energetics in the development of HCM and related phenotypes. The energy deficit may result from an aberration at any point along the pathway of ATP synthesis, transfer, regulation, and expenditure.

- Abnormalities in the handling of glycogen (e.g. phosphorylase B kinase deficiency), glucose or fatty acids (e.g. CD36 and carnitine deficiencies) reduce the substrate available for ATP production.
- The mitochondrial cytopathies and Friedreich's ataxia may interfere with ATP synthesis [14].
- Senger syndrome, characterized by HCM, congenital cataracts, and lactic acidosis, is associated with low activity of mitochondrial adenine nucleotide translocator 1, responsible for ATP transport out of the mitochondria.
- Mutations in AMP-activated protein kinase, the cellular fuel gauge, have been linked to HCM with pre-excitation, conduction system disease, and a propensity towards early cavity dilation and systolic impairment [15].
- Emerging data suggest that lysosomal storage of glycosphingolipids in Fabry disease may cause reduced activity of respiratory chain enzymes [16].
- The sarcomeric mutations have differing effects on contractility, but inefficient ATP utilization is a shared consequence.

Finally, the cellular energy deficit impairs the functioning of the sarcoplasmic reticulum calcium reuptake pump.

Table 18.1 Disease-causing genes in hypertrophic cardiomyopathy (HCM) and phenocopies

Sarcomeric mutations (?ineffective ATP utilization)
β-Myosin heavy chain
α-Tropomyosin
Troponin T
Troponin I
Myosin-binding protein C
Regulatory myosin light chain
Essential myosin light chain
Cardiac actin
Titin
α-Cardiac myosin heavy chain
Troponin C
Metabolic diseases
?Reduced substrate for ATP synthesis
Glycogen storage diseases
Phosphorylase B kinase deficiency
CD36 and carnitine deficiencies
?Reduced activity of respiratory chain enzymes
Anderson–Fabry disease
?Impaired regulation of ATP
AMP kinase
Other
Danon disease (LAMP-2 mutation)
Mitochondrial cytopathies
?Interference with ATP synthesis
MELAS, MERRF, LHON
Friedreich's ataxia (deficiency of frataxin, a key activator of mitochondrial energy conversion)
?Interference with ATP transport
Senger's syndrome
Syndromic HCM
Tyrosine phosphatase (Noonan and LEOPARD syndromes)

LEOPARD, *l*entigines, *e*lectrocardiogram abnormalities, *o*cular hypertelorism, *p*ulmonary stenosis, *a*bnormalities of the genitalia, *r*etardation of growth, and *d*eafness; LHON, Leber's hereditary optic neuropathy; MELAS, mitochondrial encephalomyopathy, lactic acidosis, stroke-like episodes; MERRF, myoclonic epilepsy and ragged red fibres.

The prolonged cytosolic calcium transient may serve as the signal that triggers cellular hypertrophy, although the exact pathway remains to be unravelled. Indeed, genetic defects that produce an HCM-like phenotype by an unknown mechanism may turn out to be components of the downstream signalling pathway. An example is tyrosine phosphatase non-receptor-type II protein, which has been implicated in both Noonan syndrome and LEOPARD syndrome (*l*entigines, *e*lectrocardiogram abnormalities, *o*cular hypertelorism, *p*ulmonary stenosis, *a*bnormalities of the genitalia, *r*etardation of growth, and *d*eafness).

The energy depletion hypothesis represents an attempt to reconcile the contrasting effects of the sarcomeric mutations on cellular contractility, and additionally succeeds in accounting for many of the cardiac phenocopies of HCM. Supporting evidence is emerging; magnetic resonance spectroscopy of mutations in β-myosin heavy chain, troponin T, and myosin-binding protein C found significant reductions in the cardiac phosphocreatine to ATP ratio, an indicator of myocardial energy status [17]. Energetic abnormalities are also observed in ischaemic heart disease and heart failure, and have been considered a consequence of hypertrophy rather than the primary defect. However, the presence of the bioenergetic deficit in non-penetrant gene carriers without hypertrophy argues against a secondary phenomenon [18]. Nevertheless, the value of any unifying paradigm is contingent on its relevance in the clinical arena. Grouping the sarcomeric mutations together remains meaningful owing to similarities in clinical presentation, risk stratification and management. Accordingly, validation of the energy depletion hypothesis awaits diagnostic and therapeutic applications. From a clinical standpoint, many disorders associated with unexplained hypertrophy have little in common with sarcomeric HCM, and are more usefully approached as distinct disease entities.

Pathophysiology

The main functional consequences of HCM are as follows.

Diastolic dysfunction

Both the active and passive phases of diastole are abnormal in HCM. Isovolumetric relaxation in early diastole requires energy-dependent calcium uptake in the sarcoplasmic reticulum and is prolonged in HCM. Myocyte disarray, cellular energy deficit and altered affinity of mutant sarcomeric proteins for Ca^{2+} are all potential factors. Increased pressures are a corollary of ventricular filling prior to completion of active relaxation. Subendocardial ischaemia is both a contributor to diastolic dysfunction and a consequence of it, since the delay in pressure decay may result in diminished endocardial coronary blood flow.

Passive relaxation during ventricular filling in late diastole is determined by compliance. Both hypertrophy and interstitial fibrosis cause increased chamber stiffness in HCM, again resulting in increased filling pressures and reduced coronary blood flow.

Limited exercise capacity is common in HCM. Decreased time for filling at high heart rates, combined with impaired compliance, leads to a reduction in end-diastolic volume.

This limits the ability of the left ventricle to augment stroke volume via the Frank–Starling mechanism. Chronotropic incompetence is common in HCM.

Ischaemia

Reduced coronary flow reserve is well recognized in HCM; baseline coronary velocity is elevated compared with normal subjects, while velocities during hyperaemia are similar [18]. Systolic extravascular compression may play a role but does not wholly account for the deficiency, since the diastolic coronary vasodilator reserve is also diminished [19]. Changes in the coronary microcirculation have been implicated: arteriolar lumen area is smaller and capillary density is less, both parameters showing an inverse relationship with LVH [18]. Increased coronary conductance is thought to be related to higher oxygen demands of LVH. However, vascular medial hypertrophy and lack of capillary growth preclude increments in coronary conductance during hyperaemia.

Left ventricular outflow tract obstruction

LVOTO, once the defining feature, is present in around 25% of HCM. Obstruction may also occur at mid-cavity level, or distally in the form of apical obliteration. Subaortic LVOTO, with systolic anterior movement (SAM) of the mitral valve, is the commonest form and the most amenable to treatment.

Mechanism of SAM

Current thinking dictates that two conditions facilitate SAM: 1) abnormal valve apparatus with sufficient slack in the leaflets to allow movement; and 2) a haemodynamic force with an anterior component during systole.

Primary structural abnormalities of the mitral valve apparatus have been observed in patients with obstructive HCM, the most important of which is anterior displacement of the papillary muscles (➲Fig. 18.2) [20]. This predisposes to SAM by: 1) reducing the posterior tension conferred by the papillary muscles on the mitral valve; 2) increasing the proximity of the leaflets to the left ventricular (LV) outflow stream; and 3) pulling the posterior leaflet upwards so that it meets the anterior leaflet near its mid-portion, thereby leaving a long portion of the distal leaflet unrestrained and susceptible to anterior forces. Incomplete coaptation of the leaflets also results in posteriorly directed mitral regurgitation. A central or anterior mitral regurgitant jet raises suspicion of intrinsic mitral valve disease.

The nature of the haemodynamic force has been subject to much debate [21]. Originally, SAM was thought to be due to the Venturi effect, which refers to the increase in velocity and concomitant decrease in pressure that occurs as fluid flows through a constriction. An object in the path of the fluid is subject to a force perpendicular to the direction of flow that pulls it into the stream. Thus, as blood is ejected into the narrow outflow tract in systole, it accelerates and a reduction in the static pressure occurs. The pressure difference thereby created pulls the mitral valve leaflet towards the septum.

Alternatively, the flow drag effect, i.e. the force exerted by a fluid in the direction of flow, may be involved. Thus, blood ejected into the LVOT pushes the free residual leaflet anteriorly. Doppler echocardiography suggests that SAM begins very early in systole, when the outflow tract velocity is normal [20]. The relatively low velocity is unlikely to generate significant Venturi forces; conversely, there will be increased contact of the flowing blood with the valve, augmenting the drag effect. Recently, it has been shown that reduction in septal thickness by alcohol ablation is associated with a decrease in LVOT and a disappearance of SAM and accompanying mitral regurgitation [30].

Abnormal vascular responses

In normal subjects, cardiac output rises during exercise. At high heart rates, filling time is reduced and augmentation of LV end-diastolic volume requires increased venous return. This is dependent on constriction in non-exercising venous capacitance beds, which compensates for the vasodilation occurring in exercising muscle. The importance of this

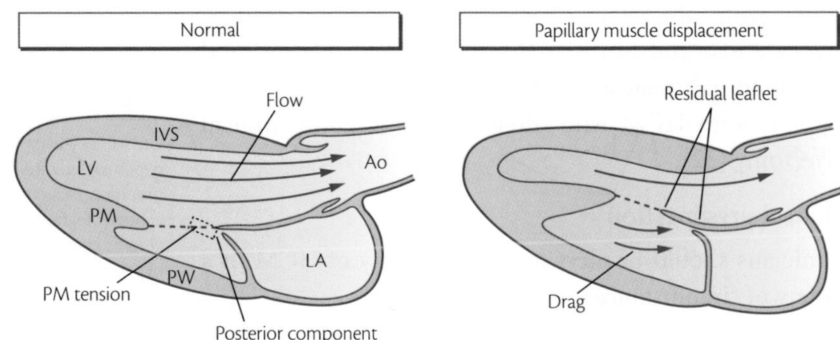

Figure 18.2 Anterior displacement of the papillary muscles in hypertrophic cardiomyopathy. Ao, aorta; IVS, interventricular septum; LA, left atrium; LV, left ventricle; PW, posterior wall. Reproduced with permission from Levine RA, Vlahakes GJ, Lefebvre *et al.* Papillary muscle displacement causes systolic anterior motion of the mitral valve. Experimental validation and insights into the mechanism of subaortic obstruction. *Circulation* 1995; **91**: 1189–95.

mechanism may be greater with HCM and diastolic dysfunction, which precludes adequate ventricular filling at high heart rates. Peripheral vasoconstriction is mediated by increased sympathetic stimulation during exercise, and partially attenuated by a number of vasodilatory influences, including stretch-induced activation of arterial baroreceptors and cardiac mechanosensitive receptors, and release of atrial and brain natriuretic peptides.

Around 30% of patients with HCM fail to increase their systolic blood pressure by ≥25mmHg during exercise, or show a paradoxical fall in blood pressure of ≥20mmHg. The inappropriate vasodilator response has been ascribed to excess stimulation of LV mechanoreceptors by abnormal wall stress and/or by an increase in LVOT with a considerable drop in cardiac output and a decrease in systolic aortic pressure [22, 30].

Arrhythmia

Triggers for ventricular arrhythmia in HCM include ischaemia, LVOTO, vascular instability and cellular energy depletion, while myocyte disarray and fibrosis provide the arrhythmogenic substrate. Non-sustained ventricular tachycardia (VT) occurs in around 20%. In contrast, sustained VT is rare and raises suspicion of a LV apical aneurysm, sometimes seen in patients with mid-cavity obstruction.

Atrial fibrillation (AF) is linked with left atrial dilation, which is often associated with diastolic dysfunction, mitral regurgitation, and LVOTO. As the most common sustained arrhythmia in HCM, chronic or paroxysmal AF is observed in 20–25%; subclinical AF may occur even more frequently. The prevalence of AF increases with advancing age.

Wall thinning and cavity dilation

A decrease in LV wall thickness was previously documented in up to 15% over 3 years [23]. Over a longer follow-up period, wall thinning ≥5mm was noted in 60% of patients with severe LVH, accounting for the rarity of marked LVH in the elderly [24]. The mechanisms underlying LV remodelling in HCM remain to be elucidated, although it is likely that ischaemia, compromised energetics and injury from abnormal haemodynamic loading lead to myocyte loss and fibrosis. However, cavity dilation and systolic impairment are infrequent, occurring in <5% of patients with HCM who often had undergone surgical myectomy [32].

Clinical presentation

Clinicians should be alert to the possibility of HCM in a variety of circumstances.

Diagnostic testing

Diagnostic testing should include a 12-lead ECG and echocardiography (➲Table 18.2). Family members will require assessment. Annual review is recommended from early adolescence, since the clinical manifestations of HCM frequently develop during pubertal growth. Relatives without evidence of disease at physical maturity were traditionally considered to be unaffected. However, growing recognition of late-onset HCM has led to the recommendation that adult relatives are offered continued evaluation on a 5-yearly basis [25]. Children below the age of puberty are usually assessed only if they are symptomatic, have a high-risk family history, participate in competitive sports, or when there is heightened parental anxiety.

The other issue pertaining to familial assessment is the need for sensitive diagnostic criteria. Systematic evaluation of

Table 18.2 Guidelines for the diagnosis of familial hypertrophic cardiomyopathy

Echocardiography
Major criteria
LV wall thickness ≥13 mm in the anterior septum or ≥15 mm in the posterior septum or free wall
Severe SAM (septum–leaflet contact)
Minor criteria
LV wall thickness of 12mm in the anterior septum or posterior wall or of 14mm in the posterior septum or free wall
Moderate SAM (no septum–leaflet contact)
Redundant mitral valve leaflets
Electrocardiography
Major criteria
Left ventricular hypertrophy and repolarization changes
T-wave inversion in leads I and aVL (≥3mm) (with QRS–T wave axis difference ≥30°), V3–V6 (≥3mm) or II and III and aVF (≥5mm)
Abnormal Q (>40 ms or >25% R wave) in at least two leads from II, III, aVF (in absence of left anterior hemiblock), V1–V4; or I, aVL, V5–V6
Minor criteria
Complete bundle branch block or (minor) interventricular conduction defect (in LV leads)
Minor repolarization changes in LV leads
Deep S V2 (>25mm)

Guidelines are applicable only to first-degree relatives of index cases with confirmed hypertrophic cardiomyopathy, all of whom have a 50% probability of carrying the mutation. Diagnosis is established in the presence of 1 major criterion, or 2 minor echocardiographic criteria, or 1 minor echocardiographic plus 2 minor electrocardiographic criteria. Other causes of left ventricular hypertrophy (e.g. athletic training and hypertension) may confound diagnosis.

LV, left ventricular; SAM, systolic anterior motion of the mitral valve.

patients with known disease-causing mutations has identified a sizeable subset (20–50%) who do not fulfil conventional echocardiographic criteria for HCM, but who nevertheless show discernible abnormalities on ECG and echocardiography. Since autosomal dominant inheritance implies a 50% probability of any first-degree relative carrying the gene, minor abnormalities are more likely to represent disease expression than in the general population (➲Table 18.2) [26].

Characteristic ECG findings in HCM are shown in ➲Fig. 18.3. Voltage criteria for LVH seldom occur in isolation in HCM, but are common in normal adolescents and young adults. Pre-excitation is a recognized feature, particularly in conjunction with mutations in AMP kinase; however, a short PR interval with a slurred QRS upstroke is not infrequently observed in HCM patients without accessory pathways.

Echocardiography is the first-line investigation for assessing wall thickness, cavity dimensions, systolic and diastolic function, and outflow tract obstruction. Exercise echocardiography is of value in patients with chest pain, dyspnoea, or presyncope for determining dynamic LVOTO. Tissue Doppler imaging is a useful adjunct for identifying regional abnormalities in systolic and diastolic function and changes in long-axis function, particularly in subclinical forms of the disease. Although the original diagnostic criteria for HCM stipulated LV wall thickness ≥15mm, any degree and distribution of LVH may be present. Considerable attention has been focused on the difficulty in distinguishing morphologically mild HCM (wall thickness 13–14mm) from hypertrophy in athletes.

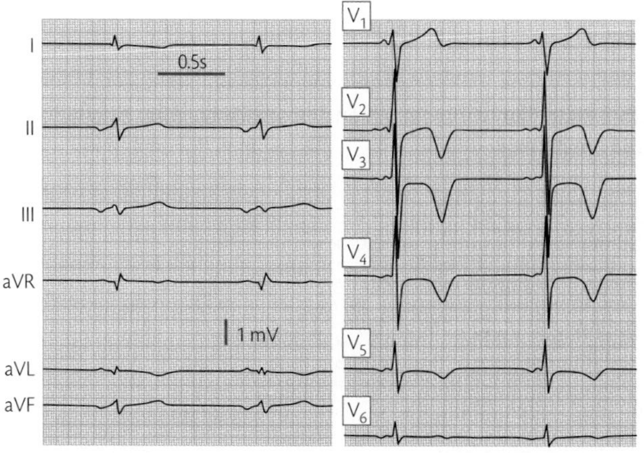

Figure 18.3 Typical ECG recording in a patient with hypertrophic cardiomyopathy. There are signs of severe LV hypertrophy with negative T-waves in V2 to V5. Giant negative T-waves can be typically seen in the apical form of hypertrophic cardiomyopathy.

Diagnosis of HCM is facilitated by the presence of repolarization abnormalities or pathological Q waves on the ECG. Echocardiography may be helpful as the LV cavity is commonly enlarged in athletes but small in HCM; diastolic function is normal or enhanced in athletes but usually impaired in HCM; and left atrial size is normal in athletes but often increased in HCM.

Patients with a confirmed diagnosis of HCM should undergo exercise testing on an annual basis. An abnormal blood pressure response is a risk factor for sudden death, although its prognostic impact appears to be greatest in patients <40 years of age. Simultaneous metabolic gas exchange measurements are useful for obtaining an objective assessment of exercise capacity. Metabolic exercise testing may be important in differentiating HCM from cardiovascular adaptation to training; athletes frequently demonstrate peak oxygen consumption >120% of predicted, while >98% of HCM patients show abnormal indices.

Holter ECG monitoring is recommended annually. Findings include paroxysmal AF, which merits antiarrhythmic therapy for suppression and/or anticoagulation, and non-sustained VT, a risk factor for sudden death. Extended monitoring with an event recorder or implantable loop recorder may be warranted in patients with symptoms suggestive of arrhythmia.

Management

Management of patients with HCM (➲Fig. 18.4) aims to alleviate symptoms, prevent complications (e.g. AF) and reduce sudden cardiac death.

Medical therapy

Asymptomatic patients with mild LVH should not receive drug therapy, whereas asymptomatic patients with severe LVH should be treated with verapamil to improve relaxation and diastolic filling thereby lowering diastolic filling pressure [27–29].

Symptomatic patients should be first treated with verapamil, a calcium-channel blocker that improves diastolic filling (positive lusitropic effect; ➲Table 18.3) and reduces systolic outflow tract obstruction (negative inotropic effect). As an alternative diltiazem may be used, although documentation is less extensive. If these drugs fail to improve symptoms, beta-blockers may be used either alone or in combination with a calcium-channel blocker. Beta-blockers reduce outflow tract obstruction by their negative chronotropic and inotropic actions. Furthermore, the decrease in heart rate increases LV size, which further reduces outflow tract gradient and increases diastolic filling time. However, these drugs exert

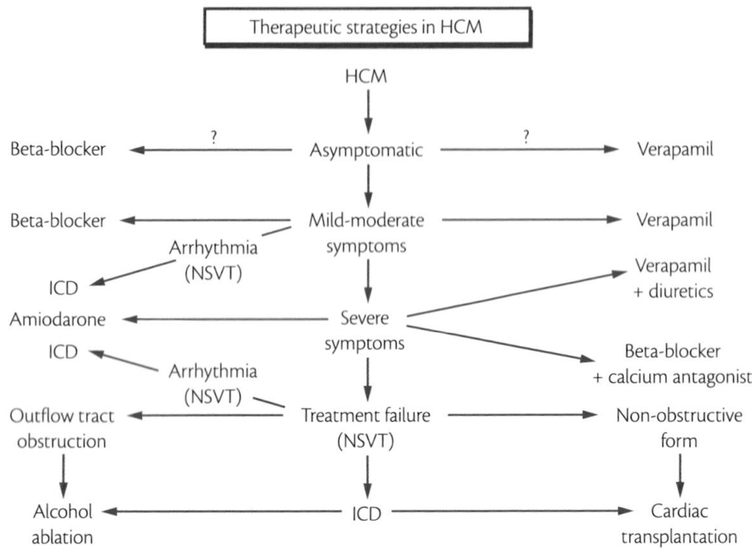

Figure 18.4 Treatment strategy in hypertrophic cardiomyopathy (HCM). ICD, implantable cardioverter defibrillator; NSVT, non-sustained ventricular tachycardia. Reproduced with permission from Hess OM, Sigwart U. New treatment strategies for hypertrophic obstructive cardiomyopathy. Alcohol ablation of the septum: the new gold standard? *J Am Coll Cardiol* 2004; **44**: 2054–5.

no positive lusitropic effect and do not effectively improve diastolic function as do calcium-channel blockers. Diuretics may be used in severely symptomatic patients to reduce filling pressure, although caution is recommended because these patients are sensitive to sudden volume changes. Volume sensitivity can be explained by the steep LV pressure–volume curve, when a small drop in filling pressure reduces stroke volume and cardiac output dramatically. Diuretics may be used in combination with a beta-blocker or calcium-channel blocker in order to reduce symptoms of pulmonary congestion.

Disopyramide, an antiarrhythmic drug that alters calcium kinetics, has been associated with symptomatic improvement and abolition of systolic pressure gradient. This effect has been attributed to its negative inotropic action and peripheral vasoconstriction. Nevertheless, long-term experience with this drug is limited.

Beta-blockers, calcium antagonists, and the conventional antiarrhythmic drugs do not appear to suppress serious ventricular arrhythmias in HCM. However, amiodarone, which prolongs action potential duration and refractoriness of cardiac fibres, is effective in the treatment of both supraventricular and ventricular arrhythmias. Although it is believed that amiodarone improves prognosis and symptoms in HCM, only limited and inconclusive data are available. Amiodarone may be used in patients with supraventricular (AF) and ventricular tachyarrhythmias, although in severe cases implantation of a defibrillator may be mandatory.

Contraindications to medical treatment with calcium-channel blockers or beta-blockers may be prolongation of the atrioventricular (AV) interval (risk of second- or third-degree AV block). Treatment with beta-blocking agents may be contraindicated in the presence of asthma bronchiale or chronic obstructive pulmonary disease.

Timing of therapy

Treatment is indicated when the patient becomes symptomatic or LVH is severe. Refractoriness to medical therapy usually indicates progression of the disease. At this point more aggressive therapies such as alcohol ablation of the septum [30] or surgical septal myectomy are indicated. Double-chamber pacing for symptomatic relief and reduction of outflow tract obstruction has been used previously but is not recommended at present. However, insertion of an implantable cardioverter-defibrillator (ICD) is strongly advised in high-risk patients with severe LVH and a history

Table 18.3 Common agents and doses for treating hypertrophic cardiomyopathy

Calcium channel blockers
Verapamil 120mg two to three times daily
Diltiazem 180mg once or twice daily
Beta-blockers
Propranolol 80mg two to three times daily
Metoprolol 100–200mg daily
Bisoprolol 5–10mg daily
Antiarrhythmic drugs
Amiodarone 100–200mg five times weekly
Disopyramide 100mg three times daily or 200mg twice daily

of non-sustained or sustained tachyarrhythmias or syncopes [31]. Patients with severe LVH, recurrent syncopes, sustained and non-sustained ventricular tachyarrhythmias, a history of familial sudden cardiac death, and a genetic phenotype for an increased risk of premature death should receive an ICD.

Surgical treatment

Until recently, septal myectomy has been considered the treatment of choice for therapy-refractory patients with obstructive HCM [32, 33]. Long-term follow-up after surgical myectomy has shown excellent results (➲Fig. 18.5) but ventricular remodelling with dilatation of the left ventricle may occur in 15–20% of patients. Alcohol ablation has changed this treatment strategy and surgical resection of the septum is reserved for selected cases with combined procedures such as coronary bypass grafting or mitral valve repair.

Alcohol ablation of the septum

Alcohol ablation of the ventricular septum can be considered to reduce LVOTO [34, 35]. Outflow tract gradients of >30–50mmHg at rest and 60–100mmHg after provocation (extrasystole, isoproterenol infusion or amyl nitrite inhalation) are considered to qualify for septal ablation. With a small over-the-wire balloon catheter, 1–3ml of pure alcohol are injected over 5min into the first or second septal branch (➲Fig. 18.6) after identification of the correct ablation site by contrast echocardiography (➲Fig. 18.7).

Alcohol injection leads to a small myocardial infarction with a rise in creatine kinase (CK) of 500–1500 U/L.

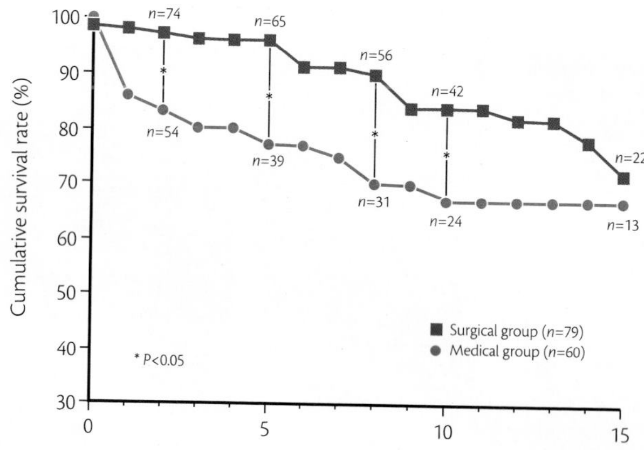

Figure 18.5 Cumulative survival rates of 139 patients with hypertrophic cardiomyopathy. Group 1, medical therapy ($n = 60$); Group 2, surgical therapy ($n = 79$). The average follow-up was 8.9 years for the entire study group, 8.2 years for Group 1 and 9.4 years for Group 2. Group 2 had higher 2-, 5-, 8- and 10-year survival rates than those of Group 1.

There is alcohol-induced septal hypokinesis, which leads to a reduction in outflow tract gradient (➲Fig. 18.8). In approximately one-third of patients the pressure gradient disappears immediately and in two-thirds after weeks or months (➲Fig. 18.9). Ventricular remodelling with a decrease in muscle mass and septal/posterior thickness takes 3–4 months.

Not all patients show a complete loss of outflow tract obstruction. Those who fail can be treated a second time. Complications include transient or permanent third-degree AV block (➲Fig. 18.10). Therefore, the procedure should not be done without a temporary pacemaker; 3–5% of all patients require definitive pacemaker implantation.

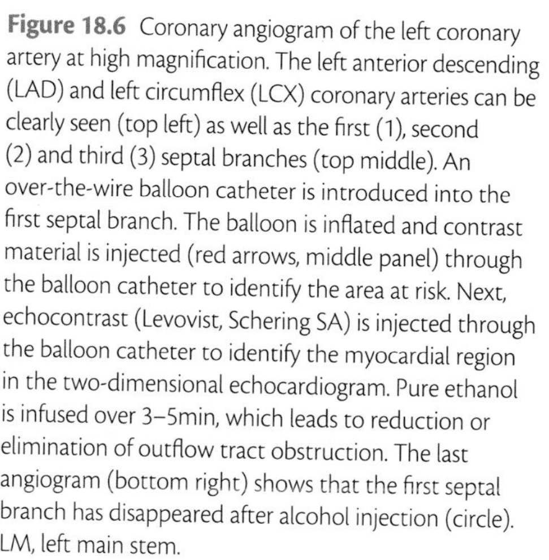

Figure 18.6 Coronary angiogram of the left coronary artery at high magnification. The left anterior descending (LAD) and left circumflex (LCX) coronary arteries can be clearly seen (top left) as well as the first (1), second (2) and third (3) septal branches (top middle). An over-the-wire balloon catheter is introduced into the first septal branch. The balloon is inflated and contrast material is injected (red arrows, middle panel) through the balloon catheter to identify the area at risk. Next, echocontrast (Levovist, Schering SA) is injected through the balloon catheter to identify the myocardial region in the two-dimensional echocardiogram. Pure ethanol is infused over 3–5min, which leads to reduction or elimination of outflow tract obstruction. The last angiogram (bottom right) shows that the first septal branch has disappeared after alcohol injection (circle). LM, left main stem.

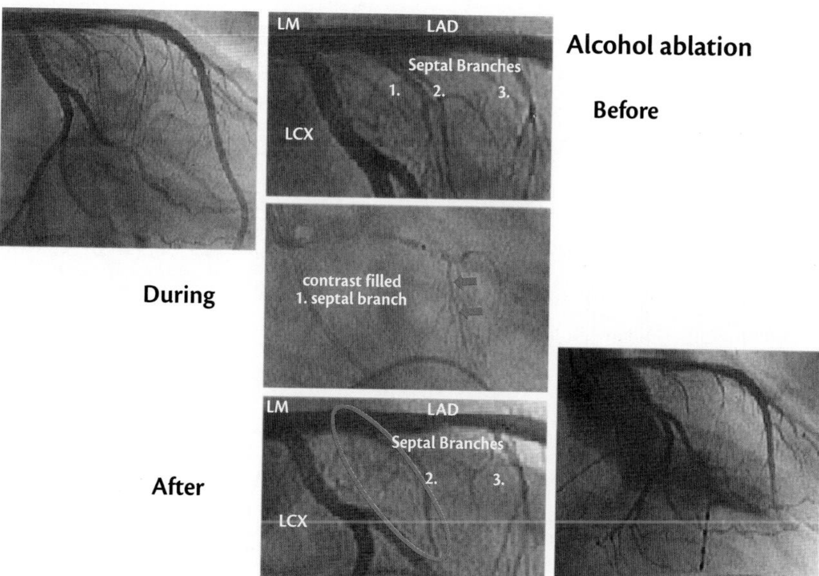

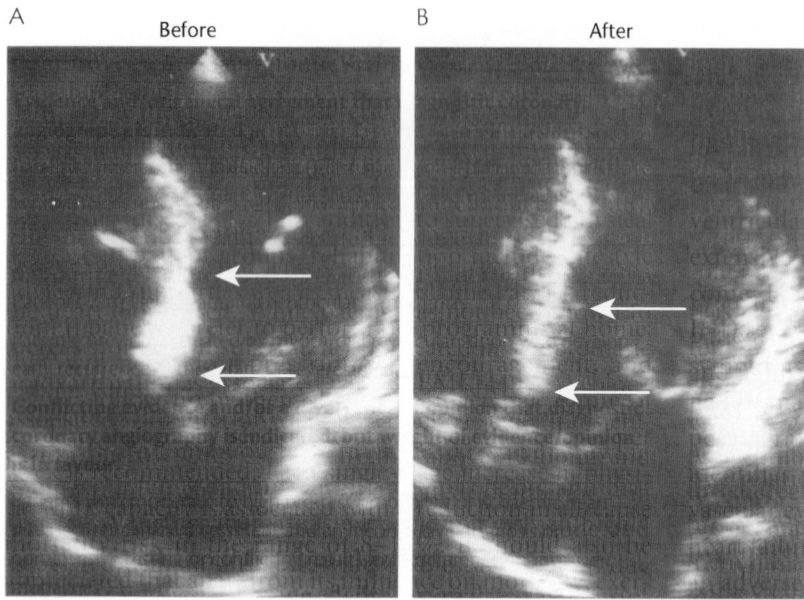

Figure 18.7 Two-dimensional echocardiogram before and after alcohol ablation. (A) Arrows indicate septal hypertrophy after injection of echocontrast medium. (B) Normalization of septal thickness 1 month after the intervention (arrows). Reproduced with permission from Faber L, Meissner A, Ziemssen P, *et al.* Percutaneous transluminal septal myocardial ablation for hypertrophic obstructive cardiomyopathy: long term follow up of the first series of 25 patients. *Heart* 2000; **83**: 326–31.

Complications

Sudden death is the most important threat for patients with HCM. Approximately 50–60% of those who die do so suddenly. Sudden death is assumed to be due to ventricular tachyarrhythmias, but haemodynamic factors and myocardial ischaemia may contribute. Young age (<30 years) and a positive family history for cardiac arrest are risk factors for sudden cardiac death [36].

Syncopes may occur as a result of either arrhythmias or a sudden increase in outflow tract obstruction. Rapid changes in body position or strenuous exercise may lead to an increase in outflow tract obstruction because of a decrease in venous return with a decrease in cardiac volumes and an increase in outflow tract obstruction ('ASH-crash') or as a result of an increase in cardiac contractility with hypercontraction of the left ventricle (increase in outflow tract obstruction) and elimination of the LV cavity (drop in cardiac output).

Strenuous exercise or competitive sports should be avoided because of the risk of sudden death. Typically, sudden death occurs during or after strenuous physical exercise.

AF as a cause of diastolic dysfunction, with increased filling pressure and dilatation of the atria, should be pharmacologically or electrically converted because of the haemodynamic consequences of the loss of atrial contraction on cardiac output. If sinus rhythm cannot be reached, oral anticoagulation is mandatory when no contraindications exist.

Infective endocarditis may occur in about 5% of patients with HCM but due to the new recommendations of the

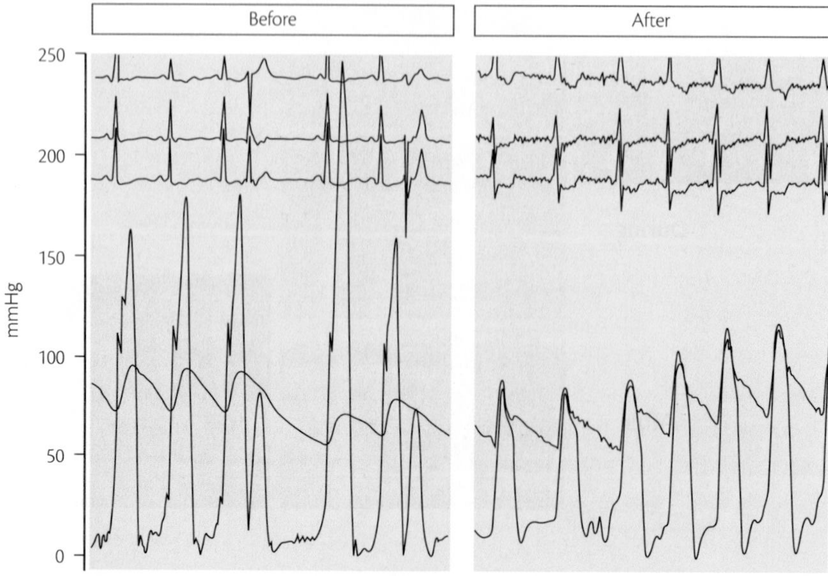

Figure 18.8 Pressure recording in a patient with hypertrophic cardiomyopathy before and after alcohol ablation of the septum. Before the intervention there is a large pressure gradient at rest (75mmHg) and after postextrasystolic potentiation (150mmHg). The systolic pressure gradient disappears completely after alcohol ablation.

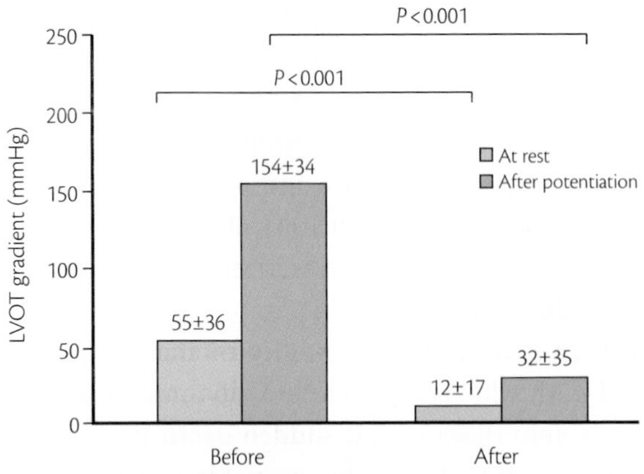

Figure 18.9 Left ventricular pressure gradient before and after alcohol ablation. Maximal pressure gradients are indicated at rest (first bar) and after post-extrasystolic potentiation (second bar). Data are shown at baseline (left bars) as well as 6 months after alcohol ablation (right bars). After the intervention there is a significant decrease in pressure gradients to one-quarter of the initial values.

American Heart Association antibiotic prophylaxis is not recommended anymore. Infection typically occurs on the aortic or mitral valve or on the septal contact site of the anterior mitral leaflet [37].

Prognosis and outcome

The clinical course in HCM is variable and may remain stable over years. However, HCM patients with risk factors such as a familial history of premature death, recurrent syncopes, septal thickness >30mm or a genetic phenotype with an increased risk of premature death may show a poor outcome [37]. Annual mortality rates have been reported to range between 2 and 3% but may be higher in children. Clinical deterioration is often slow but clinical symptoms are poorly related to the severity of outflow tract obstruction. Generally, symptoms increase with age. The occurrence of AF is an indicator of diastolic dysfunction with increased filling pressures and dilated atria. Timely conversion of atrial fibrillation is indicated.

Randomized clinical trials have not been undertaken, possibly because of the relatively low prevalence and the variability of the disease as well as the presence of symptomatic and asymptomatic patients. There is an urgent need for such randomized multicentre treatment trials.

Dilated cardiomyopathy

According to the WHO/ISFC Task Force on the Definition and Classification of Cardiomyopathies, the diagnosis of 'idiopathic' dilated cardiomyopathy (DCM) should only be made after exclusion of the specific cardiomyopathies [38]. Clinical evaluation alone does not allow reliable segregation of specific cardiomyopathies, i.e. inflammatory, ischaemic, and alcoholic cardiomyopathy, or cardiomyopathies associated with metabolic disorders [39–46].

Definition and prevalence

DCM is a chronic heart muscle disease characterized by cavity enlargement and impaired systolic function of the left or both ventricles (➲Table 18.4). The extent of myocardial dysfunction is not accounted for by abnormal loading

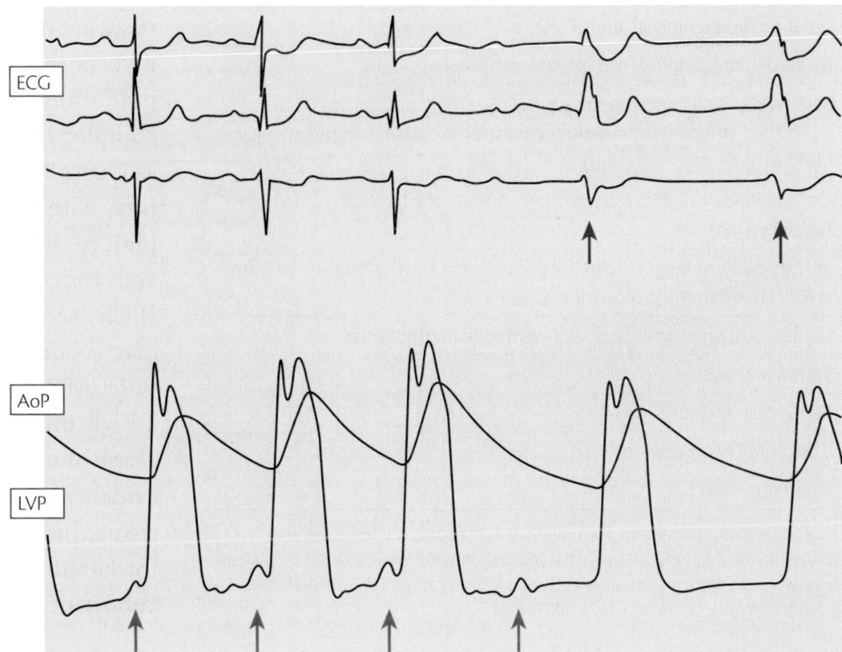

Figure 18.10 Simultaneous ECG and pressure recordings in a patient during alcohol ablation. Blue arrows indicate atrial contraction in the pressure curve (lower row). Occurrence of third-degree atrioventricular (AV) block can be seen after the fourth atrial beat, with an intermittent pacemaker rythm (red arrows). Three to four minutes after the occurrence of third-degree AV block, normal sinus rhythm was restored. AoP, aortic pressure; LVP, left ventricular pressure.

conditions such as systemic hypertension or valve disease, previous infarction, ongoing ischaemia or sustained arrhythmia. The age-adjusted prevalence of DCM in the USA is 36 per 100,000 population.

Aetiology

Once considered idiopathic or sporadic, DCM is now recognized to be genetically transmitted in at least 30–40%. Other factors linked with pathogenesis include anthracycline derivatives such as doxorubicin (➲ Chapters 11 and 20), and malnutrition, particularly thiamine and protein deficiencies. Many apparently secondary forms of DCM, notably alcoholic cardiomyopathy and hypertensive or ischaemic cardiomyopathy, probably arise when incompletely penetrant genetic disease is unmasked by an additional insult to the myocardium (alcohol) or stress upon the cardiovascular system (pregnancy).

The prevalence of familial DCM has been underestimated, because disease expression is frequently incomplete in family members. Prospective evaluation of the asymptomatic relatives of DCM patients revealed isolated LV enlargement in 20%, mild contractile impairment in 6%, and frank DCM in 3% [47]. Asymptomatic relatives with LV enlargement showed histological and immunohistochemical changes similar to those with established disease, including myocyte pleomorphism, interstitial fibrosis and markers of inappropriate immune activation [41]. A proportion of relatives with minor abnormalities progressed to overt DCM, underscoring their importance as markers of early disease. Thus, relying on the family history alone is not adequate, and clinical screening of relatives is requisite for identification of familial cases.

A further issue is the variability of the phenotype in familial DCM, which may include arrhythmia, stroke, conduction system disease, and sudden death in addition to ventricular dilation and dysfunction. Since the most common pattern of inheritance is autosomal dominant, first-degree relatives of DCM index cases have a 50% probability of being genetically affected, and the likelihood that mild unexplained features represent disease expression is high. Specific diagnostic criteria have been proposed for familial DCM [48]. Variable and age-related penetrance is a second impediment to recognition of familial cases. In one Italian series, penetrance was 10% in those <20 years old, 34% in those aged 20–30 years, 60% in those aged 30–40, and 90% in those >40 [48]. This is compounded by the fact that the families seen in clinical practice are often small. Estimation of the true prevalence of familial DCM will therefore necessitate serial assessment of extended families over lengthy follow-up periods.

In those with no family history, DCM has been thought to be due to acute myocarditis. A triphasic model has been proposed, with an initial insult to the myocardium, followed by chronic inflammation, leading to ventricular remodelling and dysfunction [49]. The primary insult is believed to be a viral infection. Enteroviruses and adenoviruses are most commonly implicated. Although acute viral myocarditis is rapidly fatal in a small subset of patients, predominantly children, the majority recover without complications. Some will develop chronic inflammation as a corollary of viral persistence or triggered autoimmunity, with endomyocardial biopsies demonstrating lymphocyte infiltration and histological markers of immune activation. Studies employing polymerase chain reaction (PCR) techniques to detect viral ribonucleic acid in cardiac tissue have reported positive findings in up to 35% of DCM patients [49]. More recently, it was reported that a high proportion of patients with the acute or healing phase of myocarditis or DCM have immunohistochemical evidence of enterovirus capsid protein VP1 in myocardial tissue, indicating translation of viral epitopes and a role for latent viral infection in pathogenesis [50]. In a small cohort of patients with LV failure and viral persistence,

Table 18.4 Diagnostic criteria for dilated cardiomyopathy

1 Left ventricular ejection fraction <0.45 (>2SD) and/or fractional shortening <25% (>2SD), as ascertained by echocardiography, radionuclide scanning or angiography *and*
2 Left ventricular end-diastolic diameter >117% of the predicted value corrected for age and body surface area, which corresponds to 2SD of the predicted normal limit + 5%
Exclusion criteria, which can lead to phenocopies
Systemic arterial hypertension (>160/100mmHg documented and confirmed at repeated measurements and/or evidence of target-organ disease)
Coronary heart disease (obstruction >50% of the luminal diameter in a major branch)
History of chronic excess alcohol consumption, with remission of heart failure after 6 months of abstinence
Clinical, sustained and rapid supraventricular arrhythmias
Systemic diseases
Pericardial diseases
Congenital heart disease
Cor pulmonale

Reproduced with permission from Mestroni L, Maisch B, McKenna WJ, *et al.* Guidelines for the study of familial dilated cardiomyopathies. Collaborative Research Group of the European Human and Capital Mobility Project on Familial Dilated Cardiomyopathy. *Eur Heart J* 1999; **20**: 93–102.

6-month therapy with β-interferon resulted in elimination of viral genomes and improvement in LV function [44]. However, the demonstration of viral presence in DCM does not amount to a causal link, particularly as enteroviral genome has also been detected in patients with ischaemic heart disease [51].

The autoimmune model of DCM invokes a central role for the immune system in causing continued myocardial injury. During the initial viral infection, an effective immune response is critical in preventing fulminant myocarditis, with clinical markers of immunity such as anti-cardiac IgG correlating with a favourable outcome [49]. Unfortunately, tissue damage during this initial insult may result in the presentation of previously sequestered myocardial peptides to the immune system. Alternatively, molecular mimicry between viral proteins and endogenous myocardial antigens may result in an organ-specific autoimmune response. A third potential mechanism involves viral-induced expression of class II major histocompatibility complex (MHC) molecules in cardiac tissue, leading to presentation of self-peptides to infiltrating T cells and activation of organ-specific immunity. Evidence for inappropriate class II MHC expression has been found in endothelial and endocardial cells from cardiac biopsies of patients with DCM. Lending further support to the autoimmune hypothesis is the presence of circulating heart-reactive antibodies in 25–30% of patients with DCM and symptom-free relatives [52]. Of note, cardiac antibodies were more commonly found among relatives who showed disease progression, but frequently became undetectable during follow-up and in advanced DCM. A possible role as early markers of disease susceptibility is therefore suggested. From a therapeutic standpoint, a 3-month course of steroids and azathioprine for immunosuppression was associated with early and lasting improvement in LV function in DCM patients with evidence of MHC upregulation on cardiac biopsy [46].

It should be noted that the familial preponderance of DCM is compatible with autoimmune pathogenesis, since susceptible self-antigens may bind more avidly to certain MHC alleles than others. The HLA-DR4 allele, for example, appears to confer a predilection for autoimmune disorders such as rheumatoid arthritis and multiple sclerosis, and does in fact show a weak association with DCM. Similarly, viruses may act as a trigger factor for the development of DCM in subjects with a genetic predisposition. The absence of viral nucleic acids in the hearts of patients with familial DCM [53] argues against this possibility, implying that viral DCM and familial DCM are indeed distinct patient populations. Furthermore, DCM behaves as a single gene disorder in many affected families, and the identification of disease-causing mutations has provided insight into its pathogenesis. Autosomal dominant transmission predominates in adult-onset DCM, although recessive, mitochondrial, and X-linked forms are also recognized.

Genetics

Elucidation of the molecular aetiology of DCM has proved challenging because of its exceptional genetic heterogeneity. One of the first major breakthroughs was the identification of dystrophin as the causative gene in X-linked familial DCM [54]. Defects in dystrophin are also responsible for Duchenne and Becker muscular dystrophy [55]. While muscular dystrophy patients frequently develop DCM, skeletal muscle involvement is rare among sufferers with X-linked DCM, although serum CK muscle isoforms are elevated in both [54] (see also ➲ Chapter 9).

A 427-kDa rod-shaped protein, dystrophin, localizes to the inner aspect of the myocyte cytoplasmic membrane (sarcolemma). Its large size is thought to predispose to a high rate of spontaneous mutations [56]. Dystrophin binds to actin at its N-terminus and to the transmembrane dystrophin–glycoprotein complex at its C-terminus (➲ Fig. 18.11), thereby providing a link between the cytoskeleton and sarcolemma. Most of the mutations isolated in X-linked DCM affect the N-terminal domain [54].

The first disease-causing gene in autosomal dominant DCM to be discovered was cardiac actin and was localized to chromosome 15q14 [55]. Actin is a sarcomeric thin filament with a dual function in myocytes: it interacts with other components of the sarcomere (β-myosin heavy chain, α-tropomyosin, troponins) and has a key role in force generation within the contracting myocyte. At its other end, actin binds to the anchoring proteins dystrophin and α-actinin (which resides in Z-bands and intercalated discs), thereby facilitating transmission of the contractile force to the sarcolemma and adjacent myocytes. Interestingly, mutations in the sarcomeric end of actin are associated with HCM [57], while defects in its anchoring end cause DCM, presumably via impaired force transmission. A similar mechanism has been invoked for the DCM-related α-tropomyosin mutations, which may cause localized charge reversal at the surface of the tropomyosin protein. This may affect stability of the tropomyosin molecule and disrupt its electrostatic interaction with actin within the thin filament [58]. The role of the thin filament in transmitting force to adjacent sarcomeres will be compromised [54]. In contrast, the tropomyosin

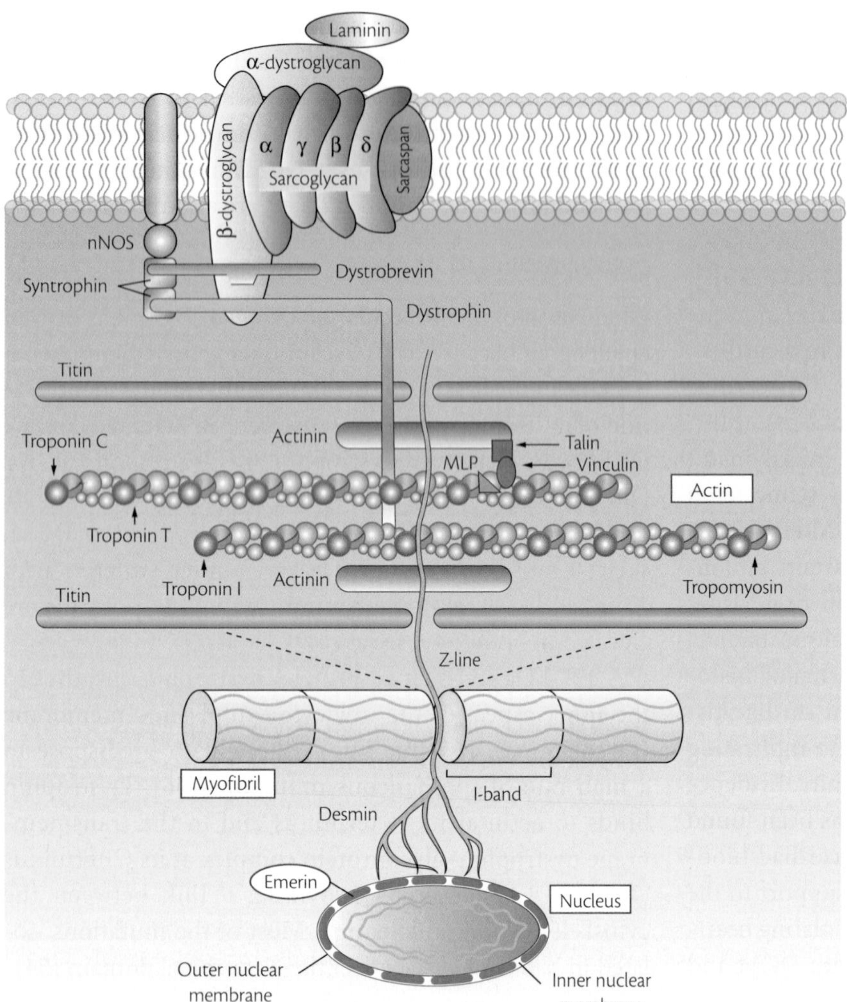

Figure 18.11 Proteins and pathways involved in the development of cardiomyopathy. nNos, neural nitric oxide synthase; MLP, muscle LIM protein. Reproduced with permission from Towbin JA, Bowles, NE. The failing heart. *Nature* 2002; **415**: 227–33.

mutations isolated in HCM cause an increase in isometric force output; inefficient sarcomeric ATP utilization is the likely consequence.

A missense mutation in the intermediate filament desmin has also been identified in a family with DCM [59]. The association of desmin, actin, and dystrophin suggests that disruption of cytoskeletal function might be the final common pathway of disease expression [59]. In line with this, DCM mutations in δ-sarcoglycan [54], β-sarcoglycan (both components of the dystrophin–glycoprotein complex), Cypher/Zasp (a Z-line protein that bridges the sarcomere to the cytoskeleton) [60] and metavinculin [59] (which connects actin filaments to the intercalated disc) have been found. Skeletal myopathy, which varies from subclinical to overt, may be an associated feature of some of these mutations.

Mutations in a number of other sarcomeric genes, including β-myosin heavy chain [61], cardiac troponin T and troponin C [62], may result in DCM. A recessive missense mutation in troponin I has also been isolated in a DCM family [63]. Early-onset disease expression and adverse prognosis have been reported in many families with sarcomeric DCM. The discovery of sarcomeric mutations in DCM raises two important issues. First, the mechanism by which these mutations induce ventricular dilation and impairment merits investigation; their functional effect is not readily explained by impaired transmission of force. Second, an explanation must be sought as to why certain sarcomeric mutations cause DCM, while other defects in the same genes produce the distinct phenotype of HCM. It has been proposed that the mutations associated with DCM may result in a deficit in force generation by the sarcomere. Conversely, the sarcomeric mutations that cause HCM may enhance mechanical function, and induce ventricular remodelling (i.e. hypertrophy) through ineffective utilization of ATP.

Impaired generation and transmission of force are therefore considered the key mechanisms underlying disease expression in DCM. Both may be relevant in the case of titin, a giant sarcomeric protein recently implicated in autosomal dominant DCM [61]. Titin binds to α-actinin, stabilizes the myosin filament and confers elasticity to the sarcomere. The position of the mutation is likely to be the main determinant of the functional effect.

Despite the remarkable diversity of molecular mechanisms in DCM, the consequences at a cellular level are similar: neuroendocrine activation and local production of cytokines, maladaptive myocyte hypertrophy, apoptosis, fibrosis, and progressive ventricular dilation and impairment. Thus, the premise of a final common pathway may hold true. Recent studies demonstrate disruption of the N-terminus of dystrophin in both DCM and ischaemic heart failure, implying that loss of cytoskeletal integrity may be central to myocyte dysfunction in the failing heart. Of note, dystrophin remodelling was reversible following support with a left ventricular assist device (LVAD), suggesting that reduction of mechanical stress is critical to recovery of cellular and cardiac function [67].

Clinical presentation

Clinical course

The natural history of DCM is heterogeneous and most patients are not critically ill. The prognosis of DCM has improved significantly in the last decades as a consequence of optimized treatment with angiotensin-converting enzyme (ACE) inhibitors and beta-blockers and, generally, is not different between sporadic or familial cases of DCM [68,69]. However, patients with DCM can be separated into two groups according to disease progression [68]:

- patients with a more favourable outcome (group 1);
- patients with a rapidly progressive downhill course, high mortality and urgent indication for heart transplantation (group 2).

More favourable outcome in DCM is associated with improvement in LV function under medical treatment, a shorter duration of clinical symptoms, younger age, a worse NYHA class, and a history of hypertension [70] (➲Fig. 18.12).

In patients with DCM, medical treatment with ACE inhibitors and/or beta-blockers improves LV pump function in 50% of cases, while normalization occurs in 16%. In the remaining 33%, however, disease progresses long term, even independent of the initial response to treatment [68]. As many as 20% of patients with DCM will die within 1 year after diagnosis [71], most frequently due to sudden death (64%), with terminal heart failure accounting for most other cases. The 8-year transplant-free survival is as follows:

- 94% in those with normalized left ventricular ejection fraction (LVEF);
- 83% in those with functional NYHA class I–II and LVEF >40%;
- 64% in those with NYHA class I–II when combined with LVEF ≤40%;
- 31% in those with persisting functional NYHA class III–IV.

Clinical symptoms

Clinical symptoms in patients with DCM are no different to those in patients with heart failure of other aetiology (see ➲Chapter 21). Most often, DCM patients are less symptomatic and present with higher exercise tolerance when compared with other cardiomyopathies. Clinical symptoms in patients with DCM and systolic dysfunction of other aetiology can be grouped into major (specific) and minor (unspecific) criteria according to the Framingham study [72] and occur at different frequencies (➲Table 18.5).

Information from physical examination and medical history are not only valid and cost-effective for management decisions in heart failure but also relevant with respect to prognosis. Because of effective medical treatment, many patients with systolic pump dysfunction present with no or minor clinical symptoms. Nevertheless, the hepatojugular reflux and the third heart sound provide clinical information

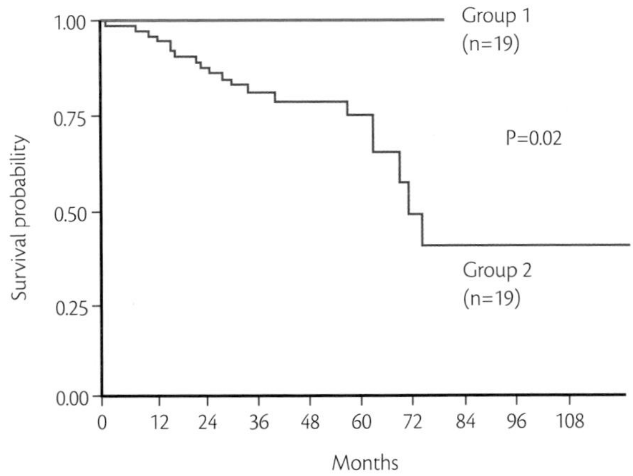

Figure 18.12 Kaplan–Meier survival curves of two groups of patients with dilated cardiomyopathy. Group 1, improvement of left ventricular ejection fraction (LVEF) with medical treatment; group 2, no improvement in LVEF. The survival probability was significantly different ($P = 0.02$).

Table 18.5 Clinical symptoms in patients with congestive heart failure: percentage occurrence of major and minor criteria

Major criteria	
Pulmonary rales	81%
Cardiomegaly	70%
Elevated jugular pressure	55%
Radiological signs of congestion	48%
Paroxysmal nocturnal dyspnoea	32%
Orthopnoea	31%
Third heart sound	19%
Minor criteria	
Exertional dyspnoea	93%
Peripheral oedema	56%
Depression	46%
Pleural effusion	32%
Hepatomegaly	14%
Nocturnal coughing	12%
Heart rate >120bpm.	4%
Weight loss <4.5kg in 6 months	2%

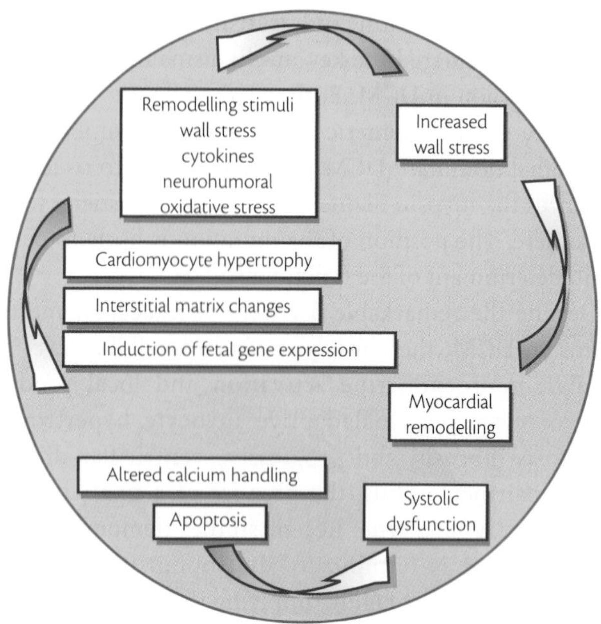

Figure 18.13 Vicious cycle in systolic dysfunction. Different remodelling stimuli induce complex cellular changes, ultimately resulting in systolic and/or diastolic dysfunction and increased wall stress, thereby promoting pathological remodelling.

on the prognosis of the individual patient even in the context of best modern medical management [73].

Pathophysiology

The initial stimuli that induce DCM are diverse: arterial hypertension, familial or genetic factors, myocarditis of viral or toxic origin, tachyarrhythmias, abnormal immune response. The consequent increased wall stress in combination with neurohumoral activation causes maladaptive changes in myocardial structure (remodelling), with complex molecular and cellular modifications. Histologically, remodelling is associated with cellular hypertrophy of cardiomyocytes, together with changes in the quantity and nature of the interstitial matrix. Biochemically, expression of the adult gene programme decreases and re-expression of fetal genes increases. Finally, the number of viable, functionally active cardiomyocytes decreases via programmed cell death (apoptosis) (➲Fig. 18.13). Several factors known to be present in the failing myocardium have been shown to cause apoptosis of cardiomyocytes *in vitro*:

- catecholamines via β-adrenergic signalling and reactive oxygen species [74];
- wall stress and angiotensin II [75];
- nitric oxide and inflammatory cytokines [76].

Thus it is not surprising that almost all the drugs used in heart failure have an antagonistic action on these pathways. All these drugs reduce and, potentially, reverse pathological cardiac remodelling and improve survival by attenuating stress signalling in the heart.

The β-adrenergic system

Prolonged increased sympathetic activity results in both desensitization and down-regulation of sarcolemmal cardiac β-adrenergic receptors. Desensitization of β-adrenergic receptors is promoted by increased β-adrenoreceptor kinase (β-ARK) expression in the failing heart; this enzyme phosphorylates the β-adrenergic receptor [77]. Phosphorylated β-adrenergic receptors are then internalized and sequestered in the failing cardiomyocyte [78]. In the transgenic dominant-negative MLP mouse model of heart failure, cardiac expression of a dominant-negative β-ARK mutant restores β-adrenergic signalling and prevents progression to heart failure in several models of animal heart failure (➲Fig. 18.14). These results suggest that the loss of β-adrenergic signalling in the failing heart is a key mechanism, although the mechanisms responsible for the salutary effects of beta-blockade still remain unclear.

Calcium homeostasis

Calcium is vital for contractile function, and therefore it is not surprising that abnormalities in calcium handling have been implicated in the systolic dysfunction of DCM. Calcium ions enter the cardiac muscle cell through L-type calcium channels during each heart beat and trigger calcium release through ryanodine receptors. This raises

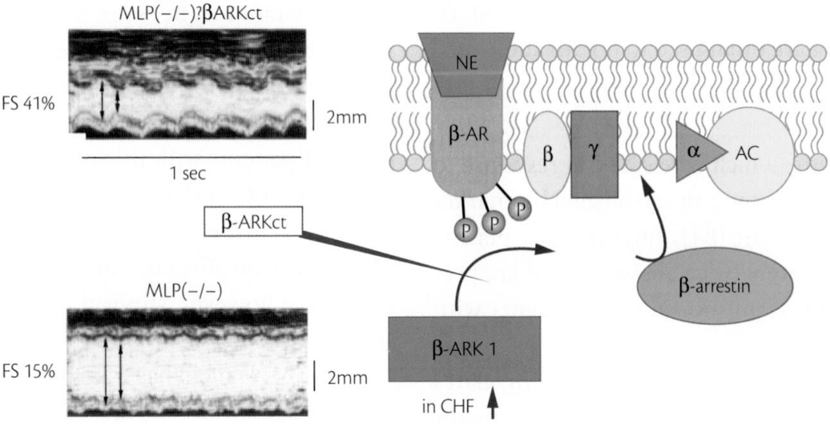

Figure 18.14 Signalling through the β-adrenergic receptor (βAR) in heart failure. βARK1 binds to the βγ-subunit of activated G-proteins, translocates to the sarcolemmal membrane and phosphorylates the agonist-occupied receptor. Phosphorylation allows binding of β-arrestin, uncoupling the receptor from further G-protein stimulation and downstream effectors such as adenylyl cyclase (AC). Both βARK1 and β-arrestin are required for homologous βAR desensitization, a phenomenon that occurs after the persistent agonist (noradrenaline, NE) stimulation characteristic of chronic heart failure. Expression of the C-terminal truncated, ineffective βARK1 in MLP (−/−) rescues myocardial function (see M-mode echocardiogram) and restores β-adrenergic responsiveness.

the intracellular calcium concentration about tenfold. Reuptake of calcium into the sarcoplasmic reticulum via the sarcoplasmic reticulum Ca^{2+}-ATPase allows cardiac relaxation. The ability of the Ca^{2+}-ATPase to pump calcium back into the sarcoplasmic reticulum is governed by its interaction with phospholamban, a small modulatory protein within the membrane of the sarcoplasmic reticulum [79] (➲Fig. 18.15). In the failing heart, calcium release and uptake is diminished owing to a decrease in expression and activity of the Ca^{2+}-ATPase, resulting in diastolic and systolic dysfunction. The notion that aberrant calcium handling contributes to the pathogenesis of systolic dysfunction in DCM is supported by the finding that in mice lacking the cardiac LIM domain (double-zinc finger domain found in Lin1, Isl1, and Mec3 protein MLP, the heart failure phenotype is completely abrogated by homozygous deletion of the gene encoding phospholamban, which allows for enhanced calcium reuptake by the sarcoplasmic reticulum. However, the apparently beneficial effects of phospholamban ablation can be observed only in a subset of mouse models of DCM and heart failure because the phospholamban knockout does not rescue cardiomyopathic hearts resulting from sarcomere abnormalities [80].

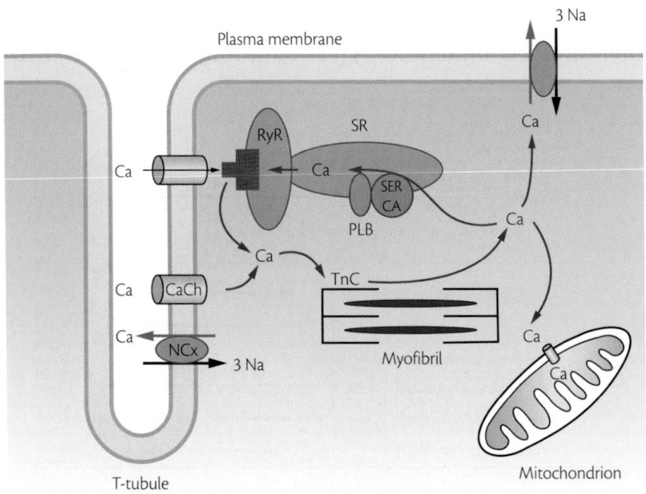

Figure 18.15 Calcium homeostasis. Membrane depolarization opens voltage-activated L-type calcium channels (CaCh), extracellular Ca^{2+} ions enter the cardiomyocyte and induce Ca^{2+} release by ryanodine receptors (RyR). Cytosolic Ca^{2+} concentration rises and intiates contraction. ATP-driven reuptake of Ca^{2+} ions into the sarcoplasmic reticulum (SR) by the sarcoplasmic Ca^{2+}-ATPase (SERCA) or extrusion of Ca^{2+} via the sodium–calcium exchanger (NCx) lowers cytosolic Ca^{2+} concentration and terminates contraction.

Natriuretic peptides

Heart failure in DCM is accompanied by the up-regulation and secretion of atrial and B-type natriuretic peptides by the heart that signal through cell-surface receptors coupled to guanylate cyclase [81]. The resultant activation of protein kinase G by cGMP has been shown to suppress fetal gene activation through mechanisms that are only beginning to be unveiled. Nevertheless, the observation that gender influences the severity of cardiomyopathic phenotypes [82] suggests the presence of other underlying but not yet identified pathogenetic mechanisms.

Diagnostic testing

Clinical examination in patients with DCM is frequently of limited value in the assessment of haemodynamics and prognosis. Therefore, plasma biomarkers and physical examinations such as echocardiography, QTc interval, or maximal exercise testing are often used to obtain additional objective information.

Neurohormones

B-type natriuretic peptide, which is released in response to myocyte stretch [83], has become an established biomarker for guiding medical treatment [84]; furthermore, plasma concentrations approximately twice above normal are predictive of increased long-term mortality in patients with heart failure.

The plasma concentration of interleukin 6 correlates with the severity of symptoms and is an identified predictor of cardiovascular mortality in stable severe chronic heart failure [85]. Plasma concentrations of noradrenaline (norepinephrine) are predictive of cardiovascular morbidity and mortality.

Electrocardiography

Electrocardiography provides no specific diagnosis in DCM. However, AF is associated with increased mortality or heart failure progression in all types of cardiomyopathy with chronic heart failure. In DCM, a decrease in heart rate variability due to chronic excessive sympathetic stimulation is related to an adverse prognosis [86], and prolonged QTc intervals predict mortality [87]. In addition, complex ventricular arrhythmias and decreased heart rate variability during 24-hour Holter monitoring, when associated with low ejection fraction (EF), place DCM patients at higher risk of death. Left bundle branch block with QRS duration of 130–150ms reflects high intra-left ventricular dyssynchrony and has been proposed as a criterion for selecting patients for resynchronization therapy.

Echocardiography

Two-dimensional Doppler echocardiography plays an important role in the assessment of dilated cardiomyopathy. Not only the size (LV end-diastolic diameter) and shape (long/short axis ratio) are important parameters for assessing LV remodelling. One of the most widely used parameters for determination of LV function is LV EF which has been used for classifying cardiomyopathies into severe (EF) ≤30%), moderate (EF 30–45%), and mild forms (EF ≥45%). Furthermore, Doppler findings like severity of mitral regurgitation predict development and severity of heart failure symptoms. Previously [87] an adverse prognosis has been reported in patients with cardiomyopathy when EF is <30%, LV filling pressure (LVEDP) ≥15mmHg and onset or worsening of mitral regurgitation is found. Mortality rate ranged between 15–20%, whereas in the moderately diseased group (EF ≥45% and LVEDP <15mmHg) annual mortality rate was between 5–8%. A restrictive physiology with high atrial filling pressures is associated with a higher mortality rate. However, if the abnormal filling is reversed into one of pseudo-normal or impaired relaxation, survival of DCM patients with this pattern is much better, whereas persistence of restrictive filling after 3 months despite optimal medical treatment is associated with a high mortality. Mitral valve insufficiency in DCM is associated with adverse prognosis; however, surgical mitral valve repair by undersized annuloplasty in combination with coaptation of the mitral valve leaflets has a favourable outcome [88]. Thus, transoesophageal echocardiography plays an important role with respect to treatment of the mitral valve disease in DCM.

Cardiopulmonary exercise testing

Cardiopulmonary exercise testing measures the adequacy of the cardiac response to strenuous exertion and is an established predictor of risk in DCM [89] (➲Fig. 18.16). In addition, VO_2 of anaerobic threshold (when <11mL/kg/min) and ventilatory efficiency (slope of Ve vs. $V\,CO_2$) >34 in combination are reliable predictors for 6-month mortality [90]. Prediction of prognosis is no different between ischaemic or dilated cardiomyopathy, although patients differ with respect to their neurohumoral profile.

Magnetic resonance imaging

Cardiac magnetic resonance (CMR) imaging has become a new standard for the assessment of ventricular volumes, EF, myocardial mass, and regional wall motion (➲Fig. 18.17). Paramagnetic contrast detects regional abnormalities in myocardial contraction [91]. In addition, late enhancement

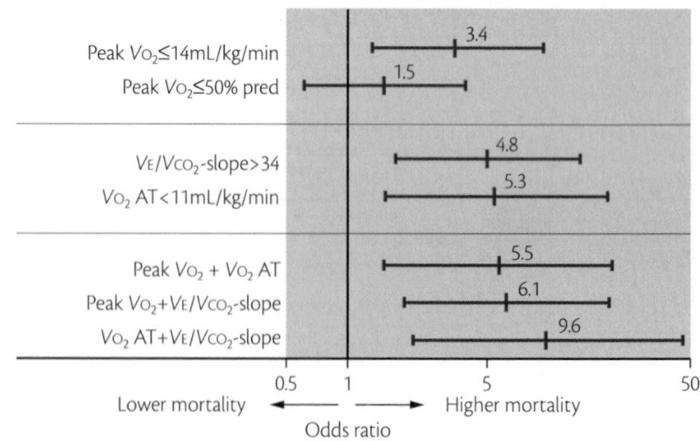

Figure 18.16 Cardiopulmonary exercise testing: predictors of death within 6 months in patients with ischaemic or dilated cardiomyopathy given as odds ratios (univariate analysis). Bars are 95% confidence intervals. Reproduced with permission from Gitt AK, Wasserman K, Kilkowski C, *et al.* Exercise anaerobic threshold and ventilatory efficiency identify heart failure patients for high risk of early death. *Circulation* 2002; **106**: 3079–84.

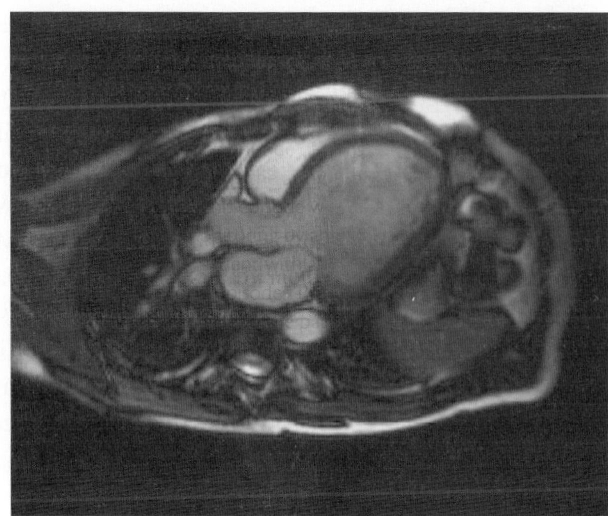

Figure 18.17 Cardiac magnetic resonance image in a patient with dilated cardiomyopathy. Horizontal transection of the dilated left ventricle with mitral jet due to mitral regurgitation.

marks areas of non-viable myocardium with higher sensitivity when compared with thallium scintigraphy [92].

Left and right heart catheterization

Coronary angiography is required to exclude coronary atherosclerosis when the diagnosis of DCM is considered. Additional information regarding cardiac output, wall stress, distensibility, compliance, and pulmonary artery pressure can be obtained, and pulmonary wedge pressure or pulmonary resistance may add to risk stratification. Cardiac catheterization should not be considered when instituting chronic therapy.

Endomyocardial biopsy

Frequently, the histology of endomyocardial specimens is non-specific, with cardiomyocyte hypertrophy, enlarged nuclei and increased interstitial fibrosis. However, most asymptomatic relatives of patients with DCM with LV enlargement have histopathological and immunopathological findings similar to those of patients with established disease [41]. In addition, *in situ* hybridization allows detection of persisting viral genome in endomyocardial biopsy and thus the diagnosis of chronic myocarditis, even when microscopic examination does not demonstrate lymphocytic infiltration.

Management

Independent of the aetiology and possible specific therapeutic options (e.g. anti-inflammatory, antiviral, or immunomodulatory agents), the general guidelines for the treatment of heart failure apply equally to DCM, i.e. ACE inhibitors, angiotensin (AT)II receptor blockers, beta-blockers, diuretics, aldosterone antagonists, digitalis and cardiac transplantation [93, 94]. The three cornerstones of heart failure therapy are:

1) ACE-inhibitors or AT1-receptor antagonists.
2) Beta-blockers (carvedilol, metoprolol, bisoprolol or nebivolol) which should be administered according to the principle: 'start low go slow'.
3) Aldosterone antagonists (cave hyperkalaemia with ACE-inhibitors or AT_1-receptor antagonists).

Potentially cardiotoxic agents (i.e. alcohol, anthracyclines) should be discontinued [95]. In addition, exercise training can contribute to alleviation of heart failure symptoms and improve prognosis [96]. Similarly, in DCM with left bundle branch block and QRS duration >120ms and NYHA III–IV, cardiac resynchronization therapy may be considered [97–99] (see ➲Chapter 21).

Cardiac transplantation remains the ultimate treatment option in patients with DCM with terminal heart failure refractory to conventional treatment [100]. LVADs may improve LV function until cardiac transplantation ('bridge to transplantation') or until sustained improvement of LV function occurs ('bridge to recovery') [101–103]. The value of partial ventriculectomy is limited [104].

Risk assessment and primary prevention of SCD is a challenge in DCM, especially since programmed ventricular stimulation has no predictive value as opposed to its use in ischaemic heart disease [105]. Aborted SCD is an indication for ICD (secondary prevention). Syncope is a strong predictor of SCD in DCM [106]. The combination of LV end-diastolic diameter >70mm and non-sustained VT on Holter monitoring, and the combination of LVEF <30% and non-sustained VT on Holter monitoring may identify patients at higher risk for SCD [107, 108]. Conventional heart failure treatment also reduces mortality due to prevention of SCD (see ➲Chapter 23) [109–111]. ICD appears superior in the primary prevention of SCD compared with amiodarone: whereas the AMIOVIRT (Amiodarone Versus Implantable Defibrillator in Patients with Nonischemic Cardiomyopathy and Asymptomatic Nonsustained Ventricular Tachycardia) study showed no significant difference between amiodarone or ICD [112], the COMPANION (Comparison of Medical Therapy, Pacing and Defibrillation in Heart Failure) trial [99], and the SCD-Heft (Sudden Cardiac Death in Heart Failure Trial) trial demonstrated the superiority of ICD [113]. Rate control and/or rhythm control should be achieved in DCM patients with AF.

Anticoagulation is indicated in DCM patients with AF [114]. In light of the thromboembolic complications in DCM patients with substantially impaired LV function [115–117], anticoagulation should be prescribed. However, evidence from the WATCH trial on the benefit of anticoagulation in DCM patients with sinus rhythm is lacking [118].

Genetic counselling is advisable in patients with familial DCM and their first-degree relatives. Since a high proportion of affected relatives are asymptomatic despite LV enlargement, screening (ECG, echocardiography) should be performed in first-degree relatives [119].

Prognosis and outcome

The 5-year survival of DCM patients averages between 36% [120] and 30% [121]. After the initial diagnosis of DCM, clinical courses are highly heterogeneous. Identification of modifiable prognostic factors and elaboration of effective interventions is important for the outcome of DCM patients. Detailed prospective investigations have been elucidated by the Heart Muscle Disease Study Group. A subgroup characterized by a rapidly progressive course with high mortality rates, need for inotropic and/or LVAD support, and urgent transplantation can be distinguished from the subgroup with more favourable outcome responding to concurrent heart failure medication (about 50% of patients). Less frequently (about 16%), healing courses can be observed [68], especially in the setting of acute DCM/fulminant myocarditis [122–124]. Transplant-free survival, as well as SCD, in DCM patients is significantly associated with the course of NYHA/LVEF improvement under optimized heart failure medication [68].

Evidence emerging confirms the decrease in mortality and hospitalization of DCM patients undergoing heart failure treatment [68, 125]. However, this treatment does not specifically target the cause of the disease, and some DCM patients do not respond. Pathogenic substrates of DCM, namely inflammation and especially cardiotropic viral persistence/viral replication, are associated with adverse outcome [126–129], whereas histological morphometric analyses have no predictive value [130, 131]. There is an emerging role for gene mutations, which are associated with a worse prognosis in DCM [132].

Restrictive cardiomyopathy

Definition and classification

Restrictive cardiomyopathy is characterized by abnormal diastolic function with either thickened or rigid ventricular walls leading to elevated filling pressures of the left- or right-sided cardiac chambers. In contrast to constrictive pericarditis, left- and right-sided diastolic filling pressures are discordant in restrictive cardiomyopathy but concordant in constrictive pericarditis. ‘Discordant’ describes the haemodynamic phenomenon of dissociation between left and right ventricular diastolic filling pressures during respiration, whereas ‘concordant’ describes parallel changes

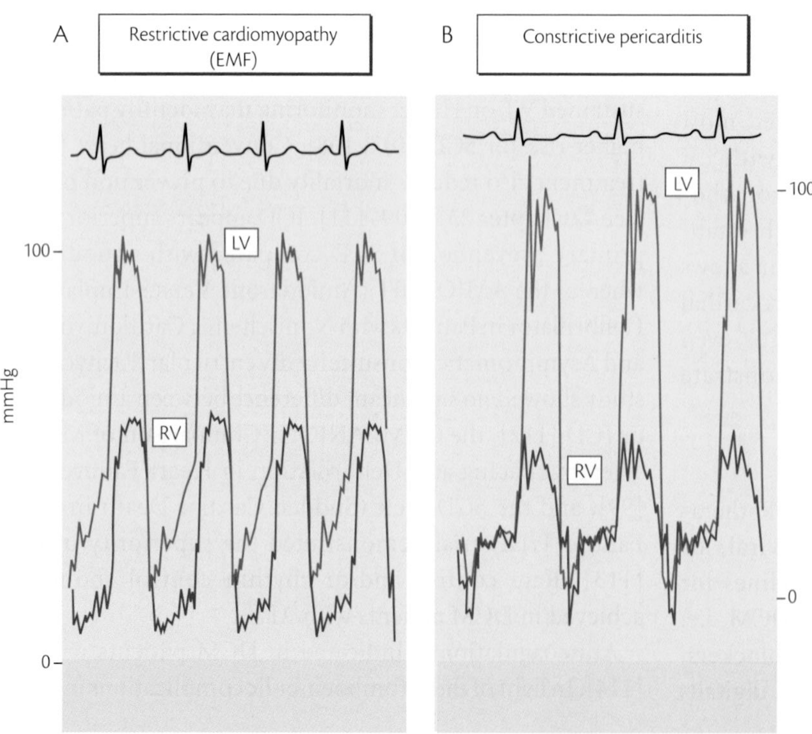

Figure 18.18 Simultaneous pressure recordings of the left ventricle (LV) and right ventricle (RV) in restrictive cardiomyopathy (A) and constrictive pericarditis (B). Diastolic pressures are discordant in (A) but concordant in (B).

in both left and right ventricular diastolic pressures during respiration (➲Fig. 18.18).

The classification of restrictive cardiomyopathy is based on aetiological and clinical findings.

- Primary forms:
  - Löffler's endocarditis;
  - endomyocardial fibrosis.
- Secondary forms:
  - infiltrative diseases;
  - storage diseases;
  - post-radiation disease.

Primary forms are associated with inflammation and hypereosinophilia and are due to chronic inflammatory processes, i.e. parasite infections, autoimmune diseases, or eosinophilic leukaemia. Primary forms are rare in Western industrialized countries but may be endemic in some African or South American countries [133–137]. Secondary forms are caused by a variety of systemic diseases which are associated with thickening of the myocardial wall by infiltration, storage, or excessive fibrosis. Secondary forms are classified by the specific type of material deposition, i.e. infiltration, storage, or replacement. Depending on the degree of infiltration or storage, clinical course in restrictive cardiomyopathy is often mitigated [137–140].

Primary forms

There are two primary forms of restrictive cardiomyopathy: the acute form, which is called Löffler's endocarditis, and the chronic form, which is termed endomyocardial fibrosis.

Löffler's endocarditis

The acute form of primary restrictive cardiomyopathy was described for the first time by Wilhelm Löffler in Zurich in 1936 [141]. He observed two patients who died from endocarditis, with extensive fibrosis of the endocardium and thrombotic thickening with severe blood eosinophilia. The fibrotic process is usually located at the apex of one or both ventricles and extends into the inflow tract, frequently involving the chordae tendineae [142–145]. These obliterations cause mitral and/or tricuspid regurgitation. Histological examination shows acute eosinophilic myocarditis involving both the endocardium and myocardium, with mural thrombosis often containing eosinophils and fibrotic thickening. The eosinophils have been recognized as pro-inflammatory effector cells which play a role in the pathogenesis of inflammation and tissue damage in eosinophile-associated diseases [146]. Patients with hypereosinophilia are often associated with an indeterminate diagnosis of hypereosinophilia of unknown etiology. This syndrome has been called hypereosinophilic syndrome (HES). This syndrome is characterized by sustained overproduction of eosinophiles and tissue infiltration, most commonly involving the heart with the development of eosinophilic endomyocardial fibrosis. The eosinophils may be primary or secondary or small granules. Eosinophils differentiate in the bone marrow from stem-cell derived CD34 progenitor cells and contain a number of T-cell derived cytokines and growth factors including IL-3, GM-CSF, and IL-5. The cytokines and growth factors are thought to induce endorgan damage through secretion of inflammatory mediators leading to tissue damage, remodelling, and fibrosis [146].

Pathophysiology

The pathophysiological mechanism is not clear but eosinophils are thought to play a major role. Any process associated with hypereosinophilia for several weeks or months may lead to eosinophilic myocarditis [139,140]. Patients may die ultimately from cardiogenic shock, thromboemboli, or renal or respiratory dysfunction. Hypereosinophilia may be due to autoimmune disease, rheumatoid arthritis, parasite infections, or eosinophilic leukaemia [147]. The patient shown in ➲Fig. 18.19 suffered from eosinophilic leukaemia that was stabilized by medical therapy. Because of severe congestive heart failure, the patient underwent LV decortication, which was associated with a dramatic clinical improvement. One year after the operation, the patient died from recurrence of eosinophilic leukaemia.

Clinical manifestations

The typical clinical symptoms include weight loss, fever, cough, rash, and congestive heart failure. Although early cardiac involvement may be asymptomatic, cardiac dysfunction can be found in >50% of all patients. Cardiomegaly may be present on the chest radiograph, with lung congestion. Mitral or tricuspid regurgitation is common in most patients. Systemic embolism is frequent and often associated with neurological and renal dysfunction. Death is usually due to congestive heart failure.

Diagnosis

Chest radiography may show cardiomegaly and pulmonary congestion, with dilatation of one or both atria. The ECG usually shows non-specific ST-segment and T-wave abnormalities. Arrhythmias are often present, especially AF [138]. The most important tool for diagnosis is echocardiography, which shows localized thickening of one or

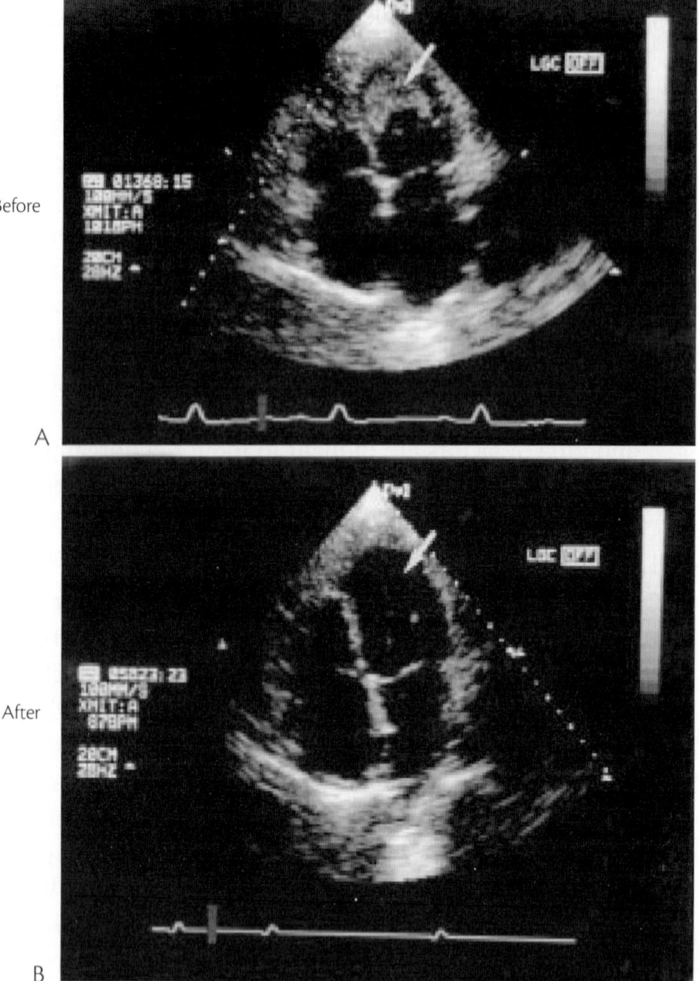

Figure 18.19 (A) Preoperative and (B) postoperative two-dimensional echocardiograms (four-chamber view) of a patient with eosinophilic leukaemia and Löffler's endocarditis of the left ventricle. Preoperatively, the left ventricle is globular and small but regains normal size with a clear decrease in left atrial chamber volume after surgical decortication.

both ventricles at the apex (➲Fig. 18.19) with involvement of the chordae tendineae. Typically the atria are enlarged, associated with mitral and/or tricuspid regurgitation. Systolic function is usually preserved, with a typical restrictive mitral inflow pattern [143]. Cardiac catheterization shows markedly elevated ventricular filling pressures in the presence of a small ventricle with typical obliterations of the apex. Most patients have mild to moderate tricuspid or mitral regurgitation. The diagnosis may be confirmed by right or left ventricular EMB.

Management

Cardiac therapy is based on treatment of restrictive cardiomyopathy, including diuretics and after-load reduction with ACE inhibitors or AT1 receptor blockers. Beta-blockers may be used for reducing heart rate, or digitalis in the case of AF. Because of the risk of cardiac embolization, low-molecular-weight heparin or oral anticoagulation is mandatory.

Medical therapy depends on the aetiology of the hypereosinophilic syndrome: autoimmune disease may be treated with corticosteroids or immunosuppressive agents, rheumatoid arthritis with antitumour necrosis factor α, or eosinophilic leukaemia with antiproliferative agents [144].

Surgical therapy may be considered in patients who remain symptomatic but have been stabilized medically (➲Fig. 18.19). Endocardial decortication of one or both ventricles may be performed and may improve cardiac symptoms and reduce cardiac mortality.

Prognosis

The classic syndrome of Löffler's endocarditis is associated with a poor prognosis and most patients die within 6–12 months. Since the cause of hypereosinophilia remains unknown in most patients, clinical outcome is often poor, although corticosteroids may suppress hypereosinophilia. Those patients with a known aetiology for hypereosinophilia may do better [145].

Differential diagnosis

In a subacute phase, Löffler's endocarditis may mimic chronic endomyocardial fibrosis. However, the clinical picture of acute illness, fever, cough, congestive heart failure, and hypereosinophilia is so typical that correct diagnosis should not be missed.

Endomyocardial fibrosis

Endomyocardial fibrosis was first described in 1968 [134]. Since then, the endemic or equatorial African and the sporadic European form have been characterized. Endomyocardial fibrosis is marked by intense endocardial thickening of the apex and subvalvular apparatus of one or both ventricles [137, 138]. The fibrotic thickening of the apex leads to obliteration of one or both ventricles, with obstruction to filling producing restrictive and, in some biventricular forms, constrictive physiology.

Three types of endomyocardial fibrosis have been described: right ventricular (10%), LV (40%), and biventricular (50%) (➲Fig. 18.20). The African form is associated with a mean age of approximately 30–40 years and a male:female ratio of 2:1. The European form is associated with a mean age of 30–50 years and a male/female ratio of 1:2.

Aetiology

The term 'primary restrictive cardiomyopathy' suggests idiopathic pathophysiology without a clear infective agent or autoimmune disease. In fact, aetiology appears to be multiple, such as parasite infections in equatorial Africa (filariasis) or autoimmune diseases associated with glomerulonephritis or rheumatoid arthritis in the sporadic European form.

The common pathophysiological pathway for both Löffler's endocarditis and endomyocardial fibrosis is probably excessive blood eosinophilia [139, 145]. Hypereosinophilia of any cause (parasite infection, autoimmune disease, eosinophilic leukaemia, etc.) may also be responsible for the occurrence of endomyocardial fibrosis. It is believed that eosinophils are mechanically destroyed in the ventricles, which release fibroblast-stimulating factors that cause the typical lesions in the inflow tract and apex. The obliteration leads to a reduction in chamber volume (➲Figs. 18.20 and 18.21) typically associated with mitral or tricuspid regurgitation because the chordae tendineae are often involved. Haemodynamically, the obliterations are associated with diastolic dysfunction and increased filling pressures, leading to lung congestion and right-sided heart failure. Typically the chambers are small but systolic contractions are maintained [137]. The clinical course is chronic and may be stable for several years or decades. However, progression to

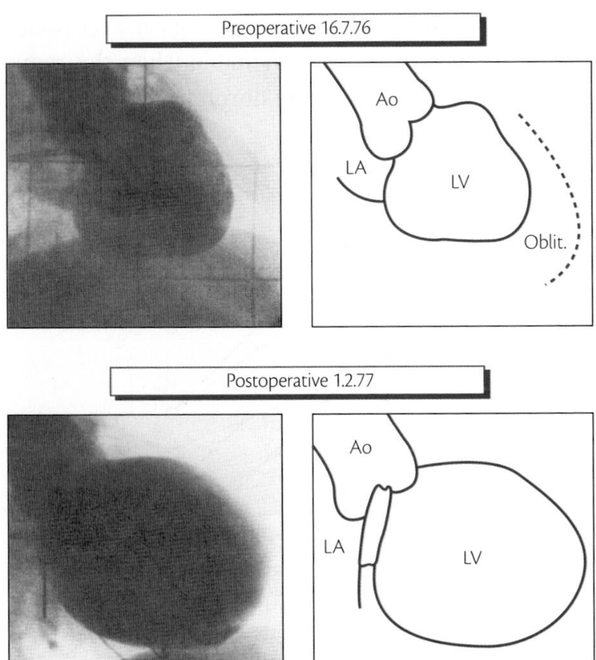

Figure 18.20 Preoperative (top) and postoperative (bottom) angiograms in a patient with biventricular endomyocardial fibrosis. The left ventricle (LV) is of globular shape with severe regurgitation into the left atrium (LA). After surgical decortication, the ventricle is significantly larger and mitral regurgitation is no longer present due to prosthetic valve replacement. Ao, ascending aorta. Reproduced with permission from Hess OM. Endomyokardfibrose. In Krayenbuehl HP, Kuebler W (eds.). *Herzkrankheiten*, 1981. Stuttgart: Thieme Verlag, pp. 4717–21.

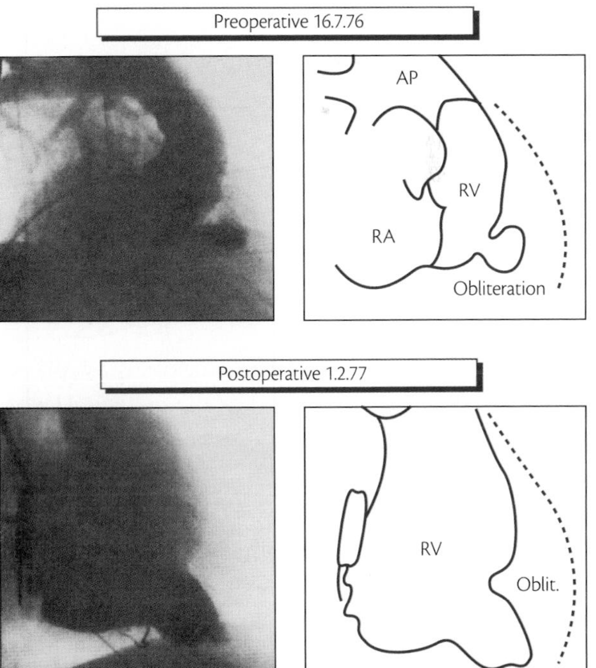

Figure 18.21 Preoperative (top) and postoperative (bottom) right ventricular angiograms in a patient with biventricular endomyocardial fibrosis (same patient as in ➲Fig. 18.20). A characteristic, almost pathognomonic finding is obliteration of the right ventricular apex with a residual bay-like formation. After decortication, the right ventricle becomes larger but the bay-like formation persists. Prosthetic valve replacement has been performed because of severe tricuspid regurgitation. AP, arteria pulmonalis; RA, right atrium; RV, right ventricle. Reproduced with permission from Hess OM. Endomyokardfibrose. In Krayenbuehl HP, Kuebler W (eds.). *Herzkrankheiten*, 1981. Stuttgart: Thieme Verlag, pp. 4717–21.

severe heart failure may be fast. The only treatment is surgical decortication [137].

Diagnosis

The most important tool for diagnosis is two-dimensional Doppler echocardiography. The typical obliterations of the LV apex can be seen (➲Fig. 18.19), with normal contractions of the basal regions. The haemodynamic consequence of diastolic dysfunction is atrial dilation, and AF may occur [143,144].

Chest radiography may not be very helpful but mild to moderate enlargement of the cardiac silhouette with signs of pulmonary congestion may be present. Pleural effusion may be seen. In patients with slow progression, diffuse calcifications of the endocardium may be found (➲Fig. 18.22).

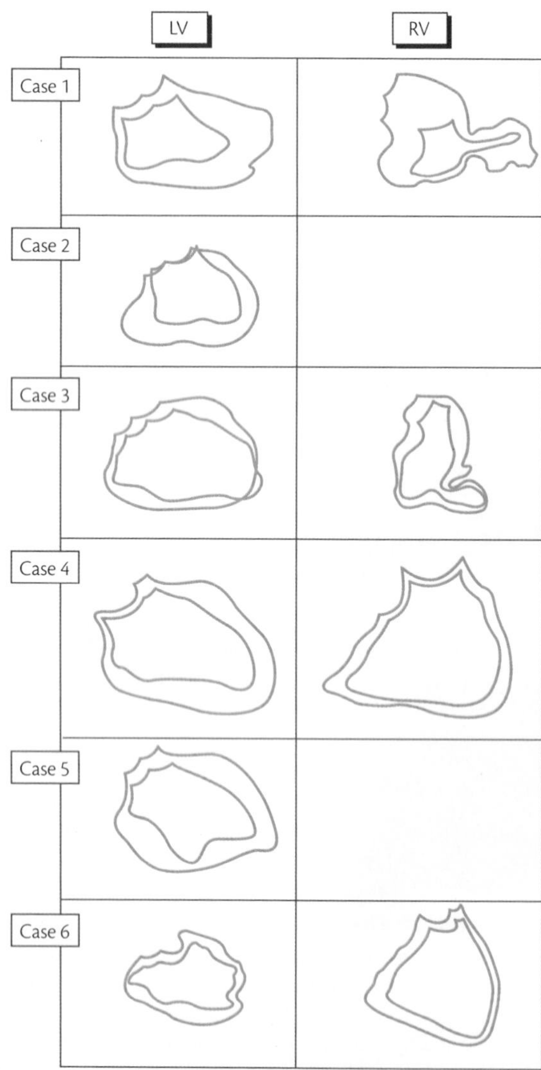

Figure 18.22 Typical angiographic findings (end-diastolic and end-systolic silhouettes) in six patients with endomyocardial fibrosis. LV silhouettes are shown on the left, RV silhouettes on the right. Please note the irregular shapes of the left and right ventricles with bay-like formations of the RV in cases 1 and 3.

Laboratory findings are usually unspectacular but there may be increased C-reactive protein, electrolyte imbalance due to diuretic treatment, and haematological changes according to the underlying disease.

Management

Heart failure treatment for diastolic dysfunction is appropriate in patients with mild to moderate restriction. Diuretics and ACE inhibitors may be helpful. Digitalis can be used in patients with atrial flutter or fibrillation. Beta-blockers are appropriate in patients with tachycardia but bradycardia is not well tolerated in these patients with small ventricles and high filling pressures.

Endocardial decortication has to be considered in advanced disease. Typically one or both ventricles are decorticated, with mitral or tricuspid valve replacement because of involvement of chordae tendineae and papillary muscles. Good to excellent surgical results have been reported by several groups but slow progression to systolic heart failure may become a problem [148–156]. After decortication most patients show an increase in cardiac volumes (➲Figs 18.20 and 18.21), with a decrease in LVEDP (➲Fig. 18.23).

Prognosis

Clinical course may be stable over years. When restriction becomes clinically apparent, a downhill course begins with a decrease in quality of life. After surgical decortication the clinical course may remain stable when the remaining myocardium is not severely fibrotic and dysfunctional.

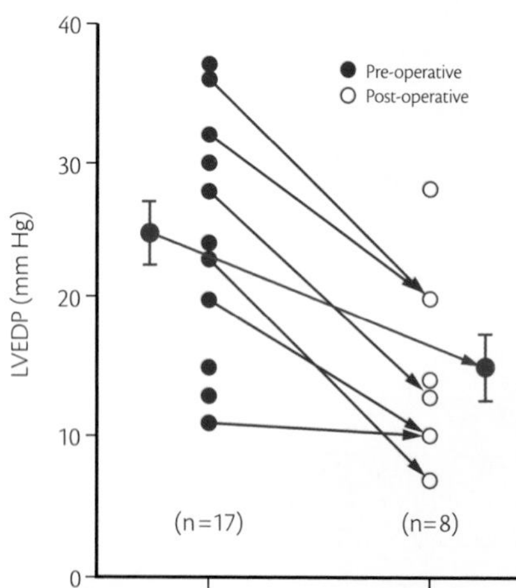

Figure 18.23 Left ventricular end-diastolic pressure (LVEDP) in 17 patients with endomyocardial fibrosis before (left) and 6–12 months after (right) successful decortication of the left ventricle (n = 8). LVEDP decreases from 25 to 15mmHg as a consequence of improved diastolic function. Reproduced with permission from Hess OM, Turina M, Egloff L, *et al.* Velauf der Endomyokardfibrose nach chirurgischer Endokarddekortikation. *Schweiz Med Wochenschr* 1984; **114**: 1595–8; and Schneider U, Jenni R, Turina, J, *et al.* Long-term follow up of patients with endomyocardial fibrosis: effects of surgery. *Heart* 1998; **79**: 362–7.

In rare cases recurrence of an acute Löffler's endocarditis may occur. At our institution a female patient developed Löffler's endocarditis, with marked blood eosinophilia and fibrotic thickening of the endocardium, 1 year after successful biventricular decortication [155]. The patient died a few days later in cardiogenic shock. Cardiac transplantation may be considered in patients with severe biventricular endomyocardial fibrosis but secondary pulmonary hypertension may be a limiting factor.

Differential diagnosis

Primary restrictive cardiomyopathy can be difficult to differentiate from post-viral constrictive pericarditis, carcinoid syndrome of the right ventricle and amyloidosis [155, 156]. There is a triad of key features of endomyocardial fibrosis:

- apical obliterations of one or both ventricles (echocardiogram or angiocardiogram);
- mild cardiomegaly with severe pulmonary congestion;
- mitral and/or tricuspid regurgitation; diastolic heart failure.

Secondary forms

Infiltrative diseases

In infiltrative diseases, a product of metabolism, inflammation, or carcinomatosis pervades the cardiac interstitium and increases stiffness of the myocardium, thereby restricting ventricular relaxation, increasing filling pressures, and reducing stroke volume.

Amyloidosis

Amyloidosis refers to a large group of disorders in which soluble extracellular proteins are misfolded and deposited as insoluble fibrils in the tissues, leading to disruption of tissue architecture and organ dysfunction. The disease may be acquired or hereditary, and is classified according to the nature of the fibril precursor protein and clinical features.

Acquired amyloidosis

In primary (or AL) amyloidosis, the fibrillar protein is composed of κ and λ immunoglobulin light chains, produced by a proliferating clone of plasma cells. A systemic disease that tends to follow a rapidly progressive course, primary amyloidosis is often seen in conjunction with plasma cell dyscrasias such as multiple myeloma or the monoclonal gammopathies.

Secondary (or AA) amyloidosis occurs in association with chronic inflammatory disorders such as rheumatoid arthritis, ankylosing spondylitis, and familial Mediterranean fever. Nephrotic syndrome and renal failure are common at presentation. The amyloid fibrils are composed of protein A.

β_2-microglobulin amyloidosis is a complication of long-term haemodialysis that usually occurs in localized peri-articular form but is occasionally systemic.

Senile systemic amyloidosis is seen in patients >60 years. The fibril precursor is normal wild-type transthyretin. Congestive heart failure, heart block, AF, and ventricular arrhythmia are recognized manifestations. Progression is slow and prognosis better than that of other acquired forms.

Hereditary amyloidosis

Hereditary amyloidosis is the result of a mutation in one of a number of fibril precursor proteins, including transthyretin, apolipoprotein AI or AII, lysozyme, fibrinogen Aα chain, gelsolin, and cystatin C. The phenotype varies according to the protein affected. Autosomal dominant inheritance is typical.

Cardiovascular involvement

Amyloidosis frequently affects the heart. The propensity for cardiovascular involvement is greatest in primary, senile systemic, and certain hereditary forms of the disease. Cardiac disease is relatively less common in AA amyloidosis but is a marker of unfavourable prognosis when present [157]. Amyloid fibrils may be deposited in the myocardium, papillary muscles, valves, conduction system, and/or vessels, with consequent clinical manifestations.

Clinical presentation of cardiac amyloidosis

Clinical suspicion of cardiac amyloidosis arises in the following circumstances:

- cardiac disease in the setting of established AL amyloidosis and/or plasma cell dyscrasia;
- ventricular dysfunction or arrhythmia and long-standing connective tissue disease or other chronic inflammatory disorder;
- any patient with restrictive cardiomyopathy of unknown aetiology;
- LVH on echocardiography but a low-voltage ECG;
- congestive heart failure of unknown cause refractory to standard medical therapy.

Diagnosis of cardiac amyloidosis

The preliminary work-up for a patient with suspected cardiac amyloidosis includes a 12-lead ECG and two-dimensional echocardiography, with or without Holter monitoring. Characteristic findings are summarized in ➲Table 18.6 [158]. A low-voltage ECG with increased septal and posterior LV wall thickness on echocardiography is specific for cardiac amyloidosis on non-invasive testing [158]. Other investigations that are of value include

Table 18.6 Clinical investigations in cardiac amyloidosis

12-lead ECG
Low voltage*
Interventricular conduction delay/bundle branch block
Varying degrees of atrioventricular block
Poor R-wave progression ('pseudo-infarct pattern')*
Left-axis deviation
Holter
Atrial fibrillation
Other tachyarrhythmia or bradyarrhythmia
Two-dimensional echocardiography
Concentric or asymmetric thickening of the left ventricular wall
Occasional thickening of the right ventricle
Sparkling/granular appearance of myocardium*
Thickened interatrial septum*
Thickened valves and/or papillary muscles
Left atrial or biatrial dilation
Pericardial effusion
Diastolic dysfunction in early disease (E/A reversal)
Restrictive physiology (E >> A)
Systolic impairment with normal end-diastolic volume
Histology
Apple-green birefringence under polarized light microscope after staining with Congo red*
Immunoperoxidase stains to differentiate light chains/transthyretin/protein A, etc.
Cardiac catheterization
Raised filling pressures
Protein electrophoresis
Serum and urine electrophoresis for presence of monoclonal protein in patients with suspected AL amyloidosis
Genetic testing
Commercially available to detect common mutations

*Features considered relatively more specific for amyloidosis.

protein electrophoresis and genetic testing. EMB is often diagnostic, although multiple specimens may have to be obtained to avoid sampling errors.

Management and outcome

Treatment is directed at both the underlying disease process and the cardiac complications. Systemic therapy is type-specific, underscoring the importance of determining the precise aetiology of amyloidosis. Prognosis of AL amyloidosis is poor; however, in subgroups of patients, combined treatment with high-dose melphalan and autologous stem cell transplantation has resulted in haematological remission, improved 5-year survival, and reversal of amyloid-related disease [159]. In contrast, senile systemic amyloidosis is characterized by slow progression not requiring alkylating agents [160]. Reactive AA amyloidosis may respond to anti-inflammatory and immunosuppressive drugs that reduce production of acute-phase reactant serum amyloid A protein.

Ventricular dysfunction secondary to amyloidosis may be difficult to treat. Diuretics and vasodilators are used judiciously owing to the risk of hypotension with excessive falls in preload. Digoxin is contraindicated because it binds to amyloid fibrils and toxicity may develop at ordinary therapeutic doses. Complex ventricular arrhythmia has been documented in patients with cardiac amyloidosis and may be a predictor of SCD. Beta-blockers are administered with caution as they may promote AV block and their negative inotropism is often poorly tolerated. Implantation of a permanent pacemaker is indicated in patients with symptomatic bradyarrhythmias or complete AV block.

Sarcoidosis

Sarcoidosis is a multisystem disease characterized by non-caseating granulomas. Familial aggregation [161] suggests that genetic factors are involved. The lungs and lymphatic system are frequently affected. Cardiac involvement is uncommon; myocardial granulomas were detected in 27% of patients in one study [162]. It should be noted that microscopic granulomas within the heart may be overlooked at autopsy, resulting in underestimation of their prevalence. Indeed, cardiac disease has been reported in 58% of patients with sarcoidosis [163]. The most common sites of sarcoid granulomas are the LV free wall (96%), septum (73%), right ventricle (46%), right atrium (11%), and left atrium (7%) [164].

Early treatment with corticosteriods and, if required, additional immunosuppressive agents improves outcome. Timely diagnosis is critical. Unfortunately, the perception that cardiac involvement is rare may lead to a delay in detection and therapy; in one study an antemortem diagnosis was made in only 65% of subjects [162]. LV diastolic dysfunction was present in 14% of patients with biopsy-proven pulmonary sarcoidosis but no other clinical features of cardiac disease [165], suggesting that subclinical sarcoid cardiomyopathy may be under-recognized.

Clinical presentation of cardiac sarcoidosis

Cardiac involvement should be considered in any sarcoidosis with symptoms of arrhythmia (i.e. palpitation, presyncope, or syncope). Also worth investigating are patients with dyspnoea out of proportion to pulmonary disease, particularly if physical signs of heart failure are present. Since sudden death may be the first manifestation of cardiac sarcoidosis, periodic screening with 12-lead ECG and echocardiography, with or without Holter monitoring, may be indicated.

Isolated cardiac sarcoidosis is rare and usually followed by systemic involvement. Alternatively, cardiac manifestations may develop after pulmonary sarcoidosis has resolved. In many cases, medical attention is not sought for mild respiratory complaints, or cough and dyspnoea are misattributed to infection or allergy. Thus, cardiac complications may be the presenting feature of sarcoidosis. In patients without a diagnosis, the following cardiac abnormalities should raise suspicion:

- the young patient with conduction system disease;
- DCM with AV block, abnormal wall thickness, regional wall motion abnormalities, or perfusion defects in anteroseptal and apical regions that improve with stress [166];
- sustained re-entrant VT [167], non-specific ECG abnormalities and echocardiogram, and angiographically normal coronary arteries;
- restrictive cardiomyopathy of unknown aetiology;
- presumed arrhythmogenic right ventricular cardiomyopathy and AV block, or signs and symptoms of chronic respiratory disease [168].

Diagnosis of cardiac sarcoidosis

The minimum work-up for any patient with suspected cardiac sarcoidosis comprises a 12-lead ECG, echocardiography and Holter monitoring (➲Table 18.7).

Management and outcome

Corticosteroids are first-line therapy for cardiac sarcoidosis. Prevention of disease progression necessitates early treatment, preferably at the time of diagnosis. Improvement or resolution of arrhythmia, conduction defects or perfusion abnormalities is well documented [169]. LV systolic impairment may respond, although steroids should ideally be commenced prior to the development of heart failure. The combination of pacemaker implantation for bradyarrhythmia and steroid therapy may improve prognosis and reduce mortality from SCD. Heart failure is now the main cause of death from cardiac sarcoidosis [170]. Once established, systolic heart failure may be treated with ACE inhibitors and/or AT2 receptor antagonists and beta-blockers. The use of beta-blockers in patients with early conduction system disease warrants careful monitoring.

Antiarrhythmic therapy for recurrent VT remains largely empirical. Placement of an ICD should be considered for all sarcoidosis patients with ventricular tachyarrhythmia. Besides offering optimal protection against sudden death, the ICD may enable control of refractory VT by antitachycardia pacing. VT storm that is resistant to drug therapy may require catheter ablation as a last resort.

Table 18.7 Clinical investigations in cardiac sarcoidosis

12-lead ECG
Non-specific depolarization or repolarization abnormalities
Poor R-wave progression ('pseudo-infarct pattern')
Varying degrees of atrioventricular block
Arrhythmia
Two-dimensional echocardiography
Mild thickening of the left ventricular wall, concentric or asymmetric
Thinning of the myocardium with or without aneurysms in later stage, resulting from fibrosis
Right ventricular hypertrophy, dilation, and/or dysfunction
Increased pulmonary artery pressure
Mitral regurgitation secondary to papillary muscle dysfunction
Pericardial effusion
Systolic and/or diastolic dysfunction
Biatrial enlargement with restrictive physiology
Holter monitoring
Frequent PVCs, sustained or non-sustained VT
Bradyarrhythmias or conduction system disease
Myocardial perfusion scan
Perfusion defects affecting the anteroseptal and apical regions that improve with stress on thallium scanning
Gallium uptake in areas of inflammation
Magnetic resonance imaging
Structural and functional changes described above
Focal enhancement following administration of gadolinium, indicating fibrosis
Chest radiography/computed tomography
Detects pulmonary features of sarcoidosis in patients with cardiac presentation
Cardiac catheterization
Angiographically normal coronary arteries in presence of perfusion defect
Coronary artery stenosis secondary to vasculitis
Increased pulmonary artery pressure
Endomyocardial biopsy
High specificity but low sensitivity because of patchy disease involvement and likelihood of sampling errors

PVC, premature ventricular contraction; VT, ventricular tachycardia.

Storage diseases

The storage disorders are inborn errors of metabolism that result in the accumulation of the substrate or byproduct of the affected pathway. The intracellular location of the metabolite distinguishes storage disease from infiltrative disorders, in which deposition is confined to the interstitium. Accretion of the abnormal metabolite in the heart is toxic to myocytes and induces either concentric (HCM-like phenotype) or eccentric (DCM-like phenotype) hypertrophy.

Haemochromatosis

Haemochromatosis refers to genetically determined disorders of iron metabolism that result in iron overload and deposition. Organ dysfunction is due to the toxic effects of redox-active iron. Most commonly affected are the liver, pancreas, joints, and heart. The adult-onset form of haemochromatosis has been linked to mutations in the *HFE* gene on the short arm of chromosome 6 and, less commonly, the gene encoding transferrin receptor 2 (*TfR2*) [171]. Autosomal recessive inheritance with variable penetrance is typical. Heterozygosity is present in 8–10% of people of European descent, while 5 in 1000 are homozygous. Overt disease expression is rare in women of child-bearing age owing to protective blood loss during menstruation.

Three stages are recognized in the natural history of adult-onset haemochromatosis. In the initial biochemical phase, iron overload is confined to the plasma compartment, with increased transferrin saturation. More than 50% of *HFE* homozygotes with the most common disease-causing mutation (C282Y) will progress to the second deposition phase, in which iron accumulates in parenchymal tissues, with concomitant elevation of serum ferritin levels. Few patients progress to the final stage, with impairment of target organ function.

This pattern of gradual iron loading is in marked contrast to juvenile hereditary haemochromatosis, in which organ dysfunction ensues by the age of 30, with hypogonadism and glucose intolerance. Cardiac complications are also common and may result in premature death from intractable heart failure. Mutations have been identified in the genes encoding hepcidin (*HAMP*) and haemojuvelin (*HJV*) [171].

Cardiovascular involvement

Although haemochromatosis seldom affects the heart in isolation, cardiac complications are occasionally the presenting feature of the disease. The site and quantity of iron deposition within the heart determines the type and extent of cardiac dysfunction. The ventricles are commonly involved, leading in most cases to DCM, although a restrictive picture may be present. Subclinical cardiac disease can be identified by echocardiography.

On histology stainable iron is localized to the sarcoplasm but is generally absent from the interstitium. Cardiac haemochromatosis is therefore a storage disorder rather than infiltration, as evidenced by the normal ventricular wall thickness [172]. Ultrastructural studies reveal the presence of iron in the cytoplasm, nucleus and mitochondria; at least part of the toxicity of iron is ascribed to oxidative damage to the mitochondrial genome, with progressive mitochondrial dysfunction [173]. Consistent with this hypothesis is the predilection of haemochromatosis for organs with high mitochondrial activity: liver, pancreas, and heart.

Of note, degenerative changes and fibrosis are minimal within the myocardium, probably accounting for the infrequency of ventricular tachyarrhythmia. Nevertheless, heart failure is often accompanied by ventricular extrasystoles or even VT, which may be difficult to treat [174]. In some patients, intravenous lidocaine (lignocaine), procainamide, and propafenone fail to terminate sustained VT, as might DC cardioversion. Amiodarone may be successful in restoring sinus rhythm [175]. In a case of haemochromatosis presenting with recurrent syncope, both spontaneous and inducible polymorphic VT was present but there was no evidence of impaired ventricular function or diabetes, although liver function tests were mildly elevated. Marked signal loss in the liver was detected on MRI, a technique also useful for monitoring myocardial iron overload [176].

Commonly observed in cardiac haemochromatosis are atrial flutter or fibrillation and supraventricular tachycardia, possibly due to iron deposition in the atrium or related to increased pressures from ventricular dysfunction. Involvement of the conduction system may manifest as varying degrees of AV block or sick sinus syndrome.

Management and outcome

Regular phlebotomy is the mainstay of treatment for cardiac haemochromatosis, and may effect partial or complete reversal of ventricular dysfunction and suppression of arrhythmia. Depletion of myocardial iron has been documented by serial EMB. CMR offers a non-invasive means of assessing the response to therapy. Blood count, serum ferritin, and transferrin saturations should also be monitored; excessively rapid mobilization of iron is thought to carry a risk of aggravating end-organ damage. Standard medical therapy is indicated for heart failure and arrhythmia.

Unfortunately, the correlation between cardiac iron load and function may decline in advanced disease [177]. It has been suggested that there is a threshold beyond which the toxic effects of iron accumulation in the myocardium result in permanent ultrastructural or metabolic derangements. Reduction in myocardial iron deposits at this stage do not result in improvement of cardiac function. Thus early diagnosis and initiation of prophylaxis or venesection remain critical. Screening of first-degree relatives for the disease is imperative and may be facilitated by increased availability of genetic testing.

Glycogen storage disease

Glycogen storage disease (GSD) is a group of inherited metabolic disorders characterized by abnormalities in the enzymes that regulate the synthesis or degradation of glycogen. Glycogen storage occurs in the liver, heart, skeletal muscle, and/or central nervous system. The heart is affected in types II, III, and IV [178]. Cardiac manifestations often include severe LVH, which may mimic HCM or demonstrate a restrictive pattern. Cavity dilation and systolic impairment develop in advanced stages, producing a DCM-like phenotype. Conduction system disease is also described.

Glycogen storage disease type II

Type II GSD, or Pompe disease, is caused by deficiency of acid α-glucosidase (acid maltase) [179], which cleaves α-1,4 and α-1,6 glycosidic linkages of glycogen. The mode of inheritance is autosomal recessive. Genetic counselling and family screening are paramount once the diagnosis has been established.

The infantile form of type II GSD usually presents in the first months of life with failure to thrive, generalized hypotonia, and weakness. Macroglossia and moderate hepatomegaly are associated features. Cardiomegaly is evident on chest radiography and may raise suspicion of the disease. Plasma CK levels are markedly elevated. The diagnosis is confirmed by enzyme assay of muscle or skin fibroblasts; acid α-glucosidase activity is virtually undetectable.

ECG findings in type II GSD include left-axis deviation, short PR interval, high-voltage QRS complexes, and repolarization abnormalities. Echocardiography confirms severe concentric biventricular hypertrophy [180], which initially resembles HCM and may be associated with LVOTO. Systolic function is normal or hyperdynamic in the initial stages, but deteriorates with disease progression as the ventricles dilate. Weakness of the diaphragm and intercostal muscles may necessitate mechanical ventilation, but high airway pressures may reduce ventricular filling and are poorly tolerated [181]. Death usually results from cardiorespiratory failure.

At post-mortem, the heart may be three times normal size. Fibroelastic thickening of the endocardium is often present. Histology reveals glycogen accumulation in cardiomyocytes, contained within membrane-bound vacuoles and free in the cytoplasm. Skeletal muscle shows a similar appearance.

In the past, infantile-onset Pompe disease was almost uniformly fatal by 1 year of age. However, enzyme replacement therapy is promising and emphasizes the importance of early recognition, since the therapeutic window is short. In limited clinical trials of recombinant human acid α-glucosidase, treated infants showed decreased cardiomegaly, motor improvement and prolonged survival [181, 182].

Late-onset type II GSD, in which disease develops after the age of 12 months, is associated with residual acid α-glucosidase activity (≤10% of normal in toddlers and children, and up to 40% in adults). Presentation in the elderly has been documented [183]. Interestingly, the clinical picture is dominated by proximal myopathy and respiratory insufficiency. Cardiac involvement is rare, suggesting that partial enzyme activity may be sufficient to protect the heart.

Glycogen storage disease type III

Type III GSD, also known as Cori or Forbe disease, is caused by deficiency of the enzyme amylo-1,6-glucosidase, which is involved in 'debranching' the glycogen molecule during catabolism. This results in arrest of glycogen breakdown when the outermost branch points are reached. Phosphorylase limit dextrin, an abnormal form of glycogen, accumulates in affected tissue [184].

Type III GSD is also transmitted in autosomal recessive fashion. The clinical heterogeneity is explained at least in part by the variety of mutations identified. Fasting hypoglycaemia and hepatomegaly predominate. While liver dysfunction usually resolves during adolescence, worsening dysfunction and cirrhosis are also described. Cardiac involvement generally takes the form of LVH resembling HCM, which may be accompanied by SAM and LVOTO [185]. Many patients with echocardiographic abnormalities are asymptomatic. However, biventricular dilation, recurrent sustained VT and sudden death have also been reported. Late gadolinium enhancement has been observed on CMR, suggesting that progressive fibrosis may be the substrate for cavity dilation and re-entrant VT.

Glycogen storage disease type IV

Type IV GSD is an autosomal recessive disorder linked to deficiency of the 'branching' enzyme amylo-1,4-1,6 transglucosidase [186]. The accumulation of polyglucosan bodies (an abnormal form of glycogen) in the liver may cause cirrhosis and hepatic failure in early childhood. However, non-progressive forms have also been documented [187]. Skeletal myopathy may occur and cardiac involvement characteristically manifests as congestive heart failure. A late-onset variant of type IV GSD is also described, with complete deficiency of branching enzyme and presentation in adolescence with DCM [188].

Fabry disease

Anderson–Fabry disease is a metabolic storage disease in which deficiency of the enzyme α-galactosidase (α-Gal A) results in progressive tissue deposition of glycosphingolipids. Glycosphingolipids are components of the cytoplasmic membrane that consist of an outer saccharide component attached to a lipid called ceramide; the B blood group antigen is an example. Their ultimate breakdown inside lysosomes requires the action of a number of hydrolytic enzymes. α-Gal A is a lysosomal hydrolase responsible for the degradation of glycolipids with a terminal α-galactosamine residue. This substrate accumulates within cells owing to lack of α-Gal A activity in Fabry disease.

The α-Gal A gene is located in the Xq22 region of the X chromosome. X-linked inheritance accounts for the male predominance, with incidence estimated at 1 in 40,000 to 1 in 60,000. Varying degrees of disease expression may nevertheless occur in female carriers as a result of random X-chromosome inactivation [189, 190].

Fabry disease predominantly affects the skin, endothelium, kidneys, liver, pancreas, and nervous system (➔Table 18.8). Cardiac involvement is also common. In the classic phenotype, clinical manifestations begin in childhood or adolescence, on average at 10 years of age. Unfortunately, the non-specific symptoms may be misattributed to 'growing pains' or rheumatological diseases. Relentless progression is usual; neurological, cardiac and renal complications develop from late adolescence to adulthood. The average lifespan of 40 years improved by about a decade following introduction of renal dialysis. However, a major advance in Fabry disease has been enzyme replacement therapy, which underscores the importance of early recognition. Clinical trials of gene-activated and recombinant human α-Gal A showed marked and rapid reduction in plasma and tissue levels of globotriaosylceramide, diminished pain, and improved renal function [189].

Atypical variants of Fabry disease may manifest after the age of 40. The phenotype is milder and may be confined to one organ system; isolated cardiac or renal manifestations are recognized. Residual enzyme activity is present in these patients, whereas α-Gal A levels are virtually undetectable in the classic form.

Table 18.8 Systemic manifestations of Fabry disease

Pain
Chronic burning tingling pain in hands and feet
Fabry crisis (acute severe pain precipitated by stress, exertion, concurrent illness/fever)
Skin
Angiokeratomas, lymphoedema
Eyes
Corneal opacity
Gastrointestinal
Diarrhoea, abdominal discomfort, vomiting
Neurological
Tinnitus, vertigo, headache, transient ischaemic attacks, cerebrovascular accidents
Pulmonary
Obstructive airways disease
Renal
Proteinuria, lipiduria, uraemia, hypertension, end-stage renal failure
Other
Reduced saliva and tear production; exercise and heat intolerance

Cardiovascular involvement

Intracellular accumulation of glycosphingolipids has been observed in the myocardium, conduction system, valves, and vascular endothelium. Myocardial involvement typically manifests as LVH resembling HCM. Concentric hypertrophy is the most frequent distribution (37%), followed by asymmetric septal hypertrophy (10%). Eccentric and distal patterns of hypertrophy occur less frequently [4, 191, 192]. The degree of hypertrophy shows a positive correlation with age and an inverse relationship with the level of α-Gal A activity; blood pressure does not appear to be a major determining factor. SAM and LVOTO may be present. As in HCM, systolic function is generally preserved, but mild to moderate diastolic impairment is common. A restrictive picture is rare. The deposits account for only around 1% of the increase in LV mass, suggesting that the metabolic derangement induces compensatory hypertrophy by a mechanism that is still to be elucidated.

Thickening of the papillary muscles and mitral valve leaflets, with mild accompanying regurgitation, occurs in over half of patients with Fabry disease. Mitral valve prolapse appears less common. Minor structural abnormalities of the aortic valve were observed in a smaller subset [191].

AF and non-sustained VT may occur in Fabry disease, although the exact prevalence is uncertain. Varying degrees of AV block are a corollary of conduction system involvement.

Preferential storage of glycosphingolipids in the endothelium of cerebral vessels is associated with premature strokes. The vertebrobasilar circulation is predominantly affected. Endothelial dysfunction of coronary capillaries contributes to subendocardial ischaemia. Hypertension and dyslipidaemia related to chronic renal failure may also predispose patients with Fabry disease to coronary artery disease. A relatively high prevalence of cigarette smokers has been reported among the Fabry population; it has been suggested that smoking may alleviate the neuropathic pain associated with the disorder.

Clinical management

Patients with Fabry disease experience the same cardiac symptoms as those with sarcomeric HCM, including anginal chest pain, exertional dyspnoea, palpitation, syncope, and presyncope. In the isolated cardiac form of Fabry disease, systemic manifestations are absent and diagnosis is dependent on enzyme assay and/or EMB. Affected males have reduced or undetectable levels of α-Gal A in plasma and peripheral leucocytes. Assessment of α-Gal A activity in 79 consecutive patients with late-onset HCM revealed a 6% prevalence of Fabry disease [4]. X-linked inheritance will raise suspicion. Routine screening for Fabry disease has therefore been advocated in male patients with HCM.

Female heterozygotes, in contrast, may have relatively high residual α-Gal A activity, limiting the value of enzyme assay in establishing the diagnosis. Confirmation of Fabry disease in a male relative is strongly suggestive. Where this is not possible, EMB may elicit the diagnosis. Among 34 consecutive women with late-onset HCM, histology and/or electron microscopy showed features consistent with Fabry disease in 12% [192]. Genetic testing may facilitate familial evaluation. Most affected families have private mutations, accounting in part for the variability in disease expression and prognosis. *De novo* mutations are uncommon.

Enzyme replacement is now the mainstay of disease-specific treatment. The cardiac manifestations of Fabry disease respond to standard management strategies.

Post-radiation disease

Radiation may cause damage to any structure, including the pericardium, myocardium, valves, conduction system, and coronary arteries. Much of our knowledge of radiotherapy-induced cardiovascular disease arose from experience with survivors of Hodgkin disease, many of whom are young and may develop sequelae. Chest irradiation is also used to treat breast cancer, lung cancer, and seminomas [193]. The clinical impact of post-radiation cardiovascular disease will become more significant as long-term survival from cancer improves.

Myocardial involvement

At least two mechanisms are thought to underlie myocardial injury from irradiation: microcirculatory damage and free-radical toxicity. Work with experimental animals suggests that the former is a three-stage process. The first acute phase occurs shortly after exposure to radiation and is characterized by acute inflammation of small and medium-sized arteries. In the latent phase that follows, damage to capillary endothelial cells causes thrombotic occlusion and ischaemia. Progressive myocyte death and fibrosis occurs over time. Experimentally, the end-result is extensive fibrosis and death. Fortunately, myocardial disease is generally milder in patients who have received radiotherapy, most of whom remain asymptomatic. Clinically overt cardiomyopathy is uncommon and generally shows a restrictive pattern. A DCM-like phenotype may occur with anthracycline derivatives, the cardiotoxicity of which is increased by radiation.

Pericarditis

Pericardial disease may occasionally present during irradiation, although delayed onset is far more common. Early acute pericarditis is usually associated with radiation-induced necrosis of a large tumour adjacent to the heart. Radiotherapy is continued and long-term sequelae are rare.

Delayed pericardial disease may present months to years after radiation exposure in two overlapping forms: 1) an acute pericarditis that evolves, in around 20% of patients, into chronic constrictive pericarditis; and 2) chronic pericardial effusion, which often resolves spontaneously over years. Patients with symptoms and/or evidence of haemodynamic compromise may benefit from total parietal pericardiectomy, which is associated with a more favourable outcome than pericardiocentesis alone.

Arrhythmia/conduction system disease

The prevalence of conduction defects after radiotherapy is unknown, and delayed onset may preclude corroboration of a causal link. However, sick sinus syndrome and varying degrees of AV block have been reported. The level of the block is commonly infranodal rather than within the AV node. Supraventricular and ventricular arrhythmia have also been documented.

Valvular disease

Among 294 asymptomatic patients previously treated with mediastinal irradiation for Hodgkin disease, 29% had valve disease of sufficient clinical importance to justify antibiotic prophylaxis. The aortic valve was more commonly affected than the mitral and tricuspid valves, owing perhaps to its proximity to the radiation field. Both regurgitation and stenosis have been reported, although their relative frequency is unresolved. The prevalence of valve dysfunction increased with the time elapsed from radiotherapy.

Coronary artery disease

Increased risk of coronary artery disease has been reported in patients previously treated with mediastinal irradiation. The left anterior descending and right coronary arteries fall within the typical radiation mantle field and are frequently affected. Proximal narrowing involving the ostia is typical [194]. Coronary artery disease generally occurs in patients with at least one other recognized risk factor besides exposure to radiation.

Clinical management

Patients with radiation-induced cardiovascular disease may present with symptoms characteristic of the particular complication. Thus, acute pericarditis is accompanied by pleuritic chest pain and fever, while myocardial disease may manifest as chronic progressive dyspnoea. However, many radiotherapy recipients are asymptomatic. Subclinical myocardial dysfunction, pericardial effusion and valvular abnormalities are far more common than overt disease. Possibly silent myocardial infarction occurs more commonly in this subgroup than in the general population, owing to damage to cardiac nerve endings by irradiation.

Periodic cardiovascular evaluation of radiotherapy recipients has been advocated in order to identify clinically occult abnormalities [195]. A non-invasive work-up should include 12-lead ECG, echocardiography, exercise testing, Holter monitoring and a fasting blood lipid profile. CMR may also be useful (see ➲Chapter 5). Risk factors for coronary artery disease should be monitored and primary prevention measures instituted where necessary. Patients with valvular dysfunction may need endocarditis prophylaxis. Pregnancy is associated with increased cardiovascular demand and women should be encouraged to undergo cardiac assessment during antenatal care.

Contemporary radiotherapy techniques that involve lower total radiation doses and which minimize cardiac exposure by subcarinal shielding may diminish the risk of most types of cardiac disease. The antioxidant and iron chelator dexrazoxane confers protection against the cardiotoxic effects of anthracyclines, while amifostine reduces radiation-induced toxicity. Concurrent administration of cardiotoxic chemotherapeutic agents during radiotherapy should be avoided if at all possible. Aggressive treatment of hypertension and hyperlipidaemia in this population may also reduce the likelihood of coronary artery disease developing in later life.

Arrhythmogenic cardiomyopathy

Definition

The 1996 WHO classification of cardiomyopathies defines arrhythmogenic right ventricular cardiomyopathy (ARVC) as a group of heart muscle diseases characterized by structural and functional abnormalities of the right ventricle due to localized or diffuse atrophy with replacement of the myocardium by fatty and fibrous tissue [38]. Preferred areas include the outflow tract, the apex and the subtricuspid area of the free wall. Usually, the ventricular septum is spared [196]. Generally, men aged 15–35 years are affected [197]. Clinically, these morphological alterations are associated with regional or global right ventricular dysfunction and life-threatening arrhythmias of right ventricular origin (e.g. premature ventricular beats, sustained VT, or ventricular fibrillation), occasionally causing SCD in young patients with apparently normal hearts [196, 198]. Since its first description by Fontaine and colleagues in 1977, considerable progress has been made in understanding its pathogenesis, morbid anatomy, and clinical presentation [199–204]. Genetic background, natural history, exact clinical diagnosis including risk stratification, and treatment of high-risk patients are still poorly defined.

Aetiology and prevalence

Progressive loss and fibrofatty replacement of right ventricular myocardium in ARVC may be due to apoptosis of cardiomyocytes [205], myocardial inflammation [196, 202, 206], genetically determined myocardial atrophy [202] and possibly viral involvement [207]. Furthermore, regional clustering in Greece or northern Italy and familial history suggests an inherited disease usually with autosomal dominant inheritance and variable penetrance and phenotypes [197, 208–210]. Because the disease is difficult to diagnose and because many patients may be asymptomatic until their first presentation with sudden death, the true incidence and prevalence of ARVC are unknown [211].

Genetics

Familial background has been demonstrated in 30–50% of ARVC cases [197]. Sporadic development or familial disease with incomplete penetrance and variable phenotypic expression may constitute for the remaining cases. Both males and females can carry the disease and transmit it. At present, ten chromosomal loci on seven chromosomes have been identified (➲Table 18.9) [212]. Three involved gene products have been identified. In a rare inherited disease with a recessive form of transmission and 90% penetrance, mapped to chromosome 17, a defect in the gene encoding the cytoskeletal protein plakoglobin has been identified [213]. Genetic analysis of a similar disease with keratoderma and woolly hair at infancy and development of heart failure during adolescence revealed a mutation on chromosome 6p23–p24 encoding for desmoplakin, a protein important

Table 18.9 Genetics of arrhythmogenic right ventricular cardiomyopathy (ARVC)

Chromosome	Gene	Reference
Autosomal dominant forms of ARVC		
14q23–q24	–	Rampazzo *et al.* [208]
1q42–q43	Ryanodine receptor	Rampazzo *et al.* [219]
14q12–q22	–	Severini *et al.* [220]
2q32.1–q32.3	–	Rampazzo *et al.* [221]
3p23	–	Ahmad *et al.* [222]
10q22.3	–	Melberg *et al.* [223]
10p12–p14	–	Li *et al.* [224]
6p24	Desmoplakin	Rampazzo *et al.* [225]
Autosomal recessive forms of ARVC		
14q24–q	Plakoglobin	Frances *et al.* [226]
17q21	(Naxos disease)	Coonar *et al.* [213]

Adapted with permission from Paul M, Schulz-Bahr E, Breithard G, *et al.* Genetics of arrhythmogenic right ventricular cardiomyopathy: status quo and future perspectives. *Z Kardiol* 2003; **92**: 128–36.

for attachment of intermediate filaments to the desmosome [214]. Mutations in the cardiac ryanodine receptor gene (chromosome 1q23–q24) may impair intracellular calcium release and trigger electrical instability and VT.

Pathophysiology

Acquired replacement of the right ventricular anterolateral free wall myocardium by fatty or fibrofatty tissue extending from the epicardium towards the endocardium in a wave-like manner is characteristic. Fatty replacement of the myocardium may be diffuse (80%) or segmental (20%). Transmural infiltration is often associated with increased wall thickness. Saccular aneurysms of the apex, infundibulum or postero-inferior wall are detected in 50% in the fibrofatty variant. Histomorphological findings with atrophic myocardium and focal myocyte necrosis in association with infiltrating lymphocytes resemble chronic myocarditis. Myocardial inflammation [206, 215], viral infections [207] and genetically determined dystrophy may be involved in the apoptotic loss of cardiac myocytes [205, 216]. Islands of surviving myocardium interspersed with fatty or fibrofatty tissue may predispose to re-entrant tachycardia.

Clinical presentation

Exercise-triggered symptomatic VT of right ventricular origin (left bundle branch block configuration) is the most common clinical presentation. Palpitations and syncope are not uncommon due to sustained or non-sustained VT. With respect to VT morphology, it may be difficult to differentiate ARVC from benign and non-familial idiopathic right ventricular outflow tract tachycardia or pre-excitated AV re-entry tachycardia. In untreated patients, prolonged VT may degenerate into ventricular fibrillation. Because many patients are asymptomatic until their first presentation with sudden death, the true incidence and prevalence of VT-derived ventricular fibrillation leading to sudden cardiac arrest remains unknown. Patients presenting with congestive heart failure with or without ventricular arrhythmias are often misdiagnosed as having DCM.

Diagnostic testing

Clinical history may provide diagnostic and prognostic information if clinical events including palpitations, dizziness, presyncope, syncope, and arrhythmias or a positive familial history are present.

ECG abnormalities are detected in up to 90%. Most commonly, right ventricular involvement is associated with T-wave inversion in V1–V3 without right bundle branch block (➲Fig. 18.24). Repolarization abnormalities in leads beyond V3 may suggest LV involvement [200]. Right bundle branch block, prolongation of QRS duration in V1–V3, and epsilon wave (➲Fig. 18.24) caused by ventricular postexcitation (in about 30%) reflect delayed right ventricular activation and are distinct ECG markers of the disease. Epsilon waves may be atypical and look like a smooth potential forming an atypical prolonged R′ wave in leads V1–V3 if increased numbers of myocardial fibres are activated with delay. Therefore, any QRS duration in V1–V3 that exceeds QRS duration in V6 by >25ms should be considered an epsilon wave [200].

Right ventricular angiography, which reveals right ventricular dilatation and regional or segmental wall movement abnormalities or dyskinesia typically detected in the infundibular, apical, and subtricuspid region (bulgings and aneurysms), is the gold standard for the diagnosis of ARVC. These features, which have a diagnostic specificity of 90%, may also be detected non-invasively by CMR imaging and echocardiography. MRI allows accurate characterization of right ventricular function and anatomy. Limitations of

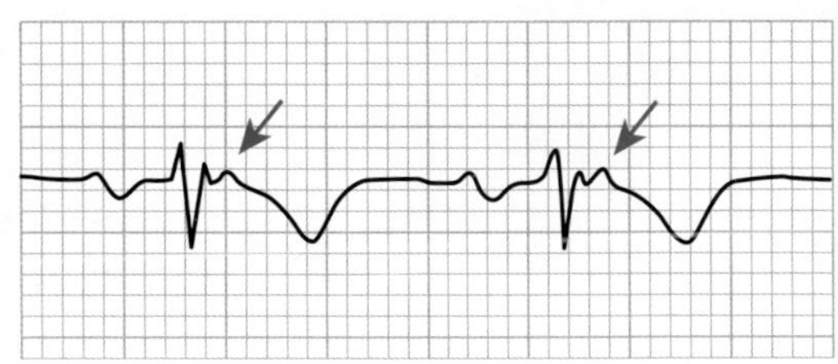

Figure 18.24 ECG lead in V1 with T-wave inversion and epsilon-wave (arrows) in a patient with arrhythmogenic right ventricular cardiomyopathy.

CMR in the detection of characteristic structural changes include exact determination of right ventricular free wall thickness and estimation of the amount of fatty tissue in comparison with the normally present epicardial and pericardial fat tissue (➲Fig. 18.25). Differential diagnostic exclusion of other heart diseases, quantification of left and right ventricular function and structural abnormalities, non-invasive serial examinations of disease progression and screening of family members constitute the enormous potential of echocardiography as the preferential first-line diagnostic procedure. In minor forms of ARVC, localized abnormalities of the right heart cavities are difficult to detect. Subtle lesions may be missed by all imaging techniques.

The *in vivo* documentation of the typical histological changes of ARVC by EMB may be of diagnostic value but is limited by low sensitivity, especially in mild forms. EMB cannot prove transmural replacement of the myocardium by fatty or fibrofatty tissue. Moreover, the focal or segmental nature of lesions, the lack of involvement of the ventricular septum and the natural content of fatty tissue in older healthy patients may contribute to the low sensitivity of biopsy-derived diagnosis. The increased content of fatty and fibrotic tissue in older individuals or other cardiomyopathic conditions also interferes with the diagnostic accuracy of MRI.

Based on clinical and morphological findings, diagnostic criteria have been established for ARVC (➲Table 18.10) [217]. The diagnosis is based on two major criteria, one major plus two minor criteria, or four minor criteria, respectively, encompassing histological, electrocardiographic and arrhythmic factors [218].

Risk stratification

Prevention of fatal arrhythmic events and SCD is the main goal of management of ARVC. The development of often stress-induced ventricular fibrillation or haemodynamically intolerable VT is difficult to predict, especially in

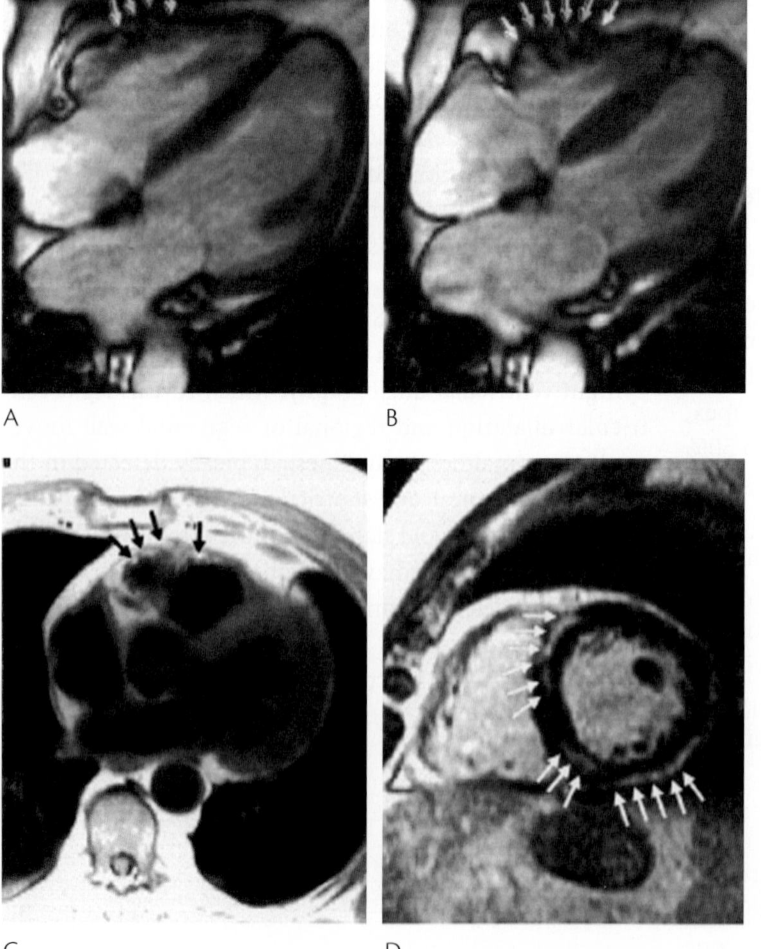

Figure 18.25 Cardiovascular magnetic resonant images in a 72-year-old man with arrhythmogenic right ventricular cardiomyopathy. Shown on the four-chamber views in diastole (A) and systole (B). Diffuse regional wall motion abnormalities can be seen in the outflow tract with mid-free wall aneurysm (arrows). In the short-axis views the myocardial fat tissue (black arrows) (C) can be seen. In the late enhancement images fibrotic changes can be seen in the septum, inferior septal region, as well as in the infrolateral wall (white arrows). Reproduced with permission from Sen-Chowdhry S, K., Prasad S, Syrris P, *et al.* Cardiovascular magnetic resonance in arrhythmogenic right ventricular cardiomyopathy revisited. *J Am Coll Cardiol* 2006; **48**: 2132–40.

Table 18.10 Major and minor criteria of arrhythmogenic right ventricular cardiomyopathy

Major criteria
Familial disease confirmed at necropsy or surgery
Epsilon wave or QRS duration >110ms in V1–V3
Severe RV dilatation and systolic dysfunction with no/mild LV involvement
Localized RV aneurysms (akinetic/dyskinetic areas with diastolic bulgings)
Severe segmental RV dilatation
Fibrofatty replacement of myocardium (endomyocardial biopsy)
Minor criteria
Family history of premature sudden death (<35years)
Family history based on clinical diagnostic criteria
Late potentials (signal-averaged ECG)
Inverted T waves in V2 and V3, no RBBB, in patients >12 years
LBBB-type tachycardia (sustained or non-sustained) on ECG, Holter monitoring or during exercise testing
Ventricular extrasystoles (>1000 in 24h) on Holter monitoring
Mild global reduced RV dilatation and/or RV dysfunction with preserved LV function
Mild segmental RV dilatation
Regional right heart hypokinesia

LBBB, left bundle branch block; LV, left ventricle; RBBB, right bundle branch block; RV, right ventricle
Adapted with permission from McKenna WJ, Thiene G, Nava A, *et al.* Diagnosis of arrhythmogenic right ventricular dysplasia/cardiomyopathy. *Br Heart J* 1994; **71**: 215–18.

asymptomatic young subjects and athletes. Guidelines for prophylactic treatment of identified patients with minor symptoms or minor morphological changes are not available. Asymptomatic patients at high risk of sudden death are characterized by familial background and complex ventricular arrhythmias at young age or during competitive sport activities, syncope, or LV involvement. In spite of ECG, Holter monitoring, exercise stress testing and signal-averaged ECG analysis, the predictive value of these non-invasive diagnostic tools for fatal events remains insufficient. Symptomatic patients should undergo a more detailed invasive analysis including LV angiography, programmed ventricular stimulation, and EMB.

Management of heart failure

Treatment of severe right ventricular or biventricular systolic dysfunction consists of current heart failure therapy, including ACE inhibitors or AT1 receptor antagonists, beta-blockers, diuretics, digitalis, spironolactone, and anticoagulants. Heart transplantation may be considered in patients with refractory congestive heart failure.

Management of arrhythmias

Since the risk of sudden death in patients with ARVC is still poorly defined, pharmacological and non-pharmacological therapy is individualized. In patients with preserved systolic ventricular function, treatment of well-tolerated and non-life-threatening ventricular arrhythmias empirically includes amiodarone, beta-blockers, or propafenone. In patients with LV dysfunction, pharmacological treatment is limited to amiodarone, possibly in combination with class I antiarrhythmics or beta-blocking agents.

The insertion of an automatic ICD is the treatment of choice in patients with syncope, cardiac arrest, documented VT or ventricular fibrillation, or positive familial history of SCD. The use of an ICD is limited by the progressive morphological changes within the right ventricular myocardium with low endocardial signals and increased pacing threshold.

Since new arrhythmic foci may develop over time due to the progressive nature of the disease, VT recurrences are reported in >50% after catheter ablation. Nevertheless, monomorphic VT may be terminated by radiofrequency ablation in unstable patients with otherwise not effectively controlled arrhythmias. Sustained VT with ineffective drug control despite ICD may require heart transplantation.

Prognosis and outcome

Biventricular dysplastic involvement resulting in substantial LV dysfunction mimicking DCM is rare. Progressive right ventricular failure may be a serious problem in a minority of patients, as may ventricular arrhythmias. Untreated sustained or non-sustained VT may be well tolerated by the majority of patients over a number of years but may degenerate to ventricular fibrillation and to sudden death (incidence of 1–2% per year) [196, 204].

Unclassified cardiomyopathy: left ventricular non-compaction

Left ventricular non-compaction (LVNC) is a myocardial disease with a genetic basis that may result in heart failure, arrhythmia, thromboembolism, and sudden death. It has only recently been recognized as a distinct cardiomyopathy and is defined by the presence of the following structural abnormalities.

- A two-layer myocardium with thin compacted myocardium adjacent to the epicardium and thicker non-compacted myocardium near the endocardium (➲ Fig. 18.26). The ventricular wall appears markedly thickened overall. Current diagnostic criteria rely on

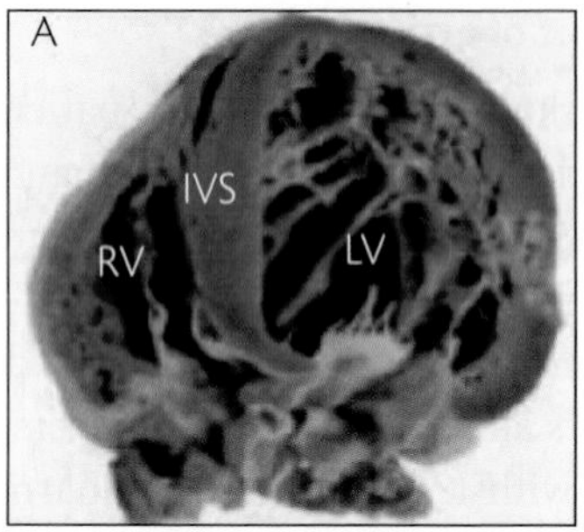

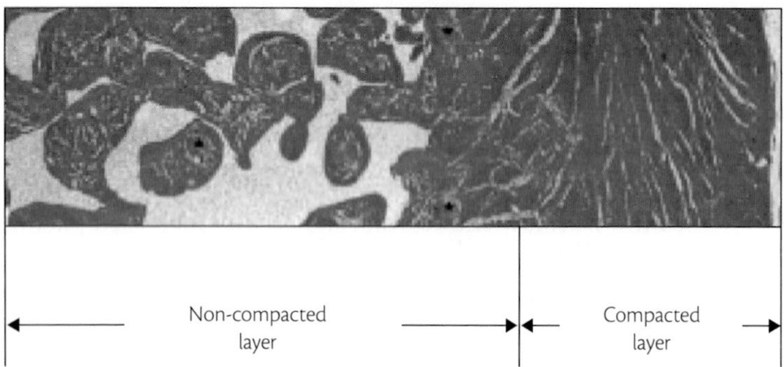

Figure 18.26 Anatomical findings (A) in a patient with left ventricular non-compaction of the infro-posterior wall. A two layer structure can be seen with a compacted epicardial band and a thicker non-compacted endocardial layer. Histological examination shows clearly the two layers with the compactec outer and the non-compacted inner layers. Modified and reproduced with permission from Jenni R, Oechslin E, Schneider J, *et al.* Echocardiographic and pathoanatomical characteristics of isolated left ventricular non-compaction: a step towards classification as a distinct cardiomyopathy. *Heart* 2001; **86**: 666–71.

measurement of the maximal end-systolic thickness of the non-compacted layer (N) and compacted layer (C). The diagnosis is confirmed with a ratio of N/C ≥2 in adults or N/C ≥1.4 in children [227]. The X/Y ratio, a measure of the relation between the depth of intertrabecular recesses and the overall wall thickness, is significantly higher in patients with LVNC compared with normal subjects; however, differentiation between the two layers in end-diastole is difficult [228].

- Prominent and excessive trabeculations (usually three or more) in the non-compacted layer.
- Deep intertrabecular recesses that fill with blood directly from the LV cavity, as demonstrated by colour flow Doppler.
- Predominant localization of non-compacted regions to the lateral, apical, and/or inferior walls of the left ventricle. The distribution is segmental rather than diffuse in LVNC. In contrast, heavy trabeculation coursing from the free wall to the septum is characteristic of normal hearts [229].
- These stipulations serve to distinguish LVNC from prominent trabeculations of normal hearts, and in association with other diseases such as hypertension, valve lesions, or DCM. Ventricular dilation and/or systolic impairment are common associated findings but are not requisite for diagnosis.

Prevalence and aetiology

Perhaps more so than any other cardiomyopathy, LVNC has been misdiagnosed as distal HCM, DCM, or LV apical thrombus [230]. It was only with the advent of superior echocardiographic technology that discrimination of two separate layers within the myocardium became possible. At lower resolutions, it is difficult to distinguish trabeculation from hypertrophy. Conversely, growing awareness of this new entity has led to over-diagnosis of prominent trabeculation or false tendons as LVNC, underscoring the need for standardized diagnostic criteria. The true prevalence of LVNC therefore remains difficult to estimate.

LVNC is thought to arise from arrest of normal myocardial maturation during embryogenesis. The early myocardium is composed of a loose network of interwoven fibres separated by deep recesses that communicate with the LV cavity. During the fifth to eighth week of development, this spongy meshwork of fibres gradually becomes 'compacted', a process that advances from the epicardium to the endocardium and from the base of the heart to the apex. At the same time, the coronary circulation is being established and the intertrabecular recesses are reduced to capillaries [231]. While it is apparent that interruption of normal myocardial compaction would produce the characteristic LVNC phenotype, evidence for this mechanism is presently lacking.

LVNC is generally distinguished from persistent intramyocardial sinusoids, which are observed in the setting of congenital obstructive lesions of the right and LV outflow tracts [232]. Ventricular pressure overload prevents regression of the embryonic sinusoids, resulting in deep recesses that communicate with both the ventricular cavity and the coronary circulation. This is considered a sporadic phenomenon. However, LVNC may occur in conjunction with congenital heart defects as a distinct inherited syndrome. Mutations in α-dystrobrevin have been identified in a Japanese family with LVNC, one or more ventricular septal defects and other congenital anomalies [233]. α-Dystrobrevin is a component of the dystrophic-associated glycoprotein complex that links the cytoskeleton of cardiac myocytes to the extracellular matrix.

Isolated LVNC, defined by the absence of coexisting cardiac abnormalities, has been linked with mutations in the gene *G4.5* at Xq28 [233], which has also been implicated in Barth syndrome [234]. Barth syndrome is an X-linked recessive disease that presents in infancy with the clinical triad of DCM, neutropenia, and skeletal myopathy. The *G4.5* gene encodes a family of proteins known as tafazzins, the function of which is still being elucidated.

Mutations in Cypher/ZASP have been identified in both familial DCM and isolated LVNC [60]. Cypher/ZASP is a novel Z-line protein found in both cardiac and skeletal muscle that appears to play a role in bridging the sarcomere to the cytoskeleton.

Pathophysiology

Examination of post-mortem and explanted hearts from patients with LVNC confirms the anatomical features observed on imaging. Histology further demonstrates focal ischaemic necrosis within the thickened endocardial layer and trabeculations, but not in the epicardial zone. Interstitial fibrosis is also observed, of varying severity. Chronic myocarditis has been reported [227].

The pathological findings suggest possible mechanisms for the arrhythmia and progressive LV failure that may accompany LVNC. The intertrabecular recesses receive blood directly from the LV cavity. However, the epicardial and endocardial layers of the myocardium, including the trabeculations themselves, rely on the coronary arteries for their blood supply [235]. Failure of the coronary microcirculation to grow in step with the numerous trabeculae will result in capillary mass mismatch. The thickened myocardium may additionally compress intramural coronary vessels. The end-result of both of these processes is diminished subendocardial perfusion despite the presence of unobstructed coronary arteries. Reduced coronary flow reserve has indeed been documented in patients with LVNC by positron emission tomography [236]. Progressive ischaemia and consequent fibrosis may lead to systolic impairment and provide a substrate for arrhythmia.

The excessive trabeculation may also contribute to diastolic dysfunction by limiting the compliance of the myocardium; restrictive physiology occurs in 35% of adults with LVNC [235]. The frequency of thromboembolic events is as high as 24%. Thromboembolism is thought to result from stagnation of blood within the intertrabecular recesses and may manifest as cerebrovascular accidents, transient ischaemic attacks, mesenteric infarction, or pulmonary embolism.

Clinical presentation

Clinical onset ranges from the neonatal period to senescence. Patients with LVNC may present with symptoms of LV failure, arrhythmia, or, less commonly, thromboembolism. Cyanosis, failure to thrive, and dysmorphic features are also described in childhood [237]. An increasing proportion of cases are identified via familial evaluation or incidentally during routine cardiac imaging.

Whether sudden death may be the first clinical manifestation of LVNC remains unresolved. LVNC is seldom represented in postmortem series of victims of SCD, possibly due to a lack of awareness of the disease. It has been speculated that LVNC may account for a proportion of deaths ascribed to myocarditis or 'sudden arrhythmic death syndrome' with a structurally normal heart.

Diagnosis

The diagnostic work-up for a patient with suspected LVNC comprises 12-lead ECG, transthoracic echocardiography and Holter monitoring. Cardiopulmonary exercise testing with metabolic gas exchange measurements may also be useful for obtaining an objective assessment of functional capacity.

Most patients with LVNC have non-specific ECG findings. Shifts in the QRS axis, high QRS voltages, intraventricular conduction delay, bundle branch block, and varying degrees of AV block have been described. Repolarization abnormalities include inverted T waves and ST-segment changes [231]. Up to 17% of paediatric patients have ECG features typical of Wolff–Parkinson–White syndrome [237], although this is rare among adults.

Considerable attention has focused on the role of cardiovascular MRI in the diagnosis of LVNC. Cardiovascular MRI is not restricted by acoustic windows and has the additional benefit of delineating areas of myocardial fibrosis following administration of gadolinium. However, two-dimensional echocardiography remains the mainstay of diagnosis. Use of intravenous contrast agents may improve definition of the endocardial border.

Management

Standard heart failure therapy is indicated for LV dysfunction. Reports of the prevalence of arrhythmia vary widely. VT may occur in up to 41% of adult patients with LVNC [235]. In contrast, VT was rare in a study of Japanese children [238]. Extrapolating from the DCM population, treatment with beta-blockers and/or amiodarone may be sufficient for those with non-sustained VT and preserved LV function. ICD placement should be considered in LVNC patients with sustained VT, recurrent unexplained syncope or LVEF <35% on optimal medical therapy and non-sustained VT on Holter monitoring.

Similar discrepancies have been observed with regard to the frequency of thromboembolic events. At present, a pragmatic approach may involve anticoagulation of LVNC patients with ventricular dilation and/or significant systolic impairment. There is less evidence to support routine anticoagulant therapy for asymptomatic patients with normal ventricular function.

The most common pattern of inheritance in LVNC is autosomal dominant [239], which translates into a 50% probability of any first-degree relative carrying the disease-causing gene. Offering prospective cardiac evaluation to family members is therefore mandatory.

Prognosis and outcome

In a series of 34 adults with LVNC the mortality rate was high at 35% after 44 months; half of these deaths occurred suddenly. One patient died from refractory sustained VT and another from pulmonary embolism. End-stage heart failure accounted for one-third of the deaths and a further 12% of the patients in this cohort underwent cardiac transplantation. Unfavourable clinical outcomes were frequent [235].

However, this does not imply that LVNC has a uniformly poor prognosis. Preliminary surveys of any newly recognized disorder tend to be dominated by experience with symptomatic index cases with clinically severe disease. Adverse events among patients with HCM, for example, are far less common in community-based populations than originally predicted from tertiary centre studies. Many patients with LVNC are asymptomatic at initial diagnosis and may remain so for extended periods. Timely detection and judicious use of ICDs may improve outcomes in the remainder. The clinical course of LVNC in large populations without selection bias is still being defined.

Inflammatory myocardial disease

Myocarditis and viral cardiomyopathy

Definition

The term 'myocarditis' was first introduced by Sobernheim in 1937. However, myocardial inflammation is no longer restricted to the early phase of 'acute myocarditis' since it is acknowledged that DCM may represent a sequel of chronic intramyocardial inflammation evoked by viral infection. With the expanding knowledge on the pathogenic link between myocarditis and DCM, the 1995 WHO/ISFC Task Force Report on the Definition and Classification of Cardiomyopathies introduced, among other specific cardiomyopathies, the new entity 'inflammatory cardiomyopathy' (DCMi), which is characterized by myocarditis in association with cardiac dysfunction [38]. Myocardial inflammation can be established by histological, immunological, and immunohistochemical criteria. Idiopathic, autoimmune, and infectious forms of DCMi are recognized.

Aetiology and prevalence

Several cardiotropic viruses have been identified in myocarditis and DCMi (➲Table 18.11). In patients with DCMi,

Table 18.11 Cardiotropic viruses involved in myocarditis and inflammatory cardiomyopathy

Coxsackie virus
Adenovirus
Parvovirus B19
Human herpesvirus type 6
Epstein–Barr virus
Cytomegalovirus
Echovirus
Mumps virus
Influenza A and B viruses
Flavovirus
Human immunodeficiency virus
Measles virus
Polio virus
Hepatitis C virus
Rabies virus
Rubella virus
Variola virus
Varicella-zoster virus

parvovirus B19, human herpesvirus type 6 (HHV-6), enteroviruses (i.e. Coxsackie virus), adenovirus and Epstein–Barr virus (EBV) are frequently detectable (➲Fig. 18.27). In the Western world, non-viral aetiologies (i.e. *Borrelia*, Chagas disesae, diphtheria) are of minor importance. Evolution from myocarditis to DCM occurs in 21% of patients within a mean follow-up of 33 months.

The annual prevalence of DCM is 29 per million persons, and the annual prevalence of viral myocarditis is 131 per million persons. Detailed epidemiological data regarding acute myocarditis are not available.

Genetics

At present, there is no evidence for monogenic inheritance of myocarditis or DCMi. It is hypothesized that a genetic predisposition might be associated with increased susceptibility for cardiotropic viruses and/or chronic myocardial inflammation in response to a viral infection. A well-investigated link is the disequilibrium of HLA haplotypes, with elevated HLA-DR4 frequencies (51% in DCM vs. 27% in controls, $P < 0.001$) and decreased HLA-DRw6 frequencies (9% in DCM vs. 24% in controls) [240]. However, the genetic inheritance of certain mutations and interference with modifier genes identified in familial cardiomyopathy does not preclude immunological pathomechanisms. In line with this, almost equally high rates of DCMi were reported in patients with familial DCM and their asymptomatic relatives and those with non-familial DCM [41].

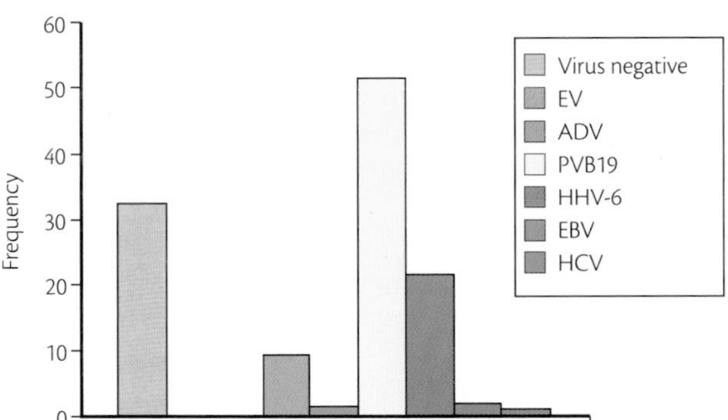

Figure 18.27 Spectrum of cardiotropic viruses in inflammatory cardiomyopathy. Frequencies of cardiotropic viruses proved by nested polymerase chain reaction in endomyocardial biopsies from patients with dilated cardiomyopathy. Results comprise in parts multiple viral infections. ADV, adenovirus; EBV, Epstein–Barr virus; EV, enterovirus; HCV, hepatitis C virus; HHV-6, human herpesvirus type 6; PVB19, parvovirus B19. Reproduced from Kühl U, Pauschinger M, Noutsias M, *et al.* High prevalence of viral genomes and multiple viral infections in the myocardium of adults with 'idiopathic' left ventricular dysfunction. *Circulation* 2005; **111**: 887–93.

Pathophysiology

Several viruses can be detected in biopsies from patients with clinically suspected myocarditis and DCMi, especially enteroviruses (i.e. Coxsackie virus), adenovirus, parvovirus B19, HHV-6, and EBV (➲Fig. 18.27) [42, 241]. The most detailed pathogenic pathways have been unravelled with respect to Coxsackie virus. The *de novo* induction

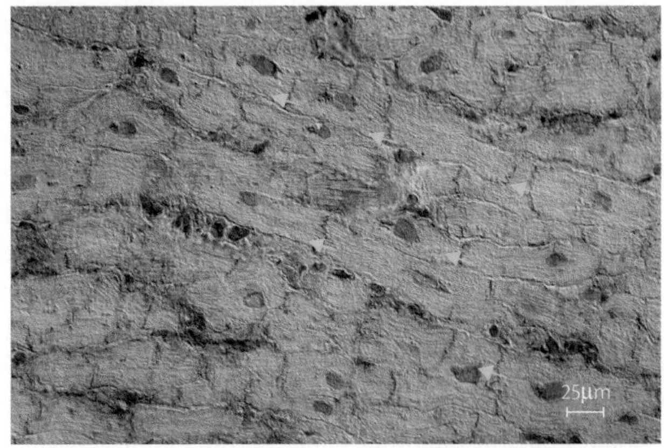

A

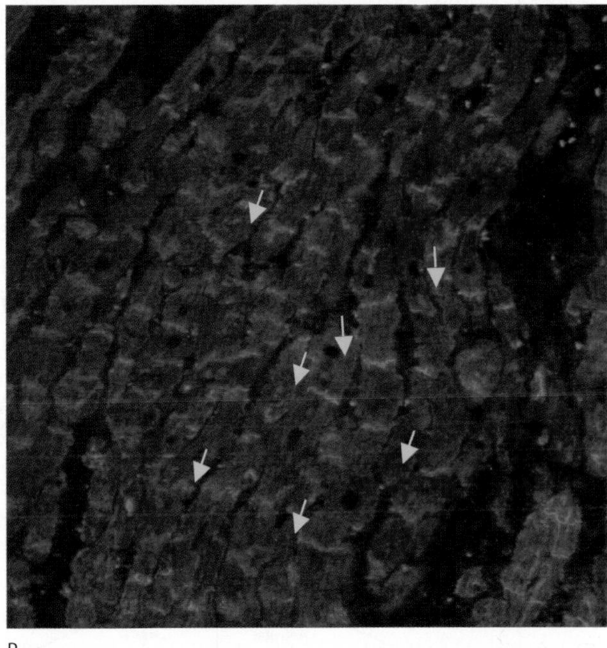

B

Figure 18.28 Coxsackie–adenovirus receptor (CAR) expression in dilated cardiomyopathy (DCM). (A) CAR induction in DCM with embryological expression pattern on the cardiomyocyte sarcolemma and the intercalated discs (arrows) (original magnification × 400). (B) Confocal laser scanning microscopy (Cy3 labelling) of CAR induction in DCM on the cardiomyocyte sarcolemma and the intercalated discs (arrows) (original magnification × 400). Reproduced with permission from Noutsias M, Fechner H, Jonge H, *et al.* Human Coxsackie–adenovirus receptor is colocalized with integrins alpha(v)beta(3) and alpha(v)beta(5) on the cardiomyocyte sarcolemma and upregulated in dilated cardiomyopathy: implications for cardiotropic viral infections. *Circulation* 2001; **104**: 275–80.

of Coxsackie–adenovirus receptor in about 60% of DCM hearts, colocalized with the co-receptors for adenovirus internalization $\alpha_v\beta_3$ and $\alpha_v\beta_5$ (➲ Fig. 18.28), indicates an important molecular determinant for the cardiotropism of both Coxsackie virus and adenovirus [242]. Basically, two different pathways of virus infection can be differentiated: 1) direct cytopathic effects; and 2) secondarily induced effects, for example Coxsackie-virus protease 2A cleaves dystrophin, leading to disruption of the cytoskeleton [243]. Even non-replicating Coxsackie viral genomes at low expression levels can exert cytopathic effects.

With regard to indirect pathways related to the host's immune response, the presentation of viral antigens evokes the antiviral immune response that aims at viral elimination and which is not necessarily detrimental to the heart. However, this immune response is a 'double-edged sword': molecular mimicry and perhaps genetically predisposing conditions can secondarily target cryptic myocardial antigens. In the case of postviral (auto)immunity, this immune response can continue despite possible elimination of the viral genome. On the other hand, chronic viral persistence maintains the anticardiac immune response. Activated B lymphocytes produce antibodies that can cross-react with myocardial antigens and may thus also contribute to impairment of cardiac contractility. Numerous autoantibodies have been identified in patients with DCM, targeting the ADP/ATP carrier, the β_1 adrenoreceptor, and further mitochondrial and contractile proteins. While the pathogenic relevance of autoantibodies may have been questioned in the past as epiphenomena of the immune response, recent experiments have proved the pathogenic principle of stimulating antibodies directed against the second extracellular β_1-receptor loop, since sera transferred from immunized rats induces DCM in healthy littermates [244]. Furthermore, results from immunoadsorption studies clearly indicate a causative role for autoantibodies in DCM [245].

Cardiodepressive cytokines induced by the immune system can directly impair cardiac contractility. Cytokines promote an imbalance between metalloproteinases (MMP) and their tissue inhibitors (TIMP), thus contributing to remodelling [246]. Preliminary results indicate a relationship between MMP/TIMP expression patterns and LV function. Moreover, cytokines induce cell adhesion molecules (CAMs) on the endothelium, which mediate transendothelial migration of immunocompetent cells into the myocardium [39]. CAM interactions are also involved in the continuous loss of cardiomyocytes, mediated specifically by cytotoxic T lymphocytes [247]. This pathogenic model of myocarditis and DCMi is illustrated in ➲ Fig. 18.29.

Clinical presentation

The clinical symptoms of myocarditis and DCMi comprise chest discomfort, heart failure symptoms, palpitations, syncope, and SCD. Patients with acute myocarditis may report a close temporal association (days to weeks) with an antecedent flu-like illness (upper respiratory or gastrointestinal tract infection) before the onset of symptoms. However, acute myocarditis, with its often subtle or virtually absent symptoms, may be frequently missed. Two different presentations of acute myocarditis can be differentiated.

- In the setting of acute fulminant myocarditis, patients complain of acute onset and rapidly progressive (within hours to days) heart failure symptoms (i.e. dyspnoea at rest, peripheral oedema). LV function is severely impaired in concert with LV dilatation, and possibly pulmonary oedema. Patients may require inotropic or mechanical support (i.e. LVAD). LV function in acute fulminant myocarditis usually improves dramatically and may even

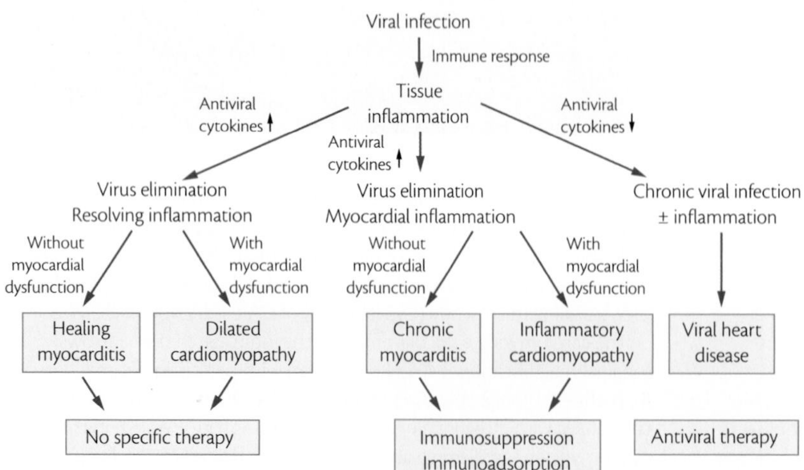

Figure 18.29 Pathophysiology of inflammatory cardiomyopathy and specific treatment options.

normalize completely at follow-up examinations [122], which is consistent with the hypothesis that LV function can improve after viral elimination and resolution of myocarditis. Acute fulminant myocarditis is less frequent than acute non-fulminant myocarditis.

- In comparison, patients with acute non-fulminant myocarditis typically present with acute onset of symptoms of angina pectoris and ST-segment elevation/depression or T-wave inversions as well as elevated CK-MB/troponin levels, mimicking acute myocardial infarction in the absence of coronary artery stenoses. Creatine phosphokinase/troponin levels usually normalize within 60 hours. C-reactive protein is often increased. Global systolic function is often preserved in acute non-fulminant myocarditis, although regional wall motion abnormalities and diastolic dysfunction can be frequently observed. Furthermore, pericardial effusions and wall oedema can be detected by echocardiography [241].

Both acute myocarditis and DCMi can present with various types of ECG abnormalities (right or left bundle branch block, ST-segment depression, Q waves, and T-wave inversions, AV block) and rhythm disturbances on Holter monitoring (sinus tachycardia/bradycardia, supraventricular/ventricular extrasystoles, atrial fibrillation/flutter, ventricular tachycardia/flutter/fibrillation). Myocarditis is a frequent cause of SCD (up to 40%), especially in the young, and is often associated with strenuous physical exertion.

Coronary artery stenoses are excluded by coronary angiography in both myocarditis and DCMi. Coronary artery vasospasm may be induced by vasoconstrictor challenge, especially in the setting of acute non-fulminant myocarditis [241, 248].

Management

In patients with clinically suspected acute myocarditis and those with DCMi, secondary causes of heart failure (i.e. coronary artery disease, arterial hypertension, significant valvular heart disease) should be excluded. The diagnostic procedures for and treatment of heart failure (i.e. ACE inhibitors, AT1 receptor blockers, betablockers, diuretics, aldosterone antagonists, digitalis; cardiac transplantation as ultimate option) apply also to myocarditis and DCMi. In addition, cardiac resynchronization and LVAD have provided substantial improvement in patients with myocarditis and DCMi. Risk stratification and primary prevention of SCD imposes a clinical challenge, especially since programmed ventricular stimulation is not predictive. Based on the recently published SCD-Heft trial, the same criteria apply to both ischaemic and non-ischaemic cardiomyopathies: chronic heart failure, NYHA >II and LVEF <35%. There are no conclusive data with respect to acute myocarditis. Patients should be monitored at least during the phase of elevated CK-MB/troponin levels. Screening of relatives in the case of positive family history can reveal early disease stages.

If patients with myocarditis/DCMi improve with heart failure regimens, patients should be monitored clinically and by non-invasive ECG, Holter, and echocardiography. Especially in patients with acute myocarditis, courses with spontaneous recovery of LV function can be observed. However, if LV function progressively deteriorates despite symptomatic heart failure medication, immunomodulatory treatment should be considered additionally (see ➲Immunomodulatory treatment strategies, p.708). EMB should be obtained in these patients and subjected to contemporary diagnostic techniques (immunohistological assessment of inflammation, molecular biological proof of cardiotropic viruses). In addition, cardiac autoantibodies and their functional activity should be ascertained.

The algorithm for the management of patients with myocarditis and DCMi is presented in ➲Fig. 18.30.

Diagnostic EMB procedures

Biopsy samples can be obtained from the right or left ventricle or from the atrial septum. Procedural complications of endomyocardial biopsies are fairly rare in experienced centres, and a fatal outcome due to perforation accounts for <0.4% in large studies [249]. EMB procedures are therefore justified, provided that a clinical impact results from investigation of the biopsy.

Histological assessment of inflammation

The Dallas criteria differentiate 'active' (interstitial infiltrates with myocytolysis) from borderline myocarditis (increased infiltrates with or without fibrosis; ➲Fig. 18.31) [250]. Myocarditis is only rarely revealed by histological assessment (5–10%, including both forms). However, histological assessment is hampered by sampling error and interobserver variability. Further characteristics of cardiomyopathies (i.e. hypertrophy, loss of myofibrils) are also detectable by histological assessment but are not pathognomonic for myocarditis or DCMi. Notwithstanding these pitfalls, histological assessment of biopsy samples is still mandatory for the diagnosis of 'active myocarditis' and also for the differentiation from other conditions such as storage diseases.

Immunohistological evaluation of inflammation

Immunohistological techniques have been established that are sensitive and specific and which provide quantification

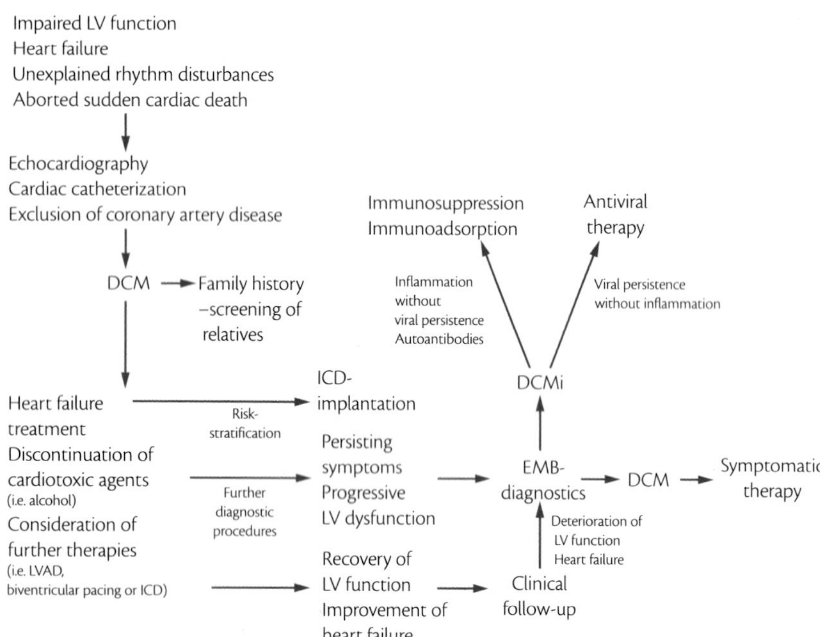

Figure 18.30 Diagnostic algorithm in DCMi and therapeutic algorithms in dilated cardiomyopathy (DCM) and inflammatory cardiomyopathy (DCMi). EMB, endomyocardial biopsy; ICD, implantable cardioverter-defibrillator; LVAD, left ventricular assist device.

and phenotypic characterization of inflammation. These techniques have numerous advantages compared with the histological Dallas criteria and have helped elucidate many of the key players of the immune response in myocarditis and DCMi.

Increased T-lymphocyte infiltration (>7/mm^2) is considered pathogenic (➲Fig. 18.32A). In addition, functional markers such as cytotoxic T lymphocytes (➲Fig. 18.32B) or activated T lymphocytes (i.e. CD45R0$^+$ or CD69$^+$) and macrophages can be specified. A further pivotal diagnostic hallmark is the endothelial abundance of CAMs, significantly related to the extent of infiltration due to specific receptor–ligand interactions; however, because of their homogeneous expression pattern, they are not prone to sampling error (➲Fig. 18.32C). Immunohistological staining can be quantified by digital image analysis, enabling observer-independent evaluation [39, 242, 249]. Commonly used target antigens for the immunohistological

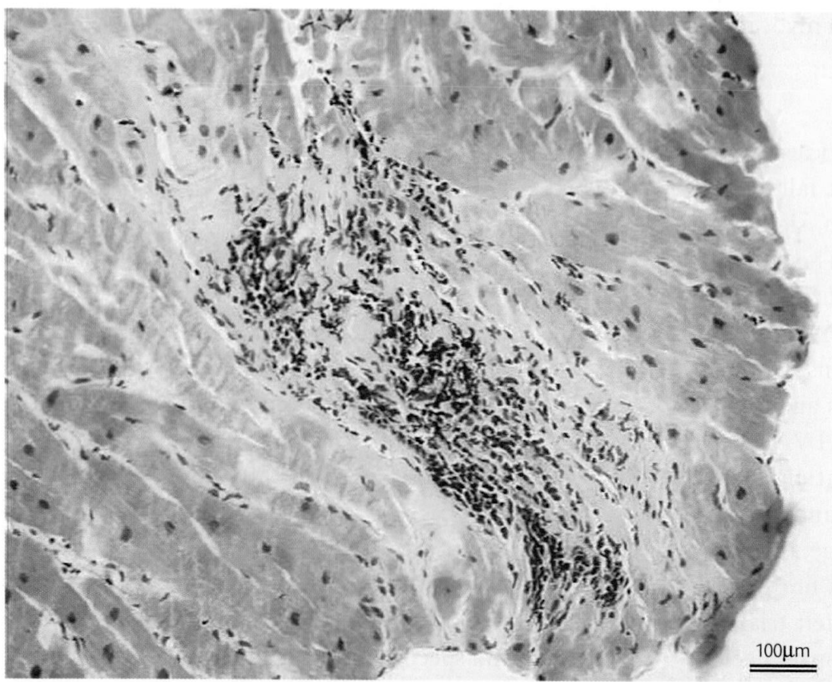

Figure 18.31 Histology of active myocarditis: focal lymphomononuclear infiltrate with adjacent myocytolysis (original magnification ×200).

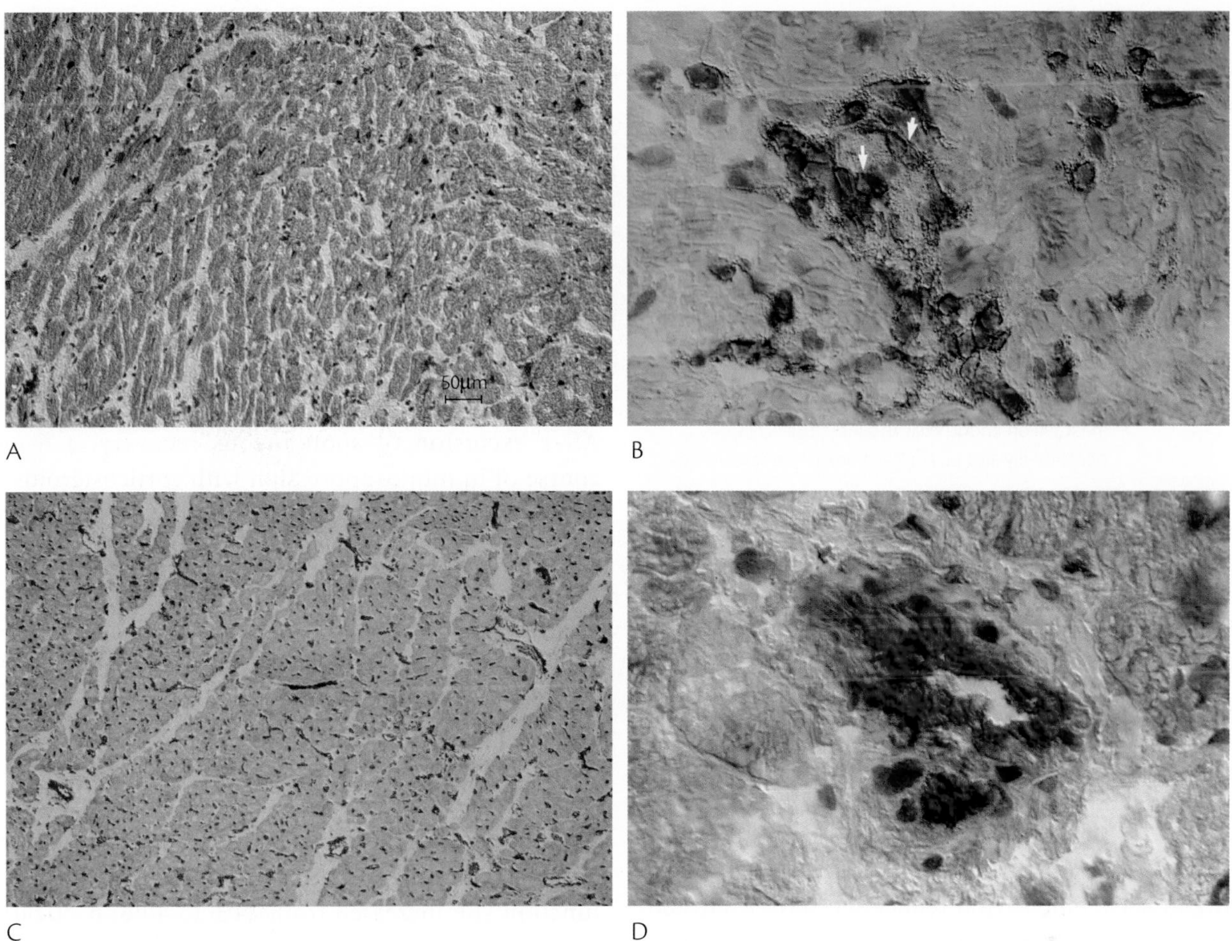

Figure 18.32 Immunohistological aspects of inflammatory cardiomyopathy (DCMi). (A) Typical diffuse infiltration pattern of LFA-1$^+$ lymphocytes in DCMi (original magnification ×200). (B) Focal cytotoxic T lymphocytes (perforin positive) encircling and entering a cardiomyocyte suggestive of myocytolysis in DCMi (original magnification ×630). (C) Homogeneous endothelial ICAM-1 abundance in DCMi (original magnification ×200). (D) Endothelial VCAM-1 expression in DCMi (original magnification ×630). Reproduced with permission from Noutsias M, Pauschinger M, Schultheiss HP, *et al.* Cytotoxic perforin+ and TIA-1$^+$ infiltrates are associated with cell adhesion molecule expression in dilated cardiomyopathy. *Eur J Heart Fail* 2003; **5**: 469–79.

evaluation of intramyocardial inflammation are summarized in ➲Table 18.12.

Molecular biological detection of viral genomes

Molecular biological detection of viral genomes is pertinent for the differentiation of DCMi. Because of low sensitivity and specificity, serology or direct virus isolation from the myocardium has a negligible diagnostic value. PCR amplification of viral genomes has confirmed viral persistence in a major proportion of patients with myocarditis and DCMi, and broadened the spectrum of cardiotropic viruses substantially.

The adverse prognostic impact of enteroviral persistence in DCMi was identified early [126] and recent results indicate the importance of the replicative infection mode in many patients with DCMi [127, 251]. There is a growing importance of other cardiotropic viruses, especially parvovirus B19, HHV-6 and EBV (➲Fig. 18.27), and preliminary data indicate that these viruses also have adverse prognostic impact in DCMi [45, 241]. In addition, retrospective analysis has confirmed that patients with persistence of these recently identified viruses (except for hepatitis C) do not improve and may even deteriorate under immunosuppression [45], which infers that myocardial persistence of these viruses may have similar prognostic impact and therapeutic implications as for Coxsackie virus infection.

In addition to nested PCR amplification of viral genomes, further methodological approaches are available to characterize viral infections. An important issue is the replicative mode of viral infection: viruses may exhibit either latent infection or active replication within the host tissue. Both infection modes have been reported in myocarditis and DCMi with respect to enteroviral infection using strand-specific PCR, with minus-strand RNA indicating active viral replication [251]. It is noteworthy that patients with

Table 18.12 Commonly used target antigens for the immunohistological evaluation of intramyocardial inflammation

Target antigen	Recognized phenotypes/expression pattern
CD3	T lymphocytes
CD11a/LFA-1	T lymphocytes, large granular lymphocytes including CTLs; counter-receptor of ICAM-1
CD45R0	Memory T cells
Perforin	Specifically CTLs
CD11b/Mac-1	Macrophages; counter-receptor of ICAM-1
27E10	Specifically early activated macrophages
HLA class I	Expressed constitutively at baseline levels, induced in DCMi on endothelial and interstitial cells, occasionally also on the cardiomyocyte sarcolemma
CD54/ICAM-1	Expressed constitutively at baseline levels, induced in DCMi on endothelial and interstitial cells, occasionally also on the cardiomyocyte sarcolemma; endothelial receptor for both LFA-1+ and Mac-1+ infiltrates
CD106/VCAM-1	Expressed exclusively on endothelial cells; no constitutive expression; *de novo* induction in DCMi

CTLs, Cytoxic T Lymphocyts; DCMi, Imflammatory cardiomyopthy; ICAM-1, intercellular adhesion molecule 1; VCAM-1, vascular cell adhesion moluclue 1.
Reproduced with permission from Noutsias M, Pauschinger M, Poller WC, *et al.* Immunomodulatory treatment strategies in inflammatory cardiomyopathy: current status and future perspectives. *Expert Rev Cardiovasc Ther* 2004; **2**: 37–51

DCMi and active enteroviral replication have a substantially worse prognosis compared with those DCMi patients showing viral latency [127]. Real-time PCR approaches are suitable for quantifying the virus load. Direct sequencing of positive PCR results allows the identification of the virus genotype. Sequence analysis should be performed from the perspective of quality control in order to exclude contamination, which may occur especially during nested PCR methods [42, 241, 248].

Immunomodulatory treatment strategies

Immunomodulatory treatment should be considered as an additional treatment option in patients with DCMi whose LV function progressively deteriorates despite heart failure medication. This approach is based on the hypothesis that heart failure treatment does not affect the underlying pathogenic mechanisms of DCMi and that tailored immunomodulation will improve the progressive course of the disease by specific interaction with these pathways.

Several recent studies have demonstrated a clear benefit of tailored immunomodulatory regimens in selected patients with DCMi when using contemporary diagnostic tools. Endomyocardial biopsies are mandatory in order to elucidate inflammation and/or viral infection, and the functional activity of autoantibodies should be assessed, since these pathogenic factors are important hallmarks for the choice of immunomodulatory strategy. According to current concepts, patients with DCMi with immunohistologically proven chronic inflammation but no viral persistence benefit from immunosuppression. Immunoadsorption is a treatment option in those patients with functionally active autoantibodies. Finally, patients with DCMi and cardiotropic viral persistence should not be subjected to immunosuppression, since these patients are candidates for antiviral treatment. At present, immunomodulation remains an option for expert centres.

Immunosuppression

After exclusion of spontaneous recovery, a 6-month course of immunosuppression with corticosteroids in 31 patients with DCMi with immunohistological diagnosis demonstrated significant positive effects on heart failure symptoms and haemodynamic measurements, paralleled by a significant decrease in infiltrates and CAM expression in 64% of the patients [252]. This substantial improvement in LVEF was observed irrespective of the initial LVEF at study entry, which implies that virtually all patients with DCMi can benefit from immunomodulatory treatment, even in cases with only slightly impaired LV function (e.g. regional LV dysfunction), since these patients demonstrated almost a normalization of LV function (EF increased from 24% to 40%, $p < 0.001$ at 6 months and 44%, $p < 0.001$ at 2 years. Sustained beneficial effects of immunosuppression on heart failure symptoms, LV dimensions and LVEF in immunohistologically biopsy-proven DCMi have been confirmed in a randomized trial with 41 patients at 2 years' follow-up after ≥3 months of treatment with corticosteroids and azathioprine [46]. Prednisone was started at a dose of 1mg/kg/day and after 12 days the dose was tapered off every 5 days by 5mg/day until reaching the maintenance dose of 0.2mg/kg/day for a total of 90 days. Azathioprine was given at a dose of 1mg/kg/day for a total of 100 days. This trial ultimately validates the diagnostic sensitivity and accuracy of CAM abundance for DCMi even in the absence of lymphocytic infiltration, possibly due to the close functional association between CAM induction and immunocompetent infiltration and cytokine induction [39], and thus constitutes an important criterion for selecting those patients who will likely benefit from immunosuppression. Furthermore, this study showed for the first time that a 3-month regimen is equally effective as previous trials that used 6 months of immunosuppression, and that beneficial effects last for an extended period of time (2 years).

Viral persistence and lack of anticardiac autoantibodies were the key discriminators of those patients with DCMi who did not respond to a 6-month course of immunosuppression [45]. These compelling insights have confirmed the hypothesis that DCMi patients with viral persistence should not be subjected to immunosuppression, since inhibition of the antiviral immune response might perpetuate viral replication, and antiviral regimens should be favoured in these patients. However, this seems to be different in cases of hepatitis C virus-induced DCMi.

Immunoadsorption

The rationale for immunoadsorption is to extract cardiodepressive antibodies from the patient's plasma. The plasma is separated by a conventional plasmapheresis unit and passed through an immunoadsorber column. Total IgG is adsorbed during repetitive sessions at defined intervals, i.e. first course comprises daily immunoadsorption session on three consecutive days, followed by four courses at 1-month intervals. After every session, plasma IgG levels must be restored by injection of 0.5g/kg polyclonal IgG.

The favourable haemodynamic results of immunoadsorption in patients with DCMi may be related to removal of functionally active cardiac autoantibodies, since immunoadsorption leads to biopsy-proven decrease in lymphocytic infiltration and CAM expression [253].

Antiviral treatment

Type I interferons such as interferon-β are pivotal for the antiviral immune response. In a phase II study, 22 patients with DCMi with biopsy-proven enteroviral persistence were treated with interferon-β for 24 weeks [44]. Complete elimination of viral genome was shown in follow-up biopsies in all patients. This was paralleled by a significant increase in LVEF (from 45% to 53%, $p < 0.001$) and amelioration of heart failure symptoms.

Prognosis and outcome

The 5-year survival of patients with DCMi is approximately 36%. Myocarditis resolves in about 80% of patients spontaneously, but prospective studies have revealed a bad prognosis for patients with myocarditis: 10-year survival rate was 45%, mostly due to the manifestations of DCMi and to sudden cardiac death [122].

The initial clinical presentation of both myocarditis and DCMi is highly variable as is their spontaneous prognosis. At present, no clinical parameter has proven prognostically useful for predicting the evolution from myocarditis to DCMi. Even LVEF, which in ischaemic heart disease serves as a strong predictor, has a seemingly inverse prognostic impact in acute myocarditis [122]. Furthermore, the maximum troponin and creatine phosphokinase levels in acute myocarditis, in contrast to myocardial infarction, have no prognostic impact.

Histological and morphometric biopsy analyses have no predictive value. In contrast, immunohistological analysis of viral persistence in particular, but also chronic intramyocardial inflammation, have been associated with adverse prognosis in patients with DCMi [126–128].

Secondary myocardial diseases

Myocardial disease that can be directly linked to an identifiable source is termed secondary. Acute ischaemia often precipitates LV failure, while chronic ischaemia may induce hibernation of the myocardium. Both states may be reversible by revascularization owing to the presence of viable myocardium. Similarly, ventricular impairment frequently occurs in conjunction with valvular abnormalities; aortic stenosis is a classic example where timely correction may normalize ventricular function. Hypertension, diabetes and excess alcohol are common causes of secondary cardiomyopathy. A rare but important entity is peripartum cardiomyopathy. Tachycardia-induced cardiomyopathy is an under-recognized entity in which control of chronic atrial or ventricular tachyarrhythmia leads to restoration of normal ventricular function. Finally, cardiac involvement in the muscular dystrophies is also included under the umbrella term of secondary myocardial disease.

Hypertensive cardiomyopathy

Hypertension is a major predisposing factor for coronary artery disease, heart failure, and cerebrovascular disease. Although LVH has been considered an adaptation to systolic overload in hypertensive patients, there is considerable evidence that it is independently associated with ventricular dysfunction, arrhythmia, and sudden death. Hypertension-induced LVH may therefore be considered a cardiomyopathy in its own right.

Histological changes in hypertensive cardiomyopathy include enlargement and proliferation of cardiac myocytes [254]. Interstitial fibrosis is a key feature, characterized in particular by accumulation of type I and type III collagen [255]. The severity of myocardial fibrosis appears to correlate with heart weight, hypertrophy and systolic blood pressure [256]. As the collagen content of the interstitium increases to two to three times normal, the myocardium becomes non-compliant and diastolic dysfunction results. Hypertension is the leading cause of diastolic heart failure in clinical practice. Further progression of fibrosis ultimately leads to systolic impairment; myocyte apoptosis may also play a role.

During the course of hypertrophy, the coronary vasculature fails to enlarge at a rate sufficient to compensate for the increased myocardial mass. Abnormalities of the microcirculation are also recognized in the hypertensive heart. Endothelial dysfunction, medial thickening, and perivascular fibrosis are all thought to contribute to diminished coronary reserve [256]. As a result, many patients with hypertensive cardiomyopathy have signs and symptoms of myocardial ischaemia despite unobstructed coronary arteries on angiography.

There is a significantly higher prevalence of AF and ventricular arrhythmia in patients with hypertension and LVH compared with the general population. Characteristic findings on Holter ECG include frequent multifocal ventricular extrasystoles and short runs of non-sustained VT; sustained ventricular tachyarrhythmia is rare [257]. However, patients with hypertensive heart disease are at increased risk of sudden death, for which LVH and high-grade ventricular arrhythmia appear to be predictors [260]. The arrhythmogenic substrate is likely to be a product of myocardial fibrosis, ischaemia, autonomic imbalance and heterogeneous prolongation of the action potential in LVH [257].

Regression of LVH is accompanied by diminished ventricular arrhythmia, improved diastolic function, preservation of systolic function and resolution of microvascular ischaemia. Lowering of LV mass during antihypertensive treatment is associated with reduced incidence of cardiovascular events, additional to the effects of blood pressure control. However, not all antihypertensives are equipotent in this regard. ACE inhibitors and AT receptor antagonists appear most efficacious. Calcium-channel antagonists also decrease LV mass. Atenolol, in contrast, has been linked with increased cardiovascular mortality in comparison with other antihypertensives [258]. The hydrophilic profile of atenolol, and consequent low permeability into the central nervous system, may account for its apparent ineffectiveness in preventing VF.

Alcoholic cardiomyopathy

Alcoholic cardiomyopathy (ACM), by definition, is a form of dilated cardiomyopathy that occurs secondary to excess long-term alcohol consumption. The concept largely predates recognition of the genetic basis of DCM. Since the prevalence of heavy alcohol intake far exceeds that of ACM, it is likely that ethanol, as a known myocardial depressant, unmasks an underlying genetic predisposition to DCM. Intake of >90g of alcohol daily for over 5 years appears to confer an increased risk of ACM [259]. The effects of alcohol on the heart appear to be dose dependent but non-linear [260]. The threshold for the development of ACM is also lower in women, although reasons underlying this increased sensitivity to alcohol have not been elucidated [261].

Two phases are recognized in the natural history of ACM: an asymptomatic stage, characterized by isolated LV enlargement with or without diastolic dysfunction; and a clinically overt stage, during which systolic impairment supervenes, together with signs and symptoms of heart failure. The incidence of AF and non-sustained VT appears similar to that of DCM. The sudden death rate is also comparable, although prognosis is noticeably more favourable in ACM patients practising abstinence [262].

In vitro experiments and animal models have suggested several potential mechanisms for the development of ACM, including ethanol-induced apoptosis of cardiac myocytes, impaired function of the mitochondria and sarcoplasmic reticulum, altered expression of sarcomeric proteins, and abnormal calcium handling. The contribution and interplay of these factors in the clinical setting remain to be clarified.

Heart failure therapy improves ventricular function in ACM, particularly in the presence of alcohol abstinence. Increased LVEF has also been documented in the context of continued heavy drinking, but pharmacological therapy does not confer any survival benefit in this subgroup [263]. The importance of abstinence in reducing mortality from ACM is therefore underscored. A recent study suggests that comparable outcomes may be achieved by controlled moderate drinking [264], although long-term follow-up data in a large cohort will be necessary before this approach can be recommended.

Metabolic cardiomyopathy

The term 'metabolic cardiomyopathy' refers to a heterogeneous group of disorders in which myocardial dysfunction occurs as a consequence of a derangement in metabolism. Covered previously in this chapter are the cardiac complications of the storage diseases and mutations in AMP kinase, the cellular fuel gauge. Nutritional deficits such as thiamine deficiency are well-known causes of a reversible DCM. Perhaps the most common form of metabolic cardiomyopathy is that seen in association with diabetes. Diabetes is a prominent risk factor for the development of ischaemic heart disease, but there is growing awareness of a direct effect on ventricular function that is independent of obstructed coronary arteries or concurrent hypertension. The prevalence of heart failure is considerably higher in diabetic patients than in age-matched controls, and

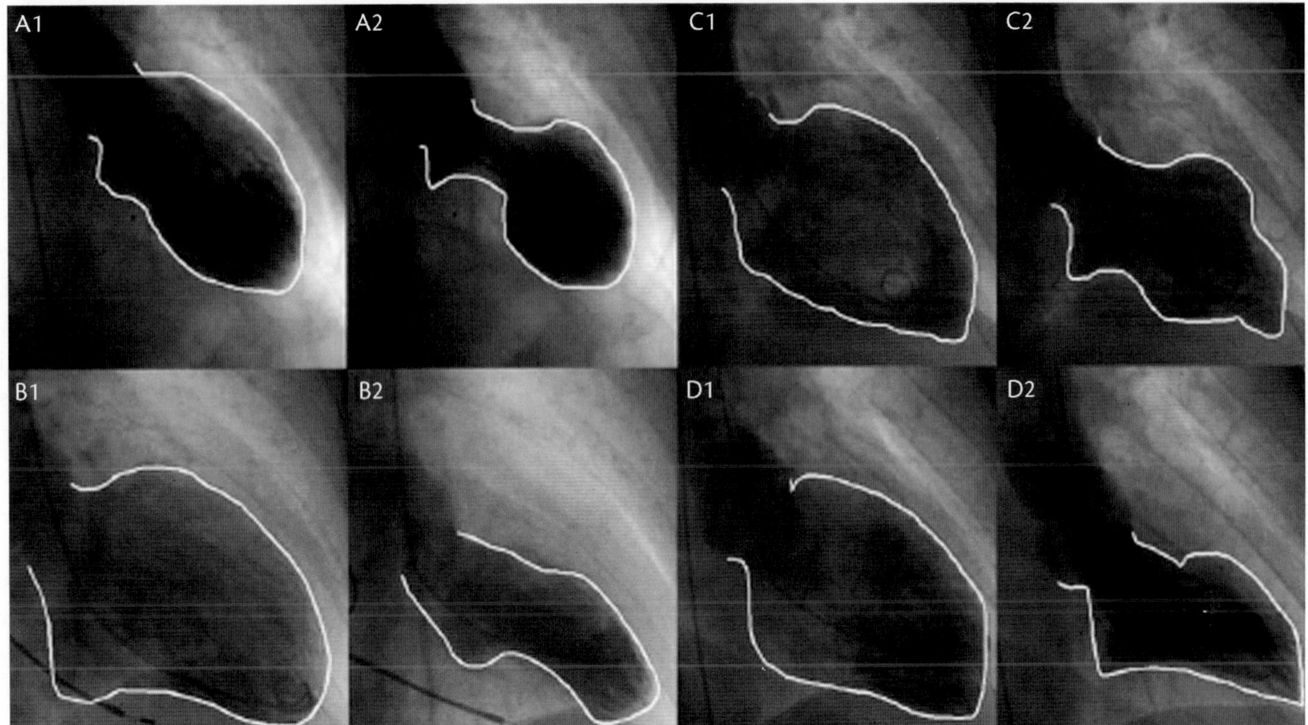

Figure 18.33 Takotsubo cardiomyopathy with typical apical ballooning pattern. Classic form of Takotsubo cardiomyopathy (A1/A2). Reverse Takotsubo with basal akinesia and apical hyperkinesia (B1/B2). Mid-ventricular type (C1/C2). Localized Takotsubo with segmental LV-ballooning (D1/D2). Reproduced from Eshtehardi P, Koestner S, Adorjan P, *et al.* Transient apical ballooning syndrome—clinical characteristics, ballooning pattern, and long-term follow-up in a Swiss population. *Int J Cardiol* 2009; **135:** 370–75.

a less favourable prognosis has also been reported [265, 266]. Diabetic cardiomyopathy may account, at least in part, for the increased risk.

Profound changes in cardiac metabolism occur in diabetes. Periodic evaluation of diabetic patients may be advisable to ensure early detection of subclinical ventricular dysfunction. Optimal glycaemic control and pharmacological therapy with ACE inhibitors/AT receptor antagonists and beta-blockers may attenuate ventricular remodelling and lead to improved survival.

Takotsubo cardiomyopathy

Takotsubo cardiomyopathy has also been termed transient apical ballooning due to its typical angiographic picture seen in this form of cardiomyopathy [267–269]. Patients are presenting with electrocardiographic changes similar for acute coronary syndrome with elevated cardiac biomarkers in the absence of significant coronary artery disease.

Prevalence and aetiology

Prevalence of Takotsubo cardiomyopathy remains largely unknown. Takotsubo cardiomyopathy is named after the original Japanese octopus trap and is characterized by LV dysfunction most commonly with preserved basal function and moderate to severe dysfunction of the mid ventricle and apical regions (➲Fig. 18.33). In the minority of patients, different patterns with preserved apical and impaired basal contractile function can be found (➲Fig. 18.33). This syndrome predominantly affects women and is often triggered by emotional or physical stress.

The pathogenesis of Takotsubo cardiomyopathy is still unknown but high catecholamine levels associated with emotional or physical stress has been suggested as inducing peripheral coronary vasospasm with severe dysfunction of the apical and mid ventricular regions of the LV. Typically, LV dysfunction is rapidly reversible within hours and days.

Clinical presentation

Mean age of this population is around 62–65 years, with a majority of 90% being women. Leading symptoms are chest pain, dyspnoea, ST-segment elevation, T-wave inversion, or QT prolongation. Patients typically suffer from ischaemic chest pain.

From the clinical picture an acute coronary syndrome is diagnosed in most cases and rapid coronary angiography is carried out for diagnostic purposes and possible percutaneous interventions. Typical for this syndrome is that coronary arteries are normal and only the left ventricle shows the typical apical ballooning. Some patients may show a reverse Takotsubo syndrome with basal akinesia and apical hyperkinesia, a mid-ventricular or localized type (➲Fig. 18.33).

Patients may present in cardiac shock and may require intravenous catecholamines to support blood pressure and to maintain cardiac output.

Management

Standard treatment includes aspirin, ACE-inhibitors or AT1 receptor antagonists when blood pressure is maintained, beta-blockers to reduce heart rate, and nitrates to reverse coronary vasospasm. Typically, LV dysfunction disappears within hours and days. EF may be as low as 30% at admission and completely normalized a few days later.

Cardiac biomarkers are mildly elevated such as troponin I or CK. Mean CK values may be as low as 240 U/L.

Prognosis and outcome

Clinical outcome is usually good and medical therapy can be reduced or even stopped after 3–6 months. Recurrence of Takotsubo cardiomyopathy has been described as high as 5%.

Prognosis of patients with Takotsubo cardiomyopathy seems to be favourable and only a slightly elevated in-hospital mortality has been reported.

Tachycardiomyopathy

Pacing at heart rates of 180-200 bpm over 3-4 weeks has been shown to induce heart failure in the experimental animal. In clinical routine, it has been known for years that patients with high heart rates such as during sustained superventricular tachycardia or tachycardic artrial fibrillation develop heart failure over time. Restoration of sinus rhythm with normalization of heart rate leads to normalization of cardiac function. Thus, reduction in heart rate is the therapeutic goal in tachycardia-associated cardiomyopathy. From this observation it became evident that heart rate reduction is an important therapeutic principle in the treatment of heart failure. Therefore, beta-blockers have been found to be efficient in the treatment of heart failure and may improve EF in the range of 5–10%.

A recent study on Ivabradine (n = 10,917), a selective blocker of the sinus node which leads to a reduction in heart rate without effecting cardiac contractility or blood pressure, showed a significant reduction in the rate of myocardial infarction in patients with a heart rate >70 bpm but not in those with a heart rate <70 bpm [270].

Muscular dystrophy cardiomyopathy

Muscular dystrophies are primary disorders of skeletal and/or cardiac muscle that have a genetic basis. Originally defined by the presence of progressive muscle wasting and weakness, the dystrophies are classified according to the distribution and severity of skeletal muscle involvement. Many forms of muscular dystrophy are accompanied by myocardial disease, which was previously attributed to processes extrinsic to the heart. Weakness of the postural musculature causes lordosis and scoliosis, which impair thoracic movement during respiration. Intrinsic disease of the intercostal muscles and diaphragm is also well described. The combined result is restrictive lung disease, which may in turn lead to pulmonary hypertension and a secondary cardiomyopathy [271].

However, cardiomyopathy in the muscular dystrophies is a consequence of intrinsic myocardial dysfunction rather than skeletal muscle disease and respiratory complications. Several lines of evidence support this inference.

- Duchenne and Becker muscular dystrophies have been linked to absolute or relative deficiency of the sarcolemmal protein dystrophin. Mutations in dystrophin have also been identified in X-linked DCM [272], underlining its role in primary myocardial disease. Molecular disruption of dystrophin in both ischaemic heart failure and DCM may be reversible by treatment with LVADs [67]. Thus it has been proposed that dystrophin remodelling may provide a final common pathway for contractile impairment in heart failure.
- Histological examination of the heart in Duchenne and Becker muscular dystrophy reveals replacement of the myocardium with connective tissue and fat [273]. Similar findings in skeletal muscle suggest a common underlying disease process.
- Equally compelling is the observation that female carriers of Duchenne and Becker muscular dystrophy may have LV dilation in the absence of significant myopathic symptoms [274].
- In some forms of muscular dystrophy, notably Emery–Dreifuss, locomotor involvement is mild and cardiac manifestations predominate [275].

➲Table 18.13 summarizes cardiac involvement in the muscular dystrophies and myotonic dystrophy. Periodic evaluation of affected patients and carriers with 12-lead ECG, two-dimensional echocardiography, and ambulatory ECG monitoring is recommended. Myotonic dystrophy may occasionally present with cardiac manifestations

Table 18.13 Cardiac involvement in muscular dystrophies

Type	Inheritance	Gene affected	Mechanism of disease expression	Extracardiac manifestations	Cardiac involvement
Duchenne	X-linked	Dystrophin gene at Xp21	Dystrophin serves as a bridge between the cytoskeletal protein actin (at the N-terminus) and the transmembrane protein β-dystroglycan (at the C-terminus). Absence of dystrophin leads to disruption of the mechanical link between the sarcolemma and the extracellular matrix	Childhood onset Progressive proximal myopathy Wheelchair-bound by teens	Dilated cardiomyopathy
Becker	X-linked	Dystrophin gene at Xp21	Dystrophin present but reduced in quantity or otherwise abnormal	Onset age 12 or later in life Proximal myopathy Slowly progressive	Dilated cardiomyopathy
Emery–Dreifuss	X-linked AD, rarely AR	STA gene at Xq28 LMNA gene at 1q21	Emerin is an integral protein of the inner nuclear membrane Lamins A and C are also nuclear envelope proteins	Contractures at ankles,elbows and neck Slowly progressive myopathy Humeroperoneal distribution	Atrial flutter/fibrillation 'Isolated atrial standstill'; low-amplitude or absent P waves; atria unresponsive to pacing. Ventricular pacing indicated Massive atrial dilation; anticoagulants advised Dilated cardiomyopathy Sudden death
Myotonic (type 1)	AD	DMPK gene at 19q13.3	Abnormal expansion of a trinucleotide cytosine-thymine-guanine sequence in the myotonin protein kinase gene (DMPK) 35 copies or less of CTG repeat in normal subjects; 50–2000 in myotonic patients May demonstrate genetic anticipation Exact function of DMPK unknown; localized to intercalated discs; can modify actin cytoskeleton	Myotonia Weakness of facial, pharyngeal and distal limb muscles Diabetes, thyroid dysfunction Cataracts	Conduction system defects (prolonged PR interval and/or wide QRS on ECG; pacing may be required) Atrial flutter/fibrillation Ventricular tachyarrhythmia Sudden cardiac death Mitral valve prolapse LV dilation and/or systolic impairment Left ventricular hypertrophy

AD, autosomal dominant; AR, autosomal recessive; LV, left ventricle.

and should be considered part of the differential diagnosis in a young patient with progressive conduction system disease. Treatment is tailored according to the nature of cardiac involvement; conduction defects may require pacing, while standard heart failure therapy is indicated for ventricular dilation and impairment. The presence of ventricular tachyarrhythmia in myotonic dystrophy may prompt the use of an ICD, as sudden death is a recognized complication.

Peripartum cardiomyopathy

Peripartum cardiomyopathy (PPCM) is defined as LV systolic impairment in the presence of the following additional criteria:

- presentation within 1 month of delivery or during the first 5 months post-partum;
- absence of pre-existing cardiac disease; and
- no other cause for cardiac dysfunction.

Table 18.14 Risk factors for the development of peripartum cardiomyopathy

Increasing maternal age
Multiparity
Multiple pregnancy
Pre-eclampsia
Gestational hypertension
Afro-Caribbean
Familial occurrence
Malnutrition
Cocaine use by mother
Long-term tocolytic therapy
Selenium deficiency
Chlamydia infection
Enterovirus infection

Data from de Beus E, van Mook WN, Ramsay, G, *et al.* Peripartum cardiomyopathy: a condition intensivists should be aware of. *Intensive Care Med* 2003; **29**: 167–74; and James, PR. A review of peripartum cardiomyopathy. *Int J Clin Pract* 2004; **58**: 363–5.

Underlying cardiac disorders that are unmasked by the haemodynamic stress of a normal pregnancy are thereby excluded [276, 277].

Prevalence and aetiology

The true incidence has not been established, although existing data suggest a frequency of between 1 in 3000 and 1 in 10,000 pregnancies [278]. This is likely to be an underestimate, as mild forms of PPCM probably remain unrecognized because of the prevalence of exertional dyspnoea and ankle oedema in the last trimester.

The aetiology of PPCM also remains uncertain (➲Table 18.14). Endomyocardial biopsies demonstrate features of myocarditis in up to 62% of cases [279], suggesting an inflammatory component. However, there does not appear to be any association between the presence of myocarditis and the clinical outcome. Malnutrition has been cited as a possible factor; women with PPCM in certain geographical areas have low plasma levels of selenium [280]. Others, however, appear to have good nutritional status. Viral infection has been postulated, although recurrence in subsequent pregnancies is less easy to explain on this basis. One intriguing possibility is that of an abnormal immune response during pregnancy [281], which has also been implicated in the pathogenesis of pre-eclampsia. Finally, familial occurrence of PPCM has been reported [282]. The most likely explanation is that PPCM is a manifestation of familial DCM, with the cardiovascular burden of pregnancy uncovering previously unrecognized subclinical disease. This possibility is supported by anecdotal evidence but warrants further prospective evaluation.

Clinical presentation

Patients with PPCM typically present with symptoms of LV failure, such as orthopnoea and paroxysmal nocturnal dyspnoea. Repetitive monomorphic VT and systemic thromboembolism have also been reported. The findings on physical examination may be difficult to interpret as a third heart sound and ejection systolic murmur are present in >90% of normal pregnant women. Similarly, slight leftward deviation of the QRS axis is a normal ECG feature during pregnancy. Non-specific ST-segment changes and supraventricular or ventricular extrasystoles are often seen in PPCM. Two-dimensional echocardiography is the principal investigation. LV systolic impairment is requisite for diagnosis, with some authors recommending strict echocardiographic criteria: LVEF <45% and/or fractional shortening <30% plus LV end-diastolic measurement of 2.7cm/m^2 body surface area. Dilation of cardiac chambers may also be present, particularly in patients presenting >1 month after delivery.

Management

Standard therapy for LV failure is employed in PPCM. Cardiogenic shock may necessitate insertion of an intra-aortic balloon pump. In the absence of significant decompensation, however, PPCM may be managed on an out-patient basis. ACE inhibitors and AT receptor antagonists are contraindicated after the first trimester owing to the potential for adverse effects on the fetus (oligohydramnios and its consequences, i.e. limb deformities, cranial ossification deficits, lung hypoplasia) and neonate (hypotension and renal failure). However, beneficial rescue therapy with a low-dose, short-acting ACE inhibitor has been reported in a small series of pregnant women with severe resistant vasoconstrictive hypertension [283]. Serial assessment of amniotic fluid volume was conducted and delivery was remote from maternal dosing. There were no fetal or neonatal complications; improved haemodynamics were observed in the mothers, with successful continuation of pregnancy. In a multicentre survey of the management of PPCM in current practice, 6% of perinatologists reported using ACE inhibitors during pregnancy [284]. In cases of severe refractory ventricular failure, the potential risks to the fetus from ACE inhibitor therapy should perhaps be balanced against the urgent need to optimize ventricular function to ensure a positive outcome for both mother and baby.

Pregnancy per se is a hypercoagulable state, and the risk of thromboembolism is further enhanced by bed rest, diuretic therapy, and impaired ventricular function. Prophylactic doses of low-molecular-weight heparin are appropriate during pregnancy; warfarin may be instituted following delivery.

Prognosis and outcome

Reports of the long-term prognosis in PPCM are highly variable. Many patients experience symptomatic improvement, accompanied by complete or partial recovery of LV function. However, a few progress to end-stage heart failure. In a retrospective series of 42 patients with PPCM followed up for an average of 8 years, death was recorded in 7% and a similar proportion underwent cardiac transplantation. LV function normalized in 43%. Earlier studies indicated a less favourable clinical outcome, with mortality rates of up to 56% [285]. Death usually results from worsening pump failure, although systemic thromboembolism and ventricular tachyarrhythmia have been documented. Predictors of high risk are lacking at present, but a combined strategy of early recognition and aggressive medical therapy is recommended.

Counselling patients with PPCM on the issue of future pregnancies poses a major clinical challenge because of potential recurrences of symptomatic heart failure. It has been suggested that subclinical ventricular dysfunction persists in many patients, and the haemodynamic burden of another pregnancy precipitates decompensation. Reactivation of a pregnancy-related disease process may also be invoked. Surveys of subsequent pregnancies in survivors of PPCM have elicited the following findings [286].

- LV dysfunction and clinical deterioration may recur in the mother.
- The incidence of complications is higher (up to 50%) in women with incomplete recovery of ventricular function. Maternal deaths are more likely to occur. An increased incidence of fetal prematurity and loss is also reported in this subgroup.
- Women in whom ventricular function has normalized prior to pregnancy are at very low risk of death. Symptomatic heart failure may nonetheless recur in around 20% and result in persistent LV impairment. Careful monitoring is therefore warranted.

Personal perspective

Myocardial diseases represent a large spectrum of inherited and acquired forms of heart muscle disease. The term 'cardiomyopathy' has been used in the past to describe primary forms of myocardial disease of unknown aetiology. However, in the past few years it has become evident that most of the primary forms are genetically transmitted, affecting the sarcomeric genes in HCM and the cytoskeleton-encoding genes in DCM. Secondary forms may represent HCM or DCM and are, as in the primary forms, most frequently genetically transmitted (e.g. amyloidosis, haemochromatosis, glycogen storage diseases, Fabry disease). True secondary forms of myocardial disease are ischaemic, alcoholic, or hypertensive heart disease, which are also genetically determined but which may mimic the cardiac phenotype of HCM or DCM. Thus most forms of myocardial disease today represent inherited forms of heart disease.

Further reading

Abraham WT, Fisher WG, Smith AL, *et al.* Cardiac resynchronization in chronic heart failure. *N Engl J Med* 2002; **346**: 1845–53.

Crilley JG, Boehm EA, Blair E, *et al.* Hypertrophic cardiomyopathy due to sarcomeric gene mutations is characterized by impaired energy metabolism irrespective of the degree of hypertrophy. *J Am Coll Cardiol* 2003; **41**: 1776–82.

Drazner MH, Rame JE, Stevenson LW, *et al.* Prognostic importance of elevated jugular venous pressure and a third heart sound in patients with heart failure. *N Engl J Med* 2001; **345**: 574–81.

Elkayam U, Tummala PP, Rao K, *et al.* Maternal and fetal outcomes of subsequent pregnancies in women with peripartum cardiomyopathy. *N Engl J Med* 2001; **344**: 1567–71.

Eshtehardi P, Koestner S, Adorjan P, *et al.* Transient apical ballooning syndrome – clinical characteristics, ballooning pattern, and long-term follow-up in a Swiss population. *Int J Cardiol* 2008 Jul 1. [Epub ahead of print.]

Faber L, Meissner A, Ziemssen P, *et al.* Percutaneous transluminal septal myocardial ablation for hypertrophic obstructive cardiomyopathy: long term follow-up of the first series of 25 patients. *Heart* 2000; **83**: 326–31.

Hess OM, Sigwart U. New treatment strategies for hypertrophic obstructive cardiomyopathy. Alcohol ablation of the septum: the new gold standard? *J Am Coll Cardiol* 2004; **44**: 2054–5.

Jenni R, Oechslin E, Schneider J, *et al.* Echocardiographic and pathoanatomical characteristics of isolated left ventricular non-compaction: a step towards classification as a distinct cardiomyopathy. *Heart* 2001; **86**: 666–71.

Kühl, U, Pauschinger, M & Noutsias, M *et al.* High prevalence of viral genomes and multiple viral infections in the myocardium of adults with 'idiopathic' left ventricular dysfunction. *Circulation* 2005; **111**: 887–93.

Maron BJ, McKenna WJ, Danielson GK, *et al.* American College of Cardiology/European Society of Cardiology Clinical Expert Consensus Document on Hypertrophic Cardiomyopathy. *Eur Heart J* 2003; **24**: 1965–91.

McCarthy RE, Boehmer JP, Hruban RH, *et al.* Long-term outcome of fulminant myocarditis as compared with acute (nonfulminant) myocarditis. *N Engl J Med* 2000; **342**: 690–5.

Piano MR. Alcoholic cardiomyopathy: incidence, clinical characteristics, and pathophysiology. *Chest* 2002; **121**: 1638–50.

Pietrangelo A. Hereditary hemochromatosis: a new look at an old disease. *N Engl J Med* 2004; **350**: 2383–97.

Skinner M, Sanchorawala V, Seldin DC *et al.* High-dose melphalan and autologous stem-cell transplantation in patients with AL amyloidosis: an 8-year study. *Ann Intern Med* 2004; **140**: 85–93.

Thiene G, Nava, A, Corrado D, *et al.* Right ventricular cardiomyopathy and sudden death in young people. *N Engl J Med* 1988; **318**: 129–33.

Towbin JA, Bowles NE. The failing heart. *Nature* 2002; **415**: 227–33.

➲ For full references and multimedia materials please visit the online version of the book (http://esctextbook.oxfordonline.com).

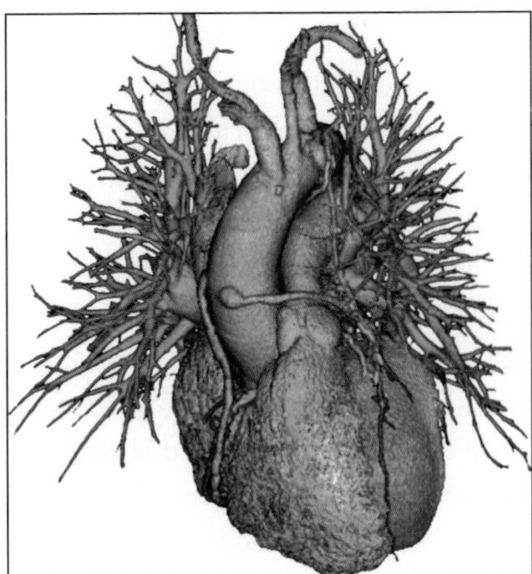

CHAPTER 19

Pericardial Disease

Jordi Soler-Soler and Jaume Sagristà-Sauleda

Contents

Summary

Pericardial diseases are not uncommon. The diagnosis is not usually difficult and the prognosis is good, but uncertainty frequently arises in relation to their management. Clinical syndromes include acute inflammatory pericarditis, pericardial effusion, cardiac tamponade, and constrictive pericarditis. These syndromes sometimes coexist. Acute pericarditis is the most frequent pericardial syndrome; accordingly, it is extensively dealt with in this chapter, with emphasis on the clinical management. The advantages and limitations of invasive pericardial procedures and sophisticated laboratory studies in pericardial fluid and tissue are discussed, and recommendations for the indications of pericardiocentesis and pericardial biopsy are provided. Pericardial effusion, either as an isolated finding or accompanying other pericardial or extra-cardiac diseases, constitutes a frequent diagnostic challenge that is discussed separately. The correct diagnosis and management of pericardial constriction is an important issue as the concept of constrictive pericarditis has recently been expanded and, on the other hand, it is a curable disease if pericardiectomy is appropriately indicated. The main characteristics and management of the most important specific types of pericarditis are discussed and, finally, some rare types of pericardial diseases are commented on.

Introduction

The pericardium is a sac with two fibroserous layers that surrounds the heart. The pericardium can be affected by a wide variety of agents and processes [1–3]. However, the response of the pericardium is relatively uniform, consisting of inflammatory clinical manifestations such as chest pain and fever, production of pericardial fluid with the possible complication of cardiac tamponade, and thickening, retraction, and calcification leading to constrictive pericarditis. From a clinical point of view, the most frequent manifestation is the acute pericardial syndrome (acute pericarditis and tamponade). Pericardial effusion accompanies many causes of pericardial diseases, but sometimes constitutes an isolated finding.

Acute pericardial syndromes

Acute pericarditis

Acute pericarditis is a clinical syndrome due to inflammation of the pericardium and is characterized by chest pain, pericardial friction rub, and typical electrocardiogram (ECG) repolarization changes. The diagnosis of pericarditis requires at least two of these three elements, although auscultation of a pericardial friction rub can be considered a pathognomonic feature. Chest pain with 'pericardial characteristics' is not sufficient per se to establish the diagnosis, an attitude unfortunately quite frequent. Acute pericarditis results from a wide range of aetiologies of very different nature (➲Table 19.1).

Table 19.1 Causes of acute pericarditis

Causes
Acute idiopathic pericarditis
Infectious pericarditis:
Viral
Tuberculosis
Bacterial
Others
Postpericardiotomy syndrome
Postmyocardial infarction pericarditis
Renal insufficiency
Neoplastic disease
Chest trauma
Irradiation
Collagen diseases
Others

Differential diagnosis

In the first few hours after onset, acute pericarditis may be confused with ST-segment elevation myocardial infarction (➲ Chapter 16). However, chest pain of myocardial infarction has a sudden onset, does not vary with respiration, and is often accompanied by vegetative symptoms. In myocardial infarction, ST-segment elevation is present in some leads while in others there is ST-segment depression (mirror image), and appearance of Q waves within a few hours. Finally, in myocardial infarction definite elevation of myocardial necrosis markers is present, although marginal elevation of troponin may occur in acute pericarditis [4]. Dissecting aortic aneurysm (➲ Chapter 31) is rarely mistaken for pericarditis since the onset of pain is very acute, very intense, and located in the back rather than in the precordial region. Pleuritic pain is located at the sides of the chest, but may coexist with pericardial pain in the frequent cases of pleuropericarditis. Chest wall pain is sensitive to local pressure. Overall, the diagnosis of acute pericarditis is easy in the vast majority of patients.

Clinical manifestations

The basic symptom of acute pericarditis is chest pain with rapid onset, but not as abrupt as in acute myocardial infarction. Pain is located in the precordial and retrosternal region, but characteristically radiates to the supraclavicular region, the back, and the trapezoid region. Usually it is exacerbated by inspiration, chest movements, and the decubitus position, and is alleviated by sitting with the trunk leaning forward. Pain is usually of moderate intensity and lasts several days. After the acute phase, patients not infrequently remain with minor symptoms for some weeks. Other common symptoms are dyspnoea, fever, cough, and asthenia. The pathognomonic sign of acute pericarditis is pericardial friction rub (60–80%) which is a scratchy superficial sound that is heard in the mesocardium and the lower left parasternal edge. Its intensity varies with respiratory movements. Typically, friction rub has three components, although sometimes only one or two components can be heard; hence, they can be confused with a murmur. Friction rub can be present with or without effusion. Auscultation of a rub permits the diagnosis of acute pericarditis to be established, although this diagnosis cannot be ruled out in its absence. When pericarditis presents with moderate/large effusion, signs of tamponade may occur.

Diagnostic techniques

ECG is abnormal in 80% of patients (➲ Chapter 2). In the most typical cases, ECG changes can be described in four stages. Stage 1 consists of a diffuse ST-segment elevation with upward concavity and positive T waves in several leads (➲ Fig. 19.1). The PR-segment may be depressed, indicating atrial injury. The concomitant presence of these two findings is pathognomonic of pericarditis. These findings may last several hours to a few days. In stage 2, ST-segment returns to the isoelectric position. Stage 3 is characterized by the appearance of negative T waves which may return to normality in a few days, although they may remain negative for several weeks. Such an evolution should not be considered a persistence of the disease. Stage 4 corresponds to normalization of the ECG. Stage 1 changes may be confused with acute myocardial infarction or the normal variant of repolarization known as 'early repolarization'. In acute myocardial infarction, no PR-segment depression occurs, ST-segment elevation is upwardly convex and may have a mirror image in some opposing leads, and Q waves appear in most cases. Early repolarization is characterized by ST-segment elevation with upward concavity and positive T waves; several differential findings have been described [5], but the most distinctive is the unchanging pattern of early repolarization pattern. When large pericardial effusion is present, the amplitude of QRS complex may decrease or follow cyclic changes (electrical alternans), particularly in patients with tamponade.

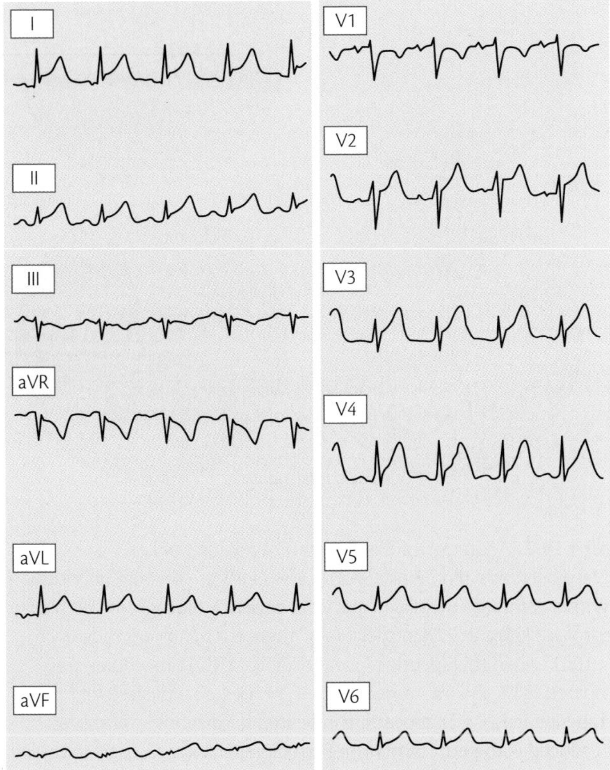

Figure 19.1 Acute pericarditis. Typical ECG pattern of stage I: diffuse ST-segment elevation with positive T waves and PR-segment depression.

Chest radiography shows cardiomegaly when effusion exceeds 250mL. Pleural effusion, particularly in the left side, is frequent in patients with pleuropericarditis.

Echocardiography is the most useful technique for the identification of pericardial effusion (➲ Chapter 4). However, echocardiographic findings should not be considered crucial for establishing the diagnosis of acute pericarditis, as effusion may be absent in 50% of patients [2]; on the other hand, pericardial effusion can have multiple other causes.

General blood analysis usually provides only non-specific information. Slightly troponin elevation may be detected in 35–50% of patients [4], indicating epicardial inflammation and involvement of adjacent myocardium.

Aetiological diagnosis approach

Once the clinical diagnosis of acute pericarditis has been established, the next step is to establish the aetiology. The strategy for aetiological diagnosis in acute pericardial disease can be quite simple. The main concepts are:

- knowledge of the epidemiological distribution and prevalence of aetiologies;
- importance of identifying some specific aetiologies;
- awareness of the diagnostic yield of the invasive procedures of the pericardium.

Acute pericardial disease can be caused by a vast array of agents or conditions [1]. However, frequency notions can considerably simplify diagnostic reasoning in most instances. Acute pericardial disease is usually either associated with an obvious clinical condition that makes a cause–effect relationship quite likely [6], or is idiopathic. The term idiopathic denotes acute pericarditis for which no specific aetiology can be found with routine diagnostic tests. Therefore 'idiopathic' pericarditis is not really a distinct entity but the failure to uncover the aetiology. In fact, when an aggressive protocol study is applied a substantial proportion of specific aetiologies (mainly viral) can be found [7, 8]. The majority of the remaining causes are very infrequent; however, in several parts of the world, some of these causes may have a different prevalence that may accordingly lead to a modified approach. Tuberculosis is a case in point. Tuberculous pericarditis is rare among immunologically-competent people in the Western world [9]. However, in developing countries or in immunologically-compromised patients, tuberculous pericarditis may be a comparatively common pericardial disease [10–12]; hence, an earlier use of invasive or blind antituberculous therapy may be justified. Unfortunately, the true prevalence of tuberculous pericarditis and other major causes of pericardial disease in different parts of the world and in different patient communities are unknown.

In Western societies, the most common cause of acute pericarditis is idiopathic (i.e. presumably viral) [9, 13–18]. This high predominance of idiopathic self-limited disease justifies restrictive indications of invasive pericardial procedures (pericardiocentesis or pericardial biopsy). The different patterns of clinical presentation of acute pericardial disease are helpful for the identification of certain aetiologies. When acute pericardial disease develops in a patient with a disease known to predispose to pericardial involvement (such as myocardial infarction (➲ Chapter 16), renal failure, widespread neoplasia, or lupus erythematosus), the likelihood of this disease being the cause for the acute pericarditis is very high [6]. An immunologically-competent patient without associated conditions has a probability of around 90% of acute idiopathic pericarditis when an acute picture of pericardial pain, characteristic ECG changes, and pericardial friction rub are present [9, 13, 15]. The probability of idiopathic disease approaches 100% when clinical features subside in the following few days. No further studies are required in such cases. The occurrence of subsequent relapses is also highly specific for idiopathic pericarditis, especially when collagen vascular disease has been ruled out.

The development of tamponade in the context of acute pericarditis renders the situation somewhat more complex. Tamponade is significantly more common in patients with specific aetiologies such as tuberculous or purulent pericarditis or neoplasia than in patients with acute idiopathic pericarditis; however, the first cause of tamponade in everyday practice is acute idiopathic pericarditis, given its much higher prevalence [9, 13].

Other features such as a sustained clinical course (i.e. over 3 weeks) may increase the likelihood of specific forms of pericarditis; however, in Western societies, idiopathic pericarditis is again the first-choice diagnosis [13]. Two exceptions to this rule are tamponade with massive haemopericardium (often caused by malignancy) [19], and severely toxic patients with high fever and leucocytosis, where purulent pericarditis should be ruled out even in the absence of predisposing conditions such as intra-thoracic infection [20].

The diagnostic yield of pericardiocentesis, pericardial biopsy, and pericardioscopy is a very important issue when the indications of these invasive procedures are considered. The major uncertainties relate to the diagnostic yield of these invasive procedures in patients free from haemodynamic compromise and in whom the procedures are indicated because of severe constitutional symptoms, insidious evolution, or large effusion. A remarkable finding of our series [7, 16] was that the diagnostic yield of both pericardiocentesis and subxiphoid pericardial drainage with biopsy was significantly higher when they were performed in patients with cardiac tamponade than when indicated for purely diagnostic purposes (35% versus 6%) (➲Fig. 19.2). Therefore, invasive pericardial procedures in the absence of clinical tamponade provide the diagnosis in only a minority of patients in the Western world; however, it should be emphasized that epidemiological data, mainly the relative prevalence of different aetiologies in specific areas, are a crucial issue when the indications of invasive diagnostic procedures are considered.

In recent years, newer methods for pericardial drainage have been introduced [22–25]. These reports claim higher sensitivity and specificity of pericardioscopy than simple pericardial drainage or biopsy, and its use has been advocated as the preferential invasive diagnostic technique. Although pericardioscopy may offer an advantage in selected patients with experienced operators, there is not enough experience to justify its routine use. On the other hand,

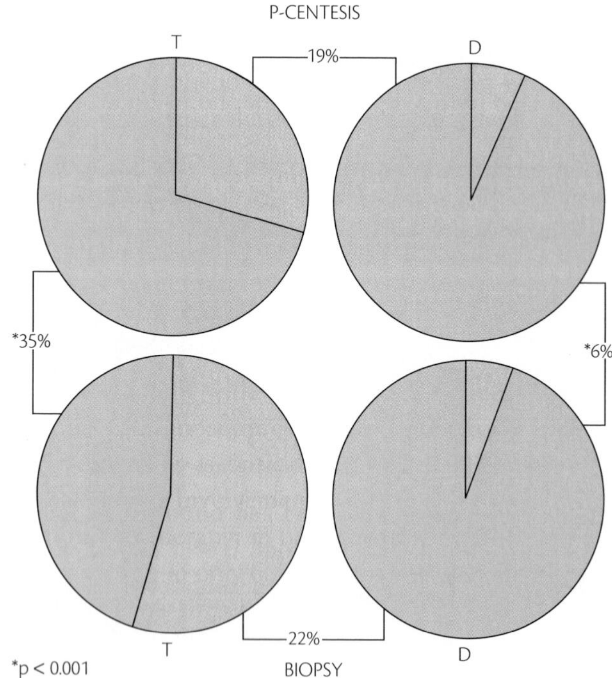

Figure 19.2 Acute pericardial disease. Diagnostic yield of pericardiocentesis and biopsy. Shades areas indicate the rate of positive diagnosis. Although the diagnostic yield of pericardiocentesis and biopsy are similar (19% and 22%, respectively), there is a significant difference (p <0.001) when therapeutic (T) and diagnostic (D) procedures are compared (35% and 6%, respectively). T, procedure indicated for therapeutic reasons; D, procedure indicated for diagnostic purposes. Reproduced with permission from Permanyer-Miralda G, Sagristà-Sauleda J, Soler-Soler J. Primary acute pericardial disease: a prospective series of 231 consecutive patients. *Am J Cardiol* 1985: **56**; 623–30.

in addition to a likely selection bias in the reports of the results of this sophisticated technique, it is not evident that a diagnosis pertinent to management could not have been achieved by simple pericardiocentesis or subxiphoid pericardial biopsy. Furthermore, the reported higher diagnostic yield of pericardioscopy does not mean it should be used without clinical features to identify the group of patients in whom specific diagnoses are more likely. These features have not yet been unequivocally established. Accordingly, it is quite likely that, at present, pericardioscopy should not modify the basic approach to the management of patients with pericardial effusion. The same considerations should also be applied to epicardial biopsy, a procedure associated with pericardioscopy [22, 25].

The shortcomings of aetiological diagnosis in a significant proportion of patients justify the adoption of a comprehensive protocol for routine clinical management [9, 14] consisting of three stages. Stage 1 includes basic laboratory studies, chest X-rays, and Doppler echocardiogram. For patients in whom clinical disease does not abate within 1 week or who have clinical features of tamponade, anti-DNA antibodies, rheumatoid factor, serologic tests for toxoplasma, legionella, and mycoplasma, and three sputa or gastric aspirate cultures for mycobacteria are carried out. If pleural effusion is present, thoracocentesis is indicated. In addition to routine cytological and biochemical studies in pleural fluid, adenosine deaminase activity is measured (a value >45UI/L suggest tuberculosis, whereas lower values point against this aetiology) and a search for mycobacteria is also made. Stage 1 also includes any other investigation (such as computed tomography, lymph node biopsy, or immunological status) warranted by the initial clinical findings to rule out associated disease. Stage 2 consists of pericardiocentesis, which is only indicated to treat cardiac tamponade and when purulent pericarditis is suspected. Pericardial fluid is studied in a similar manner to pleural fluid. Stage 3 consists of subxiphoid pericardial drainage and biopsy, with histological examination (including stains for mycobacteria) and culture of the biopsy specimen. This procedure is recommended when pericardiocentesis is ineffective or tamponade relapses, and in selected patients with active clinical disease of more than three weeks' duration and no diagnosis (➲Table 19.2 and ➲Fig. 19.3). A more aggressive protocol with wider indications of invasive pericardial procedures is proposed in the European Society of Cardiology guidelines on the diagnosis and management of pericardial diseases [7]. The appropriateness of this

Table 19.2 Indications of pericardiocentesis and surgical pericardial biopsy in acute pericardial disease

Pericardiocentesis
Clinical tamponade
Suspicion of purulent pericarditis
Surgical pericardial biopsy
Clinical tamponade not resolved with or recurrent after pericardiocentesis
Unremitting clinical course after 3 weeks of anti-inflammatory treatment

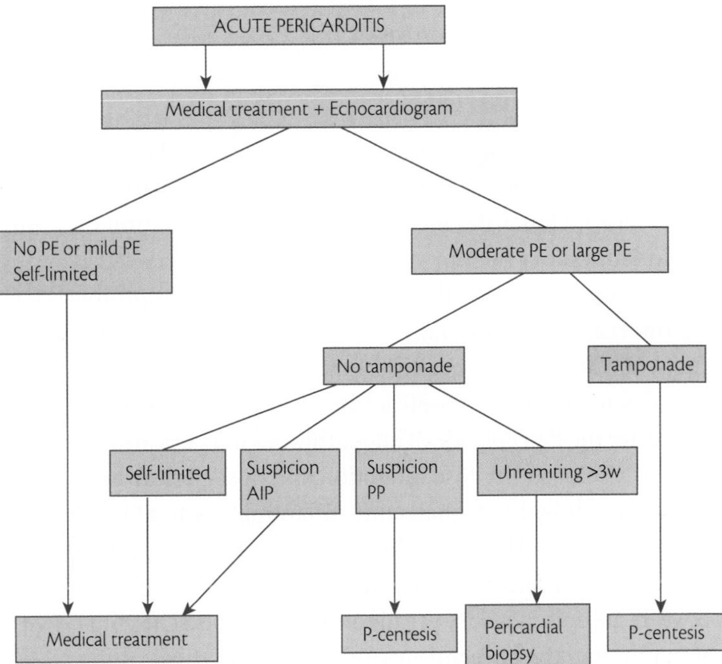

Figure 19.3 Flow chart of the management of acute pericarditis. AIP: acute idiopathic pericarditis; P-centesis: pericardiocentesis; PE: pericardial effusion; PP: purulent pericarditis; w: weeks.

approach should be balanced towards the increased costs and discomfort for the patients in relation to its diagnostic yield (mainly, documentation of aetiologies with specific treatment).

Treatment

Patients with acute idiopathic or viral pericarditis should rest in bed or an armchair while inflammatory symptoms persist. Most patients can be treated in an outpatient setting [26], with hospital admission being reserved for patients with high fever, prolonged clinical course, cardiac tamponade, large effusion, or myocardial involvement, and for immunodepressed patients or those on anticoagulant treatment. Pain and fever are usually satisfactorily managed with analgesic-antipyretic drugs, either alone or in combination. For patients with no contraindications, the first choice is aspirin (500–1000mg/6 hours) while pain and fever are present, and tapered gradually over 3–4 weeks. In non-responders to aspirin, or if aspirin is contraindicated, non-steroidal anti-inflammatory drugs (NSAIDs) can be used (indomethacin 75–225mg/day, paracetamol 2–4g/day, or ibuprofen 1600–3200mg/day), either alone or in combination. Additional administration of colchicine (1–2mg/day) has been proposed to prevent relapses [27], but more information is required before systematic use in the first episode of pericarditis can be recommended. Corticosteroids must be avoided since they are probably associated with the appearance of relapses [27]; in fact, some patients suffer repeated relapses every time they try to reduce the doses, and become corticosteroid-dependent. In some reluctant cases, administration of immunoglobulin or immunosuppressive drugs has been advocated [7].

Recurrent pericarditis

Recurrent or relapsing pericarditis is the most troublesome complication of acute pericarditis. The term recurrent pericarditis includes the incessant type (discontinuation of anti-inflammatory therapy nearly always produces a relapse in a short period) and the intermittent type (symptom-free intervals conventionally >6 weeks without therapy). Frequency of recurrences after a first episode of acute pericarditis varies between 8–80% [28]. Commonly, relapses occur after the first episode of idiopathic or viral pericarditis, but may also occur in post-infarction and post-pericardiotomy pericarditis. Inadequate anti-inflammatory treatment and corticosteroids [27] in the index attack may account for the relapses. The number of recurrences and the interval between the episodes vary greatly among patients. The clinical manifestations of recurrences are similar to those of the first episode, but quite characteristically the index attack is usually more severe, while subsequent episodes are milder [29]. Evolution to constrictive pericarditis is exceptional.

The two main goals of therapy are the treatment of acute episodes and prevention of recurrences. Each episode should be treated according to the recommendations pointed out for acute pericarditis. There is no definitively efficacious treatment for the prevention of recurrences. Colchicine (1–2mg/day) for 1 year has been proposed, but the great body of evidence is limited to observational and uncontrolled studies [30–34], and its efficacy is probably around 50% of cases. One randomized study [35] suggested that colchicine administered at the first recurrence significantly reduced the recurrence rate at 18 months (24% versus 51%, $p = 0.02$). Use of high doses of prednisone (1mg/kg/day) compared to low doses (0.2–0.5mg/kg/day) was associated with more side effects, recurrences, and hospitalizations [36]. Immunosuppressive therapy is not justified. Pericardiectomy is considered as the last resort due to its unpredictable result [29], although good long-term outcome has been reported with 'complete' pericardiectomy [37]. As mentioned, probably the most effective strategy for preventing recurrences is to avoid the administration of corticosteroids in the index episode and proceed to a gradual titration of anti-inflammatory therapy. Overall, prognosis is excellent and serious complications, apart from the disturbing recurrences, are uncommon [29, 38].

Cardiac tamponade

Cardiac tamponade is a clinical-haemodynamic syndrome of cardiac compression caused by pericardial effusion with increased intrapericardial pressure. Tamponade is not an 'all-or-nothing' condition, but a 'continuum' that ranges from a minimally increased intrapericardial pressure with no clinical repercussion to severe haemodynamic compromise that may be fatal. The consequence is a restriction of cardiac inflow that is more apparent in the right chamber cavities. Although subtle changes in arterial pressure, cardiac output, and variations in arterial pressure with inspiration can be detected with small elevations of intrapericardial pressure [39], 'haemodynamic' tamponade is present when intrapericardial pressure equals right atrial and diastolic right ventricular pressures. At this point, right transmural pressure (cavity pressure minus intrapericardial pressure) approaches zero mmHg. The consequent echocardiographic-Doppler findings are diastolic collapses of the right atrium and right ventricle, and exaggerated respiratory variations in blood flow velocity through the cardiac valves. However, many patients with 'haemodynamic' and 'echocardiographic' tamponade remain asymptomatic and do not manifest any of the signs of 'clinical' tamponade [40, 41]. Isolated right atrial collapse is a poor marker of clinical tamponade (positive predictive value of 30%), with right atrial plus right ventricular collapses being more specific (74%) [41]. In contrast, the absence of collapses precludes tamponade. Thus, as shown in ➲Fig. 19.4, many patients with significant pericardial effusion probably suffer some degree of haemodynamic tamponade, others exhibit echocardiographic signs of tamponade, while only a few have clinical tamponade. Therefore, clinical tamponade represents the tip of the iceberg of the 'continuum' of severity of cardiac tamponade.

Two pathophysiological issues of tamponade are relevant. First, elevation of intrapericardial pressure depends not only on the amount of pericardial effusion but on fluid accumulation velocity and pericardial distensibility. Small amounts of fluid may cause severe tamponade, as occurs in free wall ventricular rupture or stab wounds; in contrast, a massive chronic effusion may cause only small elevation of intrapericardial pressure. Second, intravascular volume and intracavitary pressures are important determinants in the development of tamponade. Usually, tamponade develops when intrapericardial pressure increases around 8mmHg (normal right atrial pressure). In patients with volume depletion or lower intracavitary pressure, tamponade may develop at lower intrapericardial (and intracavitary) pressure levels, the so-called low-pressure cardiac tamponade. This syndrome was initially described in a dehydrated critically ill patient [42]. We identified low pressure tamponade in 20% of patients with catheterization-based criteria of tamponade [43]. Clinical recognition may be difficult because of the absence of some typical physical findings of tamponade in most patients.

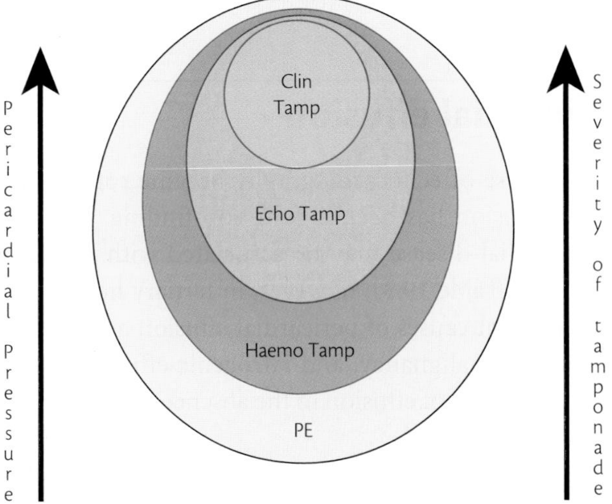

Figure 19.4 Diagram of haemodynamic-echocardiographic-clinical correlation in tamponade (Tamp). Severity of tamponade (right arrow) increases in parallel to the increase of intrapericardial pressure (left arrow). Mild degrees of tamponade are only recognized by haemodynamic (Haemo) measurements. As intrapericardial pressure increases, echocardiographic (Echo) findings of tamponade are present, and further increases of intrapericardial pressure lead to clinical tamponade (Clin). PE, pericardial effusion.

Aetiology

Tamponade can be due to any of the causes of pericardial effusion. In acute pericarditis, tamponade is proportionally more common in neoplastic, tuberculous, and purulent pericarditis but, owing to the higher prevalence of idiopathic pericarditis, in absolute terms the most common cause of tamponade in medical patients without an underlying disease is acute idiopathic pericarditis [9, 15]. These patients usually have inflammatory signs and symptoms, in contrast to tamponade in malignancy where such symptoms may be absent [6].

Clinical findings

Patients with clinical tamponade complain of chest discomfort or typical pericardial chest pain if the cause is an acute inflammatory pericarditis, and dyspnoea on exertion progressing to dyspnoea at rest and tachypnoea. Acute cardiac tamponade, as occurs in aortic and free wall ventricular rupture, may manifest with syncope and sudden collapse. Physical examination discloses tachycardia, jugular distention, hepatomegaly, pulsus paradoxus, and, in severe cases, hypotension and shock. Pulsus paradoxus is defined [7] as an inspiratory systolic drop in arterial pressure of 10mmHg or more during normal breathing. To quantify the pulsus paradoxus non-invasively [7], a cuff is inflated to 10–15mmHg above the highest systolic level and slowly deflated until the first beats are heard. Deflation is then continued till all beats are audible. The difference between these two points corresponds to the pulsus paradoxus. During inspiration, filling of the right cardiac chambers increases with a consequent further increase in intrapericardial pressure, resulting in a leftward shift of the atrial and ventricular septa that impedes left ventricular filling. Pulsus paradoxus is not pathognomonic of tamponade as it may also occur in chronic obstructive airway disease, acute asthma, tracheal compression, severe pulmonary embolism, or right ventricular infarction. On the other hand, it may be absent in patients with severe hypotension, regional post-surgical cardiac compression, severe aortic regurgitation or atrial septal defect.

Diagnosis

Tamponade should be suspected in any patient with dyspnoea, chest discomfort, tachycardia, or tachypnoea, together with signs of raised venous pressure, hypotension, and pulsus paradoxus, especially if signs of left heart failure are absent. However, jugular distention can be absent in patients with low-pressure cardiac tamponade [42, 43]. Heart sounds may be distant, but pericardial friction rub may be present. The chest radiography usually shows an enlarged cardiac silhouette with clear lungs, but cardiomegaly may be inconspicuous in acute tamponade. Echocardiographic findings (➲Fig. 19.5; 19.1) are very important in patients with a clinical picture suggestive of tamponade because the presence of moderate–large pericardial effusion, chambers diastolic collapses, and increased tricuspid and pulmonary flow velocities (>50%) with decreased mitral and aortic flow velocities (>25%) during inspiration have a very high predictive value (>90%) for the diagnosis of tamponade. By contrast, diagnosis should be reconsidered whenever these signs are absent. Haemodynamic-assisted pericardiocentesis (➲Fig. 19.6) shows the pathognomonic pattern of tamponade: increased intrapericardial pressure at the same level as right atrial and diastolic ventricular pressures; after pericardiocentesis, intrapericardial pressure drops to around zero with a parallel decrease of intracavitary pressures.

Treatment

Mild or even moderate tamponade and a clinical picture suggestive of acute idiopathic pericarditis usually respond to anti-inflammatory therapy. In patients with severe tamponade, prompt evacuation of pericardial fluid is mandatory. When pericardial drainage is not rapidly available, volume infusion has been proposed as an interim therapy; however, this manoeuvre has unpredictable haemodynamic effects and we do not recommend it [44]. Whether pericardiocentesis or surgical drainage is preferred depends on experience of the treating physician along with the hospital facilities. Our approach is to start with subxiphoid pericardiocentesis and surgical drainage is only indicated when pericardiocentesis has been ineffective or tamponade recurs. Pericardiocentesis requires an adequate technique to minimize its inherent risk [7] (19.2). Whenever possible, pericardiocentesis should be performed in the catheterization laboratory, guided by fluoroscopy and under local anaesthesia and aseptic conditions, because this allows measurement of intrapericardial and cardiac chamber pressures. If this approach is not possible, echocardiography-guided pericardiocentesis [45] is the method of choice. In any event, a recent ESG should be available, preferably performed just before the procedure. Echocardiogram and blood pressure monitoring are mandatory. The subxiphoid approach is the best. A long blunt-tip needle permitting passage of the guidewire is directed towards the left shoulder at an angle of 30° to the frontal plane. The needle slowly approaches the pericardium under steady manual aspiration. As soon as the pericardial effusion is aspirated, a soft J-tip guidewire is inserted and, after dilatation, a long introducer is inserted and the dilator is exchanged for a multi-hole pigtail catheter. Drainage should be as complete as possible. Particularly in patients with neoplastic effusion, prolonged suction drainage until the effusion volume obtained falls to <25mL per day is recommended.

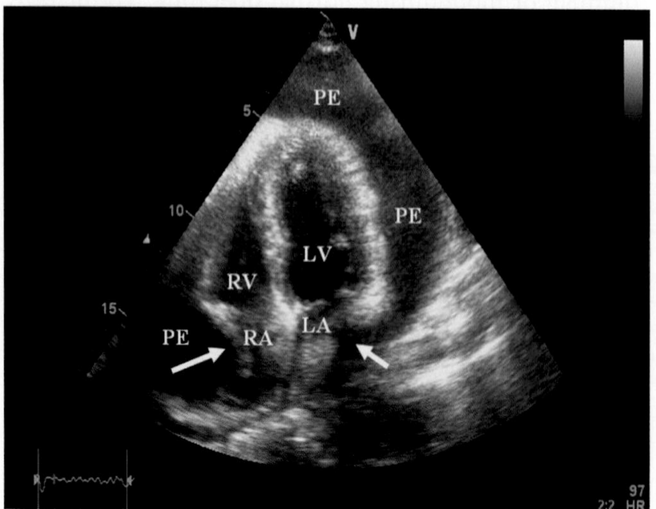

Figure 19.5 Tamponade in a patient with large circumferential pericardial effusion (PE). Arrows indicate right atrium (RA) and left atrium (LA) diastolic collapses. LV, left ventricle; RV, right ventricle.

Pericardial effusion

Since the use of echocardiography became routine, pericardial effusion has been a common finding. Any cause of pericardial disease may be associated with pericardial effusion (➲Table 19.3); however, in tertiary hospitals, the most frequent causes of pericardial effusion are idiopathic pericarditis, malignancy, and iatrogenic effusion [6]. The pathophysiology of effusion in the absence of inflammation is poorly understood.

Pericardial effusion without clinical tamponade or inflammation is asymptomatic. The prognosis of pericardial effusion is related to the underlying aetiology, provided that haemodynamic compromise is not life-threatening.

Diagnostic techniques

The classical diagnostic tools of electrocardiography and chest radiography have limited diagnostic value. Both may

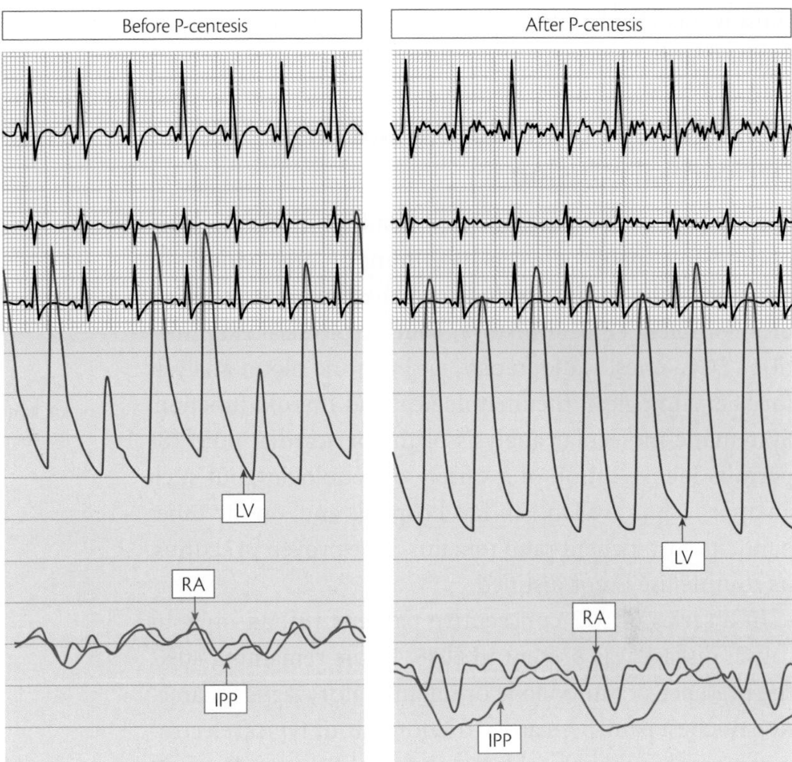

Figure 19.6 Tamponade. Before pericardiocentesis (P-centesis), wide respiratory variation of left ventricular (LV) pressure is shown together with elevation of intrapericardial pressure (IPP) (18mmHg), which equals right atrial (RA) pressure. After pericardiocentesis, intrapericardial pressure drops to near zero and right atrial pressure decreases (11mmHg).

be normal even in the presence of significant effusions, although low ECG voltage, electrical alternans, and a bottle-like cardiac silhouette on the chest radiography can be seen in large pericardial effusions.

Echocardiography is the technique of choice (➲ Chapter 4) for detecting pericardial effusion. The diagnosis is established whenever an echo-free space in the anterior or posterior pericardial sacs persists throughout the cardiac cycle. Commonly, effusions are circumferential, but may be regional; in such cases, two-dimensional echocardiography is the best technique. Arbitrarily, the amount of the effusion has been graded from mild (sum of echo-free spaces <10mm in the anterior and posterior pericardial sacs) to large (>20mm). The absence of chamber collapses is very useful to rule out tamponade.

Table 19.3 Causes of pericardial effusion

Any type of acute pericarditis
Cardiac surgery
Acute myocardial infarction
Heart failure
Chronic renal failure
Iatrogenic
Metabolic diseases
Autoimmune diseases
Trauma
Chylopericardium
Pregnancy
Idiopathic
Others

Computed tomography and magnetic resonance imaging provide precise information on the spatial location and quantity of the effusion; however, their use is only justified when the echocardiographic window is poor or the effusion is regional. The diagnostic yield of these techniques for characterization of the effusion remains to be established.

Management of mild pericardial effusion

A pericardial effusion of <10mm echo-free space is usually an incidental finding [46]. If the patient is asymptomatic and the clinical examination is normal, neither invasive procedures nor treatment are required. Long-term follow-up is not warranted if the effusion remains stable or has disappeared on a posterior echocardiographic control at 3–6 months. In symptomatic patients, pericardial effusion must be managed according to the aetiology of the underlying pericardial disease.

Management of moderate and large pericardial effusion

A wide variety of conditions may result in moderate (sum of echo-free spaces between 10–20mm) or large pericardial effusions. The initial approach to these patients consists of a complete clinical history, routine physical examination, ECG, chest radiography, and routine blood analysis for haematological, rheumatological and thyroid function. Systematic molecular analysis of the pericardial fluid [8] permits identification of a variety of aetiologies, but such an approach is available in few hospitals and, on the other hand, its cost–benefit ratio remains to be proven [47]; thus, its routine use is not justified.

In a series of 322 consecutive patients [6], an obvious causal disease was present in 60%. In the remaining 40%, the presence of tamponade or inflammatory signs (characteristic chest pain, pericardial friction rub, or typical electrocardiographic changes) was predictive of the most frequent aetiologies (➲Fig. 19.7). Inflammatory signs were predictive of acute idiopathic pericarditis (p <0.001), regardless of the size of the effusion and presence or absence of tamponade. In addition, a large effusion without inflammatory signs and no tamponade was highly predictive of chronic idiopathic pericardial effusion (p <0.001, likelihood ratio 20); on the other hand, tamponade without inflammatory signs was suggestive of neoplastic effusion. In this latter situation, evidence of a previous longstanding effusion may help to differentiate neoplastic pericarditis from chronic pericardial effusion. Although the final aetiological diagnosis depends on individual findings, these clinical clues may be helpful in the initial assessment and indication of invasive procedures.

The indications of invasive pericardial procedures in acute pericardial disease have been discussed previously. In patients without an apparent cause and without an acute inflammatory picture or tamponade, only a clinical follow-up seems appropriate; however, in some patients, a thoraco-abdominal computed tomography may be justified if the suspicion of neoplasia or lymphoma is raised.

Treatment with aspirin and NSAIDs for pain relief, and colchicine to prevent recurrences is used as in acute pericarditis. Corticosteroids should not be used, except in autoimmune diseases and post-pericardiotomy pericarditis. Oral anticoagulants must be withdrawn in patients with acute inflammatory pericarditis. Treatment of specific aetiologies is commented on at the end of this chapter (see ➲Specific types of pericardial disease, p.730).

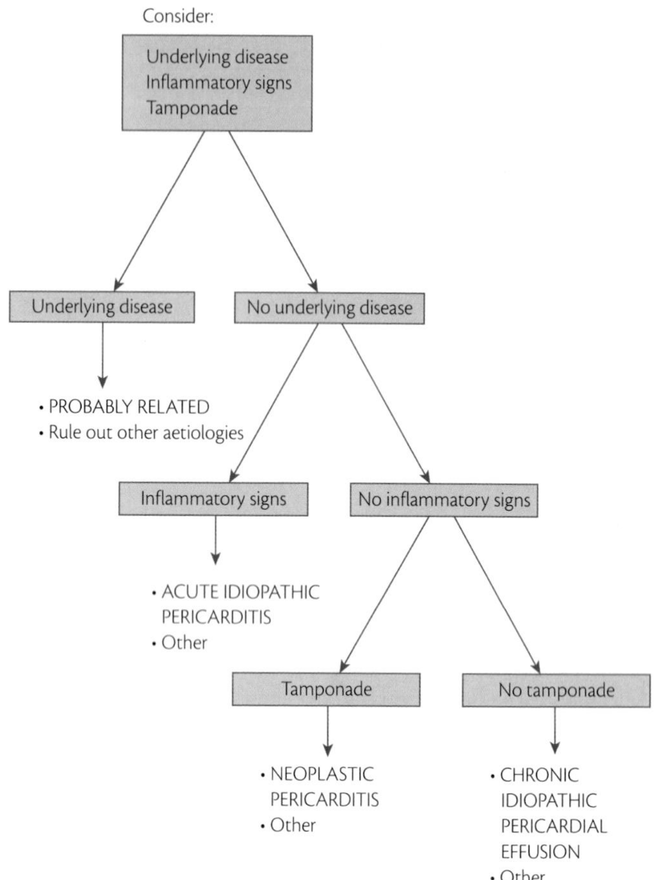

Figure 19.7 Initial clinical approach to aetiology of moderate–large pericardial effusion. Presence or absence of simple clinical data (underlying disease, inflammatory signs, and tamponade) helps to orientate the aetiological diagnosis of the most frequent aetiologies (capital letters).

Chronic pericardial effusion

Moderate–large pericardial effusions persisting >3 months are considered chronic. The effusion may be present for many years. The cause is unknown in most cases. Importantly, intrapericardial pressure is usually elevated even in asymptomatic patients [48]. In a series of 28 patients, 29% developed unexpected tamponade [48]. Taking into account the haemodynamic pattern and the unpredictable clinical evolution, pericardiocentesis is warranted in asymptomatic patients and pericardiectomy should be contemplated whenever large effusion reappears after pericardiocentesis. The long-term prognosis is excellent with this strategy. Corticosteroids and colchicine have not proved to be useful in the majority of cases.

Constrictive pericarditis

Constrictive pericarditis is the syndrome(s) due to compression of the heart caused by rigid, thickened, and frequently fused pericardial membranes. Constrictive pericarditis causes a restriction in cardiac filling that is not acting throughout diastole, as occurs in cardiac tamponade, but which is limited to the last two-thirds of diastole, while brisk and abrupt filling is preserved in early diastole, leading to the dip and plateau pressure pattern in both ventricles. Constrictive pericarditis was already known three centuries ago, but in recent years its clinical spectrum has changed. From the aetiological point of view, in the Western world there has been a decline in the incidence of tuberculous constriction and an increase in cases related to therapeutic mediastinal radiation and cardiac surgery, which account for 18% of patients in some series [49], although its prevalence is not higher than 0.2–0.3% after coronary artery bypass grafting or valvular surgery. Clinical manifestations have also changed. For instance, pericardial calcification was present in 90% of patients in a series published in 1959 [50], while in a more recent series [51] calcification was present in only 27% of cases. On the other hand, a major suspicion index and the wide availability of modern diagnostic techniques (mainly Doppler echocardiography and computed tomography) have permitted the diagnosis of less severe forms of constrictive pericarditis. In addition, the clinical-haemodynamic spectrum has been expanded with forms of constriction different from the classical calcified chronic constrictive pericarditis.

Chronic constrictive pericarditis

Chronic constrictive pericarditis is caused by a rigid, shell-like pericardial scar that restricts diastolic ventricular filling. Although different aetiological types of pericarditis may eventually end in constrictive pericarditis, histological study of the removed pericardium shows non-specific findings in the vast majority of cases. The clinical picture includes chronic fatigue and dyspnoea, jugular distension with a brisk diastolic collapse (*Y* descent) (➲ Chapter 1), proto-diastolic pericardial knock, enlarged liver, ascites, peripheral oedema, and pleural effusion. Pulsus paradoxus is usually absent. Diffuse flattened or negative T waves are usually present, and atrial fibrillation is found in half of the patients. Constrictive pericarditis should be suspected in all patients with findings suggestive of isolated right heart failure or ascites. Differential diagnosis includes cardiomyopathies with restrictive physiology [7, 52] (➲Table 19.4), right ventricular infarction, mitral stenosis (pericardial knock may be confounded with the opening snap), right atrial tumours, and liver cirrhosis. However, at present the

Table 19.4 Differential diagnosis between chronic constrictive pericarditis and restrictive cardiomyopathy

	Constrictive pericarditis	Restrictive cardiomyopathy
Physical examination	Early diastolic precordial impulse Pericardial knock No murmur	Apical impulse may be prominent Third sound may be present Regurgitant murmur common
Electrocardiography	Low voltage Frequent atrial fibrillation Normal QRS complex	Low voltage in amiloidosis Frequent atrial fibrillation Bundle branch block
Chest radiogram	Pericardial calcification possible	Non-specific cardiomegaly
Echocardiography	Normal wall thickness Pericardial thickening Diastolic notch of interventricular septum	Increased wall thickness (amyloidosis) Enlarged left and right atria
Doppler studies	e′ septal ≥8 cm/sec and normal S′ mitral annular velocity Mitral inflow increase during expiration Mitral flow propagation velocity M-mode colour ≥45cm/s Increased diastolic flow reversal in the hepatic vein with expiration	e′ septal <8cm/s and decreased mitral annular velocity Mitral inflow velocity without respiratory variation Mitral flow propagation velocity M-mode colour <45cm/s Increased diastolic flow reversal in the hepatic vein with inspiration
Cardiac catheterization	RVEDP and LVEDP usually equal RV systolic pressure <50mmHg RVEDP >one-third of RV systolic pressure	LVEDP often >5mm greater than RVEDP
Endomyocardial biopsy	Normal or non-specific changes	May reveal specific causes
CT/MR imaging	Pericardium thickened or calcified	Normal pericardium

CT, computer tomography; e′, e wave velocity by tissue velocity imaging; LVEDP, left ventricular end-diastolic pressure; MR, magnetic resonance; RV, right ventricular; RVEDP, right ventricular end-diastolic pressure.

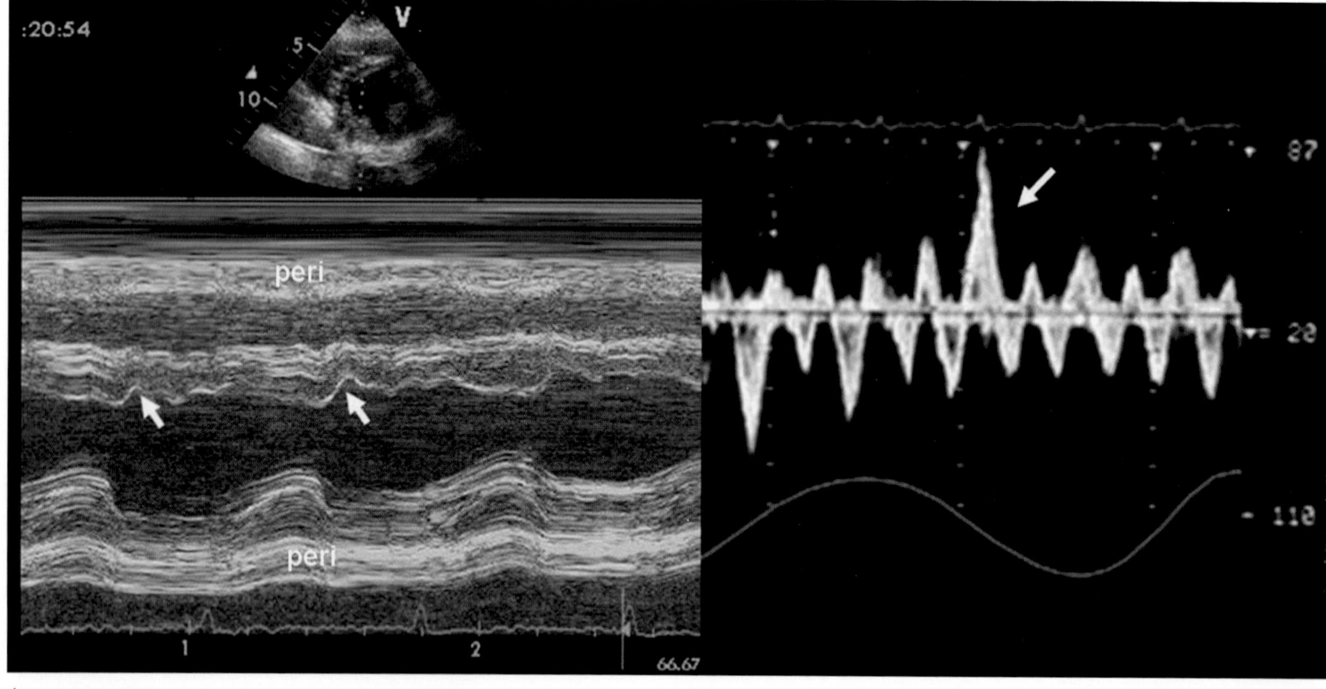

Figure 19.8 Chronic constrictive pericarditis. (A) M-mode ECG from the paraesternal window. Typical features of constrictive pericarditis are shown: thickened pericardium (peri), interventricular septal notch (arrow), and left ventricular posterior wall flattening. (B) Pulsed-wave Doppler recording from the hepatic vein. Reversal diastolic flow increases with expiration (arrow).

diagnosis is not usually difficult provided there is a good suspicion index and the availability of computed tomography and magnetic resonance imaging.

Diagnosis should be established based on the following triad: suggestive clinical findings, demonstration of a physiology of constriction/restriction, and demonstration of a thickened pericardium. The second point is mainly accomplished by Doppler echocardiography [53–55] (➲Table 19.4 and ➲Fig. 19.8), but altogether the accuracy is not 100%. A thickened pericardium can be apparent in a chest radiography in cases with pericardial calcification, or on computed tomography or magnetic resonance imaging (🎥19.3); however, the pericardium may have a nearly-normal thickness [56], hence an apparently normal imaging of the pericardium does not rule out constrictive pericarditis. The haemodynamic study shows characteristic dip-plateau morphology of diastolic ventricular pressure with equalization of end-diastolic ventricular, right atrial, and pulmonary wedge pressures. However, a haemodynamic study is rarely necessary nowadays for the diagnosis of constrictive pericarditis. Wide pericardiectomy is the only effective treatment. Once severe constrictive pericarditis has been diagnosed, surgery should not be delayed since surgical mortality (6–14%) and poor outcome increase with age and advanced functional class [49, 57], with prognosis being worse (HR 9.47) in post-radiation constrictive pericarditis [49].

Subacute elastic constriction

The term 'elastic' cardiac constriction, as opposed to the 'rigid' chronic type, was introduced to characterize the pathophysiological pattern of subacute constriction [58]. Elastic constriction would lie halfway between cardiac tamponade and classical chronic constriction. It is caused by a thickened pericardium which is not stiff but elastic, distensible enough to change in volume during the respiratory cycle. These changes result in two important features: dip-plateau morphology may be inconspicuous and pulsus paradoxus may be present. The pathological changes underlying elastic constriction are a thickened pericardium or epicardium that have not yet developed severe fibrosis or calcification. Pericardial effusion is often present. Subacute elastic constriction is usually seen in the early weeks or months after an acute inflammatory or infectious pericarditis. Sometimes it is severe enough to warrant urgent pericardiectomy, but may evolve to chronic pericardial constriction or be a transient phenomenon.

Effusive-constrictive pericarditis

Effusive-constrictive pericarditis is a clinical-haemodynamic syndrome in which there is constriction of the heart by the visceral pericardium in the presence of tense effusion in a free pericardial space. This variety of constrictive pericarditis was characterized, from the haemodynamic point of view, by Hancock [59] in his report on 13 patients who underwent pericardiectomy. The hallmark of effusive-constrictive pericarditis is the demonstration of persistence of increased right atrial and end-diastolic ventricular pressures after intrapericardial pressure has been reduced to normal levels by removal of pericardial fluid (➲ Fig. 19.9). The prevalence of this disorder is 1.3% among patients with pericardial disease and 6.8% in patients with clinical tamponade [60]. Aetiological spectrum includes idiopathic cases, chest radiation, cardiac surgery, neoplasia, and tuberculosis. Patients with effusive-constrictive pericarditis usually show a subacute clinical course, with inflammatory symptoms. On admission, clinical findings suggest tamponade; commonly, the presence of concomitant constriction is overshadowed, although some Doppler-echocardiography findings suggestive of constriction may put the clinician on the alert. After resolution of tamponade by pericardiocentesis, these findings can become more apparent together with clinical findings of constriction (prominent *Y* descent, third sound). Most cases of effusive-constrictive pericarditis will eventually evolve to persistent constriction requiring pericardiectomy, though a few cases may be transient and resolve spontaneously, especially in idiopathic cases. At surgery, special attention must be paid to the visceral pericardial layer with an adequate attempt at wide epicardiectomy (🎥 19.4).

Transient cardiac constriction

We reported [61] 16 patients from a series of 177 patients with effusive acute idiopathic pericarditis in which features of constriction were detected in the phase of pericarditis resolution, at a time when signs of activity had abated and effusion was already minimal or null. Some clinical (pericardial knock on auscultation, *Y* descent in jugular pulse) (➲ Chapter 1) and echocardiographic (early diastolic septal notch) (➲ Chapter 4) features of constriction were present in all patients, and two had overt signs of venous congestion. Cardiac catheterization (➲ Fig. 19.10) showed features of constrictive pericarditis, either at baseline or after fluid challenge (➲ Chapter 8). After a mean period of 2.7 months, the clinical and haemodynamic features of constriction had spontaneously subsided. The possible transient character of cardiac constriction is not only of theoretical interest but has a significance practical impact since conservative management may avoid some pericardiectomies. Clinical and particularly subtle echocardiographic findings of transient constriction are rather common in acute effusive idiopathic pericarditis (20%), but may also be seen in tuberculous and purulent pericarditis. In a recent series, post-pericardiotomy pericarditis was the most common cause of transient constriction [62].

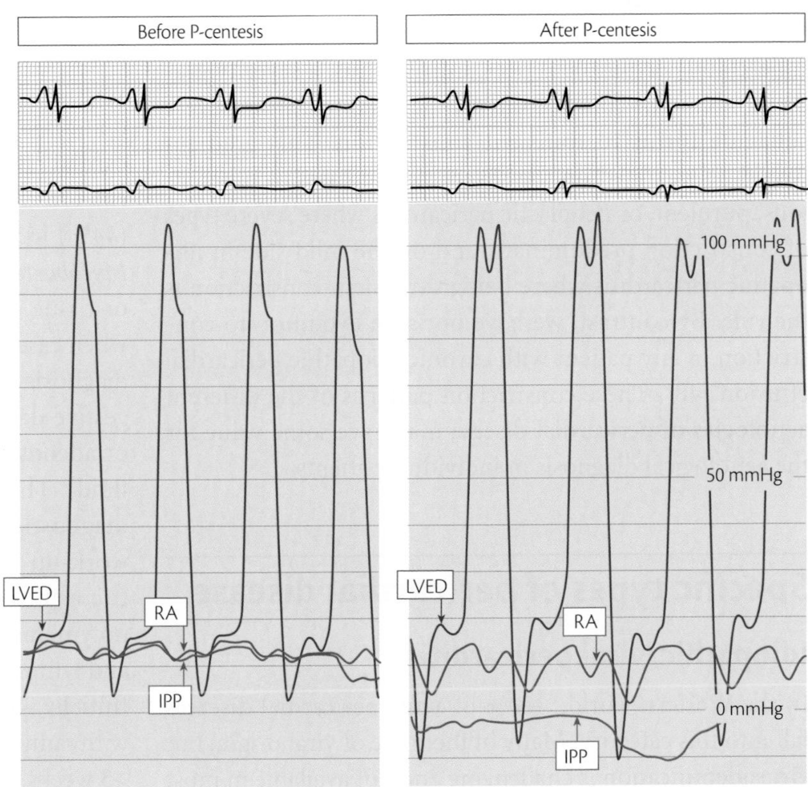

Figure 19.9 Effusive-constrictive pericarditis. Before pericardiocentesis (P-centesis), intrapericardial (IPP), right atrial (RA) and end-diastolic left ventricular (LVEP) pressures are elevated (14mmHg). After pericardiocentesis, intrapericardial pressure drops below zero whereas right atrial and left ventricular pressures remain almost unchanged and a dip-plateau morphology of left intraventricular pressure recording is apparent.

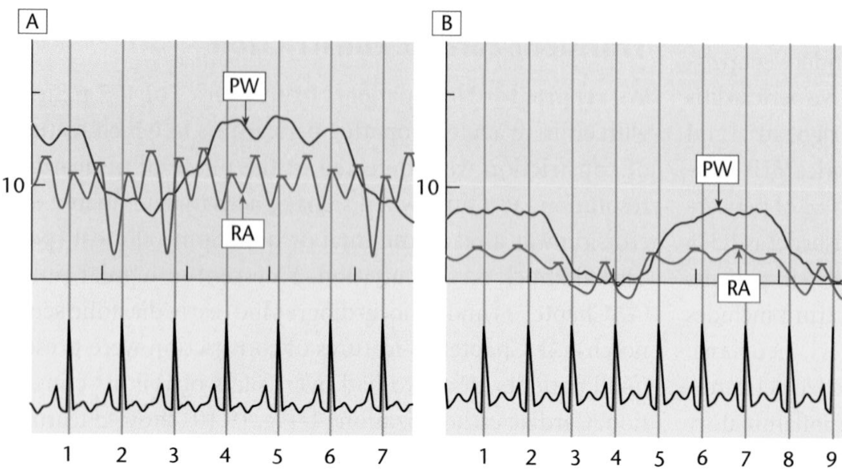

Figure 19.10 Transient cardiac constriction. (A) Pulmonary wedge (PW) and right atrial (RA) pressures are increased (10mmHg) at a similar level, and the tracing shows a 'W' morphology suggestive of constriction. (B) Four weeks later, both right atrial pressure and curve morphology are within normality.

Aetiological considerations

In a prospective follow-up of patients with acute effusive pericarditis [9], severe subacute constriction requiring pericardiectomy developed in 56%, 35%, and 17% of patients with tuberculous, purulent, or neoplastic pericarditis, respectively; in contrast, only 2 of 177 patients with acute effusive idiopathic pericarditis developed subacute effusive-constrictive pericarditis requiring pericardiectomy within the first 6 months. Thus, a patient with acute pericardial disease that develops subacute constriction is much more likely to have a specific pericarditis than an idiopathic one. On the other hand, transient constriction is much more frequent in patients with idiopathic pericarditis (with a prevalence of 20% when specifically sought) than in tuberculous or purulent pericarditis. Thus, a severity gradient of cardiac constriction can be assumed: from severe subacute forms to transient constriction. This gradient would be weighted on the severe side in cases of tuberculous, purulent, or neoplastic pericarditis where severe types of constriction predominate, and on the mild side in idiopathic pericarditis where benign transient constriction is the rule. By contrast, we have not seen evolution to constriction in any patient with chronic idiopathic pericardial effusion [48]. These constriction patterns of the different aetiologies of pericardial disease may have some value for the aetiological diagnosis in individual patients.

Specific types of pericardial disease

Idiopathic/viral pericarditis

In the Western world, >80% of acute pericardial diseases fall into this category. Many of them are of viral origin, but virus identification is challenging and not available in most institutions; on the other hand, there is no specific viral treatment to warrant further complex investigations [8]. Pericardial effusion, tamponade, and left pleural effusion are frequent. Recurrences are also frequent (20–25%), but troublesome relapsing pericarditis is rare [28]. Treatment has been discussed in the Acute pericarditis section of this chapter. Prognosis is good and evolution to chronic constriction is very rare, although transient cardiac constriction is frequent (20%).

Tuberculous pericarditis

Tuberculous pericarditis is rare in the Western world (4.4% of acute pericardial disease) [63] in contrast to developing countries [64] or in patients with human immunodeficiency virus (HIV) [65]. The initial clinical presentation varies, ranging from acute pericarditis to insidious pericardial disease. Main clinical findings are fever (94%), pericardial effusion (94%), pericardial pain (73%), pericardial rub (75%), pleural effusion (62%), and cardiac tamponade (44%) [63]. Diagnosis can be definitively established when *Mycobacterium tuberculosis* is identified in pericardial fluid or tissue, or elsewhere (sputum, pleural fluid, ganglia) or when caseating granulomas are documented. However, the diagnosis can only be suspected on the basis of highly suggestive data (chest radiography suggestive of tuberculosis or adenosine deaminase >45UI/L in pericardial or pleural fluid). The response to blind antituberculous therapy as a diagnostic method is not recommended. The diagnostic work-up includes three examinations of sputum or gastric aspirate, measurement of adenosine deaminase, and polymerase chain reaction in pleural fluid when present and lymph node biopsy in patients with lymphadenopathy. Initially, pericardiocentesis should be restricted to patients with tamponade; however, in cases with an insidious course >3 weeks, pericardial invasive procedures may establish the diagnosis. In such patients, the choice between pericardiocentesis and surgical drainage with pericardial biopsy must be individualized, although the latter provides wider information. Pericardial fluid analysis should include packed red cell volume, cytology, stain, and culture for mycobacteria, culture in ordinary media, protein, glucose, lactic dehydrogenase, adenosine deaminase content, and polymerase chain reaction to detect *M. tuberculosis* DNA. In the biopsy specimen, the studies to be performed are histology, stain for mycobacteria, and culture.

Prognosis is excellent provided that at least three antituberculous agents are administered [7, 66]. The true benefit of the addition of corticosteroids in preventing fluid re-accumulation or constriction is under debate [67, 68]. Pericardial constriction is common (45%) [63]. Usually, it is subacute (first weeks to few months) and requires early pericardiectomy with excellent outcome; sometimes is transient, in the initial phase of effusion resolution when close follow-up is mandatory before pericardiectomy is considered.

Purulent pericarditis

Purulent pericarditis is a serious disease with a high mortality (30–50%); the two main reasons for this are the presence of a severe underlying disease in most patients and an elusive diagnosis since some clinical findings can be erroneously attributed to the underlying condition. High fever, dyspnoea, and tachycardia are the most frequent findings [20]. Pericardial pain and rub may be absent. Tamponade is frequent (50%). Acute cardiac constriction may occur. Purulent pericarditis must be suspected in any patient with an intrathoracic (pneumonia, empyema, mediastinitis) or subphrenic infection or sepsis who develops any sign (jugular venous distension, cardiomegaly) or symptom (chest pain, dyspnoea) suggestive of pericardial involvement. In such patients, echocardiography is indicated and pericardiocentesis must be performed, even in the absence of tamponade. Whenever a purulent pericardial effusion is demonstrated, surgical drainage and appropriate antibiotic therapy (4–6 weeks) are mandatory. Pericardiectomy is indicated in pericardial constriction, relapsing tamponade, or lack of response to medical therapy. The additional benefit of intrapericardial streptokinase is to be proven [69]. The long-term prognosis is excellent for patients who can be discharged [20].

Post-infarction pericardial disease

Asymptomatic self-limited pericardial effusion is common (25–35%) in the early phase of myocardial infarction. It is not associated with early pericarditis, anticoagulation level, or mortality [70]. Treatment is not necessary.

Acute pericarditis occurs within the first week after Q-wave myocardial infarction and is strongly associated with infarction size [71]. Frequency is double in patients not treated with thrombolytic agents (12.0% versus 6.7%) [71]; the impact of primary percutaneous coronary intervention on further reduction of pericarditis is not known. Pericardial pain may be absent and ECG changes, if present, may not be characteristic of acute pericarditis; hence, the diagnosis is frequently established by the presence of a pericardial rub. When pain is present, the distinction between pericardial and ischaemic pain may be challenging if a pericardial rub is not heard. Full doses of aspirin are the treatment of choice. Anticoagulant therapy should not be modified. Pericardial involvement is associated with poorer outcome, but is not an independent prognostic factor.

Dressler's syndrome now is very rare [72]. It is a late event (weeks to months) occurring after an acute myocardial infarction (➲ Chapter 16), and consists of a pleuropericarditis of probable autoimmune origin. Corticosteroids are effective and prognosis is good.

Neoplastic pericarditis

Metastatic malignancy is one of the more frequent specific aetiologies of pericardial disease. The most common neoplasm is lung cancer (40–72%), followed by breast carcinoma and lymphoma. Clinical features of pericardial involvement may be the first manifestation of secondary malignancy [73, 74], although they are much more frequent in patients being treated for advanced malignancy (➲ Chapter 20). Cardiac symptoms are mainly related to the development of tamponade (50% of cases). Tamponade at presentation in the absence of inflammatory signs is highly suggestive of neoplastic pericarditis [6, 74], together with a history of malignancy and lack of response to NSAIDs. Survival is short; however, correct management is mandatory as it may alleviate painful symptoms and perhaps prolong life. The first step is to determine whether the effusion is due to malignancy or is a non-malignant effusion, which is the case in 60% of patients [75]. Imaging techniques and pericardial fluid examination are helpful to this end. The management of tamponade has two aims: to alleviate symptoms and prevent recurrences [76]. Pericardiocentesis is safe but tamponade frequently relapses. Pericardiocentesis with an in-dwelling catheter and prolonged suction drainage is more effective. Intrapericardial instillation of chemotherapeutic drugs has also been advocated [7]. Surgical drainage and pericardiectomy might be more effective, but are excessively aggressive in these patients, who usually have a poor clinical condition.

Pericardial disease in renal failure

Asymptomatic small pericardial effusion is common and does not require intervention. Pericardial disease is frequent (20%) both in patients with renal failure on chronic dialysis (dialysis-associated pericardial disease) or without/recent dialysis (uraemic pericarditis) (➲ Chapter 15). Constrictive pericarditis is very rare.

Dialysis-associated pericardial disease is common in patients on chronic dialysis, irrespective of the creatinine level. In contrast, uraemic pericarditis is less frequent. The pathophysiology and aetiology are unknown. Clinical manifestations vary from a typical picture of acute pericarditis to life-threatening tamponade. Acute intravascular depletion associated with haemodialysis may provoke tamponade at relatively low intrapericardial pressure (low-pressure tamponade). The primary treatment is intensive dialysis and pericardial drainage, if required [77, 78]. Corticosteroids and NSAIDs are of limited value when intensive dialysis fails. Indomethacin, colchicine (in just one patient) [79], and intrapericardial steroids have been used in patients with variable results [7]. Pericardiocentesis is a high-risk procedure and should be reserved for emergency situations [78]. Pericardiectomy is the procedure of choice in recurrent symptomatic effusions, but has substantial morbidity.

Pericardial involvement in HIV

In HIV patients, small pericardial effusions are frequent (10–20%) [80, 81]. Aetiology is very wide and includes the immunodeficiency virus itself. In Africa, the leading cause is tuberculosis. Effusion may be asymptomatic or complicated by tamponade (30–40%). Pericardiocentesis is recommended in large effusions, and in tamponade [82]. The presence of pericardial effusion implies poorer survival and is independent of CD4 count and albumin level [80], even if the effusion is transient. Survival in acquired immunodeficiency syndrome (AIDS) patients with effusion is decreased (36% versus 93%). The effects of highly-active anti-retroviral therapy on pericardial involvement remains unknown.

Pericardial involvement in autoimmune diseases

Almost all autoimmune diseases may lead to the development of some form of pericardial disease [83]; however, the most frequently affected are systemic lupus erythematosus (40%) [84], systemic scleroderma (40%) [85], and rheumatoid arthritis (25%) [86], with a greater prevalence in necropsy series. Very rarely, pericardial involvement is the first manifestation of the underlying disease. Usually, there is no correlation between pericardial involvement and inflammatory indices or drug therapy. Apart from the specific treatment for each autoimmune disease, the management is similar to the standard approach to pericardial disease.

Autoreactive pericarditis

Autoreactive pericarditis was the final diagnosis in 32% of a series of 260 patients with pericarditis [87]. An autoimmunological disorder should be the cause. The diagnosis of autoreactive pericarditis requires a complex work-up that includes, among several other criteria, pericardial/endomyocardial biopsies, virus culture, and exclusion of certain specific aetiologies by polymerase chain reaction and/or cultures. Many of these examinations are not available in the majority of institutions and, on the other hand, this approach implies an invasive protocol for the management of acute pericarditis which, in the majority of cases, has excellent outcome with a much easier approach [88]. In addition, treatment with intrapericardial triamcinole, though very effective in that series, caused a transient Cushing syndrome in 30% of patients. We agree with LeWinter [89] that 'the overall effectiveness of this approach is at present uncertain'.

Post-pericardiotomy pericarditis

This is a frequent complication (18%) after cardiac surgery [90], although its incidence has decreased in recent years. An autoimmune origin has been advocated [91]. It may cause bypass graft closure and fatal cardiac tamponade. The syndrome presents as a delayed pericardial/pleural reaction, characterized by fever, pleuritic pain, friction rub, and leucocytosis. Corticosteroids, ibuprofen, and indomethacin [92] are effective. Colchicine might be useful [93] and long-term prognosis is good.

Traumatic pericardial effusion

Isolated blunt chest trauma may cause pericardial effusion. Iatrogenic pericardial effusion (occasionally with tamponade) as a complication of invasive procedures occurs frequently (16%) [6]. Conservative management, pericardiocentesis, or surgery must be tailored to each patient.

Pericardial effusion in hypothyroidism

The prevalence of pericardial effusion in primary hypothyroidism varies widely (5–30%) depending on the severity of the disease; among myxoedematosous patients it is frequent but is rare in early mild hypothyroidism [94]. Tamponade is exceptional. Pericardial fluid has a high concentration of cholesterol. Effusion remits slowly with thyroid replacement therapy.

Rare causes

Radiation pericarditis

Pericardial disease may become manifest from the start of radiation to many years after it. The incidence with modern radiation techniques is around 2% [95]. Pericardial involvement may be difficult to identify owing to the underlying malignant disease. Pericardial effusion is frequent, although the most serious complication is constrictive pericarditis, with poor surgical prognosis [49, 57].

Pericardial effusion in pregnancy

Small asymptomatic pericardial effusion in the third trimester is common (40%) [96]. Other types of pericardial disease are not related to pregnancy and must be managed as in non-pregnant women, except for the administration of colchicine which is contraindicated.

Chylopericardium

This is due to a communication between the pericardium and thoracic duct and is predominantly of idiopathic origin [97] or a complication of trauma or surgery [98]. Pericardiocentesis yields a milky pericardial fluid rich in triglyceride content and negative culture. Conservative therapy usually fails. Thoracic duct ligation with pericardial window is the treatment of choice.

Fungal pericarditis

The most common organisms are *Candida*, *Aspergillus*, and *Histoplasma*. Positive culture in pericardial fluid or histological evidence of yeast establishes the diagnosis. The treatment consists of pericardial drainage and antifungal therapy. Prognosis is poor [99].

Drug- and toxin-related pericardial disease

A variety of drugs and toxic substances may produce any type of pericardial involvement [100], although its occurrence is exceptional and difficult to validate.

Primary pericardial tumours

Both benign (lipoma, fibroma) and malignant primary tumours (mainly mesothelioma) are exceptional [101]. Pericardial effusion with or without tamponade is often the first clinical manifestation. Computed tomography and magnetic resonance imaging are superior to echocardiography for diagnosis of the tumour. Surgery is indicated in benign neoplasms. Mesothelioma is fatal [102].

Congenital abnormalities

Absence of the pericardium

Complete absence is either asymptomatic or manifests with atypical chest pain, and no treatment is required. In contrast, partial absence may cause severe non-exertional chest pain, entail the risk of herniation of left atrial appendage or ventricle, and require surgery. Computed tomography and magnetic resonance imaging establish the diagnosis [103, 104].

Pericardial cysts

Pericardial cysts are benign asymptomatic malformations located in the right costophrenic angle. They are usually an incidental finding of a chest imaging technique and treatment is not required.

Personal perspective

The main challenge in the management of acute pericardial disease is to identify the aetiology since, in the majority of patients (± 80%), the cause is unknown (idiopathic). A thorough study of pericardial fluid may identify a significant number of specific aetiologies (mainly viral) or pathophysiological mechanisms (e.g. autoreactive pericarditis); however, this approach has two major limitations. First, not all pericardial diseases have a pericardial effusion large enough to be tapped safely; and second, this complex invasive approach is available at few centres. Furthermore, the final benefit is doubtful since many of the identified aetiologies lack a specific treatment. In fact, the conservative management of acute pericarditis advocated in this chapter entails very low mortality with excellent outcome in patients without associated malignant diseases, although it has to be kept in mind that epidemiological data are very important for the most appropriate management to be established in individual geographic areas. Future reliable non-invasive methods might help to unmask the underlying cause of idiopathic pericarditis, hopefully with beneficial impact on treatment.

Relapsing pericarditis is still a major issue. Although the prognosis is good, it remains a nightmare for both patient and physician. The mechanisms of recurrence and identification of patients prone to relapse are unknown.

On the other hand, the different therapies have their pros and cons. Aspirin and NSAIDs do not control the majority of cases. Corticosteroids administered during the index episode appear to favour recurrences despite very rapid control of the episode (corticosteroid paradox), but may have a role in demonstrated autoimmune cases. Colchicine has proved to be effective in many cases, but its mechanism of action, responders, and duration of therapy remain to be determined; ongoing trials may help to define its use. Finally, the role of wide pericardiectomy is unclear since the present belief of its uselessness is not based on solid data.

Further reading

Shabetai R. *The Pericardium*, 2003. Boston: Kluwer Academic Publishers.

LeWinter MM. Pericardial diseases. In Libby P, Bonow RO, Mann DL, *et al.* (eds.) *Braunwald's Heart Disease. A Textbook of Cardiovascular Medicine*, 8th edn., 2008. Philadelphia, PA: Saunders, pp.1829–53.

Soler-Soler J, Permanyer-Miralda G, Sagristà-Sauleda J (eds.). *Pericardial disease. New insights and old dilemmas*, 1990. Dordrecht: Kluwer Academic Publishers.

Spodick DH. *The Pericardium. A Comprehensive Textbook*, 1997. New York: Marcel Dekker.

Additional online material

- 19.1 Two-dimensional echocardiogram of a patient with cardiac tamponade.
- 19.2 Pericardiocentesis procedure in the catheterization laboratory.
- 19.3 Cine-RM in a patient with chronic constrictive pericarditis.
- 19.4 Surgical epicardiectomy of a patient with severe cardiac constriction.

For full references and multimedia materials please visit the online version of the book (http://esctextbook.oxfordonline.com).

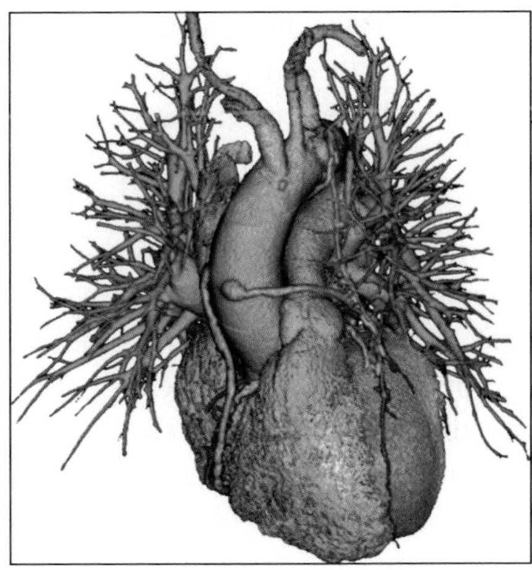

CHAPTER 20

Tumours of the Heart

Gaetano Thiene, Marialuisa Valente, Massimo Lombardi, and Cristina Basso

Contents

Summary

Tumours rarely involve the heart; secondary neoplasms (cardiac metastases from lung carcinoma, lymphoma, breast, hepatic, and kidney cancer) are much more frequent than primary neoplasms (20:1).

Ninety per cent of all primary cardiac tumours are benign. Myxoma, by far the most frequent benign tumour (70%), is typically located in the left atrium, and manifests with intracavitary obstruction, embolism, and constitutional symptoms but may also be silent and discovered incidentally by echocardiography. It is also observed in children. Papillary fibroelastoma is an endocardial papilloma, which although quite small, may become symptomatic through embolic events. Typical tumours of the paediatric age group are fibroma, rhabdomyoma, and teratoma.

Primary malignant neoplasms account for 10% of all primary cardiac tumours and are represented by sarcomas (angiosarcoma, leiomyosarcoma, fibrosarcoma, liposarcoma, rhabdomyosarcoma, undifferentiated pleomorphic sarcoma) and primary lymphomas. They usually infiltrate the cardiac walls, but may also be solely intracavitary, mimicking myxoma. Histology with immunohistochemistry of any cardiac mass is mandatory for diagnosis, therapy, and prognosis. Endomyocardial biopsy may be of help for histological investigation without thoracotomy. Malignancies may be cured with surgery and/or chemotherapy/radiotherapy.

Non-neoplastic masses may consist of thrombi and infections, which again can be identified by a thorough surgical pathology examination.

Cardiac non-invasive imaging through transthoracic and transoesophageal echocardiography easily detects heart masses. Cardiac magnetic resonance and computed tomography are helpful complementary investigations, for refining diagnosis and in the post-surgery follow-up.

Introduction

In the popular mind, the term tumour recalls the idea of 'cancer', namely an extremely aggressive biological phenomenon destined to consume the body, due to malignant infiltration and metastasis. This is not true at the cardiac level, where primary tumours are rarely malignant and their importance is mostly haemodynamic, due to obstruction of the blood circulation because of intracavitary growth and embolism following detachment of neoplastic fragments with potentially devastating ischaemic damage to several organs.

Before the advent of cardiac imaging and of open heart surgery, cardiac neoplasms were not diagnosed *in vivo* and were mostly fatal [1, 2].

The first book on cardiac tumours was published by Ivan Mahaim in 1945 [1]. It was a collection of postmortem observations and a thorough review of the literature (➲Fig. 20.1). While treating atrial myxoma ('Le polype du coeur'), the most frequent cardiac tumour (nearly two-thirds of primary heart neoplasms), he said '... *surgical resection of atrial polyp encounters apparently insurmountable difficulties. However, we should not give up because of this feeling. In any field of science, with technological progress, the impossible is just a moment during the evolution of our powers. As Mummery said about alpinism, the inaccessible peak becomes an easy route for ladies ...*'

Some years later in 1951, Goldberg and colleagues [3] for the first time successfully made a clinical diagnosis of left atrial myxoma using angiography, and in 1954, Craafoord [4] resected a myxoma using extracorporeal circulation.

Thus, the era of 'surgical pathology' started when the pathologist establishes *in vivo* the nature and histology of the neoplasm, as in any other field of oncology.

The historical watershed in the diagnosis and treatment came in the 1980s [5], with the advent of non-invasive imaging, i.e. echocardiography (➲Fig. 20.2), which, together with computed tomography (CT) and cardiac magnetic resonance (CMR), substantially improved diagnosis and subsequent treatment. It is possible to easily visualize cardiac tumours at the first onset of symptoms or even incidentally, during routine diagnostic procedures, and send the patient promptly to the surgeon for resection with a nearly 100% success in the benign forms. Before the 1980s, cardiac myxomas were a postmortem finding; thereafter they became almost exclusively a clinical and surgical observation. The role of the pathologist is now to establish the nature of the resected mass (non-neoplastic, benign, or malignant neoplasms) and, last but not least, to make the differential diagnosis with secondary neoplasms.

It is curious to recall that the first description of cardiac tumours was made by Matteo Realdo Colombo in 1559, in his book *De Re Anatomica*: '*In Rome I saw a solid tumour, large like an egg, in the left ventricle of Cardinal Gambaro of whom I was committed by the Pope to make autopsy*' [6]. Most probably it was not a neoplasm, but a mural postinfarction thrombus.

Epidemiology, classification, and nomenclature

Knowledge of the prevalence of cardiac tumours is still based on postmortem studies. In a study of 12,485 consecutive autopsies carried out in a 20-year time span from 1972–1991, Lam and colleagues [7] reported a prevalence rate of 0.056% for primary and 1.23% for secondary tumours.

Epidemiological data are strongly influenced by when and where the data have been collected. For instance, at the Mayo Clinic, USA, in the 1915–1930 period, the autopsy prevalence

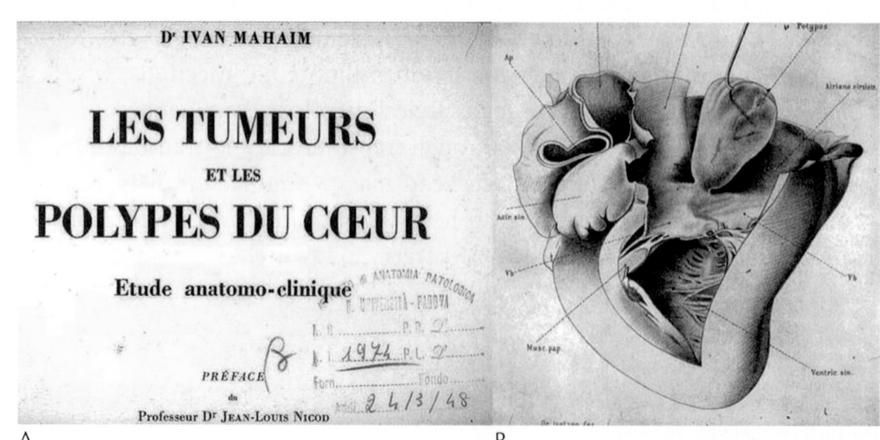
Dr IVAN MAHAIM

LES TUMEURS

ET LES

POLYPES DU CŒUR

Etude anatomo-clinique

PRÉFACE
du
Professeur Dr JEAN-LOUIS NICOD

A B

Figure 20.1 (A) The title page of *Les Tumeurs et les Polypes du Coeur: Etude Anatomoclinique* by Ivan Mahaim, published in 1945 [1] and (B) the drawing of the left atrial myxoma ('le polype du coeur'). Modified from Basso C, Valente M, Thiene G. *Tumori del cuore. Monografie di Cardiologia. Società Italiana of Cardiologia*, 2005. Novate-Millan: Arti Grafiche Color Black.

A

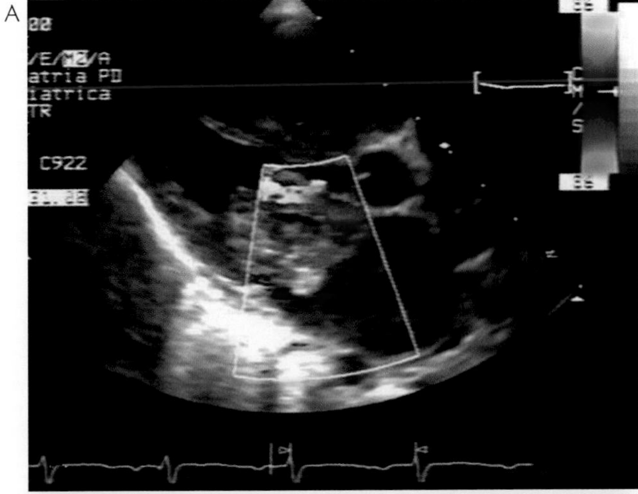

B

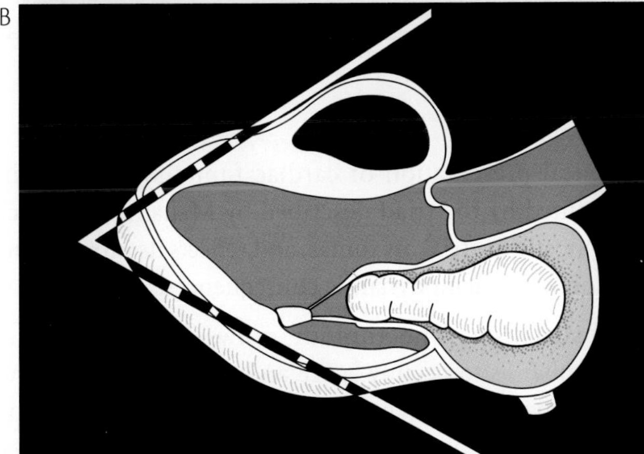

Figure 20.2 Two-dimensional echocardiography of left atrial myxoma in a 6-year-old female child with congestive heart failure. (A) Parasternal long-axis view of a left atrial myxoma with tumour prolapse into the left ventricular cavity during diastole. (B) Schematic representation.

of primary cardiac tumours was 0.05%. With the advent of cardiac surgery, the Mayo Clinic became a referral centre, thus in a more recent 15-year interval, from 1954–1970, the autopsy prevalence had increased threefold (0.17%) [5].

Regarding secondary neoplasms, a study carried out in the Institute of Pathology of the University of Padua, Italy, during 1967–1976, found that among 7460 autopsies the cause of death was due to malignancies in 1181, in which cardiac metastases occurred in 74 (1% of all the autopsies and 6% of those with any malignancy) [8].

Thus, approximately, autopsy prevalence of primary cardiac tumour is 1 in 2000 and that of secondary cardiac tumours is 1 in 100 autopsies, with a secondary/primary ratio of 20:1.

With regards to classification and nomenclature of primary tumours, the World Health Organization (WHO) recently assembled a group of pathologists to put forward a new classification as reported in ➲Table 20.1 [9].

Neoplasms are divided into benign tumours and tumour-like lesions, malignant tumours, and pericardial tumours. Although some neoplasms or tumour-like lesions have been ignored (cysts of pericardium, blood cyst of heart valves), this classification has the merit of being comprehensive and unifies the terminology. However, since cardiac tumours have been variously named, we will add the synonym for each histotype.

Concerning the epidemiology and prevalence of various histotypes, we refer to the experience of the University of Padua [8, 10]. In the time interval 1970–2004, 210 consecutive primary cardiac neoplasms were studied, 187 (89%) of which were benign and 23 (11%) malignant (➲Fig. 20.3). This is mostly a biopsy-based experience (91% of cases),

Table 20.1 WHO classification of tumours of the heart

Benign tumours and tumour-like lesions	**ICD Code**
Rhabdomyoma	8900/0
Histiocytoid cardiomyopathy	
Hamartoma of mature cardiac myocytes	
Adult cellular rhabdomyoma	8904/0
Cardiac myxoma	8840/0
Papillary fibroelastoma	
Haemangioma	9120/0
Cardiac fibroma	8810/0
Inflammatory myofibroblastic tumour	8821/1
Lipoma	8850/0
Cystic tumour of the atrioventricular node	
Malignant tumours	
Angiosarcoma	9120/3
Epithelioid haemangio-endothelioma	9133/3
Malignant pleomorphic fibrous histiocytoma (MFH)/ Undifferentiated pleomorphic sarcoma	8830/3
Fibrosarcoma and myxoid fibrosarcoma	8840/3
Rhabdomyosarcoma	8900/3
Leiomyosarcoma	8890/3
Synovial sarcoma	9040/3
Liposarcoma	8850/3
Cardiac lymphoma	
Metastatic tumours	
Pericardial tumours	
Solitary fibrous tumour	8815/1
Malignant mesothelioma	9050/3
Germ cell tumours	
Metastatic pericardial tumours	

ICD, International Classification of Diseases for Oncology.

Behaviour is coded /0 for benign tumours, /3 for malignant, and /1 for borderline or uncertain.

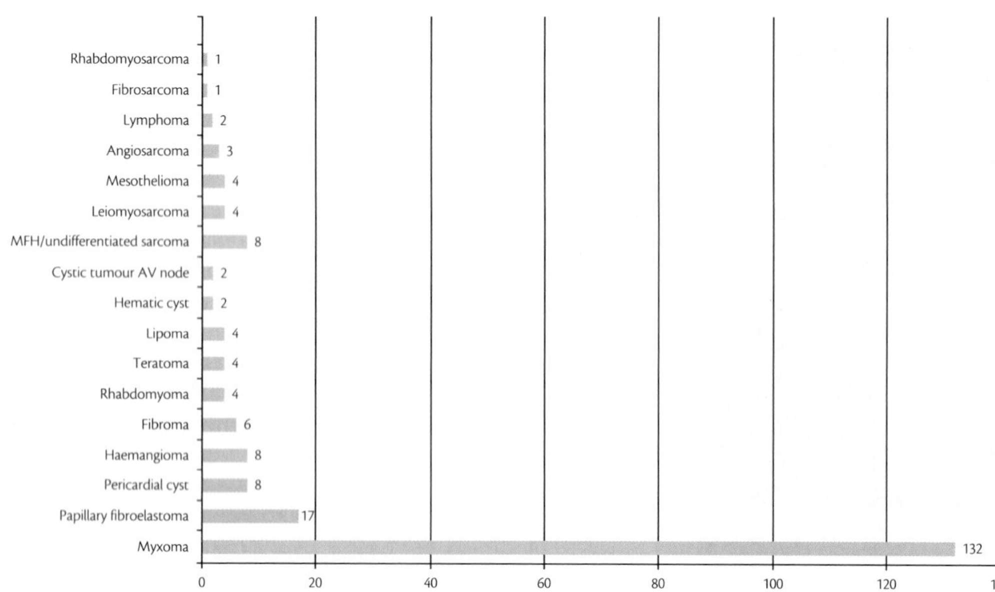

Figure 20.3 Primary cardiac and pericardial tumours at the Cardiovascular Pathology Unit, University of Padua (1970–2004): total n = 210 cases.

just to emphasize that nowadays cardiac tumour is rarely fatal, with the exception of primary malignancies.

- Among the 187 benign cardiac tumours, the majority (71%) were myxomas, followed by papillary fibroelastomas (9%). There was a female predominance (1.4:1), mean age 47 years.
- As far as malignant primary cardiac tumours were concerned, malignant pleomorphic fibrous histiocytoma, leiomyosarcoma, and malignant mesothelioma ranked first. There was a male predominance (1.3:1), mean age 51 years.
- Primary neoplasms, all benign, were also observed in the paediatric age group (<18 years) in 27 cases, and atrial myxoma was still the most frequent (30% of all paediatric cases).
- Regarding metastatic cardiac tumours, lung carcinoma was by far the most common in our experience (32.5%), especially as pericardial carcinosis with effusion, followed by lymphoma and leukaemia (16%), breast carcinoma (5%), hepatic carcinoma (5%), and kidney carcinoma (4%).

The rate of malignant cardiac tumours is often wrongly reported as up to 30% in the literature, when based on data derived from pathology tertiary centres, where the most difficult cases are sent for expert opinion [11].

Clinical presentation

Cardiac tumours may be symptomatic, although more and more frequently they are detected incidentally by echocardiography, during routine examination [12–14].

Clinical presentation of cardiac tumours is classically represented by the triad described by Mahaim [1], which refers mostly to atrial myxomas, and reflects its intracavitary position with haemodynamic consequences.

1. **Obstruction.** The tumour grows inside a cardiac chamber as to occupy space and to hinder blood flow. Lipothymia and syncope are the usual symptoms in this setting, especially when the tumour is located in the left atrium and the mass dislodges into the left ventricle during diastole. Bending or other body positions may precipitate syncope. Dyspnoea during effort and even pulmonary oedema may occur, especially when the tumour is stuck in the left atrioventricular (AV) orifice. When located in the right atrium, the tumour may account for congestive right ventricular failure. If the mass growth is associated with atrial enlargement, atrial arrhythmias, including atrial flutter and fibrillation, may develop.
2. **Embolism.** If the mass is friable, as is the villous myxoma, which consists mostly of gelatinous tissue, fragments may detach producing neoplastic embolism. Systemic embolism may be the first symptom and may be catastrophic when occurring in the cerebral circulation, with transient ischaemic attack or stroke, or in the coronary bed, with myocardial infarction and sudden death. Renal, splenic, mesenteric, and femoropopliteal embolism may also occur. A Fogarty procedure may be effective and histological examination of the removed embolism is mandatory to establish the neoplastic nature of the tissue, as well as to prompt echocardiographic investigation for detection of the cardiac source. Neoplastic embolism may

occur even in the setting of very small non-obstructive myxomas, due to the extremely friable tissue, and may lead to disappearance of the original source. On the other hand, there are exceptional cases of huge myxomas, a large part of which may detach and obstruct the aorta, with saddle embolism of the abdominal aortic carrefour. They require concomitant emergency aortic surgery and open heart tumour removal. The intracavitary tumours, located in right-sided chambers, may be the source of embolism in the pulmonary arterial circulation and account for pulmonary infarction which can be misdiagnosed as pneumonia. In rare circumstances, the embolism may be large enough to create obstruction of a main pulmonary artery or even a saddle occlusion of pulmonary trunk bifurcation. Tumours located in the right ventricle and pulmonary infundibulum may herniate into the pulmonary trunk and mimic acute pulmonary embolism with cardiogenic shock.

The tissue detaching from an intracavitary cardiac tumour may not necessarily be neoplastic. Thrombosis may occur on the surface of intracardiac tumours, including smooth myxomas. In case of papillary fibroelastoma, thrombus deposition may occur within the multiple neoplastic fronds branching out from the main stalk.

3 **Constitutional symptoms**. These consist of fatigue, fever, weight loss, and joint-muscular pains and are associated with anaemia, hypergammaglobulinaemia, and increased erythrocyte sedimentary rate. They are mostly observed in people with myxoma and are due to release of cytokines such as interleukin-6.

There are also symptoms and signs that are particularly frequent in the setting of cardiac tumours with an intramural growth, such as arrhythmias and conduction disturbances. When growing in the atrial septum, cardiac tumours may manifest with atrial arrhythmias and various degrees of AV block. When in the ventricles or septum, ventricular arrhythmias and bundle branch blocks can occur, besides systo-diastolic dysfunction.

Pericardial effusion can occur in the setting of either benign or malignant cardiac tumours, but haemorrhagic effusion, even with cardiac tamponade, is a typical manifestation of malignancies.

Finally, there are cardiac tumours which are completely silent, because of their limited size, they do not produce obstruction or embolism, and they do not provoke constitutional symptoms. Before the cardiac imaging era, they were occasional findings at autopsy. Nowadays, they are an incidental observation during routine echocardiography, and may pose intriguing problems as far as indication to surgery is concerned.

Diagnosis through interdisciplinary collaboration

Echocardiography (also see ➲Chapter 4)

In vivo visualization of the heart led to a diagnostic revolution [8, 12–15]. Angiocardiography was the first procedure employed, but had its limitations: invasive, time-consuming, left atrium visualized only after contrast injection in the right heart. Ultrasound with two-dimensional transthoracic echo imaging changed the course of *in vivo* diagnosis of cardiac tumours: prompt detection by easy and quick exploration with routine tomographic approaches (horizontal and vertical long axes, short axis including the arterial pole and semilunar valves) and additional projections (two, three chambers and subcostal views to visualize venae cavae, right ventricular inflow and outflow). Transoesophageal echo possesses a better resolution for left-sided masses, the transducer being located posteriorly just behind the left atrium and pulmonary venous pole [16]. Moreover, transoesophageal echocardiography is particularly useful as an intraoperative procedure for assessing the extent of surgical removal, the repair of cardiac valves, and the absence of residual intracardiac shunts in case of atrial septal procedures.

Overall, two-dimensional and Doppler echocardiography can easily assess the tumour site, size, shape, attachment, and mobility as well as haemodynamic consequences in terms of valve and cardiac dysfunction and presence of pericardial effusion. Even small masses are detectable and prenatal diagnosis of cardiac masses can be achieved by fetal echocardiography. However, limited information can be provided as far as pericardial infiltration and tissue composition of cardiac masses are concerned (➲Fig. 20.4). Contrast echocardiography allows visualization of intracardiac mass perfusion and better differentiation between tumour and mural thrombus.

Cardiac magnetic resonance and multislice computed tomography

CMR imaging is the best available non-invasive procedure for cardiac tumour diagnosis in terms of site, morphology, dimension, extension, topographic relations, and possible infiltration of surrounding structures [17–19]. It may also help for tissue characterization (presence of adipose

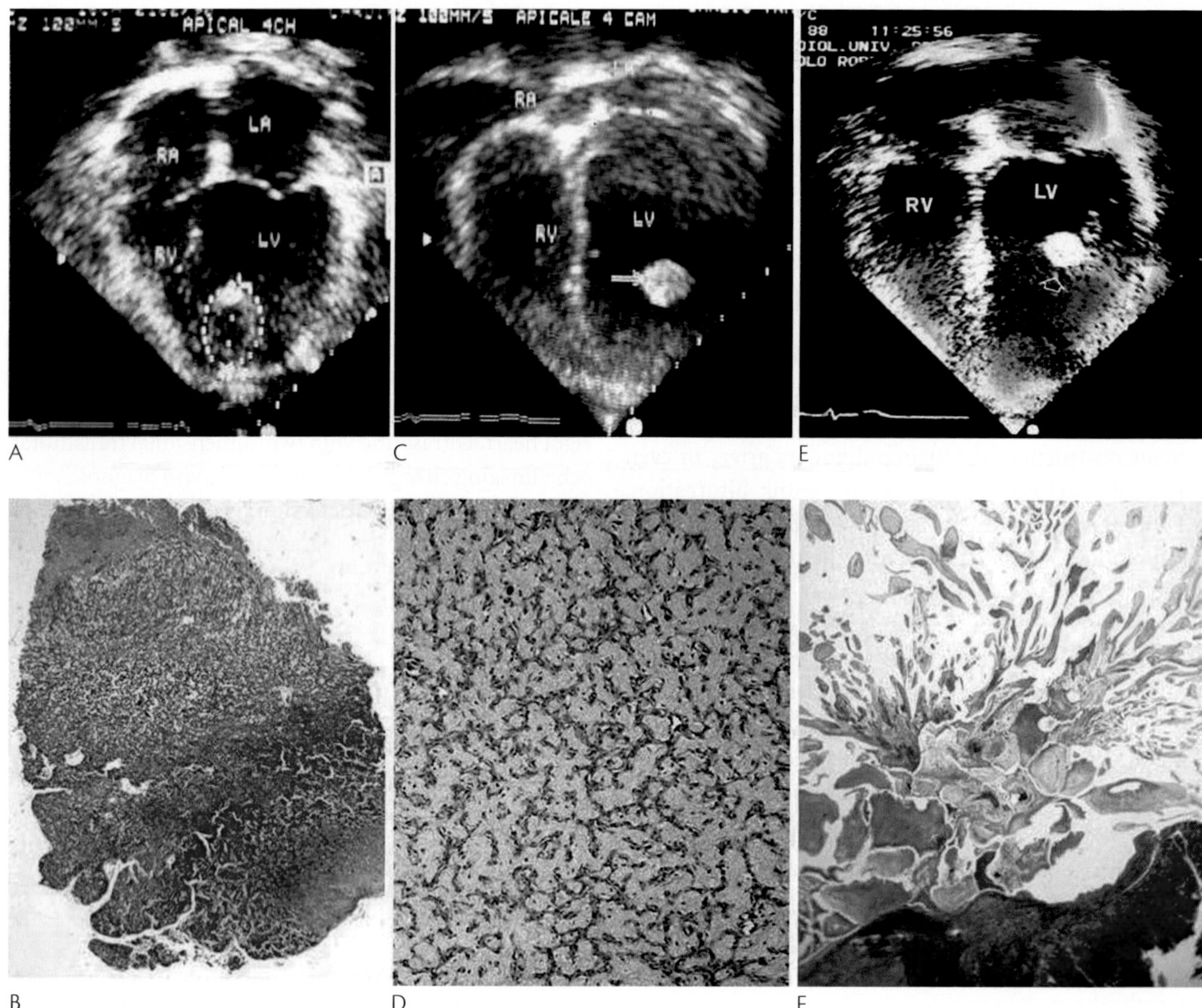

Figure 20.4 Two-dimensional echocardiography, four-chamber views, of left ventricular masses and histology of the corresponding specimens excised at surgery. Ultrasound investigation allows a precise assessment of size and location, but no tissue characterization: (A, B) thrombus; (C, D) myxoma; (E, F) papillary fibroelastoma. LA, left atrium; LV, left ventricle; RA, right atrium; RV, right ventricle.

tissue, necrosis, haemorrhage, vascularization, calcification), although the specificity is still low (➲Fig. 20.5). A 'probabilistic' histopathological diagnosis is more reliable and the provisional term 'mass' should be employed, leaving the final answer to histology. In the case of lipomas, with hyperintensity signal in T1 imaging, the precise histotype may be established by CMR, with a very high diagnostic probability (➲Table 20.2). Use of contrast medium may be of help to detect highly vascularized tumours, such as myxomas, angiomas, and angiosarcomas. In case of fibroma, delayed contrast enhancement shows homogeneous uptake of gadolinium, indicating fibrous tissue.

Multislice CT has the advantage of a better spatial resolution in cases of possible lung, pleural, and mediastinal involvement (➲Fig. 20.6) [20–22]. Moreover, calcification is easily detected within the mass and may point to a fibroma, in a case of mural mass; a myxoma in a case of an intracavitary atrial mass in the elderly; or a teratoma in a case of pericardial mass in infancy. Multislice CT is particularly indicated for detection of concomitant coronary artery disease, to plan coronary angioplasty or surgical revascularization, associated with neoplasm removal, if deemed necessary. CMR and CT can differentiate serous from haemorrhagic pericardial effusion.

However, multislice CT does not permit full investigation of the involvement of cardiac valves, and presents the limitation of high dosage radiation, which precludes its employment in the follow-up of young subjects.

Fast heart rates and arrhythmias may jeopardize the quality of imaging of both CMR and multislice CT.

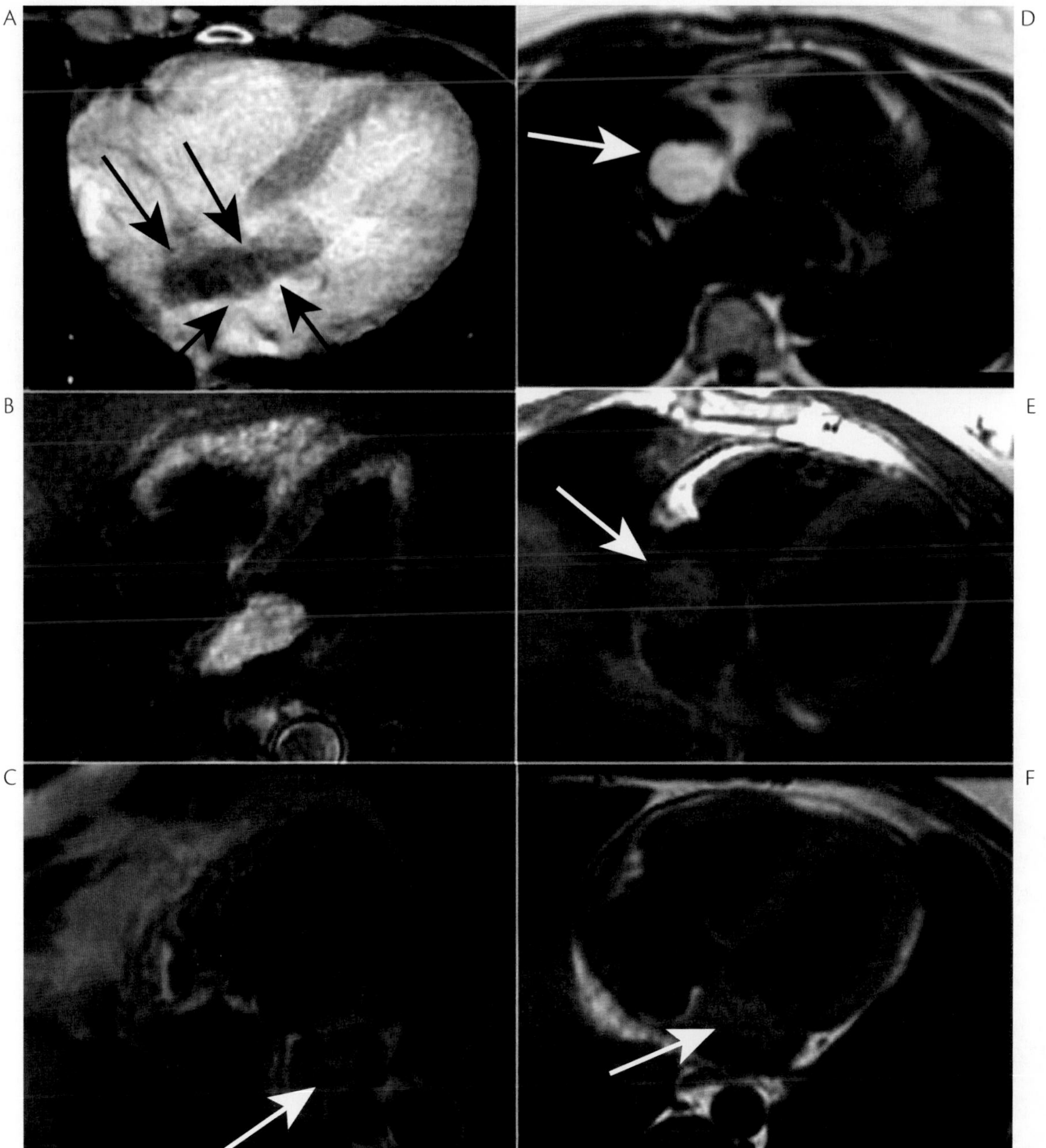

Figure 20.5 Multislice computed tomography (CT) and cardiac magnetic resonance (CMR) of left atrial masses. (A) CT scan of cardiac myxoma: a mobile left atrial mass protruding during diastole into the mitral valve orifice is visible. (B) CMR, triple-IR of cardiac myxoma: the mobile left atrial mass appears hyper-intense compared with the surrounding myocardium, a signal which is suggestive for myxoid tissue. (C) CMR, spin echo (SE) T1 image of cardiac myxoma after contrast medium (Omniscan): note the non-homogeneous signal from the atrial mass which is enhanced by contrast medium. (D) CMR, T1-weighted image of cardiac lipoma: note the diffuse hyper-intense homogenous signal which is typical of adipose tissue. (E) CMR, SE T1 image of cardiac thrombus after contrast medium (Omniscan): note the absent or scarce enhancement by contrast medium. (F) CMR, T1-weighted image of left atrial undifferentiated sarcoma. Modified from Basso C, Valente M, Thiene G. *Tumori del cuore. Monografie di Cardiologia. Società Italiana di Cardiologia*, 2005. Novate-Milan: Arti Grafiche Color Black..

Obviously, two-dimensional echocardiography remains the first diagnostic approach for detection of cardiac masses, whereas CMR and CT may be complementary tools, with their own advantages and limitations. Due to their non-invasiveness and lack of radiation, two-dimensional echocardiography and CMR are also the gold standard for follow-up studies.

Endomyocardial biopsy

In vivo histological diagnosis may be achieved through thoracoscopic or endomyocardial biopsy. The latter is particularly feasible in the setting of right-sided infiltrating cardiac masses, in which tissue samples may be taken with the bioptome introduced either through femoral or jugular

Table 20.2 *In vivo* tissue characterization of cardiac masses: cardiac magnetic resonance signal of different tissues in T1- and T2-weighted images

	T1-weighted	T2-weighted	Post-contrast enhancement
Fluid	Low (---)	High (+++)	Absent
Myxoid tissue	Low (---)	High (+++)	Scarce
Thrombus	Low (--)	Low (--)	Usually absent
Adipose tissue	High (+++)	High(++)	Absent
Necrotic areas	Low (--)	High (+++)	Absent
Fibrous tissue	Low (--)	Low/High (--/++)*	Scarce*
Calcification	Low (---)	Low (---)	Absent
Vascularized tissue	Low (--)	High (++)	Marked

*Type of signal and contrast enhancement depends on vascularization and cellularity of tissues.

veins under echocardiographic guidance (➲ Figs. 20.7–20.9) [10, 23–25].

The procedure avoids thoracotomy for diagnosis and allows therapeutic planning, including cardiac transplantation, in cases of malignant neoplasm without extracardiac metastasis. Moreover, endomyocardial biopsy can be useful in the setting of tumours which are unresectable or require histological characterization before chemotherapy is started. An adequate number and size of samples (four or five pieces, 1–2mm each) is usually enough for a thorough histological investigation, including immunohistochemistry, to achieve a precise diagnosis.

Surgical pathology

Histopathology is absolutely mandatory in any resected cardiac mass, to establish the benign or malignant nature

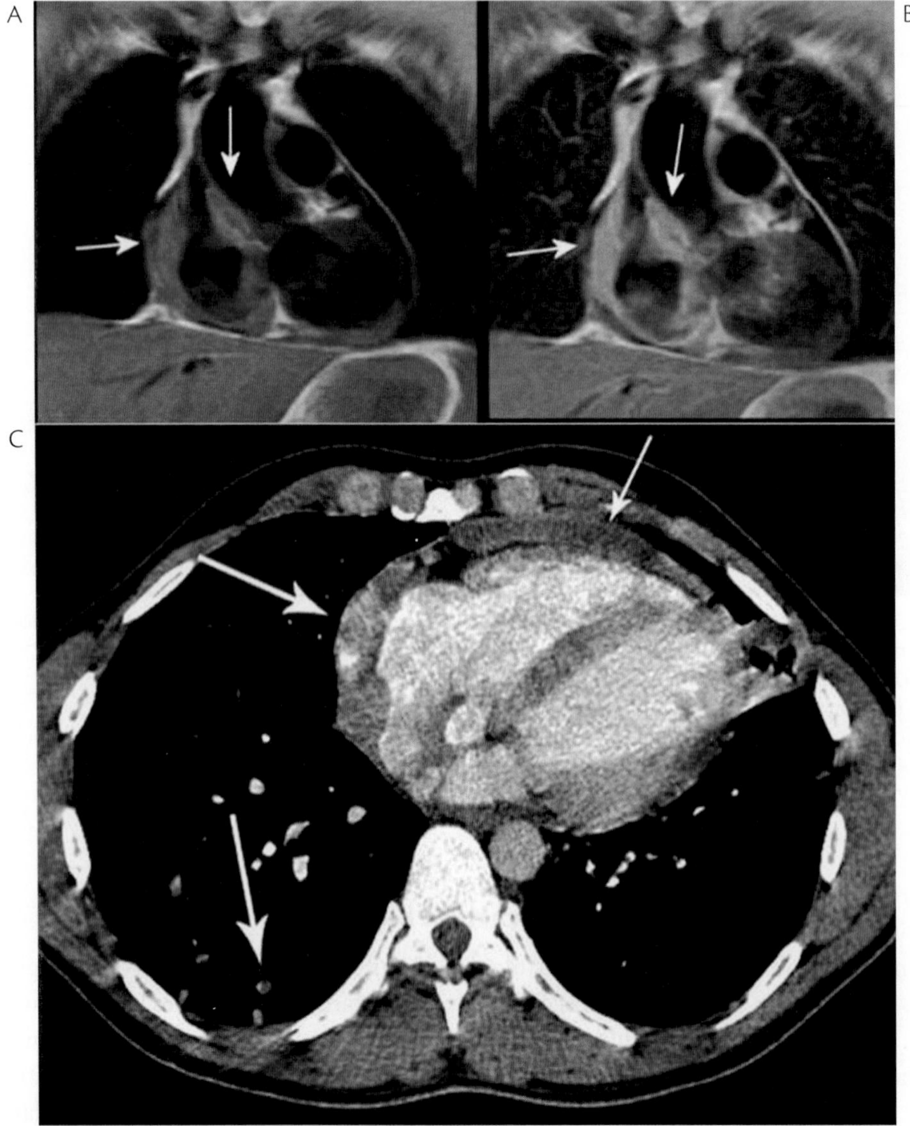

Figure 20.6 Multislice CT and CMR images of primary cardiac angiosarcomas. (A) CMR, T1-weighted images: note the slightly hyperintense areas (arrows) due to metahaemoglobin. (B) CMR, SE T1 image after contrast medium (Omniscan) (same patient): hyper-enhancement after contrast medium (arrow). (C) Multislice CT: a mass with irregular profile appears infiltrating the myocardium of the right atrium and the pericardium (arrows). A probable small metastasis is also visible in the right lung (thin arrow). Modified from Basso C, Valente M, Thiene G. *Tumori del cuore. Monografie di Cardiologia. Società Italiana di Cardiologia*, 2005. Novate-Milan: Arti Grafiche Color Black.

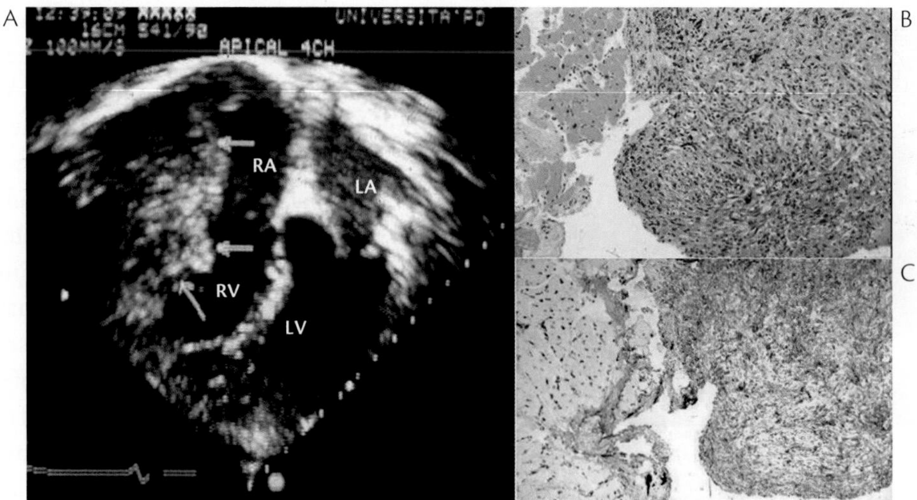

Figure 20.7 Right atrial angiosarcoma diagnosed at endomyocardial biopsy in a 36-year-old woman with dyspnoea. (A) Two-dimensional echocardiography, four-chamber view, showing an intramural, irregular mass protruding into the right atrial and ventricular cavities. Modified from Poletti A, Cocco P, Valente M, *et al.* In vivo diagnosis of cardiac angiosarcoma by endomyocardial biopsy. *Cardiovasc Pathol* 1993; **2**: 89–91, with permission from Elsevier. (B) Transvenous endomyocardial biopsy sample showing the myocardium (on the left) infiltrated by a neoplastic proliferation of pleomorphic, spindle cells with frequent mitoses, forming vascular-like structures (haematoxylin-eosin stain). (C) Immunohistochemistry shows diffuse positivity of neoplastic cells for endothelial cell markers (factor VIII). LA, left atrium; LV, left ventricle; RA, right atrium; RV, right ventricle.

and the precise histotype. This information may be crucial in case of malignancy for the choice of therapy and prognosis. Intraoperative consultation allows rapid pathological diagnosis and surgical decision making. Masses may be neoplastic, but even thrombotic, calcific, septic, or infective. The employment of traditional histological and histochemical staining should be accompanied by immunohistochemistry with a large panel of antibodies, for establishing the histotype of tumour-cell proliferation. In rare cases of cardiac sarcoma, electron microscopy may also be of help.

Benign tumours

Myxoma

Myxoma is the paradigm of benign intracavitary cardiac tumour [26]. It usually is an atrial neoplasm and for this reason is also known as atrial myxoma. The eponym is a misnomer since it refers to its mucoid component and gelatinous nature, which, however, does not reflect the precise histogenesis.

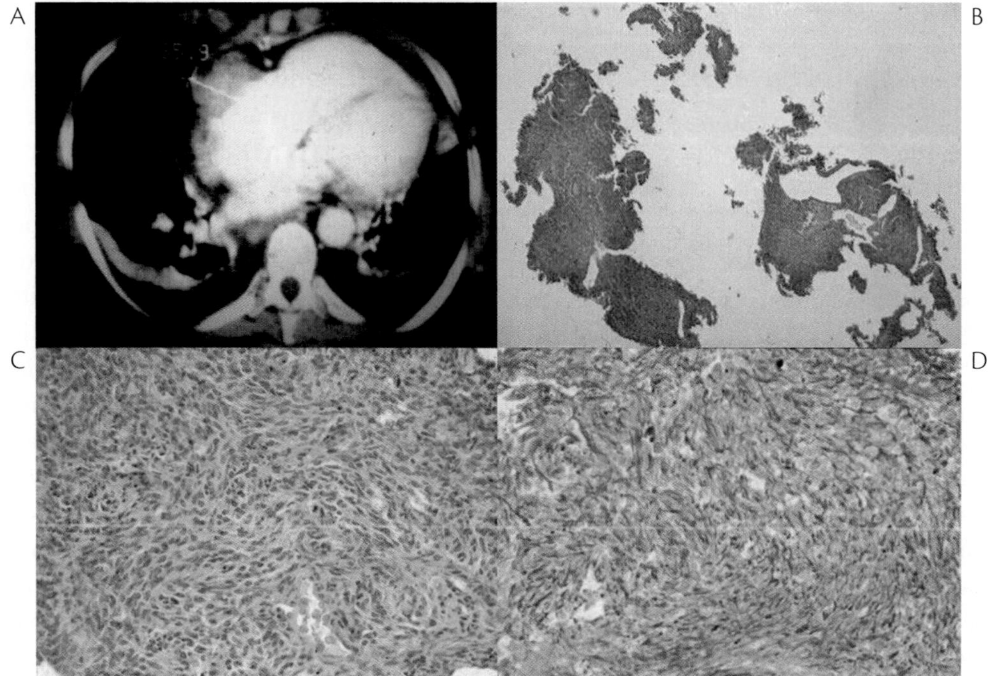

Figure 20.8 Right atrial fibrosarcoma in a 62-year-old woman with asthenia and fever diagnosed by transvenous endomyocardial biopsy. (A) CT shows an infiltrative mass of the right atrial wall. Modified from Basso C, Stefani A, Calabrese F, *et al.* Primary right atrial fibrosarcoma diagnosed by endocardial biopsy. *Am Heart J* 1996; **131**: 399–402, with permission from Elsevier. (B) Endomyocardial biopsy samples (haematoxylin eosin stain). (C) Close up of (B): note the proliferation of mesenchymal cells with fibroblastic features and the storiform, herring-bone pattern with a collagen stroma. (D) Immunohistochemistry shows the neoplastic cells positive for vimentin.

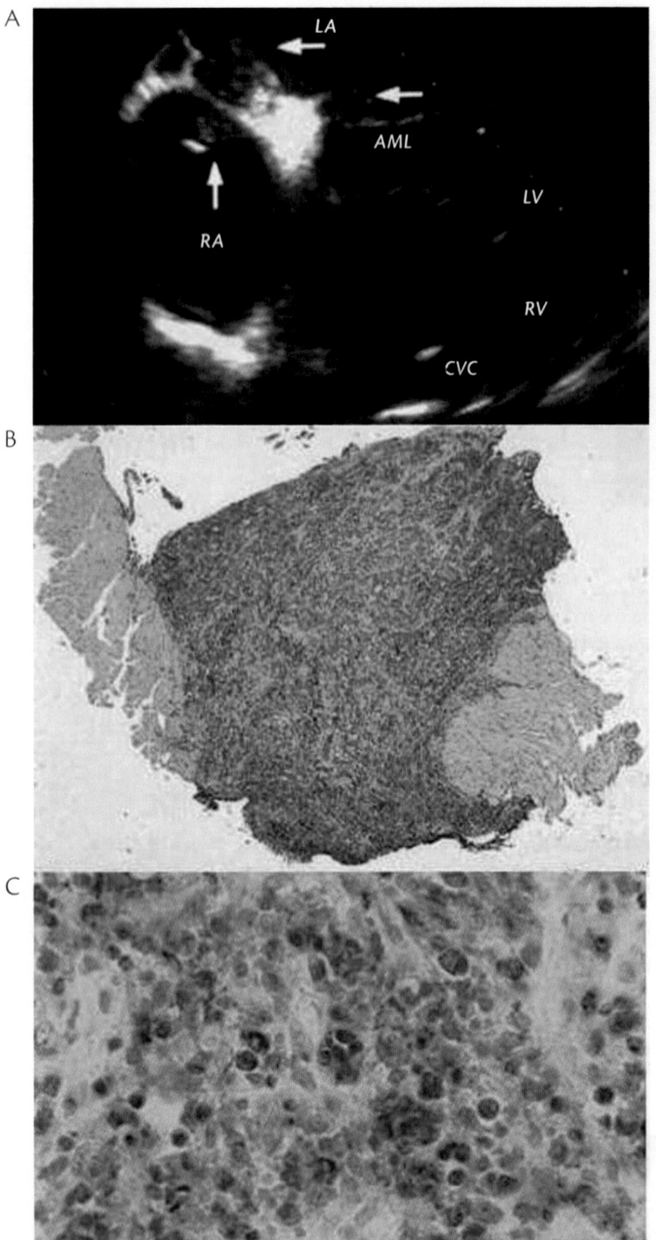

Figure 20.9 *In vivo* diagnosis through transvenous endomyocardial biopsy of cardiac metastasis of T-cell lymphoma in a 36-year-old woman. (A) Two-dimensional transoesophageal echocardiography, four-chamber view: a round mass is visible on both sides of the interatrial septum. (B) Biopsy sample showing the myocardium infiltrated by a lymphoproliferative lesion (heamatoxylin-eosin stain). (C) Immunohistochemistry reveals a T-cell lymphoma (CD3). AML, anterior mitral leaflet; CVC, central venous catheter; LA, left atrium; LV, left ventricle; RA, right atrium; RV, right ventricle. Modified from Testolin L, Basso C, Pittarello D, *et al.* Cardiogenic shock due to metastatic cardiac lymphoma: still a diagnostic and therapeutic challenge. *Eur J Cardiothorac Surg* 2001; **19**: 365–8, with permission from Elsevier.

It is now definitively established that cardiac myxoma is not an organized thrombus [27], but a true neoplasm originating from subendocardial multipotent cells, with angioblastic proliferation and mucoid secretion [28–30]. The histology indeed shows not only single, fusiform or stellate cells, but also angioblastic-like structures, surrounded by Alcian-positive mucoid substance, in keeping with a neoplastic cell able to both differentiate into vessels and produce ground substance (➲Fig. 20.10). The term myxomatous endothelioma or myxomatous angioma (pseudomyxoma) [31] is probably more correct. Glandular-like aspects have been also described [32]. Multinucleated cells can be occasionally observed and should not be interpreted as sign of malignancy. Foci of extramedullary haemopoiesis, calcifications and haemorrhage can be also seen.

In the experience of the University of Padua, the myxoma was located in the left atrium in 80% of cases and in the right atrium in 18%, and concomitant growth of the myxoma on both sides of the atrial septum ('biatrial' myxoma) was observed only twice [8, 10].

Myxoma of the right ventricle was rare (2%) and of the left ventricle exceptional (only one case, 0.5%) (➲Fig. 20.4C and D) [33, 34]. It is possible that blood flow velocity prevents growth within the ventricular chambers.

Onset of clinical presentation varies, from the paediatric age to the elderly, with a peak in the sixth decade. The prevalence in females was twice that in males.

As far as gross features are concerned, the myxoma is a soft and gelatinous tumour, often with large areas of haemorrhage and lined by thrombus, it may be both sessile or pedunculated, and, when in the atria, it is mostly attached to the fossa ovalis of the atrial septum, with residuals of embryonic cardiac jelly as a possible source. The shape was a single smooth mass in 65% and villous in 35% (➲Fig. 20.11). Lacking a fibrous axis, the villi are friable and prone to tissue fragmentation and detachment with embolism.

There is a wide range in size (1–15cm, mean 5–6cm), from very small masses, that can also be symptomatic particularly when villous and embolizing, to huge ones occupying the atrial cavity or valve orifice. The size variability is reflected by the weight range of resected myxomas, from 7–120g, with the largest ones observed in the right atrium.

According to our experience, 30% of cases presented with constitutional symptoms, 60% with obstructive symptoms, and 16% with embolism, whereas 25% were asymptomatic. Constitutional symptoms are usually linked to interleukin-6 production from myxoma cells [35].

On auscultation, in cases of left atrial myxoma a diastolic murmur may be heard, mimicking rheumatic mitral stenosis. Obstructive symptoms may include dyspnoea, lipothymia, syncope, and congestive heart failure. Sudden obstruction, with atrial myxoma entrapped in the AV orifice during diastolic ventricular sucking (➲Fig. 20.12), may account for pulmonary oedema or even sudden death. Infective endocarditis may superimpose to myxoma.

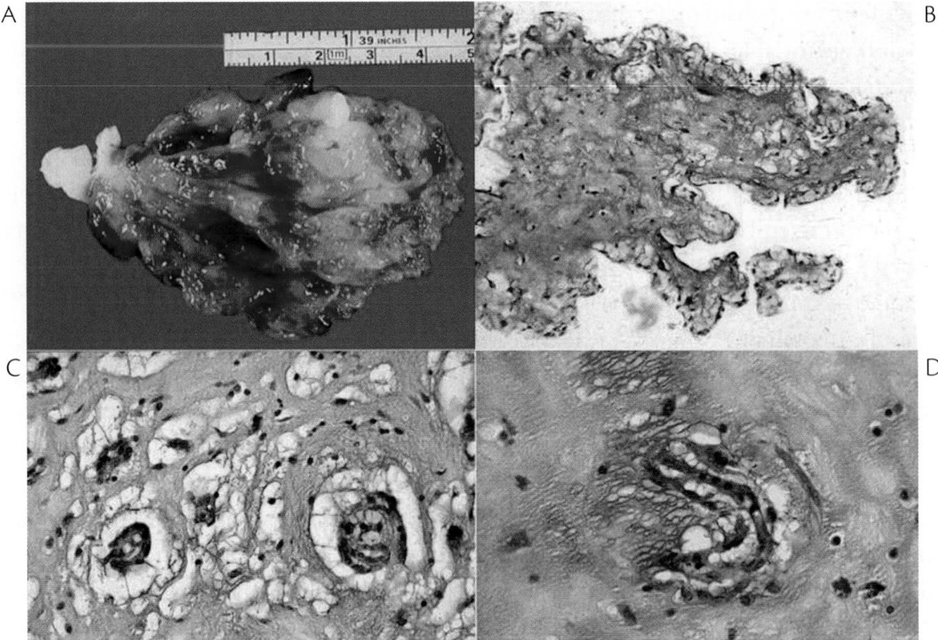

Figure 20.10 Surgically resected left atrial myxoma in a 50-year-old woman. (A) Villous, gelatinous mass. (B) Histology of a villous with mucoid extracellular matrix in the absence of a fibrous axis (Alcian PAS stain). (C, D) Angioblastic-like structures surrounded by mucoid, Alcian-positive ground substance, visible also inside the tumour cells (Alcian PAS stain).

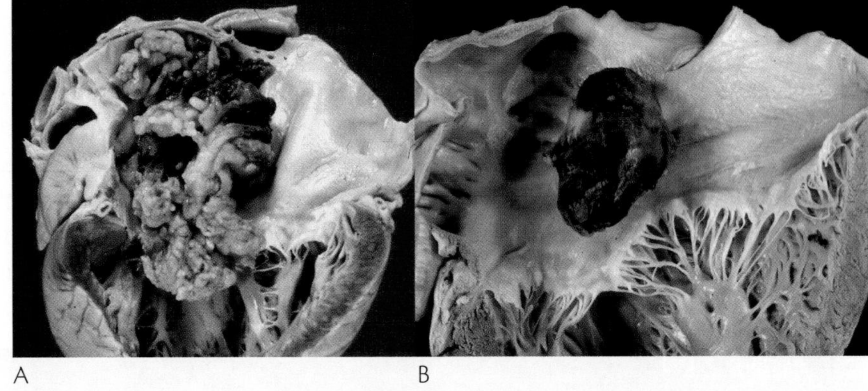

Figure 20.11 Two autopsy examples of left atrial myxomas. (A) A 51-year-old man who died due to pulmonary oedema: a giant villous left atrial myxoma herniates into the mitral orifice. (B) A 45-year-old man who died following recurrent systemic embolization: the mass is smooth and covered by thrombus. At histology, the peripheral embolus was revealed to be thrombotic. Modified from Basso C, Valente M, Thiene G. *Tumori del cuore. Monografie di Cardiologia. Società Italiana di Cardiologia*, 2005. Novate-Milan: Arti Grafiche Color Black.

Figure 20.12 Left atrial myxoma in a 47-year-old woman with syncope while bending. (A) Four-chamber two-dimensional echocardiography with a left atrial mass attached to the inter-atrial septum and prolapsing into the left ventricle during diastole. (B) Sessile myxoma with a smooth surface at surgical removal. Modified from Basso C, Valente M, Thiene G. *Tumori del cuore. Monografie di Cardiologia. Società Italiana di Cardiologia*, 2005. Novate-Milan: Arti Grafiche Color Black.

Systemic embolism may cause myocardial, cerebral, intestinal, renal, or splenic infarcts with severe sequelae such as hemiparesis, myocardial infarction, or sudden death. The detachment of a large amount of atrial myxoma may obstruct the aorta itself, usually at the abdominal carrefour. Prompt echocardiographic investigation to search for the cardiac source of the embolism easily leads to diagnosis and emergency cardiac surgery. Recently, an increased expression of matrix metalloproteinases has been demonstrated in embolic myxomas [36].

In 25% of cases in our experience, there was no sign or symptom, and the myxoma was just an incidental observation at autopsy or during routine echocardiography. Even in these circumstances, because of the embolic potential, surgical removal is indicated. In the elderly, the 'silent myxoma' may undergo calcification ('lithomyxoma') [37], like a sort of a self-healing. It appears as a 'stone' usually attached to the atrial septum.

Most cardiac myxomas are sporadic and are not transmissible to the offspring [26]. A rare familiar condition has been reported, comprising multiple myxomas of the heart and skin, hyperpigmentation of the skin (lentiginosis), and endocrine overactivity (so-called Carney complex or reported also with the acronyms NAME—Naevi, Atrial myxoma, Myxoid neurofibroma, Ephelides, or LAMB—Lentiginosis, Atrial myxoma, Mucocutaneous myxomas, Blue naevi) [38, 39]. It is a monogenic disease, with Mendelian autosomal dominant transmission (➲Chapter 9). The syndrome accounts for up to 7% of all cardiac myxomas. The subjects are younger than those with sporadic myxoma, have no female prevalence, present with a tendency to recurrence following surgery, and multiple endocrine neoplasm.

As far as genetics is concerned, in non-sporadic cardiac myxomas mutations in the gene *PRKAR1A*, located at 17q24, have been found [40]. This gene represents a putative tumour suppressor gene, coding for the regulatory R1 alpha subunit of protein kinase A.

Papillary fibroelastoma

Also known as endocardial papilloma, this is the second primary cardiac tumour following myxoma in all series [41, 42]. Some authors consider this tumour as a giant Lambl excrescence, a frequent occurrence in valve disease, originating as small thrombus on endocardial surfaces [27].

It is a small neoplasm, usually 1–2cm in size, typically intracavitary arising from the endocardium. The preferential site is the aortic valve (➲Fig. 20.13), followed by mitral, tricuspid, and pulmonary valves [43, 44]. The mural non-valvular endocardium may also be the site of growth, as well as the papillary muscles (➲Fig. 20.4E and F) and chordae tendineae.

At gross examination, the neoplasm looks like a papilloma with multiple fronds similar to a sea anemone, a shape better detectable under water. Histologically, a typical papillary shape is visible with non-vascularized, fibroelastic fronds arising from a main stalk, surrounded by myxoid tissue and covered by a single layer endocardium. Recent or organized thrombi may be observed, entrapped within the fronds. Many published cases have been wrongly reported as valvular villous 'myxoma', in the absence of histology.

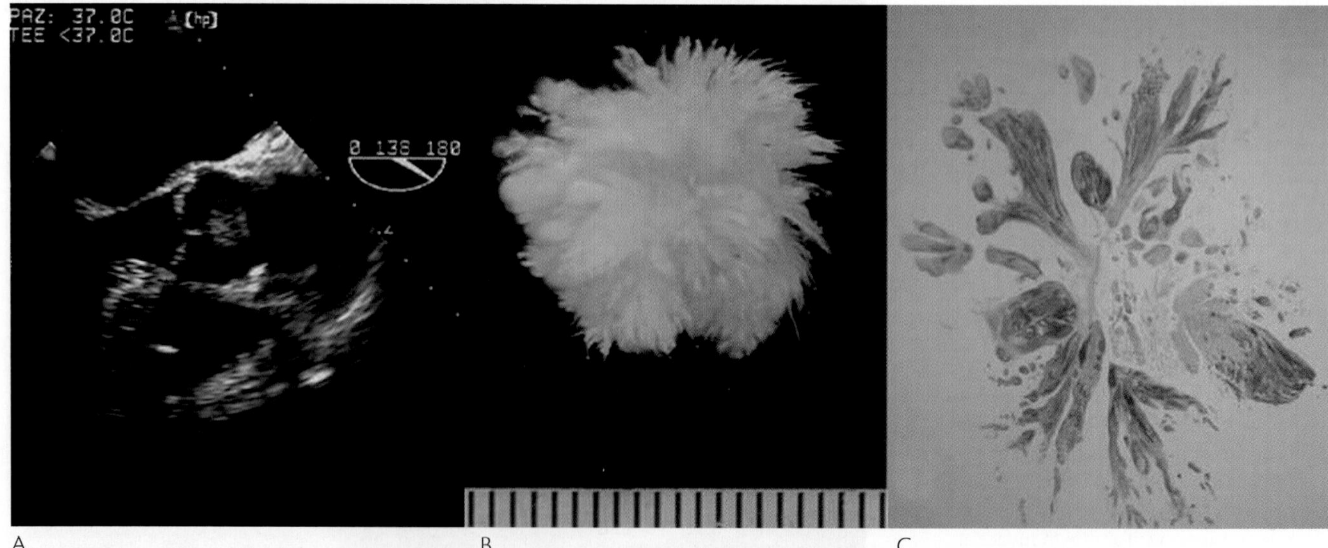

Figure 20.13 Papillary fibroelastoma of the aortic valve in an asymptomatic 77-year-old woman (incidental finding). (A) Transoesophageal echocardiography showing a small mass attached to the non-coronary aortic cusp. Modified from Basso C, Valente M, Thiene G. *Tumori del cuore. Monografie di Cardiologia. Società Italiana di Cardiologia*, 2005. Novate-Milan: Arti Grafiche Color Black. (B) The resected mass, viewed under water, resembles a sea anemone. (C) Histology shows multiple fronds with a fibroelastic axis (elastic van Gieson stain).

Because of the small size, papillary fibroelastoma rarely presents clinically with signs of obstruction. Nonetheless, systolic or diastolic murmurs may be audible.

Although, unlike myxoma, the mass is firm, rarely friable because of the fibroelastic axis of the fronds, embolism may occur and is the typical, worrisome clinical presentation, due to detachment either of part of the neoplastic mass or, more frequently, of associated thrombus. Myocardial infarction, transient ischaemic attack, and stroke are often reported as first clinical manifestations [41]. Another very rare complication, which may provoke sudden death, is represented by the wedging of the aortic valve papilloma into a coronary ostium, when located at the free edge of a coronary cusp.

Once an incidental finding at autopsy, nowadays papillary fibroelastoma is becoming a frequent observation at echocardiography, either following unexplained murmur or embolism or during an ultrasound procedure for other reasons. The potential embolic risk is such that the neoplasm should not be considered 'innocent' and indication for surgery is mandatory, at least for left-sided lesions [42–44]. On the other hand, the risk of micro-embolization into the pulmonary circulation from right-sided papillary fibroelastomas does not usually justify surgery with thoracotomy and cardio-circulatory arrest [45].

Lipoma

This is a benign tumour consisting of mature adipose tissue. Histologically, adipocytes are enmeshed in a fine fibrous collagen network [9, 11]. Two main variants exist.

Single or multiple capsulated masses, usually located in both the visceral and parietal pericardium or possibly intracavitary from the mural or valvular endocardium, have a variable size, and in some cases may cause obstruction (➲ Fig. 20.5D).

The second variant is the so-called 'lipoma of the interatrial septum', better known as lipomatous hypertrophy of the interatrial septum since the adipose tissue proliferation is not surrounded by a capsule [46–48]. It is usually observed in obese, elderly people and consists of an intracardiac extension of the subepicardial fat of the right AV sulcus, thus questioning its neoplastic nature (➲ Fig. 20.14).

Palpitations due to atrial arrhythmias (premature beats, atrial fibrillation and flutter) are the usual symptoms. AV conduction disturbances may also occur. When the lipomatous hypertrophy of the interatrial septum is so large as to obstruct the inflow of the venae cavae, congestive heart failure may appear, making surgical removal mandatory. The adipose nature of both capsulated lipomas and lipomatous hypertrophy of the interatrial septum may be easily identified by CMR because of the typical high intensity signal.

Haemangioma

This is a benign neoplastic vessel proliferation. Three patterns have been reported [9, 11, 49], according to histological features:

1) cavernous haemangioma, consisting of multiple, dilated thin-walled vessels;
2) capillary haemangioma, consisting of small vessels resembling capillaries;
3) arteriovenous haemangioma, consisting of dysplastic malformed arteries and veins (also known as cirsoid aneurysm).

Mixed forms are frequently described. The dimension of haemangiomas is variable, up to several centimetres.

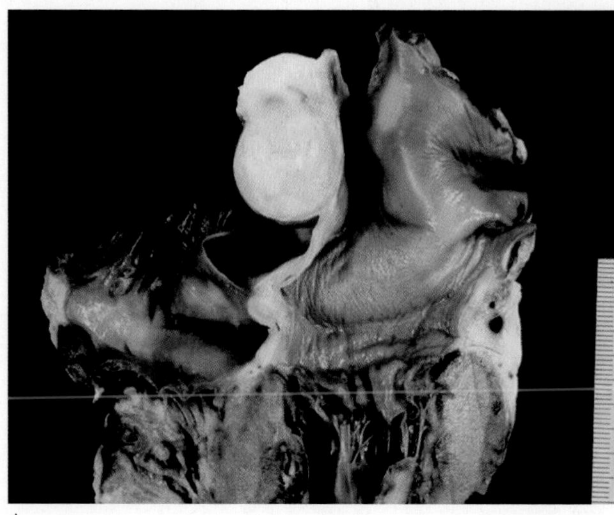

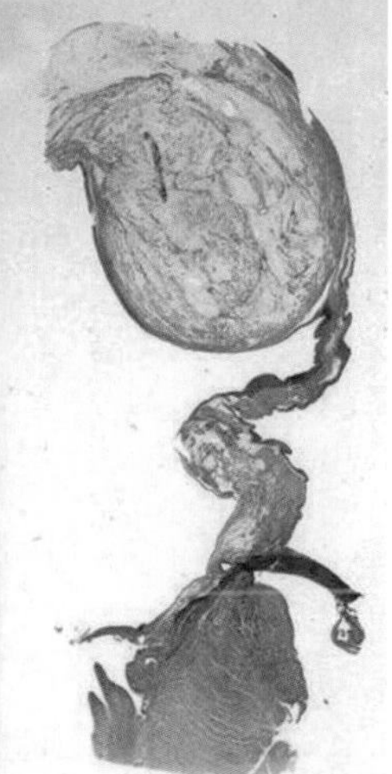

Figure 20.14 Lipomatous hypertrophy of the interatrial septum in a 74-year-old diabetic, obese woman (incidental finding at autopsy). (A) Four-chamber view of the heart specimen with lipomatosis of the interatrial septum. (B) Histology showing a non-capsulated mass consisting of mature adipocytes (Heidenhain trichrome). Modified from Basso C, Barbazza R, Thiene G. Images in cardiovascular medicine. Lipomatous hypertrophy of the atrial septum. *Circulation* 1998; **97**: 1423.

75% presents with an intramural growth and 25% are endocardial tumours that project into the atrial or ventricular cavities, sometimes mimicking myxoma (➲Fig. 20.15) [50]. The capillary haemangioma are capsulated, whereas the cavernous or arteriovenous haemangiomas, although benign, tend to be infiltrative.

The intracavitary haemangiomas may present with obstructive symptoms, the intramural ones with arrhythmias, pericardial effusion, and exceptionally with cardiac tamponade. Many may be silent and just discovered incidentally at echo or autopsy. The histotype may be suspected *in vivo* by CMR, particularly following contrast medium administration with mass enhancement, or by coronary angiography with neo-vessels visualization. The rich vascularization, however, is not specific, being frequently observed also in myxoma.

Cystic tumour of the atrioventricular node

This is also known as tawarioma (from Tawara, the discoverer of the AV node) or celothelioma (mesothelioma of the AV node) because it is thought to be of mesothelial (pericardial) 'disontogenetic' nature. Recent immunohistochemistry studies proved its origin from endodermal 'remnants', thus the term celothelioma (mesothelioma) has been abandoned.

The tumour is located exactly at the level of the AV node in the triangle of Koch, at the right side of the atrial septum, in front of the coronary sinus, with size varying from 2–20mm, and appears multicystic even with the naked eye [51, 52]. Histologically, the tumour is located on the right side of the central fibrous body, infiltrating and compressing the AV node. The cysts are filled by mucoid substance and are lined by cuboid, squamous, or transitional epithelial cells, which at immunohistochemistry strongly express cytokeratin and epithelial membrane antigen.

The mean age at clinical presentation is nearly 40 years [11]. Seventy-five per cent of patients present with complete and 15% with incomplete AV block, whereas in 10%, sudden unexpected death is the first clinical manifestation.

Histological diagnosis is usually achieved at postmortem or after cardiac transplantation through histological examination of the conduction system, but cases with *in vivo* diagnosis following surgical removal have been reported [52].

Blood cyst

These are usually small cysts of no clinical significance, located along the closure rim of the AV valves in newborns and infants, particularly <2 months of age, due to blood entrapped into leaflet crevices, covered by endocardium [11]. Exceptionally, the blood sequestration may increase and the cyst assumes such huge endocavitary dimensions, as to create obstructive symptoms and require surgery [53].

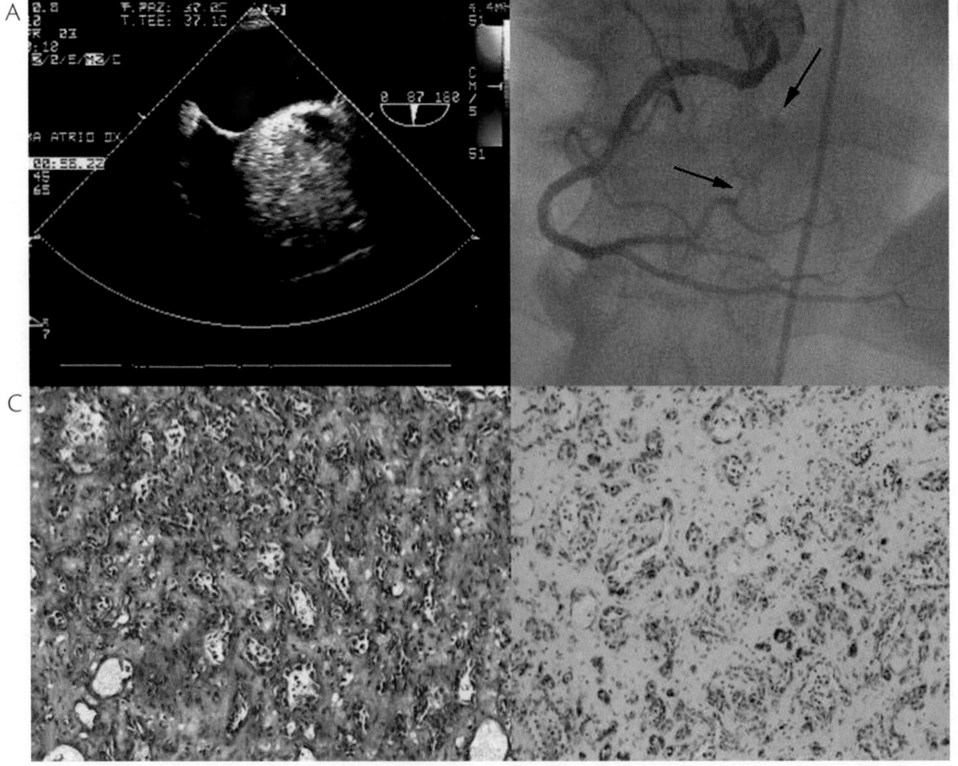

Figure 20.15 Right atrial angioma in a 62-year-old woman with effort dyspnoea. (A) Transoesophageal two-dimensional echocardiography shows a right atrial mass attached to the atrial septum, suggestive of a myxoma. (B) Coronary angiography shows tumour vascularization from the right coronary artery. (C) Histology shows multiple vascular, capillary like structures (Heidenhain trichrome stain). (D) Immunohistochemistry shows positivity for endothelial markers (CD31). Modified from Rizzoli G, Bottio T, Pittarello D, *et al.* Atrial septal mass: transesophageal echocardiographic assessment. *J Thorac Cardiovasc Surg* 2004; **128**: 767–9, with permission from Elsevier.

Pericardial cyst

This is a relatively frequent mass, most probably disontogenetic in origin, mostly detected incidentally during a chest X-ray. It consists of uni- or multiloculated cysts, full of serous liquid [8, 10, 11]. It is usually asymptomatic, but sometimes so large (up to 15cm) that it creates symptoms like chest pain, dyspnoea, cough, palpitations, and even congestive heart failure. Although most probably congenital, it becomes symptomatic in adult age because of increasing storage of fluid within the cystic cavity. Histologically, the thin wall consists of highly vascularized connective tissue covered by mesothelial lining on both sides.

Benign tumours of paediatric age

Cardiac tumours are not so rare in the paediatric age (<18 years). They represent 15% of the University of Padua's experience with primary cardiac tumours and were all benign [54–56].

Myxoma, a typically adult neoplasm, may manifest itself also during the first two decades of life (7% of all cardiac myxoma of our experience and 30% of all paediatric tumours) [57]. Their clinical presentation is similar to that in the adult, including congestive heart failure (➲Fig. 20.2) and embolism. Haemangiomas are also observed in paediatric age, with identical features as in adults. However, there are cardiac tumours which may be considered typical or exclusive to the paediatric age which deserve separate description.

Rhabdomyoma

Considered to be a non-proliferative hamartomatous lesion, it is the most common cardiac tumour in the paediatric population, but not in surgical pathology series (in our experience, only 15% of paediatric cardiac tumours were rhabdomyoma) since in many cases there is no indication for surgery [58].

The diagnosis is frequently prenatal by fetal echocardiography, in case of arrhythmias, hydrops, retarded intrauterine growth and familiarity of tuberous sclerosis. Indeed, cardiac rhabdomyomas are found in up to 80% of cases affected by tuberous sclerosis, consisting of a classical clinical triad: neuro-fibromatous lesions, mental slowing, and cutaneous lesions. Defective genes have been recently discovered in familial forms of tuberous sclerosis: *TSC1* encoding amartin (9q34) and *TSC2* encoding tuberin (16p13.3) [9, 59]. The proteins are involved in tumour suppression; however their function in cardiac mass development remains to be elucidated. Up to 50% of children with cardiac rhabdomyoma present with tuberous sclerosis.

Rhabdomyomas are single or, more frequently, multiple nodules, up to 1–2cm in diameter, usually intramural within the ventricular myocardium, but also intracavitary because of growth from the sub-endocardium (➲Fig. 20.16). The latter may create obstructive or restrictive symptoms, with fetal hydrops or neonatal respiratory distress and congestive heart failure as to require surgery. Rhabdomyoma may be a cause of severe subaortic [60] or subpulmonary stenosis in infants.

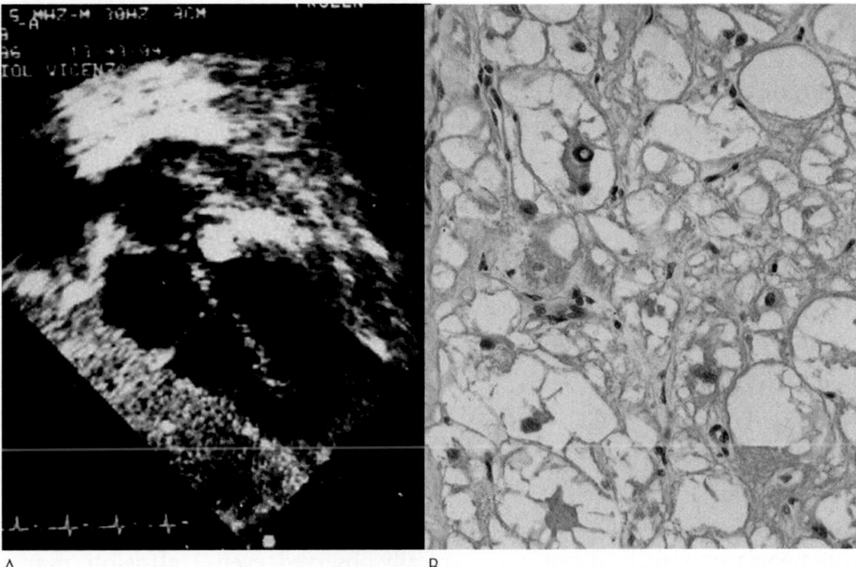

Figure 20.16 Rhabdomyoma in a 7-month-old male infant with systolic murmur. (A) two-dimensional echocardiography reveals a subaortic endocavitary round mass. (B) The resected mass was revealed to be a rhabdomyoma: note the typical 'spider' cells (haematoxylin-eosin stain). Modified from De Dominicis E, Frigiola A, Thiene G, *et al.* Subaortic stenosis by solitary rhabdomyoma. Successful excision in an infant following 2D echocardiogram and Doppler diagnosis. *Chest* 1989; **95**: 470–2.

Grossly, the neoplastic, non-capsulated, nodules are white or grey, and histologically consist of large, clear vacuolated, myocytes full of glycogen, with residual cytoplasm with myofilaments stretching from the central nucleus to the membrane, thus giving rise to a spider appearance ('spider cells'). The cells are immune-positive for myoglobin, desmin, and actin. More than a proliferation of cardiomyocytes, the rhabdomyoma is a localized storage disease of glycogen, which may account for severe contractile ventricular dysfunction.

Arrhythmias and conduction disturbances are frequent, in terms of supraventricular tachycardia, AV block, ventricular pre-excitation, and ventricular tachyarrhythmias.

Diagnosis is easily achieved by two-dimensional echocardiography, with detection of multiple homogeneous, highly echogenic round masses. A peculiar feature in the natural history is the spontaneous regression of the neoplasm, probably due to re-absorption or consumption of the glycogen stores, as to suggest in many cases a symptomatic treatment, and leaving surgery only in case of emergency obstructive or arrhythmic clinical presentation.

Fibroma

Fibromas represent nearly 20% of paediatric cardiac tumours in our experience [10, 56]. Diagnosis is usually achieved by clinical imaging during infancy or adolescence, but cases of prenatal diagnosis by fetal echo have been also reported [61, 62].

Grossly, the fibroma consists of a single (or, more rarely, multiple) oval, non-capsulate mass of the ventricular myocardium, which appears whitish and stiff (➲Fig. 20.17). It is typically intramural (ventricular septum, left or right ventricular free walls) and appears as a homogeneous mass on echocardiogram and CMR [63], the latter also showing a hypoperfused core. Size and location are the major determinants of symptoms and signs. The size may be so huge (up to 8cm) to obstruct or obliterate the ventricular cavities, thus leading to congestive heart failure. Small-sized fibromas may remain silent. Growth may interfere with intramyocardial spread of conduction impulse and create re-entry phenomena with life-threatening tachyarrhythmias, such as ventricular tachycardia and fibrillation. Sudden death has been reported as the first manifestation of the disease.

Histologically, the neoplasm consists of fibroblast proliferation with collagen bundle deposition. In neonates and infants the proliferation is seen to entrap cardiomyocytes, such as to suggest that we are dealing with a fibromatosis more than a true neoplasm. Calcific deposits are typically observed, even at X-ray or CT, and may be considered pathognomonic of fibroma in case of intramural cardiac masses.

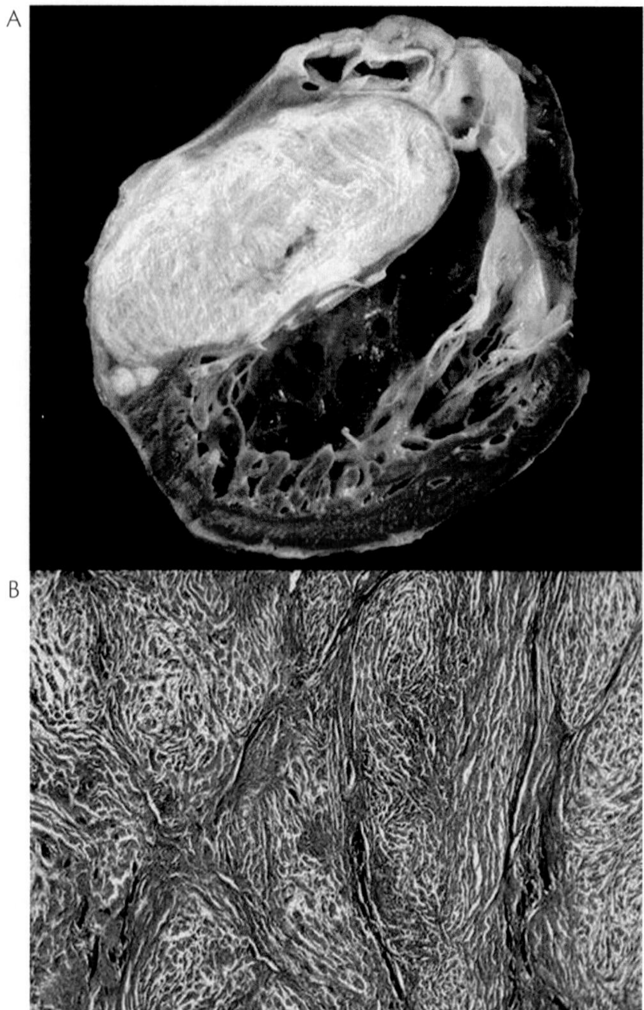

Figure 20.17 Cardiac fibroma in a 40-year-old woman who underwent cardiac transplantation due to congestive heart failure with a misdiagnosis of hypertrophic cardiomyopathy with subaortic obstruction. (A) Long-axis section of the native heart reveals an intramural huge, firm, white, oval mass and two satellite small nodules within the interventricular septum. (B) The mass at histology consists mostly of collagen bundles (Heidenhain trichrome stain). Modified from Valente M, Cocco P, Thiene G, *et al.* Cardiac fibroma and heart transplantation. *J Thorac Cardiovasc Surg* 1993; **106**: 1208–12.

Teratoma

This is a tumour of germinal cells, which in 90% of cases is located within the pericardial cavity, usually at the base of the heart (➲Fig. 20.18) [64]. Teratomas represent nearly 10% of all paediatric cardiac tumours. Diagnosis is usually achieved within 1 month of age because of severe obstructive symptoms through compression of the arterial pole and lungs, with signs of congestive heart failure and respiratory distress as to require emergency operation. Indeed, size may be so huge as to exceed the heart itself. Pericardial effusion may occur and lead to cardiac tamponade.

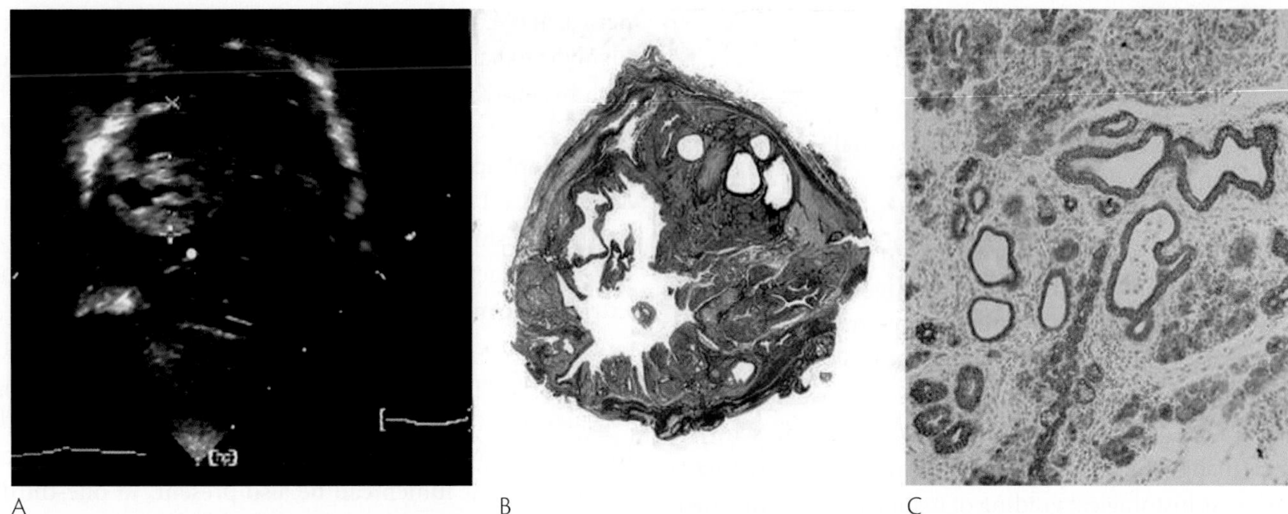

Figure 20.18 Pericardial teratoma in a 12-days-old neonate with pericardial effusion. (A) Two-dimensional echocardiography, four-chamber view, shows a non-homogeneous, cystic mass at the root of the great arteries. (B) Panoramic view at histology with cystic features (Heidenhain trichrome stain). (C) Presence of various tissues from different embryonic origin (keratin positivity in some areas). Modified from Padalino M, Basso C, Milanesi O, *et al.* Surgically treated primary cardiac tumors in early infancy and childhood. *J Thorac Cardiovasc Surg* 2005; **129**: 1358–63, with permission from Elsevier.

Due to routine use of fetal echocardiography, many cases of prenatal diagnosis have been recently reported. Grossly they appear as cystic lesions, well visible at clinical imaging (echocardiogram, CMR). Histologically, proliferation of various tissues from all three germ layers is visible (neural, glandular, and stromal structures), clearly identified by immunohistochemistry.

Histiocytoid cardiomyopathy

This is a quite rare tumour-like lesion, consisting of small, non-capsulated, whitish-yellow nodules (1–15mm in size), more frequently located in the mural subendocardium of the left ventricle. Histologically, they consist of large, foamy, round cells ('oncocytes') [65]. These cells are immune-positive for myoglobin, desmin, and myosin, but a 'spider' shape is not visible. Most probably they are specialized (Purkinje) cells of the conduction system; for this reason it is also known as Purkinjoma. Differential diagnosis with mitochondrial cardiomyopathy, which does not show discrete nodules and presents a diffuse involvement of cardiac myocytes, is needed. Histiocytoid cardiomyopathy is an arrhythmogenic lesion, accounting for tachyarrhythmias and conduction disturbances including ventricular pre-excitation, even at risk of sudden death.

Other benign tumours

Other benign tumours with rare occurrence have been recently reported and require an update of the WHO classification.

Hamartoma of mature cardiac myocytes is a single or multiple, non-capsulated lesion consisting of mature, hypertrophic cardiomyocytes with cross striations and large, bizarre nuclei and spatial disorganization ('myocardial disarray') as to mimic focal hypertrophic cardiomyopathy [66].

Adult rhabdomyoma consists of round-shaped cardiomyocytes with cross striations, which occasionally show vacuoles and 'spider' feature as seen in rhabdomyoma of infants. A 2–5cm mass, with a pseudo-capsule, has been described mostly in the mural atrial myocardium, protruding into atrial cavities. No association with tuberous sclerosis has been reported [67].

The inflammatory myofibroblast tumour is probably not a true neoplasm and it is indeed also known as plasma cell granuloma or inflammatory pseudo-tumour [68]. These tumours are very rare in the heart and any endocardial site of the heart may be involved, although it has been described mostly in the ventricles. It may reach huge dimensions, up to 8cm, and histologically consists of a proliferation of spindled myofibroblasts and fibroblasts, including chronic inflammatory cells, such as plasma cells, lymphocytes, macrophages, and eosinophils.

Other benign neoplasm or tumour-like lesions, which are no longer part of the WHO classification [9], but are still reported in the classical series of the Armed Forces Institute of Pathology (AFIP), Washington, DC are: granular cell tumour, paraganglioma (or cardiac pheochromocytoma), neurofibroma, leiomyoma, intracardiac bronchogenic cyst, thyroid heterotopy, mesothelial excrescences (MICE) [11].

Malignant tumours of the heart

Primary malignant tumours represent nearly 10% or so of all cardiac neoplasms and consist essentially of sarcomas and lymphomas [8–11, 69, 70].

The updated list refers to the latest WHO classification (➲Table 20.1) [9]. This classification introduces a new malignant entity (epithelioid haemangioendothelioma), puts together malignant fibrohistiocytoma, undifferentiated pleomorphic sarcoma, and osteosarcoma, fuses fibrosarcoma and so-called myxosarcoma, and excludes other very rare primary cardiac tumours, like malignant schwannoma, malignant rhabdoid tumour, and carcinosarcoma.

As far as histological grading of malignancy is concerned, there are no specific parameters and we have to refer to soft tissue neoplasms [71–73]. A histological grading system has been put forward by the French Fédération Nationale des Centres de Lutte Contre le Cancer (FFNCLCC), which is based upon a cumulative score deriving from three parameters, i.e. 1) tumour differentiation; 2) mitotic count; and 3) tumour necrosis.

Angiosarcoma

Angiosarcoma is the most common malignant differentiated cardiac neoplasm, with endothelial cell differentiation, also known as haemangioendothelioma, haemangiosarcoma, haemangioendothelial sarcoma, malignant haemangioendothelioma, malignant haemangioma, malignant angioendothelioma [8–11, 74].

It may be observed in individuals of any age with a peak in the fourth decade and no sex predilection. The most frequent location is the right atrial chamber, close to the AV groove, but any chamber as well as the pericardium can be involved (➲Figs. 20.6 and 20.7)

Fever, weight loss, asthenia, chest pain, supraventricular arrhythmias, and, in advanced stage, congestive heart failure and haemorrhagic pericardial effusion are the usual symptoms and signs. Lung metastases may be the first manifestation. Coexistent bleeding episodes, coagulopathy, and anaemia have been reported in a significant number of cases.

Grossly, it is a lobulated, mural, brown neoplasm, ≥2cm in size, infiltrating the wall and the pericardium, and protruding in right cardiac cavities, with invasion of the inferior vena cava and the tricuspid orifice. The site is ideal for *in vivo* diagnosis through endomyocardial biopsy (➲Fig. 20.7) [23].

An irregular echogenic mass is seen at echocardiography, associated with pericardial effusion or even direct pericardial extension. At angiography, the mass appears highly vascularized. The heterogeneity of neoplastic tissue, with haemorrhage and necrosis, is visible at contrast CMR and CT. After administration of gadolinium contrast, typical enhancement along the vascular lakes may be seen. Moreover, CT and CMR are superior to echocardiography in distinguishing pericardial involvement and invasion of adjacent structures, besides providing information about extracardiac metastases.

At histology, two-thirds of angiosarcoma are moderately to well differentiated and show an irregular, anastomosing vascular network, lined by pleomorphic, atypical cells with frequent mitoses. Chord-like structures in the absence of a clear vascular lumen can be also present. In one-thirds of cases, the tumour is poorly differentiated, without discrete vascular structures, and consists of anaplastic spindle cells within a hyaline stroma, containing focally extravascular red cells. Immunohistochemistry plays a crucial role in diagnosis, especially in undifferentiated forms, with the detection of cells expressing endothelial cell antigen (factor VIII/von Willebrand, CD31, CD34). Mutations of *TP53* and *K-ras* genes have been reported, as well as several chromosomal abnormalities [75].

Prognosis is extremely poor, usually because of delayed diagnosis, with a mean survival of 10 months even after surgical excision, with or without adjuvant therapy, or cardiac transplantation.

Epithelioid haemangioendothelioma

An usually extracardiac tumour (limbs, lung, liver), this is quite rare at heart level, originating from the AV sulcus or valves. It consists grossly of small, reddish nodules with frequent calcifications and histologically of round or oval CD34-positive cells, with small intracellular lumina, arranged in short strands and nests. The differential diagnosis with metastasis of adenocarcinoma is possible thanks to immunohistochemical positive reaction with factor VIII, CD31, and CD34. In other words, it is an angiosarcoma with epithelioid features. Occurrence of metastases is rare, as in extracardiac epithelioid haemangioendothelioma.

Malignant pleomorphic fibrous histiocytoma/undifferentiated pleomorphic sarcoma

This is a diagnosis achieved by exclusion, when all the immunohistochemical stains fail to give evidence of specific cell differentiation. Once, when immunohistochemistry was not available, undifferentiated sarcoma represented 50% of all cardiac malignancies, but in more recently published series it has almost disappeared [9, 76].

The most frequent site is the left atrium, with an endocavitary growth similar to left atrial myxoma, of which it mimics obstructive and constitutional symptoms (➲Fig. 20.19). It may also arise from the right atrium and right ventricle. Metastasis to the lymph nodes, lungs, skin, and systemic organs occur early.

The mass is easily detected at echocardiography and CMR and CT may be of great help in establishing lungs metastases, lymph node involvement, extent of excision, and recurrences.

Grossly, the mass is clearly distinguishable from myxoma because it may be multiple, whitish with a rough surface and hard consistency, in the absence of gelatinous-myxoid appearance.

Microscopically, the proliferation consists of bizarre, pleomorphic cells, frequently giant multinuclear, with high mitotic activity. The negative immunohistochemical staining, including that for histiocytes, point to an undifferentiated mesenchymal cell. Only vimentin may be positive.

The prognosis is very poor due to metastases and local recurrences, with a mean postoperative survival ranging from 5–18 months.

Areas of bone differentiation are detectable in 15% of undifferentiated pleomorphic sarcomas. They have been reported in the past as primary osteosarcoma of the heart, most of which located in the left atrium. Nowadays they are grouped within malignant pleomorphic fibrous histiocytomas/undifferentiated pleomorphic sarcomas with osteosarcomatous differentiation.

Fibrosarcoma and myxoid fibrosarcoma

Fibrosarcoma consists of a malignant proliferation of mesenchymal cells with fibroblastic features and a storiform, herring-bone pattern with a collagen stroma [24]. They represent nearly 5% of all primary cardiac malignancies. The most frequent location is in the atria (particularly the left), with both intracavitary and mural location (➲Fig. 20.8). A pericardial form does exist (solitary malignant fibrous tumour of the pericardium), which may mimic a mesothelioma. As with other sarcomas, clinical presentation depends on site and size of the tumour. Being mostly left sided, signs and symptoms of pulmonary congestion, mitral stenosis, and pulmonary vein obstruction are the most frequent.

Microscopically, the fibrosarcoma consists of a collagen stroma and monomorphic spindle cells, with variable mitotic index (➲Fig. 20.8). Pleomorphism, giant cells, and vascularization are absent.

Immunohistochemistry is positive for vimentin and frequently also for actin, in keeping with a myofibroblastic differentiation.

The prognosis is poor (mean survival 5 months), even in intracavitary cases in which surgical resection is apparently radical.

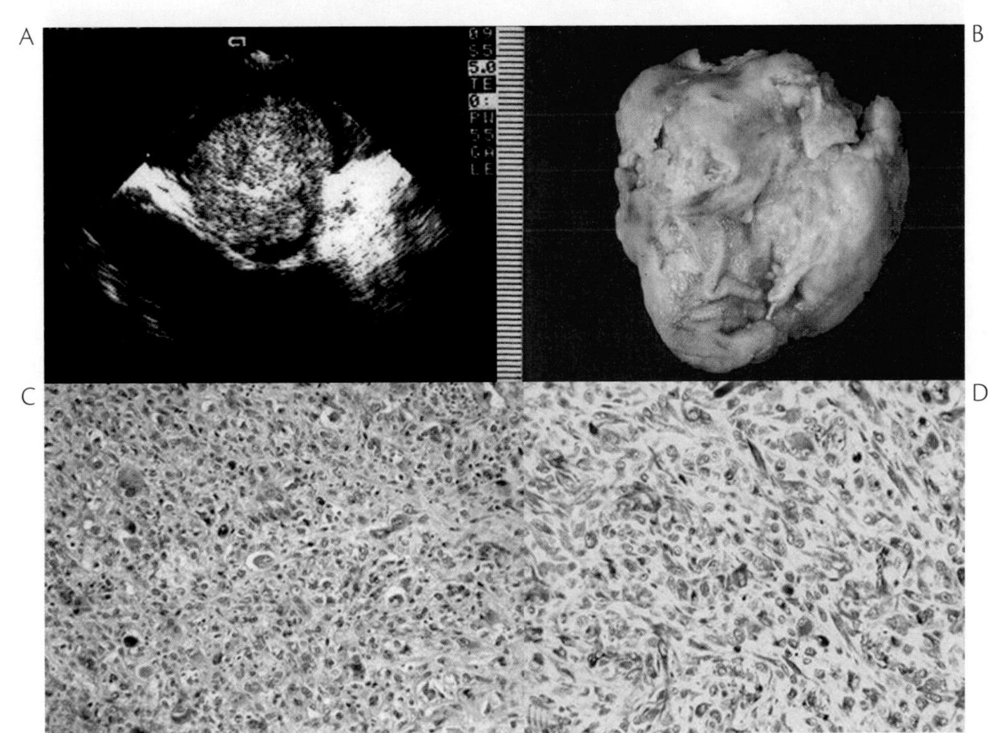

Figure 20.19 Left atrial malignant pleomorphic fibrous histiocytoma in a 68-year-old man with fever and fatigue. (A) Two-dimensional transoesophageal echocardiography shows a round, non-infiltrating, intracavitary mass in the left atrium. (B) Gross view of the resected mass: note the rough surface and non-gelatinous appearance. (C) At histology, bizarre, pleomorphic cells, frequently giant multinuclear, with high mitotic activity are visible. (D) Immunohistochemistry points to an undifferentiated mesenchymal cell (vimentin positivity). Modified from Basso C, Valente M, Thiene G. *Tumori del cuore. Monografie di Cardiologia. Società Italiana di Cardiologia*, 2005. Novate-Milan: Arti Grafiche Color Black.

Myxosarcoma is considered the myxoid variant of cardiac fibrosarcoma, from which it differs not only because of the myxoid stroma but also because of the presence of stellate or ovoid cells. Myxosarcoma should not be considered a malignant variant of myxoma, as originally thought.

In the AFIP Atlas, this term has been applied to undifferentiated cardiac malignant sarcomas with myxoid stroma. Myxoid fibrosarcoma is nowadays equivalent to the extracardiac soft tissue myxofibrosarcoma and fibromyxoid sarcoma at a low grade of malignancy, which are grouped among fibroblastic/myofibroblastic neoplasms.

Rhabdomyosarcoma

This is a mesenchymal cardiac malignancy constituted by cells with striated muscle differentiation. Thought to be the most frequent cardiac sarcoma due to its cardiomyocyte origin, it has been proven instead, with the advent of immunohistochemistry, to represent <5% of primary cardiac malignancies [8–11, 77].

Rhabdomyosarcoma is a solid intramural infiltrating tumour, originating from the atrial, ventricular, and septal myocardium, rarely protruding into the cavities.

It affects children and young adults, with male sex prevalence. Pericardial effusion, dyspnoea, conduction disturbances and extracardiac metastases are the usual presentation.

Embryonal rhabdomyosarcoma is the most frequent at cardiac level, thus explaining the younger mean age at presentation compared to other sarcomas [78]. Within a rich proliferation of round cells with frequent mitoses, periodic acid-Schiff (PAS)-positive rhabdomyoblasts are visible, either 'racket' shaped or with the typical 'tadpole' feature. The more the myoblasts, the greater the differentiation. Nuclear staining for antibodies against myogenin helps the diagnosis, as well as cytoplasmatic positivity for desmin, documenting muscular differentiation. Electron microscopy may be of help in detecting myofilaments.

Sarcoma botryoides, a form of embryonal rhabdomyosarcoma, which looks like a gelatinous mass with a typical 'grape-like' appearance and presents histologically with a rich mucoid stroma, has also been described in the heart. Genetic mutations at the level of *K-ras* exon I have been discovered.

Alveolar rhabdomyosarcoma in the heart has been reported only as a metastatic lesion.

Leiomyosarcoma

Leiomyosarcoma is a sarcoma of smooth muscle cells and account for nearly 10% of all cardiac malignancies with a peak in the fifth decade [8, 11].

There are two usual sites of origin. One is the left atrium, where it may present as a single or multinodular endocavitary mass, mimicking the left atrial myxoma (➲Fig. 20.20)

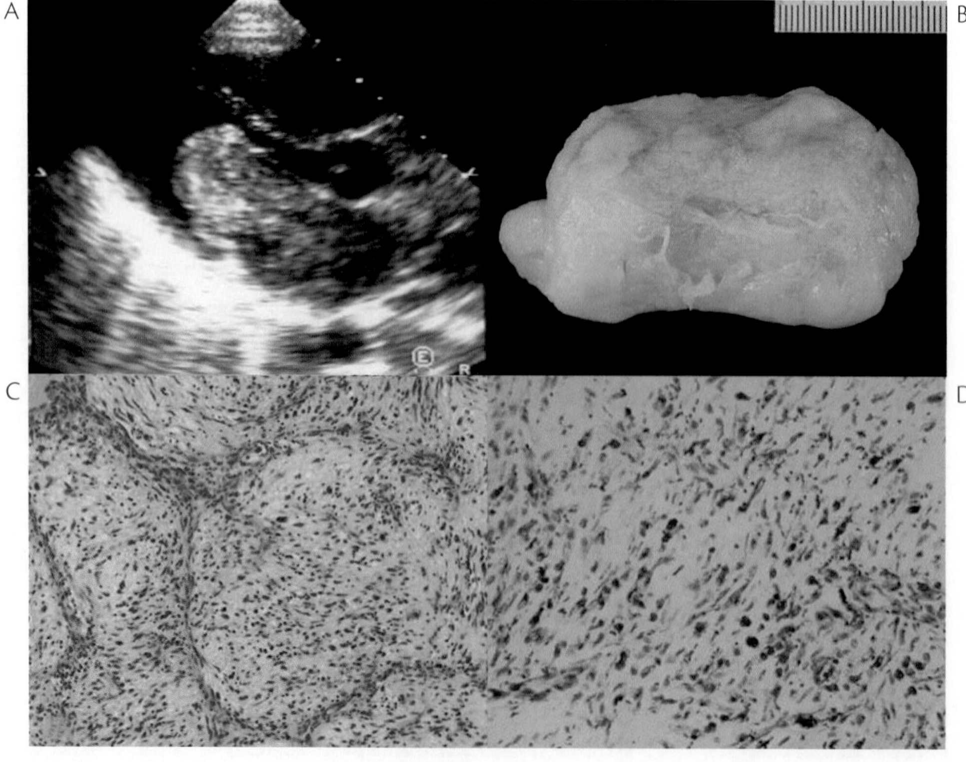

Figure 20.20 Left atrial leiomyosarcoma in a 21-year-old woman with a preoperative diagnosis of myxoma. (A) Two-dimensional echocardiography, parasternal long-axis view: note the left atrial mass prolapsing into the left ventricular cavity during diastole. (B) Macroscopic appearance of the resected mass which appears firm, not myxoid, and with a rough surface. (C) At histology, storiform proliferation of pleomorphic cells. (D) Immunohistochemistry shows diffuse positivity for smooth muscle markers (desmin). Modified from Mazzola A, Spano JP, Valente M, *et al.* Leiomyosarcoma of the left atrium mimicking a left atrial myxoma. *J Thorac Cardiovasc Surg* 2006; **131**: 224–6, with permission from Elsevier.

[79], but also infiltrating the pulmonary veins. The second typical location is the pulmonary infundibulum and artery, where it may present abruptly mimicking pulmonary embolism [80].

Grossly, the mass is irregular, whitish or grey, with a rough surface and quite solid. Histologically, fascicles of spindle cells, oriented at right angles, and with blunt-ended nuclei mitoses are visible. Pleomorphism, giant cells, and necrosis are focally present. The tumour histotype diagnosis is reached through immunohistochemical positivity for smooth muscle-specific actin and desmin. Although the prognosis is generally poor, survival up to 7 years has been reported after surgical removal followed by adjuvant chemotherapy [80].

Liposarcoma

This is a very rare cardiac mesenchymal malignant tumour of the adult, consisting of lipoblasts. It is usually a bulky endocavitary left atrial mass, mimicking myxoma [9, 11, 81].

The tumour is yellow, tender, and frequently mucoid. There are two types at cardiac level, one pleomorphic mimicking malignant fibrous histiocytoma and the other myxoid. The neoplastic cell is the lipoblast, which in the pleomorphic form is full of cytoplasmic fatty vacuoles, whereas the myxoid histotype shows a single, large cytoplasmic vacuole of fat which compress the nucleus with the shape of signet ring. The myxoid type of liposarcoma is highly vascularized. Some liposarcomas show both myxoid and pleomorphic features. At immunohistochemistry, the lipoblasts express S100 antigen. With electron microscopy, the lipid vacuoles do not exhibit a discrete membrane.

Synovial sarcoma

The name is a misnomer, since this primary neoplasm does not arise from or differentiate towards synovia [82]. In the heart, it has a typical primary location in the atria and pericardium, where in the past it has been confused with the sarcomatoid variant of malignant mesothelioma. When in the pericardium, in contrast to malignant mesothelioma which tends to grow diffusely, it is a solitary localized mass.

Grossly, it appears as a solid, whitish infiltrative mass, with areas of haemorrhage or necrosis. Histologically, it shows two variants, one 'biphasic' with both spindle and epithelioid cells with nested or glandular structures, and one 'monophasic', in which only spindle cells are present in the setting of interstitial oedema.

At immunohistochemistry the epithelioid cells express cytokeratin and the epithelial membrane antigen, whereas fusiform cells are positive for vimentin.

A definite diagnosis may be achieved only through molecular biology techniques with the detection of molecular markers, namely SS18/SSX transcripts.

Cardiac lymphoma

Extranodal lymphomas do exist with exclusive involvement of the heart and/or the pericardium [83]. Overall, they represent 10% of primary cardiac malignant neoplasms, i.e. 1% of all cardiac primary tumours. Age varies from 5–90 years (median 60), male:female ratio is approximately 3:1, and onset occurs not necessarily in immune-deficient people. Prognosis is usually fatal, with a mean survival of 7 months.

The clinical course presentation has usually an acute onset, with chest pain, pericardial effusion, congestive heart failure, arrhythmias, syncope, and even complete AV block.

Primary cardiac lymphomas may arise in any cardiac chamber, but in two-thirds of cases the right atrium is the site of involvement with an intramural, whitish infiltrating mass extended to pericardium with massive effusion. The subtype most frequently observed (80% of cases) is B-cell lymphoma with huge, CD20-positive cells, whereas the remaining 20% are CD3-positive T-cell lymphomas.

Cytology of pericardial effusion may be of help for diagnosis, by using molecular techniques to differentiate B- and T-cell lymphomas from reactive lymphocyte hyperplasia. Primary cardiac lymphomas should be promptly treated like aggressive lymphomas in other sites, since a late diagnosis is the major determinant of a poor prognosis.

Malignant tumours of the pericardium

Solitary fibrous tumour

Also known as benign mesothelioma, fibrous mesothelioma, or submesothelial fibroma, this is a well-circumscribed, even huge solid mass with local invasion [84]. Clinical presentation is related to pericardial mass effect.

Although histological variability is the rule, most tumours consist of a proliferation of spindle cells, with either fibrous or myxoid areas, which react positively to CD34 and bcl-2.

Differential diagnosis is made with malignant mesothelioma, which is diffuse and shows positive immunohistochemistry for keratin and calretinin; with low-grade fibrosarcoma, the cells of which are CD34-negative; and with monophasic synovial sarcoma, which may show focal keratin positivity. Overall, the prognosis is good despite the tendency to recurrence after resection.

Malignant mesothelioma

This derives from pericardial mesothelium and is extremely rare (1% of all malignant mesothelioma, including those of pleura and peritoneum) [85]. It is also related to asbestos exposure, although radiotherapy for mediastinal neoplasms and breast cancer may play a causative role in some cases.

It affects individuals of any age (mean 45 years) and manifests itself with haemorrhagic pericardial effusion, leading even to cardiac tamponade, and congestive heart failure due to pericardial constriction. The clinical imaging (echocardiography, but mainly CMR or CT) of diffuse pericardial thickening and masses, besides effusion, is highly suspicious. It is imperative to rule out any neoplasm, especially from lungs with secondary pericardial involvement. The gross features consist of multiple nodules plugging the pericardial cavity or of a diffuse pericardial thickening, involving both venous (venae cava) and arterial (aorta and pulmonary artery) poles.

Histologically, the tumour cells may have two distinct patterns: epithelioid, with papillary or tubular structures, or sarcomatoid. The cells are positive to calretinin and cytokeratins 5 and 6 and negative to carcinoembryonic antigen (CEA), the latter instead being positive in pericardial metastasis of adenocarcinoma. Presence of long cell microvilli at electron microscopy is also diagnostic.

The prognosis is very poor with fatal outcome within a few months from onset. Distal metastases are extremely unusual.

Malignant germinal cell tumour

The great majority of germinal cell tumours of the pericardium are benign teratomas [9]. In the framework of a benign teratoma, malignant areas may be observed with a feature of a 'yolk sac tumour', secreting alfa-fetoprotein. The prognosis depends upon the extension of these malignant areas.

A true 'yolk sac tumour' of the pericardium has been reported only once.

Cardiac metastases

In principle, any extracardiac malignant tumour may metastasize to the heart. When a patient affected by malignancy develops otherwise unexplained cardiac symptoms, a metastasis to the heart should be suspected. The postmortem rate of cardiac metastases in people with malignancy varies from 4–18% [8, 9, 11]. Bussani and colleagues [86] reported 662 patients among 7289 (9.1%), with a decreasing occurrence with age (16.8% in people aged <64 years vs. 8.5% in people >85 years), probably due to less biological aggressiveness in the elderly. Melanoma, lung carcinoma, and breast cancer show the highest cardiotropism in terms of metastases. Usually cardiac metastases occur in the setting of multiorgan secondary involvement, but early and sole metastasis to the heart may also be encountered. Cardiac involvement of lymphomas is usually intramural, with invasion and infiltration of the myocardium by a greyish lymphoproliferative mass. The cardiac involvement is higher in non-Hodgkin vs. Hodgkin lymphoma.

The metastatic localization may involve the pericardium with haemorrhagic pericardial effusion and signs and symptoms of cardiac tamponade, like paradoxical pulse and decreased QRS voltage on 12-lead ECG. Pericardiocentesis is mandatory to relieve the constriction and cytological examination of the effusion is of great help in establishing the neoplastic nature and tumour histotype. In the most advanced forms, constriction persists despite of pericardiocentesis, because of diffuse neoplastic thickening of the epicardium like a sheath.

In case of intramural myocardial metastasis, the clinical picture relies on the site and extension of neoplastic invasion: atrial and ventricular arrhythmias, including flutter and fibrillation, and conduction disturbances, when the conduction tissue is involved. In case of multiple or obstructive metastases, congestive heart failure may also occur. Endocardial metastases may be observed of such a size to create endocavitary obstruction. This is a typical behaviour of renal carcinoma and hepatocarcinoma, which diffuse alongside the inferior vena cava and may obliterate the caval orifice, right atrium, and tricuspid orifice (neoplastic 'thrombosis'). Signs of myocardial ischaemia may develop, including myocardial infarction because of outside compression from metastases or infiltration of a major coronary artery or, more rarely, because of neoplastic embolism. Even the coronary sinus may be involved. Lung carcinoma may infiltrate the pulmonary veins and invade the left atrium. When huge, the metastasis may block the mitral valve orifice. Small neoplastic metastases may be observed, scattered in the sub-endocardium of the right atrium and ventricle within the pectinate muscles and trabeculae, in the absence of any symptom. They may be the consequence of direct haematogenous dissemination. It is interesting to note the virtual absence of valvular metastases, most probably because valves lack vascularization and are in continuous movement as to hinder malignant secondary settlement.

There are four pathways of metastatic involvement of the heart: 1) direct infiltration as in the case of mediastinal and lung malignancies; 2) haematic, in the case of distant primary neoplasm; 3) lymphatic due to a spread through the trachea-mediastinal lymphatic network, especially in case of lung carcinoma (pericardial 'carcinosis'); and 4) endocavitary diffusion through the inferior vena cava and pulmonary veins.

As far as clinical diagnosis is concerned, when the primary source is known, cardiac imaging may easily detect the secondary cardiac involvement. In case of pericardial effusion and unknown extracardiac malignancy, cytology of the pericardiocentesis fluid or pericardial biopsy through thoracotomy may be of great help. Differential diagnosis with infective-inflammatory disease of the pericardium should be taken into account. In case of metastases to the pericardium of lung adenocarcinoma, the differential diagnosis is with innocent reactive mesothelial hyperplasia, observed in acute, non-neoplastic pericarditis and with malignant mesothelioma with glandular histotype. The use of immunohistochemistry is essential to this aim. Mesothelioma, in contrast to lung adenocarcinoma, is positive for vimentin and calretinin.

Endomyocardial biopsy is a useful diagnostic tool in case of endocavitary growth (➲Fig. 20.9) [25]. Again the use of immunohistochemistry is fundamental for establishing the tumour histotype.

Chemotherapy, radiotherapy, and cardiotoxicity in malignant cardiac neoplasms

Surgical resection, if feasible, and even cardiac transplantation may be accomplished in heart malignancies, in the absence of extracardiac metastases [87–91]. Otherwise, chemoradiotherapy is the only therapeutic option.

Moreover, in cases of primary sarcomas, use of radiotherapy is carried out before surgery, to facilitate complete removal, and after surgery as adjuvant support to reduce/prevent recurrences.

The prophylactic dose of 6000–6500cGy is usually employed as adjuvant whereas, in case of unresectable or residual masses, the dose is increased to 7000cGy. With a 6000cGy dose in the cardiac field, attinic pericarditis has been reported with an incidence of 40%.

Chemotherapy consists of antibiotics with cytotoxic antineoplastic activity, such as those employed in the treatment of onco-haematologic and soft tissue malignancies. Anthracyclines like epirubicin and doxorubicin are usually used for therapy of cardiac sarcomas, in association with ifosfamide, with the protocols reported in ➲Table 20.3 [92–95].

They are particularly indicated in cardiac sarcomas with high-grade malignancy, resulting from a high score of differentiation, mitosis, and tumour necrosis. In aggressive cardiac sarcomas, with residual tumour at surgery and evidence of distant metastases, chemotherapy plays a palliative role in reducing tumour mass and relieving symptoms, but unfortunately does not increase survival significantly, with a mean time survival of 11 months. We reported an exceptional long-term survival of 5 years in a patient with a low-grade malignancy case of leiomyosarcoma [79].

The therapeutic efficacy of chemotherapy is limited by cardiotoxicity with a safe threshold of 550mg/m^2 for doxorubicin and of 900mg/m^2 for epirubicin. Three types of cardiotoxicity by anthracyclines have been reported: 1) acute or subacute symptoms occurring early after infusion with transient arrhythmias, perimyocarditis syndrome, and left ventricular failure; 2) chronic toxicity occurring within 1 year in the form of dilated cardiomyopathy; and 3) ventricular dysfunction with late occurrence, years or decades after treatment, with arrhythmias and congestive heart failure [8, 96, 97].

The occurrence of cardiac decompensation is clearly dose-dependent with an incidence of 0.14% for a total dose of doxorubicin of 400mg/m^2, 7% for 550mg/m^2, and 18% for 700mg/m^2. However, recently a 26% incidence of heart failure has been reported for 550mg/m^2 doxorubicin, questioning the safety of this threshold [8]. Previous mediastinal radiotherapy may be an additional risk factor.

The myocardial injury consists of sarcolysis with loss of myofibrils. Increased release of calcium from endoplasmic reticulum with free radicals production and release of cytokines from macrophage (tumour necrosis factor

Table 20.3 Anthracyclines and ifosfamide protocols for therapy of cardiac sarcomas

	Epirubicin	**Ifosfamide**
Dose	60mg/m^2/day	1800mg/m^2/day
Frequency	1st, 2nd day/every 21 days	1st–5th day/every 21 days
	Doxorubicin	**Ifosfamide**
Dose	50mg/m^2/day	5000mg/m^2/day
Frequency	1st day/every 21 days	1st day/every 21 days
	Doxorubicin	**Ifosfamide**
Dose	25mg/m^2/day continuous infusion	2000mg/m^2/day
Frequency	1st– 3rd day/every 21 days	1st– 5th day/every 21 days

Table 20.4 Chemotherapy protocol for cardiac lymphomas

	Cyclophosphamide	Doxorubicin	Vincristine	Prednisone	Rituximab
Dose	750mg/m^2	50mg/m^2	1.4mg/m^2	100mg/m^2	375mg/m^2
Frequency	Day 1/every 21 days	Day 1/every 21 days	Day 1/every 21 days	Day 1/every 21 days	Days 1, 8, 15, 22, 43, 60, 85, 106

(TNFα) and interleukin-2 (IL-2)) have been advanced as possible mechanisms.

Continuous drug infusion instead of a bolus, use of less toxic epirubicin in place of doxorubicin, and employment of a cardioprotector like dexrazoxane for patients with a doxorubicin dose >300mg/m^2 have been recommended. Selective release of doxorubicin by liposomes into the tumour field may reduce cardiotoxicity by preserving anti-tumour efficacy [8].

For primary cardiac lymphomas, 80% of which are B-cell subtype, the chemotherapy treatment is that of extranodal lymphomas as indicated in ➲Table 20.4. Rituximab is a monoclonal antibody against CD20 antigen, chimeric for man and mouse. Cardiotoxicity of doxorubicin is limited because the dose employed is lower. Side effects are of less importance and occur in 10% of cases: hypertension, angio-oedema, bronchospasm with hypoxic spells, can easily be kept under control with appropriate therapy.

It is worthwhile pointing out that primary cardiac lymphomas, with chemotherapy, are the only malignant cardiac neoplasms to present a fairly good prognosis [8].

A special cardiotoxicity has been observed in breast cancers with cardiac mestastases, treated with transtuzumab (Herceptin®), a monoclonal antibody against the protein coded by the *HER2* (human epidermal growth factor oncogen), the overexpression of which is associated with a very poor prognosis [98]. Unlike doxorubicin toxicity, transtuzumab toxicity is less severe, not dose-related, and may be reversible. It has been postulated that this antibody may interfere with calcium inflow–outflow from T-tubules and Z bands of the sarcomere.

Non-neoplastic masses

Only histological examination may establish whether a cardiac mass is neoplastic, either benign or malignant. When seen by clinical imaging, the use of the term 'mass' is advisable, since it may have several explanations other than cardiac tumours [8].

- **Thrombi**. An isolated mass inside an atrial appendage is almost exclusively a thrombus. In the left atrium, free-floating masses 'ball thrombus'-like should point to a mitral valve pathology, usually rheumatic in origin. Small mural thrombi may be observed at the apex of the left ventricle, even in the setting of normal contractility, and misinterpreted clinically as left ventricular myxomas (➲Fig. 20.4A and B). Non-bacterial thrombotic endocarditis may mimic valve papillary fibroelastoma. Valvular and non-valvular endocardial thrombosis may be observed in antiphospholipid syndrome [99].
- **Cardiomyopathies (➲Chapter 18).** Endocardial fibroplastic Loeffler endocarditis is a restrictive (obliterative) cardiomyopathy, usually associated with eosinophilia, hypersensitivity, or eosinophilic leukaemia, consisting of a mural thrombus filling the apical and inflow portions of the ventricles to such an extent to entrap the mitral and/or tricuspid valves apparatus. Cardiac imaging may misdiagnose an apical form of hypertrophic cardiomyopathy or an endocardial tumour. Endomyocardial biopsy with tissue characterization may be of help for differential diagnosis (➲Fig. 20.21).
- **Infections (➲Chapter 22).** Valve masses may be infective vegetations mimicking papillary fibroelastoma, and sometimes at the mitral level they may be so huge as to simulate embolizing atrial myxoma. Free-floating masses may not necessarily be thrombotic, but even septic (fungal in immunosuppressed patients) (➲Fig. 20.22) [100]. Pericardial or myocardial cysts may be hydatid cysts by echinococcosis, to be treated cautiously during the surgery to avoid rupture and spread of infection.
- **Calcium**. Calcium stones, intramural or intracavitary [101], may occur and not necessarily are the outcome of dystrophic calcification of previous infections/tumours, as in the case of lithomyxoma. The phenomenon may be so massive as to transform the heart into a sort of a stone quarry. Dystrophic calcification of the mitral valve annulus can also account for misdiagnosis of an AV mass by echocardiography.

Surgical treatment

Surgical treatment of cardiac neoplasms became available with the advent of open heart surgery with cardiac arrest and extracorporeal circulation in the 1950s. There are rare conditions of pericardial tumours in which resection may be

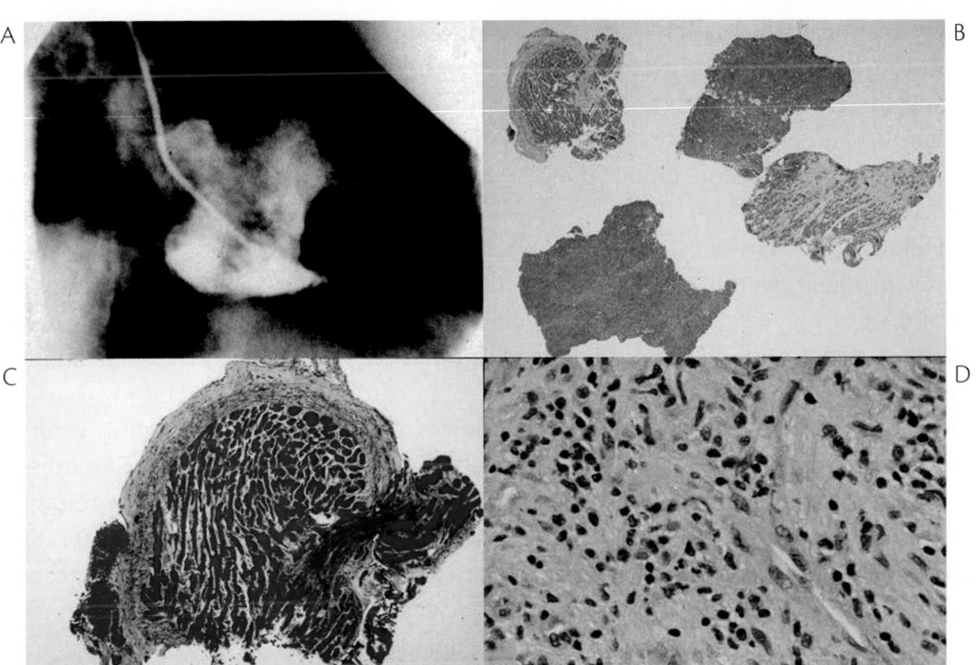

Figure 20.21 Loeffler fibroplastic endocarditis in a 61-year-old man with an apical left ventricular mass. (A) Ventricular angiography showing a round mass occupying the left ventricular apex. (B) Endomyocardial biopsy samples consist of both thrombus and myocardial tissue (haematoxylin eosin stain). (C) Endocardial fibrous thickening is visible at higher magnification (Heidenhain trichrome stain). (D) The underlying myocardium reveals inflammatory infiltrates with frequent eosinophils (haematoxylin-eosin stain). Modified from Basso C, Valente M, Thiene G. *Tumori del cuore. Monografie di Cardiologia. Società Italiana di Cardiologia*, 2005. Novate-Milan: Arti Grafiche Color Black.

accomplished with thoracotomy but without the need of circulatory arrest. Taking into consideration that 90% of primary cardiac tumours are endocavitary, they require the opening of the heart and/or great arteries to be removed [102–104].

Before the development of non-invasive cardiac imaging, the indication for surgery could erroneously be valve disease, because diagnosis was frequently accomplished by simple auscultation, X-ray, and symptoms. At the Mayo Clinic, prior to the advent of echocardiography in the 1980s, nearly 25% of surgically resected myxomas were mistakenly sent to surgery for rheumatic mitral valve stenosis [5]. Nowadays, thanks also to the speed of ultrasound examination, no patient with a cardiac mass undergoes surgery without imaging investigation. CT and CMR add further information regarding the extent of infiltration in cases of malignancies and tissue characterization. Right ventricular cardiac catheterization provides information on the pulmonary blood pressure and selective coronary angiography visualizes the coronary artery tree for detection of obstructive atherosclerotic plaques, to be surgically treated as well, and the amount of mass vascularization.

Benign tumours are usually approached through medial sternotomy and extracorporeal circulation with bicaval drainage. Because of friability of most endocavitary cardiac

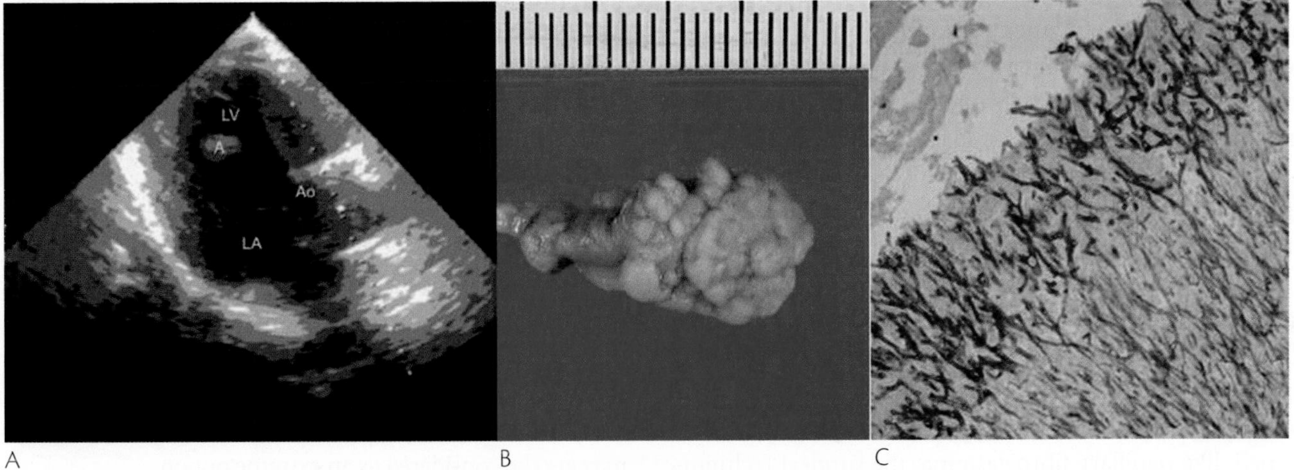

Figure 20.22 Left ventricular intracavitary aspergilloma in a 23-year-old man who underwent chemotherapy for acute myeloid leukaemia. (A) Two-dimensional echocardiography showing a mobile mass inside the left ventricular cavity. (B) Gross view of the resected elongated mass which shows a small pedicle and an irregular surface. (C) At histology, fungal ifae of aspergillus are detected (Alcian PAS stain). Modified from Vida V, Biffanti R, Thiene G, *et al.* Left ventricular mass after treatment with chemotherapic drugs. *Circulation* 2004; **109**: e300–e301.

tumours, soft manipulation of the heart is recommended ('no-touch technique'). Intraoperative transoesophageal echocardiography is of great help to define tumour localization, to guide cannulation and the opening of cardiac cavities, and to monitor tumour integrity during surgical procedures.

Following the start of extracorporeal circulation, a moderate corporeal hypothermia is induced (28°–32°C) and then the heart is separated from the systemic perfusion by clamping the ascending aorta and stopped in diastole by perfusing the coronary tree with high potassium cardioplegia, either anterogradely via coronary arteries from the aortic root, or retrogradely via the coronary sinus.

The surgical approach then varies, according to the site of the tumour, with right, left, or combined atriotomy. In any case, a thorough exploration of all cardiac chambers is advisable.

A wide surgical exposure is a 'conditio sine qua non' for en-bloc resection of the tumour, including the implant base. Aspiration of blood surrounding the tumour is not returned to the extracorporeal circulation, to avoid possible dissemination of neoplastic emboli.

As far as the left atrial myxoma is concerned, which is frequently attached to the fossa ovalis, the surgical approach may be right atrial or trans-septal. Left atriotomy may be also performed to improve mass exposure. Resection is extended at least 5mm around the base of implant to ensure radical excision of the neoplasm in order to prevent recurrence. In case of attachment of the myxoma to the free wall, the latter is removed with the tumour at full thickness or, if not possible, with a deep endomyocardial excavation. During resection the mass should be manipulated gently to prevent fragmentation. Following removal, the cardiac chambers are copiously irrigated with saline solution to remove neoplastic fragments. Exploration of the pulmonary artery and aorta, in case of right- or left-sided masses removal, is also advisable through separate arteriotomy to exclude migration of neoplastic fragments. Closure of the residual atrial septal defect is accomplished through autologous pericardial patch or with a patch of polytetrafluoretilene (PTFE).

In case of endocavitary ventricular neoplasm, a surgical approach is accomplished through an ipsilateral atriotomy, if the neoplasm is located in the ventricular inflow, or through aortic or pulmonary arteriotomy if located in the ventricular outflow. As far as valvular neoplasms are concerned, like papillary fibroelastoma, the surgical technique should try to preserve the native valve with complete tumour removal and its attachment, even using reconstructive techniques with autologous pericardium. If a conservative approach is not feasible, valve replacement is necessary using prosthetic biological or mechanical devices.

When the neoplasm is intramural in the ventricles, ventriculotomy with mass enucleation is necessary.

If risk of enucleation would result in an excessive reduction of ventricular myocardium or damage of vital cardiac structures (valves, conduction system, septa), cardiac transplantation is the extreme option [105]. Cardiomyoplasty (➲Chapter 23) has been even advanced as an alternative to heart transplantation for the therapy of large ventricular tumours [106].

After weaning from extracorporeal circulation, transoesophageal echocardiography has to be performed to assess the extent of the resection, valve integrity, and myocardial function as well as the absence of residual shunts. Histological examination of the removed mass, even in 'myxomatous' neoplasms, is mandatory to rule out malignancies.

Hospital surgical mortality for benign intracavitary tumours, like myxoma and papillary fibroelastoma, is <5% and long-term survival and quality of life are excellent in 'sporadic' benign neoplasms.

Relapses of myxoma may be the consequence of incomplete resection or of neoplastic fragment dissemination, but more frequently occur in the 'familial' form of myxomas, genetic in origin, which are often associated with multicentric lesions.

With regards to cardiac malignancies, several options may be considered. Resection, which is rarely complete in infiltrating sarcomas, may be carried out even in deep hypothermia (17°C) with circulatory arrest, to clean the operative field as more as possible. Total heart removal with *ex-vivo* repair on the bench, followed by auto-transplant, has been also carried out. The association of surgical resection with adjuvant chemotherapy may improve survival.

In selected cases of right-sided malignant tumours, Fontan-like operations like cavopulmonary or atriopulmonary anastomoses to bypass the right heart may be considered as a palliative procedure.

Orthotopic cardiac transplantation (➲Chapter 23) has also been accomplished in non-resectable cases, but this should only be considered in the absence of metastases.

The results are good when the tumour is benign. In malignancies, the mean survival is poor, as to question the indication for cardiac transplantation with such a bad prognosis considering the shortage of donor hearts. In the case of pulmonary metastases, combined heart and lung transplantation may also be considered as an extreme option.

Secondary cardiac tumour may also be helped with cardiac surgery. Palliative procedures may be carried out to relieve symptoms and achieve a diagnosis (subxyphoid pericardiotomy with external drainage and biopsy, pleura-pericardial drainage).

Subdiaphragmatic tumours, like renal carcinoma, hepatocarcinoma, and ovarian carcinoma, may invade the inferior vena cava and extend to the right atrium. Ten per cent of renal carcinomas infiltrate the inferior vena cava and 40% of them reach the right atrium. The neoplastic 'thrombus' is usually adherent to the endothelium of the vena cava or to endocardium of the right atrium. Surgery aims to combine removal of the primary lesion and its extension to the inferior vena cava–right atrium. In case of renal carcinoma, selective cannulation of the superior vena cava and ascending aorta is first made and then, during deep hypothermia and circulatory arrest, the right atrium is opened and the mass removed from both the atrium and inferior vena cava with endocardial–endothelial cleavage and smooth dissection. Transection of the renal vein and nephrectomy is carried out thereafter, checking the right atrial cavity and with blood aspiration not returned to extracorporeal circulation. Results of nephrectomy associated with inferior vena cava–right atrial resection of neoplastic thrombus are good, with 75% survival at 5-year follow-up [107, 108].

Personal perspective

The following steps forward may be expected in the near future:

Improvements in diagnosis. The neoplastic nature and histotype of a cardiac mass can be established nowadays only by histology. With technological advances, contrast echocardiography, CMR, and CT might detect pathognomonic tissue characteristics in a highly sensitive and specific manner, with fundamental diagnostic, therapeutic, and prognostic implications.

Refinements in surgical and interventional therapy. Cardiac tumours are resected at surgery through sternotomy, cardiopulmonary bypass, and open heart procedures. Mini-invasive techniques and robotic surgery are nowadays accomplished in valve and coronary surgery, to minimize surgical trauma. Invasive, non-surgical approaches are expected for small tumours, like papillary fibroelastoma, which might be removed without thoracotomy.

Progress in understanding cancer development and progression. The treatment of malignancies is generally based on histologic grade, resectability and the presence or absence of metastasis. Because interventions after the manifestation of metastases are notoriously ineffective, a great effort is being made to identify the molecular mechanisms that mediate malignant transformation and to understand the molecular basis of metastasis. Transgenic mouse models may elucidate the pathogenesis of cardiac sarcomas and allow the testing of new therapeutic approaches. Meanwhile, a less toxic chemotherapy should be tested.

Knowledge in epidemiology. Cardiac tumours, particularly primary malignant neoplasms, are rare. National and international registries are needed, to establish epidemiology, prevalence, histotypes, and therapeutic efficacy, as well as clinical trials of chemotherapy protocols with follow-up and prognosis. Central core laboratories should be established for clinical imaging and histopathology. The European Society of Cardiology should consider managing this task.

Further reading

Basso C, Valente M, Poletti A, *et al.* Surgical pathology of primary cardiac and pericardial tumours. *Eur J Cardiothorac Surg* 1997; **12**: 730–7.

Burke AP, Virmani R. *Tumours of the Heart and Great Vessels*, 3rd edn., 1996. Washington DC: Armed Forces Institute of Pathology.

Butany J, Nair V, Naseemuddin A, *et al.* Cardiac tumours: diagnosis and management. *Lancet Oncol* 2005; **6**: 219–28.

Travis WD, Brambilla E, Muller-Hermelink H, *et al. Pathology and Genetics of Tumours of the Lung, Pleura, Thymus and Heart*, 2004. Lyon: IARC Press.

➲ For full references and multimedia materials please visit the online version of the book (http://esctextbook.oxfordonline.com).

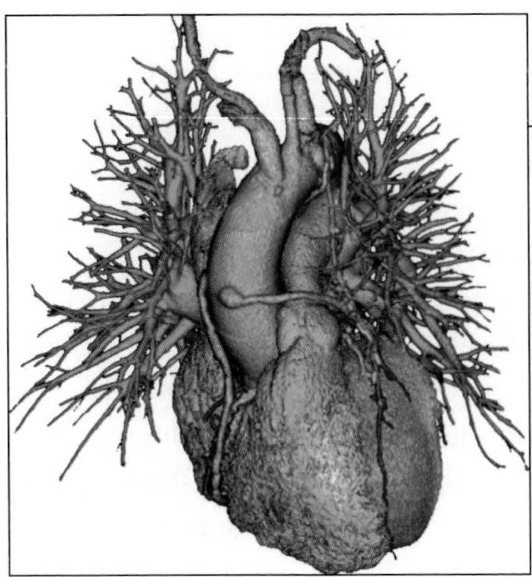

CHAPTER 21

Valvular Heart Disease

Alec Vahanian, Bernard Iung, Luc Piérard, Robert Dion, and John Pepper

Contents

Summary

Valvular heart disease (VHD), although not as common as coronary disease, heart failure, or hypertension, is an important, and challenging, clinical entity. It is of interest for the following reasons: substantial advances have been made in the understanding of its pathophysiology; important changes in patient characteristics and aetiologies have occurred over recent years; diagnosis is now largely dominated by non-invasive imaging, especially echocardiography which has become the standard to evaluate valve structure and function; and, finally, treatment has not only developed through the continuing progress in prosthetic valve technology, but also has been re-orientated by the development of conservative surgical techniques and the development of interventional cardiology.

This chapter will provide an updated review of the main aspects of each acquired valve disease in adults, and include the important sub-group of patients who have previously undergone valve surgery. It will also present principles of management with regards to diagnosis and treatment that are derived from the most recent guidelines. Useful complements to this chapter can be found in ➲ Chapters 4 (Cardiac Ultrasound), 10 (Congenital Heart Disease in Children and Adults), 22 (Infective Endocarditis), and 34 (Pregnancy and Heart Disease).

Introduction

Epidemiology

There have been important changes in the distribution of the aetiologies of VHD in Western countries over the last 50 years. The continuous decline of acute rheumatic fever explains the decrease in the incidence of rheumatic valve disease, which has been compensated by an increase in the incidence of degenerative valvular diseases.

In a study including systematic echocardiographic examinations in large randomly-selected populations from the US, the prevalence of VHDs was estimated at 2.5%, while in another patient cohort in a community study, using echocardiography when clinical signs were found, the incidence was 1.8%, underlining the fact that valve disease is still under diagnosed [1]. Prevalence did not change according to gender but was highly related to age: the figure being 13.2% after the age of 75 years (➲Fig. 21.1). In the Euro Heart Survey the mean age was 65 years in patients presenting to hospital, 38% being aged >70 years [2]. The higher prevalence in the elderly is related to the predominance of degenerative aetiologies in all types of heart valve diseases, except mitral stenosis (MS) [2]. Due to the predominance of degenerative valve diseases, calcified aortic stenosis (AS) and mitral regurgitation (MR) are the two most frequent native valve diseases, while aortic regurgitation (AR) and MS have become unusual.

The frequency of degenerative valve disease increases with increasing age. In Western countries, life expectancy and the proportion of elderly patients in the population is rising. Thus the number of patients with degenerative valve diseases is expected to grow in the future.

Despite the decrease in the incidence of rheumatic fever, with an estimated prevalence of <0.5 per 1000 in Western countries, rheumatic heart disease remains the second most frequent cause of heart valve disease in Europe [2](21.1). It is encountered either in young immigrants or in older patients originating from Western countries who were exposed to acute rheumatic fever when it was still endemic.

The incidence of infective endocarditis has been estimated at approximately 30 cases per million in France from two prospective surveys, and this did not change between 1991 and 1999 [3]. Infective endocarditis occurs in the absence of previously known heart valve disease in almost half of cases.

Congenital heart valve disease is a rare aetiology of valve dysfunction except for bicuspid aortic valve, which affects 0.5–1% of the population and is the most common reason for aortic valve surgery in patients <70 years of age.

Other less common aetiologies include inflammatory, carcinoid, drug- or radiation-related valve disease [2, 4, 5].

Another particularity of contemporary heart valve disease in Western countries is the growing proportion of previously operated patients, who accounted for 28% of patients in the Euro Heart Survey [2].

Unlike in Western countries, acute rheumatic fever remains endemic in developing countries, which explains a high prevalence of chronic rheumatic heart valve diseases. A report from the World Health Organization estimates prevalence rates between 2–15 per 1000 in school children and adolescents in Africa [6]. A survey estimated the prevalence of rheumatic valve disease at 5.7 per 1000 in Pakistan, with no decrease over time [7]. Most patients were not aware of the diagnosis and prophylaxis was underused.

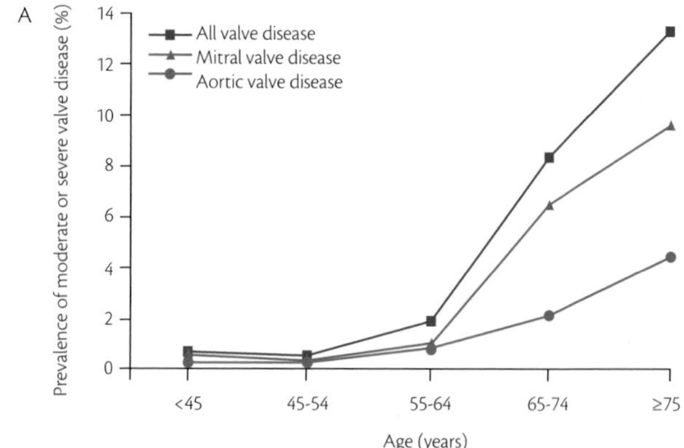

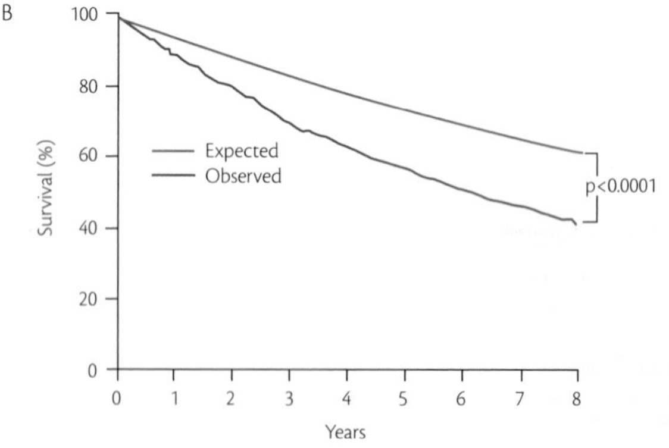

Number at risk	971	863	765	667	589	518	449	392	73
Expected survival	100%	94%	88%	83%	78%	73%	69%	65%	61%

Figure 21.1 Prevalence and consequences on outcome of valvular heart disease. (A) Prevalence of valvular heart disease by age. Population had prospectively defined echocardiographic valvular analysis. (B) Survival after detection of moderate or severe valvular heart disease. Survival in population-based studies. The blue line represents survival of 971 residents diagnosed with valve diseases between 1990 and 1995; the red line represents the expected survival in the age-matched and sex-matched population of the county. Adapted with permission from Nkomo VT, Gardin JM, Skelton TN, *et al.* Burden of valvular heart diseases: a population-based study. *Lancet* 2006; **368**: 1005–11.

These findings are likely to be underestimated when obtained only using clinical screening, since systematic echocardiographic screening provides higher prevalence rates, as shown in a recent series of 5847 children from Cambodia and Mozambique. Respective prevalences were estimated at 21.5 and 30.4 per 1000 when using systematic echocardiographic screening, whereas the corresponding estimations using clinical screening alone were 2.2 and 2.3 per 1000, respectively [8].

The number of valve procedures has not decreased in surgical registries from Western countries [9]. Surgical series analysing temporal trends over the two last decades have consistently shown that changing frequencies in aetiologies of valve disease have important implications in patient presentation and management [10].

Finally, increased age is associated with a higher frequency of comorbidity, which contributes to increased operative risk and also to decreased life expectancy, thereby rendering decision making for intervention more complex [2].

Patient evaluation

Clinical evaluation

Case history

Case history is the first contact with the patient and remains of utmost importance to assess symptoms. Dyspnoea reflects the poor tolerance of VHD and it has an important prognostic value. Except in highly disabled patients, shortness of breath may be difficult to assess because of its subjective component, particularly in patients who claim to be asymptomatic, and in the elderly, who often adapt their activity to their functional capacity. It is necessary to spend time with the patient to analyse his/her lifestyle and to search for progressive changes in daily activity. Repeated clinical evaluations are useful in this setting. Although fatigue is not specific, it may be an equivalent of dyspnoea, particularly in the elderly. Other symptoms are angina pectoris and syncope or equivalents.

The case history is also the first step in the assessment of comorbidities, which play an important role in decision making for interventions, particularly in the elderly. In patients with previously known heart valve disease, and even more so in patients who have previously undergone valve intervention, the case history may be used to assess the quality of follow-up, knowledge of endocarditis prophylaxis, and anticoagulant therapy.

It is also necessary to search for minor complications. For example, transient ischaemic attack or minor bleeding are complications that are frequently overlooked by the patient.

Clinical examination

The detection of a murmur is the most frequent way of detecting VHD in an asymptomatic patient or of relating symptoms to a valvular cause. Auscultation often gives the first clue to the severity of VHD. It should be noted that patients with heart failure can have low-intensity murmurs despite severe underlying valve disease.

Clinical signs of heart failure are usually only encountered at advanced stages of VHD. These signs have a strong prognostic utility. Clinical examination also contributes to the search for comorbidities, in particular peripheral atherosclerosis.

Electrocardiogram and chest X-ray are generally performed with clinical examination. Analysis of pulmonary vascular distribution is useful in the interpretation of dyspnoea.

Investigations

Echocardiography

Echocardiography is the cornerstone of investigations of VHD. It is indicated in the patient with a cardiac murmur, except in certain young patients who have a trivial mid-systolic murmur (i.e. innocent murmur) [11, 12].

The aim of echocardiography is to confirm the diagnosis of VHD, to assess its severity, mechanism, and consequences, and to search for associated lesions, such as associated valve disease and abnormalities of the ascending aorta.

The general rule for quantifying of the severity of valvular disease is to combine and check for the consistency of different indices and to be aware of potential errors of measurements [11–13]. Thus, examinations should be performed by experienced echocardiographers who have experience in the field of VHDs.

The assessment of valve anatomy and the mechanism of valve dysfunction are important when conservative interventions are being considered. Real-time three-dimensional echocardiography has the advantage of providing a comprehensive assessment of valve anatomy but its incremental usefulness in decision making remains to be assessed.

Measurements of left ventricular (LV) enlargement and systolic function play an important role in decision making for intervention in regurgitant valve diseases. They should be indexed to body surface area (BSA) while keeping in mind the limitations of indexing for extreme body sizes.

Transoesophageal echocardiography is not a routine investigation. It is indicated in the rare cases of suboptimal transthoracic imaging or in case of suspected thrombosis, prosthetic valve dysfunction, or endocarditis. It is also indicated to monitor the results of valve repair during surgery.

Other non-invasive investigations

Stress testing is mainly used to assess the objective tolerance of VHDs [14] and to unmask dyspnoea in patients who claim to be asymptomatic. It may also have an additional prognostic value. Exercise echocardiography can detect dynamic changes in the severity of valve disease that can occur during exercise. However, its value as a prognostic tool remains limited. Low-dose dobutamine stress echocardiography is useful to identify patients with severe AS who present with a low gradient and LV dysfunction.

Fluoroscopy is more specific than echocardiography for assessing valvular and annular calcification.

Radionuclide angiography is more reproducible than echocardiography for assessing the ventricular ejection fraction (EF) in patients in sinus rhythm.

Computed tomography (CT) has been reported to be of interest to exclude coronary artery disease (CAD) in patients at low risk of atherosclerosis. It can also quantify valve calcification and assess geometric mitral or aortic valve area.

Magnetic resonance imaging (MRI) can be used to assess cardiac chamber dimensions and contractility, and to quantitate valvular regurgitations.

In practice, CT and MRI are widely used to assess dimensions of thoracic aorta. Even if they can quantitate accurately the severity of valvular diseases or LV volumes, the limited availability of these techniques and the need for specific expertise restrict such applications.

Invasive investigation

Cardiac catheterization should not be performed routinely to measure pressures and cardiac output. It is indicated only in the rare instances when non-invasive investigations are inconclusive or discordant with clinical findings [11, 12].

In practice, the invasive investigation is most often only coronary angiography, which should be performed before surgery in men aged >40, in post-menopausal women aged >50, or in patients with coronary risk factors [11, 12].

Risk stratification

The aim of the assessment of VHD is to estimate the patients' outcome and compare it with operative mortality and late results of interventions. This comparison remains the rationale for the recommendations of interventions given the lack of randomized trials in this setting.

Ideally, spontaneous outcome should be assessed from contemporary series including prognostic variables, such as the severity of valvular disease and LVEF [15, 16]. The assessment of spontaneous outcome should also take into account comorbidities, particularly in the elderly. The Charlson comorbidity index [17] has been widely validated and more recent scoring systems are useful for identifying patients whose life expectancy is compromised more by comorbidities than by heart disease itself [18].

Multivariate risk scores are increasingly used to estimate operative mortality. The EuroSCORE is user-friendly and thus widely used. It has been validated in patients with valvular disease [19]. The EuroSCORE, however, tends to overestimate operative mortality in high-risk patients [20, 21]. Other scores have been specifically developed for valvular diseases, but are less widely used in practice than the EuroSCORE, at least in Europe [22–24]. Even if the Society of Thoracic Surgeons (STS) score appears to be more reliable than the EuroSCORE in high-risk patients, it is important to realize that no risk score is perfect. In addition, these scores have become outdated in light of ongoing improvements in surgical techniques and do not take into account the surgical results in the given institution (i.e. validation). Although scoring systems have limitations, their use is encouraged since they can reduce the subjectivity in estimating the risk:benefit ratio of interventions.

Late outcome after valvular surgery depends mainly on the stage of heart disease before surgery and prosthetic-related complications.

Final decision making relies on clinical judgement of the physician, which should combine components of risk stratification, analysis of patient's quality of life and wishes after appropriate information.

Aortic stenosis

AS is now considered to be a major societal and economic burden since it is the most common valve disease in Europe and North America [1, 2] and it is increasing in prevalence due to the ageing population. The frequency of aortic valve sclerosis is approximately 25% at 65 years of age, rising to 48% after 75 years, while the frequency of AS is 4–5% in those aged >65 [25, 26]. AS has become the most common indication for valve surgery, which explains the interest in its management.

Aetiology

AS is most often due to calcification of a normal trileaflet valve or a congenitally bicuspid valve. In surgical series, bicuspid valves account for approximately 50%, tricuspid valves 30–40%, and rare unicuspid valves <10% [27]. The frequency of AS observed on bicuspid valves is higher in patients aged <60, and then the trend is inverted afterwards. Calcification begins at the base of the cusps and progresses towards the edges, while the commissures remain open (➲Fig. 21.2; 21.2). The 'degenerative' aetiology accounts for 80% of cases in Western countries followed by rheumatic disease which is characterized by commissural fusion and fibrosis, with retraction and stiffening of the cusps [2]. Other rare causes are: familial hypercholesterolaemia, hyperuricaemia, hyperparathyroidism, Paget disease, ochronosis, Fabry disease, lupus erythematosus, and drug-induced diseases.

Pathophysiology

Calcific 'degenerative' AS has long been considered as a passive and degenerative process ('wear and tear phenomenon') but recent data has challenged this concept—in fact, AS is an active, complex, and highly regulated pathobiological process including chronic inflammation, lipoprotein deposition, renin–angiotensin system activation, osteoblastic transformation of valvular interstitial cells, and active calcification [28–32] (➲Fig. 21.3). The association with traditional atherogenic cardiovascular risk factors such as hypertension, current smoking, diabetes, cholesterol levels, and histopathological parallels have led to the hypothesis that AS is primarily an atherosclerotic-like process [25, 26, 29–31]. However, there are also important dissimilarities suggesting a more complicated picture. Several specific cell-signalling pathways regulating valvular calcification such as BMP2/RANK/runx2/Cbfa1 seem to be involved. Identification of familial clusters and recent findings implicating genetic polymorphisms of the vitamin D receptor and mutations such as in NOTCH 1 [33] in bicuspid aortic valves suggest that genetic factors may also influence valve pathogenesis [34]. These findings indicate that 'degenerative' may not be the most accurate term for this process, although it remains in common usage.

In addition, in patients with bicuspid valves, tissue abnormality is not only localized to aortic leaflets but also to the aortic arterial wall which has abnormalities resembling those of Marfan syndrome.

CAD is present in 30% of patients with mild to moderate AS and 50% with critical AS.

Normal aortic valve area is 3–4cm^2 [35]; 21.3. A gradient between the LV and aorta begins to appear once the valve area is <1.5cm^2. AS is considered severe when the area is <1cm^2 or, more accurately, 0.6cm^2/m^2 BSA. The obstruction develops gradually. Bicuspid valves are less efficient than tricuspid valves at distributing mechanical stress, leading to the more rapid development of stenosis. The obstruction of the valve imposes a pressure overload on the LV, which subsequently causes the development of concentric hypertrophy at rates that vary according to the individual. Ventricular hypertrophy is a key adaptive mechanism to counter pressure overload as it normalizes wall stress. However, it also has adverse consequences: an increase in the total collagen volume of the myocardium; a reduction of LV compliance leading to a limited preload reserve; and myocardial ischaemia, which may be present even when

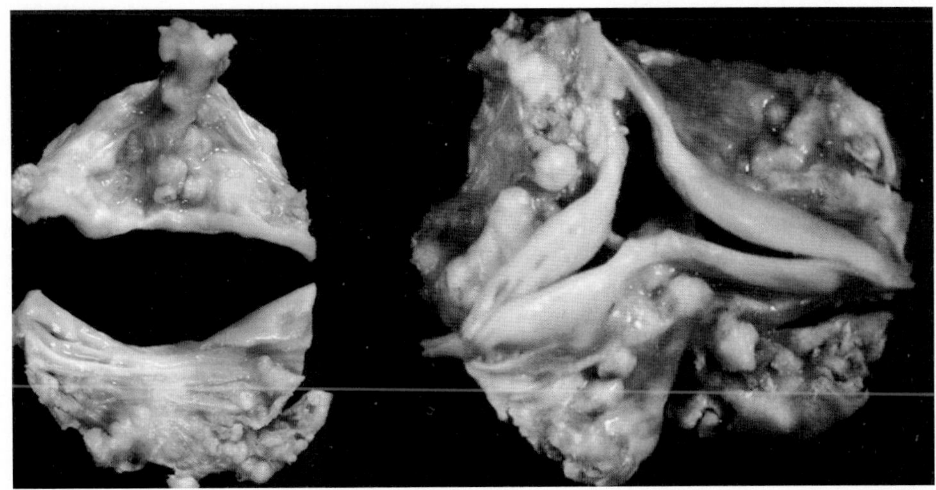

Figure 21.2 Explanted aortic valves during aortic valve replacement for AS. (A) Congenitally bicupid aortic valve. (B) Tricuspid aortic valve. Reproduced with permission from Roberts WC, Ko JM. Frequency by decades of unicuspid, bicuspid, and tricuspid aortic valves in adults having isolated aortic valve replacement for aortic stenosis, with or without associated aortic regurgitation. *Circulation* 2005; **111**: 920–5.

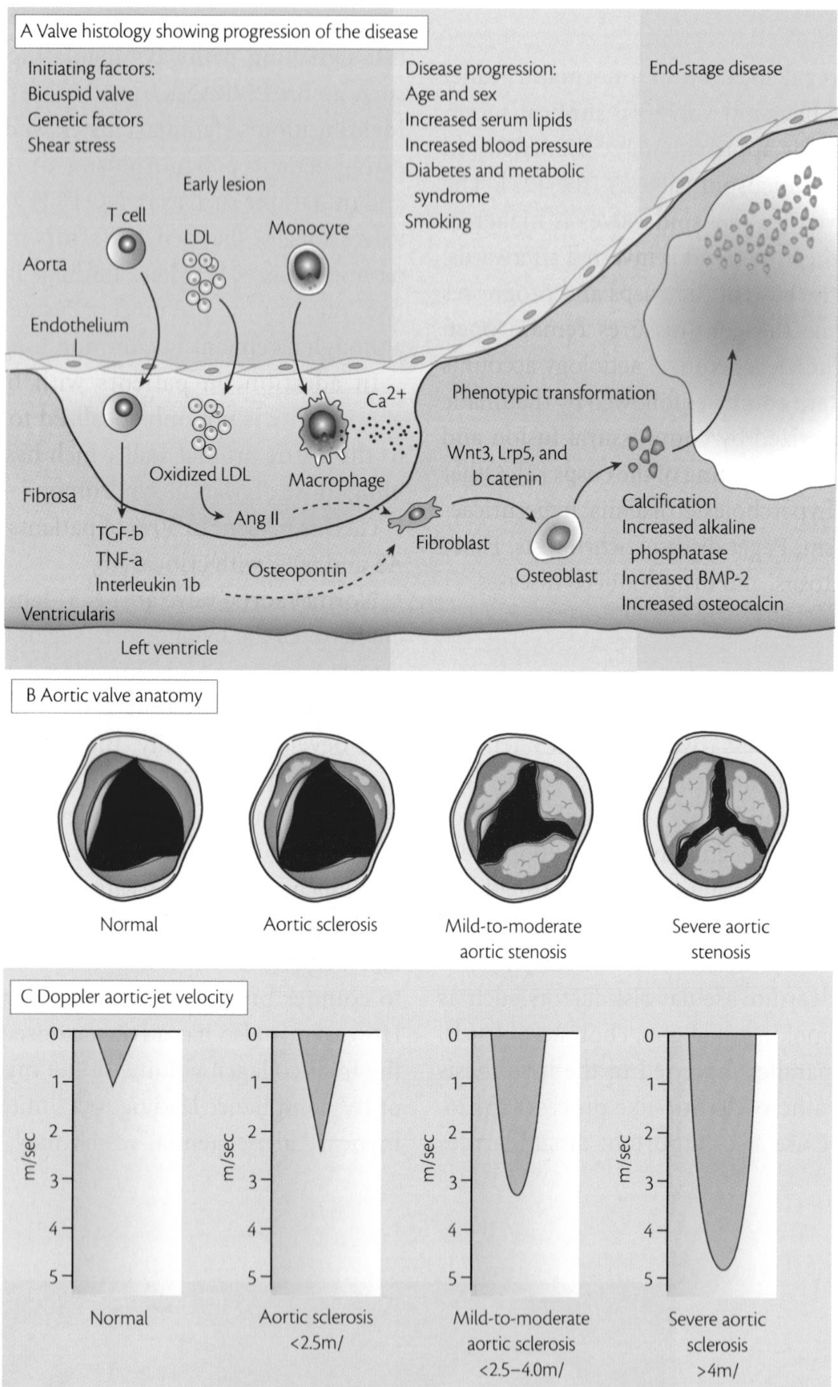

Figure 21.3 Disease progression in calcific AS, illustrating changes in aortic valve histologic features, leaflet opening in systole, and Doppler velocities. In (A) the histology of the early lesion is characterized by a subendothelial accumulation of oxidized low-density lipoprotein (LDL), production of angiotensin (Ang) II, and inflammation with T lymphocytes and macrophages. Disease progression occurs by several mechanisms, including local production of proteins, such as osteopontin, osteocalcin, and bone morphogenic protein 2 (BMP-2), which mediate tissue calcification; activation of inflammatory signalling pathways, including tumour necrosis factor α (TNF-α), tumour growth factor β (TGF-β), the complement system, C-reactive protein, and interleukin-1β; and changes in tissue matrix, including the accumulation of tenascin C, and up-regulation of matrix metalloproteinase 2 and alkaline phosphatase activity. In addition, leaflet fibroblasts undergo phenotypic transformation into osteoblasts, regulated by the Wnt3–Lrp5–β catenin signalling pathway. Microscopic accumulations of extracellular calcification (Ca^2+) are present early in the disease process, with progressive calcification as the disease progresses and areas of frank bone formation in end-stage disease. The corresponding changes in aortic valve anatomy are viewed from the aortic side with the valve open in systole (B) and in Doppler aortic-jet velocity (C). Adapted with permission from Otto CM. Calcific aortic stenosis—time to look more closely at the valve. *New Engl J Med* 2008; **359**: 1395–8.

coronary disease is not, and is caused by the combination of increased myocardial oxygen demand and limited coronary flow [36]. LV systolic performance may be impaired (even if contractility is normal) due to afterload mismatch, leftwards shift of the ventricular preload on the Starling curve, or asynchrony of the temporal sequence of contraction. In addition, reduced systemic arterial compliance is a frequent occurrence in elderly patients with AS and independently contributes to increased afterload and decreased LV function. Late in the course of the disease, the cardiac output, and therefore the transvalvular gradient, declines, whereas the pressures in the left atrium and pulmonary artery rise.

Diagnosis

History

Frequently, the diagnosis is made when a systolic murmur is detected during a routine physical examination or on an echographic examination for another cause. AS is gradually progressive and symptoms usually appear between the second and fourth decade in rheumatic AS, the fifth and sixth decade in patients with bicuspid valves, and the seventh or eighth decade in degenerative aetiology.

The most common initial symptom is exertional dyspnoea or fatigue. Exertional dyspnoea is mostly related to the increased LV end-diastolic pressure due to LV hypertrophy and/or systolic dysfunction. Angina on exertion is due to an increased oxygen demand by the hypertrophic myocardium, exacerbated by the decrease of flow in the presence of coronary stenoses. It is a poor indicator of coronary disease, as coronary disease may be present in 25% of patients without angina and in 40–80% of those with angina [37]. Syncope, or light-headedness, also occurs on exertion when elevated LV pressures stimulate baroreceptors located in the LV, inducing arterial hypotension, decreased venous return, and bradycardia. Later, dyspnoea may progress to overt heart failure. In practice, AS may be discovered during attempted diagnosis of unexplained congestive heart failure.

Besides progressive deterioration, acute decompensation may be due to precipitating factors, such as atrial fibrillation, suppressing the atrial systole, which is of utmost importance for the filling of the hypertrophic myocardium. Other factors include fever, anaemia, and endocarditis leading to acute AR which is poorly tolerated in a small hypertrophic ventricle.

In the elderly, a clear description of symptoms and their onset may be difficult to obtain. These patients frequently present with atypical presentation, with fatigue being most common. Breathlessness on exercise may be difficult to interpret in patients with only low physical activity. Finally, symptoms may be due to associated disease.

Physical examination

In severe AS, typically the prolonged LV ejection through the narrowed valve orifice yields a slow rising carotid pulse and the reduced stroke volume results in a weak and small amplitude pulse. However, this sign may be absent in patients with increased arterial stiffness such as the elderly. The murmur is related to the pressure gradient and jet velocity. It is crescendo–decrescendo and mid-systolic, with a late peaking sound in severe AS since the maximum gradient occurs later in systole when stenosis becomes severe. It is harsh and rasping at the base and is transmitted to the carotids. It often radiates towards the apex as a high-pitched murmur mimicking MR. The differential diagnosis with MR may be done on the timing of the murmur which has no early systolic components in AS. The intensity of the murmur is specific to the severity of obstruction but it has a poor sensitivity, since it may be soft if cardiac output is low, as in obese patients, or in patients with lung disease. When the murmur is of high intensity, a thrill may be palpated. In severe AS, the second heart sound may be paradoxically split, or more often single due to the inaudibility of the aortic component related to the rigidity of the thickened leaflets. The disappearance of the second aortic sound is specific to severe AS although it is not a sensitive sign. An ejection click may be heard after the first sound at the base in patients with mobile valves, and, unlike the pulmonary clicks, it does not vary with respiration. Finally, a fourth sound is frequent at the apex, related to forceful atrial contraction.

The physical examination may be misleading in patients with low output since there is no slowly rising pulse; the murmur may become softer or even disappear and auscultation could be limited to a soft murmur of functional MR and the third heart sound at the apex.

Chest radiograph

Overall cardiac silhouette and pulmonary vascular distribution are normal unless cardiac decompensation is present. Post-stenotic dilatation of the ascending aorta is frequent. Calcification of the valve is found in almost all adults with severe AS; however, fluoroscopy may be necessary to detect it.

Electrocardiogram

LV hypertrophy, with or without repolarization abnormalities, is seen in approximately 80% of patients with severe

AS. Other non-specific signs include left atrial enlargement, left axis deviation, and left bundle branch block. Atrial fibrillation can be seen at a late stage and may otherwise suggest coexisting mitral valve disease or coronary disease.

Echocardiography

Echocardiography has become the key diagnostic tool. It confirms the presence of AS, assesses the numbers of cusps, the degree and distribution of valve calcification, and the size of the annulus. Doppler echocardiography is the preferred technique for assessing severity.

The clinical evaluation of the severity of AS is mainly based on the measurements of AS maximum jet velocity, mean transaortic gradient, and valve area by continuity equation (➲Fig. 21.4). The main limitation of maximum jet velocity and transvalvular pressure gradients is that they are flow dependent. In addition, when the aorta is <30mm, which is rare in the adult population, the pressure recovery phenomenon may be misleading. Blood pressure can indirectly affect the assessment of severity through concurrent changes in transvalvular blood flow, thus ideally AS severity should be assessed at a normotensive state. Valve area measurements also have their potential inaccuracies. Therefore, for clinical decision making, valve area should be considered in combination with flow velocity, pressure gradient and ventricular function, as well as functional status [11, 12, 38].

The thresholds generally recommended for the definition of severe AS are aortic jet velocity >4m/s; mean gradient >40–50mmHg; aortic valve area <1cm^2 [11, 12]. Indexing to BSA, with a cut-off value of 0.6cm^2/m^2 BSA is particularly helpful in patients with either an unusually small or large BSA.

In the presence of low flow, usually due to depressed LV function, low pressure gradients may be encountered in patients with severe AS. As soon as mean gradient is <40mmHg, even a small valve area does not definitely confirm severe AS since mild to moderately diseased valves may not open fully resulting in a 'functionally small valve area' (pseudosevere AS) [39, 40].

In addition, it has recently been shown that in some elderly women of small stature with severe LV hypertrophy

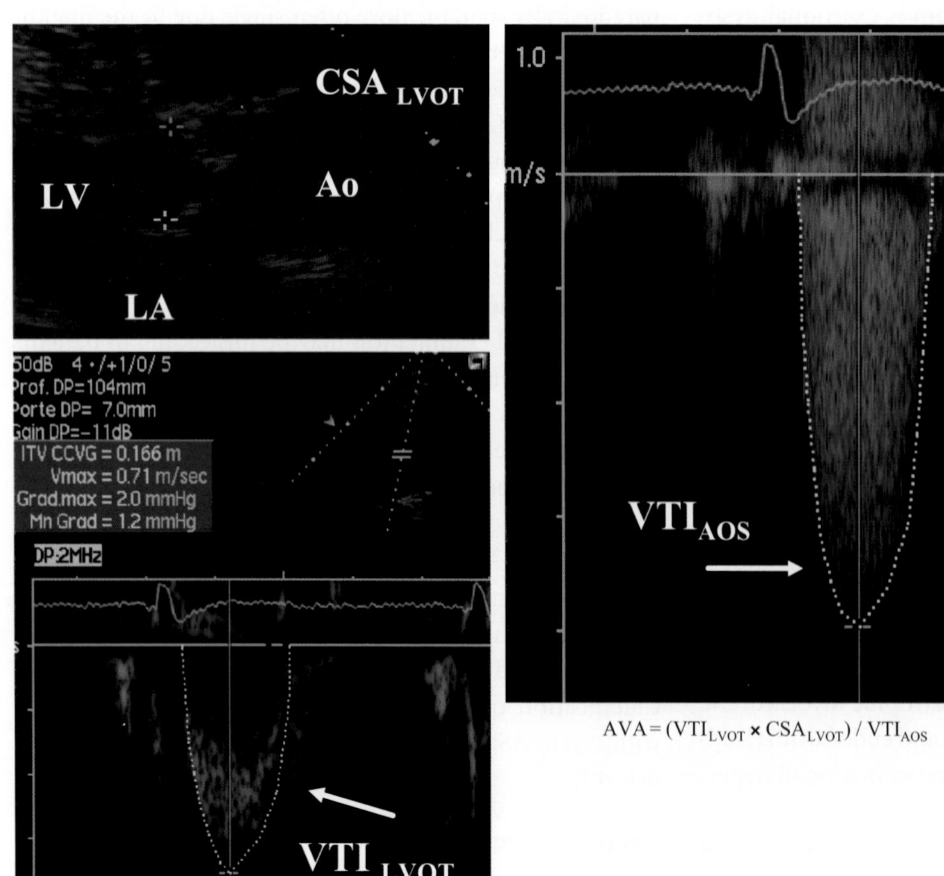

$AVA = (VTI_{LVOT} \times CSA_{LVOT}) / VTI_{AOS}$

Figure 21.4 Calcification of the aortic valve area using the continuity equation. The continuity equation is based on the conservation of energy. Flow through an orifice is equal to the area of this orifice × velocity time integral. AOS, aorta; AVA, aortic valve area (cm^2); CSA, cross-sectional area; LA, left atrium; LV, left ventricle; LVOT, left ventricular outflow tract; VTI, velocity time integral. (Courtesy of Dr E. Brochet.)

and diastolic dysfunction, the stroke volume is small, so that even when severe stenosis is present the AS velocity and mean gradient may be lower than expected for a given valve area [41].

Alternate severity measures may be used when additional information is needed such as simplified continuity equation, velocity ratio, or valve area planimetry. However, long-term longitudinal data from prospective studies are lacking for these indices.

Echocardiographic evaluation will identify coexistent valvular lesions including mitral annular calcification, mitral valve disease with a careful assessment of MR mechanism if needed, and asymmetric dynamic subvalvular obstruction, especially in elderly women. Evaluation of the aortic root anatomy and dimensions at the level of the sinuses of Valsalva and aortic root should be standard in all patients with AS.

Transoesophageal echocardiography is rarely needed, although it may provide images that are good enough to allow valve planimetry, which is useful when transthoracic visualization is poor and leaflets only moderately calcified. Transoesophageal echocardiography will also provide, if needed, additional evaluation of other mitral valve abnormalities.

Other non-invasive investigations

Exercise testing is contraindicated in symptomatic patients with AS but is useful for risk stratification and the unmasking of symptoms in asymptomatic patients with severe AS [42, 43]. In such cases, it is safe, provided it is performed under the supervision of an experienced physician while symptoms, changes in blood pressure, and electrocardiogram (ECG) are closely monitored. It is reasonable to propose it in patients >70 years who are still highly active. In the asymptomatic patient, stress tests also determine the recommended level of physical activity.

Stress echocardiography, using low-dose dobutamine, may be helpful in low-flow low-gradient AS (to distinguish the truly severe cases from the rare cases of pseudosevere AS). Truly severe AS shows only small changes in valve area (increase $<0.2\text{cm}^2$) which remains $<1\text{cm}^2$ with increasing flow rate but significant increase in gradients (maximum value of mean gradient >40mmHg), whereas pseudosevere AS shows a marked increase in valve area with a final value $>1\text{cm}^2$ but only minor changes in gradients [39, 40]. In addition, this test may detect the presence of contractile reserve (increase >20% of stroke volume during low dose dobutamine test), which has prognostic implications [35, 39].

Exercise stress echocardiography has been proposed for risk stratification in asymptomatic severe AS [44]. Although the increase in mean pressure gradient with exercise has been reported to predict outcome and provide information beyond a regular exercise test, more data is required to validate this finding and recommend its use in clinical practise.

Multislice CT [45] and MRI [46] could improve assessment of the ascending aorta. CT provides high sensitivity and specificity in the detection of high-grade coronary artery stenosis and could be useful to rule out CAD preoperatively in patients with low prevalence of CAD. Electron-beam CT (EBCT) may be useful in quantifying valve calcification, which aids in assessing prognosis [47]. It also enables the measurement of valve area, aortic annulus size, and finally the distance between the aortic cusps and the coronary ostia, which is useful prior to performing transcatheter aortic valve implantation (TAVI) [48]. More data is required to determine the full role of multislice CT in this setting and its cost–benefit value versus echocardiography.

Natriuretic peptides, in particular BNP and pro-BNP, have been shown in preliminary studies to be increased in relation to the severity of symptoms and the degree of LV dysfunction. These measurements may be a helpful adjunct in identifying patients with equivocal symptoms at risk of progression to symptoms [49]. Large prospective trials will be necessary before the use of these measures can be advocated on a routine basis to identify optimal timing of surgery.

As most patients with severe AS are elderly and have comorbidities, the preoperative assessment should also include a comprehensive search for extracardiac abnormalities and other localizations of atherosclerosis.

Invasive investigations

Retrograde LV catheterization to assess the severity of AS is only needed when echocardiography is inconclusive [11, 12] and should only be used with caution as it is not without risk [50].

Coronary angiography remains the gold standard to detect CAD and it should be performed preoperatively according to guidelines [11, 12].

Natural history

The natural history of AS has been evaluated in several recent prospective studies [25, 51–56]. The average decrease in valve area is approximately 0.1cm^2/year, the increase in gradient is 7mmHg/year, and the increase in peak aortic jet velocity is 0.25m/s. In general the rate of progression is linear, although it varies markedly among individuals. More rapid progression is associated with a higher event rate, although the specific degree of valve narrowing associated with clinical symptoms also shows considerable individual variability. Nearly all patients with bicuspid valves develop significant outflow obstruction over time, especially in the R-N type, whereas only a relatively small proportion of patients with trileaflet valve progress to severe AS [56].

Large population-based studies have shown that even aortic sclerosis has an important impact on prognosis as it was associated with a 50% increased risk of cardiovascular mortality and morbidity [25]. Mild to moderate AS is not a benign disease as it is associated with a substantial mortality rate [25, 55]. Progression to severe stenosis may be quicker than previously assumed; however, this only partially accounts for the high mortality rate as >50% of the deaths were not cardiac. The mechanism of this association is not clear and is most likely linked to the presence of atherosclerosis in the entire cardiovascular system, acting through endothelial dysfunction or other undetermined factors.

During a long latent period patients remain asymptomatic. However, the duration of the asymptomatic phase varies widely among individuals. Sudden cardiac death is a frequent cause of death in symptomatic patients but appears to be rare in asymptomatic patients (≤1% per year) [51–54]. Reported average symptom-free survival at 2 years ranges from 20% to >50%. The lower numbers must be viewed with caution since some patients underwent surgery without symptoms in these studies. Predictors of the progression of AS, and, therefore, of poor outcome in asymptomatic patients, have recently been identified. The main predictors are as follows:

- Clinical: old age, smoking, the presence of coronary disease, hypertension, or dyslipidaemia, higher body mass index, metabolic syndrome, renal failure, mitral annular calcification, initial aortic valve area [25, 52–55].
- Echocardiographic: valve calcification, peak aortic jet velocity, LVEF. In the study by Rosenhek and colleagues [54], the combination of moderate to severe calcification and rapid increase in peak velocity identified 79% of patients who either underwent surgery or became symptomatic within 2 years (➲Fig. 21.5).
- Exercise testing: symptom development on exercise testing in physically active patients, particularly those <70 years, predicts a very high likelihood of symptom development within 12 months. Recent data demonstrates a lower positive predictive value for abnormal blood pressure response, and even more so for ST segment depression, than symptoms for poor outcome [43].
- Patients with bicuspid valves are exposed to a high risk of cardiac events, concerning 40% of them at 20 years, which are mainly related to the development of AS, particularly in those with echographic valve degeneration at diagnosis. In addition, the risk of aortic complication is notable. Aortic dilatation does not depend on valve function and its rate of progression increases with aortic diameter, although it cannot be reliably predicted in any given patient [56].

Outcome is poor when any symptoms are present, with survival rates of only 15–50% at 5 years [51]. Among the elderly population the strongest predictors of poor outcome are New York Heart Association (NYHA) class III/IV, associated MR, and LV dysfunction. The combination of

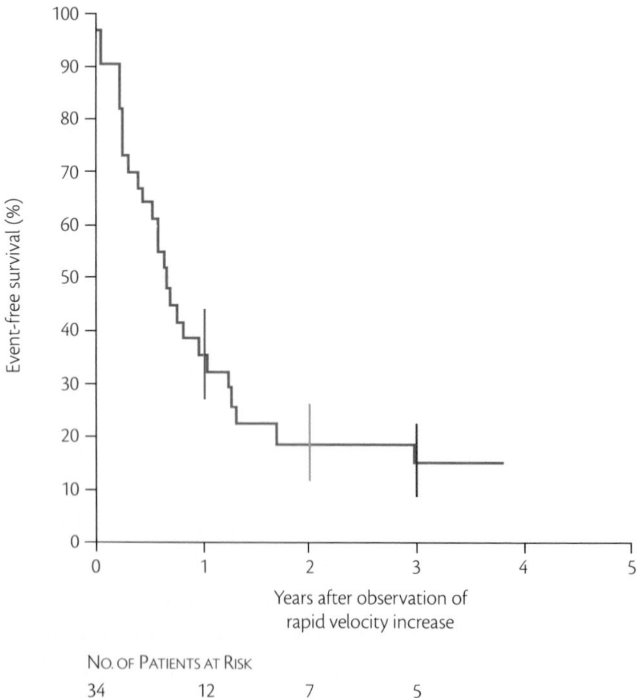

Figure 21.5 Outcome of asymptomatic patients with severe AS. Kaplan–Meier analysis of event-free survival among 34 patients with moderate or severe calcification of the aortic valve and a rapid increase in aortic-jet velocity (at least 0.3m/s within 1 year). The vertical bars indicate standard errors. Reproduced with permission from Rosenhek R, Binder T, Porenta G, *et al.* Predictors of outcome in severe asymptomatic aortic stenosis. *N Engl J Med* 2000; **343**: 611–17.

these three factors identifies a group at particular high risk since survival is only 30% at 3 years [15].

Medical treatment

Given the relationship between AS and systemic atherosclerosis it was appealing to evaluate the potential of modifying risk factors in the progression of AS. Although several retrospective reports have shown beneficial effects of statins on the progression of AS, data is still conflicting. The two randomized trials assessing the effect of statin therapy on patients who do not have other indications for statins were negative since they did not halt the progression of the disease or induce its regression either on echographic or clinical parameters [57, 58]. Until further data is available there does not seem to be an indication for statin therapy on the basis of AS alone. Further data is needed to evaluate the influence of the stage at which treatment is initiated on the effect and the potential of statins to prevent the development of AS. Similarly, the role of angiotensin-converting enzyme (ACE) inhibitors on the progression of AS still needs to be clarified.

However, the modification of atherosclerotic risk factors is strongly recommended following the guidelines on secondary prevention in atherosclerosis.

Symptomatic patients require early surgery as no medical therapy for AS is able to delay the inevitability of surgery. Patients who are unsuitable candidates for intervention may be treated with digitalis, diuretics, ACE inhibitors, or angiotensin receptor blockers if they are experiencing heart failure. Beta-blockers should be avoided in these circumstances. In selected patients with pulmonary oedema, nitroprusside can be used under haemodynamic monitoring.

Co-existing hypertension should be treated, however treatment should be carefully titrated to avoid hypotension and patients more frequently evaluated.

Maintenance of sinus rhythm is particularly important. Endocarditis prophylaxis is indicated according to guidelines [59] (see ➲ Chapter 22, Infective Endocarditis).

Surgery

Aortic valve replacement is the definitive therapy for severe AS. It uses either a mechanical prosthesis or a bioprosthesis (➲Table 21.1).

In contemporary series, operative mortality of isolated aortic valve replacement is around 2–5% in patients <70 years and 5–15% in older adults including selected octogenarians. If bypass surgery is combined with valve replacement operative mortality ranges between 5–7% [2, 9, 20, 23, 24, 60–62]. The following factors all increase the risk of operative mortality: older age, associated comorbidities, female gender, higher functional class, emergency operation, LV dysfunction, pulmonary hypertension, coexisting coronary disease, and previous bypass or valve surgery [60, 61]. After successful valve replacement long-term survival rates are close to those expected, symptoms are less marked, and quality of life is greatly improved [63]. Risk factors for late death include age, comorbidities, severe functional condition, irreversible myocardial damage, ventricular arrhythmias, and untreated coexisting CAD. In addition, poor postoperative outcome may result from prosthesis-related complications or sub-optimal prosthetic valve haemodynamic performance [64]. Finally, aortic valve replacement has also recently been shown to be cost effective for all age groups [65].

Percutaneous interventions

Percutaneous aortic valvuloplasty

The efficacy of percutaneous aortic valvuloplasty (PAV) is limited as the final valve area is only between 0.7–1.1cm^2.

Table 21.1 Type of intervention in single native left-sided valve disease

	Aortic stenosis (n = 512)	**Aortic regurgitation (n = 119)**	**Mitral stenosis (n = 112)**	**Mitral regurgitation (n = 155)**
Mechanical prosthesis (%)	49	76	58	43
Bioprosthesis (%)	50	18	4.5	10
Valve repair (%)	0	1.7	3.5	47
Homograft (%)	0.6	2.6	0	0
Autograft (%)	0.4	1.7	0	0
Percutaneous intervention (%)	0	0	34	0

Adapted with permission from Iung B, Baron G, Butchart EG, *et al.* A prospective survey of patients with valvular heart disease in Europe: the Euro Heart Survey on valvular heart disease. *Eur Heart J* 2003; **24**:1231–43.

Mortality and morbidity of the procedure are high (>10%). Restenosis and clinical deterioration occur within 6–12 months in most patients resulting in a mid-term and long-term outcome similar to natural history [66].

Transcatheter aortic valve implantation

Six years after the first implant in humans by Alian Cribier, transcatheter aortic valve implantation (TAVI) currently represents a dynamic field of research and development [67–70]: two devices have been CE marked and are being commercialized. These devices consist of three pericardial leaflets mounted in a balloon-expandable stent in one case, and in a self-expanding, nitinol stent in the other (➲Figs. 21.6 and 21.7; 21.4 and 21.5).

Over 6000 patients have been treated using TAVI. Two approaches can be used: retrograde transfemoral [67, 68] or antegrade transapical [69, 70] through a limited thoracotomy.

The patients treated were mostly >80 years old, at high risk, or with contraindications for surgery. Procedural success is closely linked to experience, and is about 90% in experienced centres. Valve function is good with a final valve area ranging from 1.5–1.8cm^2. Mortality at 30 days ranges from 5–18%. Acute myocardial infarction occurs in 2–11%. Coronary obstruction is rare (<1%). Severe AR is 5–10%. Prosthesis embolization is around 1%. The incidence of vascular complications has decreased from 10–15% to <5% with the availability of smaller devices. Stroke ranges from 3–9%. Finally, atrioventricular block occurs in 20%. Long-term results up to 2 years show a survival rate of 70–80% with a significant improvement in clinical condition in most cases with no structural deterioration of valve tissue on mid-term sequential echocardiographic studies.

In light of the current experience, bearing in mind the preliminary nature of these results and inherent limitations of any conclusions, TAVI can be said to be feasible and provides good clinical and haemodynamic results for up to 2 years. However, the technique remains challenging, in particular as regards vascular access, device sizing, and positioning. Questions need to be answered regarding the safety and long-term durability of these bioprostheses, and the feasibility of subsequent aortic valve intervention is not known [71].

Treatment strategy

Taking into account the population of patients who are now elderly with comorbidities, the selection of candidates, and especially risk assessment, should involve multidisciplinary consultation between cardiologists, surgeons, and anaesthesiologists.

A stepwise approach to the management of AS according to ESC guidelines is detailed in ➲Fig. 21.8 [11].

Symptomatic patients

Early valve replacement should be strongly recommended soon after symptom onset in all symptomatic patients with severe AS who are otherwise candidates for surgery. As long

A

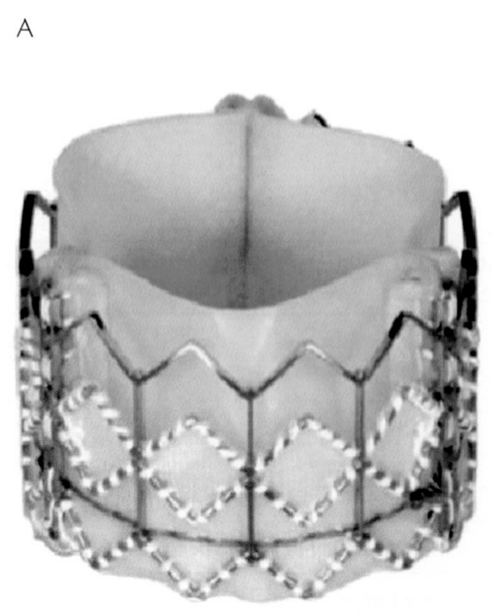

B

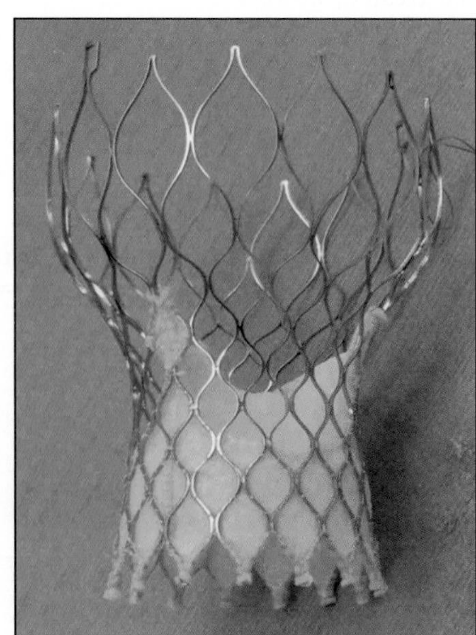

Figure 21.6 Stent-valve prostheses currently commercialized for transcatheter aortic valve implantation. (A) Edwards–Sapien valve (Edwards–Sapien Lifesciences Inc. USA) consisting of three bovine pericardial leaflets mounted with a tubular slotted stainless-steel balloon expandable stent. (B) CoreValve revalving system (CoreValve Inc Irvine CA, USA) which has three porcine pericardial leaflets, mounted on a self-expanding nitinol frame.

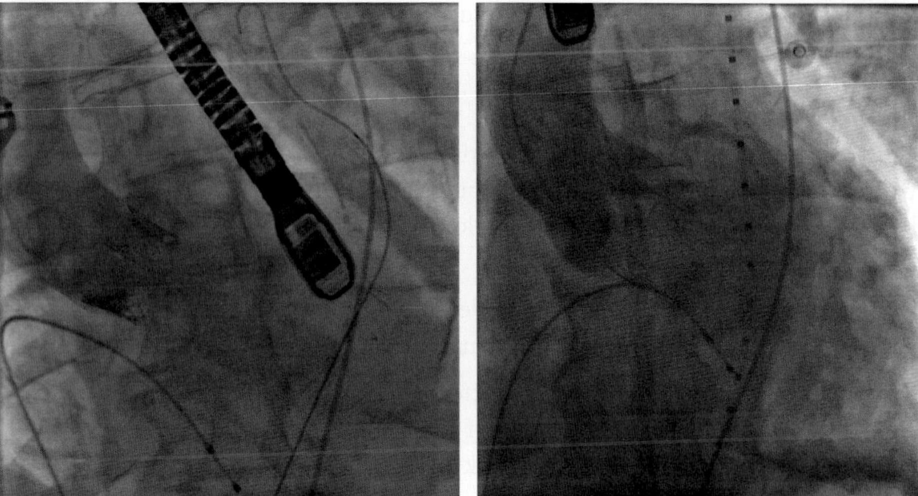

Figure 21.7 Aortography after transcatheter aortic valve implantation. Left: transcatheter aortic valve implantation using the balloon expandable stent. Right: transcatheter aortic valve implantation using self-expandable stented valve. In both cases, the prosthesis is deployed at the level of the aortic valve and coronary flow is not impeached. (Courtesy of Dr. D Himbert.)

as mean gradient is still >40mmHg, there is virtually no lower EF limit for surgery.

According to the current knowledge, TAVI can be considered if the patient has a contraindication for surgery, or if surgery is judged to be at high risk, on the condition that the patient's life expectancy is >1year, and if there are no contraindications to the technique. Such contraindications are mostly related to the size of the aortic annulus and/or size and disease of the peripheral arteries when using the transfemoral approach [71].

Indications for PAV are very limited: it may be considered as a bridge to surgery, or to TAVI, in haemodynamically unstable patients who are at high risk for intervention, or in patients with symptomatic severe AS who require urgent major non-cardiac surgery. Occasionally, PAV may be considered as a palliative measure in individual cases when intervention is contraindicated because of severe comorbidities.

Finally, it seems reasonable to manage medically patients whose life expectancy is <1 year, while acknowledging

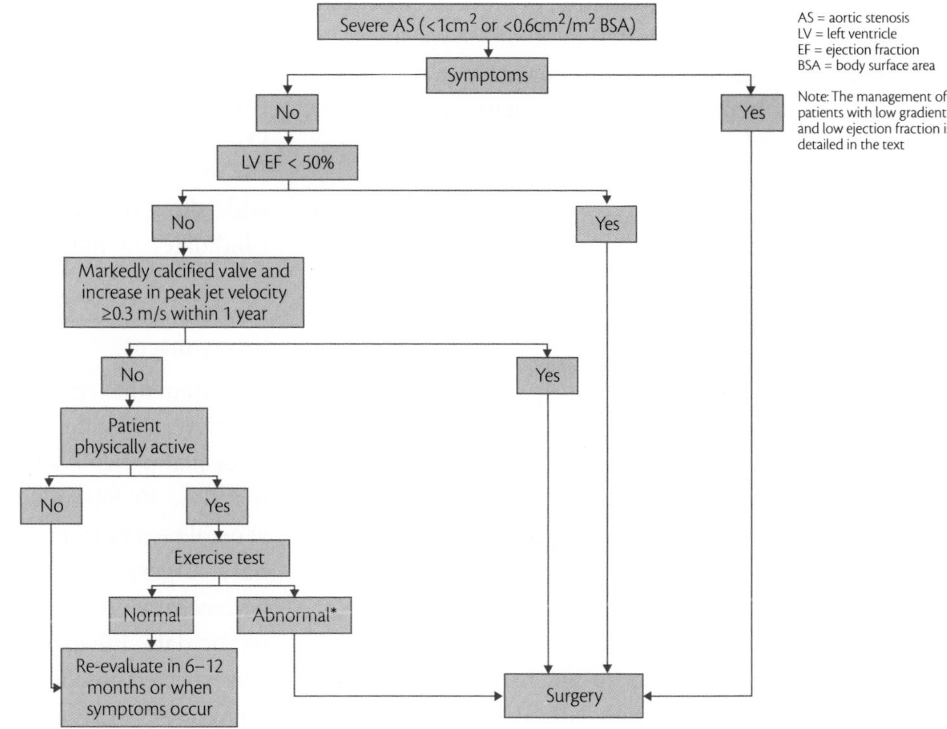

Figure 21.8 Management of patients with severe AS. *Abnormal exercise test is defined by exercise test showing symptoms on exercise, or fall in blood pressure below baseline, or complex ventricular arrhythmias. Adapted with permission from Vahanian A, Baumgartner H, Bax J, *et al.* Guidelines on the management of valvular heart disease. The Task Force on the Management of Valvular Heart Disease of the European Society of Cardiology. *Eur Heart J* 2007; **28**: 230–68.

that this should be tailored to the individual patient's condition.

Asymptomatic patients

This requires the careful weighing of risks and benefits. Early elective surgery at the asymptomatic stage can only be recommended in selected patients at low operative risk. This is the case in:

- the rare asymptomatic patients with depressed LV function (EF <50%) not due to another cause;
- those with echocardiographic predictors of poor outcome suggested by the combination of a markedly calcified valve with a rapid increase in peak aortic velocity of ≥0.3m/s per year;
- if the exercise test is abnormal, particularly if it shows symptom development, which is a strong indication for surgery in physically active patients.

Combined procedures

Patients with moderate AS who require bypass or other surgery are in most cases symptomatic. Whatever their functional status, patients with severe AS who undergo bypass surgery, aortic surgery, or other valve surgery should also undergo aortic valve replacement.

In patients with severe AS and severe coronary disease, the performance of concomitant coronary artery bypass grafting (CABG) provides a lower mortality rate than that observed in patients who do not undergo combined bypass surgery. Thus, CABG should be combined whenever possible with valve surgery. Recent studies have suggested the potential use of percutaneous coronary revascularization in place of bypass surgery in patients with AS [72]. However, currently available data is not sufficient to recommend this approach except for in selected high-risk patients with acute coronary syndromes or in patients with non-severe AS.

Concomitant treatment of a dilated aorta, in particular in the case of bicuspid valves, is recommended at the same thresholds as in AR and uses similar techniques.

When MR is associated with AS, as long as there are no morphological valve abnormalities, mitral annulus dilatation, or marked abnormalities of LV geometry, surgical intervention on the mitral valve is generally unnecessary, and functional MR often resolves after the aortic valve is replaced.

Follow-up

Asymptomatic patients who do not meet the criteria for intervention should be carefully educated about reporting symptoms as soon as they develop. Follow-up visits should include echocardiographic assessment, since the rate of haemodynamic progression is important for management decisions. In the asymptomatic patient, stress tests also determine the recommended level of physical activity.

Type and interval of follow-up should be determined on the basis of the initial examination.

In cases of moderate to severe calcification of the valve and peak aortic jet velocity >4m/s at initial evaluation patients should be re-evaluated every 6 months for the occurrence of symptoms, change in exercise tolerance or in echo-parameters. If peak aortic jet velocity has increased since the last visit (>0.3m/s per year) or if other evidence of haemodynamic progression is present, surgery should be considered. If no change has occurred and the patient remains asymptomatic, 6-monthly clinical and 6–12-monthly clinical and echocardiographic re-evaluations are recommended.

In patients who do not meet these criteria, a clinical yearly follow-up is necessary, follow-up being closer in those with borderline values. The frequency of echocardiographic examinations should be adapted to clinical findings.

Finally, genetic counselling is advisable in first-degree relatives of patients with bicuspid valves.

Special populations

Elderly

Age, per se, should not be considered as a contraindication for surgery. Decisions should be made on an individual basis taking into account patients' wishes, and cardiac and non-cardiac factors. Octogenarians, or even nonagenarians, experience higher morbidity and operative mortality; however, surgery can prolong and improve the quality of life [62, 63, 73]. Unfortunately, repeated observations worldwide show that a large proportion of potentially suitable candidates are not referred for surgery at present [74].

Moderate aortic stenosis and significant coronary artery disease

Percutaneous revascularization should be considered whenever possible. Data from retrospective analysis indicates that patients with mean gradient in presence of normal flow 30–50mmHg, and valve area 1.0–1.5cm^2 will in general benefit from valve replacement at the time of coronary surgery [75]. However, individual judgement must be recommended, considering BSA, individual haemodynamic data, life expectancy, expected progression rate of AS, expected outcome, and individual risk of valve replacement or eventual reoperation.

Aortic stenosis with low gradient, low ejection fraction

This group of patients, defined by the following three conditions: effective orifice area <1cm^2, LVEF <40%, and mean pressure gradient <30–40mmHg, is characterized by high operative risk and a dismal spontaneous prognosis. The depressed EF in many patients in this group is predominantly caused by excessive afterload and LV function usually improves after surgery [39, 40]. In patients with evidence of contractile reserve surgery should be considered. The outcome of patients without contractile reserve is compromised by a high operative mortality; however, survival is better after surgery and ventricular function often improves [76]. In view of the poor spontaneous prognosis, surgery can be performed in these patients but decision making should take into account the presence of comorbidity and the feasibility of revascularization.

Aortic regurgitation

AR may be the consequence of diverse aetiologies, the distribution of which has changed over time. The analysis of aetiology and mechanism of AR influences patient management, in particular when the ascending thoracic aorta is involved or when conservative surgery is considered.

Aetiology

Degenerative AR is the most common aetiology in Western countries, accounting for approximately half of the cases of AR in the Euro Heart Survey on VHD [2]. It is a heterogeneous entity involving leaflet lesions, which are thin and subject to prolapse, and an aneurysmal dilatation of the ascending aorta predominating at the sinuses of Valsalva. Aortic aneurysm alone may cause AR, even with normal leaflets, because changes in the geometry of the aortic root create abnormal stress on the leaflet implantation [77].

Aortic root aneurysm is encountered in Marfan syndrome and in rare degenerative diseases, such as Ehlers–Danlos disease or osteogenesis imperfecta. Aortic aneurysm is the consequence of a degeneration of the medial layer (cystic medial necrosis) which is generally caused by mutations in the gene encoding fibrillin-1 [78]. The same pattern of ascending aortic enlargement can be encountered in patients who do not have generalized tissue disease and this is known as annuloaortic ectasia [79].

Bicuspid aortic valve represented 15% of the causes of AR in the Euro Heart Survey. AR is a rarer complication of bicuspid aortic valve than AS. Its frequency may be underestimated by echocardiography since it accounted for 29% of explanted valves for AR [80]. The most frequent mechanism of regurgitation is valve prolapse, followed by a lack of valve coaptation secondary to the dilatation of the ascending aorta, and superimposed infective endocarditis. The ascending aorta is frequently enlarged and this predominates most often above the sinuses of Valsalva, the dilatation pattern differing according to valve morphology [81]. The dilated ascending aorta associated with bicuspid aortic valve is related to abnormalities of the aortic wall and is not a consequence of valve dysfunction alone [82].

Rheumatic fever has become a rare cause of AR in Europe [2], but remains common in developing countries. Central regurgitation is the consequence of thickening and retraction of aortic leaflets (21.6).

Endocarditis still represents approximately 10% of the aetiologies of AR [2]. Regurgitation is related to leaflet tearing or perforation and, in certain cases, to perivalvular abscess communicating with the aorta and the LV.

Aortitis is a heterogeneous group representing <5% of the aetiologies of AR [2]. Aortitis may be encountered in inflammatory diseases, such as ankylosing spondylitis, Takayasu's arteritis, rheumatoid arthritis, lupus erythematosus, Behçet's disease, giant cell arteritis, relapsing polychondritis, or syphilis, now a very unusual cause.

Dissection of the ascending aorta compromises commissural support and causes acute AR, which is usually well tolerated, while tamponade is the major complication.

Besides bicuspid aortic valve, AR can be associated with ventricular septal defect or subvalvular AS in which regurgitation is caused by jet lesions.

The other rare causes are traumatism, radiation therapy, and drug-induced AR.

Pathophysiology

Acute severe AR in a non-dilated LV causes an abrupt increase in end-diastolic pressure and a cardiac output. In chronic AR, progressive LV enlargement maintains LV compliance within a respectable range and therefore limits the increase in LV end-diastolic pressure. The increased LV volume enables total stroke volume to increase, thereby compensating for the regurgitant volume and helping preserve normal cardiac output. Increased afterload is compensated by eccentric LV hypertrophy. This compensation of volume and pressure overload explains why patients with chronic severe AR may remain asymptomatic for a long time [83]. In many cases, symptom onset is the consequence of systolic LV dysfunction. LV dysfunction is potentially reversible if related to afterload mismatch, but may persist after the correction of AR if related to structural myocardial injury.

Diagnosis

History

Acute AR rapidly leads to disabling dyspnoea or pulmonary oedema due to the rapid elevation of end-diastolic pressures in the non-dilated, non-compliant LV.

In chronic AR there is a long latent period and exertional dyspnoea occurs at a late stage of the disease process due to elevated LV end-diastolic pressures. Even without atherosclerotic disease angina may occur due to decreased myocardial perfusion pressure (i.e. decreased aortic diastolic pressure) and increased oxygen demand. Sudden death is rare.

Physical examination

Exaggerated arterial pulsations are related to the increased forward stroke volume and diastolic flow reversal. Widened pulse pressure is the main clinical sign for quantifying chronic AR. The classic peripheral signs of severe AR are: the Corrigan's pulse of the water hammer's type with abrupt distension and quick collapse at the level of finger nails; Musset's sign with movements of the head (i.e. head bobbing) following exaggerated carotid pulsations; Duroziez's sign with systolic and diastolic bruit heard at the level of femoral arteries. LV apical impulse is enlarged and displaced leftwards because of the LV dilatation. The holodiastolic murmur is at its maximum at the left sternal border, best heard in the sitting position. It is typically blowing, holodiastolic with an early peak and decrescendo. It is frequently associated with a mesosystolic murmur caused by the increased stroke volume. If the diastolic murmur radiates to the right sternal border, a root aetiology of the AR must be investigated. Other signs of severe AR are an apical diastolic low pitched rumble (Austin Flint) due to a jet directed toward the anterior leaflet causing vibrations and a mesosystolic sound ('pistol shot') heard at the level of femoral arteries. The second aortic sound may be louder in the case of aortic root aneurysm. When LV decompensation occurs, the pulse pressure narrows and the third heart sound may be heard at the apex.

In acute AR, patients are tachycardic and could present with clinical signs of pulmonary oedema. The diastolic murmur and peripheral signs are attenuated because the pulse pressure is narrow.

Electrocardiography

LV hypertrophy is the main feature of AR.

Chest radiograph

Cardiomegaly is the main abnormality found on chest X-ray in chronic AR. Signs of left heart failure are frequent in acute AR and are observed at an advanced stage in chronic AR. Although specific, the chest X-ray is not a sensitive examination to detect ascending aortic aneurysm.

Echocardiography

Transthoracic and/or transoesophageal echocardiography enable the anatomy of aortic leaflets and the aortic root to be accurately assessed, thereby contributing to the identification of the aetiology and mechanisms of AR. Transoesophageal echocardiography is more accurate in this setting and should be performed preoperatively when conservative surgery is considered. The mechanism of AR can be classified in three groups following the same principle as for MR: enlargement of aortic root with normal cusps (type 1); cusp prolapse or fenestration (type 2); poor cusp tissue quality or quantity (type 3) [84] (➲Fig. 21.9).

A number of indices have been proposed to quantify AR; the most frequently used with colour Doppler are the width of regurgitant jet at its origin and its extension into the LV (➲Fig. 21.10). Measurements using continuous-wave Doppler are the rate of decline of aortic regurgitant flow and diastolic flow reversal in the descending aorta. All these indices are influenced by loading conditions and the compliance of the ascending aorta and LV. Quantitative Doppler echocardiography uses the continuity equation or analysis of proximal isovelocity surface area, which is less sensitive to loading conditions. The criteria for defining severe AR are an effective regurgitant orifice (ERO) area of >0.30cm^2, regurgitant volume >60mL, or a regurgitant fraction of >50% [11–13]. Quantitative measurements are favoured but are less validated than for MR. Thus, it is necessary to combine different measurements of the severity of AR and to check for their consistency (➲Table 21.2).

Morphologic analysis of the ascending aorta is of particular importance in the case of degenerative AR or bicuspid aortic valve. Diameters should be measured at four levels: aortic annulus, sinuses of Valsalva, sino-tubular junction, and ascending aorta [85] (➲Fig. 21.11).

The reference measurement of LV dimensions is time-motion echocardiography as it was used in the prognostic studies.

Other valves should be examined since mitral valve disease may be associated in particular with Marfan syndrome or rheumatic AR.

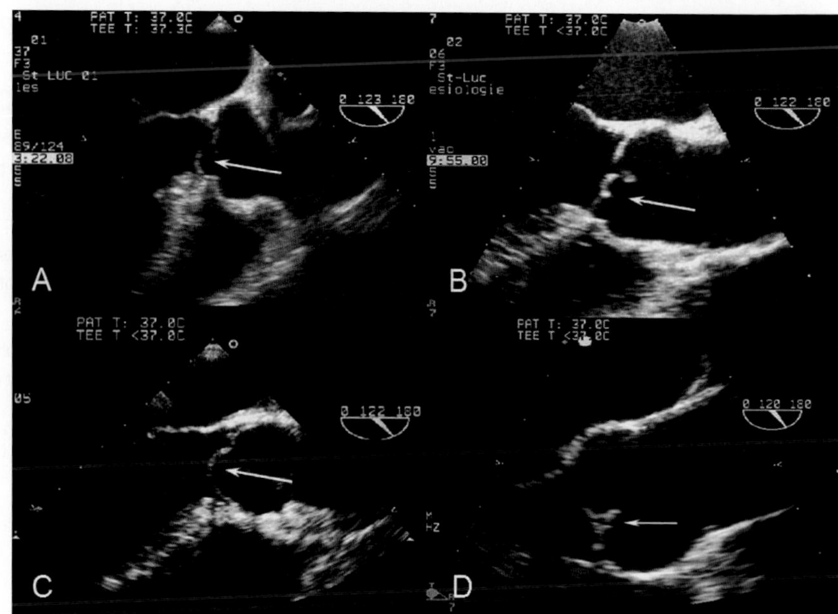

Figure 21.9 Echographic functional analysis of AR. Representative examples of the four subtypes of type 2 AR lesions. (A) Anterior cusp flail. (B) Partial cusp prolapse with mid-cusp bending. (C) Whole cusp prolapse. (D) Free edge fenestration. Adapted with permission from Le Polain de Waroux JB, Pouleur AC, Goffinet C, *et al.* Functional anatomy of aortic regurgitation. Accuracy, prediction of surgical repairability, and outcome implications of transesophageal echocardiography. *Circulation* 2007; **116**(Suppl.I): I264–I269.

Other non-invasive investigations

The main interest of exercise testing is to objectively evaluate exercise capacity. Studies of the prognostic value of exercise testing combined with ECG, echocardiography, or radionuclide ventriculography led to conflicting results, which explains why these methods are not taken into account in guidelines [11, 12].

Morphology of the ascending aorta can be analysed and accurately quantified using CT or MRI. The ability to analyse all segments of thoracic aorta is particularly important in patients with Marfan syndrome and those with bicuspid valves

MRI can also be used for AR quantification and for the measurement of LV volumes and EF [86].

Invasive investigation

Quantification of AR, LV volumes, and EF is generally obtained non-invasively using echocardiography.

Coronary angiography is required in preoperative evaluation [11, 12]. Coronary angiography may not be performed

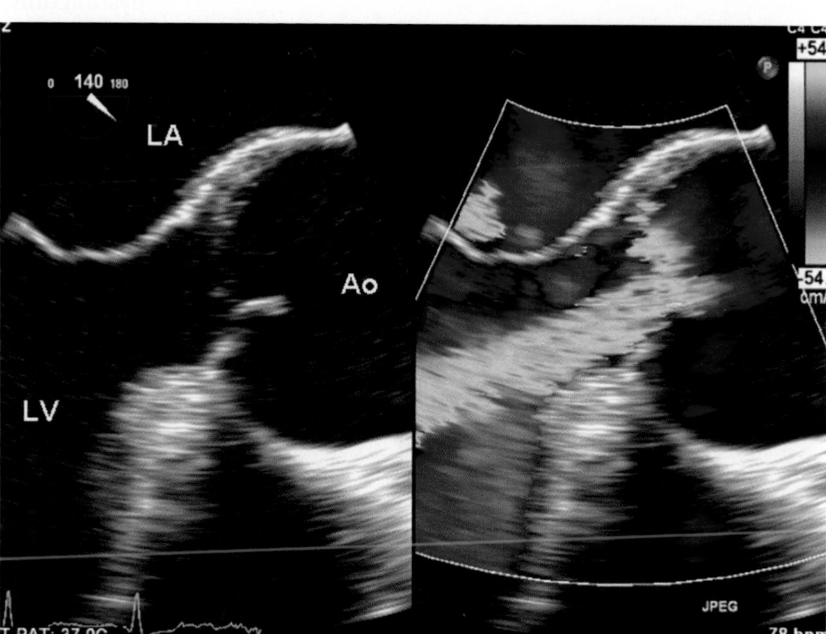

Figure 21.10 Severe AR. Transesophageal echocardiography. Colour flow imaging showing an eccentric AR due to prolapse of the non-coronary cusp. Ao, aorta; LA, left atrium; LV, left ventricle. (Courtesy of Dr E. Brochet.)

Table 21.2 Criteria for the definition of severe valve regurgitation—an integrative approach

	AR	MR	TR
Specific signs of severe regurgitation	◆ Central jet, width ≥65% of LVOT[a] ◆ Vena contracta >0.6cm[a]	◆ Vena contracta width ≥0.7cm *with* large central MR jet (area >40% of LA) or *with* a wall impinging jet of any size, swirling in LA[a] ◆ Large flow convergence[c] ◆ Systolic reversal in pulmonary veins ◆ Prominent flail MV or ruptured papillary muscle	◆ Vena contracta width >0.7cm in echo ◆ Large flow convergence[c] ◆ Systolic reversal in the hepatic veins
Supportive signs	◆ Pressure half-time <200ms ◆ Holodiastolic aortic flow reversal in descending aorta ◆ Moderate or greater LV enlargement[b]	◆ Dense, triangular CW Doppler MR jet ◆ E-wave dominant mitral inflow (E >1.2m/s[d]) ◆ Enlarged LV and LA size[e] (particularly when normal LV function is present)	◆ Dense, triangular CW TR signal with early peak ◆ Inferior cava dilatation and respiratory diameter variation <<50% ◆ Prominent transtricuspid E-wave, especially if >1m/s ◆ RA, RV dilatation
Quantitative parameters			
R vol, mL/beat	≥60	≥60	
RF, %	≥50	≥50	
ERO, cm^2	≥0.30	≥0.40	

AR, aortic regurgitation; CW, continuous wave; ERO, effective regurgitant orifice area; LA, left atrium; LV, left ventricle; LVOT, LV outflow tract; MR, mitral regurgitation; MS, mitral stenosis; MV, mitral valve; R vol, regurgitant volume; RA, right atrium; RF, regurgitant fraction; RV, right ventricle; TR, tricuspid regurgitation.

[a] At a Nyquist limit of 50–60cm/s.

[b] Large flow convergence defined as flow convergence radius of ≥0.9cm for central jets, with a baseline shift at a Nyquist of 40cm/s; cut-offs for eccentric jets are higher and should be angled correctly.

[c] Usually above 50 years of age or in conditions of impaired relaxation, in the absence of MS or other causes of elevated LA pressure.

[d] In the absence of other aetiologies of LV dilatation.

[e] In the absence of other aetiologies of LV and LA dilatation and acute MR.

Adapted with permission from Vahanian A, Baumgartner H, Bax J, *et al.* Guidelines on the management of valvular heart disease: The Task Force on the Management of Valvular Heart Disease of the European Society of Cardiology. *Eur Heart J* 2007; **28**: 230–68.

in certain cases of acute AR, in particular in aortic dissection or acute endocarditis with large vegetations.

Natural history

The severity of AR increases more rapidly for moderate rather than mild regurgitation and in patients with bicuspid valve or degenerative disease rather than in those with pure rheumatic AR [87, 88].

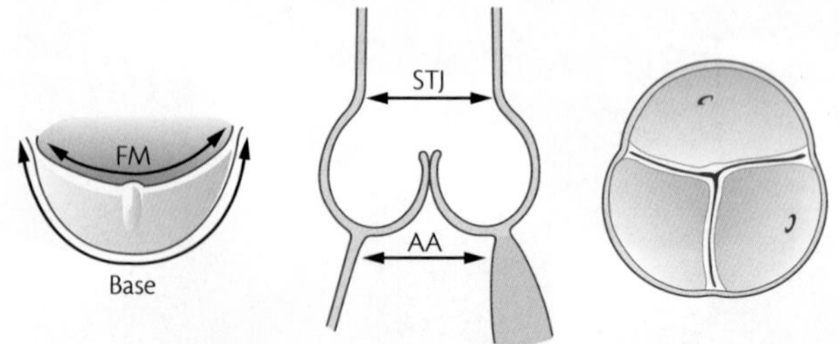

Figure 21.11 Geometric relationships of the aortic root. AA, aortic annulus; FM, free margin; STJ, sinotubular junction. Adapted with permission from David T. Aortic valve repair and aortic valve-sparing operations. In Cohn LH, Edmunds LH Jr (eds.) *Cardiac Surgery in the Adult*, 2nd edn., 2003. New York: McGraw-Hill, pp. 811–23.

In asymptomatic patients with chronic severe AR and initially normal LV function, the incidence of symptoms, LV dysfunction, or sudden death, is estimated to be between 3–6% per year [87–93]. The most frequent complication is deterioration of LV function. The risk of sudden death is low. The strongest predictor of a cardiac event is the initial LV end-systolic dimension [89]. The temporal changes of LV dimensions and function should also be taken into account. Symptom onset carries a poor prognosis and is frequently preceded by LV enlargement. Recently the volume of AR, as assessed using quantitative measurements, has been shown to predict prognosis [90].

The risk of aortic complications (dissection or rupture) depends mainly on the aortic diameter. It is estimated to be >20% per year when indexed aortic diameter is >4.25cm/m^2 of BSA [94]. In bicuspid aortic valves, the rate of progression does not depend on valve function and seems higher than in patients with tricuspid valves [95]. The risk of complications is higher in Marfan syndrome. Models have been proposed to predict the expansion rate of ascending aorta; however, they do not enable the evolution of aortic diameter to be reliably predicted for any given patient. In patients with Marfan syndrome, aortic complications are rare when the ratio between observed and predicted aortic root diameter is <1.3 [96].

Acute AR has a dismal prognosis if not corrected.

Medical treatment

The utility of vasodilators to influence the timing of surgery in patients with chronic severe AR without LV dysfunction has been investigated by randomized trials [91, 97]. Because of contradictory results their use is not advised outside the presence of systemic hypertension or overt heart failure en route to surgery [11, 12].

In patients with Marfan syndrome, beta-blockers can slow the dilatation of aortic root and decrease the risk of aortic complications [98]. Preliminary findings suggest that angiotensin-receptor blockers may slow the progression of aortic dilatation by the preservation of elastic fibres of ascending aortic wall [99]. However, their clinical benefit remains to be proven by ongoing trials.

Medical treatment of AR includes endocarditis prophylaxis [59] (see ➲Chapter 22, Infective Endocarditis).

Surgical treatment

Technique

Surgical treatment of AR is aortic valve replacement in most cases when there is no associated aortic aneurysm. When an aneurysm of the aortic root is associated with severe AR, the reference technique is the replacement of the ascending aorta using a composite graft comprising an aortic prosthesis, associated with a re-implantation of coronary arteries, according to the Bentall technique. Replacing only the supra-coronary section of the ascending aorta is technically easier and can be used when aortic enlargement is localized in the supra-coronary part of ascending aorta.

In the Ross intervention, the aortic root is replaced by the patient's pulmonary root. The durability of the valve substitute is good in the aortic position [100]. This is the technique of choice in infants and children but it is used less in adults in current practice [11].

There is now a growing interest for conservative surgery in AR (i.e. aortic valve repair), which combines different surgical techniques on the aortic valve and the ascending aorta according to a thorough analysis of the anatomy and mechanisms of AR [78, 101, 102]. The quality of the cusps is essential for repair: they should be pliable and the final length of the free margin should be 1.5 times shorter than the base of implantation. The other structures, such as the annulus and sinotubular junction can be readapted to the cusps. The surgical procedure is adapted to the mechanism of AR, which can be reliably predicted by preoperative transoesophageal echocardiography [84].

In the case of dilation of the sinotubular junction, AR can be simply treated by adjustment of the sinotubular junction to the annulus using a short Dacron® graft (➲Fig. 21.12).

In aortic root aneurysm (➲Fig. 21.13), two techniques have been proposed: firstly, remodelling of the aortic root with replacement of the Valsalva sinuses with or without annuloplasty [103], the diameter of the graft being equal to that of the ideal sinotubular junction; and secondly, reimplantation of the aortic valve inside a Dacron® conduit [104] (➲Fig. 21.14). In the presence of annulo-ectasia and in Marfan disease, the reimplantation technique is preferred above the remodelling technique because it prevents further or recurrent dilatation of the aortic annulus.

Leaflet pathology can be treated by central plication with potential reinforcement of the free margin with a Gore-Tex® thread. Patch repair can be used to treat a perforation. A bicuspid valve can be treated by resectioning the raphe of the common prolapsing cusp and by bilateral commissuroplasty to ensure sufficient coaptation [105].

In current practice, prosthetic valve replacement remains the standard and the other procedures are performed in only a small percentage of patients [2].

Results

Operative mortality in AR is low. Operative risk is strongly determined by age, degree of LV dysfunction, and comorbidity [106–113]. Recent series report low operative mortality even in patients with severe LV dysfunction [106, 107].

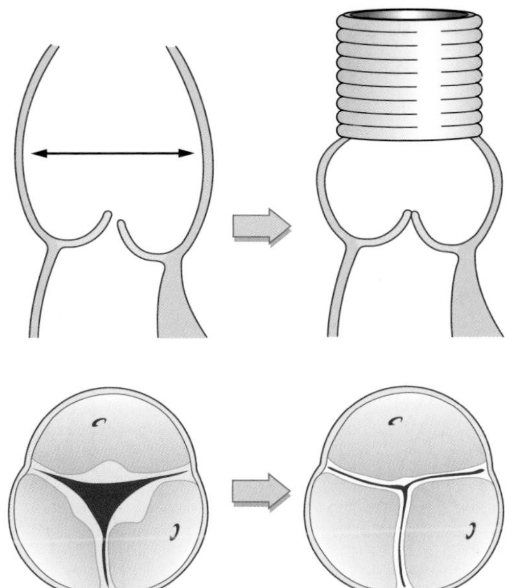

Figure 21.12 Correction of AR by replacement of the ascending aorta and adjustment of sinotubular junction. (Courtesy of Dr T. David.)

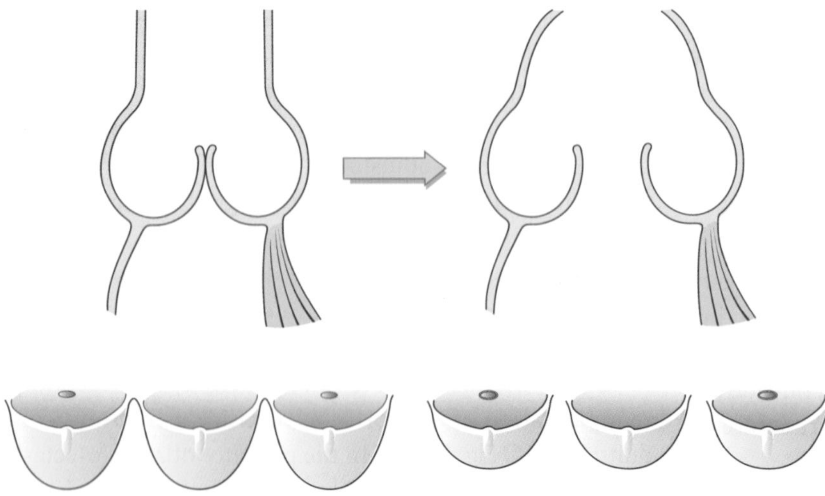

Figure 21.13 Aortic root aneurysm with annulo-aortic ectasia. Left, normal aortic annulus. (Courtesy of Dr T. David.)

Late results of valve surgery for AR are closely related to preoperative LV function [106–108]. Prospective series have identified thresholds of LV dimensions, mostly end-systolic dimension, or EF, which were related to outcome [11, 12]. Thresholds should take into account patient stature [109]: preoperative end-systolic LV dimension <25mm/m^2 BSA was associated with a good late outcome after valve replacement [110].

The aim of surgery is also to avoid aortic complications in patients who present with aortic aneurysm. Isolated aortic valve replacement does not preclude further aortic dilatation in patients who had preoperative dilatation of the ascending aorta [78, 79, 111]. Immediate and late results of the replacement of the ascending aorta using a composite graft are excellent in Marfan syndrome when performed by experienced teams on an elective basis [112]. This technique should also be favoured in annulo-aortic ectasia.

Data on conservative surgery is more limited and comes from expert centres. Yacoub has reported a 10-year freedom from valve replacement of 89% in 158 consecutive patients [103]. David, in a series of 120 patients, has reported an operative mortality of 1.6%, 10-year survival of 88%, freedom from aortic valve replacement of 99%, and freedom from at least moderate AR of 83% [104].

Treatment strategy

A stepwise approach to the management of AR according to ESC guidelines is detailed in ➲Fig. 21.15.

Symptomatic patients with chronic aortic regurgitation

Once symptoms appear or LV dysfunction ensues the prognosis worsens significantly. Thus the detection of symptoms or LV dysfunction is an indication for surgery even if there appears to be a transient improvement after medical therapy.

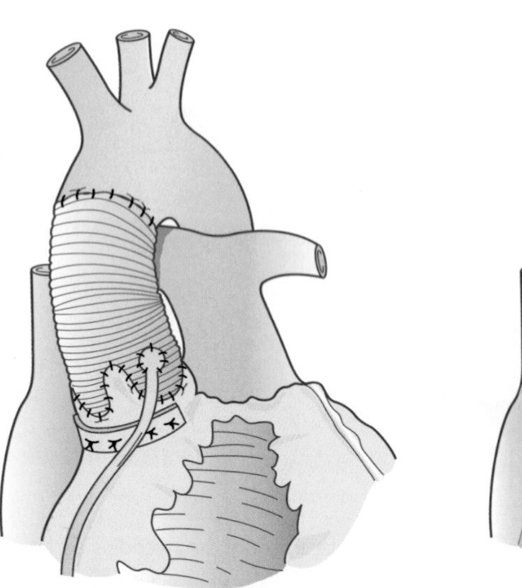

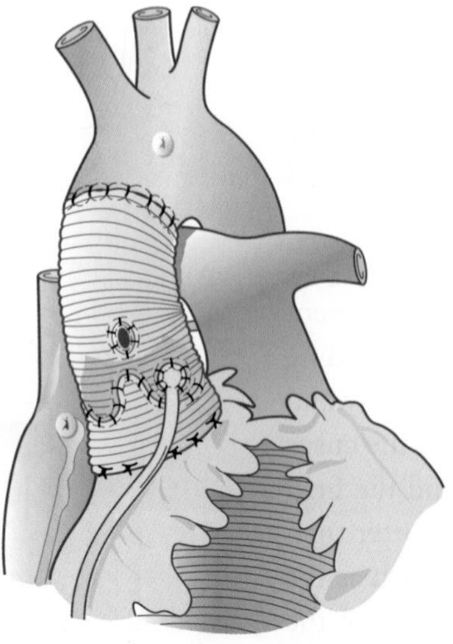

Figure 21.14 Conservative surgery techniques for aortic root aneurysm. Left: remodelling of the aortic root with aortic annuloplasty; right: re-implantation of the aortic valve inside a Dacron® graft. Reproduced with permission from David T. Aortic valve repair and aortic valve-sparing operations. In Cohn LH, Edmunds LH Jr (eds.) *Cardiac Surgery in the Adult*, 2nd edn., 2003. New York: McGraw-Hill, pp. 811–23.

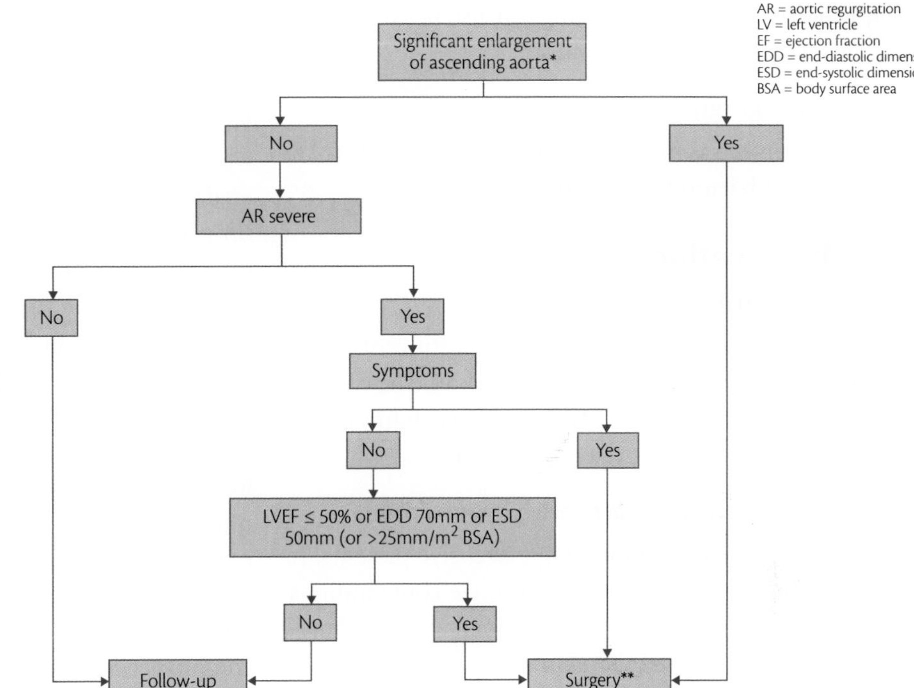

Figure 21.15 Management of AR. *Maximal aortic diameter >45mm in patients with Marfan syndrome; ≥50mm for patients with bicuspid valve; ≥55mm for all other patients. **Surgery must also be considered if significant changes occur during follow-up. Adapted with permission from Vahanian A, Baumgartner H, Bax J, *et al.* Guidelines on the management of valvular heart disease. The Task Force on the Management of Valvular Heart Disease of the European Society of Cardiology. *Eur Heart J* 2007; **28**: 230–68.

Operative mortality is relatively low, surgery improves symptoms and late outcome compares favourably with natural outcome. After surgery, patients with persisting LV systolic dysfunction should also receive optimal medical therapy according to the guidelines on heart failure, including ACE-inhibitors and beta-blockers. A study has suggested that long-term vasodilator therapy may allow for a better preservation of postoperative LV function [113].

In patients with severe LV dysfunction, the current trend is to favour aortic valve replacement over heart transplantation. However, in patients with major LV dysfunction, the final choice between valve replacement, heart transplantation, or medical therapy, is made on an individual basis.

Asymptomatic patients with chronic aortic regurgitation

Early intervention in asymptomatic patients according to LV dimensions and/or EF improves late survival and late preservation of LV function, as compared with patients operated at a more advanced stage of the disease. Surgery is indicated in asymptomatic AR when LVEF is <50% and should be considered when LV end-diastolic and end-systolic dimensions are >70mm and >50mm (25mm/m^2 BSA), respectively [11]. Indications for surgery should also take into account temporal changes in LV indices.

Thus the decision to intervene in asymptomatic patients depends on the collective assessment of measurements obtained from various imaging modalities and should also take into account the rate of change of LV dimensions, LV function, and ascending aortic diameters.

Patients with aneurysm of the ascending aorta

In patients with aortic aneurysm, intervention is advised when maximal aortic diameter is >55mm, regardless of the degree of AR; the threshold being lower in patients with bicuspid aortic valve (50mm) and with Marfan syndrome (45mm). When valve replacement is required on the basis of the severity of AR, replacement of the ascending aorta should be considered when aortic diameter is >45 to 50mm depending on the aetiology [11, 12]. The decision should be adapted according to patient age and body size, although no definite thresholds can be advised in this regard.

Beta-blockers are advised in patients with ascending aortic aneurysm and should be used systematically for Marfan's syndrome (78).

In patients who do not meet the criteria for intervention, clinical follow-up is advised on a yearly basis. The decision to perform an echocardiogram depends on the severity of AR, LV and aortic dimensions obtained at baseline or previous investigations. When LV or aortic dimensions significantly change or approach thresholds mentioned in guidelines, clinical and echocardiographic follow-up should be performed every 6 months [11].

Finally, echocardiographic screening of first-degree relatives is recommended in patients with Marfan syndrome to detect asymptomatic enlargement of the ascending aorta.

Family echocardiographic screening can also be considered in patients with bicuspid aortic valve.

Acute aortic regurgitation

Urgent intervention is indicated in most cases of acute AR because of poor haemodynamic tolerance.

Particular situations

Infective endocarditis

Severe AR is a particularly serious complication of infective endocarditis and urgent intervention should be considered, without waiting for haemodynamic instability which increases operative mortality (see ➲Chapter 22).

Aortic regurgitation associated with hypertension

Trivial or mild AR is common in hypertensive patients. It may be difficult to determine the respective contributions of hypertension and AR to LV enlargement and dysfunction, which requires a careful quantification and analysis of the mechanisms of AR after optimization of blood pressure control.

Mitral stenosis

Although the prevalence of rheumatic fever has greatly decreased in Western countries, MS still results in significant morbidity and mortality worldwide [2, 6–8]. The treatment of MS has been revolutionized since the development of percutaneous mitral balloon commissurotomy (PMC).

Aetiology

Rheumatic heart disease accounts for almost all cases of MS. The anatomic lesions combine to varying degrees: fusion of one or both commissures; thickening, fibrosis, and calcification of the valves; and shortening, thickening, and fusion of the subvalvular apparatus. Other valves are also involved in over one-third of cases, the most frequent associated lesions being tricuspid disease and AR [114]. Degenerative and congenital MS are very seldom seen [2]. Other rare aetiologies include carcinoid disease, Fabry's disease, mucopolysaccharidosis, Whipple's disease, gout, rheumatoid arthritis, lupus erythematosus, methysergide therapy, or obstruction of the valve by an atrial tumour or a large vegetation.

Pathophysiology

After a rheumatic attack, the alterations of the valve slowly progress, mostly driven by the abnormal flow dynamics caused by the initial and eventually repeated rheumatic insults.

Normal mitral valve area is 4–6cm^2. A diastolic transvalvular gradient between the left atrium and the LV appears when the valve area approaches 2cm^2 or less. MS is considered significant when the valve area is $<$1.5cm^2, or $<$1cm^2/m^2 BSA in large individuals. Valve obstruction progressively limits cardiac output and increases pressure in the left atrium, which, in turn, raises pulmonary circulation pressure. Pulmonary oedema, related to transudation from the pulmonary capillaries, occurs when mean capillary wedge pressure is approximately $>$25mmHg. The transvalvular gradient and its consequences are highly dependent on heart rate and transvalvular flow. Exercise limitation is multifactorial and heterogeneous for a given degree of stenosis. This heterogeneity may be explained by differences in the evolution of stroke volume during exercise [115] and differences in atrioventricular compliance [116]. A low net compliance is mainly the consequence of a low compliance of the left atrium and is associated, even more than at rest, with a higher pulmonary pressure at exercise and more severe symptoms. The degree of pulmonary hypertension is variable and often greater than the passive increase caused by elevated left atrial pressures. This could be due to initially reversible morphological changes in pulmonary vasculature, reactive pulmonary vasoconstriction, or reduced lung compliance [117]. Chronic pulmonary hypertension causes right ventricular (RV) hypertrophy, which, possibly exacerbated by tricuspid regurgitation (TR), causes failure of the RV.

Intrinsic LV contractility is usually preserved; however, chronic afterload elevation and preload reduction, related to MS and ventricular interactions, can cause LV dysfunction in up to 25% of cases.

Atrial fibrillation, which is not strictly linked to the severity of MS, is a consequence of left atrial dilatation and hypertrophy, as well as rheumatic insult to the atria, internodal tracts, and sino-atrial node. Atrial fibrillation causes haemodynamic compromise through decreased cardiac output due to the loss of atrial contraction and shortening of diastole. It also increases thromboembolic risk as a result of left atrial enlargement, blood stagnation, and increased concentrations of prothrombotic markers.

Diagnosis

History

Usually, symptoms appear gradually over years, with patients first reporting dyspnoea on exertion, which is the consequence of the abnormal elevation of the left atrial and capillary wedge pressure. Patients frequently adapt their level of functional capacity and deny dyspnoea despite objective effort limitation. Pregnancy, emotional stress, sexual intercourse, infection, or the onset of atrial fibrillation may all be precipitating factors of marked dyspnoea or pulmonary oedema. Haemoptysis, paroxysmal cough, as well as chest discomfort, is infrequent.

Atrial fibrillation often begins in paroxysms and eventually becomes chronic. Embolic events, which may be the presenting complaint in 20% of cases, are most often cerebral and leave sequelae in one-third of cases.

At a more advanced stage, patients may complain of fatigue due to low cardiac output, weakness, or abdominal discomfort due to hepatomegaly when RV failure is present. Hoarseness may occasionally be observed in the case of severe enlargement of the left atrium (i.e. Ortner's syndrome).

Physical examination

The main signs of auscultation are appreciated at the apex. The low-pitched rumbling diastolic murmur (typically holodiastolic, decrescendo with a presystolic accentuation in sinus rhythm) can be palpated when it is of high intensity. The loudness of the murmur depends on the level of the transmitral gradient. It may be of low intensity or even inaudible in patients with low output, emphysema, or obesity. The opening snap occurs 0.013–0.03s after the second heart sound—the more severe the stenosis, the shorter the interval, as increased left atrial pressure causes earlier opening of the mitral valve. The accentuated first heart sound (a high-pitched sound due to the fact that ventricular systole closes the mitral valve from a long moment arm) may be blunted in patients with severe calcification which alters both the opening and closing of the valve.

Pulmonary hypertension causes both a louder second heart sound at the base and a murmur of TR located at the xyphoid. This can be differentiated from a murmur of MR by its respiratory variation. In patients with RV failure, the dilated ventricle can be palpated at the xiphoid, as can a systolic impulse of the pulmonary artery at the third left intercostal space.

Pulmonary rales are present in patients with severe symptoms and at an advanced stage, and mitral facies with intermittent malar flushes, jugular distension, and peripheral cyanosis may be seen. Respiratory failure, cachexia, and the discovery of severe pulmonary hypertension dominate examination.

Auscultation should also search for a holosystolic murmur at the apex suggesting MR. Finally, it should look for an associated aortic valve disease resulting in either a mid systolic or a diastolic murmur at the level of the left sternal border.

Electrocardiography

Patients who are in sinus rhythm demonstrate signs of left atrial enlargement with a prolonged P wave and a negative deflection in lead V1 and left axial deviation of P wave. Atrial fibrillation is frequent. Signs of RV hypertrophy are usually present in cases of severe pulmonary hypertension (➲ Chapter 2).

Chest radiograph

The cardiac silhouette is only mildly enlarged during the early stages. As severity increases, signs of left atrial enlargement can be observed: (1) straightening of the left heart border; (2) double contour of the left atrium; and (3) widening of the carinal angle of the trachea. As the disease progresses, signs of RV enlargement can follow. Redistribution of pulmonary vascular flow towards the upper lung fields, a progressively enlarged pulmonary trunk, and signs of interstitial pulmonary and alveolar oedema are all indicative of the elevation of pulmonary pressures. Usually, fluoroscopy is necessary to visualize valve calcification.

Echocardiography

Echocardiography is the main method to assess the severity and consequences of MS, as well as the extent of anatomic lesions (➲ Chapter 4). Measurements of the mean transvalvular gradient from Doppler velocities are highly rate- and flow-dependent; however, they provide useful information for patients in sinus rhythm. Severity of MS should ideally be quantified using two-dimensional planimetry (the most accurate way of assessing valve area after PMC) (➲ Fig. 21.16) and the pressure half-time method, which are complementary (🎥 21.7). Continuity equation and proximal isovelocity methods are less frequently used to calculate valve area. The consistency between planimetry, the pressure half-time method, and gradient should always been checked, bearing in mind the limitations of the different measurements.

Three-dimensional echo is feasible, and improves reproducibility and accuracy measuring the valve area (🎥 21.8–10) [118].

The assessment of valve morphology is increasingly important for the selection of candidates for PMC. Scores have been developed that take into account valve thickening, mobility, calcification, and subvalvular deformity [119,120] (➲ Tables 21.3 and 21.4).

Echocardiography also evaluates pulmonary pressures, the presence of associated MR, concomitant aortic and tricuspid valve disease, and left atrial size [121].

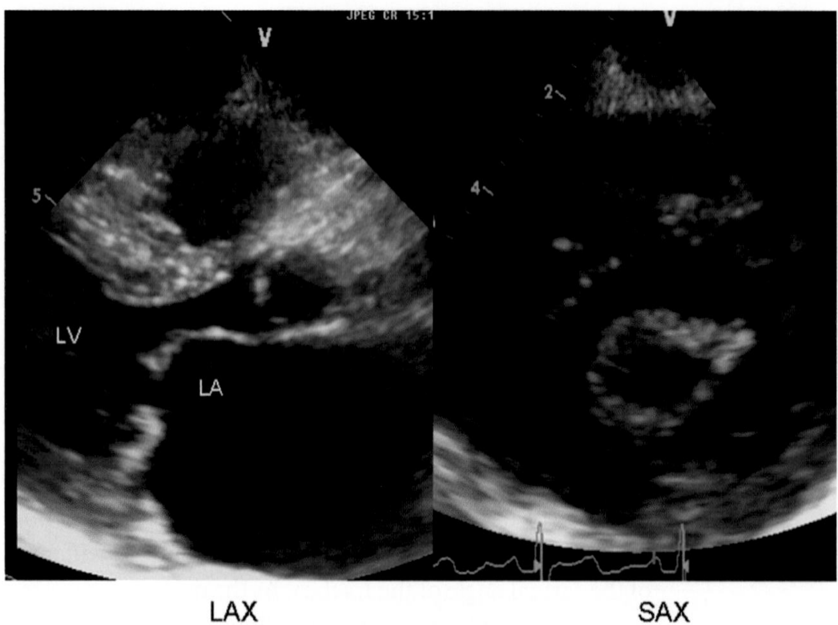

Figure 21.16 Echographic analysis of MS. Transthoracic echocardiography. Parasternal long-axis (left) and short-axis (right) views showing MS. Note on the short-axis view the bilateral commissural fusion without calcification. LA, left atrium; LAX, long-axis view; LV, left ventricle; SAX, short-axis view. (Courtesy of Dr. E Brochet.)

A transthoracic approach provides sufficient information for routine management and decision making (21.11); however, transoesophageal examination should also be performed when transthoracic visualization is suboptimal or to exclude left atrial thrombosis, in particular in the appendage, before PMC or in case of suspicion such as after an embolic complication. In addition, transoesophageal echocardiography may show the presence of spontaneous echo contrast.

Echocardiography also plays an important role in monitoring the results of PMC during the procedure and in evaluating the final results (21.12 and 21.13)

Other non-invasive investigations

Bicycle ergometry may provide a useful objective assessment of functional capacity in patients whose symptoms are equivocal or discordant with the severity of MS.

Dobutamine or, preferably, exercise echocardiography may also be used to assess the evolution of mitral gradient and pulmonary pressure in patients with doubtful symptoms. However, the added value for decision making has to be further defined [122, 123].

Preliminary reports suggest that MRI and multislice CT could be alternate techniques for planimetry when echocardiography is inconclusive [124].

Table 21.3 Grading of mitral valve characteristics from the echocardiographic examination. The total echocardiographic score was derived from an analysis of mitral leaflet mobility, valvar and subvalvar thickening, and calcification which were graded from 0–4 according to these criteria. This gave a total score of 0–16.

Grade	Mobility	Subvalvular thickening	Thickening	Calcification
1	Highly mobile valve with only leaflet tips restricted	Minimal thickening just below the mitral leaflets	Leaflets near normal in thickness (4–5mm)	A single area of increased echo brightness
2	Leaflet mid and base portions have normal mobility	Thickening of chordal structures extending to one of the chordal length	Mid-leaflets normal, considerable thickening of margins (5–8mm)	Scattered areas of brightness confined to leaflet margins
3	Valve continues to move forward in diastole, mainly from the base	Thickening extended to distal third of the chords	Thickening extending through the entire leaflet (5–8mm)	Brightness extending into the mid portions of the leaflets
4	No or minimal forward movement of the leaflets in diastole	Extensive thickening and shortening of all chordal structures extending down to the papillary muscles	Considerable thickening of all leaflet tissue (>8–10mm)	Extensive brightness throughout much of the leaflet tissue

Adapted with permission from Wilkins GT, Weyman AE, Abascal VM, *et al.* Percutaneous balloon dilatation of the mitral valve: an analysis of echocardiographic variables related to outcome and the mechanism of dilatation. *Br Heart J* 1988; **60**: 299–308.

Table 21.4 Description of the three-group grading of mitral valve anatomy, as assessed by two-dimensional echocardiography and fluoroscopy

Echocardiographic group	Mitral valve anatomy
Group 1	Pliable non-calcified anterior mitral leaflet and mild subvalvular disease (i.e. thin chordae ≥10mm long)
Group 2	Pliable non-calcified anterior mitral leaflet and severe subvalvular disease (i.e. thickened chordae <10mm long)
Group 3	Calcification of mitral valve of any extent, as assessed by fluoroscopy, whatever the state of subvalvular apparatus

Adapted with permission from Iung B, Cormier B, Ducimetière P, *et al.* Immediate results of percutaneous mitral commissurotomy. *Circulation* 1996; **94**: 2124–30.

Invasive investigation

The accuracy of echocardiography has virtually eliminated the use of invasive haemodynamic assessment of MS or associated valve disease. There are still, however, occasional indications for catheterization when clinical and echocardiographic data are discordant. Coronary angiography is required prior to surgery according to guidelines [11, 12].

Natural history

In developing countries, severe MS is commonly observed in infants or young adults, whereas in industrialized countries symptoms are usually delayed until the fifth decade of life. The rate of progression of stenosis is variable: ranging from 0.1–0.3cm^2/year, higher rates being observed in patients with severe anatomic deformity and high transmitral gradient. Studies on natural history are old and non-controlled. In asymptomatic patients, survival was 84% at 10 years; among patients with few symptoms, survival was 42% at 10 years and the incidence of heart failure was approximately 60%. Symptomatic patients had a poor prognosis with a 5-year survival of only 44% [125]. The progression was highly variable with gradual deterioration in one-half of patients, and sudden deterioration, precipitated by a complication, in the rest. Atrial fibrillation can occur in asymptomatic patients and is often preceded by supraventricular arrhythmias. The occurrence of atrial fibrillation increases with age and left atrial enlargement, and the incidence of thromboembolism is also higher with age, atrial fibrillation, larger left atrium, smaller valve area, and, most significantly, the presence of left atrial spontaneous echo contrast [126].

Medical treatment

Diuretics or long-acting nitrates transiently ameliorate dyspnoea. Beta-blockers or calcium-channel blockers are useful to slow the heart rate.

Anticoagulant therapy with a target international normalized ratio (INR) in the upper half of the range 2–3 is indicated in patients with atrial fibrillation. In patients with sinus rhythm, anticoagulation is recommended when there has been prior embolism or a thrombus is present in the left atrium, and it should be considered in patients who have an enlarged left atrium (>50–55mm in diameter) or a dense spontaneous echo contrast [11, 12, 127].

Cardioversion is not indicated before intervention in patients with severe MS, as it does not durably restore sinus rhythm. If atrial fibrillation is of recent onset and the left atrium only moderately enlarged, cardioversion should be performed soon after successful intervention.

Infective endocarditis prophylaxis is indicated as appropriate [59] (see ➲Chapter 22).

In countries with a high prevalence of rheumatic disease, rheumatic fever prophylaxis should be given to young patients and should be continued after PMC or surgical commissurotomy. The duration for which prophylactic antibiotic therapy should be continued is controversial. It seems to be rarely necessary after 21 years.

Percutaneous mitral commissurotomy

Since its introduction in the early 1980s, successful results of PMC have led to its worldwide adoption [128, 129].

Trans-septal catheterization is one of the most crucial steps of the procedure and the Inoue balloon technique has become the most popular technique (➲Fig. 21.17; 21.24).

PMC, which results in commissural splitting (➲Fig. 21.18), usually provides at least a 100% increase in valve area, with a final valve area of approximately 2cm^2. The improvement in valve function results in an immediate decrease in pulmonary pressures, both at rest and during exercise.

Failure rates range from 1–15%. Procedural mortality ranges from 0–3%, and incidence of haemopericardium varies from 0.5–12%. Embolism is encountered in 0.5–5% of cases. Severe MR, which occurs in 2–10% of patients, is a result of non-commissural leaflet tearing. Urgent surgery is seldom needed for complications (<1%). Immediately after PMC, in 40–80% of patients, colour Doppler echo shows small intra-atrial shunts, which are likely to close later in the majority of cases. The complication rate of the procedure is related to the patient's condition and the experience of the team [128–132].

Clinical follow-up data, now up to 17 years, confirms the late efficacy of PMC: event-free survival ranges from 35–70% after 10–15 years [133–137]. When the immediate results are unsatisfactory, surgery is usually required in the following months. Conversely, after successful PMC,

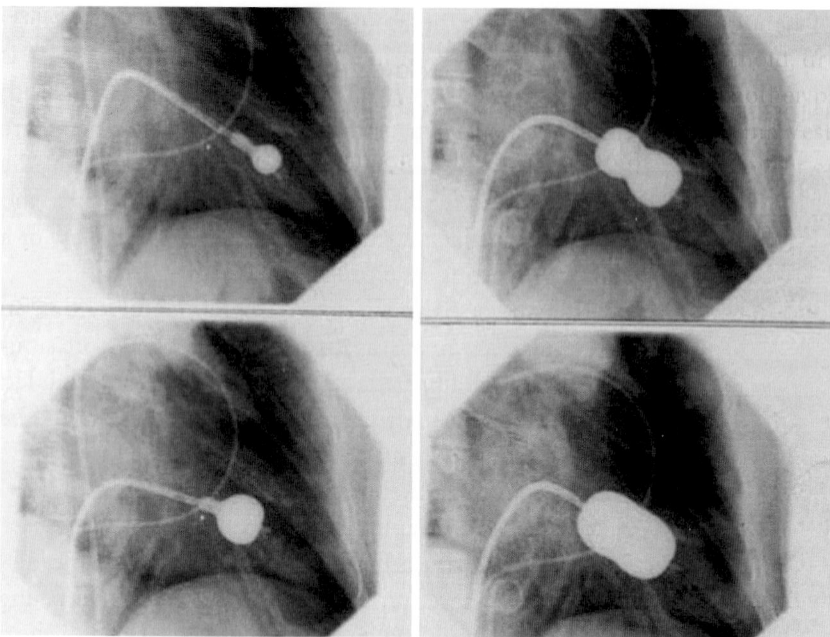

Figure 21.17 Percutaneous mitral commissurotomy using the Inoue balloon technique. Right anterior oblique view. Upper left, the distal part of the balloon is inflated with contrast in the centre of the mitral valve; lower left, the distal part is further inflated and the balloon is pulled back into the mitral orifice; upper right, inflation occurs in the central portion; lower right, at full inflation the waist on the balloon disappears.

long-term results are good in the majority of cases. When functional deterioration occurs, it is late and mainly related to re-stenosis (around 40% after 7 years). Repeat PMC can be proposed in selected patients with favourable characteristics [138]. Successful PMC has been shown to reduce embolic risk [126] while its efficacy in preventing atrial fibrillation is debatable [139].

The prediction of the long-term results of PMC is multifactorial. In addition to morphological factors, preoperative variables such as age, history of commissurotomy, functional class, small mitral valve area, and presence of TR are all independent predictors of poor results. The prediction of long-term results is also closely related to the quality of the immediate results [133, 135, 137].

Surgery

Conservative surgery

The first operation performed >50 years ago was closed mitral valve commissurotomy [140]. This operation was effective and easily accessible, which explains its high use until recently in developing countries. Today it has been replaced by open-heart mitral commissurotomy using cardiopulmonary bypass, which enables surgeons not only to correct commissural fusion, but also to act on chordal and papillary fusion, and to even improve leaflet mobility and pliability by enlarging the leaflets by using pericardial patches. The use of prosthetic rings is controversial in these cases. In young patients and with experienced operators, long-term

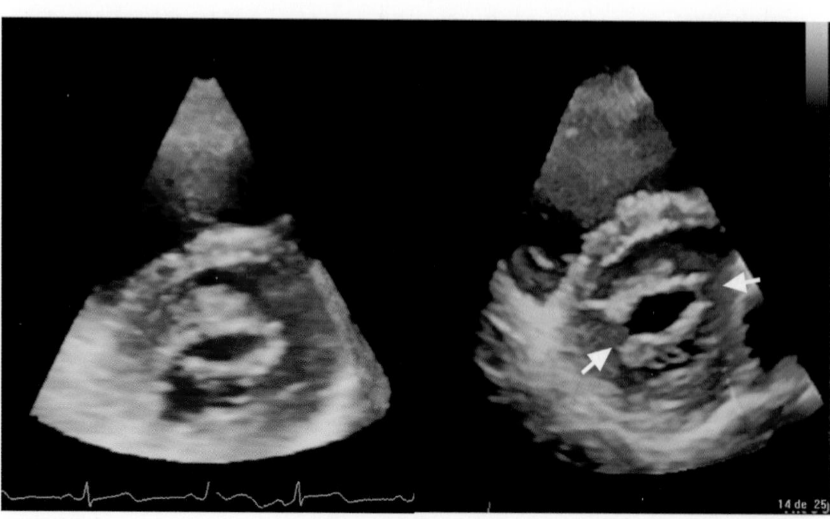

Figure 21.18 Echographic evaluation after percutaneous mitral commissurotomy (PMC). Real time three-dimensional transthoracic echocardiography before (left) and after (right) PMC. Note the well-defined opening of both commissures with real-time three-dimensional transthoracic echocardiography after PMC (white arrows). (Courtesy of Dr E. Brochet.)

results are good, with survival of 96% and freedom from valve-related complications of 92% at 15 years [141].

Valve replacement

Valve replacement uses predominantly mechanical valves because of their better durability in the mitral position and because patients may require long-term anticoagulation anyway for atrial fibrillation.

Operative mortality ranges between 3–10% and correlates with age, functional class, pulmonary hypertension, and the presence of CAD. Long-term survival is related to age, functional class, atrial fibrillation, pulmonary hypertension, preoperative LV function, and complications of the prosthetic valve, especially thromboembolism and haemorrhage [142].

The Euro Heart Survey [2] reveals that, in current practice, percutaneous intervention has almost replaced open-heart commissurotomy and valve replacement mostly uses mechanical prosthesis (➲Table 21.1).

Treatment strategy

Intervention should be performed only in patients with significant MS. A stepwise approach to the management of MS according to ESC guidelines is detailed in ➲Fig. 21.19.

Symptomatic patients

PMC is the procedure of choice when surgery is contraindicated or for patients with favourable characteristics, i.e. young patients with sinus rhythm and favourable anatomy [143, 144].

The decision to intervene in patients with unfavourable anatomy must take into account multiple factors that can influence outcomes. In addition, the respective skills of the surgical and interventional teams in the institution concerned must be considered. In such cases, PMC may achieve good long-term results and may be useful to defer surgery in selected patients with mild to moderate calcification or severe impairment of the subvalvular apparatus, who have otherwise favourable characteristics [145] (➲Fig. 21.20).

Surgery is the only alternative when PMC is contraindicated, the most important contraindication being left atrial thrombosis. A contraindication is self-evident if the thrombus is localized in the cavity, and the current guidelines still consider a thrombus localized in the appendage as a contraindication [11, 12]. Other contraindications for PMC

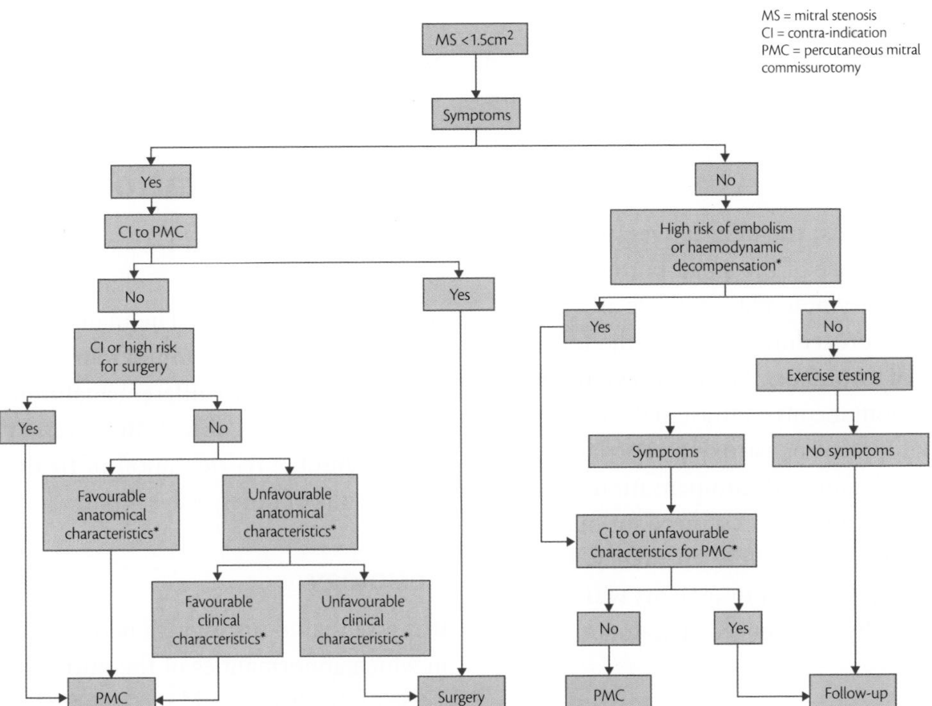

Figure 21.19 Management of severe MS. *Favourable characteristics for PMC are defined by the absence of several of the following: *clinical characteristics*: old age, history of commissurotomy, NYHA class 4, atrial fibrillation, severe pulmonary hypertension; *anatomic characteristics:* echo score >8, Cormier's score 3 (calcification of mitral valve of any extent as assessed by fluoroscopy), very small mitral valve area, severe TR. Patients at high risk of embolism or haemodynamic decompensation are defined by previous history of embolism, dense spontaneous contrast in the left atrium on transoesophageal echocardiography, recent or paroxysmal atrial fibrillation, systolic pulmonary pressure >50mm of mercury at rest, need for major non-cardiac surgery, desire of pregnancy. Adapted with permission from Vahanian A, Baumgartner H, Bax J, *et al.* Guidelines on the management of valvular heart disease. The Task Force on the Management of Valvular Heart Disease of the European Society of Cardiology. *Eur Heart J* 2007; **28**: 230–68.

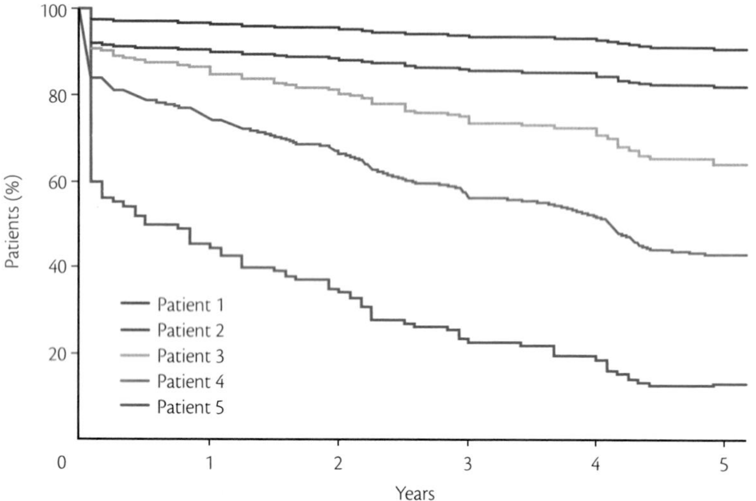

Figure 21.20 Prediction of the long-term event-free survival of percutaneous mitral commissurotomy in calcified MS. Patient 1: <50 years, NYHA class 2, sinus rhythm, mild calcification, valve area 1.2cm^2; patient 2: <50 years, NYHA class 2, sinus rhythm, moderate calcification, valve area 1cm^2; patient 3: 50–70 years, NYHA class 3, sinus rhythm, moderate calcification, valve area 1.25cm^2; patient 4: 50–70 years, NHYA class 3, atrial fibrillation, moderate calcification, valve area 1.2cm^2; patient 5: <70 years, NYHA class 4, atrial fibrillation, severe calcification, valve area 0.75cm^2. Adapted with permission from Iung B, Garbarz E, Doutrelant L, *et al.* Late results of percutaneous mitral commissurotomy for calcific mitral stenosis. *Am J Cardiol* 2000; **85**: 1308–14.

include more than mild MR, severe calcification, absence of commissural fusion, combined severe aortic or tricuspid valve disease, or coronary disease requiring bypass surgery. In such patients, valve replacement is preferred in most cases, whereas open commissurotomy may be performed by experienced teams in selected patients. Intraoperative correction of AF can be combined with valve surgery in selected cases; the benefit of this approach, however, requires further validation.

Finally, coexisting moderate aortic valve disease and functional TR are not considered as contraindications for the technique.

Asymptomatic patients

For asymptomatic patients, the alternatives are medical treatment or PMC. Because of the small but definite risk inherent in PMC, truly asymptomatic patients are not usually candidates for the procedure, except in the following cases: increased risk of thromboembolism (previous history of embolism, dense spontaneous contrast in the left atrium, or, to a lesser extent, recent or paroxysmal atrial fibrillation); risk of haemodynamic decompensation (systolic pulmonary pressure >50mmHg at rest; need for major extracardiac surgery; or finally, to allow pregnancy. In these cases, PMC should be performed in patients with favourable characteristics and by experienced operators.

Special populations

After surgical commissurotomy, re-operation almost always requires valve replacement at a somewhat higher risk. Here, PMC can delay re-operation in patients with favourable characteristics and if the predominant mechanism of restenosis is commissural refusion [138, 146]. Similarly, repeat PMC can be proposed in patients with the same characteristics if restenosis occurs several years after an initially successful PMC.

For information on MS during pregnancy see ➲Chapter 33, Pregnancy and Heart Disease.

In the elderly, when surgery is very high risk or even contraindicated but life expectancy is still >1 year, PMC is a useful option, even if only palliative. In patients with still favourable anatomy, PMC can be attempted first, resorting to surgery if results are unsatisfactory [147]. In other patients, surgery is preferable as the first option.

Mitral regurgitation

MR is the second most frequent valve disease after AS in hospitalized patients [2] and appears to be the first in the general population [1]. The main points to be covered are the complexity of the mitral valve apparatus, the various aetiologies leading to different anatomical lesions and functional mechanisms of MR, the diversity of clinical presentations, and the reorientation of treatment resulting from good results of timely valve repair.

Aetiology

It is essential to distinguish between primary organic MR, in which abnormalities of the mitral valve apparatus is the cause of the disease, and secondary (functional and ischaemic) MR, which results from LV disease and remodelling.

Primary mitral regurgitation

Reduced prevalence of rheumatic fever and increased life span in western countries have progressively changed the distribution of aetiologies.

Degenerative MR is the most common aetiology in Europe [2]. Primary mitral valve prolapse phenotypes can be diffuse myxomatous degeneration ('Barlow's disease') or primary flail leaflets accompanied by myxomatous degeneration, localized to the flail segment. Pathologic examination shows leaflet infiltration by mucopolysaccharides and accumulation of proteoglycans in the absence of inflammation. Non-specific alteration of collagen and elastin leads to increased elasticity and increased tension on the chordae tendinae which can become elongated and subsequently rupture [148]. Mitral valve prolapse (MVP) occurs in connective tissue disorders such as Marfan and Ehlers–Danlos syndromes. Although most cases of MVP are sporadic, familial MVP has been observed with autosomal dominant inheritance and genetic heterogenicity, linked to chromosomes 11, 13, 16, and the X chromosome [149, 150]. Annular calcification can be present in Barlow's disease and in elderly patients.

In rheumatic heart disease, MR is frequently associated with various degrees of MS. Regurgitation is essentially due to valvular and subvalvular retraction rather than thickening. Other causes leading to similar lesions are: rheumatoid arthritis, lupus erythematosus, the antiphospholipid syndrome, carcinoid disease, and drug-induced valve disease [5].

Infective endocarditis remains common and can result in leaflet perforation and chordal rupture.

The rupture of a papillary muscle, usually involving a head of the posteromedial papillary muscle, is a dramatic complication of acute myocardial infarction, which occurs less frequently since the use of immediate reperfusion strategies. Acute or chronic papillary muscle ischaemia or dysfunction in isolation does not result in MR.

Secondary mitral regurgitation

Ischaemic MR is increasingly prevalent but frequently unrecognized or underestimated.

Functional MR, which is frequent in patients with heart failure, is the consequence of annular dilatation and papillary muscle displacement tethering one or both leaflets, and of LV systolic dysfunction decreasing the mitral valve closing force [151]. The paradigm of a structurally normal valve in functional MR has recently been challenged, since the observation of structural changes in the mitral leaflets of patients with functional MR [152].

In all aetiologies of chronic MR, annular enlargement is a contributive factor.

Pathophysiology

MR consists of backflow—systolic regurgitation of blood from the LV to the left atrium—and results from incomplete mitral valve closure and a pressure gradient between the LV and the left atrium. MR can result from dysfunction of one or often several of the following components: the annulus, the leaflets, the chordae tendineae, the papillary muscles, and the LV. The mechanisms of regurgitation can be: valve prolapse due to redundant leaflets and elongation or rupture of chordae; loss of valvular tissue by retraction, perforation, or tethering on the leaflets (usually the posterior valve by chordal retraction); or LV remodelling causing geometric valvular distortion. The Carpentier classification [153] has subcategorized the mechanisms by leaflet movement and is useful to assess valve function (➲Fig. 21.21).

Regurgitant volume is determined by the regurgitant area, systolic pressure gradient across the MR orifice, and systolic duration. Systolic ventriculo-atrial pressure gradient is present throughout isovolumic contraction, ejection, and isovolumic relaxation. When the regurgitant orifice area is small, MR predominates in early systole [154]. The regurgitant orifice increases during systole in valve prolapse. In ischaemic MR, it peaks in early and late systole [155], and increases in parallel with LV enlargement or rise in afterload.

The ERO is dynamic, and can be modified by changes in loading conditions or contractility [154, 155].

Progression of functional MR is weakly linked to annular enlargement but more importantly to increased mitral tenting caused by LV remodelling, papillary muscle displacement, and increased chordal traction [156] (➲Fig. 21.22).

Acute mitral regurgitation

Acute MR, resulting from papillary muscle chordal rupture, leaflet tear or perforation, induces an immediate decrease in afterload. LV emptying increases, and left atrial pressure rises acutely, which is transmitted back to the pulmonary circulation. LV function is normal and EF is increased. Forward stroke volume is reduced, resulting in tachycardia to maintain cardiac output.

Chronic mitral regurgitation

MR causes LV volume overload. The total stroke volume is increased and the forward stroke volume is maintained or decreased. Diastolic function is supernormal [157]. LV remodelling is characterized by a large radius-to-thickness ratio and a small mass-to-volume ratio resulting in normal—and no longer decreased—afterload. Thus in chronic organic MR, altered LV function may coexist with normal EF. Eccentric LV hypertrophy develops and occurs from a decrease in protein degradation rather than an increase in the rate of protein synthesis [158]. Atrial compliance progressively increases. Regurgitant volume is thus handled

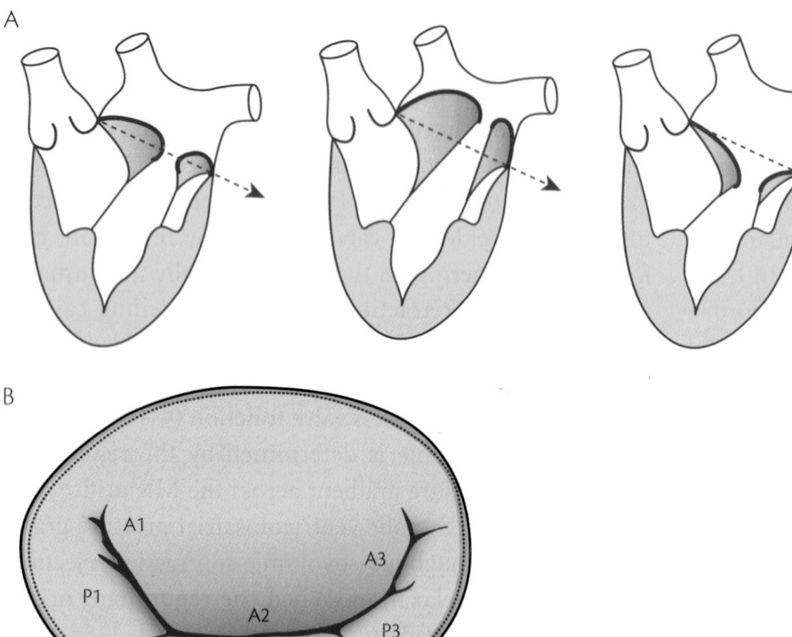

Figure 21.21 Carpentier classification in MR. (A) Functional anatomy subcategorized by leaflet movement; type I: normal leaflet motion; type II: leaflet prolapse; type III: restricted leaflet motion. (B) Anatomic location: the posterior leaflets segments are designated as P1, P2, and P3. P1 is adjacent to the anterolateral commissure, P2 is the middle scallop, and P3 is adjacent to the posteromedial commissure. The anterior leaflet has less clearly defined segments, designated as A1, A2, and A3, corresponding to the adjacent posterior leaflet segments.

without a large increase in left atrial pressure and pulmonary congestion.

The haemodynamic state may remain compensated for many years. However, as concentric hypertrophy does not develop, the increased volume is not compensated by increased thickness: the radius-to-thickness ratio remains high, which maintains increased systolic and diastolic stress.

Neurohormonal mechanisms develop [159] and sympathetic nervous system activity is especially increased.

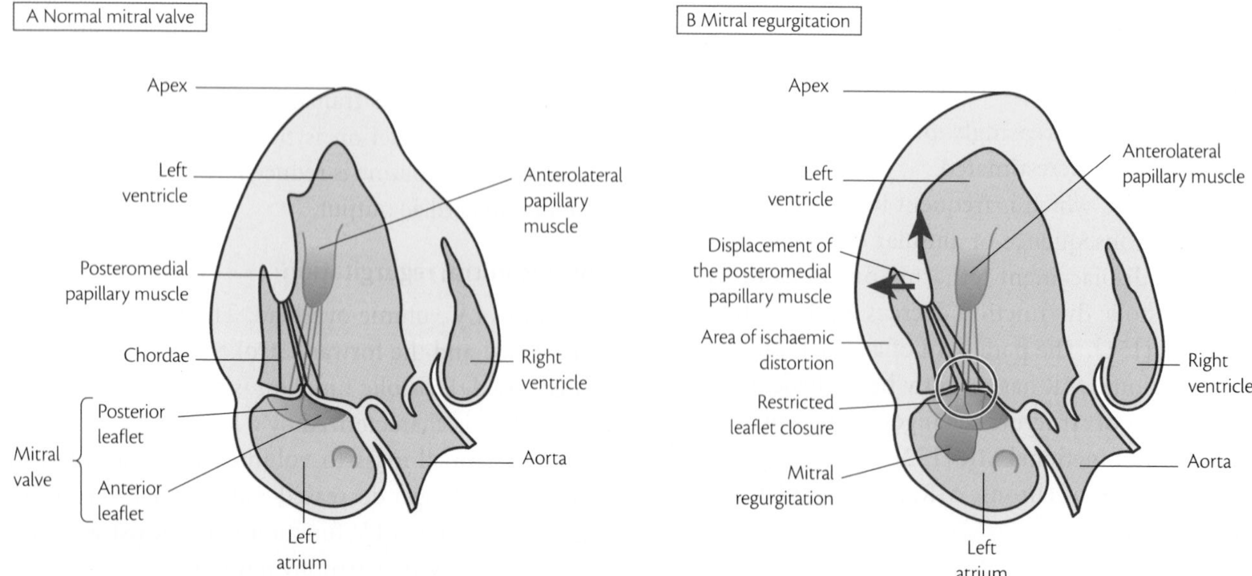

Figure 21.22 Pathophysiology of ischaemic MR. A normal mitral valve is shown in (A). Ischaemic MR, in which the leaflets cannot close effectively, is shown in (B). The orientation of the illustration is typical of ultrasound imaging. Adapted with permission from Levine RA. Dynamic mitral regurgitation—more than meets the eye. *N Eng J Med* 2004; **351**: 1681–4.

LV dysfunction can occur by loss of contractile elements, myocyte dysfunction, and abnormal calcium handling [160]. When chronic MR decompensates, afterload increases and heart failure can develop.

Diagnosis

History

Acute severe MR usually results in severe dyspnoea, acute pulmonary oedema, or congestive heart failure.

Patients with chronic severe organic MR may remain asymptomatic for years [16]. Symptoms, such as fatigue or dyspnoea, occur late when contractile dysfunction develops or at the onset of atrial fibrillation. In secondary MR, symptoms are related to the underlying disease process. MR is a dynamic condition and its severity may vary over time in relation to arrhythmias, ischaemia, hypertension, or exercise. Dynamic chronic ischaemic MR can lead to acute pulmonary oedema in the absence of acute myocardial ischaemia [161].

Physical examination

Systolic blood pressure is usually normal and pulse pressure is not increased.

In chronic severe primary MR, the apical impulse is displaced to the left. The main finding of auscultation is a systolic high-pitched murmur, loudest at the apex. It typically radiates to the axilla, but the radiation of the murmur depends on the direction of the regurgitant jet. If MR is at least moderate, the murmur is holosystolic, beginning at the onset of the first heart sound and continuing after the second heart sound. Its peak intensity is usually heard in late systole in valve prolapse. If the prolapse is not holosystolic, the typical feature is a mid- or late systolic click, generated by the tensing of the chordae and billowing of the mitral leaflets, followed by a late systolic murmur. Both click and murmur vary in intensity and timing with manoeuvres that induce changes in LV volume. The murmur of MR shows little changes in the presence of large variations of LV stroke volume which help to differentiate it from that of AS. The loudness of the murmur correlates somewhat with regurgitant severity. In severe MR, a third heart sound and a short diastolic rumble reflect the rapid and voluminous LV filling. When LV function is good, the first heart sound is masked by the holosystolic murmur, the second heart sound is normal early, then the loudness of the pulmonary component increases when pulmonary hypertension is present.

In secondary MR, auscultatory signs are highly dynamic; the murmur is usually of low intensity [162] and peak intensity is usually heard in early systole. The third heart sound is frequent.

In acute MR, the murmur is shortened by a rapid reduction in the pressure gradient between LV and left atrium; it may even be inaudible in papillary muscle rupture with low output.

Evidence of pulmonary congestion or of congestive heart failure is only seen in patients with decompensated disease.

Electrocardiography

Patients in sinus rhythm may present with LV and left atrial hypertrophy. Atrial fibrillation is common. In ischaemic MR, Q waves may be seen, most frequently in the inferior and/or lateral leads; and a left bundle branch block may be present.

Chest radiograph

Chronic severe MR leads to cardiomegaly due to LV and left atrial enlargement, and radiologic signs of left heart failure when cardiac dysfunction is present. In acute MR, heart volume may be normal, with evidence of interstitial or alveolar pulmonary oedema.

Echocardiography

Echocardiography is the cornerstone for diagnosing MR. It allows for establishing aetiology and mechanisms, quantifying severity, and assessing the reparability of the valve. Anatomic and functional assessment of MR relies on a precise description of the components of the mitral apparatus and a functional analysis of MR according to the Carpentier classification, independently of the aetiology (➲Figs. 21.23–21.25; 21.14–21.16).

In experienced hands, transthoracic echocardiography is highly accurate for a precise localization of the involved scallops in case of degenerative MR [163]. A >5mm thickness of the leaflets with tissue excess characterizes myxoid degeneration. A ratio of anterior–posterior diameter of the annulus to the length of the anterior leaflet >1.3 in diastole implies annular dilatation. The presence and severity of annular calcification should be analysed.

In ischaemic MR, the apical displacement of the leaflets can be quantitated by measuring the tenting area and the distance between the annulus and the coaptation point [164] (21.17).

Finally, in functional MR, the localization and extent of regional LV dyssynergy must be analysed (21.18).

The transoesophageal approach is not mandatory but is useful in the presence of complex lesions and/or poor transthoracic echogenicity. Preliminary studies show that real-time three-dimensional echocardiography provides precise

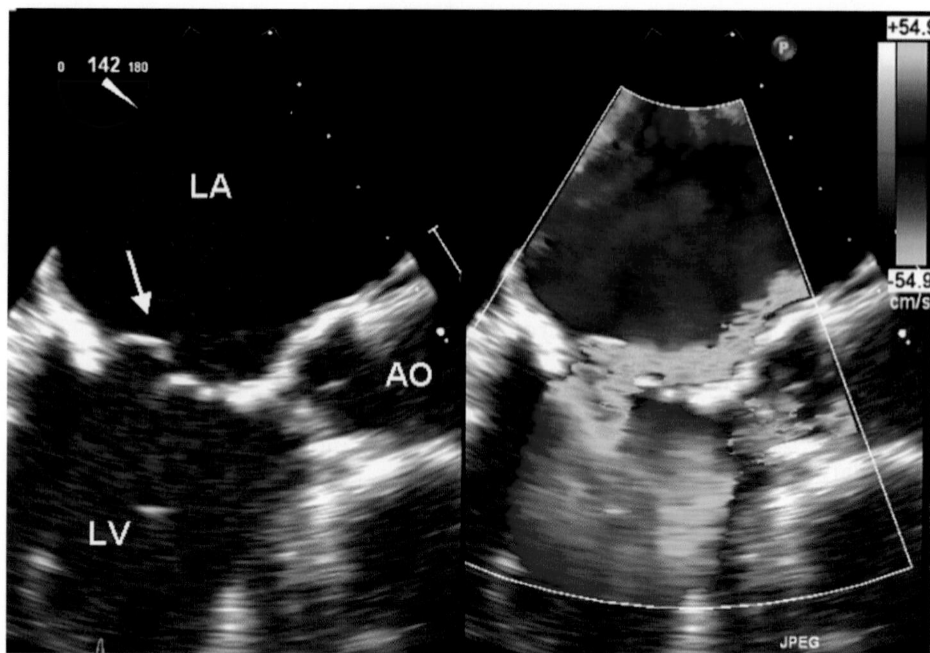

Figure 21.23 Transoesophageal echocardiography in MR. Left: severe mitral valve prolapse with a flail of posterior leaflet (P2 segment) (arrow). Right: colour flow imaging showing severe MR with an eccentric jet directed in the opposite direction to the prolapse segment. Ao, aorta; LA, left atrium; LV, left ventricle. (Courtesy of Dr E. Brochet.)

anatomical information and may be of additional value in the operating room (21.19). It may also allow quantitative assessment of structures not easily measurable by two-dimensional echocardiography such as mitral annulus [165].

The assessment of severity should not rely entirely on one single parameter, but requires an approach integrating blood-flow data from Doppler with morphologic information, and careful cross-checking of the validity of such data against the consequences on LV and pulmonary pressures (➲Table 21.2) (➲Fig. 21.26).

Several methods can be used to determine the severity of MR. Colour-flow mapping appears to be the easiest, providing the measurement of the regurgitant jet and the regurgitant jet to left atrial ratio. MR is considered severe when the jet area is >10cm^2 or >40% of the left atrial area. However, it is admitted that this method largely

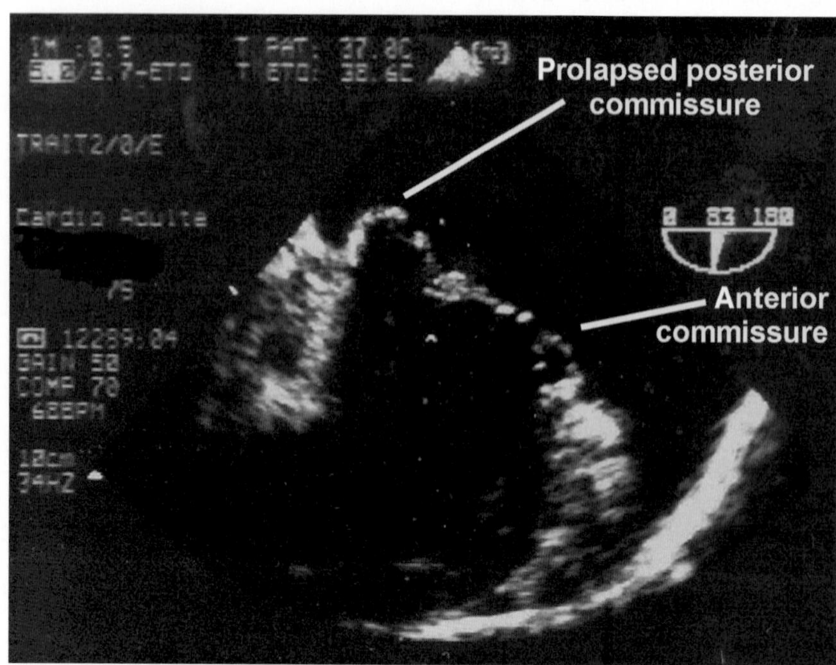

Figure 21.24 Prolapse of the posterior commissure. Transoesophageal echocardiography. (Courtesy of Dr B. Cormier.)

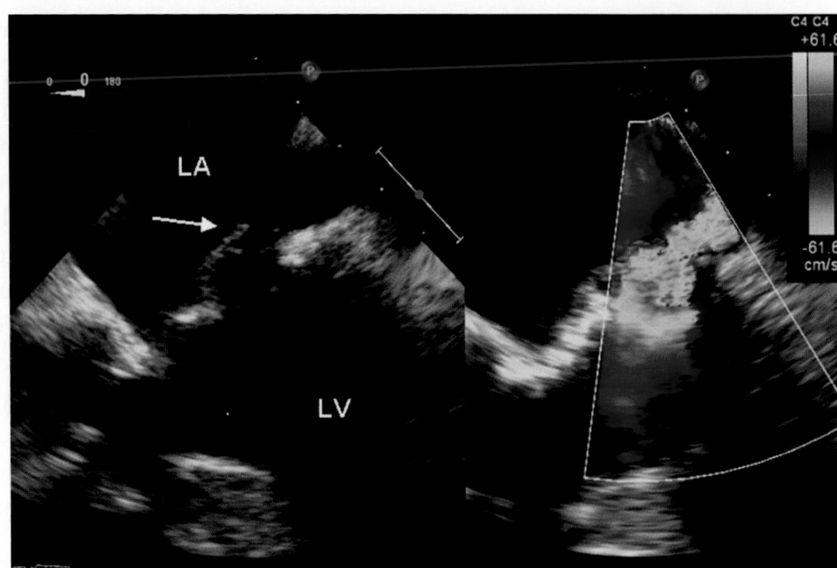

Figure 21.25 Mitral valve prolapse with a flail of anterior leaflet. Transoesophageal echocardiography. Left: severe mitral valve prolapse with a flail of posterior leaflet (P2 segment) (arrow). Right: colour flow imaging showing severe MR with an eccentric jet directed in the opposite direction to the prolapse segment. LA, left atrium; LV, left ventricle. (Courtesy of Dr E. Brochet.)

overestimates the severity of ischaemic MR and underestimates MR when the jet is eccentric and lateral. The reversal of the systolic component of the pulmonary venous flow is specific but poorly sensitive, depending not only on the severity of MR but also on jet characteristics and volume and filling pressure of the left atrium. The width of the vena contracta—the narrowest part of the jet—correlates with quantitative measurements of MR. A <3mm width corresponds to trivial or mild MR; >7mm width vena contracta corresponds to severe MR [166]. The moderate lateral resolution is, however, a limitation. Two quantitative methods are reliable and clinically applicable but require experience. The Doppler method is based on the calculation of mitral and aortic stroke volumes, and the difference between them corresponds to the regurgitant volume [167]. The second is the flow-convergence method, based on the principle of conservation of momentum using the measurements of the proximal isovelocity surface area, the aliasing velocity

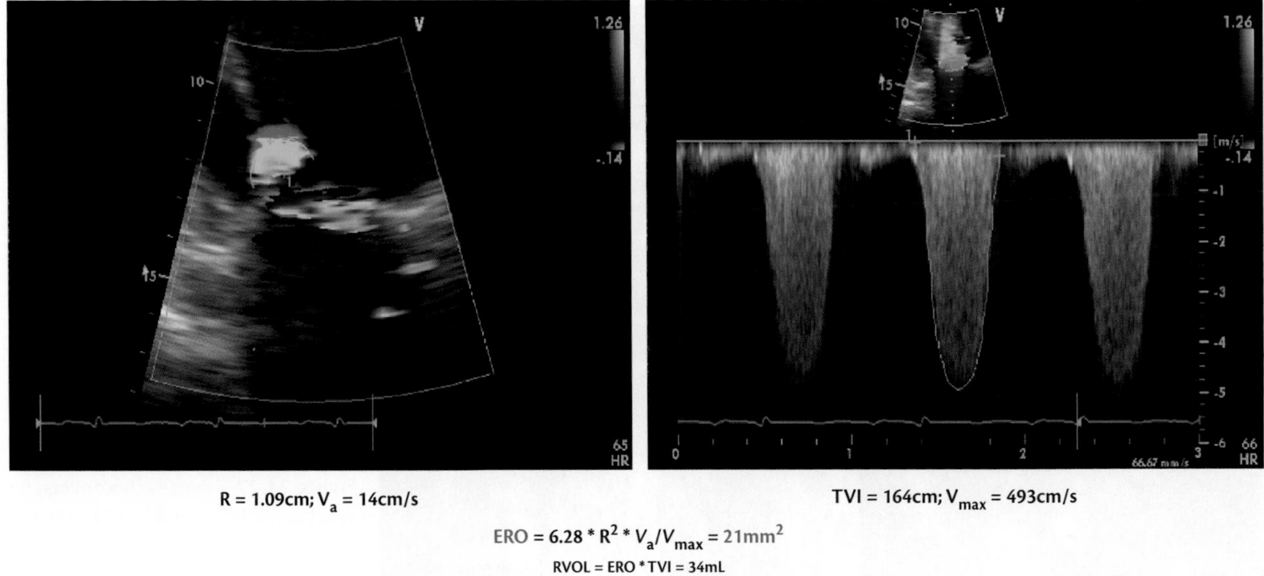

R = 1.09cm; V_a = 14cm/s
TVI = 164cm; V_{max} = 493cm/s
ERO = 6.28 * R^2 * V_a/V_{max} = 21mm^2
RVOL = ERO * TVI = 34mL

Figure 21.26 Estimation of MR severity using the PISA method. This method is based on the conservation of energy and assumes that blood flow converging towards a flat orifice forms a hemispheric isovelocity shell. ERO, effective regurgitant orifice; R, radius of the flow convergence; RVOL, regurgitant volume; TVI, time velocity integral; VA velocity of the isovelocity shell, which is arbitrarily selected by shifting the colour-flow scale baseline; V_{max}, velocity at the level of the regurgitant orifice measured in continuous wave Doppler. (Courtesy of Dr E. Brochet.)

and the maximum velocity and time velocity integral of the regurgitant flow [168] (21.20). Organic MR is considered severe when the regurgitant orifice area is ≥40mm^2 and regurgitation volume is ≥60mL [13]. In ischaemic MR, the corresponding thresholds of severity are 20mm^2 and 30mL respectively [169].

MRI also shows regurgitant jets, can reveal myocardial scars, and measure LV volumes but its role needs to be refined [86].

LV repercussions are assessed by measuring LV diameters and volumes and by calculating LVEF. As LVEF obviously includes both forward and backward flow, new less load-dependent indices of LV systolic function such as strain and strain rate, which could be earlier markers of LV dysfunction, are currently being evaluated [170].

Left atrial repercussions are too often assessed by the left atrial diameter measurement alone which is poorly reproducible. Instead, the left atrial volume should be measured (left atrium is considered dilated when >40mL/m^2).

Haemodynamic evaluation is completed with Doppler measurement of cardiac index and pulmonary pressures.

Preliminary series have suggested the value of BNP levels to evaluate the consequences of MR and as a predictor of long-term outcome, but this also needs to investigated further [171].

Other non-invasive investigations

Limitations in peak exercise oxygen consumption provide a reference with regards to functional capacity [172].

Exercise echocardiography allows the assessment of contractile reserve which has been shown to predict postoperative LV function [173]. Preliminary data suggests that exercise-induced changes in LV strain could potentially be more accurate than changes in LVEF. In ischaemic MR, quantitation of MR during exercise echocardiography is feasible, provides a good appreciation of dynamic characteristics [174], and has prognostic importance (175) (➲Fig. 21.27).

In addition, exercise may show changes in mitral valve deformation and LV synchronicity [176].

Invasive investigation

Cardiac catheterization is useful only when clinical and echocardiographic parameters are discordant. Coronary angiography is necessary prior to surgery as in other valve diseases.

Natural history

Acute mitral regurgitation

Acute MR secondary to papillary muscle rupture has a dismal short-term spontaneous prognosis. Clinical condition

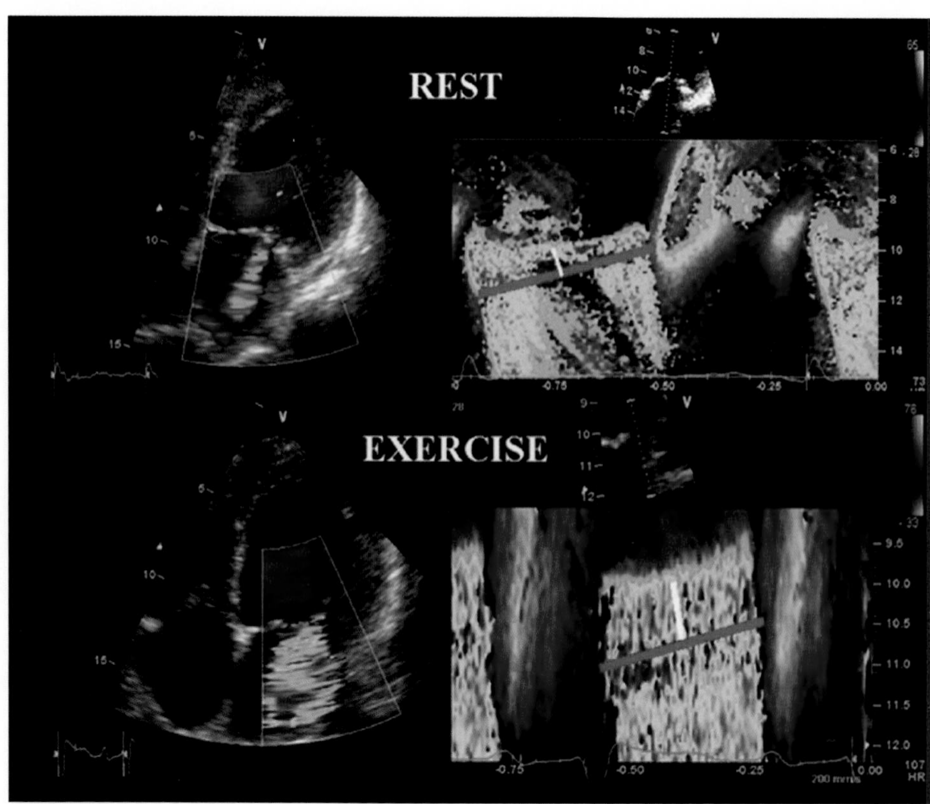

Figure 21.27 Exercise echocardiography in ischaemic MR. Apical four-chamber view showing colour-flow Doppler and colour M-mode of the proximal flow-convergence region at rest and during exercise in a patient with dynamic MR. A large exercise-induced increase in PISA radius MR is observed. (Courtesy of Dr E. Brochet.)

may stabilize after chordal rupture following an initial symptomatic period. However, it carries a poor spontaneous prognosis due to subsequent rapid development of pulmonary hypertension.

Chronic mitral regurgitation

In chronic MR, MR begets MR, and this vicious cycle has important effects on LV geometry. MR progression is observed in all clinical and anatomic subsets and is associated with more severe LV and atrial remodelling and worse outcome [177].

Chronic primary mitral regurgitation

Our knowledge of the natural history of chronic primary MR has greatly improved due to recent observational studies evaluating the bearing that clinical and echocardiographic variables have on outcome [16, 178, 179].

In symptomatic patients with flail leaflets and severe MR, there is an excess mortality overall [16].

When severe MR is present, asymptomatic patients have poor clinical outcomes with conservative management [178] (➲Fig. 21.28). The estimated 5-year rates of death from any cause, death from cardiac causes, and cardiac events (death from cardiac causes, heart failure, or new atrial fibrillation) with medical management were 22%, 14%, and 33%, respectively [178].

In addition to the appearance of symptoms, several parameters can predict poor outcome: age, atrial fibrillation [180], degree of MR (particularly ERO), left atrial dilatation, LV dilatation, and low LVEF, and recent data also suggest the predictive value of reduced functional capacity [172] and high BNP level [171].

Chronic functional mitral regurgitation

The natural history of patients with functional MR is less well known.

Overall, patients with ischaemic MR have a poor prognosis [169, 181, 182]. Following myocardial infarction complicated by LV dysfunction, heart failure, or both, baseline MR severity is associated with large LV volumes and worse LV function. Besides the prognostic importance of CAD, LV dysfunction and comorbidity, which is frequent in these patients, the presence and severity of MR, as well as its progression and dynamic component, are independently associated with increased mortality [169, 175, 182].

Quantitative studies have shown that even small volumes of MR are associated with markedly increased mortality (182). Nevertheless it remains to be demonstrated in a clinical randomized trial that suppression of MR minimizes mortality and heart failure.

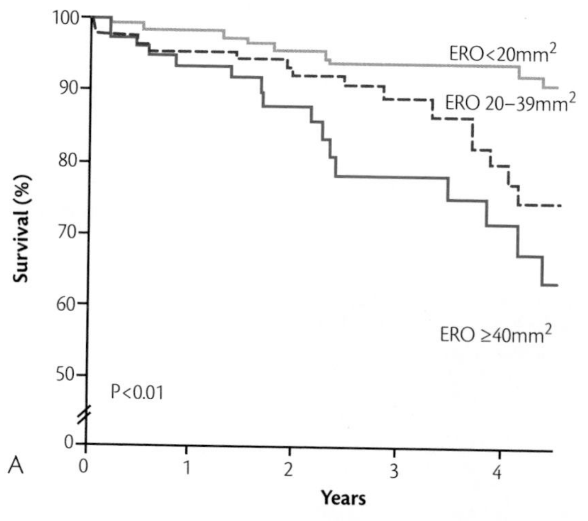

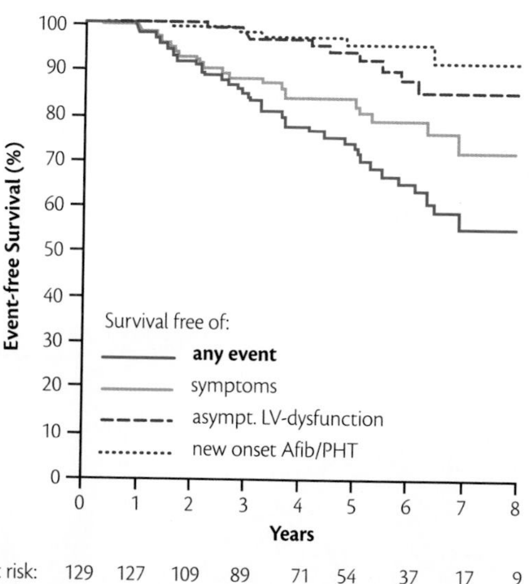

Figure 21.28 Outcome of patients with asymptomatic MR. (A) Estimates of the rate of cardiac events among patients with asymptomatic MR under medical management according to the effective regurgitant orifice (ERO). Cardiac events are defined as death from cardiac causes, congestive heart failure, or new atrial fibrillation. Values in parentheses are survival rates at 5 years. Reproduced with permission from Enriquez-Sarano M, Avierinos JF, Messika-Zeitoun D, *et al.* Quantitative determinants of the outcome of asymptomatic mitral regurgitation. *N Engl J Med* 2005; **352**: 875–83. (B) Event-free survival of patients with asymptomatic MR managed according to the guidelines. Solid green line shows survival free of any event to indicate surgery. Orange line shows survival free of symptoms. Blue dashed line shows survival free of asymptomatic (asymtp) LV dysfunction. Violet dotted line shows survival free of asymtomatic development of atrial fibrillation (Afib) and/or pulmonary hypertension (PHT) to indicate surgery. Reproduced with permission from Rosenhek H, Rader F, Klaar U, *et al.* Outcome of watchful waiting in asymptomatic severe mitral regurgitation. *Circulation* 2006; **113**: 2238–44.

Clinical outcome of functional MR due to cardiomyopathies is less well defined but data suggest that MR also plays a role in the poor outcome of these patients [183].

Medical treatment

In acute MR, reduction of filling pressures can be obtained using diuretics and nitrates. Vasodilators such as nitroprusside preferentially increase forward flow and reduce regurgitant flow through a reduction in both regurgitant orifice area and aortic impedance [184].

In chronic organic MR, the use of vasodilator therapy remains controversial in asymptomatic patients since long-term therapy has not been shown to prevent or delay LV dysfunction, and it should not be used if surgery is indicated [185]. Although beta-blockers are effective in experimental MR, human studies are lacking [184].

Patients with MR and hypertension should be treated to normalize blood pressure as hypertension increases the pressure gradient between the LV and the left atrium, and thus increases regurgitant volume.

In functional MR associated with systolic dysfunction and heart failure, ACE inhibitors and beta-blockers, which reduce MR by progressive reverse remodelling, are indicated [186]. Sublingual nitrates are useful for treating acute dyspnoea secondary to the dynamic component. Diuretics and spironolactone can also be used to treat heart failure.

Patients with persistent or paroxysmal atrial fibrillation should receive drugs for controlling heart rate and anticoagulant therapy with an INR between 2–3 [11, 12, 127]. Anticoagulant therapy is also needed if there is a history of systemic embolism, presence of left atrial thrombus, or during the first 3 months after mitral valve repair. In severe MR, maintenance of sinus rhythm after cardioversion is illusory in the absence of surgery.

Endocarditis prophylaxis is required according to recommendations [59] (see ➲Chapter 22).

Percutaneous intervention

In patients with ischaemic MR, percutaneous coronary revascularization in isolation usually leaves patients with significant residual MR [187].

Two specific interventional approaches to MR treatment are currently evaluated:

- Edge-to-edge repair mimics the surgical procedure proposed by Alfieri, creating a tissue bridge between the mitral leaflets. This approach is technically demanding since it necessitates a trans-septal approach and capture of both leaflets in systole under transoesophageal guidance (➲Fig. 21.29). The current preliminary experience in 400 patients suggests that the technique is feasible and safe in experienced centres. Two-thirds of patients can be discharged with a clip in place and MR ≤2/4. Mid term results show that two-thirds of patients remain alive without severe MR or need for surgery 3 years after an initially successful procedure. Potential limitations are related to the applicability, which is restricted to localized prolapse representing only a small proportion of patients currently operated, and also to the absence of annuloplasty which could compromise efficacy and long-term durability [188, 189].
- Annuloplasty aiming to reduce annular dilatation is also investigated using coronary sinus cinching with devices with sufficient force to obtain >20% diameter reduction in annulus diameter (➲Fig. 21.30). The procedure is easier than edge-to-edge repair. Total experience is around 200 patients with secondary MR. Feasibility and immediate safety appears acceptable. Efficacy appears encouraging even if limited. Limitations are related to the variable

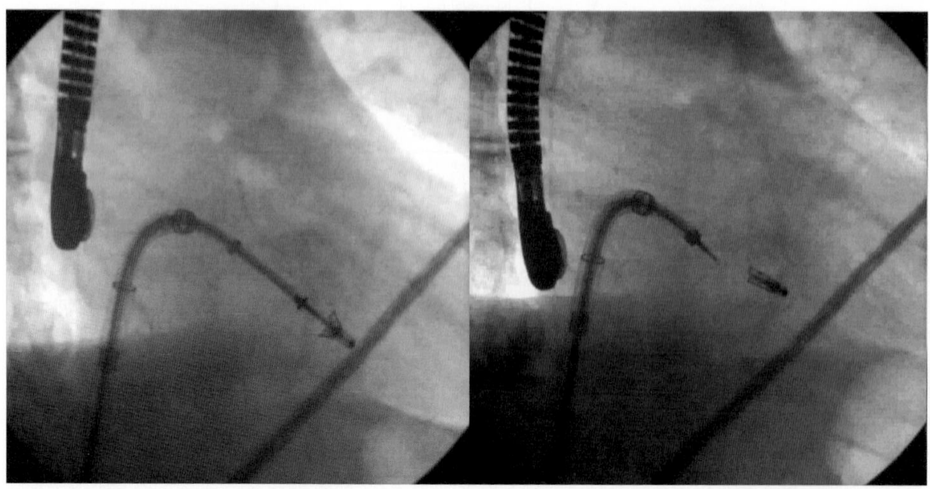

Figure 21.29 Percutaneous mitral valve repair using edge-to-edge technique (right oblique anterial view). Left: the evalve clip is deployed trans-septally in the left ventricle. It is in the open position. Right: the clip is released. (Courtesy of Dr M. Tuzcu, Cleveland Clinic.)

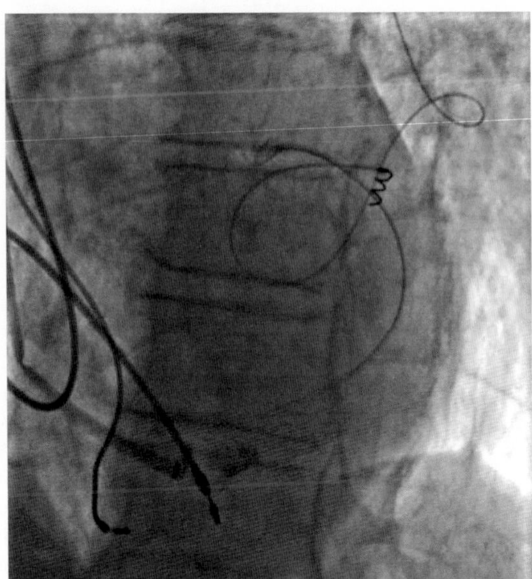

Figure 21.30 Percutaneous coronary sinus annuloplasty using the MONARC system. The device is positioned in the coronary sinus. A proximal stent is deployed in the proximal part of the coronary sinus and a distal stent in the descending cardiac vein. Both stents are linked by a nitinol bridge. (Courtesy Dr D. Himbert.)

anatomic relationship between the coronary sinus and mitral annulus, and incomplete covering of the annulus which may limit both efficacy and potential compression of the circumflex artery. Overall, these techniques are at an earlier stage of evaluation than TAVI and their future is more uncertain [189].

Cardiac resynchronization therapy

In patients with increased QRS duration, intraventricular asynchrony, and heart failure, in NYHA class III or IV despite medical treatment, cardiac resynchronization therapy increases the mitral valve closing force, and reduces MR severity [190,191].

Surgery

Technique

Valve replacement

It is now admitted that valve replacement in MR should include wherever possible the preservation of the subvalvular apparatus, as well as the chordal attachments between the leaflets and the papillary muscles, in order to better preserve postoperative LV function [192].

Conservative surgery

Valve repair may combine different techniques according to aetiology.

In degenerative MR, annuloplasty is the cornerstone of treatment. Its principle is to reduce—or remodel—the posterior annulus in order to restore an optimal surface of coaptation. It mostly uses rings, usually sized according to the area of the anterior leaflet, which can be complete or incomplete, rigid, or pliable [153].

Posterior leaflet prolapse can be treated using a variety of techniques: quadrangular resection (➲Fig. 21.31), sliding plasty (➲Fig. 21.32), transfer of normal marginal or secondary chord to the free margin of the prolapsed segment, replacement of elongated or ruptured chords using Gore-Tex® neo-chordae [193] or, in some cases, the Alfieri stitch, when the prolapsed segment is sutured to the opposite normal segment, creating a double-orifice valve.

Anterior leaflet prolapse can be treated by transferring a normal marginal or secondary chord, or a normal segment of posterior leaflet with normal chords to the free margin of the prolapsed segment, or by using chordal replacement (Gore-Tex®), papillary muscle repositioning or the Alfieri stitch [194].

The treatment of commissural prolapse is more difficult and less standardized. It includes resection plus sliding plasty, resuspension by neo-chordae, papillary muscle repositioning, or even in some cases the Alfieri technique.

In endocarditis the first step is to resect all infected tissues and then assess for repair. Leaflet perforation requires pericardial patch plasty (➲Fig. 21.33). Commissural destruction can be treated using sliding plasty, patch replacement, or in some cases by transferring the posterior leaflet of the tricuspid valve [195].

In rheumatic MR, repair uses all the artifices described for MS and cure of prolapse as described for degenerative disease. Specific techniques for rheumatic disease combine: shaving of the free margin of anterior leaflet and repositioning the marginal chords; leaflet augmentation, usually of the posterior leaflet using pericardial patches [196]; in extreme cases, resection of subvalvular apparatus and resuspension by means of neo-chordae; and finally 'oversized' annuloplasty, merely for remodelling.

In functional MR, the main technique is restrictive annuloplasty, in order to obtain a coaptation length of at least 8mm [197]. In larger LV, other techniques such as surgical ventricular restoration could be added [198, 199].

In current practice, valve repair is applied in up to 90% of patients in experienced centres [200], but only around 50% of cases in recent registries [2] (➲Table 21.1).

Anti arrhythmic surgery

Recently, additional anti arrhythmic procedures have been proposed in patients with preoperative atrial fibrillation [201] (➲Chapter 29). The limited amount of data available

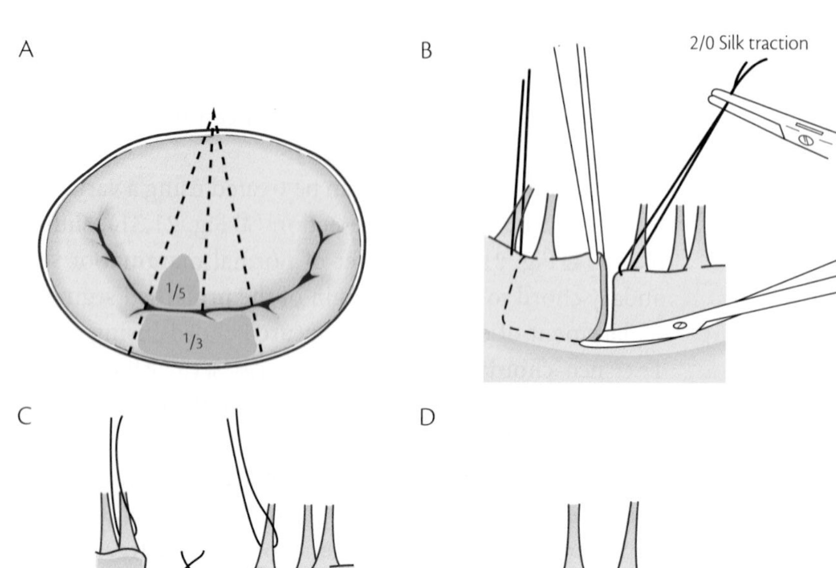

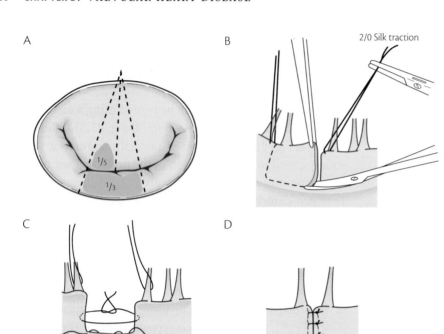

Figure 21.31 Mitral valve repair in degenerative MR. Quadrangular resection. AL, anterior leaflet; AN, annulus; PL, posterior leaflet. (A) Leaflet resection. Identification of a rectangular segment of up to one-third of the total length of the posterior leaflet that can be resected. (B) The segment of the posterior leaflet is resected close to the annulus. (C) The annulus is plicated and the continuity of the leaflet is re-established with sutures. (D) Completed repair. Reproduced with permission from Antunes MJ. *Mitral Valve Repair*, 1989. Berlin: Verlag.

suggests that the results vary according to patients (characteristics, atrial fibrillation, LV function, atrial size) and techniques (Maze or Cox techniques, cryoablation, radio frequency ablation). The definitive role of these procedures is as yet undetermined.

Results of surgery

Primary mitral regurgitation

Despite the absence of randomized comparisons between the results of valve replacement and repair and the possible inherent biases resulting from this, it is widely accepted that valve repair, when feasible, is the optimal surgical treatment in patients with severe MR [11, 12]. When compared with valve replacement, repair has a lower perioperative mortality 1–3% vs. 3–6% improved survival, better preservation of postoperative LV function, and lower long-term morbidity, (thromboembolism, endocarditis, and need for reoperation) [202–206].

Clinical outcome after surgery depends on patient-specific, and disease- and surgery-related factors.

Besides symptoms, the most important patient-related predictors of postoperative outcome are age, atrial fibrillation [207], preoperative LV function, need for combined bypass operation, and the reparability of the valve.

The best results of surgery are observed in patients with a preoperative LVEF >60%. A preoperative end-systolic diameter <40–45mm (no indexed value has been validated in MR) is also closely correlated with a good postoperative prognosis [202]. However, a value at which postoperative LV dysfunction will not occur has not been demonstrated, rendering prediction of the postoperative dysfunction difficult in the individual patient. Progressive

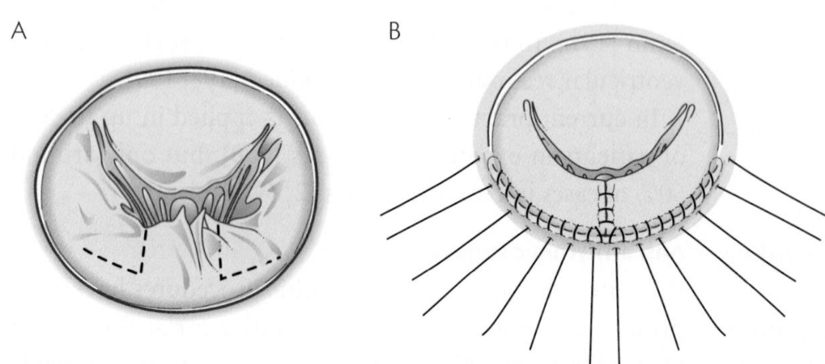

Figure 21.32 Mitral valve repair in degenerative MR. Sliding plasty technique. (A) Resection of excessive tissue in prolapsed segment of the posterior leaflet; (B) repair is completed. (Courtesy of Dr V. Jebara.)

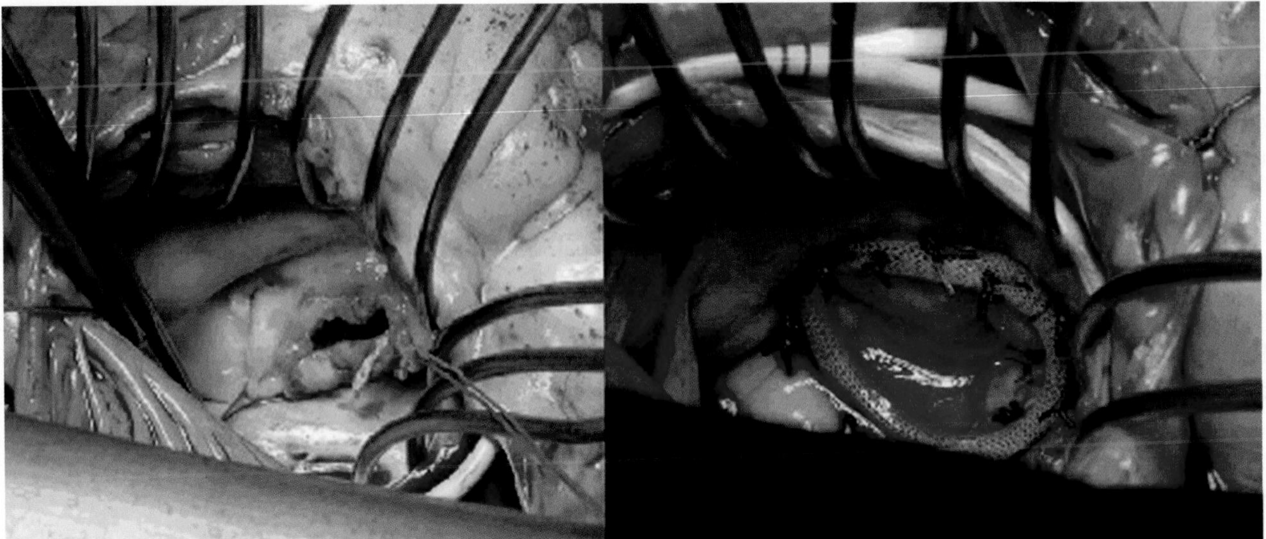

Figure 21.33 Mitral valve repair in mitral valve endocarditis. Left: abcess and perforation of the anterior leaflet, respecting the free margin of the leaflet. Right: final result after pericardial patch plasty.

development of pulmonary hypertension is also a marker for poor prognosis.

The probability of durable valve repair is of crucial importance.

Degenerative MR due to valve prolapse can usually be successfully repaired (10-year survival of 90% for valve repair compared to 74% for valve replacement [205] and cardiac event-free survival of 74% at 20 years) [206]. The reoperation rate after repair or valve replacement is not significantly different (at 19 years, 20 ± 5% for repair vs. 23 ± 5% for replacement: $p = 0.4$) [205]. In general, the results of posterior prolapse are better than those of anterior and bileaflet prolapse [208]. However, extensive annular calcification represents a surgical challenge for valve repair and probably even more so for valve replacement. Re-repair can be performed successfully in selected patients when operated on by experienced surgeons [209].

In the other aetiologies experience is more limited and results are not as consistent, even in experienced hands. In rheumatic lesions, good long-term results, with survival rates up to 82% at 20 years, were reported in selected patients [196]. A higher reoperation rate is, however, expected in young patients when there is a risk of further episodes of rheumatic fever. Limitations of repair include the absence of pliable anterior leaflet and of at least one commissure free from calcification. In endocarditis, a recent series [210] reported 78 cases, of which 63 benefited from mitral valve repair, even in acute endocarditis. Operative mortality was 3.2% and the 7-year event-free survival was 78%. Here the limitation for repair is extensive destruction of the leaflets and subvalvular apparatus.

The results of valve repair are also highly dependent on the experience of the surgeon, especially as the lesions get more complex, which is an incentive for referring these patients to experienced centres as well as for improving surgeons' training in these techniques [12, 200, 211].

Secondary mitral regurgitation

In ischaemic MR the data is more limited and heterogeneous. Outcomes after surgery remain suboptimal; operative mortality is notable (between 5–18%) depending on the degree of emergency and patients characteristics) [212]. Despite recent improvements, long-term mortality and the risk of heart failure are high [213, 214].

In patients with low EF, combined CABG and valve repair reduces postoperative MR and improve early symptoms [215] compared with CABG alone, but it has not been shown to improve long-term functional status or survival [216–219]. Recurrent MR is frequent (up to 30% at 6 months) [220], due to continued LV remodelling resulting in recurrent valve tenting, and is associated with poor survival [220–223]. Determinants of postoperative outcome are myocardial viability, preserved mitral competence and lack of advanced LV remodelling.

Postoperative outcome of secondary MR due to cardiomyopathy is mediocre and whether it is improved by repair over medical therapy is in doubt [224, 225].

Thus there is a need for better patient selection and improved repair techniques and devices. Recent series report encouraging results when using careful patient selection, and echocardiographic screening, restrictive annuloplasty, and liberal use of combined LV remodelling techniques [199], devices, and resynchronization [197, 198, 219, 226, 227]. In the series by Braun such a strategy led to only 13% recurrent MR at 4 years and excellent 5-year survival in a subgroup of patients with preoperative LV end-diastolic diameter <65mm [197].

Treatment strategy

Acute mitral regurgitation

Urgent surgery is indicated in patients with acute MR.

Rupture of a papillary muscle necessitates urgent surgical treatment after stabilization of the haemodynamic status using an intra-aortic balloon pump and vasodilators. In addition to CABG, surgery usually consists of valve replacement [228].

Chronic primary mitral regurgitation

Intervention is only indicated in patients with severe MR [11] (➲Fig. 21.34).

Symptomatic patients

Surgery is indicated in patients who have symptoms due to chronic MR, no contra-indications to surgery, and when EF is >30%. When LVEF is <30%, the decision whether to operate will take into account the response to medical therapy, comorbidity, and the likelihood of valve repair.

It is surprising that still almost 50% of symptomatic patients with severe MR are not referred for surgery [229].

Asymptomatic patients

The management of asymptomatic patients is controversial since no randomized trials exist to support any particular course of action. On the one hand, the good results of valve repair and the potential risk of postoperative LV dysfunction are incentives for early surgery. On the other hand, even in low-risk cases there is a small but definite risk of surgical mortality. The indications for surgery depend on risk stratification, the possibility of valve repair, and the preferences of the informed patient.

Indications for surgery include the presence of LV dysfunction (EF <60%, end-systolic diameter >40–45mm). In addition to the initial measurements, temporal changes in LV function should also be taken into account when making decisions about surgery. Surgery should also be considered in patients with normal LV function but with atrial fibrillation and/or pulmonary hypertension (systolic pulmonary arterial pressure >50mmHg at rest). Further proof of the validity of such a strategy in carefully followed-up patients has been provided by recent data, showing that it allows surgery at low risk and with a good long-term outcome [179]. Unfortunately, surveys in current practice

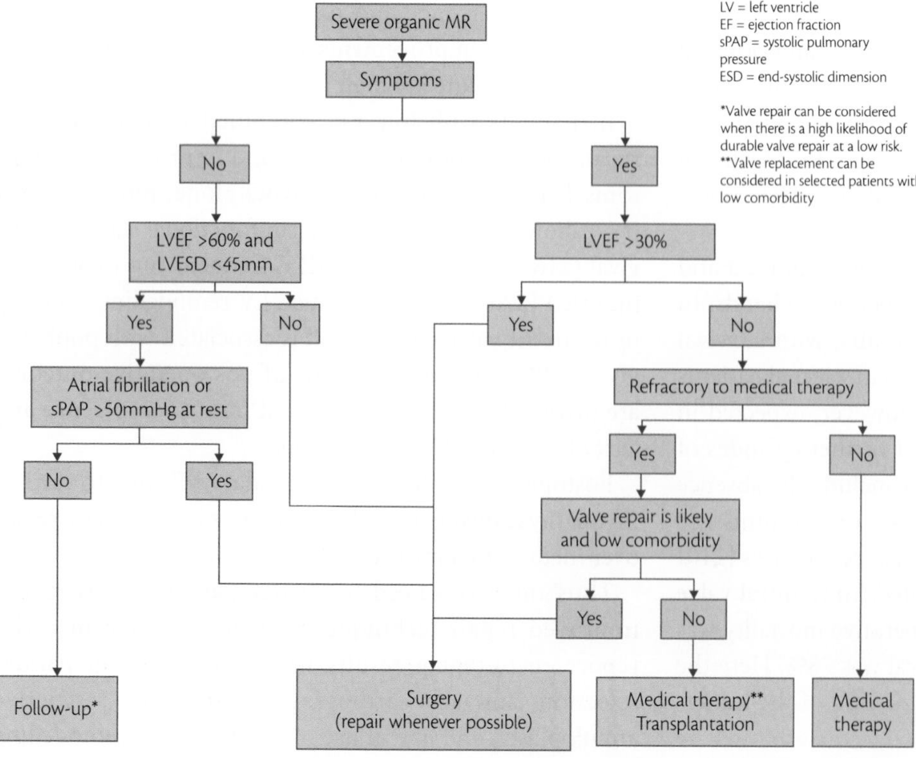

Figure 21.34 Management of severe chronic organic MR. *Valve repair can be considered where there is a high likelihood of durable valve repair at a low risk. **Valve replacement can be considered in selected patients with low comorbidity. Adapted with permission from Vahanian A, Baumgartner H, Bax J, *et al.* Guidelines on the management of valvular heart disease. The Task Force on the Management of Valvular Heart Disease of the European Society of Cardiology. *Eur Heart J* 2007; **28**: 230–68.

show that surgery is often not considered in asymptomatic patients presenting with these characteristics [230].

There is still a debate concerning the indication for surgery in asymptomatic patients with severe MR and neither signs of LV dysfunction, atrial fibrillation, nor pulmonary hypertension. Intervention may be considered if there is a high likelihood of valve repair on the basis of valve lesions, the surgeon's experience, and a low operative risk. Conversely, attentive clinical follow-up is recommended for patients at relatively high operative risk or where the feasibility of valve repair is doubtful. In this latter group of patients, operative risk and/or prosthetic valve complications probably outweigh the advantages of correcting MR. These patients should be reviewed carefully and surgery indicated when symptoms or objective signs of LV dysfunction occur [179].

Asymptomatic patients with severe MR and preserved LV function should be seen every 6 months, with echocardiography performed every 12 months—the follow-up being sooner in patients with borderline values. Asymptomatic patients with moderate MR and preserved LV function can be clinically followed-up on a yearly basis with echocardiography performed every 2 years [11, 12].

Functional mitral regurgitation

Limited data in the field of ischaemic MR results in less evidence-based management.

Severe MR should be corrected at the time of bypass surgery. There is a continuing debate on the management of moderate ischaemic MR. In such cases valve repair is preferable and the decision must be made preoperatively, since intraoperative echocardiographic assessment underestimates the severity of ischaemic MR [231].

In patients with LV dysfunction, medical therapy should be the first-line treatment.

Surgery is more likely to be considered if myocardial viability is present and if comorbidity is low. The preferred surgical procedure remains controversial, although there is a trend in favour of repair even if results are less satisfactory than in other aetiologies.

The limited data available suggest that isolated mitral valve surgery in combination with LV reconstruction techniques may be considered in selected patients with severe functional MR and severely depressed LV function. Such patients include those with coronary disease where bypass surgery is not indicated, who remain symptomatic despite optimal medical therapy, and where comorbidity is low—the aim being to avoid or postpone transplantation. Ongoing trials are expected to better define appropriate strategies. In other patients, medical therapy followed by transplantation when this fails is probably the best option. However, surgery on the regurgitant mitral valve should not be considered in 'in extremis' patients with low output, severe RV failure, and high comorbidity.

Cardiac resynchronization therapy with or without a defibrillator should be performed according to the classical recommendations.

Specific situations

Mitral regurgitation associated with Marfan syndrome

The lesions of the mitral valve are frequently complex and extensive; the association of severe annular calcification reduces the feasibility of valve repair, even in experienced hands. Since MR can be associated with lesions of the aorta, choice of treatment is also influenced by the dimensions of the ascending aorta and the reparability of the aortic valve and root.

Mitral regurgitation in infective endocarditis

See ➲Chapter 22, Infective Endocarditis.

Tricuspid valve disease

Tricuspid stenosis

Tricuspid stenosis (TS), although still present in developing countries, is rarely observed in the West. Detection requires careful attention, as it is almost always associated with left-sided valve lesions that dominate the presentation.

Aetiology

TS is often combined with TR, most frequently of rheumatic origin, and almost always associated with left-sided valve lesions, particularly MS, that dominate the presentation. The anatomical changes of rheumatic TS resemble those of MS. Carcinoid disease may cause tricuspid valve disease, frequently associated with pulmonic stenosis [232]. Other aetiologies are rare: congenital, drug-induced valve diseases, Whipple's disease, endocarditis, or large right atrial tumour.

Pathophysiology

Normal valve area is around 7–8cm^2, a pressure gradient occurs if <2cm^2. TS usually induces a small (<5mmHg) diastolic pressure gradient between the right atrium and ventricle, which increases during inspiration due to the increase of venous return, and is limited by venous compliance and reduced cardiac output. A mean pressure gradient

>5mmHg is considered indicative of significant TS and is usually associated with symptoms.

Diagnosis

History

The main symptoms are those of the other valvular lesions. Hepatalgia on exercise or after meals may be more directly a consequence of TS. Low cardiac output causes fatigue.

Physical examination

Clinical signs are often masked by those of the combined valvular lesions, especially MS. The diastolic murmur is of low intensity and increases with inspiration, preceded by a subtle opening snap. Presystolic jugular distension, Harzer's sign, systemic venous congestion, oedema, or even anasarca may be seen in the most severe cases.

Electrocardiography

In patients in sinus rhythm, the most frequent abnormality is right atrial hypertrophy or, more frequently, biatrial hypertrophy. Atrial fibrillation is present in one-half of cases.

Chest radiograph

Cardiac silhouette is enlarged with right atrial dilatation. Coexistent MS results in left atrial enlargement, but the degree of pulmonary congestion is less than usual.

Echocardiography

Echocardiography provides the most useful information, but requires careful evaluation. In rheumatic disease the leaflets are thickened with reduced motion and frequent commissural fusion, the chordae are shortened and thickened, and diastolic doming is seen. In carcinoid syndrome, retraction of leaflets and/or subvalvular apparatus towards the apex persists during systole [232]. Echocardiographic evaluation of valve anatomy is important to assess valve reparability (➲ Chapter 4).

Although there is no consensus, severe TS is generally defined by a mean gradient >5mmHg [11]. There is no relevant method to estimate tricuspid valve area [35]: the pressure half-time method has never been validated. In the absence of significant TR, the continuity equation can be used. When TR is significant, which is common, the measurement of tricuspid annulus and inflow are technically challenging, and planimetry is very difficult [233]. Real-time three-dimensional echo may be useful in this setting.

Invasive investigation

Catheterization has been replaced by echocardiography for evaluating severity.

Medical treatment

In the presence of congestive heart failure, diuretics are useful but of limited efficacy.

Percutaneous intervention

Percutaneous balloon tricuspid dilatation has been performed in a limited number of cases [66], either alone or alongside PMC, but frequently induces significant regurgitation. Data on long-term results are scarce.

Surgery

Open valvotomy usually combines commissurotomy, leaflet augmentation using pericardial patch, and annuloplasty [234]. For valve replacement, biological prostheses are usually preferred to mechanical ones because of the higher risk of thrombosis carried by the latter and the satisfactory long-term durability of the former in the tricuspid position [235].

Treatment strategy

Percutaneous balloon dilatation can be performed in the rare cases of isolated and pure TS. In most cases, surgical intervention is carried out at the time of intervention on the other valves [11]. Conservative surgery can be performed according to anatomy and surgical expertise in valve repair. However, given the lack of pliable tissue and the frequency of associated TR, prosthetic valve replacement is more frequently performed than valve repair.

Tricuspid regurgitation

The trivial form of TR is frequently detected by echocardiography in normal subjects. Pathological TR is more often functional than primary.

Aetiology

Functional tricuspid regurgitation

Functional TR is the consequence of RV pressure and/or volume overload in the presence of structurally normal leaflets. The tricuspid annulus becomes larger and also more circular and flatter than normal, which determines regurgitation due to lack of coaptation [236]. As in functional MR, valve tethering may contribute to regurgitation.

Pressure overload is most often caused by pulmonary hypertension resulting from left-sided heart disease, or, more rarely cor pulmonale, primary pulmonary hypertension, and ventricular volume overload possibly relating to atrial septal defects or intrinsic disease of the RV (ischaemic or cardiomyopathy).

Primary tricuspid regurgitation

Possible causes are infective endocarditis (especially in intravenous drug addicts) [237], rheumatic heart disease, carcinoid syndrome, myxomatous disease, endomyocardial fibrosis, Ebstein's anomaly, drug-induced valve diseases, thoracic trauma, and iatrogenic diseases.

Pathophysiology

TR induces RV and atrial dilatation, both of which tend to increase annular dilatation, which causes further increase of TR. Severe TR can also induce ventricular interdependency and reduction in both right-sided stroke volume and LV preload. Haemodynamic abnormalities increase during inspiration.

Diagnosis

History

Even severe TR may be well tolerated for a long period of time. It is most often discovered during an echocardiographic examination for another cause.

Predominant symptoms are those of associated diseases. Dyspnoea and fatigue are common. Symptoms more specifically related to TR are right-sided congestion and hepatalgia. Anorexia and weight loss may occur at a later stage.

Physical examination

Three signs are typical: (1) a soft holosystolic murmur best heard along the left sternal border and in the xyphoid region increasing with inspiration, due to the increase of the venous return (Carvalho's sign); (2) systolic jugular vein expansion; and (3) a pulsatile and enlarged liver with hepatojugular reflux. The murmur could be mild, or even absent, in severe TR when turbulent flow disappears. Peripheral cyanosis, leg oedema, or even ascitis may be observed in response to the increased right atrial pressure.

Electrocardiography

Atrial fibrillation and incomplete right bundle branch block are frequent.

Chest radiograph

Marked cardiomegaly is usually present due to enlargement of the right cavities.

Echocardiography

Echocardiography is the ideal technique to quantify TR and distinguish between functional and primary forms. The aetiology of primary TR can usually be identified from specific abnormalities: vegetations in endocarditis, leaflet retraction in rheumatic disease or carcinoid, flail leaflet in myxomatous or post-traumatic disease. TR is identified using colour flow mapping of the systolic regurgitant jet in the right atrium, inferior vena cava, and hepatic veins.

In functional TR, tricuspid valve deformation can be assessed by measuring the distance between the tricuspid annulus plane and the coaptation point, and the tethering area as the area between the annulus plane and the atrial surface of the leaflets at the time of maximal systolic closure in the apical four-chamber view. The measurement of tricuspid annulus diameter is useful for decision making, but lacks standardization (21.21 and 21.22).

The severity of TR should be based on the integration of different indices, taking into account their particularly high sensitivity to loading conditions [11]. Colour flow mapping of the regurgitant jet lacks discrimination between mild and moderate regurgitations. Systolic flow reversal in the hepatic veins identifies severe TR but lacks sensitivity for less severe regurgitations. The accuracy of continuity equation is limited due to the non-circular shape of the tricuspid annulus and the difficulties of its measurement. The width of the vena contracta seems to be the most reliable quantitative index; a vena contracta diameter >7mm is a good marker of severe TR [238]. The proximal flow convergence method has been validated in only one study, criteria for severe TR were an ERO >40mm^2 and a regurgitant volume >45mL [239]. In functional TR, the severity of the regurgitation is related to the tethering area of the tricuspid valve [240].

Measurement of systolic velocity of the regurgitant jet permits quantification of transtricuspid pressure gradient and, thus, to estimate systolic pulmonary arterial pressure. This may be inaccurate in the presence of voluminous TR, which leads to less or non-turbulent flow and equalization of RV and atrial pressures. Finally, echocardiography carefully evaluates the RV, despite the existing limitations, and the degree of the combined lesions.

MRI may provide additional information on the size and function of the RV.

Invasive investigation

Today, catheterization is not needed to diagnose TR or to estimate its severity.

Natural history

Primary TR has a poor spontaneous prognosis, even when isolated. In a series of TR due to flail leaflet, there was an excess mortality and even asymptomatic patients experienced a 10-year rate of 75% of cardiac events [241].

Functional TR may diminish or disappear as RV failure improves following the treatment of its cause. Predicting the evolution of functional TR before surgical treatment of mitral valve disease remains difficult. Reduced RV function and the diameter of tricuspid annulus are important risk factors for persistence or late worsening of TR [242]. However, TR may persist or indeed worsen even after successful correction of primary or functional MR, which may have a negative impact on survival [243–245].

Medical treatment

Diuretics improve signs of congestion. Specific therapy of the underlying disease is warranted.

Surgery

Valve replacement carries a risk of operative mortality ranging from 7–40%. Ten-year survival ranges from 30–50%, the predictors being preoperative functional class, LV and RV function, and prosthetic complications [246]. The current experience favours the use of bioprostheses over mechanical valves.

Annuloplasty, which restricts the annulus corresponding to the anterior and posterior leaflets but should respect the membranous septum at the apex of the triangle of Koch (His bundle), is key to conservative surgery. Annuloplasty may be performed using a stitch or either flexible or rigid rings (➲Fig. 21.35). Additional techniques are used according to aetiology: resection, repositioning, sliding plasty or neo-chordae in prolapse, pericardial patch in localized perforation, or leaflet augmentation for severe valve tethering in functional TR [247].

Better long-term results are observed with the ring technique than with the stitch technique [234, 248, 249]. In particular the incidence of residual TR is lower with rings and ring annuloplasty was a predictive factor of long-term survival in multivariate analysis in a series of 702 patients. Tricuspid valve tethering predicts residual TR after annuloplasty [250]. Systolic tricuspid annular velocities measured by Doppler tissue imaging can predict postoperative clinical outcome [251].

Treatment strategy

The timing of surgical intervention and the appropriate technique remain controversial. The indication is usually discussed at the time of surgical correction of left-sided valvular lesions.

In these circumstances, severe TR should be corrected [11]. In patients with moderate TR, although this is debated, there is a current trend to combine the correction of TR and left-heart valve surgery at the same time. Surgical correction can be recommended when there is pulmonary hypertension, important dilatation of the annulus (diameter >40mm or >21mm/m^2) [11], or even more so if TR is of primary origin. If technically possible, conservative surgery is preferable to valve replacement. Reoperation on the tricuspid valve when TR develops or persists after mitral valve surgery carries a high risk related to previous operations and/or irreversible RV dysfunction [252].

Surgery limited to the tricuspid valve may be required in symptomatic patients with severe primary TR, or for persistent or recurrent TR after mitral valve surgery in the absence of left-sided myocardial, valve, or severe RV dysfunction. In asymptomatic severe primary TR, surgery may be considered in patients with RV enlargement [11].

Prosthetic valve surgery

Introduction

The ideal valve substitute would mimic the haemodynamic properties of native valves, be durable, and chemically inert. In addition, it would be silent, carry no risk of thromboembolism and require no valve-specific medication. Despite the fact that >100 different types of valves have been produced for human use in the last 40 years, this goal remains elusive.

Surgical techniques and valve substitutes

Prostheses

The design of mechanical valves can be catalogued into three types (➲Fig. 21.36; 21.23–21.25). The design of biological valves (➲Fig. 21.37) can be divided into true biological valves, such as the homograft or autograft, and valves constructed of xenogeneic biological material, rendered immunologically quiescent by treatment with glutaraldehyde. Porcine valve or bovine pericardium is sewn onto an artificial stent to produce a bioprosthetic valve.

Manufacturers have developed 'supra-annular' designs to achieve as low a transvalvular gradient as possible in patients with small aortic annulus, which may be of particular concern in elderly patients.

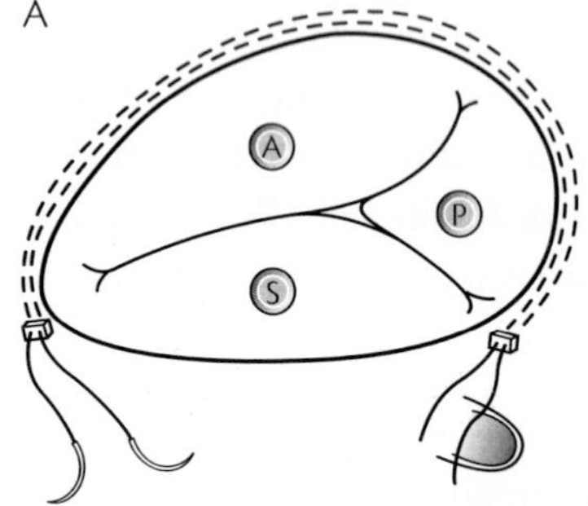

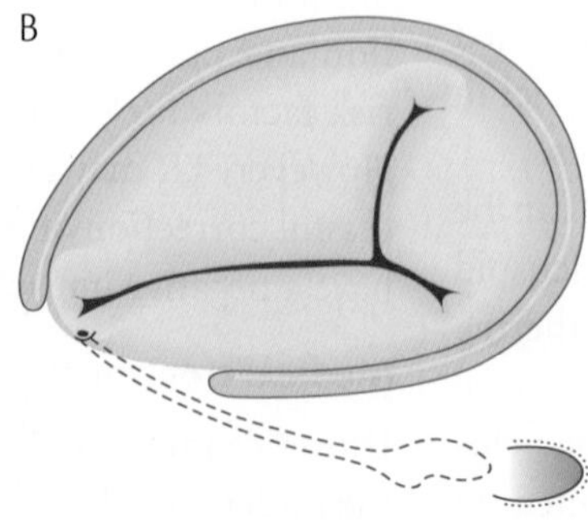

Figure 21.35 Conservative surgery for TR. (A) Tricuspid annuloplasty using stitches (De Vega). A, anterior leaflet; P, posterior leaflet; S, septal leaflet. (B) Tricuspid annuloplasty using ring (Carpentier, Cosgrove, Duran). (Courtesy of Dr D. Koolbergen.)

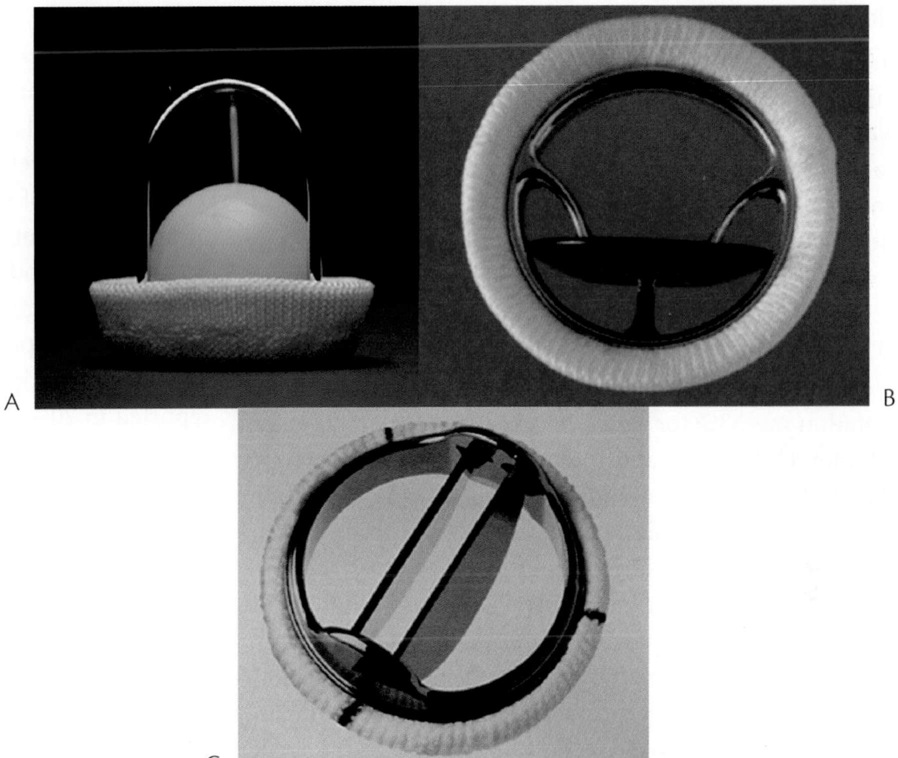

Figure 21.36 The three main designs of mechanical valve: (A) ball and cage; (B) single disk; (C) bileaflet.

The design of the stentless porcine valve was intended to reduce residual obstruction to transaortic flow by maximizing the available flow area. Better haemodynamics and a greater resolution of LV hypertrophy have been reported, but no improvement regarding long-term durability has been demonstrated so far [253]. A series reported a high deterioration rate of stentless bioprostheses beginning 8 years after follow-up, which highlights the need for a long follow-up when evaluating the durability of biological valve substitutes [254].

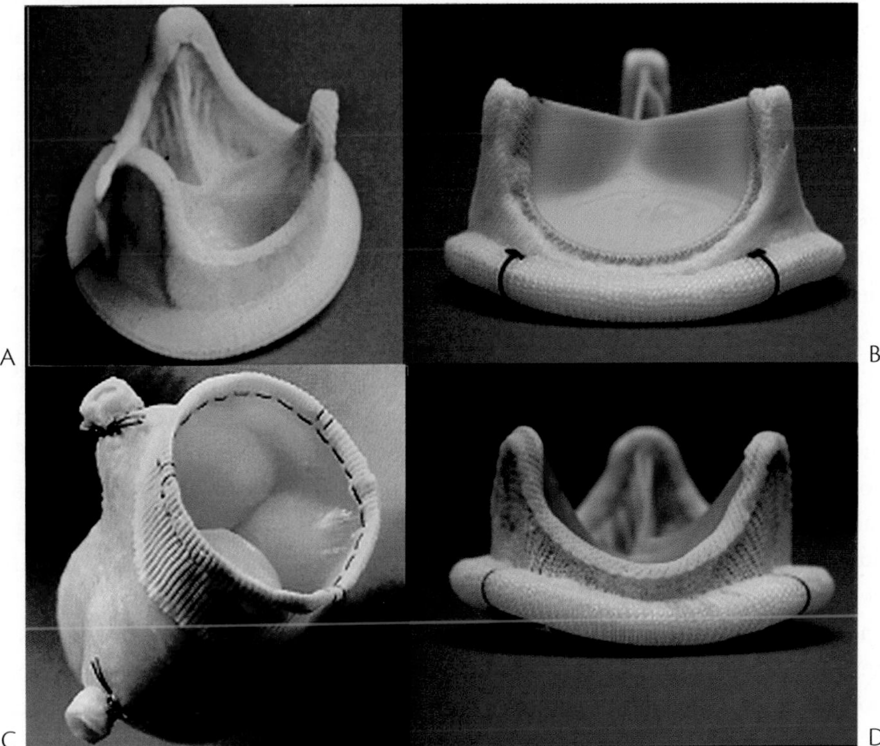

Figure 21.37 The four main designs of bioprosthetic valve: (A) porcine intra-annular valve; (B) pericardial intra-annular valve; (C) stentless porcine valve; (D) supra-annular porcine valve.

Homografts

In the early 1960s, Ross and Barratt-Boyes separately introduced the aortic homograft but only a few skilled surgeons were able to obtain predictable results with a free-sewn valve. Changes in the technique have resulted from different methods of preservation, such as cryopreservation or storage in antibiotics, and of implantation: full root or subcoronary.

One of the largest and most complete series comes from O'Brien and colleagues [255]. With cryopreserved valves the reoperation rate at 15 years for structural valve deterioration was 53% for age 1–20 years; 15% for 21–40 years; 19% for 41–60 years; and 16% for those aged >60 years. In this study, valve preservation techniques and implantation technique had no effect on the overall actuarial 20-year incidence of endocarditis, thromboembolism, structural valve deterioration, or late survival. One limitation of the technique is the shortage of high quality homografts. In addition, concerns remain regarding the possible superiority to bioprostheses in terms of durability. A study comparing propensity-matched patients who had undergone aortic valve replacement using either cryopreserved homografts or pericardial bioprostheses did not find a better durability of homografts [256]. Structural valve deterioration was the most frequent cause of reintervention and occurred earlier in patients aged <50 years, without any significant difference between homografts and pericardial bioprostheses. Finally, reoperation in patients with aortic homografts is more complex than with a bioprosthesis, in particular because of the propensity of homografts to degenerate with extensive calcification, which raises technical problems, in particular when homografts are implanted according to the mini-root technique [257].

Although not supported by controlled comparative studies, aortic homografts remain a substitute of choice for infective endocarditis with perivalvular lesions since they enable valvular and perivalvular lesions to be treated using a single biological substitute.

The pulmonary autograft

In 1967, Ross introduced the pulmonary autograft as a possible long-term biological solution for diseased aortic valves. Although it is a more complex and difficult procedure, it has the advantage in children that the valve is able to grow as the child grows. The autograft remains viable and grows in proportion with somatic growth and the annulus and sinotubular junction increase in size to the normal range. Good late results have been reported, in particular as regards the durability of the pulmonary autograft in aortic position. The main mechanism of late deterioration is the recurrence of AR mainly due to progressive aortic root enlargement without structural abnormality of aortic cusps [258, 259]. Patients with rheumatic heart disease may develop rheumatic valvulitis in the autograft. The incidence of thromboembolism is very low, as is that of infective endocarditis. Early stenosis on the pulmonary homograft is another possible complication inherent to this technique; it is generally located on the distal anastomosis with the native pulmonary artery rather than on the valve itself. Deterioration of the pulmonary homograft has been reported in 20% of patients within 1 year following intervention, requiring reintervention on the pulmonary outflow tract in 3% of all cases [260].

The exact role of the pulmonary autograft remains controversial, and it is only performed by a few surgeons in specialist centres, for children or young adults.

Given their availability, the experience of their use, and the standardization of surgical techniques, mechanical and biological prostheses are by far the most widely used valve substitutes [2].

Minimal invasive valve surgery

Minimal invasive surgery was developed at the end of the 1990s as an alternative to conventional sternotomy. The term 'minimal invasive surgery' applies to different techniques, the common characteristics of which being a smaller chest incision [189]. Certain interventions are carried out under conventional cardiopulmonary bypass while other use femoral cardiopulmonary bypass combined with an endoaortic balloon to reproduce the effect of the aortic clamp. Isolated aortic valve replacement can be performed using a partial upper sternotomy with good immediate results [261]. An endoscopic, video-assisted approach via the right chest [262], and an even more preliminary series of robotic surgery, have been reported for the treatment of mitral valve diseases [263].

Late outcome after valvular surgery

Late outcome after valve surgery depends on a number of patient-related factors, the type of intervention, and the prosthesis. The clinical performance of valvular substitutes is judged according to the 'Guidelines for Reporting Mortality and Morbidity After Cardiac Valve Intervention' [264].

The specific complications associated with cardiac valve prostheses are structural valve degeneration, non-structural dysfunction, thromboembolism and thrombosis, anticoagulant-related haemorrhage, and prosthetic valve endocarditis.

Randomized studies

Two large randomized trials have compared long-term results of valve replacement using a mechanical or a biological prosthesis. These two trials included patients who underwent valve replacement during the end of the 1970s.

The Veterans Affairs trial reported a mean 15-year follow-up of 575 randomized men, between 1987 and 1992 [142]. Mortality was lower in patients who had undergone aortic valve replacement using a mechanical prosthesis, but the difference only appeared after 10 years. Primary structural valve deterioration of bioprostheses begins to occur 5 years after mitral valve replacement and 7 years after aortic valve replacement. Bioprosthesis structural valve deterioration seldom occurred in patients aged >65 years.

In the Edinburgh Heart Valve Trial, 541 men and women were randomized between 1975 and 1979 and followed-up for up 20 years (➲Table 21.5) [265]. Major event-free survival was significantly higher in patients with a mechanical prosthesis than those with a bioprosthesis [14 ± 2% vs. 5 ± 1%, $p = 0.0007$], but there was no difference in survival.

The strength of these two studies is that they remain the only randomized controlled trials performed so far to compare mechanical and biological valve substitutes. Their consistent findings can be summarized as follows: the incidence of thromboembolism and endocarditis were not significantly different according to the type of prosthesis; bleeding rate was higher with mechanical valves; and reoperation rate was higher with bioprostheses. Nevertheless, the relevance of these findings are partially hampered by changes that occurred since the 1970s in the design of prostheses, the intensity of anticoagulant therapy, and indications for surgery which are now considered at an earlier stage of the valve disease. Patients aged >65 years represented a small sample in the two randomized trials whereas they now account for the majority of patients with valvular diseases in Western countries. Therefore, the findings from these two randomized trials have limitations regarding their practical implications for the choice of the prosthesis in an individual patient.

Non-randomized studies

Overall, late mortality rates in large series of valve replacements are high, in the order of 15–20% at 10–15 years [266–269]. There are wide variations in prognosis, even for a given type of prosthesis, which shows the importance of patient characteristics in late outcome after valve surgery, in particular: age; LV dysfunction; NYHA functional class; signs of congestive heart failure; arrhythmias; pulmonary hypertension; and comorbidity, such as CAD, diabetes, renal insufficiency, and lung disease.

The modalities of intervention also play a role, late survival being consistently lower in the case of associated coronary bypass grafting. Besides cardiac and non-cardiac variables, socioeconomic status also has an impact on long-term survival after valve replacement. A follow-up study including >50,000 patients from the UK Heart Valve Registry showed that social deprivation, as assessed by a composite index, was associated with a worse long-term survival in uni- and multivariate analysis. Survival differences according to socioeconomic status appeared only after 5 years of follow-up and were observed regardless of age and type of prosthesis [270].

Thus, comparison of different series should be cautious, in particular when comparing biological and mechanical prostheses. Differences in outcome are more likely to be the consequence of differences in patient characteristics rather than the type of prosthesis used [271]. This is illustrated by the somewhat conflicting results of recent series comparing long-term outcomes (at least 10-year follow-up) of large numbers of patients with biological and mechanical

Table 21.5 Actuarial rates (%) of events 20 years after valve replacement in the Edinburgh Heart Valve randomized trial. The 61 patients who had double valve replacement are not represented.

	Aortic prostheses			**Mitral prostheses**		
	Mechanical (n = 109)	Bioprosthesis (n = 102)	*p*	Mechanical (n = 129)	Bioprosthesis (n = 132)	*p*
Survival	28 ± 4	31 ± 5	0.57	22 ± 4	18 ± 4	0.41
Reoperation	7 ± 3	56 ± 8	<0.0001	13 ± 4	78 ± 7	<0.0001
Embolism	24 ± 6	39 ± 9	0.13	53 ± 7	32 ± 6	0.32
Bleeding	61 ± 8	42 ± 12	0.001	53 ± 8	37 ± 11	0.39
Endocarditis	8 ± 4	9 ± 6	0.71	4 ± 3	7 ± 3	0.38

Adapted with permission from Oxenham H, Bloomfield P, Wheatley DJ, *et al.* Twenty-year comparison of a Bjork–Shiley mechanical heart valve with porcine bioprostheses. *Heart* 2003; **89**: 715–21.

prostheses [267, 271–274]. In patients aged >70 years, the low rate of structural valve deterioration and the competitive risks with increased risk of death in the elderly generally favours bioprostheses in term of mortality [274] or morbidity [272]. However, in patients aged <70 years, certain series favour bioprostheses [272] whereas others report lower mortality rates in patients receiving mechanical prostheses [273, 274].

Does improved valve design result in improved clinical outcome?

Series based on the first generation of mechanical prostheses reported 10- and 20-year survival rates of 60% and 35% respectively after aortic valve replacement using the Starr–Edwards prosthesis model 1260, with an incidence of thromboembolic events of 1.4% per year [275]. The 5-year data from a prospective randomized trial reported by Murday and colleagues [276] showed no statistically significant difference in patient outcomes between the St. Jude and Starr–Edwards valves in either the aortic or mitral position.

The mortality and complication rates in patients with the use of various prosthetic devices followed up for >10 years indicate that there are no major differences in patient outcomes among the different valve substitutes. However, there may be differences in quality of life, which is more difficult to measure.

Complications of valve substitutes

Randomized trials and a large review have consistently shown that the incidence of thromboembolic events is not significantly different between mechanical prostheses and bioprostheses [142, 265, 277]. The main drawback of mechanical prostheses is increased bleeding risk while bioprostheses are associated with an increase in re-operation after 8–10 years because of structural deterioration.

Thromboembolism and anticoagulation-related haemorrhage

The analysis of the incidence of thromboembolism and bleeding in retrospective series should be cautious because of the frequent underestimation of event rates. For an evaluation to be accurate, it must be prospectively defined and repeated for the duration of follow-up. Furthermore, comparison between series may be influenced by differences in treatment, as well as patient- and prosthesis-related characteristics. Therefore, optimizing antithrombotic therapy requires randomized controlled trials.

Several randomized controlled trials have shown that in selected patients, i.e. patients with recent mechanical valve prostheses in sinus rhythm and without prior embolism, benefit from anticoagulant therapy with a target INR between 2–3 [278–280]. Randomized trials consistently showed that there was no significant increase in the thromboembolic risk of patients who had a target INR between 2–3 as compared to a target INR between 3–4.5, while there was a 30–50% decrease in the incidence of bleeding. This was confirmed by the GELIA trial, although the interpretation may be difficult because of overlapping INR target ranges [281].

There may be a further decrease in the thromboembolic risk by associating antiplatelet drugs, which should be balanced with the increase in bleeding risk. A randomized study demonstrated a decrease in the incidence of thromboembolism when low-dose aspirin was added to warfarin and the benefit remained significant when taking into account severe bleeding [282]. In the aspirin group, the main benefit was related to the decrease in sudden death and heart failure. As 30% of the population had associated CAD, the benefit of aspirin may have been due more to the prevention of atherosclerotic rather than prosthetic-related events. In a meta-analysis, the addition of an antiplatelet drug to oral anticoagulant therapy was associated with a 59% decrease in the risk of thromboembolic events, but at the expense of a 50% increase in the risk of major bleeding [283].

Endocarditis

The management of prosthetic endocarditis is detailed in ➲Chapter 22.

Structural valve deterioration

The risk of structural valve deterioration is considered 'negligible' with current models of mechanical prosthesis.

Bioprosthesis failure occurs via several mechanisms: regurgitation via leaflet tears; stenosis due to leaflet calcification; or perforations unrelated to calcification. The two main predictive factors of the risk of bioprosthesis structural valve deterioration are the site of the prosthesis and patient age [267, 277]. Structural valve deterioration occurs earlier after mitral than after aortic valve replacement because of a higher closing pressure. The older the patient at the time of surgery, the lower the rate of structural valve deterioration: <15% 15 years after aortic valve replacement in patients aged >70 years, while the corresponding 10-year rate is approximately 60% in those aged <40 years.

Non-structural dysfunction

The conditions referred to under this heading are paraprosthetic leaks, pannus, and haemolysis. Pannus refers to a membrane of material, which encroaches on the surface of the valve usually on the inflow side in either the mitral or aortic position. A retrospective study of mechanical valves in the mitral position [284] revealed a constant, but low, risk of valve obstruction due to pannus over a 14-year period. Pannus occurred more frequently, but later, than thrombus.

Paraprosthetic regurgitation has been reported in 6% of patients after aortic valve replacement and in 32% after mitral valve replacement when using systematic transoesophageal echocardiography [285]. Even mild paraprosthetic regurgitation may cause haemolysis, requiring reoperation if there is severe and recurrent anaemia. Subclinical haemolysis is frequently observed in patients with a normally functioning mechanical prosthesis.

Of 2680 patients with mechanical prosthesis, 250 required reoperation between 1970 and 1997: 133 for paravalvular leaks, 48 for obstructive pannus, and 29 for thrombotic obstruction. Reoperation rates have been estimated at 0.24 per 100 patient-years for pannus and 0.15 per 100 patient-years for thrombus [286].

Valve prosthesis–patient mismatch

Depending on its severity, valve prosthesis–patient mismatch may result in higher gradients at rest and on exercise, persistence of LV hypertrophy, impaired functional capacity, or even an increase in late morbidity and mortality.

Valve prosthesis–patient mismatch has been mainly studied in patients with aortic prostheses. It is generally defined by an effective orifice area ≤0.85cm/m^2 BSA and considered as severe when effective orifice area is ≤0.65cm^2/m^2 BSA [287]. Moderate mismatch has been reported to occur in 30–60% of patients and severe mismatch in ≤10%. Mismatch should be diagnosed using effective orifice area as assessed by echocardiography and not from values derived from manufacturers' in vitro data or the measurement of internal geometric area of the prosthesis [288]. No consensus has been reached on the impact of valve prosthesis–patient mismatch. A majority of series have reported impaired survival in patients with mismatch, in particular when severe, and the negative impact of mismatch remained significant in multivariate analysis [289, 290]. However, certain series did not find a significant impact of mismatch on survival [291], even in patients with AS and severe left ventricular dysfunction [292]. These discrepancies can be at least partly explained by the role of confounding factors. Patients with valve prosthesis–patient mismatch generally present with a more severe heart disease and/or with more frequent comorbidities [290–292], and the impact of these factors cannot be fully taken into account even with multivariate analyses. Current findings on valve prosthesis–patient mismatch support the use of prostheses with the largest effective orifice area possible, in particular in patients with small aortic annulus. Whether there is a real benefit in using complex surgical procedures to enlarge the aortic annulus remains unclear.

Less data is available after mitral valve replacement. Mitral valve prosthesis–patient mismatch is defined by an effective orifice area ≤1.2cm/m^2 BSA and considered as severe when effective orifice area is ≤0.9cm^2/m^2 BSA. Severe mismatch was reported to occur in 9% of patients and was an independent factor of late mortality in one series [293].

Choice of prosthesis for the individual patient

The choice of the type of prosthesis for any given patient should include a risk:benefit analysis of the drawbacks of the main types of valve substitutes, i.e. bleeding with mechanical prostheses and the risk of reoperation with bioprostheses. Results from randomized and non-randomized series enable these respective risks to be assessed according to patient characteristics. Age is an important issue since bleeding risk tends to increase with age, while the presumed durability of a bioprosthesis exceeds life expectancy in the elderly. However, the choice of the type of valve substitute should not over-stress patient age and should also take into account cardiac and non-cardiac patient characteristics which influence life expectancy, as well as the risk of bleeding, bioprosthesis deterioration, and reoperation. Furthermore, it is of utmost importance to inform the patient and to take into account their feeling about the prospect of reoperation versus the constraints and risks of anticoagulant therapy as well as specific wishes related to lifestyle or, for example, the desire for pregnancy. In the final analysis, the decision of which valve to use is an individual one between the patient, cardiologist, and cardiac surgeon. This is the reason why the ESC Guidelines highlight the importance of the desire of the informed patient, which is a class I recommendation for mechanical as well as biological prostheses [11] (➲Tables 21.6 and 21.7). The age after which a bioprosthesis is favoured is the range 65–70 years rather than a single threshold to show the relative relevance of an age threshold in the choice of the type of heart valve prosthesis. Age alone is only a class IIa recommendation as in ACC/AHA Guidelines [12].

Patient management after valve surgery

Modalities of follow-up

Clinical evaluation is the cornerstone of follow-up after valve surgery. During the postoperative period, repeated

Table 21.6 Choice of prosthesis: in favour of a mechanical prosthesis[a]

	Class
Desire of the informed patient and absence of contraindication for long-term anticoagulation	IC
Patients at risk of accelerated structural valve deterioration[b]	IC
Patient already on anticoagulation because of other mechanical prosthesis	IC
Patients already on anticoagulation because at high risk for thromboembolism[c]	IIaC
Age< 65-70 and long life expectancy[d]	IIaC
Patients for whom future redo valve surgery would be at high risk (due to left ventricular dysfunction, previous CABG, multiple valve prosthesis)	IIaC

CABG, coronary artery bypass grafting; LV, left ventricular; SVD, structural valve deterioration.

[a] The decision is based on the integration of several of the factors given in the table.

[b] Young age, hyperparathyroidism.

[c] Risk factors for thromboembolism: severe LV dysfunction; atrial fibrillation; previous thromboembolism; hypercoagulable state.

[d] According to age, gender, the presence of comorbidity, and country-specific life expectancy.

Adapted with permission from Vahanian A, Baumgartner H, Bax J, *et al.* Guidelines on the management of valvular heart disease: The Task Force on the Management of Valvular Heart Disease of the European Society of Cardiology. *Eur Heart J* 2007; **28**: 230–68.

clinical examination is the best way to diagnose early complications, in particular concerning tamponade or septic complications. Functional deterioration or change in auscultation during late follow-up raises the question of valve dysfunction and requires prompt echocardiographic examination. If there is suspicion of a neurologic event, transoesophageal echocardiography and CT of the brain must be carried out.

Clinical follow-up by a cardiologist is advised in all patients who have undergone valve surgery, generally on a yearly basis. There is no consensus regarding the usefulness of systematic echocardiographic follow-up, except 5–7 years after valve replacement using a bioprosthesis [11, 12]. Interpretation of follow-up echocardiography should take into account a baseline evaluation performed 6–12 weeks after surgery, since the relevance of gradients is questionable during the early postoperative period [11]. The diagnosis of prosthetic dysfunction relies more on the analysis of trends in measurements than on the comparison with predicted values for a given prosthesis, which supports the case for annual echocardiographic examination after any valve surgery. Transoesophageal echocardiography should be performed when prosthetic thrombosis or prosthetic endocarditis is suspected [11].

The main usefulness of blood tests is to detect silent bleeding in patients under anticoagulant therapy, or suffering from pathological haemolysis, or infection according to the clinical context. Although not specific, lactate dehydrogenase blood level is a good marker of the severity of haemolysis.

Table 21.7 Choice of prosthesis: in favour of a biological prosthesis[a]

	Class
Desire of the informed patient	IC
Unavailability of good quality anticoagulation (contraindication or high risk, unwillingness, compliance problems, lifestyle, occupation)	IC
Reoperation for mechanical valve thrombosis in a patient with proven poor anticoagulant control	IC
Patient for whom future redo valve surgery would be at low risk	IIaC
Limited life expectancy[b], severe comorbidity, or age >65–70 years	IIaC
Young woman contemplating pregnancy	IIbC

[a] The decision is based on the integration of several of the factors given in the table.

[b] According to age, gender, the presence of comorbidity, and country specific life expectancy.

Adapted with permission from Vahanian A, Baumgartner H, Bax J, *et al.* Guidelines on the management of valvular heart disease: The Task Force on the Management of Valvular Heart Disease of the European Society of Cardiology. *Eur Heart J* 2007; **28**: 230–68.

Anticoagulant therapy

Guidelines

Anticoagulation with a target INR between 2–3 is now advised in selected patients with an aortic prosthesis (➲Table 21.8). Higher levels of anticoagulation are recommended in patients who have mitral prosthesis or older types

Table 21.8 Target INR for mechanical prostheses

Prosthesis thrombogenicity[a]	Patient-related risk factors[b]	
	No risk factor	≥ 1 risk factor
Low	2.5	3.0
Medium	3.0	3.5
High	3.5	4.0

[a] Prosthesis thrombogenicity: Low = carbomedics (aortic position), Medtronic Hall, St Jude Medical (without Silzone); Medium = Bjork–Shiley, other bileaflet valves; High = Lillehei–Kaster, Omniscience, Starr–Edwards.

[b] Patient-related risk factors: mitral, tricuspid, or pulmonary valve replacement; previous thromboembolism; atrial fibrillation; left atrial diameter >50mm; left atrial dense spontaneous contrast; MS of any degree; LVEF <35%; hypercoagulable state.

LVEF, left ventricular ejection fraction; MS, mitral stenosis.

Adapted with permission from Vahanian A, Baumgartner H, Bax J, *et al.* Guidelines on the management of valvular heart disease: The Task Force on the Management of Valvular Heart Disease of the European Society of Cardiology. *Eur Heart J* 2007; **28**: 230–68.

of aortic prosthesis, although there are some differences according to guidelines regarding the target INR, which reflects the lack of data in the literature as regards these subgroups [11, 12, 294].

In the European guidelines [11], the combination of aspirin with vitamin K antagonists is restricted to patients with associated atherosclerosis or who experience recurrent embolism despite correct anticoagulation, while this combined therapy is recommended in all patients with a mechanical prosthesis in ACC/AHA Guidelines [12].

Recurrent thromboembolic events or severe bleeding should lead to search for an underlying cause and, if there is no additional cause, to adapt the modalities of anticoagulant therapy.

Anticoagulation monitoring

In a retrospective study, INR variability was a strong predictive factor of late survival after valve replacement [295]. The impact of insufficient or excessive anticoagulation has a particularly negative impact in the elderly [296]. Besides patient education, there are two main approaches for improving effective INR stability: anticoagulation clinics and self-monitoring. Randomized studies have shown that self-monitoring improves INR stability and decreases the incidence of thromboembolism and bleeding compared to conventional monitoring [297, 298].

The management of INR exceeding the upper target range should be adapted to the INR value and the presence or absence of active bleeding [11].

Specific situations

Postoperative period

The management of anticoagulant therapy is particularly difficult soon after valve replacement using a mechanical prosthesis because of the following factors:

- the incidence of thromboembolism is higher during the first postoperative month;
- bleeding risk is also higher and the consequences of bleeding may be particularly harmful, whether it is local bleeding requiring reintervention or gastrointestinal bleeding;
- there is a lack of comparative series in the literature enabling different anticoagulant modalities to be evaluated, which explains the absence of specific guidelines in this field and the wide heterogeneity in the practice of postoperative anticoagulant therapy.

The only randomized trial conducted during the postoperative period evaluated the addition of low-dose aspirin to conventional oral anticoagulation [299]. It showed a decrease in the incidence of thromboembolism but an increase in bleeding explaining an adverse trend on 1-year survival in patients who received aspirin, in particular because of an increased frequency of gastrointestinal bleeding.

There is an agreement to recommend the initiation of oral anticoagulant therapy during the first postoperative days [11]. The use of intravenous unfractionated heparin immediately after surgery enables effective anticoagulation to be obtained before INR reaches the target range. However, heparin therapy is difficult to manage because its efficacy is particularly unstable in the postoperative period, in particular because of inflammation, thereby requiring a particularly close monitoring.

The use of low-molecular-weight heparins can be interesting because of the better predictability and stability of their anticoagulant effect as compared with unfractionated heparin. Their use seems to be associated with a relatively low frequency of adverse events during the postoperative period but cannot be recommended in the absence of comparative controlled trials [300, 301].

There is a growing trend not to use or to shorten the use of oral anticoagulation after prosthetic valve replacement using a bioprosthesis, although there is no convincing evidence in the literature [302]. ESC and ACC/AHA guidelines still recommend a 3-month effective anticoagulant therapy after valve replacement using a bioprosthesis in the aortic or mitral position [11, 12].

Although this is also debated, a 3-month effective anticoagulant therapy is recommended after mitral valve repair [11]. Despite the lack of controlled trials, observational studies reporting thromboembolic events early after mitral repair support the use of anticoagulant therapy during the postoperative period [203].

Pregnancy

The specificity of anticoagulant therapy during pregnancy is described in ➲Chapter 33.

Management of anticoagulant therapy during non-cardiac interventions

Bleeding risk during non-cardiac interventions under anticoagulant therapy is mainly related to the type of procedure. Management of anticoagulation during non-cardiac interventions should be adapted to the type of procedure and patient risk for thromboembolism [11, 12]. Minor surgery, in particular most procedures of dental care, can be safely performed under effective anticoagulant therapy, provided the risk of thromboembolism and bleeding are carefully assessed and the procedure uses appropriate resources to prevent and, if required, to treat local bleeding [303].

Conversely, major surgery generally requires an INR <1.5 and, therefore, temporary withdrawal of oral anticoagulation [11]. It has been suggested that the thromboembolic risk can be low enough (approximately 0.1%) for a 3-day interruption [12]. However, this was the result of debatable extrapolations, and thromboembolic risk during non-cardiac interventions has been estimated at 1.6% in observational studies [304]. Thus, when major surgery requires withdrawal of oral anticoagulation in a patient with a mechanical heart valve prosthesis, heparin should be used when INR is <2 in low-risk patients or <2.5 in high-risk patients. Heparin is stopped 6 hours before surgery and resumed 6–12 hours after. Unfractionated intravenous heparin should be favoured. Low-molecular-weight heparins are an interesting alternative but their use has not been approved so far in patients with valve prosthesis [11, 305].

The modalities of perioperative anticoagulation for non-cardiac surgery in patients with mechanical heart valve prosthesis should always be discussed and planned according to a close collaboration between the cardiologist, surgeon, and anaesthesiologist.

Endocarditis prophylaxis

Infective endocarditis prophylaxis is of particular importance in patients with heart valve prosthesis, who are considered at high-risk for endocarditis in all guidelines [59]. Principles are described in ➲Chapter 22.

Treatment of specific complications

Prosthetic thrombosis

Occlusive prosthetic thrombosis is characterized by impaired motion of the mobile part of the prosthesis. This high-risk complication justifies a particular awareness in the case of thromboembolism or heart failure in a patient with a mechanical prosthesis and should lead to prompt performance of transthoracic, and most often transoesophageal, echocardiography and cinefluoroscopy [11, 306, 307]. Occlusive prosthetic thrombosis is usually treated by redo surgery, which carries a relatively high risk, particularly when patients are in poor haemodynamic condition [306] (➲Fig. 21.38). Thrombolysis is an alternative but it is associated with high mortality rates due to failure or embolic events [307]. According to recent guidelines, thrombolysis is mainly considered if surgery is contraindicated or not available in urgent situations or in rare cases of thrombolysis of a tricuspid prosthesis [11, 12]. There is a debate about the use of thrombolysis as a first-line treatment in patients with few or no symptoms and a small clot burden. However, this relies on low levels of evidence; it is not recommended in ESC guidelines and it is only a class IIb recommendation in ACC/AHA guidelines [12].

Non-occlusive prosthetic thrombosis is mainly diagnosed on transoesophageal echocardiography after an embolic event and in as much as 10–15% of patients after mitral valve replacement using a mechanical prosthesis [308] (➲Fig. 21.39). First-line treatment is intensification of anticoagulation and addition of antiplatelet drugs under close echocardiographic monitoring. Surgery can be considered in large non-occlusive prosthetic thrombosis (≥10mm), in particular if it is complicated by an embolic event or persists despite intensification of anticoagulant therapy [11]. Fibrinolysis is generally not considered to treat non-occlusive prosthetic thrombosis because of concerns related to the risks of bleeding and embolism.

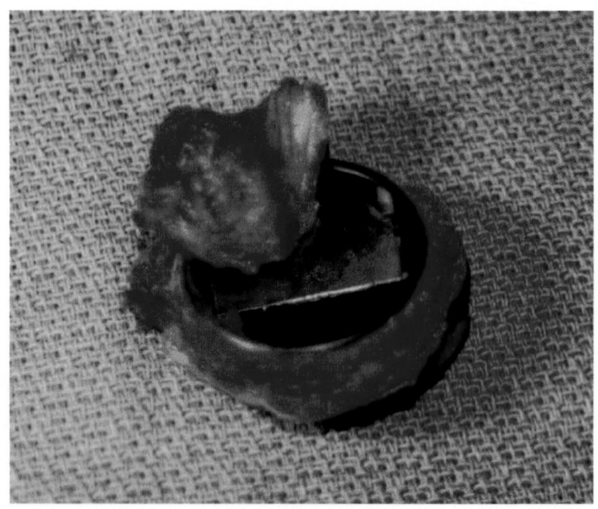

Figure 21.38 Occlusive thrombosis on a bileaflet mechanical prosthesis in the mitral position. (Courtesy of Dr I. Philip.)

Bioprosthesis failure

Reoperation is indicated in symptomatic patients in whom there is an increase in transprosthetic gradient or new significant regurgitation. Surgery should be considered early, since its risk rapidly increases in patients in NYHA class III or IV. There is no consensus in asymptomatic patients with structural valve deterioration and the decision should take into account the magnitude of the gradient or regurgitation as well as its evolution, consequences, and risk of reoperation. In the future, percutaneous implantation of a valve in a valve may be a potential attractive alternative to reoperation in such cases [309].

Non-structural dysfunction

Reoperation should be considered in patients with paraprosthetic regurgitation causing severe haemolysis requiring repeated blood transfusions or, less frequently, leading to severe symptoms. Reoperation can be associated with a prohibitive risk which may lead to strongly considering palliative treatment using beta-blockers and/or erythropoietin in certain patients. Transcatheter closure of paravalvular regurgitations is feasible [310] but complex and concerns exist regarding its efficacy. Little information is

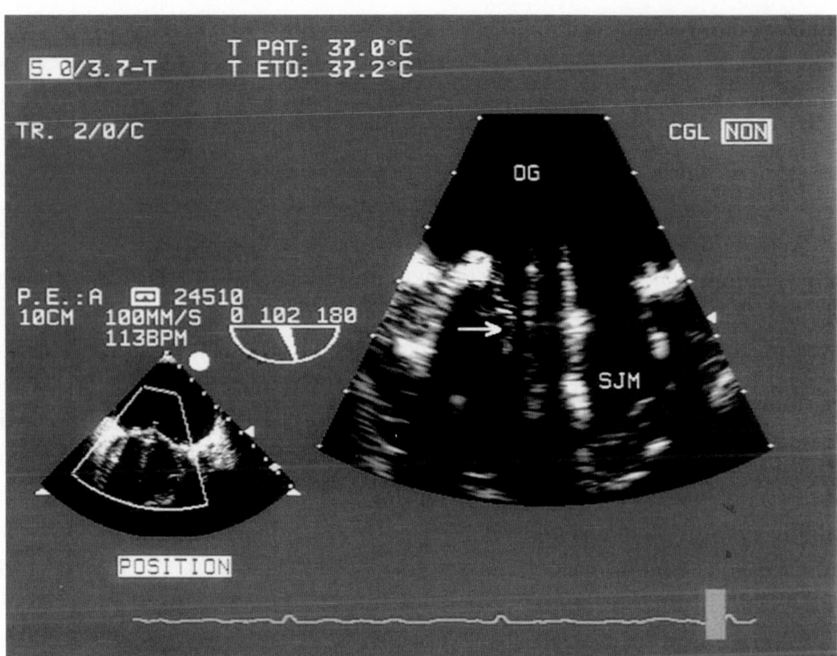

Figure 21.39 Non-occlusive prosthetic thrombosis (arrow) on the ring of a bileaflet prosthesis in mitral position. Transoesophageal echocardiography. (Courtesy of Dr B. Cormier.)

available since most evaluations of transcatheter closure of paravalvular regurgitations are case reports. A small series showed improvement of symptoms but no efficacy on haemolysis in most patients [311]. This explains why transcatheter intervention is not considered as an alternative to surgery in guidelines [11, 12].

Endocarditis

Prosthetic valve endocarditis frequently requires surgery, which should not be delayed to avoid intervening in a patient in poor haemodynamic condition. The management of prosthetic endocarditis is detailed in ➲Chapter 22.

Conclusion

Although the mortality for elective valve replacement is low, the long-term survival is far from satisfactory. This highlights the need to optimize the choice of valve substitute as well as improve education and follow-up after surgery.

Personal perspective

Valve disease will remain an increasingly important public health problem: AS will assert its presence due to population ageing and become the first indication for intervention. MR is also an emerging disease, and patients with previous valve intervention will increase.

Basic science collaboration will elucidate the cellular and molecular mechanisms of 'degenerative' valve disease and LV response to overload, and support identification of new prognostic factors and development for novel therapies. Genetic research using genomic approaches is in its infancy in the field of VHD but holds promise.

Non-invasive techniques will be improved for the evaluation of VHD, most importantly three-dimensional echocardiography, CT, and MRI. The development of less load-dependent indices, easy to obtain and to repeat, are desirable for the earlier detection of myocardial damage and optimal timing for intervention. Greater use of echo or MRI-based dynamic testing is expected as well as that of biomarkers such as BNP for decision making. Non-invasive techniques will be increasingly used for the guidance of interventional procedures and may well replace fluoroscopy in selected indications in the future.

A great challenge will be to prevent or delay degenerative AS, as was done with rheumatic disease. Prospective studies are necessary to further evaluate hypotheses concerning statins used at an early stage, ACE inhibitors, or anti-metalloproteases. There are great expectations for the use of new antithrombotic agents which are easier to use and safer than the current vitamin K antagonists in patients with a mechanical prosthesis.

Education of patients is key for the prevention of endocarditis and thromboembolism, as well as rheumatic fever which is still a major public health problem in many parts of the world.

The development and prospective evaluation of tools for better quantitative evaluation of the risks of surgery are expected to aid decision making, especially in the elderly population.

The search for the 'perfect valvular substitute' will continue. Material derived from nanotechnology and tissue engineering aided by emerging stem cell technology hold promise. Conservative techniques will gain wider acceptance in MR through their dissemination and further evaluation. The same should apply for AR but will necessitate the development and evaluation of anatomic and functional classification followed by standardization of the surgical techniques similar to what was achieved for MR.

The role of interventional cardiology will increase. PMC will remain a useful complement to valve replacement in the treatment of MS. The initial experience of TAVI opens a new era for research and potential clinical applications for AS. The technology will improve. The precise role of this new technique will most probably increase, leading to lower risk for patients in the future, after careful evaluation which is currently ongoing. The outlook for percutaneous mitral valve repair is currently uncertain—it is a great technological challenge to be evaluated in the future. These current trends in percutaneous interventions should be developed in collaboration between cardiologists, surgeons, and imaging specialists, and hold promise. Calculating the cost effectiveness of valve intervention will be an important direction of study.

Finally, in order to improve patient care in the field of VHD, well-designed trials are required to create more evidence-based guidelines, which need to be implemented and scrutinized by surveys.

Further reading

Bonow RO, Carabello BA, Chatterjee K, *et al.* Focused update incorporated into the ACC/AHA 2006 guidelines for the management of patients with valvular heart disease: a report of the American College of Cardiology/American Heart Association Task Force on Practice Guidelines (Writing Committee to Revise the 1998 Guidelines for the Management of Patients With Valvular Heart Disease): endorsed by the Society of Cardiovascular Anesthesiologists, Society for Cardiovascular Angiography and Interventions, and Society of Thoracic Surgeons. *Circulation* 2008; **118**: e523–e661.

Iung B, Baron G, Butchart EG, *et al.* A prospective survey of patients with valvular heart disease in Europe: the Euro Heart Survey on valvular heart disease. *Eur Heart J* 2003; **24**: 1231–43.

Lancellotti P, Marwick T, Piérard LA. How to manage ischaemic mitral regurgitation. *Heart* 2008; **94**: 1497–502.

Levy F, Laurent M, Monin JL, *et al.* Aortic valve replacement for low-flow/low-gradient aortic stenosis operative risk stratification and long-term outcome: a European multicenter study. *J Am Coll Cardiol* 2008; **51**: 1466–72.

Nkomo VT, Gardin JM, Skelton TN, *et al.* Burden of valvular heart diseases: a population-based study. *Lancet* 2006; **368**: 1005–11.

Oxenham H, Bloomfield P, Wheatley DJ, *et al.* Twenty-year comparison of a Bjork–Shiley mechanical heart valve with porcine bioprostheses. *Heart* 2003; **89**: 715–21.

Rosenhek R, Binder T, Porenta G, *et al.* Predictors of outcome in severe asymptomatic aortic stenosis. *N Engl J Med* 2000; **343**: 611–17.

Rosenhek H, Rader F, Klaar U, *et al.* Outcome of watchful waiting in asymptomatic severe mitral regurgitation. *Circulation* 2006; **113**: 2238–44.

Tornos P, Sambola A, Permanyer-Miralda G, *et al.* Long-term outcome of surgically tretaed aortic regurgitation. Influence of guideline adherence toward early surgery. *J Am Coll Cardiol* 2006; **47**: 1012–17.

Vahanian A, Baumgartner H, Bax J, *et al.* Guidelines on the management of valvular heart disease: The Task Force on the Management of Valvular Heart Disease of the European Society of Cardiology. *Eur Heart J* 2007; **28**: 230–68.

Vahanian A, Alfieri O, Al-Attar N, *et al.* Transcatheter valve implantation for patients with aortic stenosis: a position statement from the European Association of Cardio-Thoracic Surgery (EACTS) and the European Society of Cardiology (ESC), in collaboration with the European Association of Percutaneous Cardiovascular Interventions (EAPCI). *Eur Heart J* 2008; **29**: 1463–70.

Zoghbi WA, Enriquez-Sarano M, Foster E, *et al.* Recommendations for evaluation of the severity of native valvular regurgitation with two-dimensional and Doppler echocardiography. *J Am Soc Echocardiogr* 2003; **16**: 777–802.

Online resources

- Francophone society of oral medicine and oral surgery, with the collaboration of the French society of cardiology. Guidelines for management of patients under antivitamin K treatment in oral surgery. Available at: http://www.societechirbuc.com/Recommandations/recommandations_avk_gb.pdf
- US Society of Thoracic Surgeons National Database. Available at: http://www.sts.org/section/stsdatabase

Additional online material

- 21.1 Typical rheumatic aortic and mitral valve.
- 21.2 Moderate aortic stenosis.
- 21.3 Normal aortic valve.
- 21.4 Implantation of a balloon expandable aortic valve
- 21.5 X-plane real-time three-dimensional transoesophageal echocardiography during aortic prosthesis deployment (Edwards–Sapien prosthesis) in aortic stenosis.
- 21.6 Severe rheumatic aortic regurgitation.
- 21.7 Severe mitral stenosis.
- 21.8 Mitral stenosis: bi-commissural opening after percutaneous mitral commissurotomy.
- 21.9 Mitral stenosis: view of the medial commissure.
- 21.10 Mitral stenosis: view of the lateral commissure.
- 21.11 Mitral stenosis.
- 21.12 Real-time three-dimensional transoesophageal echocardiography imaging showing frontal view of mitral stenosis from the left atrium perspective.
- 21.13 Real-time three-dimensional transoesophageal echocardiography imaging showing balloon positioning and inflation during percutaneous balloon commissurotomy of mitral stenosis.
- 21.14 Severe organic mitral regurgitation due to a flail of the posterior leaflet with rupture of chordae; transoesophageal echocardiography; 6°.
- 21.15 Severe organic mitral regurgitation due to a flail of the anterior leaflet with rupture of chordae: transoesophageal echocardiography; 0°.
- 21.16 Typical rheumatic mitral regurgitation.
- 21.17 Functional mitral regurgitation: moderate to severe mitral regurgitation.
- 21.18 Functional mitral regurgitation.
- 21.19 Real-time three-dimensional transoesophageal echocardiography imaging: frontal view of the mitral valve from the left atrium perspective showing prolapse of the posterior valve (P_2 segment) with ruptured chordae.
- 21.20 Severe organic mitral regurgitation: colour Doppler.
- 21.21 Functional tricuspid regurgitation.
- 21.22 Functional mitral and tricuspid regurgitation.
- 21.23 Bileaflet mechanical prosthetic valve.
- 21.24 Bileaflet mechanical prosthetic valve: colour Doppler.
- 21.25 Ball-and-cage mechanical prosthetic valve.

For full references and multimedia materials please visit the online version of the book (http://esctextbook.oxfordonline.com).

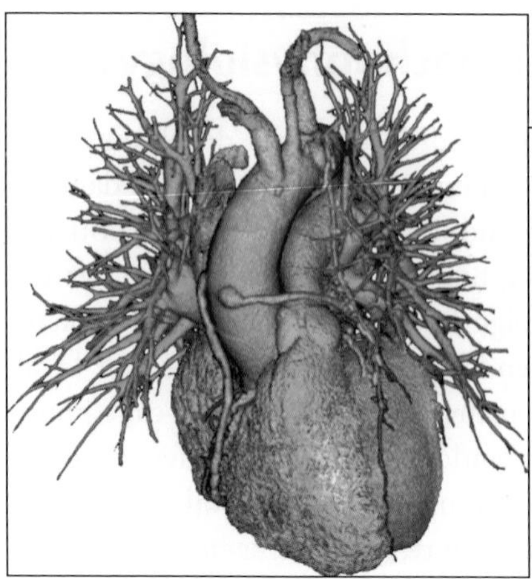

CHAPTER 22

Infective Endocarditis

Werner G. Daniel and Frank A. Flachskampf

Contents

Summary

This protean disease, whose salient features have been known for centuries, continues to pose major diagnostic and therapeutic challenges. Infective endocarditis predominantly affects cardiac valves and leads to local destruction with subsequent regurgitation. Embolism, especially to the brain, is the most feared extracardiac complication. Diagnosis rests on positive blood cultures and demonstration of vegetations by echocardiography. The rise of aggressive pathogens and the frequency of unfavourable clinical circumstances, such as presence of prosthetic valves or compromised immunocompetence, have resulted in more frequent and earlier surgical therapy. Although endocarditis is no longer uniformly fatal, outcomes are still characterized by high morbidity and mortality. The upcoming European Society of Cardiology recommendations for endocarditis prophylaxis hopefully will further improve disease prevention and management of patients at increased risk.

Definition

Infection of valvular tissue or cardiovascular endothelium by a variety of pathogens constitutes infective endocarditis. Although endocarditis mostly involves the cardiac valves, it may also manifest as endarteritis (e.g. in aortic coarctation) or develop on foreign bodies such as intravenous lines, pacemaker leads, conduits, etc. Former classifications of endocarditis as subacute, acute, or chronic have been discarded. A newer classification based on European Society of Cardiology (ESC) task force recommendations [1] is provided in ➲Table 22.1.

Epidemiology

The incidence of infective endocarditis in the general population is estimated at 14–31 per million persons and year [2–5]. Subgroups such as immunocompromised persons and addicts of intravenous drugs have a much higher incidence of endocarditis. The incidence increases with age and is higher in men than in women.

Table 22.1 ESC recommendations on classification and terminology of infective endocarditis [1]

Infective endocarditis may be classified by:
Activity
Active/healed
Recurrence
Recurrent, if a relapse occurs within a year of eradication/operation; persistent, if no eradication has occurred
Confidence of diagnosis
Definite, if vegetations are demonstrated in the presence of systemic infection (with or without positive blood cultures)
Suspected, if clinically strongly suggested
Possible if clinical suspicion is less strong (e.g. differential diagnosis of fever)
Special circumstances
Prosthetic endocarditis (early if within 1 year of valve replacement, otherwise late), pacemaker endocarditis, and endocarditis in a patient with intravenous drug abuse
According to the site of involvement
Aortic, mitral, tricuspid, pulmonary, right heart, left heart
According to the causative agent
E.g. staphylococcal endocarditis

Pathology and pathophysiology

The initial necessary condition for the development of infective endocarditis is endocardial or endothelial damage. Such damage may be induced by regurgitant, stenotic, or shunt lesions creating high-velocity blood jets, (micro-) trauma, surgery, foreign bodies, etc. Adherence of platelets to the injured endothelium leads to a small local, initially sterile fibrin-platelet aggregate, the so-called non-bacterial thrombotic endocarditis, which then becomes infected by pathogens circulating in the blood. Conversely, intact endothelium is very resistant to bacterial colonization. Bacteraemia most often originates from the skin and oropharynx. The ability of microorganisms to adhere to the initial thrombus, to colonize it, and to grow, differs widely and depends, among other factors, on their ability to bind to fibronectin, a surface glycoprotein found on many cells, including endothelial cells. If the initial microthrombus is colonized and to the degree in which cellular and humoral host defences are overcome, rapid growth ensues and within days a macroscopically detectable vegetation is formed, which contains staggering amounts of bacteria (in the order of 10^{10}/g), thrombus, and leucocytes, together with tissue debris. The vegetation is the hallmark of infective endocarditis (➲Fig. 22.1). It may grow from nearly

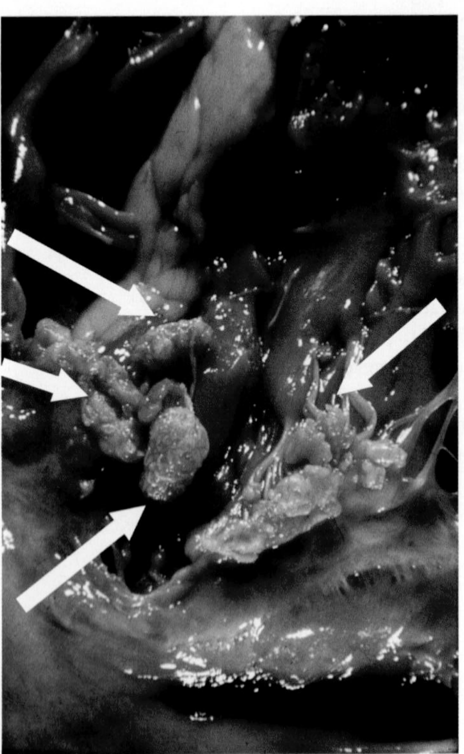

Figure 22.1 Large vegetations (arrows) on the tricuspid valve in candida endocarditis.

invisible to several centimetres in length and is most often (though not exclusively) attached on the low-pressure side of the underlying structure, i.e. the atrial side of atrioventricular valves and the low-pressure side of shunt lesions, due to the endothelial damage secondary to high-velocity jets at these sites.

Vegetations may lead to valve incompetence, or, rarely, obstruction. Bacterial invasion may also lead to direct damage of valve structures, such as leaflet defects or tears, chordal rupture, to the development of fistulae between heart cavities, or to perivalvular abscess formation. A rare form of an endocarditic abscess is the so-called pseudoaneurysm of the mitral aortic intervalvular fibrosa [6], which is a ring abscess located in the section of the aortic and mitral valve circumference which are contiguous. These outpouchings may communicate with the left ventricle or left ventricular outflow tract and, after rupture, create a fistula to the left atrium. Tissue invasion may lead to conduction abnormalities such as complete atrioventricular block, and to pericardial effusion.

Prosthetic valves are high-risk lesions for endocarditis. In mechanical valves usually the sewing ring is affected, with a high incidence of periprosthetic leaks and abscesses. In bioprostheses, both the ring and the leaflets themselves can be affected. Intravenous lines and pacemaker leads may develop adherent vegetations and infection may spread to contiguous tissue.

Vegetations are prone to embolization, in particular if they are large and mobile. Clinically, embolism is found in one-third to one-half of cases, but the true incidence is much higher due to often silent embolism. Left heart endocarditis embolizes predominantly to the brain, the spleen, and the kidneys, as well as the limbs. Metastatic abscesses may ensue. Right heart endocarditis embolizes to the lung with consecutive lung abscess or pneumonia. Aortic vegetations prolapsing into the left ventricle may create secondary infection of the anterior mitral leaflet by direct contact during diastole ('kissing lesions').

Renal involvement in infective endocarditis includes septic renal embolism, immune-complex mediated glomerulonephritis, and interstitial nephritis due to antimicrobial therapy. Renal involvement in infective endocarditis is associated with impaired prognosis [7].

Infective endocarditis leads to a constant, often low-grade bacteraemia. Frank sepsis often ensues, especially with aggressive organisms such as staphylococci. Infective endocarditis is believed to be uniformly fatal if not treated.

Infective endocarditis may also arise in extracardiac locations, mostly the cerebral and thoracic large arteries, and create so-called mycotic aneurysms, which may rupture.

Risk factors

Congenital and acquired valvular heart diseases are strong risk factors for infective endocarditis. It is estimated that approximately one-half of patients with endocarditis have some form of underlying heart disease, most often bicuspid aortic valve, mitral valve prolapse, other degenerative valvular disease, ventricular septal defect, hypertrophic obstructive cardiomyopathy, aortic coarctation, and others. Prosthetic heart valves, both of the mechanical and biological type, are prone to infection, as are other foreign bodies such as central venous lines, pacemaker and ICD leads, intravenous ports, ventriculo-atrial shunts, Dacron patches or conduits (see ➲Table 22.2). Of note, while ventricular septal defects carry a high risk of endocarditis, atrial septal defect of secundum type or patent foramen ovale do not entail an elevated risk. Furthermore, immunosuppression, dialysis, intravenous drug abuse, HIV infection, and long-term intensive care treatment all increase the risk of acquiring infective endocarditis, in particular in the presence of a pre-existent cardiovascular lesion. Whereas previously all patients with risk lesions were considered candidates for endocarditis prophylaxis whenever they underwent procedures inducive of bacteraemia (such as oropharyngeal procedures or surgery, dental procedures, lower digestive tract procedures (in particular with biopsy), and others) (➲Tables 22.2 and 22.3), the recent corresponding guidelines by the American Heart Association have completely revised this standpoint, as outlined in ➲'Prophylaxis and prevention', p.831 [8].

Table 22.2 Lesions conferring elevated risk of acquiring infective endocarditis*

Acquired or congenital valvular heart disease, including bicuspid aortic valve and mitral valve prolapse
Presence of a valvular prosthesis or surgically created conduit
Previous endocarditis
Immunosuppression (e.g. after organ transplantation)
Hypertrophic obstructive cardiomyopathy
Ventricular septal defect
Complex, especially cyanotic, congenital heart disease
Shunt lesions (congenital or surgically constructed) except atrial septal defects of secundum type
Aortic coarctation

*However, note that endocarditis prophylaxis is regarded mandatory by recent guidelines in only some of these lesions (see text).

Data from Dajani AS, Taubert KA, Wilson W, *et al.* Prevention of bacterial endocarditis. Recommendations by the American Heart Association. *Circulation* 1997; **96**: 358–66.

Table 22.3 Interventions and procedures potentially associated with bacteraemia

Dental procedures that cause oral bleeding (e.g. dental extraction, removal of tartar)
Oropharyngeal surgery including tonsillectomy
Oesophageal dilatation, sclerotherapy of oesophageal varices, and endoscopic retrograde cholangiography with biliary obstruction
Gall bladder surgery, appendectomy, colectomy
Genitourinary procedures including catheterization and cystoscopy in the presence of urinary tract infection, transurethral prostate resection
Abscess surgery

*However, note that endocarditis prophylaxis is regarded mandatory by recent guidelines in only some of these lesions (see text).

Data from Dajani AS, Taubert KA, Wilson W, *et al.* Prevention of bacterial endocarditis. Recommendations by the American Heart Association. *Circulation* 1997; **96**: 358–66.

Causative pathogens

Almost all known pathogenic bacteria have been implied in cases of infective endocarditis. In practice, however, a limited variety of organisms are significant. Only the most frequent pathogens will therefore be discussed. Remarkably, infective endocarditis is most often a disease produced by Gram-positive bacteria, especially cocci.

Streptococcal disease

These bacteria are still the most frequent cause of infective endocarditis and typically produce the classic protracted or 'subacute' course of endocarditis. The origin of streptococci is most often the oropharynx. They are mostly, but not always susceptible to penicillin G. *Streptococcus gallolyticus* (formerly *Streptococcus bovis*) endocarditis has been found to be frequently associated with adenoma and adenocarcinoma of the colon, making colonoscopy advisable if *Streptococcus gallolyticus* bacteraemia is documented [9, 10].

Staphylococci

Staphylococcal endocarditis has increased substantially in frequency and staphylococci are now the second most common, and in some series the most common, aetiologic agents in native valve endocarditis. *Staphylococcus aureus*, an extremely aggressive and destructive organism, causes 90% of all cases of staphylococcal endocarditis. *Staphylococcus epidermidis* is the most frequent cause of early prosthetic valve endocarditis. Staphylococci often produce beta-lactamase and are therefore resistant to many, if not all beta-lactam antibiotics, i.e. penicillins and cephalosporins. Vancomycin and teicoplanin remain effective. The origin of staphylococci is most frequently the skin. Hospital-acquired staphylococcal infections via catheters and intravenous lines are also frequent.

Q fever endocarditis

Q fever, a zoonosis caused by the intracellular rickettsia *Coxiella burnetii*, is endemic worldwide but particularly frequent in France. Its natural sources are cattle, sheep, goats, and others. An estimated 10% of cases affect the heart. *Coxiella burnetii* does not grow on culture media. Diagnosis is by serology or polymerase chain reaction (PCR). Doxycycline in combination with rifampicin is the recommended antibiotic therapy.

Enterococci

Enterococcus faecalis is the most frequent pathogen of this group, typically originating in the gastrointestinal tract. Antibiotic resistance in these organisms is variable, although they are usually susceptible to the combination of a beta-lactam antibiotic and an aminoglycoside as gentamicin.

Fungi

Fungal infections are typical for immunocompromised patients or following long-term intravenous therapy. Treatment usually requires surgery.

Symptoms and signs

Clinical signs

Fever, chills, malaise, night sweats, arthralgias, and weight loss are unspecific systemic symptoms of infectious endocarditis, in particular the more protracted forms formerly designated as 'subacute'. It should be noted that in the elderly these symptoms, including temperature elevation, may be mitigated or absent. In immunosuppressed patients, clinical signs of generalized infection may also be inapparent. Haemofiltration may suppress temperature elevation. However, endocarditis without at least a minor degree of temperature elevation is very rare. A warm dry skin, tachycardia, and spleen enlargement (in particular in protracted endocarditis) are additional physical signs of systemic inflammation.

The classical specific physical signs of endocarditis are largely signs of destructive (valvular regurgitation murmurs and heart failure) or embolic (although in part immunologically mediated) complications of endocarditis and thus signal advanced disease.

Cardiac signs include:

- *In mitral endocarditis:* a new or greatly increased typical holosystolic murmur of mitral regurgitation, best heard over the apex and radiating to the left axilla, associated with dyspnoea, pulmonary congestion, or oedema, and other signs of left heart backward failure;
- *In aortic endocarditis:* a new typical diastolic murmur of aortic regurgitation, best heard over the left sternal border, low diastolic blood pressure, associated with dyspnoea, pulmonary congestion, or oedema, and other signs of left heart backward failure;
- *In tricuspid endocarditis:* a new typical soft parasternal systolic murmur of tricuspid regurgitation increasing with inspiration, together with jugular vein distention, a prominent systolic jugular vein pulse, and liver enlargement.

Systemic embolism from left heart (or arterial) endocarditis is often the first clinical sign of endocarditis, and may manifest as

- Neurologic impairment, ranging from transient symptoms to fatal massive stroke. Intracranial haemorrhage in infective endocarditis occurs in 5% of patients, may be due to secondary bleeding into an infarcted zone or to rupture of a mycotic aneurysm of a cerebral artery (➲Fig. 22.2). Meningitis may develop due to a septic cerebral abscess. Neurologic complications in infective endocarditis are ominous and predict dramatically increased mortality.
- Limb, abdominal (kidney, spleen), or even coronary ischaemia (rare).

All of these sites may develop septic abscesses. Right heart endocarditis in the majority of cases leads to—sometimes clinically silent—septic pulmonary embolism and may present with signs of pneumonia and pleuritis. For typical cutaneous signs of endocarditis see ➲Table 22.4 and Fig. 22.3. Fundoscopy may reveal retinal haemorrhage with a pale centre (Roth spots; see ➲Fig. 22.4). It cannot be overemphasized that, in spite of the wealth of time-honoured clinical signs and symptoms of infective endocarditis, this is a notoriously difficult disease to diagnose. This holds particularly true for the early stages, before destructive or embolic events have occurred. It may also explain why in a large multicentre registry [11], average time from onset of symptoms to hospital admission was 29 days!

Table 22.4 Cutaneous signs of infective endocarditis (mediated by microembolism, haemorrhage, or immunologic responses) (see ➲Fig. 22.3)

Petechiae (extremities, conjunctivae, buccal mucosa);
Splinter haemorrhages (subungual)
Osler nodes (small, tender, purple, subcutaneous nodules on the palmar side of the digits)
Janeway lesions (erythematous non-tender macular lesions on palms and soles)

Laboratory signs

There is no specific laboratory marker of infective endocarditis. Laboratory abnormalities include leucocytosis with granulocytosis with a left shift (or even leucopoenia, especially in overt sepsis), elevated sedimentation rate, elevated C-reactive protein and gamma globulin levels. Anaemia of infection with low serum iron levels is a cardinal sign of endocarditis. Circulating immune complexes and occasionally a positive rheumatoid factor are detectable. Importantly, urinalysis is very frequently pathologic even without manifest septic embolism to the kidney. Haematuria (often only

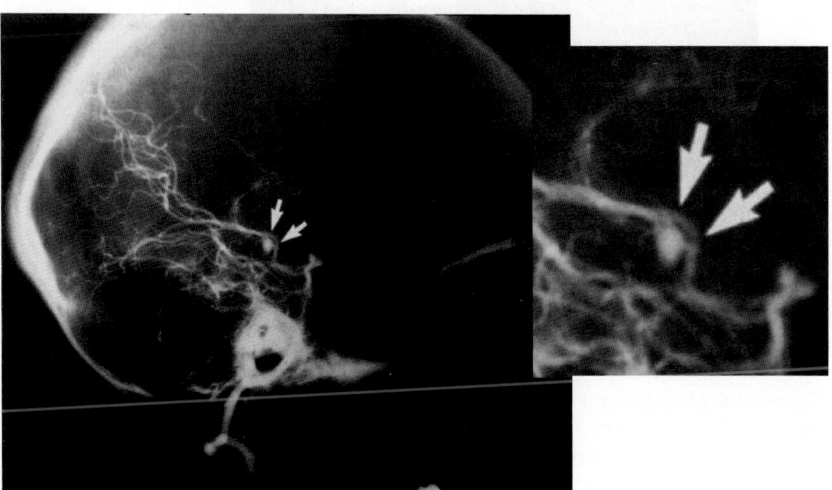

Figure 22.2 Mycotic aneurysm (arrows) of the left posterior cerebral artery.

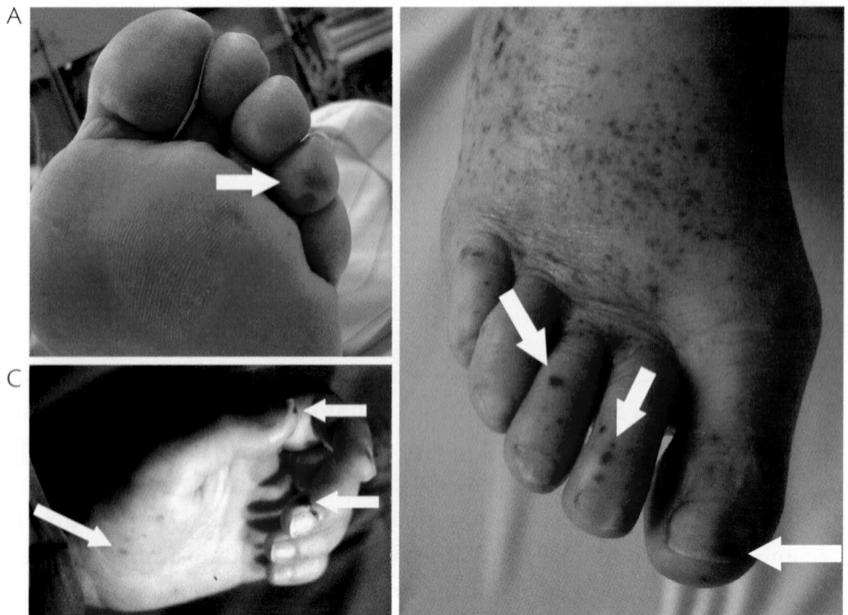

Figure 22.3 Macular petechial and embolic skin lesions (arrows) in three different patients with infective staphylococcal endocarditis. (Images of patient A and B, courtesy of Dr. Christian Schlundt, Department of Cardiology, University Clinic Erlangen.)

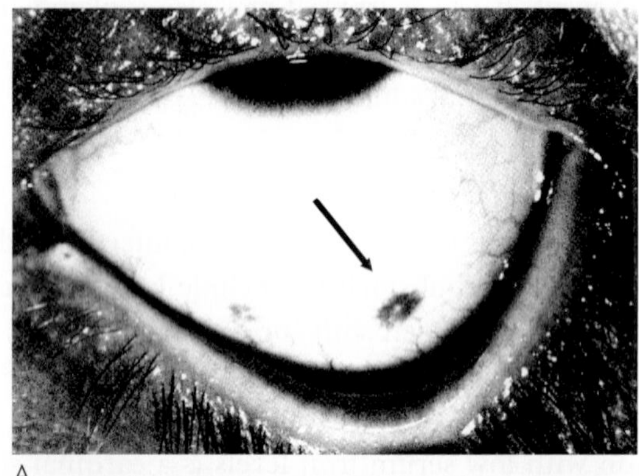

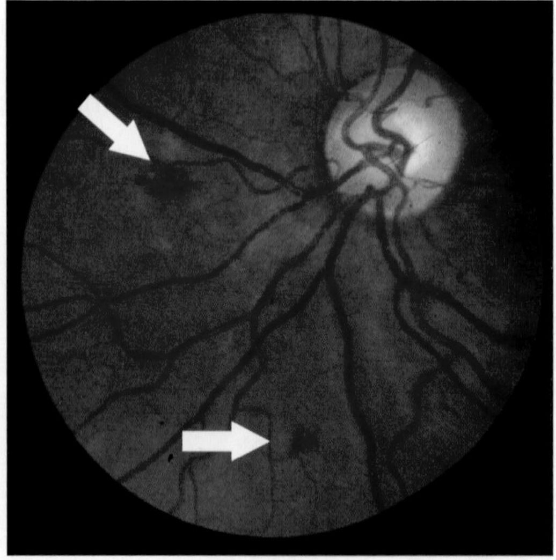

Figure 22.4 (A) Bulbar conjunctival petechial haemorrhage and (B) Roth spots (arrows) in streptococcal endocarditis. Fundoscopy of the left eye. Both reproduced, with permission, from Gahl K (ed.). *Infektiöse Endokarditis*, 2nd edn.,1994. Darmstadt: Steinkopff.

microscopic) and proteinuria, and particularly red blood cell casts are present. However, the most important laboratory test is unquestionably the blood culture.

Infective endocarditis usually leads to a continuous bacteraemia, such that (in the absence of pre-treatment with antibiotics) blood cultures are very sensitive to detect the disease and may be drawn at any time independent from the time course of fever. It has been reported that one of the first two separate blood cultures was positive in 98% of patients with infective bacterial endocarditis in patients not receiving antibiotics [12]. For proper technique, see ➲Table 22.5. However, if the patient is already treated with antibiotics the diagnostic yield decreases drastically. Furthermore, some pathogens are fastidious or don't grow at all on usual culture media, necessitating a close cooperation with the microbiologist in such cases. ➲Table 22.6 provides a list of difficult-to-identify pathogens and techniques to identify them.

Table 22.5 Properly obtaining blood cultures in suspected endocarditis

Three separate sets from three different venepunctures over 24 hours, at least 1 hour apart
If possible before antibiotic therapy or after cessation of antibiotic therapy (3–7 days, depending on previous therapy duration)
Each set contains one aerobic and one anaerobic flask, to each of which 5–(preferably)10mL blood are added
Rapid processing or storage at appropriate temperature (check with laboratory); notify laboratory of the clinical suspicion of infective endocarditis

Table 22.6 Culture-negative endocarditis: difficult-to-identify pathogens and tests to detect them

Coxiella burnetii (Q fever): serology or PCR
Bartonella spp.: acridine orange staining of blood cultures, extended subculturing, serology, PCR
Brucella spp.: serology, PCR
Legionella spp.: serology, PCR
Fungi other than *Candida* spp.: lysis-centrifugation and culturing on special fungal media
'HACEK' pathogens (*Haemophilus, Actinobacillus, Cardiobacterium, Eikenella, Kingella* spp.): prolonged culturing

PCR, polymerase chain reaction.

Pathogens can, and should, also be cultured or identified by PCR from excised material, e.g. valves or emboli, especially if blood cultures remain negative, to guide appropriate antibiotic therapy, in particular after surgery. This technique may also identify specific pathogenic strains and thus elucidate their source [13–15].

Diagnosis

The definitive diagnosis of endocarditis rests on two pillars: the positive blood culture and evidence of vegetations, usually by echocardiography. ➲Table 22.7 lays out the accepted criteria for the diagnosis of infective endocarditis, the so-called Duke criteria [16]. These criteria are helpful for epidemiology and standardization of diagnosis but may not be sufficient to make management decisions or to confirm or reject the diagnosis in unclear cases. Echocardiography is the imaging technique of choice and its findings are pivotal for patient management. Transoesophageal echocardiography has a well-documented superior sensitivity to transthoracic echo to diagnose endocarditic vegetations, destructive complications, and abscesses [17–21]. Whenever there is a strong clinical suspicion of endocarditis and the transthoracic echo is inconclusive or negative, transoesophageal echocardiography should be performed. Conversely, a negative transoesophageal echo argues strongly against infective endocarditis. However, if the clinical suspicion is substantial (e.g. positive blood cultures of a typical pathogen), transoesophageal echocardiography should be repeated after a few days, in particular in the presence of underlying heart disease, e.g. a prosthetic heart valve. It has been shown that repeat negative transoesophageal echocardiography carries a very high negative predictive value for infective endocarditis and may be the clinical 'gold standard' for excluding infective endocarditis [22]. Because of the increasing frequency of 1) antibiotic pre-treatment, leading to false negative blood cultures, and 2) prosthetic valve endocarditis, with its attendant difficulty of visualization of vegetations, it has been proposed to modify the Duke criteria to include patients with clear vegetations on echo and systemic inflammatory signs, but negative blood cultures, if they have had antibiotic pre-treatment, and to require a repeat negative transoesophageal echo study to exclude endocarditis in patients with prosthetic valves. Furthermore, Q fever endocarditis should be routinely ruled out serologically, since blood cultures remain negative in this disease [23].

Table 22.7 The 'Duke criteria' [16] for the diagnosis of infective endocarditis

'Definite' diagnosis—established by:
Pathology (histologic evidence of active endocarditis in an endocarditic lesion or identification of microorganisms in a vegetation or abscess), *or*
Clinically:
two major
or
one major + three minor
or
five minor criteria
Major criteria:
Positive blood culture (>one) of typical pathogens
Vegetation, abscess, or prosthesis dehiscence on echo
New valvular regurgitation
Minor criteria:
Predisposition (predisposing heart disease or intravenous drug use), fever ≥38°C, embolic events, immunologic/embolic signs (conjunctival haemorrhages, Janeway lesions*, Osler nodes*, Roth spots, glomerulonephritis, rheumatoid factor), serology consistent with endocarditis, positive blood culture which is not typical for infective endocarditis
Possible diagnosis
Neither definite nor rejected
Rejected diagnosis
Firm alternative diagnosis for symptoms suggestive of endocarditis, resolution of symptoms after <4 days of antibiotic treatment, no pathologic evidence of endocarditis during surgery or autopsy.

*For definition, see ➲Table 22.4.

Echocardiographic signs of infective endocarditis

Conceptually, these can be divided into additional structures due to the disease (vegetation, abscess, pseudoaneurysm)

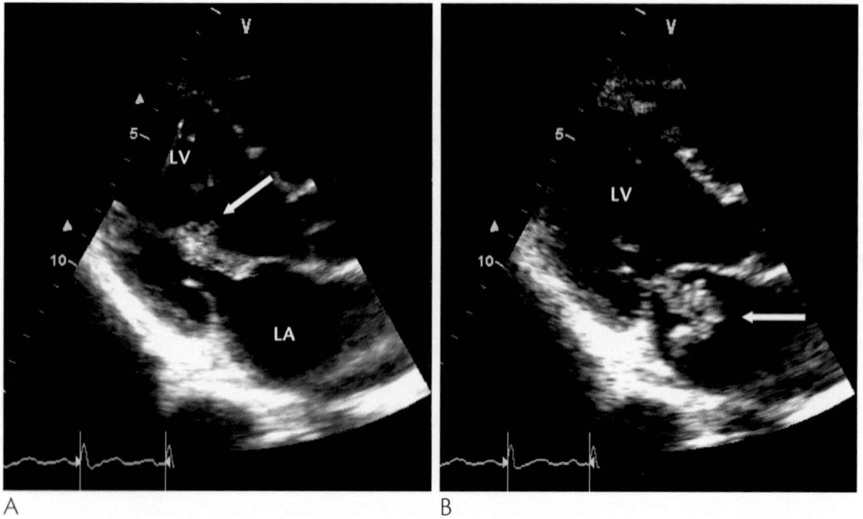

Figure 22.5 Large, mobile vegetation on the mitral valve. The vegetation is in the left ventricle (LV) during diastole (A) and prolapses into the left atrium (LA) in systole (B). There was also severe mitral regurgitation. Also see 🎥 22.1 and 22.2.

and defects (regurgitant lesions, perforations, fistulae). The hallmark of endocarditis on echo is the identification of a vegetation, appearing as a mobile, irregular mass with jagged edges attached to a valvular structure (➲Figs. 22.5–22.8; 🎥 22.1 and 22.2). Size may vary from few millimetres to several centimetres. Vegetations typically arise from the low-pressure side of a valve leaflet (e.g. the atrial side of the mitral valve) and are highly mobile. They may prolapse through the valve with the blood flow. Their echodensity is relatively low (similar to myocardium) in the early stages and increases over time. Highly echogenic, 'fibrous' or 'calcified' vegetations usually indicate that the vegetation is old, with lower embolic risk. If vegetations are large, in rare cases obstruction may occur.

Typically, endocarditis causes valvular regurgitation by several mechanisms: defects in the valvular tissue, rupture of chordae, and interposition of vegetations between the leaflet tips. Valvular regurgitation due to endocarditis is very frequent and often severe and dramatic (🎥 22.3). All typical echocardiographic signs of acute severe mitral or aortic regurgitation may be present. Endocarditis may progress to invasion of the tissue with central necrotization, i.e. abscess formation. This is typical of aortic and prosthetic endocarditis and aggressive pathogens such as staphylococci. On echocardiography, abscesses are perivalvular zones of abnormal tissue thickening, sometimes with central echolucency and possible flow in and out of an abscess cavity (➲Figs. 22.9 and 22.10; 🎥 22.6–22.8). They are recognized better and much more frequently by transoesophageal echocardiography [19]; recognition is important because formation of an abscess not rarely predicts failure of conservative antibiotic treatment. A special form of abscess is the mitral valve pseudoaneurysm (➲Fig. 22.11), a localized outpouching of a mitral leaflet or the intervalvular fibrous tissue between aortic and mitral valve, often with a perforation and regurgitation [6].

Other imaging modalities, such as magnetic resonance imaging, multidetector computed tomography (CT), or

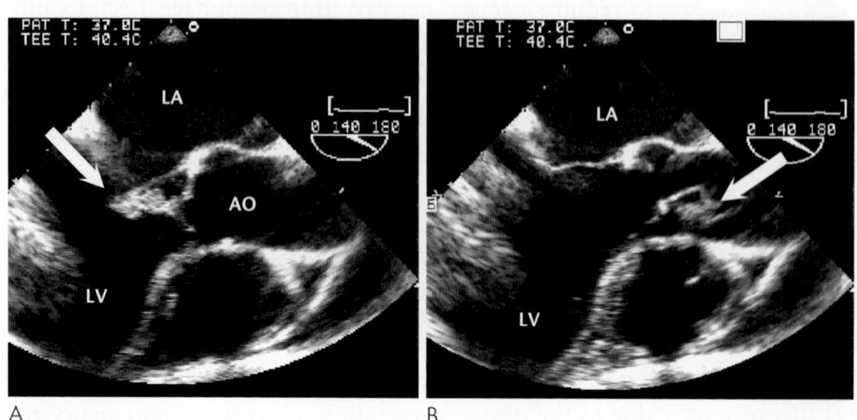

Figure 22.6 Long, mobile vegetation (arrows) attached to the right coronary cusp of the aortic valve. Transoesophageal long-axis views of the aortic valve in diastole (A), with the vegetation prolapsing into the left ventricular (LV) outflow tract, and in systole (B), with the vegetation in the aortic root (AO). Transoesophageal echocardiogram.

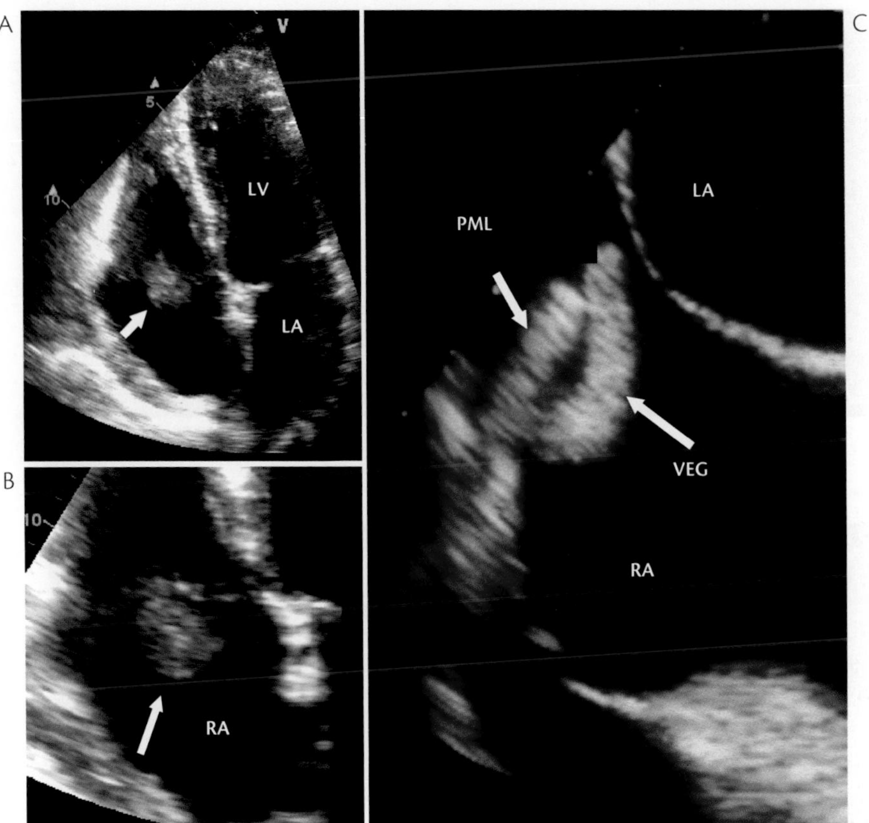

Figure 22.7 Vegetation (VEG, arrows) attached to the atrial site of the tricuspid valve (A, B) and to a pacemaker lead (C, transoesophageal echocardiogram). Both patients had infective staphylococcal endocarditis. LA, RA, left and right atrium; LV, left ventricle; PML, pacemaker lead. Also see 22.9 and 22.10.

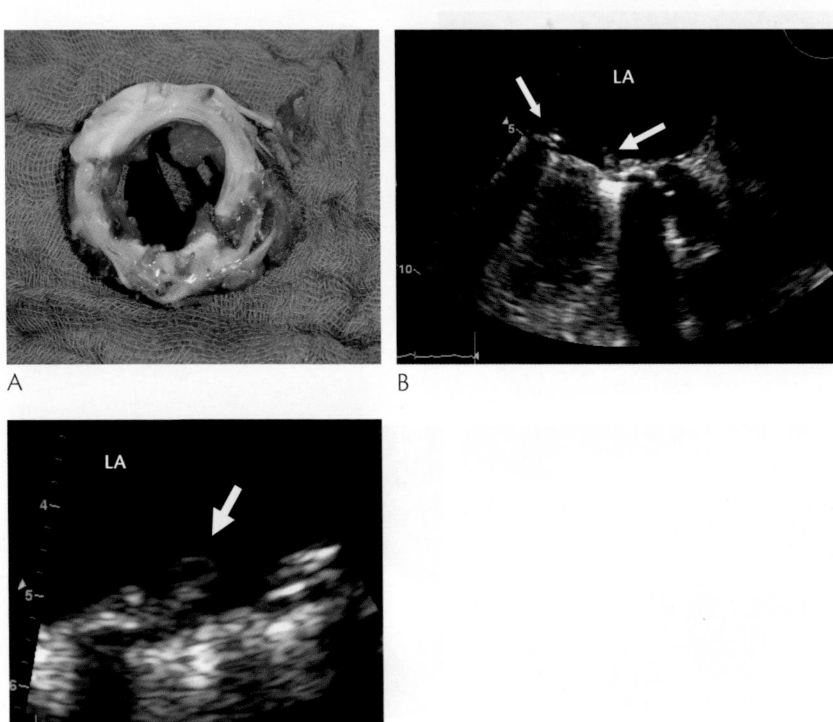

Figure 22.8 (A) Explanted bileaflet mechanical mitral valve prosthesis showing large vegetations due to staphylococcal infection (courtesy of Prof. Dr. M. Weyand, Department of Heart Surgery, University Clinic Erlangen). (B) and (C) Vegetations (arrows) are clearly visualized on the transoesophageal echocardiogram. LA, left atrium. Also see 22.11 and 22.12.

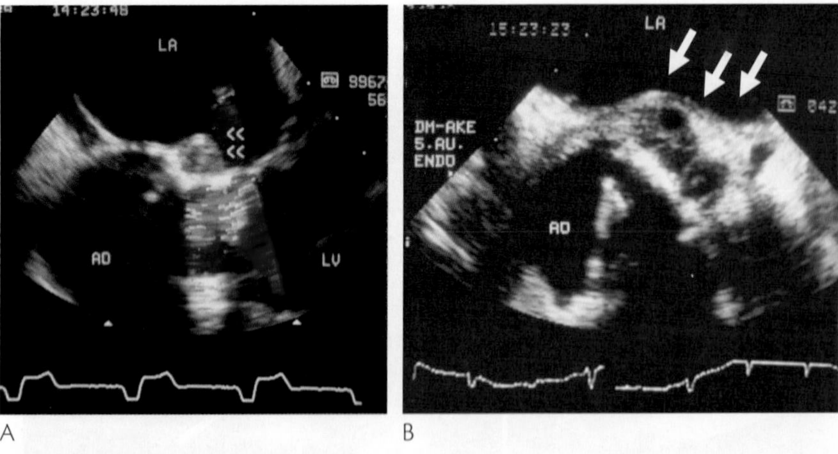

Figure 22.9 (A) Small abscess region (arrows) attached to the ascending aorta at the connection to the anterior mitral valve leaflet in a patient with mitral and aortic valve endocarditis. (B) Large abscess area (arrows) at the posterior ascending aorta in a patient with *Staphylococcus aureus* infection of a mechanical prosthetic valve in aortic position. Both images are transoesophageal echocardiographic views. AO, ascending aorta; LA, left atrium; LV, left ventricle.

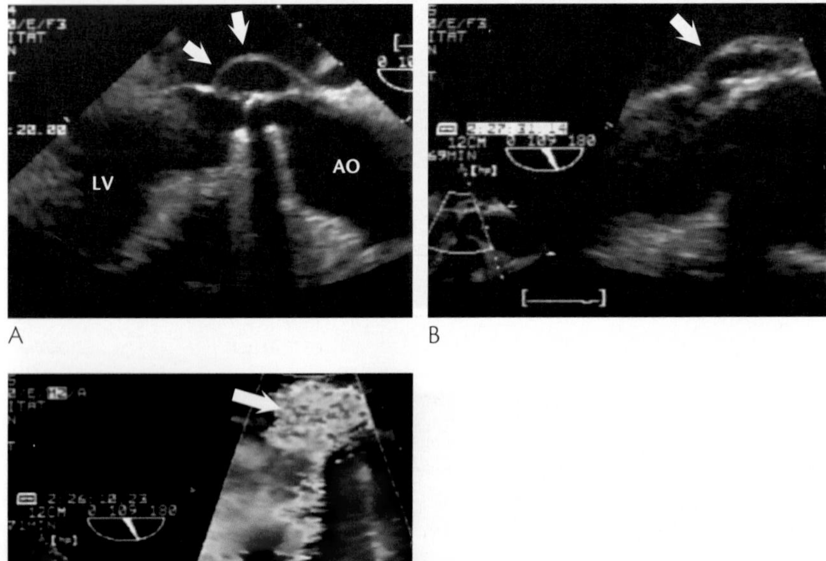

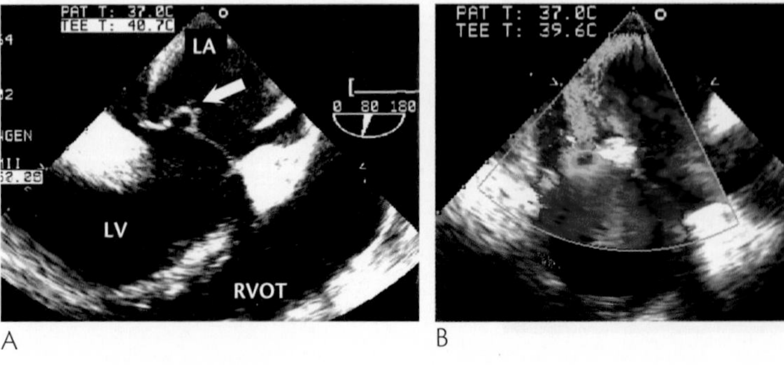

Figure 22.10 Para-aortic abscess cavity in the presence of an aortic valve prosthesis. (A) Transoesophageal long-axis view of the aortic valve. The arrows point at the abscess cavity. (B) Close-up of (A), with visible entry (arrow) into the abscess cavity from the left ventricular (LV) outflow tract. (C) During systole, the cavity fills with turbulent flow (colour Doppler; arrow). AO, ascending aorta.

Figure 22.11 (A) Streptococcal endocarditis with pseudoaneurysm of the anterior mitral leaflet with two small attached vegetations (arrow). The patient had also severe mitral regurgitation, as evidenced by colour Doppler (B). RVOT, right ventricular outflow tract.

scintigraphy with radioactively labelled leucocytes, are currently inferior in diagnosing infective endocarditis, when compared to echocardiography.

Problems in the diagnosis of infective endocarditis

The widespread use of antibiotics in the presence of signs of systemic inflammation, e.g. fever, often without a clear diagnosis of the type of infection, greatly impairs the sensitivity of blood cultures. In one large registry [11], at least 23% of patients were treated with antibiotics before blood cultures were obtained, and without recognizing endocarditis as the underlying disease. Thus, one is often left with a clinical picture compatible with infective endocarditis, but negative blood cultures. This situation would not qualify as 'definite endocarditis' applying the Duke criteria strictly, and a corresponding modification of the Duke criteria has been advocated, as outlined earlier [23]. There is now consensus that if in the presence of systemic inflammatory signs clear-cut echocardiographic evidence of fresh vegetations or abscess can be obtained, these patients should be managed as having acute infective endocarditis. However, the situation remains problematic if morphologic evidence is less clear, e.g. in the presence of degenerative valvular changes, in prosthetic valves, or pacemaker leads without unequivocal vegetations, or if old endocarditic changes are present. In these cases, often the course of the disease and changes in valve appearance over time have to be awaited in order to make a clear diagnostic decision.

Prosthetic valve endocarditis

Infective endocarditis in a patient with a prosthetic valve is conceptually classified into early endocarditis, which is perceived as nosocomial disease originating in the surgical valve replacement, occurring up to 1 year after surgery, and late (usually community-acquired) prosthetic valve endocarditis. The risk is highest in the first weeks and months after surgery, and mortality in early prosthetic endocarditis has been reported to be extremely high. While the absolute number of patients with prosthetic valves is increasing, the relative incidence of prosthetic endocarditis has declined in recent years and is now well under 0.5% per year for late prosthetic endocarditis [24]. Early prosthetic endocarditis is characterized by preponderance of *Staphylococcus epidermidis* as a causative agent, while the pathogens of late endocarditis are similar to native valve endocarditis. Prosthetic endocarditis tends to be more severe than native valve endocarditis, is difficult to diagnose due to echocardiographic imaging problems with prostheses (22.4 and 22.5), and almost always necessitates repeat surgery [25, 26]. In staphylococcal prosthetic valve endocarditis, mortality has been reported to be 75% (!) with medical treatment and still 25% with surgical treatment [27]. In mechanical prostheses, the disease is almost exclusively located along the sewing ring of the prosthesis, creating paravalvular leaks, fistulae, and abscesses, while in bioprostheses both the ring and the leaflets may be colonized by bacteria. Transoesophageal examination is extremely useful and should always be performed.

Infective endocarditis in addicts of intravenous drugs

Several features set this type of infective endocarditis apart from the general picture. Infections are often mixed, involving *Staphylococcus aureus* in >50%, and predominantly affect the tricuspid valve (because of the venous entry site of the infection). The majority of patients are HIV infected or otherwise immunocompromised, but mostly have no underlying heart disease. The prognosis of tricuspid endocarditis of intravenous drug addicts is relatively good under conservative treatment, but recurrence is common due to patients' lifestyles.

Therapy

Antibiotic treatment is mandatory and should be instituted immediately by intravenous route after a sufficient number of blood cultures have been taken (see Table 22.5) and the diagnosis is clear or probable. Susceptibility testing should always be obtained if a pathogen is identified. Vancomycin and aminoglycoside therapy may be optimized by drug serum level determinations. Table 22.8 lists typical antibiotic regimens for different clinical situations and causative agents. Duration of therapy is somewhat arbitrary and should be guided by the course of the disease, but 4 weeks of intravenous therapy are a usually considered the minimum. Response to treatment is best monitored by clinical status, in particular course of fever, and by C-reactive protein. C-reactive protein and leucocyte count should fall rapidly and may remain slightly, but not markedly, elevated if the patient responds to therapy [1].

Table 22.8 Antibiotic therapy of infective endocarditis

I Native valve endocarditis due to penicillin-sensitive streptococci
Penicillin G IV 3–6 million units every 6 hours for 4 weeks
+ gentamicin IV 1mg/kg every 8 hours over 2 weeks
II Empirical therapy of culture-negative native valve endocarditis
Vancomycin IV 15mg/kg every 12 hours over 4–6 weeks
+ gentamicin IV 1mg/kg every 8 hours over 2 weeks; some recommendations add IV ampicillin or amoxycillin to this regimen
Empirical therapy of culture-negative prosthetic valve endocarditis:
As in I + rifampicin PO 300–450mg every 8 hours over 4–6 weeks
III Staphylococcal native valve endocarditis
If methicillin-susceptible:
Oxacillin IV 2–3g every 6 hours over 4 weeks
+ gentamicin IV 1mg/kg every 8 hours over 3–5 days
If methicillin-resistant:
Vancomycin IV 15mg/kg every 12 hours over 6 weeks
IV Staphylococcal prosthetic valve endocarditis
If methicillin-susceptible:
Oxacillin IV 2–3g every 6 hours over 6 weeks
+ gentamicin IV 1mg/kg every 8 hours over 2 weeks
+ rifampicin IV 300mg every 8 hours, over 6 weeks
If methicillin-resistant:
Vancomycin IV 15mg/kg every 12 hours over 6 weeks
+ gentamicin IV 1mg/kg every 8 hours over 6 weeks
+ rifampicin IV 300mg every 8 hours over 6 weeks

IV, intravenous

Note that in prosthetic valve endocarditis, surgery is recommended. Vancomycin may be replaced by teicoplanin.

Modified with permission from the ESC recommendations where further regimens for special clinical situations may be looked up: Horstkotte D, Follath F, Gutschik E, *et al.* Guidelines on prevention, diagnosis and treatment of infective endocarditis executive summary; the task force on infective endocarditis of the European society of cardiology. *Eur Heart J* 2004; **25**: 267–76.

Echo follow-up examinations are important for later comparisons and detection of complications.

Indications, timing, and type of surgery

Traditionally, infective endocarditis has been seen as a disease amenable to antibiotic therapy, which in case of complications necessitated surgery. The typical complications were heart failure due to severe acute regurgitation or sepsis, and systemic embolism. This view was supported by the frequency of streptococcal endocarditis of native valves with its relatively protracted, subacute course; indeed, this led to the term 'endocarditis lenta', or slow endocarditis. This type of endocarditis responds relatively well to penicillin therapy. Unfortunately, today the physician often confronts more aggressive infections, in particular staphylococcal endocarditis, and often the disease arises in immunocompromised patients or patients with implanted devices, such as prosthetic valves, pacemaker electrodes, central venous lines, port access lines, etc. Moreover, the focus of attention has shifted to prevent, rather than treat, catastrophic complications such as embolism and valvular destruction. Thus, in referral centres nowadays surgery is used earlier and much more frequently than previously [28–32]. ➲Table 22.9 lists accepted indications for surgery in infective endocarditis. Although the decision must always be individualized, indications for surgery include heart failure from valvular dysfunction, a high risk of embolism (large mobile vegetations), presence of an abscess, and treatment-resistant sepsis. Prosthetic valve endocarditis is usually an indication for surgery, especially in the presence of prosthetic malfunction and in the first year after valve replacement, but sometimes late bioprosthetic endocarditis can be managed conservatively. The most difficult problem in the decision to proceed to surgery revolves around preventing embolism or recurrence of embolism. While it is generally accepted that large (usually defined as >10mm) mobile vegetations pose a grave embolic threat and should therefore be removed surgically as soon as possible [33–36], there are conflicting data on how to treat smaller vegetations. Particularly difficult clinical decisions have to be made after a cerebral embolic event. Several retrospective analyses have suggested that immediate operation on cardiopulmonary bypass with its profound anticoagulation entails a substantial risk of haemorrhagic transformation of an embolic insult and subsequent aggravation of neurological damage [37]. Traditionally, therefore, an interval of 2–3 weeks after a cerebral embolism has been recommended before surgery. However, recently there has been some support for early operation (within 72 hours) after an embolic insult if no haemorrhage is detectable on cerebral CT [1, 38]. Because of the critical importance of

Table 22.9 Indications for surgery in infective endocarditis

Congestive heart failure due to valvular regurgitation
Untreatable sepsis, ineffective antibiotic therapy (e.g. in fungi)
Large (>10mm maximal diameter) mobile vegetation or recurrent embolism
Endocarditic abscess or other evidence of local tissue invasion, e.g. fistula
Involvement of a valve prosthesis (especially within 12 months after valve replacement or in the presence of prosthetic malfunction), or other foreign body

cerebral embolism in the decision for surgery, it is advisable to obtain a preoperative cerebral CT in all patients undergoing surgery for endocarditis. If concomitant coronary artery disease is suspected, coronary angiography may be performed, but should not delay surgery for endocarditis; in the presence of mobile aortic vegetations, coronary angiography should be withheld. Non-invasive coronary angiography by multidetector CT has become an acceptable alternative in these patients. Surgically, it is usually necessary to replace the valve if disease is extensive or destruction has occurred. Operation may become even more extensive if surrounding tissue is affected, e.g. in the case of aortic abscess. In some cases, valve repair or vegectomy (removal of vegetations leaving the valve intact) suffices [38, 40, 41]. Valve replacement may be done with any kind of prosthetic valves, although some authors have found homografts to be particularly successful [42].

Anticoagulation

It has been hypothesized that anticoagulatory or antiaggregatory drugs might be beneficial in reducing the growth of vegetations [43]. However, there is no clinical evidence for such measures, and anticoagulation may even be hazardous in view of the potential for haemorrhagic complications after cerebral embolization. Thus, anticoagulation or aspirin in the setting of infective endocarditis is not recommended, unless there is a compelling independent reason for anticoagulation (e.g. a mechanical prosthetic valve) [44].

Prognosis

In spite of antibiotic and surgical therapy, infective endocarditis is not a easily treatable disease. Mortality in large series ranges between 15–20% [5, 11]. Mortality is highest in staphylococcal and fungal endocarditis, and in (especially early) prosthetic endocarditis. The disease also entails a tremendous morbidity from neurologic events and from valvular damage. It is estimated that approximately 30–50% of patients with endocarditis undergo early heart surgery [5, 11], and many sustain a permanent neurologic damage.

Prophylaxis and prevention

The concept of antibiotic prophylaxis is to abolish or mitigate bacteraemia arising predictably from certain procedures in patients who are considered at risk for infective endocarditis by administering one or two properly timed doses of antibiotics. In 2007, the American Heart Association (AHA) has issued new recommendations that were innovative, clear, simple, and associated with a major departure from previous guidelines used for many years [8]. Initial steps into a similar direction had been suggested by the French recommendations in 2002 [45, 46] and by the British Society for Antimicrobial Chemotherapy recommendations in 2006 [47]. The AHA recommendations may be summarized in the following three points:

- Endocarditis prophylaxis is only recommended in high-risk patients. Importantly, high-risk patients here are defined not primarily on the basis of an increased risk to develop endocarditis, but rather on the risk of a particularly severe morbid outcome in case they really develop endocarditis. This group includes patients with 1) prosthetic cardiac valve; 2) previous infective endocarditis; 3) complex congenital heart disease; and 4) valuvulopathy following cardiac transplantation (details given in ➲Table 22.10).
- Endocarditis prophylaxis prior to dental procedures is only recommended if they involve manipulations in gingival tissue or the periapical region of the teeth or perforation of the oral mucosa. Nevertheless, oral hygiene is considered of critical importance to reduce the risk of endocarditis. Prophylaxis is reasonable for patients who undergo an invasive procedure of the respiratory tract that involves incision or biopsy, such as tonsillectomy or adenoidectomy.

Table 22.10 Cardiac conditions associated with the highest risk of adverse outcomes from endocarditis for which prophylaxis with dental procedures is reasonable

Condition
Prosthetic cardiac valve or prosthetic material used for cardiac valve repair
Previous infective endocarditis
Congenital heart disease (CHD)
Unrepaired cyanotic CHD, including palliative shunts and conduits
Complex repaired congenital heart defect with prosthetic material or device, either placed by surgery or by catheter intervention, during the first 6 months after the procedure*
Repaired CHD with residual defects at the site or adjacent to the site of a prosthetic patch or prosthetic device (which inhibit endothelialization)
Cardiac transplant recipients who develop cardiac valvulopathy

* Endothelialization of prosthetic material occurs within 6 months after the procedure.

Modified from Wilson W, Taubert KA, Gewitz M, *et al.* Prevention of infective endocarditis: guidelines from the American Heart Association: a guideline from the American Heart Association Rheumatic Fever, Endocarditis, and Kawasaki Disease Committee, Council on Cardiovascular Disease in the Young, and the Council on Clinical Cardiology, Council on Cardiovascular Surgery and Anesthesia, and the Quality of Care and Outcomes Research Interdisciplinary Working Group. *Circulation* 2007; **116**: 1736–54. Source: American Heart Association.

- Endocarditis prophylaxis is no longer recommended prior to gastrointestinal or genitourinary procedures.

Primary reasons leading the committee to revise earlier recommendations [48] and issue the 2007 version of the AHA guidelines for infective endocarditis prophylaxis were [8]:

- Infective endocarditis is much more likely to result from frequent exposure to bacteraemias associated with daily activities (e.g. tooth brushing) than from bacteraemia caused by a single dental, gastrointestinal, or genitourinary tract procedure.
- Prophylaxis may prevent only an exceedingly small number of cases of infective endocarditis, if any, in individuals who undergo a dental, gastrointestinal, or genitourinary tract procedure.
- The risk of antibiotic-associated adverse events exceeds the benefit, if any, from prophylactic antibiotic therapy.
- Maintenance of optimal oral health and hygiene may reduce the incidence of bacteraemia from daily activities and is more important than prophylactic antibiotics for a dental procedure to reduce the risk of endocarditis.

Furthermore, over the years AHA guidelines (as well as those of other nations) on endocarditis prophylaxis had become overly complicated, hampering their application by physicians and patients. And finally, previous guidelines and recommendations were based primarily on expert opinion and a few case–control and descriptive studies. There has not been a single controlled, randomized study that evaluated the concept of preventing infective endocarditis by antimicrobial prophylaxis administered prior to dental, gastrointestinal, or genitourinary tract procedures. Based on currently used evidence criteria for guidelines and recommendations, previous endocarditis prophylaxis recommendations would belong to Class IIb (i.e. usefulness/efficacy is less well-established by evidence/opinion) with a Level of Evidence C (only consensus opinion of experts, case studies, or standard of care) [8].

Current recommendations of the AHA for chemoprophylaxis of infective endocarditis in adults are listed in ➲Table 22.11.

Table 22.11 Regimens for prophylaxis against endocarditis recommended by the AHA for adults

Situation	Agent	Single dose for adults 30–60min before procedure
Standard oral	Amoxicillin	2g
Unable to take oral medication	Amoxicillin or cefazolin or ceftriaxone	2g IM or IV 1g IM or IV
Allergic to penicillins or ampicillin—oral	Cephalexin*† *or* clindamycin *or* azithromycin *or* clarithromycin	2g 600mg 500mg
Allergic to penicillins or ampicillin, and unable to take oral medication	Cefazolin or ceftriaxone† *or* clindamycin	1g IM or IV 600mg IM or IV

IM, intramuscular; IV, intravenous.

* Or other first- or second-generation oral cephalosporin in equivalent adult dosage.

† Cephalosporins should not be used in an individual with a history of anaphylaxis, angio-oedema, or urticaria with penicillins or ampicillin

Modified from Wilson W, Taubert KA, Gewitz M, *et al.* Prevention of infective endocarditis: guidelines from the American Heart Association: a guideline from the American Heart Association Rheumatic Fever, Endocarditis, and Kawasaki Disease Committee, Council on Cardiovascular Disease in the Young, and the Council on Clinical Cardiology, Council on Cardiovascular Surgery and Anesthesia, and the Quality of Care and Outcomes Research Interdisciplinary Working Group. *Circulation* 2007; **116**: 1736–54. Source: American Heart Association.

The AHA guidelines for prevention of infective endocarditis have caused considerable concern among physicians and dentists. There is uncertainty if patients might be exposed to a larger risk of acquiring endocarditis by discarding previously accepted rules for endocarditis prophylaxis that also included patients at intermediate risk (e.g. patients with mitral valve proplapse and mitral insufficiency, with aortic regurgitation, etc.) and various non-dental procedures (e.g. genitourinary and gastrointestinal interventions). The ESC guidelines for prevention of infective endocarditis are currently under revision and will be published in 2009.

Personal perspective

Despite the substantial advances made in the past in diagnosis (e.g. transoesophageal echocardiography, PCR) and treatment (early surgery, new and better antibiotics) of infective endocarditis, its toll remains depressingly high. The wide spectrum of clinical symptoms, from fever of unexplained origin to stroke and to congestive heart failure implies that very often the physician first confronting the patient is not a cardiologist, and therefore the entire medical community must be better prepared to recognize the disease. To keep infective endocarditis in mind as a differential diagnosis in cases with unexplained fever or infection is the most important step in the diagnostic work-up of the disease. Furthermore, much would be gained if antibiotic therapy in unclear cases of serious infection was not instituted before blood cultures are drawn.

While improvements in diagnostic imaging and in therapy are likely to be rather incremental in the near future (e.g. three-dimensional ultrasound or even intracardiac imaging for better assessment of prostheses), the ability to rapidly detect and identify pathogens may improve dramatically by the use of molecular methods (e.g. PCR). In addition, recommendations for endocarditis prophylaxis are currently undergoing major changes, and it can be speculated that recent and upcoming guidelines will further simplify and improve the preventive management of patients who run a particularly high morbidity and mortality risk if they develop endocarditis after exposure to bacteraemia-associated interventions.

Finally, infective endocarditis will continue to be a field where a multidisciplinary approach with intensive, repeated, and close interaction between cardiologists, cardiac surgeons, and microbiologists is of the utmost importance for the patient's sake.

Further reading

Horstkotte D, Follath F, Gutschik E, *et al*. Guidelines on prevention, diagnosis and treatment of infective endocarditis executive summary; The Task Force on Infective Endocarditis of the European Society of Cardiology. *Eur Heart J* 2004; **25**: 267–76.

Moreillon P, Que YA. Infective endocarditis. *Lancet* 2004; **363**: 139–49.

Mylonakis E, Calderwood SB. Infective endocarditis in adults. *N Engl J Med* 2001; **345**: 1318–30.

Wilson W, Taubert KA, Gewitz M, *et al*. Prevention of infective endocarditis: guidelines from the American Heart Association: a guideline from the American Heart Association Rheumatic Fever, Endocarditis, and Kawasaki Disease Committee, Council on Cardiovascular Disease in the Young, and the Council on Clinical Cardiology, Council on Cardiovascular Surgery and Anesthesia, and the Quality of Care and Outcomes Research Interdisciplinary Working Group (erratum appears in *Circulation* 2007; **116**: e376–e377). *Circulation* 2007; **116**: 1736–54.

Additional online material

- 22.1 Large, mobile vegetation on the mitral valve.
- 22.2 A close-up of 22.1.
- 22.3 Bicuspid aortic valve and mitral valve endocarditis, with perforation of aortic leaflet.
- 22.4 Staphylococcal endocarditis of aortic bioprosthesis: transoesophageal short-axis view.
- 22.5 Same case as 22.4. Staphylococcal endocarditis of aortic bioprosthesis: transoesophageal long-axis view.
- 22.6 Enterococcal endocarditis of mechanical aortic valve prosthesis in the presence of a valved conduit.
- 22.7 Para-aortic abscess cavity in the presence of an aortic valve prosthesis.
- 22.8 Two-dimensional image of 22.7.
- 22.9 Vegetation attached to the atrial side of the tricuspid valve; staphylococcal endocarditis.
- 22.10 Close-up of 22.9.
- 22.11 Surgically confirmed staphylococcal vegetation on the atrial side of a mechanical mitral bileaflet prosthesis. Transoesophageal view.
- 22.12 Close-up of 22.11.

For full references and multimedia materials please visit the online version of the book (http://esctextbook.oxfordonline.com).

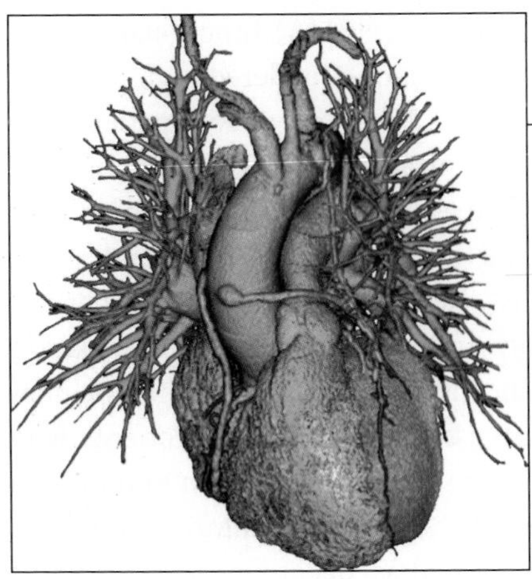

CHAPTER 23

Heart Failure

John McMurray, Mark Petrie, Karl Swedberg, Michel Komajda, Stefan Anker, and Roy Gardner

Contents

Summary

Although morbidity and mortality are improving, heart failure continues to present major challenges to healthcare systems. This affliction of mainly the elderly may be falling in incidence but is probably growing in prevalence, in part due to greater longevity resulting from evidence-based drug and device therapy for patients with a low ejection fraction (EF). New guidelines emphasize the combination of an angiotensin-converting enzyme inhibitor and beta-blocker as the cornerstone of therapy, with the addition of either an angiotensin receptor blocker or aldosterone antagonist as the third disease-modifying agent in patients who remain symptomatic. An implanted cardioverter defibrillator should also be added in patients with a persistently low EF and life expectancy of reasonable quality of ≥12 months. In patients in sinus rhythm, New York Heart Association class III–IV, and a QRS duration ≥120ms, cardiac resynchronization therapy has substantial additional morbidity and mortality benefits. This evidence-based care should be delivered through an organized and seamless multidisciplinary framework with a focus on the patients' and carers' needs. Apart from transplantation, the place of any other surgical intervention remains uncertain. Unfortunately the success of treatment in low EF heart failure has not been replicated in patients with heart failure and a preserved EF, and treatment of these patients remains empirical. The same is largely true for the treatment of patients with acute heart failure, with no treatment yet shown to be superior to empirical therapy with diuretic, oxygen, and nitrates. In particular the role of inotropes remains uncertain.

Introduction

Heart failure is the term used to describe a common clinical syndrome arising, in ways that are incompletely understood, as a consequence of reduced cardiac pump function. The term 'syndrome' merely describes a constellation of symptoms and signs and, therefore, heart failure is not a diagnosis as such. Unfortunately, the typical symptoms (breathlessness and fatigue) and signs (e.g. oedema) of heart failure are relatively non-specific, making clinical confirmation of the syndrome difficult. The syndrome of heart failure itself can arise as a result of almost any abnormality of the structure, mechanical function, or electrical activity of the heart, each of which may require quite different treatments, emphasizing the importance of appropriate investigation of patients with suspected heart failure.

Many of the typical clinical symptoms and signs of heart failure do not arise directly as a result of the cardiac abnormality but rather from secondary dysfunction of other organs and tissues, e.g. the kidneys, bone marrow, and muscles. These secondary consequences of pump failure are myriad and their causes are not fully elucidated. Dysfunction of tissues and organs remote from the heart cannot, however, be explained solely by reduced perfusion and it is generally believed that other systemic processes (e.g. neurohumoral activation) are involved. In other words, the pathophysiology of heart failure is complex and incompletely understood and, consequently, so is the pathophysiological basis of treatment. Although it has proved difficult to agree a simple definition of heart failure, a pragmatic approach has been advocated (➲Table 23.1) [1]. The terms used to describe different types of heart failure can also be confusing. Generally the term 'heart failure' is used to describe the symptomatic syndrome (graded according to the New York Heart Association (NYHA) functional classification), although a patient can be rendered asymptomatic with treatment (➲Table 23.2). In our view, a patient who has never exhibited the typical signs or symptoms of heart failure is better described as having asymptomatic left ventricular systolic dysfunction (or whatever the underlying cardiac abnormality is). Recently, however, the American College of Cardiology and American Heart Association have adopted a classification of heart failure that includes asymptomatic patients (➲Table 23.2) [2]. Patients who have had heart failure for some time are often said to have 'chronic heart failure'. If chronic heart failure deteriorates the patient may be described as 'decompensated' and this may happen suddenly, i.e. 'acutely', usually leading to hospital admission, an event of considerable prognostic importance [3]. New (*'de novo'*) heart failure may also present acutely, for example as a consequence of acute myocardial infarction (or in a subacute or acute on chronic fashion,

Table 23.1 Definition of heart failure

Heart failure is a clinical syndrome in which patients have the following features:
◆ **Symptoms typical of heart failure** (breathlessness at rest or on exercise, fatigue, tiredness, ankle swelling)
and
◆ **Signs typical of heart failure** (tachycardia, tachypnoea, pulmonary rales, pleural effusion, raised jugular venous pressure, peripheral oedema, hepatomegaly)
and
◆ **Objective evidence of a structural or functional abnormality of the heart at rest** (cardiomegaly, third heart sound, cardiac murmurs, abnormality on the echocardiogram, raised natriuretic peptide concentration)

Table 23.2 Classification of heart failure by symptoms relating to structural capacity (NYHA) or by structural abnormality (ACC/AHA)

NYHA functional classification	ACC/AHA stages of heart failure
Severity based on symptoms and physical activity	**Stage of heart failure based on structure and damage to heart muscle**
Class I No limitation of physical activity. Ordinary physical activity doses not cause undue fatigue, palpitation, or dyspnoea.	**Stage A** At high risk for developing heart failure. No identified structural or functional abnormality; no signs or symptoms.
Class II Slight limitation of physical activity. Comfortable at rest, but ordinary physical activity results in fatigue, palpitation, or dyspnoea.	**Stage B** Developed structural heart disease that is strongly associated with the development of heart failure, but without signs or symptoms.
Class III Marked limitation of physical activity. Comfortable at rest, but less than ordinary activity results in fatigue, palpitation, or dyspnoea.	**Stage C** Symptomatic heart failure associated with underlying structural heart disease
Class IV Unable to carry on any physical activity without discomfort. Symptoms at rest. If any physical activity is undertaken, discomfort is increased.	**Stage D** Advanced structural heart disease and marked symptoms of heart failure at rest despite maximal medical therapy.

ACC, American College of cardiology; AHA, American Heart Association; NYHA, New York Heart Association.

Adapted with permission from Dickstein K, Cohen-Solal A, Filippatos G, *et al.* ESC guidelines for the diagnosis and treatment of acute and chronic heart failure 2008: the Task Force for the diagnosis and treatment of acute and chronic heart failure 2008 of the European Society of Cardiology. Developed in collaboration with the Heart Failure Association of the ESC (HFA) and endorsed by the European Society of Intensive Care Medicine (ESICM). *Eur Heart J* 2008; **29**: 2388–442.

for example in a patient who has had asymptomatic cardiac dysfunction for an often indeterminate period) and may resolve (the patient may become 'compensated') or persist [1, 4]. 'Congestive heart failure' is a term still used commonly in the USA and may describe acute or chronic heart failure with evidence of congestion, i.e. sodium and water retention. Congestion, though not some symptoms of heart failure (e.g. fatigue), may resolve with diuretic treatment. Many or all of these terms may be accurately applied to the same patient at different times, depending on what stage of their illness they are in.

Epidemiology

The epidemiology of symptomatic heart failure in developed countries is well understood, especially in Europe (➲Fig. 23.1) [5–14]. Approximately 2% of the adult population has heart failure, although the syndrome mainly afflicts the elderly, affecting 6–10% of people over the age of 65 years [5–15]. In Europe and North America, the lifetime risk of developing heart failure is approximately one in five for a 40-year-old [16, 17]. The age-adjusted incidence of heart failure appears to have remained stable or even decreased over the past 20 years [18–20]. Prevalence is thought to be increasing, partly because survival is increasing [20, 21]. Approximately two in 1000 of the adult population are discharged from hospital with heart failure each year and heart failure accounts for about 5% of all medical and geriatric admissions and is the single most common cause of such admissions in those >65 years [22–31]. Age at admission (and at death) seems to be increasing, suggesting that preventive treatments, such as antihypertensives, and secondary prevention after myocardial infarction are delaying the development of heart failure [22–31]. Hospital discharges include patients developing heart failure suddenly, *de novo*, as a consequence of another cardiac event (usually myocardial infarction); patients presenting for the first time with decompensation of previously unrecognized cardiac dysfunction; and patients with established, chronic heart failure who have suffered worsening sufficiently severe to lead to hospital admission (though it is recognized that the 'threshold' for admission to hospital may vary substantially between countries). Some of these admissions are unavoidable, reflecting the progressive natural history of heart failure whereas others may be avoidable (e.g. as a result of non-adherence to treatment, failure of prompt recognition, and treatment of early decompensation) [32]. After years of steady increase, age-adjusted rates of admission for heart failure seem to have reached a plateau, or even decreased, in Europe and North America (➲Fig. 23.2) though absolute numbers of admissions continue to increase and heart failure is still an enormous burden on health services and a cost to society, accounting for approximately 2% of all healthcare spending [22–31, 33]. Hospital admissions account for the main part of this expenditure, typically about 70%. Even in primary care, heart failure accounts for more consultations than angina (➲Fig. 23.3), reflecting the limiting symptoms and reduction in well-being experienced by patients with heart failure [34]. Indeed, quality of life has, consistently, been shown to be reduced more by heart failure than by other chronic illnesses (➲Fig. 23.4) [35].

Heart failure is deadly as well as disabling. Community-based surveys indicate that 30–40% of patients die within 1 year of diagnosis and 60–70% die within 5 years, mainly

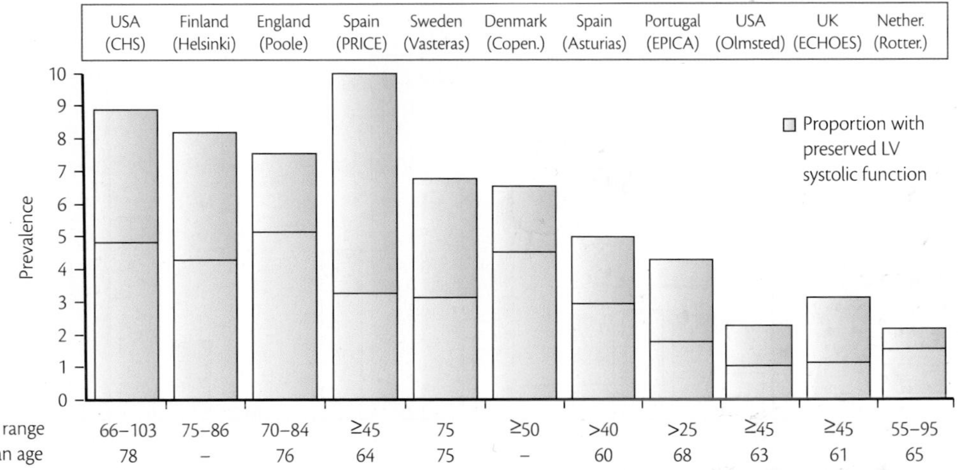

Figure 23.1 Prevalence of heart failure in cross-sectional population echocardiographic studies: proportion of subjects with preserved left ventricular systolic function. Adapted with permission from McMurray JJ, Pfeffer MA. Heart failure. *Lancet* 2005; **365**: 1877–89.

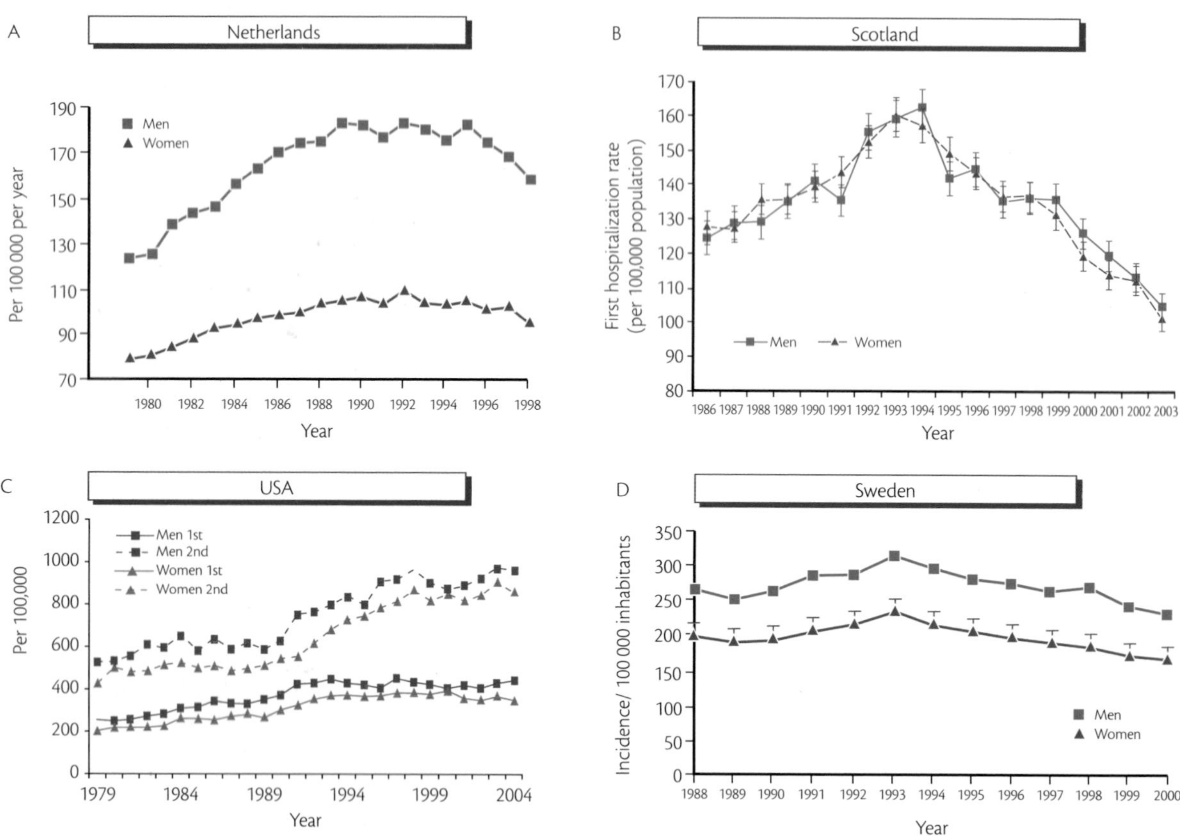

Figure 23.2 Trends in hospital admissions for heart failure demonstrating recent plateau or decline. (A) Age-adjusted discharge rate for heart failure in men and women. Reproduced with permission from Mosterd A, Reitsma JB, and Grobbee DE. Angiotensin converting enzyme inhibition and hospitalisation rates for heart failure in The Netherlands, 1980 to 1999: the end of an epidemic? *Heart* 2002; **87**: 75–6. (B) Age-adjusted trends in discharges for a first hospitalization for heart failure according to sex. Reproduced with permission from Jhund PS, Macintyre K, Simpson CR, *et al.* Long-term trends in first hospitalization for heart failure and subsequent survival between 1986 and 2003: a population study of 5.1 million people. *Circulation* 2009; **119**: 515–23. (C) Trends of age-adjusted hospitalization rates for heart failure (per 100,000) among patients with heart failure as the first listed or additional (second to seventh) diagnosis for men and women. Blue squares, men first; dotted blue squares, men second; red triangles, women first; dotted red triangles, women second. National Hospital Discharge Survey 1979–2004. Adapted with permission from Fang J, Mensah GA, Croft JB, *et al.* Heart failure-related hospitalization in the U.S., 1979 to 2004. *J Am Coll Cardiol* 2008; **52**: 428–34. (D) Age-adjusted annual incidence of first-ever hospitalization for heart failure as the principal diagnosis. Reproduced with permission from Schaufelberger M. *et al.* Decreasing one-year mortality and hospitalization rates for heart failure in Sweden. *Eur Heart J* 2004; **25**: 300–7.

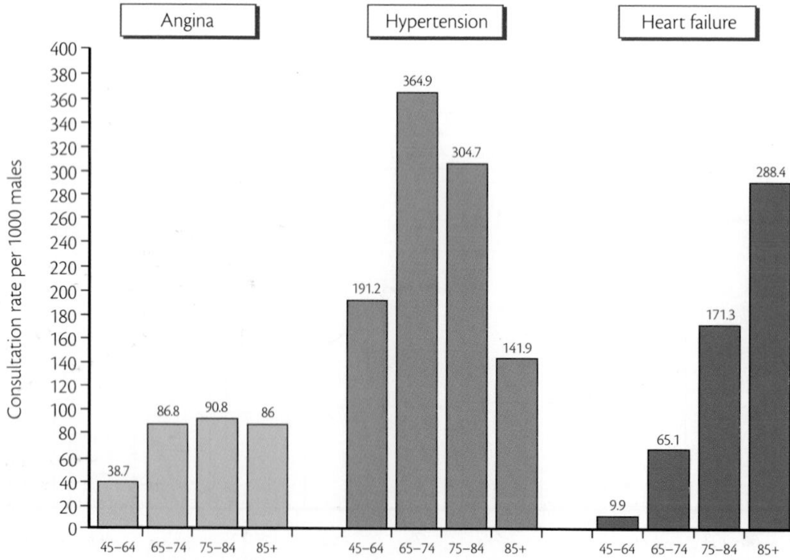

Figure 23.3 Age-stratified primary-care consultation rates per 1000 population for heart failure, angina and hypertension in men. Reproduced from Murphy NF, Simpson CR, McAlister FA, *et al.* National survey of the prevalence, incidence, primary care burden, and treatment of heart failure in Scotland. *Heart* 2004; **90**: 1129–36, with permission from BMJ Publishing Group Ltd.

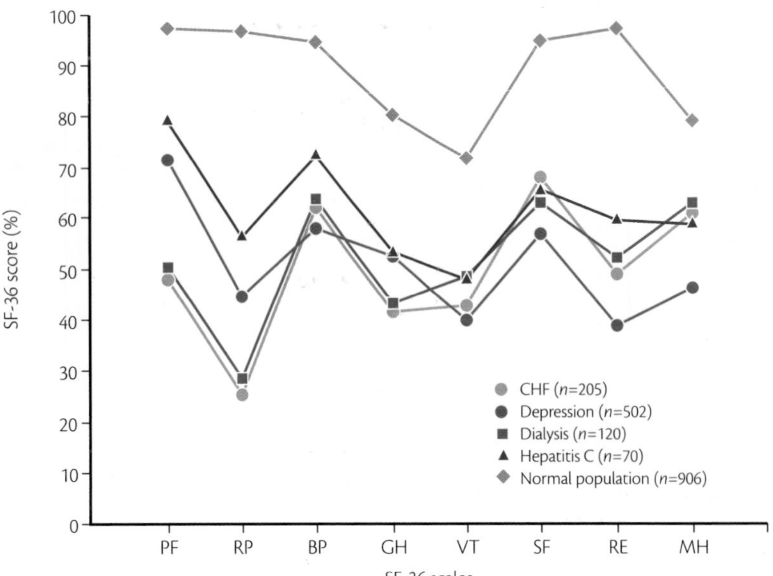

Figure 23.4 Quality of life in patients with congestive heart failure compared to other chronic illnesses and the normal population. The eight scales of the SF-36 short-form health survey instrument are physical functioning (PF), role limitations due to physical limitations (RP), bodily pain (BP), general health perceptions (GH), vitality (VT), social functioning (SF), role limitations caused by emotional problems (RE), and mental health (MH). A lower score equates to worse quality of life. Reproduced with permission from Juenger J, Schellberg D, Kraemer S, *et al.* Health related quality of life in patients with congestive heart failure: comparison with other chronic diseases and relation to functional variables. *Heart* 2002, **87**: 235–41.

from worsening heart failure or suddenly (probably because of a ventricular arrhythmia) [15, 17, 19, 36, 37]. Thus an adult living to age 40 has a one in five risk of developing heart failure and, once apparent, a one in three chance of dying within a year of diagnosis. Mortality is even higher in patients requiring hospital admission, exceeding that of most cancers (➲ Fig. 23.5), though a number of recent studies indicate that prognosis may be improving (➲ Fig. 23.6) [23–31, 38–43].

Left ventricular function has also been measured in a number of population-based echocardiographic studies, notably in Europe, enabling estimation of the prevalence of heart failure with a low and preserved EF, as well as the prevalence of asymptomatic left ventricular systolic and diastolic dysfunction (➲ Fig. 23.1) [44–54]. Synthesis of these epidemiological surveys suggests that approximately half of patients with symptomatic heart failure in the community have a low EF (and half have a preserved EF) [44]. The epidemiology of symptomatic heart failure with reduced EF differs from that of heart failure with preserved EF in that patients with preserved EF are, on average, older, are more often women, have more comorbidity, and have a better age-adjusted survival (➲ Fig. 23.7) [31–55]. The causes of heart failure in patients with preserved EF also differ from those with a low EF [31–55].

Because about half of patients with a low left ventricular EF are asymptomatic the argument has been made for screening for symptomless cases although no consensus

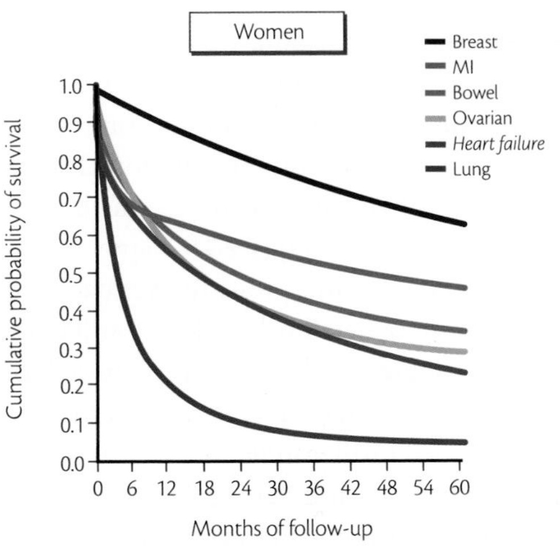

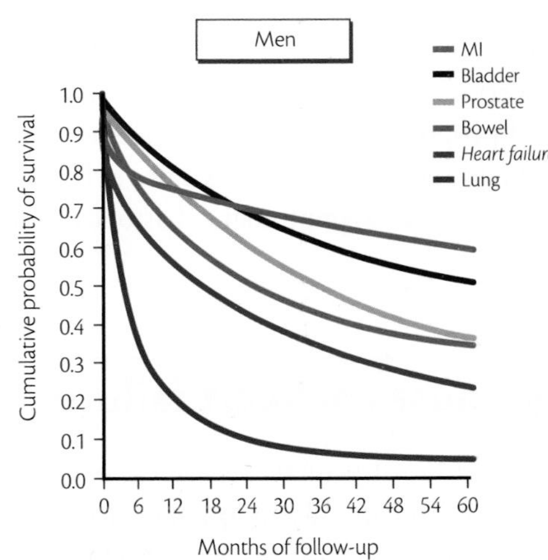

Figure 23.5 Five-year survival following a first admission to any Scottish hospital in 1991 for heart failure, myocardial infarction, and the four most common sites of cancer specific to men and women. Reproduced with permission from Stewart S, MacIntyre K, Hole DJ. More 'malignant' than cancer? Five-year survival following a first admission for heart failure. *Eur J Heart Fail* 2001; **3**: 315–22.

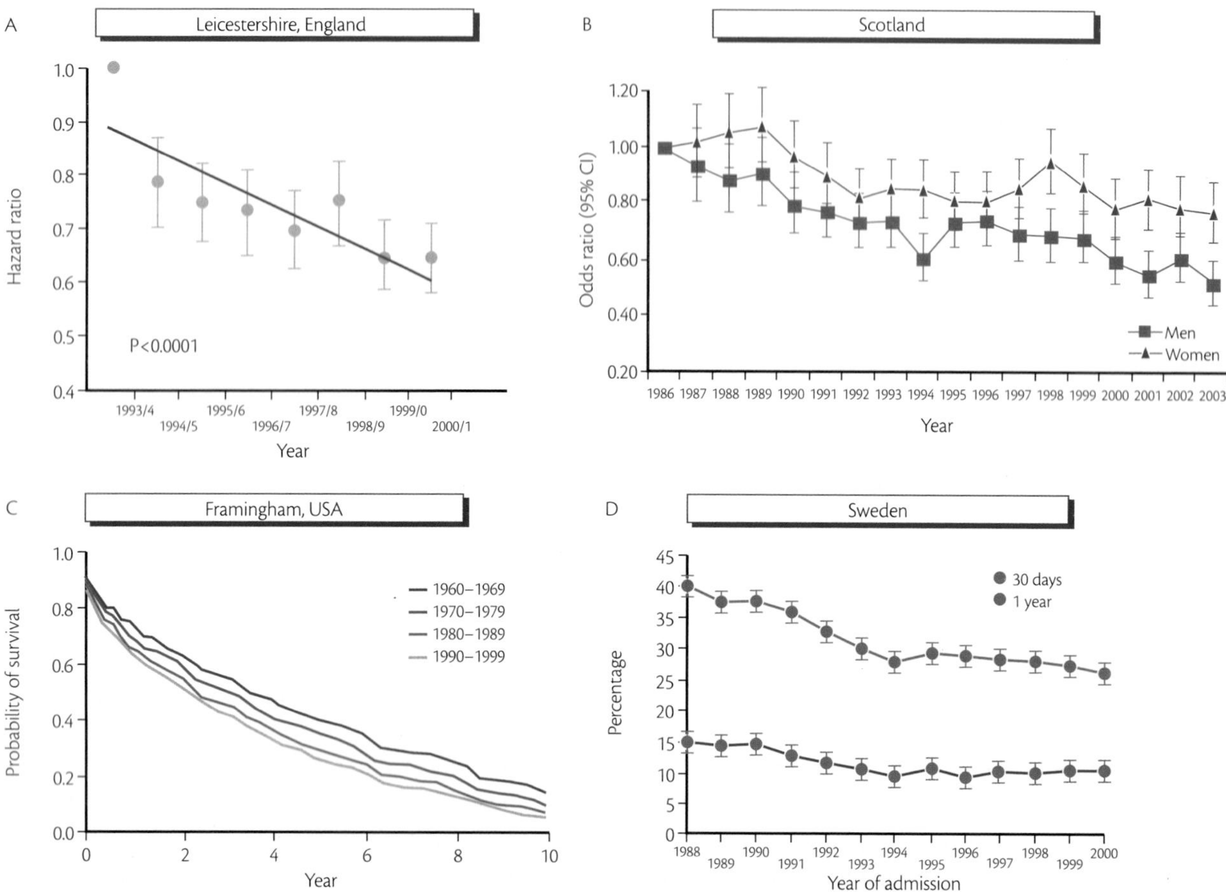

Figure 23.6 Evidence of improving survival from heart failure in the general population. (A) Hazard ratio and 95% confidence intervals for all-cause mortality in patients having a first admission for heart failure, according to year of admission (adjusted for age, gender, comorbidity, and social deprivation). Hazard ratio for first year of study (1993/1994) set at 1. Reproduced with permission from Blackledge HM, Tomlinson J, and Squire IB. Prognosis for patients newly admitted to hospital with heart failure: survival trends in 12,220 index admissions in Leicestershire 1993–2001. *Heart* 2003; **89**: 615–20. (B) Adjusted 30-day mortality according to sex and year of admission. Error bars represent 95% CIs. Reproduced with permission from Jhund PS, Macintyre K, Simpson CR, *et al.* Long-term trends in first hospitalization for heart failure and subsequent survival between 1986 and 2003: a population study of 5.1 million people. *Circulation* 2009; **119**: 515–23. Odds ratio for first year of period of study (1986) set at 1. (C) Age-adjusted survival after the onset of heart failure in men. Values were adjusted for age (< 55, 55 to 64, 65 to 74, 75 to 84, and ≥ 85 years). Estimates are shown for men who were 65 to 74 years of age. Similar trends were observed in women. Reproduced with permission from Levy, D *et al.* Long-term trends in the incidence of and survival with heart failure. *NEJM* 2002; **347**: 1397–1402. (D) Standardized 30-day and 1-year case fatality rates (%) for women with a first admission to hospital for heart failure. Reproduced with permission from Schaufelberger M, *et al.* Decreasing one-year mortality and hospitalization rates for heart failure in Sweden. *Eur Heart J* 2004; **25**: 300–7.

has been reached on this point [56, 57]. Recent studies have reported very disparate prevalence rates of diastolic dysfunction and proportions of symptomatic and asymptomatic individuals and no conclusions can yet be drawn about the epidemiology of asymptomatic diastolic dysfunction [44–52, 54, 58].

Aetiology: causes of heart failure

As already mentioned, any structural, mechanical, or electrical abnormality of the heart can cause it to fail (➲Table 23.3). Similarly, heart failure can be caused by ischaemic, metabolic, endocrine, immune, inflammatory, infective, genetic, and neoplastic processes, by failure of the heart to develop properly, and even by pregnancy. The potential causes of heart failure are, therefore, legion, vary geographically, and have changed over time. Rheumatic valvular disease remains a common cause in many developing countries whereas this diagnosis is now uncommon in developed countries; in the latter, degenerative valvular disease in the elderly is now more common [42, 59–63] (see ➲Chapter 17). Valve disease may lead to volume and pressure overload of the heart, as described in more detail below. Endocardial disease is very rare in Europe but much less so in parts of Africa, where it can cause what is referred to as a restrictive cardiomyopathy, as described further in the rest of this section [59–63].

In the developed world, ventricular dysfunction is the commonest underlying problem and is caused, mainly, by myocardial infarction (leading to systolic ventricular dysfunction, i.e. failure of normal contraction and emptying of the heart), hypertension (causing systolic dysfunction, diastolic dysfunction,

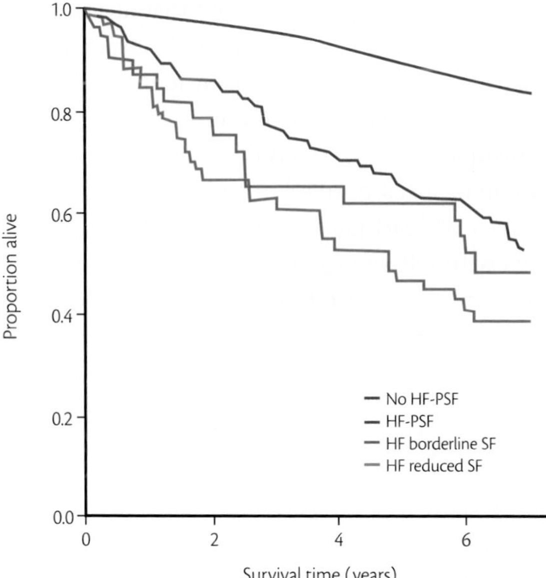

Figure 23.7 Unadjusted Kaplan–Meier survival curves for participants with heart failure (HF) based on left ventricular function from The Cardiovascular Health Study. Preserved systolic function (PSF), Systolic function (SF). Reproduced with permission from Gottdiener JS, McClelland RL, Marshall R, *et al.* Outcome of congestive heart failure in elderly persons: influence of left ventricular systolic function. The Cardiovascular Health Study. *Ann Intern Med* 2002; **137**: 631–9.

i.e. failure of normal relaxation and filling of the heart or both) or, often, both infarction and hypertension (see Chapter 17). These causes are becoming more important in some parts of the developing world [63]. Whether persisting systolic dysfunction is caused by coronary artery disease in the absence of infarction is uncertain. The converse, i.e. whether treatment of ischaemia and a state known as 'hibernation' (where chronic poor perfusion results in non-contracting but viable myocardium) improves systolic function, is also a question of great current interest, addressed by ongoing studies of coronary 'revascularization' [64].

In Europe, North America, and Australasia, hypertension was once the principal cause of heart failure whereas now that position is filled by coronary heart disease (or more exactly, myocardial infarction); this is also increasingly the case in many developing countries [63].

While myocardial infarction is a much more important individual risk factor than hypertension, the population-attributable risk due to hypertension is probably still more important [65, 66]. Both causal factors also interact to augment the risk of heart failure, with concomitant hypertension greatly increasing the risk of failure after myocardial infarction [65, 66]. By the time heart failure presents, prior hypertension may no longer be present. Both of these factors probably result in underestimation of the role of hypertension in causing heart failure. Hypertension is a more common aetiology in women than men.

Table 23.3 Aetiology of heart failure

There is no agreed or satisfactory classification for the causes of heart failure with much overlap between potential categories, e.g. dilated cardiomyopathy may be variously regarded as idiopathic, genetic, caused by a remote virus infection or the result of current or previous excessive alcohol consumption.
Myocardial disease ◆ coronary artery disease ◆ hypertension ◆ immune/inflammatory viral myocarditis Chagas' disease ◆ metabolic/infiltrative thiamine deficiency haemochromatosis amyloidosis sarcoidosis ◆ endocrine hypothyroidism phaeochromocytoma thyrotoxicosis ◆ toxic alcohol cytotoxics (e.g. trastuzumab) negatively inotropic drugs (e.g. calcium-channel blockers) ◆ idiopathic cardiomyopathy (dilated, hypertrophic, restrictive, peri-partum)
Valvular disease ◆ mitral stenosis/regurgitation ◆ aortic stenosis/regurgitation ◆ pulmonary stenosis/regurgitation ◆ tricuspid stenosis/regurgitation
Pericardial disease ◆ effusion ◆ constriction
Endocardial/endomyocardial disease ◆ Löffler endocarditis ◆ endomyocardial fibrosis
Congenital heart disease ◆ e.g. atrial or ventricular septal defect
Genetic ◆ e.g. familial dilated cardiomyopathy
Arrhythmias (brady- or tachy-) ◆ atrial ◆ ventricular
Conduction disorders ◆ sinus node dysfunction ◆ second-degree atrioventricular block ◆ third-degree atrioventricular block
High output states ◆ anaemia ◆ sepsis ◆ thyrotoxicosis ◆ Paget's disease ◆ arteriovenous fistula
Volume overload ◆ renal failure ◆ iatrogenic

'Idiopathic' dilated cardiomyopathy remains the only other cause of systolic dysfunction commonly encountered, perhaps accounting for 15–20% of cases of heart failure with reduced systolic function. These cases probably have multiple causes and an increasing number of genetic causes are being identified [67]. Prior viral infection is a recognized cause and recent research studies suggest that persisting virus infection may be identified (by endomyocardial biopsy) in a high proportion of patients with dilated cardiomyopathy. Whether this is of prognostic significance or requires therapeutic intervention is currently uncertain [68]. Current or previous excessive alcohol consumption may also cause a dilated cardiomyopathy, as can exposure to other toxins, including chemotherapeutic agents used in cancer treatment such as anthracyclines and trastuzumab [69]. These must always be considered when a patient presents with an unexplained dilated cardiomyopathy. If angiography is not carried out to exclude coronary disease, it may also be wrongly concluded that the patient has an 'idiopathic' dilated cardiomyopathy. Chagas disease, caused by the protozoan parasite *Trypanosoma cruzi*, can also cause systolic dysfunction. Though rarely encountered in Europe it is a relatively common cause of heart failure in South America and is now recognized in Central and North America [59, 61].

It is not clear whether diabetes mellitus should be considered an aetiological factor or a comorbidity in heart failure. Its potential role in causation of systolic and diastolic dysfunction is uncertain [70]. Diabetics have a higher prevalence of heart failure. Diabetes accelerates the development of coronary atherosclerosis and is often associated with hypertension. Whether it directly causes a specific cardiomyopathy is, however, uncertain. Diabetes is also associated with a higher risk of developing heart failure in patients with other causes, e.g. acute myocardial infarction. It is believed that diabetes promotes the development of myocardial fibrosis and diastolic dysfunction. Diabetes is also associated with more autonomic dysfunction and worse renal, pulmonary, and endothelial function, as well as worse functional status and a worse prognosis. Conversely, heart failure increases the risk of developing diabetes [70].

Although it is associated with diabetes, hypertension, and coronary artery disease, obesity also seems to be an independent risk factor for developing heart failure [71].

Atrial fibrillation is both an aetiological factor and comorbidity. It can cause heart failure directly as a consequence of the loss of the atrial contribution to cardiac output and reduced diastolic filling as a result of tachycardia [72, 73]. Patients with underlying structural or functional cardiac disease are more likely to develop failure as a consequence of these effects with the onset of atrial fibrillation. There is, however, a growing belief that atrial fibrillation can cause a dilated cardiomyopathy the exact mechanism of which is uncertain, though persistent tachycardia may play a role (i.e. atrial fibrillation may cause a 'rate-related cardiomyopathy') [74]. Heart failure also increases the risk of developing atrial fibrillation and this risk increases with the severity of heart failure. Consequently, when a patient presents with left ventricular dilatation, systolic dysfunction, and atrial fibrillation it can be difficult to determine which came first.

Comorbidity

It is important to appreciate that heart failure does not occur in isolation. It is caused by an underlying cardiac defect in, usually, elderly individuals frequently treated for other medical problems with multiple medications. Consequently, the patient with heart failure often has comorbidity related to the underlying cardiac problem or its cause (e.g. angina, hypertension, diabetes, smoking-related lung disease) and age (e.g. osteoarthritis), as well as a consequence of heart failure (e.g. arrhythmias) and its treatment (e.g. gout from diuretics) [75]. Some common comorbidities have multiple causes (e.g. renal dysfunction, see ➲Cardiorenal syndrome, p.842), whereas others are not fully explained (e.g. anaemia, depression, disorders of breathing, and cachexia) [75–80]. The existence of multiple comorbidities creates the potential for drug intolerance (e.g. angiotensin-converting enzyme (ACE) inhibitor and renal dysfunction), drug interactions (e.g. non-steroidal anti-inflammatory drugs (NSAIDs) and ACE inhibitors), worsening of heart failure as a specific adverse effect (e.g. thiazolidinediones), and makes the management of heart failure very complex [1, 70, 81–83]. This is especially true of renal dysfunction, the importance of which is increasingly recognized by a growing use of the term 'cardiorenal syndrome' [84, 85] to describe concurrent heart and renal failure.

Cardiorenal syndrome

This syndrome arises from multiple interactions between the age-related decline in glomerular filtration, the effects of treatment for heart failure (diuretics, ACE inhibitors, angiotensin receptor blockers (ARBs), and aldosterone antagonists) and other conditions (e.g. NSAIDs for arthritis), comorbidity (e.g. hypertension, diabetes, atherosclerosis), reduced renal blood flow and the actions on the kidneys of the array of neurohumoral pathways activated in heart failure [84, 85]. The prevalence of severe renal dysfunction in heart failure is often underestimated because serum creatinine concentration may not be greatly elevated because of the reduction in skeletal muscle mass in advanced heart failure. Renal dysfunction may contribute to the high prevalence of anaemia in patients with heart failure. The blood concentrations of creatinine, urea (blood urea nitrogen), and estimated glomerular filtration rate are powerful independent predictors of prognosis and deterioration in renal function during an episode of worsening heart failure (e.g. an increase in creatinine concentration of ≥0.3mg/dL or 27μmol/L) is associated with higher morbidity and mortality [86].

Anaemia

Anaemia is another important comorbidity and can be both the cause and, it seems, consequence of heart failure [76, 87–89]. Anaemia is common (especially in more severe heart failure) and is associated with worse symptoms, increased risk of hospital admission, and reduced survival. The causes are unknown but may include haemodilution, renal dysfunction, poor nutrition, inflammation, blood loss related to medication, and reduced production of (or response to) erythropoietin.

Catabolic/anabolic imbalance and cachexia

Patients with heart failure often exhibit some degree of muscle wasting which is restricted to the lower limbs (disuse atrophy) [77, 90, 91]. This loss of tissue may become more extensive in some patients, usually when their heart failure is more advanced, and may affect all body compartments (muscle, fat, and bone tissue). This general wasting is referred to as cardiac cachexia. The underlying metabolic causes are complex and differ from patient to patient. Three important contributors are, probably, dietary deficiency (exacerbated by anorexia), loss of nutrients through the urinary or digestive tracts (malabsorption), and metabolic dysfunction (including an imbalance of anabolic and catabolic factors and inflammation). The development of cachexia is an ominous sign [77, 90].

It is important to appreciate that it is comorbidity, along with the key pathophysiological processes in heart failure, i.e. left ventricular remodelling and activation of systemic pathways (and age), that are the principal determinants of prognosis.

Pathophysiology

We have only limited knowledge of the pathophysiology of heart failure, and that of left ventricular systolic dysfunction is best understood. Much of our understanding comes from studies of myocardial infarction (➲ Fig. 23.8) [92, 93]. Following an initial injury to the myocytes and cytoskeleton, heart failure may develop immediately, in the short term (over days or weeks), over a longer time period (months to years), or not at all. The factors leading to the development of heart failure acutely after myocardial infarction (e.g. size of infarction, concomitant hypertension [66], etc.), the important pathophysiological mechanisms operating (e.g. cardiac remodelling), and the time-course of this complication of infarction are fairly well established. On the other hand, the natural history of asymptomatic left ventricular systolic dysfunction is less well understood, as are the pathophysiological mechanisms causing progression from the asymptomatic to the symptomatic state. Once symptomatic heart failure has developed we believe that the pathophysiology is again better understood, at least in patients with systolic dysfunction. One thing is certain: the syndrome is characterized by progressive worsening of the patient's symptoms, of cardiac function, and of the function of other tissues (e.g. skeletal muscle, bone marrow) and organs (e.g. the kidneys).

The progression of left ventricular systolic dysfunction (and the heart failure syndrome), because of 'remodelling'

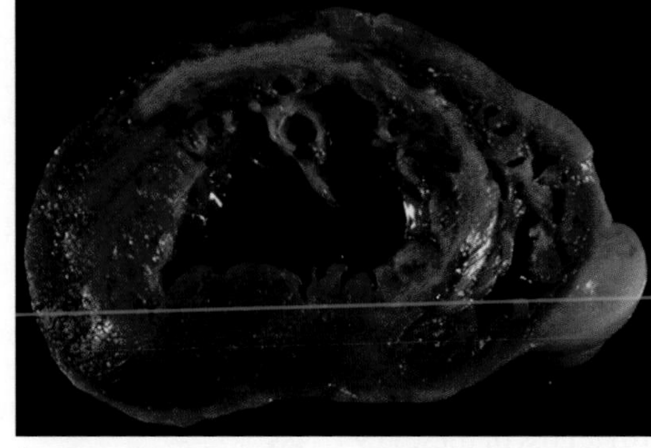
A

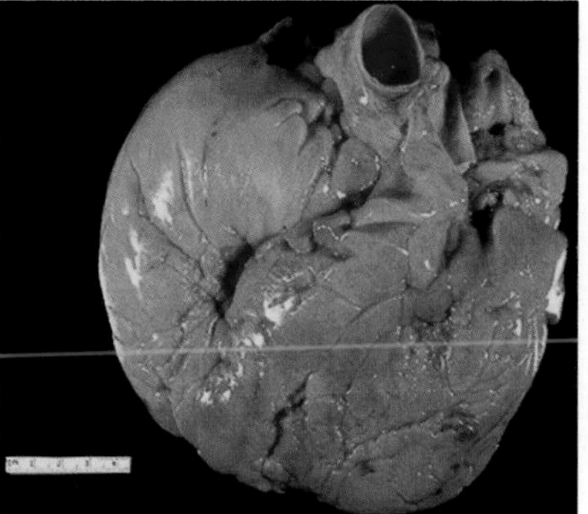
B

Figure 23.8 Gross pathological appearance of (A) an anteroseptal myocardial infarction, with wall thinning and endocardial fibrosis, in a patient with a background of left ventricular hypertrophy due to hypertension, and (B) a heart in idiopathic dilated cardiomyopathy characterized by four chamber enlargement.

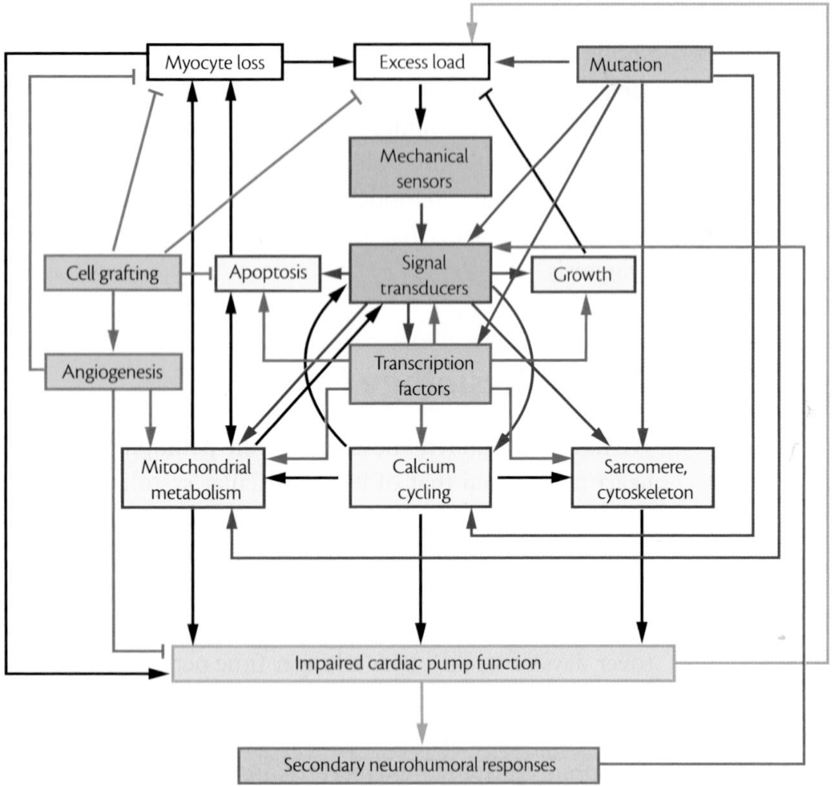

Figure 23.9 A partial wiring diagram of biological circuits for heart failure. Impaired pump function after myocyte death from myocardial infarction or abnormal loading conditions such as found in hypertension (white) activate a biomechanical stress-dependent signalling cascade (purple). The responsible targets of altered signal transduction cascades in heart failure include transcription factors, coactivators and co-repressors for cardiac gene expression (green) as well as the effector mechanisms like calcium cycling, metabolism, growth and apoptosis (yellow) that culminate in ventricular dysfunction (orange) and secondary neurohumoral responses (grey) such as adrenergic drive and intramyocardial growth factors. Inherited mutations for cardiomyopathy (blue) affect proteins at many of these points and are thought to engage a similar cascade of events to elicit the full myopathic phenotype. Cell-based therapies (red), although often envisioned working chiefly or wholly by replacing dead myocytes, probably improve ventricular performance through a combination of mechanisms, including angiogenesis, paracrine signals for myocyte protection, and conceivably augmenting host self-repair. Reproduced with permission from Benjamin, IJ, Schneider, MD. Learning from failure: congestive heart failure in the postgenomic age. *J Clin Invest* 2005; **115**: 495–9.

of the left (and right) ventricle (as a result of the loss of myocytes and maladaptive changes in the surviving myocytes and extracellular matrix), probably occurs in two main ways [92–97]. One is because of intercurrent cardiac events (e.g. myocardial infarction [98]) and the other is as a consequence of the local processes (e.g. the autocrine pathway and molecular adaptations, including, perhaps, apoptosis) and systemic processes (e.g. neurohumoral pathways) that are activated as a result of reduced systolic function (➲Fig. 23.9) [92–97]. These systemic processes, which are discussed in detail in later sections, also have detrimental effects on the functioning of the lungs, blood vessels, kidneys, bone marrow, muscles, and probably other organs (e.g. the liver), and contribute to a pathophysiological vicious cycle (➲Fig. 23.10). The molecular, structural, and functional changes in the heart and these systemic processes, coupled with electrolyte imbalances, result in electrical as well as mechanical dysfunction of the heart. In addition, cardiac metabolism is altered in the failing heart and some believe that a state of relative energy starvation exists [93, 99].

It is important to remember that atrial function, synchronized contraction of the left ventricle, and normal interaction between the right and left ventricles are also important in preserving stroke volume [93, 100, 101]. Loss of these key

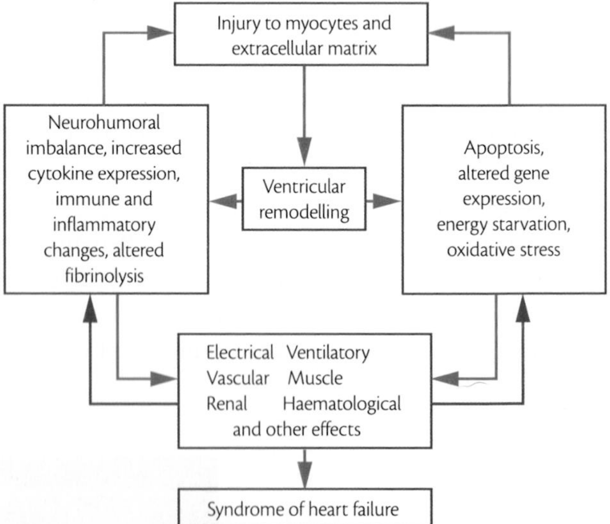

Figure 23.10 Pathophysiology of heart failure as a result of left-ventricular systolic dysfunction. Damage to the myocytes and extracellular matrix leads to changes in the size, shape, and function of the left ventricle and heart more generally ('remodelling'). These changes, in turn, lead to electrical instability, systemic processes resulting in many effects on other organs and tissues, and further damage to the heart. These vicious cycles, along with intercurrent events, such as myocardial infarction, are believed to cause progressive worsening of the heart-failure syndrome over time. Adapted with permission from McMurray JJ, Pfeffer MA. Heart failure. *Lancet* 2005; **365**: 1877–89.

mechanical interactions is often secondary to disturbances of conduction arising as a consequence of cardiac fibrosis.

Dilated cardiomyopathy

The term 'cardiomyopathy' is used to define a myocardial disorder in which the heart muscle is structurally and functionally abnormal, in the absence of coronary artery disease (hence the term 'ischaemic cardiomyopathy' should be avoided), hypertension, valvular disease, and congenital heart disease sufficient to cause the observed myocardial abnormality [67, 102]. Myocyte necrosis whether caused by infarction or by other injury has a common consequence. Whether diffuse or focal, myocyte loss leads to replacement fibrosis, hypertrophy of the remaining myocytes and dilatation of the affected cardiac chamber [67, 93, 102–104]. How these molecular and cellular changes affect the left ventricle macroscopically (by causing remodelling) is discussed in more detail in later sections. The resulting anatomical and pathophysiological picture is, however, identified by clinicians as a dilated cardiomyopathy. Certain inherited cardiomyopathies result in a similar phenotype. Poor contraction and emptying of the ventricle are usually referred to as systolic dysfunction. Other cardiomyopathic phenotypes occur (➲Fig. 23.11).

Systolic versus diastolic dysfunction

Systolic and diastolic dysfunction are terms used to describe whether the principal abnormality of the myocardium is an inability of the ventricle to contract and expel blood or to relax and fill normally, respectively (though in reality these two abnormalities frequently coexist). Systolic dysfunction is the result of reduced shortening of sarcomeres, which is a consequence of a global or regional reduction of contractility or greatly increased impedance to left ventricular ejection. An increase in preload can provide short-term compensation (via the ➲Frank–Starling mechanism, see p.847) for a reduction in contractility or increases in impedance. However, long-term compensation usually involves myocardial hypertrophy, which is the result of laying down new sarcomeres that increase the width (concentric) or the length (eccentric) of myocytes [93, 105–110]. Remodelling also contributes to reduced sarcomere shortening. All these factors causing reduced fibre shortening and eventually lead to a decrease in the left ventricular ejection fraction (LVEF). Hence, end-systolic volume increases.

Rapid filling during systole is assisted by active, energy-dependent, relaxation of the ventricle [93, 105–110]. Primary myocardial diseases may affect this process. Ventricular relaxation also depends on myocardial mass, collagen content, and extrinsic forces (e.g. the pericardium) [93, 105–110]. The hallmark of diastolic dysfunction is elevation in left ventricular end-diastolic pressure or left arterial pressure in the absence of systolic dysfunction [93, 105, 110].

Restrictive cardiomyopathy and pericardial constriction

Infiltrative processes in the myocardium may cause a restrictive cardiomyopathy (➲Fig. 23.12) [111, 112] (see ➲Chapter 17). The principal consequence is impaired ventricular filling with normal or decreased diastolic volume of either or both ventricles, akin to the diastolic dysfunction described earlier. Systolic function is typically maintained during the early stages of the disease and wall thickness is

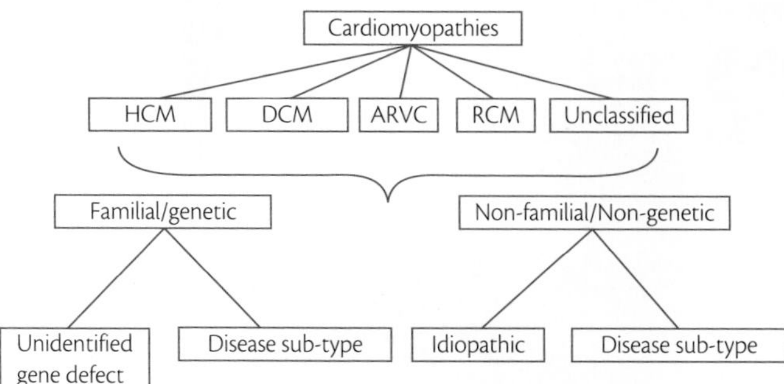

Figure 23.11 Summary of proposed classification system. ARVC, arrhythmogenic right ventricular cardiomyopathy; DCM, dilated cardiomyopathy; HCM, hypertrophic cardiomyopathy; RCM restrictive cardiomyopathy. Reproduced from Elliott P, Andersson B, Arbustini E, *et al.* Classification of the cardiomyopathies: a position statement from the European Society Of Cardiology Working Group on Myocardial and Pericardial Diseases. *Eur Heart J* 2008; **29**: 270–6, with permission from Oxford University Press.

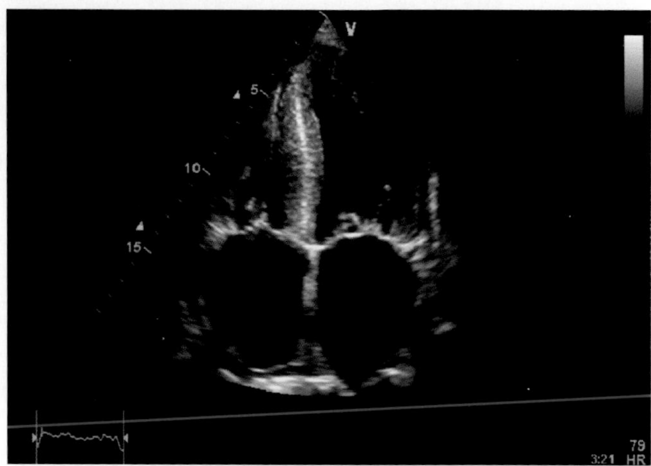

Figure 23.12 Transthoracic four-chamber echocardiogram of patient with cardiac amyloidosis.

normal or increased. The main problem is that increased stiffness of the myocardium causes pressure within the ventricle to rise precipitously with only small increases in volume. Restrictive cardiomyopathy may affect either or both ventricles. Elevated jugular venous pressure, peripheral oedema, and ascites are often prominent features. Pericardial constriction has similar pathophysiological effects and causes a similar clinical picture but can be hard to diagnose. Clinical suspicion may be raised by a history of prior tuberculosis, radiotherapy, cardiothoracic surgery, etc. Special investigations, including cardiac computed tomography (CT) scanning and simultaneous right and left heart pressure measurements at catheterization are often necessary [113, 114].

Valve disease: pressure and volume overload

Arterial hypertension and aortic stenosis cause a sustained increase in systolic wall stress during left ventricular ejection leading to concentric hypertrophy of the left ventricle because of myocyte hypertrophy and extracellular matrix overgrowth [115].

Conversely, mitral and aortic regurgitation result in an increased volume load on the ventricle. The resultant ventricular remodelling is characterized by dilatation, representing, at least in part, lengthening of the cardiac myocytes [116, 117].

Other terms sometimes used when describing heart failure

Right and left heart failure

These terms are not useful and are reminiscent of the now discarded terminology of 'backwards' and 'forwards' heart failure. The term right heart failure is often used to describe patients in whom there are prominent signs of peripheral 'congestion', e.g. a raised jugular venous pressure, hepatomegaly, and peripheral oedema (➲Fig. 23.13), on the basis that these findings reflect right ventricular failure; in fact all of

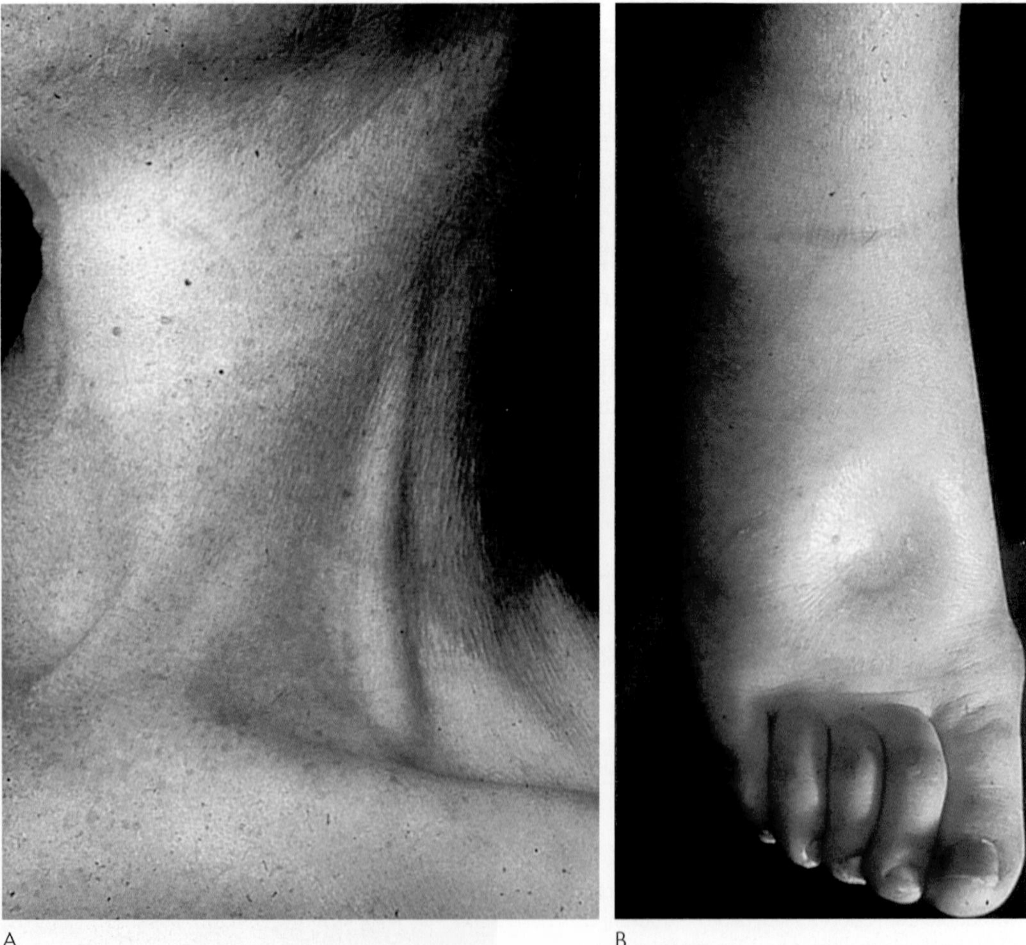

Figure 23.13 (A) A raised jugular venous pressure (JVP) reflects an elevation in right atrial pressure as occurs in heart failure. However this can also be seen in pericardial disease, tricuspid stenosis, superior vena cava obstruction, reduced compliance of the right ventricle, and hypervolaemia. (B) Pitting pedal oedema as seen in a patient with heart failure. This can also be seen in hypoalbuminaemia, nephrotic syndrome, chronic venous insufficiency and myxoedema.

these signs are also found in patients with predominantly left ventricular involvement. The description pulmonary heart disease is used to depict patients who do have isolated right heart failure as a result of primary lung disease and has generally replaced the term 'cor pulmonale'.

High- and low-output heart failure

A more useful pathophysiological classification is to distinguish between high- and low-output heart failure, although the former is uncommonly encountered in Western clinical practice. Cardiac index is normally 2.2–3.5L/min/m^2. Low-output cardiac failure implies that cardiac output fails to rise adequately during exercise or that it is inadequate even at rest. This prototypical form of heart failure is seen in cases of heart failure as a result of left ventricular systolic dysfunction. High-output cardiac failure, on the other hand, implies that although the pumping action of the heart is intact other factors make it difficult for the heart to deliver oxygen commensurate with the needs of the metabolizing tissues, either because of increased tissue demand (e.g. as a result of anaemia, hyperthyroidism, or pregnancy) or reduced oxygen-carrying content of the blood (e.g. anaemia). This type of heart failure can also be caused by arteriovenous shunting.

Cardiac responses to ventricular injury and reduced stroke volume

Frank–Starling mechanism

The Frank–Starling law describes an intrinsic mechanism that helps maintain stroke volume when the heart is acutely injured and may also play a compensatory role in chronic heart failure, though this is less certain [118]. Together with neurohumoral activation (an extrinsic mechanism), the Frank–Starling law is an adaptive phenomenon that comes into play within minutes of cardiac injury. The resultant acute fall in the volume of blood ejected by the ventricle (the stroke volume) leads to a rise in left ventricular end-diastolic volume (and pressure). Through the Frank–Starling mechanism this rise in preload increases the force of contraction, thereby helping restore stroke volume. The mechanism whereby increased stretch of the myocyte causes increased force of contraction is also referred to as the law of heterometric autoregulation. In the chronic setting, sodium retention, water retention, and venoconstriction may represent continuing attempts by the body to use the Frank–Starling mechanism by increasing left ventricular filling pressure and preload.

These adaptations may, however, lead to abnormally high pulmonary capillary and artery pressures, probably contributing to the shortness of breath experienced by patients with heart failure. Furthermore, arterial constriction and stiffening (as a result of sodium and water retention in the vascular wall) increase afterload and will eventually cause the injured left ventricle to fail further because it is especially sensitive to increases in afterload (law of homeometric regulation).

Ventricular remodelling

The heart attempts to compensate for increased preload (e.g. because of increased extracellular fluid volume and venous return) and afterload (e.g. because of systemic arterial constriction) in several ways. One is the development of ventricular hypertrophy in an attempt to maintain systolic wall stress within normal limits [92–97, 119, 120]. Pressure overload tends to lead to concentric hypertrophy, whereas volume overload tends to lead to ventricular dilatation [92–97, 119, 120]. Both entities are distinct at the molecular level. Pressure overload is associated with parallel replication of myofibrils and thickening of individual myocytes. Volume overload, on the other hand, leads to replication of sarcomeres in series and elongation of myocytes. The two types of haemodynamic overload are presumed to activate distinct signalling pathways.

Compensated remodelling results in relatively little change in ventricular dimensions, shape, function, and wall thickness. However, these compensatory adaptations only seem to be capable of maintaining pump function over a limited period of time and a ventricle subjected to an elevated load for a prolonged period will ultimately fail. Ventricular dilatation may lead to stretching of the mitral valve ring and cause valvular incompetence (➲Fig. 23.14). This may further increase the load on the failing ventricle; this is an example of another 'vicious cycle' that develops and which may drive progression of heart failure.

An initial stress-induced increase in sarcomere length yields an optimal overlap between myofilaments [92–97, 119–121]. Severe haemodynamic overload eventually yields depression of myocardial contractility. In patients with mild disease, this depression is manifested by reduced velocity of shortening of the myocardium or by a reduction in the rate of force development during isometric contraction. More severe stages are accompanied by a decline in isometric force development and shortening as well. EF and cardiac output during exercise decline [92-97, 119–121].

Our understanding of the molecular mechanisms behind these changes is still limited and can only be touched upon

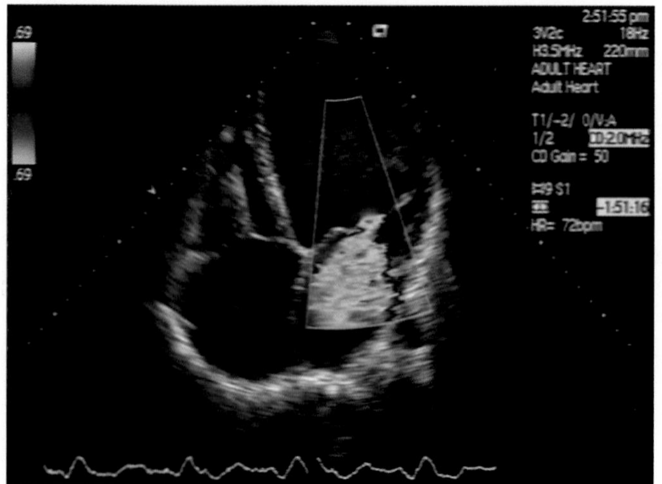

Figure 23.14 Colour-flow Doppler study of a patient with mitral regurgitation as a result of left ventricular dilatation seen in the apical four-chamber view.

briefly (➲Fig. 23.9). They comprise myocyte loss by necrosis and apoptosis, alterations in excitation–contraction coupling, and alterations in composition of the extracellular matrix [119–120]. Myocyte loss as a result of necrosis is a well-understood process which is localized after myocardial infarction but more diffuse in patients with dilated cardiomyopathy or myocarditis. Apoptosis, or programmed cell death, on the other hand, results from the induction of a genetic programme that leads to degradation of nuclear DNA (➲Fig. 23.9) [92–97, 119–122]. Several recent reports have described apoptotic cells in the failing myocardium. It may be relevant that several substances, such as angiotensin II, reactive oxygen species, nitric oxide (NO), and pro-inflammatory cytokines may induce apoptosis experimentally in cardiac myocytes. However, the precise frequency of occurrence and role of apoptosis in the failing myocardium remains unclear [122]. Changes in the extracellular matrix are usually manifested by an increase in collagen content though both degradation and synthesis (and the activity of the enzymes controlling these processes) may be increased [93, 95]. While this change in collagen content may contribute to impaired systolic contraction it may be even more important in reducing ventricular compliance and impaired ventricular filling.

Systemic responses

Neurohumoral responses

The human body responds to the haemodynamic changes in patients with heart failure in a highly complex way. Many neurohumoral systems appear to be involved to varying degrees and at different stages. It has been suggested that these are initially activated in a manner appropriate to haemorrhage or some other crisis threatening vital organ perfusion [93, 123, 124]. Their sustained activation in heart failure, however, is not only inappropriate but probably detrimental (➲Fig. 23.10). Moreover, at some stage during the progression of heart failure, haemodynamic abnormalities may cease to be the main trigger of neurohumoral activation. Instead, a number of other self-sustaining pathophysiological vicious cycles may develop.

The predominant effects of the neurohumoral systems activated in heart failure are to cause vasoconstriction, sodium and water retention, and abnormal cell growth. Two exceptions are the natriuretic peptides [93, 125] (secreted mainly by the failing heart, ➲Fig. 23.15) and adrenomedullin (secreted mainly from blood vessels) [126].

The neurohumoral pathways activated in heart failure are thought to be particularly important because they appear to explain how many of the successful pharmacological treatments for heart failure work (and offer the potential for more such therapeutic interventions). Neurohumoral activation seems to be much less marked in patients with heart failure and preserved EF, compared to those with a low EF [127].

Sympathetic nervous system

It has long been recognized that an increased activity of the sympathetic nervous system and parasympathetic withdrawal are prototypical characteristics of heart failure [93, 128–130]. Elevated levels of plasma norepinephrine (noradrenaline) are a common finding in patients with heart failure. Increased sympathetic nerve traffic and enhanced spill-over of norepinephrine from the synaptic cleft account for this, and are particularly pronounced in the heart, kidney, and skeletal muscle [93, 128–131]. Raised plasma norepinephrine concentrations predict higher mortality rates [130, 131]. Heart failure is also characterized by reductions in myocardial norepinephrine stores and in myocardial beta-receptor density. These again reflect generalized adrenergic activation [93, 128–131].

It is believed that enhanced sympathetic activity initially increases myocardial contractility and heart rate (leading to an increase in cardiac output). Sympathetic activation also promotes renin release, sodium retention, and vasoconstriction thereby increasing preload and activating the Frank–Starling mechanism (see ➲Frank–Starling mechanism, p.847). These responses are capable of maintaining ventricular performance and cardiac output for a limited period of time. In part this may be because the increase in afterload caused by arterial constriction (to which the failing ventricle is particularly sensitive) leads to a further fall in

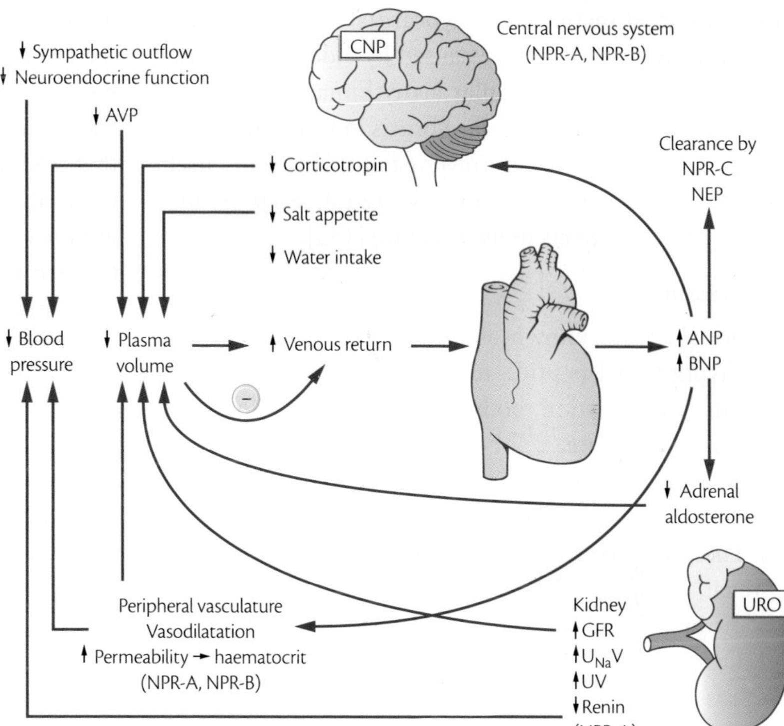

Figure 23.15 Physiological effects of the natriuretic peptides in heart failure. Increased secretion of the natriuretic peptides reduces blood pressure and plasma volume through coordinated actions in the brain, adrenal gland, kidney, and vasculature. Urodilatin (URO); neutral endopeptidase (NEP); C-type natriuretic peptide (CNP); natriuretic peptide receptors A, B and C (NPR-A, NPR-B, and NPR-C respectively); arginine vasopressin (AVP); atrial and brain natriuretic peptides (ANP and BNP); glomerular filtration rate (GFR); urinary sodium excretion ($U_{Na}V$); urinary volume (UV); blood pressure (BP). Reproduced with permission from Levin, ER, Gardner, DG, Samson WK. Mechanisms of disease: Natriuretic peptides. *N Engl J Med* 1998; **339**: 321–8.

stroke volume. Sympathetic overdrive probably alters myocardial metabolism and catecholamines may also even be directly toxic to cardiomyocytes [93, 130]. Excessive adrenergic activity (and reduced vagal activity) also increases the electrical instability of the heart. As well as having complex and changing effects on myocardial contractility and structure, activation of the sympathetic nervous system leads to redistribution of regional blood flow and even to changes in the structure of the vasculature [129].

The precise cause of sympathetic activation in heart failure is unknown. Reduced stimulation of stretch-activated baroreceptors in the carotid arteries and the aorta from decreased arterial pressure and stroke volume may contribute (in an analogous way to haemorrhage). Another factor suggested is structural and functional abnormalities of afferent receptors. Other neurohumoral systems may also activate the sympathetic nervous system and augment its actions, i.e. many neurohumoral systems act in concert, synergistically reinforcing each other.

Renin–angiotensin–aldosterone system

Increased activity of the renin–angiotensin–aldosterone system (RAAS) also produces deleterious effects on the cardiovascular system (and other organs and tissues) and contributes to the poor prognosis in heart failure [93, 123, 124, 132–134]. The plasma components of this system are usually increased in patients with heart failure and a low serum sodium concentration is a marker for particularly excessive activation of the RAAS [134]. The increase in renin release is mediated by decreased stretch of the glomerular afferent arteriole and reduced delivery of chloride to the macula densa. Although the sympathetic nervous system also stimulates renin release, the two systems are independently regulated. One puzzle about heart failure is why the sodium and volume overload that characterizes the syndrome does not suppress renin release, as would normally occur.

The increased secretion of renin leads to an augmented production of angiotensin II, which, it is believed, has mostly deleterious effects in heart failure (although its efferent glomerular arteriolar action may help maintain glomerular filtration). Angiotensin II not only induces vasoconstriction, but also salt and water retention directly and via aldosterone. Moreover, it mediates myocardial cell hypertrophy and fibrosis and these effects may contribute to the maladaptive remodelling and progressive loss of myocardial function in heart failure. Angiotensin II may also cause activation of the sympathetic nervous system, prothrombotic actions, and augment the release of arginine vasopressin.

Plasma aldosterone levels are also increased in heart failure, and release of this hormone is influenced by angiotensin and other stimuli such as potassium and corticotropin. Aldosterone is an independent and harmful component of the RAAS [135]. It causes sodium and water retention and, importantly, potassium wastage. Potassium loss, along with autonomic dysfunction and myocardial fibrosis (both of which are also thought to be caused by aldosterone), may increase the risk of ventricular arrhythmias. Aldosterone may also contribute to vascular fibrosis in heart failure.

There is recent interest in the possibility that renin itself, acting through a specific renin/pro-renin receptor, may have detrimental effects in heart failure [136].

Vasopressin

Vasopressin (also known as antidiuretic hormone) is a neurohypophysial peptide involved in the regulation of free water reabsorption, body fluid osmolality, blood volume, blood pressure, cell contraction, cell proliferation, and adrenocorticotropin secretion [137, 138]. Vasopressin binds to three different specific G protein-coupled receptors. These are currently classified as V1 (or V1A)-vascular, V2-renal, and V3 (or V1B)-pituitary subtypes. All subtypes have distinct pharmacological profiles and intracellular second messengers. As well as reducing renal water excretion, vasopressin is one of the most powerful vasoconstricting substances known. It also stimulates blood platelet aggregation, coagulation factor release, and cellular proliferation. This profile of action is clearly unattractive in heart failure.

Elevated circulating levels of vasopressin are often, but not invariably, found in patients with chronic heart failure. It appears that vasopressin release from the posterior pituitary in heart failure is largely non-osmotic, although, normally, increased serum osmolality is the major physiological stimulus for its secretion.

Natriuretic peptides

A-type (atrial) natriuretic peptide (ANP) and B-type (brain) natriuretic peptide (BNP) are released in response to atrial and ventricular wall stretch and, as their names suggest, serve to maintain sodium homeostasis by enhancing renal sodium and water excretion (➲Fig. 23.15) [93, 125, 139–142]. These peptides also have haemodynamic effects, dilating arteries and, especially, veins. They also suppress the RAAS and, possibly, the sympathetic nervous system. There is some evidence that natriuretic peptides inhibit arginine vasopressin and endothelin-1 release and the biological actions of these peptides. Consequently, the natriuretic peptides are thought to play an important protective role in heart failure, countering the actions of the other vasoconstricting and anti-natriuretic neurohumoral systems which are activated in heart failure.

Circulating levels of both ANP and BNP are greatly increased in heart failure. This is the consequence of an increased synthesis and release of these hormones. In humans, BNP is mostly secreted from the ventricles in both healthy individuals and patients with heart failure. ANP secretion, on the other hand, is mainly from the atria in healthy individuals but from both the atria and the ventricles in patients with heart failure. Therefore, it appears that BNP is the only natriuretic peptide that is specific to the ventricles. Pro-BNP, the precursor of BNP, is stored in granules in myocytes. Pro-BNP is activated by a protease to form its biologically active form, BNP, and N-terminal (NT)-proBNP.

BNP levels vary according to sex and age in healthy subjects [141]. Female patients display higher plasma concentrations than male patients with heart failure. Advancing age and declining renal function are associated with increases in BNP levels.

C-type natriuretic peptide (CNP), which was originally believed to be of endothelial origin, may also be produced by the failing heart. A D-type (Dendroaspis) natriuretic peptide and a renal specific peptide (urodilatin) has also been described recently, though the origin and actions of each in humans are not yet well defined [142].

As well as having important physiological effects, the various A-type and B-type natriuretic peptides and related fragments can be used to aid the diagnosis of heart failure and to provide prognostic information.

Relaxin

Relaxin is a pregnancy-related hormone with vasodilator activity which has been shown to improve haemodynamic indices in heart failure [145, 146].

Adrenomedullin, apelin, and urocortin

These three more recently described neurohumoral factors have vasodilator and inotropic properties, as well as other actions [126, 143, 144]. Apelin is unusual in that blood and tissue concentrations are reduced in heart failure [143]. The pathophysiological role, if any, that these factors play in heart failure is presently uncertain as is any therapeutic potential that might exist. [126, 143, 144].

The endothelium, nitric oxide, and endothelin-1

The principal product of the endothelium, NO, plays a central role in vascular homeostasis. Endothelial dysfunction, which is characterized by reduced production and action of NO, occurs as a result of ageing, as well as in a number of chronic conditions related to heart failure, such as hypercholesterolaemia, atherosclerosis, as well as in heart failure itself [147]. Endothelium-dependent dilatation of coronary and peripheral resistance vessels is blunted in patients with heart failure. This probably contributes to the impaired reactive hyperaemia in various vascular beds, an impairment in tissue perfusion and, perhaps, reduced muscular function [148]. There has even been speculation that NO might be a key regulator of lung function and that exercise-induced dyspnoea may be related to impaired pulmonary vasodilatation resulting from reduced NO production compared to healthy subjects. Endothelial dysfunction in heart failure may be partly the result of increased oxidative stress.

Although lack of NO is associated with the development of endothelial dysfunction, its overproduction by the inducible isoform of NO synthase (iNOS) may also be detrimental [148]. Increased iNOS activity is thought to lead to increased free radical formation and to depression of myocardial activity [93]. Increased iNOS expression may result from the actions of inflammatory cytokines.

The endothelins are another important product of the endothelium and endothelin-1 is one of the most powerful vasoconstrictor peptides known [149]. It is also a mitogen and generally shares the potentially detrimental properties of angiotensin II and vasopressin in heart failure. Plasma concentrations of endothelin-1 are increased in heart failure, probably because of increased secretion, both by blood vessels and the failing myocardium. The importance of this is, however, uncertain because specific antagonists have not improved outcome in heart failure.

Oxidative stress, xanthine oxidase, and uric acid

Oxygen free radicals have a number of potentially detrimental actions in heart failure [93, 150, 151]. They inactivate NO, depress myocardial contractility, and may induce apoptosis [93, 152]. One source of the superoxide anion radical is NADPH oxidase which is activated by angiotensin II and aldosterone [93, 153]. Xanthine oxidase may be another source of increased free oxygen radical load in heart failure and is normally involved in the last step of purine breakdown which yields uric acid. Hyperuricaemia is a consistent finding in patients with heart failure, may reflect impairment of oxidative metabolism, and is a predictor of worse outcome [152]. Oxidative stress may be part of the generalized inflammatory state that characterizes at least some patients with heart failure. The importance of oxidative stress is, however, uncertain because specific antagonists (oxypurinol and vitamin E) did not improve pathophysiological measures or clinical outcomes in heart failure [155, 156].

Inflammatory responses

Inflammation may also be a factor contributing to the progression of heart failure although its role has not been 'confirmed' in the same way as neurohumoral activation, i.e. by the demonstration of improved outcomes with blocking agents [93, 157]. Several cytokines have been studied in detail. Different cell types secrete cytokines for the purpose of altering either their own function (autocrine) or that of adjacent cells (paracrine). Some cytokines also act as circulating hormones (i.e. have an endocrine action). Tumour necrosis factor-α (TNF-α), interleukin-1, and interleukin-6 are thought to be the most important pro-inflammatory cytokines that may be implicated in heart failure progression. The cause of cytokine activation in heart failure remains unclear. Pro-inflammatory cytokines may be secreted by mononuclear cells, hypoxic peripheral tissue, or even by the myocardium itself. Catecholamines may augment myocardial cytokine production, one of several possible links between neurohumoral activity and inflammation. It has also been hypothesized that increased bowel wall oedema may lead to translocation of bacterial endotoxin or lipopolysaccharide from the gut which may cause pro-inflammatory cytokine production from blood monocytes and possibly other tissues [157, 158].

Plasma TNF-α and TNF receptor (TNFR) concentrations are increased in some patients with heart failure, especially in those whose disease is severe, and they are independent predictors of poor prognosis. Although TNF-α has several potentially untoward effects that could contribute to the progression of heart failure, studies of TNF antagonists to date have not shown benefit in this syndrome [159, 160].

Diagnosis: symptoms, signs, and investigations

It is symptoms and signs that usually alert the patient (and physician) to the presence of a cardiac disorder. However, neither the symptoms nor signs commonly recognized as suggesting the presence of heart failure are specific for this syndrome. Therefore confirmation of heart failure requires objective tests to confirm that the patient's symptoms and the physical findings are the result of abnormal cardiac function and not of another cause (see ➲ Simple investigations, p.854) [1, 2].

Symptoms

Fatigue is a key symptom reported by patients with heart failure. Its origins are not clearly understood but probably include low cardiac output and skeletal muscle abnormalities (see ➲ Pathophysiology, p.843). Fatigue is very non-specific and is found in the population at large, as well as in many non-cardiovascular disorders.

Dyspnoea or breathlessness is another cardinal symptom of heart failure. Dyspnoea is usually first manifested on exertion and the level of exertion which causes breathlessness is useful in gauging heart failure severity and monitoring the patient's progress. Though it is more specific than fatigue, dyspnoea is still caused by many other disorders such as pulmonary disease, obesity, and anaemia, which are common in the elderly population and may coexist with heart failure. Even ageing itself is associated with dyspnoea on exercise. The origin of dyspnoea in heart failure is also probably multifactorial. It may be related to elevated pulmonary pressures, abnormalities in pulmonary compliance, respiratory dysfunction, accentuated respiratory drive, increased airway resistance, abnormal chemical and mechanical muscle reflexes [161–166], and even low haemoglobin. It is notable that there is a poor correlation between dyspnoea and left ventricular function at rest [161–166].

Orthopnoea is defined as dyspnoea which occurs in the recumbent position and is usually relieved by sitting upright or by the addition of pillows. In extreme cases, the patient is unable to lie down and may spend the night in the sitting position. Orthopnoea results from the return of venous blood which has pooled in the lower extremities while the patient is ambulatory. The failing heart may be unable to cope with return of this blood from the legs on adoption of the recumbent position and pulmonary oedema may occur.

Paroxysmal nocturnal dyspnoea is characterized by acute episodes of suffocation usually occurring while recumbent at night. It has the same causes as orthopnoea. Paroxysmal nocturnal dyspnoea may manifest as cough or wheezing, possibly because increased pressure in the bronchial arteries (and resultant increase in their diameter), along with interstitial pulmonary oedema, leads to increased airways resistance. Sometimes these patients are described as having 'cardiac asthma', which must be differentiated from primary asthma and pulmonary causes of wheezing.

Both orthopnoea and paroxysmal nocturnal dyspnoea are relatively specific for heart failure but are usually only encountered in untreated or advanced heart failure and are uncommon in most patients with mild to moderate heart failure taking diuretics [161–166]. Treated patients developing either symptom should be advised to report this to their physician/nurse as soon as possible. Paroxysmal nocturnal dyspnoea requires urgent treatment.

Cerebral symptoms such as confusion, disorientation, sleep or mood disturbances may be observed in advanced heart failure, particularly in the presence of hyponatraemia. These symptoms can be the first manifestation of heart failure in elderly patients. Sometimes sleep disturbances can be associated with ventilatory abnormalities (including central and obstructive sleep apnoea and Cheyne–Stokes respiration) which occur in advanced heart failure and may be reported by the patient's spouse or partner [167].

Nausea and abdominal discomfort may occur when there is marked congestion of the liver and gastrointestinal tract (although the former may also be caused by digitalis glycosides). Congestion of the liver and stretching of its capsule may cause pain in the right upper quadrant of the abdomen.

Oliguria is usually present in advanced heart failure as the result of reduced renal perfusion and avid sodium and water retention.

Functional classification

This has been alluded to earlier (➲Table 23.2). We prefer to use the NYHA functional classification [168]. Although it is subjective and has a large interobserver variation, it is used worldwide and, most importantly, has been employed as an entry criterion in almost all important clinical trials in heart failure.

At the individual patient level it is useful to measure functional limitation (and monitor progress) by way of the distance the patient can walk on the level, the number of steps that can be climbed, and ordinary activities that can (or cannot) be carried out, e.g. washing, bed-making, vacuum-cleaning, sweeping, shopping, etc. Because there is a poor correlation between symptoms and cardiac dysfunction, it must be emphasized that mild symptoms do not imply minor cardiac dysfunction or a good prognosis. Patients with very different EFs can experience quite similar degrees of functional limitation and treatment with a diuretic may lead to a marked improvement in symptoms without having any effect on cardiac function [169].

The Killip classification may be used to assess the severity of heart failure in the acute context, e.g. in myocardial infarction [170].

Quality of life

'Quality of life' assessments have been used to assess the impact of heart failure on patient well-being in a more complete way than just measuring specific symptoms or functional limitations. Various dimensions of quality of life including those reflecting physical, social, sexual, and professional activities can be measured, along with indices of mood, emotions, and mental health. Various questionnaires or visual scales have been proposed but none has been universally accepted. One of the most widely used is the Minnesota Living with Heart Failure questionnaire which includes a list of 21 questions, each answered on a scale of 0 to –5 [171]. More recently, the Kansas City Cardiomyopathy

Questionnaire has been used [172]. These measures are more often used in clinical trials than in clinical practice.

Signs

Clinical examination, including observation of the patient and palpation and auscultation of the heart, is essential in the assessment of an individual with suspected heart failure. Percussion of the heart is seldom performed although it can provide an accurate assessment of cardiac size; percussion of the lung fields is valuable [165, 166, 173].

General examination

Patients with advanced heart failure are sometimes severely dyspnoeic even when speaking and have peripheral oedema, cachexia, or cyanosis. Conversely, the general appearance of a patient presenting with mild to moderate heart failure is often normal.

Systolic blood pressure is usually reduced in heart failure because of left ventricular systolic dysfunction, especially if severe or treated. Sometimes blood pressure may be elevated, especially if hypertension is the cause of heart failure and particularly if systolic function is preserved. Blood pressure can be markedly increased during an episode of acute pulmonary oedema. It is important to distinguish between low blood pressure (hypotension) which may be unimportant per se and hypoperfusion of the vital organs, i.e. where there are symptoms such as dizziness or confusion, renal dysfunction, or myocardial ischaemia, which is always important and requires attention.

Sinus tachycardia is a non-specific sign which is caused by increased sympathetic activity and can be absent in the presence of conduction disturbances (or if the patient is taking beta-adrenergic blocker therapy). Some patients may also have tachycardia because of atrial fibrillation (or another supraventricular arrhythmia) or, rarely, ventricular tachycardia.

Peripheral vasoconstriction with coldness, cyanosis, and pallor of extremities is also caused by increased sympathetic activity.

Peripheral oedema is a key manifestation of heart failure but is non-specific and usually absent in patients already treated with diuretics (➲ Fig. 23.13). It is related to extracellular volume expansion, is accompanied (and even preceded) by weight gain, and is progressive. It is usually bilateral and symmetrical, painless, pitting, and occurs first in the lower extremities in ambulatory patients, namely the feet and the ankles. In bedridden patients, oedema may instead be found over the sacrum and scrotum. Even oedema to mid-calf may reflect an increase of ≥2L in extracellular fluid volume. Long-standing leg oedema may be associated with indurated and pigmented skin. If untreated, oedema may become generalized (anasarca), with the development of hepatic congestion, ascites, and hydrothorax (pleural effusions). At this stage there is usually clear jugular venous distension (➲ Fig. 23.13—see ➲ Cardiac signs, p.853). Generalized oedema is often accompanied by resistance to oral diuretic treatment. Patients should be warned to be observant for progressive increases in weight, accompanied by ankle swelling and, especially, increasing dyspnoea. Daily weight monitoring is important to identify sodium and water retention episodes and initiate early therapy. A prompt (and often temporary) increase in diuretic therapy may resolve worsening congestion in this situation.

Hepatomegaly is an important but uncommon sign in patients with heart failure. The liver is usually tender except in long-standing heart failure and can pulsate during systole in the presence of tricuspid regurgitation. Firm and continuous compression of the right upper abdominal quadrant for 30s to 1min may exhibit hepato-jugular reflux, i.e. an increase in jugular distension that is sustained during and after compression (see ➲ jugular venous distension in Cardiac signs, p.853). Examination should be made on a patient lying comfortably with their head resting on a pillow.

Cardiac signs

Jugular venous distension, detected by inspection of the internal jugular veins, may identify an elevated right atrial pressure and by inference (and in the absence of tricuspid and pulmonary valve disease) left atrial pressure (➲ Fig. 23.13). Although, estimates of jugular venous pressure by physical examination correlate poorly with invasive measurement of right atrial pressure and interobserver reproducibility is low among non-specialists, elevation of jugular venous pressure is of prognostic importance [165, 166, 173–177]. Giant 'V waves' indicate the presence of tricuspid incompetence.

A third heart sound is usually only heard when there is left ventricular dilatation and systolic dysfunction, but interobserver agreement on this sign is low. A third heart sound is more common in severe heart failure and is associated with poor prognosis [165, 166, 173, 175].

A systolic murmur as because mitral or tricuspid regurgitation can be present, even in the absence of primary valve disease, when the left or right ventricle is markedly enlarged, leading to a dilatation of the mitral or the tricuspid annulus. In the latter case, the tricuspid murmur is selectively increased in loudness following inspiration (Carvallo's sign).

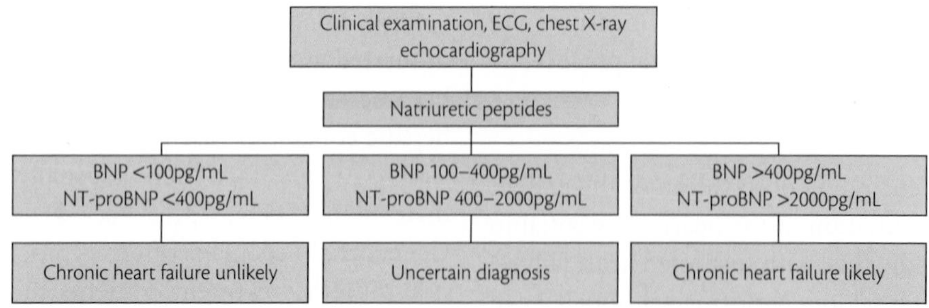

Figure 23.16 Flow chart for the diagnosis of heart failure with natriuretic peptides in untreated patients with symptoms suggestive of heart failure. Adapted with permission from Dickstein K, Cohen-Solal A, Filippatos G, *et al.* ESC guidelines for the diagnosis and treatment of acute and chronic heart failure 2008: the Task Force for the diagnosis and treatment of acute and chronic heart failure 2008 of the European Society of Cardiology. Developed in collaboration with the Heart Failure Association of the ESC (HFA) and endorsed by the European Society of Intensive Care Medicine (ESICM). *Eur Heart J* 2008; **29**: 2388–442.

The degree of mitral regurgitation can be dynamic and increase on exertion.

Lung examination

Pulmonary crackles (crepitations or rales) result from the transudation of fluid from the intravascular space into the alveoli. The presence of crackles at the lung bases is suggestive of pulmonary congestion but the positive predictive value of this sign is low and the interobserver variability is high [165, 166, 173]. Moreover, the origin of crackles can be difficult to assess in smokers who may also have chronic pulmonary disease (or in patients at risk of pulmonary disease for some other reason). In acute pulmonary oedema, bubbling crackles may be accompanied by expectoration of frothy sputum which is blood stained. Patients with long-standing heart failure may become resistant to developing pulmonary oedema and only do so at very high left atrial pressures. Pleural effusions can also be detected in patients with heart failure; they are normally bilateral and usually associated with marked dyspnoea and generalized congestion.

Overall, the presence of several of the aforementioned symptoms and signs, particularly in the context of a history of previous cardiac disease, is suggestive of heart failure, if not its precise cause. The declining skill of physicians in clinical examination, the lack of sensitivity and specificity of most signs (and the large interobserver variability in their detection), and the subjective nature of clinical assessment highlight the need for objective assessment of cardiac function. This objective assessment is also essential for diagnosis of the cause of heart failure and, therefore, treatment tailored to aetiology.

Simple investigations

Electrocardiogram

A resting 12-lead electrocardiogram (ECG) is one of the most useful investigations in a patient with suspected heart failure and is recommended as a first-line diagnostic test in the European Society of Cardiology (ESC) guidelines (➲Fig. 23.16) [1]. The ECG provides diagnostic and prognostic information and helps in choosing treatment. ECG changes are frequent in heart failure and a normal ECG virtually excludes left ventricular systolic dysfunction [1,177]. Various abnormalities may be present, such as abnormal Q waves (➲Fig. 23.17), left bundle branch block (➲Fig. 23.18) and other conduction disturbances, left atrial or left ventricular hypertrophy (➲Fig. 23.19),

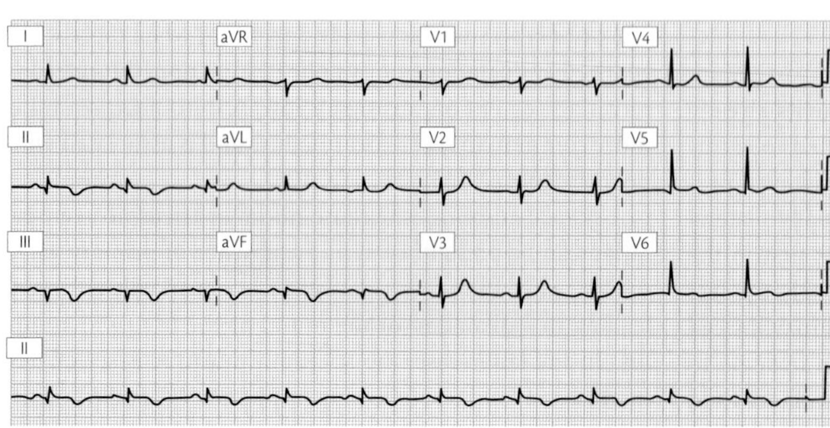

Figure 23.17 Twelve-lead ECG depicting an established transmural inferior myocardial infarction—there are Q-waves and T-wave inversion seen in leads II, III, and aVF.

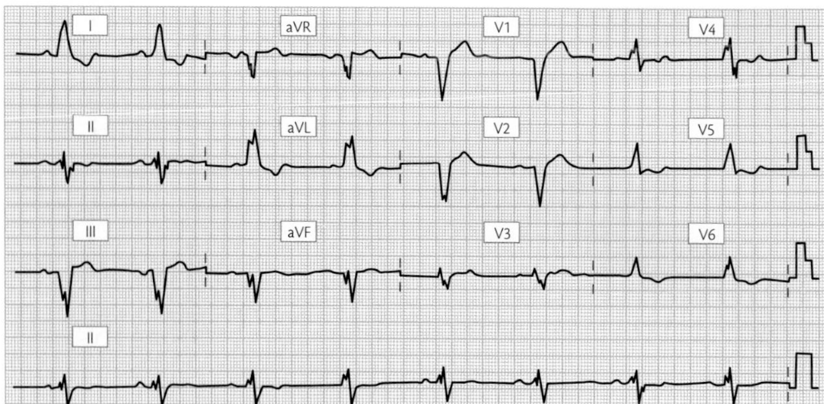

Figure 23.18 Twelve-lead electrocardiogram depicting left bundle branch block (LBBB).

atrial or ventricular arrhythmias may suggest a specific aetiology or precipitating factor. Some abnormalities provide prognostic information and help in choosing treatment, e.g. bundle branch block is predictive of a worse prognosis (178, 179) in patients with left ventricular systolic dysfunction and may also identify patients who benefit from a specific treatment (cardiac resynchronization therapy). The same is true of atrial fibrillation where there may be an indication for warfarin.

Chest X-ray

The chest X-ray (or radiograph) is also recommended as a first-line investigation (➲ Fig. 23.16). It may identify a non-cardiac cause for the patient's symptoms. It also provides information on the size and shape of the cardiac silhouette and the state of the pulmonary vasculature [180]. This information is, however, of limited value [181]. The absence of cardiomegaly (➲ Fig. 23.20) does not exclude valve disease or left ventricular systolic dysfunction (heart size is more often normal in patients with left ventricular diastolic dysfunction and in acute compared to chronic heart failure). Even if cardiomegaly is present (➲ Fig. 23.20), the chest X-ray does not identify the cause of cardiac enlargement. The relationship between central haemodynamic and pulmonary vascular radiological abnormalities is also variable and some patients with long-standing severe heart failure may not show pulmonary venous congestion or oedema (➲ Fig. 23.20) despite a very high pulmonary capillary pressure [182].

Haematology and biochemistry

Several laboratory investigations are recommended in the ESC guidelines as part of the routine diagnostic evaluation of patients with suspected heart failure: complete blood count, electrolytes, glucose, urea, creatinine, hepatic enzymes, and urinalysis [1]. Myocardial biomarkers such as troponin T or I are important during an acute episode to rule out myocardial infarction, although some degree of troponin elevation occurs in around a third of patients hospitalized with acute heart failure and is a powerful predictor of outcome [183, 184]. Other tests including serum uric acid, C-reactive protein, and thyroid stimulating hormone are optional. It is important to repeat some of these tests during follow-up and after the initiation of certain treatments (or dose changes), e.g. urea, creatinine, and potassium.

Electrolyte disturbances are uncommon in untreated mild to moderate heart failure.

Hyponatraemia is sometimes found in severe heart failure and its cause is complex and probably multifactorial. Impaired free water excretion, sodium restriction, and diuretic therapy (especially thiazide diuretic treatment or excessive use of loop diuretics) are thought to be important. Hyponatraemia may identify patients with an elevated plasma concentration of arginine vasopressin (AVP) and a particularly activated RAAS [134, 137]. AVP antagonists may have a therapeutic role in patients with hyponatraemia [185].

Potassium concentration is usually normal but may be reduced by the use of kaliuretic agents such as loop diuretics, or increased in patients with end-stage heart failure with markedly reduced glomerular filtration rate, particularly in the presence of concomitant renal disease, treatment with an inhibitor of the RAAS (e.g. some combination of an ACE inhibitor, angiotensin II receptor blocker, or spironolactone) [185]. Nephrotoxic drugs such as NSAIDs may also precipitate hyperkalaemia.

Elevation of creatinine and urea is common in treated heart failure, especially if severe. A significant reduction in glomerular filtration rate may be present despite a normal urea and creatinine, especially in patients with reduced muscle mass. Several causes are recognized: (1) reduced glomerular filtration rate in advanced heart failure; (2) excessive treatment with diuretics alone or in combination with

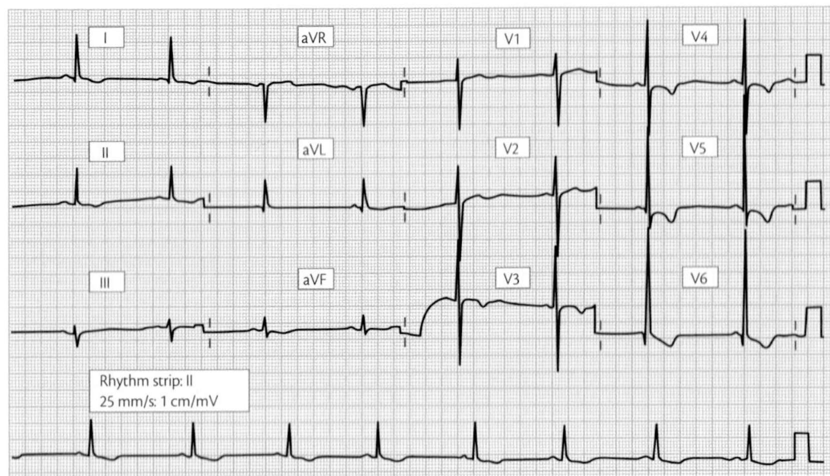

Figure 23.19 Twelve-lead electrocardiogram depicting left ventricular hypertrophy.

inhibitors of the RAAS (e.g. some combination of an ACE inhibitor, angiotensin II receptor blockerl or spironolactone); (3) ageing; and (4) primary renal disease, including renal artery stenosis.

Impaired renal function and worsening renal function are associated with a poor outcome in chronic heart failure though, paradoxically, drugs which improve prognosis, particularly inhibitors of the RAAS, may cause some deterioration in renal function (although this is usually mild).

Elevation of liver enzymes and other markers, including aspartate aminotransferase (AST) and alanine aminotransferase (ALT) and of serum bilirubin is often observed in heart failure. These changes may be caused by reduced hepatic blood flow as much as by liver congestion and are prognostically important [187, 188].

Anaemia may be the cause or consequence of heart failure. It is common, especially in advanced heart failure, and is associated with a worse prognosis.

Urinalysis is important for the detection of proteinuria or glycosuria, indications of underlying renal disease and diabetes mellitus, respectively.

Thyroid function tests are indicated if either hyper- or hypothyroidism is suspected.

Natriuretic peptides

The use of plasma natriuretic peptides as a tool for the diagnosis of heart failure has developed in recent years, particularly in primary care and emergency units (➲Fig. 23.21) [189]. Both BNP and N-terminal pro-BNP are available as commercial assays. In clinical practice, both are used as 'rule out' tests, i.e. a normal concentration of either peptide in an untreated patient means that it is very unlikely that heart failure is present [189]. Conversely, an elevated concentration identifies a patient who merits comprehensive cardiac examination including echocardiography. Natriuretic peptides may, therefore, offer a cost-effective means of ensuring the efficient use of echocardiography. One important caveat is that prior treatment may reduce natriuretic peptide concentrations to within the normal range.

Age and female gender both increase plasma concentration of natriuretic peptides and must be considered when defining 'normal' cut-off values which are also assay-specific [189]. Plasma levels are also increased in other conditions including renal dysfunction, pulmonary embolism, left ventricular hypertrophy, acute ischaemia, and hypertension (but reduced in obesity). Because these various cardiac and non-cardiac disorders lead to a moderate increase in plasma concentrations of natriuretic peptides, a 'grey zone' exists and is the reason why natriuretic peptides are used as a 'rule out' (rather than a 'rule in') test.

In heart failure with preserved EF, plasma levels of BNP, although generally higher than in patients without heart failure, are significantly lower than in patients with left ventricular systolic dysfunction (➲Fig. 23.21) [127]. In a general population, the ability of plasma natriuretic peptides to detect left ventricular hypertrophy appears limited [190]. Patients with relaxation abnormalities and mild symptoms or who are asymptomatic may have normal levels of natriuretic peptides. Thus low levels may not exclude a diagnosis of heart failure with preserved EF although those with more severe diastolic dysfunction seem to have higher natriuretic peptide concentrations [106, 127].

Doppler echocardiography

Transthoracic Doppler echocardiography (or ultrasound) is recognized by the ESC guidelines as the most important investigation for the patient with suspected heart failure.

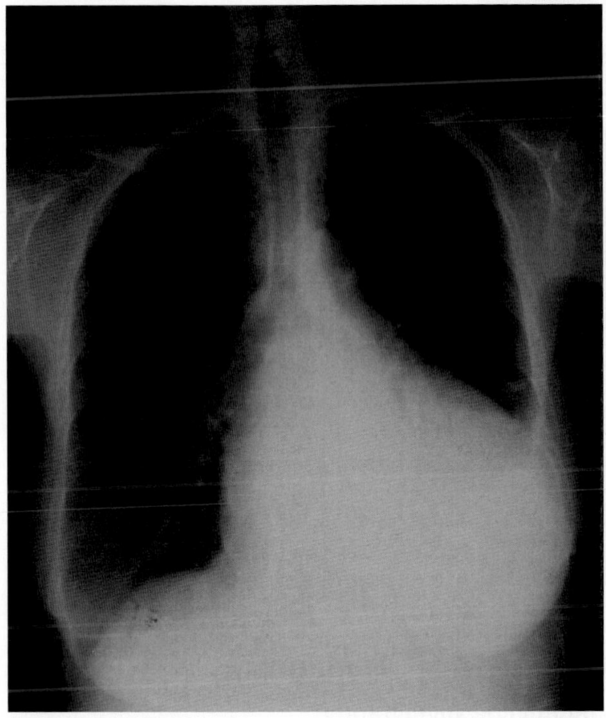

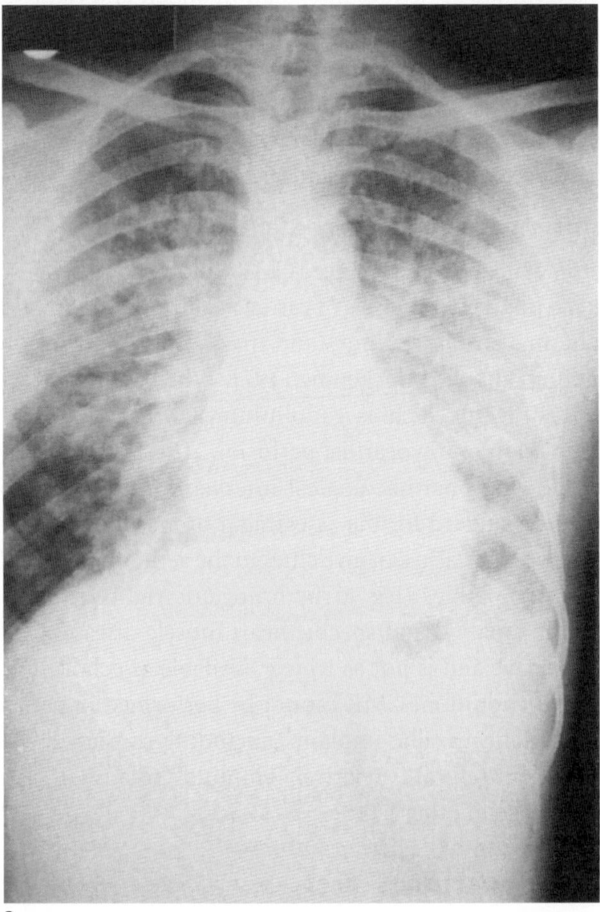

Figure 23.20 Posteroanterior chest X-rays of (A) a patient with left ventricular systolic dysfunction showing marked cardiomegaly; (B) a patient in acute pulmonary oedema. There is evidence of 'bat's wings pulmonary oedema', upper lobe venous diversion, as well as fluid in the horizontal fissure.

Echocardiography is a widely available, rapid, non-invasive, and safe technique which provides extensive information on chamber dimensions, wall thickness, and measures of systolic and diastolic function. Disappointingly, despite the value of Doppler echocardiography, surveys in Europe commonly show that cardiac function is only evaluated in approximately 50% of patients treated for suspected heart failure [191, 192]. The recent development of portable echocardiography machines, together with the potential of remote analysis of echocardiograms, may help improve this situation.

Determination of the LVEF is a key measure of left ventricular systolic function and has been used to enrol patients in almost all important clinical trials. Systolic function is usually considered to be reduced when the LVEF is <0.40 and 'preserved' if >0.50. This clearly leaves a 'grey area' in the range 0.40–0.50. Furthermore, LVEF is a crude method for the evaluation of systolic function and is dependent not only on the intrinsic inotropic state of the myocardium, but also on the loading conditions of the heart.

The most widely recommended approach to the accurate measurement of LVEF is the modified Simpson's method, using apical biplane summation of discs (➲ Fig. 23.22) [193]. It is, however, dependent on reliable endocardial detection. Other methods are less accurate, particularly in the presence of regional hypokinesia or akinesia. Other measures are, however, used including fractional shortening, sphericity index, and left ventricular wall motion index.

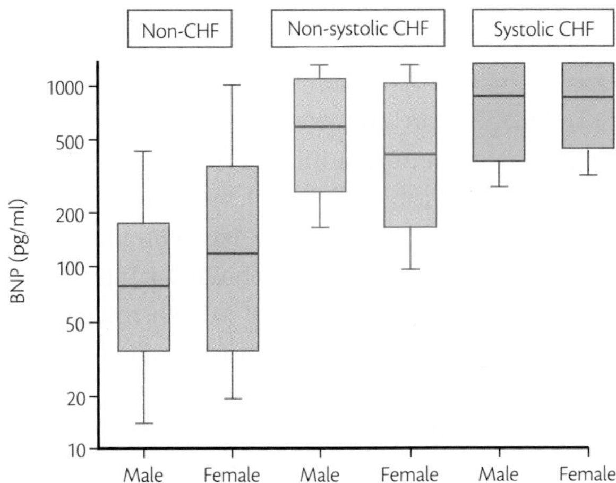

Figure 23.21 Box plots showing median levels of B-type natriuretic peptide (BNP) measured in men and women over 70 years of age with dyspnoea not caused by heart failure, and those with an adjudicated final diagnosis of heart failure, subdivided into those with systolic and those with non-systolic congestive heart failure. CHF, congestive heart failure. Reproduced with permission from Maisel AS, McCord J, Nowak RM, *et al.* Bedside B-type natriuretic peptide in the emergency diagnosis of heart failure with reduced or preserved ejection fraction: Results from the Breathing Not Properly Multinational Study. *J Am Coll Cardiol* 2003; **41**: 2010–17.

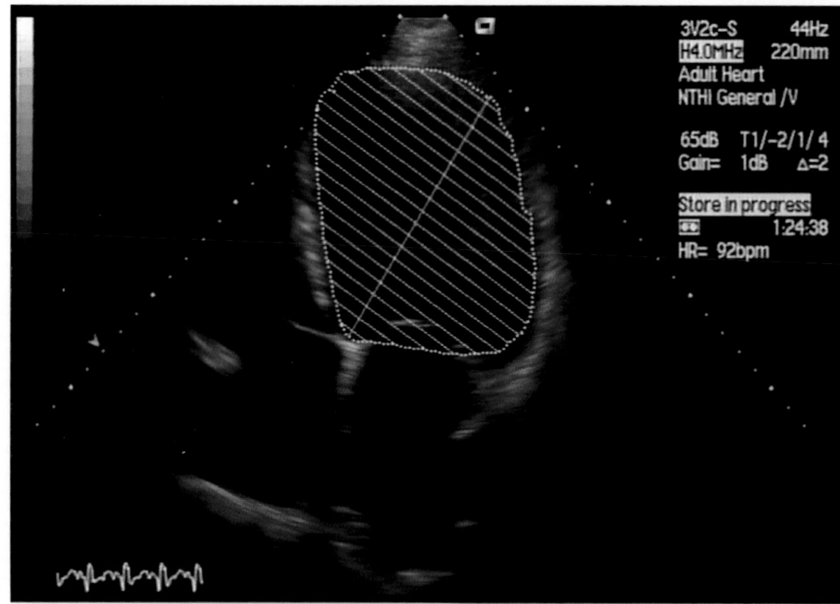

Figure 23.22 Measurement of ejection fraction using Simpson's biplane method. Only the apical four-chamber view at end-diastole is shown here. This young man has a dilated cardiomyopathy, with a left ventricular end-diastolic diameter of 9.7cm.

Identification of diastolic dysfunction is more difficult and requires evidence of abnormal left ventricular relaxation (➲Fig. 23.23) or diastolic distensibility or diastolic stiffness. Which measures to use in daily practice are still debated [106, 194].

The finding of morphological changes such as left atrial dilatation or left ventricular hypertrophy, as well as abnormal measures of left ventricular diastolic function, is particularly helpful in determining whether diastolic dysfunction is clinically important. Abnormal diastolic function has prognostic as well as diagnostic significance [106, 195].

It is important to appreciate that the terms heart failure with preserved EF and heart failure as a result of diastolic dysfunction ('diastolic heart failure') describe overlapping but not identical syndromes.

Valve function can also be assessed by Doppler echocardiography, e.g. semi-quantitative evaluation of mitral regurgitation is possible (➲Fig. 23.14), as is calculation of pulmonary artery systolic pressure (based on the velocity of tricuspid regurgitation). Doppler echocardiography may also be repeated during the follow-up of patients receiving treatment, to assess changes in cardiac structure and function.

Other new ultrasound techniques, such as three-dimensional echocardiography, are still being evaluated clinically.

Stress echocardiography

Dobutamine (or exercise) stress echocardiography (➲Chapter 4) may be used to detect ischaemia as a cause of cardiac dysfunction and to assess myocardial viability in the presence of marked hypokinesia or akinesia. It may be used to identify myocardial stunning and hibernating myocardium [196].

Other imaging techniques

Radionuclide angiography

This technique provides information on left and right ventricular volumes and EF but is not widely available. It does not provide information on valve function but is generally more accurate than echocardiography for measuring right ventricular function. The reproducibility of this technique is also better than that of echocardiography.

Cardiac magnetic resonance (also see ➲Chapter 5)

Cardiac magnetic resonance (CMR) allows comprehensive and reproducible analysis of cardiac anatomy and function, including cardiac volumes and mass, global and regional function, and wall thickening [197]. When combined with contrast agents such as gadolinium, CMR also provides information on myocardial perfusion at rest (➲Fig. 23.24) or following pharmacological intervention. CMR is now the gold standard for the assessment of mass volumes and wall motion. It also can give clues to the aetiology of specific cardiomyopathies (e.g. arrhythmogenic right ventricular cardiomyopathy) and specific heart muscle diseases. CMR is expensive and is not as widely available as echocardiography. In addition, CMR cannot be performed in patients with certain metallic implants, including cardiac devices, and patient refusal is relatively common because of claustrophobia and other factors.

Other functional tests

Exercise testing (also see ➲Chapter 25)

Treadmill or bicycle testing can be used to determine the maximum level of exercise which can be achieved. Recent

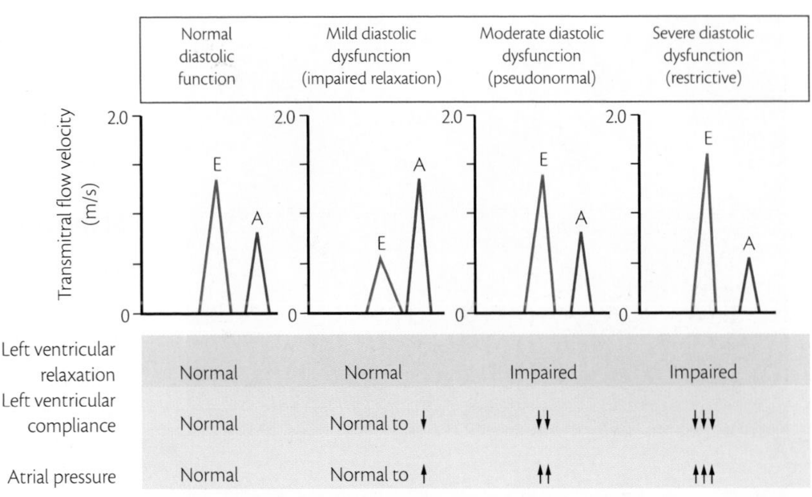

Figure 23.23 Patterns of left ventricular diastolic filling as shown by standard Doppler echocardiography. The abnormal relaxation pattern (mild diastolic dysfunction) is brought on by abnormally slow left ventricular relaxation, a reduced velocity of early filling (E wave), an increase in the velocity associated with atrial contraction (A wave), and a ratio of E to A that is lower than normal. In more advanced heart disease, when left atrial pressure has risen, the E-wave velocity and E: A ratio is similar to that in normal subjects (the pseudonormal pattern). In advanced disease, abnormalities in left ventricular compliance may supervene (called the restrictive pattern because it was originally described in patients with restrictive cardiomyopathy). Reprinted with permission from Aurigemma GP, Gaasch WH. Diastolic Heart Failure. *N Engl J Med* 2004; **351**: 1097–105..

recommendations on testing have been published [198]. Small increments in workload are recommended. As well as exercise duration, gas exchange is often measured. Peak oxygen uptake (VO_2) and the anaerobic threshold are useful indicators of the patient's capacity to exercise. There is a poor correlation between exercise capacity and EF. Peak VO_2 has been used also for prognostication and selection of patients for heart transplantation. A peak VO_2 >14mL/kg/min is associated with a relatively good prognosis unlikely to be improved by heart transplantation. Patients with a VO_2 max of <14mL/kg/min have been shown to have a better survival if transplanted than if treated medically. This latter threshold is part of the criteria used for listing patients for heart transplantation [195]. It should be noted that the survival studies on which this threshold is based were carried out before the advent of modern treatments for heart failure, such as beta-blockers and cardiac resynchronization therapy.

Pulmonary function testing

Pulmonary function testing is indicated in patients in whom the origin of dyspnoea is unclear, to determine whether it is of cardiac or pulmonary origin or both. Heart failure itself is associated with abnormalities of pulmonary function [200]. These include reductions in vital capacity, pulmonary diffusion at rest (and on exercise), and pulmonary compliance. Conversely, airway resistance is usually increased.

Invasive investigations

Pulmonary arterial catheterization is usually only used in acute or emergency situations, especially in patients not responding to appropriate medical therapy and is not routinely indicated [201]. This procedure allows close monitoring of haemodynamic changes following medical intervention. It is also indicated in patients with valvular heart disease who are candidates for valve replacement or repair and in the assessment of patients for transplantation.

Coronary angiography is indicated in patients with heart failure and angina or evidence of myocardial ischaemia, if revascularization is being considered. However, the role of revascularization in the treatment of heart failure, including in patients with hibernating myocardium, remains to be determined [64, 202].

Coronary angiography may also be indicated in acute heart failure with shock that is not responding to initial therapy.

Many also believe that coronary angiography is indicated as a diagnostic test in patients with heart failure or left ventricular systolic dysfunction of unknown origin.

Endomyocardial biopsy of the left or the right ventricle is only indicated when a specific myocarditis or a specific myocardial disease is suspected and during the follow-up of patients after cardiac transplantation to detect graft rejection [203].

Overall, the indication for invasive procedures in heart failure has declined. They are not necessary to establish the presence of heart failure but may be helpful on an individual basis to determine the aetiology and for the monitoring of patients in acute or difficult situations.

Ambulatory ECG monitoring

Ambulatory monitoring is valuable in the assessment of patients with symptoms suggestive of an arrhythmia (e.g. palpitations and syncope) and in monitoring ventricular rate control in patients with atrial fibrillation.

Asymptomatic ventricular premature beats and non-sustained ventricular tachycardia are frequent in heart failure but do not appear to be predictive of sudden death or of selecting treatment to reduce sudden death.

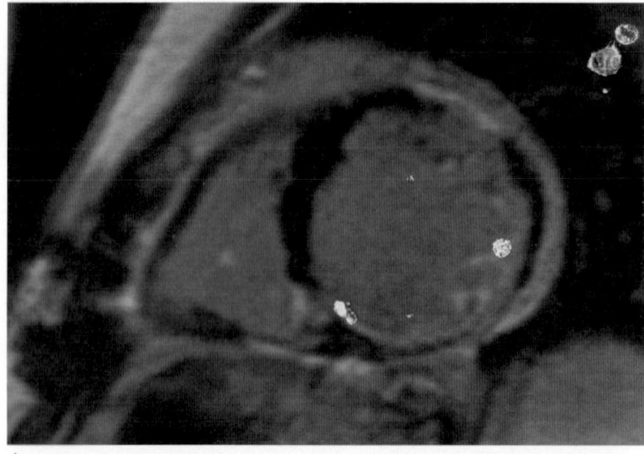
A

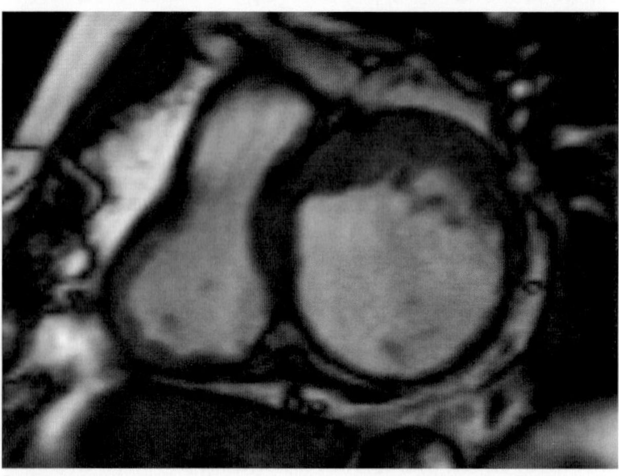
B

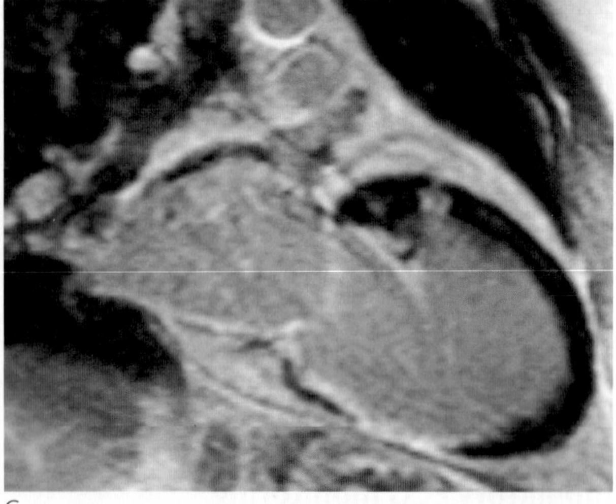
C

Figure 23.24 (A)Short-axis contrast-enhanced CMR demonstrating extensive inferior myocardial infarction indicated by late gadolinium enhancement. There is also a smaller anterior infarct. (B) Non-contrast still end-diastolic cine image showing marked wall thinning in the inferior wall corresponding with the area of infarction. There is marked ventricular dilatation and systolic dysfunction. (C) Vertical long-axis view of the same patient demonstrating both a large inferior infarct and a much smaller apical anterior infarct. (Courtesy of Dr Patrick Mark, Western Infirmary, Glasgow.)

An approach to the diagnosis of a patient with suspected heart failure

The following describes a stepwise approach to the diagnosis of the patient with suspected heart failure (➲Table 23.4).

Step 1: establish the presence of heart failure

This requires the presence of signs and symptoms suggestive of heart failure at rest or on exercise and also objective evidence of a cardiac abnormality, preferably by Doppler echocardiography. Doppler echocardiography may not be necessary in previously untreated patients with a normal plasma natriuretic peptide concentration and these patients should be investigated for another cause of their symptoms or signs (➲Fig. 23.16). Other essential first-line diagnostic tests should be performed, including an ECG, chest X-ray, and blood tests. Pulmonary function and exercise testing may help when the diagnosis remains doubtful.

The diagnosis of heart failure with preserved EF can be particularly difficult. Although often described as a diagnosis of exclusion, i.e. other possible causes of the patient's symptoms and signs must be ruled out, this type of heart failure may co-exist with other relevant comorbidities, e.g. chronic lung disease and anaemia. ➲Figs. 23.25 and 23.26 show an approach to this problem.

Step 2: evaluation of the patient's clinical status

This step includes:

- The assessment of clinical profile: patients may present with acute new-onset heart failure, e.g. after acute myocardial infarction, acute or subacute decompensation of chronic heart failure, or acute or subacute onset of heart failure in a patient with previously asymptomatic cardiac dysfunction. The clinical presentation may be in primary care or to hospital. The patient may have breathlessness, fatigue, or both with few clinical signs. Alternatively, the patient may have these symptoms and peripheral oedema or may present as an emergency with frank pulmonary oedema. The clinical profile of patients with preserved systolic function may be different from that of patients with systolic dysfunction: on average, the former patients are older and are more likely to be women. They are also more likely to have hypertension but are less likely to have a third heart sound [106]. It is important to assess the severity of symptoms, with the Killip and NYHA classifications being the most widely used in the acute and chronic setting, respectively. In acute new-onset heart failure, the patient may be

Table 23.4 Stepwise approach to the diagnosis of heart failure

Step 1: Diagnosis
Signs and symptoms of heart failure
History of cardiac disease
First-line tests: ECG, X-ray, BNP or NT-proBNP
Documentation of cardiac dysfunction: Doppler echocardiography
Nuclear angiography/Nuclear magnetic resonance
Step 2: Clinical profile
Clinical presentation: acute *de novo*/decompensated/chronic heart failure
Left/right side heart failure
Comorbidities
Age and severity
Step 3: Aetiology
Consider other diagnostic tests (coronary angiography, central haemodynamics, etc.)
Step 4: Precipitating factors
Anaemia
Infection (pulmonary infection)
Tachycardia (atrial fibrillation)
Bradycardia
Pulmonary embolism
Hypertensive crisis
Acute myocardial ischaemia
Poor compliance (diet and/or drugs)
Thyroid disorders
Medications (NSAIDs, cyclooxygenase-2 inhibitors, glitazones, class I antiarrhythmics, corticosteroids, tricyclic antidepressants)
Valve disorders
Acute myocardial ischaemia
Step 5: Prognostic evaluation
Clinical factors (e.g. age, sex)
Biological factors (e.g. blood pressure, ejection fraction)
Neurohumoral factors and cytokines
Electrical variables (e.g. bundle branch block, arrhythmias)
Imaging variables
Exercise testing
Central haemodynamic indices
Genetic factors
Comorbidities (e.g. diabetes mellitus)
Step 6: Treatment and follow-up

hypotensive if there has been a haemodynamic catastrophe, e.g. rupture of a mitral valve papillary muscle or interventricular septum (➲Fig. 23.27).

- In advanced heart failure, another system of classification has been advocated. This is based on the presence/absence of signs of congestion and adequate/inadequate perfusion. Four categories have been proposed: dry–warm; wet–warm; dry–cold; and wet–cold [1, 204]. Wet patients with or without hypoperfusion are at higher risk than dry patients.
- It is also important to identify comorbidities such as stroke, chronic obstructive pulmonary disease, asthma, diabetes mellitus, and renal failure, which can complicate patient management and modify outcome. The proportion of patients presenting with multiple comorbidities increases with age. In the Euro Heart Failure Survey, 9% had had a previous stroke, 10% a previous transient ischaemic attack, 27% were reported to have diabetes mellitus, 12% had dementia, 17% a renal dysfunction, and 32% a pulmonary disease [191].

Step 3: identify underlying aetiology

Ischaemic heart disease and hypertension are the commonest causes of heart failure in Western countries and their contribution to heart failure is also rapidly expanding in the developing countries. In the Euro Heart Failure Survey, ischaemic heart disease was the commonest cause of heart failure, 40% of patients having myocardial infarction and 51% a history of angina; 53% of the patients also had hypertension [191]. The extent of investigation to identify the underlying cardiac disease should be decided on an individual basis taking into consideration the patient profile (age, severity of heart failure and comorbidities) and the potential reversibility of cardiac dysfunction (such as valvular heart disease and reversible ischaemia).

Step 4: identify precipitating factors

It is also important to identify precipitating factors: decompensation of heart failure is frequently associated with comorbid factors which:

- increase body metabolic requirements such as fever, infection (hence the recommendation that influenza and pneumococcal immunization/vaccination is offered to patients with heart failure) [1] or hyperthyroidism;
- decrease cardiac output due to a rapid tachycardia or marked bradycardia;

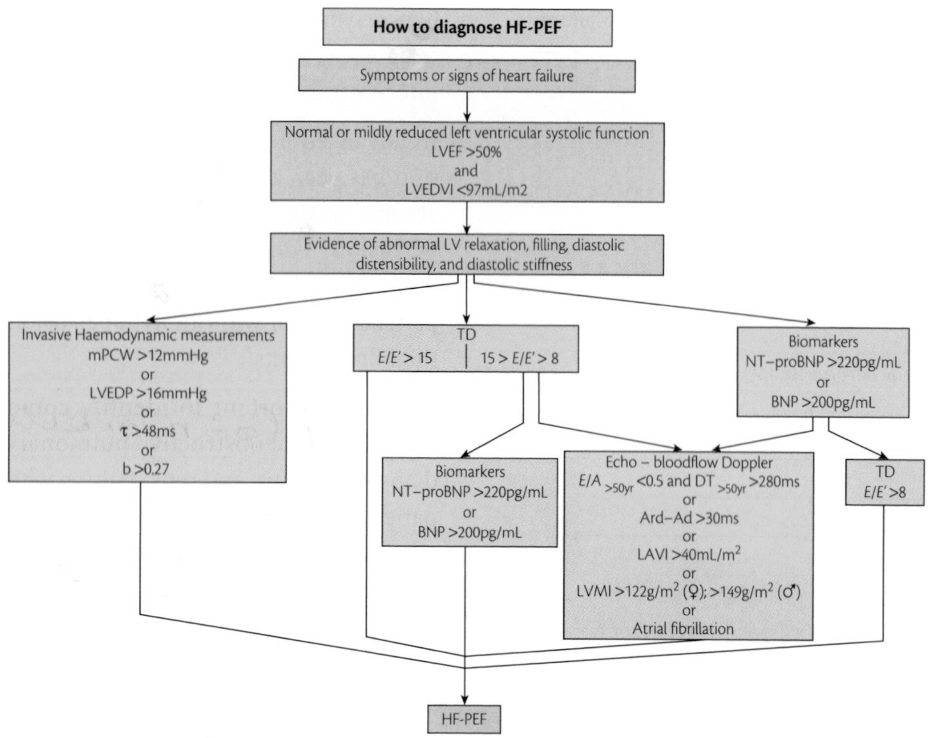

Figure 23.25 Diagnostic flowchart on 'How to diagnose HF-PEF' in a patient suspected of HF-PEF. LVEDVI, left ventricular end-diastolic volume index; mPCW, mean pulmonary capillary wedge pressure; LVEDP, left ventricular end-diastolic pressure; τ, time constant of left ventricular relaxation; b, constant of left ventricular chamber stiffness; TD, tissue Doppler; E, early mitral valve flow velocity; E', early TD lengthening velocity; NT-proBNP, N-terminal-pro brain natriuretic peptide; BNP, brain natriuretic peptide; *E/A*, ratio of early (*E*) to late (*A*) mitral flow velocity; DT, deceleration time; LVMI, left ventricular mass index; LAVI, left atrial volume index; Ard, duration of reverse pulmonary vein atrial systole flow; Ad, duration of mitral valve atrial wave flow. Reproduced with permission from Paulus WJ, Tschope C, Sanderson JE, *et al.* How to diagnose diastolic heart failure: a consensus statement on the diagnosis of heart failure with normal left ventricular ejection fraction by the Heart Failure and Echocardiography Associations of the European Society of Cardiology. *Eur Heart J* 2007; **28**: 2539–50.

- reduce the oxygen transport capacity (anaemia) or oxygen exchange (pulmonary infection);
- induce a sudden haemodynamic overload (pulmonary embolism or hypertensive crisis) or water and sodium overload (excessive sodium intake, poor compliance with diet, and heart failure medications)
- ischaemic episodes (➲Table 23.4).

Air pollution and seasonal temperature changes are more recently described factors associated with risk of decompensation and hospitalization [200, 201].

Among arrhythmias, a new episode of atrial fibrillation can be particularly harmful because it combines both an increase in ventricular rate (with a risk of myocardial ischaemia and reduced time for diastolic filling) and loss of atrial contraction [205, 206].

Step 5: prognostic evaluation

Prognostic assessment in heart failure remains difficult. Indeed the number of clinical, aetiological, comorbid, biological, haemodynamic, structural, functional, electrical, and neurohumoral variables independently associated with poor outcome is high and suggests that there is no simple method to assess the risk of death or rehospitalization in patients with this syndrome (➲Table 23.5) [209, 210]. Most studies have been performed in populations of patients with systolic dysfunction and little is known about prognostic evaluation in patients with preserved systolic function.

The assessment of prognosis has also been conducted differently in acute and in chronic heart failure: in acute heart failure, in-hospital and short-term (3–6 months) mortality or readmission have usually been evaluated whereas in chronic heart failure, long-term (>1 year) prognosis and rehospitalization rates have normally been considered.

Furthermore, factors which predispose to overall mortality or pump failure mortality do not necessarily apply to sudden death.

An additional problem is that extrapolation of risk assessment based on a small series of selected patients exposed to conventional therapy (including low rate of prescription of ACE inhibitors and beta-blockers) to the overall

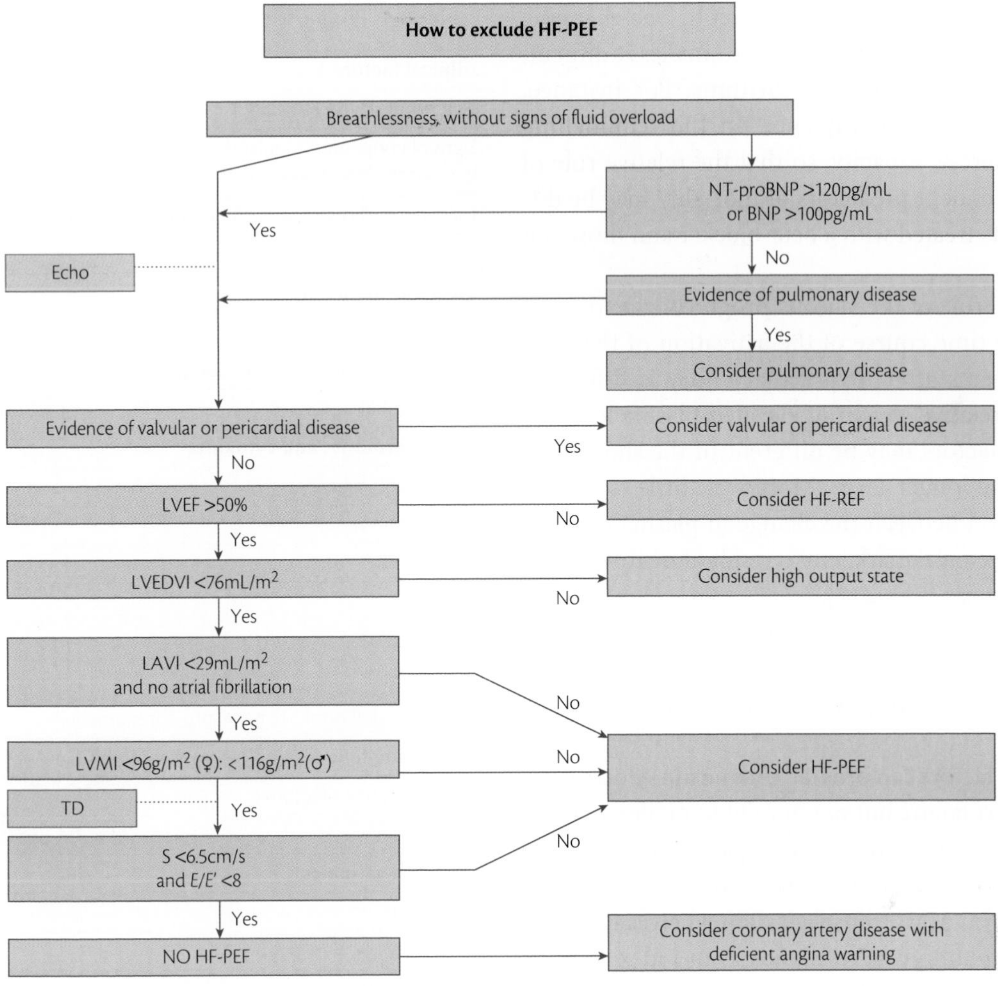

Figure 23.26 Diagnostic flow chart on 'How to exclude HF-PEF in a patient presenting with breathlessness and no signs of fluid overload. S, TD shortening velocity; TD, tissue Doppler. Reproduced with permission from Paulus WJ, Tschope C, Sanderson JE, *et al*.. How to diagnose diastolic heart failure: a consensus statement on the diagnosis of heart failure with normal left ventricular ejection fraction by the Heart Failure and Echocardiography Associations of the European Society of Cardiology. *Eur Heart J* 2007; **28**: 2539–50.

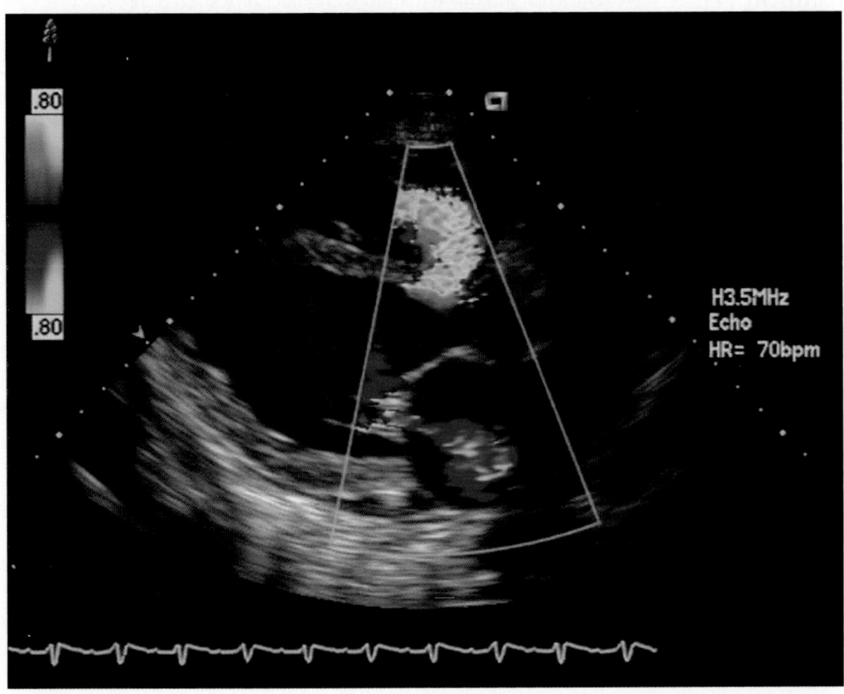

Figure 23.27 Colour flow Doppler of mitral regurgitation and a ventricular septal rupture post-myocardial infarction in the parasternal long-axis view.

current heart failure population is difficult. The changing background therapy of heart failure also makes it difficult to provide simple prognostic algorithms. For instance, beta-blockers have more influence on the remodelling process than exercise capacity, so that the relative role of these two independent predictors of mortality may be different in patients treated with a beta-blocker and those not so treated.

The temporal role of the various prognostic factors can be variable: the time course of the activation of the neurohumoral systems after myocardial injury is different. Therefore, the relative weight of elevated plasma levels of neurohumoral factors may be different in the short term compared to the longer term. Moreover, little is known about the relation between the change in plasma concentrations of biochemical markers as a result of treatment and long-term prognosis [211, 212].

The multivariable analyses reported so far usually include only a limited number of parameters and these may lose their predictive power in more comprehensive analyses.

Finally, some factors can provide prognostic information in advanced heart failure but not in mild to moderate heart failure: severely reduced functional capacity, measured by VO_2, is a recognized index for the selection of patients who might benefit from heart transplantation whereas elevated, non-reversible, pulmonary resistance is an index of poor outcome after heart transplantation or implantation of a ventricular assist device [199].

Step 6: treatment and management

Full diagnosis is a prerequisite for optimal treatment [1]. Often, however, a diuretic may be required before a full diagnostic work-up is completed. The further treatment of heart failure depends on the underlying aetiology (e.g. valve replacement for aortic stenosis), functional status (e.g. spironolactone for severely symptomatic patients), comorbidity (e.g. warfarin if atrial fibrillation), and the results of investigations (e.g. cardiac resynchronization therapy if a broad QRS on the ECG). Each of these may contraindicate treatments as well as indicate them (e.g. caution with ACE inhibitors in aortic stenosis, beta-blockers if atrioventricular block, spironolactone if renal dysfunction etc.).

Table 23.5 Prognostic factors

Clinical factors
Age, ethnicity, NYHA class
Signs of congestion, jugular vein pressure, third heart sound, low systolic blood pressure
Diabetes mellitus, renal dysfunction, depression
Ischaemic aetiology
Biochemical factors
Serum sodium
Serum creatinine/creatinine clearance
Haemoglobin
Neurohormones and cytokines
Plasma renin activity
Angiotensin II
Aldosterone
Galectin-3
Norepinephrine
Endothelin-1
Adrenomedullin/mid-regional pro-adrenomedullin
B type natriuretic peptide/N-terminal pro-BNP
Tumour necrosis factor-α
Vasopressin
Electrical variables
QRS width
Left ventricular hypertrophy
Atrial fibrillation
Complex ventricular arrhythmia
Heart rate variability
Imaging variables
Left ventricular internal dimensions and fractional shortening
Cardiothoracic ratio X-ray (normal <0.55)
Wall motion index (various*)
Ejection fraction (normal >0.40)
Restrictive filling pattern/short deceleration time (various*)
Right ventricular function (various*)
Mitral regurgitation
Estimated pulmonary artery pressure
Exercise test/haemodynamic variables (rest/exercise)
Vo_2 max/peak (normal >20mL/kg/min†)
6-minute walk distance (normal >600 m†)
Cardiac index (normal >2.5 L/min/m^2)
Left ventricular end-diastolic pressure/pulmonary artery wedge pressure (normal <12mmHg)

* Various measures/classifications can be used and no single threshold for normal/abnormal can be given; † functional capacity varies greatly according to prior fitness, age and sex; values given are a guideline for older (>65 years) adults.

Treatment

The goals of treatment for patients with heart failure are relief of symptoms, avoidance of hospital admission, and prevention of premature death.

Heart failure with a low left ventricular ejection fraction

Pharmacological treatment

Drugs are the mainstay of the treatment of patients with heart failure based upon a series of key randomized controlled trials (➲Table 23.6). However, devices and surgery have an important and increasing role, particularly in patients with more severe heart failure (➲Fig. 23.28). How care is structured and delivered is also important. Although lifestyle measures are also considered important, the evidence base for these interventions is less robust.

Diuretics

Mechanism of action

Diuretics act by blocking sodium reabsorption at specific sites in the renal tubule, thereby enhancing urinary excretion of sodium and water.

Clinical benefits

Although not proven to improve mortality and morbidity in large trials, diuretics are required in nearly all patients with symptomatic heart failure to relieve dyspnoea and the signs of sodium and water retention ('congestion'), i.e. peripheral and pulmonary oedema [213, 214]. No other treatment relieves symptoms and the signs of sodium and water overload as rapidly and effectively. Once a patient needs a diuretic, treatment is usually necessary for the rest of the patient's life, though the dose and type of diuretic may vary.

Practical use

The key principle is to prescribe the minimum dose of diuretic needed to maintain an oedema-free state ('dry weight') [213]. Excessive use can lead to electrolyte imbalances, such as hyponatraemia, hypokalaemia (with the risk of digitalis toxicity), hyperuricaemia (with the risk of gout), and uraemia. The risk of renal dysfunction is increased by concomitant use of NSAIDs. Diuretic-induced hypovolaemia may also cause symptomatic hypotension and pre-renal uraemia. Restriction of dietary sodium intake may help reduce, but not eliminate, the requirement for diuretics. Diuretic dosing should be flexible with temporary increases for evidence of fluid retention (e.g. increasing symptoms, weight gain, oedema) and decreases for evidence of hypovolaemia (e.g. as consequence of increased electrolyte loss owing to gastroenteritis, decreased fluid intake, or both).

In some patients with milder symptoms of heart failure (NYHA class II), a thiazide diuretic such as bendroflumethiazide may suffice. In more severe heart failure or in patients with concomitant renal dysfunction, a loop diuretic such as furosemide is often needed. Loop diuretics cause a rapid onset of an intense but relatively short-lived diuresis, compared with the longer-lasting but gentler effect of a thiazide diuretic. The timing of administration of a loop diuretic, which need not be taken first thing every morning, can be adjusted according to the patient's social activities. The dose may be postponed or even temporarily omitted if the patient has to travel or has another activity that might be compromised by the prompt action of the diuretic. In severe heart failure, the effects of long-term administration of a loop diuretic may be diminished by increased sodium reabsorption at the distal tubule. This problem can be offset by use of the combination of a loop diuretic and a thiazide or thiazide-like diuretic (e.g. metolazone), which acts in synergy with a loop diuretic by blocking sodium reabsorption in different segments of the nephron [215]. This combination requires more frequent monitoring of electrolytes and renal function for diuretic-induced hyponatraemia, abnormalities of the serum potassium level, and prerenal uraemia.

A period of intravenous loop diuretic, given either as bolus injections or by continuous infusion, may be required in patients who become resistant to the action of oral diuretics [216]. Why this resistance develops is uncertain, but factors thought to be important include impaired absorption of oral diuretics owing to gut oedema, hypotension, reduced renal blood flow, and adaptive changes in the nephron. In cases of severe resistant volume overload, mechanical removal of fluid using ultra-filtration may be considered [217].

Patients with severe failure (NYHA class III–IV) should usually also be treated with an aldosterone antagonist, such as spironolactone, which increases excretion of sodium but not potassium [218]. Patients receiving a combination of diuretics require careful monitoring of blood chemistry and clinical status. The use of a potassium sparing diuretic or aldosterone antagonist along with an ACE inhibitor or ARB (*treatment with all three is not recommended*) requires particular care and surveillance for hyperkalaemia [219].

Although highly effective in relieving symptoms and signs, diuretics alone are not a sufficient treatment for heart failure. The addition of other disease-modifying treatments is essential to slow pathophysiological progression, better maintain clinical stability, and reduce the risk of hospital admission and premature death.

ACE inhibitors

Mechanism of action

These drugs act by inhibiting the enzyme that converts the inactive decapeptide angiotensin I to the active octapeptide

Table 23.6 Positive randomized controlled trials[*] in patients with symptomatic heart failure and a low left ventricular ejection fraction

Treatment, trial, year published	N	Severity of heart failure	Estimated first year placebo/ control group mortality	Background treatment[**]	Treatment added	Trial duration (years)	Primary endpoint	RRR (%)[***]	Events prevented per 1000 patients treated[††]		
									Death	HF Hosp.	Death or HF Hosp.
ACE inhibitors											
CONSENSUS 1987	253	End-stage	52	Spiro	Enalapril 20mg BID	0.54[†]	Death	40	146	–	–
SOLVD-T 1991	2569	Mild–severe	15.7	–	Enalapril 20mg BID	3.5	Death	16	45	96	108
Beta-blockers											
CIBIS-2 1999	2647	Moderate–severe	13.2	ACE-I	Bisoprolol 10mg QD	1.3[†]	Death	34	55	56	–
MERIT-HF 1999	3991	Mild–serve	11.0	ACE-I	Metoprolol CR/XL, 200mg QD	1.0[†]	Death	34	36	46	63
COPERNICUS 2001	2289	Severe	19.7	ACE-I	Carvedilol 25mg BID	0.87[†]	Death	35	55	65	81
SENIORS 2005	2128	Mild–severe	8.5	ACE-I + Spiro	Nebivolol 10mg QD	1.75	Death or CV Hosp.	14	23	0	0
ARBs											
Val-HeFT 2001	5010	Mild–severe	8.0	ACE-I	Valsartan 160mg BID	1.9	CV Death or Morbidity	13	0	35	33[†††]
CHARM-Alternative 2003	2028	Mild–severe	12.6	BB	Candesartan 32mg QD	2.8	CV Death or HF Hosp.	23	30	31	60
CHARM-Added 2003	2548	Moderate–severe	10.6	ACE-I +BB	Candesartan 32mg QD	3.4	CV Death or HF Hosp.	15	28	47	39
Aldosterone blockade											
RALES 1999	1663	Severe	25	ACE-I	Spirolactone 25–50mg QD	2.0[†]	Death	30	113	95	–
H-ISDN											
V-HeFT-1 1986	459	Mild–severe	26.4	–	Hydralazine 75mg TID–QID ISDN 40mg QID	2.3	Death	34	52	0	–
A-HeFT 2004	1050	Moderate–severe	9.0	ACE-I+BB + Spiro	Hydralazine 75mg TID ISDN 40mg TID	0.83[†]	Composite	–	40	80	–
n-3 PUFA											
GISSI-HF 2008	6975	Mild–severe	9.0	ACE-I + BB + Spiro	n-3 PUFA 1g QD	3.9	Death Death or CV Hosp.	9 8	18	0	–

Digitalis glycosides											
DIG 1997	6800	Mild–severe	11.0	ACE-I	Digoxin	3.1	Death	0	0	79	73
Exercise											
HF-ACTION 2009	2331	Mild–severe	6.0	ACE-I + BB + Spiro	Exercise	2.5	Death or CV Hosp.	11	0	–	–
CRT											
COMPANION 2004	925	Moderate–severe	19.0	ACE-I + BB + Spiro	CRT	1.35†	Death or Any Hosp.	19	38	–	87
CARE-HF 2005	813	Moderate–severe	12.6	ACE-I + BB + Spiro	CRT	2.45	Death or CV Hosp.	37	97	151	184
CRT-D											
COMPANION 2004	903	Moderate–severe	19.0	ACE-I + BB + Spiro	CRT-ICD	1.35†	Death or Any Hosp.	20	74	–	114
ICD											
SCD-HeFT 2005	1676	Mild–severe	7.0	ACE-I + BB	ICD	3.8	Death	23	–	–	–
VAD											
REMATCH 2001	129	End-stage	75	ACE-I + Spiro	LVAD	1.8	Death	48	282	–	–

* excluding active–controlled trials (patients with preserved LVEF as well as low LVEF were included in CONSNSUS and SENIORS).; ** in >1/3 of patients: ACE-I + BB means ACE-Is used in almost all patients and BB in the majority. Most patients also taking diuretics and many digoxin (except in DIG). Spironolactone was used at baseline in 5% Val-HeFT, 8% MERIT-HF, 17% CHARM-Added, 19% SCD-HeFT, 20% COPERNICUS, and 24% in CHARM Alternative. *** relative risk reduction in primary endpoint. HF hosp., patients with at least one hospital admission for worsening HF; some patients had multiple admissions.; † stopped early for benefit.; †† individual trials may not have been designed or powered to evaluate effect of treatment on these outcomes.; ††† primary endpoint which also included treatment of HF with intravenous drugs for 4 hours or more without admission and resuscitated cardiac arrest (both added small numbers).

ACE-I, angiotensin-converting enzyme inhibitor; ARB, angiotensin receptor blocker; BB, beta-blocker; CRT, cardiac resynchronisation therapy (biventricular pacing); CRT-D, CRT device that also defibrillates; CV,cardiovascular; hosp., hospital admission; ICD, implantable cardioverter defibrillator; ISDN, isosorbide dinitrate; LVAD, left ventricular assist device; pub., published; RRR, relative risk reduction; spiro, spironolactone; VAD, ventricular assist device.

A-HeFT, African-American Heart Failure Trial; CARE HF, Cardiac Resynchronization-Heart Failure; COPERNICUS, Carvedilol Prospective Randomized Cumulative Survival; CIBIS, Cardiac Insufficiency Bisoprolol Study COMPANION, Comparison of Medical Therapy, Pacing, and Defibrillation in Heart Failure; CONSENSUS, Cooperative North Scandinavian Enalapril Survival Study; DIG, Digitalis Investigation Group; GISSI-HF, Gruppo Italiano per lo Studio della Sopravvivenza nell'Infarto Miocardico -Heart Failure; HF-ACTION, Heart Failure- A Controlled Trial Investigating Outcomes Exercise TraiNing; MERIT-HF, Metoprolol CR/XL Randomized Intervention Trial in congestive heart failure; RALES, Randomized Aldactone Evaluation Study; REMATCH, Randomized Evaluation of Mechanical Assistance for the Treatment of Congestive Heart Failure; SENIORS, Study of Effects of Nebivolol Intervention on Outcomes and Rehospitalization in Seniors with Heart Failure; SOLVD-T, Studies of Left Ventricular Dysfunction Treatment; V-HeFT, Vasodilator Heart Failure Trial; Val-HeFT, Valsartan Heart Failure Trial.

Adapted with permission from McMurray JJ, Pfeffer MA. Heart failure. *Lancet* 2005; **365**: 1877–89.

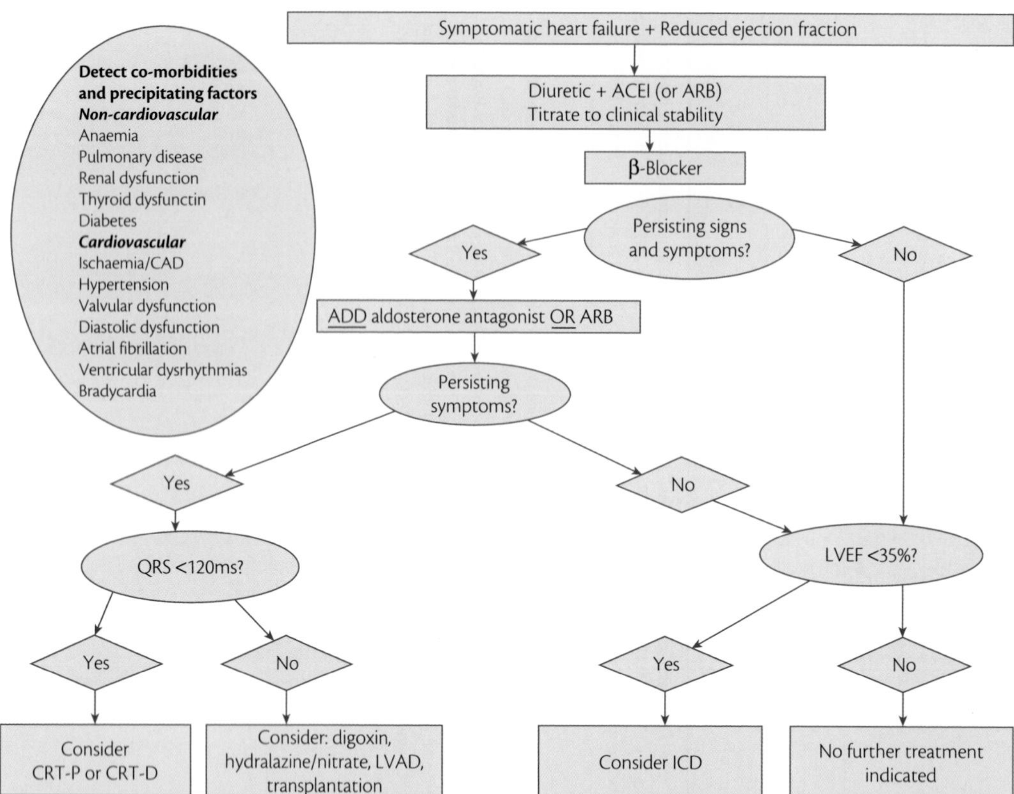

Figure 23.28 A treatment algorithm for patients with symptomatic heart failure and reduced ejection fraction. ACE-I, angiotensin-converting enzyme inhibitor; ARB, angiotensin receptor blocker; CAD, coronary artery disease; CRT, cardiac resynchronization therapy (D, with defibrillator function; P, pacing only); ICD, implantable cardioverter defibrillator; LVAD, left ventricular assist device; LVEF, left ventricular ejection fraction. Dickstein K, Cohen-Solal A, Filippatos G, *et al.* ESC Guidelines for the diagnosis and treatment of acute and chronic heart failure 2008: The Task Force for the Diagnosis and Treatment of Acute and Chronic Heart Failure 2008 of the European Society of Cardiology. Developed in collaboration with the Heart Failure Association of the ESC (HFA) and endorsed by the European Society of Intensive Care Medicine (ESICM). *Eur Heart J* 2008; **29**: 2388–422. Copyright ©ESC, 2008.

angiotensin II. Excessive angiotensin II is thought to exert the myriad of harmful actions described earlier by stimulating the angiotensin II type 1 receptor subtype (AT_1R)—see ➲ Pathophysiology, p.843. ACE inhibitors also reduce the breakdown of bradykinin (as ACE is identical to kininase II) and the resultant accumulation of bradykinin is directly or indirectly responsible for two of the specific adverse effects of ACE inhibitors: cough and angio-oedema. Bradykinin may, however, also have beneficial effects (vasodilation, inhibition of adverse cardiovascular remodelling, and antithrombotic actions), though the importance of these bradykinin-mediated actions to the clinical benefits of ACE inhibition is uncertain.

Clinical benefits

When added to diuretics and digoxin, treatment with an ACE inhibitor decreases left ventricular size, improves systolic function, reduces symptoms and hospital admissions, and prolongs survival (➲ Table 23.6; Fig. 23.29) [220, 221]. These agents also reduce the risk of developing myocardial infarction and possibly atrial fibrillation [222]. Consequently, treatment with an ACE inhibitor is recommended for all patients with systolic dysfunction, irrespective of symptom severity or aetiology. ACE inhibitors are not a substitute for a diuretic but mitigate diuretic-induced hypokalaemia.

Practical use

ACE inhibitors should be introduced as early as possible in a patient's treatment [219]. The only contraindications are current symptomatic hypotension, severe aortic stenosis, and bilateral renal artery stenosis; the latter is often associated with a prompt and marked increase in serum levels of blood urea and creatinine when renal perfusion is reduced precipitously by inhibiting the production and actions of angiotensin. Treatment should be started in a low dose (➲ Table 23.7) and gradually increased toward that proven to be of benefit in a clinical trial (➲ Table 23.8). The patient should be evaluated for symptomatic hypotension, uraemia, and hyperkalaemia after each dose increment; these adverse effects are uncommon and can usually be resolved by reduction in the dose of diuretic (if the patient is oedema free) or concomitant hypotensive or nephrotoxic medications (e.g. nitrates, calcium-channel blockers, or NSAIDs). A dry, non-productive cough occurs in approximately 15% of patients treated with an ACE inhibitor and, if troublesome, substitution of an ARB is recommended [223]. In the rare cases of angio-oedema, the ACE inhibitor should be stopped and not used again; an ARB can be cautiously substituted.

Angiotensin receptor blockers

Mechanism of action

Instead of inhibiting the production of angiotensin II through ACE, ARBs block the binding of angiotensin II to the AT_1R. This distinct mechanism of action may be important because angiotensin II is also believed to be produced by other enzymes such as chymase. ARBs do not inhibit kininase II or the breakdown of bradykinin, so they do not cause cough or angio-oedema.

Clinical benefits

When used as the *sole* RAAS blocking agent in addition to a diuretic and digoxin, ARBs produce similar benefits to ACE inhibitors and can be substituted for them in patients who have cough or angio-oedema with ACE inhibitors [223, 224]. When used in clinically-effective doses, other adverse effects such as hypotension, renal dysfunction, and hyperkalaemia are encountered as frequently as with an ACE inhibitor. As with an ACE inhibitor, the specific agents, dosing regimens, and target doses that were of demonstrable benefit in clinical trials are recommended (➲Table 23.7).

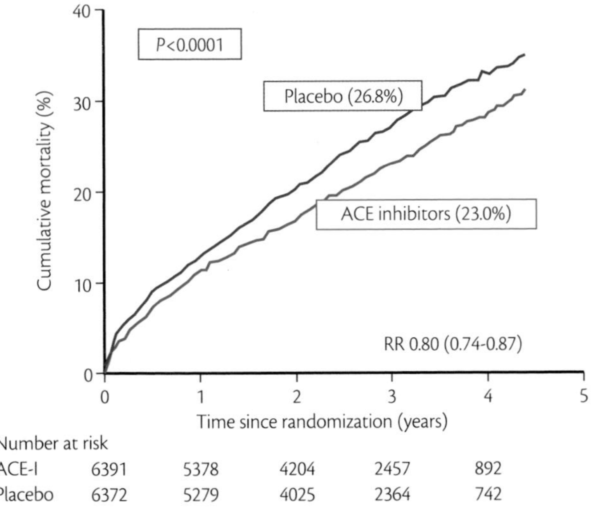

Figure 23.29 Meta-analysis of long-term (> 1-year duration) placebo-controlled trials (> 1000 patients) of angiotensin-converting enzyme (ACE) inhibitors in chronic heart failure or left ventricular dysfunction after a recent myocardial infarction. RR, relative risk. Reproduced with permission from Flather, MD, Yusuf, Køber L, *et al.* Long-term ACE-inhibitor therapy in patients with heart failure or left-ventricular dysfunction: a systematic overview of data from individual patients. ACE-Inhibitor Myocardial Infarction Collaborative Group. *Lancet* 2000; **355**: 1575–81.

An ARB used in *combination* with an ACE inhibitor (and beta-blocker) further improves LVEF, relieves symptoms, reduces the risk of hospital admission for worsening heart failure, and can also reduce the risk of cardiovascular death (➲Table 23.6) [225–228]. Consequently, the addition of an ARB to both an ACE inhibitor and a beta-blocker should be considered in any patient with persisting symptoms (NYHA class II–IV). There is, however, also strong evidence that adding an aldosterone antagonist to an ACE inhibitor is of benefit in patients with advanced (NYHA class III–IV) heart failure (see ➲ Aldosterone antagonists, Clinical benefits, p.874), but the efficacy and safety of the four-drug combination of an ACE inhibitor, beta-blocker, ARB, and aldosterone antagonist are uncertain [218, 229]. *Consequently, either an ARB or an aldosterone antagonist, but not both, should be added to an ACE inhibitor and a beta-blocker in such patients.*

The approach to initiation, titration, and monitoring of an ARB is similar to an ACE inhibitor (➲Table 23.9). The adverse effects, with the exception of cough and angio-oedema, are similar. Use of multiple inhibitors of the RAAS requires even more diligent monitoring, especially in patients at higher risk of uraemia, hypotension, or hyperkalaemia (i.e. patients ≥75

Table 23.7 Dosages of commonly used drugs in heart failure

	Starting dose (mg)	Target dose (mg) ACE-I
Captopril	6.25 TID	50–100 TID
Enalapril	2.5 BID	10–20 BID
Lisinopril	2.5–5.0 OD	20–35 OD
Ramipril	2.5 OD	5 BID
Trandolapril	0.5 OD	4 OD
ARB		
Candesartan	4 or 8 OD	32 OD
Valsartan	40 BID	160 BID
Aldosterone antagonist		
Eplerenone	25 OD	50 OD
Spironolactone	25 OD	25–50 OD
Beta-blocker		
Bisoprolol	1.25 OD	10 OD
Carvedilol	3.125 BID	25–50 BID
Metoprolol succinate	12.2/25 OD	200 OD
Nebivolol	1.25 OD	10 OD

ACE-I, angiotensin-converting enzyme inhibitor; ARB, angiotensin receptor blocker; BID, twice daily; OD, once daily;TID, three times daily.

Adapted with permission from Dickstein K, Cohen-Solal A, Filippatos G, *et al.* ESC guidelines for the diagnosis and treatment of acute and chronic heart failure 2008: the Task Force for the diagnosis and treatment of acute and chronic heart failure 2008 of the European Society of Cardiology. Developed in collaboration with the Heart Failure Association of the ESC (HFA) and endorsed by the European Society of Intensive Care Medicine (ESICM). *Eur Heart J* 2008; **29**: 2388–442. Copyright © ESC 2008.

Table 23.8 Practical guidance on the use of ACE inhibitors in patients with heart failure due to left ventricular systolic dysfunction

Why?

Two major randomized trials (CONSENSUS I and SOLVD-T) and a meta-analysis of smaller trials have conclusively shown that ACE inhibitors increase survival, reduce hospital admissions, and improve NYHA class and quality of life in patients with *all* grades of symptomatic heart failure. Other major randomized trials in patients with systolic dysfunction after acute myocardial infarction (SAVE, AIRE, TRACE) have shown that ACE inhibitors increase survival. In patients with heart failure (ATLAS), the composite endpoint of death or hospital admission was reduced by higher doses of ACE inhibitor compared to lower doses. ACE inhibitors have also been shown to delay or prevent the development of symptomatic heart failure in patients with *asymptomatic* LVSD

In whom and when?

Indications:

Potentially *all* patients with heart failure

First-line treatment (along with beta-blockers) in patients with NYHA Class II–IV HF; start as early as possible in course of disease. ACE inhibitors are also of benefit in patients with asymptomatic LVSD (NYHA class I)

Contraindications:

History of angioneurotic oedema

Severe aortic stenosis

Known bilateral renal artery stensis

Cautions/seek specialist advice:

Significant hyperkalaemia (K^+ >5.0mmol/L)

Significant renal dysfunction (creatinine 221μmol/L or >2.5mg/dL)

Symptomatic or severe asymptomatic hypotension (systolic BP <90mmHg)

Drug interactions to look out for:

K^+ supplements/K^+ sparing diuretics e.g. amiloride and triamterene (beware combination preparations with furosemide).
Aldosterone antagonists (spironolactone and eplerenone)

Aldosterone antagonists (spironolactone, eplerenone), angiotensin receptor blockers, NSAIDS*

'Low salt' substitutes with a high K^+ content

Where?

In the community for most patients

Exceptions—see 'Cautions/specialist advice'

Which ace inhibitor and what dose?

	Starting dose (mg)	Target dose (mg)
Captopril	6.25 TID	50 TID
Enalapril	2.5 BID	10–20 BID
Lisinopril	2.5–5.0 OD	20–35 OD
Ramipril	2.5 OD	5 BID or 10 OD
Trandolapril	0.5 OD	4 OD

How to use?

Start with a low dose (see above)

Double dose at *not less than* 2-weekly intervals

Aim for target dose (see above) or, failing that, the highest tolerated dose

Remember *some* ACE inhibitor is better than no ACE inhibitor

Monitor blood pressure and blood chemistry (urea/BUN, creatinine, K^+)

Check blood chemistry 1–2 weeks after initiation and 1–2 weeks after final dose titration

When to stop up-titration/reduce dose/stop treatment—see 'Problem solving'

A specialist heart failure nurse may assist with patient education, follow-up (in person/by telephone), biochemical monitoring, and dose up-titration

Advice to patient?

Explain expected benefits (see 'Why?')

Treatment is given to improve symptoms, to prevent worsening of heart failure leading to hospital admission, and to increase survival

Table 23.8 *(continued)* Practical guidance on the use of ACE inhibitors in patients with heart failure due to left ventricular systolic dysfunction

Advice to patient?
Symptoms improve within a few weeks to a few months of starting treatment
Advise patients to report principal adverse effects i.e. dizziness/symptomatic hypotension, cough—see 'Problem solving'
Advise patients to avoid NSAIDs* not prescribed by a physician (self-purchased 'over-the counter') and salt substitutes high in K^+— see 'Problem solving'
Problem solving
Asymptomatic low blood pressure:
Does not usually require any change in therapy
Symptomatic hypotension:
If dizziness, light-headedness and/or confusion, and a low blood pressure reconsider need for nitrates, calcium-channel blockers**, and other vasodilators
If no signs/symptoms of congestion consider reducing diuretic dose
If these measures do not solve problem seek specialist advice
Cough:
Cough is common in patients with heart failure, many of whom have smoking-related lung disease
Cough is also a symptom of pulmonary oedema which should be excluded when a new or worsening cough develops
ACE inhibitor-induced cough rarely requires treatment discontinuation
When a very troublesome cough does develop (e.g. one stopping the patient sleeping) and can be proven to be due to ACE inhibition (i.e. recurs after ACE inhibitor withdrawal and rechallenge) substitution of an ARB should be made (➲Table 23.9)
Worsening renal function:
Some rise in urea (BUN), creatinine, and potassium is to be expected after initiation of an ACE inhibitor; if an increase is small and asymptomatic no action is necessary
An increase in creatinine of up to 50% above baseline, or 266μmol/L (3mg/dL), which ever is the smaller, is acceptable
An increase in potassium to <5.5mmol/L is acceptable
If urea, creatinine, or potassium do rise excessively consider stopping concomitant nephrotoxic drugs (e.g. NSAIDs*), other potassium supplements/retaining agents (triamterene, amiloride, spironolactone/eplerenone***) and, if no signs of congestion, reducing the dose of diuretic
If greater rises in creatinine or potassium than those outlined above persist despite adjustment of concomitant medications the dose of the ACE inhibitor should be halved and blood chemistry rechecked within 1–2 weeks; if there is still an unsatisfactory response specialist advice should be sought
If potassium rises to >5.5mmol/L or creatinine increases by >100% or to above 310μmol/L (3.5mg/dL) the ACE inhibitor should be stopped and specialist advice sought
Blood chemistry should be monitored frequently and serially until potassium and creatinine have plateaued

NB it is very rarely necessary to stop an ACE inhibitor and clinical deterioration is likely if treatment is withdrawn—ideally, specialist advice should be sought before treatment discontinuation.

* avoid unless essential.; ** calcium-channel blockers should be discontinued unless absolutely essential (e.g. for angina or hypertension).; *** The safety and efficacy of an ACE inhibitor used with an ARB *and* spironolactone (as well as beta-blocker) is uncertain and the use of all 3 inhibitors of the renin-angiotensin-aldosterone system together is not recommended. ACE, angiotensin-converting enzyme; ARB, angiotensin receptor blocker; AIRE, Acute Infarction Ramipril Efficacy; ATLAS, Assessment of Treatment with Lisinopril And Survival; BID, twice a day; BUN, blood urea nitrogen; CONSENSUS, Cooperative North Scandinavian Enalapril Survival Study; LVSD, left ventricular systolic dysfunction; OD, once a day; SOLVD-T, Studies of Left Ventricular Dysfunction Treatment; SAVE, Survival and Ventricular Enlargement; TID, three times a day; TRACE, TRAndolapril Cardiac Evaluation.

Adapted with permission from McMurray J, Cohen-Solal A, Dietz R, *et al.* Practical recommendations for the use of ACE inhibitors, beta-blockers, aldosterone antagonists and angiotensin receptor blockers in heart failure: putting guidelines into practice. *Eur J Heart Fail* 2005; **7**: 710–21.

years of age or with a systolic blood pressure <100mmHg, diabetes, or renal impairment) [219, 230, 231].

As with ACE inhibitors, beta-blockers and aldosterone antagonists, treatment with ARBs should be indefinite unless there is intolerance.

Beta-blockers

Mechanism of action

Beta-blockers are believed to counteract the many harmful effects of sympathetic nervous system hyperactivity described earlier—see ➲Pathophysiology, p.843.

Table 23.9 Practical guidance on the use of ARBs in patients with heart failure due to left ventricular systolic dysfunction

Why?

When added to standard therapy, including an ACE inhibitor, in patients with all grades of symptomatic heart failure, the ARBs valsartan and candesartan have been shown, in two major randomized trials (Val-HeFT and CHARM), to reduce heart failure hospital admissions, improve NYHA class, and maintain quality of life. The two CHARM low LVEF trials (CHARM Alternative and CHARM-Added) also showed that candesartan reduced all-cause mortality. In patients *previously intolerant of an ACE inhibitor,* candesartan has been shown to reduce the risk of the composite outcome of cardiovascular death or heart failure hospitalization, the risk of heart failure hospital admission, and to improve NYHA class. These findings in heart failure are supported by another randomized trial in patients with left ventricular systolic dysfunction, heart failure, or both complicating acute myocardial infarction (VALIANT) in which valsartan was as effective as the ACE inhibitor captopril in reducing mortality and cardiovascular morbidity.

In whom and when?

Indications:

- Potentially *all* patients with heart failure
- First-line treatment (along with beta-blockers) in patients with NYHA class II–IV HF intolerant of an ACE inhibitor
- Second-line treatment (after optimization of ACE inhibitor and beta-blocker*) in patients with NYHA class II–IV heart failure

Contraindications:

- Known bilateral renal artery stenosis
- Severe aortic stenosis
- Cautions/seek specialist advice:
- Significant hyperkalemia (K^+ >5.0mmol/L)
- Significant renal dysfunction (creatinine 221μmol/L or >2.5mg/dL)
- Symptomatic or severe asymptomatic hypotension (systolic BP <90mmHg)

Drug interactions to look out for:

- K^+ supplements/K^+-sparing diuretics, e.g. amiloride and triamterene (beware combination preparations with furosemide) Aldosterone antagonists (spironolactone and eplerenone), ACE inhibitors, NSAIDS**
- 'Low salt' substitutes with a high K^+ content

Where?

In the community for most patients

Exceptions—see 'Cautions/specialist advice'

Which ARB and what dose?

	Starting dose (mg)	Target dose (mg)
Candesartan	4 or 8mg OD	32mg OD
Valsartan	40mg BID	160mg BID

How to use?

Start with a low dose (see above)

Double dose at *not less than* 2-weekly intervals

Aim for target dose (see above) or, failing that, the highest tolerated dose

Remember *some* ARB is better than no ARB

Monitor blood pressure and blood chemistry (urea/BUN, creatinine, K^+)

Check blood chemistry 1–2 weeks after initiation and 1–2 weeks after final dose titration

When to stop up-titration/reduce dose/stop treatment—see 'Problem solving'

A specialist heart failure nurse may assist with patient education, follow-up (in person/by telephone), biochemical monitoring, and dose up-titration

Advice to patient?

Explain expected benefits (see 'Why?')

Treatment is given to improve symptoms, prevent worsening of heart failure leading to hospital admission, and to increase survival

Symptoms improve within a few weeks to a few months of starting treatment

Advise patients to principal adverse effect, i.e. report dizziness/ symptomatic hypotension—see 'Problem solving'

Advise patients to avoid NSAIDs** not prescribed by a physician (self-purchased 'over-the-counter') and salt substitutes high in K^+—see 'Problem solving'

Table 23.9 *(continued)* Practical guidance on the use of ARBs in patients with heart failure due to left ventricular systolic dysfunction

Problem solving
Asymptomatic low blood pressure:
Does not usually require any change in therapy
Symptomatic hypotension:
If dizziness, light-headedness and/or confusion, and a low blood pressure reconsider need for nitrates, calcium-channel blockers***, and other vasodilators
If no signs/symptoms of congestion consider reducing diuretic dose
If these measures do not solve problem, seek specialist advice
Worsening renal function:
Some rise in urea (BUN), creatinine and potassium is to be expected after initiation of an ARB; if the increase is small and asymptomatic no action is necessary
An increase in creatinine of up to 50% above baseline, or 266μmol/L (3mg/dL), which ever is the smaller, is acceptable
An increase in potassium to < 5.5mmol/L is acceptable
If urea, creatinine, or potassium do rise excessively consider stopping concomitant nephrotoxic drugs (e.g. NSAIDs**), potassium supplements/ retaining agents (triamterene, amiloride, spironolactone/eplerenone*), and, if no signs of congestion, reducing the dose of diuretic
If greater rises in creatinine or potassium than those outlined above persist despite adjustment of concomitant medications, the dose of the ARB should be halved and blood chemistry rechecked within 1–2 weeks; if there is still an unsatisfactory response specialist advice should be sought. If potassium rises to >5.5mmol/L or creatinine increases by >100% or to above 310μmol/L (3.5mg/dL) the ARB should be stopped and specialist advice sought. Blood chemistry should be monitored frequently and serially until potassium and creatinine have plateaued

NB it is very rarely necessary to stop an ARB and clinical deterioration is likely if treatment is withdrawn—ideally, specialist advice should be sought before treatment discontinuation.

* The safety and efficacy of an ARB used with an ACE inhibitor *and* spironolactone (as well as beta-blocker) is uncertain and the use of all three inhibitors of the RAAS together is not recommended.; ** avoid unless essential.; *** calcium-channel blockers should be discontinued unless absolutely essential (e.g. for angina or hypertension).

ACE, angiotensin-converting enzyme; ARB, angiotensin receptor blocker; BID, twice a day; BUN, blood urea nitrogen; CHARM, Candesartan in Heart failure: Assessment of Reduction in Mortality and Morbidity; LVEF, left ventricular ejection fraction; OD, once a day; Val-HeFT, Valsartan Heart Failure Trial; VALIANT, VALsartan In Acute myocardial iNfarcTion.

Adapted with permission from McMurray J, Cohen-Solal A, Dietz R, *et al.* Practical recommendations for the use of ACE inhibitors, beta-blockers, aldosterone antagonists and angiotensin receptor blockers in heart failure: putting guidelines into practice. *Eur J Heart Fail* 2005; **7**: 710–21.

Clinical benefits

The long-term addition of a beta-blocker to an ACE inhibitor (and diuretic and digoxin) further improves left ventricular function and symptoms, reduces hospital admissions, and improves survival, strikingly (➲Table 23.6; Fig. 23.30). Consequently, a beta-blocker is recommended for all patients with symptomatic systolic dysfunction, irrespective of aetiology and severity. The combination of a beta-blocker with an ACE inhibitor is now the cornerstone of the treatment of symptomatic heart failure (➲Fig. 23.28) [232–239].

Practical use

The major contraindications to using a beta-blocker in heart failure are asthma (though it is important to note that the dyspnoea caused by pulmonary congestion can be confused with reactive airway disease) and second- or third-degree atrioventricular block [219]. Initiation of treatment during an episode of acute decompensated heart failure should also generally be deferred until the patient is stabilized and recovering (but, ideally, treatment should be commenced before discharge). In addition, caution is advised in patients with a heart rate <60 beats per minute (bpm) or a systolic blood pressure <100mmHg. It is recommended that a beta-blocker shown to produce benefits in a randomized trial be used (➲Table 23.7).

As with ACE inhibitors, beta-blockers should be introduced as early as possible in a patient's treatment, started in a low dose (➲Table 23.7) and increased gradually toward the target dose used in a clinical trial (the 'start low–go slow' approach). The patient should be checked for symptomatic hypotension and excessive bradycardia after each dose increment, but both of these side effects are uncommon, and hypotension can often be resolved by reduction in the dose of other non-essential blood pressure-lowering medications, e.g. nitrates and calcium-channel blockers (➲Table 23.10). Bradycardia is more likely in patients who are also taking digoxin, ivabradine, or amiodarone and the necessity for the simultaneous use of these agents should be reviewed if excessive bradycardia occurs. Occasionally, symptomatic worsening and fluid retention (i.e. weight gain or oedema) may occur after initiation of a beta-blocker or

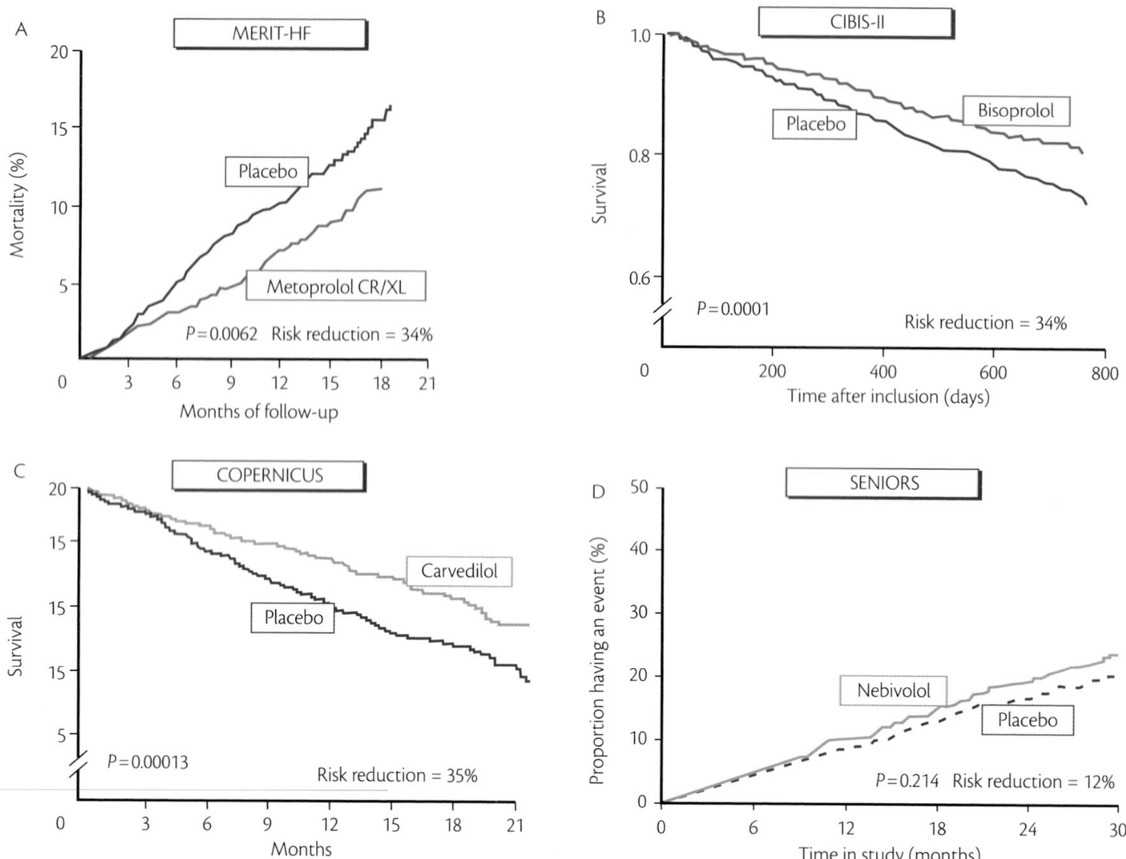

Figure 23.30 Kaplan–Meier curves of the three major survival studies with beta-blocker therapy: (A) Metoprolol CR/XL Randomized Intervention Trial (MERIT-HF); (B) Cardiac Insufficiency Bisoprolol Study II (CIBIS-II); (C) Carvedilol Prospective Randomized Cumulative Survival (COPERNICUS) study. (D) SENIORS (Study of the Effects of Nebivolol on Outcomes and Rehospitalisation in Seniors with heart failure). Reproduced with permission from MERIT-HF Study Group Effect of metoprolol CR/XL in chronic heart failure: Metoprolol CR/XL Randomised Intervention Trial in Congestive Heart Failure (MERIT-HF). *Lancet* 1999; **353**: 2001–7; CIBIS-II Investigators and Committees. The Cardiac Insufficiency Bisoprolol Study II (CIBIS-II): a randomised trial. *Lancet* 1999; **353**: 9–13; Packer,M, Coats AJ, Fowler MB *et al.*; Carvedilol Prospective Randomized Cumulative Survival Study Group. Effect of carvedilol on survival in severe chronic heart failure. *N Engl J Med* 2001; **344**: 1651–8.

during dose up-titration; these side effects usually can be resolved by a temporary increase in the diuretic dose without necessitating discontinuation of the beta-blocker.

Treatment with a beta-blocker should be given for life, though the dose may need to be decreased or temporarily discontinued during episodes of acute decompensation if the patient shows signs of circulatory hypoperfusion or refractory congestion.

Aldosterone antagonists

Mechanism of action

These agents block the undesirable actions of aldosterone described earlier and act as potassium sparing diuretics.

Clinical benefits

The aldosterone antagonist spironolactone (➲Table 23.6) improves symptoms, reduces hospital admissions, and increases survival when added to an ACE inhibitor (and diuretics and digoxin) in patients with a reduced LVEF and severely symptomatic heart failure (➲Fig. 23.31) [218]. Eplerenone, another aldosterone antagonist, reduces mortality and morbidity when added to both an ACE inhibitor and beta-blocker in patients with a reduced LVEF and heart failure or diabetes after a recent myocardial infarction (➲Table 23.7). Consequently, an aldosterone antagonist should be considered in patients who remain in severe heart failure (NYHA class III or IV) despite treatment with a diuretic, ACE inhibitor (or ARB), and beta-blocker. When begun, it should be given indefinitely. The value of an aldosterone antagonist in patients with milder heart failure is uncertain but is under investigation. The combination of an ACE inhibitor, an ARB, and an aldosterone antagonist has not been adequately evaluated and is *not recommended.*

Treatment with an aldosterone antagonist should be initiated with a low dose (➲Table 23.7) with careful monitoring of serum electrolytes and renal function (➲Table 23.11). Hyperkalaemia and uraemia are the adverse effects of greatest concern (as with ACE inhibitors and ARBs) and an aldosterone antagonist should not be given to patients with a serum potassium concentration of >5mmol/L, serum creatinine >221μmol/L (>2.5mg/dL) or other evidence of markedly

Table 23.10 Practical guidance on the use of beta-blockers in patients with heart failure due to left ventricular systolic dysfunction

Why?

Several major randomized controlled trials (i.e. USCP, CIBIS II, MERIT-HF, COPERNICUS) have shown, conclusively, that certain beta-blockers increase survival, reduce hospital admissions, and improve NYHA class and quality of life when added to standard therapy (diuretics, digoxin, and ACE inhibitors) in patients with *stable* mild and moderate heart failure and in some patients with severe heart failure. In the SENIORS trial which differed substantially in design from the aforementioned studies (older patients, some patients with preserved left ventricular systolic function, longer follow-up), nebivolol appeared to have a smaller treatment effect, though direct comparison is difficult. One other trial (BEST) did not show a reduction in all cause mortality but did report a reduction in cardiovascular mortality and is otherwise broadly consistent with the aforementioned studies. The COMET trial showed that carvedilol was substantially more effective than a low dose of short-acting metoprolol tartrate[*] (long acting metoprolol succinate was used in MERIT-HF).

In whom and when?

Indications:
- Potentially *all* patients with *stable* mild and moderate heart failure; patients with severe heart failure should be referred for specialist advice
- First-line treatment (along with ACE inhibitors) in patients with *stable* NYHA class II–III heart failure; start as early as possible in course of disease

Contraindications:
- Asthma
- Second- or third-degree atrioventricular block

Cautions/seek specialist advice:
- Severe (NYHA class IV) heart failure
- Current or recent (<4 weeks) exacerbation of heart failure, e.g. hospital admission with worsening heart failure
- Heart block or heart rate <60bpm.
- Persisting signs of congestion, hypotension/low blood pressure (systolic <90mmHg), raised jugular venous pressure, ascites, marked peripheral oedema

Drug interactions to look out for:
- Verapamil/diltiazem (should be discontinued)[**]
- Digoxin, amiodarone

Where?

In the community in stable patients (NYHA class IV/severe heart failure patients should be referred for specialist advice)
Not in unstable patients hospitalised with worsening heart failure
Other exceptions—see 'Cautions/seek specialist advice'

Which beta-blocker and what dose?

	Starting dose (mg)	**Target dose (mg)**
Bisoprolol	1.25 OD	10 OD
Carvedilol	3.125 BID	25–50 BID
Metoprolol CR/XL	12.5–25 OD	200 OD[*]
Nebivolol	1.25 OD	10 OD

How to use?

Start with a low dose (see above)
Double dose at *not less than* 2-weekly intervals
Aim for target dose (see above) or, failing that, the highest tolerated dose
Remember *some* beta-blocker is better than no beta-blocker
Monitor heart rate, blood pressure, clinical status (symptoms, signs—especially signs of congestion, body weight)
Check blood chemistry 1–2 weeks after initiation and 1–2 weeks after final dose titration
When to stop up-titration/reduce dose/stop treatment—see 'Problem solving'
A specialist heart failure nurse may assist with patient education, follow-up (in person/by telephone), and dose up-titration

Advice to patient?

Explain expected benefits (see 'Why?')
Treatment is given to improve symptoms, prevent worsening of heart failure leading to hospital admission, and to increase survival
Symptomatic improvement may develop slowly after starting treatment, taking 3–6 months or longer
Temporary symptomatic deterioration *may* occur during initiation/up-titration phase; in long-term beta-blockers improve well-being
Advise patient to report deterioration (see 'Problem solving') and that deterioration (tiredness, fatigue, breathlessness) can usually be easily managed by adjustment of other medication; patients should be advised not to stop beta-blocker therapy without consulting their physician
To detect and treat deterioration early, patients should be encouraged to weigh themselves daily (after waking, before dressing, after voiding, before eating) and to increase their diuretic dose should their weight increase, persistently (>2 days), by >1.5–2.0kg[***]

(Continued)

Table 23.10 *(continued)* Practical guidance on the use of beta-blockers in patients with heart failure due to left ventricular systolic dysfunction

Problem solving
Worsening symptoms/signs (e.g. increasing dyspnoea, fatigue, oedema, weight gain): If increasing congestion increase dose of diuretic and/or halve dose of beta-blocker (if increasing diuretic doesn't work) If marked fatigue (and/or bradycardia—see below) halve dose of beta-blocker (rarely necessary) Review patient in 1–2 weeks; if not improved seek specialist advice If serious deterioration halve dose of beta-blocker or stop this treatment (rarely necessary); seek specialist advice Low heart rate: If <50bpm and worsening symptoms—halve dose beta-blocker or, if severe deterioration, stop beta-blocker (rarely necessary) Review need for other heart rate slowing drugs, e.g. digoxin, amiodarone, diltiazem/verapamil** Arrange ECG to exclude heart block Seek specialist advice
Asymptomatic low blood pressure: *Does not usually require any change in therapy* Symptomatic hypotension: If dizziness, light-headedness and/or confusion, and a low blood pressure reconsider need for nitrates, calcium-channel blockers** and other vasodilators If no signs/symptoms of congestion consider reducing diuretic dose or ACE inhibitor If these measures do not solve problem seek specialist advice

NB beta-blockers should not be stopped suddenly unless absolutely necessary (there is a risk of a 'rebound' increase in myocardial ischaemia/infarction and arrhythmias)—ideally specialist advice should be sought before treatment discontinuation.

* metoprolol tartrate should not be used in preference to an evidence-based beta-blocker in heart failure.; ** calcium-channel blockers should be discontinued unless absolutely necessary and diltiazem and verapamil are generally contraindicated in heart failure.; *** this is generally good advice for all patients with heart failure. ACE, angiotensin-converting enzyme; BD, twice a day; BEST, Beta-Blocker Evaluation Survival Trial; CIBIS, Cardiac Insufficiency Bisoprolol Study; COMET, Carvedilol or Metoprolol European Trial; COPERNICUS, Carvedilol Prospective Randomized Cumulative Survival; MERIT-HF, Metoprolol CR/XL Randomized Intervention Trial in congestive heart failure; OD, once a day; SENIORS, Study of the Effects of Nebivolol on Outcomes and Rehospitalisation in Seniors with heart failure; USCP, US Carvedilol heart failure Program.

Adapted with permission from McMurray J, Cohen-Solal A, Dietz R, *et al.* Practical recommendations for the use of ACE inhibitors, beta-blockers, aldosterone antagonists and angiotensin receptor blockers in heart failure: putting guidelines into practice. *Eur J Heart Fail* 2005; **7**: 710–21.

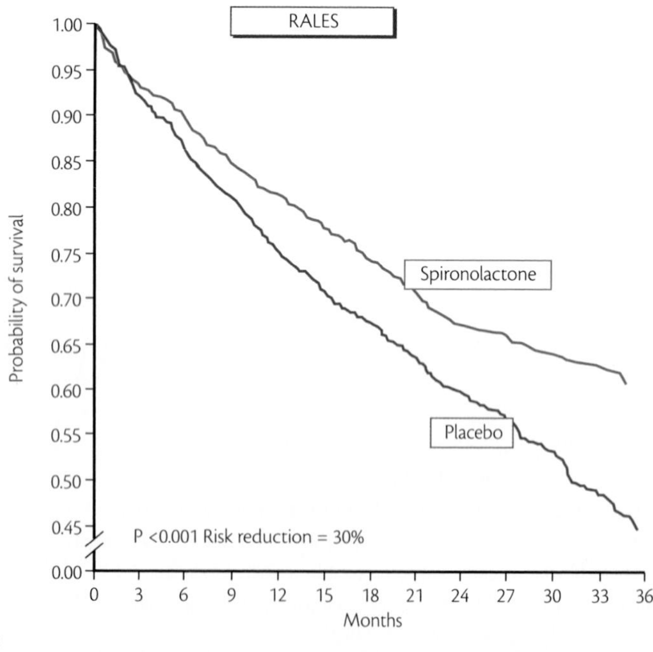

Figure 23.31 Effect of spironolactone in severe chronic heart failure: findings from RALES (Randomized Aldactone Evaluation Study). Risk reduction 0.70; 95% CI 0.62–0.80; $P < 0.001$. Reproduced with permission from Pitt B, Zannad F, Remme WJ, *et al.* The effect of spironolactone on morbidity and mortality in patients with severe heart failure. Randomized Aldactone Evaluation Study Investigators. *N Engl J Med* 1999; **341**: 709–17.

Table 23.11 Practical guidance on the use of spironolactone in patients with heart failure due to left ventricular systolic dysfunction

Why?

The RALES study showed that low-dose spironolactone increased survival, reduced hospital admissions, and improved NYHA class when added to standard therapy (diuretic, digoxin, ACE inhibitor, and, in a minority of cases, a beta-blocker) in patients with severe (NYHA class III or IV) heart failure. These findings in heart failure are supported by another randomized trial in patients with left ventricular systolic dysfunction and heart failure (or diabetes) complicating *acute* myocardial infarction (EPHESUS) in which another aldosterone antagonist, eplerenone, increased survival and reduced hospital admissions for cardiac causes.

In whom and when?

Indications:

Potentially all patients with symptomatically moderately severe or severe HF (NYHA class III/IV)

Second-line therapy (after ACE inhibitors and beta-blockers*) in patients with NYHA class III–IV heart failure; there is no evidence of benefit in patients with milder heart failure

Cautions/seek specialist advice:

Significant hyperkalaemia (K^+ >5.0mmol/L)**

Significant renal dysfunction (creatinine >221μmol/L or 2.5mg/dL)**

Drug interactions to look out for:

K^+ supplements/K^+-sparing diuretics, e.g. amiloride and triamterene (beware combination preparations with furosemide)
Aldosterone antagonists (spironolactone and eplerenone), ACE inhibitors, ARBs, NSAIDS***
'Low salt' substitutes with a high K^+ content

Where?

In the community or in hospital

Exceptions—see 'Cautions/seek specialist advice'

Which dose?**

	Starting dose (mg)	**Target dose (mg)**
Spironolactone	25 OD or on alternate days	25–50 OD
Eplerenone	25 OD	50 OD

How to use?

Start with a low dose (see above)

Check blood chemistry at 1, 4, 8, and 12 weeks; 6, 9, and 12 months; 6-monthly thereafter

If K^+ rises above 5.5mmol/L or creatinine rises to 221μmol/L (2.5mg/dL) reduce dose to 25mg on alternate days and monitor blood chemistry closely

If K^+ rises to >6.0mmol/L or creatinine to > 310μmol/L (3.5mg/dL) stop spironolactone immediately and seek specialist advice

A specialist heart failure nurse may assist with patient education, follow-up (in person/by telephone), biochemical monitoring, and dose up-titration

Advice to patient?

Explain expected benefits (see 'Why?')

Treatment is given to improve symptoms, prevent worsening of heart failure leading to hospital admission and to increase survival

Symptom improvement occurs within a few weeks to a few months of starting treatment

Avoid NSAIDs*** not prescribed by a physician (self-purchased 'over-the-counter') and salt substitutes high in K^+

If diarrhoea and/or vomiting occurs patients should stop spironolactone and contact their physician

Problem solving

Worsening renal function/hyperkalaemia:

See 'How to use?'

Major concern is hyperkalaemia (>6.0mmol/L); although this was uncommon in RALES it has been seen more commonly in clinical practice: conversely, a high normal potassium may be desirable in heart failure patients, especially if taking digoxin

It is important to avoid other K^+-retaining drugs (e.g. K^+-sparing diuretics such as amiloride and triamterene) and nephrotoxic agents (e.g. NSAIDs***)
The risk of hyperkalaemia and renal dysfunction when an aldosterone antagonist is given to patients already taking an ACE inhibitor *and* ARB is higher than when an aldosterone is added to just an ACE inhibitor or ARB given singly; close and careful monitoring is mandatory*

Some 'low salt' substitutes have a high K^+ content
Male patients treated with spironolactone may develop breast discomfort and/or gynaecomastia (these problems are significantly less common with eplerenone)

* the safety and efficacy of spironolactone used with an ACE inhibitor *and* an ARB (as well as beta-blocker) is uncertain and the use of all 3 inhibitors of the RAAS together is not recommended.; ** it is extremely important that these cautions and doses are adhered to in the light of recent evidence of serious hyperkalaemia with spironolactone in usual clinical practice in Ontario, Canada.; *** avoid unless essential. ACE, angiotensin-converting enzyme; ARB, angiotensin receptor blocker; EPHESUS, Epleronone Post-Acute Myocardial Infarction Heart Failure Efficacy and Survival Study; OD, once a day; RALES, Randomized Aldactone Evaluation Study.

Adapted with permission from McMurray J, Cohen-Solal A, Dietz R, *et al.* Practical recommendations for the use of ACE inhibitors, beta-blockers, aldosterone antagonists and angiotensin receptor blockers in heart failure: putting guidelines into practice. *Eur J Heart Fail* 2005; **7**: 710–21.

impaired renal function. The importance of patient selection and dose are underscored by reports of a worrisome incidence of serious hyperkalaemia in community practice settings. Spironolactone can have antiandrogenic effects, especially painful gynaecomastia, in men. Since eplerenone does not block the androgen receptor, it is a reasonable substitute in patients who experience this adverse effect [240].

Digitalis glycosides (including digoxin)

Mechanism of action

Digitalis glycosides inhibit the cell membrane sodium–potassium adenosine triphosphatase (ATP) pump, thereby increasing intracellular calcium and myocardial contractility. In addition, digoxin is thought to enhance parasympathetic and reduce sympathetic nervous activity, as well as inhibit renin release [241].

Clinical benefits

Only one large randomized placebo-controlled trial examined the effects of starting (as opposed to withdrawing) digoxin on mortality and morbidity in patients with heart failure in sinus rhythm [241, 242]. In that trial, digoxin did not reduce mortality but did decrease the risk of admission to hospital for worsening heart failure when added to a diuretic and an ACE inhibitor (➲Table 23.6). In patients in sinus rhythm, addition of digoxin is recommended only for patients whose heart failure remains symptomatic despite standard three-drug treatment with a diuretic, ACE inhibitor, beta-blocker, and either an ARB or aldosterone antagonist. In patients with atrial fibrillation, digoxin may be used at an earlier stage if a beta-blocker fails to control the ventricular rate (ideally <80bpm at rest and <110–120bpm during exercise; see ➲Chapter 29). Digoxin can also be used to control the ventricular rate when beta-blocker treatment is being initiated or up-titrated.

Digoxin should be avoided in patients with second-degree or greater atrioventricular block and pre-excitation syndromes; it should be used with caution in patients with sick-sinus syndrome. Hypokalaemia should be corrected before digoxin is administered. A loading dose of digoxin is generally not needed in stable patients in sinus rhythm. A single daily oral maintenance dose of 0.25mg is commonly used in adults with normal renal function. In the elderly and in those with renal impairment, a dose of 0.125mg or 0.0625mg may suffice. If the effect of digoxin is needed urgently, loading with 10–15mcg/kg *lean* body weight, given in three divided doses, 6 hours apart, may be used. The maintenance dose should be one-third of the loading dose. Smaller maintenance doses (e.g. one-quarter the loading dose and not more than 62.5mcg/day) should be used in the elderly and in patients with reduced renal function, as well as in patients with a low body mass. Monitoring of the serum digoxin concentration is recommended because of the narrow therapeutic window. A steady state is reached 7–10 days after starting treatment; blood should be collected at least 6 hours (and ideally 8–24 hours) after the last dose. The currently recommended therapeutic range is 0.6–1.2ng/mL (approximately 0.77–1.54nmol/L) [1, 2, 243].

Digoxin can cause anorexia, nausea, sinoatrial and atrioventricular block, arrhythmias, confusion, and visual disturbances (including xanthopsia), especially if the serum concentration is >2.0ng/mL. Hypokalaemia increases susceptibility to the adverse effects. The dose of digoxin should be reduced in the elderly and patients with renal dysfunction. Certain drugs increase serum digoxin concentration, including amiodarone, verapamil, and diltiazem.

Hydralazine and isosorbide dinitrate

Mechanism of action

Hydralazine is a powerful direct acting, arterial vasodilator. Its mechanism of action is not understood, though it may inhibit enzymatic production of superoxide, which neutralizes NO and may induce nitrate tolerance. Nitrates dilate both veins and arteries, thereby reducing preload and afterload by stimulating the NO pathway and increasing cyclic GMP in vascular smooth muscle. Neither drug on its own nor any other direct acting vasodilator has been demonstrated to be beneficial in heart failure.

Clinical benefits

Although this combination has been known for some time to improve systolic function and probably reduce death in NYHA class II–IV heart failure compared with placebo, a head-to-head comparison showed an ACE inhibitor was superior for improving survival (➲Table 23.6) [244, 245]. Nevertheless, based on subgroup analyses suggesting that African Americans responded better to hydralazine and isosorbide dinitrate, a subsequent randomized controlled trial showed that the addition of hydralazine and isosorbide dinitrate in African Americans, most of whom were receiving an ACE inhibitor and beta-blocker and many of whom were on spironolactone, further reduced mortality and hospital admissions for heart failure and improved quality of life [246]. A fixed combination of 37.5mg of hydralazine and 20mg of isosorbide dinitrate was used in the trial; one tablet was given and if tolerated a second was given 12 hours later. One tablet was then prescribed three times daily for 3–5 days, at which point the dose was increased to the target maintenance of two tablets three times daily, i.e. a daily dose of 225mg hydralazine and 120mg isosorbide dinitrate. Because of the limited inclusion criteria of this trial, however, it is uncertain whether this combination of vasodilators is an effective addition in other patient populations.

Practical use

Other than for African Americans, the main indication for hydralazine and isosorbide dinitrate is as a substitute in patients with intolerance to an ACE inhibitor and an ARB. Hydralazine and isosorbide dinitrate should be used as additional treatment in African Americans and considered, on an empirical basis, for other patients who remain symptomatic on other proven therapies. The main dose-limiting adverse effects with hydralazine and isosorbide dinitrate are headache and dizziness. A rare adverse effect of higher doses of hydralazine, especially in slow acetylators is a systemic lupus erythematosus-like syndrome.

Omega-3 polyunsaturated fatty acids

A recent study showed that treatment with 1g of omega-3 polyunsaturated fatty acids (n-3 PUFA) (850–852mg eicosapentaenoic acid and docosahexaenoic acid as ethyl esters in the average ratio of 1:1.2) per day led to a small reduction in cardiovascular morbidity and mortality in patients with heart failure (➲Table 23.6) [247]. The exact mechanism of action of this treatment is uncertain, although it may have beneficial, anti-inflammatory and electrophysiological effects (the latter reducing the risk of arrhythmias).

Other drug treatments tested in heart failure

It is important to note that the aforementioned treatments are the only pharmacological agents shown to be of benefit in patients with heart failure and a low LVEF. Many other treatments have been tested in randomized trials and shown to have a neutral (e.g. amlodipine) [248] or uncertain (e.g. alpha-adrenoceptor blockers, bosentan, and etanercept) [249–252] effect on mortality and morbidity. Some also increased mortality and have either been withdrawn from the market or should be avoided in heart failure (e.g. dronedarone, milrinone, flosequinan, vesnarinone, and moxonidine) [253–257].

Other pharmacological treatments

Other therapies of proven value for cardiovascular conditions underlying or associated with heart failure have not been specifically tested in heart failure (e.g. antiplatelet treatment in patients with coronary heart disease, see ➲Chapter 16) or may not be as clearly beneficial in heart failure (e.g. statins) [258, 259]. In patients with advanced systolic heart failure of ischaemic aetiology, statins did not reduce the primary outcome of cardiovascular death, myocardial infarction, or stroke (or all-cause mortality) but did reduce the number of cardiovascular hospitalizations [258]. A vitamin K antagonist, e.g. warfarin, is indicated in patients with atrial fibrillation provided there is no contraindication to its use (➲Chapters 11 and 29). Warfarin may also be used in patients with evidence of intra-cardiac thrombus (e.g. detected during echocardiographic examination) or systemic thromboembolism. Warfarin's many interactions with other drugs, including with some statins and amiodarone (➲Chapter 11), must always be considered when initiating warfarin or another drug in a patient taking warfarin. Low-molecular-weight heparin prophylaxis (➲Chapter 37) against deep venous thrombosis is indicated when patients with heart failure are bed-bound, for example during hospital admission, although heparin can cause hyperkalaemia and the dose must be reduced in patients with renal impairment.

Vaccination against influenza and pneumococcal infection is advised in all patients with heart failure because the stress of infection can lead to clinical deterioration [1].

Drugs to use with caution in heart failure

Patients with heart failure, especially if severe, often have renal and hepatic dysfunction, so any drug excreted predominantly by the kidneys or metabolized by the liver may accumulate [75, 83–85, 187, 188]. Similarly, because of their extensive comorbidity, patients with heart failure are inevitably treated with multiple drugs, thereby increasing the risk of drug interactions.

Drugs that should be avoided, if possible, in heart failure include most antiarrhythmic drugs including dronedarone [257] (with the exception of amiodarone and dofetilide), most calcium channel blockers (with the exception of amlodipine), corticosteriods, NSAIDs, COX-2 inhibitors, and many antipsychotics (e.g. clozapine) and antihistamines. Thiazolidinediones (because of the risk of fluid retention) should be used with caution [70, 81–83, 260]. The use of metformin is usually not recommended because of the risk of lactic acidosis although this may be overstated [70]. Some salt substitutes contain substantial amounts of potassium and must be used cautiously. Other dietary constituents (e.g. grapefruit and cranberry juice) and supplements such as St. John's Wort can interact with drugs taken by patients with heart failure, especially warfarin and digoxin [1, 2].

Organization of care

Several studies have shown that organized, nurse-led, multidisciplinary care can improve outcomes in patients with heart failure, particularly by reducing recurrent hospital admissions [261–263]. The most successful approach seems to involve education of the patients, their families, and caregivers about heart failure and its treatment (including flexible diuretic dosing and reinforcing the importance of adherence), recognizing (and acting upon) early deterioration (dyspnoea, weight gain, oedema), and optimizing proven pharmacological treatments (see ➲General measures, p.913) (➲Table 23.12). A home-based rather than clinic-based approach may be best, though trials are needed to compare these types of interventions directly. Even telephone follow-up is of value. New technology enabling non-invasive home telemonitoring of physiological measures (e.g. heart rate and rhythm, blood pressure, temperature, respiratory rate, weight, and estimated body water content) and implanted devices, which collect similar data and may be interrogated remotely, are also being tested as aids to monitoring and management [264, 265].

Education

Education of the patient, family, and caregivers is invaluable (➲Table 23.12) [1, 2, 266]. Detection of early signs and symptoms of deterioration provides for earlier intervention. Counselling on the proper use of therapies, with an emphasis on adherence, is critical.

Useful patient and carer orientated material is available from the Heart Failure Association of the European Society of Cardiology in several languages (currently English, French, German, and Spanish) and from the Heart Failure Society of America and other organizations (see ➲Online resources, p.892).

Medication use counselling

When appropriate, a patient should be taught how to adjust the dose of diuretic within individualized limit—see ➲Diuretics, p.865. The dose should be increased (or a supplementary diuretic added) if there is evidence of fluid retention (symptoms of congestion), and decreased if evidence of hypovolaemia (e.g. increased thirst associated with weight loss or postural dizziness, especially during hot weather or an illness causing decreased fluid intake or sodium and water loss). If hypovolaemia is more marked, the doses of other medications (e.g. ACE inhibitors, spironolactone) also will have to be reduced.

The expected effects, beneficial and adverse, of other drugs should also be explained in detail (e.g. possible association of cough with ACE inhibitor). It is useful to inform patients that improvement with many drugs is gradual and

Table 23.12 Essential topics in patient education with associated skills and appropriate self-care behaviours

Educational topics	Skills and self-care behaviours
Definition and aetiology of heart failure	Understand the cause of heart failure and why symptoms occur
Symptoms and signs of heart failure	Monitor and recognize signs and symptoms
	Record daily weight and recognize rapid weight gain
	Know how and when to notify healthcare provider
	Use flexible diuretic therapy if appropriate and recommended
Pharmacological treatment	Understand indications, dosing, and effects of drugs
	Recognize the common side effects of each drug prescribed
Risk factor modification	Understand the importance of smoking cessation
	Monitor blood pressure if hypertensive
	Maintain good glucose control if diabetic
	Avoid obesity
Diet recommendation	Sodium restriction if prescribed
	Avoid of excessive fluid intake
	Modest intake of alcohol
	Monitor and prevent malnutrition
Exercise recommendations	Be reassured and comfortable about physical activity
	Understand the benefits of exercise
	Perform exercise training regularly
Sexual activity	Be reassured about engaging in sex and discuss problems with healthcare professionals
	Understand specific sexual problems and various coping strategies
Immunization	Receive immunization against infections such as influenza and pneumococcal disease
Sleep and breathing disorders	Recognize preventive behaviour such as reducing weight of obese, smoking cession, and abstinence from alcohol
	Learn about treatment options if appropriate
Adherence	Understand the importance of following treatment recommendations and maintaining motivation to follow treatment plan
Psychosocial aspects	Understand that depressive symptoms and cognitive dysfunction are common in patients with heart failure and the importance of social support
	Learn about treatment options in appropriate
Prognosis	Understand important prognostic factors and make realistic decisions
	Seek psychosocial support if appropriate

Adapted with permission from Dickstein K, Cohen-Solal A, Filippatos G, *et al.* ESC guidelines for the diagnosis and treatment of acute and chronic heart failure 2008: the Task Force for the diagnosis and treatment of acute and chronic heart failure 2008 of the European Society of Cardiology. Developed in collaboration with the Heart Failure Association of the ESC (HFA) and endorsed by the European Society of Intensive Care Medicine (ESICM). *Eur Heart J* 2008; **29**: 2388–442. Copyright © ESC 2008.

may become fully apparent only after several weeks or even months of treatment. It is also important to explain the need for gradual titration with ACE-inhibitors, ARBs, and beta-blocking drugs to a desired dose level, which again may take weeks or even months to achieve. Patients should be advised not to use NSAIDs without consultation and to be cautious about using herbal or other non-proprietary preparations.

Adherence

Education and counselling of the patient, caregiver, and family promotes adherence, which is associated with better outcomes [267]. Drug adherence can also be helped by certain pharmacy aids such as dose allocation ('Dosette') boxes.

Exercise

The recent Heart Failure: A Controlled Trial Investigating Outcomes of Exercise TraiNing (HF-ACTION) trial also showed that a programme of tailored, structured, aerobic exercise is safe, improves functional capacity and quality of life, and may also reduce cardiovascular mortality and heart failure hospitalization [268, 269]. The regimen used was, however, labour intensive (➲Table 23.13) and, on average, patients did not attain the target level of exercise, especially during the home-maintenance phase.

Diet, nutrition, and alcohol

Most guidelines advocate avoidance of foods containing relatively high salt content in the belief that this may reduce the need for diuretic therapy, although there is little evidence from clinical trials to support this recommendation [1]. Some also believe that excess sodium intake can be a precipitant of clinical decompensation. Certain salt substitutes have a high potassium content, which can lead to hyperkalaemia.

Restriction of fluid intake is indicated only during episodes of decompensation associated with peripheral oedema or hyponatraemia. In these situations, daily intake should be restricted to 1.5–2L to help facilitate elimination of excess extracellular fluid volume and avoid hyponatraemia.

Reducing excessive weight will reduce the work of the heart and may lower blood pressure and is recommended in those who are obese (body mass index >30kg/m^2). Conversely, malnutrition is common in severe heart failure, and the development of cardiac cachexia is an ominous sign [77, 90, 91]. Sometimes reduced food intake is caused by nausea (e.g. related to digoxin use or hepatosplenic congestion) or abdominal bloating (e.g. due to ascites). In these cases, small frequent meals and high protein and calorie liquids may be helpful. In severe decompensated heart failure, eating may be difficult because of dyspnoea.

Moderate alcohol intake (up to 10–20g/day, e.g. 1–2 standard glasses of wine is permissible) is not thought to be harmful in heart failure, although excessive intake can cause cardiomyopathy and atrial arrhythmias in susceptible individuals. In patients with suspected alcoholic cardiomyopathy, abstinence from alcohol may improve cardiac function and is recommended.

Smoking

Smoking causes peripheral vasoconstriction, which is detrimental in heart failure [1, 2]. Nicotine replacement therapy is believed to be safe in heart failure. The safety of bupropion and varenicline in heart failure are uncertain.

Sexual activity

Sexual activity need not be restricted in patients with compensated heart failure, though dyspnoea may be limiting [1, 2]. Sublingual nitrate may be used as prophylaxis against chest pain and dyspnoea caused by sexual activity.

Table 23.13 HF-ACTION trial exercise training programme

Training phase	Location	Week*	Weekly sessions	Aerobic duration (min)	Intensity (percentage of HRR)	Mode of exercise
Initial, supervised	Clinic	1–2	3	15–30	60	Walk or cycle
Supervised	Clinic	3–6	3	30–35	70	Walk or cycle
	Clinic/Home	7–12	3/2	30–35	70	Walk or cycle
Maintenance	Home	13 to end of treatment	5	40	60–70	Walk or cycle

HRR, heart rate recovery.

* Week intervals shown are goals and may vary for individual patients. Reproduced with permission from Whellan, DJ, O'Connor, CM, Lee, KL *et al*; HF-ACTION Trial Investigators. Heart failure and a controlled trial investigating outcomes of exercise training (HF-ACTION): design and rationale. *Am Heart J* 2007; **153**: 201–11.

In men with erectile dysfunction, treatment with a cyclic guanine monophosphate phosphodiesterase type V inhibitor, such as sildenafil, can be useful, but these drugs must not be taken within 24 hours of prior nitrate use, and nitrates must not be restarted for at least 24 hours afterwards [270].

Driving

Patients with heart failure can continue to drive provided their condition does not induce undue dyspnoea, fatigue, or other incapacitating symptoms [1, 2]. Patients with recent syncope, cardiac surgery, percutaneous coronary intervention, or device placement may be restricted from driving, at least temporarily, according to local regulations. Patients holding an occupational or commercial licence may be subject to additional restrictions.

Travelling and flying

Short flights are unlikely to cause problems for a patient with compensated heart failure [1, 2]. Cabin pressure is generally maintained to provide an oxygen level no lower than equivalent to 6000 feet above sea level, which should be well tolerated in patients without severe pulmonary disease or pulmonary hypertension. Longer journeys may cause limb oedema and dehydration, thereby predisposing to venous thrombosis. Adjustment of the dose of diuretics and other treatments should be discussed with the patient wishing to travel to a warm climate or a country where the risk of gastroenteritis is high. It is also advisable for heart failure patients to carry a list of medications and contact information for their healthcare provider.

Treatment considerations related to comorbidity

Angina

Beta-blockers are of benefit in both angina and heart failure. Nitrates relieve angina but, on their own, are not of proven value in chronic heart failure. Calcium-channel blockers should generally be avoided in heart failure as they have a negative inotropic action and cause peripheral oedema; only amlodipine has been shown to have no adverse effect on survival [248]. Trimetazine, ranolazine, and nicorandil are available in certain countries but their safety in heart failure is uncertain. Ivabradine is an inhibitor of the I_f current in the sinoatrial node, reduces heart rate, and is an effective antianginal agent. It has been evaluated in patients with coronary heart disease and an EF <40% many of which had heart failure and most of which were treated with an ACE inhibitor/ARB and beta-blocker. In the morBidity-mortality EvAlUaTion of the I_f inhibitor ivabradine in patients with coronary disease and left-ventricULar dysfunction (BEAUTIFUL) trial, ivabradine did not reduce the primary composite endpoint of cardiovascular death, myocardial infarction, or heart failure hospitalisation. However, no safety concerns were identified [271]. Percutaneous and surgical revascularization are also of value in relieving angina in selected patients with heart failure.

Atrial fibrillation

The recent Atrial Fibrillation and Congestive Heart Failure (AF-CHF) trial showed that there is no evidence to support a strategy of restoring sinus rhythm over one of controlling the ventricular rate (coupled with thromboembolism prophylaxis) in most patients with heart failure [272]. Exceptions include patients in which new-onset atrial fibrillation has caused myocardial ischaemia, hypotension, or pulmonary oedema and where pharmacological rate control is not rapidly achieved; in these patients, prompt electrical or pharmacological cardioversion may be indicated. In the routine setting, a beta-blocker alone or in combination with digoxin should be used to control the ventricular rate. The patient should be supervised closely after the initiation of these treatments because underlying sinus node dysfunction may raise the risk of bradycardia. Atrioventricular node ablation and pacing may be required to control ventricular rate in resistant cases. There is current interest in catheter ablation to cure atrial fibrillation in patients with heart failure, though this approach remains experimental [273]. There is a strong indication for thromboembolism prophylaxis with warfarin in patients with heart failure and atrial fibrillation.

Ventricular arrhythmias

Sustained ventricular tachycardia causing syncope or haemodynamic instability and ventricular fibrillation is an indication for an implantable cardioverter defibrillator (ICD) for 'secondary prevention' of sudden arrhythmic death. Amiodarone can be used to suppress recurrent arrhythmias and reduce ICD firing. General measures to reduce the substrate for arrhythmias are also important, including institution of an optimal combination of evidence-based pharmacological treatment (ACE inhibitor, beta-blocker, and either an ARB and aldosterone antagonist) used in optimal doses, correction of electrolyte imbalances, amelioration of myocardial ischaemia, cessation of pro-arrhythmic drugs etc. Catheter ablation may also be useful in selected cases [274].

Asthma/reversible airways obstruction

Asthma is a contraindication for use of a beta-blocker but most patients with COPD can tolerate a beta-blocker. Pulmonary congestion can mimic COPD. Systemic administration of a corticosteroid to treat reversible airways obstruction may cause sodium and water retention and exacerbate heart failure, whereas inhalation therapy is better tolerated [200].

Diabetes mellitus

Beta-blocker treatment is not contraindicated and is of benefit in patients with diabetes and heart failure. Thiazolidinediones cause sodium and water retention and may lead to decompensation [70, 81, 260]. Metformin may cause lactic acidosis [70]. As a result, neither drug is recommended in patients with severe heart failure.

Abnormal thyroid function

Amiodarone can also induce both hypothyroidism and hyperthyroidism, the latter being particularly difficult to diagnose [275].

Gout

Hyperuricaemia and gout are common in heart failure and, in part, are caused by diuretic treatment. Allopurinol may prevent gout. Acute attacks are better treated with colchicine or intra-articular steroids, rather than NSAIDs, COX-2 inhibitors, or oral steroids.

Renal dysfunction

Most patients with heart failure have a reduced glomerular filtration rate (GFR) [83–86]. ACE inhibitors, ARBs, and aldosterone antagonists often cause a further small reduction in GFR and rise in serum urea/blood urea nitrogen (BUN) and creatinine levels, which, if limited, should not lead to discontinuation of treatment (➲Tables 23.8, 23.9, and 23.11). Marked increases in BUN and creatinine, however, should prompt consideration of underlying renal artery stenosis. Renal dysfunction may also be caused by sodium and water depletion leading to relative hypovolaemia (e.g. due to excessive diuresis, diarrhoea and vomiting) or hypotension [83–86]. Nephrotoxic agents such as NSAIDs and certain antibiotics such as trimethoprim are also a common cause of renal dysfunction in heart failure [83–86].

Prostatic obstruction

For prostatic disease, a 5-alpha-reductase inhibitor may be preferable to an alpha-adrenoceptor antagonist, which can cause hypotension and salt and water retention [276]. Prostatic obstruction should also be considered in male patients with deteriorating renal function.

Anaemia

A normocytic, normochromic anaemia is common in heart failure, in part because of the high prevalence of renal dysfunction. Malnutrition and blood loss may also contribute. The roles of iron replacement and erythropoietic-stimulating substances in treating the anaemia of heart failure are under investigation and these are not currently recommended treatments [76, 87–89, 277].

Depression

Depression is common in patients with heart failure, perhaps partly owing to disturbance of the hypothalamic pituitary axis and other neurochemical pathways, but also as a result of social isolation and the adjustment to chronic disease. Depression is associated with worse functional status, reduced adherence to treatment, and poor clinical outcomes [78, 278]. Both psychosocial interventions and pharmacological treatment are helpful. Selective serotonin reuptake inhibitors are believed to be the best tolerated pharmacological agents, whereas tricyclic antidepressants should be avoided because of their anticholinergic actions and potential to cause arrhythmias [78].

Cancer

Many anticancer drugs, particularly anthracyclines, cyclophosphamide, and trastuzumab (Herceptin®) can cause myocardial damage and heart failure, as can mediastinal radiotherapy [69, 279]. Pericardial constriction can be a result of previous radiotherapy, and malignant pericardial involvement can cause effusion and tamponade.

Devices and surgery

ICDs for primary prevention of sudden death

About half of patients with heart failure die suddenly, mainly as the result of a ventricular arrhythmia. The relative risk of sudden death, as opposed to death from progressive heart failure, is greatest in patients with milder heart failure. In patients with more advanced heart failure, progressive pump failure deaths are relatively more common. Antiarrhythmic drugs have not been shown to improve survival in heart failure, but ICDs (➲Fig. 23.32) reduce the risk of death in selected patients after myocardial infarction (➲Chapter 30) and improve survival in patients with NYHA class II–III heart failure due to systolic dysfunction of both ischaemic and non-ischaemic aetiology who were otherwise treated with optimal medical therapy (➲Fig. 23.33) [280–282]. As a result, all patients with NYHA class II and III heart failure, irrespective of aetiology, and LVEF ≤35% without other conditions greatly limiting life expectancy (i.e. anticipated survival ≥1 year) or the quality of life should be considered for an ICD (➲Fig. 23.28). The guidelines recognize that there is more evidence of benefit from ICDs in patients with heart failure of an ischaemic [274, 280, 281] compared to non-ischaemic aetiology [283] (➲Table 23.14).

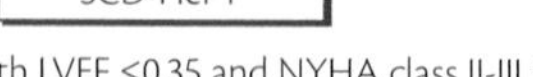

Figure 23.33 Sudden Cardiac Death in Heart Failure Trial (SCD-HeFT): Implantable cardioverter defibrillator vs. amiodarone vs. placebo. Reproduced with permission from Bardy GH, Lee KL, Mark DB, *et al.* Amiodarone or an implantable cardioverter-defibrillator for congestive heart failure. *N Engl J Med* 2005; **352**: 225–37.

Cardiac resynchronization therapy

Between a quarter and a third of patients with heart failure have substantial prolongation of the QRS duration on the surface ECG, which is a marker of abnormal electrical activation of the left ventricle causing dyssynchronous contraction, less efficient ventricular emptying, and, often, mitral regurgitation [276]. Atrioventricular coupling may also be abnormal, as reflected by a prolonged PR interval, as may interventricular synchrony. One recent study showed that 10% of patients develop substantial new widening of the QRS each year, suggesting regular ECG review is worthwhile [283]. Cardiac resynchronization therapy (CRT) with atriobiventricular or multisite pacing optimizes atrioventricular timing and improves synchronization of cardiac contraction. In selected patients with severe heart failure, CRT improves pump function, reduces mitral regurgitation, relieves symptoms, and significantly prolongs exercise capacity. In two major trials, CRT reduced the composite of death or hospital admission in patients with severe heart failure (➲Table 23.6) by >35%, and in one trial it also reduced the relative risk of death from any cause by 36% (and absolute risk by 10%) (➲Fig. 23.34) [284, 285]. Many other outcome measures, including quality of life, were also improved. The current debate focuses on how best to select patients who will benefit from CRT. The key trials to date selected patients on the basis of a markedly prolonged QRS duration, usually manifest as left bundle branch block and a QRS duration of >120ms (➲Table 23.14). Although tissue Doppler echocardiography and other imaging techniques have been advocated as tools to identify patients likely to benefit from CRT, the evidence does not support such approaches [286, 287]. Whether patients with right bundle branch block, atrial fibrillation, milder heart failure, or with dyssychrony without marked QRS prolongation are helped by CRT is uncertain [288, 289]. There is no consensus yet about whether (or in whom) CRT pacing alone, i.e. CRT-P (➲Fig. 23.35) or a CRT device with an ICD function i.e. CRT-D (➲Fig. 23.36) should be used.

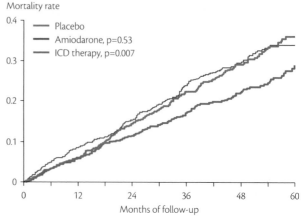

There is also uncertainty about how CRT devices should be 'optimized' [290].

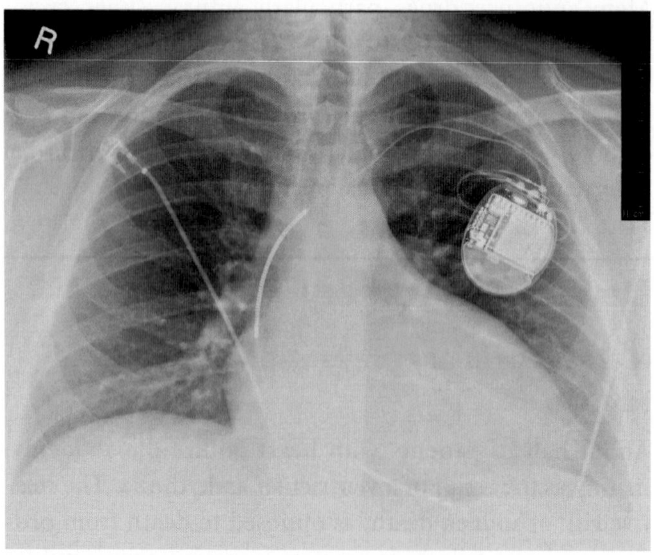

Figure 23.32 Chest radiograph showing an ICD *in situ*.

Table 23.14 Class I recommendations for devices in patients with left ventricular systolic dysfunction

ICD	
Prior resuscitated cardiac arrest	Class I, Level A
Ischaemic aetiology and >40 days of myocardial infarction	Class I, Level A
Non-ischaemic aetiology	Class I, Level B
CRT	
NYHA class III/IV and QRS >120ms	Class I, Level A
To improve symptoms/reduce hospitalization	Class I, Level A
To reduce mortality	Class I, Level A

ICD, implantable cardioverter defibrillator; CRT, cardiac resynchronization therapy.
Adapted with permission from Dickstein K, Cohen-Solal A, Filippatos G, *et al.* ESC guidelines for the diagnosis and treatment of acute and chronic heart failure 2008: the Task Force for the diagnosis and treatment of acute and chronic heart failure 2008 of the European Society of Cardiology. Developed in collaboration with the Heart Failure Association of the ESC (HFA) and endorsed by the European Society of Intensive Care Medicine (ESICM). *Eur Heart J* 2008; **29**: 2388–442. © ESC 2008.

The combination of multiple neurhohumoral inhibitors (in patients with mild–moderate symptoms) and CRT (in patients with severe symptoms) has led to stepwise improvements in survival over the past two decades (➲Figs. 23.37 and 23.38).

Surgery

With the exception of cardiac transplantation (and possibly ventricular assist devices), there are no generally accepted criteria for surgical intervention [199, 291]. There are very few sizeable clinical trials of surgical strategies in patients with heart failure. The largest to date did not show any benefit of surgical ventricular reconstruction [292]. Use of operative procedures is, therefore, very variable among centres and greatly dependent on local experience and expertise. Expert imaging and detailed haemodynamic and functional assessments are usually required when any patient with heart failure is considered for surgery, and close liaison between the relevant experts in these fields is essential. The collective expertise in surgical centres is often used to make highly individualized decisions about whether to operate and what procedures will be attempted. 'Established' operative treatments for patients with heart failure include coronary artery bypass grafting (CABG), surgery for valvular disease, left ventricular remodelling surgery (including aneurysmectomy), implantation of ventricular assist devices, and heart transplantation. 'Experimental' approaches include ventricular constraint devices and intramyocardial cell transplantation.

PCI or CABG

PCI or CABG (see ➲Chapter 17), when appropriate, is indicated for relief of angina or reversible ischaemia that contributes to the heart failure syndrome. The extent of ischaemia and myocardial viability can be assessed using non-invasive assessments such as dobutamine echocardiography (see ➲Chapter 4), cardiac MRI (see ➲Chapter 5), or PET scanning (see ➲Chapter 7) in patients with impaired LVEF. Whether CABG is beneficial in patients with coronary artery disease but without angina is uncertain, but it is postulated that improvement of coronary blood flow to viable but non-contracting ('hibernating') myocardium may improve ventricular function and clinical outcomes even in patients without inducible ischaemia. A large clinical trial comparing surgery (CABG and/or surgical ventricular reconstruction) and medical therapy has completed enrolment and will report initial findings in 2009/2010 [64].

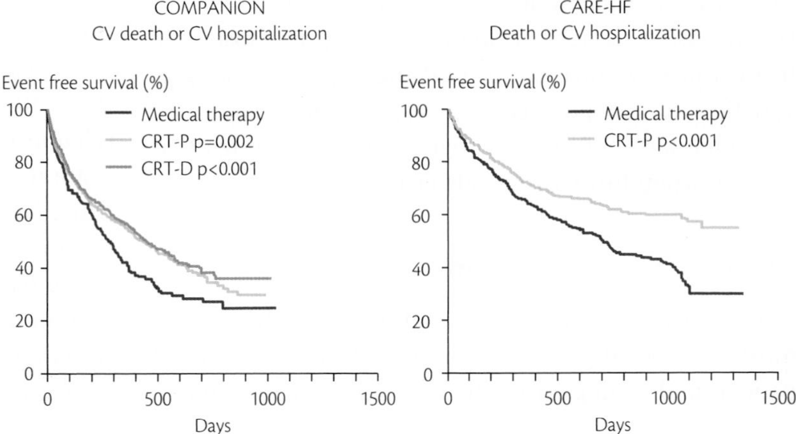

Figure 23.34 Cardiac resynchronization therapy for severe heart failure: two pivotal trials. Reproduced with permission from Bristow MR, Saxon LA, Boehmer J, *et al.*; Comparison of Medical Therapy, Pacing, and Defibrillation in Heart Failure (COMPANION) Investigators. Cardiac-resynchronization therapy with or without an implantable defibrillator in advanced chronic heart failure. N Engl J Med 2004; 350: 2140–50; and Cleland JG, Daubert JC, Erdmann E, *et al.*; Cardiac Resynchronization-Heart Failure (CARE-HF) Study Investigators. The effect of cardiac resynchronization on morbidity and mortality in heart failure. *N Engl J Med* 2005; **352**: 1539–49.

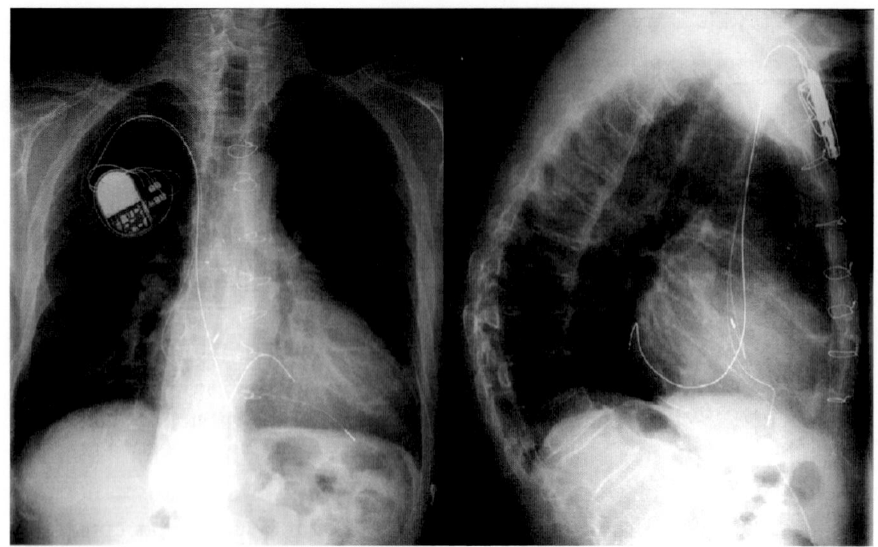

Figure 23.35 CRT-P device *in situ* showing right and left ventricular pacing leads.

Left ventricular assist devices

One randomized controlled trial showed that long-term use of a left ventricular assist device (LVAD) led to a short but significant prolongation of survival in patients which had end-stage heart failure and were ineligible for transplantation (➲Table 23.6) [291]. After 2 years of follow up, all patients in both the LVAD and medical therapy arms were dead. Device complications (e.g. due to infection and thromboembolism) were frequent. Such devices are also very expensive, as is the healthcare infrastructure required to support their use [293]. Despite this, in some centres, patients with severe heart failure are receiving these devices both as a 'bridge to transplantation' and as 'destination therapy', i.e. as the permanent, definitive, procedure [294, 295]. Short-term LVADs are also used, increasingly, as a 'bridge to decision' in the management of patients with acute heart failure who cannot be stabilized on inotropes and intra-aortic balloon pumps. Patients can be supported to cardiac transplantation, 'upgraded' to long-term ventricular assist devices or sometimes (e.g. in those with myocarditis) weaned to medical therapy. There is large variation in these practices between and within countries. There has also been some progress in LVAD design that might warrant further controlled trials.

Cardiac transplantation

Cardiac transplantation (➲Chapter 18) remains the most accepted surgical intervention in heart failure. Most patients undergoing cardiac transplantation in the modern era are those presenting with acute severe heart failure [199, 296]. Some ambulatory patients with severe cardiac dysfunction and unacceptable symptoms also warrant consideration of listing. Conventional selection criteria for this group were developed in the era before beta-blockers, spironolactone, ICDs, and CRT, and up-to-date risk stratification tools are needed.

Heart failure with preserved left ventricular ejection fraction

Most of the randomized controlled trials underpinning the evidence-based treatment of heart failure included only patients with a low LVEF (➲Table 23.6). Treatment of this heart failure syndrome is, therefore, mainly empirical. Treatment of the underlying cardiovascular and other disorders thought to contribute to the development of heart failure with preserved LVEF (HF-PEF), such as hypertension, myocardial ischaemia, and diabetes, should be given as usual [297]. In patients with atrial fibrillation, control of the ventricular rate with a beta-blocker or a rate-limiting calcium-channel blocker (i.e. verapamil or diltiazem) (or restoration of sinus rhythm) is important (➲Chapter 29). Diuretics are used, empirically, to treat sodium and water retention, according to the same principles as in heart failure with a low LVEF. Two small studies in patients in sinus rhythm showed that the alcium-channel blocker verapamil can improve symptoms and exercise capacity in patients with heart failure and preserved LVEF, possibly by reducing

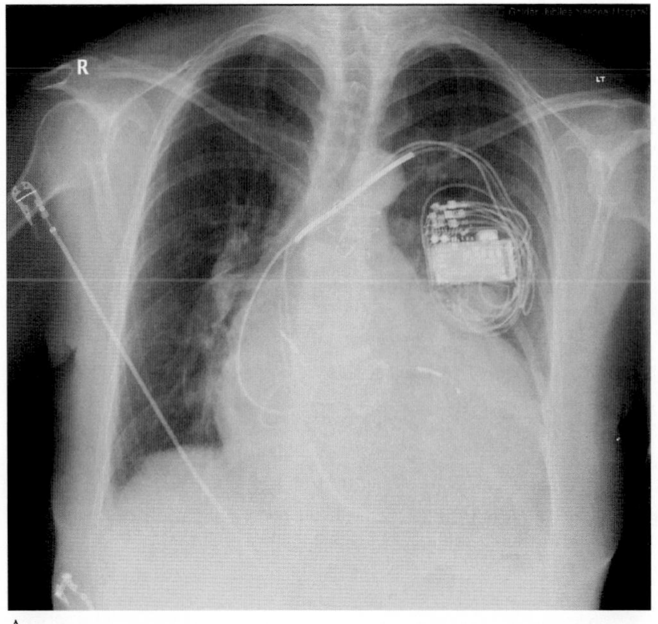

A

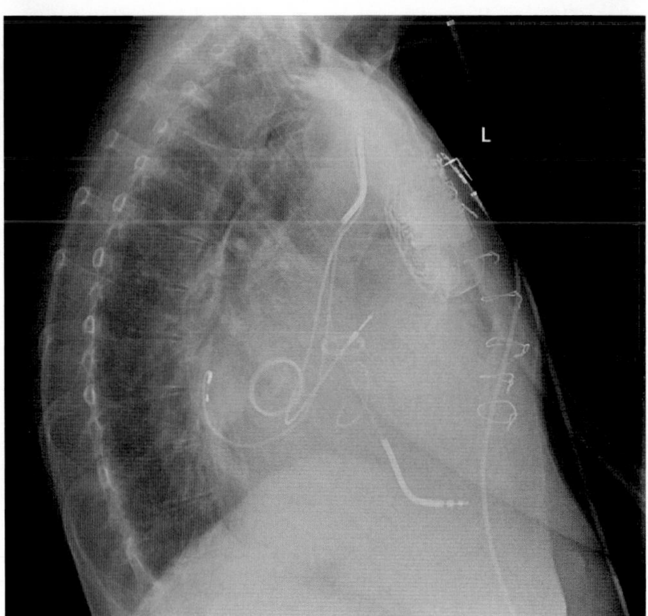

B

Figure 23.36 CRT-D device *in situ*.

heart rate, and thereby increasing the duration of diastolic left ventricular filling, as well as by directly enhancing myocardial relaxation [298]. There are, however, no prospective randomized controlled mortality–morbidity trials with this drug in patients with heart failure and preserved LVEF. One medium-sized trial with an ACE inhibitor and two large trials with ARBs failed to show a clear-cut benefit on NYHA class, quality of life, or morbidity/mortality with drugs that block the RAAS [299–301].

Heart failure due to valvular heart disease

Heart failure also can arise as a result of regurgitant and stenotic valve disease. The objective of treatment of primary valve disease is the prevention of heart failure by surgical repair or replacement of the diseased valve or valves (➲Chapter 21). The development of overt heart failure is an ominous sign, sometimes requiring urgent valve replacement (e.g. aortic stenosis) but occasionally indicating that valve replacement may no longer be possible (e.g. because of severe pulmonary hypertension).

Aortic stenosis

Evaluation of the aortic valve can be difficult in patients with poor left ventricular systolic function. Such patients may have insufficient cardiac output to generate a gradient across even a severely stenotic valve. Conversely, a calcified and degenerate but non-stenotic aortic valve may appear stenosed simply because it does not open normally in patients with very low cardiac output. Valve area provides a better assessment of whether there is significant aortic stenosis in these patients. Stress echocardiography may help assess the potential for ventricular recovery following relief of aortic stenosis (and the patient's operative risk). Consideration should also be given to the occurrence of reversible depression of systolic function due to concomitant myocardial ischaemia resulting from coronary artery disease. There is a great deal of current interest in the potential of transcatheter valve replacement for aortic stenosis.

Mitral regurgitation

Sometimes it can be difficult to determine whether mitral regurgitation is primary or secondary in a patient with heart failure and left ventricular dilatation, though a prior history of known valve disease or rheumatic fever may suggest a primary valve problem. Surgery sometimes will result in clinical improvement but some patients will have such advanced left ventricular dysfunction that they will not achieve substantial benefit (e.g. mitral valve surgery in a patient with long-standing severe mitral regurgitation). Valve repair or annuloplasty may, however, have a role in the treatment of some carefully selected patients with secondary mitral regurgitation caused, or exacerbated, by left ventricular dilatation. Valve repair is generally preferable

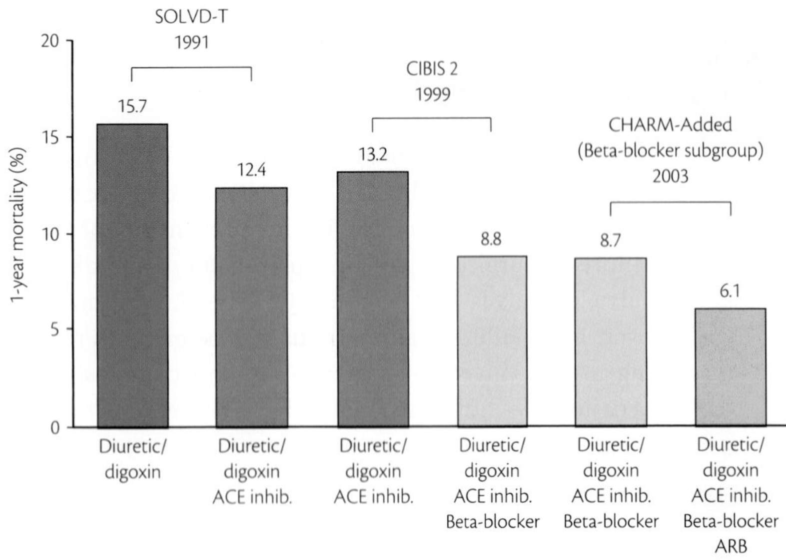

Figure 23.37 Cumulative benefit of polypharmacy in mild–moderate heart failure

to valve replacement. As with aortic stenosis, surgical treatment is largely empirical and there is a need for randomized clinical trials to provide evidence-based management.

Heart failure due to dilated cardiomyopathy

Patients with heart failure and normal coronary arteries should be evaluated for possible reversible causes. Untreated hypertension is now an unusual cause of dilated cardiomyopathy in developed countries but hypertension was once a leading cause in Europe and the USA and still remains a major consideration in many parts of the world. Infiltrative cardiomyopathies (e.g. haemochromatosis, amyloidosis, sarcoidosis) sometimes have specific recommended therapies. Chagas disease must be considered in patients from endemic areas. However, most cases of dilated cardiomyopathy will be 'idiopathic' (i.e. no specific aetiology is apparent). Possible inherited causes should be considered (➲Chapter 18) and these patients should otherwise be treated in the same way as patients whose dilated, poorly contracting, left ventricle is a result of coronary artery disease [67, 102–104].

Heart failure due to hypertrophic cardiomyopathy

Heart failure can arise in patients with hypertrophic cardiomyopathy because of predominant diastolic dysfunction,

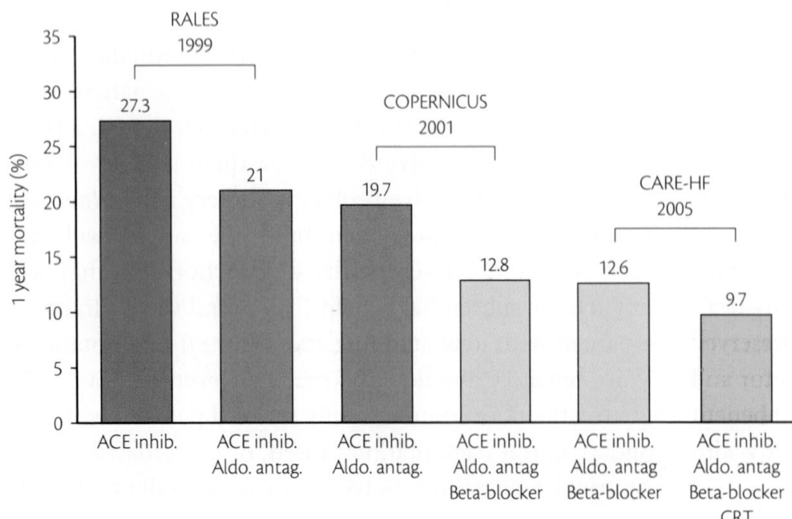

Figure 23.38 Cumulative benefit of polypharmacy (and cardiac resynchronization therapy) in severe heart failure.

left ventricular outflow tract obstruction (by either the septum or anterior mitral valve leaflet), associated mitral incompetence, or the development of systolic dysfunction. The management of hypertrophic cardiomyopathy and its complications is quite different than that of dilated cardiomyopathies and is discussed in ➲Chapter 18 [67, 102–104].

Acute heart failure and pulmonary oedema

Patients presenting with acute heart failure include those who develop heart failure '*de novo*' as a consequence of another cardiac event, usually a myocardial infarction, and those who present for the first time with decompensation of previously asymptomatic and often unrecognized cardiac dysfunction (patients previously in NYHA class I). However, due to frequent recurrences, most episodes of acute decompensation occur in patients with established, chronic heart failure that has worsened because of the unavoidable natural progression of the syndrome, an intercurrent cardiac (e.g. arrhythmia) or non-cardiac (e.g. pneumonia) event, or as a consequence of an avoidable reason such as non-adherence with treatment or use of an agent that can alter renal function. Although not always identified, searching for a reversible precipitant is an important aspect of the initial therapy plan (➲Table 23.4).

Most patients with acute heart failure require admission to the hospital, especially if pulmonary oedema is present. In contrast to chronic heart failure, randomized controlled trials showing benefits of therapy are generally not available in acute heart failure. The principal goals of management are to relieve symptoms, the most important of which is extreme dyspnoea, and maintain or restore vital organ perfusion [1, 2, 303]. An intravenous bolus or infusion of a loop diuretic, and, in hypoxaemic patients, oxygen are the key first-line treatments. Non-invasive ventilation improves symptoms but does not reduce mortality [302]. Intravenous infusion of a nitrate is also valuable in patients with a systolic blood pressure ≥100mmHg (➲Fig. 23.39) Intravenous nesiritide (human BNP) which is available

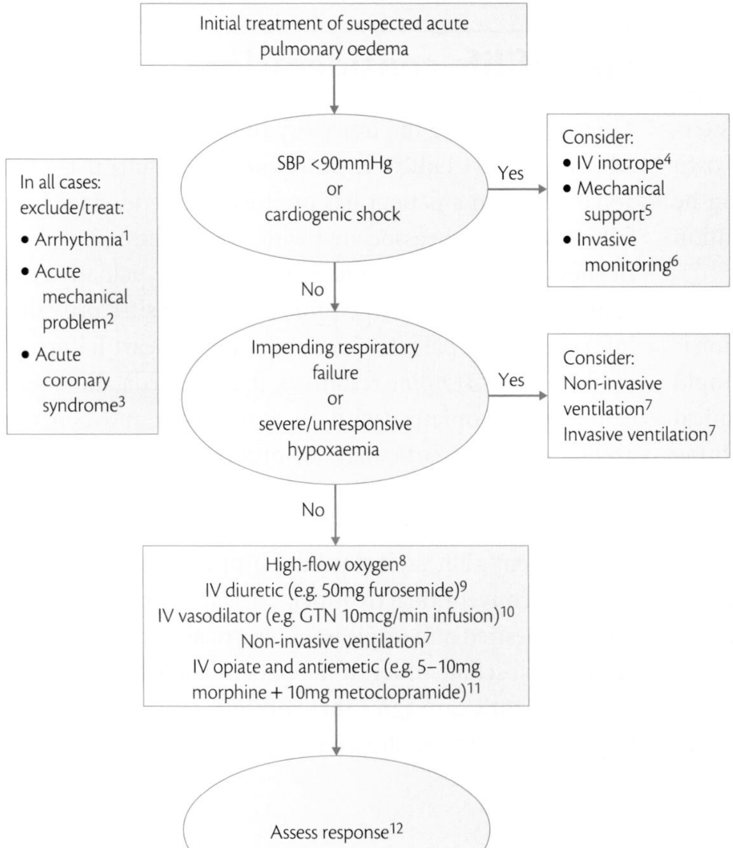

[1]Causal arrhythmia, e.g. ventricular tachycardia. It can be difficult to determine whether atrial fibrillation is a primary cause of acute pulmonary oedema or secondary to it. An ECG is an essential investigation.

[2]Acute mechanical problems include ventricular septal rupture and mitral valve papillary muscle rupture. Mechanical support (e.g. an intra-aortic balloon pump) and urgent surgery should be considered. An echocardiogram should be performed as soon as possible, especially in a patient without a prior diagnosis of heart failure or other relevant heart disease, e.g. prior myocardial infarction or valve disease.

[3]Emergency revascularization should be considered.

[4]An IV infusion of dobutamine may be started at a dose of 2.5mcg/kg/min, doubling every 15min according to response and tolerability (dose titration is usually limited by excessive tachycardia, arrhythmias or ischaemia). A dose >20mcg/kg/min is rarely needed.

[5]For example, an intra-aortic balloon pump.

[6]Consider pulmonary artery catherization and arterial line.

[7]Continuous positive airways pressure (CPAP) and non-invasive intermittent positive pressure ventilation (NIPPV) are valuable in severe pulmonary oedema, especially if associated with hypoxaemia. Endotracheal intubation and mechanical ventilation should be considered in patients with persisting hypoxaemia and an inability to generate an adequate tidal volume.

[8]Oxygen causes an increase in systemic vascular resistance and a reduction in heart rate and cardiac output; it should be administered only to patients with hypoxaemia.

[9]Dose of diuretic depends on prior diuretic use and renal function—a lower dose may suffice in patients with preserved renal function and no prior diuretic use.

[10]An IV infusion of glycerytrinitrate should be started at a dose of 10mcg/min and doubled every 10min according to response and tolerability (usually dose up titration is limited by hypotension). A dose of >100mcg/min is rarely needed.

[11]Consider if patient agitated/distressed/in pain; may cause respiratory depression and dose should be reduced in the very elderly.

[12]Should see improvement in symptoms, peripheral perfusion, and urine output—patient should be monitored closely, and usually a response will occur within 30min. Bladder catheterization may help in monitoring urine output.

Figure 23.39 Treatment algorithm for suspected acute pulmonary oedema.

in some countries may reduce the pulmonary capillary wedge pressure more promptly than intravenous glyceryltrinitrate, but the effect of this short-term therapy on other clinical outcomes is controversial. Levosimendan has both vasodilator and inotropic actions. An intravenous opiate is also valuable in excessively anxious or distressed patients and those in pain (➲Fig. 23.39). In volume overloaded patients with severe heart failure unresponsive to diuretics, ultrafiltration is an option at specialized centres [304].

In patients with marked hypotension or other evidence of organ hypoperfusion, an inotropic agent such as dobutamine a phosphodiesterase inhibitor (e.g. milrinone), or levosimendan should be considered, although none of these treatments has been shown to reduce in-hospital deaths or readmission [1]. In general, potent inotropic agents should be used at the lowest clinically effective dose and for the shortest duration possible in a setting with close cardiac monitoring. Low-dose dopamine may be administered in an attempt to improve renal function, although there are limited data in support of this benefit [305].

In more critically ill patients, mechanical support, for example with an intra-aortic balloon pump, may also be considered. As alluded to earlier, short-term use of a mechanical assist device is sometimes also used in this setting. The aim of treatment is to support the patient's circulation and vital organ function until either their own heart recovers or a definitive operative procedure can be performed (e.g. transplantation or long-term implantation of a ventricular assist device) [291–295].

In patients admitted to hospital, discharge planning and subsequent management to reduce the risk of readmission is important. Ideally, an effective oral diuretic regimen should have been identified, and fluid-volume and biochemical stability should have achieved. This optimization of volume status and development of a stable oral regimen prior to discharge is thought to reduce the risk of early readmission. Treatment with an ACE inhibitor, beta-blocker, and ARB or aldosterone antagonist, as appropriate, should also be started and titrated in the stabilized patient prior to discharge [306, 307]. Outpatient follow-up should be arranged to ensure that any of those treatments that have not been started, prior to discharge are initiated after discharge, and that the dose of each drug is increased, as tolerated, to the appropriate target [308].

Outpatient follow-up

The key to successful follow-up is the careful tracking of clinical symptoms and patient weights, which often involves interviewing not only the patient, but also family members, who may be more aware of changes in status than the patient. Continuity of care and seamless transitions from the inpatient to outpatient setting are crucial aspects of optimal management. Patients with severe heart failure and patients requiring frequent hospitalization require special care. Programmes that provide telephone-based tracking of daily weights and symptoms may detect deterioration in time to intervene before the need for hospitalization [261, 264]. Although these programmes may be costly, several evaluations have found them to be cost-effective [309]. Because the management of these patients requires considerable experience and expertise, specialized heart failure disease-management programmes and clinics have been developed and may provide additional benefit compared with traditional care [263].

End-of-life considerations

Though predicting the trajectory of illness in patients with advanced heart failure is notoriously difficult, it is often apparent when a patient has progressed to end-stage heart failure, commonly associated with renal failure [310–312]. In these circumstances, the expertise of the palliative care team may be especially helpful. Useful websites providing information on palliative care relevant to heart failure are available (see ➲Online resources, p.892). Medications such as parenteral opiates (with an antiemetic) and benzodiazepines may be particularly helpful in relieving dyspnoea, anxiety, and pain that arises from ascites, hepatic congestion, lower limb oedema, and pressure points. At this stage in the patient's illness, it may be appropriate to discuss withdrawal of conventional treatment, deactivation of an ICD to avoid undesired and unpleasant electrical discharges, and a 'do not resuscitate order' if the patient and others involved in the patient's care agree that comfort-care is appropriate. Hospice care may be chosen by some at this point.

Personal perspective

The past two decades have seen almost unimaginable improvements in morbidity and, especially, mortality in patients with heart failure and a low EF. Remarkably, these have been brought about by only a handful of drugs (from among the many tested) and two devices. These treatments (ACE inhibitors, beta-blockers, ARBs, aldosterone antagonists, ICDs, and CRT) have changed the natural history of heart failure and created new problems bringing new challenges. This is no more apparent than in the emergence of the 'cardiorenal anaemia' syndrome in elderly patients surviving with advanced heart failure. New treatments targeting renal dysfunction (adenosine antagonists) and new applications of a treatment used for anaemia in chronic kidney disease (erythropoiesis-stimulating agents) are currently being evaluated in these patients. But this is even more the era of devices, with unresolved questions (CRT-P or CRT-D?) and potentially broader application (e.g. CRT in less symptomatic patients or those with narrower QRS) being evaluated. While the prospect of new treatments is always exciting, we can still do better in applying the very effective treatments currently available to us and this may be aided by better information technology and perhaps by using biochemical markers such as natriuretic peptides to encouraging physicians to optimize therapy. Assessing the role of monitoring (either biochemically or technologically) to detect earlier deterioration (or pre-empt it) continues to be a priority as does the development of affordable and effective ventricular assist or even replacement devices. Transcatheter valve replacement and ablation therapy may yet improve outlook for patients with aortic stenosis and atrial fibrillation.

We also have to recognize, however, that the success of treatments for low EF heart failure has led to a growing population of very elderly patients with end-stage heart failure and that we need to help these patients die better having allowed them live better. We will need to apply the skills and resources of palliative care services to this new population.

Finding an effective treatment for HF-PEF has proved remarkably difficult and only spironolactone is presently being tested in a large-scale study in this type of heart failure. Similarly, bettering diuretics and nitrates has not been possible in acute heart failure although a very large trial is currently evaluating nesiritide in these patients. Although impressive recovery of myocardial function is now routinely seen in patients treated with multiple neurohumoral antagonists (and in some receiving ventricular assist devices), this is not universal and the dream of replacing scar tissue with new myocytes continues to drive research with cell therapies although when, if ever, a therapeutic breakthrough will occur is uncertain. To repeat the therapeutic triumphs of the past two decades in the next two is hugely challenging but equally rewarding if we can do it.

Acknowledgement

The authors would like to thank Dr Davide Castagno for his valuable contribution to this chapter.

Further reading

Arnold JM, Liu P, Demers C, *et al.* Canadian Cardiovascular Society consensus conference recommendations on heart failure 2006: diagnosis and management. *Can J Cardiol* 2006; **22**: 23–45. Erratum in: Can J Cardiol 2006; 22: 271.

Arnold JM, Howlett JG, Dorian P, *et al.* Canadian Cardiovascular Society Consensus Conference recommendations on heart failure update 2007: Prevention, management during intercurrent illness or acute decompensation, and use of biomarkers. *Can J Cardiol* 2007; **23**: 21–45.

Braunwald E. Biomarkers in heart failure. *N Engl J Med* 2008; **358**: 2148–59.

Dickstein K, Cohen-Solal A, Filippatos G, *et al.* ESC guidelines for the diagnosis and treatment of acute and chronic heart failure 2008: the Task Force for the diagnosis and treatment of acute and chronic heart failure 2008 of the European Society of Cardiology. Developed in collaboration with the Heart Failure Association of the ESC (HFA) and endorsed by the European Society of Intensive Care Medicine (ESICM). *Eur Heart J* 2008; **29**: 2388–442.

Hunt SA, Abraham WT, Chin MH, *et al.* ACC/AHA 2005 Guideline Update for the Diagnosis and Management of Chronic Heart Failure in the Adult: a report of the American College of Cardiology/American Heart Association Task Force on Practice Guidelines (Writing Committee to Update the 2001 Guidelines for the Evaluation and Management of Heart Failure): developed in collaboration with the American College of Chest Physicians and the International Society for Heart and Lung Transplantation: endorsed by the Heart Rhythm Society. *Circulation* 2005; **112**: e154–e1235.

Jessup M, Brozena S. Heart failure. *N Engl J Med* 2003; **348**: 2007–18.

Krum H, Jelinek MV, Stewart S, *et al.* Guidelines for the prevention, detection and management of people with chronic heart failure in Australia 2006. *Med J Aust* 2006; **185**: 549–57.

Liew CC, Dzau VJ. Molecular genetics and genomics of heart failure. *Nat Rev Genet* 2004; **5**: 811–25.

Maisel A, Mueller C, Adams K, Jr., *et al.* State of the art: using natriuretic peptide levels in clinical practice. *Eur J Heart Fail* 2008; **10**: 824–39.

Malcom J, Arnold O, Howlett JG, *et al.* Canadian Cardiovascular Society Consensus Conference guidelines on heart failure – 2008 update: best practices for the transition of care of heart failure patients, and the recognition, investigation and treatment of cardiomyopathies. *Can J Cardiol* 2008; **24**: 21–40.

McAlister FA, Ezekowitz J, Hooton N, *et al.* Cardiac resynchronization therapy for patients with left ventricular systolicdysfunction: a systematic review. *JAMA* 2007; **297**: 2502–14.

McMurray JJ, Pfeffer MA. Heart failure. *Lancet* 2005; **365**: 1877–89.

Mosterd A, Hoes AW. Clinical epidemiology of heart failure. *Heart* 2007; **93**: 1137–46.

Paulus WJ, Tschöpe C, Sanderson JE, *et al.* How to diagnose diastolic heart failure: a consensus statement on the diagnosis of heart failure with normal left ventricular ejection fraction by the Heart Failure and Echocardiography Associations of the European Society of Cardiology. *Eur Heart J* 2007; **28**: 2539–50.

Stewart S, McAlister FA, McMurray JJ. Heart failure management programs reduce readmissions and prolong survival. *Arch Intern Med* 2005; **165**: 1311; author reply 1311–12.

Zipes DP, Camm AJ, Borggrefe M, *et al.* ACC/AHA/ESC 2006 guidelines for management of patients with ventricular arrhythmias and the prevention of sudden cardiac death – executive summary: A report of the American College of Cardiology/American Heart Association Task Force and the European Society of Cardiology Committee for Practice Guidelines (Writing Committee to Develop Guidelines for Management of Patients with Ventricular Arrhythmias and the Prevention of Sudden Cardiac Death) Developed in collaboration with the European Heart Rhythm Association and the Heart Rhythm Society. *Eur Heart J* 2006; **27**: 2099–140.

Online resources

Useful patient and carer orientated material is available from the following, and other, organizations:

- Heart Failure Association of the European Society of Cardiology in several languages: http://www.heartfailurematters.org/English_Lang/Pages/index.aspx
- Heart Failure Society of America: http://www.hfsa.org/hf_modules.asp
- American Heart Association: http://www.americanheart.org/presenter.jhtml?identifier=1486)
- National Gold Standards Framework (GSF) Centre England: http://www.goldstandardsframework.nhs.uk/index.php
- Scottish Partnership for Palliative Care: http://www.palliative carescotland.org.uk/publications/HF%20final%20document.pdf

For full references and multimedia materials please visit the online version of the book (http://esctextbook.oxfordonline.com).

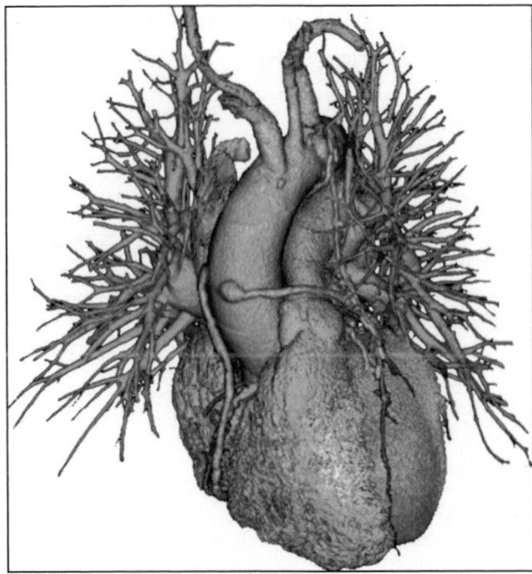

CHAPTER 24

Pulmonary Hypertension

Nazzareno Galiè and Alessandra Manes

Contents

Summary

Pulmonary hypertension (PH) is a haemodynamic and pathophysiological state that can be found in multiple clinical conditions which have been classified into six diagnostic groups with specific histological, clinical, and therapeutic features. Despite possible comparable elevations of pulmonary pressure in the different clinical groups, the underlying mechanisms, the diagnostic approaches, and the prognostic and therapeutic implications are completely different.

Group 1, defined as pulmonary arterial hypertension (PAH), includes rare conditions which share comparable clinical and haemodynamic pictures and virtually identical pathological changes in the lung microcirculation. PAH comprises the idiopathic and familial forms and the forms associated with connective tissue diseases, congenital heart defects with systemic-to-pulmonary shunts, portal hypertension, and human immunodeficiency virus (HIV) infection. A sequential diagnostic approach is suggested to identify and characterize the different types. Three classes of drugs (prostanoids, endothelin-receptor antagonists, phosphodiesterase type-5 inhibitors) have proven to be effective in this severe condition and an evidence-based treatment algorithm is presented. Specific clinical and therapeutic characteristics of each PAH type are also discussed. Lung transplantation is indicated in case of medical treatments failure.

Group 2 includes patients with PH due to left heart disease. In these cases the treatment is addressed to the underlying heart condition and specific medications approved for PAH have not proven to be convincingly effective.

Group 3 includes cases of PH due to lung diseases in which the use of specific medications approved for PAH is not recommended on the basis of their minimal clinical efficacy and because they may impair pulmonary gas exchange.

Group 4 comprises patients with chronic thromboembolic PH where treatment of choice is pulmonary endarterectomy, and group 5 includes a miscellanea of rare conditions.

Definition and classification of pulmonary hypertension

PH is a haemodynamic and pathophysiological condition defined by a mean pulmonary artery pressure (PAP) ≥25mmHg at rest by right heart catheterization [1]. The definition of PH on exercise is not supported by convincing published data and no specific limits are therefore given.

The haemodynamic classification of PH is shown in ➲Table 24.1. According to various combinations of values of pulmonary wedge pressure (PWP), pulmonary vascular resistance (PVR), and cardiac output (CO), different haemodynamic definitions of PH are shown. Precapillary PH includes the clinical groups 1, 3, 4, and 5, while post-capillary PH includes clinical group 2 (➲Table 24.2).

The more updated clinical classification of PH is presented in ➲Table 24.2 [2]. Clinical conditions with PH are classified into six groups according to similar pathological, pathophysiological, and therapeutic characteristics. Despite possible comparable elevations of PAP and PVR in the different clinical groups, the underlying mechanisms, the diagnostic approaches, and the prognostic and therapeutic implications are completely different. The features of each clinical group are discussed in specific sections, with particular attention to clinical group 1, defined as PAH in which PH represents the leading pathophysiological feature.

Pathology and pathobiology of pulmonary hypertension

Different pathological [3] and pathobiological features [4] characterize the diverse clinical PH groups.

Table 24.1 Haemodynamic definitions of pulmonary hypertension

Definition	Characteristics	Clinical group(s)*
Precapillary pulmonary hypertension	Mean PAP ≥25mmHg PWP ≤15mmHg CO normal or reduced*†	1, 3, 4, 5
Postcapillary pulmonary hypertension	Mean PAP ≥25mmHg PWP >15mmHg CO normal or reduced*†	2
Passive	TPG <12mmHg	
Reactive	TPG >12mmHg	

CO, cardiac output; PAP, pulmonary arterial pressure; PH, pulmonary hypertension; PVR, pulmonary vascular resistance; PWP, pulmonary wedge pressure; TPG, transpulmonary pressure gradient (mean PAP – mean PWP)

* According to ➲Table 24.2. †High cardiac output can be present in cases of hyperkinetic conditions such as systemic-to-pulmonary shunts, anaemia, hyperthyroidism, etc.

Table 24.2 Updated clinical classification of pulmonary hypertension in six groups (Dana Point, 2008)

1. Pulmonary arterial hypertension (PAH)
1.1 Idiopathic PAH
1.2 Heritable
1.2.1 BMPR2
1.2.2 ALK1, endoglin (with or without HHT)
1.2.3 Unknown
1.3 Drugs and toxins induced
1.4 Associated with (APAH):
1.4.1 Connective tissue diseases
1.4.2 HIV infection
1.4.3 Portal hypertension
1.4.4 Congenital heart diseases
1.4.5 Schistosomiasis
1.4.6 Chronic haemolytic anaemia
1.5 Persistent pulmonary hypertension of the newborn
1' Pulmonary veno-occlusive disease and/or pulmonary capillary haemangiomatosis
2. Pulmonary hypertension due to left heart disease
2.1 Systolic dysfunction
2.2 Diastolic dysfunction
2.3 Valvular disease
3. Pulmonary hypertension due to lung diseases and/or hypoxia
3.1 Chronic obstructive pulmonary disease
3.2 Interstitial lung disease
3.3 Other pulmonary diseases with mixed restrictive and obstructive pattern
3.4 Sleep-disordered breathing
3.5 Alveolar hypoventilation disorders
3.6 Chronic exposure to high altitude
3.7 Developmental abnormalities
4. Chronic thromboembolic pulmonary hypertension
5. PH with unclear multifactorial mechanisms
5.1 Haematologic disorders: myeloproliferative disorders splenectomy.
5.2 Systemic disorders: sarcoidosis, pulmonary Langerhans cell histiocytosis lymphangioleiomyomatosis, neurofibromatosis, vasculitis
5.3 Metabolic disorders: glycogen storage disease, Gaucher's disease, thyroid disorders
5.4 Others: tumoural obstruction, fibrosing mediastinitis, chronic renal failure on dialysis.

ALK-1, activin receptor-like kinase 1 gene; APAH, associated pulmonary arterial hypertension; BMPR2, bone morphogenetic protein receptor 2; HHT, hereditary haemorrhagic telangiectasia; PAH, pulmonary arterial hypertension.

Group 1 and Group 1' (➲Fig. 24.1)

Pathologic lesions affect particularly the distal pulmonary arteries (<500μm) and are characterized by medial hypertrophy

(➲Fig. 24.1A), intimal fibrosis (concentric, eccentric) (➲Fig. 24.1B), adventitial thickening (➲Fig. 24.1C) with moderate peri-vascular inflammatory infiltrates, complex lesions (plexiform (➲Fig. 24.1D), dilated lesions), and thrombotic lesions. Pulmonary veins are usually unaffected. Group1': include mainly pulmonary veno-occlusive disease which involves septal veins and preseptal venules (constant involvement) with occlusive fibrotic lesions, venous muscularization, common capillary proliferation (patchy), pulmonary oedema, occult alveolar haemorrhage, lymphatic dilatation and lymph node enlargement (vascular transformation of the sinus), and inflammatory infiltrates. Distal pulmonary arteries are affected by medial hypertrophy, intimal fibrosis, and uncommon complex lesions.

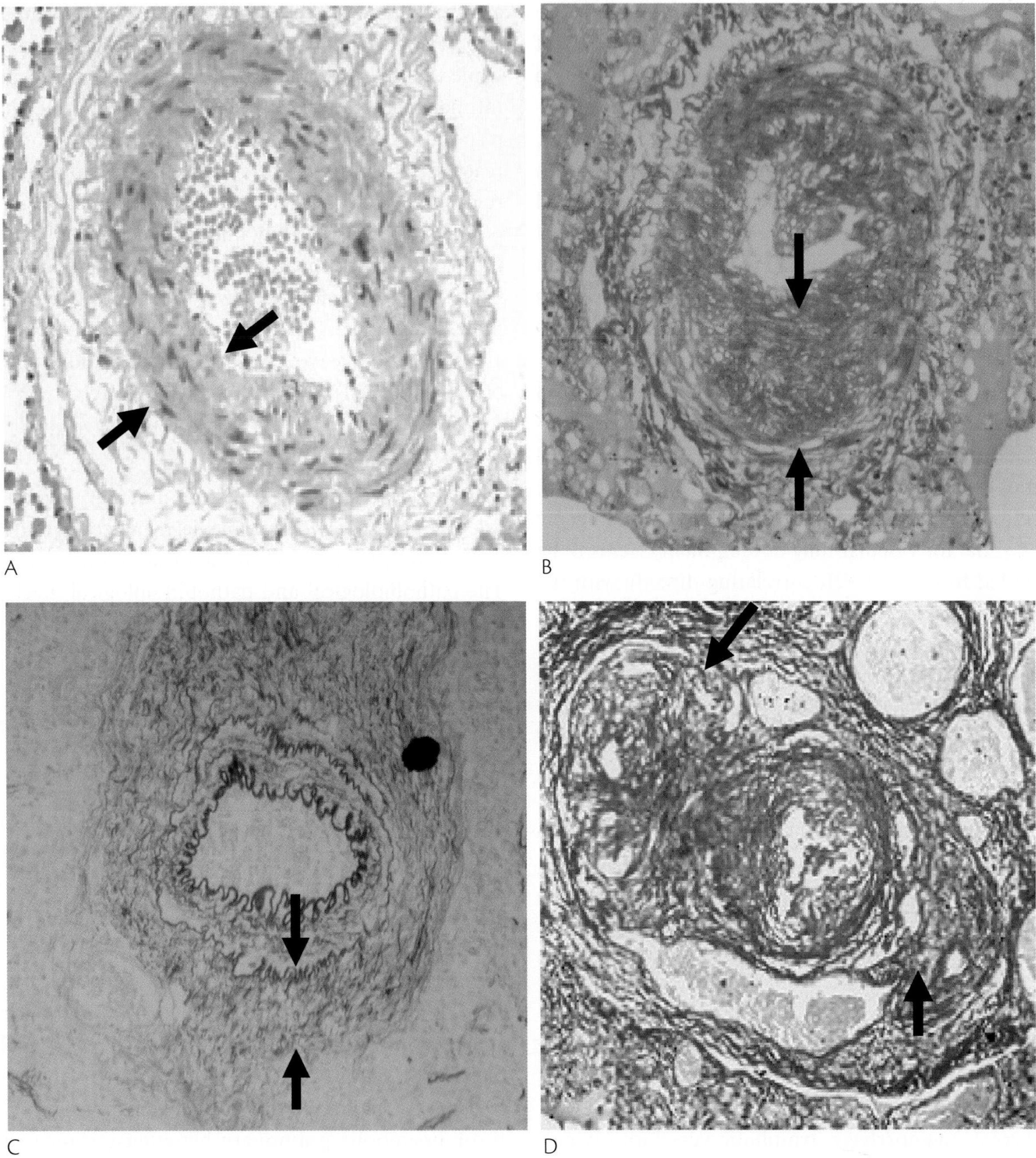

Figure 24.1 Histopathological features of pulmonary arterial hypertension. Pulmonary arteriopathy in intra-acinar pulmonary arteries: (A) Medial hypertrophy: increase in the cross sectional area of the media (between arrows) due to both hypertrophy and hyperplasia of smooth muscle fibres as well as increase in connective tissue matrix and elastic fibres. (B) Intimal thickening (between arrows): eccentric non-laminar thickening due to fibroblasts, myofibroblasts, smooth muscle cells, connective tissue matrix, and elastic fibres. (C) Adventitial thickening (between arrows) with its typical ill-defined boundaries. (D) Plexiform lesion: focal proliferation of endothelial channels (arrows) lined by myofibroblasts, smooth muscle cells, and connective tissue matrix.

The exact processes that initiate the pathological changes seen in PAH are still unknown even if it is recognized that PAH has a multifactorial pathobiology that involves various biochemical pathways and cell types. The increase in PVR is related to different mechanisms, including vasoconstriction, proliferative and obstructive remodelling of the pulmonary vessel wall, inflammation, and thrombosis. Pulmonary vasoconstriction is believed to be an early component of the pulmonary hypertensive process. Excessive vasoconstriction has been related to abnormal function or expression of potassium channels in the smooth muscle cells and to endothelial dysfunction. Reduced plasma levels of a vasodilator and antiproliferative substance such as vasoactive intestinal peptide have been demonstrated in patients with PAH. Endothelial dysfunction leads to chronically impaired production of vasodilator and antiproliferative agents such as nitric oxide and prostacyclin, along with over-expression of vasoconstrictor and proliferative substances such as thromboxane A2 and endothelin-1. Many of these abnormalities both elevate vascular tone and promote vascular remodelling by proliferative changes that involve several cell types, including endothelial, smooth muscle, and fibroblast. In addition, in the adventitia there is increased production of extracellular matrix including collagen, elastin, fibronectin, and tenascin. Angiopoietin-1, an angiogenic factor essential for vascular lung development, seems to be up-regulated in cases of PH, correlating directly with the severity of the disease.

Inflammatory cells and platelets may also play a significant role in PAH. In fact, inflammatory cells are ubiquitous in the pathological changes of PAH and pro-inflammatory cytokines are elevated in the plasma of PAH patients. Alteration in the metabolic pathways of serotonin, a pulmonary vasoconstrictor substance stored in the platelets, has also been detected in PAH patients. Prothrombotic abnormalities have been demonstrated in PAH patients and thrombi are present in both the more distal small pulmonary arteries and in the proximal elastic pulmonary arteries.

Group 2

Pathological changes in PH due to left heart disease are characterized by enlarged and thickened pulmonary veins, pulmonary capillary dilatation, interstitial oedema, common alveolar haemorrhage, lymphatic vessel and lymph node enlargement. Distal pulmonary arteries may be affected by medial hypertrophy and intimal fibrosis. The mechanisms responsible for the increase in PAP are multiple and include the passive backward transmission of the pressure elevation (postcapillary passive PH; ➲Table 24.1). In these cases the transpulmonary pressure gradient (mean PAP – mean PWP) and PVR are within the normal range. In other circumstances the elevation of PAP is greater than that of PWP (increased transpulmonary pressure gradient) and an increase in PVR is observed (postcapillary reactive PH; see ➲Table 24.1). The elevation of PVR is due to an increase in pulmonary artery vasomotor tone and/or to fixed structural obstructive remodelling of the pulmonary artery resistance vessels [5]: the former component of reactive PH is reversible under acute pharmacological testing while the latter, characterized by medial hypertrophy and intimal proliferation of the pulmonary arteriole, does not respond to the acute challenge [6]. Which factors lead to reactive PH and why some patients develop the acutely reversible vasoconstrictive or the fixed obstructive components or both is poorly understood. Pathophysiological mechanisms may include vasoconstrictive reflexes arising from stretch receptors localized in the left atrium and pulmonary veins, and endothelial dysfunction of pulmonary arteries that may favour vasoconstriction and proliferation of vessel wall cells.

Group 3

Pathological changes in cases of pulmonary hypertension due to lung diseases include medial hypertrophy and intimal obstructive proliferation of the distal pulmonary arteries. The pathobiological and pathophysiological mechanisms involved in this setting are multiple and include hypoxic vasoconstriction, mechanical stress of hyperinflated lungs, inflammation, and toxic effects of cigarette smoking. There are also data supporting an endothelium-derived vasoconstrictor–vasodilator imbalance.

Group 4

Chronic thromboembolic PH is characterized by organized thrombi in the elastic pulmonary arteries which are tightly attached to the pulmonary arterial medial layer, replacing the normal intima, and can completely occlude the lumen or form different grades of stenosis, webs, and bands [7]. Interestingly, in the non-occluded areas, a pulmonary arteriopathy indistinguishable from that of PAH (including plexiform lesions) can develop [8]. Pulmonary thromboembolism (➲Chapter 37) or in situ thrombosis in chronic thromboembolic pulmonary hypertension may be initiated or aggravated by abnormalities in either the clotting cascade, endothelial cells, or platelets, all of which interact in the coagulation process [9]. Platelet abnormalities and biochemical features of a procoagulant environment within the pulmonary vasculature support a potential role for thrombosis in initiation of the disease in some patients. In most cases, however, it remains unclear whether thrombosis and platelet dysfunction are a cause or consequence of the disease. Inflammatory infiltrates are commonly detected in the endarterectomy specimens. Thrombophilia studies have shown that lupus anticoagulant may be detected in approximately 10% of such patients, and 20% carry anticardiolipin antibodies, lupus anticoagulant, or both. A recent study [10] has demonstrated that the plasma level of factor VIII, a protein associated with both primary and recurrent venous thromboembolism, is elevated in 39% of patients with chronic thromboembolic pulmonary hypertension. No abnormalities of fibrinolysis have been detected. The lesion observed in non-obstructed areas may be related to a variety of factors, such as shear stress, pressure, inflammation, and the release of cytokines and vasculotrophic mediators.

Group 5

This group includes heterogeneous conditions with different pathologic and pathobiologic pictures and for which the aetiology is unclear or multifactorial.

Genetics and epidemiology

Group 1

PAH may occur in different clinical contexts, depending on associated clinical conditions [11]. Idiopathic PAH corresponds to sporadic disease, without any familial history of PAH or known triggering factor. When PAH occurs in a familial context, germline mutations in the bone morphogenetic protein receptor 2 (*BMPR2*) gene are detected in at least 70% of cases [11]. *BMPR2* mutations can also be detected in 11–40% of apparently sporadic cases. *BMPR2* mutation thus represents the major genetic predisposing factor for PAH [12]. The *BMPR2* gene encodes a type 2 receptor for bone morphogenetic proteins (BMPs), which belong to the TGF-beta superfamily. Among several biological functions, BMPs are involved in the control of vascular cell proliferation. Mutations in TGF-beta receptors, activin-receptor-like kinase 1 (ALK-1), and endoglin have been identified in PAH patients with a personal or family history of hereditary haemorrhagic telangiectasia (i.e. Osler–Weber–Rendu syndrome) [13].

Recent registries have described the epidemiology of PAH [14, 15]. The low estimate of the prevalence of PAH and idiopathic PAH are 15 and 5.9 cases/million adult inhabitants respectively. The low estimate of PAH incidence is 2.4 cases/million adult inhabitants/year. Recent data from Scotland and other countries have confirmed that PAH prevalence ranges 15–50 subjects per million inhabitants in Europe [14]. In the French registry, 39.2% of patients had idiopathic PAH and 3.9% familial PAH. In the subgroup of PAH associated with other conditions, 15.3% had connective tissue diseases (mainly systemic sclerosis), 11.3% congenital heart diseases, 10.4% portal hypertension, 9,5% anorexigen-associated PAH, and 6.2% HIV infection.

Group 2

Even if constitutional factors may play a role in the development of PH, no specific genetic linkages have been identified. The prevalence of PH in patients with chronic heart failure increases with the progression of the functional class impairment. Up to 60% of patients with severe left ventricular (LV) systolic dysfunction and up to 70% of patients with isolated LV diastolic dysfunction may present with PH [16].

Group 3

No genetic factors have been involved in the development of PH in this group. On the basis of published series, the incidence of significant PH in chronic obstructive pulmonary disease (COPD) patients with at least one previous hospitalization for exacerbation of respiratory failure should be around 20%. In advanced COPD, PH is highly prevalent (>50%) [17], although in general it is of only mild severity. In interstitial lung fibrosis, the prevalence of PH ranges between 32–39% [18].

Group 4

No specific genetic mutations have been linked to the development of chronic thromboembolic PH. Even if more recent papers suggest a chronic thromboembolic PH prevalence of up to 5% in survivors of acute PE [19], most experts believe that the true incidence of chronic thromboembolic PH after acute PE is 0.5–2%. Chronic thromboembolic PH can be found in patients without any previous clinical episode of acute pulmonary embolism or deep venous thrombosis (up to 50% of different series).

Pulmonary arterial hypertension (Group 1)

The clinical group 1 defined as PAH comprises apparently heterogeneous conditions that share comparable clinical and haemodynamic pictures and virtually identical pathological changes of the lung microcirculation [3]. PAH includes idiopathic PAH (IPAH, formerly termed primary pulmonary hypertension), heritable PAH (HPAH) [20], and PAH associated with various conditions such as connective tissue diseases, congenital heart defects with systemic-to-pulmonary shunts, portal hypertension, HIV infection, drugs, and toxins. Even if many pathobiological mechanisms have been identified in the cells and tissues of patients with PAH (see ➲ Group 1 and Group 1', p.894), the exact interactions between them in initiating and progressing the pathological processes are not well understood. The consequent increase in PVR leads to right ventricular (RV) overload, hypertrophy and dilatation, and eventually to RV failure and death. The importance of the progression of RV failure on the outcome of IPAH patients is testified by the prognostic impact of right atrial pressure, cardiac index, and mean PAP [21], three main determinants of RV pump function. The depression of myocardial contractility seems to be one of the primary events in the progression of heart failure in a chronically overloaded RV. In fact, changes in the adrenergic pathways of RV myocytes leading to reduced contractility have been shown in IPAH patients [22]. However, afterload mismatch remains the leading determinant of heart failure in patients with PAH and chronic thromboembolic PH because its removal, as after successful pulmonary endarterectomy or lung transplantation [23], leads almost invariably to sustained recovery of RV function. Therefore, the haemodynamic changes and the prognosis of patients with PAH are related to the complex pathophysiological interactions between the rate of progression (or regression) of the obstructive changes in the pulmonary circulation and the response of the overloaded RV, which may also be influenced by genetic determinants [24].

Diagnostic strategy

The evaluation process of a patient with PH requires a series of investigations intended to make the diagnosis, clarify the clinical group of PH and the type of PAH, and evaluate the functional and haemodynamic impairment. After the description of each examination, an integrated algorithm will be presented.

Clinical presentation

The symptoms of PAH include breathlessness, fatigue, weakness, angina, syncope, and abdominal distension [25]. Symptoms at rest are reported only in very advanced cases. The physical signs of PAH include left parasternal lift, accentuated pulmonary component of the second heart sound (S_2), pansystolic murmur of tricuspid regurgitation, diastolic murmur of pulmonary insufficiency, and RV third heart sound (S_3) [25]. Jugular vein distension, hepatomegaly, peripheral oedema, ascites, and cool extremities characterize patients in a more advanced state. Lung sounds are usually normal.

Electrocardiogram

The electrocardiogram (ECG) may provide suggestive or supportive evidence of PH by demonstrating RV hypertrophy and strain, and right atrial dilation (➲Fig. 24.2) (see ➲Chapter 2). RV hypertrophy on ECG is present in 87% and right axis deviation in 79% of patients with IPAH [25]. The ECG has inadequate sensitivity (55%) and specificity (70%) to be a screening tool for detecting significant PH. Supraventricular arrhythmias may be present in advanced stages, in particular atrial flutter which invariably leads to a further clinical deterioration.

Chest radiograph

In 90% of patients with IPAH the chest radiograph is abnormal at the time of diagnosis [25]. Findings include central pulmonary arterial dilatation, which contrasts with 'pruning' (loss) of the peripheral blood vessels (➲Fig. 24.3). Right atrial and ventricular enlargement may be seen and it progresses in more advanced cases. The chest radiograph allows associated moderate to severe lung disease or pulmonary venous hypertension due to left heart abnormalities to be reasonably excluded (see ➲ High-resolution CT of the lung, p.900).

Pulmonary function tests and arterial blood gases

Pulmonary function tests and arterial blood gases will identify the contribution of underlying airway or parenchymal lung disease. Patients with PAH usually have decreased lung diffusion capacity for carbon monoxide (D_LCO) (typically in the range of 40–80% predicted) and mild to moderate reduction of lung volumes. Arterial oxygen tension (P_aO_2) is normal or only slightly lower than normal and arterial carbon dioxide tension (P_aCO_2) is decreased as a result of alveolar hyperventilation. COPD, as a cause of hypoxic PH, is diagnosed on the evidence of irreversible airflow obstruction together with increased residual volumes, reduced D_LCO, and normal or increased P_aCO_2. A decrease in lung volume together with a decrease in D_LCO may indicate a diagnosis of interstitial lung disease (ILD). The severity of emphysema and of ILD can be diagnosed using high-resolution computed tomography (CT). If clinically suspected, screening overnight oximetry will exclude significant obstructive sleep apnoea/hypopnoea.

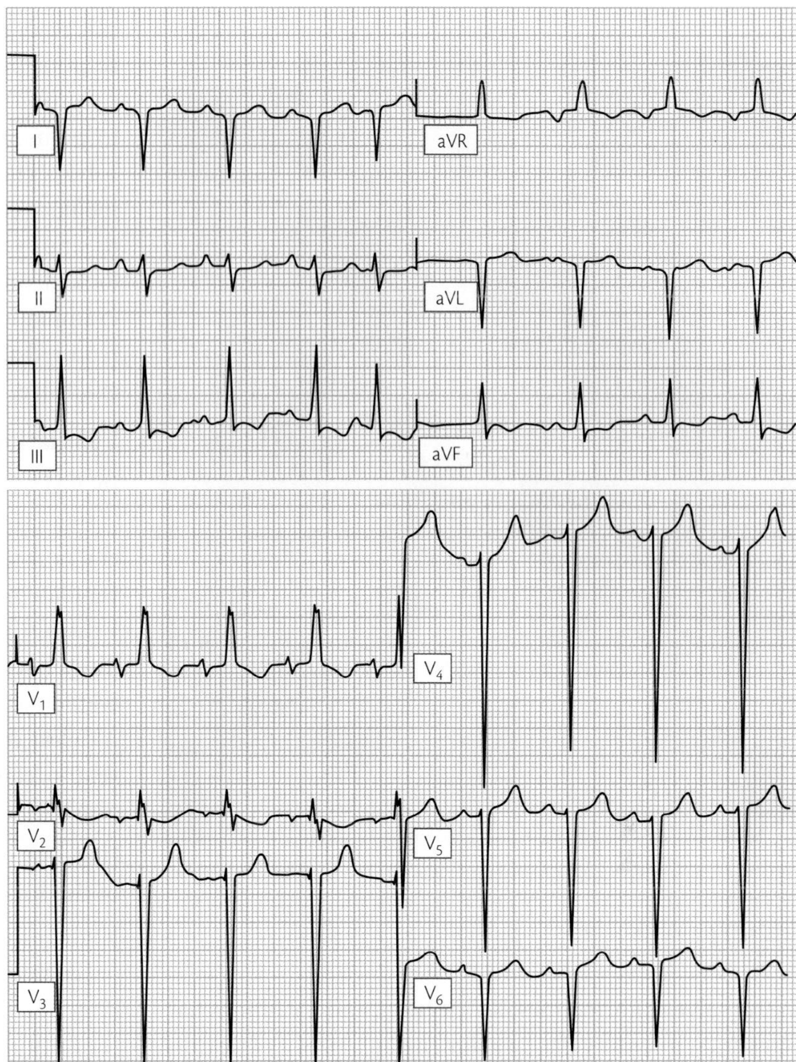

Figure 24.2 ECG of a patient with severe pulmonary arterial hypertension: right atrial enlargement, right axis deviation, right ventricular hypertrophy, and strain can be noted.

Echocardiography

Transthoracic echocardiography (➲Chapter 4) is an excellent non-invasive screening test for the patient with suspected PH. Transthoracic echocardiography estimates pulmonary artery systolic pressure (PASP) and can provide additional information about the cause and consequences of PH. PASP is equivalent to RV systolic pressure in the absence of pulmonary outflow obstruction. RV systolic pressure is estimated by measurement of the systolic regurgitant tricuspid flow velocity and an estimate of right atrial pressure (RAP) (➲Fig. 24.4A,B). Tricuspid regurgitant jets can be assessed in 74% of patients with PH [26]. According to data obtained in normal subjects [27], possible PH as estimated by Doppler echocardiography can be defined as a PASP of approximately 37–50mmHg or a resting tricuspid regurgitant velocity of 2.8–3.4m/s (assuming a normal RAP of 5mmHg). It should also be noted that with this definition a number of false-positive diagnoses can be anticipated, especially in aged and obese subjects. PH as estimated by Doppler echocardiography is likely if tricuspid regurgitation velocity is >3.4m/s. Confirmation with right heart catheterization of the presence of PH is required in particular in symptomatic patients (WHO/NYHA functional class II/III/IV) and if the use of specific PAH drugs is considered. In asymptomatic subjects (WHO/NYHA functional class I) with possible PH, a concomitant connective tissue diseases should be excluded and echocardiography should be repeated in 6 months. Also the possibility of false negative Doppler echocardiographic results should be considered in cases of high clinical suspicion [28].

The use of Doppler exercise echocardiography to identify cases of 'latent' PH is still investigational and should not be utilized in clinical practice for management decision making. Additional echocardiographic and Doppler parameters are important for the confirmation of diagnosis and assessment of the severity of PH, including RV dimensions (enlarged) and function (reduced), LV dimensions (reduced) (➲Fig. 24.4C), and function (normal), tricuspid, pulmonary, and

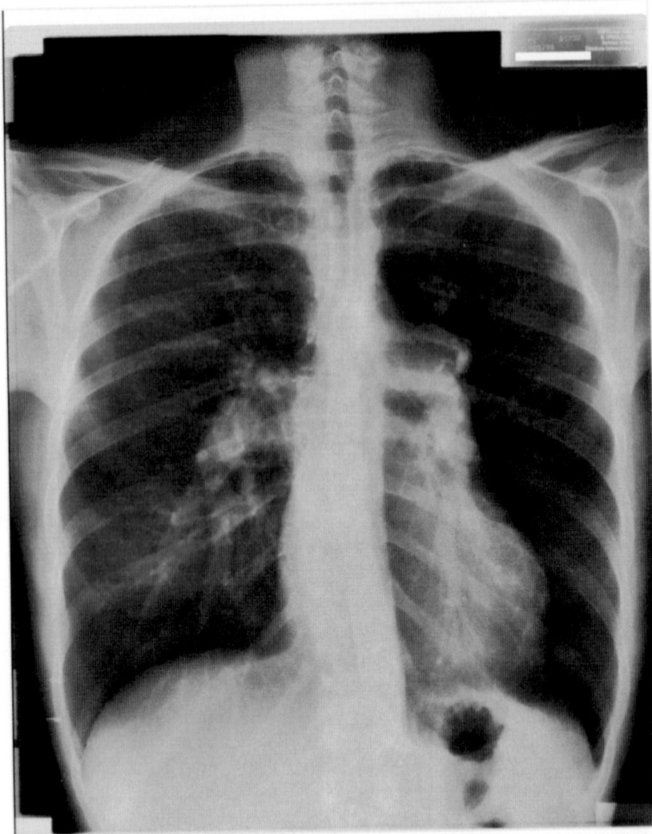

Figure 24.3 Chest radiograph of a patient with severe pulmonary arterial hypertension: central pulmonary arterial dilatation and 'pruning' (loss) of the peripheral blood vessels can be noted.

mitral valve abnormalities, RV ejection, and LV filling characteristics, inferior vena cava dimensions, size of pericardial effusion [29, 30], and the tricuspid annular plane systolic excursion [31]. Besides identification of PH, transthoracic echocardiography also allows a differential diagnosis of possible causes. In fact, transthoracic echocardiography can recognize left heart valvular and myocardial diseases responsible for pulmonary venous hypertension (clinical group 2), and congenital heart diseases with systemic-to-pulmonary shunts can be easily identified (clinical group 1.4.4). The venous injection of agitated saline as contrast medium can help the identification of patent foramen ovale or sinus venosus-type atrial septal defects that can be overlooked on the standard transthoracic echocardiography examination. Transoesophageal echocardiography is rarely required and is used to confirm the presence, and assess the exact size, of atrial septal defects.

Ventilation–perfusion (*V*[Lt]/*Q*[Lt]) lung scan

In PAH, lung *V*[Lt]/*Q*[Lt] scans may be entirely normal (➲Fig. 24.5A). However, they may also show small peripheral non-segmental defects in perfusion. These are normally ventilated and thus represent *V*[Lt]/*Q*[Lt] mismatch. Lung *V*[Lt]/*Q*[Lt] scan provides a means of diagnosis of chronic thromboembolic PH (clinical group 4), showing lobar and segmental defects in the perfusion image (➲Fig. 24.5B). A caveat is that unmatched perfusion defects are also seen in veno-occlusive disease. In patients with parenchymal lung disease the perfusion defects are *matched* by ventilation defects.

High-resolution CT, contrast-enhanced spiral CT of the lung, and pulmonary angiography

High-resolution CT provides detailed views of the lung parenchyma and facilitates the diagnosis of interstitial lung fibrosis (ILD) (➲Fig. 24.6A) and emphysema. High-resolution CT may be indicated in cases where there is interstitial marking on the chest radiograph without evidence of LV failure. In these cases the confirmation of a diffuse, central, ground-glass opacification and thickening of interlobular septa suggest pulmonary veno-occlusive

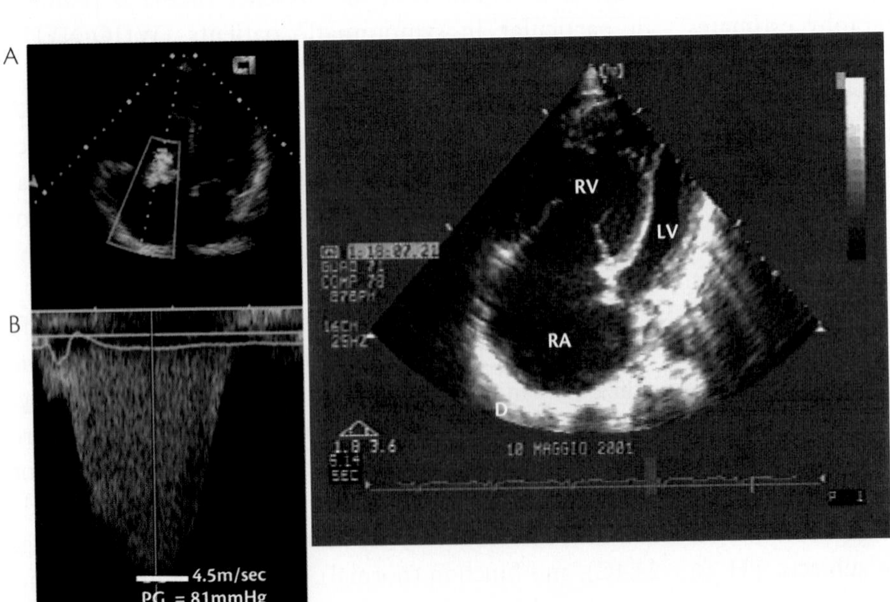

Figure 24.4 Doppler-echocardiography in pulmonary arterial hypertension. (A) Continuous-wave Doppler beam guided by colour-coded Doppler visualization of the jet of tricuspid regurgitation. (B) Doppler measurement of the peak velocity of the jet of tricuspid regurgitation. According to the Bernoulli equation, a velocity of 4.5m/s indicates a maximum systolic pressure gradient between the right ventricle and the right atrium (PG) of 81mmHg. (C) Apical four-chamber view: enlarged right ventricle (RV) and right atrium (RA) and reduced left ventricle (LV) are shown.

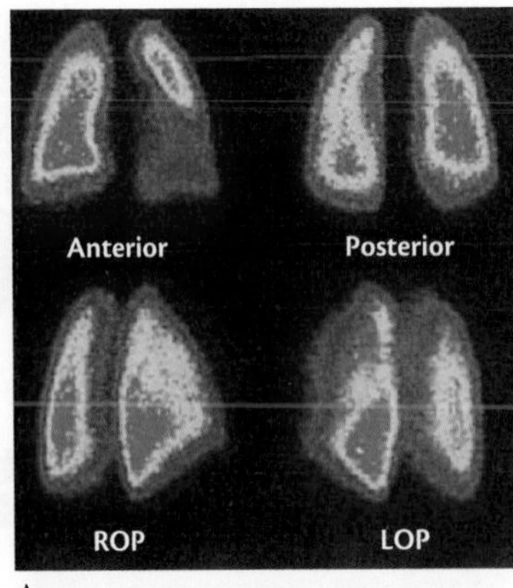

A

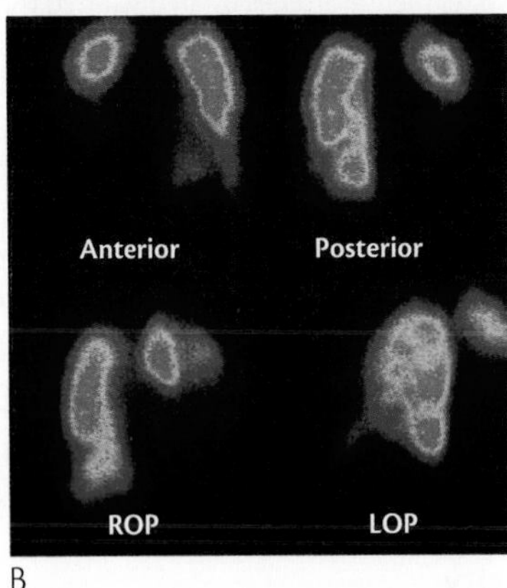

B

Figure 24.5 Perfusion lung scan. (A) Normal perfusion lung scan of a patient with pulmonary arterial hypertension according to the anterior, posterior, right (ROP), and left (LOP) oblique posterior views. (B) Lobar and segmental perfusion defects in a patient with chronic thromboembolic pulmonary hypertension.

disease (➲Fig. 24.6B); additional findings are lymphadenopathy, pleural shadows, and effusions [32].

Contrast-enhanced spiral CT is indicated in patients with PH when *V*[Lt]/*Q*[Lt] lung scintigraphy shows segmental defects of perfusion with normal ventilation and may demonstrate central chronic pulmonary thromboemboli. CT features of chronic thromboembolic disease include complete occlusion of pulmonary arteries, eccentric filling defects consistent with organized thrombi, recanalization, and stenoses or webs [33] (➲Fig. 24.7). With this technique, collaterals from bronchial arteries can be identified (➲Fig. 24.7C). Traditional pulmonary angiography is still required in the work-up of chronic thromboembolic pulmonary hypertension to better identify patients who can benefit from the intervention of endarterectomy [7] (Fig. 24.8A). Pulmonary angiography is more accurate in the identification of distal obstructions (➲Fig. 24.8B) and is indicated also in cases of inconclusive contrast-enhanced spiral CT in patients with clinical and lung perfusion scan suspicion of chronic thromboembolic PH .

Magnetic resonance imaging

Cardiac magnetic resonance (CMR) (➲Chapter 6) provides (➲Fig. 24.9) a direct evaluation of RV size, morphology, and function and allows non-invasive assessment of blood flow including stroke volume, CO, distensibility of PA and of RV muscle mass [34]. There is good correlation between right heart catheterization and CMR suggesting that CMR data could be used as a surrogate for right heart haemodynamics. A decreased stroke volume, an increased RV end-diastolic volume, and a decreased LV end-diastolic volume measured at baseline are associated with a poor prognosis. Among the triad of prognostic signs, the increasing RV end-diastolic volume appears to be the most straightforward and appropriate marker of progressive RV failure [35].

Blood tests and immunology

Routine biochemistry, haematology and thyroid function tests are required. Connective tissue diseases are diagnosed primarily on clinical and laboratory criteria and an autoimmune screen consists of antinuclear antibodies, including anti-centromere antibodies, anti-SCL70 and RNP. About one-third of patients with IPAH have positive but low antinuclear antibody titre (<1:80 dilutions).

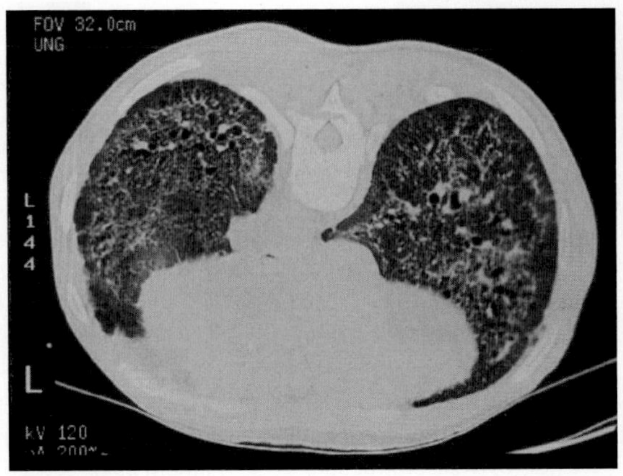

A

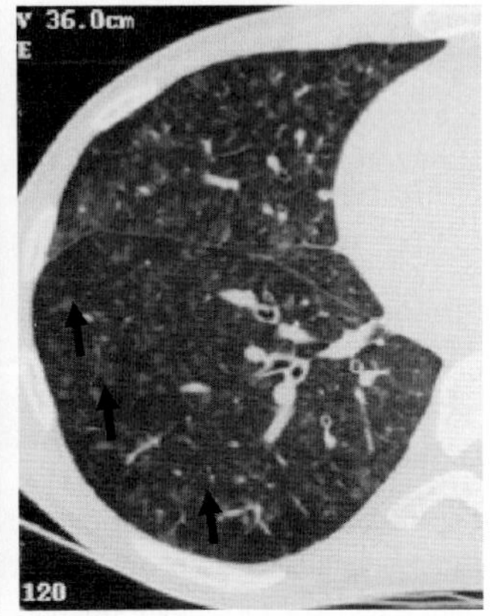

B

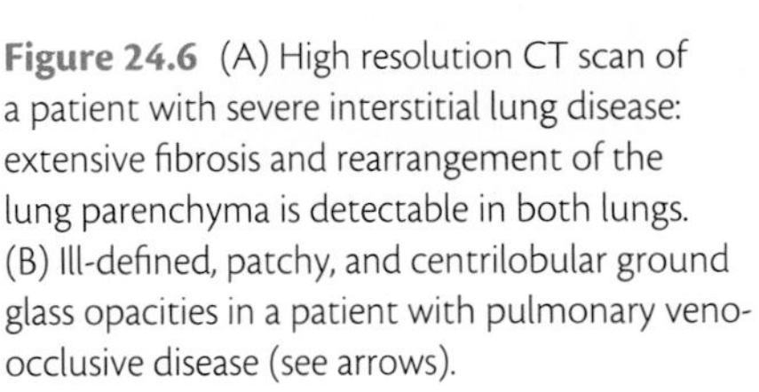

Figure 24.6 (A) High resolution CT scan of a patient with severe interstitial lung disease: extensive fibrosis and rearrangement of the lung parenchyma is detectable in both lungs. (B) Ill-defined, patchy, and centrilobular ground glass opacities in a patient with pulmonary veno-occlusive disease (see arrows).

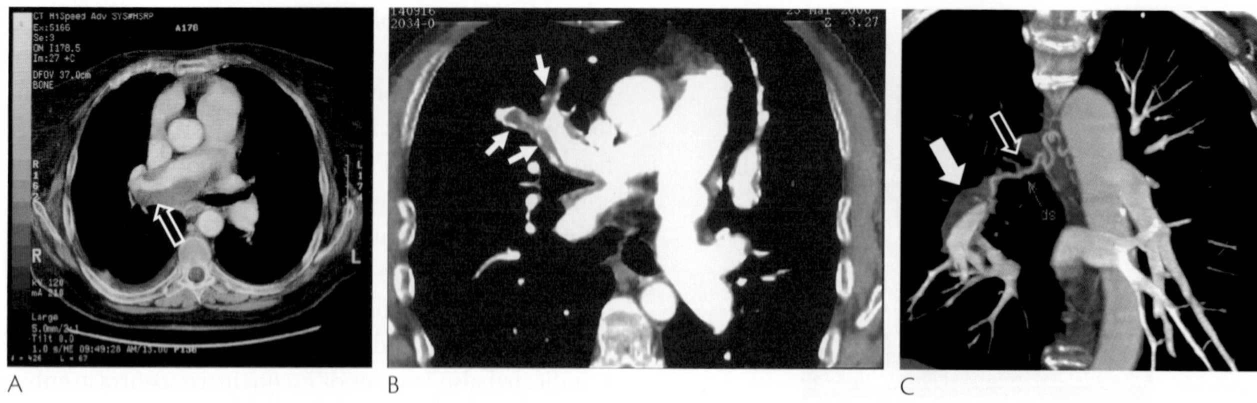

Figure 24.7 Contrast enhanced spiral CT of the lungs of patients with chronic thromboembolic pulmonary hypertension. (A) Severe reduction of calibre of the right main pulmonary artery by an organized thrombus (open arrow). (B) Obstruction of two segmental arteries by an organized thrombus which extends proximally to a lobar branch (arrows). (C) Collaterals from a dilated bronchial artery (open arrow) perfuse the right lower lobe pulmonary artery which is proximally obstructed (filled arrow) by an organized thrombus.

Patients with substantially elevated antinuclear antibodies and/or suspicious clinical features require further serological assessment and rheumatology consultation. Finally, consent of all patients should be obtained and an HIV serology test undertaken.

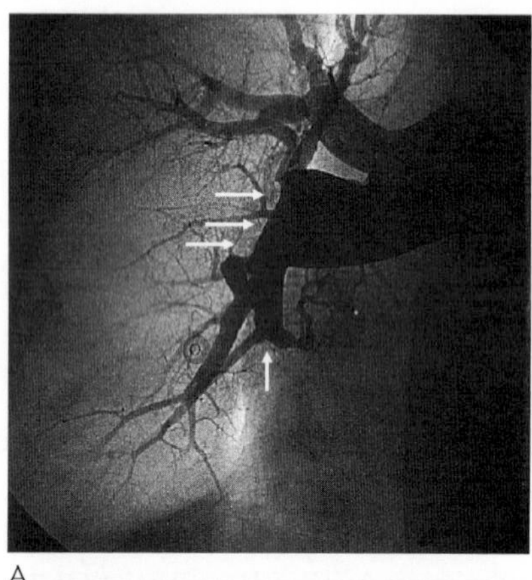

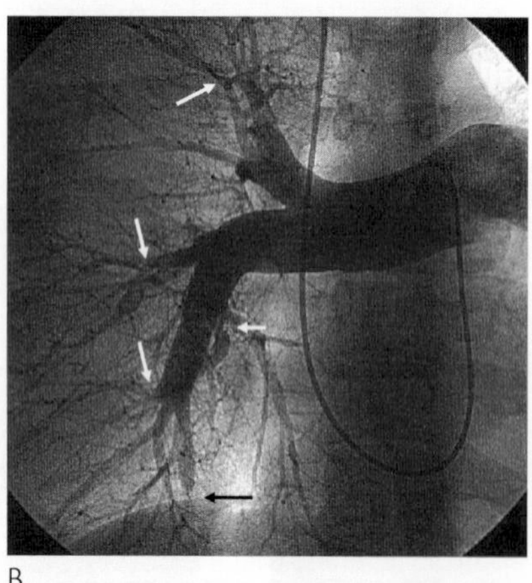

Figure 24.8 Pulmonary angiography of patients with chronic thromboembolic pulmonary hypertension. (A) Proximal obstructions of middle and lower lobe right pulmonary arteries. (B) Distal obstruction/stenosis of multiple segmental and subsegmental right pulmonary arteries.

Abdominal ultrasound scan

Liver cirrhosis and/or portal hypertension can be reliably excluded by the use of abdominal ultrasound. The use of contrast agents may improve the diagnosis. Portal hypertension can be confirmed by the detection of an increased gradient between free and occluded (wedge) hepatic vein pressure at the time of right heart catheterization [36].

Exercise capacity

The objective assessment of exercise capacity in patients with PAH is an important instrument for evaluating disease severity and treatment effect. The most commonly used exercise tests for PH are the 6-minute walk test (a normal middle-aged individual can walk >500m in 6min) and cardiopulmonary exercise testing with gas exchange measurement. [37]

Right heart catheterization and vasoreactivity

Right heart catheterization is required to confirm the diagnosis of PAH, to assess the severity of the haemodynamic impairment, and to test the vasoreactivity of the pulmonary circulation. PAH is defined by a mean PAP ≥25mmHg at

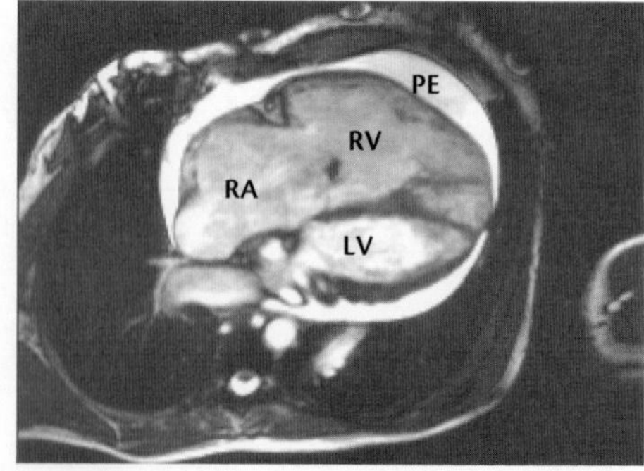

Figure 24.9 Magnetic resonance imaging of the heart of a patient with pulmonary arterial hypertension. Enlarged right ventricle (RV) and right atrium (RA), reduced left ventricle (LV), and pericardial effusion (PE) are shown. (Courtesy of Anton Vonk Noordegraaf.)

rest, by a pulmonary wedge (occluded) pressure (PWP) ≤15mmHg (precapillary PH; see Table 24.1), Left heart catheterization is required in the rare circumstances in which a reliable PWP cannot be measured. The assessment of PWP may allow the distinction between arterial and venous PH in patients with concomitant left heart diseases. Right heart catheterization is also important in patients with definite moderate to severe PAH because the haemodynamic variables have prognostic relevance [21]. Elevated mean RAP, mean PAP, and reduced CO and central venous oxygen saturation identify IPAH patients with the worst prognosis. An acute vasodilator challenge performed during right heart catheterization [38] can identify patients who may benefit from long-term treatment with calcium-channel blockers. Acute vasodilator testing should only be done using short-acting pulmonary vasodilators at the time of the initial right heart catheterization in experienced centres in order to minimize the potential risks. Currently the agent more used in acute testing is nitric oxide [38]; based on older experiences [39–41] intravenous epoprostenol could also be used and intravenous adenosine may also be used. A positive acute vasoreactive response (positive acute responders) is defined as a reduction of mean PAP ≥10mmHg to reach an absolute value of mean PAP ≤40mmHg with an increased or unchanged CO. Generally, only about 10% of patients with IPAH will meet these criteria [39, 42].

Diagnostic algorithm

The various investigative tests can be combined in a diagnostic algorithm (Fig. 24.10), which for practical purposes can be divided into four phases.

- *Suspicion*: clinical suspicion of PH should be aroused when there are symptoms such as breathlessness without overt signs of specific heart or lung disease, in cases of screening in predisposing conditions or in cases of incidental findings.
- *Detection*: the detection of PH requires investigations able to confirm the diagnosis, e.g. clinical examination, ECG, chest radiograph, and transthoracic echocardiography.
- *Group identification*: the next step is the identification of the clinical group (see Table 24.1) [2]. This is accomplished by the use of essential investigations such as pulmonary function tests, arterial blood gases, and ventilation–perfusion lung scan. In particular circumstances, additional tests can be performed such as high-resolution CT of the chest, contrast-enhanced spiral CT of the lung, and pulmonary angiography.
- *Evaluation*: after the diagnosis of PAH (clinical group 1), additional investigations are required for the exact identification of the type and for the assessment of exercise capacity and haemodynamics.

Evaluation of severity

The variables that have been shown to predict prognosis in IPAH when assessed at baseline or after targeted treatments are listed in Table 24.3. Very little information is available in other conditions, such as PAH associated with connective tissue diseases, congenital systemic-to-pulmonary shunts, HIV infection, or portal hypertension. In these circumstances, additional factors may contribute

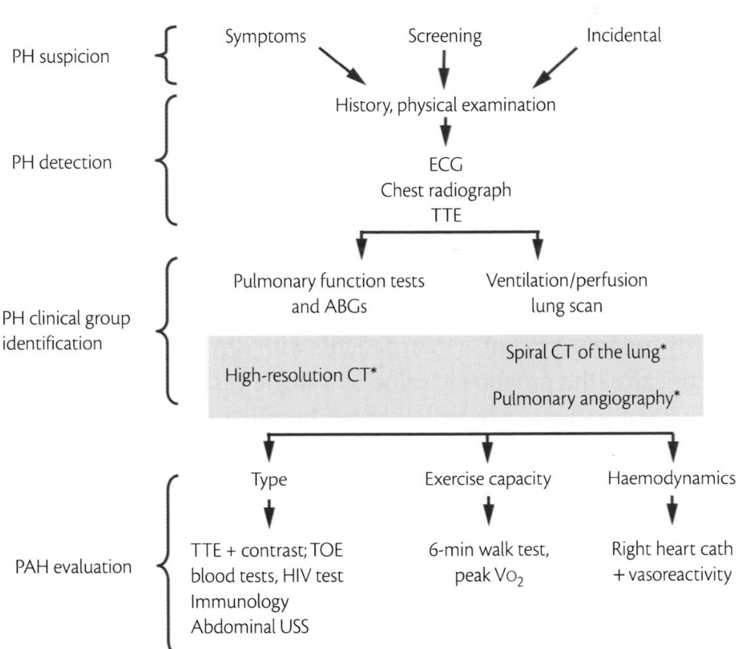

Figure 24.10 Diagnostic algorithm of pulmonary hypertension. ABGs, arterial blood gases; CT, computed tomography; PAH, pulmonary arterial hypertension; PH, pulmonary hypertension; TOE, transoesophageal echocardiogram; TTE, transthoracic echocardiogram; USS, ultrasound scan. *Required in specific circumstances, see text.

Table 24.3 Prognostic parameters in patients with idiopathic pulmonary arterial hypertension

Clinical parameters
Baseline WHO/NYHA functional classification [21]
WHO/NYHA functional class on chronic epoprostenol treatment [44;45]
History of right heart failure [46]
Exercise capacity
Baseline 6MWT distance [47]
6MWT distance on chronic epoprostenol treatment [46]
Baseline peak VO_2 [43]
Echocardiographic parameters
Pericardial effusion [48]
Right atrial size [48]
Left ventricular eccentricity index [48]
Doppler right ventricular (Tei) index [43]
Tricuspid annular plane systolic excursion [31]
Haemodynamics
Right atrial pressure [21]
Mean PAP [21]
Cardiac output [21]
Mixed venous oxygen saturation [21]
Positive acute response to vasoreactivity tests [39, 41]
Fall in pulmonary vascular resistance <30% after 3 months of epoprostenol [46]
Blood tests
Hyperuricaemia [43]
Baseline brain natriuretic peptide [43]
Brain natriuretic peptide after 3 months of therapy [43]
Troponin: detectable, especially persistent leakage [49]
Plasma norepinephrine [43]
Plasma endothelin-1 [50]

6MWT: 6-Minute walk test; WHO/NYHA: World Health Organization/New York Heart Association; PAP: pulmonary arterial pressure.

to the overall outcome. In fact, PAH associated with connective tissue diseases has a worse prognosis than that of patients with IPAH, whereas patients with PAH associated with congenital systemic-to-pulmonary shunts have a more slowly progressive course than patients with IPAH. In clinical practice, the prognostic value of a single variable in the individual patient may be less than the value of multiple concordant variables.

Comprehensive prognostic evaluation

Regular evaluation of patients with PAH should focus on variables with established prognostic importance as outlined in ➲Table 24.3. Treatment decisions should be based on parameters that reflect symptoms and exercise capacity and that are relevant in terms of predicting outcome. Not all parameters regularly obtained in PAH patients are equally well suited to assess disease severity. For example, the PAP is measured on a regular basis, either by right heart catheterization or by echocardiography. The magnitude of the PAP, however, correlates poorly with symptoms and outcome as it is determined not only by the degree of PV obliteration but also by the performance of the RV. Not all parameters listed in ➲Table 24.3 need to be assessed at every single visit but in order to obtain a clear picture it is important to look at a panel of data derived from clinical evaluation, exercise tests, biochemical markers, echocardiographic and haemodynamic evaluation. It is crucial not to rely just on a single parameter as several assessments may provide divergent results.

Definition of clinical status

Based on the clinical, non-invasive and invasive findings patient's conditions can be defined as stable and satisfactory, stable but not satisfactory, unstable and deteriorating [51]:

- *Stable and satisfactory*: Absence of clinical signs of RV failure; stable WHO/NYHA functional class I or II without syncope; a 6-min walk distance >500m [3, 4], depending on the individual patient; a peak VO_2 >15mL/min/kg [2]; normal or near-normal brain natriuretic peptide (BNP)/N-terminal prohormone BNP (NT-proBNP) plasma levels [6, 7]; no pericardial effusion; tricuspid annular plane systolic excursion >2.0cm; a right atrial pressure (RAP) <8mmHg; and a cardiac index >2.5L/min/m^2.
- *Stable and not satisfactory*. This is a patient who although stable has not achieved the status which patient and treating physician would consider desirable. Some of the limits described earlier for a satisfactory condition are not fulfilled. These patients require re-evaluation and consideration for additional or different treatment following full assessment in the expert centre.
- *Unstable and deteriorating*. These are patients that have evidence of RV failure; progression of symptoms and signs; worsening WHO/NYHA functional class, i.e. from II to III or III to IV; a 6-min walk distance of <300m; rising BNP/NT-proBNP plasma levels; evidence of pericardial effusion; tricuspid annular plane systolic excursion <1.5cm; a RAP that is >15mmHg and rising; and a cardiac index that is <2L/min/m^2 and falling. Clinical warning signs are increasing oedema and/or the need to escalate diuretic therapy; new onset or increasing frequency/severity of angina which can be a sign of deteriorating right RV function; and the new occurrence

or increasing frequency of syncope, which is often a grim prognostic sign and requires immediate attention as it heralds low CO heart failure.

Treatment goals and follow-up strategy

Treatment goals for PAH patients may be considered as those listed in the 'Stable and satisfactory' definition given in the previous section. However, target values and treatment goals should be adjusted to the individual patient according, for example, to the age and the presence of comorbidities. For example, a 6-min walk distance >400m is usually considered acceptable in middle-aged PAH patients.

Established follow-up strategies for patients with PAH after a complete baseline assessment include re-evaluation at 3-month intervals, usually by clinical assessment and non-invasive tools.

There is no universally accepted recommendation about when and how often to perform follow-up right heart catheterization. In general, right heart catheterization in PAH is indicated for confirmation of PAH diagnosis and when PAH specific medications are considered; it should be considered for confirmation of efficacy of PAH specific medications, and it should be considered for confirmation of clinical deterioration and as baseline for the evaluation of the effect of treatment escalation and/or combination therapy.

Treatment

Treatments for PAH will be reviewed individually. Level of evidence and grade of recommendation [52] for each of them are reported in ➲Table 24.4 and a treatment algorithm is described in ➲Fig. 24.11 [51].

General measures

- *Physical activity*: patients should avoid excessive physical activity that leads to distressing symptoms, but when physically deconditioned may undertake supervised exercise rehabilitation.
- *Pregnancy and, birth control*: pregnancy is associated with a 30–50% mortality in patients with PAH and as a consequence PAH is a contraindication to pregnancy. Barrier contraceptive methods are safe but with an unpredictable effect. Progesterone-only preparations such as medroxyprogesterone acetate and etonogestrel are effective approaches to contraception and avoid potential issues of oestrogens. The patient who becomes pregnant should be informed of the high risk of pregnancy and termination of pregnancy discussed. Those patients who chose to continue pregnancy should be referred to an expert multidisciplinary team.

Table 24.4 Grading of recommendations and level of evidence for efficacy in idiopathic PAH

Measure/treatment	Classes of recommendation: level of evidence		
	WHO/ NYHA-FC II	WHO/ NYHA-FC III	WHO/ NYHA-FC IV
General measures			
Avoid excessive physical exercise	III: C	III: C	III: C
Birth control	I: C	I: C	I: C
Psychosocial support	IIa: C	IIa: C	IIa: C
Respiratory infection prevention	I: C	I: C	I: C
Supportive therapy			
Oral anticoagulants	IIa: C*	IIa: C*	IIa: C*
Diuretics	I: C	I: C	I: C
Digoxin	IIb: C	IIb: C	IIb: C
Oxygen†	I: C	I: C	I: C
Supervised rehabilitation	IIa: B	IIa: B	–
Calcium-channel blockers	I: C‡	I: C‡	–
Epoprostenol (intravenous)	–	I: A	I: A
Treprostinil (subcutaneous)	–	I: B	IIa: C
Treprostinil (intravenous)	–	IIa: C	IIa: C
Treprostinil (inhaled)**	–	I: B	IIa: C
Iloprost (inhaled)	–	I: A	IIa: C
Iloprost (intravenous)	–	IIa: C	IIa: C
Beraprost	–	IIb: B	–
Bosentan	I: A	I: A	IIa: C
Sitaxsentan	IIa: C	I: A	IIa: C
Ambrisentan	I: A	I: A	IIa: C
Sildenafil	I: A	I: A	IIa: C
Tadalafil††	I: B	I: B	IIa: C
Combination therapy	IIa: C	IIa: B	IIa: B
Balloon atrial septostomy	–	I: C	I: C
Lung transplantation	–	I: C	I: C

* IIa for idiopathic PAH, IIb for other associated PAH conditions.
† If arterial oxygen saturation <90% except for Eisenmenger's syndrome.
‡ Only in patient responders to acute reactivity tests, I for idiopathic PAH, IIa for other associated PAH conditions.
††Under regulatory review in the European Union
** Under regulatory review in the European Union and in the USA

- *Air travel* (➲*Chapter 38*): flight oxygen administration should be considered for patients in WHO/NYHA functional class III and IV and those with an arterial oxygen saturation <92%.

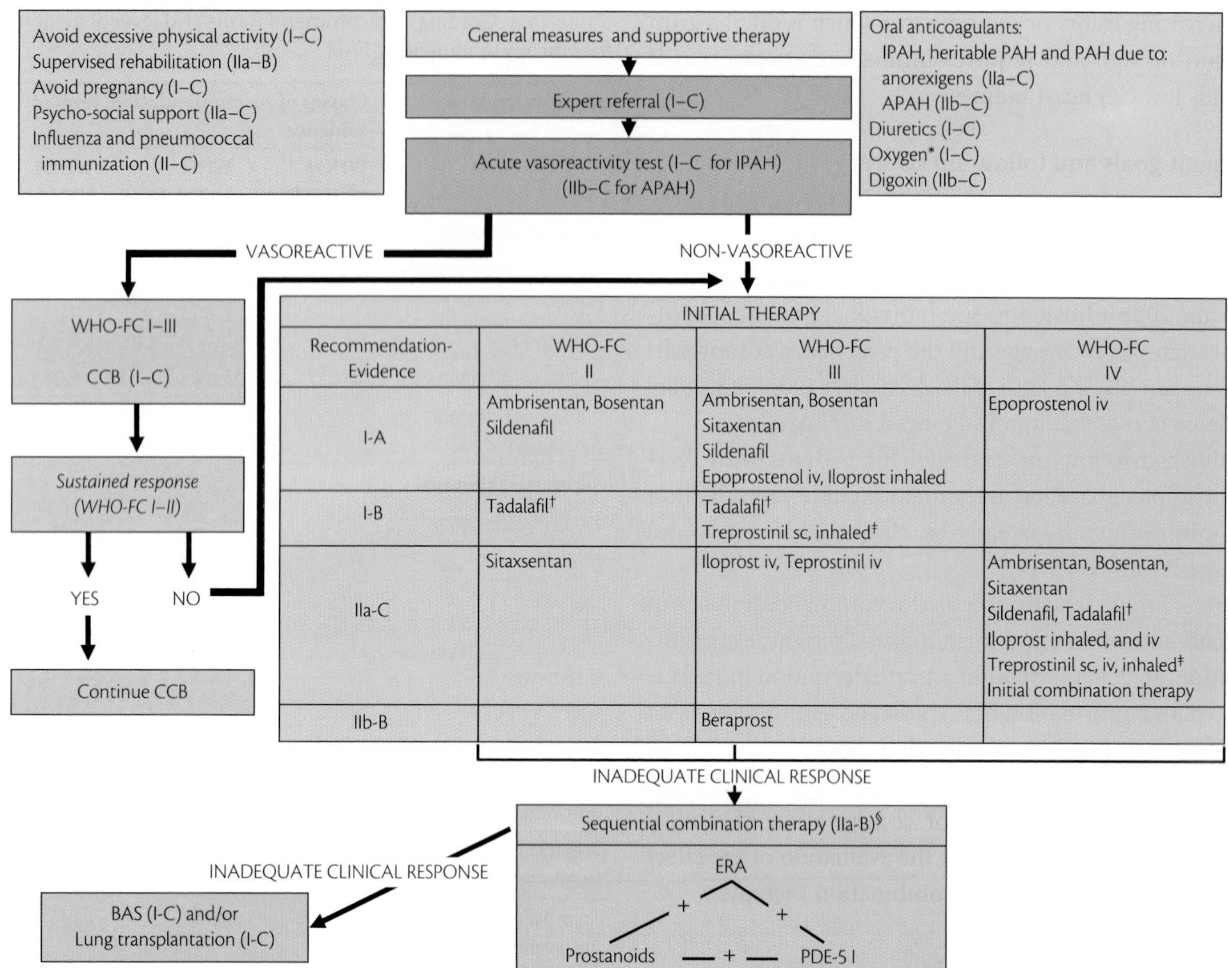

Recommendation-Evidence	WHO-FC II	WHO-FC III	WHO-FC IV
I-A	Ambrisentan, Bosentan Sildenafil	Ambrisentan, Bosentan Sitaxentan Sildenafil Epoprostenol iv, Iloprost inhaled	Epoprostenol iv
I-B	Tadalafil†	Tadalafil† Treprostinil sc, inhaled‡	
IIa-C	Sitaxsentan	Iloprost iv, Teprostinil iv	Ambrisentan, Bosentan, Sitaxentan Sildenafil, Tadalafil† Iloprost inhaled, and iv Treprostinil sc, iv, inhaled‡ Initial combination therapy
IIb-B		Beraprost	

Figure 24.11 Evidence-based treatment algorithm for pulmonary arterial hypertension patients (for group1 patients only). *To maintain arterial blood O2 pressure ≥8kPa (60mmHg). † Under regulatory review in the European Union. ‡ Under regulatory review in the European Union and in the USA. § IIa-C for WHO-FC II. APAH: associated pulmonary arterial hypertension; BAS balloon atrial septostomy; CCB: calcium channel blockers; ERA: endothelin receptor antagonist; IPAH: idiopathic pulmonary arterial hypertension; iv: intravenous; PDE5 I: phosphodiesterase type-5 inhibitor; sc: subcutaneous; WHO-FC: World Health Organization functional class.

- *Psychosocial support*: many PAH patients develop anxiety and depression leading to impairment in quality of life. Timely referral to a psychiatrist or psychologist should be made when appropriate.
- *Infection prevention*: patients with PAH are susceptible to developing pneumonia which is the cause of death in 7% of cases. Whilst there are no controlled trials it is sensible to recommend vaccination against influenza and pneumococcal pneumonia.
- *Elective surgery*: elective surgery is expected to have an increased risk in patients with PAH. It is not clear as to which form of anaesthesia is preferable but epidural is probably better tolerated than general anaesthesia.
- *Concomitant medications:* there is potential for clinical significant drug interactions in patients with PAH: ketoconazole and cyclosporine increase the plasma levels of bosentan and sitaxsentan and coadministration of these drugs is contraindicated. Coadministration of bosentan and glyburide is also contraindicated. Sitaxentan co-prescription with warfarin requires a reduction in warfarin dose of about 80%. Sildenafil plasma levels are increased by erythromycin, ketoconazole, cimetidine, and HIV protease inhibitors such as ritonovir and saquinovir. Nitrates are contraindicated in patients receiving phospherodiesterase-5 (PDE-5) inhibitors. Finally, care is needed when PAH-targeted medications are coadministered with antihypertensive drugs such as beta-adrenoceptor blockers, angiotensin-converting enzyme (ACE) inhibitors, etc., to avoid excessive hypotensive effects.

Supportive therapy

- *Oral anticoagulant treatment*: the evidence for the favourable effects of oral anticoagulant treatment in patients with IPAH or PAH associated with use of anorexigens is based on retrospective analysis of single-centre studies [41, 53]. The target international normalized ratio (INR) in patients with IPAH varies somewhat, being 1.5–2.5 in most centres in North America and 2.0–3.0 in European centres. The evidence supporting anticoagulation in patients with IPAH may be extrapolated to other patients with PAH provided that the risk:benefit ratio is carefully considered in presence of bleeding risks factors in particular in patients with portopulmonary hypertension and connective tissue diseases.

- *Diuretics*: patients with decompensated right heart failure develop fluid retention that leads to increased central venous pressure, abdominal organ congestion, peripheral oedema, and, in advanced cases, ascites. Appropriate diuretic treatment in right heart failure allows clear symptomatic and clinical benefits in patients with PAH. High doses may be required in cases of reduced intestinal absorption.
- *Oxygen*: no consistent data are currently available on the effects of long-term oxygen treatment in PAH. Although improvement in PH with low-flow supplemental oxygen has been reported in some PAH patients, this has not been confirmed in controlled studies. However, it is generally considered important to maintain oxygen saturations at >92% at all times.
- *Digitalis and dobutamine*: short-term intravenous administration of digoxin in IPAH produces a modest increase in CO and a significant reduction in circulating noradrenaline (norepinephrine) levels [54]; however, no data are available on the effects of long-term treatment. Patients with end-stage PAH are treated with intravenous dobutamine in most expert centres [55].
- *Supervised rehabilitation*: there is growing evidence supporting loss of peripheral muscle mass in patients with advanced PAH and this may be corrected by a defined supervised rehabilitation program [56].

Calcium-channel blockers

Favourable clinical and prognostic effects of high doses of calcium-channel blockers in vasoreactive patients with IPAH have been shown in single-centre, non-randomized, non-controlled studies [38, 41]. However, it would appear unethical to withhold therapy with high-dose calcium-channel blocker in a patient with a consistent reduction in PAP by acute pharmacological testing and to perform a placebo-controlled clinical trial in these subjects [57]. Empirical treatment with calcium-channel blockers without an acute vasoreactivity test is strongly discouraged due to possible severe adverse effects. The calcium-channel blockers that have been predominantly used are nifedipine, diltiazem, and amlodipine with particular emphasis with the first two. The doses of these drugs that have shown efficacy in IPAH are relatively high, i.e. up to 120–240mg/day for nifedipine, 240–720mg/day for diltiazem [41], and up to 20mg of amlodipine. It is advisable to start with reduced doses (i.e. 30mg of extended-release nifedipine BID, or 60mg of diltiazem TID, or 5mg of amlodipine OD) and then increase cautiously and progressively in the subsequent weeks to the maximal tolerated regimen. About 10% of patients with IPAH will meet the criteria for a positive acute vasoreactive response and only about half of these will also be clinical and haemodynamic long-term responders to treatment with calcium-channel blockers. It is commonly accepted that only in these cases is continuation of calcium-channel blockers as a single treatment warranted. Vasodilator responsiveness does not appear to predict a favourable long-term response to calcium-channel blocker therapy in patients with PAH in the setting of connective tissue diseases and tolerance of high dose calcium-channel blockers is unusual in such patients.

Synthetic prostacyclin and prostacyclin analogues (prostanoids)

Prostacyclin is produced predominantly by endothelial cells and induces potent vasodilatation of all vascular beds studied. This compound is the most potent endogenous inhibitor of platelet aggregation and it also appears to have both cytoprotective and antiproliferative activities [58]. Dysregulation of the prostacyclin metabolic pathways has been shown in patients with PAH as assessed by reduction of prostacyclin synthase expression in the pulmonary arteries and of prostacyclin urinary metabolites [59].

Epoprostenol

Epoprostenol (synthetic prostacyclin) is available as a stable freeze-dried preparation that needs to be dissolved to allow intravenous infusion. Epoprostenol has a short half-life (3–5min) and is stable at room temperature for only 8 hours; this explains why it needs to be administered continuously by means of infusion pumps and permanent tunnelled catheters. The efficacy of continuous intravenous administration of epoprostenol has been tested in three unblinded randomized controlled trials in patients with IPAH [60, 61] and in those with PAH associated with the scleroderma spectrum of diseases [62]. Epoprostenol improves symptoms, exercise capacity, and haemodynamics in both clinical conditions, and is the only treatment shown to improve survival in IPAH in a randomized study.

Long-term treatment with epoprostenol is initiated at a dose of 2–4ng/kg/min, with doses increasing at a rate limited by adverse effects (flushing, headache, diarrhoea, leg pain). Optimal dose is variable between individual patients, ranging in the majority between 20–40ng/kg/min [45, 46]. Serious adverse events related to the delivery system include pump malfunction, local site infection, catheter obstruction, and sepsis. Abrupt interruption of the epoprostenol infusion should be avoided as this may, in some patients, lead to a rebound worsening of their PH with symptomatic deterioration and even death.

Treprostinil

Treprostinil is a tricyclic benzidine analogue of epoprostenol, with sufficient chemical stability to be administered at ambient temperature. These characteristics allow administration of the compound by the intravenous as well as the subcutaneous route. The subcutaneous administration of treprostinil can be accomplished by micro-infusion pumps and small subcutaneous catheters. The effects of treprostinil in PAH were studied in the largest worldwide randomized controlled trial performed in this condition, and showed improvements in exercise capacity, haemodynamics, and symptoms [63]. The greatest exercise improvement was observed in patients who were more compromised at baseline and in subjects who could tolerate upper quartile dose (>13.8ng/kg/min). Infusion site pain was the most common adverse effect of treprostinil, leading to discontinuation of the treatment in 8% of cases on active drug and limiting dose increase in an additional proportion of patients. Among the 15% of patients who continued to receive subcutaneous treprostinil alone, survival appears to be improved [64]. In another long-term, open-label study, a sustained improvement in exercise capacity and symptoms with sc treprostinil was reported in patients with IPAH or chronic thromboembolic pulmonary hypertension, with a mean follow-up of 26 months [65]. Treprostinil has been approved in the USA also for intravenous use in patients with PAH: the effects appear to be comparable with epoprostenol but at a dose which is between two to three times higher. It is more convenient for the patient because the reservoir can be changed every 48 hours as compared to 12 hours with epoprostenol. A phase III randomized controlled trial of inhaled treprostinil was recently completed and preliminary data show improvements in exercise capacity. Oral treprostinil is currently being evaluated in randomized controlled trials and in PAH.

Beraprost

Beraprost is the first chemically stable and orally active prostacyclin analogue. Two randomized controlled studies [66, 67] with this compound have shown an improvement in exercise capacity that unfortunately persists only up to 3–6 months.

Iloprost

Iloprost is a chemically stable prostacyclin analogue available for intravenous, oral, and aerosol administration. Inhaled therapy for PAH is an attractive concept that has the theoretical advantage of being selective for the pulmonary circulation. Inhaled iloprost has been evaluated in one randomized controlled trial in which daily repetitive iloprost inhalations (six to nine times, 2.5–5mcg/inhalation, median 30mcg daily) were compared with placebo inhalation in patients with PAH and chronic thromboembolic PH [68]. The study showed an increase in exercise capacity and improvement in symptoms, PVR, and clinical events in enrolled patients. A second randomized controlled trial on 60 patients already treated with bosentan has shown increase in exercise capacity in the subjects randomized to the addition of inhaled iloprost in comparison with placebo. Overall, inhaled iloprost was well tolerated. Continuous intravenous administration of iloprost appears to be as effective as epoprostenol in a small series of patients with PAH and chronic thromboembolic pulmonary hypertension [69].

Endothelin-1 receptor antagonists

Activation of the endothelin (ET)-1 system has been demonstrated in both plasma and lung tissues of PAH patients [70]. Although it is not clear if the increases in ET-1 plasma levels are a cause or a consequence of PH [71], studies on tissue ET system expression support a prominent role for ET-1 in the pathogenesis of PAH [50].

Bosentan

Bosentan is an oral active dual ET_A and ET_B receptor antagonist and is the first molecule of this class of drugs to be synthesized. Bosentan has been evaluated in PAH in five randomized controlled trials that have shown improvement in exercise capacity, functional class, haemodynamics, echocardiographic and Doppler variables, and time to clinical worsening [72–76]. Two randomized controlled trials have enrolled exclusively patients with WHO/NYHA functional class II [75] or patients with Eisenmenger's syndrome [76]. Long-term observational studies have demonstrated the durability of the effect of bosentan over time [9]. Increases in hepatic aminotransferases occurred in 10% of the subjects but were found to be dose dependent and reversible after dose reduction or discontinuation. For these reasons, liver function tests should be performed at least monthly in patients receiving bosentan.

Sitaxsentan

Sitaxsentan, a selective orally active ET_A receptor antagonist, has been assessed in two randomized controlled trials on patients with WHO/NYHA class II/III PAH [77, 78]. Aetiology included IPAH and PAH associated with connective tissue diseases or congenital heart diseases. The studies demonstrated improvements in exercise capacity and haemodynamics. A 1 year, open-label observational study has demonstrated the durability of the effects of sitaxsentan over time [79]. Incidence of abnormal liver function tests, which reversed in all cases, was 3–5% for the approved dose of 100mg (monthly checking is required). Interaction with warfarin requires the reduction of the dose of the anticoagulant by about 80% to avoid INR increases.

Ambrisentan

Ambrisentan is a non-sulfonamide, propanoic acid-class, ET receptor antagonists that is selective for the ET_A receptor. Ambrisentan, has been in evaluated in a pilot study [80] and in two large randomized controlled trials which have demonstrated efficacy on symptoms, exercise capacity, haemodynamics, and time to clinical worsening [81]. The open label continuation study has demonstrated the durability of the effects of ambrisentan for at least 1 year [81]. Ambrisentan has been approved also for the treatment of WHO/NYHA -FC II patients. The current approved dose is 5mg OD which can be increased to 10mg OD in case the drug is tolerated with the initial dose.

Incidence of abnormal liver function tests is ranging from 0.8–3%. However, even in patients treated with ambrisentan, liver function tests are required at least monthly. Caution is suggested for the coadministration of ambrisentan with ketoconazole and cyclosporine.

Phosphodiesterase type-5 inhibitors

Sildenafil

Sildenafil is an orally active, potent and selective inhibitor of PDE-5 that exerts its pharmacological effect by increasing the intracellular concentration of cGMP. A number of uncontrolled studies have reported favourable effects of sildenafil in IPAH, PAH associated to connective tissue diseases and to congenital heart diseases, and in chronic thromboembolic PH [82–84]. A pivotal randomized controlled trial on 278 PAH patients treated with sildenafil 20, 40, or 80mg TID has confirmed favourable results on exercise capacity, symptoms, and haemodynamics [85]. Even if the approved dose is 20mg TID, the durability of effect up to 1 year has been demonstrated only with the dose of 80mg TID. In clinical practice, up-titration beyond 20mg TID (mainly 40–80mg TID) is frequently needed. Most side effects of sildenafil were mild to moderate and mainly related to vasodilation.

Tadalafil

Tadalafil is an OD dosing, selective PDE-5 inhibitor, currently approved for the treatment of erectile dysfunction. A pivotal randomized controlled trial on 406 PAH patients treated with tadalafil 5, 10, 20, or 40mg OD has shown favourable results on exercise capacity, symptoms, haemodynamics, and time to clinical worsening for the largest dose [86]. Side effect profile was similar to sildenafil.

Combination therapy

Combination therapy is the simultaneous use of more than one PAH-targeted class of drugs, e.g. ET receptor antagonists, PDE-5 inhibitors, prostanoids, and novel substances. Although long-term safety and efficacy have not yet been extensively explored, numerous case series have suggested that various drug combinations appear to be safe and effective. Different randomized controlled studies have shown the efficacy of the combination of bosentan and epoprostenol [74], of the addition of inhaled iloprost to patients on background therapy with bosentan [87], of bosentan in patients on background therapy with sildenafil [75], of sildenafil in patients on background treatment with epoprostenol [88], of inhaled treprostinil in patients with background treatment with either bosentan or sildenafil and of tadalafil in patients on background treatment with bosentan. Different additional trials are ongoing also with novel compounds. There are many open questions regarding combination therapy including the choice of combination partners and the optimal timing. Candidates for combination therapy are patients which status is defined as stable but unsatisfactory or unstable and deteriorating (see ➲ Definition of clinical status, p.904). For the complexities related to combination therapy, it is recommended that candidates are referred to expert centres.

Balloon atrial septostomy

The role of balloon atrial septostomy in the treatment of patients with PAH is uncertain because its efficacy has been reported only in small series and case reports [23]. In addition to symptomatic and haemodynamic improvement, an increase in survival as compared with historical control groups has also been shown. In most circumstances, this intervention has been performed in severely ill patients as a palliative bridge to lung transplantation, which may explain a procedure mortality rate of 5–15%. In expert centres this procedure is now performed in cases of failure of available medical treatments.

Lung transplantation

Lung and heart–lung transplantation in PAH has been assessed only in prospective uncontrolled series, since formal randomized controlled trials are considered unethical in the absence of alternative treatment options [23]. The 3-year and 5-year survival after lung and heart–lung transplantation is approximately 55% and 45% respectively [89]. Both single and bilateral lung transplantation have been performed for IPAH and these operations have been combined with repair of cardiac defects in Eisenmenger's syndrome (➲Chapter 10). Recipient survival rates have been similar after single and bilateral lung transplantation and after heart–lung transplantation for PAH. However, many transplant centres currently prefer to perform bilateral lung transplantation. Lung and heart–lung transplantation are indicated in PAH patients with advanced WHO/NYHA class III and class IV symptoms that are refractory to available medical treatments. The unpredictability of the period on the waiting list and donor organ shortage complicate the decision making regarding the appropriate timing of listing for transplantation.

Treatment algorithm

A treatment algorithm for PAH patients is shown in ➲Fig. 25.11 [51]. The Grade of Recommendation and Level of Evidence for the PAH treatments [52] are reported in ➲Table 24.4. Definition of Clinical Response to Treatments is reported in ➲Table 24.5.

- The treatment algorithm is not appropriate for patients with other clinical groups and in particular for patients with PH associated with left heart diseases or with parenchymal lung diseases.
- General measures and initiation of supportive therapy need to be initiated after PAH diagnosis.
- Due to the complexity of the additional evaluation and the treatment options available, it is strongly recommended that patients with PAH are referred to a specialized centre.
- Acute vasoreactivity testing should be performed and high-dose calcium-channel blocker therapy performed as appropriate.
- Non-responders to acute vasoreactivity testing who are in WHO/NYHA-FC II should be treated with an endothelin receptor antagonist or a PDE-5 inhibitor.
- Non responders to acute vasoreactivity testing, or responders who remain in (or progress to) WHO/NYHA-FC III should be considered candidates for treatment with either an ET receptor antagonist, or a PDE-5 inhibitor, or a prostanoid. As head-to-head comparisons among different compounds are not available, no evidence-based first-line treatments can be proposed. In this case, the choice of the drug is dependent on a variety of factors, including the approval status, the route of administration, the side effect profile, patient's preferences, and physician's experience. Some authors still use first-line intravenous epoprostenol in WHO/NYHA -FC III patients, due to its demonstrated survival benefits.
- Continuous intravenous epoprostenol may be considered as first-line therapy for WHO/NYHA-FC IV PAH patients because of the demonstrated survival benefit in this subset. Intravenous. and subcutaneous treprostinil have been also approved for the treatment of WHO/NYHA-FC IV patients in the USA. Although no randomized controlled trials have been performed with the intravenous delivery of iloprost, this PGI2 analogue has been approved in New Zealand. Although both ET receptor antagonists and PDE-5 inhibitors are considered as a second line for severely ill patients, in WHO/NYHA-FC IV patients initial combination therapy may also be considered.
- In case of inadequate clinical response (➲Table 24.5), sequential combination therapy can be considered. Combination therapy can either include a prostanoid plus an ET receptor antagonist or an ET receptor antagonist plus a PDE-5 inhibitor or a prostanoid plus a PDE-5 inhibitor. Appropriate protocols for timing and dosing to limit possible side effects of the combination have still to be defined.
- Balloon atrial septostomy and/or lung transplantation are indicated for PAH with inadequate clinical response (➲Table 24.5) despite optimal medical therapy or where medical treatments are unavailable. These procedures should be performed only in experienced centres.

Table 24.5 Definition of inadequate response to PAH treatments

Inadequate clinical response for patients who were initially in WHO/NYHA functional class II or III:
1. Resulting clinical status defined as stable and not satisfactory
2. Resulting clinical status defined as unstable and deteriorating
Inadequate clinical response for patients who were initially in WHO/NYHA functional class IV:
1. No rapid improvement to WHO/NYHA functional Class III or better
2. Resulting clinical status defined as stable and not satisfactory

See also Definition of clinical status, p.904.

Specific pulmonary arterial hypertension types

Paediatric PAH

Paediatric PH is similar to adult disease even if in a growing child the lungs are still developing. The worse prognosis in children with a median survival estimated at 10 months compared to 2.8 years in the adult [21], has not been confirmed. The exact incidence and prevalence of PH in children is not known. Persistent PH of the neonates is also classified in the PAH group 1 but natural history, treatment, and outcome are sufficiently different to justify its exclusion from this discussion. No clear differences have been identified among the mechanisms involved in the development of PAH in children and adults. Also, the incidence of vasoreactivity is similar to adults. Children often present sicker than adults. A similar diagnostic work-up as in the adult is suggested. The response to therapy is difficult to predict with some patients having dramatic response and some requiring rapid escalation of therapy. The therapeutic algorithm used for children is similar if not identical to the one used in adults even if evidence-based studies are lacking.

Therapy should include close follow-up; treat rapidly any upper or lower airway infections as these may induce a rapid deterioration. The use of anticoagulation is controversial as no studies are available in children. Calcium-channel blockers are used in responders but close follow up is mandatory as several patients may fail long-term therapy. Only a few studies have been performed to confirm the exact dosage of new therapies to be applied in children. Data are available with bosentan, pharmacokinetics has been assessed in one study [90]. Several uncontrolled studies have shown positive results similar to adults with survival around 80–90% at 1 year [91]. Data with selective ET_A antagonists are not available so far. Sildenafil has shown some efficacy [92] and a randomized controlled study is underway. Indications for epoprostenol is similar to adults. An increasing number of paediatric patients are on combination therapy. Atrial septostomy is possible in children with good results as well as the possibility of a Pott's shunt [93]. As in adults, cure is only obtained with lung transplant but lack of suitable donors is a major problem.

PAH associated with congenital cardiac shunts

PAH associated with congenital cardiac shunts (➲Chapter 10) is included in group 1 of the PH classification (➲Table 24.2). A clinical classification (➲Table 24.6) and a pathologic pathophysiologic classification (➲Table 24.7) are useful to better define each individual patient [2].

Table 24.6 Clinical classification of congenital systemic-to-pulmonary shunts associated with PAH

A) Eisenmenger's syndrome
Includes all systemic-to-pulmonary shunts due to large defects, leading to a severe increase of PVR and resulting in a reversed (pulmonary-to-systemic) or bidirectional shunt. Cyanosis, erythrocytosis, and multiple organs involvement are present.
B) PAH associated with systemic-to-pulmonary shunts
In these patients with moderate to large defects the increase of PVR is mild to moderate, systemic-to-pulmonary shunt is still largely prevalent and no cyanosis is present at rest.
C) PAH with small defects
In these cases with small defects (usually ventricular septal defects <1cm and atrial septal defect <2cm of effective diameter assessed by echo) the clinical picture is very similar to idiopathic PAH.
D) PAH after corrective cardiac surgery
In these cases congenital hart disease has been corrected but PAH either is still present immediately after surgery or has recurred several months or years after surgery in the absence of significant postoperative residual lesions.

The prevalence of PAH in adult CHD appears to be 5–10% [94]. The persistent exposure of the pulmonary vasculature to increased blood flow as well as increased pressure may results in the pulmonary obstructive arteriopathy (identical to idiopathic PAH) that leads to the increase of PVR and if it approaches or exceeds systemic resistance, the shunt is reversed (Eisenmenger's syndrome).

The clinical picture of Eisenmenger's syndrome (➲Chapter 10) includes multiple organ involvement progressively deteriorating over time. The signs and symptoms are characterized by central cyanosis, dyspnoea, fatigue, haemoptysis, syncope, and right heart failure in advanced stages. Survival of patients with Eisenmenger's syndrome is clearly reduced as compared to the general population but appears to be better than that of subjects with idiopathic PAH with comparable functional class.

The treatment strategy for patients with PAH associated with congenital systemic-to-pulmonary shunts and in particular for subjects with Eisenmenger's syndrome is mainly based on the clinical experience of experts rather than formally evidence based. A treatment algorithm similar to the one in ➲Fig. 25.11 has been recently proposed [95]. General measures include recommendations for physical activity, pregnancy and birth control, infections prevention, travel and altitude, elective surgery, and psychological assistance. Phlebotomies are required only if relevant symptoms of hyperviscosity are present and usually when haematocrit is >65%. The use of supplemental oxygen therapy is controversial and should be prescribed only in cases in which it

Table 24.7 Anatomic-pathophysiologic classification of congenital systemic-to-pulmonary shunts associated to pulmonary arterial hypertension

1. Type
1.1 Simple pre-tricuspid shunts
1.1.1 Atrial septal defect (ASD)
1.1.1.1 Ostium secundum
1.1.1.2 Sinus venosus
1.1.1.3 Ostium primum
1.1.2 Total or partial unobstructed anomalous pulmonary venous return
1.2 Simple post-tricuspid shunts
1.2.1 Ventricular septal defect (VSD)
1.2.2 Patent ductus arteriosus
1.3 Combined shunts
Describe combination and define predominant defect
1.4 Complex CHD
1.4.1 Complete atrioventricular septal defect
1.4.2 Truncus arteriosus
1.4.3 Single ventricle physiology with unobstructed pulmonary blood flow
1.4.4 Transposition of the great arteries with VSD (without pulmonary stenosis) and/or patent ductus arteriosus
1.4.5 Other
2. Dimension (specify for each defect if more than one congenital heart defect)
2.1 Haemodynamic (specify Qp/Qs)*
2.1.1 Restrictive (pressure gradient across the defect)
2.1.2 Non-restrictive
2.2 Anatomic
2.2.1 Small to moderate (ASD ≤2cm and VSD ≤1cm)
2.2.2 Large (ASD >2cm and VSD >1cm)
3. Direction of shunt
3.1 Predominantly systemic-to-pulmonary
3.2 Predominantly pulmonary-to-systemic
3.3 Bidirectional
4. Associated cardiac and extracardiac abnormalities
5. Repair status
5.1 Unoperated
5.2 Palliated (specify type of operation/s, age at surgery)
5.3 Repaired (specify type of operation/s, age at surgery)

*Ratio of pulmonary (Qp) to systemic (Qs) blood flow

Modified from Venice 2003.

produces a consistent increase in arterial oxygen saturation. Oral anticoagulant treatment with warfarin can be initiated in patients with pulmonary artery thrombosis and absent or only mild haemoptysis. Three classes of drugs, targeted to the correction of the endothelial dysfunction abnormalities, have been recently approved for the treatment of PAH: prostanoids, ET receptor antagonists, and PDE-5 inhibitors. The efficacy and safety of these compounds have been confirmed also in patients with PAH associated with corrected and uncorrected congenital systemic-to-pulmonary shunts and in subjects with Eisenmenger's syndrome (➲Chapter 10) by uncontrolled studies. One randomized, controlled trial has reported the short- and long-term favourable results of the treatment with the orally active dual ET receptor antagonist bosentan in Eisenmenger's syndrome patients [76]. There is no published data on combination therapy, but there is a rationale as in IPAH. Lung transplantation with repair of the cardiac defect or combined heart–lung transplantation is an option for patients with Eisenmenger's syndrome who have markers of a poor prognosis.

PAH associated with connective tissue diseases

PH is a well-known complication of connective tissue diseases such as systemic sclerosis [96], systemic lupus erythematosus, mixed connective tissue diseases, and to a lesser extent, rheumatoid arthritis, dermatopolymyositis, and primary Sjögren's syndrome. In these patients, PH may occur in association with interstitial fibrosis or as a result of an isolated pulmonary arteriopathy. In addition, pulmonary venous hypertension from left heart disease can be present. It is imperative to determine which mechanism is operative, as treatment may be substantially different for each process. Systemic sclerosis, particularly in its limited variant previously defined as CREST syndrome, represents the main connective tissue diseases associated with PAH. The prevalence of haemodynamically proved PAH in large cohorts of patients with systemic sclerosis ranges between 7–12% [96, 97]. Histopathological changes in PAH associated with connective tissue diseases are generally indistinguishable from those of classical IPAH. The pathophysiologic mechanisms leading to PAH in patients with connective tissue diseases remain unknown. The presence of antinuclear antibody, rheumatoid factor, immunoglobulin-G, and complement fractions deposits in the pulmonary vessels wall suggest a role for an immunologic mechanism. Compared with patients with IPAH, patients with PAH associated with connective tissue diseases are mainly women, are older, and have a significantly lower CO. Symptoms and clinical presentation are very similar to IPAH and occasional patients can be identified as having an associated connective tissue disease by immunology screening tests. The mortality was confirmed to be higher than that seen with IPAH (40% 1-year mortality for those with advanced disease), and the predictors of outcome were the same as for IPAH (RAP, PAP, and cardiac index). Echocardiographic screening for the detection of PH has been suggested to be performed yearly in asymptomatic patients with the scleroderma spectrum of diseases and only in presence of symptoms in other connective tissue diseases. As in other forms of PAH, right heart catheterization is recommended in all cases of suspected PAH associated with connective tissue diseases to confirm the diagnosis, determine severity, and rule out left-sided heart disease. Treatment of patients with PAH associated with connective tissue diseases appears more complex as compared to IPAH. Immunosuppressive therapy seems to be effective only in a minority of patients mainly suffering from conditions other than scleroderma. The rate of acute vasoreactivity and of a long-term favourable response to CCB treatment is lower compared to IPAH. Also the risk:benefit ratio of oral anticoagulation is not well understood.

Subgroup analysis of patients with scleroderma enrolled in the randomized controlled trials performed with bosentan [73], sitaxentan [98], and sildenafil [99], have shown favourable effects with all these medications. Subcutaneous treprostinil has been shown to increase exercise capacity, symptoms of PAH, and haemodynamics in patients with connective tissue diseases [100]. Continuous epoprostenol therapy has been shown to improve exercise capacity, symptoms, and haemodynamics in a 3-month randomized controlled trial of patients with the scleroderma spectrum of the disease [62]. Some retrospective analysis show that the effect of intravenous epoprostenol on survival of IPAH patients seem to be better as compared to scleroderma patients.

Portopulmonary PAH

PAH is a well-recognized complication of chronic liver diseases [101, 102]. Portal hypertension, rather than the hepatic disorder itself, seems to be the main determining risk factor for developing PH [101]. Two recent studies carried out in patients undergoing liver transplantation found a prevalence of PH of 4% and 3.5%, respectively. The mechanism whereby portal hypertension facilitates the development of PAH remains unknown [101]. The presence of portosystemic shunt might allow vasoconstrictive and vasoproliferative substances, normally cleared by the liver, to reach the pulmonary circulation. The clinical picture of patients with portopulmonary hypertension may be indistinguishable from that of IPAH or may include a combination of symptoms and signs of the underlying liver disease [101]. Echocardiographic screening for the detection of PH in patients with liver diseases is appropriate in symptomatic patients and/or in candidates for liver transplantation. A right heart catheterization should be performed in all cases with increased systolic PAP in order to clarify the underlying haemodynamic changes and define prognostic and therapeutic implications. Haemodynamically, compared with patients with IPAH, patients with portopulmonary hypertension have a significantly higher CO and significantly lower systemic vascular resistance and PVR. In a retrospective study [101], patients with portopulmonary hypertension had a better rate of survival than patients with IPAH, although there is some debate on this issue. Beta-adrenoceptor blockers, often used in patients with portal hypertension to reduce the risk of variceal bleeding, worsen haemodynamics and exercise capacity in portopulmonary hypertension patients. The treatment of portopulmonary hypertension has not been thoroughly studied and a few studies have been performed with targeted treatments [103–105]. However, the treatment algorithm (➲ Fig. 25.11) can be used also in this setting. Anticoagulant therapy should be avoided in patients at increased risk of bleeding. Careful monitoring should be performed if endothelin receptor antagonist treatment is initiated for the hepatoxicity of these compounds. Patients with portopulmonary hypertension seem to respond favourably to chronic intravenous epoprostenol. Significant PAH can substantially increase the risk associated with liver transplantation and usually PAH is a contraindication if mean PAP is ≥35mmHg and/or PVR is ≥250 dynes.s.cm^{-5} [106]. A series of combined lung and liver transplantation has been reported [107].

PAH associated with HIV infection

PAH is a rare but well-documented complication of HIV infection. In a large case–control study, 3349 HIV-infected patients over a period of 5.5 years demonstrated a cumulative incidence of PH of 0.57%, resulting in an annual incidence of 0.1% [108]. These data have been recently confirmed [109]. The mechanism of the development of PAH is unknown. HIV-related PAH shows similar clinical, haemodynamic, and histological findings as IPAH and it does not appear to be related to the route of HIV transmission nor to the degree of immunosuppression. Echocardiographic screening for the detection of PH in patients with HIV infection is required in symptomatic patients. A careful exclusion of other causes for PH such as left heart and parenchymal lung and liver diseases are necessary. Right heart catheterization is recommended in all cases of suspected PAH associated with HIV infection to confirm the diagnosis, determine severity, and rule out left-sided heart disease. PAH is an independent predictor of mortality in this patient population [108]. Therapeutic options are not well established and oral anticoagulation is often contraindicated because of bleeding risk factors, poor compliance, and potential drug interactions. Different open label studies have confirmed the efficacy of targeted PAH treatments also in this setting. It is then reasonable to utilize the treatment algorithm (➲Fig. 25.11) also in this setting.

Pulmonary veno-occlusive disease

Both pulmonary veno-occlusive disease and pulmonary capillary haemangiomathosis are uncommon conditions, but they are increasingly recognized as causes for PAH [110]. They have been classified in a specific subgroup of the clinical classification (➲Table 24.2, group 1) for the pathologic, clinical, and therapeutic differences with the other forms included in group 1. Fewer than 200 cases of pulmonary veno-occlusive disease and PCH, combined, have been reported in the literature. Pulmonary veno-occlusive disease and pulmonary capillary haemangiomathosis are similar in some respects, particularly in relation to the changes in the pulmonary parenchyma, i.e. pulmonary haemosiderosis, interstitial oedema, and lymphatic dilatation, and to pulmonary arterial intimal fibrosis and medial hypertrophy [3]. Clinical presentation of these patients is often indistinguishable from that of patients with IPAH. However, physical examination can demonstrate findings suggestive of a diagnosis other than IPAH, such as digital clubbing and/or basilar rales on chest auscultation. Case series indicate that pulmonary veno-occlusive disease/pulmonary capillary haemangiomathosis is associated with more severe hypoxemia and reduction of single-breath D_LCO, while spirometry and lung volume measurements are generally within normal limits. Haemodynamic data are similar between pulmonary veno-occlusive disease/pulmonary capillary haemangiomathosis and IPAH, although in some patients, the hypoxemia is out of proportion to the degree of PAH and right heart dysfunction. Interestingly, PWP is often normal despite the postcapillary involvement. Indeed, the pathological changes usually occur in the venules, often without involvement of the larger veins. The static column of blood produced during the measurement of PWP is unaffected by the changes in the small pulmonary veins as long as a connection is maintained with the larger, unaffected pulmonary veins which is where the pressure will be measured in the occluded arterial segment. Radiological data may be of great help in detecting pulmonary veno-occlusive disease/pulmonary capillary haemangiomathosis [111]. The presence of Kerley B lines, pleural effusion, and patchy irregularities on a standard chest roentgenogram may provide important clues that suggest the diagnosis. Thin-section CT of the chest has characteristic changes (➲Fig. 24.8B): the most commonly reported findings are a patchy centrilobular pattern of ground-glass opacities, thickened septal lines, pleural effusion, and mediastinal adenopathy. Compared with IPAH, pulmonary veno-occlusive disease/pulmonary capillary haemangiomathosis was characterized by significantly elevated broncho-alveolar lavage cell counts with an increased number of haemosiderin-laden macrophages. Pulmonary veno-occlusive disease and pulmonary capillary haemangiomathosis probably requires similar management as other PAH subgroups. However, the prognosis seems worse, with a more rapid downhill course. In addition, vasodilators and especially epoprostenol have to be used with great caution because of the high risk of pulmonary oedema [112]. However, there are reports of sustained clinical improvement in individual patients treated with these medications. There are no data regarding the use of newer medical therapies such as ET receptor antagonists in the treatment of pulmonary veno-occlusive disease/pulmonary capillary haemangiomathosis. Atrial septostomy may be considered but is limited by hypoxemia. The only curative therapy for pulmonary veno-occlusive disease/pulmonary capillary haemangiomathosis is lung transplantation, and similar to IPAH there are no reports of recurrence of disease following transplantation.

Pulmonary hypertension associated with left heart disease (Group 2)

Pathology, pathophysiology, and epidemiology of this condition are discussed in the appropriate section in ➲Pathology and pathobiology of pulmonary hypertension, p.894 and Genetics and epidemiology, p.897.

Diagnosis

PH carries a poor prognosis for patients with chronic heart failure: in one study mortality rate after 28 months of follow-up was 57% in patients with moderate PH compared to 17% in patients without PH. In addition, patients who have a PVR exceeding 6–8 Wood units have an increased risk of postoperative RV failure following heart transplantation When the PVR can be lowered pharmacologically (e.g. with IV nitroprusside) this risk is generally thought to be reduced [113]. The diagnostic approach to PH due to left heart diseases is similar to PAH, Doppler echocardiography being the best tool for screening purposes. Diastolic dysfunction should be suspected in the presence of a dilated left atrium, atrial fibrillation, abnormal mitral outflow pattern, and LV hypertrophy [114]. Although increased left-sided filling pressures can be estimated by Doppler echocardiography [115], invasive measurements of PWP or LV end-diastolic pressure may be necessary to confirm the diagnosis of PH due to left heart diseases. PWP and LV end-diastolic pressure can be 'pseudonormal', especially when patients have been treated with diuretics. In this setting, volume challenge has been proposed to identify LV dysfunction but this diagnostic tool requires further standardization. An elevated transpulmonary gradient (mean PAP – PWP) >12mmHg is suggestive of intrinsic changes in the pulmonary circulation overriding the passive increase in PWP. In some patients, it may be difficult to distinguish PAH from PH associated with LV dysfunction, in particular in patients with borderline values of PWP (15–18mmHg). The role, significance, and setting of pharmacologic testing remain unclear in PH due to left heart diseases, although it is recommended in heart transplant candidates to identify patients at higher risk of acute postoperative RV failure [116]. In this latter case, the absence of consensus on a standardized protocol leads to the use of various agents for testing the responsiveness of the pulmonary circulation, including inotropic agents, vasodilators, prostanoids, nitric oxide, and PDE-5 inhibitors.

In heart transplant candidates, persistent increase in PVR >2.5 Wood units and/or transpulmonary pressure gradient >15mmHg are associated with up to a threefold increase in risk of RV failure and early post transplant mortality [9]. Acute postoperative RV failure may also be observed in patients with normal baseline pulmonary haemodynamics, suggesting that other mechanisms may be involved.

Therapy

Currently, there is no specific therapy for PH due to left heart diseases. A number of drugs (including diuretics, nitrates, hydralazine, ACE inhibitors, beta-blockers, nesiritide, and inotropic agents) or interventions (LV assist device implantation, valvular surgery, resynchronization therapy, and heart transplantation) may lower PAP more or less rapidly through a drop in left-sided filling pressures [117]. Therefore, management of PH due to left heart diseases should primarily aim at treating the underlying disease, and there is no drug for heart failure contraindicated because of PH. Few studies have examined the role of drugs currently recommended in PAH. Randomized-controlled trials evaluating the effects of a chronic use of epoprostenol [118]and bosentan [119] in advanced heart failure have been terminated early due to an increased rate of events in the investigational drug-treated group compared with conventional therapy. A small-sized study recently suggested that sildenafil may improve exercise capacity and quality of life in patients with PH due to left heart diseases [120]. However, the history of medication for LV failure is full of examples where drugs had positive effects on surrogate endpoints but eventually turned out to be detrimental, including PDE-3 inhibitors. Thus, the use of PAH-specific drugs is not recommended until robust data from long-term studies are available. A sustained reduction of PH is expected in weeks to months in most patients successfully operated for mitral valve disease, even if PH represents a risk factor for surgery [6].

Pulmonary hypertension associated with lung diseases (Group 3)

Pathology, pathophysiology, and epidemiology of this condition are discussed in the appropriate section in ➲ Pathology and pathobiology of pulmonary hypertension, p.894 and Genetics and epidemiology, p.897.

Diagnosis

Clinical symptoms and physical signs of PH may be difficult to identify in patients with respiratory disorders. In addition, in COPD peripheral oedema may not be a sign of RV failure, since it rather results from the effects of hypoxemia and hypercapnia on the renin–angiotensin–aldosterone system. Furthermore, concomitant left heart disease, which is commonly associated with chronic respiratory diseases, may also contribute to raise PAP.

As in other forms of PH, echocardiography is the best screening tool for the assessment of PH. Nevertheless, its diagnostic performance in advanced respiratory diseases is lower than in PAH. Reliable assessment of systolic PAP is only feasible in a limited number of cases; an elevated proportion of systolic PAP measurements are inaccurate; and the specificity of systolic PAP in detecting PH is low, although with an acceptable negative predictive value [121, 122]. Accordingly, indications of echocardiography for the screening of PH in COPD and interstitial lung fibrosis include: 1) rule-out significant PH; 2) evaluation of concomitant left heart diseases; and 3) select patients who may undergo right heart catheterization.

A definite diagnosis of PH relies on measurements obtained at right heart catheterization. Their indications in advanced lung disease are: 1) proper diagnosis of PH in candidates to surgical treatments (transplantation, lung volume reduction); 2) suspected disproportionate PH potentially amenable with targeted PAH therapy; 3) frequent episodes of RV failure; and 4) non conclusive echocardiographic study in high suspicion cases.

Therapy

Currently there is no specific therapy for PH associated with COPD or interstitial lung fibrosis. Long-term oxygen administration has been shown to partially reduce the progression of PH in COPD. Nevertheless, with this treatment PAP rarely returns to normal values and the structural abnormalities of pulmonary vessels remain unaltered [123]. In interstitial lung fibrosis, the role of long-term oxygen therapy is less clear. Treatment with conventional vasodilators is not recommended because they may impair gas exchange due to the inhibition of hypoxic pulmonary vasoconstriction [124, 125] and their lack of efficacy after long-term use [126, 127]. Published experience with targeted PAH therapy is scarce and consists essentially in the assessment of their acute effects [128, 129] or uncontrolled studies in small series [130–134].

Accordingly, the treatment of choice for patients with COPD or interstitial lung fibrosis and associated PH who are hypoxemic is long-term oxygen therapy. In the subgroup of patients with disproportionate PH (with dyspnoea insufficiently explained by lung mechanic disturbances and mean PAP >40–45mmHg), targeted PAH therapy could be considered. Consultation with an expert PH centre is strongly recommended, as these patients might be appropriate for clinical trials. The use of specific PAH drugs therapy in patients with COPD or interstitial lung fibrosis and moderate PH is currently discouraged because there is no systematic data regarding its safety or efficacy.

Chronic thromboembolic pulmonary hypertension (Group 4)

Pathology, pathophysiology, and epidemiology of this condition are discussed in the appropriate section in ➲Pathology and pathobiology of pulmonary hypertension, p.894 and Genetics and epidemiology, p.897.

Diagnosis

Any patient with unexplained PH should be evaluated for the presence of chronic thromboembolic PH (➲Chapter 37). Suspicion should be high when the patient presents with a history of previous venous thromboembolism. Survivors of PE should be followed after the acute episode to detect signs or symptoms of chronic thromboembolic PH. Patients with acute PE showing signs of PH or RV dysfunction at any time during their hospital stay should receive a follow-up echocardiography after discharge to determine whether or not PH has resolved.

In patients with unexplained PH, lung perfusion scan (➲Fig. 24.5B) is recommended to exclude chronic thromboembolic PH. A normal perfusion scan rules out chronic thromboembolic PH. Multi-row CT angiography (➲Fig. 24.7) is indicated when the scintigraphy is indeterminate or reveals perfusions defects. Even in the era of modern multi-row CT scanners there is not yet enough evidence to suggest that a normal CT angiography excludes the presence of operable chronic thromboembolic PH. Once perfusion scanning and/or CT angiography show signs compatible with chronic thromboembolic PH, the patient should be referred to a centre with expertise in the medical and surgical management of these patients. To determine the appropriate therapeutic strategy, invasive tools including right heart catheterization and traditional pulmonary angiography (➲Fig. 24.8) are usually required.

Therapy

Patients with chronic thromboembolic pulmonary hypertension should receive life-long anticoagulation, usually with vitamin K antagonists adjusted to a target INR between 2–3.

Pulmonary endarterectomy is the treatment of choice for patients with chronic thromboembolic PH. Detailed preoperative patient evaluation and selection, surgical technique and experience, and meticulous postoperative management are essential prerequisites for success after this intervention [33]. The selection of patients for surgery depends on the extent and location of the organized thrombi in relation to the degree of PH. Proximal thrombi represents the ideal indication (➲Fig. 24.8A) while more distal obstructions may prevent a successful procedure (➲Fig. 24.8B). After an effective intervention a dramatic drop of PVR can be expected with a near-normalization of pulmonary haemodynamics. A centre can be considered having sufficient expertise in this field if it performs at least 20 pulmonary endarterectomy operations per year with a mortality rate <10%. Targeted medical therapy may play a role in selected chronic thromboembolic PH patients, mainly for three different scenarios: 1) if patients are not considered candidates for surgery, 2) if preoperative treatment is deemed appropriate to improve haemodynamics, and 3) if patients present with symptomatic residual PH after PEA surgery. Several uncontrolled clinical studies suggest that prostanoids, ET receptor antagonists, and PDE-5 inhibitors may exert haemodynamic and clinical benefits in patients with chronic thromboembolic PH, regardless of whether these patients were considered operable or inoperable [135–140]. However, the only randomized, placebo-controlled clinical trial with bosentan has shown a reduction in the PVR but no change in 6-min walk distance, functional class, or time to clinical worsening. Given these limited data, further studies are necessary to obtain reliable long-term data on the effects of medical therapies in patients with chronic thromboembolic PH. Lung transplantation can also be performed in the more advanced cases.

Personal perspective

Despite the availability of an evidence-based treatment algorithm, the current treatment strategy for patients with PAH remains inadequate because the mortality rate continues to be high and the functional and haemodynamic impairments are still extensive in many patients. The non-equivocal progresses observed recently in the medical treatments of this condition are not yet sufficient. Additional efforts are required to explore new options including randomized controlled trials with initial combination therapy, with new classes of drugs, and with new designs including morbi-mortality end-points and prolonged observation periods. New classes of drugs include tyrosine kinase inhibitors, direct stimulators of guanosine cyclase, vasoactive intestinal peptide, non-prostanoid stimulators of prostacyclin receptors, RHO kinase inhibitors, tissular dual ERA: for each of these compounds phase II or III studies have been completed or are ongoing. New avenues for the treatment of PAH are related to the development of both gene therapy and regenerative medicine. Transfection of genes involved in both the nitric oxide and the prostacyclin pathway has been successfully tested in the monocrotaline-model of PH in rats. Stem cell therapy has proven to be effective in the same animal model and is currently been tested in a proof of concept and dose-finding protocols in PAH patients. Favourable data have been also shown in a small study from a Chinese group. These future treatment strategies will hopefully become available in the next 2–5 years.

The rate of inclusion in clinical trials in this field has been reduced in recent years due to several reasons including the availability of approved compounds and the treatment of patients in small centres not involved clinical research. Therefore, it is mandatory to optimize the currently available resources, implementing the usual strategies for rare diseases including the referral to centres of excellence, international collaboration, and support from patients' associations.

Further reading

Farber HW. The status of pulmonary arterial hypertension in 2008. *Circulation* 2008; **117**: 2966–8.

Galiè N, Hoeper M, Humbert M, *et al.* Guidelines on diagnosis and treatment of pulmonary hypertension: The Task Force on Diagnosis and Treatment of Pulmonary Hypertension of the European Society of Cardiology and of the European Respiratory Society. *Eur Heart J* 2009; in press.

Hoeper MM. Observational trials in pulmonary arterial hypertension: low scientific evidence but high clinical value. *Eur Respir J* 2007; **29**: 432–4.

Humbert M, Sitbon O, Simonneau G. Treatment of pulmonary arterial hypertension. *N Engl J Med* 2004; **351**: 1425–36.

Humbert M, Mc Laughlin VV (eds.). Proceedings of the 4th World Symposium on Pulmonary Hypertension. *J Am Coll Cardiol* 2009; in press.

Additional online material

24.1 Apical four-chamber view: enlarged, hypertrophic and hypokinetic right ventricle with altered movements of the interventricular septum. Enlarged right atrium and reduced left ventricle are also shown.

➲ For full references and multimedia materials please visit the online version of the book (http://esctextbook.oxfordonline.com).

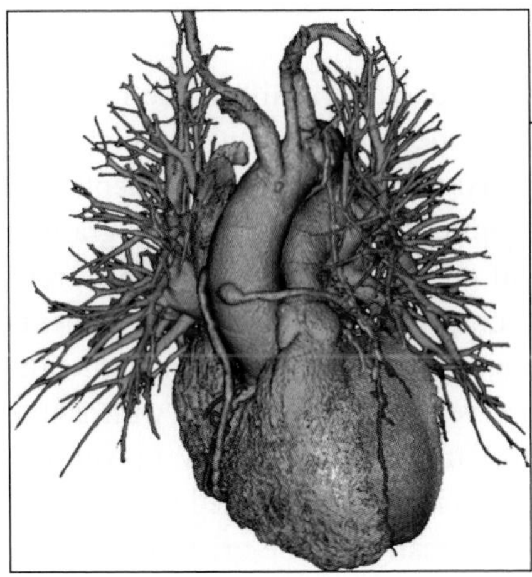

CHAPTER 25

Cardiac Rehabilitation

Stephan Gielen, Alessandro Mezzani, Rainer Hambrecht, and Hugo Saner

Contents

Summary

While many of the sophisticated interventional techniques in cardiovascular medicine applied today are symptomatic therapies, cardiac rehabilitation (CR) offers a highly effective causative treatment of atherosclerotic coronary and peripheral disease. The lifestyle and risk factor modifications achieved by CR have been shown to halt disease progression, and to reduce cardiovascular mortality and the rate of non-fatal myocardial infarction in patients with stable coronary artery disease.

This evolution from the traditional exercise training programme to facilitate return to work after a cardiovascular event into a comprehensive multidisciplinary intervention to improve patient prognosis is also reflected in the new definition of CR as *coordinated, multifaceted interventions designed to optimize a cardiac patient's physical, psychological, and social functioning, in addition to stabilizing, slowing, or even reversing the progression of the underlying atherosclerotic processes, thereby reducing morbidity and mortality.*

In addition to this preventive approach, exercise-based intervention programmes are effectively used as an adjuvant therapy in a number of cardiovascular diseases, most notably chronic heart failure (CHF). Since exercise intolerance in CHF is primarily related to the degree of peripheral changes (such as muscle atrophy, reduced peripheral perfusion due to endothelial dysfunction, abnormalities in ventilation, etc.), pharmacological treatment alone sometimes fails to significantly improve exercise capacity. Regular aerobic endurance training in stable CHF has been shown to improve peak oxygen uptake by 15–25%, to reduce peripheral vascular resistance, to retard or reverse muscle wasting, and to reduce morbidity.

Despite its documented clinical effectiveness, rehabilitation/prevention interventions are still widely underutilized in the clinical context. However, it becomes increasingly clear that the use of interventional and surgical procedures—for example, in stable coronary artery disease—is suboptimal therapy in the absence of simultaneous lifestyle modification, including regular physical exercise and aggressive treatment of cardiovascular risk factors.

Definition of cardiac rehabilitation within preventive cardiology

Definition of rehabilitation

In 1993, the World Health Organization (WHO) defined CR as the 'sum of activity and interventions required to ensure the best possible physical, mental, and social conditions so that patients with chronic or post-acute cardiovascular disease may, by their own efforts, preserve or resume their proper place in society and lead an active life' [1].

The WHO definition of CR laid special emphasis on the restoration of physical performance to premorbid levels. However, over the next decade it was realized that comprehensive rehabilitation can also favourably alter the course to the underlying cardiovascular disease process. This is reflected in the 2005 definition of the American Association of Cardiovascular Prevention and Rehabilitation (AACVPR): 'The term cardiac rehabilitation refers to coordinated, multifaceted interventions designed to optimize a cardiac patient's physical, psychological, and social functioning, in addition to stabilizing, slowing, or even reversing the progression of the underlying atherosclerotic processes, thereby reducing morbidity and mortality. As such, cardiac rehabilitation/secondary prevention programs provide an important and efficient venue in which to deliver effective preventive care' [2].

Goals of cardiac rehabilitation as a part of preventive cardiology

This new definition of CR stresses that the goals of CR have shifted from the prevention of disability resulting from coronary disease to the prevention of subsequent cardiovascular events, hospitalization, and death from cardiac causes. In other words, CR has become an essential part of the secondary prevention strategy after a first cardiovascular event. In the context of comprehensive secondary prevention important goals of comprehensive CR include:

1. patient education about the cardiovascular disease;
2. psychological adaptation to the chronic disease process;
3. induction of lifestyle changes with favourable influence on long-term survival;
4. optimized medical therapy of cardiovascular risk factors.

Comprehensive CR has well-documented effects on the symptoms, exercise tolerance, blood lipid levels and global risk profile, cigarette smoking, psychosocial well-being, progression of atherosclerosis, and subsequent coronary events resulting in reduced hospitalization and decreased morbidity and mortality [3].

Target population

As a consequence of the paradigm shift in the rationale for CR outlined earlier, the target patient population is no longer strictly limited to post-infarction patients and patients recovering from coronary artery bypass grafting (CABG). Other patient groups who clearly derive a prognostic benefit from comprehensive CR include patients with established coronary artery disease (CAD) with/without percutaneous intervention and patients with stable CHF/post-heart transplantation. Secondary prevention through CR programmes is now recognized as an essential component of the optimal guideline-oriented management of patients with CAD and with heart failure [3–6]. A clear symptomatic improvement of exercise tolerance was observed in patients with stable valvular heart disease or those post-valve replacement/repair.

The demographic change with increasing numbers of older and multimorbid patients is already felt in CR institutions. In an interdisciplinary effort with geriatricians, exercise-based CR can significantly delay the need for home care and prolong independent living.

The last 5 years have also witnessed an expansion of cardiac rehabilitative care to patients once considered to be too high risk for structured rehabilitation programmes (e.g. patients with residual myocardial ischaemia, New York Heart Association (NYHA) III heart failure, serious arrhythmias, and implantable cardioverter defibrillators, ICDs), who require more gradual and more protracted titration of exercise interventions and often start training under supervision.

Programme components

There is convincing evidence that the combination of regular exercise with interventions for lifestyle changes and modification of risk factors favourably alters the clinical course of cardiovascular diseases. Exercise interventions are therefore combined with disease education, nutritional counselling, behavioural strategies, and other psychosocial interventions and vocational counselling strategies to assist the patient to achieve coronary risk reduction and other cardiovascular health-related goals so that these programmes function as comprehensive secondary prevention services (see ➲Tables 25.1 and 25.2) [4, 5].

Organization of cardiac rehabilitation interventions

To achieve lifestyle modifications, CR and all efforts related to secondary prevention are long-term interventions.

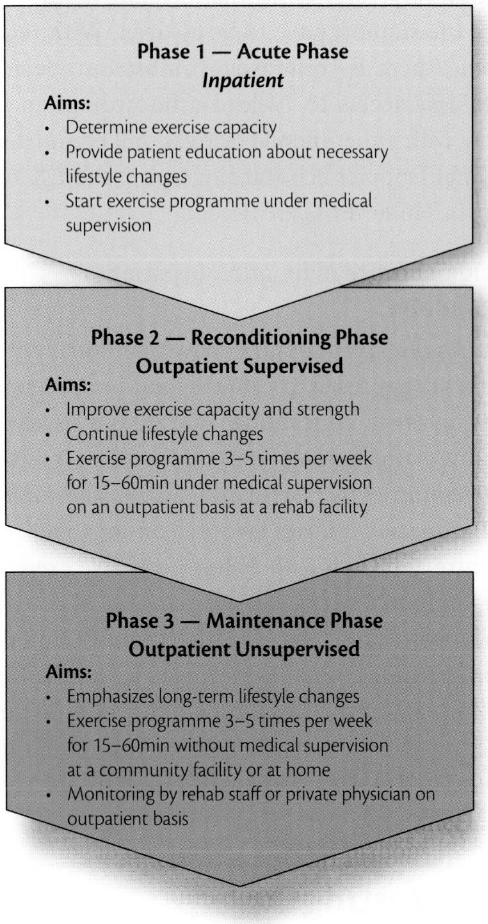

Phase 1 — Acute Phase
Inpatient
Aims:
- Determine exercise capacity
- Provide patient education about necessary lifestyle changes
- Start exercise programme under medical supervision

Phase 2 — Reconditioning Phase
Outpatient Supervised
Aims:
- Improve exercise capacity and strength
- Continue lifestyle changes
- Exercise programme 3–5 times per week for 15–60min under medical supervision on an outpatient basis at a rehab facility

Phase 3 — Maintenance Phase
Outpatient Unsupervised
Aims:
- Emphasizes long-term lifestyle changes
- Exercise programme 3–5 times per week for 15–60min without medical supervision at a community facility or at home
- Monitoring by rehab staff or private physician on outpatient basis

Figure 25.1 According to the World Health Organization (WHO) cardiac rehabilitation (CR) programmes are structured in three phases: the acute phase, when CR is usually administered in an inpatient setting at a rehabilitation institution; the reconditioning phase after the sequelae of the cardiac event have subsided, and the CR programme can safely be continued on an outpatient basis; and finally the maintenance phase in which the long-term prognostic benefits of CR are assured by an outpatient unsupervised programme. From phase 1 to phase 3 the degree of supervision and the healthcare expenses for CR decrease and the individual responsibility for continuing the lifestyle changes increases [7].

Table 25.1 General indications for the use of exercise testing in cardiovascular medicine

CAD diagnosis in subjects with no history of ischaemic heart disease, especially in adults with intermediate pre-test CAD probability and interpretable electrocardiogram (ECG)
New onset-CAD diagnosis in patients with history of ischaemic heart disease, previous revascularization procedures, and interpretable ECG
Differentiation of cardiac vs. pulmonary causes of exercise-induced dyspnoea and/or impaired exercise capacity*
Prognostic stratification of patients with: ◆ Suspected or known CAD ◆ Recent acute myocardial infarction (MI) ◆ CHF*
Functional evaluation of patients with: ◆ Suspected or known CAD ◆ Recent acute MI ◆ Previous revascularization procedures ◆ Valvular heart disease ◆ CHF* ◆ Previous heart transplantation
Exercise prescription for patients with: ◆ Suspected or known CAD ◆ Recent acute MI ◆ Previous revascularization procedures ◆ Valvular heart disease ◆ CHF ◆ Previous heart transplantation
Evaluation of therapy efficacy in patients with: ◆ Suspected or known CAD ◆ Recent acute MI ◆ Previous revascularization procedures ◆ Exercise-induced arrhythmias ◆ CHF
Evaluation of heart rhythm response/disorders in patients with: ◆ Rate-responsive pacemakers ◆ Known or suspected exercise-induced arrhythmias
Evaluation of normal subjects: ◆ Functional evaluation ◆ Prognostic stratification ◆ Exercise prescription

*Indicates conditions/diseases in which cardiopulmonary exercise testing should be performed.

As proposed by the WHO, CR is structured into three phases:

1 the acute phase;
2 the reconditioning phase;
3 the maintenance phase (➲Fig. 25.1) [7].

Integration of acute care and in- and outpatient CR programmes

For optimal results of CR programmes, comprehensive CR should start immediately after the acute event. The two main reasons for an early begin of phase 1 CR are (1) that the willingness for substantial lifestyle changes (e.g. smoking cessation) is greatest after the psychological trauma of a potentially life-threatening cardiac event, and (2) that early mobilization helps to avoid the deconditioning associated with prolonged bed-rest.

As a consequence, responsibility for CR can no longer be deferred to rehabilitation institutions but needs to be integrated into the acute care setting of every hospital dealing with cardiological emergencies. Ideally, acute post-event CR intervention, formal rehabilitation, and life-long secondary prevention with continued support to maintain the achieved lifestyle changes form an integrated approach to the patient. As a consequence, programmes should be

Table 25.2 Guideline-oriented specific indications for exercise testing [127]

Class 1 (clear indication)
Patients with suspected or proven CAD
1. Patients with exercise-related complaints of palpitations, dizziness, or syncope (diagnosis)
2. Men with atypical symptoms (diagnosis)
3. Patients with chronic stable angina or post-MI (prognosis, functional evaluation)
4. Symptomatic exercise-induced arrhythmias
5. Evaluation after revascularization procedure
Class 2 (test may be indicated)
1. Women with typical or atypical angina pectoris
2. Functional capacity evaluation to monitor cardiovascular therapy in patients with CAD or heart failure
3. Evaluation of patients with variant angina
4. Follow-up of patients with known CAD
5. Evaluation of asymptomatic men over 40 who are in special occupations (pilots, firefighters, police officers, bus or truck drivers, railroad engineers), or who have two or more atherosclerotic risk factors or who plan to enter a vigorous exercise programme
Class 3 (test probably not indicated)
1. Evaluation of patients with isolated premature ventricular beats and no evidence of CAD
2. Multiple serial testing during the course of CR programme
3. Diagnosis of CAD in patients, who have pre-excitation syndrome or complete left bundle branch block or are on digitalis therapy
4. Evaluation

coordinated between acute care, rehabilitation hospitals/institutions, and subsequent outpatient care.

Formal requirements for in- and outpatient CR programmes

CR/secondary prevention programmes should be delivered under the guidance of a cardiologist experienced in the exercise testing and exercise training of patients with various forms of cardiovascular disease suitable for such programmes, with a specific knowledge in all important aspects of rehabilitative and secondary preventative care. The staff should include a cardiologist, physiotherapists or sport teachers, nutrition counsellors or dieticians, psychologists or psychiatrists, and preferably also a social worker or vocational counsellor. There are no formal requirements on an international level for equipment, logistics, and certification; however, there are national guidelines and recommendations in most European countries. Although life-threatening cardiovascular complications are rare during formal CR programmes, a well-designed and regularly controlled emergency concept is crucial for each programme. Staff members should be regularly trained in cardiopulmonary resuscitation (CPR) and basic life support, an alarm system has to be established and also regularly tested, and very early defibrillation and rapid access to advanced life support have to be assured. With regards to equipment, there is consensus in most European countries that easy access to 12-lead echocardiogram (ECG), ergometry with either bicycle or treadmill ergometer, two-dimensional Doppler echocardiography, chest X-ray, and telemetry or Holter ECG are needed.

Worldwide practice of in- and outpatient CR programmes

While the Anglo-Saxon countries have traditionally preferred an ambulatory approach to CR with long-term exercise programmes to which educational, social, and psychological programme components may be added, continental European countries like Germany, Austria, and some of the eastern European countries favoured an inpatient rehabilitation centre approach with a short intensive exercise programme for up to 4 weeks. Comprehensive CR components like nutritional counselling, disease education, and psychological programme components are begun on the first days of the CR programme. The cultural differences do not seem to impact on the effectiveness of the CR programmes and are more related to spa traditions of Germany and Austria.

Exercise testing in cardiovascular medicine

Introduction

Exercise testing is extensively used in cardiovascular medicine, as functional assessment has become an integral component of cardiac evaluation [8]. This is due to the fact that exercise cardiopulmonary measurements allow an overall estimate of cardiac diseases pathophysiology far more reliable than resting ones. As a consequence, several indications for exercise testing are now accepted in cardiovascular medicine (➲Tables 25.1 and 25.2).

Exercise tests can be performed using different protocols, distinguished in incremental and constant-power according to workload progressive increase or constancy during the test, respectively [9]. Incremental tests are aimed at reaching a maximal stress of the cardiovascular system and are routinely used in the clinical setting, whereas constant-power ones are usually performed at submaximal effort intensities and are mainly utilized for research purposes. Among incremental protocols, the ramp-like ones are increasingly used due to their advantages as to patients' tolerance and test interpretation [10], and should be preferred to non-ramp-like incremental tests whenever possible (➲Fig. 25.2).

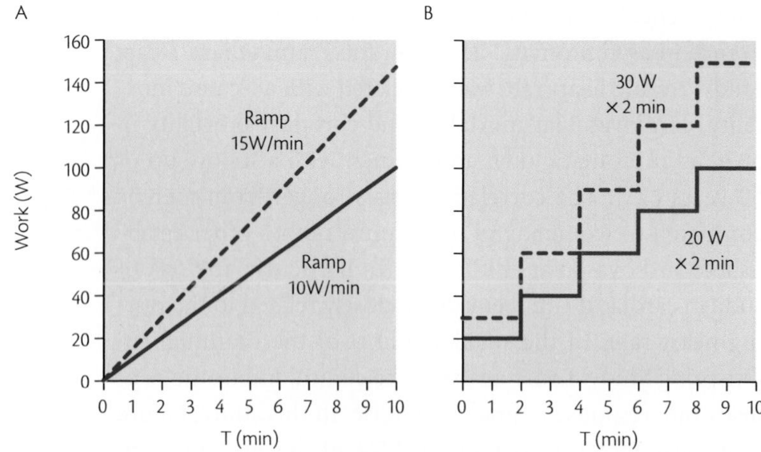

Figure 25.2 Among incremental protocols, the ramp-like protocols (A) are increasingly used due to their advantages as to patient's tolerance and test interpretation [10], and should be preferred to non-ramp-like incremental tests (B) whenever possible.

Exercise tests can be carried out on different kinds of ergometers, i.e. cycle ergometer or treadmill, the advantages and disadvantages of which are summarized in ➲Table 25.3 [9]. Finally, analysis of ventilation, oxygen consumption (VO_2), and carbon dioxide production (VCO_2) can be added to conventional exercise testing measurements in cardiopulmonary exercise testing (CPET) when a thorough evaluation of the of the O_2 transport and/or utilization efficiency is required for clinical or research purposes [9, 11, 12].

Physiology of incremental exercise testing

Cardiovascular response to incremental exercise

In the early phases of incremental exercise, up to around 50% of maximal effort, cardiac output rises as a result of an increase in both heart rate and stroke volume, whereas at higher work intensities the increase in cardiac output depends largely on increases in heart rate [9]; these adaptations lead to a four- to sixfold rise of cardiac output at maximal effort (➲Table 25.4).

Systolic and mean blood pressures rise in parallel during incremental exercise, while diastolic blood pressure remains unchanged or decreases (➲Table 25.4). Moreover, a redistribution of cardiac output occurs, induced by selective vasoconstriction of mesenteric/splanchnic arteries and vasodilatation in muscle-supplying arteries; when a large skeletal muscle mass is involved in exercise, a significant decrease in systemic vascular resistance is observed at both submaximal and maximal effort (➲Table 25.4).

Both resting heart rate and the increase of the heart rate with increasing exercise level (i.e. the chronotropic

Table 25.3 Comparison of treadmill and cycle ergometer for exercise testing

	Treadmill	Cycle ergometer
Higher peak VO_2	X	
Quantification of external work		X
Higher ECG quality		X
Ease of obtaining blood specimens		X
Higher safety		X
Possible use in supine position		X
Smaller size		X
Lower noisiness		X
Lower cost		X
Ease of move		X
Familiarity of exercise	X	
Greater experience in Europe		X
Greater experience in the United States	X	

Table 25.4 Physiological response to incremental exercise

	Rest	Peak exercise	Fold increase versus resting condition
HR (bpm)	70	180	2.6
SV (mL)	80	140	1.7
CO (L/min)	5.6	25	4.5
SBP (mmHg)	120	180	1.5
DBP (mmHg)	80	80	1
MAP (mmHg)	93	113	1.2
TPR (mmHg/L/min)	16.6	4.5	0.27
Δa-vO_2 (mL/dL)	5	16	3.2
VO_2 (mL/min)	280	4000	14.3
Vt (mL)	500	1800	3.6
BF (breaths/min)	12	40	3.3
VE (L/min)	6	72	12

HR, heart rate; SV, stroke volume; CO, cardiac output; SBP, systolic blood pressure; DBP, diastolic blood pressure; MAP, mean arterial pressure; TPR, total peripheral resistances; Δa-vO_2, arterio-mixed venous oxygen concentration difference; VO_2, oxygen consumption; Vt, tidal volume; BF, breathing frequency; VE, ventilation.

competence) were shown to have clear prognostic relevance in asymptomatic adults: in the Framingham Heart Study, resting heart rate was associated with all-cause mortality, cardiovascular mortality, and coronary mortality in 5070 asymptomatic men and women with a follow-up of 30 years [13]. The correlation was stronger from men as compared to women, and it was unrelated to other established cardiovascular risk factors. In particular, the risk of sudden cardiac death seems to be closely related to the resting heart rate. In the smaller cohort of the Framingham Offspring Study, Lauer analysed the clinical implications of heart rate response to graded exercise. In this study, failure to achieve target heart rate (i.e. 85% of the age-predicted maximum heart rate), a smaller increase in heart rate with exercise, and the chronotropic response index were all predictive of total mortality and incidence of CAD [14].

It is not only the exercise-induced increase in heart rate which is regarded as an important indicator of cardiac health; heart rate recovery immediately after exercise is also closely related to the baseline training status of the patient and their cardiovascular health. Cole [15] followed 2428 consecutive adults without a history of cardiac disease for 6 years. Study participants completed a symptom-limited exercise test; heart rate recovery was defined as the decrease in heart rate from peak exercise to 1min after the cessation of exercise, and a reduction lower than 13bpm was defined as pathologic. A low value for heart rate recovery was strongly predictive of death (relative risk (RR) 4.0, confidence interval (CI) 3.0–5.2), even after adjustments for age, sex, medication, standard cardiac risk factors, and resting heart rate [15]. The close relation between exercise-induced changes in heart rate/heart rate recovery after exercise and cardiovascular mortality underline the clinical relevance of routine exercise testing for prognostic reasons.

Ventilatory response to incremental exercise

The ventilatory response to exercise is accurately measured during CPET, when ventilation per minute and expiratory PO_2 and PCO_2 are measured by use of a face mask with an attached air-flow transducer and gas analyser. Because of its technical complexity, CPET is not routinely used for measurement of exercise capacity but it adds important physiologic insight in special patient populations (e.g. functional evaluation of patients with heart failure, respiratory disease, in transplant candidates, or in patients with exercise intolerance of unknown cause). ➲Table 25.5 provides a brief overview of important abbreviations and technical terms used in CPET:

Table 25.5 Abbreviations used in cardiopulmonary exercise testing

Abbreviation	Explanation	Unit
VE	Ventilation per minute	L/min
VO_2	Oxygen uptake per minute	L/min
VCO_2	Carbon dioxide output per minute	L/min
PO_2	Oxygen partial pressure	mmHg
PCO_2	Carbon dioxide partial pressure	mmHg
V_T	Tidal volume	L
V_D	Dead space volume	L
EELV	End-expiratory lung volume	L
$PETO_2$	End-tidal oxygen partial pressure (i.e. at the end of the expiratory phase)	mmHg
$PETCO_2$	End-tidal carbon dioxide partial pressure (frequently used as an approximation of arterial PCO_2)	mmHg
VAT	Ventilatory anaerobic threshold (or if adjusted for body weight mL/min·kg)	mL/min
Peak VO_2	Peak oxygen uptake as a measure of individualmaximal exercise capacity (or if adjusted for body weight mL/min·kg)	mL/min

The ventilatory response during incremental exercise increases at a rate required to remove the CO_2 produced by energetic metabolism [9]. The excess CO_2 produced above anaerobic threshold by buffering (see ➲Skeletal muscle metabolic response to incremental exercise) increases ventilatory drive, keeping the ventilation (VE) vs. VCO_2 relationship linear and the end-tidal CO_2 pressure ($PETCO_2$) value constant (i.e. the subject does not hyperventilate with respect to the volume of CO2 metabolically produced). However, in the final phase of incremental exercise hyperventilation occurs with respect to CO_2 as a respiratory compensation of exercise-induced metabolic acidosis, making VE/VCO_2 increase and $PETCO_2$ decrease [9]. The actual ventilation required to eliminate a given amount of CO_2 is described by the modified alveolar equation [9]:

$$VE = 863 \times VCO_2/PaCO_2 \times (1 - V_D/V_T)$$

where V_D/V_T is the physiological dead space/tidal volume ratio.

Skeletal muscle metabolic response to incremental exercise

During incremental exercise, an energy requirement is reached, termed 'anaerobic threshold', above which blood lactate concentration increases at a progressively steeper rate [9]. This is due to anaerobic glycolysis activation, which occurs as the oxygen supply rate is not rapid enough to reoxidize cytosolic NADH + H^+. Almost all of the H^+ generated in the cell from lactic acid (La) dissociation is buffered by bicarbonate according to the following reaction:

$$H^+ La^- + HCO_3^- \leftrightarrows H_2O + CO_2 + La^-$$

Such production of CO_2, in excess of that produced by aerobic metabolism (excess CO_2), makes the VCO_2 vs. VO_2 relationship become steeper. By measuring at the mouth gas exchange modifications induced by metabolic changes, the 'ventilatory anaerobic threshold' (VAT) can be determined analyzing the slope of the VCO_2 vs. VO_2 relationship as the point of transition of the VCO_2 vs. VO_2 slope from <1 (activation of aerobic metabolism alone) to >1 (anaerobic plus aerobic metabolism) (➲Fig. 25.3). When expressed relative to measured peakVO_2, VAT occurs at around 50–60% of peakVO_2 in most normal subjects and cardiac patients, with a trend towards higher percentages of peakVO_2 in patients with CHF [16].

Criteria for maximal effort attainment

Achievement of truly maximal effort during incremental exercise testing is crucial for both functional and prognostic evaluation of cardiac patients, and can be assumed in the presence of one or more of the following criteria [17]:

- failure of VO_2 and/or heart rate to increase with further increases in work rate;
- peak respiratory exchange ratio (VCO_2/VO_2) ≥1.10–1.15;
- post-exercise blood lactate concentration ≥8mmol/dL (used in athletes, rarely achieved by patients);
- rating of perceived exertion ≥8 (on the 10-point Borg scale; ➲Table 25.6);

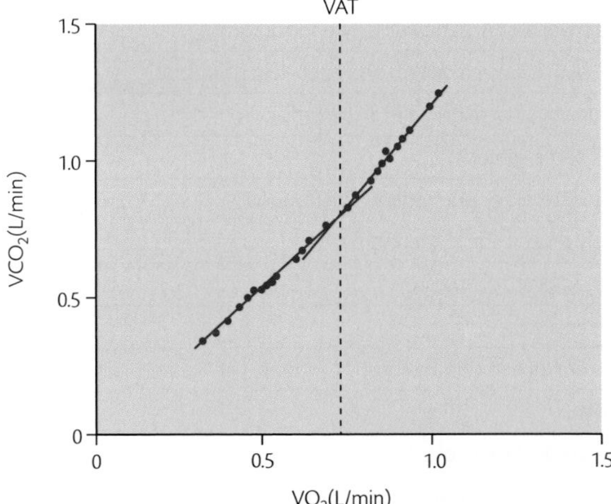

Figure 25.3 By measuring at the mouth gas exchange modifications induced by metabolic changes, the 'ventilatory anaerobic threshold' (VAT) can be determined analyzing the slope of the VCO_2 vs. VO_2 relationship as the point of transition of the VCO_2 vs. VO_2 slope from <1 (activation of aerobic metabolism alone) to >1 (anaerobic plus aerobic metabolism).

- patient's appearance (exhaustion).

However, one should keep in mind that all indices of physical exercise capacity are by nature imprecise and are approximations of the true voluntary maximal exercise capacity. In most cardiologic patients the exercise test has to be terminated before one of these criteria is reached because of cardiac symptoms (i.e. symptom-limited exercise test). Maximal exercise capacity as measured, e.g. by maximal oxygen uptake, depends on three key physiologic systems: (1) the efficacy of the gas exchange by the lungs; (2) the maximal cardiac output; and (3) the aerobic metabolic capacity of the working skeletal muscle.

Safety aspects of exercise testing

Indications/contraindications for exercise testing

Over the last decades the risk:benefit ratio of exercise testing has been systematically evaluated in a number of disease entities. As a result, the indications and contraindications of exercise testing are now clearly established and laid down in guidelines of the American Heart Association (AHA) and European Society of Cardiology (ESC) (see ➲Tables 25.1 and 25.2) [8].

In the context of CR, exercise testing is a valuable tool not only to prove/exclude exercise-induced myocardial ischaemia but also to determine the patient's fitness level prior to initiation of a training programme. It is indispensable to recommend a training heart rate for aerobic endurance training and to exclude potential risks during physical exertion such as exercise-induced arrhythmias or excessive blood pressure increase. Formal indications for exercise testing are to be found in ➲Tables 25.1 and 25.2.

Table 25.6 Borg scale of perceived exertion

0	Nothing at all
0.5	Extremely light
1	Very light
2	Light
3	Moderate
4	Somewhat heavy
5	Heavy
6	
7	Very heavy
8	
9	
10	Extremely heavy
•	Maximal

Large epidemiological studies clearly indicate a relation between cardiovascular fitness and mortality (see Physical activity and all-cause mortality) [18, 19] and exercise testing is widely used to objectively assess disease-related exercise intolerance for risk-stratification of heart failure patients.

Statistical risks of adverse events during incremental exercise testing

Despite its undisputed clinical value, maximal exercise testing confers a certain measurable statistical risk of adverse events. In an unselected patient population referred for exercise testing, mortality is reported to be <0.01% and morbidity <0.05% [20]. When performed in patients within 4 weeks of an acute MI, mortality rises to 0.03% and the rate of non-fatal MI or need for cardiac resuscitation reaches 0.09% [21].

In patients with stable compensated CHF no additional risk of maximal exercise testing has been reported with no major complications reported in one study of 1286 bicycle ergometer tests [22].

The absolute risk of major complications during exercise testing can be greatly minimized by strictly adhering to the established standards with regard to patient selection, careful history and clinical examination, and close monitoring with 12-lead ECG and blood pressure recordings during and in the minutes (minimum 3min) immediately after exercise.

Formal requirements for exercise testing facilities

Although rare in absolute numbers, major complications of exercise testing can be expected to occur from time to time in high-throughput testing facilities. Everything necessary for CPR must be available at the testing facility, including standard emergency drugs, a defibrillator, and equipment for endotracheal intubation. The exercise test must be supervised either by a trained physician or by specially trained assistant personnel with a physician present in calling distance. Regular drills with CPR procedures should be performed to ascertain adequate and quick response in emergency situations. A telephone with emergency numbers on it must be available to call additional assistance.

Criteria for termination of a maximal exercise test

To balance the diagnostic purpose and the inherent risks of maximal exercise testing, a comprehensive catalogue of criteria for test termination has been developed (➲Table 25.7). Moreover, contraindications to exercise testing are clearly established and laid down in available guidelines (➲Table 25.8) [8]. It is essential to implement these criteria in clinical practice, as their neglect may have legal consequences in case of adverse event.

Table 25.7 Criteria for exercise test termination

Muscle fatigue
Severe dyspnoea, especially when disproportionate to effort intensity
Moderate to severe angina pectoris
Horizontal or down sloping ST segment depressions >3mm as compared to baseline
ST segment upsloping >1mm with respect to baseline in leads different from V1 and aVR, in the absence of Q waves
Complex arrhythmias (II and III degree atrioventricular block, atrial fibrillation, paroxysmal supraventricular tachycardia, ventricular tachycardia)
Exercise-induced complete bundle branch block, especially when indistinguishable from ventricular tachycardia
Systolic and/or diastolic blood pressure: >240mmHg and/or 120mmHg, respectively
Systolic blood pressure fall >10mmHg with respect to baseline, especially when associated to other signs/symptoms of myocardial ischaemia
Increasing atypical chest pain
Signs of peripheral hypoperfusion (pallor, cyanosis, cool sweating, etc.)
Neurological signs/symptoms (ataxia, vertigines, lightheadness, phosphenes, etc.)
Lower limb(s) claudication
Orthopaedic limitation
Technical impossibility of ECG monitoring
Patient request

Table 25.8 Contraindications to exercise test

Absolute
Ongoing or recent acute MI
Decompensated heart failure
Unstable angina
Acute myocarditis, pericarditis, or endocarditis
Acute pulmonary embolism and deep vein thrombosis
Complex atrial or ventricular arrhythmias
Severe aortic stenosis
Severe systemic or pulmonary hypertension
Severely dilated aortic aneurysm
Acute extracardiac disease
Severe anaemia
Severe orthopaedic limitations
Relative
Moderate aortic stenosis
Severe proximal stenosis of left coronary branches
Severe subaortic hypertrophic stenosis
Advanced atrioventricular block
Electrolytic disorders
Psychical disorders

Methodological aspects of exercise testing in the clinical context

Exercise testing in coronary artery disease (ergometry)

Exercise testing is extensively used for diagnosis of obstructive CAD, most frequently caused by coronary atherosclerosis: this applies to diagnosis of both previously unknown CAD and CAD progression in native coronary vessels or coronary by-pass grafts of patients with previous coronary events and/or revascularization procedures [8].

The possible ECG changes induced by obstructive CAD during effort are shown in ➲Fig. 25.4. A horizontal or downsloping depression of the ST segment is the most common ECG sign of exercise-induced myocardial ischaemia, and is considered diagnostic when reaching at least 1mm with respect to baseline at 80ms from J point of QRS complex [23]. However, several causes of both false positive and false negative exercise test have been described (➲Table 25.9); moreover, the predictive accuracy of the exercise test is known to increase with increasing pre-test probability of CAD in the patient under examination [8]. As a consequence, sensitivity and specificity values ranging between 50–90% and predictive accuracy values ranging from 65–75% have been reported for exercise testing in different patient populations [8].

Table 25.9 Causes of false-positive and false-negative exercise test

False-positive
Left ventricular hypertrophy
Resting repolarization abnormalities (left bundle branch block, WPW pre-excitation, etc.)
Non-ischaemic cardiomyopathy
Digoxin
Systemic hypertension
Mitral valve prolapse
Pericardial disease
Hypokalaemia
Anaemia
Female sex
Interpretative error
False-negative
Lack of ischaemic threshold attainment
Lack of appreciation of symptoms or non-ECG signs possibly associated with CAD
Significant obstructive CAD well compensated by collateral circulation
Interpretation error

Exercise testing in chronic heart failure (cardiopulmonary exercise testing) (➲Chapter 2)

A reduced ability to perform aerobic exercise is the hallmark of the CHF pathophysiologic picture, related to changes in both peripheral (skeletal muscle, endothelium, regional blood flow, and reflex cardiopulmonary control systems) and central (lung and heart) links of the O_2 transport chain from ambient air to the skeletal muscle [24, 25]. CPET is thus increasingly utilized in this population, as it provides not only a precise and repeatable evaluation of functional capacity but also strong prognostic indicators currently used in heart transplantation work-up [26]. Oxygen consumption at peak incremental effort (peak VO_2) has traditionally

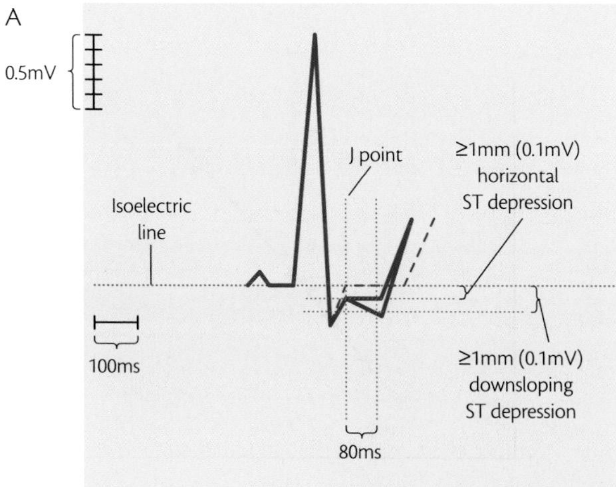

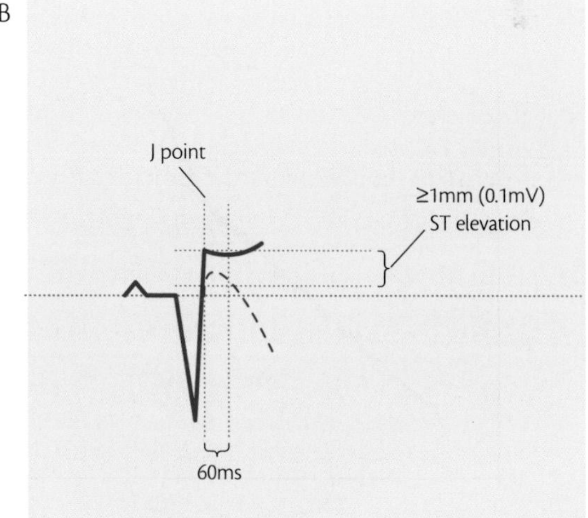

Figure 25.4 (A) A down sloping of the ST segment is the most common ECG sign of exercise-induced myocardial ischaemia, and is considered diagnostic when reaching at least 1mm with respect to baseline at 80ms from J point of QRS complex. (B) ST segment upsloping >1mm 60ms after the J point with respect to baseline in leads different from V1 and aVR in the absence of significant Q waves is also regarded as indicative of a severe ischaemic response and should lead to immediate exercise test termination.

been used as a prognostic marker in CHF patients [27] and normal subjects [28], with values ≤10mL/kg/min used as a decisional cut-off for indication to heart transplantation in CHF patients both on and off beta-blockers [27]. In patients with peak VO_2 values >10mL/kg/min, other parameters besides peak VO_2 can be used for prognostic stratification; among these, ventilation-related indexes, such as VE/VCO_2 slope and VO_2/VE relationship (➲Fig. 25.5) seem to be the most powerful predictors, offering the advantage to be assessable also at submaximal levels of effort in case of exercise test premature termination [12]. In fact, several prospective follow-up studies indicate that VE/VCO_2 slope is a more powerful predictor of cardiovascular mortality than peak VO_2. Finally, CPET is a precious tool in the rehabilitative setting for prescription of the intensity of aerobic training and evaluation of its effects [12].

Exercise testing in peripheral artery disease (treadmill walking test)

Exercise testing can be used in patients with known lower limbs peripheral artery disease (PAD) and claudication to objectively document the magnitude of functional limitation and its improvement in response to therapeutic interventions and exercise training [29]. Exercise testing should be performed on treadmill, with protocols providing less intense workload increments than commonly used for healthy individuals or patients with CAD (e.g., the Gardner–Skinner, Hiatt, or Naughton protocols) [30]. Time of onset of leg symptoms, laterality and specific muscle group(s) involved, and total walking time are the relevant indexes to be recorded [29]. Moreover, exercise testing can be useful for diagnostic purposes in the case of suspected lower limb(s) PAD by measuring the ankle–brachial index (ABI) at rest and immediately after exercise. The ABI is the ratio of the systolic blood pressure from the dorsalis pedis and/or the posterior tibial arteries and that from the brachial artery [31]. In normal subjects, the brachial and ankle blood pressures rise together and maintain their normal relationship during exercise; in contrast, in patients with lower extremity PAD, exercise-induced vasodilation in the claudicating limb(s) is associated with development of a significant blood pressure gradient across the arterial stenosis, and the postexercise ABI will fall from its baseline value.

Physical activity, physical fitness, and cardiovascular diseases

Modern epidemiological studies have confirmed the concept that physical fitness is inversely related with all-cause mortality—mostly as a consequence of reduced prevalence of ischaemic heart disease. However, there is a growing body of evidence that the incidence of other chronic diseases is also reduced by exercise: type 2 diabetes mellitus, osteoporosis, obesity, depression, and even certain malignancies (breast cancer, colon cancer).

Different implications of physical activity and physical fitness

Physical activity and physical fitness represent different approaches to measuring compliance to a healthy lifestyle. Traditionally, in large epidemiological studies the amount of leisure-time physical activity was calculated from

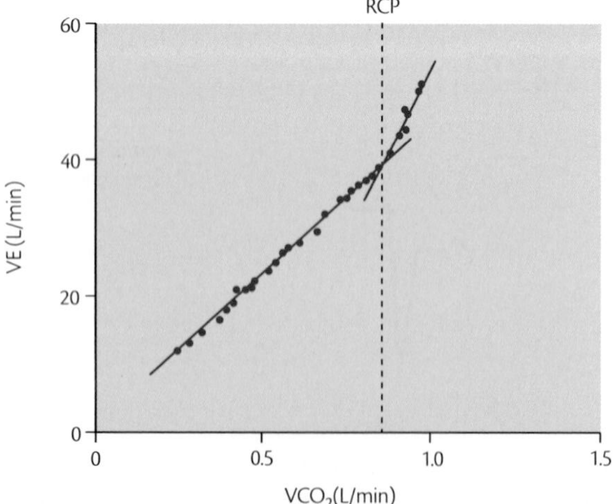

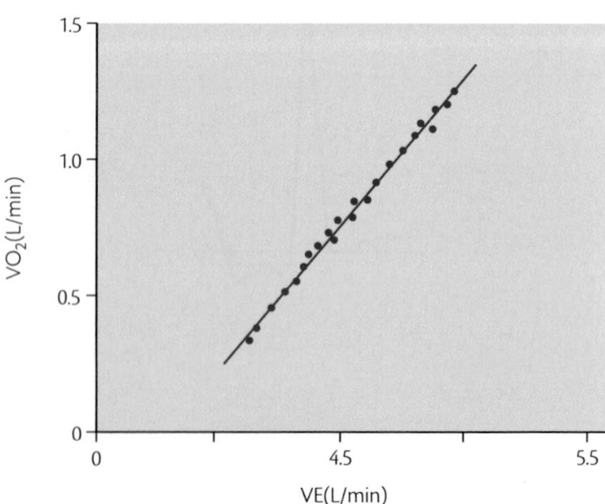

Figure 25.5 In patients with peak VO_2 values higher than 10mL/kg/min, other parameters besides peak VO_2 can be used for prognostic stratification; among these, ventilation-related indexes, such as slopes of VE vs. VCO_2 and VO_2 vs. VE relationships seem the most powerful, offering the advantage to be assessable also at submaximal levels of effort in case of exercise test premature termination [12]. RCP, respiratory compensation point.

questionnaires or recalls typically based on the patient's own information. These instruments have, however, a considerable range of error:

- patients tend to overestimate the time devoted to physical activity;
- they may be biased as a result of health education following a cardiac event;
- the calculation of energy expenditure for different types of physical activities is a very rough estimate of real physical activity.

Generally, physical activity is classified as moderate if performed at an intensity of 3–6 metabolic equivalents (METs), and vigorous at >6 METs. New approaches to direct measurement of physical activity by pedometers coupled to three-dimensional accelerometers may provide more accurate measurements in the future.

Assessment of physical fitness, on the other hand, is typically done in the form of a maximal exercise test (ergometry, CPET) and provides an objective measure of exercise capacity. The degree of inaccuracy is certainly lower as compared to physical activity measures. Over the last 15 years a number of studies were able to document a clear relation between individual levels of physical fitness and survival.

Physical activity and all-cause mortality

First hints of a beneficial prognostic impact of regular physical exercise were derived from a number of long-term observational studies: Morris [32], Paffenbarger [33, 34], and Slattery [35] were able to document that increased levels of average daily physical activity were correlated to a reduced incidence of CHD, reduced cardiac and all-cause mortality. The relative mortality reduction reached up 30–40% in moderately active persons (1000kcal/week) [35].

These and other studies led to the conclusion that men and women should engage in at least 30–45min of moderate physical activity every day [38]. Exercise intensity should be at 60–80% of the maximal age-adjusted heart rate. Some studies suggest a correlation between exercise intensity and mortality reduction [33, 39, 40] but the benefits of vigorous exercise should be weighted against the increased risk of trauma and chronic orthopaedic damage.

Traditionally, it has been recommended that a minimum of 1000kcal of physical activity energy expenditure should be generated per week to obtain a prognostic benefit. New studies suggest that there is an inverse association between relative intensity of physical activity (the individual's perceived level of exertion) and risk of CAD, even among men not satisfying the 1000kcal/week activity recommendations. Recommendations

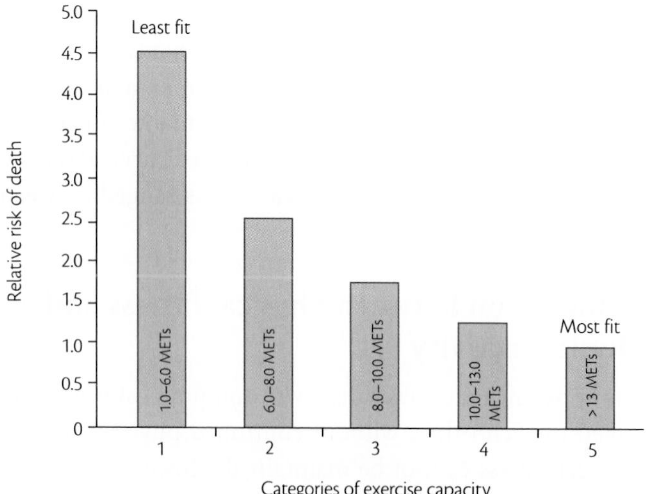

Figure 25.6 In a prospective follow-up study for 6.2 ± 3.7 years consecutive men referred for treadmill exercise testing age-adjusted mortality rates in healthy men were categorized by level of fitness. The range of values for exercise capacity (METs) for each category are represented within each bar. A clear relation between fitness level and all-cause mortality is obvious. Reproduced with permission from Myers J. Cardiology patient pages. Exercise and cardiovascular health. *Circulation* 2003; **107**: e2–e5.

may therefore need to consider individual fitness levels instead of globally prescribing activities of ≥3 METs [39].

Physical fitness and all-cause mortality

These observations for physical activity levels were confirmed by studies which analysed the relation between maximal exercise capacity (as measured by bicycle ergometry) and mortality during long-term follow-up [36, 37]. A reduced physical fitness was clearly identified as an independent predictor of mortality in men (RR 1.52, 95% CI 1.28–1.82) and in women (RR 2.10, 95% CI 1.36–3.21—equal in importance to smoking or hypertension. An increase of exercise capacity by just 1MET conferred a mortality reduction of 12% (➲Fig. 25.6) [18]. One metabolic equivalent was defined as the average resting metabolic rate (3.5mL O_2/min·kg). In an average 70kg man, an exercise intensity of 25W equals 1.6METs (➲Table 25.10).

In clinical studies, physical fitness (after adjustment for age and sex) proved to be a stronger predictor of all-cause mortality and cardiovascular morbidity than other established cardiovascular risk factors such as hypertension, smoking, hyperlipidaemia, and diabetes. Even compared with other

Table 25.10 Metabolic equivalents (METs)

Exercise intensity	METS	Watt (70kg)	kcal/min
Low	<3	<40	<4
Moderate	3–6	40–100	4–8
Vigorous	>6	>100	>8

parameters derived from exercise testing (ST depression, exercise-induced symptoms, haemodynamic response to exercise) the fitness level defined as maximal exercise capacity in Watt remained the strongest marker for future events [18, 41–43]. The extent of improved survival related to a 1-MET increment of physical fitness ranged between 10–25% [44].

Comparison between physical fitness and physical activity

It is apparent that physical activity and physical fitness are linked to each other: without continued physical activity physical fitness cannot be maintained. However, contrary to physical activity as a behavioural parameter physical fitness carries an important genetic component. As a result it has been debated whether physical activity determines fitness and thereby survival, or whether fitness levels predict mortality independently from activity patterns [37].

A recent meta-analysis compared the dose–response relationships between leisure-time physical activity and fitness and their association with cardiovascular events; Williams [28] found that (1) the risk reduction per 10% increment in physical fitness showed a sharp drop for fitness between the 15th and 25th percentile of fitness while there was a steady decline over the entire range of physical activity levels; and (2) for all percentiles >25th the relative risk reduction is greater for fitness than for physical activity (➲Fig. 25.7). These novel data suggest that the health benefits of exercise training are most pronounced in the subjects and patients with the lowest baseline fitness levels. Therefore, public health benefits may be greater for small improvements in physical activity levels achieved among completely sedentary subjects than for larger improvements in moderately fit subjects.

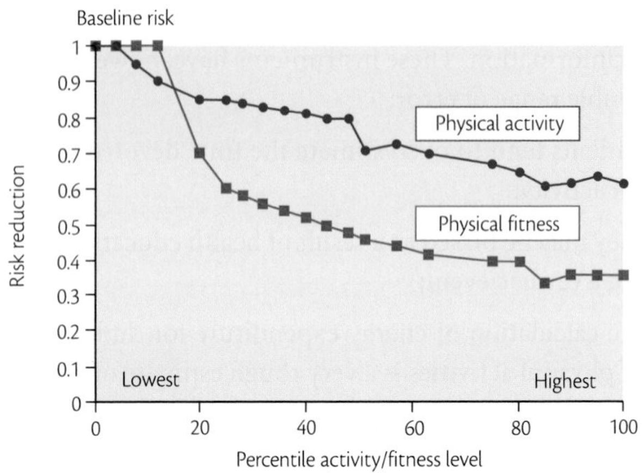

Figure 25.7 A recent meta-analysis comparing the dose-response relationships between leisure-time physical activity and fitness and their association with cardiovascular events Williams [28] found that the risk reduction per 10% increment in physical fitness showed a sharp drop for fitness between the 15th and 25th percentile of fitness while there was a steady decline over the entire range of physical activity levels. This indicates the potential of a 'threshold effect' for a minimal physical fitness to reduce one's cardiovascular risk. The meta-analysis included a total of eight fitness cohorts with >300,000 person years and 30 physical activity cohorts with >2,000,000 person years. Reproduced with permission from Williams PT. Physical fitness and activity as separate heart disease risk factors: a meta-analysis. *Med Sci Sports Exerc* 2001; **33**: 754–61.

Exercise intolerance in cardiovascular diseases

Exercise intolerance as a key symptom of cardiovascular diseases

Exercise intolerance is the major clinical symptom of the cardiac patient and the main reason for seeking medical advice. Both in CAD and in heart failure the degree of exercise limitation by either angina pectoris or dyspnoea serves as a tool for classifying disease severity and urgency of medical treatment (Canadian Cardiovascular Class (CCS); NYHA). The sensitivity of exertional dyspnoea in suspected heart failure is as high as 66% with a specificity for heart failure of 52%. Additionally, functional classifications based on symptom-limited exercise intolerance carry a strong prognostic implication and help to identify high-risk patient subgroups.

Cardiac causes of exercise intolerance

Cardiovascular causes of exercise intolerance are related to:

- the inability of the heart to increase cardiac output in line with the demand. This can be caused by a reduction in systolic contractile function, diastolic ventricular filling, chronotropic incompetence, or valvular heart disease;
- an obstruction of a significant proportion of the arterial tree can cause a critical reduction in cardiac output, i.e. in pulmonary embolism;
- vasomotor disturbances with either exaggerated vasoconstriction or vasorelaxation.

The cardiac causes of exercise intolerance are assessed by ergometry with monitoring of heart rate, blood pressure, and 12-lead ECG. The most common reasons for cardiac exercise intolerance are exercise-induced myocardial ischaemia and left ventricular (LV) systolic or diastolic dysfunction.

Peripheral causes of exercise intolerance

Peripheral causes of exercise intolerance tend to be overlooked in traditional ergometry and are very important in chronic disease processes e.g. heart failure and ageing. Here, a combination of endothelial dysfunction with attenuated flow-mediated vasodilation, weakness of the respiratory muscles, ventilatory disturbances such as oscillatory ventilation, and peripheral metabolic changes in the skeletal muscle determine a large proportion of the whole body exercise tolerance.

These systems are better examined by CPET which measures total oxygen consumption—a parameter which integrates oxygen uptake by ventilation, oxygen transport by the cardiovascular system, and energy generation by oxidation in the muscle tissue.

Exercise-based interventions in cardiac rehabilitation and secondary prevention

General indications and contraindications for exercise training

In general, the contraindications for regular physical exercise training are the same as for exercise testing. Patients should generally be in a stable clinical situation prior to starting a training programme.

Candidates for CR services historically were patients who recently had had a MI or had undergone CABG surgery, but candidacy has been broadened to include patients who: have undergone percutaneous coronary interventions (PCIs); are heart transplantation candidates or recipients; or have stable CHF, PAD with claudication, or other forms of CVD. In addition, patients who have undergone other cardiac surgical procedures, such as those with valvular heart disease, also may be eligible [2].

The problem of underuse of CR is still very prevalent in the US and parts of Europe—depending on the health insurance system. In the US, <20% of potential candidates for CR finally participate in a structured programme, in Europe the figures are somewhat better, ranging between 20–50%. What are the causes? One important factor relates to the perception of CR as optional adjunctive therapy as opposed to the life-saving interventions in the acute-care setting. This view, as unjustified as it is, may explain the low referral rates from acute care centres—particularly of women, older adults, and ethnic minority patients. Other factors include: poor patient motivation; inadequate third-party reimbursement for services; and geographic limitations to accessibility of programme sites. In fact, we could probably save more lives in cardiovascular medicine by guideline-oriented application of CR and secondary prevention than by the introduction of additional high-tech interventional procedures.

Exercise therapy in cardiovascular diseases

Historical development of exercise interventions: from rehabilitation to prognostic indication

After years of enthusiasm for percutaneous coronary intervention (PCI) several landmark trials have led to disillusionment over the last years, especially in patients with stable coronary artery disease:

- The Occluded Artery Trial (OAT) showed that a strategy of routine PCI for total occlusion of the infarct-related artery 3 to 28 days after acute MI did not reduce the occurrence of a death, reinfarction, or NYHA class IV heart failure. Rather, there was a trend to increased reinfarction rates in the intervention group at 4-year follow-up (1.16; 95% CI 0.92–1.45; $p = 0.20$) [45]. In addition to these findings, the TOSCA 2 trial documented a lack of benefit of PCI regarding improvement of LV ejection fraction in a similar patient group [46].
- A recent meta-analysis of clinical trials comparing PCI versus optimized medical therapy (OMT) in patients with stable CAD concluded that there was a 12% increase in the RR of cardiac death or MI associated with PCIs, as well as a 22% increase in the RR of non-fatal MI. Cumulative analysis favoured OMT over PCIs as early as 1997, but recent studies such as the AVERT study and the COURAGE study have increased confidence in this finding [47]. Nonetheless, future clinical studies and registries will have to confirm the validity and generalizability of these results from highly selected patient cohorts.

The growing evidence in favour of OMT in stable patients with CAD supports the basic concept of CR that it is more important to influence the course of the underlying atherosclerotic disease than to treat a single symptomatic coronary stenosis by PCI (➲Figs. 25.8 and 25.9). The understanding of how both OMT and physical activity influence the endothelium and the plaque development has provided a firm pathophysiological framework to understand and to apply CR strategies in these patients most effectively.

In stable CAD, exercise therapy has long been used for rehabilitation purposes following an acute MI. A Cochrane meta-analysis revealed a significant 27% reduction of total mortality among training patients and a significant 31% reduction in cardiac mortality (➲Figs. 25.10 and 25.11) [3]. Four mechanisms are considered important mediators of the reduced cardiac event rate: improvement of endothelial function; reduced progression of coronary lesions; reduced

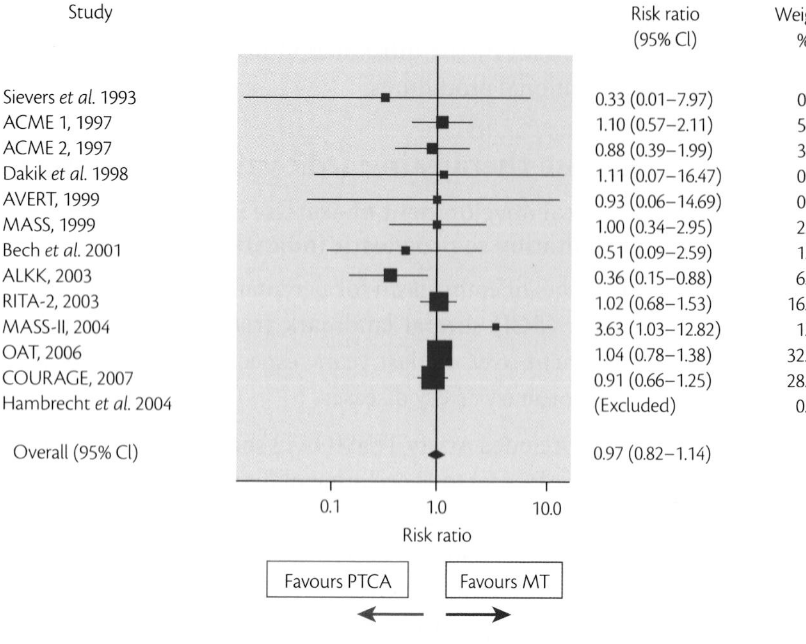

Figure 25.8 Effects on mortality. As indicated by a recent meta-analysis interventional therapy of stable CAD does not confer a survival benefit as compared to optimal medical therapy including secondary prevention with statin-lowering and platelet aggregation inhibitors. Reproduced with permission from Cecil WT, Kasteridis P, Barnes JW, Jr, *et al.* A meta-analysis update: percutaneous coronary interventions. *Am J Manag Care* 2008; **14**: 521–8.

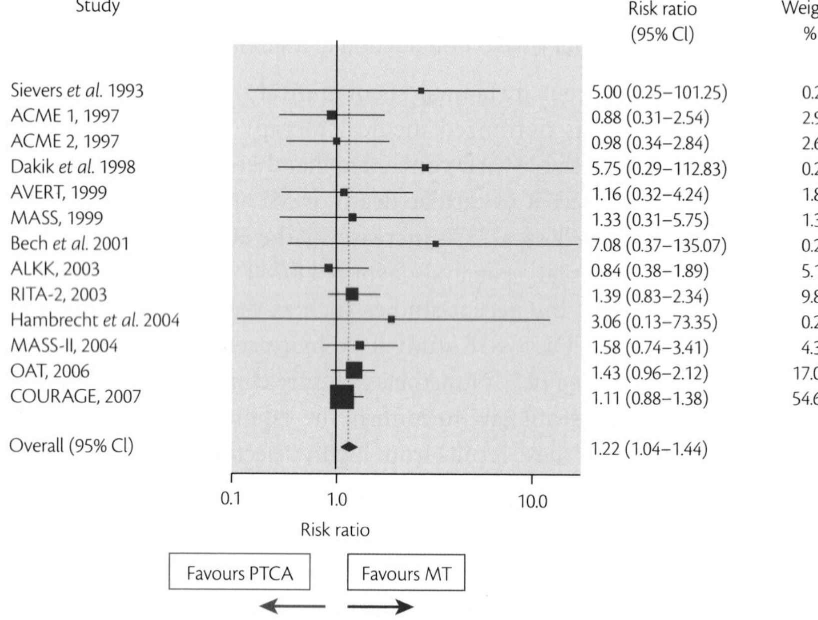

Figure 25.9 Effects on non-fatal myocardial infarction. In the same meta-analysis as in Fig. 25.8, a trend towards lower rates of non-fatal myocardial infarction was evident in the optimal medical therapy group. Keeping in mind that coronary interventions have only symptomatic effects in stable CAD, these data should encourage a more judicious use of percutaneous coronary interventions in stable CAD patients. Reproduced with permission from Cecil WT, Kasteridis P, Barnes JW, Jr, *et al.* A meta-analysis update: percutaneous coronary interventions. *Am J Manag Care* 2008; **14**: 521–8.

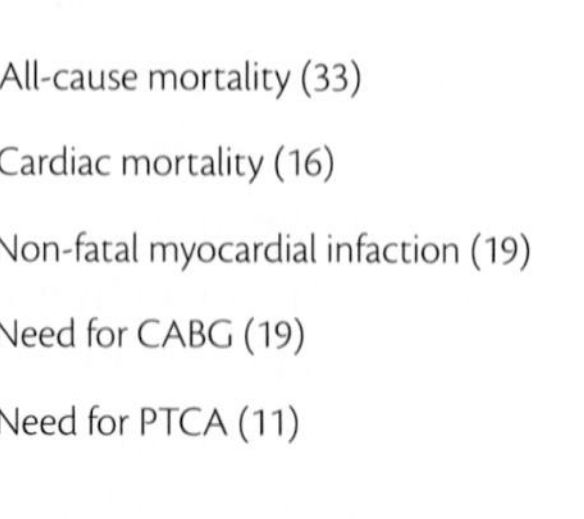

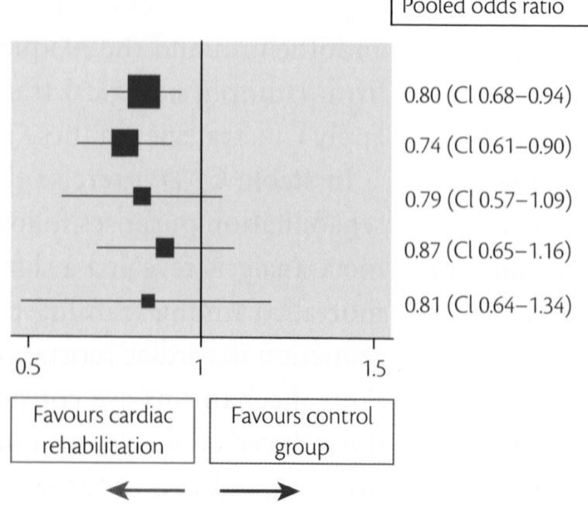

Figure 25.10 The evidence-base for cardiac rehabilitation is strengthened by a recent meta-analysis showing a reduction of clinical event in patients with coronary artery disease. Modified with permission from Taylor RS, Brown A, Ebrahim S, *et al.* Exercise-based rehabilitation for patients with coronary heart disease: systematic review and meta-analysis of randomized controlled trials. *Am J Med* 2004; **116**: 682–92.

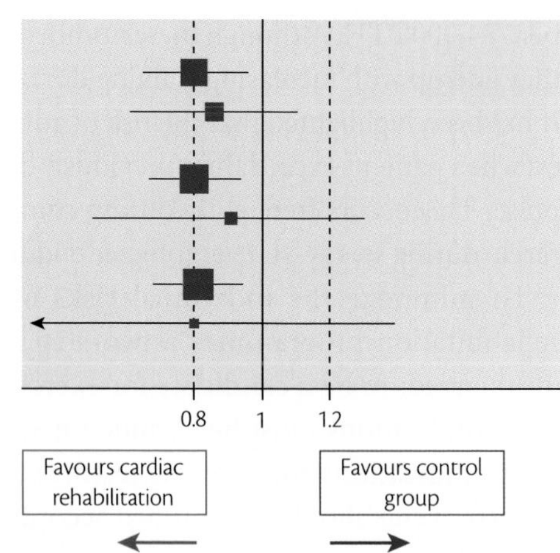

Figure 25.11 Subgroup analyses reveal that the benefit of cardiac rehabilitation is somewhat diminished in women and patients without previous MI (i.e. lower risk CAD patients). Importantly, older patients >60 years seem to benefit to a similar degree from CR as compared to those <60 years. Modified with permission from Taylor RS, Brown A, Ebrahim S *et al.* Exercise-based rehabilitation for patients with coronary heart disease: systematic review and meta-analysis of randomized controlled trials. *Am J Med* 2004; **116**: 682–92.

thrombogenic risk; and improved collateralization. The therapeutic benefit of regular physical exercise has also been confirmed in direct comparison with an interventional strategy: A 12-month exercise therapy in stable CAD patients was associated with a higher event-free survival as compared to conventional PCI (➲Fig. 25.12) [48] These results remain significant in favour of exercise training for up to 5 years' follow-up.

Over the last two decades the clinical application of physical exercise as a therapeutic strategy has evolved from rehabilitation to exercise treatment of cardiovascular diseases. This shift in clinical application was accompanied by a more systematic research approach of the involved mechanisms and the objective clinical assessment of sport

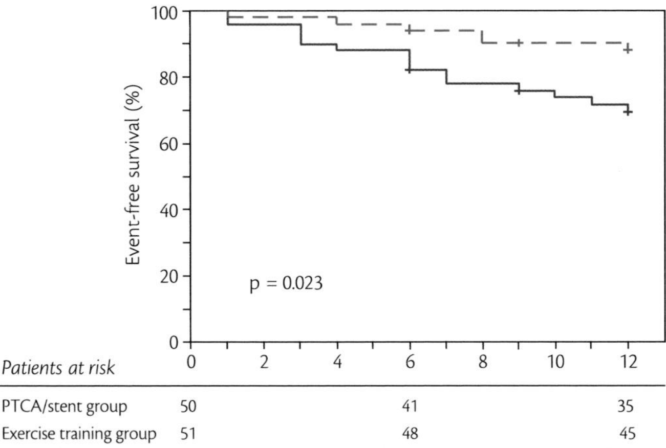

Figure 25.12 In a prospective clinical trial Hambrecht *et al.* [48] compared the event-free survival in patients with stable angina and a significant coronary stenosis randomized to either percutaneous coronary intervention or 12 months of exercise training. Event-free survival after 12 months was significantly superior in the exercise training group versus the PTCA/stent group (p = 0.023 by log rank test). Reproduced with permission from Hambrecht R, Walther C, Mobius-Winkler S, *et al.* Percutaneous coronary angioplasty compared with exercise training in patients with stable coronary artery disease: a randomized trial. *Circulation* 2004; **109**: 1371–8.

interventions using prospective randomized clinical trials. This ongoing process established physical exercise as an evidence-based and guideline-oriented treatment option.

In stable CHF physical activity was traditionally discouraged—with negative consequences for the patients: Exercise intolerance worsened, the progression of disease-related muscular atrophy accelerated. A carefully-designed exercise programme at 50–70% of the maximal oxygen uptake was effective in improving exercise capacity by 12–32%. In a recent meta-analysis exercise therapy reduced the RR of CHF-mortality by 35% and CHF-related hospitalizations by 28% [49].

Exercise therapy in stable CAD, after percutaneous transluminal coronary angioplasty, and after MI with preserved ejection fraction

Exercise interventions differ with regard to several aspects:

- **Location**: in-hospital versus outpatient;
- **Supervision**: supervised versus non-supervised;
- **Training form**: endurance versus resistance; steady state versus interval training.

The diversity has brought with it the necessity to decide which training programme is best suited for the individual patient. The aims of CR in patients with recent MI or with stable CAD are to improve the patients angina-free functional capacity and quality of life (symptomatic goals), and to prevent future cardivascular events (prognostic goal). To separate the patients concerned from those with heart failure, CAD patients should have a LV ejection fraction >40%.

Indications/contraindications

Starting a training programme in patients with overt CAD is not risk-free: Based on large clinical databases one can expect one cardiac arrest per 112,000 patients training hours (PTH), one MI per 294,000 PTH, and one cardiac death per 784,000 PTH. Although these numbers appear to be small they add up with increasing training duration and frequency. It has been highlighted that the risk of adverse events is highest when patients exceed their previously determined training pulse. This occurs frequently during competitive games and rarely during steady-state ergometer endurance training.

To minimize the individual risks of participating in rehabilitation programmes a two-step assessment is recommended: to be a candidate for exercise training certain contraindications must be excluded first (in parallel to the contraindications for exercise testing). Then the risk for adverse events should be stratified according to the patient's medical history and functional parameters (➲Figs. 25.13 and 25.14). While both low- and high-risk patients may participate in training programmes the degree of supervision and monitoring which is required will be different.

Initiation of training therapy

Based on the risk stratification, different baseline assessments are required for patients entering an exercise-based rehabilitation programme. For most patients (low to moderate risk) history, clinical examination, resting ECG, and a reliable exercise test (ergometry with 3-lead ECG, 6-min walk test) are adequate. Complete exercise testing with 12-lead ECG and baseline echocardiography are recommended for high risk patients or high intensity exercise training.

With regard to the type of exercise, submaximal strictly aerobic endurance training at 50–80% of the peak oxygen uptake is generally regarded as the gold standard. The prognostic benefits described in the earlier section 'Indications/contraindications' are only established for endurance type training programmes. Recently, resistance training is increasingly applied as an additional training modality. It appears to be safe in low-risk populations but further studies are necessary to determine the risk:benefit ratio in moderate to high-risk patients.

Among four studies comparing high intensity and moderate–low intensity exercise, three found no difference in mortality, morbidity, physical, and psychological outcomes. Therefore, aerobic moderate intensity exercise training is recommended in patients with CAD. Based on

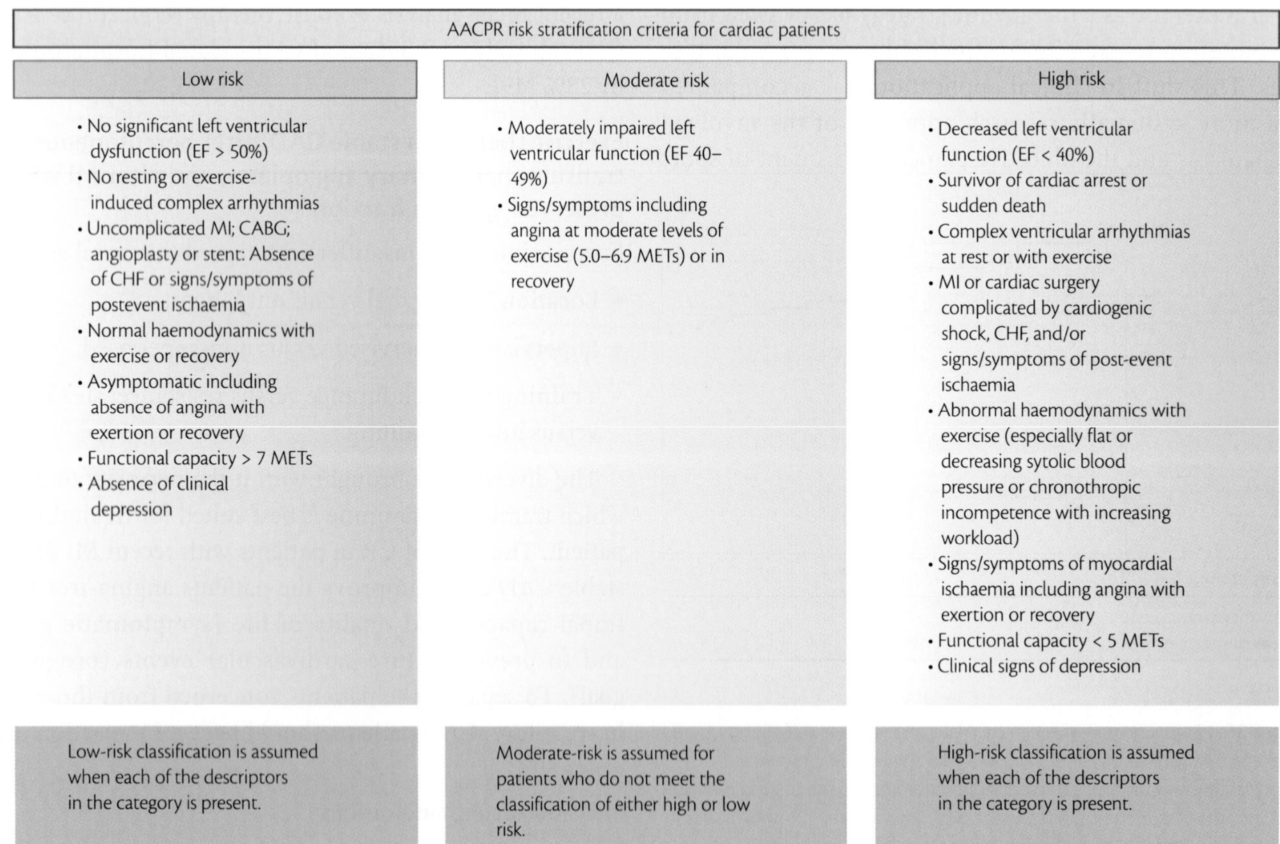

Figure 25.13 Several models for risk stratification of patients scheduled for exercise-based CR been proposed. The Risk Stratification Criteria of the American Association for Cardiopulmonary Rehabilitation (AACPR) distinguish three risk groups based on the degree of left ventricular dysfunction, exercise-induced symptoms, and the presence of ventricular arrhythmias. Modified with permission from *AACPR, Guidelines*, 3rd edn, 1999. Champaign, IL: Human Kinetics, 1999.

Risk class A (healthy persons)

1. Children, adolescents, males under the age of 45, women under the age of 55 without cardiac symptoms or without known heart disease or without any main risk factors (smoking, diabetes, hypertension, high cholesterol) for CAD
2. Males over 45 and women over 55 without cardiac symptoms or without known heart disease and less than two main risk factors
3. Males younger than 45 and women younger than 55 without cardiac symptoms or without known heart disease and with two or more than two main risk factors

Risk class B (stable cardiovascular disease, low risk for complications during severe physical stress)

1. Patients with CAD (myocardial infarction, PTCA, bypass-operation, pathological stress test, and coronary angiogram) in a stable condition and clinically characterized as stated below
2. Patients with valvular disease (severe stenosis or regurgitation ruled out) clinically characterized as stated below (congenital heart disease necessitates a special individual evaluation)
3. Patients with a cardiomyopathy (EF ≥30%) with stable CHF (except HCM or recent myocarditis <6 months)
4. Patients with a pathological stress test that is not classified as class C

Clinical characterization includes all the following points:

1. NYHA-Class I or II
2. Performance capacity ≥6METS/ ≥ 1.4W/kg body weight
3. No clinical signs of heart failure
4. No signs of myocardial ischaemia or angina pectoris either at rest or in a stress test at ≤6 METS/ ≤ 1.4W/kg body weight
5. Adequate rise in blood pressure during exercise
6. No ventricular tachycardia at rest or during exercise
7. Ability for self-appraisal with respect to stress intensity

Risk class C (moderate to high risk for cardiac complications during physical stress and/or inability for self-appraisal/self-adjustment with respect to the level of physical activity)

1. to 3. As in Class B, at 3. EF <30%

4. With complex ventricular arrhythmias refractory to therapy

Clinical characterization by one of the following points:

1. NYHA-Class III
2. Stress test results:
   - Performance capacity <6METS/<1.4Wkg body weight
   - Angina pectoris or signs of ischaemia during exercise <6 METS/<1.4W/kg body weight
   - A fall in systolic blood pressure during exercise
   - Non-sustained ventricular tachycardia during exercise
3. One episode of primary sudden death already survived (i.e. not during a myocardial infarction or a cardiac intervention)
4. A medical problem that a treating physician has classified as potentially life threatening

Risk class D (unstable patients; physical activity for training contraindicated)

1. Patients with unstable angina pectoris
2. Severe and symptomatic valvular stenosis or regurgitation (congenital heart disease necessitates a special individual evaluation)
3. Signs of heart failure, especial NYHA class IV
4. Arrhythmias refractory to therapy
5. Other clinical entities that worsen during exercise

Figure 25.14 A risk stratification scheme proposed by the American Heart Association (AHA) proposes four risk classes based on the presence of risk factors, overt coronary artery disease, valvular heart disease, reduced left ventricular ejection fraction, and ventricular arrhythmias. Modified with permission from Fletcher GF, Balady GJ, Amsterdam EA *et al.* Exercise standards for testing and training: a statement for healthcare professionals from the American Heart Association. *Circulation* 2001; **104**: 1694–740.

published studies, three to four moderate intensity exercise training sessions per week, with a duration of 30–40min each, are necessary to obtain optimal results in phase 3.

Clinical effects of exercise in CAD

Based on large meta-analyses, exercise-based CR is associated with a 27% reduction in total mortality and 31% reduction in cardiac mortality. On the symptomatic level, training interventions led to significant improvements of maximal exercise capacity and muscle strength, and increases the angina pectoris threshold.

The beneficial effect of exercise-only interventions on psychological functioning and social adaptation is less well documented but has been confirmed by observational studies. A number of clinical trials have documented an increased return to work among participants of standard comprehensive rehabilitation programmes [50, 51]; however, the efficacy is disputed [52]. Therefore, new training programmes, which simulate elements of work, were developed and seem to have a certain potential for improving return to work in cardiac patients [53, 54].

Molecular mechanisms of exercise therapy in CAD

The mechanisms responsible for mediating the beneficial effects of training in CAD can be found on different levels: modification of established risk factors; neurohormonal effects; and molecular vascular mechanisms of improved vasomotor function and regional perfusion.

Modification of established risk factors

The majority of atherosclerotic cardiovascular diseases are caused by the unhealthy sedentary lifestyle in the developed world, with food abundance and physical inactivity. As a consequence of the mismatch between our genetic background as hunter-gatherers in an environment characterized by food scarcity which required continuous activities for survival and today's lifestyle, a large proportion of the population develop diseases or conditions known as cardiovascular risk factors: hypertension, glucose intolerance and diabetes mellitus, obesity, hyperlipidaemia and others.

All of these are, to a large degree, the consequences of physical inactivity and hence are beneficially influenced by exercise training. In a meta-analysis of endurance training involving 72 trials and 105 study groups, Fagard described training-induced significant net reductions of resting and daytime ambulatory blood pressure of 3.0/2.4mmHg and 3.3/3.5mmHg, respectively. The reduction of resting blood pressure was more pronounced in the 30 hypertensive study groups (–6.9/–4.9) than in the others (–1.9/–1.6).

In this meta-analysis bodyweight decreased by 1.2kg, waist circumference by 2.8cm, percentage body fat by 1.4% and the homeostatic model assessment (HOMA) index of insulin resistance by 0.31 units. High-density lipoprotein-cholesterol increased by 0.032mmol/L [55]. Resistance training has been less well studied. A meta-analysis of nine randomized controlled trials (12 study groups) on mostly dynamic resistance training revealed a weighted net reduction of diastolic blood pressure of 3.5mmHg associated with exercise and a non-significant reduction of systolic blood pressure of 3.2mmHg [55].

Neurohormonal effects

Regular endurance training leads to a reduction in sympathicoadrenergic tone and to a concomitant increase in vagal tone at rest. These changes in the autonomic nerve system have a number of beneficial effects on the cardiovascular system: the reduced resting heart rate leads to a reduced myocardial oxygen demand and to a longer myocardial perfusion time as a result of the increase in diastolic duration. The ventricular fibrillation threshold is reduced as a consequence of lower circulating catecholamine levels. In addition, a given workload can be achieved with a lower heart rate and blood pressure after the training-associated recalibration of the autonomic balance.

With regard to the renin–angiotensin–aldosterone system a beneficial training effect on plasma renin activity with reductions as high as 20% was documented [55].

Molecular vascular mechanisms of improved vasomotor function and regional perfusion

Basically, regional myocardial hypoperfusion in CAD results from a combination of several pathogenetic components: vascular stenosis, endothelial dysfunction, and microrheology/ haemostasis. All three components may be affected by exercise training in stable CAD.

- **Vascular stenosis**: the initial hypothesis that training would lead to a regression of coronary artery stenosis was not substantiated in the majority of patients. Only those with vigorous training programmes were able to actually reverse the process of atherosclerosis. However, training was effective in retarding disease progression.
- **Endothelial dysfunction**: with increasing knowledge about the importance of vascular endothelial dysfunction as an obligatory step for the initiation of atherosclerosis interactions between training, shear stress, and vascular function have received growing attention. Hambrecht was able to show that 4 weeks of training improved coronary vasomotion in patients with stable CAD [56] (➲Fig. 25.15) and were associated with increased expression and activity of the endothelial NO synthase in samples of the left internal mammary artery harvested during bypass surgery. Because of the documented prognostic significance of endothelial dysfunction for occurrence of cardiovascular events the improvement of endothelium-dependent vasodilation after exercise may represent an important mechanism contributing to the prognostic benefits of training (➲Fig. 25.16).

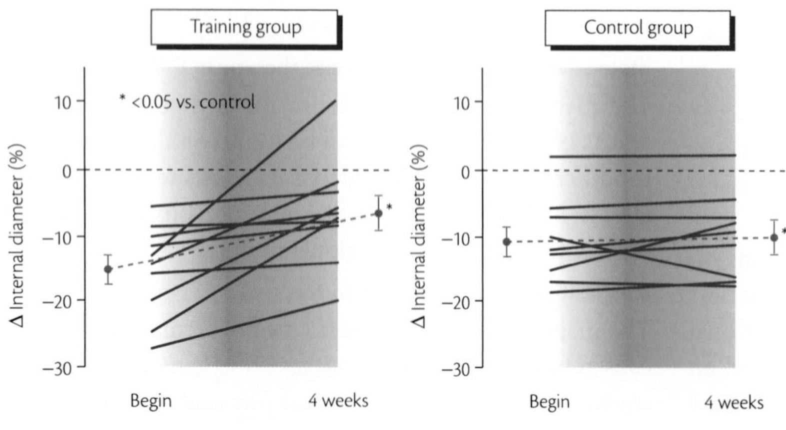

Figure 25.15 Four weeks of exercise training were associated with a significant attenuation of pathologic vasoconstriction in patients with stable coronary artery disease. This finding confirmed the beneficial effect of training on coronary endothelial function and myocardial perfusion. Reproduced with permission from Hambrecht R, Wolff A, Gielen S *et al.* Effect of exercise on coronary endothelial function in patients with coronary artery disease. *N Engl J Med* 2000; **342**: 454–60.

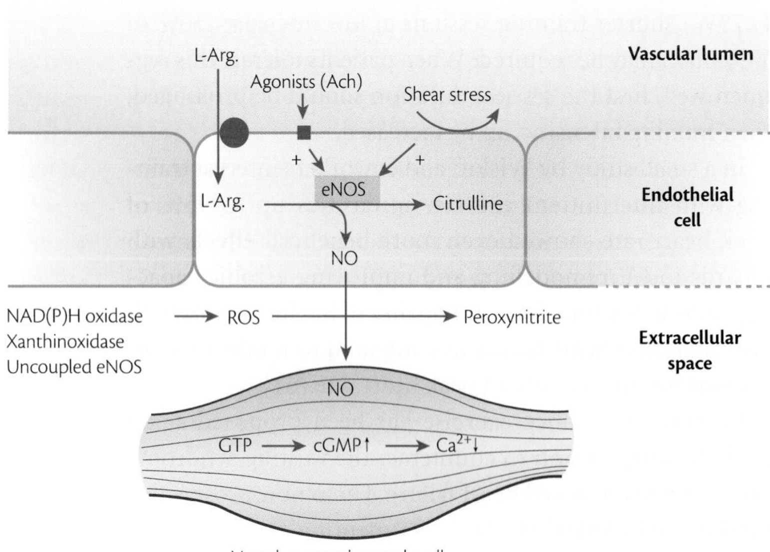

Figure 25.16 Intact vascular endothelial function depends on several steps ultimately leading to the generation of the vasodilatory mediator nitric oxide (NO) in the endothelium: L-arginine, the precursor molecule of NO, is actively transported into the endothelial cell and may be stored in intracellular vesicles until used as a substrate by the key enzyme of NO production: the endothelial nitric oxide synthase (eNOS). This enzyme can be activated by phosphorylation in response to agonists like acetylcholine or to mechanical stimuli such as laminar shear stress. NO reaches the vascular smooth muscle cell by diffusion. However, on this way it may be degraded by reactive oxygen species produced by endothelial enzyme systems e.g. the NAD(P)H oxidases, xanthinoxidases, or uncoupled eNOS, which converts molecular oxygen to ROS in the absence of the cofactor tetrahydrobiopterin. In the vascular smooth muscle cell NO leads to activation of the guanylatcyclase with increased cGMP production. This reduces intracellular calcium concentration and induces the smooth muscle cell relaxation.

- **Microvascular function**: exercise training increases resistance vessel sensitivity and maximal responsiveness to adenosine. Long-term exercise training induces not only functional but also morphologic changes of the microvasculature by increasing the total vascular bed cross sectional area by up to 37% after 16 weeks. As a consequence, vascular resistance decreases and maximal flow reserve rises. In recent years it has been demonstrated that exercise training mobilizes endothelial progenitor cells from the bone marrow, which integrate and home into areas of diseased endothelium (thereby improving endothelial function) or to form entirely new vessels in a process called angiogenesis [57, 58].
- **Blood viscosity**: chronic endurance training has been shown to attenuate the post-exercise potentiation of platelet function, to increase platelet cGMP content, and to suppress coagulability. In summary, a net reduction of thrombogenic risk in CAD by chronic exercise training has been documented. Improvements of blood rheology by reduced viscosity add to these beneficial training effects.

Exercise therapy and chronic heart failure

Any form of strenuous exercise was traditionally discouraged in CHF—a consequence of the concern that any extra haemodynamic workload would lead to further deterioration of cardiac function. However, this concept was shattered by the lack of any correlation between LV function and exercise capacity in CHF patients. In the 1990s it became increasingly clear that peripheral factors potentially amenable to exercise therapy contribute to exercise intolerance: peripheral hypoperfusion due to impaired endothelium-dependent vasodilation, reduced strength of respiratory muscles, and profound morphologic, metabolic, and functional alterations in the skeletal muscles.

Indications/contraindications

Patients with CHF have higher mortality and morbidity rates as compared to most other forms of heart disease (especially stable CAD). Therefore, current guidelines stratify CHF patients as a high-risk group for training interventions. As indicated earlier this implies a more detailed diagnostic evaluation before initiation of exercise training which includes echocardiography and a 12-lead ergometry.

In prospectively conducted exercise training studies in stable CHF patients, adverse events are, however, surprisingly low with postexercise hypotension, atrial or ventricular arrhythmias, and worsening heart failure symptoms being the most common complications.

The same contraindications to exercise as in CAD are also applicable for CHF. Although the risk of patients with ventricular arrhythmias during training interventions has never been prospectively evaluated most studies excluded patients with evidence of ventricular arrhythmias (>Lown grade IV during Holter ECG). Training post ICD implantation appears to be safe and feasible [59, 60].

Although vigorous uncontrolled exercise may precipitate cardiac decompensation in CHF patients there are no reports of an increased rate of pulmonary oedema in long-term submaximal training trials in stable CHF patients.

Initiation of training therapy

Training interventions in CHF are based on aerobic steady state exercise sessions at 50–80% of the peak oxygen uptake for 15–30min, 3–5 times per week. In highly symptomatic patients with very low symptom-free exercise tolerance (<75W) shorter training sessions at low intensity (50% of VO_2 max) may be required. When patients tolerate this regimen well, first the session duration should be prolonged, then training intensity can be increased.

In a small study by Wisloff and coworkers interval training with intermittent exercise intensities up to 95% of peak heart rate showed even more beneficial effects with regards to LV remodelling and improving aerobic capacity, endothelial function, and quality of life in patients with postinfarction heart failure as compared to moderate continuous training at 70% of peak heart rate [61].

Recently, resistance exercise has been proposed as an anabolic intervention to counteract the wasting syndrome often seen in advanced heart failure. Up to now prospective randomized clinical studies documenting the safety and efficacy of resistance training in advanced CHF are missing. Based on observational studies, single-limb short-term resistance exercise seems to be safe.

Clinical effects of exercise in chronic heart failure

The results of the EXTRA-MATCH meta-analysis of the ESC with a total of 801 CHF patients documented a significant reduction of total mortality by 35% (odds ratio 0.65; CI 0.46–0.92, p = 0.015), and of hospitalization by 28% (odds ratio 0.72; CI 0.56–0.93, p = 0.018; ➲Fig. 25.17) [49]. These favourable results stimulated the initiation of a prospective randomized controlled multicentre trial on the efficacy and safety of exercise training as a treatment modality in patients with CHF with the primary endpoint of all-cause mortality or hospitalization at 2 years' follow-up. The HF-ACTION study enrolled a total of 2331 patients who were randomized to either 120min of endurance exercise training or usual care. In the HF-ACTION trial the reduction of mortality and hospitalization did not quite reach significant levels (➲Figs. 25.18–25.20), most likely as a result of the poor adherence to the prescribed training intensity in this unsupervised protocol: After the first year average training duration declined to about 50min/week, less than half of the prescribed training duration [62]. In light of these data, exercise training is safe to perform in CHF patients; however, its efficacy clearly depends on compliance with the prescribed training protocol.

With regard to symptomatic benefit, a recent meta-analysis of randomized controlled trials by the European Heart

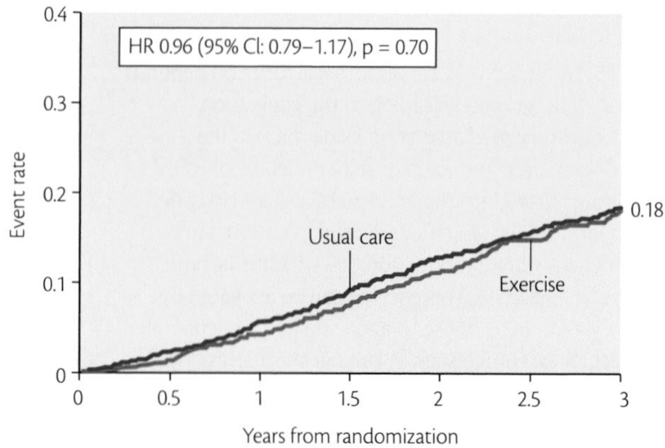

Figure 25.18 All cause mortality was not significantly reduced by the 2-year training intervention in patients with stable CHF according to data from the HF-ACTION study. Reproduced with permission from O'Connor CM, Whellan DJ, Lee KL, *et al.* Efficacy and safety of exercise training in patients with chronic heart failure. HF-ACTION randomized controlled trial. *JAMA* 2009; **301**: 1439–50.

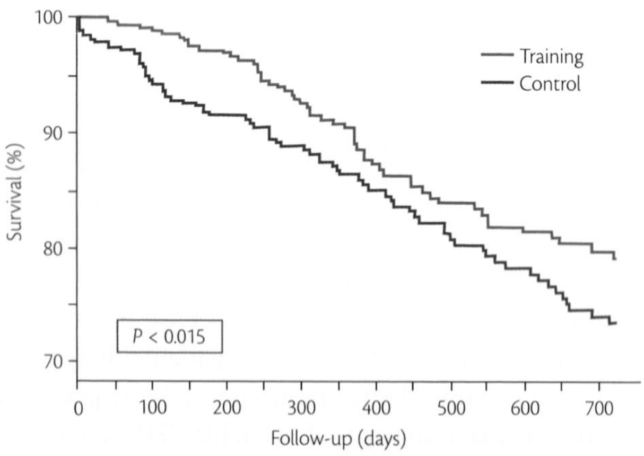

Figure 25.17 In a meta-analysis [49] of 801 CHF patients randomized to either training or control group long-term follow up was obtained and a significant mortality reduction could be documented in the intervention group. Reproduced with permission from Piepoli MF, Davos C, Francis DP, *et al.* Exercise training meta-analysis of trials in patients with chronic heart failure (ExTraMATCH). *BMJ* 2004; **328**: 189.

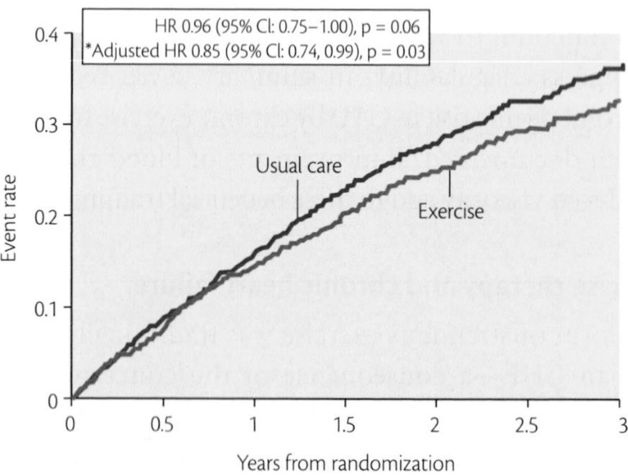

Figure 25.19 For the secondary end-point of cardiovascular mortality or heart failure-related hospitalization the HF-ACTION study [62] showed a modest 15% risk reduction in the exercise group according to the adjusted hazard ratio. This difference was statistically significant. Reproduced with permission from O'Connor CM, Whellan DJ, Lee KL, *et al.* Efficacy and safety of exercise training in patients with chronic heart failure. HF-ACTION randomized controlled trial. *JAMA* 2009; **301**: 1439–50.

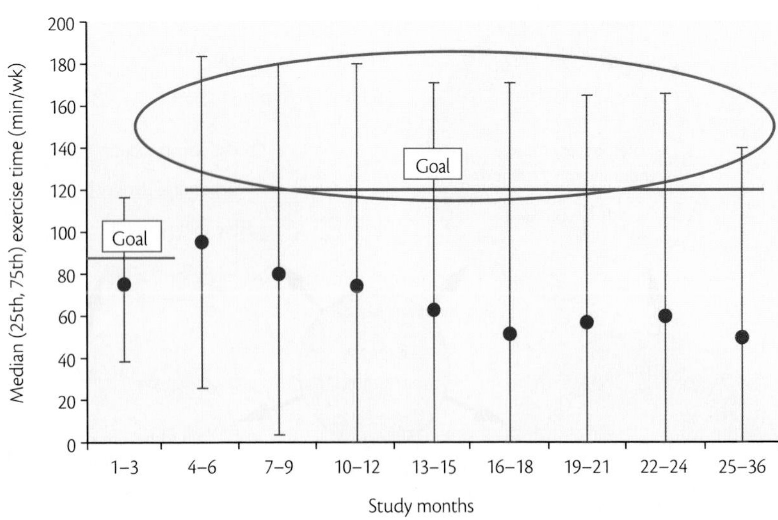

Figure 25.20 HF-ACTION Study, Adherence to training protocol. The disappointing result that the primary endpoint of reduced all cause mortality or hospitalization was not met by the HF-ACTION [62] study is most likely due to a poor training programme adherence over the 2-year period: after 1 year <60% of patients reached the prescribed exercise duration of 90min per week. Even the target duration of endurance training per week was significantly less than in most of the studies included in the Piepoli meta-analysis. Reproduced with permission from Whellan DJ, O'Connor CM. Efficacy and safety of exercise training as a treatment modality in patients with chronic heart failure: results of a randomised controlled trial investigating outcomes of exercise training (HF-ACTION). Presentation at the AHA Scientific Sessions, 2008.

Failure Training Group revealed an improvement of peak VO_2 by up to 2mL/kg.min^{-1} with a range of +14 to +31% increase versus control patients. Although modest in absolute terms this increase of about 20% translates into a considerably better quality of life for most patients.

Cardiac function is not worsened by exercise training; rather there was a small but significant improvement of ejection fraction and reduction in cardiomegaly observed in one prospective randomized trial (➲Fig. 25.21) [63].

With increasing experience in CR of heart failure patients the programmes have been expanded to include patients with ICDs, and patients in advanced stages of CHF at NYHA stage III [64]. At the same time more vigorous training programmes were tested for efficacy in heart failure involving interval training and resistance training [61]. No increased rates of adverse events were reported for these interventions.

Molecular mechanisms of exercise therapy in CHF

How does exercise training in stable CHF achieve these beneficial results? Training is a non-specific intervention which affects several functional systems: (1) vascular endothelial function; (2) central haemodynamics; (3) the level of neurohumoral activation; (4) the respiratory system; and, of course, (5) skeletal muscle metabolism and function (➲Fig. 25.22).

1 Training improves systemic endothelium-dependent vasodilation especially during exercise in CHF patients [65, 66]. This leads to a reduced cardiac afterload and enhanced peripheral perfusion. In response to a supervised exercise training program, patients with CHF showed increased levels of circulating endothelial progenitor cells which are supposed to be endogenous mediators of vascular regeneration and repair and may partially explain the improvement in endothelial function after training [67].

2 Most likely as a consequence of the afterload reduction a small improvement of cardiac function was observed after a 6-month training programme [63]. So far, no

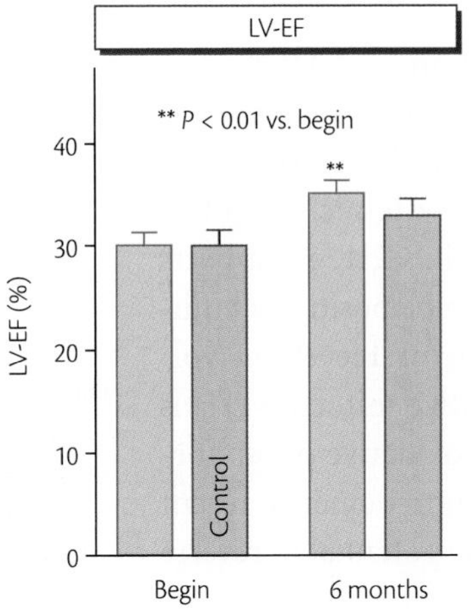

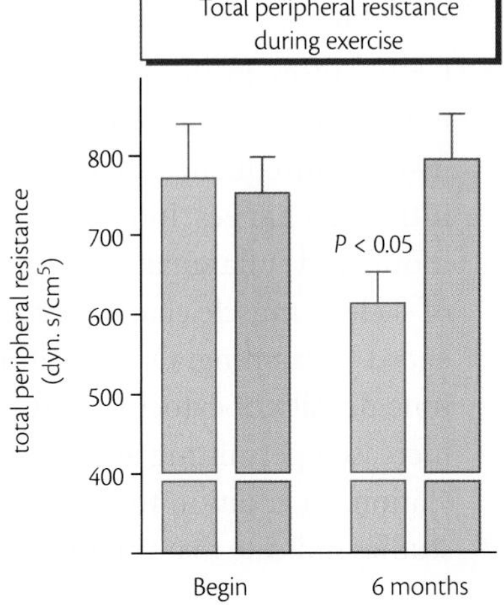

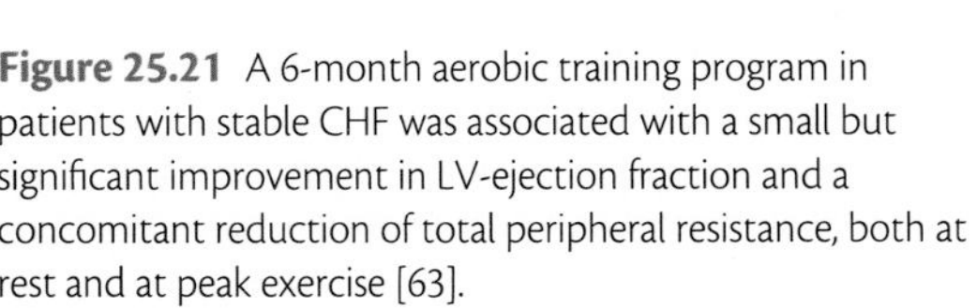
Figure 25.21 A 6-month aerobic training program in patients with stable CHF was associated with a small but significant improvement in LV-ejection fraction and a concomitant reduction of total peripheral resistance, both at rest and at peak exercise [63].

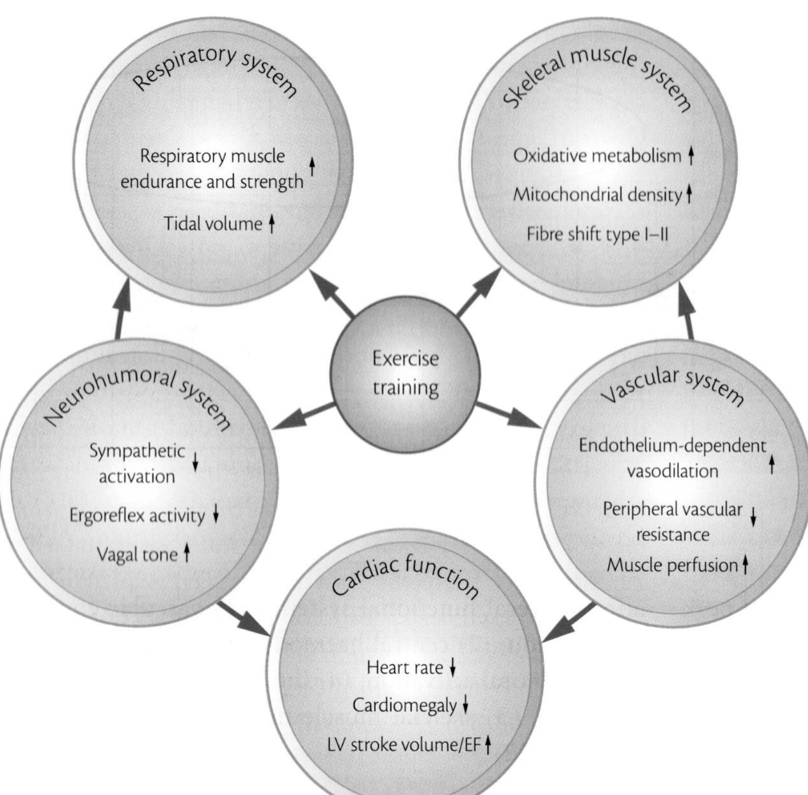

Figure 25.22 Effects of exercise training on different organ systems in CHF. Note that the effects on cardiac function are probably mediated by decreased neurohormonal activation and reduced afterload. Reproduced with permission from Gielen S, Schuler G, Hambrecht R. Benefits of exercise training for patients with chronic heart failure. *Clin Geriatrics* 2001; **9**: 32–45.

direct training-induced cardiac changes have been reported in CHF patients.

3 Training leads to 25–32% reduction in circulating levels of angiotensin II, aldosterone, and atrial natriuretic petide (➲Fig. 25.23) [68].

4 In CHF patients, it has been found that dyspnoea is related to the activity and strength of inspiratory muscles, which are significantly weaker in heart failure patients. Both systemic exercise training and selective respiratory muscle training improve ventilation dynamics and exercise performance. Additionally, oscillatory ventilation which may occur in HF as a pathologic ventilation pattern is significantly improved by endurance training.

5 CHF causes profound alterations in skeletal muscle morphology, metabolism, and function, which are not just a consequence of deconditioning but represent intrinsic changes induced by the systemic neurohumoral and inflammatory response in CHF. All aspects of skeletal muscle characteristics can be positively influenced by training: On the ultrastructural level, the volume density of cytochrome-C positive mitochondria is increased permitting an enhanced oxidative phosphorylation. In addition to metabolic improvements, recent studies indicate that training has the potential to reverse the inflammatory activation with increased expression of cytokines like TNF-alpha, IL-1 beta, and IL-6 in the skeletal muscle [69]. These changes might also attenuate the pro-apoptotic environment with reduced IGF-I in the skeletal muscle [70, 71]. It has become evident that the activated protein catabolism via the ubiquitin–proteasome system can also be attenuated by endurance training.

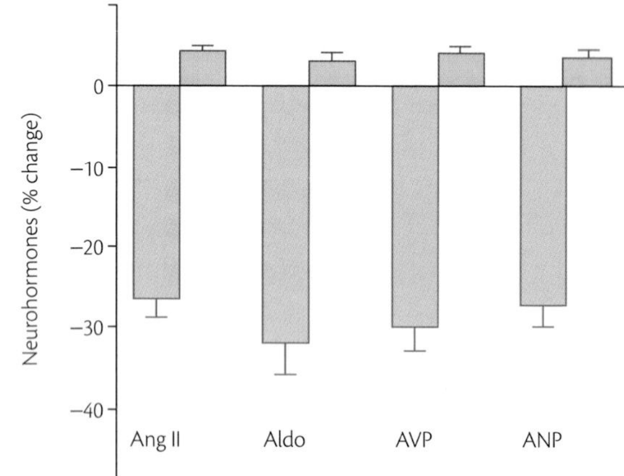

Figure 25.23 Braith and colleagues [68] described dramatic reductions in circulating neurohormones after long-term exercise training in CHF (red boxes, training group; blue boxes, control group, all changes are statistically significant at p <0.05 versus control group). Aldo, aldosterone; Ang II, angiotensin II; AVP, ANP, atrial natriuretic peptide; arginine vasopressin.

Exercise therapy after cardiac surgery

As opposed to the situation in stable CAD/CHF, patients after cardiac surgery are confronted with several additional problems: open chest surgery is frequently associated with reduced ventilatory capacity in the immediate post-operative period; pain during respiration and lifting of the arms; weight reduction due to the catabolism associated with major trauma; and reduction in muscle strength as a consequence of immobilization.

While the objective in CAD/CHF was to improve exercise capacity to levels above baseline levels, CR post cardiac surgery first aims at regaining the pre-surgery levels of physical and social functioning after correction of the exercise-limiting cardiac disorder and at preventing post-operative complications such as pneumonia or deep vein thrombosis. After the completion of wound healing, however, exercise training should be continued to fully recruit the extended cardiovascular exercise capacity.

Indications/contraindications

Limited physical exercise starts immediately after surgery in the form of mobilization on the intensive care unit. In this highly supervised and monitored setting there are very few contraindications to exercise: severe cardiac arrhythmias; overt cardiac decompensation; and paralysis or musculoskeletal disorders prohibiting exercise. Even in the presence of mild acute illnesses, i.e. postoperative infections, supervised mobilization/respiratory training can be continued.

To start with, exercise training indications/contraindications as described in an earlier section need to be observed. Patients should be in stable clinical condition. Risk assessment is according to the low, moderate, and high risk criteria.

Initiation of training therapy

Mobilization including active/passive exercise, respiratory exercise, and walking may start immediately after surgery. Formal exercise training with aerobic endurance exercise may be initiated when wound healing is adequately advanced. To counteract the loss of muscle strength/mass associated with prolonged bed rest resistance exercises may be introduced into the training programme.

Clinical effects of exercise after surgery

Of the three randomized trials of exercise-based CR after bypass surgery none was powered to analyse prognostic benefits of exercise training. However, exercise capacity and maximal oxygen uptake were significantly improved after training while serum lipids remained unchanged.

Although the number of studies is limited, training seems to be particularly beneficial in patients after cardiac transplantation due to the extensive peripheral alterations that persist after transplant if not treated by exercise.

Exercise therapy in patients with rhythm disorders

Pacemaker-dependent patients

In patients in whom the pacemaker activity is not triggered by a spontaneous supraventricular rhythm, different sensors can measure the patient's physical activity level so that the pacemaker can adapt the heart rate accordingly (simulating chronotropic competence). However, some of the sensors may require stimuli which certain training modes do not provide, for example when training a patient with an accelerometer sensor on a stationary bicycle, rate adaptation may be absent as opposed to the same patient training on a treadmill.

CHF patients with ICDs

Heart failure patients with ICDs belong to a subgroup of patients considered to be at a high risk for ventricular arrhythmias and sudden cardiac death. For a long time CR institutions were reluctant to include ICD patients in their training programmes. This was due to the fears that (1) exercise-related increase in heart rate may trigger inadequate shock delivery, and (2) that exercise-induced arrhythmias may be more common among ICD patients as compared to all CHF patients. A large retrospective observational study of 92 ICD patients who participated in a 3-month CR programme at 60–90% of the heart rate reserve 3 × 90min per week confirmed that: (1) only 1/92 patients received an inadequate shock during the training programme, and (2) indeed exercise-related arrhythmias with appropriate ICD intervention were more common in the ICD group (5/92) but without any serious sequelae. The authors concluded that endurance training was both safe and effective in ICD patients when the exercise programme is started under medical supervision for 6 weeks [60].

Exercise therapy in valvular heart disease

As opposed to CAD and CHF only a few studies have specifically evaluated training interventions in patients with valvular heart disease. Therefore, recommendations are necessarily less reliable and are based on pathophysiological considerations rather than on hard clinical evidence.

Indications/contraindications

Clear contraindications to exercise training include all critical and highly symptomatic valvular lesions on the edge to cardiac decompensation. In addition, a stable aortic stenosis with a valvular orifice area $<0.75\text{cm}^2$ and a peak pressure gradient >50mmHg is also generally regarded as a contraindication to training programmes. Specific risks for special valvular lesions include:

- **Mitral valve prolapse**: although considered a benign abnormality occurring in up to 5% in the general population, sudden death has been reported as a rare complication. Exercise is considered safe in patients without significant arrhythmias at rest and during exercise, without a family history of sudden cardiac death, and without any previous thromboembolic event or syncope.
- **Mitral regurgitation**: in patients with CHF, relative mitral regurgitation is frequent and does not preclude the initiation of training therapy provided the patient is in stable condition (NYHA II-III).
- **Mitral stenosis**: patients with a mitral valve orifice >1.5cm^2 may safely participate in normal exercise training sessions. Those with moderate to severe mitral stenosis (<1.5cm^2) are usually limited by exercise-induced dyspnoea and can only tolerate low levels of physical exertion. In these symptomatic patients, treatment of mitral stenosis by balloon valvuloplasty or valve repair replacement should be performed prior to starting a training program.
- **Aortic regurgitation**: patients with mild to moderate aortic regurgitation may engage in training without problems. However, LV diameters need to be reassessed every 3–6 months to watch for worsening of the valve disease.

Initiation of training therapy

In valvular heart disease, changes in afterload or preload associated with changes in peripheral resistance may greatly affect cardiac output. Therefore, resistance training of large muscle groups is generally discouraged in valvular heart disease. Endurance training sessions —preferably with ECG and blood pressure monitoring during the initial phase—are more reproducible with regard to haemodynamic load.

Clinical effects of exercise in valvular heart disease

Among patients with valvular heart disease, no prognostic benefit of exercise training has so far been documented. The symptomatic benefits of training are not well established either and are mostly based on anecdotal rather than systematic reports. It therefore seems prudent to opt for curative surgical treatment of the valvular heart disease wherever possible and start training programmes after the intervention.

Special challenges for exercise therapy

Impact of the demographic change

Over the next decades Europe is facing an unprecedented demographic change: between the years 2010–2030 the number of elderly people aged between 65–79 years will increase by 37.4%; the increase in those aged 80 years and older will reach 57.1% in the same time interval (➲Figs. 25.24 and 25.25). To cope with this challenge strategies need to be developed to avoid disability and to support independent living as long as possible. The number of elderly people as cardiovascular patients will also increase, since diseases such as heart failure and CAD are highly prevalent above the age of 65.

Exercise therapy in the elderly

Among key factors for disability in older people are mental depression, low aerobic fitness levels, low skeletal muscle mass, and presence of orthopaedic comorbidities. Despite these factors the elderly benefit equally from CR; however, they do so from a lower baseline. Evaluation prior to exercise follows the guidelines described in earlier sections. Due to the higher prevalence of heart failure in older patients, a baseline echocardiography is recommended.

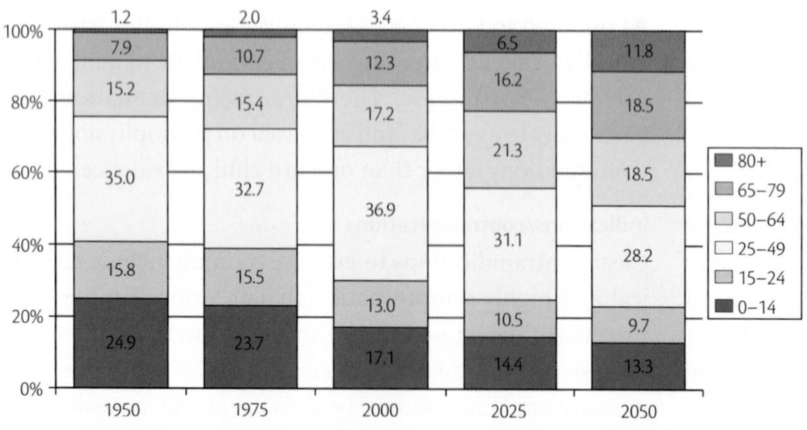

Figure 25.24 This projection of the demographic change for the European Union until the year 2050 published by EuroStat indicates the size of the problem that lies ahead: by 2050 30.3% of the people will be above the age of 65 years—this approximates to one-third of society. Reproduced with permission from Green Paper *Confronting demographic change: a new solidarity between the generations* 2005. Brussels: Commission of the European Communities.

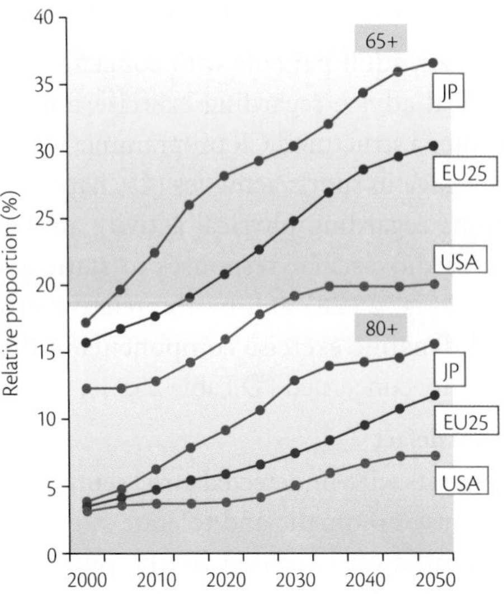

Figure 25.25 Currently, the age groups 65+ and 80+ are the fastest growing age groups in our societies doubling every 25–30 years. Data from EuroStat 2004. Reproduced with permission from Green Paper *Confronting demographic change: a new solidarity between the generations* 2005. Brussels: Commission of the European Communities.

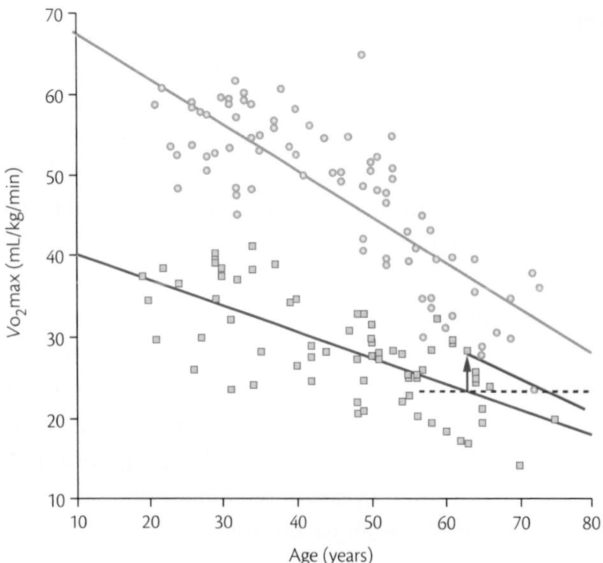

Figure 25.26 In both trained (orange circles) and untrained healthy individuals (red squares) maximal exercise capacity declines by approximately 10% per decade during the ageing process. Although the decline in peak oxygen uptake is steeper in trained individuals their exercise capacity is significantly higher than that of their untrained age-matched counterparts. Exercise interventions increase individual VO_2 max (green arrow). When we consider an exercise capacity equivalent to an oxygen uptake of 22ml/kg min as a prerequisite for leading a self-determined life (dotted green line) an exercise intervention with even minor gains in exercise capacity may significantly prolong a self-determined life (to the point where natural decline in VO_2 max (green line) crosses the dotted blue line). Adapted from Tanaka H, Seals DR. Dynamic exercise performance in Masters athletes: insight into the effects of primary human ageing on physiological functional capacity. *J Appl Physiol* 2003; **95**: 2152–62.

When initiating aerobic exercise the exercise intensity should be carefully weighted against a higher risk of injuries with higher workloads. Even workloads as low as 60–65% of maximal heart rate have documented effects on exercise capacity. To counteract the loss of muscle mass, endurance exercises are often supplemented by moderate intensity resistance training (e.g. elastic bands) with 8–10 set repetitions at 40–60% of the one-repetition maximum.

Over a period of 3 months, 34–53% increases in exercise capacity may be expected by endurance training rehabilitation. The effect of resistance training is similar to the results in younger population with a 35% increase in leg extension strength.

Although more research in this area needs to be done, current evidence suggests that CR in the elderly is cost effective because even small improvements in exercise tolerance and physical coordination may permit maintenance of self-determined living and prevent hospitalization (➲Fig. 25.26).

Impact of the obesity epidemic

Studies in obese patients suggest that exercise-based rehabilitation (optimally combined with diet programmes) is effective in reducing weight, improving exercise capacity, and in normalizing lipid status (low-density lipoprotein (LDL) levels decrease, high-density lipoprotein (HDL) levels increase) [72]. As compared to normal weight rehabilitation participants the gain in exercise capacity was lower in obese patients (+27% versus +39%). This may be a consequence of orthopaedic comorbidities, lower baseline fitness, or greater difficulties in motivation for starting to exercise.

Gender issues in exercise therapy

Despite the advances in cardiac medicine MI in women continues to be associated with higher short- and long-term mortality, reinfarction rates, and development of congestive heart failure within 6 months as compared to men. The 'old view that CAD is a male disease contributes to the gender differences in cardiac morbidity and mortality and also affects participation in rehabilitation programmes. Only approximately 20% of participants in rehabilitation programs are female while women represent close to 40% of patients with acute MI. Women are significantly less likely to be formally informed about rehabilitation interventions and are even more rarely receiving a referral to a rehabilitation institution by their treating physicians [73]. Among plausible reasons for this gender difference are medical aspects (e.g. the higher prevalence of orthopaedic problems such as osteoporosis) and social factors (e.g. lack of own car, caring for husband).

The differences in rehabilitation participation are especially unwelcome since women have more modifiable risk factors than men and are less likely to be physically active.

Exercise therapy in women

The preconditions for exercise are different in men and women: Women have a lower aerobic capacity, a greater proportion of body fat, and smaller muscle cross-sectional areas as compared to men. Nonetheless, women benefit equally as men from exercise-based CR with regard to exercise capacity: an increase in VO_2 max ranging from 15–30% may be expected.

Exercise effects on lipids are less conclusive in women—partially as a consequence of menopausal status: since oestrogen is associated with lower LDL levels hormonal status affects the extent of training-induced LDL-changes. One long-term study, however, revealed a significant 20% increase in HDL after 5 years of rehabilitation [74]. A combination of diet plus exercise training is effective for weight reduction in overweight women (a loss of 5.1kg within 1 year in a prospective controlled trial) [75] (➲Chapter 33).

Congenital heart disease and exercise intolerance

With an estimated prevalence of 0.8% of all live births, the likelihood of encountering patients with congenital heart disease in the context of CR/exercise is higher than expected. In close cooperation with a paediatric cardiologist the evaluation of these patients should focus on the family history (e.g. history of sudden cardiac death, heart failure, deafness, syncope etc.) and on current symptoms.

The degree of exercise intolerance clearly depends on the type of congenital heart disease, on the sequelae on pulmonary circulation, and on the correction by surgical interventions. Patients with Eisenmenger syndrome are usually most intolerant to physical activity, while patients with a corrected tetralogy of Fallot may experience few limitations (➲Fig. 25.27).

Exercise recommendations in congenital heart disease

In most cases, adult patients with congenital heart disease seek medical advice regarding exercise not because they want to enter a structured CR programme, but because they want to engage in sports activities (➲Chapter 10). Recommendations regarding physical activity are based on the different cardiovascular responses to static and dynamic exercise (➲Fig. 25.28) and by the relative proportion of static and dynamic exercise components in the particular sports activity concerned (➲Table 25.11).

Atrial septal defect

Young patients with undetected atrial septal defects (ASDs) are usually asymptomatic and tolerate strenuous activities. Exercise limitation is caused by the pulmonary volume overload and pulmonary hypertension as a consequence of left-to-right shunting. While children will have normal exercise capacities after correction, later repairs in adulthood may leave residual haemodynamic abnormalities (mostly persistent pulmonary hypertension).

Current recommendations indicate that patients with small ASDs without pulmonary hypertension can participate in all sports. If pulmonary hypertension or significant left-to-right shunting is present (Q_p:Q_s>1,5:1), or mean resting pulmonary artery pressure exceeds 20mmHg, only low-intensity sports are permitted. In marked pulmonary hypertension competitive sports need to be discouraged [76].

Ventricular septal defects

Ventricular septal defects (VSDs) are the most common congenital cardiac defects (15–20%). They are grouped into four categories depending on the left-to-right shunt ratio and the pulmonary vascular resistance (PVR). In small defects without haemodynamic significance (normal PVR)

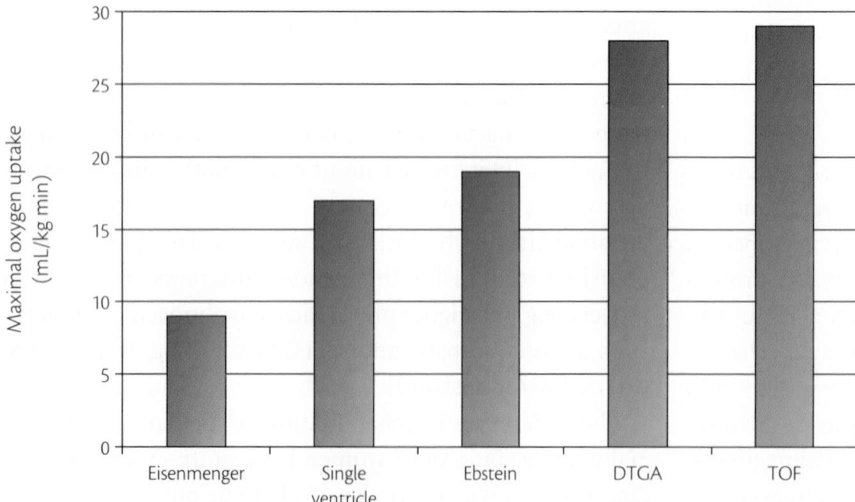

Figure 25.27 Exercise capacity in selected congenital heart defects as measured by cardiopulmonary exercise testing. Please note the large difference between patients affected by fixed pulmonary hypertension and those who are protected from volume overload of the lungs by either surgical correction or the degree of pulmonary stenosis. DTGA, D-transposition of the great arteries; TOF, tetralogy of Fallot. Reproduced with permission from Aboulhosn J, Perloff JK. Exercise and athletics in adults with congenital heart disease. In Perloff JK, Child JS, Aboulhosn J, (eds.) *Congenital heart disease in adults*. 3rd edn., 2009. Philadelphia, PA: Saunders Elsevier, p. 250.

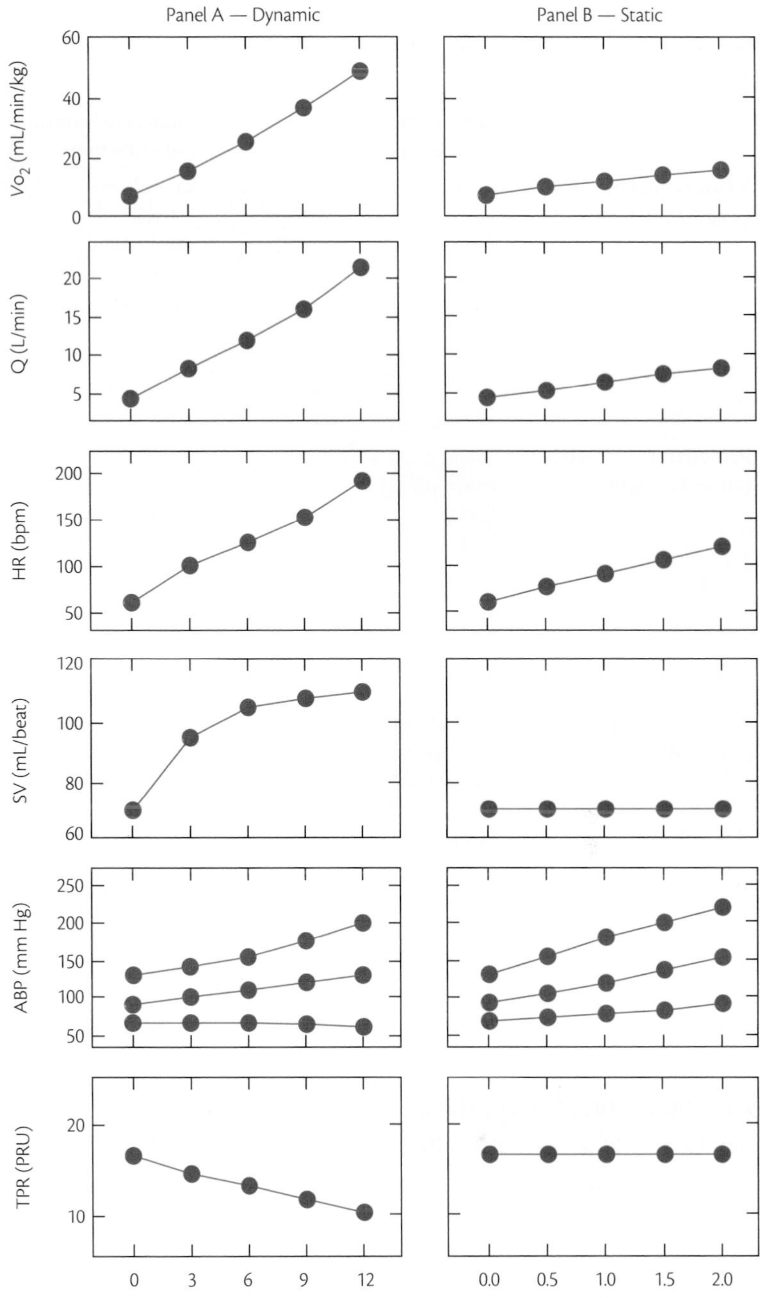

Figure 25.28 This diagram compares the haemodynamic effects of dynamic and static exercises. In dynamic isotonic exercise there is a steady rise in oxygen uptake, cardiac output, heart rate, and stroke volume. These changes are accompanied by a decrease in total peripheral resistance as a result of peripheral vasodilatation to improve muscle perfusion. In static exercise with dominant isometric activities of the peripheral arteries are compressed by muscle contracture. Therefore total peripheral resistance does not increase but remains stable or even shows slight increases. As a result stroke volume and cardiac output showed little changes while arterial blood pressure may show excessive rises. Adapted with permission from Mitchel JH, Raven PB, Cardiovascular adaptations to physical activity. In Bouchard C (ed.) *Physical Activity, Fitness and Health: International Proceedings and Consensus Statement*, 1994. Champain, Il. Human Kinetics.

patients may participate in all sports when ventricular size and function is normal and no pulmonary hypertension is present. Patients with moderately restrictive VSDs may participate in low intensity isotonic sports. Following successful surgical closure (≥6 months post surgery) patients with normal pulmonary pressures, normal ventricular function, and no evidence of arrhythmias during ergometry and Holter ECG may engage in all sports types.

Coarctation of the aorta

The main danger of coarctations of the aorta regarding physical exercise lie in the risk of excessive hypertension in the part of the circulatory bed proximal to the aortic narrowing with stroke, aortic aneurysm, and LV hypertrophy/failure as main complications. Examination should include measurement of blood pressure on all limbs, echocardiography, and chest radiograph. Patients with low gradients (≤20mmHg), normal resting blood pressure, systolic blood pressure during exercise <230mmHg, no aortic aneurysm, and no large collaterals may engage in all sports. Those with >20mmHg gradients, hypertension, systolic blood pressure during exercise >230mmHg, and aortic aneurysm or wall thinning should be restricted to low intensity exercises (≤3METs). After surgical

Table 25.11 Estimates of the proportion of isometric versus isotonic exercise for different activities. See also Tables 12.5 (p. 421) and 32.1 (p. 1216). To give adequate recommendations for sports participation in patients with congenital heart disease, it is advisable to consider the types of sports with more isotonic exercise components for patients with afterload-dependent shunts.

	Low isotonic (<40% max_2)	Moderate isotonic (40–70% max_2)	High isotonic (>70% max_2)
I. Low isometric (<20% MVC)	Billiards Bowling Cricket Golf Riflery	Baseball Softball Table tennis Tennis (doubles) Volleyball	Badminton Cross-Country skiing (classic) Field hockey* Race walking Racquetball Running (long distance) Soccer* Squash Tennis (singles)
II. Moderate isometric (20%–50% MVC)	Archery Auto racing*† Diving*† Equestrian*† Motorcycling*†	Fencing Field events (jumping) Figure skating* Football (American)* Rodeo*† Rugby* Running (sprint) Surfing*† Synchronized swimming†	Basketball* Ice hockey* Cross-country skiing (skating) Football (Australian rules)* Lacrosse* Running (middle distance) Swimming Team handball
III. High isometric (>50% MVC)	Bobsledding*† Field events (throwing) Gymnastics*† Karate/judo*† Sailing*† Rock climbing*† Waterskiing*† Weight lifting*† Windsurfing*†	Body building*† Downhill skiing*† Wrestling	Boxing* Canoeing/kayaking* Cycling*† Decathlon Rowing Speed skating

* Indicates danger of bodily collision, † indicates an increased risk of accidents when syncope occurs. Reproduced with permission from Aboulhosn J, Perloff JK. Exercise and athletics in adults with congenital heart disease. In Perloff JK, Child JS, Aboulhosn J, (eds.) *Congenital heart disease in adults.* 3rd edn., 2009. Philadelphia, PA: Saunders Elsevier, p. 249. Also see Table 12.5, p. 421 and Table 32.1, p. 1216.

correction sports (except static exercise, i.e. weight lifting) may be started ≥6 months after surgery when no residual hypertension at rest and during exercise is present. In patients with residual gradients >20mmHg, aneurysms, or aortic wall thinning only low intensity exercise is recommended.

Tetralogy of Fallot

The physiologic consequences of the tetralogy of Fallot depend to a large degree on the right ventricular outflow tract obstruction and on the systemic vascular resistance (SVR). In unoperated Fallot patients, isotonic exercise leads to a decrease in SVR with increased right-to-left shunting and subsequent central cyanosis. The clinical hallmark for a Fallot in this situation is squatting, which increases pulmonary perfusion by elevating SVR [77] (Chapter 10).

While the increase in SVR may be beneficial, after isotonic exercise isolated isometric exercise can induce a critical rise in SVR with reduced flow from the right ventricle into the aorta. This can lead to syncope and in rare cases even sudden cardiac death. It is therefore recommended that patients with unrepaired Fallot avoid all but low-intensity isometric activities.

The restriction of physical activities after successful repair of the defect depends on the age at operation and the degree of residual right ventricular outflow tract obstruction, and shunting. If these are absent, ventricular size and function are normal, and no exercise-induced arrhythmias are detected no limitations for exercise are imposed [78, 79].

Athlete's heart (Chapter 32)

In athletes competing at very high intensity levels of endurance exercise (>3 hours/week) the cardiac adaptations may lead to morphological changes summarized as 'athlete's heart': LV enlargement; increased stroke volume; LV hypertrophy; increased LV muscle mass (Fig. 25.29) [80]. These morphologic changes are regarded as appropriate compensation for the chronic mild volume overload associated with high-intensity training. However, as compared with normal values established in sedentary people, 45% of athletes exceeded the upper limits for end-diastolic diameter (55mm) in a study of

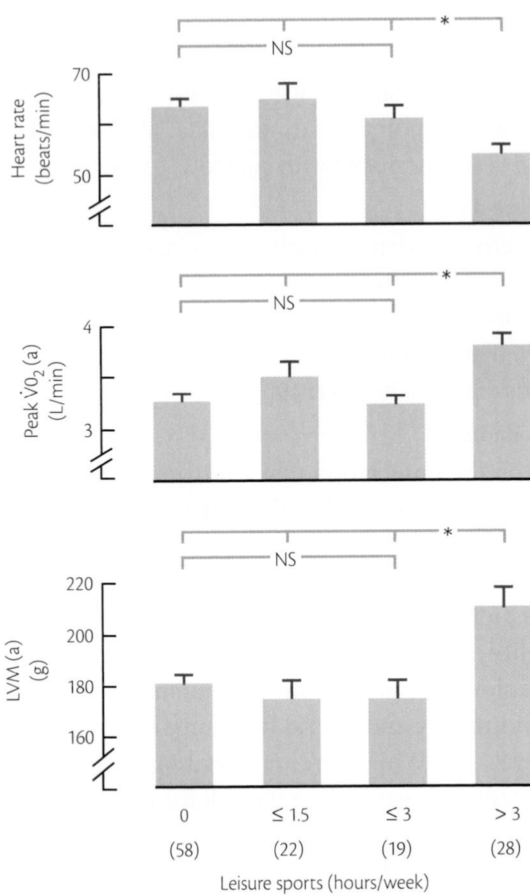

Figure 25.29 Heart rate, peak oxygen uptake, and left ventricular mass in 127 18- to 34-year-old men according to weekly hours of sports activity. An (a) indicates adjustment for height and weight. Reproduced with permission from Fagard R. Athlete's heart. *Heart* 2003; **89**: 1455–61.

1309 athletes [81]. LV systolic function remains normal and diastolic filling is improved with higher peak early diastolic filling velocities.

An association between the type of sport and specific characteristics of cardiac adaptation was first suggested by Morganroth [82]. He found increased LV dimensions without changes in LV wall thickness in endurance athletes, while isometric sports was related to increased wall thickness in the presence of unchanged LV diameter. Follow-up studies in athletes who stopped training suggest that these changes are rapidly reversible with a decrease of 15–33% in LV wall thickness within 1–13 weeks.

The key issue in athlete's heart is the task to distinguish it from structural heart disease (hypertrophic cardiomyopathy, beginning dilated cardiomyopathy, hypertensive heart disease etc.). Thomas suggested the following morphologic upper normal limits for echocardiography in healthy athletes: wall thickness <13mm; septal-to-posterior wall thickness <1.3; LV end-diastolic diameter ≤60mm; LV mass ≤294g in men and ≤198g in women [83].

Comprehensive rehabilitation and risk factor management

Definition

Current clinical guidelines recommend that CR should be integrated in a multifactorial, comprehensive, long-term process that includes clinical assistance and optimized medical or interventional treatment to relieve symptoms, appropriate cardiovascular risk evaluation, exercise training, education and counselling regarding risk reduction, and lifestyle changes including the use of appropriate behavioural interventions and involvement of family members to achieve these changes, vocational counselling, and adequate follow-up, assure long-term compliance and motivation for adherence to recommended lifestyle changes and pharmacological treatments [1, 5, 84, 85].

Patient education on heart disease

The behavioural approach to coronary risk reduction encourages and enables coronary patients to manage their illness, adopt and maintain healthy lifestyles, and improve adherence to medications and other recommended regimens. Meta-analyses of 28 controlled trials of patient education showed that 'education programs have demonstrated a measurable impact on blood pressure, mortality, exercise, [and] diet' and that other parameters are positively affected, although less consistently [86] (➲Chapter 17).

Dietary counselling

Epidemiology of overweight/obesity

In many countries, more than half the adult population is overweight and 20–30% of adults are categorized as clinically obese in Europe, where prevalence has doubled or even risen threefold in less than two decades [87].

Obesity, particularly abdominal obesity, is a substantial risk factor for cardiovascular diseases. In addition, factors such as elevated fasting blood triglycerides, low levels of HDL cholesterol, high fasting blood glucose, and hypertension are accentuated markedly by weight gain.

The driving force behind the obesity epidemic and the consequent widespread metabolic syndrome is a diet dominated by an excess of energy-dense foods, high in fat, sugar (and in addition salt), combined with an insufficient consumption of fruits and vegetables. This dysfunctional diet is compounded by predominantly sedentary lifestyles and reduced opportunities for physical activity.

Overweight and obesity in patients with CHD

Overweight and obesity are highly prevalent among CAD patients [88]. Treating overweight patients poses a real challenge to healthcare professionals because they are more likely to have inadequate blood pressure and cholesterol level control.

Primary prevention of CHD by dietary recommendations

Although the relation between overweight/obesity and CHD is well-established research about the effects of specific dietary habits is often difficult. Based on the discovery that increased serum cholesterol predicted risk of CHD in human populations in the early 1950s, the classic diet–heart hypothesis was developed, which postulated a primary role of dietary saturated fat and cholesterol in the cause of atherosclerosis and CHD in humans [89]. The diet–heart hypothesis gained further support from ecological correlations relating saturated fat intake to rates of CHD in cohorts from different countries and from studies of migrants from low- to high-risk countries [90].

Until recently, most epidemiologic and clinical investigations of diet and CHD have been dominated by the diet–heart hypothesis. However, the original hypothesis was overly simplistic because the effects of diet on CHD can be mediated through multiple biological pathways other than serum total cholesterol or LDL cholesterol.

Experimental research was essential to understand the mechanisms by which genes, hormones, and diet interact to regulate the serum cholesterol level. LDL cholesterol levels can be increased by saturated fatty acids, especially those with 12–16 carbon atoms, and by trans fatty acids.

Mediterranean diet

Common traits of a Mediterranean-style diet are the emphasis on fruits, vegetables, bread, other forms of cereals, potatoes, beans, nuts, seeds, olive oil as an important fat source, and dairy products, fish, and poultry. In addition, wine is consumed in low to moderate amounts. The Mediterranean-style Step I diet used in the Lyon Diet Heart Study was comparable to this pattern but uniquely different in that it was high in α-linolenic acid [91]. Subjects following the Mediterranean-style diet had a 50–70% lower risk of recurrent heart disease. Adherence to a Mediterranean diet has been related to decreased mortality from cardiovascular disease and from cancer in a Greek population [92].

Omega-3 fatty acids

The fact that omega-3 fatty acids exert cardioprotective effects via multiple mechanisms (i.e. decrease synthesis of cytokines and mitogens, stimulate endothelial-derived nitric oxide, and are antithrombotic) suggest that they could have accounted for the cardioprotective effect observed. In prevention trials, subjects who took fish oil had a lower rate of primary endpoint (death, non-fatal MI, or stroke) over 1.0–3.5 years compared with controls [93, 94].

High fibre diet

In numerous epidemiological studies increasing fibre intake was associated with a lower risk of heart disease—possibly as a result of lower LDL levels and improved insulin sensitivity. This relation did not persist after adjustment for CAD risk factors, however [95].

Antioxidants

Based on the observation that antioxidants like vitamin C can acutely improve endothelial function by reducing reactive oxygen species (ROS)-related NO breakdown it was hypothesized that they could also modify the long-term progression of atherosclerosis and reduce cardiovascular mortality and morbidity. However, pathophysiological studies showed that 6 months of vitamin C administration did not improve endothelial function or decrease oxidized LDL levels [96] While there are at least some hints that high-dose vitamin C may reduce the risk for major CAD events [97], there is no clear evidence that the progression of the disease is affected. In fact, mortality was increased for vitamin A, vitamin E, and beta carotene supplementation [98].

Smoking cessation

Smoking as a cardiovascular risk factor

The causative relationship between smoking and CHD is well established, with RRs or odds ratios (ORS) estimated between 1.5–3 or higher [99–101]. Observational studies have estimated that smoking cessation reduces the risk of subsequent mortality an further cardiac events among patients with CHD by as much as 50% [102].

In a systematic review from 2003, a 36% reduction in crude RR of mortality for patients with CHD who quit compared with those who continued smoking (RR, 0.64; 95 CI, 0.58–0.71) was documented [103].

Smoking cessation strategies

Smoking cessation strategies are described in Chapter 12. In patients with CHD, quitting smoking is associated with a substantial reduction in risk of all-cause mortality (RR 0.64, 95% CI 0.58–0.71) and with a considerable reduction of non-fatal MI (RR 0.68, 95% CI 0.57–0.82) [104]. Numerous organizations also provide self-help manuals designed to assist smokers who wish to quit. In addition, consulting a therapist may enhance the effectiveness of this method. Standard instructions have been found to be less effective than personalized instructions tailored for a group of smokers. Overall, instructions on smoking cessation are considered useful and more effective than attempting to quit without instructions (➲Table 25.12).

During the last 20 years, nicotine replacement therapy (NRT) has been used by some 30 million smokers and has been tested in over 34,800 smokers in more than 108 studies [105]. Treatment of the dependent smoker with NRT (in the form of transdermal patches, chewing gum, nasal sprays, sublingual tablets, or oral inhalers) can therefore be implemented without any safety concerns. Two other widely used pharmacological interventions to aid smokers in cessation include the antidepressant bupropion and the nicotine receptor partial agonist varenicline. NRT, bupropion, and varenicline all provide therapeutic effects in assisting with smoking cessation. Direct and indirect comparisons identify a hierarchy of effectiveness [106].

Table 25.12 Assessment of non-drug treatment modalities to promote smoking cessation, compiled from the Cochrane Database

	Odds ratio	Assessment
Group therapy (behavioural therapy)	2.19 (1.42–3.37)	a
Aversion therapy (aversive stimulation)	2.66 (1.00–2.78)	b
Physician counselling	1.68 (1.45–1.98)	a
Individual counselling (short counselling session; booklet, etc.)	1.62 (1.35–1.94)	a
Nurse-managed counselling	1.50 (1.29–1.73)	a
Self-help interventions	1.24 (1.07–1.45)	a
Self-help intervention with telephone counselling	—	—
Exercise interventions	d	b
Training by healthcare professionals	d	—
Aversion therapy (general)	1.15 (0.77–1.82)	—
Acupuncture	1.22 (0.99–1.49)	c
Hypnotherapy	d	—
Reduced smoking	—	c

a Claim (e.g. on efficacy) supported by several suitable, valid clinical studies (e.g. randomized clinical trials) or by one or more valid meta-analyses or systematic reviews. Positive claim clearly confirmed.

b Claim (e.g. on efficacy) supported by at least one suitable, valid clinical study (e.g. randomized clinical trial). Positive claim confirmed.

c Negative claim (e.g. on efficacy) supported by one or more suitable, valid clinical studies (e.g. randomized clinical trials) or by one or more valid meta-analyses or systematic reviews. Negative claim clearly confirmed.

d No usable studies.

Psychological risk factors and behavioural support

Background

In large cohort studies psychosocial factors are associated with the prevalence of CAD. This evidence is largely composed of data relating CAD risk to five specific psychosocial domains:

1 depression;

2 anxiety;

3 personality factors and character traits;

4 social isolation;

5 chronic life stress.

Pathophysiological mechanisms underlying the relationship between these entities and CAD can be divided into behavioural mechanisms, whereby psychosocial conditions contribute to a higher frequency of adverse health behaviour, such as poor diet and smoking, and direct pathophysiological mechanisms, such as neuroendocrine or platelet activation and endothelial dysfunction [107] (➲Chapter 35).

Depression

In the past years five out of six community surveys have observed an increased risk of CAD among depressed persons [108]. Research in post-MI patients has documented that depression increases the risk of mortality from two to seven times. For clinical purposes and indication for specialized treatment, it may be useful to distinguish minor and major depressive episodes according to the established criteria.

Anxiety

Increasing evidence links anxiety disorders to the development of cardiac events in the general population with the excess mortality being confined to sudden cardiac death [109, 110]. The association between anxiety and sudden death but not MI suggests that ventricular arrhythmias may be the mechanism for cardiac death among individuals with anxiety disorders due to an alteration in cardiac autonomic tone.

Personality factors and character traits

Although type A behaviour characterized by competition, hostility, and exaggerated commitment to work continues to receive attention, a series of studies have reported no correlation between type A behaviour and CAD risk [111].

Hostility, a major attribute of the type A behaviour pattern, has received considerable attention as a potential ‘toxic’ element in this personality construct. The potential for hostility (i.e. aggressive verbal or physical responses when angry) was consistently found to be related to CAD, predicting restenoses and recurrent events. Hostile subjects manifest higher heart rate and blood pressure responses to physiological stimuli, such as mental tasks, as well as higher ambulatory blood pressure levels during daily-life activity. Preliminary data suggest that hostile individuals may manifest diminished vagal modulation of heart function and increased platelet reactivity.

Social isolation and life stress

An inverse relation has been reported between the magnitude of social support and the incidence of CAD and/or future cardiac events [112, 113]. Low socio-economic status is a significant contributor to increased risk in healthy persons and a contributor to poor prognosis in patients with established CAD.

The effects of acute stress on heart disease are well supported by epidemiological studies regarding life stresses such as bereavement (with a twofold higher risk for men and threefold higher risk for women), anger (twofold increased relative risk of MI), earth quakes, and terrorist activities [114].

Takotsubo cardiomyopathy, also known as transient apical ballooning, apical ballooning cardiomyopathy, or stress-induced cardiomyopathy, is a type of non-ischaemic cardiomyopathy in which there is a sudden temporary weakening of the myocardium. This weakening can be triggered by emotional stress, a phenomenon which is seen predominantly in women [115].

Chronic life stress at work or at home are also important cardiovascular risk factors for men and women with some gender related differences according to the INTERHEART study [116].

Primary prevention

The prevalence of psychosocial risk factors in the general population can be estimated to be 5%. There is no reliable evidence proving the benefit of interventions on psychosocial risk factors in primary prevention. However, patients often know that their lifestyle and psychosocial problems may affect their health, but when physicians do not take these problems seriously, patients are likely to conclude that such problems are not important.

Secondary prevention

Depression and other psychosocial risk factors are highly prevalent in populations with known CAD and vary from 15–25% [107]. It has been estimated that psychosocial interventions designed to modify psychosocial risk factors may reduce fatal and non-fatal cardiac events by 30–50% with follow-up intervals equal to or more than 2 years.

The results from meta-analyses [117] suggest that these programmes yielded a 37% reduction in cardiac mortality, a 29% reduction in recurrence of MI, and significant positive effects on blood pressure, cholesterol, body weight, smoking behaviour, physical exercise, and eating habits. At the clinical level, it is recommended to routinely include psychosocial components in CR programmes such as stress management, and to offer counselling in selected cases. First results of the Sertraline and Depression in Heart Attack Study (SADHART) suggest a beneficial effect of the antidepressant drug on events and overall clinical well-being over 6 months' follow-up in post-acute MI patients [118].

Sexual problems

Sexual dysfunction is highly prevalent in both sexes and adversely affects patients' quality of life and well being [119]. Studies have reported erectile dysfunction (ED) rates of 68.3% in patients with hypertension and 40% in patients with coronary artery disease. The ED in these cases is usually due to the vascular disease itself but may also be secondary to the intake of angiotensin-converting enzyme (ACE) inhibitors, diuretics, beta-blockers, and other antihypertensive drugs [120]. Treatment options for men with ED include psychosexual therapy, oral sildenafil or vardenafil, transurethral alprostadil, intracavernous alprostadil, vacuum constriction device, surgical treatment (prosthesis), and vascular surgery. The elucidation of the nitric oxide-cyclic GMP pathway for ED and the development of sildenafil and vardenafil have been the most recent advances. However, although their incidence is small, serious cardiovascular events, including significant hypotension, can occur in certain populations at risk. The co-administration of nitrates and sildenafil/tardalafil significantly increases the risk of potentially life-threatening hypotension and must be strictly avoided.

Return to work

Despite the well-documented effects of CR on functional capacity and psychological well-being, there is contradictory evidence regarding whether rehabilitation programmes can influence the resumption of gainful employment. In theory, rehabilitation constitutes a pathway from total temporary inability to work to a substantially normal return to the previous habits.

The goals of vocational rehabilitation are to evaluate whether returning to work is safe and realistic and to expedite the resumption of gainful employment, while assisting individuals to remain at work. It is estimated that up to 80% of patients with uncomplicated MI will return to work. Moreover, the time for returning to work and resuming full activities for these patients has decreased from 4 months

Table 25.13 Programme components of cardiac rehabilitation

Programme component	Tasks	Goals
Initial evaluation	◆ Take medical history and perform physical examination ◆ Measure risk factors ◆ Obtain ECGs at rest and during exercise ◆ Determine level of risk ◆ Assess occupational status and prepare vocational counselling	Preventive plan in collaboration with primary care physician
Physical activity counselling and exercise training	◆ Assess current physical activity and exercise tolerance with monitored exercise stress test ◆ Identify barriers to increased physical activity ◆ Provide advice regarding increasing physical activity ◆ Develop an individualized regimen of aerobic and resistance training, specifying frequency, intensity, duration, and types of exercise	Increases in regular physical activity, strength, and physical functioning; more simply, at least 30min of submaximal work or moderate exercise daily is recommended. Greater benefit however can be achieved by further increasing physical activity.
Management of lipid levels	◆ Assess and modify diet, physical activity, and drug therapy	Primary goal: LDL cholesterol level <100mg/dL (<2.6mmol/L); secondary goals: HDL cholesterol level >45mg/dL (>1.16mmol/L), triglyceride level <200mg/dL (<2.26mmol/L)
Management of hypertension	◆ Measure blood pressure on ≥2 visits ◆ If resting systolic pressure is 130–139mmHg or diastolic pressure is 85–89mmHg, recommend lifestyle modifications, including exercise, weight management, sodium restriction, and moderation of alcohol intake; if patient has diabetes or chronic renal or heart failure, consider drug therapy ◆ If resting systolic pressure is ≥140mmHg or diastolic pressure is ≥90mmHg, recommend drug therapy ◆ Monitor effects of intervention in collaboration with primary care physician	Blood pressure <140/90mmHg (or <130/85mmHg if patient has diabetes or chronic heart or renal failure)
Smoking cessation	◆ Document smoking status (never smoked, stopped smoking in remote past, stopped smoking recently, or currently smokes) ◆ Determine patient's readiness to quit; if ready, pick date ◆ Offer nicotine-replacement therapy, bupropion, or both ◆ Offer behavioural advice and group or individual counselling	Long-term abstinence
Weight reduction	◆ Consider for patients with body mass index >25 or waist circumference >100cm (in men) or >90cm (in women), particularly if associated with hypertension, hyperlipidaemia, or insulin resistance or diabetes ◆ Provide behavioural and nutritional counselling with follow-up to monitor progress in achieving goals	Loss of 5–10% of body weight and modification of associated risk factors with long-term adherence
Management of diabetes	◆ Identify candidates on the basis of the medical history and baseline test ◆ Develop a regimen of dietary modification, weight control, and exercise combined with oral hypoglycaemic agents and/or insulin therapy ◆ Monitor glucose control before exercise sessions and communicate results to primary care physician ◆ For newly detected diabetes, refer patient to primary care physician for evaluation and treatment	Normalization of fasting plasma glucose level (80–110mg/dL, 4.4–6.1mmol/L) *or* glycosylated haemoglobin level (< 7.0%) and control of associated obesity, hypertension, and hyperlipidaemia
Psychosocial management	◆ Identify psychosocial problems such as denial, depression, anxiety, social isolation, anger, and hostility by means of an interview, standardized questionnaire, or both ◆ Provide individual or group counselling, or both, for patients with clinically significant psychosocial problems ◆ Provide stress-reduction classes for all patients ◆ Provide family members interventions	Improvement of clinically significant psychosocial problems and acquisition of stress-management skills

after an event in 1970 to approximately 60–70 days in 1990. Nevertheless, the socioeconomic consequences of failure to return to work for such a prevalent disease are significant.

Long-term adherence to lifestyle changes and medication

Secondary prevention interventions through CR are generally effective in the short term. Long-term adherence to a healthy lifestyle and medication is less good. The GOSPEL trial demonstrated positive effects for the first time of a long-term 3-year rehabilitation strategy on quality of care and prognosis in a large cohort of patients after MI [121].

Personal perspective

CR has made great progress over the last years: pathophysiological studies have increased our knowledge about the mechanisms by which both exercise-based and comprehensive rehabilitation achieves its goal of retarding the progression of cardiovascular diseases and improving exercise tolerance and general well-being. We are witnessing a new era of clinical research in CR with the first large-scale multicentre mortality trials on exercise-based rehabilitation in CHF being finished. At the same time there is growing consensus among cardiologists that optimized medical therapy together with secondary prevention interventions may prove to be more effective in reducing mortality and infarction rates among patients with stable CAD than an interventional strategy. Finally, there is a growing demand both from political opinion leaders and the general public for guidance on how to lead a heart-healthy life.

Despite these encouraging developments the gap between CR knowledge and implementation continues to grow. Currently, between 14–43% of potential candidates participate in formal CR programmes [122, 123] and less than half of those who participate maintain the prescribed lifestyle changes for 6 months or longer [124, 125]. Why are these figures so important? They identify an area of clinical and research activity in which a huge health benefit may be achieved with comparatively low investment. The established rehabilitation strategies and the knowledge about their efficacy are there, the key is now implementation. It is therefore a timely effort that the Cochrane Collaboration has started a formal protocol for a report on 'Promoting patient uptake and adherence in CR'. Interventions to improve patient motivation and programme adherence may range from a formal written patient commitment to optimized education interventions, formal coordination of post-discharge care, and continued reinforcement by either a nurse or the physician [126].

Some patient groups are especially underrepresented in rehabilitation programmes: patients with a migration history, women, very elderly patients, and patients from a disadvantaged social background are all less likely to benefit from rehabilitation interventions.

It takes a joint effort by cardiac societies across Europe and the world, by insurance companies, health policy makers, and by us as cardiologists to implement preventive cardiology and secondary prevention into our practice just as well as other guidelines on surgical and pharmaceutical interventions. CR should not be an option but standard of care for all patients with coronary heart disease, heart failure, and other cardiac disorders. Much still needs to be done—let us start today!

Further reading

Abuolhosn J, Perloff JK. Exercise and athletics in adults with congenital heart disease. In Perloff JK, Child JS, Aboulhosn J (eds.) *Congenital Heart Disease in Adults*, 3rd edn, 2009. Philadelphia, PA: Saunders Elsevier Inc.

Arena R, Myers J, Williams MA, *et al.* Assessment of functional capacity in clinical and research settings. A Scientific Statement From the American Heart Association Committee on Exercise, Rehabilitation, and Prevention of the Council on Clinical Cardiology and the Council on Cardiovascular Nursing. *Circulation* 2007; **116**: 329–43.

Balady GJ, Williams MA, Ades PA, *et al.* Core components of cardiac rehabilitation/secondary prevention programs: 2007 update. A scientific statement from the American Heart Association Exercise, Cardiac Rehabilitation, and Prevention Committee, the Council on Clinical Cardiology; the Councils on Cardiovascular Nursing, Epidemiology and Prevention, and Nutrition, Physical Activity, and Metabolism; and the American Association of Cardiovascular and Pulmonary Rehabilitation. *Circulation* 2007; **115**: 2675–82.

Conwell JA. Exercise in children after surgery for congenital heart disease. In Thompson PD (ed.) *Exercise and Sports Cardiology*, 2009. New York: McGraw-Hill.

Ellestad MH. *Stress testing: principles and practice*, 2003. Oxford: Oxford University Press.

Froelicher VF, Myers J (eds.) *Exercise and the Heart.* Philadelphia, PA: Elsevier Inc.

Gibbons RJ, Balady GJ, Bricker JT *et al.* ACC/AHA 2002 guideline update for exercise testing: a report of the American College of Cardiology/American Heart Association Task Force on Practice Guidelines (Committee on Exercise Testing). *J Am Coll Cardiol* 2002; **40**: 1531–40.

Leon AS, Franklin BA, Costa F *et al.* Cardiac Rehabilitation and Secondary Prevention of Coronary Heart Disease. An American Heart Association Scientific Statement From the Council on Clinical Cardiology (Subcommittee on Exercise, Cardiac Rehabilitation, and Prevention) and the Council on Nutrition, Physical Activity, and Metabolism (Subcommittee on Physical Activity), in Collaboration With the American Association of Cardiovascular and Pulmonary Rehabilitation. *Circulation* 2005; **111**: 369–76.

Maron BJ, Chaitman BR, Ackerman MJ *et al.* Recommendations for Physical Activity and Recreational Sports Participation for Young Patients With Genetic Cardiovascular Diseases. *Circulation.* 2004; **109**: 2807–16.

Perk J, Mathes P, Gohlke H, *et al.* (eds.) *Cardiovascular Prevention and Rehabilitation*, 2007. London: Springer Inc.

Thomas RJ, King M, Lui K *et al.* AACVPR/ACC/AHA 2007 Performance Measures on Cardiac Rehabilitation for Referral to and Delivery of Cardiac Rehabilitation/Secondary Prevention Services. *Circulation* 2007; **116**: 1611–42.

Wasserman K, Hansen JE, Sue SY, *et al. Principles of Exercise Testing and Interpretation.* 4th edn., 2005. Philadelphia, PA: Lippincott Williams & Wilkins.

Whaley MH, Brubaker PH, Otto RM (eds.) *ACSM's Guidelines for Exercise Testing and Prescription*, 7th edn., 2006. Philadelphia, PA: Lippincott Williams & Wilkins.

Williams MA, Haskell WL, Ades PA, Resistance Exercise in Individuals With and Without Cardiovascular Disease: 2007 Update: A Scientific Statement From the American Heart Association Council on Clinical Cardiology and Council on Nutrition, Physical Activity, and Metabolism. *Circulation* 2007; **116**: 572–84.

➲ For full references and multimedia materials please visit the online version of the book (http://esctextbook.oxfordonline.com).

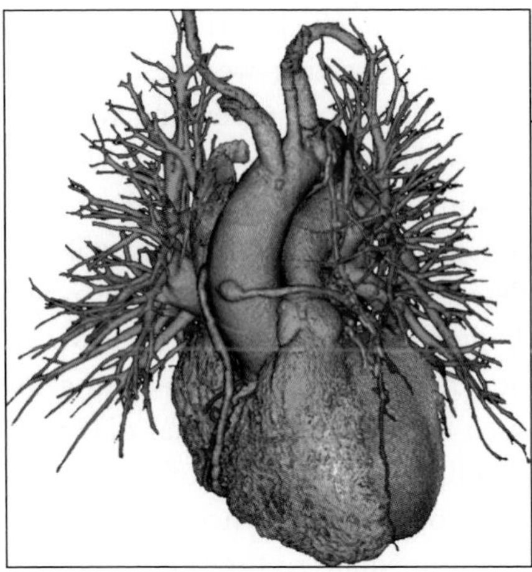

CHAPTER 26

Syncope

Michele Brignole, Jean-Jacques Blanc, Richard Sutton, and Angel Moya

Contents

Summary

Syncope is a transient loss of consciousness due to global cerebral hypoperfusion characterized by rapid onset, short duration, and spontaneous complete recovery. The starting point for evaluation of syncope is the 'initial evaluation', which consists of history, physical examination, standard electrocardiogram and (if appropriate) echocardiogram, orthostatic challenge, and carotid sinus massage. The initial evaluation has two objectives: to assess the specific risk for the patient (death, severe adverse events, or recurrence of syncope) and to identify the specific cause of the faint in order to address an effective mechanism-specific treatment.

Differentiating true syncope from other 'non-syncopal' conditions associated with real or apparent transient loss of consciousness is generally the first diagnostic challenge and influences the subsequent diagnostic strategy. Patients at high short-term risk require immediate hospitalization or early intensive evaluation. Others should be evaluated mostly as out-patients or day cases, and preferably referred to a specialized syncope facility (so-called 'syncope unit') if available. In the less severe forms, no further investigation is usually necessary and patients can be educated and reassured on the benign nature of their symptom.

The strategy of evaluation varies according to the severity and frequency of the episodes and to the presence or absence of heart disease. In general, the absence of suspected or certain heart disease excludes a cardiac cause of syncope. Conversely, the presence of heart disease at the initial evaluation is a strong predictor of a cardiac cause of syncope, but its specificity is low because about half of patients with heart disease have a non-cardiac cause of syncope. Determining the mechanism of syncope is a prerequisite to developing an effective mechanism-specific treatment. Most patients with syncope require only reassurance and education regarding the nature of the disease and the avoidance of triggering events.

Definition

Syncope is a transient loss of consciousness due to global cerebral hypoperfusion characterized by rapid onset, short duration, and spontaneous complete recovery. This definition of syncope differs from others in including the cause of unconsciousness, i.e. transient global cerebral hypoperfusion. Without that addition, the definition of 'syncope' becomes wide enough to include disorders such as epileptic seizures and concussion; in fact, the definition then becomes that of '*transient loss of consciousness*' (T-LOC), a term purposely meant to encompass all disorders with several similar presenting features. T-LOC is divided into traumatic and non-traumatic forms. Concussion causes LOC by definition; as the presence of a trauma is usually clear there is limited chance of diagnostic confusion. Non-traumatic T-LOC is divided into syncope, epileptic seizures, functional T-LOC, and rare miscellaneous causes (➲Fig. 26.1).

Syncope is a symptom, not a disease (neither is it a 'diagnosis'), and the mechanism has to be identified to allow a nosological diagnosis to be made. In some forms of syncope there may be a premonitory period in which various symptoms (e.g. light-headedness, nausea, sweating, weakness, and visual disturbances) offer warning of an impending syncopal event. Often, however, loss of consciousness occurs without warning. An accurate estimate of the duration of syncope episodes is rarely obtained. However, typical syncopal episodes are brief. Complete loss of consciousness in vasovagal syncope is usually no longer than 20s in duration. However, rarely syncope duration may be longer, even lasting for several minutes. In such cases, the differential diagnosis between syncope and other causes of loss of consciousness can be difficult. Recovery from syncope is usually accompanied by almost immediate restoration of appropriate behaviour and orientation. Retrograde amnesia, although believed to be uncommon, may be more frequent than previously thought, particularly in older individuals. Sometimes the post-recovery period may be marked by fatigue [1, 2].

'Presyncope' or 'near-syncope' is used often to describe a state that resembles the premonitory phase of syncope but which is not followed by loss of consciousness; doubts may remain whether the mechanisms involved are the same as in syncope. The term 'presyncopal' is used to indicate signs and symptoms that occur before unconsciousness in syncope, so its meaning is more literal and it is a synonymous of 'warning' and 'prodromal'.

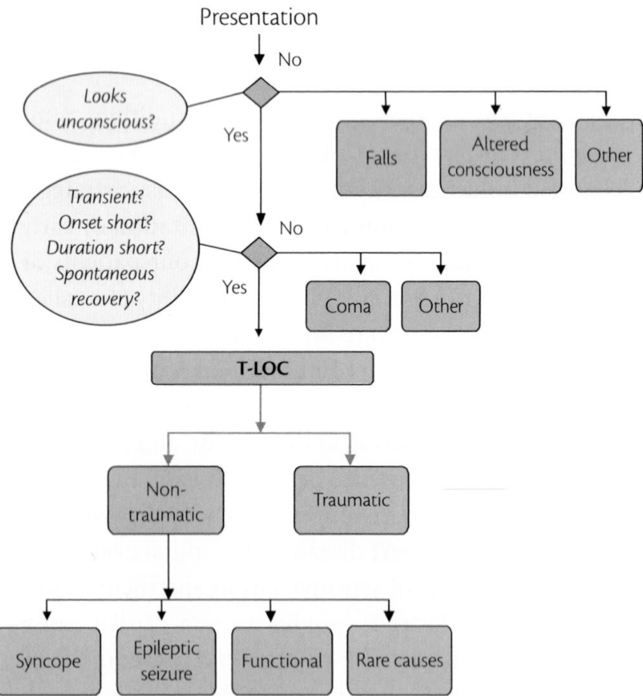

Figure 26.1 The context of transient loss of consciousness (T-LOC) is shown. Two decision nodes separating T-LOC from other conditions are whether or not consciousness appeared lost or not, and whether the four features defining the presentation of T-LOC were present. Whereas 'coma' is usually reserved for long-lasting forms, there is no common name for disorders with a duration of unconsciousness intermediate between T-LOC and coma. Examples are metabolic derangements such as hypoglycaemia and various intoxications.

Epidemiology

Syncope is extremely frequent in the general population and probably >50% of the general population complains of an episode of T-LOC of suspected syncopal nature during life. Approximately 30–40% of young adults experience at least one episode of T-LOC with a peak between the ages of 10–30 years. T-LOC also becomes increasingly frequent over the age of 60. In the Framingham study [3], the 10-year cumulative incidence of syncope was 6%. However, the incidence was not constant, but increased rapidly starting at the age of 70 years. The 10-year cumulative incidence of syncope was 11% for both men and women at age 70–79, and 17% and 19% respectively for men and women at age ≥80. In brief, there is a very high prevalence of first faints in patients in the age group between 10–30 years; first faint is uncommon in middle aged adults; there appears to be a peak above the age of 65 years [4, 5] (➲Fig. 26.2). However, only a small fraction of these subjects present in a clinical setting and an even smaller proportion deserve some specialized evaluation [6] (➲Fig. 26.3).

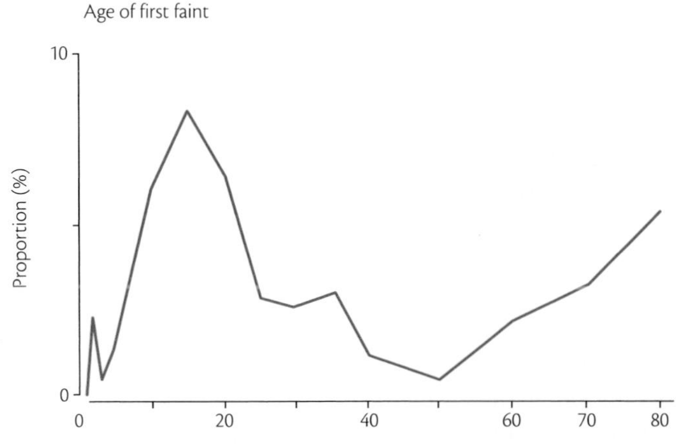

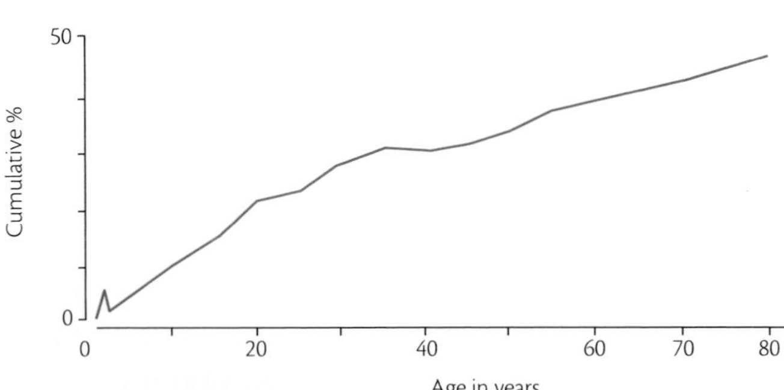

Figure 26.2 Schematic presentation of the distribution of age and cumulative incidence of first episodes of syncope in the general population in subjects up to 80 years old.

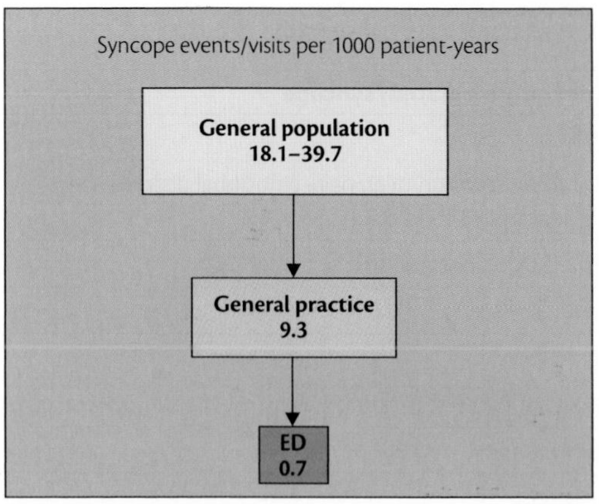

Figure 26.3 Syncope events/visits per 1000 patient-years in The Netherlands. ED, Emergency Department. Reproduced with permission from Olde Nordkamp LAR, van Dijk N, Ganzeboom KS, *et al.* Syncope prevalence in the ED compared to that in the general practice and population: a strong selection process. *Am J Emerg Med* 2009; **27**: 271–9.

Classification and pathophysiology

➲Table 26.1 provides a pathophysiological classification of the principal known causes of syncope. Several disorders may resemble syncope in two different ways. In some, consciousness is truly lost, but the mechanism is different from cerebral hypoperfusion. Examples are epilepsy, several metabolic disorders (including hypoxia and hypoglycaemia), and intoxications. In several other disorders, consciousness is only apparently lost; this is the case in 'psychogenic pseudo-syncope', cataplexy, and drop attacks. In psychogenic pseudo-syncope, patients may pretend to be unconscious when they are not. This condition can be seen in the context of factitious disorders, malingering, and conversion. Finally, some patients may voluntarily trigger true syncope in themselves to attract attention, as a game, or to obtain some other advantage. ➲Table 26.2 lists the most common conditions misdiagnosed as the cause of syncope. A differentiation such as this is important because the clinician is usually confronted with patients with sudden loss of consciousness (real or apparent) which may be due to causes not associated with decreased cerebral blood flow, such as seizure and/or conversion reaction.

Syncope classification (➲Table 26.1) emphasises large groups of disorders with a common presentation associated with different risk profiles. A distinction along pathophysiological lines centres on a fall in systemic blood pressure as the basis for syncope. Systemic blood pressure is the product of cardiac output and total peripheral vascular resistance and a dysfunction of either can cause syncope, but a combination of both mechanisms is often present, even if their relative contributions vary considerably. ➲Fig. 26.4 shows the pathophysiological underpinning of the classification with low blood pressure at the centre, and low peripheral resistance and low cardiac output next to it. A low peripheral resistance can be due to inappropriate reflex activity in the next ring, known as the *vasodepressor type* of reflex syncope in the outer ring. Other causes of a low peripheral resistance are functional and structural impairments of the autonomic nervous system with drug-induced, primary, and secondary autonomic failure in the outer ring. The causes of low cardiac output are threefold; the first is a reflex causing bradycardia known as *cardioinhibitory type* of reflex syncope. The second is purely cardiac, due to arrhythmia, structural cardiac diseases, or to pulmonary embolism. The third is inadequate venous return, due to volume depletion or venous pooling. Note that the possible mixture of causes is most apparent in reflex syncope. The main groups of the classification are shown outside the ring system; for reflex syncope and orthostatic hypotension, they span the two main pathophysiological categories.

A decrease of blood flow below critical levels causes loss of consciousness and of voluntary motor control, at a time

Table 26.1 Classification of syncope

Reflex (neurally mediated) syncope
Vasovagal:
Mediated by emotion (fear, pain, emotional distress, instrumentation, blood phobia)
Mediated by orthostatic stress
Situational:
Cough, sneeze
Gastrointestinal stimulation (swallow, defecation, visceral pain)
Micturition (post-micturition)
Post-exercise
Postprandial
Others (e.g. brass instrument playing, weightlifting)
Carotid sinus
Atypical forms (without apparent triggers and/or atypical presentation)
Syncope due to orthostatic hypotension
Primary autonomic failure:
Pure autonomic failure, multiple system atrophy, Parkinson's disease with autonomic failure, Lewy body dementia
Secondary autonomic failure:
Diabetes, amyloidosis, uraemia, spinal cord injuries
Drug-induced orthostatic hypotension
Volume depletion:
Haemorrhage, diarrhoea, vomiting, etc.
Excessive venous pooling:
Orthostatic stress, etc.
Cardiac syncope
Arrhythmia as primary cause:
Bradycardia:
Sinus node dysfunction (including bradycardia/tachycardia syndrome)
Atrioventricular conduction system disease
Implanted device malfunction
Drug-induced
Tachycardia:
Supraventricular
Ventricular (idiopathic, secondary to structural heart disease or to channelopathies, drug-induced 'torsade de pointes')
Structural disease:
Cardiac:
Cardiac valvular disease
Acute myocardial infarction/ischaemia
Hypertrophic cardiomyopathy
Cardiac masses (atrial myxoma, tumours, etc.)
Pericardial disease/tamponade
Congenital anomalies of coronary arteries
Others:
Pulmonary embolus
Acute aortic dissection
Pulmonary hypertension

when the electroencephalogram (EEG) shows slowing. Prolonged hypoperfusion causes flattening of the EEG. In children with vagally mediated asystole, induced by eyeball pressure, EEG flattening occurs only after a minimum duration of asystole of 9s. It then lasted longer as asystole lasted longer [7]. Experience from tilt testing showed that a decrease in systolic blood pressure to 40–60mmHg is associated with syncope [8]. The integrity of a number of control mechanisms is crucial to maintain sufficient arterial pressure and cerebral perfusion including: arterial baroreceptor-induced adjustments of heart rate, cardiac contractility, and systemic vascular resistance, which modulate circulatory dynamics with arterial pressure as the controlled variable; renin–angiotensin and vasopressin vasoconstriction; renal–body-fluid pressure control system; cerebrovascular 'autoregulatory' capability, which permits cerebral blood flow to be maintained over a relatively wide range of arterial pressures.

Reflex syncope (synonym: neurally mediated syncope)

Reflex syncope traditionally refers to a heterogeneous group of conditions in which cardiovascular reflexes that are normally useful in controlling the circulation become

Table 26.2 Conditions commonly misdiagnosed as syncope

Disorders with partial or complete loss of consciousness
Metabolic disorders, including hypoglycaemia, hypoxia, hyperventilation with hypocapnia
Epilepsy
Intoxications
Vertebrobasilar transient ischaemic attack (TIA)
Disorders which mimic impairment of consciousness
Falls
Cataplexy
Drop attacks
Psychogenic pseudo-syncope
TIAs of carotid origin

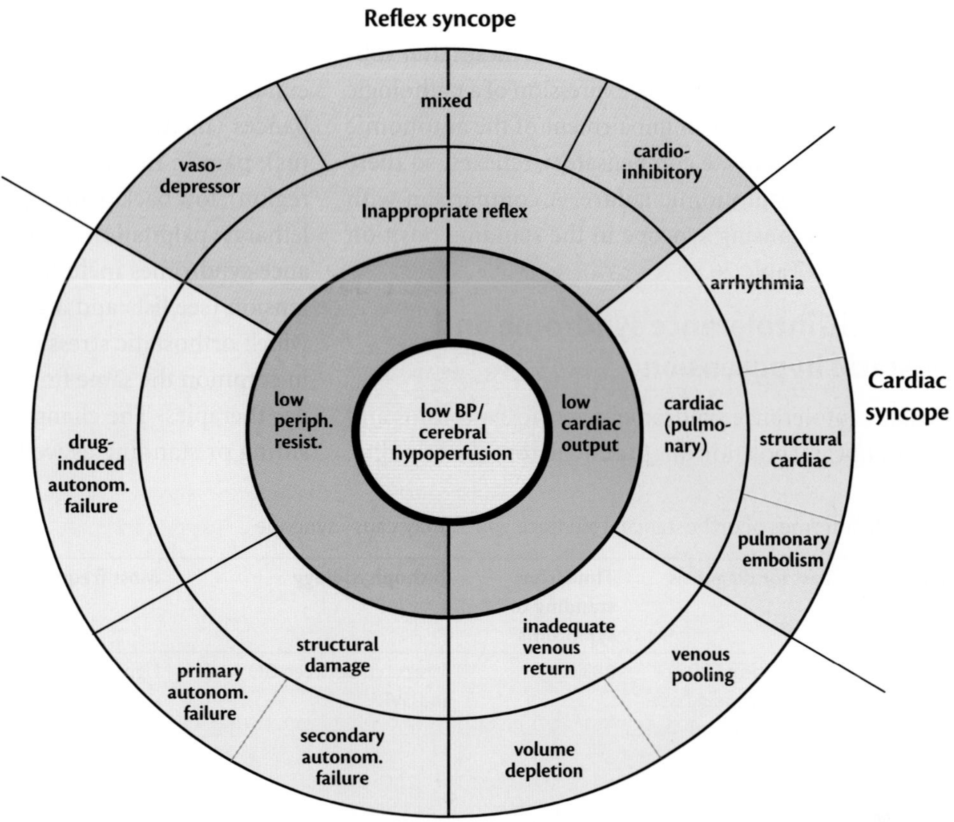

Figure 26.4 Pathophysiological basis of syncope classification (see text for discussion).

overactive, resulting in vasodilatation and bradycardia and thereby in a fall of arterial blood pressure and cerebral perfusion. A prerequisite for reflex syncope is therefore that the autonomic nervous system is intact. The term 'vasodepressor type' is commonly used if vasodilatation predominates. 'Cardioinhibitory' is used when bradycardia or asystole predominate and 'mixed' is used if both mechanisms come into play.

Reflex syncope may also be classified based on its trigger, i.e. the afferent pathway. The triggering situations vary considerably in and between individual patients. Knowing the various triggers is clinically important, as recognizing them may be instrumental in diagnosing syncope. 'Vasovagal syncope', also known as the 'common faint', is mediated by emotion (fear, pain, emotional distress, instrumentation, blood phobia) or by orthostatic stress. It is usually preceded by prodromal symptoms of 'autonomic activation' (sweating, pallor, nausea). 'Situational' syncope traditionally referred to reflex syncope associated with some specific circumstances (e.g. micturition, coughing, defecating, etc.), but there is no cause or need to set one set of triggers apart from others. 'Carotid sinus syncope' deserves special mention: in its rare 'spontaneous' form it is triggered by accidental mechanical manipulation of the carotid sinuses. This should be distinguished from 'carotid sinus hypersensitivity', which refers to a response to carotid sinus massage as a diagnostic test, and which is linked to apparently spontaneous syncope in the elderly: carotid sinus syndrome.

Reflex syncope may occur with uncertain or even apparently absent triggers. The diagnosis then rests less squarely on history taking alone, and more on the exclusion of other causes of syncope (absence of structural heart disease) and on reproducing similar complaints with tilt testing or through carotid sinus massage, (i.e. 'induced carotid sinus syndrome'). Such less clear presentations overlap with clear-cut occurrences within patients; together with the observation that syncope may be precipitated by different afferent pathways in the same subjects, this supports the concept that reflex syncope represents a tendency to respond in the central or efferent pathways rather than in an abnormality of afferent pathways.

Nonetheless, the classical form of emotional vasovagal syncope, which usually starts in young subjects as an isolated manifestation, should be distinguished from forms, frequently with a non-classical presentation, which start in old age and are often associated with cardiovascular or neurological disorders, and other disturbances such as orthostatic or postprandial hypotension. In these latter subjects, reflex syncope appears as an expression of a pathologic process, mainly related to an impairment of the autonomic nervous system to activate compensatory reflexes, so there is an overlap with autonomic failure. A comparison with other conditions causing syncope in the standing position is presented in Table 26.3.

Orthostatic intolerance syndrome and orthostatic hypotension

'Orthostatic intolerance syndrome' refers to symptoms and signs in the upright position due to a circulatory abnormality. Syncope is one symptom, and others are dizziness/light-headedness; visual disturbances (including blurring, enhanced brightness, and tunnel vision); hearing disturbances (including impaired hearing, crackles, and tinnitus); pain in the neck (occipital/paracervical and shoulder region); low back pain or precordial pain; weakness, fatigue, lethargy; palpitations and sweating [9]. Orthostatic intolerance syndromes include all the forms of orthostatic hypotension (see list) and also those forms of reflex syncope in which orthostatic stress is the main trigger. Since they have in common the same final mechanism, they also share similar therapies. The change in position may involve lying to sitting or standing as well as sitting to standing; note that

Table 26.3 Syndromes of orthostatic intolerance which may cause syncope

Classification	Test for diagnosis	Time from standing to symptoms	Pathophysiology	Most frequent symptoms	Most frequent associated conditions
Initial OH	Beat-to-beat SBP on lying-to-standing test (active standing)	0–30s	Mismatch between CO and SVR	Light-headedness/dizziness, visual disturbances a few seconds after standing up (syncope rare)	Young subjects with asthenic habitus Old age, drug-induced (alpha-blockers), carotid sinus syndrome
Classical OH (classical autonomic failure)	Lying-to-standing test (active standing) or tilt table	30s–3min	Impaired increase in SVR in autonomic failure resulting in pooling of blood/or severe volume depletion overriding reflex adjustments	Dizziness, presyncope, fatigue, weakness, palpitations, visual and hearing disturbances (syncope rare)	Old age Drug-induced (any vasoactive drug)
Delayed (progressive) OH	Standing Tilt table	3–30min	Progressive fall in venous return: low CO, diminished vasoconstriction capacity (failing adaptation reflex), no reflex bradycardia)	Prolonged prodromes (dizziness, fatigue, weakness, palpitations, visual and hearing disturbances, hyperidrosis, low back pain, neck or precordial pain) frequently followed by rapid syncope	Old age Autonomic failure Drug-induced (any vasoactive drug) Comorbidities
Delayed (progressive) OH + reflex syncope	Tilt table	3–45min	Progressive fall in venous return (as above) followed by vasovagal reaction (active reflex including reflex bradycardia and vasodilation)	Prolonged prodromes (dizziness, fatigue, weakness, palpitations, visual and hearing disturbances, hyperidrosis, low back pain, neck or precordial pain) always followed by rapid syncope	Old age Autonomic failure Drug-induced (any vasoactive drug) Comorbidities
Reflex syncope (VVS) triggered by standing	History of orthostatic stress Tilt table	3–45min	Initial normal adaptation reflex followed by rapid fall in venous return and vasovagal reaction (active reflex including reflex bradycardia and vasodilation)	Clear prodromes ('classic') and triggers always followed by syncope	Young healthy, female dominance
POTS	Tilt table	Variable	Uncertain: severe deconditioning, inadequate venous return or excessive blood venous pooling advocated	Symptomatic marked heart rate increases (>30bpm) and instability of blood pressure. No syncope	Young female

CO, cardiac output; OH, orthostatic hypotension; POTS, postural orthostatic tachycardia syndrome; SBP, systolic blood pressure; SVR, systemic vascular resistances; VVS, vasovagal syncope.

it is the upright position that is important, not the change per se.

It is of direct clinical relevance to make a distinction between three main types of orthostatic hypotension (➲Table 26.3):

- *Classically, orthostatic hypotension* is a physical sign defined as a decrease in systolic blood pressure of ≥20mmHg and/or 10mmHg in diastolic pressure within 3min of standing. Such decreases have been described in patients with pure autonomic failure or other forms of autonomic failure. In such patients, the rate of fall of blood pressure is highest directly after standing up, and slows thereafter to reach a stable level as long as patients remain in the same position. This state need not be reached within 3min.
- *Initial orthostatic hypotension* [10, 11] is caused by a blood pressure decrease immediately upon standing up. Blood pressure then spontaneously normalizes again, so the period of decreased blood pressure and symptoms is short (<30s). The cause is thought to be a temporal mismatch between cardiac output and vascular resistance. In view of its rapidity, only continuous beat-to-beat blood pressure measurement during an active standing-up manoeuvre can document this condition. A transient fall >40mmHg in systolic pressure or >20mmHg in diastolic pressure is reported as the arbitrary cut-off. Passive tilting has no diagnostic value, as only standing up actively causes the condition.
- *Delayed (progressive) orthostatic hypotension* [11–15] is commonly seen in elderly persons because of age-related impairments in compensatory reflexes. It is characterized by a slow progressive decrease in systolic blood pressure on assuming the standing position. Typically, these patients remain asymptomatic initially after standing and only develop hypotensive symptoms that cause orthostatic intolerance after a few minutes of standing. This form is frequently diagnosed by tilt testing, which shows the typical patterns of decrease of systolic blood pressure over several minutes without a steady state blood pressure period, whereas it may remain undetected using the classic 3-min criteria for the diagnosis of orthostatic hypotension. The absence of a clear bradycardic reflex (vagal) differentiates delayed orthostatic hypotension from vasovagal syncope. Sometimes, delayed orthostatic hypotension is followed by reflex bradycardia providing overlap with pure vasovagal syncope. The reflex bradycardia during a vasovagal faint in the elderly differs from that in the young in that the fall in blood pressure is less steep.
- *Autonomic failure* refers to an inadequacy of the autonomic nervous system to control one or more of its functions adequately: it tries but fails. In the context of syncope the term is limited to cardiovascular control defects. The failure then concerns sympathetic vasomotor pathways, unable to increase total peripheral vascular resistance in response to the upright position (standing, walking, and even sitting). It is important to realise that gravitational stress in combination with vasomotor failure results in venous pooling of blood below the diaphragm, resulting in a decrease in venous return and consequently in cardiac output. Heart rate control may also be affected; if so, orthostatic hypotension is not accompanied by a rise in heart rate, but remains fixed. Autonomic failure can be primary, secondary, or medication-induced [16, 17]. Examples of *primary autonomic failure* include pure autonomic failure (PAF), multiple system atrophy (MSA), and Parkinson's disease with autonomic failure. *Secondary autonomic failure* refers to autonomic failure due to diseases that primarily affect organs other than the autonomic nervous system, such as diabetic neuropathy or amyloid neuropathy. While in both these types the dysfunction is due to structural damage to the autonomic nervous system (either central or peripheral), the failure is functional in nature in drug-induced autonomic failure. Exercise and food intake can induce low blood pressures in patients with autonomic failure.

Arrhythmia

Cardiac arrhythmias can cause a decrease in cardiac output, which usually occurs irrespectively of circulatory demands. Nonetheless, syncope is often multifactorial in arrhythmias, including type of arrhythmia (atrial or ventricular), heart rate, the status of left ventricular function, posture, and the adequacy of vascular compensation (see ➲Chapters 27, 28, and 30). The latter include baroreceptorial neural reflexes as well as responses to orthostatic hypotension induced by the arrhythmia. Regardless of such contributing effects, an intrinsic cardiac arrhythmia is the primary cause of syncope, determining clinical decisions. The different clinical presentation helps to differentiate cardiac from reflex and orthostatic syncopes (see ➲Identifying the mechanism of T-LOC: the diagnostic strategy based on the initial evaluation, p.965).

Structural heart disease

Structural heart disease can cause syncope when circulatory demands outweigh the impaired ability of the heart to increase its output. Nonetheless, in several cases, syncope is not solely the result of restricted cardiac output, but may be in part due to an inappropriate reflex or orthostatic hypotension. The importance of appropriately recognizing the heart as the cause of the problem justifies the oversimplification.

Evaluation of a patient with T-LOC

There are two main reasons for evaluating a patient with T-LOC: one is to identify the specific cause of the faint in order to address an effective mechanism-specific treatment strategy; the other is to identify the specific risk for the patient (either death, severe adverse events, or recurrence of syncope). The prognosis, i.e. the risk of future adverse clinical events to which the patient is subjected, is either directly related to the faint or more generally related to the underlying disease, of which syncope is only an ominous finding or one of the clinical manifestations. Physicians should be aware not to confound the prognostic significance of syncope with that of the underlying disease. The treatment of syncope frequently differs from the treatment of the underlying disease. Therapy should be aimed either to eliminate the cause of syncope or to cure the underlying disease which predisposes to syncope. Therapeutical decisions of both situations greatly depend on the estimation of the relative prognostic significance that physicians attribute to syncope and to underlying disease.

Assessing the risk

With regard to the prognosis (i.e. risk stratification) associated with syncope, two important elements should be considered: 1) risk of death and life-threatening events and 2) risk of syncopal recurrence.

Risk of death and life-threatening events

Structural heart disease is a major risk factor for sudden death and overall mortality in patients with syncope. Conversely, young patients without structural heart disease and patients affected by neurally mediated syncope or orthostatic hypotension have an excellent prognosis with respect to mortality. Life-threatening diseases (e.g. acute coronary event, pulmonary embolism, acute heart failure) are suspected by non-invasive initial assessment, the presence of signs and symptoms such as chest pain or dyspnoea in addition to syncope suggesting those conditions. These situations require prompt and targeted confirmatory testing which should be done urgently. Most of the deaths and many detrimental outcomes seemed to be related to the severity of the underlying disease rather than to syncope per se. Life-threatening diseases may also include severe arrhythmias (e.g. third-degree atrioventricular (AV) block or ventricular tachyarrhythmias). Several clinical factors able to predict outcome have been identified in some prospective population studies involving a validation cohort (➲Table 26.4).

Few studies have directly evaluated the short-term risk (within a few days). In the San Francisco Syncope Rule [18], an abnormal electrocardiogram (ECG) result (defined as new changes or non-sinus rhythm), shortness of breath, systolic blood pressure ≤90mmHg, haematocrit ≤30%, and congestive heart failure (by history or examination) predicted the likelihood of serious adverse event within 7 days of Emergency Department (ED) evaluation (defined as death, myocardial infarction, arrhythmia, pulmonary embolism, stroke, subarachnoid haemorrhage, significant haemorrhage, or any condition causing a return ED visit and hospitalization for a related event) with a sensitivity of 98% and a specificity of 56%. However, these results could be only partially confirmed by three other external validation studies [19–21] which showed a high rate of false positive and false negative results (➲Table 26.4). The risk of life-threatening conditions in the next few days following referral is obviously the main reason for immediate hospital admission and exhaustive evaluation.

More studies have evaluated the long-term (1-year or more) risk (➲Table 26.4). In the pivotal study of Martin *et al.* [22], an abnormal ECG (defined as rhythm abnormalities, conduction disorders, hypertrophy, old myocardial infarction, and AV block), history of ventricular arrhythmia, history of congestive heart failure, or age more than 45 years were found to be predictors of severe arrhythmias (sustained ventricular tachycardia, symptomatic supraventricular tachycardia, pauses >3s, AV block, pacemaker malfunction) or 1-year mortality. The event rate (clinically significant arrhythmia or arrhythmic death) at 1 year ranged from 0% for those with none of the four risk factors to 27% for those with three or four risk factors. In the OESIL study [23], 1-year predictors of mortality were found to be age >65 years, history of cardiovascular diseases, lack of prodromes, and abnormal ECG (defined as rhythm abnormalities, conduction disorders, hypertrophy, old myocardial infarction, possible acute ischaemia, and AV block) In the OESIL risk score the mortality within 1 year increased progressively from 0% for no factor, to 57.1% for four factors. The EGSYS score [24], although specifically designed to identify cardiac syncope, was also proved to be able to predict a 2-year mortality of 21% in those with a score ≥3 compared with 2% in those with a score <3. In the STePS study [25],

Table 26.4 Risk stratification at initial evaluation in some prospective population studies including a validation cohort

Study	Risk factors	Score	Outcome	Results (validation cohort)
San Francisco Rule [18]	Abnormal ECG* Congestive heart failure Shortness of breath Haematocrit <30% Systolic blood pressure <90mmHg	No risk = 0 items Risk = ≥1 item	Serious events* at 7 days	98% sensitive and 56% specific [18] 89% sensitive and 42% specific [19] 76% sensitive and 37% specific [20] 74% sensitive and 57% specific [21]
Martin *et al.* [22]	Abnormal ECG* History of ventricular arrhythmia History of congestive heart failure Age >45 years	0 to 4 (1 point each item)	1-year severe arrhythmias* or arrhythmic death	0% score 0 5% score 1 16% score 2 27% score 3 or 4
OESIL score [23]	Abnormal ECG* History of cardiovascular diseases Lack of prodromes Age >65 years	0 to 4 (1 point each item)	1-year total mortality	0% score 0 0.6% score 1 14% score 2 29% score 3 53 score 4
EGSYS score [24]	Palpitations before syncope (+4) Abnormal ECG and/or heart disease (+3) Syncope during effort (+3) Syncope while supine (+2) Absence of autonomic prodromes[a] (−1) Absence of predisposing and/or precipitating factors[b] (−1)	Sum of + and − points	2-year total mortality -------------------- Cardiac syncope probability	2% score <3 21% score ≥3 -------------------- 2% score <3 13% score 3 33% score 4 77% score >4

* See text for explanation.
[a] Warm crowded place/prolonged orthostasis/fear, pain, emotion; [b] nausea/vomiting.

the long-term severe outcome was correlated with an age >65 years, history of neoplasms, cerebrovascular diseases, structural heart diseases, and ventricular arrhythmias. This finding is likely to reflect the importance of comorbidities, as suggested by long-term risk factors such as cardiac and cerebrovascular diseases and neoplasms.

In summary, age, an abnormal ECG, a history of cardiovascular disease, especially ventricular arrhythmia, heart failure, syncope occurring without prodrome or during effort or supine, were found to be predictors of arrhythmia and/or 1-year mortality. Risk stratification tools have been developed from these data. Again, similar to the short-term events, most of the deaths and of serious outcomes seemed to be correlated to the severity of the underlying disease rather than to syncope per se. High-risk patients need to be followed closely; optimal therapy and management must be provided. However, the presumption that an immediate in-hospital evaluation improves a patient's long-term clinical outcome has never been demonstrated and alternative strategies could be considered.

Risk of syncopal recurrence

In population studies, approximately one-third of patients have recurrences of syncope at 3 years of follow-up. Number of episodes of syncope during life and their frequency are the strongest predictors of recurrence. In 'low-risk' patients with uncertain diagnosis (see ➲ Management according to risk stratification, p.964), a history of fewer than three syncopes yields a probability of recurrence of syncope of 20% during the next 2 years, whereas a history of three syncopes yields a probability of recurrence of syncope of 42% during the same period (➲ Table 26.5). A psychiatric diagnosis and

Table 26.5 Prognosis of patients aged >40 years with *uncertain diagnosis and low risk* (see ➲ Management according to risk stratification, p.964) in the 590 patients pooled from the ISSUE 1 and 2 studies

Number of syncopes during lifetime	Risk of recurrence of syncope after the index episode		
	Actuarial risk 1 year	Actuarial risk 2 years	Estimated risk 4 years*
1–2	15.4%	19.7%	28.2%
3	36.5%	41.7%	52.2%
4–6	37.0%	43.8%	57.4%
7–10	37.5%	43.7%	56.2%
>10	44.3%	56.4%	80.7%

*Assuming a linear increase.

age <45 years are also associated with higher rates of syncopal recurrence. Conversely, sex, tilt-test response, severity of presentation, and presence or absence of structural heart disease have minimal or absent predictive value.

Major morbidity such as fractures and motor vehicle accidents were reported in 6% of patients and minor injury such as laceration and bruises in 29%. In patients presenting to an ED minor trauma were reported in 29.1% and major trauma in 4.7% of cases; the highest prevalence (43%) was observed in elderly patients with carotid sinus hypersensitivity [26]. Recurrent syncope is associated with fractures and soft-tissue injury in 12% of patients. The risk of events (i.e. trauma) is higher if syncope recurrence is unpredictable and in the absence of prodromes [25].

In general, the risk related to recurrence of syncope is higher (and it generally calls for precise diagnosis and specific treatment) in the following settings:

- where syncope is very frequent, e.g. alters the quality of life;
- where syncope is recurrent and unpredictable (absence of premonitory symptoms) and exposes patients to a 'high risk' of trauma;
- where syncope occurs during the prosecution of a 'high-risk' activity (e.g. driving, machine operation, flying, competitive athletics).

Management according to risk stratification

The management flow-chart of the European Society of Cardiology (ESC) Guidelines on Syncope is reported in ➲Fig. 26.5. According to the 2009 Guidelines on Syncope of the ESC, the patients at high short-term risk who require immediate hospitalization or early intensive evaluation can be identified after the initial evaluation (➲Table 26.6). In particular:

- Patients with an established indication for an implantable cardioverter defibrillator (ICD) should, according to current guidelines on ICD, go straight on to this therapy before the evaluation of the mechanism of syncope.
- Patients with previous myocardial infarction and preserved systolic function should undergo an electrophysiological study which includes premature ventricular stimulation; an implantable loop recorder (ILR) should be considered only at the end of a negative complete work-up.
- Patients with clinical or electrocardiographic features which suggest an arrhythmic mechanism for syncope should undergo in-hospital prolonged telemetric monitoring and eventually an electrophysiological evaluation; ILR should be considered at the end of a negative complete work-up.

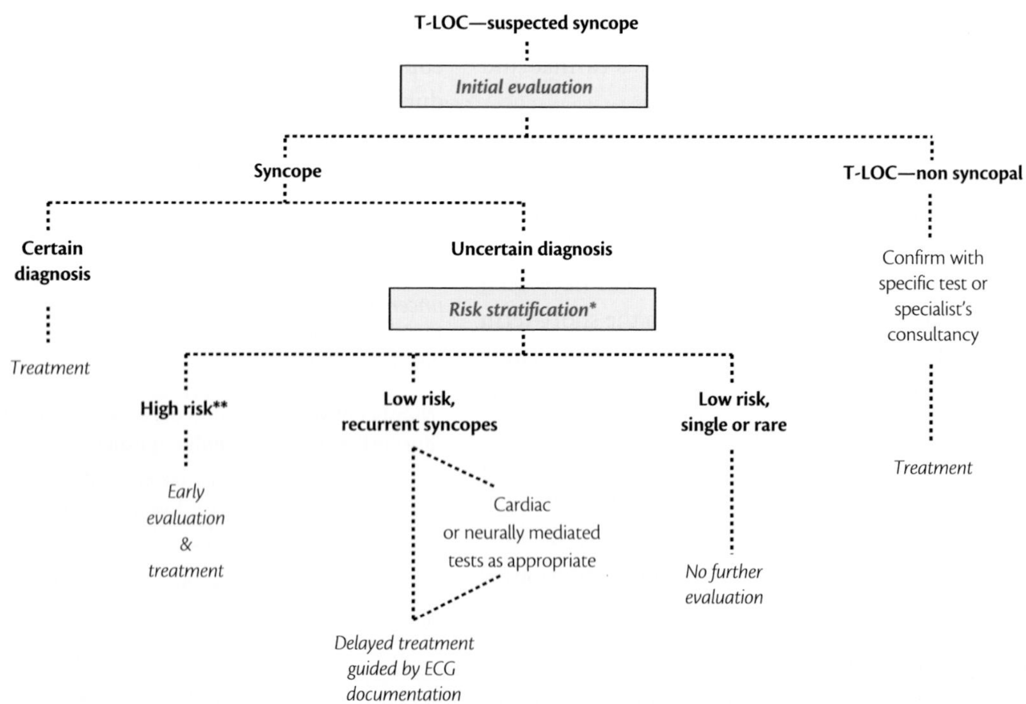

Figure 26.5 The management flow-chart of the ESC Guidelines on Syncope (2009). * May require laboratory investigations. ** Risk of short-term serious events.

Table 26.6 Risk stratification. Short-term high-risk criteria which require immediate hospitalization or early intensive evaluation as appropriate

Situations in which there is a clear indication for ICD or pacemaker treatment independently of a definite diagnosis of the cause of syncope according to ESC guidelines on ICD/CRT
◆ **Severe structural cardiovascular or coronary artery disease** (heart failure or low ejection fraction or previous myocardial infarction)
◆ **Clinical or ECG features suggesting an arrhythmic syncope:** - Syncope during exertion or supine - Palpitations at the time of syncope - Family history of sudden death - Non-sustained ventricular tachycardia - Bundle branch block (QRS duration ≥0.12 sec) - Inadequate sinus bradycardia (<50 bpm) or sinoatrial block in the absence of negatively chronotropic medications and physical training - Pre-excited QRS complexes - Prolonged or short QT interval - Right bundle branch block pattern with ST-elevation in leads V1–V3 (Brugada syndrome) - Negative T waves in right pericardial leads, epsilon waves and ventricular late potentials suggestive of arrythmogenic right ventricular cardiomyopathy
◆ **Important comobidities** (severe anaemia, electrolytic disdurbance, etc.)

If, at the end of the intensive evaluation, the work-up is negative (i.e. not persistent severe co-morbidities and no diagnosis of the cause of syncope) the patient can be evaluated as those at low risk.

When the high-risk features are absent or, if present, the subsequent work-up is negative, the risk of life-threatening events is low and the evaluation is aimed at prevention of syncopal recurrences. The patients who have a severe presentation of syncope (because of high risk of trauma or high frequency of episodes) which can benefit from a mechanism-specific therapy should be evaluated mostly as out-patients or day cases preferably referred to a specialized syncope facility (so-called 'syncope unit') if available.

Knowledge of what occurs during a spontaneous event is ideally the gold standard for evaluation. An electrocardiographic documentation of a spontaneous syncope can be achieved by in-hospital telemetry, ambulatory Holter, external (ELRs) and implantable loop recorders (ILRs). Since the diagnostic yield depends on the duration of the monitoring period, ILR is by far the most powerful and useful tool among them. However, in-hospital telemetry (or Holter monitoring, see ➲Chapter 2) has been shown to be useful when applied in selected patients referred in urgency for syncope because the probability of documenting a relapse in the 'hot phase' of the disease is high in this setting [27, 28] and ELRs are of some utility in patients with recurrent syncopes with an inter-symptom interval ≤4 weeks. Two recent randomized controlled trials showed that an early ILR strategy was safe and had a higher diagnostic yield than laboratory test strategy [29, 30]. In the less severe forms, no further investigation is usually necessary and patients can be educated and reassured on the benign nature of their symptom.

Identifying the mechanism of T-LOC: the diagnostic strategy based on the initial evaluation

The *initial evaluation* of a patient presenting with T-LOC consists of careful history, physical examination including orthostatic blood pressure measurements, and 12-lead ECG (➲Chapter 2). In patients with suspected heart disease, echocardiography is recommended as first evaluation step. In older patients without suspicion of heart or neurological disease and recurrent syncope, carotid sinus massages is recommended as first evaluation step. When loss of consciousness is related to standing position, orthostatic challenge (lying-to-standing orthostatic test and/or head-up tilt test) is recommended as first evaluation test (➲Table 26.7).

Table 26.7 Initial evaluation

To all:
History
Physical examination
Standard ECG
In selected cases (when appropriate):
Echocardiogram
In-hospital telemetric monitoring
Orthostatic challenge
Carotid sinus massage
Neurological evaluation

Three key questions should be addressed during the initial evaluation:

1) *Is loss of consciousness attributable to syncope or not?* Differentiating true syncope from 'non-syncopal' conditions associated with real or apparent T-LOC is generally the first diagnostic challenge and influences the subsequent diagnostic strategy. In most cases this can be accomplished during the initial evaluation. ➲Fig. 26.6 shows a history-based flow-chart for differential diagnosis between syncopal and non-syncopal causes of T-LOC. Note that it is based on the presence or absence of the clinical features reported on the definition of syncope (see ➲Definition, p.956).
2) *Are there features in the history that suggest the diagnosis?* Accurate history-taking alone is a key stage and often leads to the diagnosis or may suggest the strategy of evaluation.
3) *Is heart disease present or absent?* The absence of signs of suspected or overt heart disease virtually excludes a cardiac cause of syncope, with the exception of syncope accompanied by palpitations which could be due to paroxysmal tachycardia (especially paroxysmal supraventricular tachycardia). Conversely, the presence of heart disease at the initial evaluation is a strong predictor of cardiac cause of syncope, but its specificity is low as about half of patients with heart disease have a non-cardiac cause of syncope [31].

The initial evaluation may lead to certain or uncertain diagnosis (➲Fig. 26.5).

Certain diagnosis

Initial evaluation may lead to a certain diagnosis based on symptoms, physical signs, or ECG findings. Under such circumstances, no further evaluation may be needed and treatment, if any, can be planned. The results of the initial evaluation are most often diagnostic of the cause of syncope in the following situations:

- *Classical vasovagal syncope* is diagnosed if precipitating events such as fear, severe pain, emotional distress, instrumentation, or prolonged standing are associated with typical prodromal symptoms.
- *Situational syncope* is diagnosed if syncope occurs during or immediately after urination, defecation, coughing, or swallowing.
- *Orthostatic syncope* is diagnosed when there is documentation of orthostatic hypotension (defined as a decrease in systolic blood pressure ≥20mmHg or a decrease of systolic blood pressure to <90mmHg) associated with syncope or presyncope.
- *Cardiac ischaemia-related syncope* is diagnosed when symptoms are present with ECG evidence of acute ischaemia with or without myocardial infarction. However, in this case, the further determination of the specific ischaemia-induced aetiology may be necessary (e.g. neurally mediated hypotension, tachyarrhythmia, and ischaemia-induced AV block).
- *Arrhythmia*-related syncope is diagnosed by ECG when there is:
    - *sinus* bradycardia <40bpm or repetitive sinoatrial blocks or sinus pauses >3s in the absence of medications known to have negative chronotropic effect;

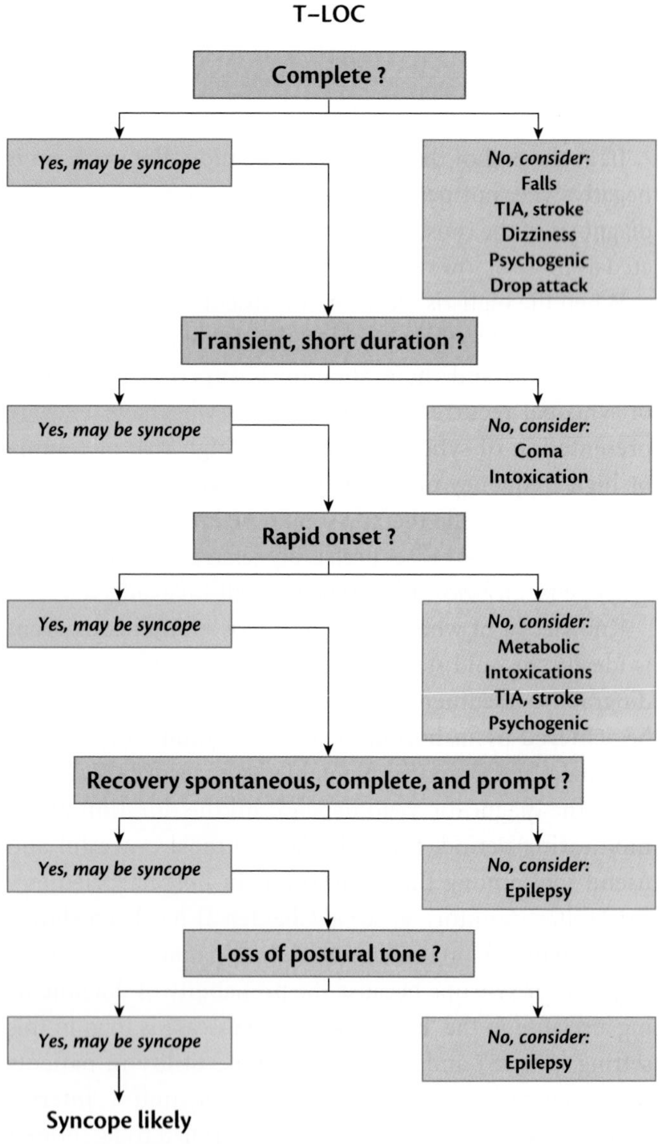

Figure 26.6 A history-based flow-chart for differential diagnosis between syncopal and non-syncopal causes of T-LOC. Note that it is based on the presence or absence of the clinical features reported on the definition of syncope (see ➲Definition, p.956).

- *second*-degree Mobitz II or third-degree AV block;
- alternating left and right bundle branch block;
- rapid paroxysmal supraventricular tachycardia or ventricular tachycardia;
- pacemaker malfunction with cardiac pauses.

However, it is important to bear in mind that syncope is often multifactorial; this is especially true in older individuals. Thus, careful consideration should be given to multiple, potentially interacting factors (e.g. diuretics in older patients already susceptible to orthostatic hypotension and myocardial ischaemia in the setting of moderate aortic stenosis).

Uncertain diagnosis

Commonly, the initial evaluation leads to a suspected diagnosis when one or more of the features listed in Tables 26.8 and 26.9 are present. The patients with an EGSYS score >4 (Table 26.4) yielded a 77% predictive value having an established diagnosis of cardiac syncope. The patients with an EGSYS score <3 yielded a 98% predictive negative value for cardiac syncope and low risk of death (24).

Table 26.8 Clinical features suggestive of specific causes of syncope

Reflex (neurally mediated) syncope
Absence of cardiac disease
Long history of syncope
After sudden, unexpected, unpleasant sight, sound, smell, or pain
Prolonged standing or crowded, hot places
Nausea, vomiting associated with syncope
During or in the absorptive state after a meal
With head rotation, pressure on carotid sinus(as in tumours, shaving, tight collars)
After exertion
Syncope due to orthostatic hypotension
After standing up
Temporal relationship with start of medication leading to hypotension or changes of dosage
Prolonged standing especially in crowded, hot places
Presence of autonomic neuropathy or Parkinsonism
After exertion
Cardiac syncope
Presence of severe structural heart disease
During exertion, or supine
Preceded by palpitation or accompanied by chest pain
Family history of sudden death

The presence of suspected or certain heart disease is associated with a higher risk of arrhythmias and mortality. In these patients, cardiac evaluation (echocardiography, stress testing, electrophysiological study, and prolonged ECG monitoring including loop recorder) is recommended. If cardiac evaluation does not show evidence of arrhythmia as a cause of syncope, evaluation for neurally mediated syndromes is recommended only in those with recurrent or severe syncope. It includes tilt testing, carotid sinus massage, and ECG monitoring, and often further necessitates implantation of an ILR. The majority of patients with single or rare episodes in this setting have a high likelihood of neurally mediated syncope, and tests for confirmation are usually not necessary.

Neurologic disease may cause T-LOC (e.g. certain seizures), but is almost never the cause of syncope. Thus, neurologic testing may be needed to distinguish seizures from syncope in some patients, but these should not be considered as essential elements in the evaluation of the basis of true syncope. The possible contribution of electroencephalography (EEG), computed tomography (CT) and magnetic resonance imaging (MRI) of the brain is to disclose abnormalities due to epilepsy; there are no specific EEG findings for any loss of consciousness other than epilepsy. Accordingly, several studies conclusively showed that EEG monitoring was of little use in unselected patients with syncope. Thus, EEG is not recommended for patients in whom syncope is the most likely cause for a T-LOC. Carotid TIAs are not accompanied by loss of consciousness. Therefore, carotid Doppler ultrasonography is not required in patients with syncope (Table 26.10).

If the cause of syncope is undetermined once the evaluation is completed, *reappraisal* of the work-up is needed

Table 26.9 ECG abnormalities suggesting arrhythmic syncope

Bifascicular block (defined as either left bundle branch block or right bundle branch block combined with left anterior or left posterior fascicular block)
Other intraventricular conduction abnormalities (QRS duration ≥0.12s)
Mobitz I second-degree AV block
Asymptomatic sinus bradycardia (<50bpm) or sinoatrial block
Pre-excited QRS complexes
Prolonged QT interval
Right bundle branch block pattern with ST-elevation in leads V1–V3 (Brugada syndrome)
Negative T waves in right precordial leads, epsilon waves, and ventricular late potentials suggestive of arrhythmogenic right ventricular cardiomyopathy
Q waves suggesting myocardial infarction

Table 26.10 Most useful and less useful tests

	Test	Suspected diagnosis
Most useful	Carotid sinus massage	Neurally mediated
	Tilt testing	Neurally mediated
	Echocardiogram	Cardiac
	Electrophysiological test	Cardiac
	Exercise stress testing	Cardiac
	Holter/external loop monitoring	Neurally mediated and cardiac
	ILR	Neurally mediated and cardiac
Less useful (indicated only in selected cases)	EEG	Epilepsy and TIA
	Brain CT	Epilepsy and TIA
	Brain MRI	Epilepsy and TIA
	Carotid Doppler sonography	Epilepsy and TIA
	Coronary angiography	Cardiac
	Pulmonary CT/ scintigraphy	Cardiopulmonary diseases
	Chest X-ray	Cardiac
	Abdominal ultrasound examination	Comorbidities

CT, computed tomography; EEG, electroencephalography; ILR, implantable loop recorder; MRI, magnetic resonance imaging; TIA, transient ischaemic attack.

because subtle findings or new historical information may change the strategy. Reappraisal may consist of obtaining additional details of history and re-examining the patient, placement of an ILR if not previously undertaken, as well as review of the entire work-up. If new clues to possible cardiac or neurological disease are yielded, further cardiac and neurological assessment are recommended. In these circumstances, consultation with appropriate specialists may be useful. Psychiatric assessment is recommended in patients with frequent recurrent syncope who have multiple other somatic complaints and in whom initial evaluation raises concerns about stress, anxiety, and possible other psychiatric disorders. If no diagnosis can be established at the end of the complete work-up as described here, the syncope is termed unexplained.

Diagnostic tests

Echocardiogram

Echocardiography (➲Chapter 4) is diagnostic of the cause of syncope in the presence of severe aortic stenosis and atrial myxoma. This investigation also provides information about the type and severity of underlying heart disease. If moderate-to-severe structural heart disease is found, evaluation is directed towards a cardiac cause of syncope, whereas in the presence of minor abnormalities the probability of cardiac cause of syncope is low and the evaluation proceeds as in patients without structural heart disease.

Carotid sinus massage

Carotid sinus syndrome is diagnosed in patients who have an abnormal response to carotid sinus massage (carotid sinus hypersensitivity) and an otherwise negative work-up for syncope. Carotid sinuses (alternatively right and left) are firmly massaged for 5–10s. The site for massage is the anterior margin of the sternocleomastoid muscle at the level of the cricoid cartilage. Both a cardioinhibitory reflex and a vasodepressor reflex are usually evoked with the massage (mixed form) but their relative contribution varies. A correct determination of the vasodepressor component of the reflex is of practical importance for the choice of pacing therapy, which is more effective in dominant cardioinhibitory forms (➲Fig. 26.7). A positive response is defined as a ventricular pause >3s and/or a fall in systolic blood pressure >50mmHg. However, abnormal responses are frequently observed in patients without syncope [32]. The specificity of the test increases if reproduction of spontaneous syncope during carotid massage is a requisite for positivity of the test [33, 34]. The syndrome is misdiagnosed in half of the cases if the massage is not performed in the upright position [33, 35]. There is a relationship between carotid sinus hypersensitivity and spontaneous, otherwise unexplained, syncope [36, 37]. Carotid sinus syndrome is a frequent cause of syncope, especially in elderly men, ranging from 4% in patients aged <40 years to 41% in patients >80 years. In a large population of 1719 consecutive patients with syncope uncertain after the initial evaluation (mean age 66 ± 17 years), carotid sinus hypersensitivity was found in 56% and syncope was reproduced in 26% of cases [33]. The response was cardioinhibitory in 46% of patients, mixed in 40%, and vasodepressor in 14%. The main complication of carotid sinus massage is neurological, i.e. TIA and stroke, its incidence ranging in three studies between 0.17–0.45% [33, 38, 39]. If there is a risk of stroke (➲Chapter 15) due to carotid artery disease, massage should be avoided. Therefore, carotid sinus massage is recommended in patients over the age of 40 years with syncope of unknown aetiology after the initial evaluation.

Orthostatic challenge

On changing from supine to erect posture, there is a large gravitational shift of blood from the chest to the venous capacitance system below the diaphragm. Failure of compensatory reflexes to orthostatic stress causes the clinical features of the syndrome of orthostatic intolerance listed

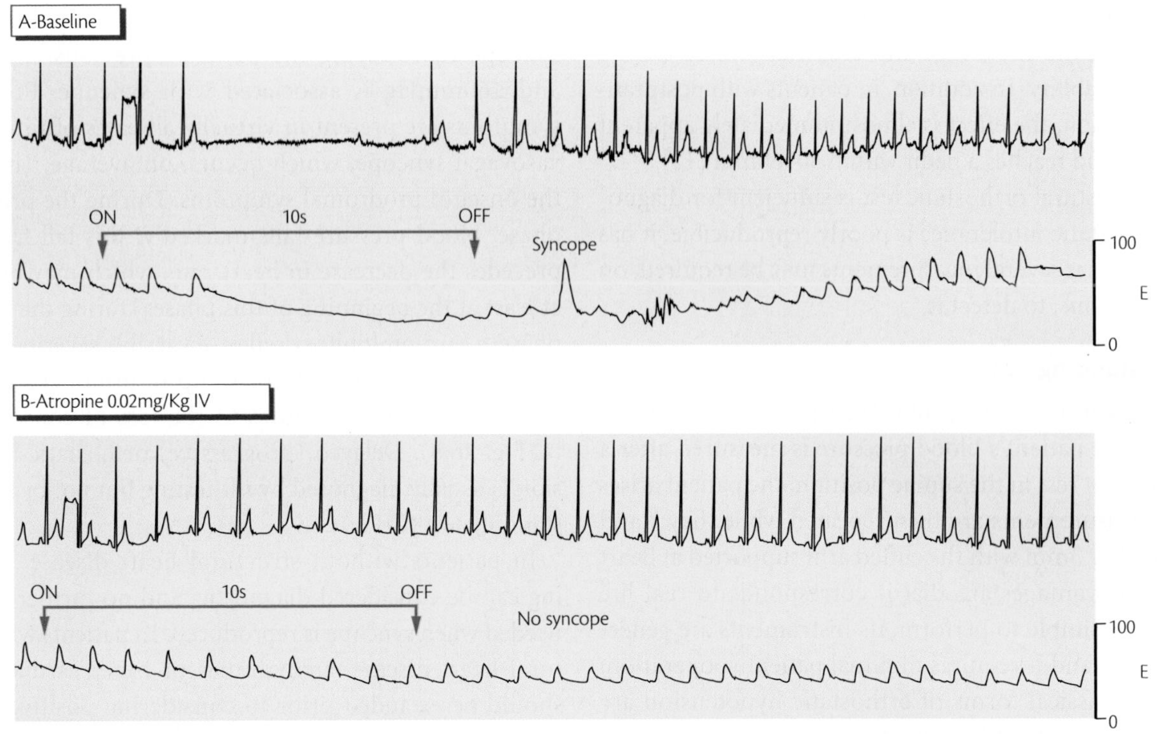

Figure 26.7 Dominant cardioinhibitory form of carotid sinus syndrome diagnosed by carotid sinus massage performed according to the 'method of symptoms' [8, 9]. (A) The massage was performed during beat-to-beat electrocardiographic (top trace) and systemic blood pressure monitoring (bottom trace) with the patient lying on a tilt table in an upright 60° position (arrows). The massage was continued for 10s. A 6.5-s asystole was induced soon after the beginning of the massage. The systolic blood pressure felt below 50mmHg; the vasodepressor reflex persisted longer than the cardioinhibitory reflex. Syncope occurred after the end of the massage when heart rhythm had already recovered. (B) In order to determine the relative contribution of the two components of the reflex, the cardioinhibitory component was suppressed by means of IV infusion of 0.02mg/kg atropine and the massage repeated. Despite a marked blood pressure fall, syncope could not be reproduced, thus showing that the cardioinhibitory component of the reflex was the major determinant of syncope in this patient.

in ➲Table 26.3. Two orthostatic challenges [12] are widely applied in practice to diagnose the forms of orthostatic hypotension and the form of vasovagal syncope triggered by prolonged standing syndrome of orthostatic intolerance: the lying-to-standing test and the head-up tilt test. Tests involving simulated orthostatic stress by applying lower body negative pressure are mainly used in research settings.

The anaeroid sphygmomanometer is used for routine clinical testing because of its reliability and simplicity. This is the standard method to which other non-invasive devices of blood pressure measurement are validated. Automatic arm-cuff devices, as they are programmed to repeat and confirm measurements when discrepant values are recorded, are at a disadvantage in following the rapidly dropping blood pressure during orthostatic hypotension and are discouraged. Beat-to-beat non-invasive blood pressure measurement is widely used in research and tilt laboratories and is recommended when tilt testing is performed. The most favoured devices are those which utilize the method of Penaz to record the arterial waveform indirectly from a finger. Studies on its accuracy have suggested little systematic bias versus intra-arterial pressure but substantial variability. In combined data from 20 published studies [40] the average systolic bias was 2.2 ± 12.4mmHg. Heart rate recording is integral to orthostatic challenge and is indispensable to the differentiation between certain clinical syndromes.

A marked day-to-day variability of postural response is well documented with both lying-to-standing test and tilt testing. In one study the day-to-day reproducibility of classic orthostatic hypotension in the elderly was only 67% [41]. The reproducibility of tilt testing has been widely studied. The overall reproducibility of an initial negative response (85–94%) is higher than the reproducibility of an initial positive response (31–92%) [42–44]. Data from controlled trials showed that approximately 50% of patients with a baseline positive tilt test became negative when the test was repeated with placebo [45]. Moreover, postural responses show diurnal (worse in the morning) and seasonal (worse during summer) variability. In addition, in patients with postprandial hypotension, the effect is almost immediately apparent after a meal and reaches a nadir within 30–60min [12].

A single postural orthostatic test is sufficient for diagnosis. As orthostatic intolerance is poorly reproducible, it has been shown that several measurements may be required, on several occasions, to detect it.

Lying-to-standing test

A frequently utilized protocol is the short, bedside orthostatic test: the patient's blood pressure is measured after a few minutes of rest in the supine position; the patient arises and the measurements are then repeated while they stand motionless for 3min with the cuffed arm supported at heart level. The advantages are that it corresponds to real-life situations, is simple to perform, its instruments are generally available, and it requires minimal patient cooperation. Initial and classical forms of orthostatic hypotension are usually diagnosed by this method.

Tilt testing

The widely accepted protocols [46–53] consist of:

- supine pre-tilt phase of at least 5min when no venous or arterial cannulation is performed, and at least 20min when cannulation is undertaken;
- tilt angle of 60–70°;
- passive phase ≥20min and ≤45 min;
- use of either intravenous isoproterenol or sublingual nitroglycerine for drug provocation if the passive phase has been negative; drug challenge phase duration should be 15–20min;
- for isoproterenol, an incremental infusion rate from 1mcg up to 3mcg/min, in order to increase average heart rate by about 20–25% over baseline, should be administered without returning the patient to the supine position;
- for nitroglycerine, a fixed dose of 300–400mcg nitroglycerine sublingually should be administered in the upright position;
- end-point of the test is the reproduction of syncope or completion of the planned duration of tilt, including drug provocation.

Experience from tilt testing [54, 55] showed that the vasovagal reaction lasts roughly ≤3min before loss of consciousness. A decrease in systolic blood pressure to ≤90mmHg is associated with symptoms of impending syncope reproducing the patient's previous experience, and ≤60mmHg is associated with syncope. Prodromal symptoms are present in virtually all cases of tilt-induced vasovagal syncope, which occurs, on average, 1min after the onset of prodromal symptoms. During the prodromal phase, blood pressure falls markedly; this fall frequently precedes the decrease in heart rate, which may be absent at least at the beginning of this phase. During the syncopal phase, a cardioinhibitory reflex of variable severity (ranging from slight heart rate decrease up to prolonged asystole) is frequent and contributes to the loss of consciousness (➲ Fig. 26.8). Delayed (progressive) orthostatic hypotension is usually diagnosed by tilt testing but not by lying-to-standing test (➲ Fig. 26.9).

In patients without structural heart disease, tilt testing can be considered diagnostic, and no further tests are needed when syncope is reproduced. In patients with structural heart disease, arrhythmias or other cardiac causes should be excluded prior to considering positive tilt test results. The clinical meaning of abnormal responses other than induction of syncope is unclear.

It should be kept in mind, however, that the relationship between symptoms occurring during an orthostatic test, essentially representative of a laboratory phenomenon, and symptoms occurring in a patient's natural ambience is not always clear [56]. The mechanism of tilt-induced syncope was frequently different from that of the spontaneous syncope recorded with the ILR in some studies [57, 58]. These data show, in addition to those of weak reproducibility, that the use of tilt testing for assessing the effectiveness of different treatments has important limitations.

Electrocardiographic monitoring (external and implantable)

In general, ECG monitoring (➲ Chapter 2) is indicated only when there is a high pre-test probability of identifying an arrhythmia responsible for syncope. These conditions are listed in ➲ Tables 26.8 and 26.9. ECG monitoring is diagnostic when a correlation between syncope and electrocardiographic abnormality (brady- or tachyarrhythmia) is detected. Conversely, ECG monitoring excludes an arrhythmic cause when there is a correlation between syncope and no rhythm variation. Presyncope may not be an accurate surrogate for syncope in establishing a diagnosis and, therefore, therapy should not be guided by presyncopal findings. In the absence of such correlations, additional testing is recommended with the possible exception of a ventricular pause >3s or periods of Mobitz II or third-degree AV block

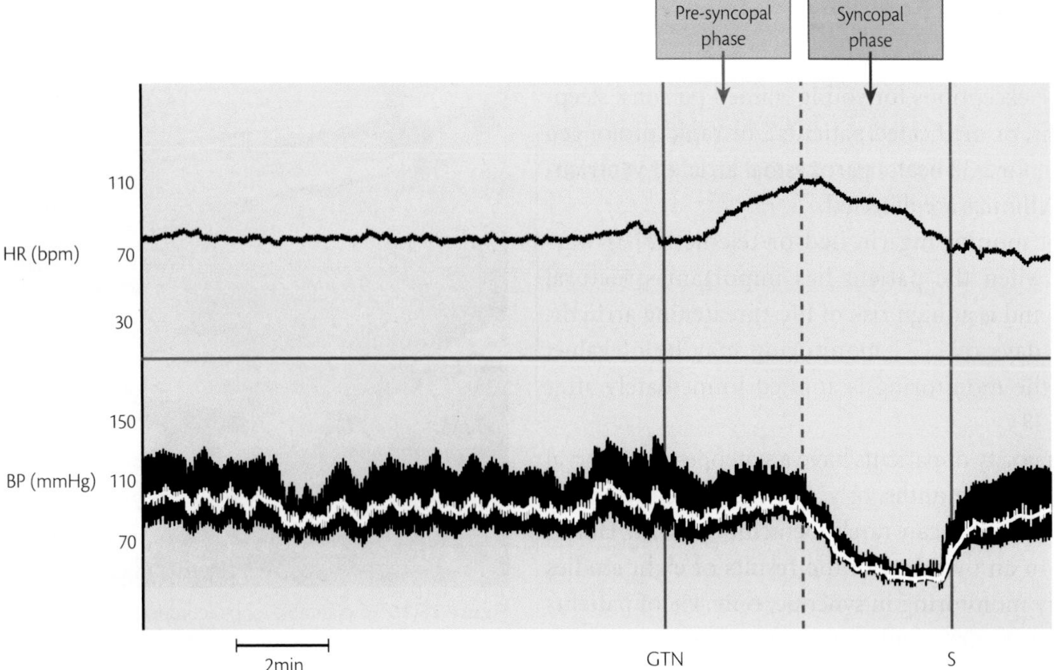

Figure 26.8 A case of classical (vasovagal) syncope, mixed pattern, occurring during nitroglycerine (GTN) challenge. The figure is expanded and the first part of the passive phase of the tilt testing is not shown. The top trace shows the heart rate curve; the bottom trace shows systolic, diastolic, and mean blood pressure curves. Immediately after the administration of 0.4mg of TNG, there is a mild decrease in blood pressure as a consequence of the haemodynamic effect of the drug. The presyncopal phase lasts about 2min and is characterized by an increase in diastolic blood pressure of 15mmHg, which indicates a full compensatory reflex adaptation with peripheral vasoconstriction. The heart rate rises approximately 35bpm. The vertical dashed line indicates the time of onset of the vasovagal reaction, which is characterized by a rapid fall in both blood pressure and heart rate that leads to syncope in about 3mm. BP, blood pressure; HR, heart rate; S, syncope; GTN, nitroglycerine.

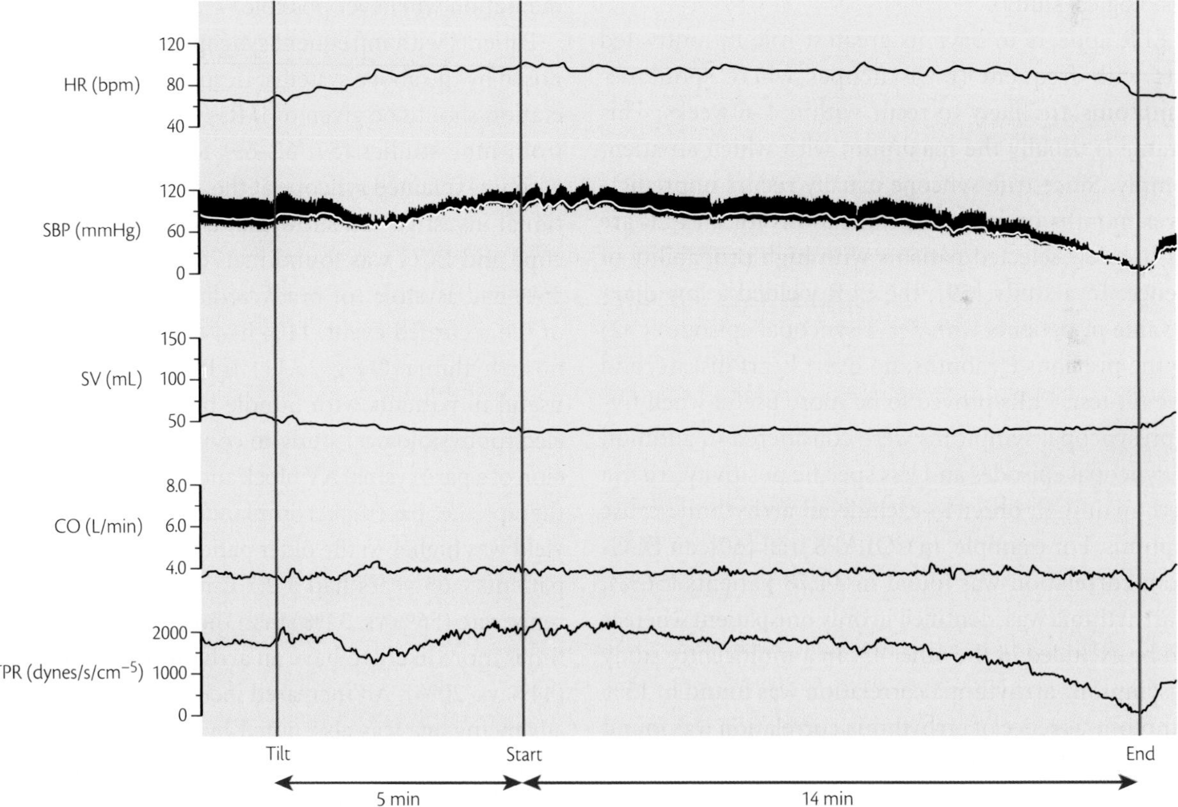

Figure 26.9 Haemodynamic pattern of a patient with progressive orthostatic hypotension syndrome. The reflex reaction starts a few minutes after standing and the following hypotensive phase is prolonged. After 5min from standing (Start), blood pressure (BP) decreases progressively, together with total vascular resistances, up to a critical value which causes pre-syncope (End). Stroke volume (SV) and cardiac output (CO) show minor variations. HR, heart rate; TPR, total peripheral vascular resistance.

(with possible exceptions for young trained persons, sleeping conditions, or medicated patients), or rapid prolonged (i.e. ≥160bpm for >32 beats) paroxysmal atrial or ventricular tachyarrhythmias are detected.

In-hospital monitoring (in bed or telemetric) is warranted only when the patient has important structural heart disease and is at high risk of life-threatening arrhythmias. A few days of ECG monitoring may be of value, especially if the monitoring is applied immediately after syncope [27, 28].

The vast majority of patients have a syncope-free interval measured in weeks, months, or years, and therefore symptom-ECG correlation can rarely be achieved with Holter monitoring. In an overview of the results of eight studies of ambulatory monitoring in syncope, only 4% of patients (range between 1–20%) had correlation of symptoms with arrhythmia. The true yield of conventional ECG monitoring in syncope may be as low as 1–2% in an unselected population. Therefore, Holter monitoring is indicated only in patients who have very frequent syncopes or presyncope. Holter monitoring may also be useful in patients who have the clinical or ECG features suggesting an arrhythmic syncope in order to guide subsequent examinations (i.e. electrophysiological study).

The ELR appears to have its greatest role in motivated patients with frequent (pre)syncopes where spontaneous symptoms are likely to recur within 4–6 weeks. This time frame is usually the maximum with which a patient can comply. Since true syncope usually recurs unpredictably over months or years, the indications for an ELR are limited to a few selected patients with high probability of recurrence. In a study [59], the ELR yielded a low diagnostic value in patients with 3 ± 4 syncopal episodes (>2) during the previous 6 months, no overt heart disease, and negative tilt test. ELRs proved to be more useful when frequent presyncopal symptoms were considered in addition to true syncopal episodes and less specific positivity criteria are used, mainly in order to exclude an arrhythmic cause of symptoms. For example, in COLAPS trial [60], an ECG-symptom correlation was found in 44/78 patients (56%), but an arrhythmia was identified in only one patient whereas it could be excluded in the other 43. In a multicentre study [61], a symptom-arrhythmia correlation was found in 15% and symptom-absence of arrhythmia correlation was found in another 25% of 51 patients. With the new auto-triggered devices, many asymptomatic tachyarrhythmias are usually recorded [61]. It should be stressed that, in the absence of a study of correlation with syncopal events, their positive predictive value is unknown, and monitoring should be continued until diagnosis is confirmed by symptom documentation whenever possible.

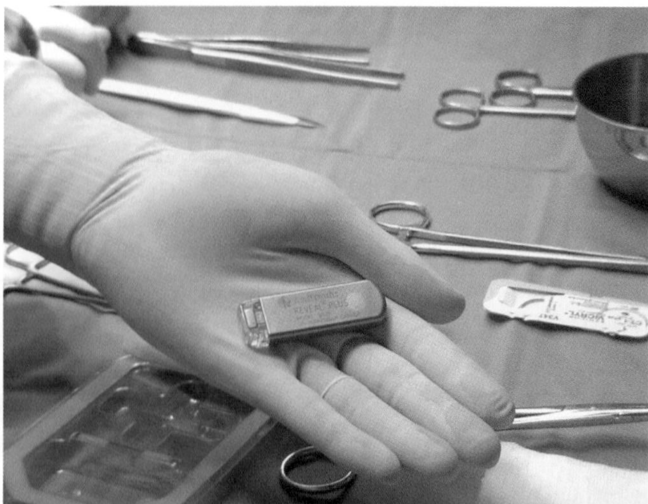

Figure 26.10 Implantable loop recorder (ILR). The ILR (Reveal®) is placed subcutaneously under local anaesthesia, and has a battery life of 36 months. The device has a solid-state loop memory, and the current version can store up to 42min of continuous single-lead ECG. Retrospective ECG allows activation of the device after consciousness has been restored. Automatic activation is also available in case of occurrence of predefined arrhythmias.

Patients with infrequent syncopes are unlikely to be diagnosed by the above systems. In such circumstances, consideration should be given to ILRs (➲Fig. 26.10). Pooled data from nine studies [57, 62–69] for a total of 506 patients with unexplained syncope at the end of a complete conventional investigation show that a correlation between syncope and ECG was found in 176 patients (35%); of these 56% had asystole (or bradycardia in few cases) at the time of the recorded event, 11% had tachycardia, and 33% had no arrhythmia (➲Fig. 26.11). ILRs proved to be particularly useful in patients with bundle branch block and negative electrophysiological study to confirm or exclude the suspicion of a paroxysmal AV block and guide subsequent specific therapy, i.e. pacemaker implantation [65]. The diagnostic yield was higher in the older patients. In one study [70], the patients >65 years had a 2.7 times higher syncope recurrence rate (56% vs. 32%) than those <65 years and were 3.1 times more likely to have an arrhythmia at time of syncope (44% vs. 20%). An increased incidence of bradycardia with advancing age was also noted by Krahn *et al.* [71]. On the contrary, the diagnostic yield was similar in patients with and without structural heart diseases (including abnormal ECG) [72]. Two randomized trials [29, 30] showed that an early ILR implantation in low risk patients (as defined elsewhere) is safe and yields a higher diagnostic value than

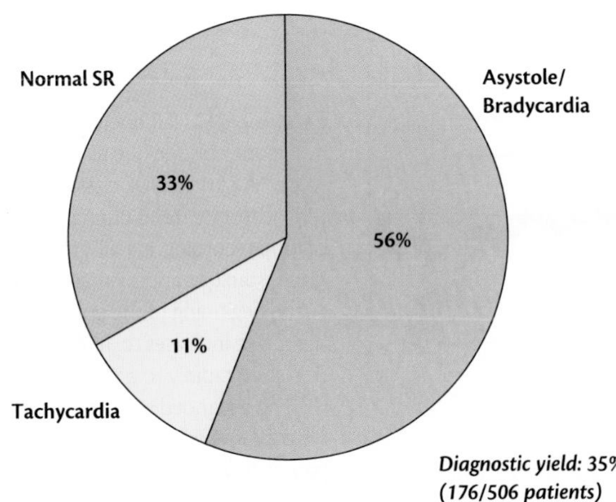

Figure 26.11 Mechanism of syncope in patients with unexplained syncope and ILR inserted at the end of the conventional work-up (pooled data of 509 patients from nine studies). The vast majority of asystole/bradycardia episodes were asystolic.

conventional investigations. Finally, the ILR implantation in an early phase of the diagnostic work-up was proven to be useful in patients at low risk with suspected neurally mediated syncope in order to understand the exact mechanism and to guide specific therapy [70].

Therefore, when the mechanism of syncope remains unclear after full evaluation, an ILR is indicated in patients who have clinical or ECG features suggesting arrhythmic syncope (➲Tables 26.8 and 26.9). An ILR may also be indicated in an initial phase of the work-up instead of the completion of conventional investigations. This is particularly the case for patients with recurrent syncope of uncertain origin who have a likely recurrence within battery longevity of the device (i.e. three or more syncopal episodes during the last 2 years) and absence of high-risk criteria which require immediate hospitalization or intensive evaluation (i.e. those listed in ➲Table 26.6).

An ILR may also be indicated to confirm suspected bradycardia before embarking on cardiac pacing in patients with suspected or certain neurally mediated syncope presenting with frequent or traumatic syncopal episodes [73]. Finally, an ILR may be indicated in selected 'difficult' cases of patients with T-LOC of uncertain syncopal origin in order to definitely exclude an arrhythmic mechanism [74].

Because of the heterogeneity of findings and the wide variety of rhythm disturbances recorded with ILR at the time of syncope, the ISSUE investigators have proposed a classification that aims to group the observations into homogeneous patterns in order to define an acceptable standard useful for future studies and clinical practice (➲Table 26.11) [75]. Type 1 (asystole) was the most frequent finding which was observed in 63% of patients; type 2 (bradycardia) was observed in 5% of patients; type 3 (no or slight rhythm variations was observed in 18% of patients; and type 4 (tachycardia) was observed in 14% of patients. This classification has become widely used and validated by others [74, 76, 77]. The ISSUE classification has some pathophysiological implications which are helpful to distinguish different types of arrhythmic syncope and have potential different diagnostic, therapeutic and prognostic implications. In types 1A, 1B, and 2 the findings of progressive sinus bradycardia, most often followed by ventricular asystole due to sinus arrest, or progressive tachycardia followed by progressive bradycardia and, eventually, ventricular asystole due to sinus arrest suggest that the syncope is probably neurally-mediated (➲Fig. 26.12). In type 1C, the finding of prolonged asystolic pauses due to sudden-onset paroxysmal AV block with concomitant increase in sinus

Table 26.11 The simplified ISSUE classification of ECG-documented spontaneous syncope

Classification	Mechanism
Type 1: asystole. RR pause ≥3	
Type 1A: sinus arrest:	Probably vasovagal
Progressive sinus bradycardia or initial sinus tachycardia followed by progressive sinus bradycardia until sinus arrest	
Type 1B: sinus bradycardia plus AV block:	Probably vasovagal
Progressive sinus bradycardia followed by AV block (and ventricular pause/s) with concomitant decrease in sinus rate	
Sudden onset AV block (and ventricular pause/s) with concomitant decrease in sinus rate	
Type 1C: AV block:	Probably intrinsic
Sudden onset AV block (and ventricular pause/s) with concomitant increase in sinus rate	
Type 2: bradycardia. Decrease of heart rate >30% or <40bpm for >10s	Probably vasovagal
Type 3: no or slight rhythm variations. Variations of heart rate <30% and heart rate >40 bpm	Uncertain
Type 4: tachycardia. Increase of heart rate >30% or >120bpm	
Type 4A: progressive sinus tachycardia	Uncertain
Type 4B: atrial fibrillation	Cardiac arrhythmia
Type 4C: supraventricular tachycardia (except sinus)	Cardiac arrhythmia
Type 4D: ventricular tachycardia	Cardiac arrhythmia

Data from Brignole M, Moya A, Menozzi C, *et al.* Proposed electrocardiographic classification of spontaneous syncope documented by an implantable loop recorder. *Europace* 2005; **7**:14–18.

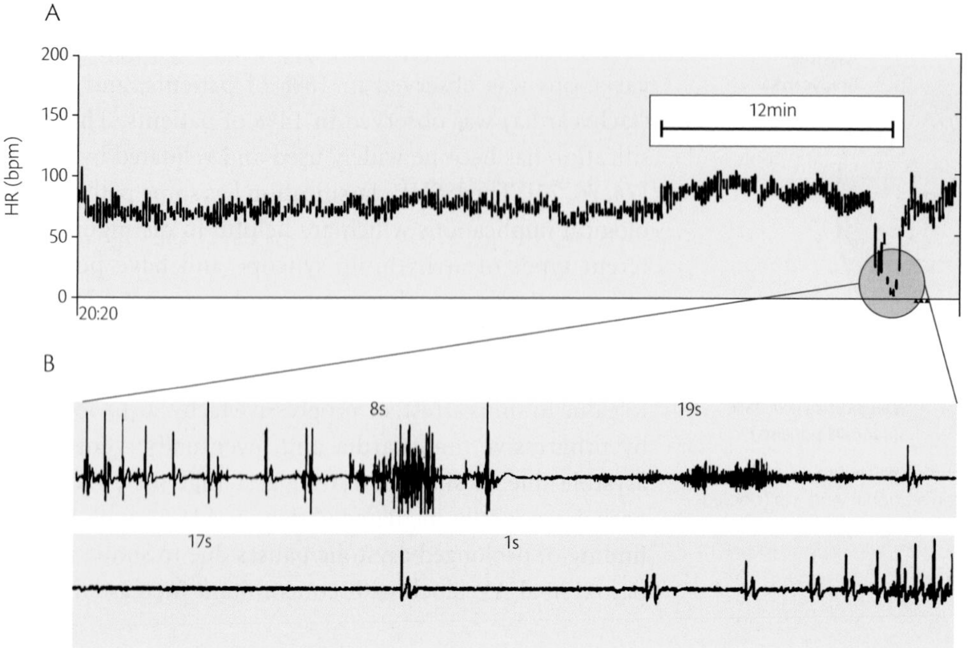

Figure 26.12 ILR documentation of a syncope episode due to sinus arrest (type 1A of the ISSUE classification). (A) Heart rate trend during 42min of loop recording. Initially, the heart rate is stable at approximately 70bpm; at the beginning of the episode the heart rate increases to 100bpm, then decreases rapidly to a very low rate. (B) The expanded ECG at the time of syncope shows prolonged multiple pauses due to sinus arrest. The noise recorded during the pauses of 8s and 19s of asystole probably reflects jerking movements of the patient. The finding of initial sinus tachycardia, progressive sinus bradycardia, frequently followed by sinus arrest has been regarded as highly suggestive of a neurally mediated mechanism.

rate suggests another mechanism, namely intrinsic disease of the His-Purkinje system as observed in Stokes–Adam attacks (➲Fig. 26.13). In types 4B, 4C, and 4D a primary cardiac arrhythmia is typically responsible for syncope. In the other types (3 and 4A), in which no arrhythmia is detected, the exact nature of syncope remains uncertain because of the lack of contemporary recording of blood pressure; however, the finding of progressive heart rate increase and/or decrease at the time of syncope suggests a (primary or secondary) activation of the cardiovascular system and a possible hypotensive mechanism.

Since prolonged asystole is the most frequent finding at the time of syncope recurrence, cardiac pacing was the specific therapy most used in ILR populations ranging from 12% in patients with neurally mediated syncope [73] to 44% in patients with bundle branch block [65]. ICD and catheter ablation were also consistently used in about 1% of the patients. Few data are available on the subsequent outcome of the patients treated with pacing. Cardiac pacing was very effective in reducing syncopal recurrences, especially in patients with type 1C pattern [76]. However, syncope still recurred in 12% (range 3–18%) of the patients during

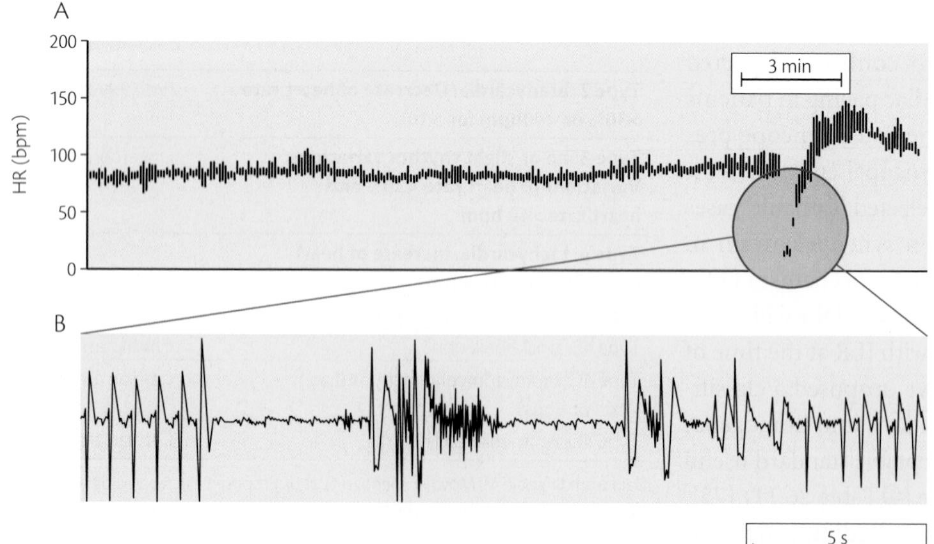

Figure 26.13 ILR documentation of a syncope episode due to a paroxysmal AV block (type 1C of the ISSUE classification). (A) Heart rate trend during the whole 21-min loop recording. Initially, the heart rate is stable at approximately 80bpm and suddenly falls at the time of the syncope. (B) The expanded ECG shows blocked P waves with two main pauses of 5s and 6s duration. The sinus rate increases during AV block. The noise recorded during the second pause probably reflects jerking movements of the patient. The sudden onset AV block (and ventricular pause) with concomitant increase in sinus rate suggests an intrinsic disease of the His–Purkinje system as observed in the Stokes–Adams attacks.

the long-term follow-up (2–3.6 years), especially in those patients more likely to be affected by neurally mediated syncope (type 1A or 1B), probably accounting for the coexistence of some vasodepressor reflex which cannot be overcome by pacing [70, 73, 76]. In patients with neurally mediated syncope [73] the 1-year burden of syncope decreased from 0.83 ± 1.57 episodes per patient/year in the control group of patients without any ILR-guided specific therapy to 0.05 ± 0.15 episodes per patient/year in the patients treated with a pacemaker (87% relative risk reduction, $p = 0.001$).

Key points for use of ILR and ELR

- Exclude high-risk patients, i.e. those with a clear indication for ICD, pacemaker, or other treatments, independently of a definite diagnosis of the cause of syncope.
- Include only those patients with a high probability of recurrence of syncope in a reasonable time period (➲Table 26.6).
- Be aware that the pre-test selection of the patients influences the subsequent findings.
- Your ideal goal should be to obtain a correlation between ECG findings and syncope. Weaker end-points are ECG-presyncope correlation or asymptomatic arrhythmias.
- Due to the unpredictability of syncope recurrence, be prepared to wait even for a long time before obtaining such a correlation.

Electrophysiological testing

The diagnostic efficiency of the invasive electrophysiological study is not only highly dependent on the degree of suspicion of the abnormality (pre-test probability) but also on the protocol (➲Table 26.12) and the criteria used for diagnosing clinically significant abnormalities. Positive results at electrophysiological study occur almost exclusively in patients with overt heart disease or conduction defects. It must be emphasized that normal electrophysiological findings cannot completely exclude an arrhythmic cause of syncope. When an arrhythmia is likely, further evaluations (e.g. loop recording) are recommended. Finally, depending on the clinical context, even apparently abnormal electrophysiological findings (e.g. relatively long HV interval, inducible ventricular fibrillation with aggressive stimulation) may not be diagnostic of the cause of syncope [78–80].

There are four areas of particular pertinence to electrophysiological testing in syncope patients: suspected sinus node disease (➲Chapter 27), bundle branch block (impending high-degree AV block) (➲Chapter 27), suspected supraventricular tachycardia (➲Chapter 28), and suspected ventricular tachycardia (➲Chapter 30).

Table 26.12 Minimal suggested electrophysiological protocol for diagnosis of syncope

Measurement of sinus node recovery time and corrected sinus node recovery time by repeated sequences of atrial pacing for 30–60s with at least one low (10–20bpm higher than sinus rate) and two higher pacing rates.*
Assessment of the His–Purkinje system includes measurement of the HV interval at baseline and His–Purkinje conduction with stress by incremental atrial pacing. If the baseline study is inconclusive, pharmacological provocation with slow infusion of ajmaline (1 mg/kg IV), procainamide (10 mg/kg IV), or disopyramide (2 mg/kg IV) is added unless contraindicated.
Assessment of ventricular arrhythmia inducibility performed by ventricular programmed stimulation at two right ventricular sites (apex and outflow tract), at two basic drive cycle lengths (100 or 120bpm and 140 or 150bpm), with up to two extrastimuli.**
Assessment of supraventricular arrhythmia inducibility by any atrial stimulation protocol.

*When sinus node dysfunction is suspected, autonomic blockade may be applied, and measurements repeated.

**A third extrastimulus may be added. This may increase sensitivity, but reduces specificity. Ventricular extrastimulus coupling intervals below 200ms also reduce specificity.

Suspected sinus node disease

The pre-test probability of a transient symptomatic bradycardia as the cause of syncope is relatively high when there is asymptomatic sinus bradycardia (<50bpm) or sinus pauses in the absence of negatively chronotropic medications. Sinus node dysfunction can be demonstrated by abnormal beat-to-beat variability and chronotropic incompetence, and by a prolonged sinus node recovery time. The prognostic value of a prolonged sinus node recovery time is largely unknown. It is widely accepted that, in presence of an SNRT >2s or corrected SNRT >1s, sinus node dysfunction may be the cause of syncope [81, 82].

Bundle branch block

In patients with syncope and bifascicular block, an electrophysiological study is diagnostic and, usually, no additional tests are required when the baseline HV interval is ≥100ms, second- or third-degree His–Purkinje block is demonstrated during incremental atrial pacing, or high-degree His–Purkinje block is provoked by intravenous administration of ajmaline (1mg/kg), procainamide (10mg/kg), or disopyramide (2mg/kg). An electrophysiological study is highly sensitive (>80%) in identifying patients with intermittent or impending high-degree AV block, but, when negative, it cannot rule out paroxysmal AV block as the cause of syncope [83–89].

This block is the likely cause of syncope in most cases but not of the high mortality rate observed in these patients, which is mainly related to underlying structural heart disease and ventricular tachyarrhythmias. Unfortunately, ventricular programmed stimulation does not seem to be able correctly to identify these patients, and the finding of inducible ventricular arrhythmia should therefore be interpreted with caution [90].

Suspected supraventricular tachycardia

Supraventricular tachycardia (➲Chapter 28) presenting as syncope without accompanying palpitations is probably a rare event. The induction of rapid supraventricular arrhythmia that reproduces hypotensive or spontaneous symptoms is usually considered diagnostic. The combination of supraventricular tachycardia and orthostasis may be responsible for syncope.

Suspected ventricular tachycardia

The outcome largely depends on the clinical features of the patients. Inducibility of sustained monomorphic ventricular tachycardia (➲Chapter 30) and/or very depressed systolic function are the two strongest predictors of life-threatening arrhythmic cause of syncope; conversely, their absence suggests a more favourable outcome.

Electrophysiological study with programmed electrical stimulation is an effective diagnostic test in patients with coronary artery disease, markedly depressed cardiac function, and unexplained syncope [91, 92]. For example, in the ESVEM trial [93], syncope associated with induced ventricular tachycardia at electrophysiological testing indicated high risk of death, similar to that of patients with documented spontaneous ventricular tachyarrhythmias. On the contrary, the induction of polymorphic ventricular tachycardia and ventricular fibrillation has low specificity and is of no value in risk stratification and therapeutical decisions [94].

Programmed ventricular stimulation has a low predictive value in patients with non-ischaemic dilated cardiomyopathy [95].

Exercise testing

Exercise testing (➲Chapter 2 and 25) should be performed in patients who have experienced episodes of syncope during or shortly after exertion.

The following two situations should be separately considered. Syncope occurring during exercise in the presence of structural heart disease is likely to have a cardiac cause. Tachycardia-related (phase 3), exercise-induced, second- and third-degree AV block has been shown to be invariably located in the His–Purkinje system and is an ominous finding of progression to chronic AV block. The resting ECG frequently shows an intraventricular conduction abnormality [96]. In the absence of structural heart disease, syncope occurring during exercise may be a manifestation of an exaggerated reflex vasodilatation [97]. By contrast, post-exertional syncope is almost invariably due to autonomic failure or to a neurally mediated mechanism [98]. Syncope in athletes may be an important problem (➲Chapter 32). However, in the absence of structural heart disease, syncope occurring during or immediately after exercise in athletes is a benign condition, with a good long-term outcome. The likely final diagnosis is neurally mediated [97].

Coronary angiography

In patients with syncope suspected to be due, directly or indirectly, to myocardial ischaemia, coronary angiography (➲Chapter 8) is recommended in order to confirm the diagnosis. However, angiography alone is rarely diagnostic of the cause of syncope.

ATP test

The test requires the rapid (<2s) injection of a 20-mg bolus of ATP (adenosine triphosphate) during electrocardiographic monitoring. The induction of AV block with ventricular asystole lasting >6s, or the induction of an AV block lasting >10s, are considered abnormal. ATP testing produced an abnormal response in patients with syncope of unknown origin (especially elderly female patients without structural heart disease), but not in controls, thus suggesting that paroxysmal AV block could be the cause of unexplained syncope [99–101]. Unfortunately, some recent studies showed no correlation between AV block induced with ATP test and the electrocardiographic findings (documented by means of implantable loop recorder) during spontaneous syncope [58, 77, 102]. Thus, the low predictive value of the test excludes any potential utility in selecting patients for cardiac pacing. The role of endogenus adenosine release in triggering some forms of syncope due to otherwise unexplained paroxysmal AV block (the so-called 'adenosine-sensitive AV block') still remains under investigation.

Neurological tests

Neurological disease may cause transient loss of consciousness (e.g. certain seizures), but is almost never the cause of syncope. Thus, neurological testing may be needed to distinguish seizures from syncope in some patients, but these should not be considered as essential elements in the evaluation of the basis of true syncope. The possible contribution of an EEG, CT, and MRI of the brain is to disclose abnormalities due to epilepsy; there are no specific EEG findings for any loss of consciousness other than epilepsy. Accordingly, several studies conclusively showed that EEG monitoring was of little use in unselected patients with syncope. Thus, EEG is not recommended for patients in whom syncope is the most likely cause of transient loss of consciousness [103–107].

Carotid TIAs are not accompanied by loss of consciousness. Therefore, carotid Doppler ultrasonography is not required in patients with syncope.

Diagnostic yield and prevalence of causes of syncope

➲Table 26.13 shows the comparative prevalence of the causes of syncope as determined by pooling data from six older population studies [108–113] performed in the 1980s (total 1499 patients) with that of four more recent population-based studies [31, 114–116] performed in the 2000s (total 1640 patients) and with that of the EGSYS study [27], which was a prospective systematic evaluation aimed at assessing the management of syncope on strict adherence to the Guidelines on Syncope of the ESC. Although difficult to reproduce in actual practice, the results of the EGSYS study probably assess the current standard for the management of syncope.

Reflex (neurally mediated) and orthostatic hypotension were the most frequent causes of T-LOC and their frequency increased in recent years, probably owing to a better knowledge of diagnostic criteria and to a more extensive use of carotid sinus massage and tilt testing. Cardiac syncope was the next most frequent cause of T-LOC and its frequency remained stable over the years. The proportion of T-LOC of suspected syncopal nature (neurological and psychiatric) at the initial evaluation was not very high and decreased slightly over time. The proportion of unexplained syncope dramatically decreased.

In general, the initial evaluation established a diagnosis in about 50% of cases in all studies. Apart from the initial evaluation, in the EGSYS study [27] a mean of 1.9 ± 1.1 appropriate tests per patient was necessary for diagnosis. The rate of appropriate indications and the diagnostic value of the most frequently used tests are reported in ➲Table 26.14. Hospitalization was appropriate in 25% of patients, but it was required for other reasons in a further 13% of cases. The median in-hospital stay was 5.5 days.

Table 26.13 Causes of T-LOC: secular trend

Diagnosis	1980s*	2000s**	2006***
Reflex and orthostatic	37%	56%	76%
Cardiac arrhythmias	13%	11%	11%
Structural cardiopulmonary	4%	3%	5%
Non-syncopal T-LOC	10%	9%	6%
Unexplained	36%	20%	2%

*Data pooled from six population-based studies (1499 patients).

**Data pooled from four population-based studies (1640 patients).

***Data from EGSYS 2 study (465 patients).

Treatment

There are two main reasons for treatment of a patient with syncope; one is to prevent recurrence by an effective mechanism-specific treatment strategy, the other is to apply an effective treatment of the underlying disease which could cause severe events unrelated to syncopal recurrence. Physicians should be aware not to confound therapy for prevention of syncopal recurrences from that of the underlying disease.

Table 26.14 Diagnostic yield of the most frequent tests in the 465 patients of the EGSYS study

	Appropriate indications (% patients)	Diagnostic yield (% tests)	NND
Standard ECG	100%	7%	14
Tilt testing	16%	61%	1.6
Carotid sinus massage	14%	28%	3.6
Basic blood chemistry tests	11%	40%	2.5
Echocardiogram	11%	10%	10
Holter/in-hospital monitoring	8%	48%	2.1
Brain CT scan and/or MRI scan	4%	23%	4.3
EP study	3%	33%	3.0
EEG	3%	31%	3.2
Exercise test	2%	30%	3.3
Coronary angiography	2%	62%	1.6
Carotid Echo-Doppler	0%	0%	∞
Chest X-ray	0%	0%	∞
Abdominal echography	0%	0%	∞

NND = number needed for diagnosis

Modified from Brignole M, Menozzi C, Bartoletti A, *et al.* A new management of syncope: prospective systematic guideline-based evaluation of patients referred urgently to general hospitals. *Eur Heart J* 2006; **27**:76–82.

Unexplained syncope in patients with high risk of death

In most patients at high short- and long-term risk of death (see Assessing the risk), a disease-specific treatment is warranted in order to reduce the risk of death and of life-threatening events even if the mechanism of syncope is still unknown at the end of a complete work-up.

In particular, the following conditions are to be considered:

- The risk of death in a patient with acute or chronic coronary artery disease is directly proportional to the severity of left ventricular dysfunction. This necessitates an evaluation for ischaemia and, if indicated, revascularization. However, the arrhythmia evaluation, i.e. electrophysiological study which includes premature ventricular stimulation, is still needed because, when present, the substrate for ventricular tachycardia and lethal ventricular arrhythmias may be not ameliorated by revascularization (➲Chapter 16 and 17).
- The patients with heart failure and an established indication for ICD according to current guidelines (as, for example, those of the ESC), should receive therapy before and independently of the evaluation of the mechanism of syncope [117–119] (➲Chapter 23). This is the case, for example, of the patients with ischaemic or dilated cardiomyopathy and low ejection fraction (<30% or 35% and NYHA class ≥2). A recent analysis of the SCD-HeFT trial [120] has shown that appropriate ICD shocks are more likely in patients with syncope; yet ICD did not protect against syncope recurrence nor against the risk of death. Patients with syncope and heart failure carry a high risk of death regardless of the origin of syncope [121].
- When syncope is closely associated with surgically addressable lesions (e.g. valvular aortic stenosis ➲Chapter 21, atrial myxoma ➲Chapter 20, congenital cardiac anomaly ➲Chapter 10), a direct corrective approach is often feasible. Also acute severe conditions like aortic dissection or pulmonary embolism must be immediately and intensively treated. On the other hand, when syncope is caused by certain difficult to treat conditions such as primary pulmonary hypertension (➲Chapter 24) or restrictive cardiomyopathy (➲Chapter 18), it is often impossible to ameliorate adequately the underlying problem
- Syncope is a major risk factor for subsequent sudden cardiac death in hypertrophic cardiomyopathy (relative risk >5) (➲Chapter 18), particularly if it is repetitive or occurs with exertion. However, in addition to self-terminating ventricular arrhythmias (➲Chapter 30), many other mechanisms can cause syncope in hypertrophic cardiomyopathy, including supraventricular arrhythmias (➲Chapter 28), severe outflow-tract obstruction, bradyarrhythmias (➲Chapter 30), decreased blood pressure in response to exercise, and reflex syncope. The presence or absence of other sudden cardiac death risk factors such as family history of sudden death, frequent non-sustained ventricular tachycardia, or marked hypertrophy may help in the determination of risk. Observational studies have demonstrated that implantable defibrillator therapy is effective in high-risk patients with hypertrophic cardiomyopathy [122–125].
- Unexplained syncope is regarded as an ominous finding in patients with arrhythmogenic right ventricular cardiomyopathy and inherited cardiac ion channel abnormalities (long QT syndrome, Brugada syndrome, short QT syndrome, polymorphic ventricular tachycardia, see ➲Chapter 9) and an ICD should be carefully considered in the absence of another competing diagnosis or when a ventricular tachyarrhythmia cannot be excluded as a cause of syncope. Nevertheless, the mechanism of syncope may be heterogeneous, being caused by life-threatening arrhythmias in some, but being of a more benign origin, i.e. vasovagal, in many others. Therefore, in these settings, it seems that syncope does not necessarily carry a high risk of major life-threatening cardiac events and yields a lower sensitivity than a history of documented cardiac arrest [126–129]. The differential diagnosis between benign and malign forms is usually very difficult in the setting of an inherited disease based on conventional investigations. Consequently, in many patients there is a rationale for more precise diagnosis (i.e. ILR documentation) of the mechanism of syncope before embarking on ICD therapy.
- Severe anaemia and other important comorbidities of which syncope is often a marker of severity should be carefully investigated and treated accordingly.

It is important to bear in mind, however, that even if an effective specific treatment of the underlying disease is found, patients may remain at risk of syncopal recurrences. For example, ICD-treated patient may remain at risk for fainting because only the sudden-death risk is being addressed and not the cause of syncope. An analysis of the SCD-HeFT trial [120] has shown that ICD did not protect patients against syncope recurrence compared with those treated with amiodarone or placebo. This implies the need of a precise identification of the mechanism of syncope and their specific treatment.

Cardiac syncope

Cardiac arrhythmias as primary cause

Syncope due to documented cardiac arrhythmias must receive treatment appropriate to the cause in all patients.

Cardiac pacing, ICDs, and catheter ablation are the usual treatments of syncope due to cardiac arrhythmias, depending on the mechanism of syncope.

In general, cardiac pacemaker therapy (➲Chapter 27) is indicated and has proved highly effective in patients with sinus node dysfunction when bradyarrhythmia has been demonstrated to account for syncope or by means of ECG documentation (see Electrocardiographic monitoring) or as consequence of abnormal sinus node recovery time (see Electrophysiological testing) [130–134]. Although formal randomized controlled trials have not been performed, it is clear from several observational studies that pacing is able to improve survival in patients with heart block as well as prevent syncopal recurrences [135, 136]. A logical inference, but not proven, is that pacing may also be life saving in patients with bundle branch block and syncope in whom the mechanism of the faint is suspected to be an intermittent AV block (see Electrophysiological testing) [84].

Owing to its curative effect, catheter ablation (see ➲Chapter 28 and 29) is the first-choice therapy for the most common forms of atrial arrhythmias causing syncope. The efficacy of conventional antiarrhythmic drugs when atrial arrhythmia is presenting with syncope is not satisfactory.

Iatrogenic atrial and ventricular arrhythmias are cured by eliminating the underlying responsible causes.

ICDs are the therapy of choice in patients with structural heart disease in whom ventricular tachycardia and ventricular fibrillation (➲Chapter 30) has been demonstrated to account for syncope or by means of ECG documentation (see Electrocardiographic monitoring) or as consequence of their induction by means of ventricular premature stimulation (see Electrophysiological testing). Several non-randomized studies have evaluated the utility of ICDs in highly selected patients with severe ischaemic and non-ischaemic cardiomyopathy and undocumented syncope suspected to be due to ventricular tachyarrhythmia: in general a high rate of appropriate shocks was observed which suggested a potential benefit in regard of survival [137–144]. ➲Table 26.15 provides commonly accepted indications for ICD therapy for the prevention of sudden death in patients with syncope. Catheter ablation is warranted in patients without structural heart disease. On the contrary, the efficacy of conventional antiarrhythmics is not satisfactory.

Structural cardiac or cardiopulmonary disease

Treatment is best directed at amelioration of the specific structural lesion or its consequences.

Table 26.15 Situations in which ICD therapy is likely to be useful

Documented syncopal ventricular tachycardia or fibrillation without correctable causes (e.g. drug-induced)
Undocumented unexplained syncope likely to be due to ventricular tachycardia or fibrillation:
Inducible sustained monomorphic ventricular tachycardia with severe haemodynamic compromise, in the absence of another competing diagnosis as a cause of syncope
Very depressed left ventricular systolic function according to current guidelines
Hypertrophic obstructive cardiomyopathy, established long QT syndrome, Brugada syndrome, arrhythmogenic right ventricular cardiomyopathy, in the absence of another competing diagnosis for the cause of syncope or when a ventricular tachyarrhythmia cannot be excluded as cause of syncope

Reflex (neurally mediated) syncope

Patients who seek medical advice after having experienced a vasovagal faint require reassurance and education regarding the nature of the disease and the avoidance of triggering events. In general, education and reassurance are sufficient for most patients. Modification or discontinuation of hypotensive drug treatment for concomitant conditions is another first-line measure for the prevention of syncope recurrence [145]. Treatment is not necessary for patients who have sustained a single or rare episode and are not having syncope in a high-risk setting. Additional treatment may be necessary in high-risk or high-frequency settings (see Risk of syncopal recurrence).

Non-pharmacological 'physical' treatments are emerging as a new front-line treatment of vasovagal syncope. Two recent clinical trials [146, 147] have shown that isometric counter-pressure manoeuvres of the legs (leg crossing), or of the arms (hand grip and arm tensing), are able to induce a significant blood pressure increase during the phase of impending vasovagal syncope that allows the patient to avoid or delay losing consciousness in most cases (➲Fig. 26.14). The results have been confirmed in a randomized multicentre prospective trial [148] which assessed the effectiveness of physical counter-pressure manoeuvres in daily life in 223 patients, aged 38 ± 15 years, with recurrent vasovagal syncope and recognizable prodromal (i.e. warning) symptoms: 117 patients were randomized to standardized conventional therapy alone, and 106 patients received conventional therapy plus training in counter-pressure manoeuvre. The median yearly syncope burden during follow-up was significantly lower in the group trained in physical counter-pressure manoeuvre (PCM) than in the control group ($p < 0.004$); overall 51% of the patients with conventional treatment and 32% of the patients trained in PCM experienced a syncopal

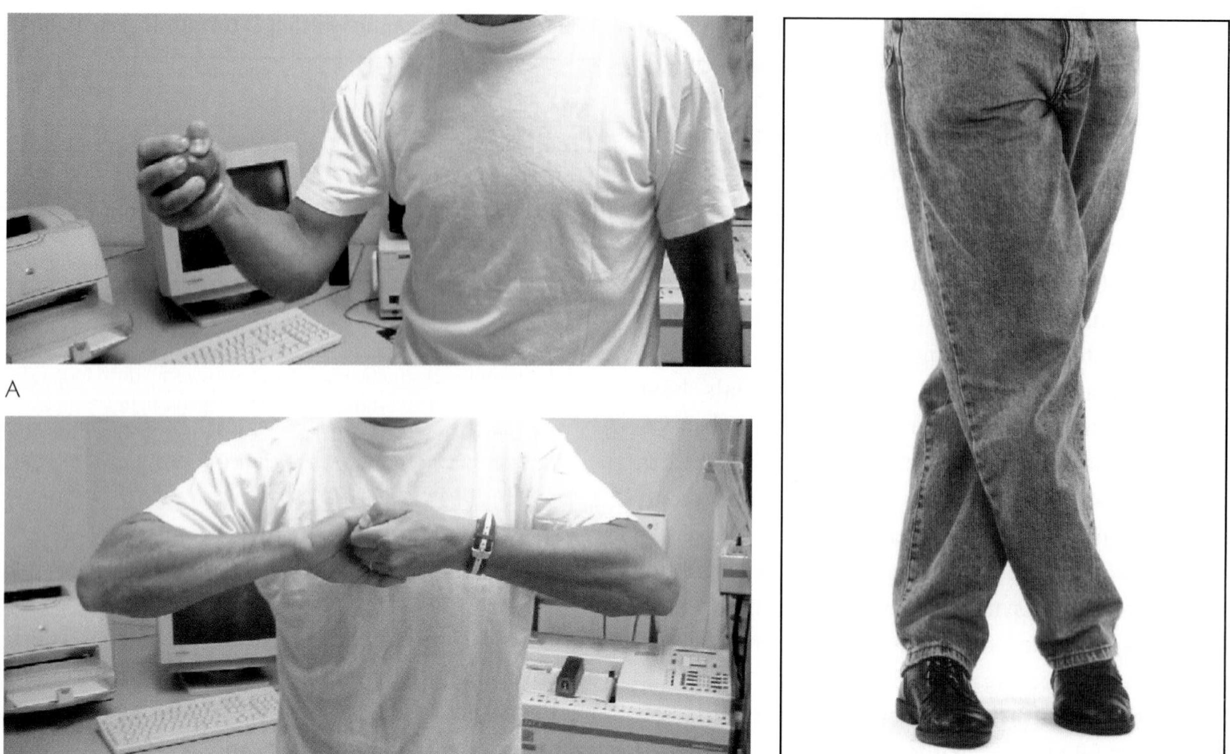

Figure 26.14 Most common counter-pressure manoeuvres. Patients should be instructed to use them as preventive measures when they experience any symptoms of impending fainting. (A) Handgrip consists of the maximal voluntary contraction of a rubber ball (approximately of 5–6cm diameter) taken in the dominant hand for the maximum tolerated time or till to complete disappearance of symptoms. (B) Arm-tensing consists of the maximum tolerated isometric contraction of the two arms achieved by gripping one hand with the other and contemporarily abducting (pushing away) the arms for the maximum tolerated time or till to complete disappearance of symptoms. (C) Leg crossing consists of leg crossing combined with tensing of leg, abdominal, and buttock muscles for the maximum tolerated time or until complete disappearance of symptoms.

recurrence ($p < 0.005$). Actuarial recurrence-free survival was better in the treatment group (log-rank $p < 0.018$), resulting in a relative risk reduction of 39% (95% confidence interval, 11–53%). No adverse events were reported.

In highly motivated young patients with recurrent vasovagal symptoms triggered by orthostatic stress, the prescription of progressively prolonged periods of enforced upright posture (so-called 'tilt training') may reduce syncope recurrence [149–151]. However, this treatment is hampered by the low compliance of patients in continuing the training programme for a long period and two randomized controlled trials failed to confirm short-term effectiveness of tilt training in reducing the positive response rate of the tilt test [152–155].

Many drugs have been used in the treatment of vasovagal syncope (beta-blockers, disopyramide, scopolamine, clonidine, theophylline, fludrocortisone, ephedrine, etilefrine, midodrine, serotonin reuptake inhibitors, etc.). In general, although the results have been satisfactory in uncontrolled trials or short-term controlled trials, long-term placebo-controlled prospective trials have failed to show any benefit of the active drug over placebo. Beta-adrenergic blocking drugs have failed to be effective in five of six long-term follow-up controlled studies [156–161]. Vasoconstrictor drugs are potentially more effective in orthostatic hypotension caused by autonomic dysfunction than in the neurally mediated syncope [162–164]. However, etilefrine proved to be ineffective in a large randomized double-blind trial [45]. To date, there are insufficient data to support the use of any other pharmacological therapy for vasovagal syncope.

Pacing for vasovagal syncope has been the subject of five major multicentre randomized controlled trials which gave contrasting results [165–169]; in all the patient the pre-implant selection was based on tilt-testing response. Adding together the results of the five trials, 318 patients were evaluated; syncope recurred in 21% of the paced patients and in 44% of unpaced patients ($p < 0.001$). The sub-optimal results are not surprising if we consider that pacing may affect the cardioinhibitory component of the vasovagal reflex, but will have no effect on the vasodepressor component, which is often dominant. The ISSUE 2 study [27] hypothesized that spontaneous asystole and not tilt test results should form the basis for patient selection for pacemaker therapy. This study followed 392 patients with presumed vasovagal syncope with an ILR. Of the 102 patients with a symptom-rhythm correlation, 53 underwent loop recorder guided therapy, predominantly pacing for asystole. These patients experienced a striking reduction in recurrence of syncope compared with non-loop recorder guided therapy (10% vs. 41%, p = 0.002). In summary, pacing plays a minimal role in therapy for vasovagal syncope, unless spontaneous bradycardia is detected during prolonged monitoring.

Cardiac pacing appears to be beneficial in carotid sinus syndrome [170–173] and, although only two relatively small randomized controlled trials have been undertaken, pacing is acknowledged to be the treatment of choice when bradycardia has been documented [32, 174]. Single-chamber atrial pacing is not appropriate for carotid sinus syndrome and dual-chamber pacing is generally preferred over single-chamber ventricular pacing [175, 176].

Orthostatic hypotension and orthostatic intolerance syndromes

Although there is a range of aetiologies that lead to orthostatic intolerance (see ➲Table 26.3), the global strategy aims to counteract the orthostatic stress which is the common denominator leading to symptoms. Since they have the same final mechanism in common, they also share similar therapies. Contrary to reflex syncope in which syncope and pre-syncope are largely the prevalent symptoms, the syndromes of orthostatic intolerance are characterized by frequent non-syncopal posture-related symptoms (dizziness, fatigue, weakness, palpitations, hearing disturbances, etc.) and syncope occurs less frequently. The goal of therapy is primarily prevention of recurrence and associated injuries, and improvement in quality of life.

In general, initial treatment comprises education regarding awareness and possible avoidance of triggers (e.g. hot crowded environments, volume depletion), early recognition of premonitory symptoms, and performing manoeuvres to abort the episode (e.g. supine posture, PCMs as described in Reflex syncope). Drug-induced autonomic failure is probably the most frequent cause of orthostatic hypotension. The principal treatment strategy is elimination of the offending agents, mainly diuretics and vasodilators. Alcohol is also commonly associated with orthostatic intolerance.

Additional treatment principles, used alone or in combination, are appropriate for consideration on an individual patient basis:

- chronic expansion of intravascular volume by encouraging a higher than normal salt intake and fluid intake of 2–2.5L/day [177];
- tilt training in young patients with recurrent vasovagal symptoms triggered by orthostatic stress (see Reflex syncope);
- fludrocortisone in low dose (0.1–0.2mg/day) [178];
- raising the head of the bed on blocks to permit gravitational exposure during sleep [178, 179];
- reduce vascular volume into which gravitation-induced pooling occurs by use of abdominal binders and/or waist-height support stockings or garments [13, 180];
- use of drugs which increase peripheral resistance (midodrine, 5–15mg three times a day) [181, 182].

Personal perspective

In the evaluation of patients with syncope, the critical first step is initial evaluation. A diagnostic strategy based on initial evaluation is warranted. In this regard, the development and evaluation of thoughtful, evidence-based (when possible), diagnostic guidelines for the evaluation of syncope patients has been of great support.

The ultimate goal of diagnostic testing is to establish a sufficiently strong correlation between syncope and detected abnormalities. Knowledge of what occurs during a spontaneous syncopal episode is ideally the gold standard for syncope evaluation. For this reason, it is likely that prolonged electrocardiographic monitoring (external and implantable) will become increasingly important in the assessment of the syncope patient and their use will increasingly be appropriate instead of, or before, many current conventional investigations. This early monitoring approach implies the need for careful initial risk stratification in order to exclude from such a strategy patients with potential life-threatening conditions. Ultimately, technology may allow recording of multiple signals in addition to the ECG (e.g. blood flow or pressure and EEG) and the automatic immediate wireless transmission of pertinent data to a central monitoring station. Such advances will permit greater emphasis on the documenting and characterizing of spontaneous episodes. Conversely, they will result in less reliance for current diagnostic testing techniques which are largely designed to assess susceptibility to the provocation of syncope in the laboratory.

Nevertheless, despite the implementation of several clinical guidelines and technological advances, current strategies for the assessment of T-LOC of suspect syncopal nature vary widely among physicians and among hospitals. Evaluation and treatment of T-LOC are often haphazard and unstratified. This results in inappropriate use of diagnostic tests and in a number of misdiagnosed and still unexplained syncope. It is the view of the European Society of Cardiology Syncope Task Force that a cohesive, structured care pathway—either delivered within a single syncope facility or as a more multifaceted service—is the optimal for quality service delivery. Furthermore, considerable improvement in diagnostic yield and cost effectiveness (i.e. cost per reliable diagnosis) can be achieved by focusing skills and following well defined, standardized care pathways.

Where possible, relying on controlled clinical trials confirmed observations is the most reliable approach to the care of patients, including those with apparent T-LOC/syncope. Clinical trials in recent years have reported important clinical evidence in several areas. Some of these are:

- Further evidence of failure of pharmacological therapy to prevent syncopal recurrences in patients with vasovagal syncope.
- Efficacy of physical counter-pressure therapies in preventing syncopal recurrences in patients with vasovagal syncope. Uncertainty still persists for tilt-training
- Efficacy of specific therapy guided by ILRs in preventing syncopal recurrences in patients with suspected neurally mediated syncope.

While the current knowledge on pathophysiology and diagnosis of syncope is satisfactory, we still have few evidence-based data on prognosis and efficacy of treatment. In particular future research fields should focus on:

- Assessing the prognostic value determined by occurrence of syncope in patients with inherited syndromes (e.g. long QT syndrome, Brugada syndrome, etc.) and the benefit of specific therapy, i.e. ICD, by means of controlled trials.
- Assessing the prognostic value determined by occurrence of syncope in patients with structural heart disease and the benefit of specific therapy, i.e. ICD, by means of controlled trials.
- Evaluating the efficacy of any therapy of reflex syncope by means of double-blind randomized controlled trials.

Further reading

Benditt DG, Blanc JJ, Brignole M (eds.) *et al. The Evaluation and Treatment of Syncope. A Handbook for Clinical Practice*, 2nd edn., 2006. New York: Blackwell Futura.

Brignole M, Alboni P, Benditt D, *et al.* Guidelines on management (diagnosis and treatment) of syncope: Update 2004. *Europace* 2004; **6**: 467–537.

Brignole M, Alboni P, Benditt D, *et al.* Guidelines on management (diagnosis and treatment) of syncope: Update 2004. Executive summary and recommendations. *Eur Heart J* 2004; **25**: 2054–72.

Brignole M, Vardas P, Hoffman E, *et al.* EHRA Position Paper: Indications for the use of diagnostic implantable and external ECG loop recorders. *Europace* 2009; **11**: 671–87.

Huff JS, Decker WW, Quinn J, *et al.* Clinical policy: critical issues in the evaluation and management of adult patients presenting to the emergency department with syncope. *Ann Emerg Med* 2007; **49**: 431–44.

Linzer M, Yang EH, Estes NA 3rd, *et al.* Diagnosing syncope. Part II: Unexplained syncope. *Ann Intern Med* 1997; **127**: 76–86.

Moya A, *et al.* Guidelines on management (diagnosis and treatment) of syncope. *Eur Heart J* in press.

Vardas PE, Auricchio A, Blanc J-J, *et al.* Guidelines for cardiac pacing and cardiac resynchronization therapy. The Task Force for cardiac pacing and cardiac resynchronization therapy of the European Society of Cardiology. Developed in collaboration with the European Heart Rhythm Association. *Eur Heart J* 2007; **28**: 2256–95.

Zipes DP, Camm AJ, Borggrefe M, *et al.* ACC/AHA/ESC 2006 guidelines for management of patients with ventricular arrhythmias and the prevention of sudden cardiac death. *Eur Heart J* 2006; **27**: 2099–140.

➲ **For full references and multimedia materials please visit the online version of the book (http://esctextbook.oxfordonline.com).**

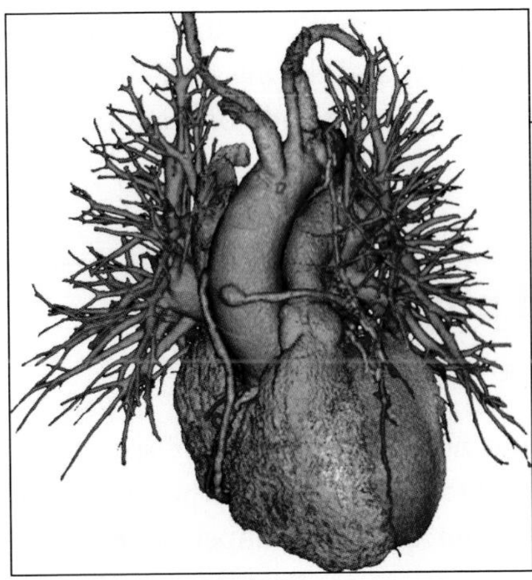

CHAPTER 27

Bradycardia

Panos E. Vardas, Hercules E. Mavrakis, and William D. Toff

Contents

Summary

Bradycardia is a common clinical finding, which requires careful and thorough assessment to correctly establish the underlying diagnosis and determine the appropriate therapy. Bradycardia is often a benign condition requiring no intervention, but when it gives rise to symptoms or results from conduction abnormalities that are associated with an adverse prognosis, cardiac pacing may be required unless a reversible and remediable cause can be identified. An accurate electrocardiographic diagnosis, consideration of the clinical context, and confirmation of a temporal association with any symptoms are the essential first steps to determine the appropriate therapy.

When permanent pacing is required, selection of the appropriate pacing mode and careful attention to pacemaker programming are needed to ensure an optimal clinical outcome. New insights from randomized trials have provided an evidence base to guide pacemaker mode selection and paved the way for increasingly physiological pacing, preserving whenever possible the natural sequence of cardiac activation and contraction. With an increasingly vast array of sophisticated pacemakers and pacing functions, sound clinical experience and judgement are essential to ensure the delivery of effective therapy and to minimize the risk of complications. Appropriately treated, the vast majority of patients can expect to enjoy full relief of symptoms and return to normal activity with a good quality of life and no adverse impact on life expectancy.

Introduction

The word bradycardia, like so many in the medical lexicon, has its origins in the ancient Greek language. Etymologically, it is a compound of the adjective 'brady', meaning slow, and the word 'cardia', meaning heart. Today, the term 'bradycardia' is used to encompass all disturbances of cardiac rhythm that result in a reduction of the normal heart rate. Detailed study and improved understanding of impulse generation and the conduction system of the heart have enriched our knowledge and enabled the classification of bradycardia into different types, according to the location of the disturbance of electrical impulse formation or propagation (abnormalities of automaticity, conduction, or both).

In daily medical practice, bradycardia is a common finding that ranges from the usually benign sinus bradycardia to sinus arrest and complete atrioventricular block. It therefore represents a considerable clinical challenge for the physician, since its consequences cover the wide range from none to a fatal outcome. Before suitable therapy can be chosen for the individual patient, it is essential to perform a thorough diagnostic work-up to establish the type of bradycardia, to evaluate associated symptoms, to identify potentially reversible causes, and to estimate the risk of severe consequences.

Cardiac pacing has been used in the treatment of bradycardia since the early 1950s, and during that time both clinical practice and an impressive body of research have confirmed its effectiveness.

Anatomy and physiology of the basic rhythm of the heart

The wedge-shaped sinus node is a collection of specialized cells lying beneath the epicardial surface in the right atrial sulcus terminalis, at the junction of the superior vena cava and the right atrium (➲Fig. 27.1). Regular spontaneous depolarization (automaticity) of its P (pacemaker) cells leads via T (transition) cells to a coordinated electrical impulse that initiates depolarization, activation, and subsequent contraction of the surrounding atrial myocardial cells. The electrical impulse propagates through the atrial tissue and pathways of preferential conduction from the right atrium to the atrioventricular node as well as to the left atrium. The blood supply of the sinus node usually originates from the proximal right coronary artery [1–5].

The atrioventricular node is a subendocardial anatomical structure located in the low atrial septum, anterior to the ostium of the coronary sinus and directly above the insertion of the septal leaflet of the tricuspid valve, in the

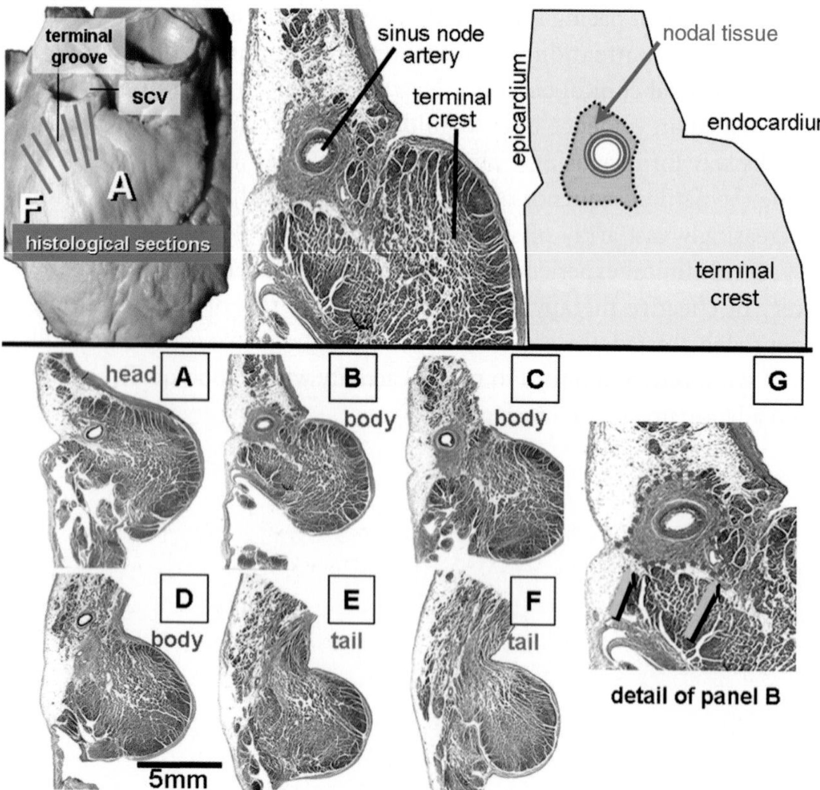

Figure 27.1 (Top) Gross specimen and example of a histological section accompanied by a diagram indicating the extent of the nodal tissue. (Bottom) Histological sections (Masson trichrome stain) taken through the levels A–F indicated on the gross specimen. (G) The red dotted line delineates the nodal boundaries. Note the irregular contour of the node and the extensions towards the neighbouring myocardium (arrows). SCV, superior caval vein. Reproduced from Sánchez-Quintana D, Cabrera JA, Farré J, *et al.* Sinus node revisited in the era of electroanatomical mapping and catheter ablation. *Heart* 2005; **91**: 189–94, with permission from BMJ Publishing Group Ltd.

anatomically defined triangle of Koch. It receives its blood supply from the atrioventricular nodal artery, a branch of the posterior descending artery, which arises from the right coronary artery in about 80% of cases, and from the circumflex coronary artery in the remainder. Automatic impulse formation may also occur in the atrioventricular node and gives rise to a junctional escape rhythm if the sinus node fails [4].

From the atrioventricular node, impulses are conducted to the bundle of His, which passes through the annulus fibrosus and penetrates the membranous interventricular septum, before separating into the left and right bundle branches (➲Fig. 27.2). The bundle of His is predominantly supplied by the atrioventricular nodal artery, but also receives a contribution from septal perforators arising from the left anterior descending coronary artery [5].

The right bundle branch crosses the anterior part of the interventricular septum and reaches the apex of the right ventricle and the base of the anterior papillary muscle. The left bundle branch, which is anatomically less discrete, typically subdivides into an anterosuperior and a postero-inferior fascicle, thereby creating a bifascicular system. Finally, the bundle branches ramify, giving rise to the endocardially located terminal Purkinje fibres, which ensure the activation of both ventricles [5].

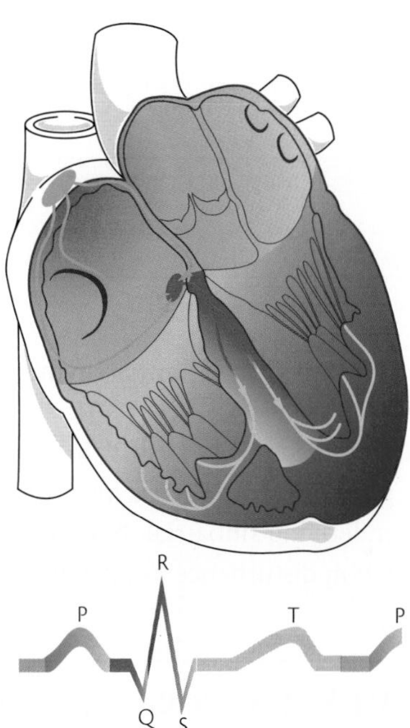

Figure 27.2 Electrical conduction system of the heart. The sinus node is located in the upper part of the right atrium between the superior vena cava and the right atrial appendage. Impulses from the sinus node are conducted to the atrioventricular node. From the atrioventricular node, impulses are conducted through the bundle of His. Below the bundle of His, the conduction system divides into the right and left bundle branches. While the right bundle is quite distinct the left bundle branch divides into one anterior and one posterior hemibranch.

The conduction system is richly innervated by the sympathetic and parasympathetic nervous systems at all levels (sinoatrial and junctional); these systems exert autonomic effects that ensure balanced control of the heart rate and intracardiac conduction [6–8]. Parasympathetic tone decreases sinus node automaticity and slows atrioventricular nodal conduction, while the sympathetic output increases automaticity and enhances conduction. An imbalance in the neurological control of the heart, as observed during vagal stimulation manoeuvres, after the administration of sympathomimetic or parasympathomimetic drugs, or as a consequence of central nervous system damage, prolonged ischaemia or infection, may therefore result in the development of bradyarrhythmias or tachyarrhythmias.

Definition of bradycardia

The baseline heart rate in an individual patient is determined predominantly by the balance between the parasympathetic and the sympathetic nervous systems. The 'normal' heart rate has been defined arbitrarily as 60–100 beats per minute (bpm) at rest, although a range of 50–90bpm has also been suggested [9]. Interestingly, the 'intrinsic' rate of the sinus node, after sympathetic and vagal blockade, is around 110bpm [10]. The heart rate may vary from patient to patient depending on age, training status, and the time of the observation [11]. In a healthy asymptomatic population, the 'normal' range of heart rates in the afternoon was found to be 46–93bpm in men and 51–95bpm in women [12–14], nocturnal rates being lower. At rest or during sleep, heart rates as low as 40bpm may be normal, even in healthy subjects. In contrast, sinus or atrial bradycardia <40bpm may be of concern in patients with sinus node dysfunction, especially if symptomatic [14]. The heart rate should fluctuate physiologically during respiration, with the Valsalva manoeuvre, and with other vagal influences, confirming normal autonomic control of the sinus node.

Bradycardia is a frequent finding in trained athletes (➲Chapter 32), and heart rates below 40bpm are often observed at rest [15–17]. Sinus pauses of up to 2.5s have been found in 10% of normal healthy individuals, pauses of >2s in 20% of athletes [15], and pauses of 2–3s in 37% of athletes during sleep [17]. However, even in athletes, pauses of >3s require further assessment, especially if associated with a history of syncope [18].

Another important component of the definition of bradycardia is the chronotropic response to exercise, which reflects the ability of the heart to accelerate according to the degree of exertion (➲Chapters 2 and 25). Chronotropic incompetence is characterized by an impaired heart rate response to exercise and is generally defined as failure to achieve 85% of the age-predicted maximum heart rate (defined as 220 minus age in years) at peak exercise. Chronotropic incompetence strongly suggests that a relative bradycardia may require further attention [9, 19–21].

During atrial fibrillation (➲Chapter 29), the ventricular rate is determined by atrioventricular nodal refractoriness. Affected patients warrant special consideration, as they exhibit greater beat-to-beat variability than patients in sinus rhythm [22]. During atrial fibrillation, daytime pauses of up to 2.8s and night-time pauses of up to 4.0s may be considered as within acceptable limits, if well tolerated by the patient [23].

Reflecting on these points, at the individual patient level, bradycardia may be defined as an inappropriately low heart rate in relation to age, gender, activity level, and physical training status. Clinical attention is required only if bradycardia is associated with symptoms, at rest or during exercise, that are troublesome or put the patient at risk.

Causes of bradycardia

Bradycardia may be caused by a variety of intrinsic and extrinsic influences on the heart or by damage to the sinus node or conduction system. Numerous causes have been identified, as shown in ➲Table 27.1. When the pathophysiology is judged to be fully reversible—for example in the case of drug effects (the most frequently identified form of reversible bradycardia) or electrolyte disturbances—or most likely reversible, as in myocardial ischaemia or inflammation, bradycardia should be treated initially without permanent implantable device therapy. Of course, in daily practice, the nature of disturbances of impulse formation and conduction are often ambiguous and the permanence of the condition may be unclear. However, early identification of a potentially reversible cause of bradycardia is the first step towards treatment. Drug interactions and competition for metabolic pathways or elimination routes may promote the negatively chronotropic and bathmotropic effects of drugs. Bathmotropic, (derived from the Greek word 'bathmos', meaning degree or threshold), refers to modification of the degree of excitability of heart musculature. Drugs that have a negative bathmotropic effect include beta-blockers, quinidine, and other class IA antiarrhythmic agents, and calcium channel blockers.

Even locally instilled drugs, such as beta-blockers for the treatment of glaucoma, may cause bradycardia and reveal or aggravate underlying sinoatrial dysfunction or atrioventricular conduction disturbance in susceptible patients [24].

Table 27.1 Causes of bradycardia

Intrinsic causes
Idiopathic degeneration (ageing)
Ischaemic heart disease
Infiltrative diseases: sarcoidosis [25, 26], amyloidosis [27], haemochromatosis [28]
Collagen vascular diseases: systemic lupus erythematosus [29], rheumatoid arthritis, [30], scleroderma
Myotonic muscular dystrophy
Surgical trauma: valve replacement, heart transplantation [31], arteriography
Congenital diseases, including sinus node and atrioventricular node disease
Infectious diseases: Chagas' disease [32, 33], diphtheria, endocarditis, Gram-negative sepsis, typhoid fever [33]
Extrinsic causes
Physical training (sports), possibly via increased vagal tone
Vagal hypertonicity: vasovagal syncope, carotid-sinus hypersensitivity
Vagal hyper-reactivity: coughing, micturition, defecation, vomiting, eye surgery
Negatively chronotropic and/or bathmotropic drugs: beta-blockers, calcium channel, blockers, clonidine, digoxin, lithium, antiarrhythmic agents (amiodarone, propafenone), including topical application [24]
Drug abuse: cocaine [34]
Electrolyte imbalance: hypokalaemia or hyperkalaemia
Metabolic disorders: hypothyroidism, hypothermia, anorexia nervosa [35, 36]
Neurological disorders: increased intracranial pressure, central nervous system
Neurological disorders: increased intracranial pressure, central nervous system tumours
Obstructive sleep apnoea [37, 38]

Clinical and electrocardiographic findings in patients with bradycardia

Signs and symptoms

Bradycardia is a frequent finding in daily medical practice. The clinical challenge is to separate those patients who are symptomatic, at risk of complications (low cardiac output, heart failure, syncope), and in need of further investigation from those who are healthy, in whom the bradycardia is physiological [12–15, 18].

Eventual symptoms depend on cardiac output, defined as the product of left ventricular stroke volume and heart rate. As long as changes in stroke volume compensate for the decrease in heart rate, even patients with profound bradycardia may remain asymptomatic, the disorder only being detected as an incidental finding on clinical examination or on an electrocardiogram (ECG) performed for other reasons [16, 17].

At the other end of the clinical spectrum, the patient with bradycardia may present with a variety of signs and symptoms. The most dramatic symptom is syncope or near syncope, although cardiac standstill of >6s is generally required before complete loss of consciousness will occur [39]. However, symptoms are often non-specific and chronic: for example, transient dizziness, light-headedness or confusional states, reflecting cerebral hypoperfusion due to decreased cardiac output, or episodes of fatigue or muscular weakness with exercise intolerance. Overt heart failure, at rest or on exercise, may also result from underlying bradycardia, especially in patients with impaired left ventricular function. Bradyarrhythmia may also present with palpitation, which simply means a perception of the beating heart. The patient may describe 'pauses' or 'strong beats', which are often manifestations of premature beats or just increased awareness of the action of the heart during a period of emotional sensitivity.

Whatever the patient's presenting symptoms, a causal relationship should only be inferred from the temporal coincidence of documented bradyarrhythmic episodes and the symptoms, whether these are specific or not. This is of particular importance with regard to patients' expectations of treatment benefits.

Sinus node disease

Sinus node disease, also known as sick sinus syndrome, is a common cause of bradycardia and designates a spectrum of sinoatrial dysfunction that ranges from the usually benign sinus bradycardia to sinus arrest or to the so-called bradycardia–tachycardia syndrome. The latter, is characterized by the development of paroxysmal atrial tachyarrhythmias alternating with periods of slow atrial and ventricular rates in patients with sinus bradycardia or sinoatrial block [40, 41].

Other manifestations of sinus node disease include: serious, persistent, and otherwise inexplicable sinus bradycardia; sinus arrest with ectopic atrial or nodal escape rhythms; paroxysmal or persistent atrial fibrillation secondary to sinus arrest; sinoatrial exit block; and inadequate chronotropic response to exercise. More than one of these conditions may be recorded in the same patient on different occasions. Sinus node disease, as a clinical entity, encompasses not only disorders of the sinus node impulse formation or its conduction to the right atrium, but also a more widespread intra-atrial conduction abnormality that is the substrate for the development of atrial tachyarrhythmias. In addition, some patients with sinus node dysfunction may also present atrioventricular node conduction abnormalities, in which case the term 'bi-nodal disease' is used [42, 43]. In order to define the structural basis of the sick sinus syndrome and its various clinical and electrocardiographic manifestations, there is a need for adequately controlled pathological studies that are presently lacking. The sinus node tissue is widely distributed at the junction between the superior vena cava and the right atrium, which suggests that the development of significant sinus node disease may require a diffuse disturbance of atrial architecture.

Sinus bradycardia is defined by sinus node depolarization at a rate <60bpm, with normal P waves before each QRS complex. Sinus bradycardia is a common and usually benign finding. Transient sinus bradycardia may be observed in patients after myocardial infarction and also following resuscitation from cardiac arrest, in which context it is associated with a poor prognosis [44].

Sinus pauses (standstill of >150% of cardiac cycle length) may be due to failure of impulse formation in the sinus node (sinus arrest) or a failure of conduction out of the nodal region to the surrounding atrium (sinoatrial exit block). In pauses due to sinoatrial exit block, the P–P interval during the pause is typically a multiple of the basic P–P interval, whereas in sinus arrest no such relationship is seen (➲Fig. 27.3A).

Although sinus pauses or arrest may have no intrinsic clinical significance, the emergence of surrogate atrial or nodal pacemaker escape rhythms to prevent ventricular asystole increases the risk of atrial fibrillation or flutter, thromboembolic events [45], and bradycardia–tachycardia syndrome. The latter, is usually symptomatic, since the overdrive suppression of sinus automaticity during the tachycardic phase [46] may result in long pauses due to increased sinus node recovery time and syncope when tachycardia terminates. In addition, attempts to decrease the rapid heart rate (e.g. with beta-blockers or digitalis) may further depress the sinus node or atrioventricular conduction and accentuate the abnormality.

Sinus node disease is not thought to have an adverse effect on survival unless other prognostically important

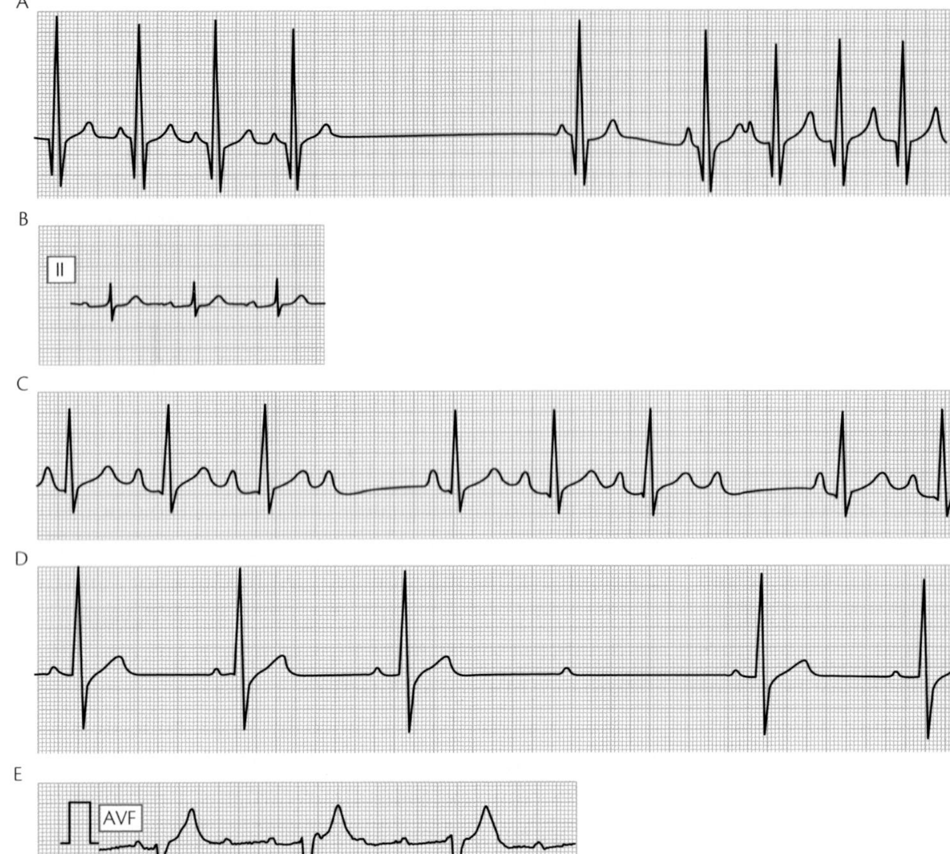

Figure 27.3 ECG appearance in sinus node disease and different types of atrioventricular block. (A) Sinus arrest. (B) First-degree atrioventricular block. (C) Mobitz type I second-degree atrioventricular block. (D) Mobitz type II second-degree atrioventricular block. (E) Third-degree atrioventricular block.

conditions are present, such as myocardial ischaemia, heart failure or systemic embolism. Permanent pacing is thus only required for the relief of symptoms that are due to bradycardia [43, 47].

Atrioventricular conduction disturbances

Atrioventricular conduction disturbances may occur at any level, from the atrioventricular junction down to the intraventricular conduction system. They include varying degrees of block in the atrioventricular node, the His bundle, the right or left bundle branches, and/or the anterior and posterior divisions of the left bundle branch (left anterior or left posterior fascicular block). Block may either occur at a single site or affect two or more components of the conduction system [48]. The atrioventricular node and the His bundle are particularly sensitive to ischaemia and traumatic injury, as they constitute a narrow preferential conduction pathway between the atria and the ventricles.

In atrioventricular block, atrial activation is conducted to the ventricles with a delay, or is not conducted at all, during a period when the atrioventricular conduction pathway (atrioventricular node or His–Purkinje system) is not expected to be refractory. Traditionally, based on electrocardiographic criteria, atrioventricular block is classified as first-, second-, or third-degree, while depending on the anatomical point at which the conduction of the activation wave front is impaired, it is described as supra-Hisian, intra-Hisian, or infra-Hisian.

Atrioventricular block

In first-degree atrioventricular block, every atrial stimulus is conducted to the ventricles, but the PR interval is prolonged to >200ms (➲Fig. 27.3B). The conduction delay may occur at the level of the atrioventricular node or the His–Purkinje system. If the QRS complex is narrow, the conduction delay is usually in the atrioventricular node and rarely within the His bundle. If the QRS complex is wide, the conduction delay may be either in the atrioventricular node or in the His–Purkinje system and only a His bundle electrogram can locate it precisely. First-degree atrioventricular block does not cause bradycardia unless it progresses intermittently to second- or third-degree block, or is associated with sinus node dysfunction. In patients with an anterior myocardial infarction and a conduction disturbance located below the bundle of His, first-degree block may progress to complete infra-Hisian block and lead to ventricular asystole, whereas inferior infarction is more often associated with the relatively benign intranodal and atropine-sensitive block [48–52].

Second-degree atrioventricular block is characterized by the failure to conduct one or more atrial stimuli to the ventricles. It is classified as either Mobitz type I (Wenckebach) or type II:

- Mobitz type I second-degree atrioventricular block (or Wenckebach block) is characterized by PR intervals that increase progressively until a P wave is not conducted (➲ Fig. 27.3C). During the following cycle, the PR interval resumes its original value and progressively increases again until the next P wave is blocked. Observation of the jugular venous pulse may reveal repetitive sudden loss of the 'v' wave, corresponding to the ventricular pause, despite the persistence of an 'a' wave. This type of block rarely manifests with syncope. The delay is usually in the atrioventricular node and deterioration to a higher degree of atrioventricular block is uncommon. However, in cases with a wide QRS complex an electrophysiological study is needed to determine the level of the block [53, 54].
- Mobitz type II second-degree atrioventricular block is characterized by abrupt conduction failure and, provided there is normal sinus rhythm, the PR interval is constant before and after the blocked P wave (➲ Fig. 27.3D). Mobitz type II block generally originates from an infra-Hisian lesion, may be associated with a wide QRS complex, often progresses abruptly to complete atrioventricular block, and frequently manifests with syncope [53, 54].

Third-degree atrioventricular block (complete heart block) is characterized by the complete dissociation of atrial and ventricular activity, each following its own rhythm. In this type of block no atrial stimulus is conducted to the ventricles and the ventricles are depolarized by an escape rhythm (➲ Fig. 27.3E). Usually symptomatic, the patient may have signs and symptoms related to reduced cardiac output, such as syncope or dyspnoea.

Although the escape rate may have significance for the development of symptoms, the site of escape rhythm origin (i.e. in the atrioventricular node, intra-, or infra-Hisian) is of major importance for the patient's safety. The nature of the escape rhythm may provide an indication of the location of the block: a sustained rhythm between 40–60bpm with narrow QRS complexes suggests a junctional rhythm associated with supra-Hisian block, whereas wide QRS complexes at a slower heart rate suggest block at a lower level in the His–Purkinje system and a more urgent need for therapeutic intervention [53, 54].

In the case of third-degree atrioventricular block, there is clinical evidence that permanent cardiac pacing improves survival [53], especially in patients who experience episodes of syncope, since third-degree atrioventricular block can also lead to aborted sudden cardiac death and/or torsade de pointes.

Intraventricular block

Intraventricular conduction delay (bundle branch block) at any level of the His–Purkinje system leads to the loss of synchronous ventricular activation and contraction. Intraventricular block may be fascicular (left anterior or left posterior hemiblock) leading to left intraventricular dyssynchrony, or it may affect the bundle branch itself (left or right bundle branch block) leading to interventricular dyssynchrony. The term 'bifascicular block' refers to an electrocardiographic picture of complete right bundle branch block with anterior or posterior left hemiblock, or complete left bundle branch block alone. The term 'trifascicular' block means impaired conduction in all three branches at the same time, or at different times, while it has also been used to describe bifascicular block together with first-degree atrioventricular block. The term 'alternating bundle branch block' refers to electrocardiographically demonstrated block of all three branches on the same or successive ECG recordings [53, 54].

Different types of block may be isolated or combined, rate dependent or not, and may indicate an increased risk for the development of high-degree atrioventricular block [55]. However, in the absence of demonstrated atrioventricular block or unexplained symptoms suggestive of bradycardia, isolated unifascicular or bifascicular block is not usually a major concern. The annual incidence of progression to high-degree atrioventricular block in unselected patients with delayed conduction in the left or right bundle branches is estimated to be 1–4% [56, 57–60], while syncope has been found to be the sole predictive factor. The annual incidence of progression is 5–11% in syncopal patients, but just 0.6–0.8% in patients without syncope [61, 62].

In patients with bi- or trifascicular block the results of studies that employed an electrophysiological study have shown that the finding of a His–ventricular conduction time >100ms, or the demonstration of intra- or infra-Hisian block during incremental atrial pacing at a rate <150bpm, is highly predictive for the development of high-grade atrioventricular block, but the prevalence of these findings is very low and hence so is their sensitivity [55, 60, 63, 64].

Diagnostic approach to the bradycardic patient

Successful management of bradycardia depends on identification of the right treatment for the right patient, always remembering the option not to treat if there is no need. The aim of the diagnostic work-up is to identify those patients in whom bradycardia impacts upon quality of life and/or puts them at risk of potentially severe complications, such as syncope, heart failure, arrhythmias with embolic risk, or sudden death.

Patient evaluation begins with a detailed history, including an attempt to identify potentially reversible causes of bradycardia (with a specific focus on drug treatments, including non-cardiovascular drugs), followed by physical examination, including careful cardiac auscultation. Commonly reported symptoms include palpitation, presyncope or syncope, and dyspnoea or fatigue. These symptoms may be paroxysmal or chronic, may be triggered or aggravated by physical exercise, or may occur only in specific situations (e.g. during the night). The standard baseline 12-lead ECG completes the initial diagnostic phase and may usefully be combined with a Valsalva manoeuvre, carotid sinus massage, and tilt testing, which may give more detailed information about autonomic function [39]. Exercise testing is often useful, as it may reveal chronotropic incompetence or reversibility of second-degree atrioventricular block in younger patients [19–21].

In patients with symptoms thought to be due to bradycardia, an important determinant of future therapeutic decisions will be to establish a causal relationship between symptoms and bradycardic episodes. The hierarchy of diagnostic testing depends upon sound clinical judgement, as some tests may be more appropriate than others to achieve a prompt and accurate diagnosis.

Long-term ECG recording

Holter recording

Ambulatory ECG recording (see ➲Chapter 2) over 24–48 hours is appropriate for patients with suspected intermittent symptomatic bradycardia in order to correlate the symptoms with the bradycardic episodes [65, 66]. Frequently identified forms of bradycardia, such as sinus bradycardia, first-degree atrioventricular block, and even second-degree Mobitz I (Wenckebach) atrioventricular block, may be considered as normal in young and/or well-trained subjects. However, the same findings may be considered as pathological if, for example, their appearance precipitates left ventricular decompensation with symptoms of heart failure. In contrast, evidence of sinus node disease, bradycardia–tachycardia syndrome, Mobitz II second-degree atrioventricular block, or third-degree atrioventricular block with ventricular pauses >3s, although less frequently seen, are always pathological. During atrial fibrillation, daytime pauses of up to 2.8s and night-time pauses of up to 4.0s may be considered as within acceptable limits, if well tolerated by the patient [23].

Event recorders and implantable loop recorders

Holter recording, even if prolonged to 48 hours, often fails to identify the cause of the patient's symptoms, especially if bradycardic episodes are intermittent, with prolonged periods of normal sinus rhythm and/or a paucity of symptoms. Two other diagnostic devices may help in such cases:

- Transient-event recorders may be kept for a month or more, allowing digital recording of the ECG for up to 30s initiated by the patient at the time he or she experiences symptoms. Despite the fact that this presupposes the patient remains conscious at the onset of the symptoms, the technique has been shown to be more efficacious and cost-effective than Holter recording in patients with intermittent palpitation [67]. Most modern loop recorders have the ability to record up to three ECG channels and are also capable of automatic triggering of event storage for bradycardic and arrhythmic events and automatic event transmission via Bluetooth mobile phone technology.
- Implantable loop recorders (➲Chapter 26) may be particularly useful in the investigation of infrequently recurring symptoms, especially if Holter and transient-event recorders have failed to establish the diagnosis. Implantable loop recorders allow patients to be monitored over a prolonged period, increasing the diagnostic yield to as much as 85% in syncope that is difficult to diagnose [68]. Because of the extended period of observation that it enables, exceeding 3 years in some instances, the implantable loop recorder has become a key contributor in establishing the temporal correlation with syncope in patients suspected to have infrequent underlying arrhythmia (➲Fig. 27.4). It has

been shown to be most useful in patients with infrequent unexplained syncope when non-invasive testing is negative [69].

Electrophysiological testing

Unexplained syncope may be due to sinus node dysfunction or atrioventricular block and is an indication for electrophysiological testing (➲Chapters 28 and 30) if non-invasive assessment fails to identify the aetiology [70]. Although the cause of syncope is identified in more than 50% of patients by non-invasive means (history, physical examination, ECG, Holter, loop recording), electrophysiological studies may be indicated in order to establish the cause in the remainder, especially in patients with known heart disease [71]. However, intermittent conduction disturbances are, by their nature, difficult to identify, even by electrophysiological testing [72], and the diagnosis may occasionally be inferred by exclusion of all other potential causes of syncope of cardiac origin.

Electrophysiological testing of sinus node function measures the sinus node recovery time, which is then corrected for the spontaneous sinus rate by subtraction of the sinus cycle length. The normal corrected sinus node recovery time (cSNRT) is <550ms and a longer recovery time is observed in patients with sinus node dysfunction. The prognostic value of prolonged sinus node recovery time is unknown. However, it is accepted that if cSNRT exceeds 800ms, sinus node disease may be the cause of syncope [53]. In all patients, the His bundle electrogram should be recorded to evaluate atrioventricular conduction, and the basic

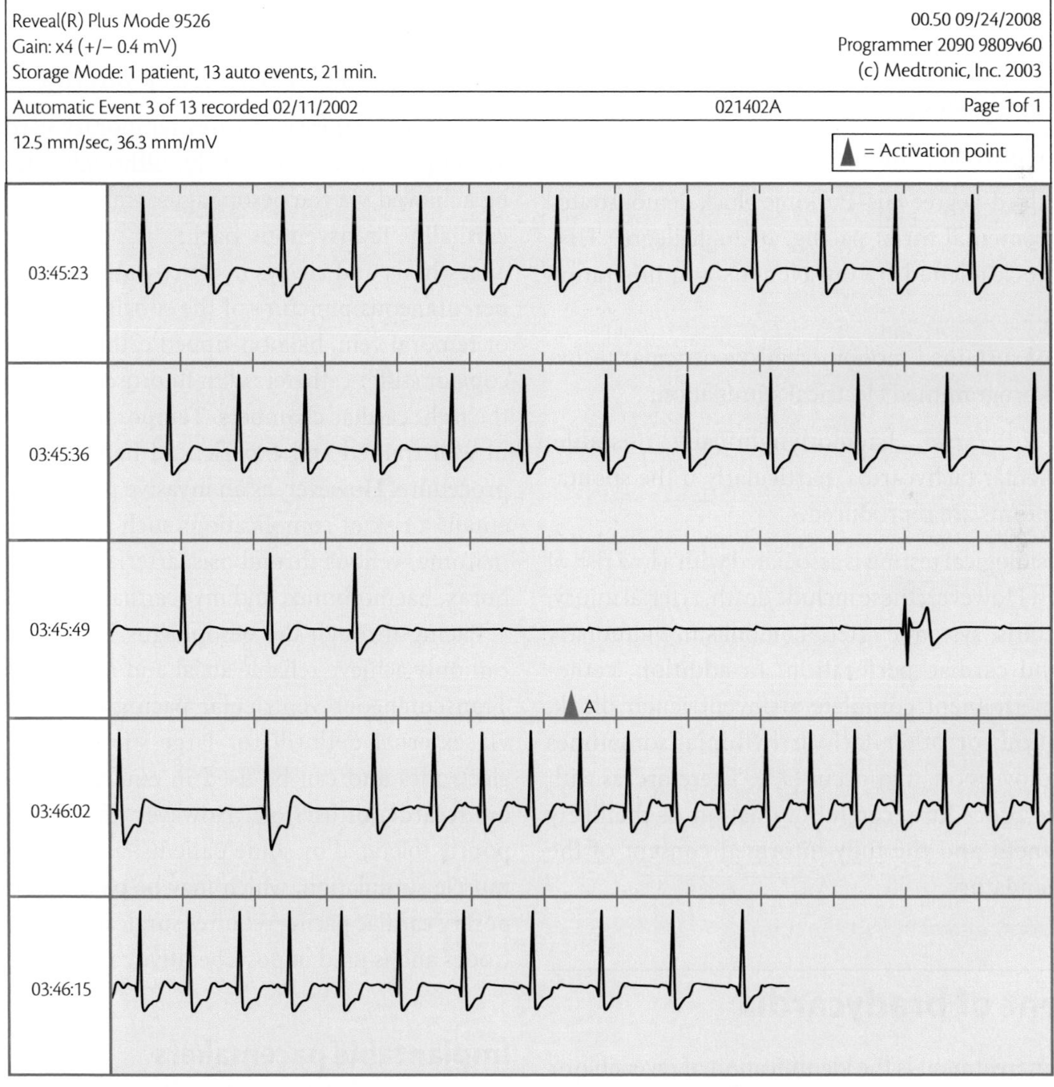

Figure 27.4 Implantable loop recordings showing third-degree atrioventricular block in a 68-year-old female patient with a 3-year history of recurrent syncopal episodes and negative electrophysiological study.

atrial–His (AH) and His–ventricular (HV) intervals should be measured since coexisting conduction disturbances are frequent. The normal values of AH and HV intervals in adults range from 60–125ms and 35–55ms, respectively.

Electrophysiological testing may be used for the elucidation of atrioventricular or intraventricular conduction disturbances when the level of the block cannot be established from the ECG. Electrophysiological studies may help to identify patients at high risk of progression to complete atrioventricular block, in whom implantation of a pacemaker may be required. Thus, in asymptomatic patients with bifascicular or trifascicular block, permanent pacing is considered appropriate only in those who exhibit intermittent second- or third-degree atrioventricular block, or signs of a severe conduction disturbance below the level of the atrioventricular node (HV >100ms, or intra- or infra-Hisian block during rapid atrial pacing) during an electrophysiological study (➲Fig. 27.5).

An electrophysiological study is considered normal in the absence of all the following:

- abnormal sinus node recovery time;
- baseline HV interval ≥70ms;
- second- or third-degree His–Purkinje block demonstrated during incremental atrial pacing, or high-degree His–Purkinje block elicited by intravenous administration of ajmaline;
- induction of sustained monomorphic ventricular tachycardia with programmed electrical stimulation;
- induction of rapid, haemodynamically unstable, supraventricular tachycardia, particularly if the spontaneous symptoms are reproduced.

Electrophysiological testing is associated with a low risk of complications. However, these include death, arterial injury, thrombophlebitis, systemic arterial embolism, pulmonary embolism, and cardiac perforation. In addition, catheter-induced permanent complete atrioventricular block, atrial fibrillation, or other tachyarrhythmia, sometimes requiring cardioversion, may occur [73]. Therefore, as with every invasive procedure, careful evaluation of the likely diagnostic benefit and the fully informed consent of the patient are mandatory.

Treatment of bradycardia

The first step in treatment is the identification of reversible or situational bradycardia and the elimination of causal drugs or other provocative factors whenever possible. In the absence of a remediable cause, drug therapy or treatment with a temporary or permanent pacemaker may be required.

Drug therapy

Treatment is usually not necessary in patients with sinus bradycardia, sinus bradyarrhythmia, sinus pauses, or sinus arrest shorter than 3s. For more significant bradycardia, intravenous atropine (0.5mg, repeated if necessary) or isoprenaline may be used to accelerate the heart rate and improve cardiac performance in the acute setting, although paradoxical reactions may rarely occur [74, 75]. Some patients with sick sinus syndrome may experience relief from bradycardic symptoms with oral theophylline [76] but this is rarely a reliable long-term therapy. Patients presenting with symptomatic sinus node disease and/or atrioventricular conduction disturbance should therefore be considered and evaluated for the implantation of a temporary or permanent artificial pacemaker.

Techniques of temporary pacing

In the vast majority of cases temporary cardiac pacing is accomplished transvenously, although pacing may also be achieved via the oesophagus, transcutaneously, or epicardially. Transvenous pacing is performed under local anaesthesia and always in strictly aseptic conditions. After percutaneous puncture of the subclavian, internal jugular, or femoral vein, balloon-tipped catheters without fluoroscopy or stiffer catheters with fluoroscopy are advanced into the right cardiac chambers. Temporary transvenous pacing in well-trained and experienced hands is a relatively safe procedure. However, as an invasive procedure, it inevitably entails a risk of complications such as infection, local haematoma, venous thrombosis, arterial puncture, pneumothorax, haemothorax, and myocardial perforation.

Pacing through the oesophagus is simple and safe but can only achieve reliable atrial and not ventricular pacing. Transcutaneous ventricular pacing can be accomplished via external defibrillator large-surface, high-impedance electrodes and can be used in emergency cases of severe bradycardia or asystole. However, this mode of pacing is poorly tolerated by some patients, as it also causes skeletal muscle stimulation, which may be painful. Epicardial temporary cardiac pacing requires surgical implantation of electrodes and is used in postoperative cardiac surgical patients.

Implantable pacemakers

Since the early 1950s, when pacemakers were large external devices used principally to ensure survival, implantable

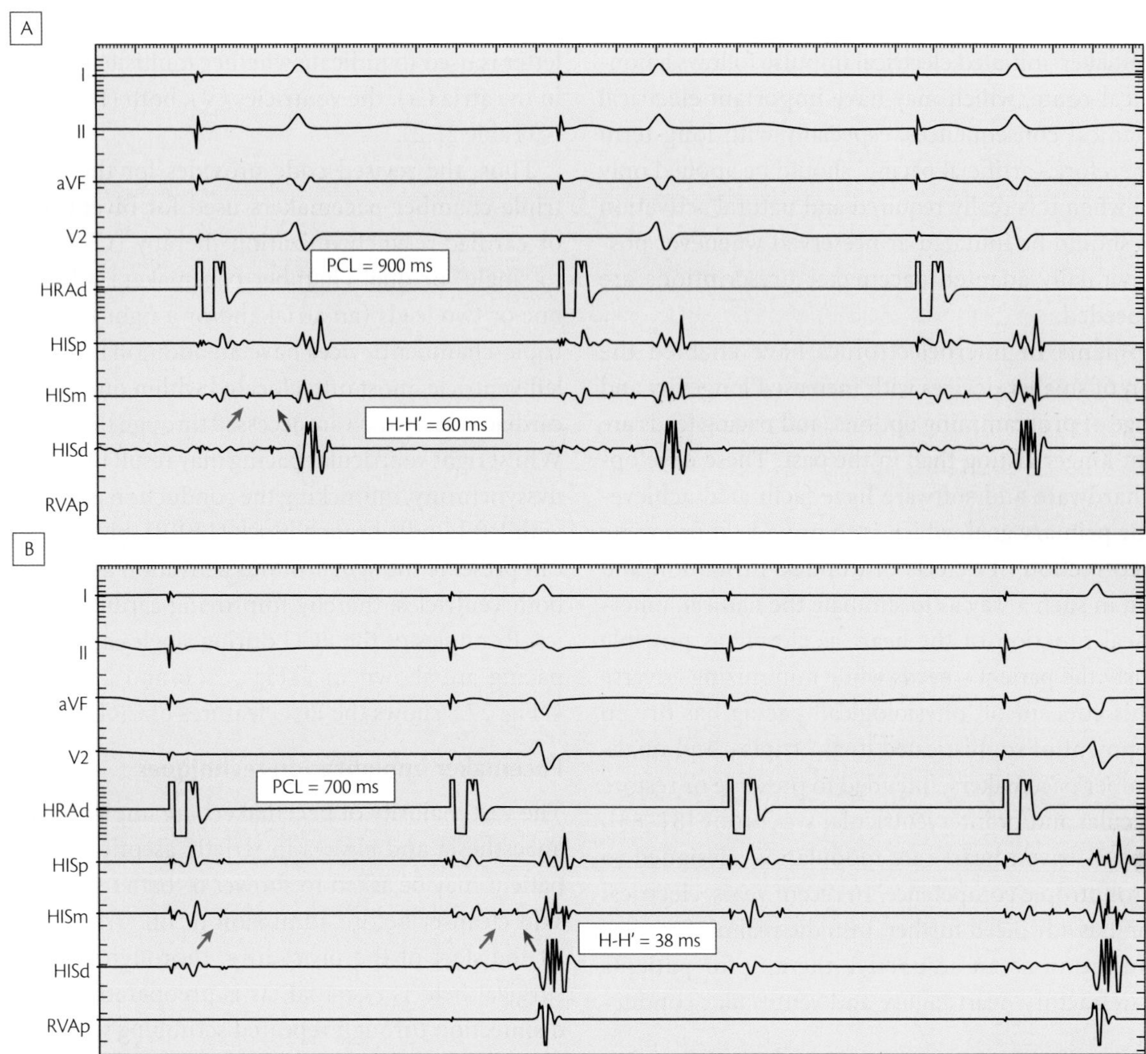

Figure 27.5 Electrophysiological study recordings showing intra-Hisian block provoked by rapid atrial pacing. Each panel shows four surface leads and intracardiac electrograms recording the high right atrium (HRAd), His-bundle region (proximal [HISp], mid [HISm], distal [HISd]), and right ventricular apex (RVAp). The H (green arrow) and H' (blue arrow) potentials are indicated. PCL = paced cycle length. (A) With an atrial paced cycle length of 900ms, split His potentials (H–H′) with an A–H interval of 75ms, H–H′ interval of 60ms, and H′–V interval of 42ms are seen. (B) With an atrial paced cycle length of 700ms, split His potentials are seen during conducted beats, but only the initial component (H) is present in during blocked beats, indicating intra-Hisian AV block. Reproduced with permission from Bilchick KC, Rade JJ, Marine JE. Change in H–H' interval during intrahisian block: What is the mechanism? *Heart Rhythm* 2007; **4**: 104–5.

pacemakers have become the gold standard for the treatment of symptomatic bradycardia with selected indications. The first pacemaker implantation into a human was performed in 1958 by Elmqvist and Senning [77], followed swiftly by the implantation of the first endocardial lead by Furman and Robinson [78]. In the two decades after the first successful implantation, the focus of research was on the development of more reliable power sources and leads. Today, millions of patients worldwide have an implanted pacemaker, and with increasingly sophisticated technology. According to a recently published world survey of cardiac pacing, there were >540,000 new pacemaker implantations in 2005 in the 43 countries involved and the number of new implants is continuing to rise [79]. However, there is considerable variability in the implant rate at both national and regional level. In the USA in 2007, there were approximately 880 new implants per million population, while in Western Europe, figures ranged from 419 per million (Ireland) to 1200 per million (Germany) [80]. These variations may partly reflect differences in the age distribution and morbidity of the relevant populations, but may also be related to the availability of resources, financial parameters, and variations in the implementation of published guidelines.

Implantable pacemakers deliver localized electrical stimulation of the cardiac tissue that propagates and activates the myocardium, leading to muscle contraction. The spread of the pacemaker-initiated electrical impulse follows a non-physiological route, which may have important electrical and mechanical consequences, especially with long-term pacing. Therefore, 'artificial pacing' should be applied only where and when it is really required and natural activation sequences should be imitated or preserved whenever possible. Individually-adapted pacemaker prescriptions are therefore needed.

Developments in microelectronics have enabled the production of smaller devices with increased longevity and a wide range of programming options, and pacing leads are thinner but longer lasting than in the past. These developments in hardware and software have facilitated achievement of the primary goal, which is to provide appropriate electrical correction of defects of impulse formation and conduction in such a way as to simulate the natural, inherent electrical function of the heart as closely as possible and to satisfy the patient's needs while minimizing adverse effects. This concept of 'physiological' pacing has driven the development of sophisticated dual-, triple-, and quadruple-chamber pacemakers, intended to preserve or restore atrioventricular and/or interventricular synchrony [81–83], and of sensor-driven heart rate modulation, designed to restore chronotropic competence. In recent years, electrical stimulation has advanced further, into the realm of cardiac resynchronization as an adjunctive therapy for patients with drug-refractory heart failure and ventricular conduction delay.

Current pacemaker nomenclature

The five-letter code for identifying pacemakers and pacing modes (NBG code) was established by the North American Society of Pacing and Electrophysiology (NASPE) and the British Pacing and Electrophysiology Group (BPEG) in 1987 [84] and revised in 2002 [85].

The first letter indicates the heart chamber(s) being paced (A, atrium; V, ventricle; D, both), the second letter the chamber(s) being sensed, and the third letter the response of the pacemaker upon sensing (T, triggered; I, inhibited; D, both). Thus, an AAI pacemaker paces in the atrium, senses in the atrium, and inhibits pacing if spontaneous electrical activity is sensed. A DDD pacemaker paces and senses both in the atrium and the ventricle and reacts in a dual fashion: an impulse sensed in the atrium inhibits atrial pacing and triggers ventricular pacing after a delay, mimicking the physiological atrioventricular conduction sequence. The fourth letter indicates the presence (R) or absence (O) of an adaptive-rate mechanism (rate responsiveness), which modulates the heart rate independently of intrinsic cardiac activity (e.g. during exercise). The fifth letter is used to indicate whether multisite pacing is present in the atria (A), the ventricles (V), both (D), or neither (O) (➲Table 27.2).

Thus, the revised code provides for the description of triple-chamber pacemakers used for biventricular pacing or cardiac resynchronization therapy (CRT). In contrast to single- or dual-chamber pacemakers, which have only one or two leads (an atrial and/or a right ventricular lead), triple-chamber devices have an additional lead to pace the left ventricle, most often located within one of the overlying cardiac veins, which are accessed through the coronary sinus. Whilst right ventricular pacing may result in interventricular dyssynchrony, mimicking the conduction pattern associated with left bundle branch block (LBBB), biventricular pacing can preserve the synchronous activation and contraction of both ventricles, thereby improving cardiac haemodynamics. Examples of the ECG during single- and dual-chamber pacing are shown in ➲Figs. 27.6 and 27.7, respectively. ➲Fig. 27.8 shows the ECG features of CRT.

Pacemaker implantation techniques

The vast majority of pacemakers are implanted under local anaesthesia and always in strictly aseptic conditions. The patient may be asked to shower or bath using an antiseptic skin cleanser before admission or on arrival on the ward. At the start of the procedure, thorough cleansing of the surgical field is essential, as is preoperative surgical hand disinfection through repeated scrubbing with an appropriate antiseptic. Perioperative systemic antibiotic prophylaxis is commonly used and may reduce the incidence of serious infective complications [86]. In patients who have cardiac

Table 27.2 NBG pacemaker code

I: chamber(s) paced	II: chamber(s) sensed	III: response to sensing	IV: rate modulation	V: multisite pacing
O, none	O, none	O, none	O, none	O, none
A, atrium	A, atrium	T, triggers pacing	R, rate modulation	A, atrium
V, ventricle	V, ventricle	I, inhibits pacing		V, ventricle
D, dual (A and V)	D, dual (A and V)	D, dual (T and I)		D, dual (A and V)
S*, single (A or V)	S*, single (A or V)			

* Used by manufacturers only and indicates that the device can be used in the atrium or the ventricle.

NBG is an acronym of the North American Society of Pacing and Electrophysiology, the British Pacing and Electrophysiology Group, Generic.

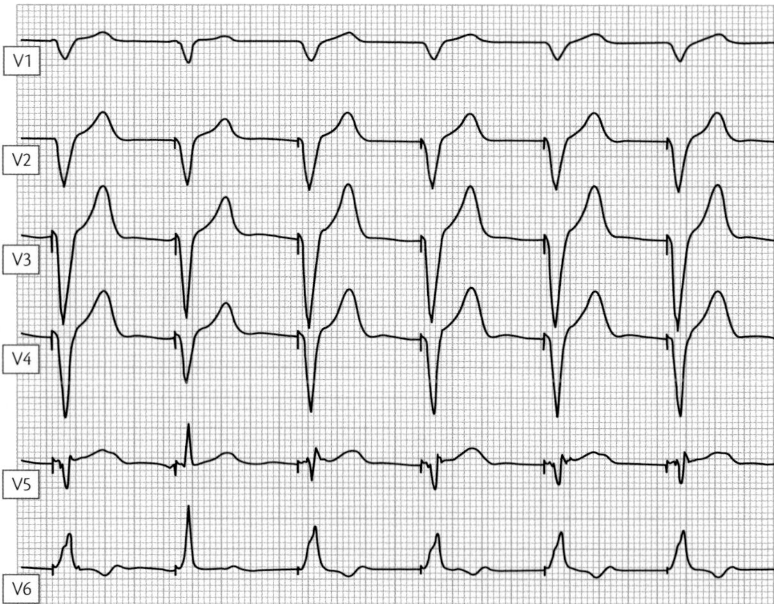

Figure 27.6 ECG during single-chamber ventricular pacing.

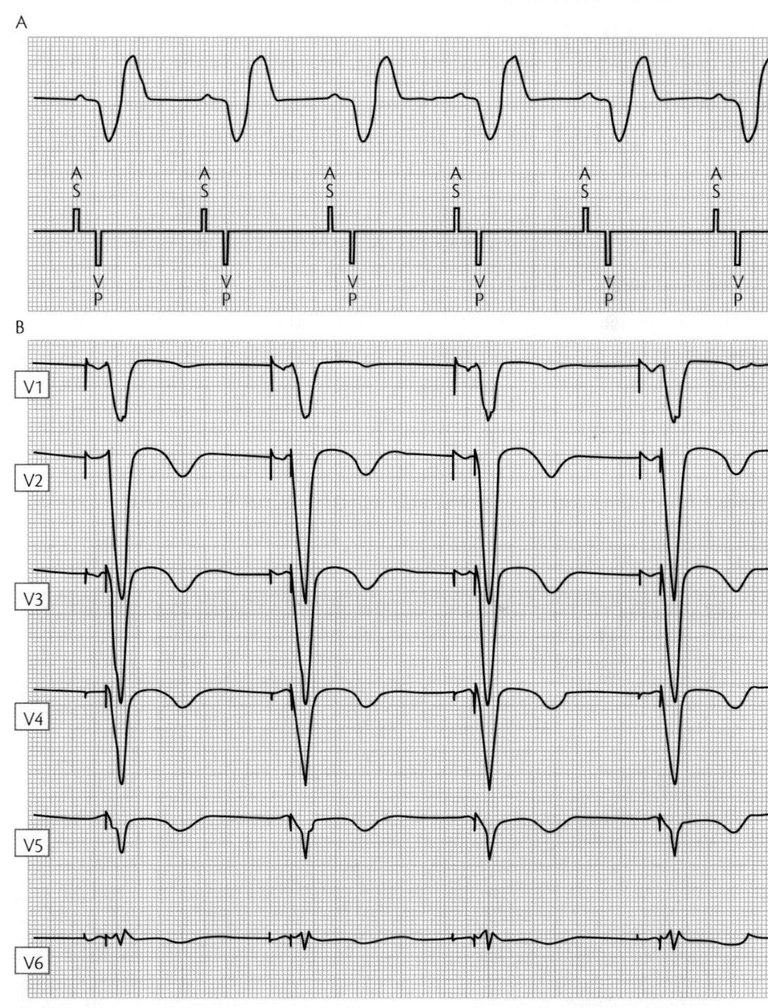

Figure 27.7 ECG during dual-chamber pacing. (A) ECG with simultaneous recording of pacemaker event markers showing atrial sensing (AS) of sinus rhythm and synchronized ventricular pacing (VP). (B) ECG showing synchronized atrial and ventricular pacing.

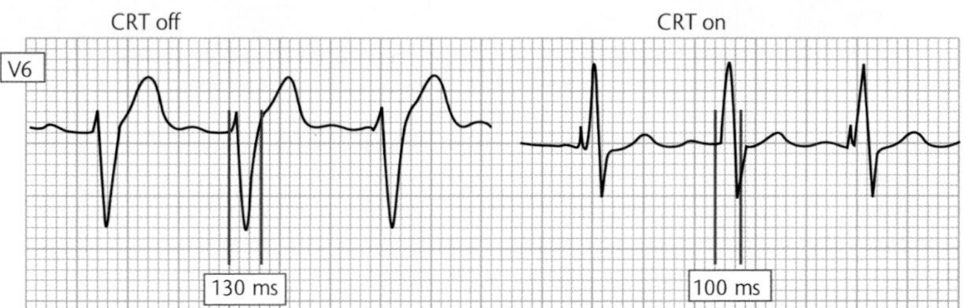

Figure 27.8 ECG features of cardiac resynchronization therapy (CRT), showing shortening of the QRS width.

valve prostheses or valve disease, chemoprophylaxis with suitable antibiotics is mandatory (for further details see ➲Chapter 22). The pacemaker is inserted into a subcutaneous pocket, which is fashioned in the anterior upper chest wall over the pectoralis major muscle. In patients without significant adipose tissue overlying the pectoralis major muscle, the sub-pectoral region can be used for pacemaker implantation [87]. The pacemaker leads are implanted transvenously using either exposure and cutdown of the cephalic vein or blind puncture of the subclavian vein, if the size of the cephalic vein is not sufficient to accommodate all of the pacing leads. Although the technique of blind subclavian puncture is potentially more hazardous than cephalic vein cutdown, in well-trained and experienced hands it is relatively safe [88]. This technique requires the initial insertion of a flexible guidewire followed by a subclavian vein introducer. Subsequently, special peel-away sheaths are used for the introduction of the pacemaker leads. The subclavian approach permits the easy implantation of two leads and reduces the duration of the implantation procedure. However, if pacemaker leads are inserted via medial subclavian puncture there is a possibility of compression damage (subclavian crush) due to the fact that the costo-clavicular angle is tight. Other possible complications of blind subclavian puncture are pneumothorax or haemothorax (<2% of implants), air embolism, subcutaneous emphysema, thoracic duct injury, and nerve injury [89, 90].

Another approach that can be used for transvenous pacemaker lead insertion is the axillary approach, in which the axillary vein is entered at the medial border of the pectoralis minor muscle. Since the axillary vein is extrathoracic, there is no risk of pneumothorax or haemopneumothorax. In certain cases, where transvenous access to the right ventricle is impossible (e.g. because of a congenital anomaly or the presence of a tricuspid valve prosthesis), epicardial leads may be used.

After implantation of the pacemaker leads, several intraoperative measurements are necessary. The most important are determination of the atrial and ventricular pacing thresholds and measurement of the lead impedance, and the amplitudes of atrial and ventricular electrograms. In addition, high voltage pacing (10V) should be used to assess possible diaphragmatic stimulation from the atrial or ventricular leads. Blood pressure measurement during ventricular pacing is also important in order to determine the possibility of pacemaker syndrome.

After the pacemaker implantation, upright anteroposterior and lateral chest radiographs are mandatory in order to confirm correct positioning of the pacing leads and rule out pneumothorax (➲Fig. 27.9). Before hospital discharge, a 12-lead ECG and a full pacemaker interrogation should be performed to confirm proper atrial and ventricular pacing and sensing.

Indications for pacemaker implantation

Although temporary or external pacemakers can be used for initial stabilization or, in the short term, for reversible or potentially reversible bradycardic episodes, the therapeutic

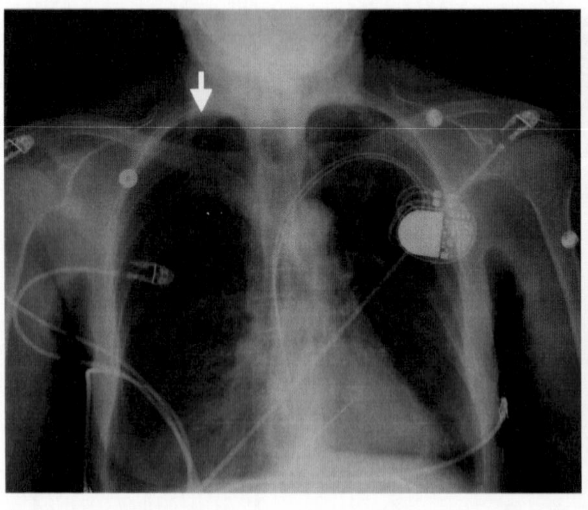

A

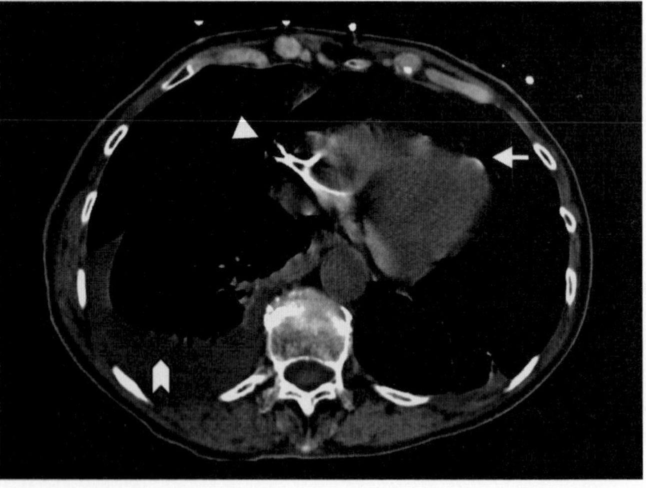

B

Figure 27.9 (A) Chest X-ray showing right pneumothorax (arrow) 8 hours after placement of a left-sided permanent dual-chamber pacemaker for symptomatic bradycardia. (B) Computed tomography scan of the chest showing extrusion of the helix of the atrial lead through the right atrial appendage (arrowhead) causing pneumopericardium (arrow). Right pleural effusion (chevron) is also seen. Reproduced with permission from Srivathsan K, Byrne RA, Appleton CP, *et al.* Pneumopericardium and pneumothorax contralateral to venous access site after permanent pacemaker implantation. *Europace* 2003; **5**: 361–3.

challenge is to identify the patient who will benefit from an implanted permanent pacemaker. The indications for permanent pacing are reviewed extensively in the guidelines for cardiac pacing and CRT published by a task force of the European Society of Cardiology (ESC) and developed in collaboration with the European Heart Rhythm Association [53] (➲Tables 27.3, 27.4, and 27.5). Similar guidelines have also been published by a joint task force sub-committee of the American College of Cardiology (ACC) and the American Heart Association (AHA) [91].

Evidence-based choice of optimal pacing mode

Once the decision to implant a pacemaker is made, the appropriate pacing mode and type of pacing system must be selected. The choice will be influenced by the primary indication for pacing and by the patient's general health status and anticipated level of activity.

Each indication encompasses a wide variety of patients and the therapeutic goal is to provide the most appropriate device and optimal programming for each individual patient. Cardiologists, electrophysiologists, and engineers have developed increasingly sophisticated devices, often exploring the frontiers of physiological knowledge while pushing back the limits of the technical possibilities. The clinical benefit of pacemaker therapy, when first introduced for the treatment of Morgagni–Adams–Stokes attacks [92], was dramatic. Today the indications for permanent pacing have broadened and there has been a proliferation of device types, pacing modes and programming options. This has heralded an era in which the effect magnitudes of new developments have become less dramatic, albeit still of potential clinical relevance. Continuing improvements in technology and optimized treatment options will result from innovative thinking and the accumulation of evidence from well-designed randomized clinical trials.

For patients with normal atrial activity, dual-chamber atrioventricular synchronous pacing (DDD) has been shown to be haemodynamically superior to ventricular pacing (VVI), mainly as a result of the preservation or restoration of the atrial contribution to left ventricular filling. This leads to increased stroke volume and improved cardiac output through optimization of the cardiac cycle, with timely closure of the atrioventricular valves. In the absence of atrioventricular synchrony, the coincidence of atrial and ventricular contraction may lead to an abrupt fall in blood pressure and a variety of symptoms, comprising the pacemaker syndrome (discussed in later sections). However, not all patients develop pacemaker syndrome with VVI pacing and some patients have no increase in cardiac output with DDD pacing, observations which may be explained, at least partially, by inter-individual variation in left ventricular filling pressure and the ability of stroke volume to adapt rapidly [93]. In daily practice, however, DDD pacing has been perceived as the best option for most patients, with regard to functional capacity and quality of life.

Table 27.3 Recommendations for cardiac pacing in sinus node disease according to the ESC guidelines for cardiac pacing and cardiac resynchronization therapy [53]

Class	Clinical indication	Level of evidence
Class I	1. Sinus node disease manifests as symptomatic bradycardia with or without bradycardia-dependant tachycardia. Symptom-rhythm correlation must have been: ◆ spontaneously occurring; ◆ drug-induced where alternative drug therapy is lacking. 2. Syncope with sinus node disease, either spontaneously occurring or induced at electrophysiological study. 3. Sinus node disease manifests as symptomatic chronotropic incompetence: ◆ spontaneously occurring; ◆ drug-induced where alternative drug therapy is lacking.	C
Class IIa	1. Symptomatic sinus node disease, which is either spontaneous or induced by a drug for which there is no alternative but no symptom rhythm correlation has been documented. Heart rate at rest should be <40bpm 2. Syncope for which no other explanation can be made but there are abnormal electrophysiological findings (cSNRT >800ms)	C
Class IIb	1. Minimally symptomatic patients with sinus node disease, resting heart rate <40bpm while awake and no evidence of chronotropic incompetence.	C
Class III	1. Sinus node disease without symptoms including use of bradycardia-provoking drugs. 2. ECG findings of sinus node dysfunction with symptoms not due directly or indirectly to bradycardia. 3. Symptomatic sinus node dysfunction where symptoms can reliably be attributed to non-essential medication	C

Note: when sinus node disease is diagnosed atrial tachyarrhythmias are likely even if not yet recorded, implying that serious consideration should be given to anticoagulant therapy.

Reproduced with permission from Vardas PE, Auricchio A, Blanc JJ, *et al.* Guidelines for cardiac pacing and cardiac resynchronization therapy: The Task Force for Cardiac Pacing and Cardiac Resynchronization Therapy of the European Society of Cardiology. Developed in Collaboration with the European Heart Rhythm Association. *Eur Heart J* 2007; **28**: 2256–95.

Table 27.4 Recommendations for cardiac pacing in acquired atrioventricular block according to the ESC guidelines for cardiac pacing and cardiac resynchronization therapy [53]

Class	Clinical indication	Level of evidence
Class I	1. Chronic symptomatic third or second degree (Mobitz I or II) atrioventricular block.	C
	2. Neuromuscular diseases (e.g. myotonic muscular dystrophy, Kearns–Sayre syndrome, etc.) with third-degree or second-degree atrioventricular block.	B
	3. Third or second degree (Mobitz I or II) atrioventricular block: ◆ after catheter ablation of the atrioventricular junction; ◆ after valve surgery when the block is not expected to resolve.	C
Class IIa	1. Asymptomatic third or second degree (Mobitz I or II) atrioventricular block.	C
	2. Symptomatic prolonged first degree atrioventricular block.	C
Class IIb	1. Neuromuscular diseases (e.g. myotonic muscular dystrophy, Kearns–Sayre syndrome, etc.) with first degree atrioventricular block.	B
Class III	1. Asymptomatic first degree atrioventricular block.	C
	2. Asymptomatic second degree Mobitz I with supra-Hisian conduction block.	C
	3. Atrioventricular block expected to resolve.	C

Reproduced with permission from Vardas PE, Auricchio A, Blanc JJ, *et al.* Guidelines for cardiac pacing and cardiac resynchronization therapy: The Task Force for Cardiac Pacing and Cardiac Resynchronization Therapy of the European Society of Cardiology. Developed in Collaboration with the European Heart Rhythm Association. *Eur Heart J* 2007; **28**: 2256–95.

Table 27.5 Recommendations for cardiac pacing in chronic bifascicular and trifascicular block according to the ESC guidelines for cardiac pacing and cardiac resynchronization therapy [53]

Class	Clinical indication	Level of evidence
Class I	1. Intermittent third-degree atrioventricular block. 2. Second-degree Mobitz II atrioventricular block. 3. Alternating bundle branch block. 4. Findings on electrophysiological study of markedly prolonged HV interval (≥100ms) or pacing-induced infra-His block in patients with symptoms.	C
Class IIa	1. Syncope not demonstrated to be due to atrioventricular block when other likely causes have been excluded, specifically ventricular tachycardia.	B
	2. Neuromuscular diseases (e.g. myotonic muscular dystrophy, Kearns-Sayre syndrome, etc.) with any degree of fascicular block.	C
	3. Incidental findings on electrophysiological study of markedly prolonged HV interval (≥100ms) or pacing- induced infra-His block in patients without symptoms.	C
Class IIb	None.	–
Class III	1. Bundle branch block without atrioventricular block or symptoms. 2. Bundle branch block with first-degree atrioventricular block without symptoms.	B

Reproduced with permission from Vardas PE, Auricchio A, Blanc JJ, *et al.* Guidelines for cardiac pacing and cardiac resynchronization therapy: The Task Force for Cardiac Pacing and Cardiac Resynchronization Therapy of the European Society of Cardiology. Developed in Collaboration with the European Heart Rhythm Association. *Eur Heart J* 2007; **28**: 2256–95.

During right ventricular pacing the electrical impulse is usually delivered to the apex of the ventricle, from where it depolarizes the slowly-conducting surrounding myocardium (instead of progressing through the fast-conducting His–Purkinje fibres), thus mimicking LBBB. Patients with LBBB have been shown to have a lower ejection fraction and shorter diastolic filling time compared to patients without LBBB [94], and ejection fraction has been shown to be lowest with ventricular pacing, intermediate with atrioventricular sequential pacing and best preserved with atrial pacing and ventricular activation via the intrinsic pathways [95]. Adverse consequences associated with pacing at the right ventricular apex include pacing-induced mitral regurgitation, decreased ejection fraction, redistribution of myocardial adrenergic innervation, and alterations in regional myocardial blood flow, protein expression, glucose uptake, and oxygen consumption, together with regional wall motion and structural abnormalities similar to those observed in patients with intrinsic LBBB [96–99]. Right ventricular pacing may be considered as causal in the development of interventricular dyssynchrony and its clinical consequences. Therefore, part of the beneficial effect on cardiac output resulting from atrioventricular synchrony in the DDD mode may be offset by the interventricular dyssynchrony induced by pacing at the right ventricular apex.

During the last two decades, several randomized trials with clinical endpoints have increased our knowledge and together with developments in pacemaker design, this has expanded the possibilities for optimal pacing therapy. The principal endpoints of the trials, comparing atrial with ventricular based pacing, were mortality, atrial fibrillation, frequency of thromboembolic episodes and stroke, heart failure, pacemaker syndrome, and the patients' quality of life. The patients included suffered mostly from symptomatic bradycardia due to sinus node disease with or without normal atrioventricular conduction [100], although one trial focused specifically on elderly patients with

Table 27.6 Randomized clinical trials of pacemaker mode selection

Reference (study name)	Year	Pacing modes	N	Indication	Mean age (years)	Duration (years)
Andersen *et al.* [102]	1994	AAI vs. VVI	225	SND with normal AV conduction	76	3.3
Andersen *et al.* [42]	1997	—				5.5
Nielsen *et al.* [103]	1998	—				
Andersen *et al.* [104]	1999	—				
Lamas *et al.* [105] (PASE)	1998	DDD(R) vs. VVI(R)	407	SND and AV block	76	2.5
Connolly *et al.* [106] (CTOPP)	2000	AAI(R) or DDD(R)* vs. VVI(R)	2568	SND and AV block	73	3.0
Skanes *et al.* [107] (CTOPP)	2001	—				3.0
Newman *et al.* [108] (CTOPP)	2003	—				N/A
Kerr *et al.* [106] (CTOPP)	2004	—				6.4
Lamas *et al.* [110] (MOST)	2002	DDD(R) vs. VVI(R)	2010	SND	74	2.7
Toff *et al.* [101] (UKPACE)	2005	DDD(R) vs. VVI(R)	2021	AV block	80	4.6

* 95% of the patients were paced DDD(R).

AV, atrioventricular; PASE, PAcemaker Selection in the Elderly; CTOPP, Canadian Trial of Physiologic Pacing; MOST, MOde Selection Trial in sinus-node dysfunction; SND, sinus node dysfunction; UKPACE, United Kingdom Pacing and Cardiovascular Events.

high-grade atrioventricular block [101]. The key features of the study designs and patients included are shown in ➲Table 27.6.

All-cause and cardiovascular mortality

The only randomized trial comparing purely atrial pacing (AAI) with purely ventricular pacing (VVI) in patients with sinus node disease, normal atrioventricular conduction, and normal QRS complexes was published in 1994 by Andersen *et al.* [102]. At the end of a 5.5-year period, the patients who were paced in AAI mode had a significantly lower incidence of atrial fibrillation, thromboembolic events, heart failure, cardiovascular mortality, and total mortality, compared with those paced in VVI mode [42]. Two things were unique about this study: it was the only randomized study to date that compared pure AAI and VVI modes over a long follow-up period; and it was also the only one to show a clear benefit in terms of all the clinical parameters examined, and primarily in mortality, for patients who had atrial pacing. The remaining clinical trials compared atrial-based pacing (predominantly DDD(R)) with VVI(R) pacing and found no significant difference in all-cause or cardiovascular mortality between groups after 2.5–4.6 years of treatment [101, 105, 106, 110] nor in the follow-up extension of one trial after 6.4 years [109] (➲Fig. 27.10A).

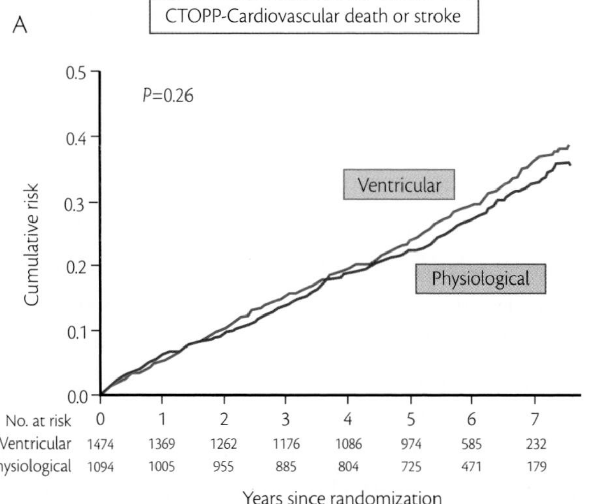

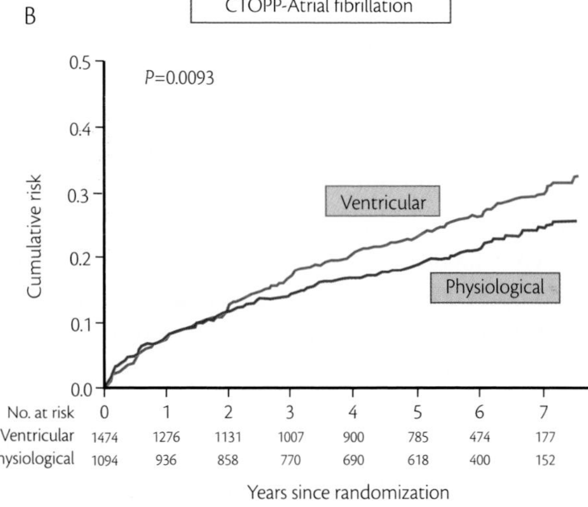

Figure 27.10 Incidence of primary end-point and atrial fibrillation in CTOPP trial (extended follow-up). Reproduced with permission from Kerr CR, Connolly SJ, Abdollah H, *et al.* Canadian Trial of Physiological Pacing: effects of physiological pacing during long-term follow-up. *Circulation* 2004; **109**: 357–62.

Thromboembolism or stroke in relation to pacing modality

Similar observations apply to the risk of thromboembolism and stroke. In patients with sick sinus syndrome, Andersen *et al.* reported a significantly greater number of thromboembolic events in the VVI group compared with the AAI group after 3.3 years of observation (20/115 vs. 6/110 events, p = 0.0083) [102], confirmed after 5.5 years (39/115 vs. 19/110 events, p = 0.0065) [42]. The risk of arterial thromboembolism was primarily associated with the presence of the bradycardia–tachycardia syndrome at randomization and with ventricular pacing, whereas it was small in atrial-paced patients in whom atrial fibrillation had never been documented [104]. No significant differences in thromboembolism or stroke were found in the other trials, comparing DDD(R) with VVI(R) pacing, neither after 2.5–3 years of treatment [101, 105, 106, 110] nor in the follow-up extension of one trial after 6.4 years [109]. The annual rates of stroke ranged from 1% in CTOPP [106] to 2.2% in MOST [110], two of the largest endpoint trials published to date in patients with permanent pacemakers. Taking into account the fact that stroke has multiple possible cardiogenic and non-cardiogenic aetiologies in elderly patients and the variable use of antiplatelet therapy, even large clinical trials may lack the power to establish adequately whether one pacing mode is superior to the other with regard to the risk of stroke.

Can pacing prevent or provoke atrial fibrillation?

The incidence of atrial fibrillation (see ➲Chapter 29) was generally found to be greater in VVI(R)-paced patients than in patients with atrial-based pacing (AAI(R) or DDD(R)), although no significant difference was observed in the UKPACE trial [101]. In the trial reported by Andersen *et al.* [102], 23% of the VVI-paced patients developed atrial fibrillation after 3 years compared with 14% of the AAI-paced patients, an observation that did not reach statistical significance, probably due to the small number of patients included (n = 225). However, atrial fibrillation occurred significantly less frequently in the atrial-based pacing group than in the VVI(R)-paced group in CTOPP [106] and the relative risk of developing atrial fibrillation was significantly reduced by 21% (p = 0.008) over 2.7 years in the DDD(R)-paced group compared with the VVI(R)-paced group in MOST [110]. This relative risk reduction was consistent with the 20.1% risk reduction (p = 0.009) observed after 6.4 years in the extension of CTOPP [109] (➲Fig. 27.10B) and the relative risk reduction for chronic atrial fibrillation of 27.1% (p = 0.016) in favour of atrial-based pacing in the same trial [107]. The following risk predictors for chronic atrial fibrillation were identified: age ≥74 years, sinoatrial node disease and prior episodes of atrial fibrillation [107]. However, in those patients with an intrinsic heart rate ≤60bpm, i.e. those most likely to have a predominantly paced rhythm, the benefit of DDD pacing for reduction of atrial fibrillation was even more pronounced [111].

There is, therefore, consistent evidence that atrial-based pacing reduces the risk of atrial fibrillation in patients with sinus node disease. Several mechanisms have been proposed, such as the suppression of premature atrial beats that might trigger the development of sustained atrial fibrillation, and the maintenance of optimal ventricular diastolic filling through the preservation of appropriately timed atrial contraction. Indeed, the follow-up observations of Andersen *et al.*, 5.5 years after pacemaker implantation, showed that the left atrial diameter increased significantly less in the AAI-paced than in the VVI-paced group [103], a finding consistent with an increased risk of atrial fibrillation in VVI-paced patients. When atrial arrhythmias are not suppressed simply by raising the atrial rate both at rest and, if necessary, on effort, recent pacemaker designs offer a host of atrial antitachycardia preventive and therapeutic pacing algorithms. These have been shown to be of benefit in some patients but clinical trials [112–117] have failed to provide convincing evidence of their efficacy.

Pacemaker syndrome

Classically, pacemaker syndrome reflects the loss of atrioventricular synchrony, resulting in loss of the atrial contribution to cardiac output during ventricular pacing. However, pacemaker syndrome is now recognized as being the result of a complex interaction of neurohumoral, autonomic and vascular changes. It is characterized by:

- congestive symptoms and signs mimicking heart failure, such as dyspnoea, orthopnoea, distended neck veins, rales, hepatomegaly, and oedema of the lower limbs;
- hypotensive symptoms and signs, such as syncope (or presyncope) at the onset of pacing, with a drop in blood pressure (➲Fig. 27.11); and
- non-specific symptoms such as fatigue and dizziness.

In clinical studies where crossover to the alternate pacing mode (from VVI to either AAI or DDD) required re-intervention, pacemaker syndrome was reportedly rare, with rates of 1.8% over 5.5 years [42] and 5% over 3 years [106]. In contrast, in clinical studies where crossover required only non-invasive transcutaneous reprogramming of the pacing mode, pacemaker syndrome was reported in 18.3% over 2.7 years [110] and 26% over 2.5 years [105], using a definition based on haemodynamics (elevated right or left filling pressures or hypotension with ventricular

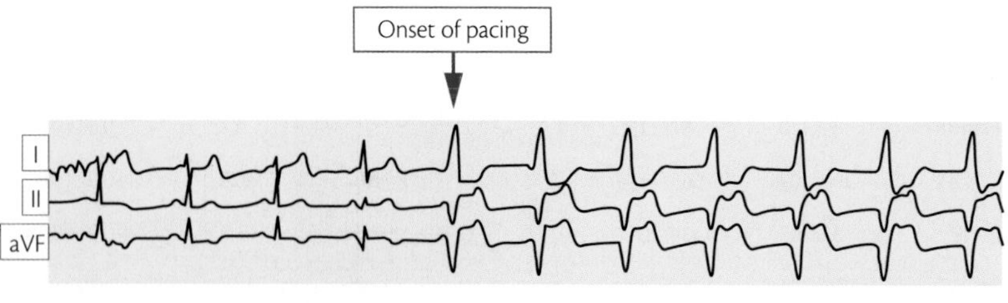

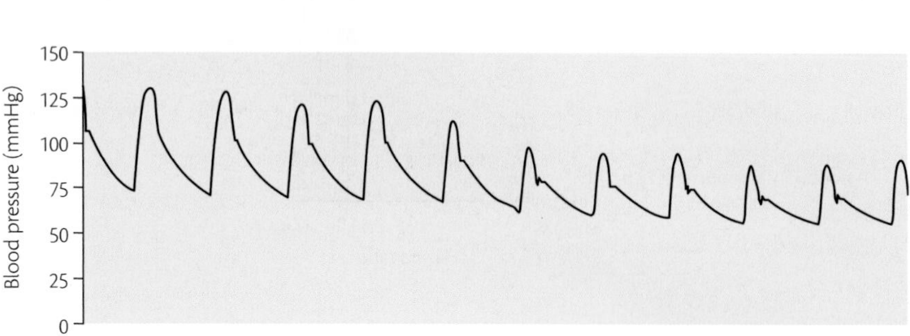

Figure 27.11 Pacemaker syndrome: simultaneous ECG and femoral arterial blood pressure recording in a 64-year-old man presenting with intermittent dizziness, palpitation, and dyspnoea 3 years after implantation of a VVI pacemaker for sinus node disease. Arterial blood pressure dropped from 131/72 to 88/55mmHg with the onset of VVI pacing during slowing of the sinus rate (arrow). Retrograde P waves are discernible after the paced QRS complexes. Reproduced from Ahn Y, Cho JG. Pacemaker syndrome. *Heart* 2004; **90**: 58 with permission of the BMJ Publishing Group.

pacing). Use of the more common operating definition of pacemaker syndrome (i.e. intolerance of ventricular pacing) would presumably have generated even higher numbers. Figures as high as 83% have been reported with VVI pacing, when patients were given the option to directly compare it with DDD pacing [118].

Quality of life

While virtually all patients implanted with a pacemaker have experienced a significant increase in quality of life versus baseline (i.e. before implantation), large-scale clinical trials published to date have not shown superiority of one pacing mode over another with regard to improvements in generic measures of quality of life [105, 108]. However, small single-centre crossover studies using disease-specific instruments have shown improvement in quality of life with physiological pacing [119, 120] and improvements in exercise tolerance have also been reported [121, 122].

Summary of clinical trial results

Summarizing the results of the above prospective, randomized studies, as well as meta-analyses and systematic reviews [123, 124], we can conclude that in patients with sinus node disease the incidence of atrial fibrillation is lower in those who are given atrial or dual-chamber pacemakers than in those treated with ventricular pacing alone. Moreover a meta-analysis of patient data from five of the trials (the Danish Trial, PASE, CTOPP, MOST, and UKPACE) demonstrated a reduction in atrial fibrillation and in stroke with atrial-based pacing (➲Fig. 27.12) [125]. In the Cochrane review, which included five parallel and 26 crossover randomized controlled trials, there was a statistically significant trend towards dual-chamber pacing being more favourable in terms of exercise capacity and pacemaker syndrome [126].

With regard to heart failure and mortality, the available evidence suggests that there is no difference between single-chamber ventricular pacing and dual-chamber pacing. However, single-chamber atrial pacing in isolated sinus node disease and the avoidance of unnecessary ventricular pacing may confer an advantage.

Patient-based choice of pacing mode

As a general rule, a patient with isolated sinus node dysfunction and no atrioventricular conduction disturbance may be considered for a single-chamber AAI(R) pacemaker, as the annual incidence of second- or third-degree atrioventricular block has been shown to be <1% [42, 43]. The ongoing DANPACE trial will ultimately provide further information about the relative merits of atrial and dual-chamber pacing in this context [127]. For a patient with sinus node dysfunction and concomitant conduction disturbance, a dual-chamber pacing system is most appropriate, with DDD pacing if the chronotropic competence of the sinus node is preserved and DDD(R) pacing if it is not. If sinus node disease is associated with the bradycardia–tachycardia syndrome, DDI(R) pacing or a device with mode-switching capability (i.e. automatically switching from an atrial-tracking mode to VVI on detection of atrial tachyarrhythmia) is preferred in order to avoid rapid paced ventricular rates in response to the tracking of high atrial rates [128].

Nowadays, the trend is towards dual-chamber pacing with minimization of right ventricular stimulation (in order to avoid changes leading to desynchronization of the ventricles as a result of their being depolarized from the

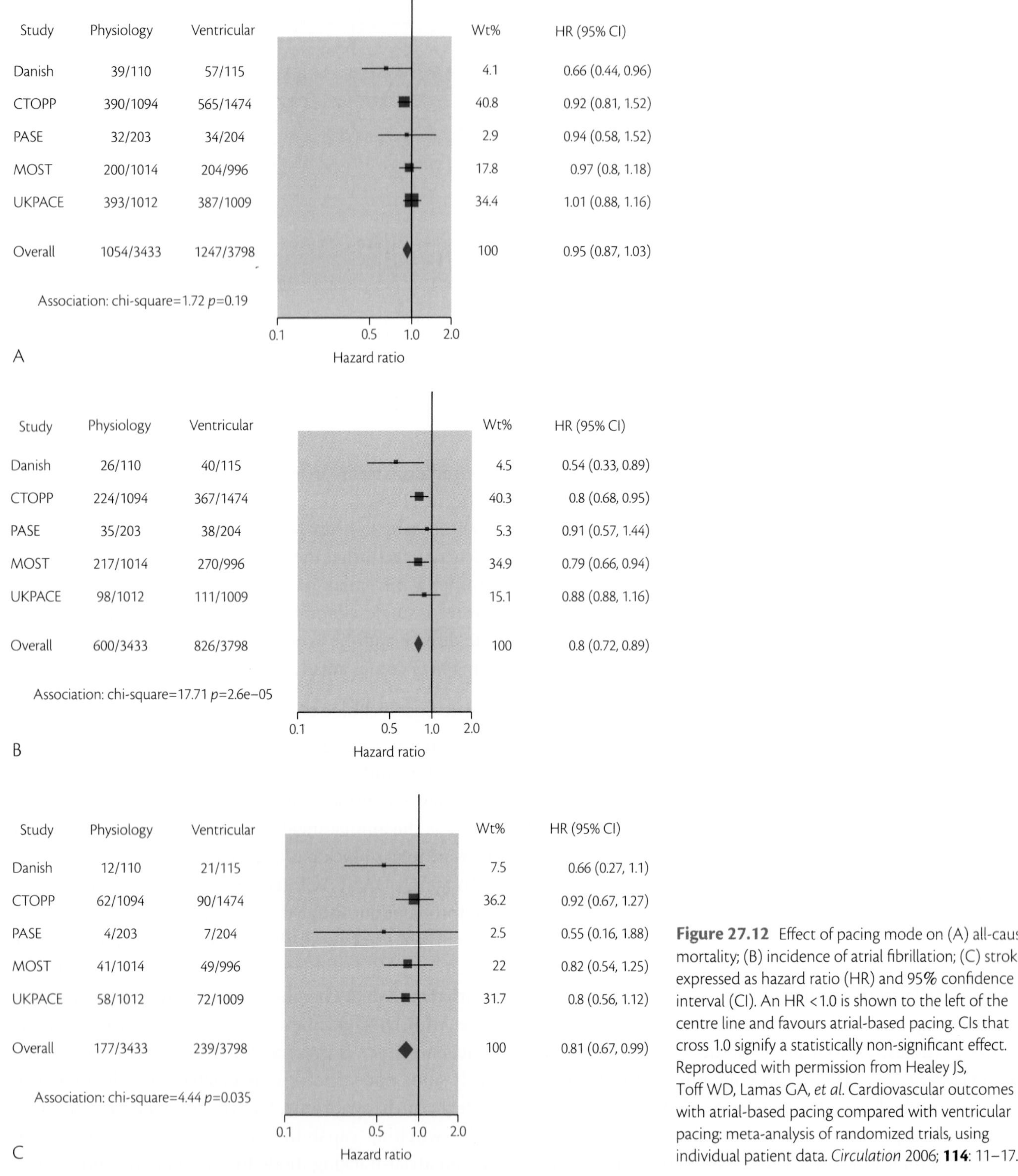

Figure 27.12 Effect of pacing mode on (A) all-cause mortality; (B) incidence of atrial fibrillation; (C) stroke expressed as hazard ratio (HR) and 95% confidence interval (CI). An HR <1.0 is shown to the left of the centre line and favours atrial-based pacing. CIs that cross 1.0 signify a statistically non-significant effect. Reproduced with permission from Healey JS, Toff WD, Lamas GA, *et al.* Cardiovascular outcomes with atrial-based pacing compared with ventricular pacing: meta-analysis of randomized trials, using individual patient data. *Circulation* 2006; **114**: 11–17.

right ventricular apex) and a panoply of antitachycardia algorithms, possibly combined with stimulation of the atria from the septum rather than the appendage. However, no consistent data from large randomized trials support the use of alternative single-site atrial pacing, multisite right atrial pacing, or biatrial pacing in patients with sinus node disease. Pacemaker mode selection in the latter patients, according to the ESC guidelines for cardiac pacing and CRT, is shown in ➲Fig. 27.13.

In a patient with atrioventricular or multifascicular block, a dual-chamber device with DDD or DDD(R) pacing is appropriate, although VVI(R) pacing may be an acceptable

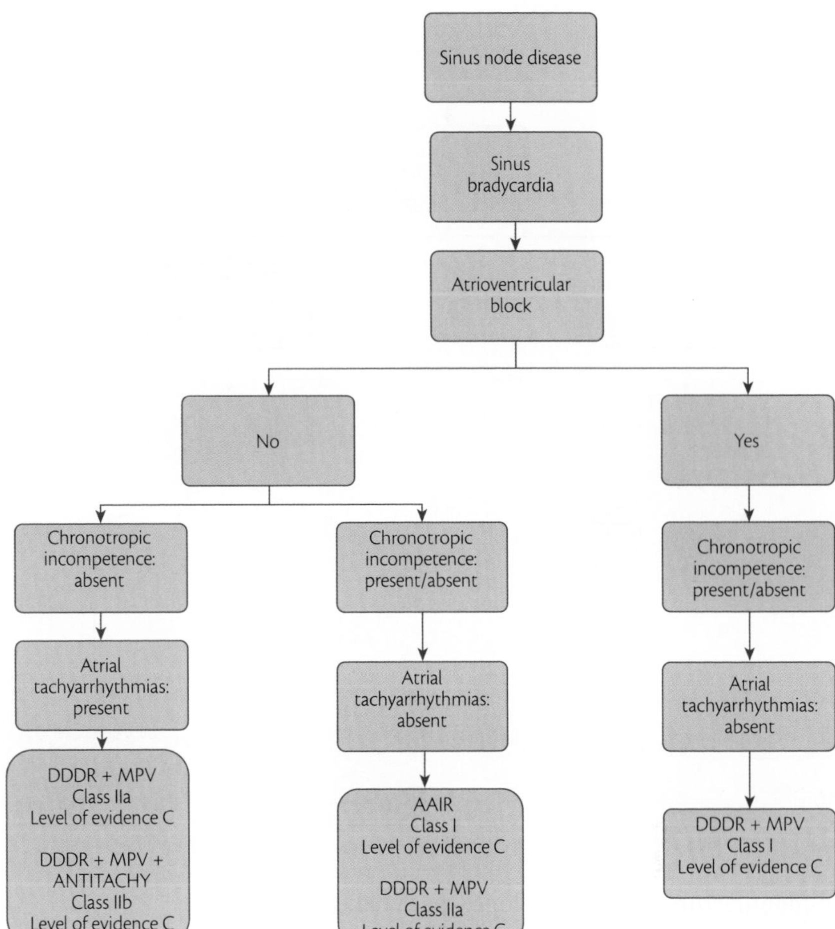

Figure 27.13 Pacemaker mode selection in sinus node disease. ANTITACHY, antitachycardia algorithms in pacemaker; MPV, minimization of pacing in the ventricles. *Note:* in sinus node disease VVIR and VDDR modes are considered unsuitable and are not recommended. Where atrioventricular block exists, AAIR is inappropriate. Reproduced with permission from Vardas PE, Auricchio A, Blanc J-J, *et al.* Guidelines for cardiac pacing and cardiac resynchronization therapy: The Task Force for Cardiac Pacing and Cardiac Resynchronization Therapy of the European Society of Cardiology. Developed in Collaboration with the European Heart Rhythm Association *Eur Heart J* 2007; **28**: 2256–95.

alternative in the elderly [101]. In the presence of permanent atrial fibrillation, a single-chamber ventricular pacemaker with VVI or VVI(R) pacing should be used. There is no universal pacing mode that suits all patients, and careful selection of the appropriate pacing system, with individualized programming to match each patient's needs, is of crucial importance. Not surprisingly, literature on the customization of individual patient settings is scarce and there is no substitute for clinical expertise. Pacemaker mode selection in acquired atrioventricular block, chronic bifascicular and trifascicular block, according to the ESC guidelines for cardiac pacing and CRT, is shown in ➲Fig. 27.14.

Two additional considerations may influence the approach to a patient-based choice of pacing mode:

- Right ventricular apical pacing has been shown to promote electrical remodelling of the heart and to induce interventricular dyssynchrony, both of which may have deleterious effects on cardiac haemodynamics and may lead to the development of new or worsening heart failure [103, 110]. In the DAVID trial, patients with ejection fraction ≤40% but no indication for cardiac pacing, who were implanted with an implantable cardioverter defibrillator (ICD) capable of dual-chamber rate-adaptive pacing, were randomly assigned to dual-chamber rate-adaptive pacing at 70bpm or backup ventricular pacing at 40bpm. After a 1-year follow up, the incidence of the composite endpoint of death or hospitalization for heart failure was significantly greater in the dual-chamber paced group (HR 1.61; 95% CI 1.06–2.44) [129]. Similarly, in a subgroup analysis of the MADIT II trial, which included patients with ischaemic cardiomyopathy and left ventricular ejection fraction (LVEF) ≤30% and evaluated the benefit of a prophylactic ICD, patients who were predominantly paced had a higher incidence of new or worsening heart failure [130]. These findings suggest that, in addition to maintaining atrioventricular synchrony, physiological pacing requires maximal preservation of intrinsic rather than paced ventricular activation. The ideally configured pacing system is one that paces only when needed but always when needed. Many pacemaker patients have only transient bradyarrhythmia, with an adequate unpaced heart rate much of the time, and are not pacemaker-dependent. Recently, several

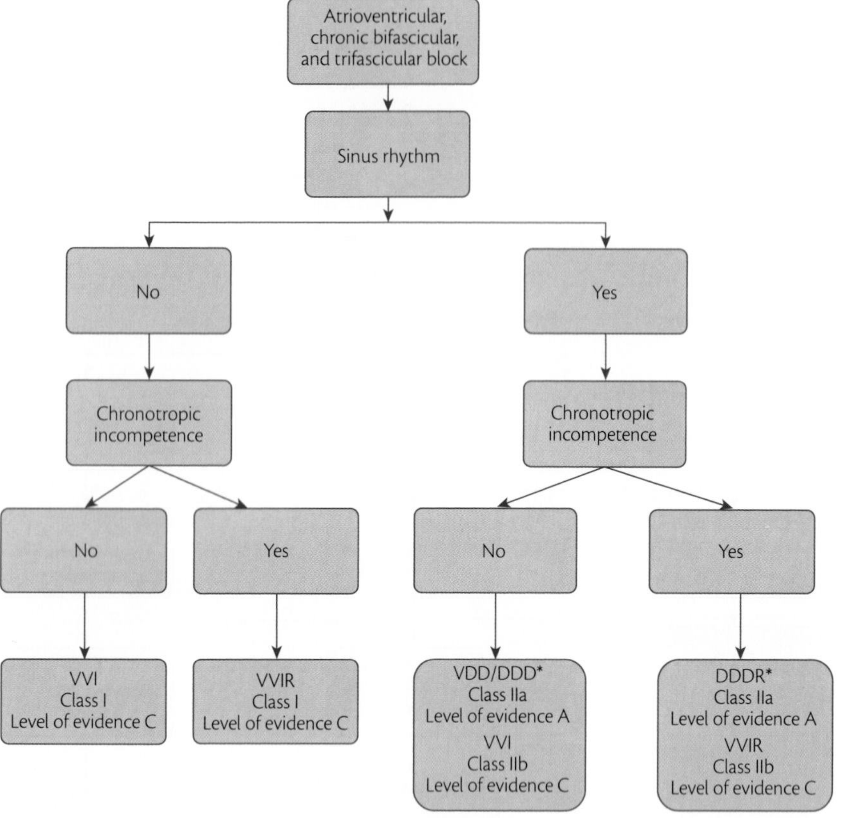

Figure 27.14 Pacemaker mode selection in acquired atrioventricular block, chronic bifascicular and trifascicular block. When atrioventricular block is not permanent, pacemakers with algorithms for preservation of native atrioventricular conduction should be selected. * VVIR could be an alternative, especially in patients who have a low level of physical activity and in those with a short expected lifespan. Reproduced with permission from Vardas PE, Auricchio A, Blanc J-J, *et al.* Guidelines for cardiac pacing and cardiac resynchronization therapy: The Task Force for Cardiac Pacing and Cardiac Resynchronization Therapy of the European Society of Cardiology. Developed in Collaboration with the European Heart Rhythm Association *Eur Heart* J 2007; **28**: 2256–95.

manufacturers have developed pacemakers with algorithms that have been shown to be effective in minimizing ventricular pacing and maximizing intrinsic cardiac conduction [131, 132] (➲Fig. 27.15). The recently published SAVE PACe trial, after a mean follow up of 1.7 years, revealed that in patients with sinus node disease and normal atrioventricular conduction there is a lower incidence of atrial fibrillation with the use of atrioventricular search hysteresis and minimal ventricular pacing algorithms than with conventional dual-chamber pacing ($p = 0.009$) [133]. However, further clinical trials are needed and are already in progress to evaluate the efficacy of these new algorithms [134–136].

- In heart failure patients (see ➲Chapter 23) who remain symptomatic and in NYHA class III–IV despite optimal pharmacological treatment, with low ejection fraction (LVEF ≤35%), left ventricular dilatation, normal sinus rhythm, and a wide QRS complex (≥120ms), there is a Class I, Level of Evidence A, indication for CRT to reduce morbidity and mortality [53]. In this context, CRT with cardioverter defibrillator back-up is also an appropriate option to consider for patients who have an expectation of survival with a good functional status for more than 1 year: Class I, Level of Evidence B [53]. CRT, with or without integrated cardioverter-defibrillator capability, has been

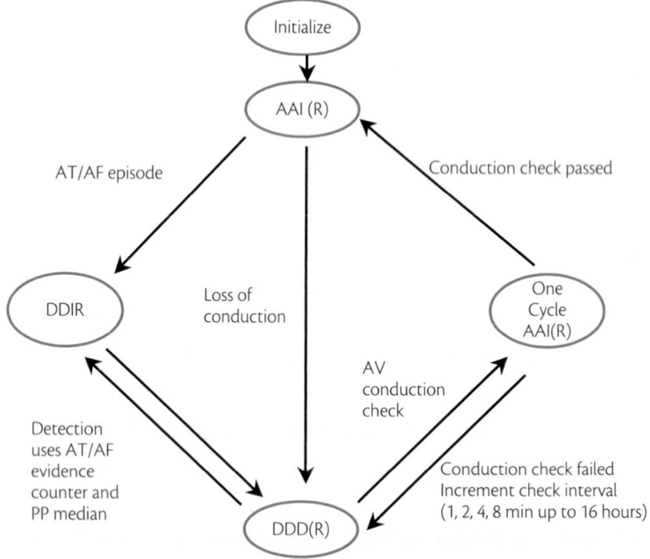

Figure 27.15 Managed ventricular pacing (MVP) mode provides functional AAI/R pacing with the safety of dual chamber ventricular support in the presence of transient or persistent loss of conduction and promotes AV conduction by reducing unnecessary RV pacing. The MVP mode is designed to convert to the appropriate mode of operation in the presence of AT/AF. Reproduced with permission from Medtronic Inc. (http://www.medtronic.com/).

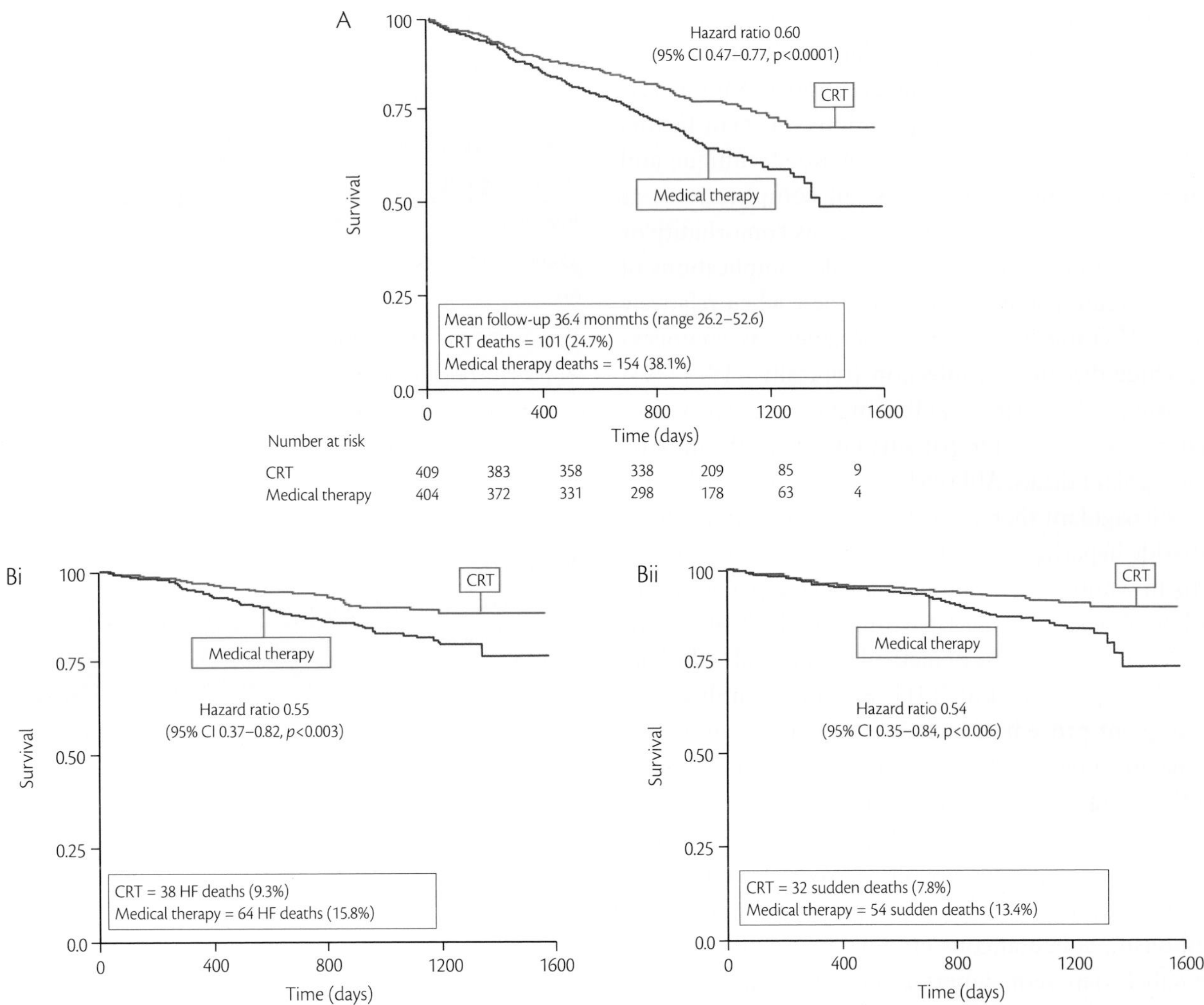

Figure 27.16 The CArdiac REsynchronization-Heart Failure (CARE-HF) trial extension phase. (A) The Kaplan–Meier estimates of the time to death from any cause. (B) The Kaplan–Meier estimates of the time to death from worsening heart failure (i) or sudden death (ii). Reproduced with permission from Cleland JG, Daubert J-C, Erdmann E, *et al.* Longer-term effects of cardiac resynchronization therapy on mortality in heart failure [the CArdiac REsynchronization-Heart Failure (CARE-HF) trial extension phase]. *Eur Heart J* 2006; **27**: 1928–32.

shown to improve NYHA functional class, 6-min walking distance, quality of life, and peak oxygen consumption. Dramatic reductions in heart failure hospitalization [137,138] and in the combined risk of death or hospitalization for any cause [139] have also been reported, as has a reduction in total and cardiac mortality [140] (➲Fig. 27.16). In heart failure patients with NYHA class III–IV symptoms, low ejection fraction (LVEF ≤35%), left ventricular dilatation, and a concomitant indication for permanent pacing (first implant or upgrading of a conventional pacemaker) there is a Class IIa, Level of Evidence C, indication for CRT [53]. The lower level of evidence reflects the fact that patients with conventional indications for pacing were excluded from the major trials evaluating CRT. There is, however, evidence of benefit in paced patients with heart failure who were upgraded to CRT in observational and crossover studies [141–143].

Encouraging results have also been obtained in small studies comparing CRT with conventional pacing at first implant. [144–146]. By avoiding the intraventricular and interventricular dyssynchrony associated with pacing at the right ventricular apex, CRT may reduce the risk of worsening or new onset heart failure. Ongoing trials are further examining the role of CRT as an alternative to conventional pacing in patients with and without left ventricular impairment and/or heart failure at the time of implantation [147, 148]. CRT is considered further in ➲Chapter 23.

Complications of pacemaker treatment

Pacemaker implantation in well-trained and experienced hands is a relatively safe procedure. However as an invasive procedure, it inevitably entails a risk of complications and failures, mainly in the perioperative period but also in the longer term. There is the potential for all of the general complications of any surgical intervention and for a variety of procedure-specific complications. Human factors related to the implanter, such as operator technique and experience, may influence the risk of complications, as may factors related to the patient, such as comorbidity or concomitant drug therapy. The possible complications of pacemaker treatment are many and varied, albeit relatively infrequent (➲Table 27.7). General perioperative complications include discomfort, infection (typically <1% [149]) and bruising or haematoma at the implant site. The risk of haematoma is increased in patients taking antithrombotic or anticoagulant drugs. Although it is customary to discontinue anticoagulant therapy 3–5 days before implantation and provide heparin cover until a few hours before surgery, patients in whom this would pose an unacceptable risk of thromboembolism may be safely implanted whilst anticoagulated, subject to the use of meticulous surgical technique by a skilled operator [150, 151]. Specific complications of the implant procedure include traumatic pneumothorax or haemo-pneumothorax (typically <2% of implants) [89, 90], brachial plexus injury, arterial puncture and left ventricular incursion or injury, which is associated with an additional risk of thromboembolism. Myocardial perforation with pericardial effusion or, more rarely, tamponade, air embolism, subcutaneous emphysema, or thrombosis of the subclavian vein, superior vena cava, right atrium, or right ventricle may also occur. Venous thrombosis may rarely lead to pulmonary embolism or the superior vena cava syndrome.

Amongst the procedure-specific complications, lead dislodgement (more usually of the atrial lead when screw-in technology is not used), loose lead connection to the pacemaker, lead fracture, or insulation break deserve special attention. Lead dislodgement has been reported in up to 4.2% of dual-chamber compared with 1.4% of single-chamber pacemaker implantations [106]. As expected, inadequate pacing and sensing was also more frequent with dual-chamber than single-chamber pacemakers. Supraventricular and ventricular arrhythmias are not uncommon during pacemaker implantation but are rarely of clinical consequence. Endless-loop tachycardia, a form of pacemaker-mediated tachycardia, is a well-recognized complication of dual-chamber pacing but is less commonly seen with modern devices and may usually be avoided by careful programming. Diaphragmatic pacing may occur due to phrenic nerve stimulation from a laterally

Table 27.7 Complications of pacemaker treatment

Perioperative
General
Haemorrhage/bruising/haematoma
Pain/discomfort
Infection
Wound dehiscence
Specific
Pneumothorax/haemothorax/haemomediastinum
Arrhythmia (asystole, atrial/ventricular arrhythmia)
Air embolism/subcutaneous emphysema
Myocardial perforation/tamponade
Left-sided lead misplacement
Brachial plexus injury
Mechanical
Lead-related
Lead dislodgement
Conduction break
Insulation failure
Twiddler's syndrome
Venous thrombosis/superior vena cava syndrome/ pulmonary embolism
Device-related
Erosion (➲Fig. 27.17)
Migration
Traumatic injury/damage
Functional
Electrical
Diaphragmatic pacing
Pectoral muscle stimulation
Intrinsic electromagnetic interference (myopotential sensing)
Extrinsic electromagnetic interference
Over-sensing
Under-sensing
Threshold rise
Premature battery depletion
Pacemaker failure
Rhythm-related
Pacemaker-mediated tachycardia
Haemodynamic
Pacemaker syndrome
Autonomic dysregulation
Psychological
Anxiety/depression/adjustment problems

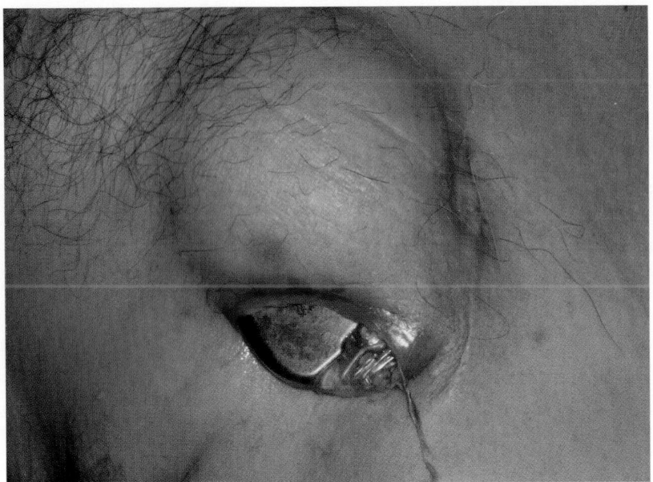

Figure 27.17 Infection and erosion of a pacemaker pocket.

placed atrial lead, or to direct activation because of proximity of the ventricular lead. The problem may be resolved by decreasing the output voltage (subject to a satisfactory safety margin) or lead repositioning. Pectoral stimulation may be due to incorrect orientation of the pacemaker with its active surface in contact with the muscle, or to a current leak from a lead insulation failure or exposed connector.

Organization of a pacemaker implantation laboratory

Requirements for implanting pacemakers and CRT devices have been articulated in detail in the ESC guidelines for cardiac pacing and CRT [53]. The following section outlines practical and technical aspects related to: 1) requirements for the operating theatre, and 2) personnel requirements for pacemaker implantation.

1) A suitable operating room for pacemaker implantation should have the following equipment and facilities:
   - Radiation exposure shielding of personnel and patients.
   - Ceiling suspended and/or floor mounted radiation shielding.
   - High-quality fixed or mobile fluoroscopic equipment capable of performing oblique projections.
   - Complete haemodynamic monitoring (12-lead ECG, invasive and non-invasive arterial blood pressure measurement, oxygen saturation monitoring).
   - Immediate availability of an external defibrillator.
   - Pacing system analyser and programmer for the implanted device.
   - Oxygen, suction, and intubation facilities.
   - Easy and quick access to an intensive care unit.

Continuous anaesthesiology support is not obligatory but prompt anaesthesiology assistance must be available if a critical clinical situation develops. A cardiac surgery unit need not be within the same hospital structure, but must be easily accessible.

2) Expert recommendations are that centres intending to implant pacemaker and CRT devices should fulfil the following conditions:
   - Two or more cardiologists qualified for device implantation and management.
   - All physicians should possess knowledge and experience of haemodynamic monitoring and administration of cardiovascular support, including positive inotropic drugs, experience in cardiovascular resuscitation and handling of low-output syndromes and life support.
   - Ideally, two nurses are required. One nurse monitors patient status and manages all necessary therapeutic interventions including the administration of intravenous drugs. A second nurse provides implant assistance.
   - Technical radiological assistance is strongly advised and in some countries is mandatory.
   - Continuing medical education for physicians, nurses, and technicians is mandatory.
   - A minimum operator caseload of at least 20 CRT device implantations per year is strongly advised [53]. A log book with 100 implantations performed as first operator (including 70 pacemakers, 20 ICDs, 10 CRT devices) performed during a period of 3 years is required for any physician who wants to apply for European Heart Rhythm Association accreditation.

Pacemaker follow-up

Apart from the successful placement of the lead(s) and generator, today's advanced pacemaker technology, along with the increased cost of sophisticated devices, requires methodical long-term follow up in order that the patient may receive the maximum benefit from pacing and the treatment may be as cost effective as possible [152, 153]. The long-term follow up of a paced patient requires a well-organized pacing clinic, whose infrastructure, know-how, and staff are sufficient to ensure a reliable periodic assessment of the patient in general and the pacemaker function in particular. The goals of such a pacing clinic are shown

Table 27.8 The goals of a pacemaker clinic

Evaluation of the overall clinical condition of the paced patient
Timely recording of failures or abnormalities of the pulse generator, leads, and correction of any problems identified
Recording of problems or complications related to the surgical procedure and placement of generator and lead(s)
Proper sensing tests and relevant optimum programming
Threshold testing and output programming, with a view to adjusting pacing to the needs of the patient and maximizing generator longevity
Non-invasive programming, utilizing the full range of programmable options in order to optimize device function for an individual's specific needs
Correct evaluation of the end of life of the pulse generator, avoiding unnecessary and premature replacement
Organization of a database containing details of each patient's pacing system, for monitoring the performance and reliability of the pulse generator and leads
Provision of education and support—medical and psychological—to the paced patient
Provision of education and training to doctors, technicians, and nurses with regard to permanent pacing

Reproduced with permission from Vardas PE, Auricchio A, Blanc JJ, *et al.* Guidelines for cardiac pacing and cardiac resynchronization therapy: The Task Force for Cardiac Pacing and Cardiac Resynchronization Therapy of the European Society of Cardiology. Developed in Collaboration with the European Heart Rhythm Association. *Eur Heart J* 2007; **28**: 2256–95.

in ➲Table 27.8. The staff should include well-trained nursing personnel, a part-time or full-time pacemaker technician, and a specialized cardiologist, experienced not only in device implantation but also in programming and pacemaker troubleshooting. A log book documenting follow-up of a total of 200 procedures (including 140 pacemakers, 40 ICDs, 20 CRT devices) performed during a period of 3 years is required for any physician who wants to apply for European Heart Rhythm Association accreditation. The staff are also responsible for evaluation of the patient's drug therapy, since several anti-arrhythmic drugs (especially class IC agents, such as propafenone and flecainide) can increase pacing and sensing thresholds.

The clinic should aim to ensure optimal pacemaker function matched to the patient's needs, to maximize device longevity, to identify any problems or complications related to the pacing system, and to ensure prompt recognition of battery depletion, enabling elective device replacement to be scheduled. The clinic is also responsible for informing official national organizations or the European pacemaker registry about pacemaker implantation rates, failures, and recalls. The organization of the clinic requires a suitable space, adequate secretarial support, facilities for conventional and electronic archiving of patients' records, and the necessary equipment and facilities (➲Tables 27.9 and 27.10).

Table 27.9 Logistical needs for a pacemaker follow-up clinic

Equipment:
Multi-channel electrocardiograph with real-time rhythm strip recording capability
Electronic device for the measurement and assessment of pulse duration and inter-stimulus interval
Magnet
Programmers corresponding to the devices monitored by the centre. The range should be more extensive if the clinic performs checks on transient patients (from other regions or countries)
A broad variety of pacemaker and programmer manuals
External defibrillator, transcutaneous pacing system, and resuscitation apparatus
Well-organized databases with telephone numbers of all relevant pacemaker providers and technicians
Facilities:
Easy access to an X-ray laboratory
A full spectrum of non-invasive cardiac diagnostics
24-hour telephone answering response

Reproduced with permission from Vardas PE, Auricchio A, Blanc JJ, *et al.* Guidelines for cardiac pacing and cardiac resynchronization therapy: The Task Force for Cardiac Pacing and Cardiac Resynchronization Therapy of the European Society of Cardiology. Developed in Collaboration with the European Heart Rhythm Association. *Eur Heart J* 2007; **28**: 2256–95.

The frequency and type of follow-up visit may be influenced by the type of pacemaker implanted (e.g. single- or dual-chamber), the patient's clinical status (e.g. symptoms, comorbidity, pacemaker dependency), and the original indication for implantation. A typical schedule would include a pre-discharge check, a follow-up visit at 4–8 weeks after discharge, and a further visit after 3–6 months. Thereafter, an annual visit is generally sufficient until the

Table 27.10 Functional aspects of a pacemaker clinic

Appropriately updated patient file including the following data: demographics, medical history, electrocardiographic and electrophysiological details, X-ray implantation features, long-term changes in programmed sensing, and pacing parameters
Archiving of information concerning generators, leads, and programmers
Editing of European Pacemaker registration card for each patient
Up-to-date training for all clinical personnel
Periodic briefing and education of patients
Adequate briefing of all care physicians concerning the paced patient
Informing official national organizations about pacemaker implantations, failures, and recalls

Reproduced with permission from Vardas PE, Auricchio A, Blanc JJ, *et al.* Guidelines for cardiac pacing and cardiac resynchronization therapy: The Task Force for Cardiac Pacing and Cardiac Resynchronization Therapy of the European Society of Cardiology. Developed in Collaboration with the European Heart Rhythm Association. *Eur Heart J* 2007; **28**: 2256–95.

time of predicted or observed battery depletion, when follow-up visits will again become more frequent (e.g. 3-monthly or less) until the pulse generator is replaced. For complex dual-chamber pacemakers, additional visits may occasionally be needed during the first 6 months after implantation, for optimization or fine-tuning of the programmed atrioventricular delay and other parameters.

As a supplement to the above, trans-telephonic monitoring (TTM) may be of value. When facilities for TTM are available, more frequent checks may be made (e.g. 3-monthly). This service provides the opportunity for frequent assessment of the pacing system's performance, as well as allowing the pacing clinic to receive and record the cardiac rhythm during symptoms such as dizziness and palpitation. TTM is particularly useful for patients who live far away from the follow-up centres in remote areas, or who have limited mobility, since it enables confirmation of satisfactory pacemaker function, estimation of battery longevity, and detection of any arrhythmia. Clinic visits are essential for wound assessment, for full evaluation of the patient or the device, and for troubleshooting problems detected on TTM.

In recent years, developments in technology have made possible the construction and clinical implementation of remote, wireless, patient-independent monitoring systems. These systems have the capability of home device interrogation and transmission of data via special cell phone-like instruments, providing a comprehensive review of heart rhythm-related information, as well as device diagnostics and function. A number of clinical studies are under way and others have already assessed the feasibility, safety, and effectiveness of remote follow-up in patients with pacemakers and ICDs [154–156]. The results of these studies reveal that this methodology is easy to use and is accepted with satisfaction by both patients and clinicians.

Moreover, clinicians are able to identify the occurrence of clinically important events (e.g. new-onset atrial tachycardia or atrial fibrillation, device loss-of-capture, and significant changes in lead impedance or in the pacing voltage threshold) more quickly than with conventional follow-up visits and trans-telephonic device monitoring. Remote wireless strategies are likely to have an increasing role in pacemaker follow-up and interrogation.

Practical considerations for the patient with a pacemaker

The latest developments in the technology of pacing devices and leads permit paced patients to lead a normal active life, including return to most forms of employment and even sports, as long as there is no danger of injury or overstretching in the pacemaker region. Driving is also permitted, usually 1 week after device implantation, provided there are no additional disabling factors or unless there are local regulations that dictate otherwise [157]. Patients should be informed of the risk of electromagnetic interference (EMI) and encouraged to avoid strong electromagnetic fields and specific known hazards, such as arc-welding machines. The sources of EMI can be broadly divided into two categories: those encountered outside the hospital, such as cellular phones and electronic article surveillance equipment, and those that occur in the hospital environment as a result of diagnostic or therapeutic procedures.

Possible effects of EMI include inappropriate pacemaker inhibition or triggering, asynchronous pacing, alteration of programmed settings, or damage to the device circuitry, which may lead to a sudden increase in pacing rate, known as 'runaway pacemaker'. In strong magnetic fields there is also the possibility of closure or distortion of magnetic reed switches, displacement of the pacemaker or lead, and heating of the lead tip. The clinical consequences will depend on many factors, the most important being the extent to which the patient is pacemaker-dependent [158].

Domestic household appliances rarely give rise to any problems, unless faulty [159]. Cellular phones do have the potential to affect pacemakers when in close proximity (<15cm), although clinically significant EMI is unlikely during normal use. Patients should be advised to use the ear opposite to the side of the implant and not to carry the telephone in a pocket overlying the pacemaker, since only minimal interference has been detected when the patient uses the ear opposite to the site of the implant [160]. Electronic article surveillance (EAS) systems, as used in many shops and libraries and airport metal detector gates (AMDG), may also affect pacemakers. However, the possibility of significant adverse effects is low if the patient passes rapidly through any EAS or AMDG field. For this reason, patients are advised to always carry with them their pacemaker ID card, to walk quickly through EAS and AMDG gates, and to avoid leaning on or lingering near them [158,161].

There are a number of potential hazards for pacemaker patients in the medical and therapeutic environment [162]. Magnetic resonance imaging is contra-indicated and should be avoided unless absolutely essential, in which case the patient should be carefully monitored throughout and the pacemaker checked after the procedure. ➲Table 27.11 summarizes recently published safety concerns and recommendations regarding magnetic resonance imaging in patients with pacemakers or ICD systems [163].

Extracorporeal shock wave lithotripsy, in the treatment of nephrolithiasis or cholelithiasis, entails a risk arising from

Table 27.11 Magnetic resonance imaging and pacemakers: safety concerns and guidelines

Patients are divided into three groups:	
(1) Pacemaker-dependent patients (very high risk)	If underlying rhythm is too slow—reconsider indication. The threshold for imaging and the safety requirements are higher, but no absolute contraindication
(2) ICD patient (non-dependent)* (high risk)	The patient must have a documented extremely serious, life-threatening, or severely quality-of-life limiting condition
(3) Pacemaker patient (non-dependent) (low risk)	The patient must have a documented very serious, life-threatening, or severely quality-of-life limiting condition

* Because of the higher degree of interaction between MR imaging and ICD, the threshold for imaging is higher than for pacemakers.

Reproduced with permission from Roguin A, Schwitter J, Vahlhaus C *et al.* Magnetic resonance imaging in individuals with cardiovascular implantable electronic devices. *Europace* 2008; **10**: 336–46.

both electromagnetic interference and mechanical damage from the hydraulic shock wave that is generated. It is, however, relatively safe provided the pacemaker is not in an abdominal position and the shock wave is synchronized to the ECG [164]. In dual-chamber devices, where the shock is synchronized to the atrial pacing pulse, inhibition of the ventricular channel may occur, but this may be avoided by reprogramming to VVI or VOO mode, or by enabling safety pacing. Rate rises in activity-sensing devices may be avoided by temporarily disabling the rate-responsive function. Careful follow-up of the pacemaker over several months is advisable to ensure that there has been no damage to the reed switches.

Ionizing radiation in therapeutic doses may cause cumulative damage to the semiconductor circuitry of the pacemaker and the device should be shielded to provide protection during radiotherapy. If the device lies within the field requiring irradiation (e.g. in a patient with ipsilateral breast malignancy), it may be necessary to relocate it, as shielding might compromise effective radiation therapy. Betatron therapy may cause severe EMI and should be avoided [165, 166].

For patients requiring surgery, it is important that the surgeon and anaesthetist are aware of the presence and type of the device, the underlying pathology, and the possible hazards in the perioperative period [167]. Surgical diathermy and electrocautery are well-recognized sources of EMI. Their use and power output should be kept to the minimum required, using short bursts, and avoiding close proximity to the device. With unipolar cautery systems, the indifferent electrode should be placed well away from the pacemaker (e.g. on the posterior thigh), so that the pacemaker does not lie between the electrodes. Bipolar cautery is less hazardous but EMI may still occur. If electrocautery is to be used in a pacemaker-dependent patient, preoperative reprogramming of the device to an asynchronous or triggered mode should be considered. In all other cases, a programmer or magnet should be immediately available to enable the activation of asynchronous fixed-rate pacing in case of pacemaker inhibition. Disabling the rate-adaptive function may also be advisable to avoid the risk of idiosyncratic rate acceleration.

Similar considerations apply to catheter ablation, since almost all procedures nowadays are performed using radiofrequency current at a frequency of 400–500kHz [168]. Prior to radiofrequency ablation, the implanted pulse generator should be interrogated and the settings recorded. On completion of the procedure further interrogation of the device will determine whether reprogramming is necessary. In patients who require external cardioversion or defibrillation, the use of anteroposterior paddle positions will reduce the risk of damage to the device or myocardial injury. The pacemaker should always be checked after a shock has been delivered.

New indications for cardiac pacing

The foregoing discussion has focused on the use of pacemakers in the treatment of bradycardia caused by sinus node disease, atrioventricular block, or chronic bifascicular and trifascicular block. In recent years, a variety of new indications have emerged and it is now clear that cardiac pacing may be of benefit in selected patients with other conditions, even in the absence of bradycardia.

- CRT for selected heart failure patients has already been mentioned and is considered further in ➲Chapter 23.
- In patients with hypertrophic obstructive cardiomyopathy (see ➲Chapter 18), pacing-induced pre-excitation of the right ventricular apex may reduce the left ventricular outflow tract gradient and clinical improvement has been reported in randomized trials [169–171]. Although there is clear evidence that some patients derive a benefit from pacing, there is to date no certain way to predict the response and the clinical benefit does not correlate well with gradient reduction. Patients with drug-refractory hypertrophic cardiomyopathy with significant resting or provoked left ventricular outflow tract gradient and contraindications for septal ablation or myectomy have a Class IIb, Level of Evidence A, indication for pacing [53].
- In patients with severe carotid sinus syndrome, the role of pacing is well established [172]. It is also recommended for patients with recurrent syncope without clear

provocative events but in whom there is a hypersensitive cardio-inhibitory response to carotid sinus massage [53]. The use of pacing in severe vasovagal syndrome with a cardio-inhibitory response to head-up tilt testing is more controversial. Although some trials have shown a reduction in syncope with pacing, using a specialized rate-drop sensing algorithm [173] or rate hysteresis [174], more recent studies designed to control for a possible placebo effect have shown no clear benefit [175, 176]. Pacemaker implantation is recommended (Class IIa, Level of Evidence C) only in patients over 40 years of age with recurrent severe vasovagal syncope who show prolonged asystole during ECG recording and/or tilt testing, after failure of other therapeutic options and being informed of the conflicting results of trials [53].

- In patients with sleep-apnoea syndrome who were already paced for conventional indications, atrial overdrive pacing at a rate higher than the mean nocturnal heart rate has been used for the reduction of apnoeic episodes. However, the results of the available clinical trials are conflicting and more studies are needed to clarify the possible effect of atrial pacing on sleep apnoea and to determine in which subgroups of patients this approach might be beneficial [177–179].
- In the long-QT syndrome (see ➲Chapters 9 and 30), pacing is indicated in patients with coincident 2:1 or third-degree atrioventricular block, symptomatic bradycardia (spontaneous or due to beta-blocker), or pause-dependent ventricular tachycardia, as an adjunct to beta-blockade [53, 180] (Class IIa, Level of Evidence C).

Detailed consideration of these new indications for pacing is beyond the scope of this discussion but they are considered elsewhere in this book in the chapters dealing with the specific conditions.

Concluding remarks

Rapid developments in biomedicine and microelectronics, and the introduction of remote, wireless, patient-independent monitoring systems have provided a tremendous boost to the diagnostic and therapeutic capabilities of the pacemaker physician. Pacing devices are becoming ever smaller, with increased reliability and longevity, and offer a host of sophisticated algorithms and programming and diagnostic options. However, the role of the cardiologist is still definitive and fundamental. Clinical insight and judgement, aided by appropriate diagnostic methods, will lead to the correct diagnostic approach to bradycardia, the choice of suitable therapy, and the selection of the most appropriate device and mode if a pacemaker is indicated. Invaluable in this task are the conclusions of randomized clinical trials and the published guidelines for cardiac pacing. However, the key factors in the success of treatment are the experience, knowledge, and skill of the pacemaker physician [181], which will determine patient satisfaction and well-being at all stages of treatment and follow-up.

Personal perspective

Implantable pacemakers are now the established gold standard for the treatment of symptomatic bradycardia. A half century of clinical and technological innovation has resulted in the development of highly sophisticated devices and in recent years, the evidence base for pacing practice has been strengthened by the findings of numerous randomized trials. The trial results have often differed from expectations and demonstrated that technological enhancements do not always translate into improved clinical outcomes. They have also highlighted the fact that physiological pacing requires the preservation or restoration not only of atrioventricular synchrony but also of inter- and intraventricular synchrony. During the next decade, attention is likely to focus on minimizing dyssynchrony by avoiding unnecessary pacing and improving the cardiac activation sequence during pacing by the use of alternative sites, such as the atrial septum and the septal aspect of the right ventricular outflow tract. In some cases, pacing at multiple ventricular sites may be needed to ensure cardiac synchronization and this will require the development of more specialized endocardial leads and the possible use of epicardial approaches using thoracoscopic techniques. Novel technologies may offer an alternative to conventional leads and preliminary data on the use of ultrasound energy to achieve cardiac stimulation have already been reported [182]. The integration of anatomic data from multiple imaging modalities with electrical activation maps may facilitate targeted lead placement to achieve optimal paced cardiac function. More immediate developments are likely to include the introduction of pacing systems that are compatible with magnetic resonance imaging [163] and increased use of remote programming and monitoring of device function along with a range of haemodynamic and clinical parameters. The incorporation of haemodynamic and other biosensors into the pacing system may also facilitate automated and dynamic optimization of programmed parameters. In the longer term, gene therapy and stem cell techniques may enable the development of biological pacemakers that might ultimately replace the artificial systems that are currently in use [183]. Whatever the direction of future developments, the expertise and care of the cardiologist, informed by the results of well-designed and carefully conducted clinical trials, will remain paramount in patient selection and tailoring pacemaker therapy to optimize clinical outcomes.

Further reading

Benditt D, Blanc J-J, Brignole M, *et al.* *The Evaluation and Treatment of Syncope. A Handbook for Clinical Practice*, 2nd edn., 2006. The ESC Education Series. Oxford: Blackwell Publishing.

Brignole M, Alboni P, Benditt DG, *et al.* Task Force on Syncope, European Society of Cardiology. Guidelines on management (diagnosis and treatment) of syncope – update 2004. Executive Summary. *Eur Heart J* 2004; **25**: 2054–72.

Cleland JG, Daubert J-C, Erdmann E, *et al.* The effect of cardiac resynchronization on morbidity and mortality in heart failure. *N Engl J Med* 2005; **352**: 1539–49.

Healey JS, Toff WD, Lamas GA, *et al.* Cardiovascular outcomes with atrial-based pacing compared with ventricular pacing: meta-analysis of randomized trials, using individual patient data. *Circulation* 2006; **114**: 11–7.

Knight BP, Gersh BJ, Carlson MD, *et al.* Role of permanent pacing to prevent atrial fibrillation: Science advisory from the American Heart Association Council on Clinical Cardiology [Subcommittee on Electrocardiography and Arrhythmias] and the Quality of Care and Outcomes Research Interdisciplinary Working Group, in collaboration with the Heart Rhythm Society. *Circulation* 2005; **111**: 240–3.

Roguin A, Schwitter J,Vahlhaus C, *et al.* Magnetic resonance imaging in individuals with cardiovascular implantable electronic devices. *Europace* 2008; **10**: 336–46.

Sweeney MO, Bank AJ, Nsah E, *et al.* Minimizing ventricular pacing to reduce atrial fibrillation in sinus-node disease. *N Engl J Med* 2007; **357**: 1000–8.

Vardas PE, Auricchio A, Blanc J-J, *et al.* Guidelines for cardiac pacing and cardiac resynchronization therapy: The Task Force for Cardiac Pacing and Cardiac Resynchronization Therapy of the European Society of Cardiology. Developed in Collaboration with the European Heart Rhythm Association. *Eur Heart J* 2007; **28**: 2256–95.

➲ **For full references and multimedia materials please visit the online version of the book (http://esctextbook.oxfordonline.com).**

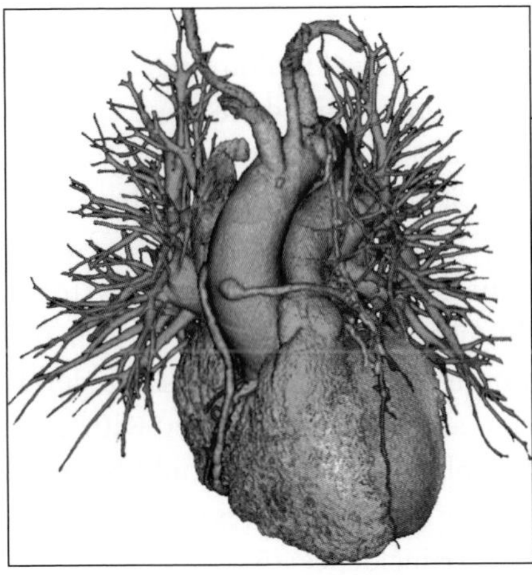

CHAPTER 28

Supraventricular Tachycardias

Jerónimo Farré, Hein J.J. Wellens, José M. Rubio, and Juan Benezet

Contents

Summary

Supraventricular arrhythmias comprise atrial extrasystoles, supraventricular tachycardia (SVT), and atrial fibrillation (AF). SVT includes atrial tachycardia and atrioventricular junctional tachycardia. Atrial flutter is the most common form of macro-re-entrant atrial tachycardia. Atrial extrasystoles are the most prevalent supraventricular arrhythmias, followed by AF, and atrial flutter. While the life expectancy of patients with paroxysmal SVT is often normal, their quality of life may be poor. Patients with the Wolff–Parkinson–White syndrome frequently develop paroxysmal SVT or AF; exceptionally, they may die suddenly if AF supervenes and degenerates into ventricular fibrillation due to a very short anterograde refractory period of the accessory pathway. Non-paroxysmal forms of SVT are rare. Among the latter, permanent SVTs can result in a tachycardiomyopathy with systolic left ventricular dysfunction that is usually reversible after abolishing the arrhythmia. The 12-lead electrocardiogram (ECG), combined with vagal or pharmacological manoeuvres, is essential for establishing the type of SVT. Paroxysmal SVT can be terminated by vagal manoeuvres, antiarrhythmic drugs, DC-shock cardioversion, and pacing. Paroxysmal atrial flutter usually is terminated by DC-shock cardioversion or overdrive atrial pacing. Although paroxysmal and permanent SVTs have various sites of origin and mechanisms, they can usually be cured by catheter ablation techniques. Electro-anatomic mapping and navigation systems facilitate the ablation of complex forms of atrial tachycardia. Surgery has no role today in the treatment of SVT. Patients in whom ablation cannot be performed may require the use of chronic antiarrhythmic drug therapy to prevent recurrences of SVT.

Introduction

Supraventricular arrhythmias and supraventricular tachycardia

Supraventricular arrhythmias are disorders in the generation of the heart impulse in which structures above the division of the bundle of His are essential for their occurrence. Supraventricular tachyarrhythmias—characterized by impulse formation more rapid than expected—include SVT and AF. SVT comprises atrial tachycardia (AT) and atrioventricular (AV) junctional tachycardias, and excludes AF. Atrial flutter (AFL) is the most prevalent form of macro-re-entrant AT. Sinus tachycardia is a physiological reactive response, except for the so-called inappropriate sinus tachycardia (IST) and the postural orthostatic tachycardia syndrome (POTS). AV junctional tachycardias include: AV nodal reciprocating tachycardia (AVNRT); AV reciprocating tachycardia (AVRT) incorporating an accessory pathway (AP); non-paroxysmal junctional tachycardia (NPJT); and the permanent junctional reciprocating tachycardia (PJRT) utilizing an AP with long conduction times as retrograde limb of the circuit [1]. Supraventricular arrhythmias also encompass atrial and AV junctional extrasystoles, sinus node disorders, wandering sinus pacemaker, and low atrial rhythms.

During the last 40 years catheter mapping and stimulation studies have defined the site of origin and pathway of SVTs, finding new electrocardiographic signs for their diagnosis, and resulting in the development of ablation techniques—first with surgery and then with catheters [2, 3]. Recently, electro-anatomic catheter mapping and navigation systems have enabled 3-dimensional reconstructions of the heart chambers, merging these morphologic models with the cardiovascular anatomy obtained with magnetic resonance (MR), multislice computerized tomography (CT), or rotational fluoroangiographic imaging examinations. Positioning electrode-catheters in the heart can be achieved without fluoroscopic control and there are tools for catheter navigation with remote control.

Mode of presentation of supraventricular tachyarrhythmias

'Paroxysmal' refers to SVT presenting as a sudden, usually recurrent, episode. 'Non-paroxysmal' is applied to a phasically ongoing supraventricular tachyarrhythmia that can be 'secondary' (related to incidental triggers), like NPJT, or 'primary' (occurring without precipitating factors) such as primary permanent SVT. 'Permanent' or 'incessant' are those SVTs that are constantly present or phasically ongoing for >50% of the time during prolonged monitoring. Sustained are SVT lasting >30s and non-sustained are those episodes with a shorter duration. Patients with permanent SVT may develop systolic left ventricular dysfunction (tachycardiomyopathy) [1, 4].

Epidemiologically speaking, only atrial extrasystoles, AF (not covered in this chapter) (see ➲Chapter 29), and AFL are relatively common arrhythmias. The risk for developing supraventricular arrhythmias changes with ageing. Incidences using Kaplan–Meier plots would be more meaningful than the usually available figures on 'incidence', 'prevalence', or 'cumulative incidence' [5].

Atrial and atrioventricular junctional extrasystoles

Definition and epidemiology

Atrial extrasystoles or atrial premature beats (APBs) are depolarizations generated at the atrial myocardium that occur earlier than the expected normal sinoatrial activation wavefront (➲Fig. 28.1). APBs are different from AV junctional echo beats where structures beyond the atria are essential for their development. APBs usually originate at areas other than the normal sinus node pacemaker and are also referred to as 'atrial ectopics'. APBs can be isolated or occur as couplets (two consecutive atrial extrasystoles), or may elicit a run of repetitive atrial responses, AF, AFL, or more rarely, any form of SVT.

The APB is the most common supraventricular arrhythmia. Low density APBs are registered in Holter recordings in ≈60% of young healthy males and females and are almost constantly present after the fifth decade of life [6–8]. Their frequency increases with age, presence of structural heart disease, and conditions prone to develop AF (hyperthyroidism, hypertension, smoking, alcohol intoxication, heart failure). In patients with 'focal AF' APBs are habitually registered during periods of sinus rhythm [9]. While ABPs are common early after a successful electrical cardioversion of AF, it is controversial if their density predicts subsequent AF recurrence [10, 11]. Frequent APBs in a 24-hour ECG of patients with an acute ischaemic stroke and undocumented episodes of AF, are markers for an increased risk of subsequent documentation of AF [12].

AV junctional premature beats (AVJPBs) are premature depolarizations arising from the AV node and His bundle. They should also be differentiated from the AV junctional echoes. They are less common than atrial or ventricular extrasystoles.

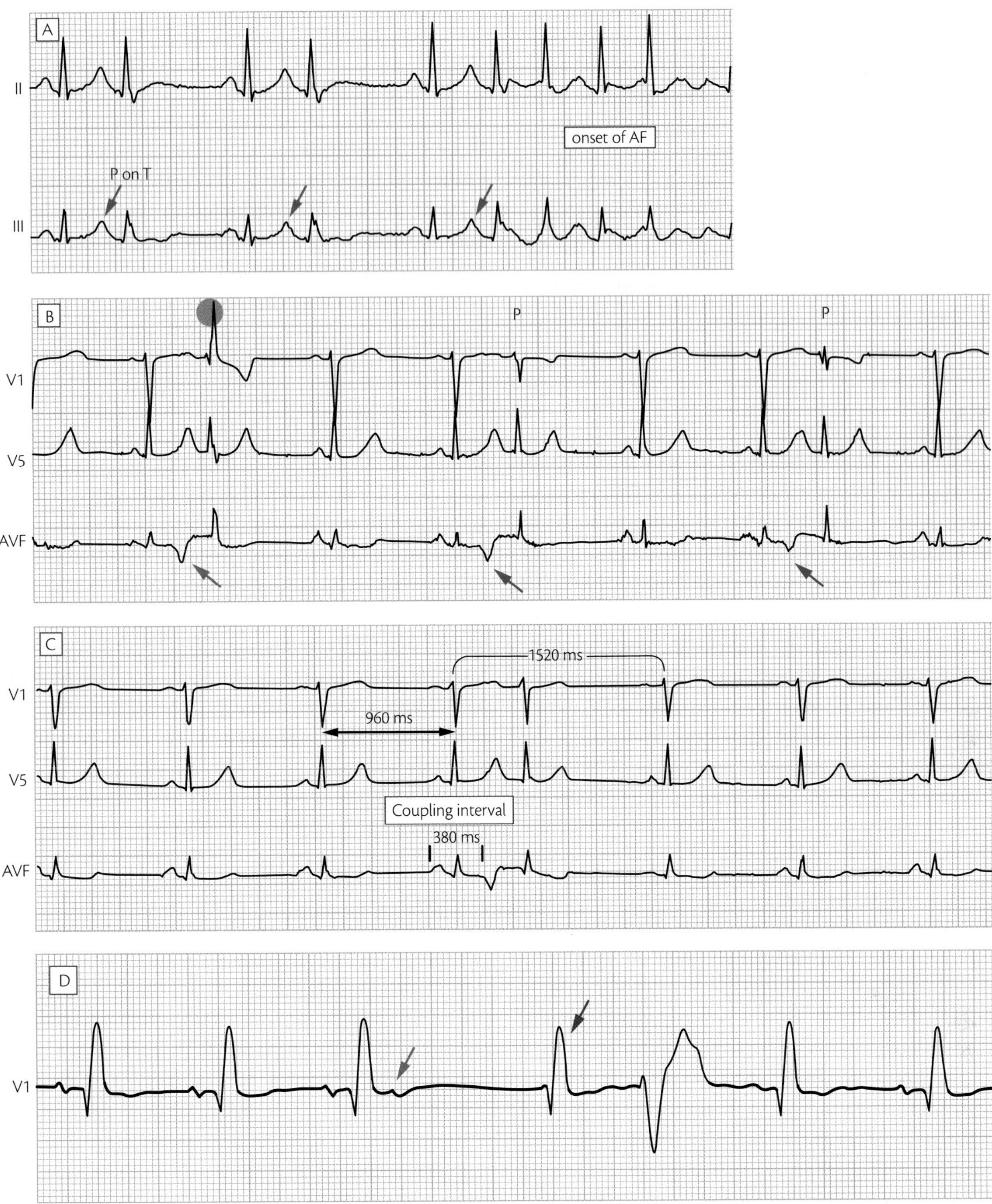

Figure 28.1 (A) Bigeminal early APBs (P-on-T) precede onset of atrial fibrillation. (B) An APB (red arrow) is conducted to the ventricles with RBBB aberrancy (red circle). In lead AVF the repolarization preceding the early ventricular depolarizations (arrows), independently of the morphology of the QRS complex, is very different to that observed in cardiac cycles not followed by a premature beat. The last two APBs (green arrows) are followed by a narrow QRS complex whose contour is different than that of ventricular complexes following normal sinus P waves. (C) (same patient as panel A) An APB with a coupling interval of 380ms is followed by a QRS complex identical in morphology to those after sinus P waves. The post-extrasystolic pause is non-compensatory (see text). (D) A blocked APB (red arrow) produces an 'unexpected' pause. Note the change in configuration of the ventricular repolarization containing the blocked APB. The post-extrasystolic pause in this case is followed not by a normally conducted sinus P wave, but by an AV junctional escape (blue arrow).

Pathogenesis

APBs originate as a result of enhanced and abnormal automaticity, triggered activity, or re-entry. APBs due to re-entry should not be confused with AV junctional reciprocal echo beats developing when a sinus impulse returns to the atria through a slow AV nodal pathway or a concealed slow-conducting bypass tract. Exercise-related APBs could suggest an adrenergic dependence, while a higher prevalence at night or rest would indicate a vagal mechanism. AVJPBs are due to increased automaticity or triggered focal activity.

Diagnosis

APBs are frequently asymptomatic or may be perceived as a missed beat, a precordial palpitation or thump, a neck strike, or the need of coughing [13]. Symptomatic APBs are usually noticed at rest. APBs with a very short coupling interval result in an atrial contraction that coincides with the mechanical ventricular systole (P-on-T phenomenon) producing 'cannon waves' in the jugular venous pulse noticed as neck thumps. Some people with symptomatic APBs become extremely worried and develop panic attacks with sweating, dyspnoea, chest discomfort, dizziness, and numbness or tingling sensations due to hyperventilation. APBs tend to be asymptomatic in elderly people, particularly with sick hearts. The AV conduction time following the atrial extrasystole, and the psychological profile of the patients, also influence their symptoms. Patients in whom SVT has been ablated may refer a feeling 'as if the tachycardia was going to start' due to APBs. Thereafter these sensations disappear either due to reassurance in relation with their cure or because the actual density of APBs is reduced. Symptomatic APBs frequently have a periodic presentation during several minutes or even hours for some weeks or months a year.

Electrocardiographically, an APB manifests itself as a premature P wave whose contour is usually different to that of the normal sinus beat. The coupling interval of the APB is the time from the onset of the atrial extrasystole to the beginning of the preceding sinus P wave (➲Fig. 28.1C). Most APBs reset the sinus node, so that the pause following the atrial extrasystole is less than compensatory (the interval from the sinus P wave preceding the APB to the sinus P wave following it is less than twice the sinus cycle length) (➲Fig. 28.1C). When an APB fails to reset the sinus node due to entry block into this structure, or to a long distance between the origin of the APB and the sinus node, the post-extrasystolic pause will be compensatory. When there is a marked sinus arrhythmia the pause following an APB may be more than compensatory.

In APBs with short coupling intervals, the ectopic P wave is coincidental with the preceding T wave. This 'P-on-T' phenomenon may herald the development of AF (➲Fig. 28.1A). The shorter the coupling interval of the APB, the shorter is the atrial refractory period, and the higher the vulnerability of the atrial myocardium to fibrillation [9].

APBs are usually conducted to the ventricles. The QRS complex following an APB may be identical, slightly different, or overtly aberrant as compared with the ventricular complexes following sinus beats (➲Fig. 28.1B–D). Aberrant wide QRS complexes may result from the development of a functional bundle branch block, or the existence of an AP, as in Wolff–Parkinson–White (WPW) syndrome. APBs may reveal the presence of a non-evident form of pre-excitation. APBs can be blocked in the AV conduction system resulting in 'pauses without apparent cause' in the ECG. It is important to look for deformities in the ST–T segment to identify the APBs in these cases (➲Fig. 28.1D).

The P-wave morphology of the APB is determined by its site of origin and the presence of atrial conduction disturbances due to atrial dilation, catheter and surgical interventions, fibrosis, and the influence of antiarrhythmic drugs. APBs with a short coupling interval are obscured by the preceding T wave. Left atrial APBs can be negative in lead I and AVL and usually positive in V1 except for those from a low septal and coronary sinus (CS) origin that produce a negative P wave in the inferior leads, and a positive or isoelectric P wave in lead I and AVL. APBs from the pulmonary veins and superior vena cava may trigger AF. APBs from the left superior and right superior pulmonary veins are positive in leads II, III, and AVF, negative in AVL, and predominantly positive in V1 (➲Fig. 28.2). Anatomic slices of the heart as those shown in ➲Fig. 28.2 have been obtained using the 'Visible Human Slice and Surface Server' with data sets of the 'Visible Human Male and Female Project' [14]. Criteria to differentiate right from left pulmonary vein APBs are a P-wave duration <120ms, a P-wave amplitude in lead I >0.05mV, and a P-wave amplitude ratio in leads II/III >1.25. An origin in the superior rather than in the inferior pulmonary veins is suggested if the sum of the P-wave amplitudes in all the inferior leads is >0.3mV but this criterion is of limited value [15]. APBs from the superior caval vein frequently have a biphasic or isoelectric P wave in lead V1, or a biphasic P wave in AVL [16].

Symptoms due to AVJPBs are similar to those of ventricular premature beats and not very different from those of APBs. The coupling interval is measured from the onset of the premature QRS complex to the onset of the preceding ventricular depolarization. The QRS complex is narrow, either identical to that of normal sinus beats, or

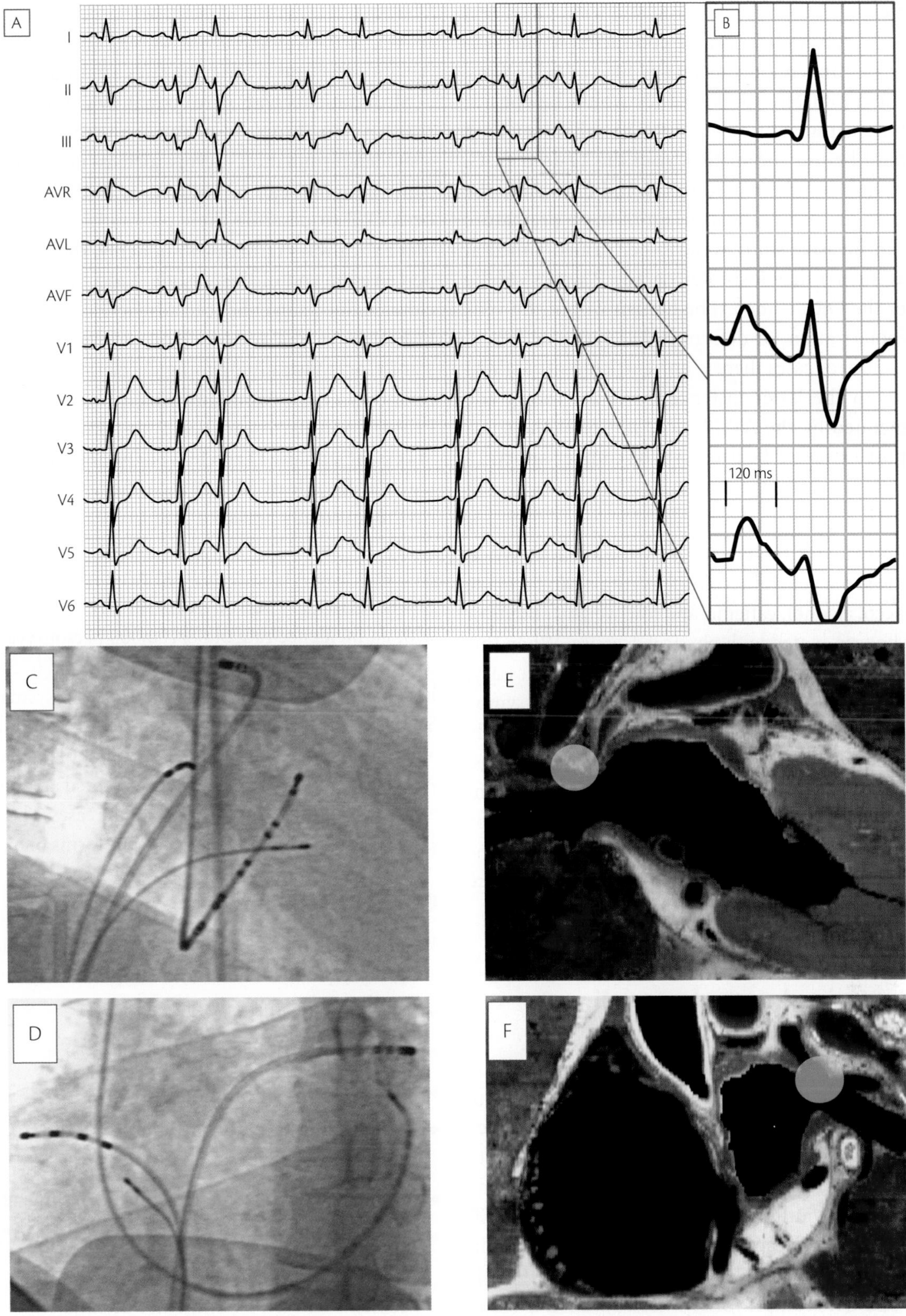

Figure 28.2 (A) APBs from the junction between left superior pulmonary vein and left atrium. Ectopic P waves are flat in lead I, negative in AVL and AVR, positive and with similar amplitudes in II and III, and positive in V1. The sum of P-wave amplitudes in II and III is 0.55mV. (B) Magnification of the green vignette shown in (A). Extrasystolic P-wave duration is 120ms. (C, D) Fluorographic frames in right anterior oblique and left anterior oblique (RAO, LAO) projections showing the site of ablation of these ectopic beats (the patient also had AT from this site). (E, F) Computer-generated sections of the heart in RAO and LAO projection, respectively. Yellow circles represent the ablation site. (EPFL's Visible Human Surface Server, ©EPFL, 1998) [14].

slightly different in configuration but still with a duration <120ms. Although AVJPBs can be conducted to the ventricles with aberrant conduction and a QRS width ≥120ms, electrocardiographically speaking they would be considered as ventricular in nature since distinction between both origins would be too speculative from the 12-lead ECG. Intracardiac His-bundle recordings would determine the ventricular or supraventricular origin of these premature beats, but an invasive study is never performed aimed at establishing such a diagnosis. Retrograde P waves can be visible after the QRS complex, be hidden within the ventricular depolarization, or deform its late terminal forces. In some 30–50% of cases there is no ventriculo-atrial (VA) conduction. In the latter instance, or if the retrograde P wave generated by the AVJPB does not reset the sinus node, the post-extrasystolic pause will be compensatory.

Treatment

APBs are untreated if the patient is asymptomatic. When symptomatic some general recommendations can be made (avoid tobacco, alcohol, caffeine, and lose weight). Bouts of APBs may be terminated with physical exercise. When this fails, beta-blocking agents may be tried and, if necessary, class I antiarrhythmic drugs. Most patients with symptomatic APBs are relatively young and have structurally normal hearts and may be safely treated with class IC drugs. The same can be said in relation to AVJPBs. Long-term heavy sport practice is a risk factor for developing AF or AFL in males over 30 years [17]. Some of these people complain of palpitations at rest due to APBs and should replace the enduring sportive practice for a less intense exercise.

Supraventricular tachycardia

Definition and epidemiology

SVT is a tachyarrhythmia in which structures above the division of the bundle of His are essential for its maintenance and comprises AT, AFL, AVNRT, AVRT incorporating one or more APs, NPJT, and the primary permanent SVTs [1, 18]. The width of the QRS complex during SVT is usually 80–100ms. Exceptionally, ventricular tachycardia (VT) may have a QRS complex duration <120ms [19, 20]. Conversely, the QRS complex of SVT has a duration ≥120ms if the patient has a permanent left or right bundle branch block (LBBB, RBBB); if during tachycardia a functional BBB (aberrancy) develops; or if AV conduction during tachycardia is over an AV bypass tract. The ventricular rate during SVT is usually >120bpm and frequently 140–250bpm. The atrial rate may be higher than the ventricular rate in AT, in AFL, and exceptionally in AVNRT. In AVRT utilizing an AP, the atrial and ventricular rates are always the same.

Most patients with paroxysmal SVT notice palpitations that have an abrupt onset and frequently, but not always, a sudden termination. Terms such as 'neck pounding' and 'shirt flapping' can be utilized by patients with AVNRT or AVRT to describe their palpitations. While paroxysmal SVT always terminates suddenly, the patient may not perceive the end of the episode if the ensuing sinus rate is elevated due to an enhanced adrenergic drive for emotional or haemodynamic reasons. Non-paroxysmal SVTs are constantly or phasically ongoing accelerated rhythms whose rates may be <100bpm but usually between 120–190bpm. Primary non-paroxysmal SVT are termed 'permanent' or 'incessant' and are characterized by runs of SVT that alternate during at least 50% of the time with the normal sinus rhythm or totally replace it [18].

The estimated prevalence of paroxysmal SVT, excluding AFL and also AT, is 2.25/1000 persons and the incidence rate is 35/100,000 person-years [21]. AFL is more common with an incidence rate of 88/100,000 person-years, ranging from 5/100,000 in individuals <50 years old to 587/100,000 in subjects aged >80 years [22]. Non-paroxysmal forms of SVT are less frequent. In patients undergoing a catheter ablation intervention, AVNRT, AVRT utilizing an AP, and AFL are the most commonly encountered arrhythmias (AF excluded) and account for ≈90% of the cases. The remaining 10% represents AT and the incessant forms of SVT.

Quality of life and life expectancy

While most patients with SVT have a normal life expectancy, their quality of life may be impaired due to:

- the symptoms during SVT;
- the frequency and duration of the attacks;
- the need to seek hospital treatment;
- the apprehension to participate in certain sports or professional activities;
- the panic of having an attack during driving; and
- the feeling of prolonged tiredness after a SVT episode [23, 24].

Problems derived from the use of antiarrhythmic drugs are minimized if SVT is cured by radiofrequency catheter ablation (RFCA). In a general population the probability of recurrences of paroxysmal SVT excluding AFL is of 20% at 2 years, most of the relapses occurring within the first year [21].

Exceptionally, SVT can compromise life expectancy either because of direct consequences of the arrhythmia, or indirectly as a result of antiarrhythmic drug therapy, complications of catheter ablation procedures, or associated conditions leading to sudden arrhythmic death. Paroxysmal SVT can be fatal when:

- syncopal and the patient suffers a life-threatening trauma;
- degenerates into ventricular fibrillation (VF);
- a severe embolism occurs (as in AF or AFL);
- precipitates acute pulmonary oedema, as in patients with systolic or diastolic left ventricular dysfunction; and
- induces myocardial ischaemia in patients with underlying coronary artery disease.

Permanent SVT can shorten life expectancy if the patient develops a tachycardiomyopathy—a form of left ventricular dysfunction usually reversible after abolishing the arrhythmia with RFCA [25–28]. Sudden death can also be an outcome in patients with tachycardiomyopathy [29].

Degeneration of AF into VF in patients with WPW syndrome is not the only situation in which sudden death can occur during SVT. An enhanced AV nodal conduction facilitates the degeneration of SVT into VF. SVT excluding AF, can be the underlying triggering mechanism responsible for 5–8% of aborted sudden deaths [30, 31] and in <50% of these cases is an AP involved [30]. This complication is more frequent in patients with structural heart disease. Syncope during SVT may be of vasovagal origin and not always related to very fast ventricular rates [32]. Patients with the Brugada syndrome can develop AF—or more rarely AVNRT or AVRT—and sudden death due to VF could occur due to the ventricular electrical abnormalities, not to the SVT itself [33].

The 12-lead ECG (also see ➲ Chapter 2)

A 12-lead ECG must be obtained during episodes of SVT. Most of the available applications for digital ECG storage on computerized hospital information systems only permit saving a 10-s view of the ECG in four three-lead sets of 2.5s each, plus a bottom rhythm strip in either II or V1. This ECG presentation and storage is correct for the outpatient clinic but not for SVT diagnosis and treatment, including vagal, pharmacological, or pacing manoeuvres.

The 12-lead ECG during tachycardia which should be compared with that obtained during sinus rhythm, serves to localize the origin and pathway of the arrhythmia. Experienced cardiologists may identify AVNRT, AVRT, PJTR, isthmus-dependent AFL, and AT, and even suspect the site of origin in focal AT and differentiate the latter from a macro-re-entrant AT. In patients with recurrent palpitations the ECG during sinus rhythm may demonstrate signs that are markers for a high probability of SVT such as:

- pre-excitation or signs consistent with a non-evident form of WPW syndrome;
- Bachmann bundle block defined by P waves ≥110ms, bimodal in various leads, and with a biphasic contour in the inferior leads where they have a wide positive initial part, and a narrow negative terminal component; this finding is a marker for an increased risk of developing AF, macro-re-entrant AT, and AFL (➲Fig. 28.3) [34, 35].

Ambulatory ECG recordings (also see ➲ Chapter 2)

Ambulatory 24-hour to 1-month ECG recordings are used to evaluate symptoms potentially due to arrhythmias—palpitations, dizziness, syncope, cerebral ischaemic attacks, or sudden dyspnoea at rest. Holter monitoring is of little practical use when symptoms occur infrequently and its yield is greatest when the patient's complaints appear on daily basis, something common for APBs but rare in patients with SVT [36, 37]. For patients with infrequent symptoms and without pre-excitation, 1-month ECG monitoring, intermittent event recorders, or even an implantable loop recorder, may be more appropriate [38, 39]. The diagnosis of inappropriate sinus tachycardia rests on Holter recordings. Patients with the WPW syndrome may show a previously undocumented intermittent pre-excitation during a Holter recording. In permanent SVT, Holter recordings may show that the arrhythmia is phasically ongoing or is constantly present [18].

Exercise electrocardiography (also see ➲ Chapters 2 and 25)

An exercise ECG can be performed when the patient's symptoms develop during physical activity. Induction of SVT during exercise is rare. An exercise test is also used for risk stratification in patients with WPW syndrome and during the post-ablation follow-up in patients with permanent SVT.

Electrophysiological studies

Catheter mapping and stimulation studies are indicated to define the origin and pathway of SVT when the patient is a candidate for RFCA, or to evaluate the cause of paroxysmal palpitations in patients with undocumented arrhythmias if the symptoms are severe or impair their quality of life. In WPW syndrome electrophysiological studies are still used

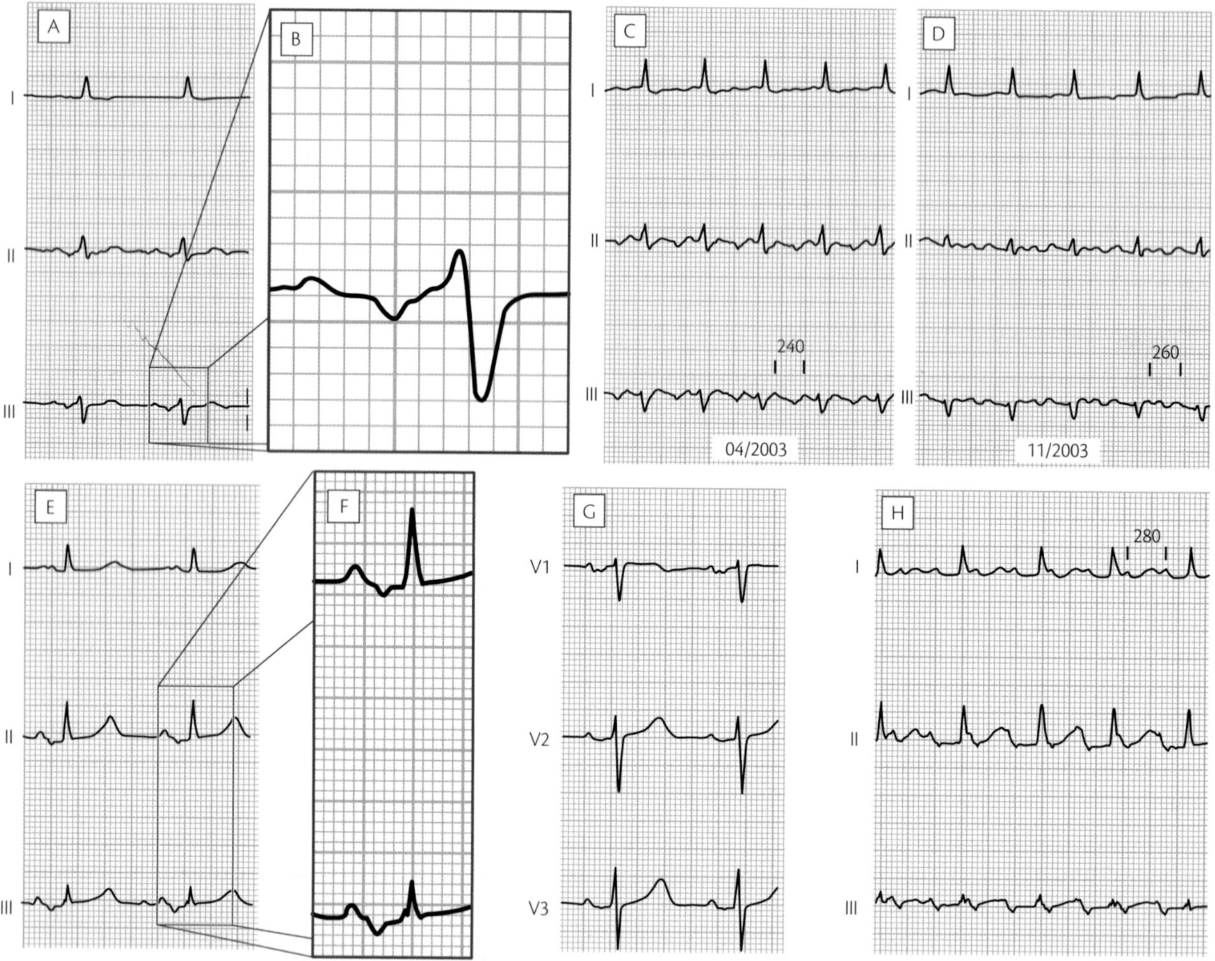

Figure 28.3 Intra-atrial block and macro-re-entrant AT. (A) Leads I, II, and III in a patient with chronic obstructive lung disease. (B) Magnification from lead III depicting a wide P wave (180ms) with a negative terminal component also observed in lead II in A. (C, D) Recordings during two episodes of palpitations on amiodarone treatment. The patient was shown to have isthmus-dependent AFL and underwent catheter ablation. In C AFL is of the common counterclockwise type and D shows an uncommon clockwise AFL. (E–H) Female patient with a mitral valve mechanical prosthesis; (E) sinus rhythm; (F) magnification of leads II and III depicting wide sinus P waves (140ms) with a negative terminal component typical of Bachmann bundle block; (G) leads V1, V2, and V3 in sinus rhythm; (H) leads I, II, and III during left macro-re-entrant AT (atypical flutter) around the left atrial atriotomy scar.

for risk stratification. An electrophysiological study may differentiate sinus tachycardia from a permanent AT in patients with a dilated cardiomyopathy. Paroxysmal tachycardias in patients without structural heart disease are usually supraventricular, although in a few cases an idiopathic right or left VT might be initiated. Electrophysiological studies differentiate AFL that depends on the cavo-tricuspid isthmus (CTI) from other types of flutters or macro-re-entrant AT requiring more complex ablation procedures.

Vagal and pharmacological manoeuvres

Vagal manoeuvres and the infusion of certain drugs are used for diagnostic and therapeutic reasons in patients with SVT. Carotid sinus massage is preferred over ocular globe compression. For carotid sinus massage the patient must lie in supine position with the neck extended, ideally with a pillow under the shoulders and the head looking at the side opposite to the approached carotid artery. A continuous ECG recording should be available and visible to the physician. A firm massage is applied for some 5s first at the right and then at the left side, with a 1-min interval between massages, using the thumb or the index and middle fingers together over the point of maximal carotid pulsation at the medial border of the sternocleidomastoid muscle. Carotid sinus massage should not be performed in patients with a cerebrovascular accident in the past 3 months or a carotid bruit on auscultation. The diagnostic and therapeutic effect of carotid sinus massage is limited by a high sympathetic tone.

Verapamil, adenosine, and ATP are used intravenously for diagnostic and acute therapeutic purposes in patients with paroxysmal SVT [40]. Adenosine is infused in very rapid boluses followed by a 20-mL saline flush. An initial dose of 3mg is followed every 2min, if required, by a second dose of 6mg, and a third dose of 12mg (in adults we can start with a 6mg dose). The 12mg dose might be repeated but doses >12mg are not recommended. If the patient has a history of asthma or of chronic obstructive lung disease, verapamil should be used instead unless the patient is in heart failure, has severe systolic left ventricular dysfunction, or is on beta-blocking agents. In adults we utilize 5–10mg of intravenous verapamil over 1min and in children we start with a 0.15mg/kg dose. The effect of adenosine is very short-lived and that of verapamil lasts for 30min so that a second dose should not be given during this period of time.

Catheter ablation

Catheter ablation interventions have replaced surgery in the treatment of SVT and are, in many instances, the treatment of choice for the majority of these patients. Complications associated with catheter ablation depend on the experience of the interventional team, the type of SVT, and the technological facilities available at each institution. Radiation exposure complications are minimized using well maintained X-ray equipment, with low-rate pulsed fluoroscopy, and avoiding fluorographic acquisition, and lateral or LAO projections. Flat-panel systems and well filtered X-ray sources have further reduced the exposure risks for patients and operators. Electro-anatomical navigation systems permit intracardiac catheter manipulation without fluoroscopic control. The incidence of pneumothorax is minimized by avoiding a subclavian vein puncture although a jugular vein approach may also result in this complication. Catheter manipulation may rarely produce:

- cardiac perforation with acute or delayed tamponade requiring drainage in the fully anticoagulated patient;
- valvular damage, exceptional with the usual gentle handling of catheters;
- dislodgment of thrombotic or atheromatous material with embolization;
- trapping of the catheter in the Chiari network requiring maintained traction for a few minutes;
- vascular dissection partially avoided using long arterial sheaths in elderly people;
- transient but prolonged mechanical A–V block due to trauma on the AV node or on the right bundle branch in patients with LBBB;
- mechanical block of an AP that may interfere with its ablation.

Even more unusual is applying RF current inside a coronary artery believing to be at the ventricular side of the AV groove, a complication avoided by carefully watching the intracardiac electrograms. RFCA may produce permanent AV block in patients with perinodal AT, AVNRT, or with septal APs (peri-Hisian, perinodal, or superior-paraseptal), and exceptionally in CTI AFL. Vagal reflexes inducing AV block and coronary artery spasm have also been observed in rare instances. Although catheter ablation should result in no mortality some fatalities have occurred, most of them unreported [1]. Vascular access problems such as haematomas, femoral vein thrombosis, arteriovenous fistula, and femoral pseudoaneurism depend on the physicians' skills but also on the intensity of the anticoagulation regimen during and after the procedure. Vascular problems are the most prevalent complications and may be severe in patients receiving anticoagulants. Careful and prolonged compression immediately after the procedure and surveillance of the inguinal region with palpation, auscultation, and eventually ultrasound examination thereafter, are mandatory measures for early identification of problems requiring more specific treatments.

Atrial tachycardia

Definition

AT is a rapid atrial impulse formation at rates of 110–240bpm, exclusively maintained by the atrial myocardium. P waves during AT are separated by an isoelectric baseline. This definition is meant to exclude AFL, a distinction that is artificial. AFL is the most frequent form of macro-re-entrant AT and is described in a separate section for didactic reasons. AT, not including AFL, is the least prevalent type of SVT. The increasing number of RFCA procedures in patients with AF is resulting in a rise of post-ablation AT due to macro-re-entry, focal re-entry, and enhanced automaticity. Some of these post-ablation ATs 'look like flutters' in the ECG.

Pathogenesis

Paroxysmal, non-paroxysmal, and permanent AT can be focal or macro-re-entrant. AT is termed 'focal' when the activation wavefront begins in a relatively circumscribed area from which the rest of the atrial myocardium is depolarized. Some patients present multiple atrial foci [41]. Focal does not mean automatic. Focal AT induced and interrupted with programmed electrical stimulation is due to triggered focal activity or re-entry and is designated 'non-automatic focal AT' [42]. The remaining forms of focal ATs are most likely due to enhanced or abnormal automaticity.

Sinus node reciprocating tachycardia (SNRT) is a non-automatic paroxysmal focal AT whose re-entry pathway remains unidentified. Its atrial breakthrough is high in the terminal crest, close to the right atrial exit of the normal sinus node impulse. IST is a rare form of non-paroxysmal AT due to an increased automaticity of the sinus node, or a disturbance on its autonomic balance eventually caused by circulating anti-beta adrenergic receptor antibodies [43, 44]. POTS is a condition that shares autonomic abnormalities with IST. These patients develop symptoms and sinus tachycardia in the upright position in the absence of orthostatic hypotension [1].

Focal AT originates along the terminal crest, in the vicinity of the tricuspid annulus including: the perinodal region; at the venous side of different veno-atrial junctions (superior vena cava–right atrium, CS–right atrium, pulmonary veins–left atrium); at the left atrial roof and mitral annulus; and finally, at the right and left atrial appendages (➲Fig. 28.4A) [41, 45–58].

Macro-re-entrant AT is based on a circus-movement around an anatomically or functionally determined obstacle (➲Fig. 28.4B). AFL is the most common form of macro-re-entrant AT rotating around a right atrial obstacle that in part is functional rather than anatomical (➲Fig. 28.4C). While CTI AFL uses a circuit present in all hearts, other forms of macro-re-entrant AT develop around or through atrial scars due to fibrosis of diverse aetiologies, including surgery or catheter ablation for AF. The term 'incisional' is applied to macro-re-entrant AT developing in relation to scarring after congenital heart disease surgical repair (atrial septal defect closure, Mustard or Senning procedures (➲Chapter 16) for D-transposition of the great arteries, Fontan operation for tricuspid atresia), or mitral valve operations (also see ➲Chapter 21). Some of these arrhythmogenic substrates are very complex and more than one AT circuit may be present [59–61].

Paroxysmal and permanent AT may develop after AF ablation procedures and are due to macro-re-entry, focal re-entry, or enhanced automaticity depending in part on the type of approach to ablate AF [62–69]. 'Segmental pulmonary vein isolation' may result in a focal AT from reconnected pulmonary vein ostia whose mechanism, re-entry, or ectopic firing, is debatable [62–67]. The 'encircling circumferential approach' can generate macro-re-entrant ATs (peri-mitral, peri pulmonary vein ostia, or in relation to incomplete roof or posterior left atrial wall ablation lines) [64–66]. AF ablation targeting 'complex fractionated electrograms' may create macro-re-entrant and focal ATs [68]. In some instances the development of post-ablation left AT is facilitated by class IC antiarrhythmic drugs or amiodarone. The various surgical approaches currently used for the treatment of AF can also build the substrate for AT occurrence. Focal and macro-re-entrant ATs have been described after Maze procedures or intraoperative left atrial radiofrequency ablation [69–70].

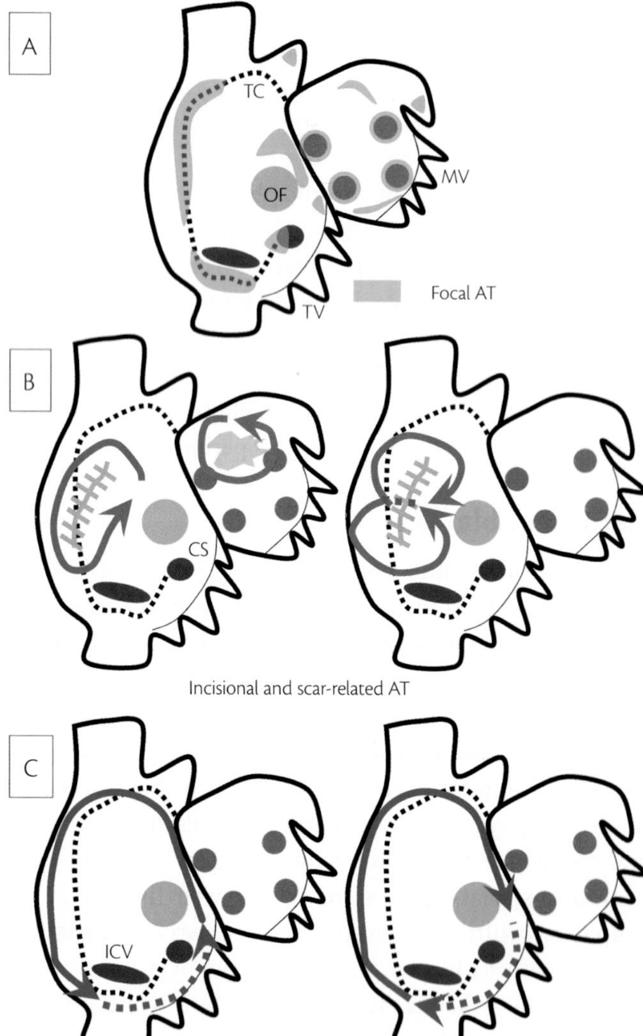

Figure 28.4 (A) Focal AT locations (in light blue). CS, coronary sinus; ICV, inferior caval vein; MV, mitral valve; OF, oval fossa; TC, terminal crest; TV, tricuspid valve. The terminal crest is represented by a dotted line extending laterally and inferiorly from the interatrial septum towards the inferior isthmus and the CS. Focal AT locations: along the TC, tricuspid and mitral annuli, perinodal region, ostium of the CS, interatrial septum, pulmonary veins and left atrial junctions, roof of the left atrium, and right and left atrial appendages. (B) Scar-related and incisional macro-re-entrant AT. Macro-re-entrant AT develops around an anatomic obstacle, either a patch of atrial fibrosis (left vignette inside the left atrium), or a post-surgical scar. Incisional re-entry may develop around a surgical scar (right atrium, left vignette) or through-the-scar (right vignette). (C) Counterclockwise CTI-dependent AFL (left vignette) and clockwise CTI-dependent AFL (right vignette).

Diagnosis

Clinical characteristics

AT can be paroxysmal and non-paroxysmal, either permanent or as repetitive runs of the arrhythmia. The main symptoms in paroxysmal AT are palpitations, anxiety, and occasionally, dyspnoea, dizziness, or syncope. In permanent AT the patient may be asymptomatic, even when a depressed ejection fraction and a certain degree of left ventricular dilation are present, or refer dyspnoea on exertion and, more rarely, overt signs of heart failure.

Paroxysmal non-automatic focal AT usually arises in patients without structural heart disease and is most prevalent in females (>70%) aged over 40 years. SNRT generally occurs in females (80%) and the occasional patient may also present an AVNRT. Focal automatic AT is usually observed in patients without structural heart disease and may be paroxysmal and sustained, non-paroxysmal in frequent repetitive runs of various durations, or strictly permanent. Primary incessant focal AT is rare—usually observed in children and young adults—and may result in a tachycardiomyopathy [18, 56–58, 71, 72]. A permanent AT should be excluded during an electrophysiological study in patients with systolic left ventricular dysfunction and an apparent sinus tachycardia because the P wave in some permanent focal ATs may mimic the sinus P wave. This occurs in AT originating at the junction superior caval vein–the right atrium, the right atrial appendage, the superior part of the terminal crest, and the right and left superior pulmonary veins. The atrial rate during incessant AT is 110–300bpm and it can vary within the same subject depending on the autonomic tone. Some patients show no evidence of sinus rhythm during Holter monitoring while others present a sinus rhythm at rest, sleep, or the induction of anaesthesia.

Macro-re-entrant AT developing after congenital heart disease surgery causes morbidity and eventually mortality. These incisional re-entrant ATs may be paroxysmal but are frequently permanent and tend to be slower in rate than the CTI AFL, with atrial rates between 150–250bpm (➲Figs. 28.4B and 28.5). When paroxysmal, because of this relatively slow atrial rate, patients may develop episodes of 1:1 AV conduction with haemodynamic deterioration [59–61]. Within the first few months after ablation for AF, a focal or macro-re-entrant AT may develop with atrial rates between 200–300bpm [65]. These ATs may spontaneously fade away with time or after withdrawal of antiarrhythmic agents.

Macro-re-entrant AT has been described in relation to electrically silent areas of atrial fibrosis unrelated to surgery or ablation [41, 73, 74]. A scar-related macro-re-entrant AT may develop after mitral valve repair or replacement (➲Fig. 28.3B). Some of the latter patients, after many years in AF, may present an AT as an expression of an extremely diseased left atrium.

Adenosine infusion terminates or transiently suppresses many forms of focal AT and produces no effect on macro-re-entrant AT. Adenosine-insensitive focal AT accounts for <10% of all focal ATs, arises close to the pulmonary vein ostia or from the right atrium, and may be due to a small re-entry circuit. Adenosine-sensitive focal AT originates from a wide distribution of locations in both atria [75–76].

Multifocal AT or chaotic atrial rhythm is rare and usually develops in elderly patients with obstructive lung disease, sometimes as a manifestation of theophylline toxicity [77, 78]. It is very infrequent in infants, children, and young adults. Infants with multifocal AT may have respiratory or structural heart disease [79]. In children it may be incessant and tends to resolve spontaneously, but if persistent the patient may develop a tachycardiomyopathy [18]. In adults with obstructive lung disease multifocal AT is transient in nature and frequently converts in AF or AFL [80].

IST usually appears in females <50 years of age and more rarely in males and elderly people. Patients with IST complain of palpitations and/or fatigue or dyspnoea with a minimal exercise. Not infrequently patients also refer headaches, atypical chest pains, apprehension, dizziness, and more rarely syncopal episodes. The average heart rate is >90bpm in a 24-hour ambulatory ECG recording with an exaggerated response to minimal physical activities [81]. In the primary form of IST the heart is structurally normal and there are not potential causes of persistent sinus tachycardia (anaemia, hyperthyroidism, hypoxaemia etc.). IST may temporarily emerge after RFCA interventions close to the compact AV node such as ablation of the fast AV nodal pathway or a peri-Hisian AP [82–84].

POTS is seen both in males and females that refer a heart-pounding sensation while standing. The sinus rate increases >30bpm, or above 120bpm, during the first 10min after adopting the upright position. In some patients POTS occurs without any noticeable past history event but others refer the onset of symptoms after a viral infection, pregnancy, trauma, a surgical intervention, or cancer. Diabetic patients may also develop POTS symptoms.

Electrocardiographic characteristics

The 12-lead ECG, combined with vagal or pharmacological manoeuvres during tachycardia, enables us:

- to establish the atrial nature of the arrhythmia;
- to postulate a focal automatic, non-automatic, or even a macro-re-entrant mechanism;

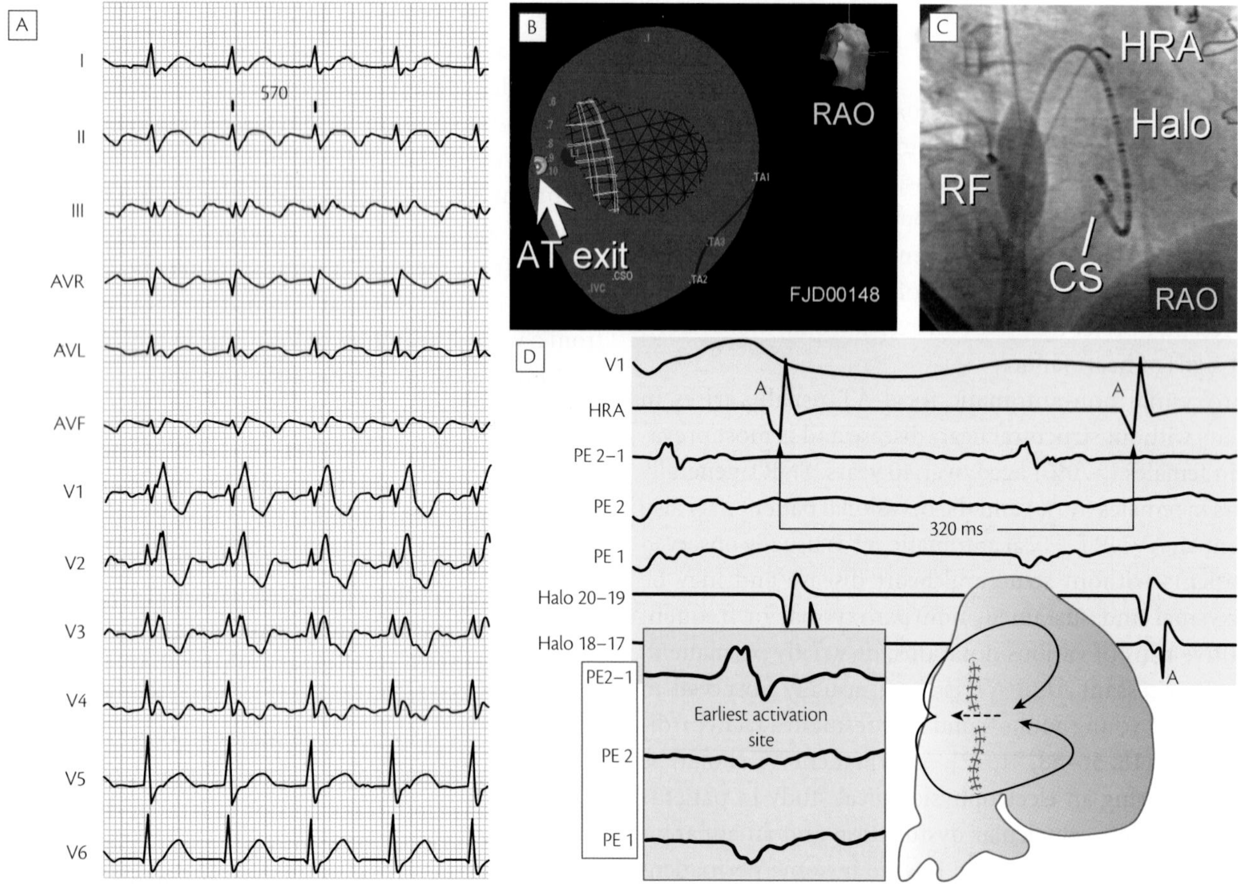

Figure 28.5 Incisional AT 18 years after repair of an *ostium secundum* atrial septal defect. (A) The surface ECG during this AT should not be confused with an isthmus-dependent AFL. The RR interval is 570ms (105bpm). P waves are caudo-cranial, like in counterclockwise isthmic AFL. During the electrophysiological study AT could not be entrained from the CTI indicating am isthmus-independent mechanism. (B, C) With a non-contact mapping system (Ensite, Endocardial Solutions) AT was shown to have a localized onset of activation from which the rest of the right atrium was depolarized. (C) The probing electrode (RF) is at the site of earliest atrial activation (posterolaterally in relation to the surgical atriotomy). Other catheters depicted in this RAO view of the right atrium are a quadripolar CS catheter, a 20-pole Halo catheter, and a high right atrial catheter (HRA). (D) Lead V1 is simultaneously displayed with recordings from HRA, probing electrode (PE), and Halo catheter. The AT cycle length is 320ms (188bpm). At the middle of the atrial incision there was a narrow isthmus electrically communicating both sides of the surgical scar so that the PE recorded the earliest activation during AT.

- to locate a likely atrial exit site in the focal forms. Amplification of the electrocardiographic signals may facilitate P-wave identification.

In automatic focal AT the initial P wave is identical to subsequent tachycardia P waves and after its start we may observe a progressive acceleration over a few beats ('warming-up' phenomenon). Preceding the termination of automatic and non-automatic AT there may be a progressive rate decrease ('cooling down'). The AV relation during AT can be 1:1, 2:1, or show higher degrees of AV block, depending on the atrial rate, the AV nodal function, or the effect of drugs on the AV node. Paroxysmal AT with block, once considered a typical arrhythmia of digitalis intoxication, is rarely related today to digitalis (➲Fig. 28.6). When the AV ratio is 1:1, the RP interval is usually longer than the PR (long-RP tachycardia) (➲Figs. 28.6A and 28.7) [1, 85, 86] (➲Table 28.1). However, a PR >RP during AT may be observed after the administration of drugs prolonging AV nodal conduction times, because of coexisting AV nodal disease, or in the presence of dual AV nodal pathways. When the AV ratio is 1:1, positive P waves in leads I, II, and III exclude an AV junctional origin. If P waves are negative in lead I, and positive in lead III, an AVRT incorporating a left free-wall AP cannot be ruled out. An AT can be diagnosed if vagal or pharmacological manoeuvres induce AV block and the tachycardia persists at the atrial level. Vagal stimulation in some patients with AT may lengthen the P–P interval, and atropine can accelerate the tachycardia [85, 86]. Adenosine terminates many focal AT before inducing AV block, in

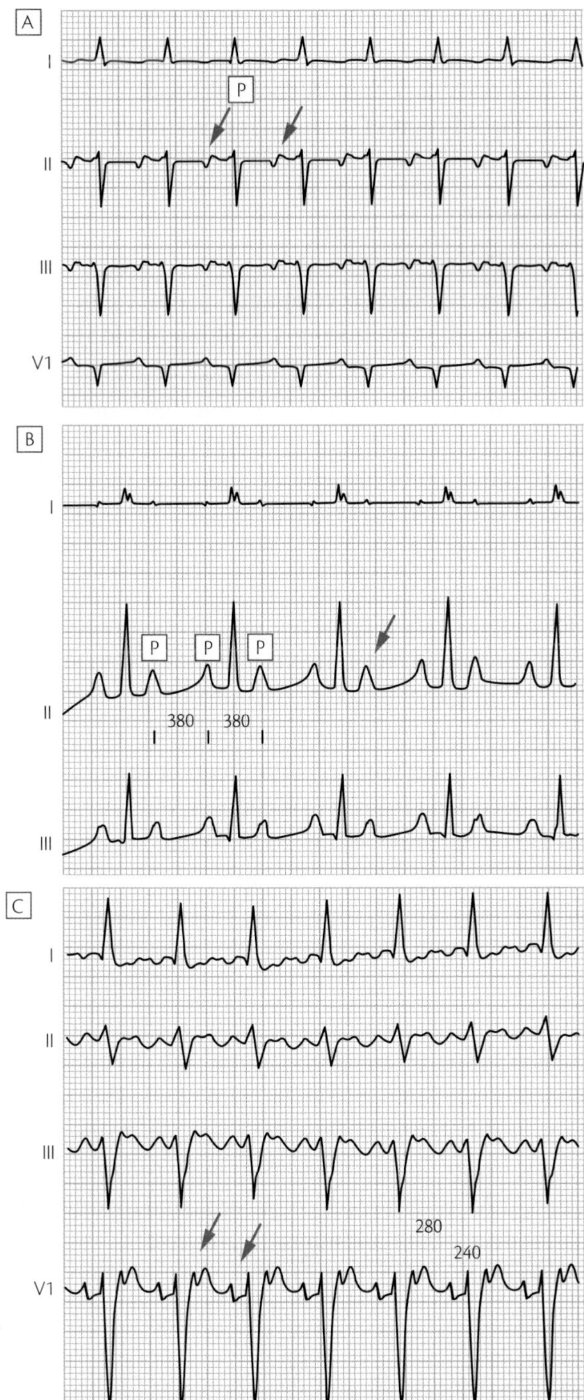

Figure 28.6 (A) Focal AT with 1:1 conduction and a PR<RP pattern. The atrial breakthrough was at the low atrial septum, above the ostium of the CS where this AT was ablated. P waves during AT are negative–positive in leads II and III, and positive in V1. (B) AT with 2:1 AV block unrelated to digitalis; PP intervals are constant (380ms). The pattern of atrial activation is cranio-caudal. There is an isoelectric baseline between consecutive P waves. (C) AT with 2:1 AV block in a patient with chronic obstructive lung disease and digitalis intoxication. Atrial activation is cranio-caudal (positive P waves in leads II and III) and there is ventriculo-phasic atrial arrhythmia (PP intervals including a QRS complex 40ms shorter than PP intervals not embracing a ventricular depolarization). This phenomenon can be seen in AT unrelated to digitalis.

which case differentiation with a mechanism involving the AV junction will not be possible.

The presence of AV block during SVT strongly suggests an atrial origin. When there is a 2:1 AV ratio, the identification of two consecutive P waves within the R–R cycle is diagnostic of AT (➲Figs. 28.6B–C, 28.8, and 28.9). P–P intervals sandwiching a QRS complex may be 20–40ms shorter than PP cycles not comprising a ventricular activation. This phenomenon, known as ventriculophasic P–P alternation or ventriculophasic atrial arrhythmia, in the past was considered associated with digitalis intoxication [87], but it can be seen in AT with 2:1 AV block under no digitalis (➲Figs. 28.6C and 28.9C).

The origin in focal AT can be suspected by examining the P-wave configuration in the 12-lead ECG. Structural heart disease, atrial dilation, and natural or drug-induced intra-atrial conduction disturbances, may interfere with a correct location of the origin of focal AT from the surface ECG. Certain rules are useful in this regard [15, 16, 45–58]:

- P waves during AT similar in configuration to those of sinus rhythm suggest a SNRT, or an AT from the upper terminal crest, or from the superior caval vein close to the right atrium. In ATs coming from the superior caval vein the P-wave V1 is not biphasic, but positive. P waves of SNRT are frequently indistinguishable from sinus P waves. P waves of AT from the superior half of the terminal crest may be slightly different to sinus P waves but still biphasic in V1.
- Focal ATs originating from the right and left superior pulmonary veins result in P waves that are positive in leads I, II, III, and AVF; negative in AVR and AVL; and positive and monophasic in V1; the P-wave is of low amplitude or flat in lead I in AT from the left superior pulmonary vein (➲Fig. 28.2). The P-wave duration may be <120ms in AT from the right superior pulmonary vein (➲Fig. 28.8).
- A deep negative P wave in II, III, and AVF with a positive P in V1 suggests a proximal CS origin; a similar configuration but with a negative P wave in V1 supports an origin from the body of the CS; when the P is biphasic, negative–positive, in the inferior leads and positive in V1, the AT may come from the region above the ostium of the CS in the low atrial septum (➲Fig. 28.6A).
- P waves of AT originating in the lower part of the terminal crest are negative in III, AVF, and V1; flat in II; and positive in I and AVL.
- Focal AT from tricuspid or mitral annulus produces variable P-wave contours. Inferior tricuspid annulus

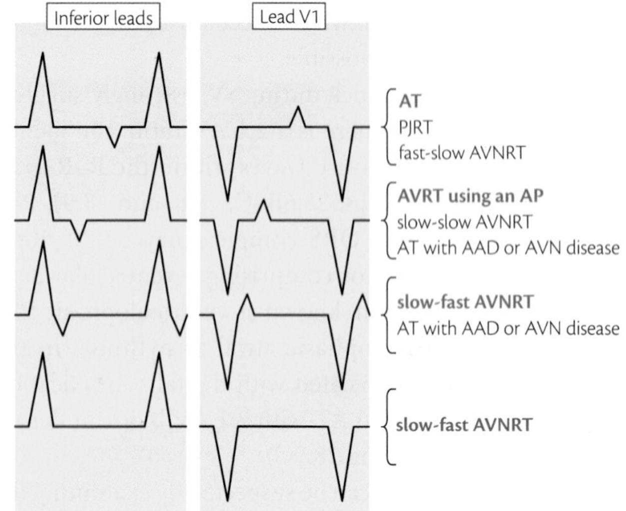

Figure 28.7 Relation between P wave and ventricular complex during narrow-QRS SVT with 1:1 AV ratio. Left column: ECG in inferior leads; middle column: ECG in lead V1. On the right, the types of SVT that can originate each of the electrocardiographic patterns (in red and bold font the most typical one).

focal AT generates negative P waves in inferior leads and from V1–V6. Superior and anterosuperior tricuspid annulus locations produce negative P waves in V1 and various patterns of polarities and contours of P waves in the frontal plane, not infrequently, positive in I, II, and sometimes in III or AVF. Focal AT coming from the posterior (formerly called lateral) area of the left AV groove are positive in lead III and AVF, negative in I and AVL, and negative–positive in V1.

In multifocal AT, P waves have three or more different morphologies, an isoelectric line between consecutive P waves, irregular PP cycle lengths at 150–220 bpm, and variable PR intervals. The RR cycle lengths are also variable.

The ECG of macro- re-entrant AT has two major manifestations: P waves more or less similar in contour to those of CTI AFL (with caudo–cranial or cranio–caudal atrial activations) (➲Fig. 28.5); or P waves with very low voltage in the limb leads [1, 41]. An isoelectric line may be present between consecutive P waves, but a true flutter-like pattern can also be observed.

Electrophysiological studies

Electrophysiological studies enables us to differentiate:

- AT from other varieties of SVT [18, 41–43, 45–69, 70, 72–76, 88, 89];
- automatic from non-automatic forms of AT;
- focal from macro-re-entrant AT, and
- macro- re-entrant AT unrelated to the CTI from isthmus-dependent AFL.

In patients with a dilated cardiomyopathy it may be worth excluding the existence of an incessant AT mimicking sinus tachycardia. The induction of focal AT frequently requires the infusion of isoprenaline or atropine.

Treatment

IST is usually first treated with beta-blockers although some patients may respond to verapamil or diltiazem. POTS is usually relieved by increasing the salt and fluid intake and by aerobic exercise training. The intake of alcohol and the consumption of vasodilating drugs must be avoided [1].

The management of patients with paroxysmal AT comprises termination of the episode and prevention of recurrences. In sustained paroxysmal AT, carotid sinus massage should be tried and if it does not terminate the arrhythmia, adenosine is used unless contraindicated. Adenosine usually terminates focal AT but not macro re-entrant AT [75]. AT is diagnosed if vagal or pharmacological manoeuvres induce AV block while the tachycardia persists at the atrial level. The role of verapamil in terminating AT is not well studied. SNRT is terminated with verapamil and adenosine. Some ATs coming from the pulmonary veins are also suppressed by verapamil (➲Fig. 28.8). When adenosine fails, intravenous propafenone or flecainide can be administered or intravenous amiodarone if the patient has systolic left ventricular dysfunction. DC-shock cardioversion can be considered if AT persists after the use of antiarrhythmic drugs or if there is a history of previous drug failures [1].

Vagal manoeuvres, short-acting intravenous drugs (adenosine, verapamil, or diltiazem), and DC-shock cardioversion, are of no practical use if AT is in the form of repetitive runs, except for testing sensitivity to calcium-channel blockers. If AT is sensitive to verapamil, oral treatment with the latter drug or diltiazem may be effective.

Various antiarrhythmic drugs have been used to prevent recurrences of AT or to control incessant AT [90–93] but their success rate is low. In patients with IST beta-blocking agents, verapamil, and diltiazem have little success. Ivabradine, a selective *If*-current blocker, may be tried in these patients [94]. In SNRT and in some focal ATs coming from the terminal crest, verapamil may suppress the arrhythmia and prevent its recurrences. Some left or right ATs, such as those originating in the vicinity of the AV node, are sensitive to calcium-channel blockers [94–97]. There are no good studies on the efficacy of amiodarone in paroxysmal and permanent AT. Because many arrhythmologists prefer not to use interventional therapies in children, most of the current literature on antiarrhythmic drugs and AT comes from the paediatric patient population [98].

Catheter ablation

The treatment of choice for symptomatic recurrent paroxysmal or permanent AT is catheter ablation [41, 42, 47, 49, 51–56, 99–104]. The success rate of RFCA in AT depends on the experience of the ablation team, the technology available for the ablation, and the type of AT (➲Table 28.1).

In patients with IST not responding to drugs, the results of RFCA are conflicting with poor long-term results even with three-dimensional electro-anatomical mapping or endo-epicardial approaches [105–108]. Improved outcomes have been obtained using intracardiac ultrasound to achieve transmural lesions, or with saline-cooled catheter ablation of all P-wave morphologies elicited by isoproterenol after complete autonomic blockade [109, 110]. The difficulties to ablate IST reflect that the sinus node is protected against RFCA by

- a the dense matrix of connective tissue in which sinoatrial cells are packed;
- the cooling effect of the nodal artery; and
- the thick terminal crest interposed between the endocardium and the sinoatrial tissue [111].

In focal AT, experienced centres report catheter ablation success rates in excess of 90%, with <8% of recurrences [1, 41, 42, 45–47, 49–58, 99, 112–117].

RFCA is also the treatment of choice for macro-re-entrant AT. Flecainide, propafenone, or amiodarone by slowing conduction velocity, may facilitate rather than prevent recurrences of macro-re-entrant AT whose atrial rate is then slower than in the basal situation. RFCA in macro reentrant AT requires identification of a

Table 28.1 Characteristics of supraventricular tachycardia

Type of SVT	Varieties	Presentation	Gender dominance	Adenosine	RFCA success	A:V ratio	PR/RP in AV 1:1	QRS complex
AT	Focal	Paroxysmal Permanent	Females	Stops ≈90% of episodes	>90%	1:1 or higher	PR <RP PR = RP PR >RP*	Narrow Wide if BBB
AT	Macro-re-entrant	Paroxysmal Permanent	Even	No effect	60–80%	2:1 or higher	NA	Narrow Wide if BBB RBBB if ASD
AFL	CTI CCW and CW	Paroxysmal Permanent	Males	No effect	>98%	2:1 or higher	NA	Narrow Wide if BBB
AFL	Non-CTI	Paroxysmal Permanent	Even	No effect	60–80%	2:1 or higher	NA	Narrow Wide if BBB
AVNRT	Slow-fast	Paroxysmal	Females	Stops	≈99%	1:1 2:1 **	PR >>RP***	Narrow Wide if BBB
AVNRT	Fast-slow	Paroxysmal Permanent	Females	Stops	≈99%	1:1	PR <RP	Narrow Wide if BBB
AVNRT	Slow-slow	Paroxysmal Permanent	Females	Stops	≈99%	1:1	PR >RP	Narrow Wide if BBB
AVRT	Orthodromic Conventional	Paroxysmal	Males	Stops	≈95–99%	1:1	PR >RP	Narrow Wide if BBB
AVRT	Antidromic Conventional	Paroxysmal	Males	Stops	≈95–99%	1:1	PR = RP PR <RP	Wide, maximally pre-excited
PJRT	Orthodromic	Permanent	Males	Stops	≈95–99%	1:1	PR <RP PR = RP	Narrow Wide if BBB
AFRT	Antidromic	Paroxysmal	Males	Stops	≈95–99%	1:1	PR >>>RP****	Wide (LBBB), maximally pre-excited
DART	Antidromic	Paroxysmal	(?)	Stops	≈95–99%	1:1	PR >>>RP****	Wide (RBBB), maximally pre-excited

AFL, atrial flutter; AFRT, atriofascicular reciprocating tachycardia; ASD, atrial septal defect; AT, atrial tachycardia; AVNRT, AV nodal reciprocating tachycardia; AVRT, AV reciprocating tachycardia utilizing an accessory pathway; BBB, bundle branch block (either organic or due to aberrant conduction); CCW, counterclockwise; CW, clockwise; DART, decremental antidromic reciprocating tachycardia; LBBB, left bundle branch block (configuration); PJRA, permanent junctional reciprocating tachycardia; RBBB, right bundle branch block; RFCA, radiofrequency catheter ablation; SVT, supraventricular tachycardia; * PR >RP if concomitant drugs acting on the AV node, if associated AV nodal disease, or if AV conduction over a slow AV nodal pathway; ** 2:1 ratio in AVNRT exceptional in the clinical scenario; *** P waves during slow–fast AVNRT are either hidden within the QRS complex or visible as a continuation of the QRS mimicking terminal s waves in inferior leads or r' waves in V1. **** P waves usually are hidden within the QRS complex during tachycardia.

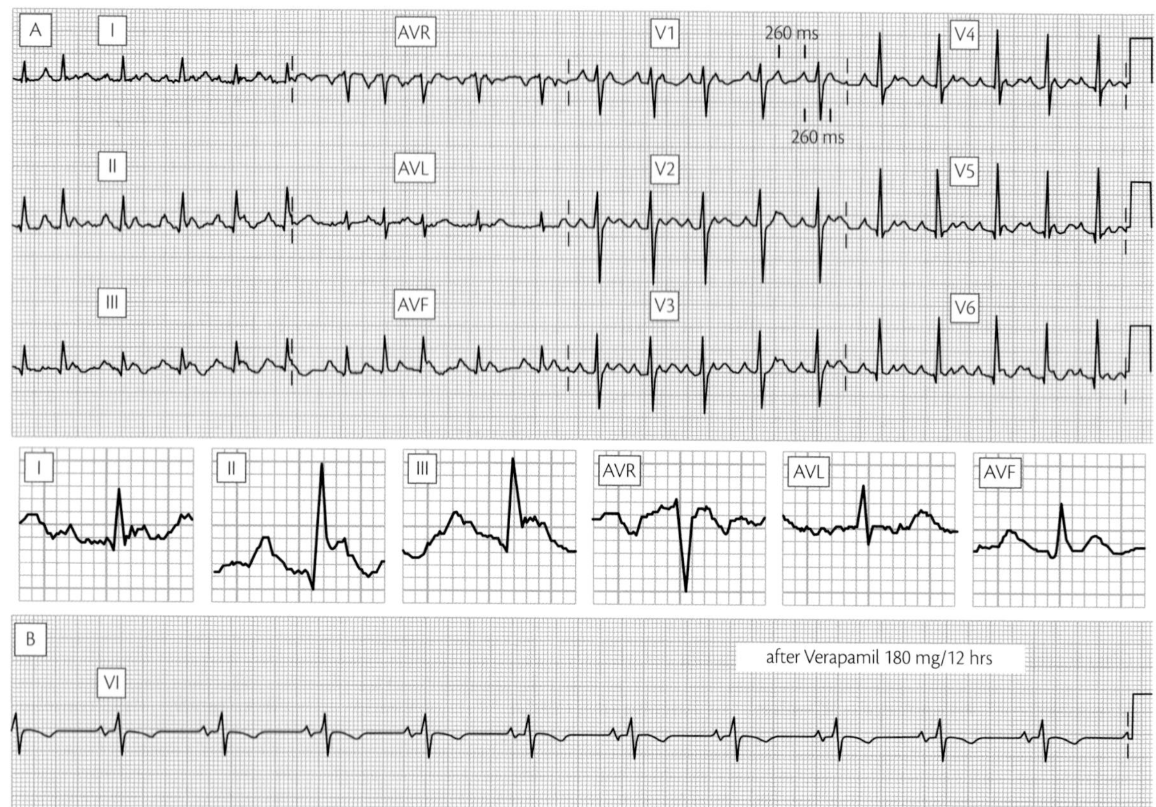

Figure 28.8 Verapamil sensitive AT from the right superior pulmonary vein in an octogenarian lady. (A) 12-lead ECG during AT with a magnified view of the tachycardia P waves in the limb leads (lower vignettes). AT cycle lengths are constant (260ms). AT P waves are: positive in leads I, II, III, and AVF,; negative, bimodal, and of low amplitude in AVL; and positive in V1 to V6. This P-wave configuration suggests a right superior pulmonary vein origin. P-wave duration during tachycardia is 120ms in lead II but is narrower in I, III, and AVF. ATs from this location may have P waves <120ms. This AT, not totally suppressed with flecainide, was completely abolished after verapamil (B).

critical isthmus of conduction between anatomical barriers, or an isolated diastolic potential shown to belong to the circuit by entrainment pacing, or a narrow gap in the scar. Electro-anatomical mapping systems facilitate the ablation of these complex ATs (➲Fig. 28.5) [41, 59, 61, 74, 118–123].

In the past, patients with incessant AT were treated with antiarrhythmic drugs, usually amiodarone, flecainide, or propafenone, with a variable success rate [1, 18, 91–93]. The treatment of choice today for incessant AT is RFCA [26, 27, 47–58,124]. Patients with an asymptomatic permanent AT with normal ventricular function should be followed-up for early identification of tachycardiomyopathy. When there are signs of systolic left ventricular dysfunction, RFCA should be performed and the ejection fraction usually recovers within a few months.

Treatment of multifocal AT

Infants with multifocal AT can be treated with digoxin and many of these tachycardias resolve spontaneously [77]. Class I drugs are of limited therapeutic success [75, 77, 79, 80, 125]. Amiodarone may be effective in these patients but the information is scanty [126]. In adults, if amiodarone does not suppress the arrhythmia, it can be used for rate control, with or without verapamil or diltiazem, particularly in elderly patients with chronic obstructive lung disease where beta-blocking agents are avoided. Successful treatment of multifocal AT has been reported on with ibutilide [127]. Modification of the AV node with RFCA techniques can be used in symptomatic patients not amenable to antiarrhythmic drug treatment [101].

Treatment of AT after AF ablation

ATs developing after ablation for AF usually disappear spontaneously or after withdrawing all antiarrhythmic agents if the patient was receiving them at the time of presentation of these arrhythmias. If AT develops on no antiarrhythmic drugs, propafenone, flecainide, or amiodarone can be used for a few months until these ATs cease. In some of these patients antiarrhythmic drugs must be maintained permanently. In the latter patients, or when antiarrhythmic drugs fail, a repeat intervention must be planned to ablate post-ablation AT [65].

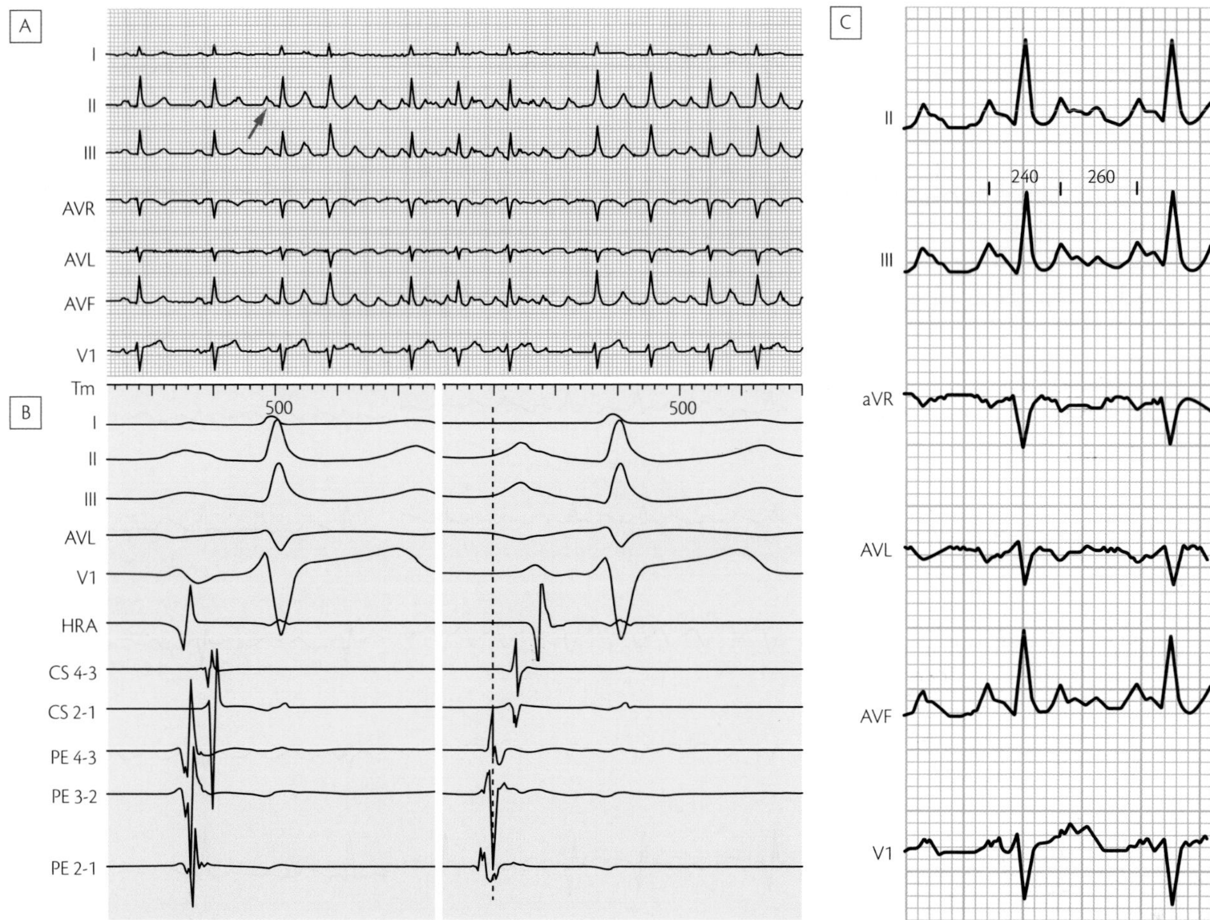

Figure 28.9 (A) Phasically ongoing incessant focal left AT originating at the vicinity of the left superior pulmonary vein. AT was automatic in nature and started with a late atrial ectopic depolarization (green arrow) followed by a rapid firing (mean atrial rate of 240bpm). (B) Catheter-electrode mapping during sinus rhythm (left) and during one of the ectopic beats initiating AT (right). From above to below time marks (Tm), leads I, II, III, AVL, and V1, and bipolar intracardiac recordings from the HRA, CS, and the quadripolar probing electrode (PE). At PE 2-1 (distal pair of electrodes) the atrial electrogram is inscribed before the onset of the ectopic P wave in the surface ECG leads (dotted red line). Application of radiofrequency current at this site resulted in the cure of the AT (not shown). (C) P–P cycles containing a QRS-complex are 20ms shorter than PP intervals not sandwiching a ventricular depolarization (ventriculophasic atrial arrhythmia). Ectopic P waves are 120ms wide, have a notched appearance in the inferior leads, and are positive in II, III, and AVF, negative in AVL, and positive in V1.

Atrial flutter

Definition and epidemiology

Traditionally, AFL was defined by a fast regular atrial rate of 240–350bpm and the absence of an isoelectric baseline separating atrial deflections (➲Fig. 28.10). Neither the first nor the second condition is actually required for flutter to exist. Thus, a common isthmus-dependent AFL can have atrial rates of 190–220bpm and an isoelectric baseline between consecutive P waves in three circumstances: a very diseased right atrium; under the effect of drugs reducing atrial conduction velocity (propafenone, flecainide, or amiodarone); and in AFL developing after a failed RFCA attempt of the flutter itself.

As already stated, AFL is in fact the most common form of macro-re-entrant AT but is considered under a separate heading for didactic reasons and because the available epidemiological data refer to AFL as diagnosed from its ECG appearance, and not to isthmus-related AFL alone.

AFL has been classified as common and uncommon [85]. In common AFL, also known as class 1 and counter-clockwise CTI-dependent AFL, atrial activation pattern is caudo-cranial (➲Fig. 28.10A, B). Uncommon or clockwise isthmus-dependent AFL has a cranio-caudal pattern of atrial activation (➲Fig. 28.10C). This classification, valid for the clinical cardiologist, does not distinguish right from left AFL, and isthmus-dependent from isthmus-independent AFL. CTI-dependent AFL can be of four types: counter-clockwise

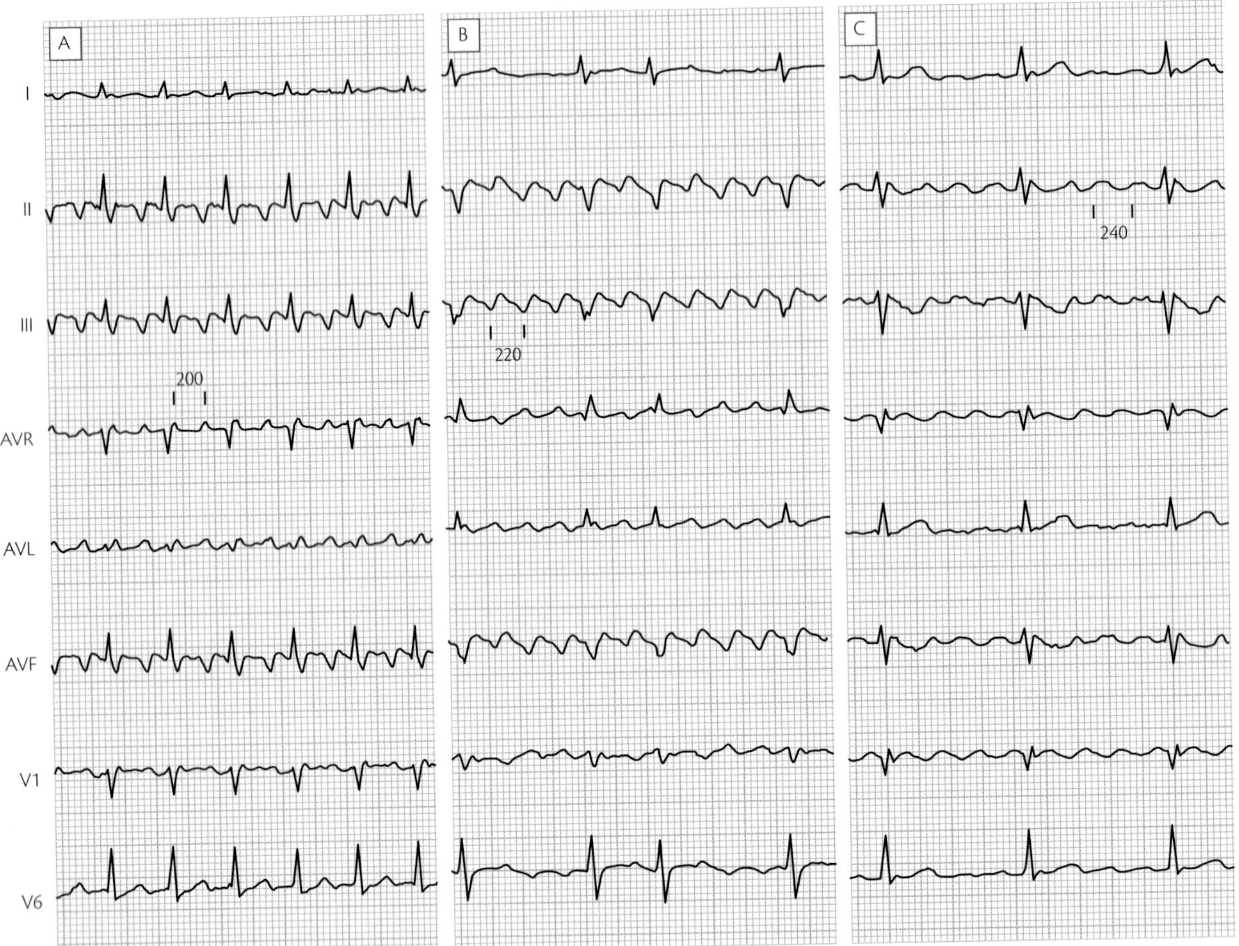

Figure 28.10 (A) Common CTI AFL with a caudo-cranial atrial activation pattern. P waves (F waves) in the inferior leads have an initial negative component, followed by a positive terminal element, and are positive in V1. The AV ratio is 2:1 and the atrial rate is 300bpm. (B) Common AFL with typical saw-tooth waves clearly seen because there is a higher degree of AV block. Note the negative initial component of the F waves in the inferior leads followed by a terminal positive deflection. F waves are positive in V1 and negative in V6. The AFL cycle length is 220ms. (C) Cranio-caudal, clockwise AFL with positive F-waves in the inferior leads. In V1 the F waves have an initial negative component followed by a terminal positive deflection. The atrial rate is 250bpm (cycle length 240ms) and the AV ratio is 4:1.

AFL; clockwise AFL; double-loop re-entry AFL; and intra-isthmus re-entry. Non-isthmian AFLs are the upper-loop re-entry right AFL, and macro-re-entrant ATs related to surgical or non-surgical scarring [128].

AFL is an 'organic' arrhythmia usually associated with cardio-pulmonary disease. 'Lone' AFL in the absence of hypertension, lung disease, or structural heart problems, is rare except for people engaged in active sport practice, or drinking alcohol on daily basis [129], or in patients with hyperthyroidism. Former athletes present AFL more frequently than the general population [130]. CTI AFL is more prevalent than other types of SVT [22] and its incidence is increasing because of the progressive ageing of the population. Left AFL is also becoming more prevalent due to the rise of catheter and surgical ablation procedures for AF and the increased survival of patients with past mitral valve surgery.

Pathogenesis

Right atrial CTI AFL

The common counterclockwise CTI-dependent AFL accounts for about 85% of the total forms of AFL and is a macro-re-entrant AT whose pathway is determined by anatomical and functional right atrial barriers. The key anatomical link of the common AFL circuit is the CTI, a corridor limited anteriorly by the tricuspid orifice and posteriorly by the inferior caval vein and the Eustachian valve and ridge (➲Figs. 28.4C and 28.11) [131]. In counterclockwise CTI AFL, the activation wavefront proceeds in a caudo-cranial direction along the septal aspect of the right atrium, and returns cranio-caudally down the terminal crest and pectinate muscles, towards the CTI. The same circuit can be used in a reverse manner, leading to the clockwise CTI AFL (➲Figs. 28.4C, 28.10C, and 28.12). In CTI AFL, the terminal crest acts as a barrier to conduction in which block

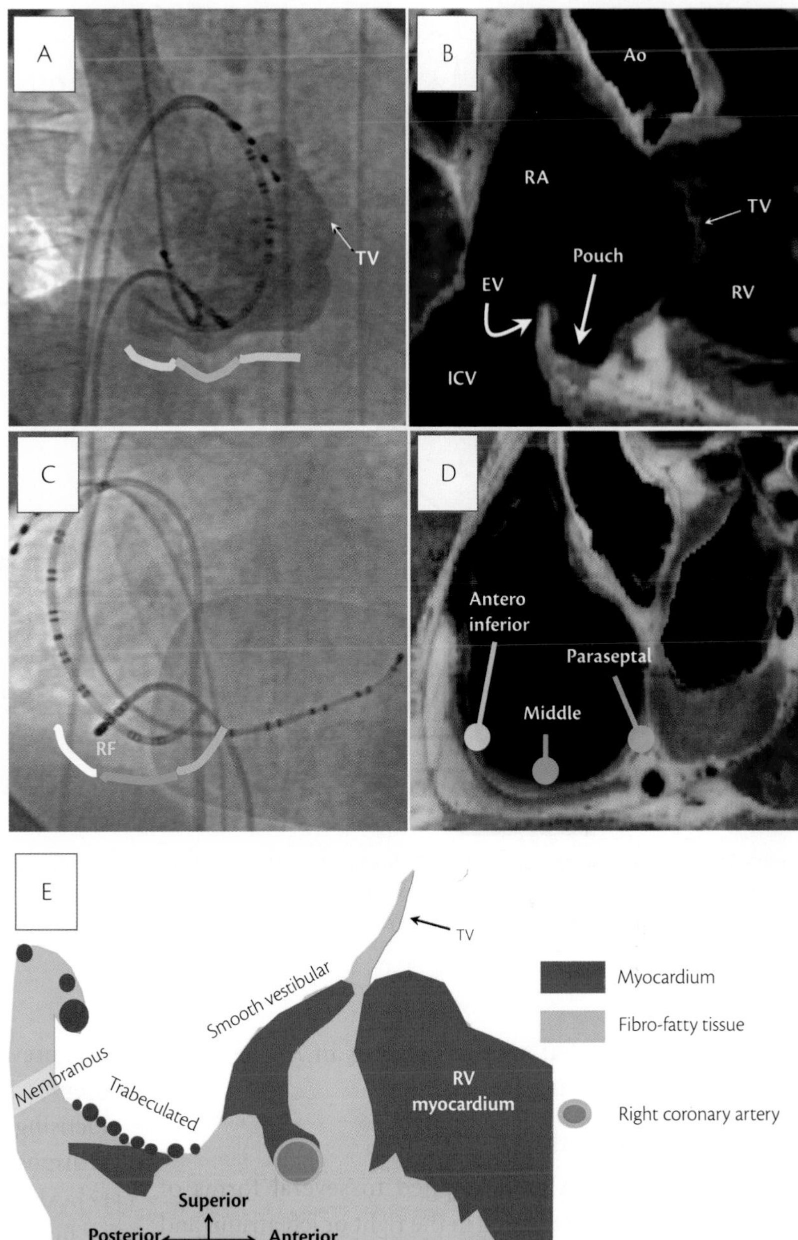

Figure 28.11 (A) Right atrial angiogram in the RAO projection showing three regions in the CTI (membranous in yellow, trabeculated in cyan, and vestibular in pink). TV, tricuspid valve. (B) Anatomic slice in RAO projection [14]. Ao, aorta; RA, right atrium; RV, right ventricle. Anterior and inferior to the Eustachian valve (EV) there is a pouch-like formation that more anteriorly continues with the smooth-walled vestibule of the tricuspid valve. This pouch (cyan in A) and the vestibule of the tricuspid valve (pink in A) can be depicted in a right atrial angiography in the RAO projection. (C) Fluorographic view of the catheters in LAO projection showing three areas along which the ablation line can be traced in the CTI: anteroinferior (white), middle (green), paraseptal (orange). (D) Anatomic slice in LAO projection [14] also depicting the three regions of the inferior isthmus. The so-called middle area (green) can be considered at the 6:00 o'clock in the LAO projection. (E) Representation of the architecture of the inferior isthmus as observed in an anatomic slice obtained in the RAO projection (as in B). The posterior sector is membranous and usually contains no myocardial fibres of very scanty and slender muscular bundles. The pouch or intermediate sector is trabeculated due to myocardial bundles that are a continuation of the pectinate muscles. Finally, the smooth anterior vestibular area also contains atrial myocardium.

is functionally rather than anatomically determined [132, 133]. Rarely, the CTI is utilized in the 'lower-loop CTI AFL' in which the circus-movement is established around the inferior vena cava [134]. A lower-loop mechanism has also been demonstrated in some apparently clockwise CTI AFL [135]. The 'double-wave re-entry' AFL is not a clinically occurring condition. It develops at the electrophysiology laboratory when an atrial premature stimulus is introduced during AFL at a time when the impulse is able to propagate in one direction but not in the opposite, in a manner that the interplay of conduction velocities and refractory periods in the re-entry pathway permits to contain two circulating wavefronts within the circuit [136]. A form of CTI-dependent AFL utilizes a re-entry pathway confined to the septal area of the CTI and the ostium of the CS [137].

The re-entry circuit of clockwise and anticlockwise CTI AFL exists in all hearts but the arrhythmia develops only when the right atrium can accommodate a circulating wavefront not colliding with the tail of refractoriness. This requires some degree of right atrial dilation and/or certain reduction of conduction velocity in the AFL pathway, generally the CTI. Using right atrial angiography, the dimensions of the right atrium and the CTI are greater in patients with common AFL than in controls without

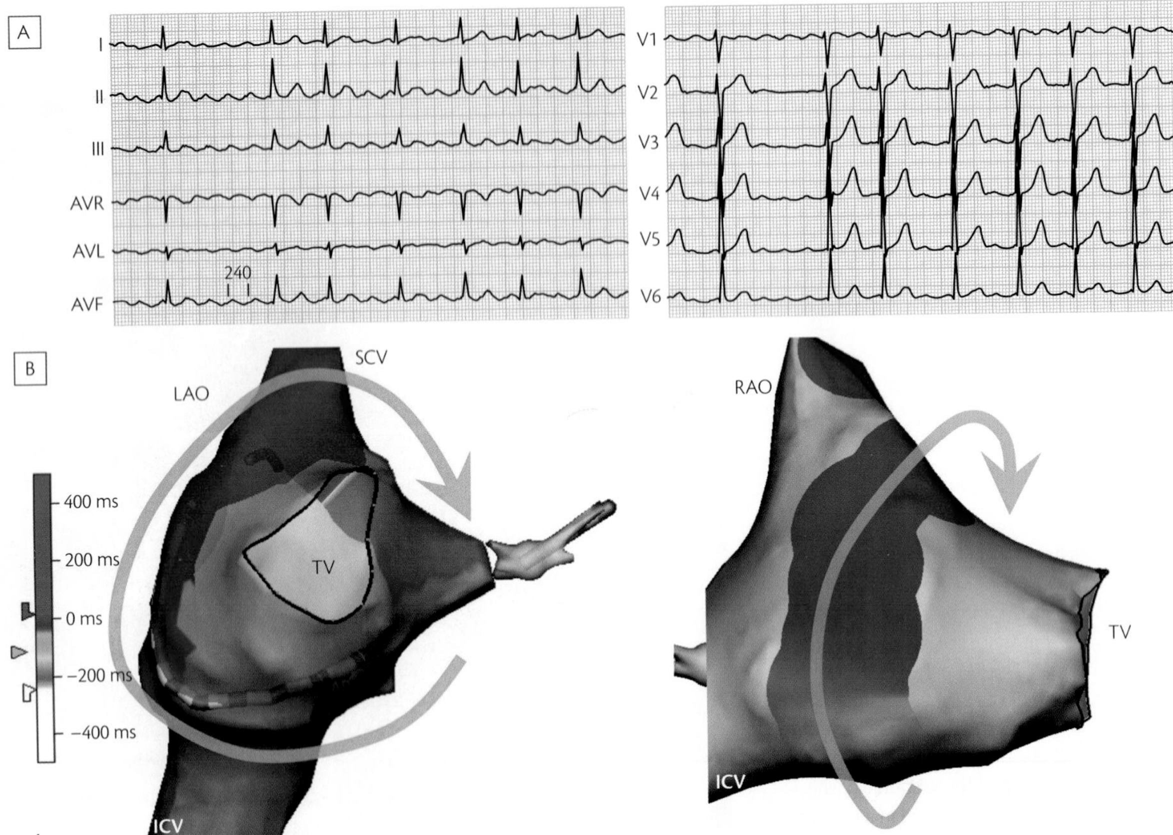

Figure 28.12 (A) Cranio-caudal, clockwise CTI-dependent AFL in a patient with chronic obstructive pulmonary disease. AFL cycle length is 240ms (250bpm). (B) Three-dimensional reconstruction of the right atrium in LAO and RAO projections showing its electro-anatomical map as displayed using the 'EnSite NavX Navigation and Visualization' system. The AFL wavefront propagates in a clockwise rotation through the right atrium. CS, coronary sinus; ICV, inferior caval vein; SCV, superior caval vein; TV, tricuspid valve.

flutter, differences that are even greater in AFL patients with structural heart disease [138].

Atypical atrial flutters

The term 'atypical AFL' is applied to several forms of macro-re-entrant AT localized in the right or left atrium and related to scars produced by surgery or ablation, or areas of atrial fibrosis of undetermined aetiology [41, 121, 139]. They are the same type of arrhythmias labelled in this chapter as macro reentrant AT [41, 73, 140]. Also atypical is the 'upper-loop right AFL' which turns around the superior vena cava through the terminal crest in a clockwise direction [41, 140, 141]. The definition of the re-entry pathway of 'atypical AFL' requires a detailed electro-anatomical mapping.

Diagnosis

Clinical characteristics

Although common AFL is usually paroxysmal, some patients are found to be in chronic AFL without having noticed any symptoms. Common CTI AFL is 2.5 times more prevalent in males than in females and is very seldom observed in patients aged <50 years except for individuals practising heavily sports. Long-term vigorous exercise may predispose to AF but also to the development of CTI AFL [17]. AFL incidence increases with ageing, chronic obstructive lung disease, hypertension, obesity, atrial septal defect (even after repair), mitral valve disease, and systolic and/or diastolic left ventricular dysfunction of various aetiologies. CTI common AFL can also develop in relation to surgical interventions, respiratory infections, and, more rarely, acute myocardial infarction. In patients with rheumatic mitral valve disease, AFL, particularly when cranio-caudal, must be regarded as left atrial in origin until proved otherwise (➲Table 28.1) [22]. Lone AFL without cardiovascular or pulmonary disease is rare, accounting for <2% of AFL documented in the general population [22]. AFL in adults tends to recur or becomes chronic. Patients with AF may develop AFL either spontaneously or after treatment with class IC drugs or amiodarone (class IC AFL). In infants, AFL is extremely rare, is generally associated with cardio-respiratory events, and does not tend to recur unless associated with a congenital heart disease [142]. Rarely, systolic left ventricular dysfunction in patients with chronic AFL reflects a tachycardiomyopathy state [143].

Patients with paroxysmal AFL usually complain of palpitations and/or nervousness sometimes associated with polyuria [144], dyspnoea, fatigue, or chest pain, either at rest or during daily physical activities. Paroxysmal AFL may result in acute heart failure in patients with systolic and/or diastolic left ventricular dysfunction. Exceptionally, if the AV ratio is 1:1, AFL may be syncopal and even fatal. Such an event may occur under sympathetic discharge (as during intense physical exercise) usually in combination with enhanced AV nodal conduction, WPW syndrome, or more frequently, the use of class I antiarrhythmic drugs [145–147]. Class IC antiarrhythmic drugs, by reducing atrial conduction velocity, facilitate the development of a form of AFL with relatively slow atrial rates (190–240bpm). Patients with class IC AFL with 2:1 AV ratio may be asymptomatic or complain of nervousness. During exercise, and because flecainide and to a lesser extent propafenone do not prolong much the AV nodal refractory period, the patient with class IC AFL may develop a life-threatening 1:1 AV conduction. Although a 'slow AFL' can also develop on amiodarone, the AV ratio is usually 2:1 or more because of the effects of the drug on AV nodal conduction.

The risk for thromboembolic events in AFL was thought to be low because of a relatively preserved atrial mechanical function. Transoesophageal echocardiography has shown left atrial thrombi and spontaneous echo contrast in a variable proportion of patients with AFL (➲Fig. 28.13) [148–152]. Left atrial appendage thrombi are rare in the absence of a previous embolic episode, a history of past AF, concomitant mitral valve disease, heart failure, or left ventricular dysfunction [153]. In spite of the lack of good studies on this matter and of some conflicting results, it seems wise to adopt in AFL precautions similar to those in patients with AF, particularly considering that both arrhythmias may coexist at different times in the same patient [1].

Electrocardiographic characteristics

In counterclockwise CTI AFL the atrial waves (F waves or P waves) in the inferior leads have a predominant negative deflection (➲Figs. 28.10A, B and 28.13B, D). The initial negative inferior wave, followed by a positive terminal portion without a baseline between consecutive F waves, produces the characteristic 'saw-tooth' morphology (➲Figs. 28.10B and 28.13D). The terminal positive deflection of the F waves in the inferior leads is due to late cranio-caudal activation of the lateral right atrial wall [154]. In counterclockwise CTI AFL, F waves are usually positive in V1 and negative in V6 and the atrial rate is ≈300bpm, being slower in patients with dilated or diseased right atria, or on class I drugs or amiodarone, and faster in young people or children (➲Fig. 28.10A, B). The slower the flutter rate, the higher the probability of having a brief horizontal baseline between consecutive atrial deflections. In the uncommon clockwise CTI AFL, the atrial F waves in the inferior leads have positive initial forces that may be followed by a terminal negative component, and are negative in V1 and positive in V6; if the P waves are positive in V1 a non-isthmian flutter must be suspected. The atrial rate in CTI clockwise AFL is frequently ≈250bpm or even slower (➲Figs. 28.10C and 28.12A).

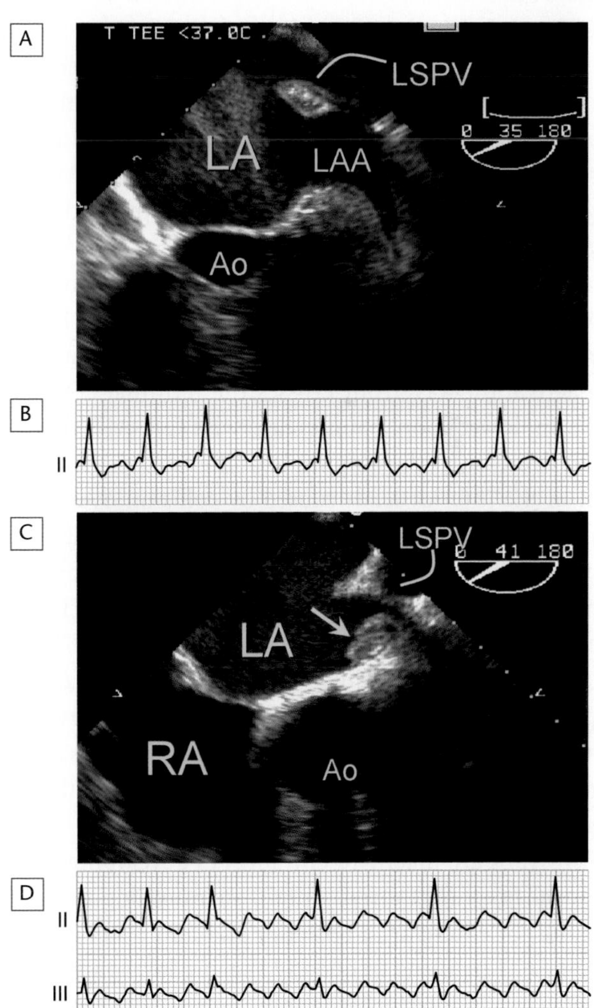

Figure 28.13 (A) and (B) are from a patient with CTI-dependent AFL and a history of hypertension and chronic obstructive lung disease. The transoesophageal echocardiogram (A) shows marked spontaneous echo contrast in the left atrial cavity. Ao, aorta; LA, left atrium; LAA, left atrial appendage; LSPV, left superior pulmonary vein. (C) and (D) belong to another patient aged 76 years, also with a CTI-dependent atrial flutter, systolic left ventricular dysfunction, and a previously documented episode of AF. In this patient the transoesophageal echocardiogram (C) showed a thrombus inside the left atrial appendage (arrow). RA, right atrium.

The AV ratio during AFL is usually 2:1. AV ratios >2:1 may be induced temporarily by vagal manoeuvres, or the intravenous infusion of adenosine, or verapamil. An AV ratio >2:1 on chronic basis can be observed in patients on drugs acting on the AV node (beta-blocking agents, calcium-channel blockers, or amiodarone), or because of the concomitant effects of ageing or disease on the AV node (➲Figs. 28.10B, C, 28.12A, and 28.13D). Exceptionally, the AV ratio during AFL may be 1:1, most frequently as a complication of class I antiarrhythmic drugs in which case we observe a tachycardia with very wide QRS complexes and a ventricular rate ranging from 190–250bpm because class IC drugs slow down the AFL rate and induce use-dependent bundle branch block.

CTI AFL developing after ablation for AF frequently exhibits atypical electrocardiographic manifestations because of altered conduction and activation pattern of the left atrium [155]. Although CTI AFL after AF ablation may electrocardiographically mimic atypical non-isthmian flutters, negativity of the P waves in the inferior or precordial leads suggests a CTI rather than a left atrial or CS AFL [155].

'Lower-loop' CTI AFL is electrocardiographically similar to counterclockwise or clockwise CTI AFL [134, 135] but the final contour of the F waves depends on the site where the activation wavefront crosses the terminal crest [140, 141]. In 'lower-loop' counterclockwise CTI AFL there is a slight decrease in the amplitude of the late positive deflection in the inferior leads caused by collision over the lateral right atrium that cancels the late cranio-caudal lateral wavefront [141]. Activation of the atrial septum and left atrium during 'lower-loop' counterclockwise CTI AFL is the same as during common counterclockwise CTI AFL, thus explaining the similar ECG manifestation of both. 'Upper loop re-entry' AFL circulating in a clockwise direction around the right superior caval vein, produces an ECG similar to that of clockwise CTI AFL [141] but with flat or negative F waves in lead I [156].

Left AFLs are macro-re-entrant ATs developing around the oval fossa (left atrial septal), surrounding the mitral annulus, or encircling a posterior scar and result in a variety of ECG patterns frequently sharing low amplitude or flat P waves in inferior leads and a tachycardia cycle length of 260–320ms [73, 141]. P waves in V1 and V2 are positive in left AFL around the oval fossa or the mitral annulus, and biphasic, positive–negative, in AFL around a left atrial posterior wall scar [141]. In AFL developing around a left atrial atriotomy scar after mitral valve surgery, the P waves are usually biphasic in the inferior leads with an initial positive or negative component depending on the rotation pattern of the activation wavefront [157].

Electrophysiological studies

Catheter mapping and stimulation studies enable us to differentiate isthmus-dependent from non-isthmian AFLs and macro-re-entrant ATs [1, 41, 59–69, 73–75, 118–123, 132–137]. Patients with AFL unrelated to the CTI or with other forms of macro-re-entrant AT should be referred to experienced centres if they are considered candidates for RFCA.

Treatment

Treatment of the acute episode

Vagal stimulation, intravenous adenosine or verapamil, will generally not terminate AFL but simply increase the AV block ratio so that the flutter waves become more apparent. Class III drugs such as ibutilide or dofetilide interrupt AFL more frequently than class I agents. Intravenous ibutilide restored sinus rhythm in 64–76% of AFL as compared with a 0–14% conversion rate with intravenous procainamide [158, 159]. Intravenous ibutilide is superior to amiodarone in the acute conversion of AFL (87% vs. 29%) [160]. Ibutilide can be used for pharmacological cardioversion of AFL in patients on class IC antiarrhythmic drugs or amiodarone with a similar incidence of *torsades des pointes* as in subjects without concomitant antiarrhythmic drug medication [161–164]. Attenuation of ibutilide-induced QT prolongation has been observed in some patients pre-treated with class IC agents [161]. Although development of AFL during pregnancy is extremely rare, ibutilide can safely terminate the arrhythmia in such a patient [164]. As of writing, ibutilide is not available in all European countries. Class III drugs may produce *torsades de pointes* and their use is not advocated in patients with systolic left ventricular dysfunction, prolonged QT interval, or underlying sinus node disease.

Class I drugs, and particularly those with a class IC profile (flecainide and propafenone), by reducing atrial conduction velocity prolong the AFL cycle length, increase the chances for developing a 1:1 AV conduction, particularly during exercise or under adrenergic stimulation. These drugs as well as amiodarone have a low probability of converting AFL into sinus rhythm.

To terminate paroxysmal AFL, most cardiologists use DC-shock cardioversion or atrial overdrive pacing. The level of energy required for electrical cardioversion of AFL is 50–100J using monophasic or biphasic waveforms. In patients with AFL, biphasic waveforms have not been shown to be clearly superior to monophasic DC-shocks in terms of success rate which is ≈97% with both [165]. Using monophasic waveforms the initial energy level should be 100J to diminish the total number of shocks for rhythm conversion and the risk of inducing AF that may be as high as 11% with a first shock of 50J [166]. AFL occurring after cardiac surgery can be terminated by overdrive pacing using the temporary atrial leads customarily left in place by most cardiovascular surgeons. In patients with respiratory failure, atrial overdrive pacing is preferred to DC-shock cardioversion since deep sedation poses additional risks. A spontaneous AV ratio >2:1 suggests coexistent AV nodal disease and a potential association with sinus node dysfunction and sinus pauses on restoring sinus rhythm should be anticipated.

The anticoagulation guidelines for patients with AF (➲Chapter 28) should be extended to those with AFL [1, 4, 167]. Cardioversion, by electrical, pharmacological, or ablation methods, without previous anticoagulation can be considered if AFL is <48 hours in duration. For patients with AFL of ≥48 hours or of unknown duration, elective cardioversion should be planned after ≥3 weeks of oral anticoagulation (INR between 2.0–3.0), even if thromboembolic risk factors are absent. Ventricular rate control is required during this anticoagulation period, something that is not easy in patients with AFL if AV conduction is normal.

An alternative approach is to exclude the presence of a left atrial thrombus with transoesophageal echocardiography followed by cardioversion. The transoesophageal echocardiogram must be performed after full anticoagulation is achieved with intravenous heparin or subcutaneous low-molecular-weight heparin. If enoxaparin is used we recommend an initial intravenous dose of 30mg, followed by 1mg/kg subcutaneously every 12 hours if renal function is normal, maintained during 5 days of concomitant therapy with oral anticoagulants. As with the conventional approach, the patient should receive oral anticoagulants during 1 month after cardioversion in all cases or permanently if the patient has one high risk or two or more intermediate risk factors for thromboembolic events [167]. Oral anticoagulation can be discontinued 6–12 months after ablation of AFL if the patient remains free from recurrences, does not suffer episodes of AF, and there is no history of previous embolic events, mitral stenosis, or mechanical valve prosthesis. Limitations of the transoesophageal echocardiogram are patient discomfort and potential procedural complications [167].

Adequate rate control of AFL with drugs acting on the AV node is difficult if the AV nodal function is normal, particularly in patients in cardiac or respiratory failure or in the presence of post-surgical anaemia. This is why the controversy 'rate versus rhythm control' does not exist in the field of AFL. Most paroxysmal AFLs become recurrent and after the second episode it is justified to consider the patient as a candidate for RFCA, particularly in CTI-dependent AFL. Also candidates for ablation are patients with AFL of unknown duration that have signs of systolic left ventricular dysfunction even if asymptomatic, for the potential of representing a tachycardiomyopathy state. Symptomatic chronic AFL should also be referred for catheter ablation. A randomized study in patients with ≥two episodes of symptomatic AFL within the last 4 months has shown that ablation is superior to conventional antiarrhythmic drug therapy in terms of maintaining sinus rhythm, quality of life, lower occurrence of AF, and lower need for rehospitalization [168]. Catheter ablation is also superior to amiodarone therapy after the first episode of AFL in patients aged >69 years, with fewer recurrences of flutter, a similar risk of subsequent AF, and lower incidence of side effects [169].

Role of catheter ablation in CTI AFL

Ablation techniques are aimed at creating a line of bidirectional block between the tricuspid annulus and the inferior vena cava or Eustachian ridge (➲Fig. 28.11) [131, 138, 169–171]. The central, most inferior, area of the CTI (6 o'clock region on a fluoroscopic LAO view) is thinner in myocardial content and shorter in length than the paraseptal and inferolateral sectors of the isthmus (➲Fig. 28.13). The paraseptal isthmus has the thickest myocardial content and is close to the posterior extensions of the AV node and its arterial supply [131].

Both RFCA and cryoablation of CTI-dependent AFL can be performed with various techniques. For RFCA of CTI AFL irrigated-tip and 8-mm tip ablation catheters are superior to 4-mm tip electrodes because they produce deeper and larger lesions on the isthmus [172–180]. The reported success rate has ranged from 100% [176] to 77% [178] with recurrences rates <5%. Cryoablation techniques have also been used with comparable results to those of RFCA in CTI AFL [181–186]. Cryoablation requires fewer applications than RFCA, is less painful for the patient, and can be performed with shorter fluoroscopy times. One study has reported a lower success rate with cryoablation as compared with RFCA using an 8-mm tip electrode [185].

Catheter ablation of the CTI in patients with AF

In patients with AF developing AFL only after having received class IC drugs or amiodarone, ablation of the CTI combined with antiarrhythmic drug treatment may serve to maintain the patient free of AF recurrences [187]. But many patients with AFL undergoing a CTI ablation procedure develop AF during follow-up [188–192]. The presence of a previous documentation of AF is the greatest predictor for the development of this arrhythmia after AFL ablation occurring in >60% of the patients. In patients without preablation, AF the incidence of post-procedural AF ranges between 7–50% [187–192].

Catheter ablation in CTI-independent atrial flutters

If the non-isthmus dependent AFL is due to atrial macro-re-entry, RFCA is directed to create a continuous ablation line along a critical corridor between anatomical barriers, or a narrow gap in the scar. These catheter ablation interventions should be performed with the aid of electro-anatomical mapping and navigation systems [1, 41, 73, 118–123, 139–140].

Management of patients in whom AFL ablation cannot be performed

Chronic antiarrhythmic drug treatment must be used in patients refusing RFCA. Dofetilide may reduce by 50% the risk of recurrence of AFL as compared with placebo [193]. The role of dronedarone in patients with AFL is not very clear and may not be safe in patients with a history of heart failure [194]. Dronedarone reduces the rates of recurrence of AF or AFL but there are no data on how effective this drug is in each of these two arrhythmias [195]. The ability of class IC drugs and amiodarone to prevent AFL recurrences is probably very limited [1].

Atrioventricular nodal reciprocating tachycardia

Definition

AVNRT is a re-entrant SVT utilizing the approaches to the AV node and the compact AV node itself. Traditional views on AVNRT considered that AV nodal conduction is functionally dissociated into a fast and a slow pathway with different electrophysiological properties. Three major forms of AVNRT exist. The common AVNRT utilizes the slow pathway anterogradely and the fast pathway retrogradely (slow–fast). The rare forms are the fast–slow, and the slow–slow AVNRT (➲Fig. 28.14). AVNRT rate ranges between 100–250bpm, usually 140–220bpm.

Pathogenesis

AVNRT is the most common paroxysmal SVT in patients without pre-excitation excluding AFL. The fast and slow AV nodal pathways are functionally and anatomically different. It is possible to ablate them at separate topographic sites in the triangle of Koch, without producing AV block. The slow AV nodal pathway is most likely represented by the right and left posteroinferior nodal extensions whose fibres run from the CS and along the tricuspid side of the triangle of Koch merging to form the compact AV node at the anterosuperior apex of the triangle (➲Fig. 28.14) [196–198]. The fast pathway may be formed by transitional fibres connecting the interatrial septum near the superior apex of the triangle of Koch with the compact AV node [199].

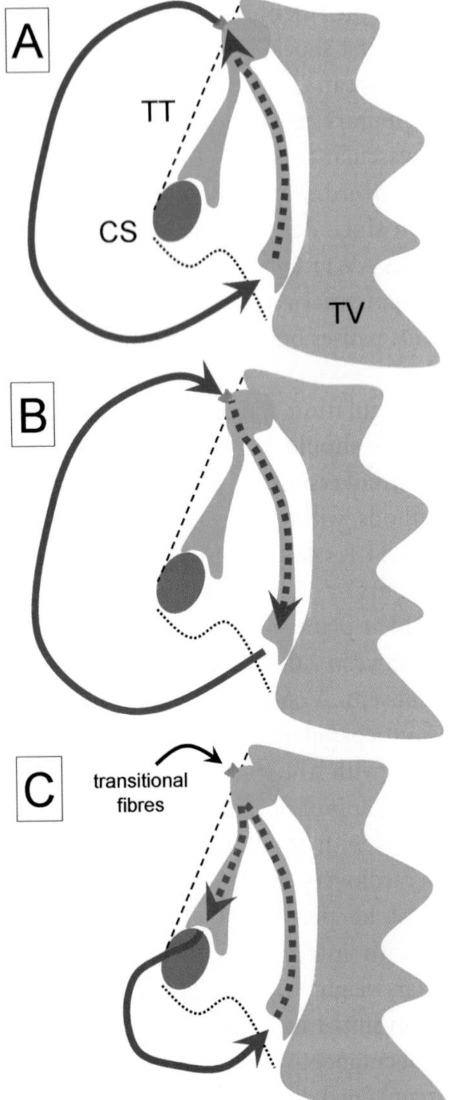

Figure 28.14 Triangle of Koch and mechanisms of AVNRT. CS, coronary sinus orifice; TT, tendon of Todaro; TV, tricuspid valve (septal leaflet). The AV node is represented with its inferior extensions. The triangle of Koch is located in the inferior paraseptal right atrial region and contains the AV node, its inferior extensions, and the transitional fibres that approach the compact nodal area. Its lateral margins are the Eustachian ridge containing the tendon of Todaro, and the attachment of the septal leaflet of the tricuspid valve. The base of the triangle is the orifice of the CS and the region from the CS to the tricuspid valve. (A) Common type of AVNRT using the slow AV nodal pathway as anterograde limb of the circuit and the fast pathway retrogradely. The slow pathway most likely is represented by the inferior extensions of the compact AV node, one coming from the CS, and the other along the tricuspid annulus. The fast AV nodal pathway (in light transparent red) may be an atrionodal or atrio-Hisian tract consisting of transitional fibres, although at least in some patients with AVNRT the fast pathway may have a fully intranodal course. (B) Uncommon fast–slow AVNRT. (C) Slow–slow AVNRT.

One area of uncertainty is if the upper link necessary to complete the re-entry loop by connecting the fast and slow nodal pathways is atrial myocardium or an upper common 'intranodal' pathway. Retrograde 2:1 block during an AVNRT favours an intranodal upper common link between the fast and slow pathways but is only exceptionally observed [88, 200]. Variations and irregularities in atrial activation with a fixed timing of His bundle depolarization, showing that the circuit is independent of the timing of atrial activation, can rarely be observed during AVNRT [201]. The lower common pathway is the bundle of His and occasionally the more distal AV node as evidenced by AVNRT with 2:1 AV ratio having the block distal and more rarely proximal to the His bundle (➲Fig. 28.15) [88–89].

The common slow–fast AVNRT is induced when the fast pathway has an anterograde refractory period that is longer than that of the slow pathway so that an APB is blocked in the fast pathway while conduction through the slow pathway is possible. On reaching the lower common pathway of the circuit, the wavefront returns retrogradely to the atria via the fast pathway. The reverse fast–slow AVNRT is rare as a clinical arrhythmia; occasionally it develops after performing RFCA on the slow pathway in patients previously suffering a common slow–fast AVNRT. The fast–slow AVNRT is elicited when the anterograde refractory period of the slow pathway is longer than that of the fast pathway and an APB can be conducted to the His bundle via the fast pathway, returning to the atria through the slow pathway. Patients frequently have more than

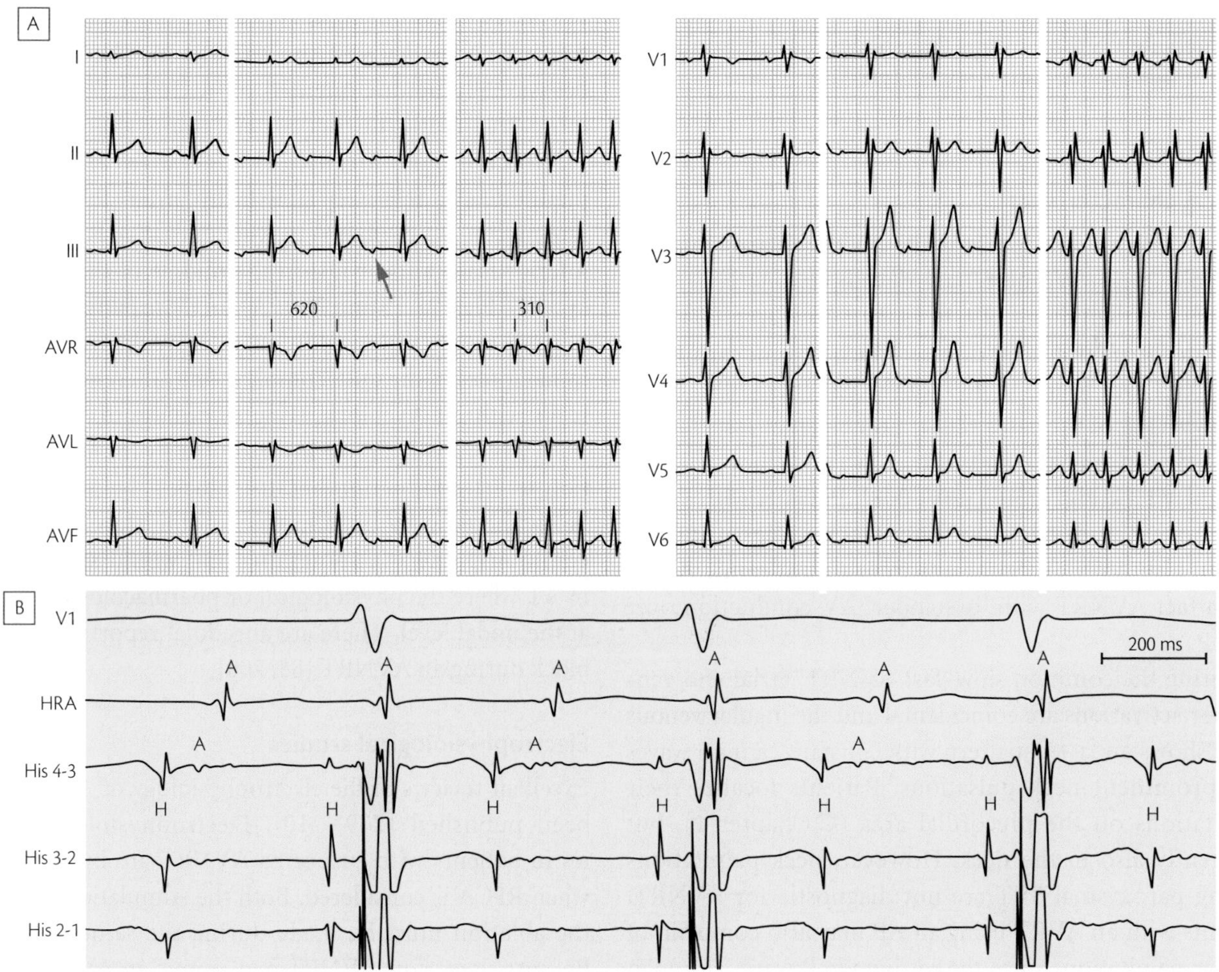

Figure 28.15 (A) ECG during sinus rhythm and AVNRT. The first tachycardia is AVNRT with 2:1 AV block and has a ventricular rate of 97bpm (cycle length 620ms). The red arrow signals the blocked retrograde P wave that is just in the middle of the interval between two consecutive QRS complexes. The second tachycardia, at 194bpm (cycle length 310ms) is AVNRT with 1:1 AV ratio. Due to the relatively fast rate of this AVNRT, there is beat-to-beat voltage alternans (see leads I, II, III, AVL, AVF, and V5). This is a non-specific finding that can be observed both in AVNRT and in AVRT using an AP. During AVNRT with 1:1 AV ratio the P wave in this case is totally hidden within the QRS-complex. The 'r' wave' in V1 is real and belongs to the ventricular complex due to an incomplete RBBB also present during sinus rhythm. (B) Intracardiac recordings from the high right atrium (HRA) and the bundle of His during the episode of AVNRT with 2:1 AV block showing that the site of block is below the His bundle.

one functional slow pathway. This probably accounts for the persistence in some patients of a slower slow pathway not sustaining the tachycardia after ablation of the slow pathway. The slow–slow AVNRT is also rare, but more common than the fast–slow AVNRT. Retrograde conduction times in slow–slow AVNRT are longer than in slow–fast AVNRT, so that P waves are recorded immediately after the QRS complex, thus mimicking the ECG pattern typical of a concealed AP. In addition, the retrograde atrial breakthrough of slow–slow AVNRT is located near or within the CS [202].

The reasons why AVNRT is more common in females than males are obscure. The proximal portion of the CS in patients with AVNRT is wider than that of controls. Females with AVNRT have the widest terminal CS which adopts a funnel-like shape in venographic studies. Males without AVNRT have the narrowest terminal CS, which has a tubular shape. Males with AVNRT have intermediate CS dimensions and shapes that are similar to those of females without ANVRT [203].

Diagnosis

Clinical characteristics

Some 70% of patients with AVNRT are females (➲Table 28.1). Women start developing AVNRT at a younger age than men (29 ± 16 vs. 39 ± 16 years) [204]. An associated structural heart disease, which in some early series of AVNRT was found in 46% of the patients [205], exists in only ≈15% of the cases [204]. Coincidental associations exist between AVNRT and AFL [206], and idiopathic left or right VT (➲Fig. 28.16) [207, 208]. Patients with WPW syndrome may develop not only tachycardias using the AP but also AVNRT. Some apparently antidromic AVRT are in fact AVNRT with 'bystander' AV conduction over the AP.

During the common slow–fast AVNRT, atrial and ventricular activations are coincidental and the jugular venous pulse shows an 'a + c' pattern with constant cannon waves and prominent neck pulsations. Patients localize their palpitations on the precordial area (➲Chapter 1), but frequently also in the neck. However, neck palpitations during paroxysmal SVT are not diagnostic for AVNRT. Patients with an AVRT using an AP may also complain of jugular palpitations since the retrograde P wave, although registered after the QRS complex, occurs during mechanical ventricular systole and gives rise to an 'a + v' jugular venous pattern. During episodes of AVNRT, patients may also complain of polyuria, dizziness, chest pain, and even syncope.

Electrocardiographic characteristics

During the common slow–fast AVNRT, retrograde P waves are hidden within the ventricular complex (25%) or are recorded at the end of the QRS, mimicking terminal 's waves' in inferior leads or more frequently 'pseudor' waves' in lead V1 (60%) (➲Figs. 28.7, 28.15, 28.16, and 28.17). Exceptionally, P waves may be registered just before the onset of the ventricular complex, simulating initial inferior 'q waves' (2%) or after the QRS offset (8%) as during the slow–slow AVNRT whose ECG mimics that of an AVRT utilizing an inferior paraseptal AP (➲Fig. 28.18) [85, 86, 202]. The remaining 5% is represented by the fast–slow AVNRT in which the P wave precedes the QRS complex with a PR <RP pattern, thus mimicking an AT or a PJRT (➲Figs 28.7 and 28.17E). The P wave during all kinds of AVNRT is negative in leads II, III, and aVF, and biphasic with a terminal positive component in V1 (➲Figs. 28.15, 28.17, and 28.18).

The AV ratio during AVNRT is usually 1:1. At the initiation of a fast AVNRT the AV ratio may be 2:1. This can occasionally be documented on a Holter recording and more frequently during an electrophysiological study. Electrocardiographically, AVNRT with 2:1 AV block manifests as a relatively slow tachycardia (the ventricular rate may be 90–120bpm) in which negative P waves in the inferior leads appear just in the middle of the ventricular cycle (➲Figs. 28.15 and 28.17A). In these patients it may be possible to identify an additional P wave deforming the terminal forces of the QRS complex. The differential diagnosis is AT with 2:1 AV block. Long recordings of AVNRT with 2:1 AV block will almost invariably show the abrupt transition to 1:1 conduction because block is below the His or below the slow AV nodal pathway (at the level of the lower common pathway), something that would seldom occur in AT where the physiological or pharmacological block is at the nodal level. There are anecdotal reports of a 2:1 VA block during an AVNRT [88, 200].

Electrophysiological studies

Excellent reviews of the electrophysiology of AVNRT have been published [209, 210]. Electrophysiological studies in patients with suspected AVNRT are indicated only when RFCA is considered. Both the stimulation study and the ablation must be made during the same procedure. Because slow–slow AVNRT may mimic an AVRT utilizing a concealed inferior paraseptal AP, and because the ablation approaches are different in both situations, special attention should be paid to making the correct diagnosis. A slow–slow AVNRT is diagnosed if a ventricular premature beat introduced during tachycardia when the His

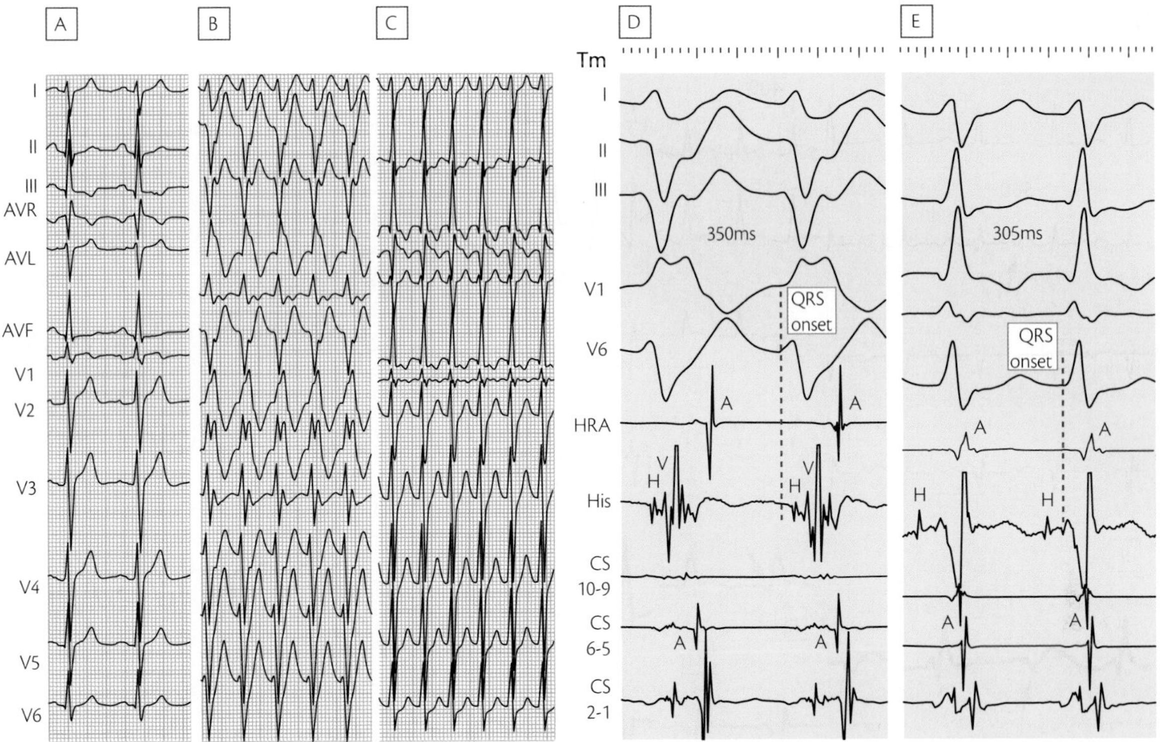

Figure 28.16 Association of an idiopathic fascicular VT and an AVNRT in the same patient. Both types of tachycardia had been documented clinically. (A) ECG during sinus rhythm. (B) ECG during a wide QRS complex regular tachycardia with a RBBB configuration and a superior axis (−15°) in the frontal plane. (C) ECG during a narrow QRS complex regular tachycardia in which P waves are not clearly identified. (D, E) Five surface ECG leads (I, II, III, V1, and V6) are displayed together with bipolar intracardiac electrograms from the high right atrium (HRA), His bundle region, and at three levels inside the CS. In (D) a His bundle potential (H) is recorded after the onset of the QRS complex (discontinuous line) thus demonstrating that this tachycardia (cycle length 350ms) was of ventricular origin. In (E) the His potential precedes the QRS complex during AVNRT (cycle length 305ms). During AVNRT the atrial electrograms are hidden within the QRS complex and P waves are not identified in the surface ECG (C).

bundle is refractory does not advance the subsequent atrial activity, as would occur in AVRT utilizing an inferior paraseptal AP [202]. The presence of dual AV nodal pathway physiology, defined by a sudden jump of ≥50ms in the AH interval for a 10-ms decrease in the coupling interval of the extrastimulus, is of no diagnostic help since dual AV nodal pathways are not always present in patients with AVNRT and may be found in patients with other forms of SVT.

In the common slow–fast AVNRT the earliest retrograde atrial activation is usually recorded close to the superoanterior apex of the triangle of Koch, whereas in the atypical slow–slow or fast–slow AVNRT the earliest retrograde atrial activation is registered close to the ostium of the CS, or inside the CS [211–214]. An eccentric sequence of retrograde atrial activation cannot therefore be taken as the sole diagnostic criterion to identify a retrogradely-conducting left-sided AP.

Treatment

Treatment of the acute episode

Paroxysmal AVNRT can be terminated, but not always, by vagal manoeuvres. Intravenous adenosine or verapamil nearly always terminate AVNRT. These interventions terminate AVNRT by inducing block in the anterograde slow AV nodal pathway. Verapamil and diltiazem should be avoided in patients using beta-blockers. The intravenous administration of class I antiarrhythmic drugs can also interrupt an AVNRT by blocking the retrograde fast pathway.

The treatment of choice for AVNRT, independently of its variety, is RFCA of the slow AV nodal pathway. For patients with frequent episodes of AVNRT who temporarily or permanently refuse RFCA, class IC drugs (flecainide or propafenone) are particularly effective due to their use-dependent effect on the retrograde fast pathway [215, 216]. Flecainide (200–300mg/day) or propafenone (600–900mg/day) prevent recurrences of AVNRT in 65% of patients. If the latter drugs are contraindicated beta-blockers, verapamil, diltiazem, or amiodarone can be used. An associated sinus node disease would prevent the use of antiarrhythmic drugs. Verapamil, diltiazem, beta-blockers, and digoxin, might prevent recurrences when the slow pathway is the weakest link of the AVNRT but can have the opposite effect if the fast pathway is the weakest

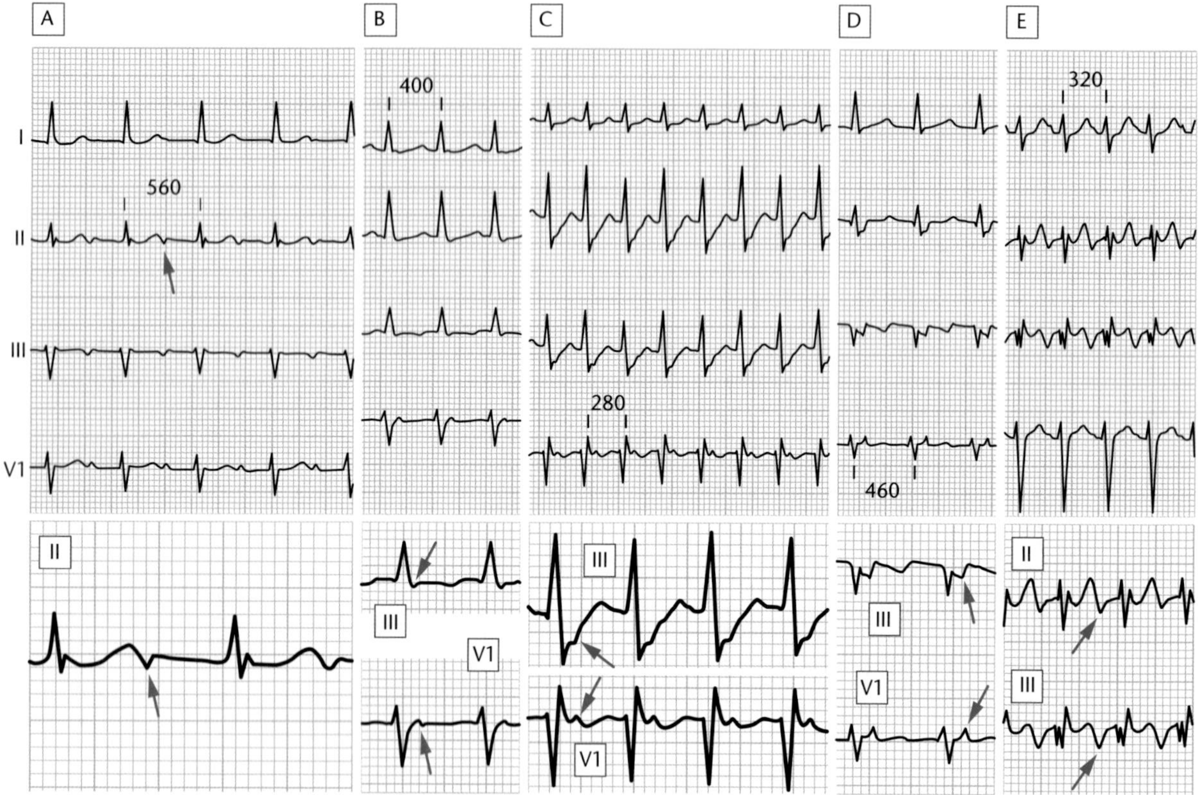

Figure 28.17 (A) AVNRT with 2:1 AV block; the ventricular rate is relatively slow (107bpm) and there is a P wave just in the middle between two consecutive QRS complexes (arrow). P waves are predominantly negative in the inferior leads and positive in lead V1. The bottom vignette shows a magnified detail of lead II. (B) AVNRT in which the retrograde P waves (arrows) mimic 'pseudo s waves' in the inferior leads and 'pseudo r′ waves' in V1. The rate of this AVNRT is 150bpm. (C) Relatively fast AVNRT (214bpm) with voltage alternans of consecutive QRS complexes. Although this finding has been said to suggest an AVRT incorporating an AP, it is a non-specific sign depending on the rate of the tachycardia. Retrograde P waves (negative in inferior leads and positive in V1) are visible just following the QRS complex. (D) Relatively slow AVNRT (130bpm) in a 72-year-old woman. P waves are visible just following the QRS complex (arrows). (E) Example of the rare fast–slow AVNRT at a rate of 188bpm. P waves with a PR interval slightly shorter than the RP time are clearly seen (arrows).

link of the circuit. Under physical or psychological stress the latter drugs may lose their efficacy. Amiodarone is a pharmacological option if all other drugs cannot be used or have failed but its long-term use is hampered by side effects [1, 217–220].

In patients with infrequent, well tolerated, but prolonged episodes of AVNRT and in whom self-performed vagal manoeuvres are ineffective or impossible, the so-called 'pill-in-the-pocket' approach has been advocated. A single oral dose of flecainide (≈3mg/kg) was not much superior to placebo in one study that demonstrated the superiority of the combination of oral propranolol (80mg) and diltiazem (120mg) over flecainide and placebo [221]. Since hypotension and sinus bradycardia are potential complications of this approach, its use is not recommended in elderly people. In patients with infrequent episodes, the use of chronic antiarrhythmic drug therapy is not acceptable because drugs do not guarantee prevention of recurrences.

Radiofrequency catheter ablation

RFCA is the treatment of choice for AVNRT after its first recurrence but if the tachycardia is very symptomatic and the patient enjoys a very active life, the physician may offer a well informed explanation of the benefits and risks of an ablation procedure without waiting to a second episode. The fear of suffering an episode of AVNRT deteriorates the quality of life of these patients and this may be an indication for catheter intervention. Females in child-bearing age should not take antiarrhythmic drugs permanently, and benefit from a permanent cure with catheter ablation.

The ablation of the slow pathway during sinus rhythm is the preferred approach (➲Fig. 22.18). In experienced centres, slow-pathway ablation can be performed with an almost negligible risk of inducing AV block (<0.5%) and with a success rate of 98% [222]. It is controversial if atypical AVNRT (fast–slow, or slow–slow) exhibiting an eccentric retrograde pattern of atrial activation (earliest atrial electrograms during VA conduction recorded 5–15mm inside

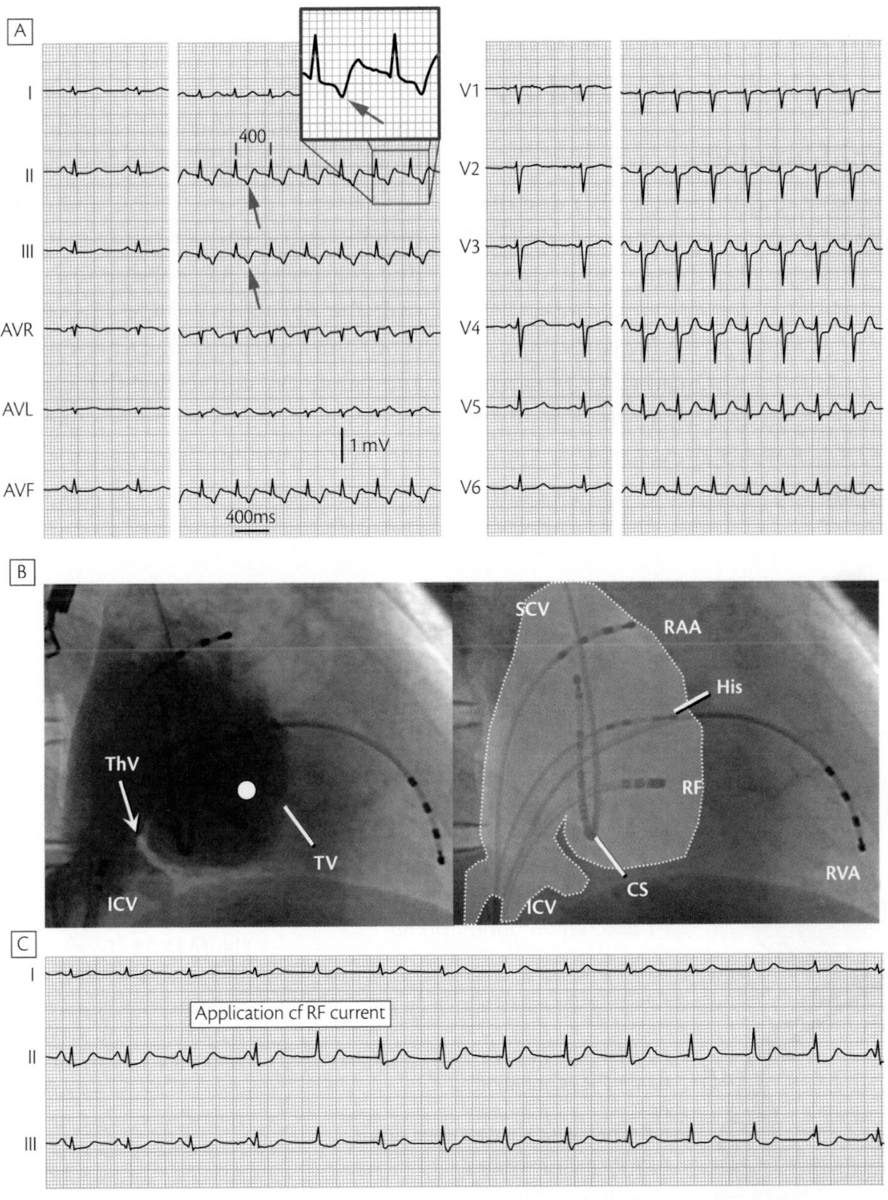

Figure 28.18 Slow–slow AVNRT. (A) ECG during sinus rhythm and during tachycardia. Electrocardiographically, this form of AVNRT cannot be differentiated from an AVRT utilizing a concealed inferior paraseptal AP. Retrograde P-waves start after the end of the QRS complex with a PR >RP pattern. The insert shows a magnification of lead II during tachycardia depicting the retrograde negative P waves after the QRS complex (arrows). (B) Right atrial angiogram in this patient depicts the limits of the right atrium and the triangle of Koch (left vignette). ICV, inferior caval vein; TV, tricuspid valve; ThV, Thebesian valve. Right fluorographic image with the ablation catheter (RF) positioned at the site of block of the slow pathway (right vignette). This point is represented as a white circle on the right atrial angiogram. A transparent contour of the right atrium and the tricuspid valve is superimposed on the fluorographic view on the right. (C) During the RF application that resulted in the ablation of the slow AV nodal pathway and in the abolition of this tachycardia, an accelerated AV junctional rhythm was induced. CS, coronary sinus; RAA, right atrial appendage; RVA, right ventricular apex; SCV, superior caval vein.

the CS) is best ablated inside the CS or with a conventional approach to the slow pathway on the triangle of Koch [211–214]. Recurrences of AVNRT after slow-pathway ablation are observed in <2% and all of them can usually be cured in a repeat procedure [1, 3, 222]. More pessimistic views from a single centre have been published [224]. The results of the arrhythmia unit of referral should be known by the referring physicians.

Elimination of AVNRT can be obtained in 100% of patients if the fast pathway is approached in those in whom the slow pathway cannot be ablated [223]. The risk of inducing AV block during fast pathway ablation is higher than that approaching the slow pathway. With experience, starting with very low temperatures that are very slowly increased, this risk is minimal and lower than the initially reported figure of 5% [223].

Accessory pathways, pre-excitation syndromes, and their tachycardias

Definition and epidemiology

In 1930, Wolff, Parkinson, and White (WPW) described in 11 healthy young people the association of a short PR interval and a wide QRS complex during sinus rhythm, with a tendency to develop paroxysmal tachycardia [225]. Classical WPW syndrome (➲ Fig. 28.19) is due to the existence of relatively fast-conducting anomalous AV fibres connecting atria and ventricles at sites where they should be electrically isolated [226]. Epicardial excitation mapping, programmed electrical stimulation, and intracardiac catheter electrode mapping techniques not only demonstrated the existence of AP in WPW syndrome but led to the development of 'curative' ablative approaches, first with surgery and then with percutaneous catheter electrode intracardiac procedures [2, 3].

The term 'pre-excitation' indicates that in WPW syndrome ventricular activation starts earlier than expected due to shorter AV conduction times via the AP than over the normal AV node–His axis [227]. Pre-excitation syndromes include all situations in which there is an anomalous AV connection that can conduct anterogradely, including instances without actual pre-excitation in which the AV conduction times over the AP are not shorter than via the normal AV node–His pathway (➲ Fig. 28.19).

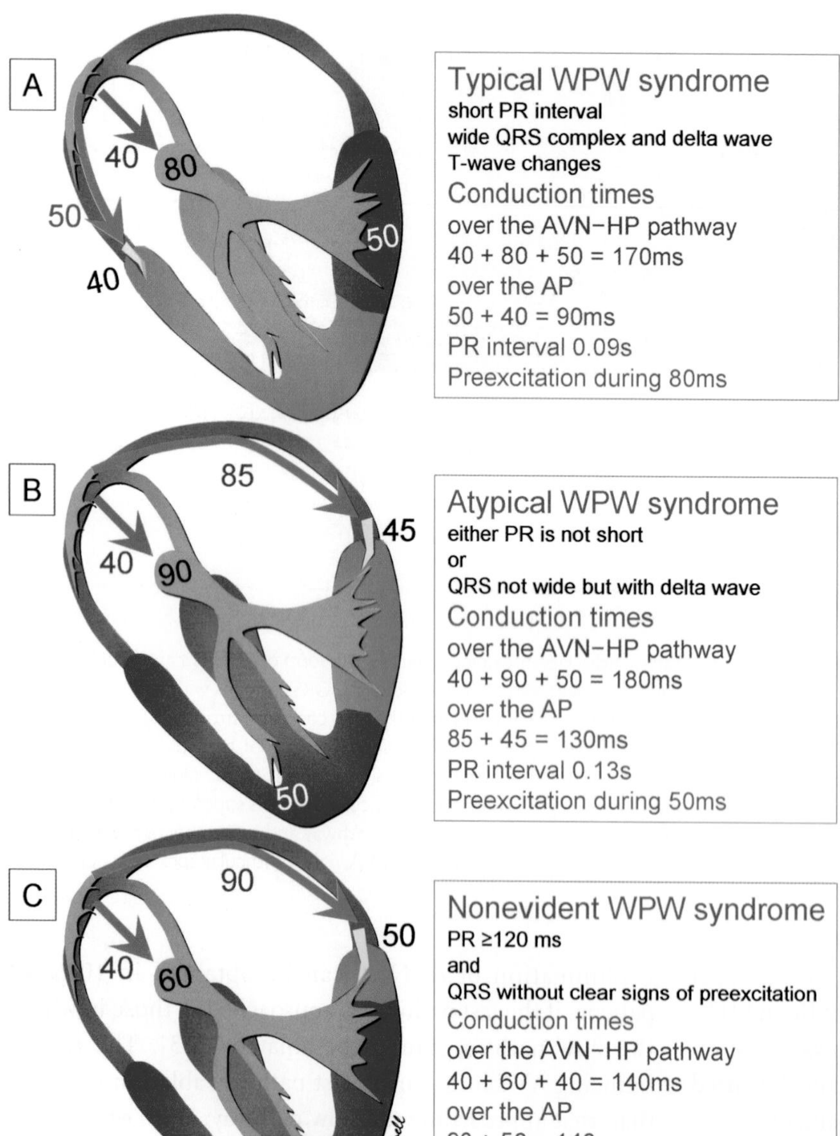

A
40
80
50
50
40
Typical WPW syndrome
short PR interval
wide QRS complex and delta wave
T-wave changes
Conduction times
over the AVN–HP pathway
40 + 80 + 50 = 170ms
over the AP
50 + 40 = 90ms
PR interval 0.09s
Preexcitation during 80ms
B
85
45
40
90
50
Atypical WPW syndrome
either PR is not short
or
QRS not wide but with delta wave
Conduction times
over the AVN–HP pathway
40 + 90 + 50 = 180ms
over the AP
85 + 45 = 130ms
PR interval 0.13s
Preexcitation during 50ms
C
90
50
40
60
40
Nonevident WPW syndrome
PR ≥120 ms
and
QRS without clear signs of preexcitation
Conduction times
over the AVN–HP pathway
40 + 60 + 40 = 140ms
over the AP
90 + 50 = 140ms
PR interval 0.14s
Preexcitation during 0ms

Figure 28.19 Typical, 'atypical', and 'non-evident' pre-excitation in WPW syndrome. The green arrow represents conduction times from the sinus node to the atrial insertion of the AP and the blue arrow conduction times from the sinus node to the AV node. (A) Right-sided AP resulting in a typical WPW pattern. AV conduction times over the AP are 80ms shorter than those over the normal axis. Pre-excitation (difference between AV conduction times via the AP and over the normal axis) occurs during 80ms, meaning that during 80ms the ventricles are activated through the wavefront of depolarization initiated at the ventricular insertion of the AP (represented in light transparent green). (B) 'Atypical' WPW pattern in a heart with a left-sided free-wall AP. The atypical feature here is a PR interval of 130ms. However, because AV conduction times over the AP are 50ms shorter than via the normal AV nodal–His pathway, pre-excitation is patent and the configuration of the QRS complex enables us to diagnose a WPW syndrome. (C) 'Non-evident' pre-excitation in a heart with a left-sided, free-wall AP. AV conduction times via the AP and over the AV node–His axis are the same (140ms in both instances). The PR interval is not short, and the QRS complex is not wide because only a very small amount of ventricular myocardium at the vicinity of the ventricular insertion of the AP will be depolarized by the wavefront arriving to the ventricles through the bypass tract. In this case the diagnosis of pre-excitation during sinus rhythm may be impossible.

APs can be patent or concealed. Patent (overt) APs conduct in AV direction and have the potential to produce ECG manifestations during sinus rhythm or atrial pacing. They are involved in WPW syndrome and in a form of pre-excitation initially thought to be due to nodoventricular Mahaim fibres but that is caused by an atriofascicular bypass tract [228, 229]. Patients with APs can develop paroxysmal SVT based on re-entry utilizing the AP, or less frequently due to other mechanisms in which the AP acts as a bystander, as when AF supervenes.

Concealed APs are those that only conduct in retrograde (VA) direction so that during sinus rhythm there are no signs of ventricular pre-excitation. These patients develop a paroxysmal AVRT utilizing the AP as retrograde limb of the re-entry circuit. A special type of concealed AP with long conduction times and decremental conducting properties is responsible for an incessant junctional reciprocating tachycardia known as permanent junctional reciprocating tachycardia (PJRT) [230].

Epidemiological data with regard to APs and ventricular pre-excitation are scanty. The prevalence of the WPW ECG pattern is ≈0.1–3/1000 tracings [231], a figure that underestimates the reality due to the existence of intermittent and non-evident forms of pre-excitation. In a recent study the annual incidence of new cases of WPW syndrome was 4.4/100000, with more than twice as many males (6.8/100,000) as females (2.2/100,000) [232].

Pathogenesis

Developmental and genetic factors leading to anomalous AV pathways

APs are generated by congenital defects in AV segmentation and in the development of the fibrous AV rings. Right-sided APs are related to an ill-formed tricuspid annulus, and left-sided pathways probably skirt the mitral annulus [226]. While the majority of patients with APs have no other associated cardiac abnormalities, patients with Ebstein's anomaly of the tricuspid valve or L-transposition of the great arteries frequently have anomalous AV connections [233]. Nearly 20% of patients with Ebstein's anomaly (➲Chapter 10) have a WPW syndrome, some 50% of them with multiple APs at electrophysiological study (➲Fig. 28.20) [234]. Some patients with tuberous sclerosis, with or without an associated rhabdomyoma, may also have an AP and eventually pre-excitation [235]. A CS diverticulum has been found in some patients with inferior paraseptal (formerly posteroseptal) APs [236].

In a very small number of patients, ventricular pre-excitation is associated with a form of left ventricular hypertrophy not due to sarcomeric-protein gene disorders like in classic hypertrophic cardiomyopathy (➲Chapter 18), but to mutations in *LAMP2* or *PRKAG2* genes regulating glycogen metabolism. Clinical features associated with defects in *LAMP2* (lysosome associated protein) or 'Danon disease' include male gender, severe hypertrophy, onset between 8–17 years of age, ventricular pre-excitation, and elevations of CK and sometimes of cTnI. These patients may also suffer a skeletal myopathy and mental retardation. Mutations in the *PRKAG2* gene encoding the regulatory γ-subunit of AMP-activated protein kinase (AMPK), cause another glycogen-storage disease phenotypically mimicking hypertrophic cardiomyopathy in which hypertrophy is associated with ventricular pre-excitation, progressive cardiac conduction system disease (sinoatrial or AV bock eventually requiring pacing), AF, and even sudden death. Cardiac hypertrophy in patients with *PRKAG2* gene mutations may evolve to a dilated cardiomyopathy pattern with systolic dysfunction and progressive heart failure [237–239]. In a transgenic mouse model expressing a human *PRKAG2* mutation, the development of APs but not of cardiomyopathy or conduction system degeneration, was reversible through transgene suppression techniques during early postnatal development [240].

A familial occurrence of WPW has been reported in ≈3% of patients with electrophysiologically demonstrated APs [241]. First-degree relatives of patients with APs have a 0.55% prevalence of a WPW pattern—a proportion higher than that in the general population (➲Chapter 9). The inheritance pattern is autosomal dominant in these patients [241].

Anatomical types of accessory pathways

Patent and concealed APs with 'short' conduction times are usually composed of ordinary working myocardium [226]. In the form of pre-excitation today termed 'Mahaim physiology', the AP is a long anomalous parallel AV conduction system in the free-wall tricuspid annulus consisting of a proximally decrementally conducting structure (like the AV node) that continues with an anomalous His which, through a Purkinje bundle, connects distally with the normal right bundle branch or directly with the apical right ventricular myocardium [229]. This AP frequently, but not always, is an atriofascicular bundle. The AP involved in PJRT may be a tortuous fibro-myocardial bundle whose anisotropic properties may account for slow and decremental conduction [242].

Bidirectional or unidirectional conduction over accessory pathways

APs may conduct only in anterograde direction, have bidirectional AV and VA conduction, or exclusively

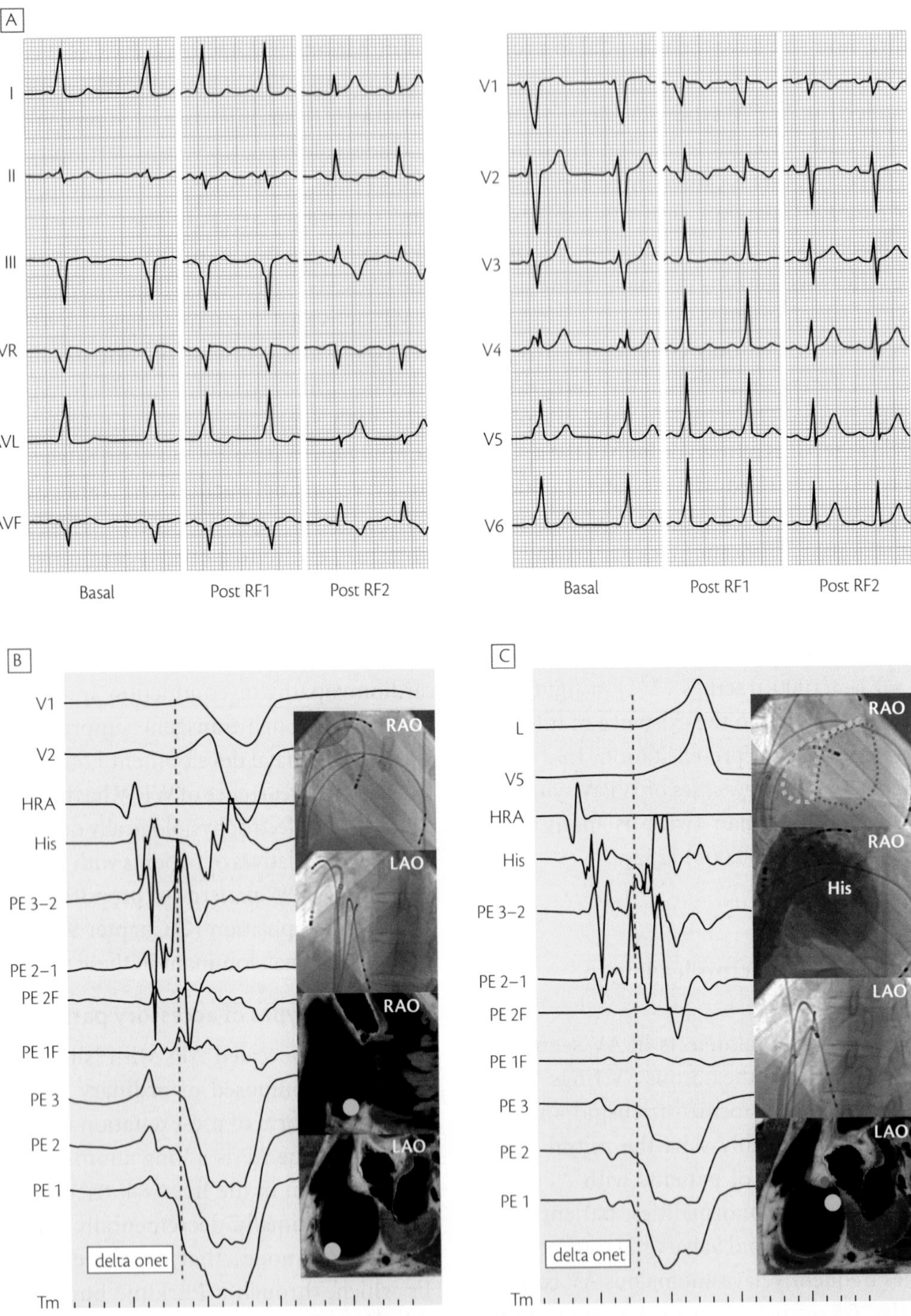

Figure 28.20 (A) ECG of a patient with an Ebstein's anomaly of the tricuspid valve showing a typical WPW pattern (basal) due to an AV right inferior AP. After ablating this AP a second ventricular pre-excitation pattern appeared (post RF1) similar to the initial one in the frontal plane leads, but very different in the precordial leads. This second AP was septally located and was abolished by RFCA. Note the normal PR interval and QRS width after this second ablation (post RF2) and that the T waves in the inferior leads are inverted due to cardiac electric memory. (B) Electrograms at the site of ablation of the right inferior AP. Leads V1 and V2 are registered with intracardiac leads from the HRA, His bundle, and the probing electrode (PE). The fluoroscopic frames in the RAO and LAO projections are displayed together with anatomic slices in RAO and LAO projections [14]. (C) Recordings at the site of ablation of the second AP (septally located). On right atrial angiogram note the downward displacement of the tricuspid valve due to Ebstein's disease. Superimposed on the RAO view of the catheters, the theoretical triangle of Koch is displayed in yellow, whereas the ventricularly displaced septal leaflef of the tricuspid valve is represented in red. The location of the His bundle (red dot) above the site of ablation of this second AP (yellow circle) is shown at the LAO anatomic slice in the bottom vignette.

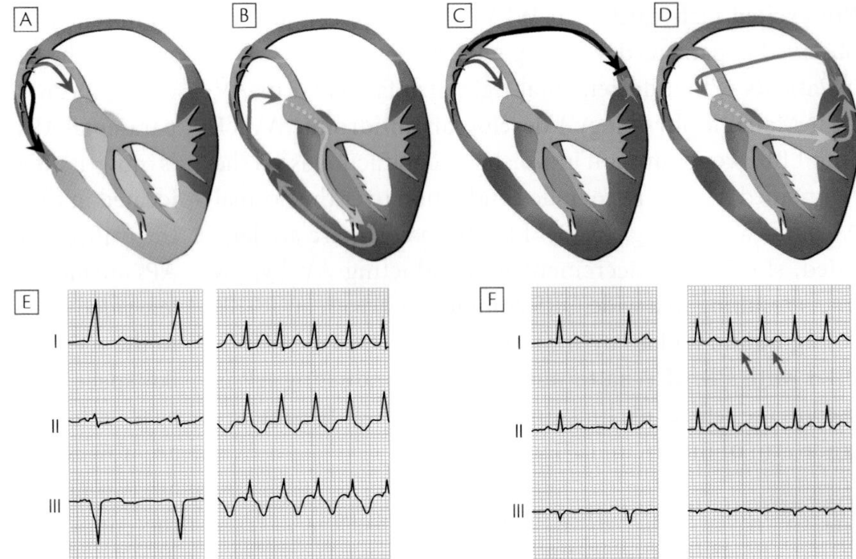

Figure 28.21 Representation of the ECG during sinus rhythm and orthodromic AVRT in a bidirectionally conducting right free-wall AP (A, B) and in a concealed left-sided AP (C, D). (E, F) Actual ECG recordings in I, II, and III of the same situations. The mechanism of AVRT is identical in both instances, but because the concealed AP only conducts in VA direction, during sinus rhythm there are no signs of ventricular pre-excitation (F). T waves during AVRT in E are negative in lead III due to cardiac electric memory. Note the negative P wave in lead I in F, expression of VA conduction through a left-sided AP.

conduct retrogradely. The anterograde and retrograde conducting properties of APs with bidirectional conduction, as well as their response to antiarrhythmic drugs, are frequently different. The reasons for directionally-dependent conduction discrepancies in APs are not clear and may be due to 'mismatch impedance' [243] or to interactions among branches at the proximal and/or distal insertions of the AP.

AVRT utilizing an accessory pathway

In patients with bidirectional AP conduction or with a concealed AP, the most frequent arrhythmia is the orthodromic AVRT that utilizes the AP as the retrograde limb of the circuit (➲Fig. 28.21). In both instances, an orthodromic AVRT can be induced by an APB that is anterogradely blocked in the AP so that its activation wavefront is conducted to the ventricles via the AV node–His axis. On activating the ventricle the wavefront returns to the atria via the AP. Alternatively, orthodromic AVRT can be induced by ventricular premature beats retrogradely conducted to the atria only via the AP so that the impulse comes back to the ventricles via the AV node–His axis. Orthodromic means that ventricular activation during AVRT is via the normal AV node–His axis, and thereby without ventricular pre-excitation.

A few patients with WPW syndrome develop the antidromic AVRT that uses the AP as anterograde limb of the circuit and the normal AV nodal axis, or a second AP, retrogradely (➲Fig. 28.22). Some of these apparently antidromic AVRT in WPW syndrome actually are AVNRT with AV conduction over an AP. In the latter case, abolition of conduction over the AP (that acts as a bystander) will not prevent tachycardia.

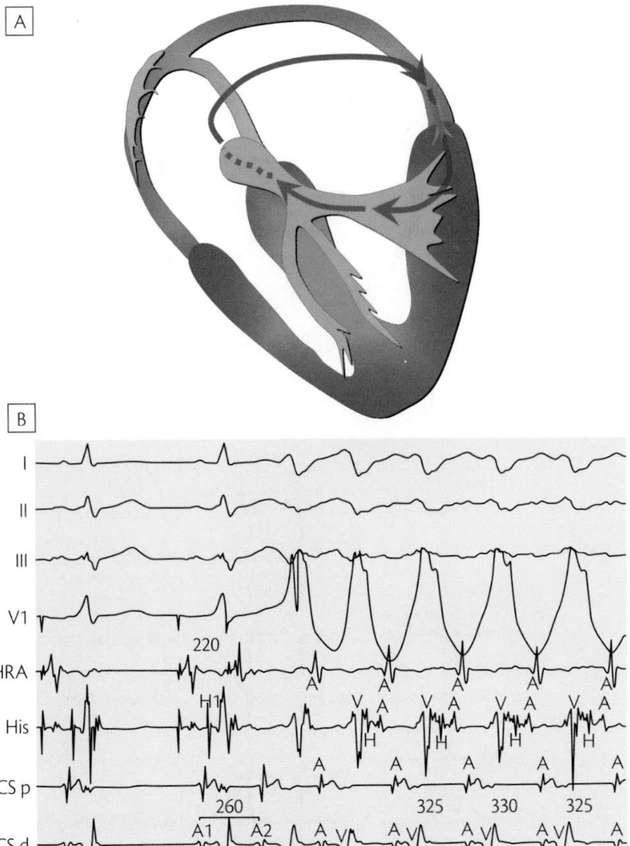

Figure 28.22 (A) Antidromic AVRT via a left-sided AP. (B) Leads I, II, III, and V1 are simultaneously displayed with intracardiac bipolar recordings from the HRA, His, and CS. A premature atrial extrastimulus with a coupling interval of 220ms is conducted to the ventricles through the AP and returns back to the atria via the normal His–AV node axis. Retrograde atrial activation starts at the His bundle lead and is preceded by a His bundle potential (H).

Pre-excited tachycardias in WPW syndrome can also be observed in patients developing AT, AFL, or AF.

Patients with a decremental right atriofascicular or AV AP ('Mahaim physiology') develop an antidromic AVRT with LBBB configuration in which AV conduction is via the right-sided AP and retrograde conduction over the normal AV node axis (➲ Fig. 28.23). Exceptionally, there are left-sided, slowly, and decrementally-conducting AV bypass tracts resulting in a wide QRS complex SVT with an RBBB configuration and an inferior axis (➲ Fig. 28.24) [244]. In PJRT with PR <RP pattern, the slowly conducting AP is used as the retrograde limb and the AV node as the anterograde arm of the circuit (➲ Fig. 28.25).

Topographic classification of accessory pathways

Initial classifications of AP locations distinguished five broad regions: right free wall; left free wall; posteroseptal; anteroseptal; and intermediate septal. Catheter mapping and ablation techniques led to the definition of a more comprehensive topographic classification of APs in agreement with the fluoroscopic locations of the ablation sites (➲ Fig. 28.26) [245]. The pyramidal space contains septal and paraseptal APs [170, 171, 198]. The old term 'posteroseptal' is now named 'inferior paraseptal'. Midseptal APs are located in the pyramidal space between the His bundle and the orifice of the CS. In the new nomenclature, midseptal APs are named true-septal or septal but there are right- and left-sided septal APs (➲ Fig. 28.26). Some APs are unrelated to the AV rings, such as those coursing within the pyramidal space, or connecting the right or left atrial appendages with their ipsilateral ventricle. Old anteroseptal APs are now termed 'superior paraseptal'. In this region there are two kinds of APs: peri-Hisian APs that course between the endocardium and the AV node–His bundle to insert distally at the superior summit of the muscular ventricular septum; and superior paraseptal APs whose ventricular insertion is at the supraventricular crest, beyond the ventricular septum.

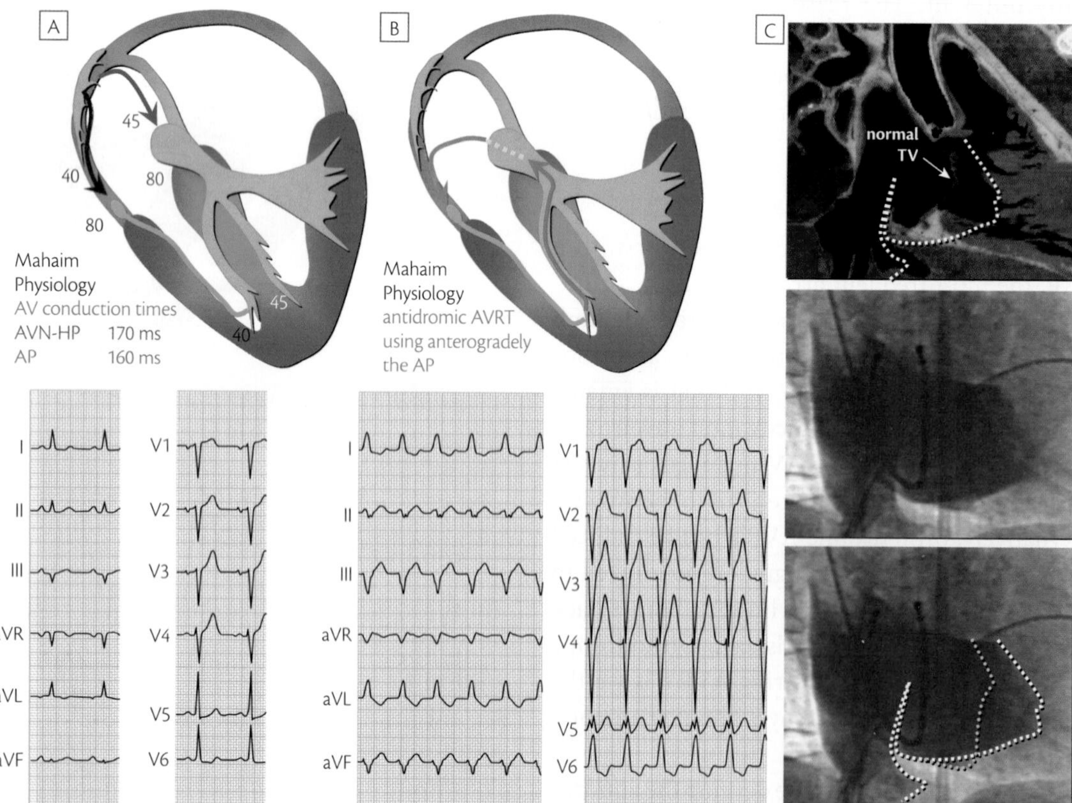

Figure 28.23 Right atriofascicular AP in a patient with Ebstein's anomaly of the tricuspid valve. (A) AV conduction times via the normal AV node–His axis and through the atriofascicular pathway. Below the ECG during sinus rhythm showing a PR interval of 160ms and not very evident signs of pre-excitation. (B) Representation of the tachycardia circuit and below the actual tachycardia with a LBBB QRS configuration. (C) Anatomic slice in RAO projection depicting the normal tricuspid valve location (TV) and the displacement of the septal leaflet of this valve towards the ventricle (dotted line) to replicate the limits of the tricuspid valve in this patient as evidenced in the right atrial angiogram. In the angiographic frame at the bottom, the white dotted line draws the contour of the septal leaflet of the tricuspid valve, the Eustachian valve, and the inferior caval vein, and the cyan dotted line delineates the theoretical expected level of the normal septal tricuspid valve leaflet.

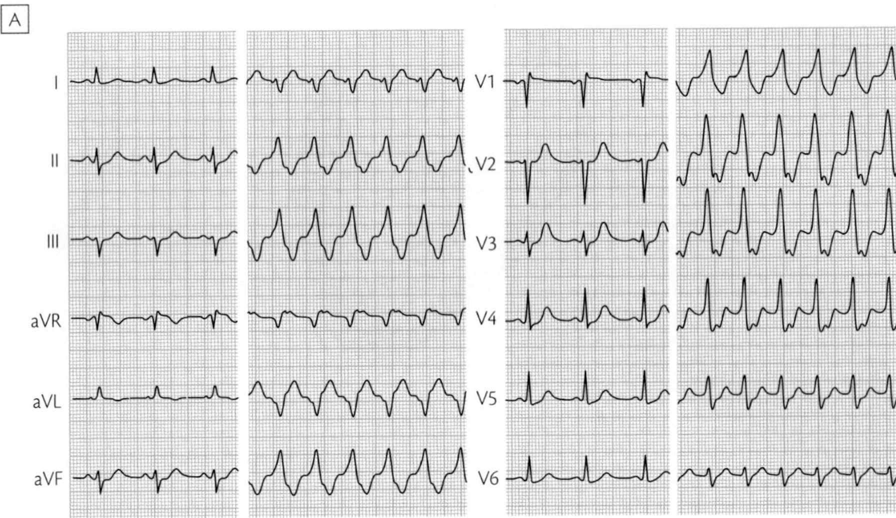

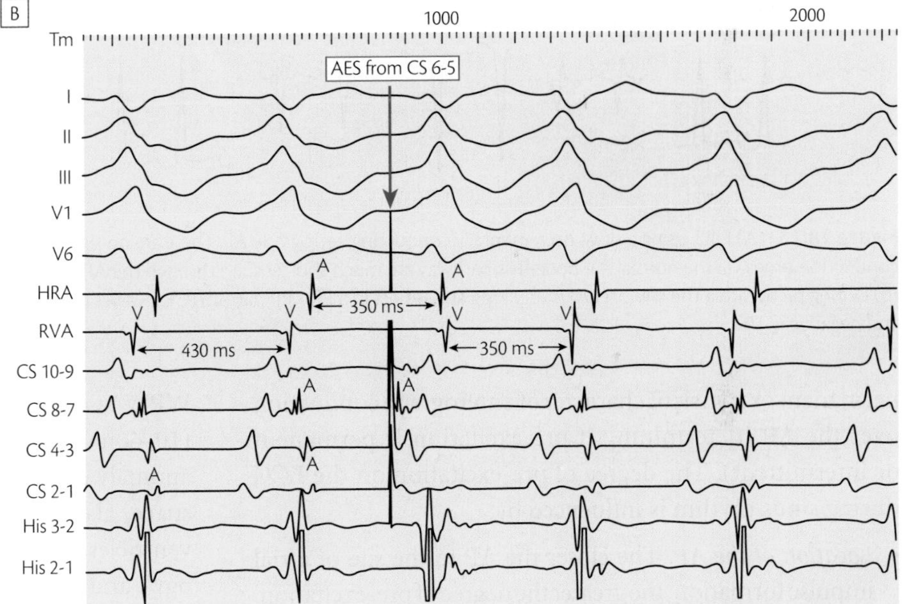

Figure 28.24 Left-sided, slow, and decrementally conducting AP participating as anterograde arm of an antidromic AVRT incorporating the AV node–His axis as retrograde limb of the circusmovement. (A) ECG during sinus rhythm and during the antidromic AVRT. The QRS complex during tachycardia is wide and with a RBBB configuration. (B) Leads I, II, III, V1, and V6 are simultaneously displayed with intracardiac recordings from the HRA, right ventricular apex (RVA), CS, and His bundle region. An atrial extrastimulus (AES) introduced during tachycardia from the CS captures the atria (the A–A interval following the extrastimulus is 350ms while the tachycardia cycle length is 430ms) and also advances the subsequent ventricular activity in an identical proportion (V–V interval after this APB 350ms). This finding proves that the atria participate in the tachycardia circuit.

Wolff–Parkinson–White syndrome

Definition

Reserving the name WPW syndrome for patients with the typical ECG in sinus rhythm and a history of palpitations is inaccurate. Not all the 11 patients in the original publication had paroxysmal tachycardia [225] and not all patients with WPW syndrome have a short PR interval and a QRS complex ≥120ms. WPW syndrome embraces patients with APs with short conduction times that conduct in the AV direction, with or without a history of palpitations. A current asymptomatic status in patients with the 'WPW electrocardiographic pattern' does not exclude the development of tachycardia or even sudden death in the future. Patients with and without symptoms at the time of diagnosis in whom pre-excitation in sinus rhythm is persistent or intermittent, evident or non-evident, are hereafter included under the umbrella of WPW syndrome. Because the definition of the varieties of WPW syndrome is mainly electrocardiographic, we describe in the next section the ECG during sinus rhythm in these patients.

ECG during sinus rhythm in WPW syndrome

In WPW the QRS complex during sinus rhythm is a fusion of two activation wavefronts, one proceeding over the normal AV node–His axis and the other via the AP (➲Fig. 28.19). The ECG manifestations of an anterogradely conducting AP during sinus rhythm depend on: the differences in AV conduction times over the normal AV node–His axis and the AP (which determine if the WPW is typical or atypical, and evident or non-evident); and the

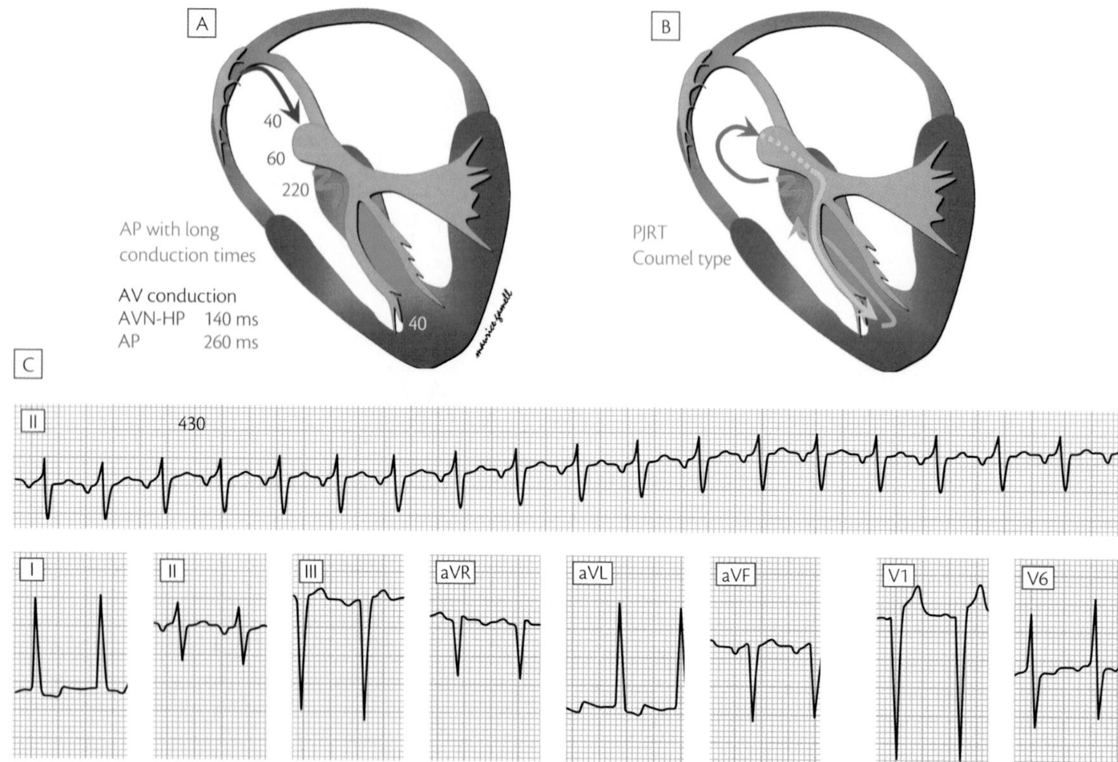

Figure 28.25 (A) PJRT using a slow, decrementally conducting, retrograde AP. There are no signs of pre-excitation during sinus rhythm because AV conduction times via the normal AV node–His pathway are much shorter than through the AP or because the AP only conducts in the VA direction. (B) During tachycardia the VA interval is very long and results in a PR <RP pattern (C). P waves during PJRP are negative in the inferior leads, positive in V1 and negative in V6.

permanent or transient character of anterograde conduction over the AP (determining if pre-excitation is permanent or intermittent). The degree of pre-excitation on the ECG during sinus rhythm is influenced by:

- *Location of the AP*. The closer the AP to the site of atrial impulse formation, the greater the degree of pre-excitation. Right free-wall APs usually result in very typical forms of pre-excitation (short PR intervals and widely pre-excited QRS complexes) (➲Figs. 28.20 and 28.21E). Left free-wall APs can result in an atypical ECG during sinus rhythm with a normal PR interval and minimal or absent signs of ventricular pre-excitation. In these patients pre-excitation becomes evident by pacing close to the atrial insertion of the AP (➲Figs. 28.19 and 28.27).
- *Intra-atrial conduction times*. Enlarged or diseased atria may result in non-evident pre-excitation in patients with a left free-wall AP because it takes too long for the sinoatrial activation wavefront to reach the atrial insertion of the bypass tract.
- *Conduction times over the AP*. The time spent by the impulse in travelling from the atrial to the ventricular insertion of the AP depends on the length and conduction velocity of the anomalous bundle. APs involved in WPW syndrome usually have short conduction times (10–60ms) that may be longer in patients with Ebstein's anomaly or in APs related to the base of the pyramidal space, also in those connecting atrial appendages and ventricles, in atriofascicular tracts with 'Mahaim physiology', and in some other anterogradely conducting APs with long conduction times and decremental conducting properties (➲Figs. 28.23 and 28.24).
- *Conduction times over the normal AV node–His axis*. When an AP coexists with AV block (usually congenital), pre-excitation is maximal since ventricular activation is exclusively over the bypass tract. Conversely, in some patients with enhanced AV nodal conduction and short AH intervals, combined or not with HV intervals in the low range, particularly when the AP is left superior or left posterior, the degree of pre-excitation may be minimal or almost absent (non-evident WPW).
- *Site of impulse formation of the driving atrial pacemaker*. In patients with left atrial rhythms permanently supplanting the activity of the normal sinus pacemaker, pre-excitation through a lateral left-sided AP is maximal due to the proximity of the site of impulse formation and the atrial insertion of the AP. During APBs close to the

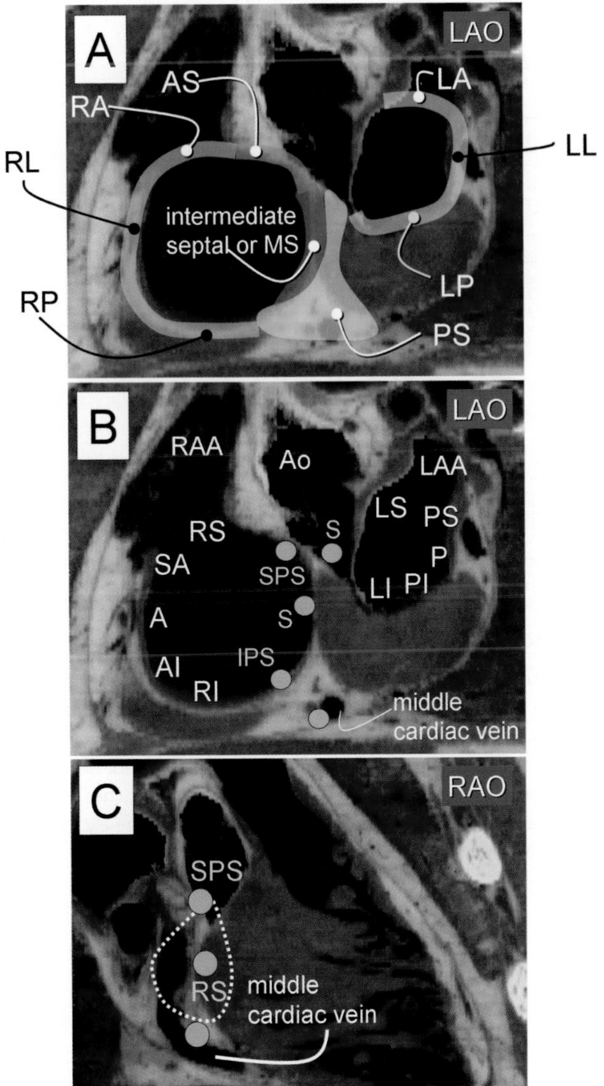

Figure 28.26 Traditional surgical (A) and current attitudinal fluoroscopic (B) nomenclatures to localize AP insertions. Both panels show a heart slice in a 45° LAO projection. (A) Right free-wall (green), left free-wall (blue), posteroseptal (yellow), anteroseptal (orange), and intermediate sepal (subsequently termed midseptal) (purple) surgical locations. These regions were subdivided by electrophysiologists in various areas: AS, anteroseptal; LA, left anterior; LL, left lateral; LP, left posterior; MS, midseptal; PS, posteroseptal; RA, right anterior; RL, right lateral; RP, right posterior. (B) A, anterior; AI, anteroinferior; Ao, aorta; IPS, inferior paraseptal; LAA, left atrial appendage; LI, left inferior; LS, left superior; P, posterior; PI, posteroinferior; PS, posterosuperior; RAA, right atrial appendage; RI, right inferior; RS, right superior; S, septal; SA, superoanterior; SPS, superior paraseptal. (C) RAO section of the heart showing the triangle of Koch (dotted white line), and the location of superior paraseptal (SPS), right septal (RS), and middle cardiac vein APs. The new nomenclaure for AP location does not consider APs connecting the atrial appendages with the ventricles and is too broad in relation to septal locations. There are right and left septal APs, and anomalous tracts related to the CS and its branches, as the middle cardiac vein, and the neck of CS diverticula. The superior paraseptal (SPS) location should differentiate peri-Hisian from cristal APs.

atrial insertion of the AP pre-excitation also becomes maximal.

Typical, atypical, and non-evident WPW syndrome

In typical WPW syndrome the PR interval is short (<120ms) and the QRS complex wide (≥120ms), with slow initial forces (delta wave) and repolarization changes (➲Figs. 28.20A and 28.21). Left-sided APs usually show lesser degrees of pre-excitation than right free-wall bypass tracts. Maximally pre-excited QRS complexes in patients with a left free-wall AP can be seen: when there is a conduction defect in the normal AV node–His pathway, and when the atrial driving rhythm is not sinus in origin but left atrial.

WPW syndrome is 'atypical' if the PR interval is ≥0.12s or the QRS complex is <0.12s although pre-excitation is evident at least for the experienced electrocardiographer (➲Figs. 28.19B and 28.28). Pre-excitation is 'non-evident' when not only the PR interval is not short but also there is no clear evidence of ventricular pre-excitation, a situation that should not be confused with a concealed AP (➲Figs. 28.19C and 28.27). In 'non-evident pre-excitation' the AP conducts in anterograde direction but AV conduction times over the bypass tract and via the normal AV node–His axis are similar so that ventricular pre-excitation is not evident. Non-evident pre-excitation does not mean that the AP cannot allow very rapid ventricular rates during AF [246]. Concealed APs do not conduct in anterograde direction, not even during pacing close to their atrial insertion.

Intermittent pre-excitation

Ventricular pre-excitation is 'intermittent' when QRS complexes with and without pre-excitation coexist on the same ECG tracing (➲Fig. 28.29) or on ECG recordings obtained on different occasions. In beats without pre-excitation the repolarization may be abnormal due to 'cardiac electric memory', a phenomenon that can also be observed during the usual orthodromic AVRT, and in the ECG following ablation of the AP (➲Figs. 28.20, 28.21, and 28.29) [247].

Diagnosis

Clinical characteristics

Patients with WPW syndrome may be asymptomatic, or complain of symptoms with various degrees of severity [248]. The ECG pattern of pre-excitation may be an incidental finding in an asymptomatic patient or be discovered because of a history of palpitations or syncope. Syncope may be related to a fast tachycardia rate but also to a vasovagal mechanism, and therefore lacks prognostic significance in WPW syndrome [249, 250]. Sudden death—which

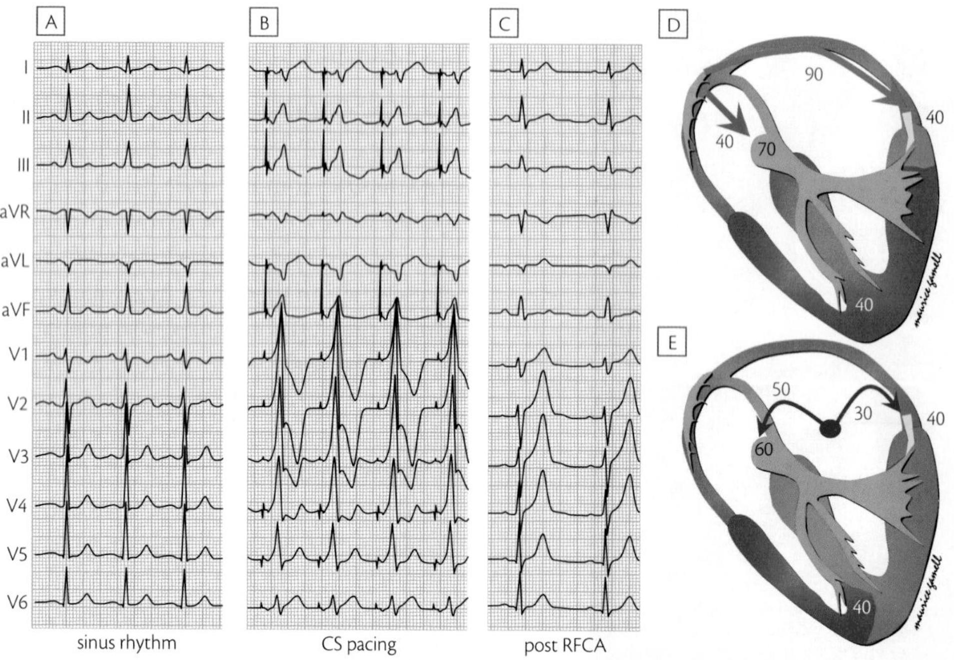

Figure 28.27 (A) During sinus rhythm there are not clear-cut electrocardiographic signs of ventricular pre-excitation ('nonevident' WPW). (B) Atrial pacing from the CS discloses the existence of a left posterior (formerly called left lateral) AP. (C) ECG after RFCA of this AP. (D) Schematic explanation for non-evident pre-excitation in this case. AV conduction times via the AP are only slightly shorter that through the AV node–His axis. The PR interval is not short (130ms) and only the basal portions of the posterior left ventricle are activated earlier than expected during 20ms accounting for the minor differences in QRS complex contour before and after ablation. (E) CS pacing results in maximal pre-excitation since the atrial wavefront reaches the AP very soon (in 30ms) so that AV conduction times via the AP are 70ms as compared to 150ms via the normal AV node–His axis. Non-evident pre-excitation is more frequently observed in left posterior or left superior APs because their atrial insertion is distant from the sinus node.

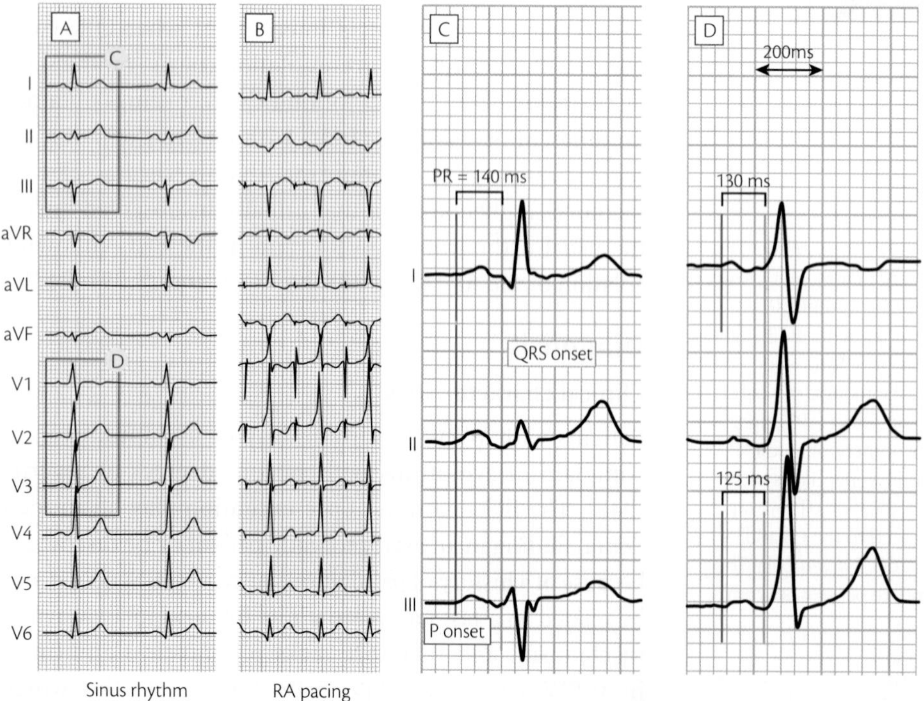

Figure 28.28 Atypical WPW. The PR interval is not short but ventricular pre-excitation is apparent during sinus rhythm from V1 to V3 (A). During right atrial pacing (B) pre-excitation becomes more evident because AV conduction times over the AV node are prolonged while those over the AP are maintained constant. (C, D) Enlarged details of panel (A) demonstrating that the PR interval in the limb leads measures 140ms and in the precordial leads from 125–130ms.

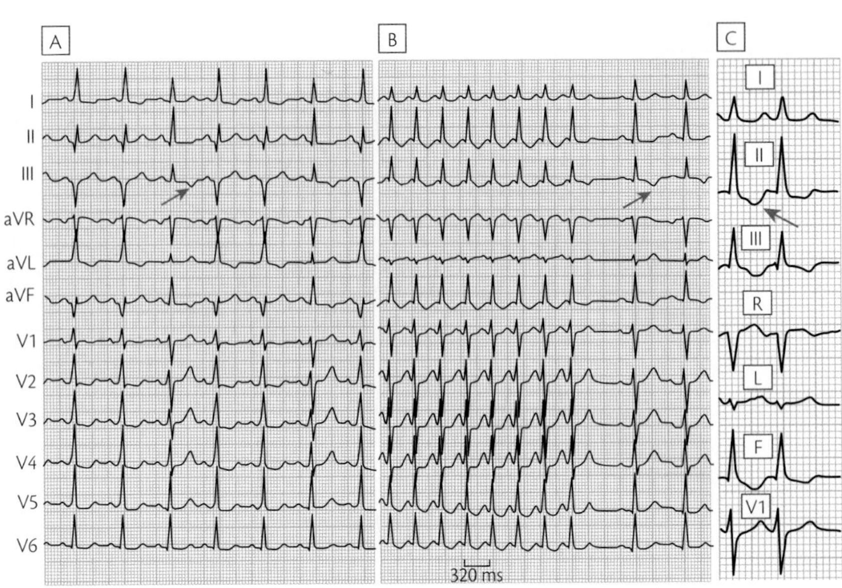

Figure 28.29 (A) Intermittent pre-excitation. Pre-excited QRS complexes coexist with ventricular depolarizations without pre-excitation. QRS complexes without pre-excitation are followed by an abnormal repolarization with negative T waves in III and AVF (arrow) (cardiac electric memory). (B) ECG during orthodromic AVRT that uses the normal AV node–His axis in anterograde direction and the AP retrogradely. During AVRT retrograde P waves are visible after the QRS complex and are negative in the inferior leads. The AP had a left inferior paraseptal location. (C) Detail showing the spontaneous termination of AVRT by block over the AP. The last QRS of the tachycardia is not followed by a negative P wave in leads II and III (the arrow is pointing to the retrograde P wave in the penultimate QRS of the AVRT).

exceptionally occurs in patients with WPW syndrome—is related to degeneration of AF into VF due to a fast ventricular response over one or more APs with a short anterograde refractory period [246, 250].

Risk evaluation in symptomatic and asymptomatic WPW patients

Sudden death has been estimated to occur in 1/1000 WPW subjects per year and may be the first manifestation in a few patients with this syndrome [250–252]. Risk evaluation must be conducted both in symptomatic and asymptomatic WPW patients. Risk factors for sudden death in WPW syndrome are:

- the presence of multiple APs;
- the development of both AF and AVRT;
- the shortest pre-excited RR interval during AF (≤260ms);
- an Ebstein's anomaly;
- the use of certain antiarrhythmic drugs;
- an incidental myocarditis;
- the age of the patient (➲Fig. 28.30) [246, 250–258].

In patients with WPW, intravenous digitalis, verapamil, diltiazem, and adenosine may increase the ventricular response over the AP during AF thus facilitating the development of VF. Myocarditis may be involved in some sudden deaths in young patients with WPW syndrome [257]. In patients with WPW syndrome, AF is rare under the age of 13 years and sudden death exceptional below 8 years. Children with WPW and documented AF have ages between 10–18 years [258].

Signs that have been said to indicate a low risk of sudden death in WPW are: spontaneous or exercise-induced sudden disappearance of pre-excitation in one beat; and, less convincingly, loss of pre-excitation after intravenous infusion of class I drugs (procainamide, ajmaline, flecainide, propafenone). Gradual disappearance of pre-excitation during exercise is of no prognostic value because it is difficult to differentiate actual AV rate-dependent AP block from non-evident pre-excitation due to adrenergic-mediated shortening of AV nodal conduction times [259, 260]. Disappearance of pre-excitation after intravenous infusion of class I drugs has been suggested to identify patients with a 'safe' and relatively long AV refractory period of the AP [261], but its prognostic significance is debatable [251]. Dose and infusion rate of the drug, and precocity and duration of the induced AP block, may play a role in the variable clinical interpretation of these tests.

Electrophysiological studies are performed for risk evaluation to determine:

- AV refractory period of the AP;
- inducibility of tachycardia;
- presence of multiple APs;
- ventricular rate after the induction of AF.

Incidence of tachycardia in WPW

The incidence of tachycardia in the WPW population is unclear. In a prospective population survey, 49% of patients with an electrocardiographic pre-excitation pattern were asymptomatic [232]. An AVRT was documented in 17% of the patients and AF in 8%. The mean age for the first

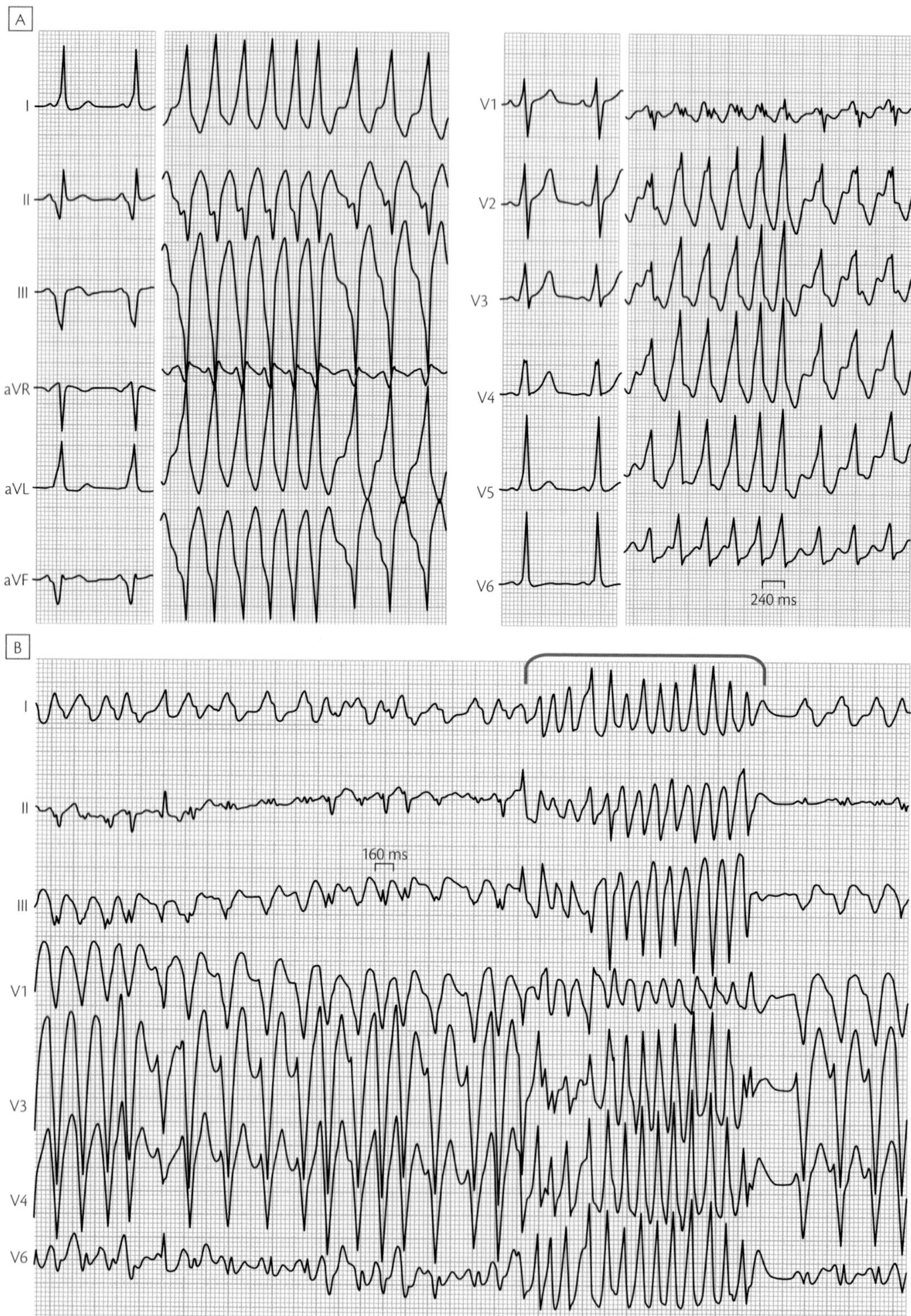

Figure 28.30 Episodes of AF in two different patients with WPW syndrome. (A) 12-lead ECG during sinus rhythm and maximally pre-excited AF from a patient with an inferior paraseptal AP related to the mid cardiac vein. The shortest RR interval during AF was 240ms. (B) Same patient as in ➲Fig. 28.20. During AF a very fast ventricular response was observed (shortest pre-excited RR interval 160ms). During 2.16s (red bracket) a non-sustained episode of VF was recorded. This patient had two APs.

episode of AVRT and AF was 31 and 52 years, respectively. During a mean follow-up of 4.5 years, there were no sudden deaths and 4% of previously asymptomatic patients became symptomatic. In 238 military aviators with WPW syndrome aged 17–56 years, only 18% had an initial history of SVT, but after a mean follow-up of 22 years sudden cardiac death occurred in one case and 15% of the originally asymptomatic became symptomatic [264]. In a study of 212 asymptomatic WPW patients, 84% remained asymptomatic during a relatively brief follow-up of about 3 years, and 16% developed symptoms. In 13% of the patients, pre-excitation disappeared after 5 years [265].

Location of the AP using the ECG during sinus rhythm

Various algorithms to localize the AP from the ECG during sinus rhythm have been developed [233, 264–269]. Limitations of these algorithms are:

- insufficient degrees of pre-excitation in some WPW patients during sinus rhythm (➲Fig. 28.27);
- presence of more than one AV-conducting AP (➲Fig. 28.31);
- an oblique AP course relative to the AV groove (lack of concordance between atrial and ventricular AP insertions);
- presence of structural heart disease or chest deformities;
- dubious reproducibility of the fluoroscopic interpretation of the AP location in the absence of angiographic or electroanatomic mapping aids;
- flaws of the current attitudinal nomenclature for septal and paraseptal APs that is too broad and overlooks several different anatomic locations of relevance for RFCA (➲Figs. 28.26, 28.32, 28.33, 28.34);
- none of the algorithms has considered connections between the atrial appendages and the ventricles.

Despite these limitations, it is frequently possible to predict the location of the AP from the surface ECG. In brief, pre-excited QRS complexes predominantly positive in V1

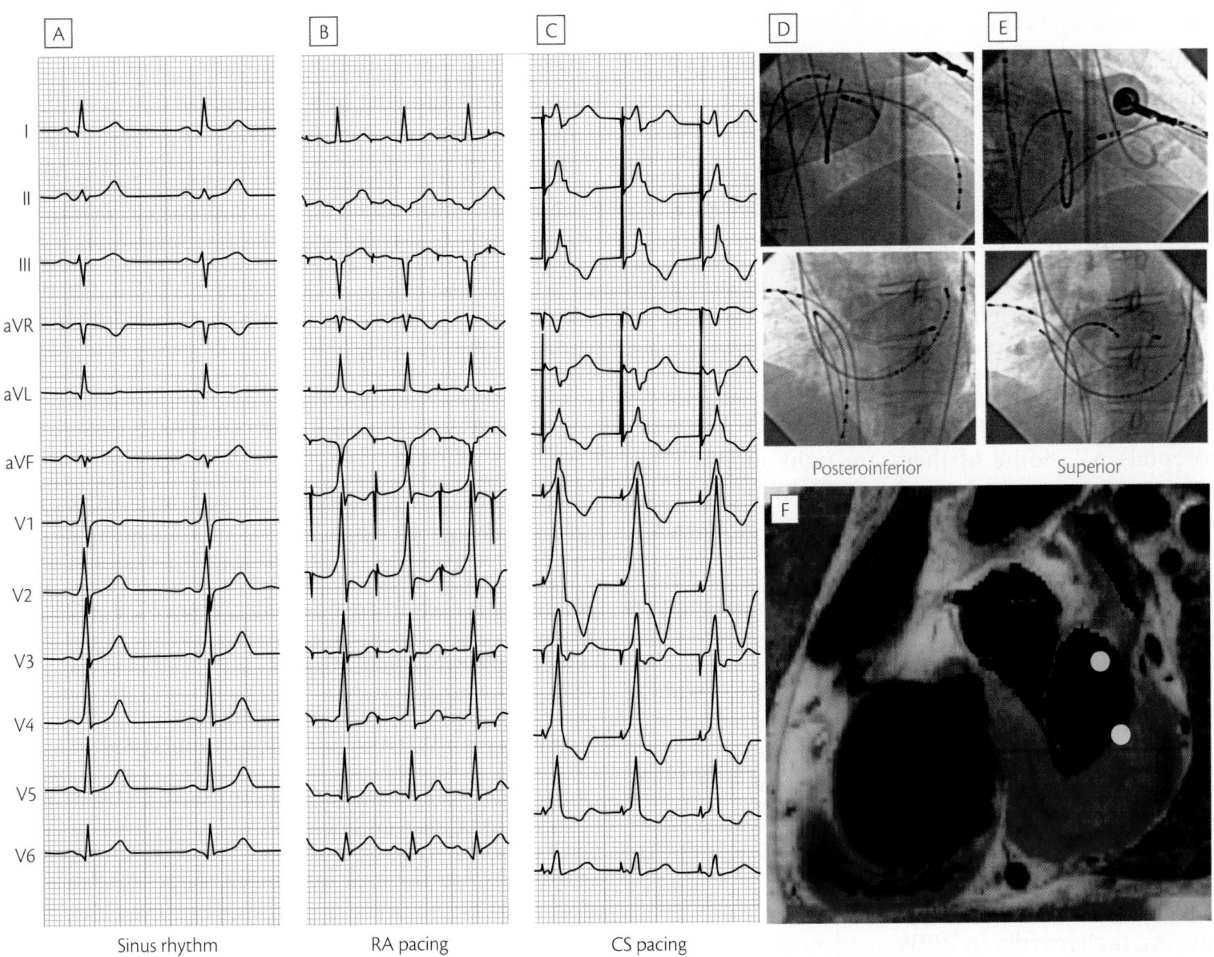

Figure 28.31 (A) Localizing the AP during sinus rhythm in this patient with WPW syndrome is hampered by the existence of two left-sided APs, one left posteroinferior (yellow in F) and the other left superior (blue in F). (B) Right atrial pacing increases the degree of pre-excitation; the initial forces are negative in inferior leads which is consistent with a left inferior or posteroinferior AP. (C) CS sinus pacing produces maximally pre-excited QRS complexes consistent with a posterosuperior AP. (D) Site of ablation of the inferoposterior AP. (E) Site of ablation of the posterosuperior AP.

are due to left-sided APs. Then, if the QRS complex is negative in the inferior leads, the AP is left paraseptal or left inferior (formerly called posterior) (➲Figs. 28.28, 28.29, 28.31, and 28.32). The more superiorly located a left-sided AP, the more positive the initial forces in inferior leads. Left posterior, left posterosuperior and left superior APs produce predominantly negative QRS complexes in aVL and positive ventricular deflections in II, III, and aVF (➲Figs. 28.27 and 28.31). The last three left-sided AP locations may result in minor degrees of pre-excitation due to their distance from the sinus node region. Also, these posterior and superior (formerly left lateral) left-sided APs may not produce predominantly positive QRS complexes in V1 unless pacing is performed from the left atrium (➲Fig. 28.27). Well pre-excited QRS complexes predominantly negative in V1 are due to inferior paraseptal, septal, superior paraseptal, and right free-wall APs. Inferior paraseptal and septal APs produce predominantly negative QRS complexes in leads II, III, and aVF with an initial Q wave (➲Fig. 28.32). A 'w-shaped' or Qr morphology in V1 would then suggest a septal (formerly midseptal) location (➲Figs. 28.20 and 28.33). A well-developed initial R wave in lead V1 (although the QRS complex is predominantly negative) would suggest a right inferior paraseptal ventricular insertion of the AP (➲Fig. 28.32). A low-amplitude initial r wave in V1 with little progression from V1 to V3 suggests a right inferior AP (➲Fig. 28.20). A well-evident right-sided pre-excitation pattern with positive QRS complexes in I and II, and a QR or qR configuration in III, suggests a right anterior (formerly lateral) AP location (➲Fig. 28.35). An evident right-sided pre-excitation pattern with positive QRS complexes in leads I, II, and III suggests a right superior or right paraseptal (formerly anteroseptal) AP. Some of them are right superior and insert in the supraventricular crest apart from the AV node and His bundle, while others are close to the normal conduction system. They usually have an initial, low-amplitude, relatively broad r wave in V1–V2. The QRS complex of some peri-Hisian APs has three ECG characteristics:

1 although evidently pre-excited, it may be not as wide as in superior right free-wall APs;
2 it is predominantly negative in V1 and V2 and positive in I, II, III;
3 it adopts a characteristic deep negative 'w' shape in V1 and sometimes in V2 as well (➲Figs. 28.33 and 28.34).

ECG during tachycardia in WPW syndrome

Orthodromic AVRT has a rate generally from 140–240bpm. The QRS complex is usually narrow, in which case P waves can be visible after the end of the ventricular complex with an RP <PR pattern (➲Figs. 28.21 and 28.29). In superior and posterior left-sided APs (formerly anterolateral or lateral), the retrograde P wave is negative in leads I and AVL, and positive or isobiphasic in the inferior leads [85]. In inferior paraseptal, right inferior, and left inferior APs, the P-waves are negative in II, III, and AVF. T waves may also be negative in these leads for the same AP locations due to 'cardiac electric memory'. While AVRT using a left-sided AP has a predominant positive P wave in V1, those utilizing a right-sided bypass have a negative and bimodal P in V1 [270]. When AVRT has a wide QRS complex due to aberrant conduction or concomitant organic bundle branch block, P waves are usually hidden within the terminal forces of the QRS complex (➲Fig. 28.36). The AVRT cycle length may prolong during BBB aberrancy that is ipsilateral to the AP location because the circuit is longer (➲Fig. 28.36) [271, 272]. Antidromic AVRT is maximally pre-excited and P waves are either not visible or precede the QRS complex (➲Fig. 28.22).

The ECG of WPW patients during AF varies according to the electrophysiological properties of the AP and the AV node, the sympathetic tone, the number of APs, and the concomitant antiarrhythmic medication (➲Fig. 28.30). There are patients showing only pre-excited QRS complexes (not infrequently with various degrees of pre-excitation), while others present a conventional AF with no signs of pre-excitation. In many instances, AF manifests electrocardiographically as an irregular tachyarrhythmia with wide, pre-excited QRS complexes and a variable number of narrow ventricular activations. 'Capture' beats in a predominantly pre-excited recording of AF are not premature, as in VT, but usually late as compared with the pre-excited QRS complexes.

VT is very rare in WPW syndrome. Bundle branch re-entry VT exceptionally develops in patient with Ebstein's anomaly of the tricuspid valve. In a few patients with WPW syndrome, an AF with very rapid ventricular response via the AP can degenerate into VF, particularly when more than one AV-conducting AP is present (➲Fig. 28.30B).

Electrophysiological studies

Catheter-electrode mapping and stimulation studies in patients with WPW syndrome are aimed at:

- confirming the existence of an AP in patients with non-evident WPW syndrome;
- establishing the location and number of APs;
- studying the AV and VA electrophysiological properties of the AP;
- investigating the mechanism of tachycardia;
- evaluating the potential risk to the patient.

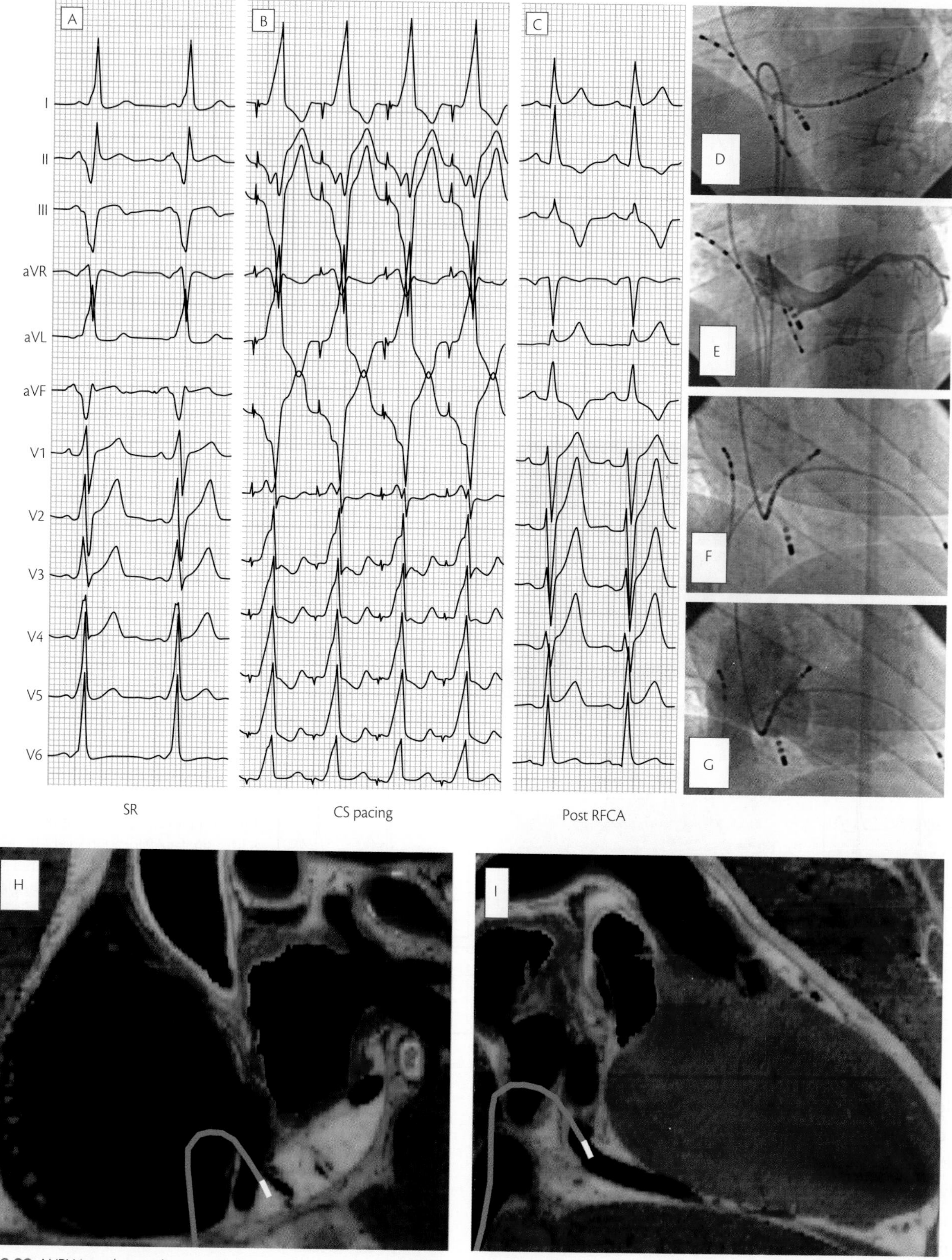

Figure 28.32 WPW syndrome due to an inferior paraseptal AP whose insertion was localized inside the middle cardiac vein. Same patient as in ➲Fig. 28.34A. ECG during sinus rhythm (A), CS pacing (B), and after RFCA (C). (D) The ablation catheter at the site of AP block in the LAO projection. (E) CS venogram showing that the ablation catheter is not against the wall of the great cardiac vein. (F) Ablation catheter in the RAO projection. (G) Right atrial angiogram in RAO projection demonstrating that the ablation catheter is 'outside' the right atrium because it was inside the middle cardiac vein. (H, I) Anatomical slices in LAO and RAO projections indicating where the ablation catheter was located at the site of block of the AP during RF application.

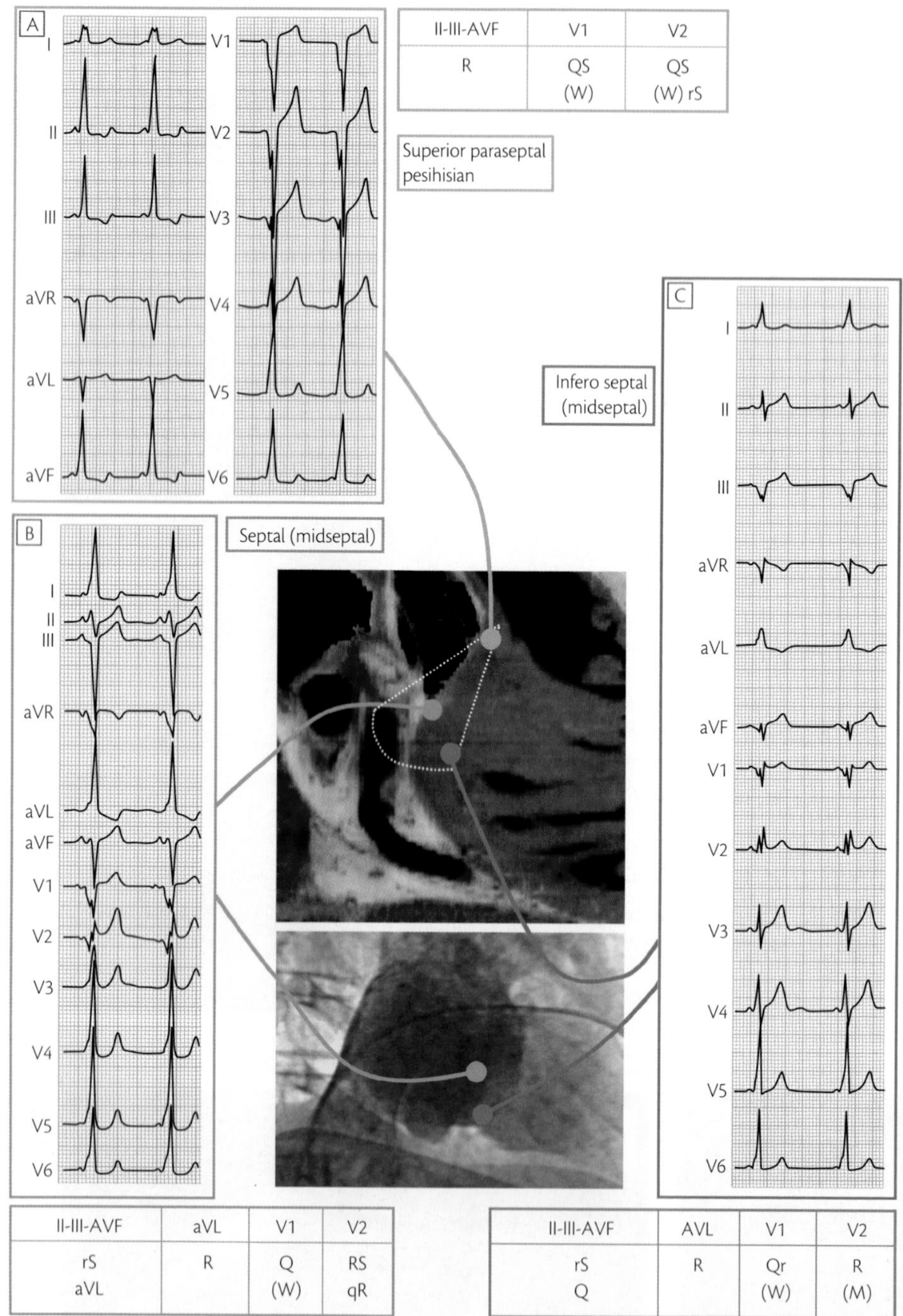

A
II-III-AVF
R
V1
QS (W)
V2
QS (W) rS
Superior paraseptal pesihisian
B
Septal (midseptal)
C
Infero septal (midseptal)
II-III-AVF
rS aVL
aVL
R
V1
Q (W)
V2
RS qR
II-III-AVF
rS Q
AVL
R
V1
Qr (W)
V2
R (M)

Figure 28.33 (A) ECG of a peri-Hisian AP. Although there is evident prexcitation, QRS complexes are not as wide as with pre-excitation due to a right free-wall AP. The QRS complex is positive in I, II, III, and AVF, and negative 'W- shaped' in V1 and V2 (also in V3 in this case). Other cases with this AP location might eventually show rS ventricular complexes in V2. (B) Septal AP located in the centre of the triangle of Koch resulting in 'rS' ventricular complexes in II and AVF, QS in III, positive R waves in AVL, and QS complexes, also 'W-shaped', in V1. In this example the QRS complex in V2 is QR but other cases with a similar AP location might have an RS or qR contour. (C) Septal AP located in the inferior tricuspid border of the triangle of Koch (also embraced within the formerly termed midseptal AP). The morphology of the QRS complex is RS in lead II, rS in AVF, QS in III, and R in AVL. In V1 it has a Qr configuration with a 'W-shaped' contour and in V2a positive bimodal 'M- shaped' morphology.

Electrophysiological studies to test the effect of antiarrhythmic drugs on the AP, or for routine evaluation of patients that have undergone a catheter ablation, are no longer performed. Only patients who after RFCA continue to complain of palpitations with a sudden onset should undergo an electrophysiological study to elucidate the nature of these symptoms.

Treatment

The initial acute treatment of an episode of orthodromic AVRT consists of vagal manoeuvres. If the patient is known to have WPW syndrome, the physician may prefer not to use adenosine because it may induce AF [255]. Intravenous flecainide, propafenone, or procainamide can be used instead. In patients with AF or pre-excited tachycardias, intravenous flecainide, propafenone, procainamide, or ibutilide are the drugs of choice. Alternatively, it is possible to proceed to DC-shock cardioversion directly. If there are not associated risk factors for systemic embolization and AF has <48 hours of duration, electrical cardioversion does not require anticoagulation. Otherwise guidelines for anticoagulation as in other AF patients should be followed [1, 4, 167]. In patients with

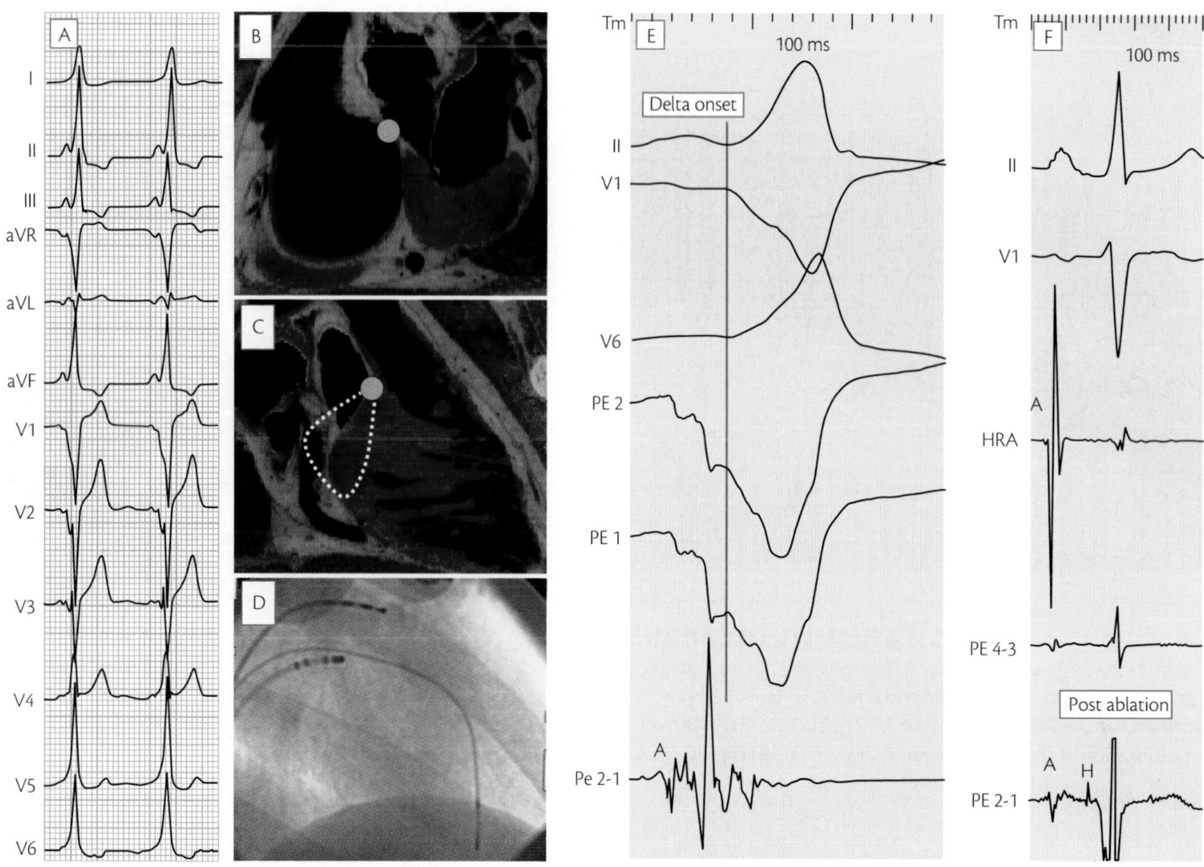

Figure 28.34 Peri-Hisian AP. (A) The ECG shows positive QRS complexes in I, II, III, and AVF, negative in AVL and AVR, and negative in V1 and V2 ('W-shaped' in V2). (B, C) Heart slices in LAO and RAO projections. The cyan circle represents the location of a peri-Hisian AP. In (C) the triangle of Koch limits are represented by the white-dotted line. (D) RAO fluorographic image showing the ablation catheter at the site of block of the AP. (E) Leads II, V1, and V6 simultaneously displayed with the unfiltered unipolar recordings from the distal two electrodes of the ablation catheter (PE2 and PE1) and the filtered bipolar lead from this pair of electrodes (PE 2-1). Before the onset of the delta-wave in the surface ECG and after the local atrial electrogram in the bipolar PE 2-1 lead, there is a fragmented electrogram most likely representing the activation through the AP. (F) At the ablation site, immediately after the radiofrequency application, a His bundle potential [H] is recorded from the distal pair of electrodes of the probing ablation electrode (PE 2-1) preceding the non-pre-excited QRS complex. HRA, high right atrium; PE, probing electrode.

pre-excited tachycardias, AV nodal-acting drugs should not be used.

The treatment of choice to prevent tachycardia recurrence in WPW patients is catheter ablation. Until this intervention is performed, or in patients refusing the procedure, class IC drugs, amiodarone, or sotalol can be used if the frequency and duration of the attacks, or the severity of symptoms during the tachyarrhythmia, justify constant pharmacological treatment [1, 261]. In the selection of drugs, factors such as age and presence of associated cardiac disorders should be considered. Digitalis, verapamil, and diltiazem should be avoided in patients with WPW syndrome [253, 254, 256]. The ability of beta-blockers to prevent tachycardia recurrences in WPW syndrome has not been studied but these agents do not act on the AP and the patient would not be protected if AF supervenes [1]. Class I antiarrhythmic drugs and amiodarone may prolong the anterograde refractory period of the AP, with little change in its retrograde refractory period. This situation can facilitate the induction of orthodromic AVRT and the patient may experience an increased number or episodes of palpitations, which although being slower may be more prolonged [256].

In certain situations, catheter ablation is the only reasonable therapeutic option, such as:

- patients with infrequent symptomatic episodes or who have already had recurrences or adverse effects on antiarrhythmic drugs;
- women considering pregnancy;
- people with professions or lifestyles of risk;
- those with severely symptomatic episodes or who have been resuscitated from a cardiac arrest.

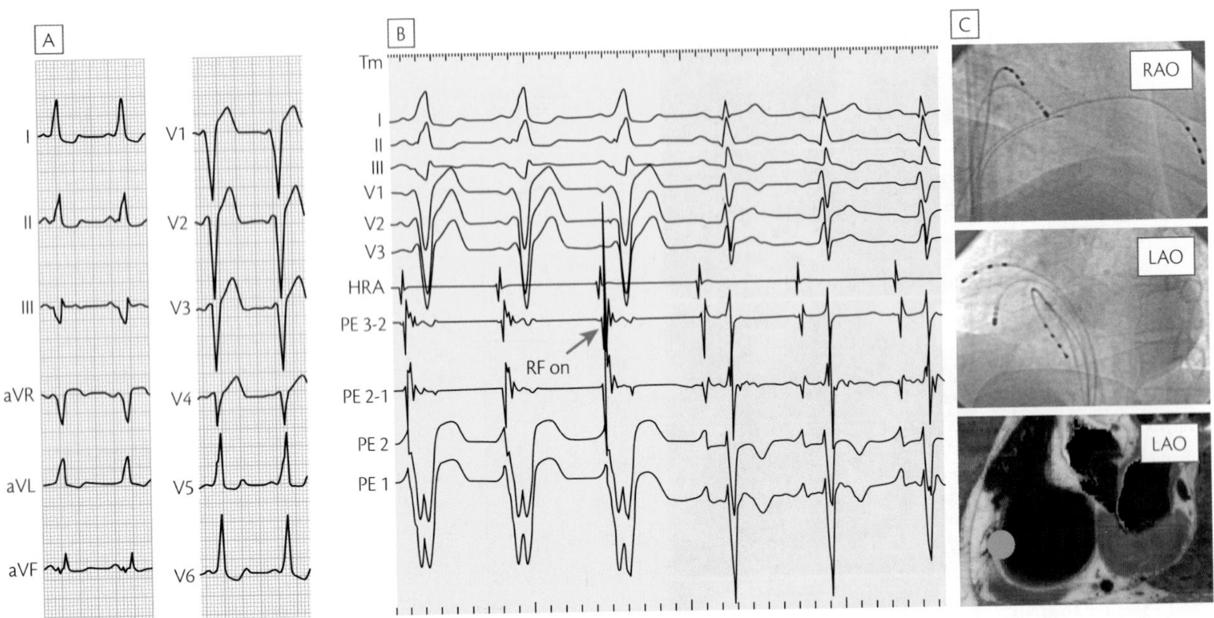

Figure 28.35 (A) ECG during sinus rhythm in a WPW syndrome due to a right-anterior AP. (B) Time marks, leads I, II, III, V1, V2, V3, and intracardiac recordings from the HRA, and the probing electrode (PE). Pre-excitation disappears <1s after the start of the radiofrequency pulse (arrow). T waves in lead III are negative after the loss of pre-excitation (cardiac electric memory). (C) Fluorographic frames in RAO and LAO projection showing the position of the ablation catheter at the site of block of the AP. The bottom vignette is an anatomic slice of the heart in LAO projection showing the tricuspid ring and the approximate location of the AP at the site of ablation (green circle).

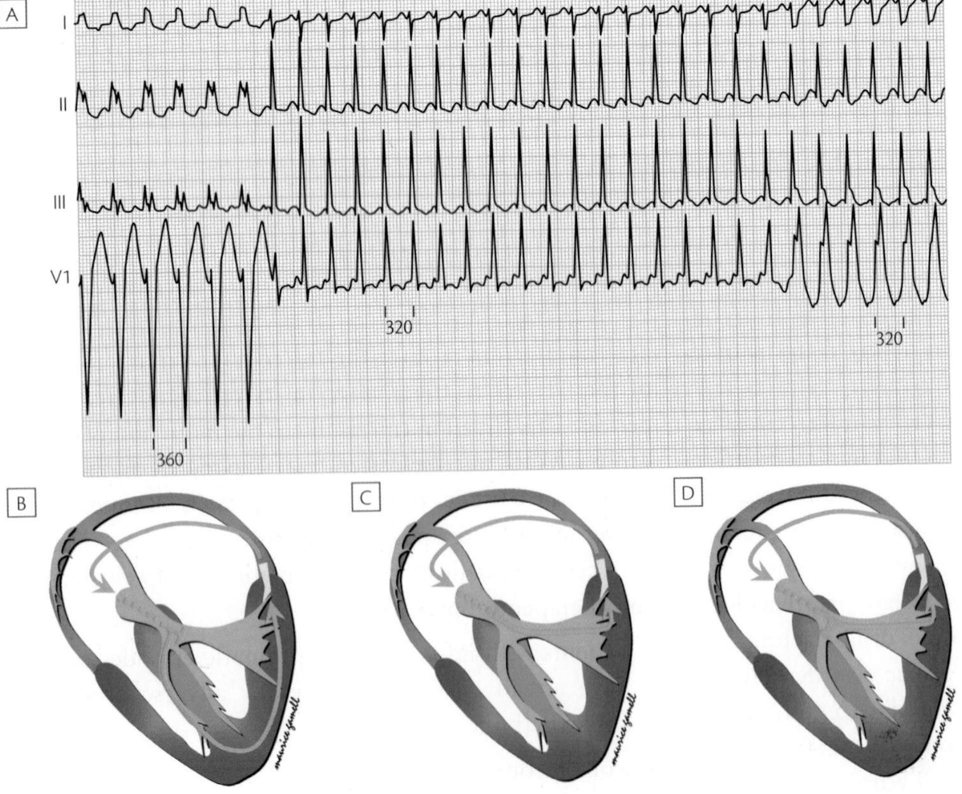

Figure 28.36 (A) Leads I, II, III, and V1 during an orthodromic AVRT using a left free-wall AP. AVRT starts with LBBB aberrancy, continues with normal intraventricular conduction, and ends with RBBB aberrancy. All these changes occurred spontaneously. The tachycardia cycle length during LBBB aberrancy is 40ms longer than during normal intraventricular conduction or RBBB aberrancy. During LBBB aberrancy the AVRT wavefront has to travel through a longer circuit (B), as compared to the pathway during normal intraventricular conduction (C), or RBBB aberrancy (D).

Radiofrequency catheter ablation

RFCA can 'cure' most patients with WPW syndrome (➲Table 28.1; ➲Figs. 28.20, 28.31–28.35, 28.37, and 28.38) [222, 273–282]. Single- and multicentre studies, and registry reports on RFCA of APs, have shown that this technique safely and effectively abolishes conduction over the bypass tract. The success rate in experienced centres is >95%, with a recurrence rate of ≈2–3%, with no mortality and minimal morbidity. Less experienced centres may not be able to offer the same results particularly in certain locations (peri-Hisian, septal AP related to the pyramidal space, or AP connecting the atrial appendages), or if there are associated structural heart problems (Ebstein's anomaly, dextrocardia, L-transposition), or simply an advanced age. Patients in whom difficulties can be advanced or with a failed previous RFCA attempt should be referred to experienced ablation centres. Also complex can be RFCA in patients with multiple APs, or with additional mechanism for tachycardias (usually AVNRT or AFL). Connections between the atrial appendages and the ventricles can be ablated with conventional endocardial catheter techniques. In difficult, usually failed cases, non-fluoroscopic 3-dimensional electroanatomical mapping and a combined endo-epicardial approach facilitate a successful ablation. Surgery is no longer needed in WPW syndrome.

Left-sided APs can be ablated using a retrograde aortic approach or with a left-atrial trans-septal method. RFCA of APs related to the left atrial appendage requires trans-septal catheterization. Septal, superior paraseptal, and right-sided APs are ablated from the right side of the heart. Inferior paraseptal APs related to the ostium, proximal portions of the CS, and middle cardiac vein or diverticula, can be ablated from the right side. The rest of the inferior paraseptal APs and exceptionally some septal (midseptal) APs are best ablated from the left side of the heart. The presence of a CS diverticulum in WPW syndrome does not imply that the AP is anatomically related to this structure. A venous diverticulum may be seen in WPW patients with an inferior paraseptal AP, but also in association with a right inferior or left inferior AP.

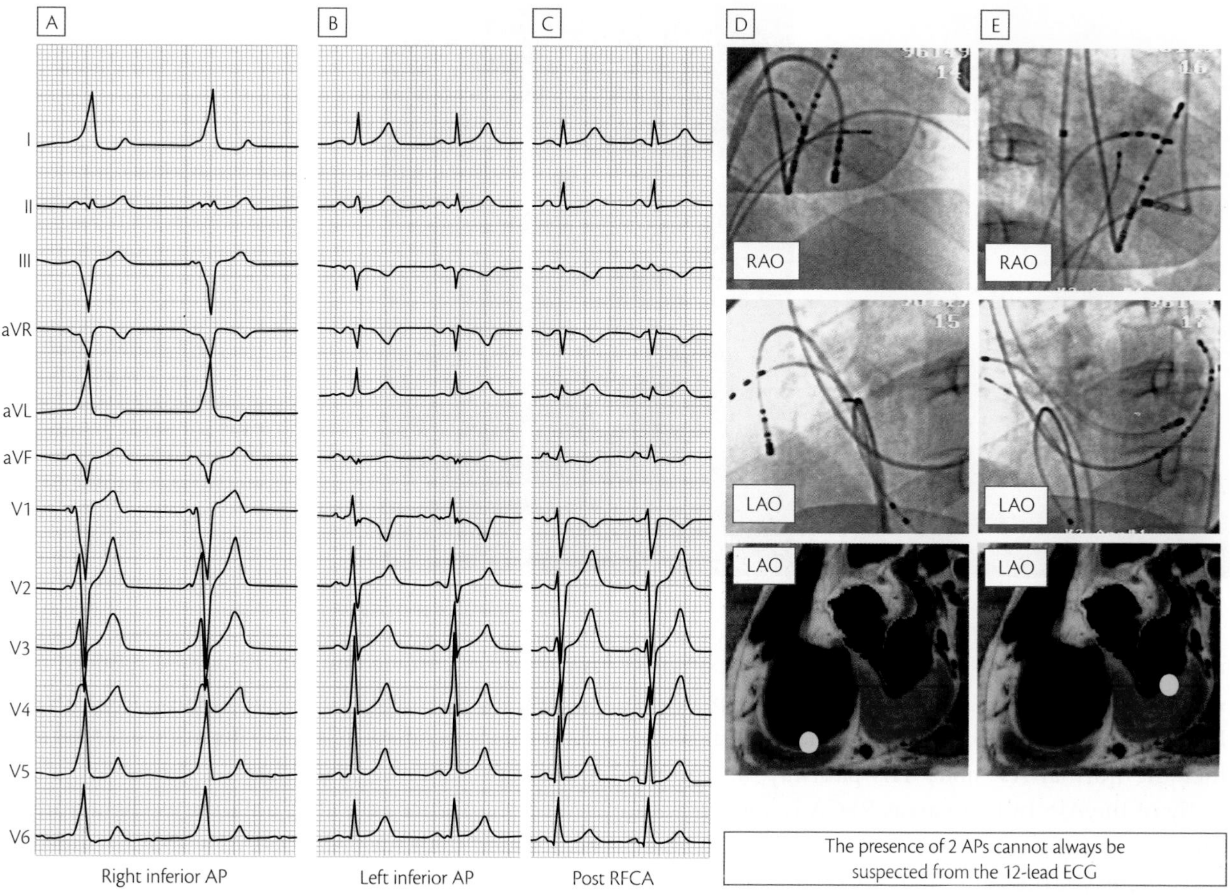

Figure 28.37 (A) ECG showing a pre-excitation pattern consistent with a right inferior, free-wall AP. This AP was ablated (panel D) and a second pre-excitation pattern appeared (B) corresponding to a left inferior AP. This second AP could not be anticipated from the initial ECG. After ablating this AP (panel E) pre-excitation disappeared completely (C).

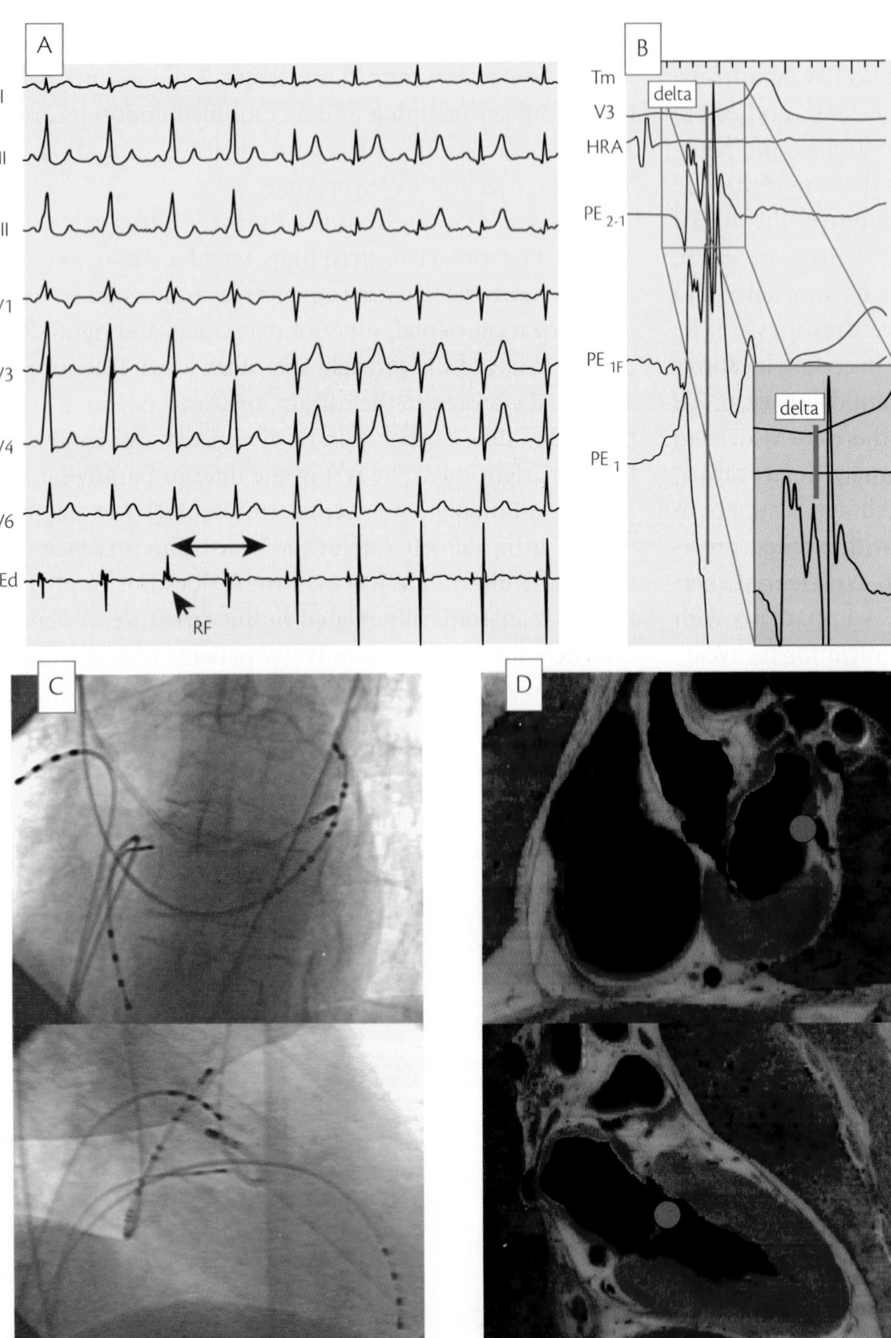

Figure 28.38 (A) Ablation of a left posterior AP; pre-excitation disappears 1s after the onset of the RF pulse (arrow). (B) Electrograms at the ablation site. The vertical dotted lines signal the onset of the delta wave in the surface ECG. The insert is a magnification of the filtered bipolar recording and the onset of the delta wave. (C) LAO and RAO fluorographic images documenting the position of the catheter at the site of ablation. This site is represented with a yellow circle in D on anatomic LAO and RAO sections at the level of the left AV groove. PEd, probing electrode distal; other abbreviations as in previous figures.

Major complications in relation to RFCA in patients with APs are rare (0.6%) [222]. In superior paraseptal and peri-Hisian APs it is possible to induce mechanical block of either the normal AV node–His pathway, and more frequently of the AP. In these areas RFCA is applied with extreme care, starting with temperatures of 40–42°C that are slowly increased thereafter in 0.5°C incremental steps. Potential complications of RFCA procedures have already been discussed [1, 222, 273–282]. In left-sided procedures anticoagulation with unfractionated heparin is used and the incidence of cardiac tamponade can be reduced by maintaining the activated plasma thromboplastin time between 2–3 times the control value. No heparin is needed for right-sided approaches.

The recurrence rate after ablation is slightly higher for right-sided than for left-sided APs and for superior paraseptal than for septal bypass tracts. Also slightly higher chances for recurrence have APs related to the pyramidal space. Successful RFCA of the AP prevents the recurrence of AVRT. AF recurrences are also prevented with RFCA in relatively young patients with WPW syndrome but less efficiently in subjects ablated at ages >50 years [283].

Therapeutic approach in asymptomatic WPW

Ablation of asymptomatic patients with a WPW ECG pattern is controversial. Patients engaged in competitive sports or with certain professions (pilots, divers) prefer to be cured. If pre-excitation is persistent and conduction over the AP remains patent during exercise, an electrophysiological study can be performed to evaluate the risk profile (anterograde AP refractory period, tachycardia inducibility, presence of multiple APs, and shortest pre-excited RR interval during AF). In one study tachyarrhythmias were inducible in 29% of asymptomatic WPW patients, and 15% developed AVRT or AF during follow-up. Two of the eight patients developing AF had a resuscitated cardiac arrest and one died suddenly; all three having inducible AVRT and multiple APs [263]. Asymptomatic but inducible WPW patients aged ≤35 years were randomized to RFCA of the AP or no treatment. During a median follow-up of 27 months, 5% of the ablated patients and 60% of controls had arrhythmic events [284]. Asymptomatic WPW children aged 5–12 years with inducible AVRT or AF during an electrophysiological study have also been randomized to ablation and no treatment. During follow-up, arrhythmic events occurred in 5% of children in the ablation group and in 12% of controls. Two children in the control group had VF, and a 10-year-old boy died suddenly. Arrhythmic events also occurred during follow-up in 8% of the patients without inducible AVRT or AF [285]. As discussed elsewhere [286], it is difficult, particularly in children, to determine if some WPW patients are asymptomatic or if certain apparently non-specific symptoms are due to tachyarrhythmias. Before sending an asymptomatic WPW patient to ablation the general cardiologist should know the success and complication rates of the referral centre, information seldom available in a transparent manner. ESC/AHA/ACC guidelines consider as a class IIa indication catheter ablation in asymptomatic WPW patients with a B level of evidence [1]. In children >5 years this indication has been viewed as class IIb by the NASPE Expert Consensus Conference, and class III (not indicated) if aged ≤5 years [287].

Pre-excitation due to 'Mahaim physiology'

Definition and pathogenesis

In 1971 Wellens described an 8-year-old boy with wide QRS-complex tachycardia with LBBB configuration that during sinus rhythm had a PR interval of 0.12s with minor 'type B' pre-excitation. A nodoventricular Mahaim tract was postulated to be the basis of this form of pre-excitation [288]. Subsequently, it has been demonstrated that the AP in these patients usually consists of a right free-wall anomalous node that continues with an accessory His–Purkinje system distally inserting at the normal right bundle branch or directly at the right ventricular myocardium. The term 'Mahaim physiology' used for this condition is a misnomer, since Mahaim described nodoventricular and fasciculoventricular connections [289] and here we are dealing with atriofascicular or AV bypass tracts. This form of pre-excitation represents <1% of all cases of patients with APs studied in the electrophysiology laboratory, is more often encountered in patients with Ebstein's anomaly of the tricuspid valve, and is more common in females than in males (➲ Fig. 28.23) [290].

Diagnosis

Atrial pacing at increasing rates results in progressive ventricular pre-excitation finally reproducing the QRS morphology observed during tachycardia. Because the proximal insertion of the AP is in the right atrium, maximal pre-excitation is obtained with right atrial pacing at slower rates than with left atrial pacing, and pre-excitation may disappear during CS left atrial pacing. The degree of pre-excitation of the QRS complex progressively increases and AV conduction times become gradually longer after APBs, thus showing the decremental conducting properties of the AV bypass [288].

There are two electrocardiographic patterns of this form of pre-excitation during sinus rhythm; one with 'non-evident pre-excitation' and the other with a normal PR interval and incomplete LBBB pattern with a small delta wave slurring the initial forces of the QRS complex (➲ Figs. 28.23 and 28.39). Tachycardia in all these patients is an antidromic AVRT using the slow and decrementally conducting AP in AV direction and the normal His–AV nodal axis retrogradely (➲ Fig. 28.23), or may be due to a coexisting AVNRT using the decrementally conducting AP as an anterograde bystander. Exceptionally an AVRT may use the decrementally conducting AP in anterograde direction and a second, conventional, anomalous AV pathway retrogradely. These antidromic AVRTs have cycle lengths between 220–450ms, QRS axis of 0 to –75°, QRS widths ≤150ms, R-waves in lead I, rS waves (or QS) in V1, and a precordial transition to a predominantly positive QRS complex after V4 (➲ Figs. 28.23 and 28.39) [290–292]. Patients with this syndrome may also develop AF that usually presents AV conduction over the AP with maximally pre-excited QRS complexes.

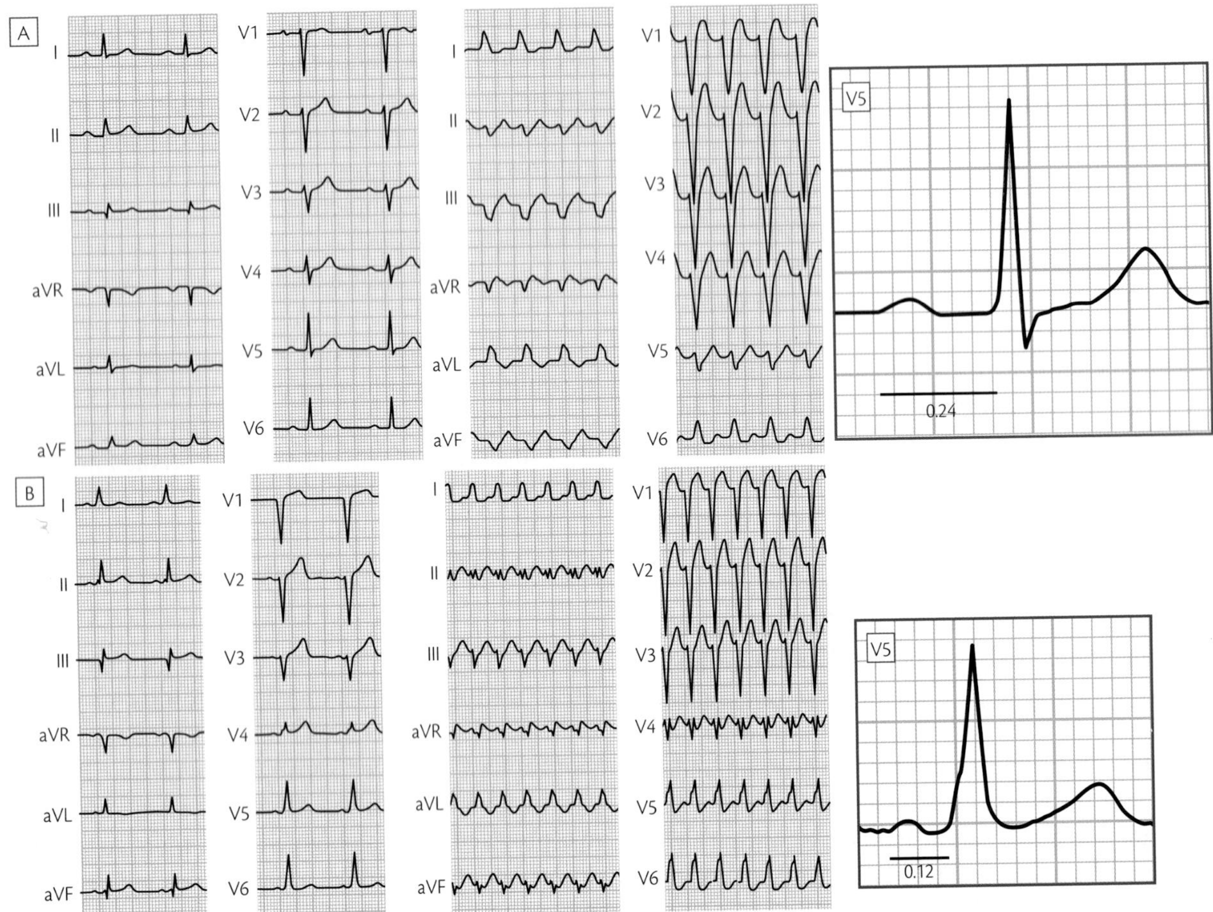

Figure 28.39 Right atriofascicular APs with 'Mahaim physiology'. (A, B) Two different patients showing during sinus rhythm 'nonevident' (A) and 'atypical' (B) pre-excitation. The ECG in lead V5 has been amplified on the right showing that the PR interval in A is 0.24s and the QRS complex is narrow. In B the PR interval is 0.12s and the QRS complex shows a kind of incomplete LBBB with a slurring of the initial forces (see detail of V5 on the right). In both instances the patient developed tachycardias that had a wide QRS complex with LBBB configuration and left axis deviation.

Retrograde conduction over the AP is typically absent although a patient has been reported in whom a right-sided, slow and decrementally conducting AP gave rise to the typical LBBB antidromic AVRT and to a narrow orthodromic AVRT in which the VA conduction times were long. The earliest site of retrograde atrial activation during orthodromic AVRT was at the same location where an atriofascicular AP potential was recorded during sinus rhythm, and RFCA at this site abolished the inducibility of both tachycardias [293].

The site of earliest ventricular activation during right ventricular mapping is generally found at the apical one-third of the right aspect of the interventricular septum. At various distances from this site and towards the right free-wall AV ring, it is possible to register fast 'Purkinje-like' deflections (referred to as 'Mahaim potentials') preceding the onset of the QRS complex. Mapping the proximal insertion of the AP from the atrial side of the tricuspid annulus can result in catheter-induced block of the anomalous bundle that may persist for several hours even after isoprenaline infusion [294].

Treatment

The treatment of choice in these patients is RFCA at the site of induction of mechanical block of the AP, or better at locations where 'Mahaim potentials' are recorded [294–296]. Segments of the AP close to its ventricular exit probably branch and are inappropriate targets for RFCA, with only temporary success [295]. Approaching the atrial insertion frequently provokes long-lasting mechanical block, thus making the ablation procedure more difficult [294]. Performing the ablation at sites where the 'Mahaim potential' precedes the onset of a maximally pre-excited QRS complex by ≥20ms avoids the more proximal areas that may be encased by a shield of connective tissue and the more distal, potentially branching, portions. Ablation at these sites permanently blocks the AP without inducing RBBB.

Concealed accessory pathways

Definition

Patients with an AP that only conducts in the retrograde direction have no pre-excitation during sinus rhythm but develop an AVRT that utilizes the AV bypass tract as retrograde limb of a re-entry circuit. AVRT using a concealed AP is the underlying mechanism of 27% of the tachycardias in patients with paroxysmal SVT without pre-excitation during sinus rhythm [297].

Pathogenesis

The reasons why an AP conducts only in retrograde direction are a matter of debate. 'Mismatch impedance' and interactions among the branches of bypass tracts at their atrial and ventricular insertions may play a role in the pathogenesis of permanent unidirectional anterograde block in concealed APs [243, 298].

Diagnosis

AVRT utilizing a concealed AP is slightly more prevalent in males than in females, and the age of onset of symptoms is 25 ± 17 years [204]. Most patients have no organic heart disease except for the occasional patient with Ebstein's disease or L-transposition. The ECG during sinus rhythm is normal or shows a short PR interval due to concomitant enhanced AV nodal conduction [297]. Tachycardia usually has a narrow QRS complex and lacks of T-wave changes related to 'cardiac electric memory'. P waves may be identified following the QRS complex, with RP <PR (➲Figs. 28.21 and 28.36). P-wave morphology during AVRT depends on the AP location (see WPW). Concealed APs are more frequently left- than right-sided. The differential diagnosis of this tachycardia is the rare slow–slow AVNRT (➲Fig. 28.18). There may be ST-segment depression, particularly if the rate is >160bpm. RR intervals may all be the same or present alternating cycle lengths. The amplitude of the QRS complex may be constant or show voltage alternans. RR or voltage alternans is more frequently observed in AVRT using an AP than in AVNRT, but its presence does not exclude the latter, particularly if the rate is >170bpm (➲Fig. 28.17C).

Treatment

If vagal manoeuvres do not terminate the tachycardia, intravenous adenosine should be administered. In this case, the possibility of AF induction is of no concern since the AP does not conduct in AV direction. RFCA is the treatment of choice for the prevention of recurrences. Although there are some technical differences in the ablation of patent and concealed APs, the results and complications are practically the same. In patients refusing to undergo RFCA oral propafenone, flecainide or amiodarone are used to prevent recurrences, something that is only obtained in about 50% of the cases [1]. If the weakest link of the AVRT pathway is the AV node, beta-blocking agents may prevent recurrences. Amiodarone is the last resort when a chronic pharmacological approach is adopted. Propafenone and flecainide may be less appropriate in elderly patients. The 'pill-in-the-pocket' approach is less effective in patients with concealed APs than in those with AVNRT. When episodes of AVRT using a concealed AP are very long-lasting, the conductivity of the AV node and of the AP is usually very good and less sensitive to the effects of antiarrhythmic agents.

Permanent junctional reciprocating tachycardia

Definition

In 1967 Coumel *et al.* described an almost constantly ongoing SVT with a PR <RP pattern due to AV junctional re-entry, in which the retrograde limb of the circuit had long conduction times and decremental conducting properties (➲Fig. 28.25) [230]. PJRT is an unusual arrhythmia. Both genders are equally affected and patients with this tachycardia are usually identified at ages <50 years.

Pathogenesis

PJRT, initially thought to be a fast–slow AVNRT [299], was finally demonstrated to incorporate as retrograde limb of the AV junctional re-entry an inferior paraseptal AV bypass tract with long conduction times and decremental conducting properties [300]. A fibromuscular bundle with a long tortuous course has been found in the only reported necropsy specimen of PJRT [242]. These APs are usually 'concealed' but they may have potential for anterograde conduction which usually does not manifest itself during sinus rhythm due to their very long anterograde conduction times [242]. Exceptionally, a slowly and decrementally conducting AP in the VA direction, responsible for a PJRT, conducts with 'normal' short AV conduction times anterogradely, thus showing more or less typical pre-excitation during sinus rhythm (➲Fig. 28.40). In some patients, these APs only conduct in VA direction and it is possible to demonstrate that a ventricular premature beat during sinus rhythm at a time when the His bundle is refractory can result in VA conduction via the retrograde

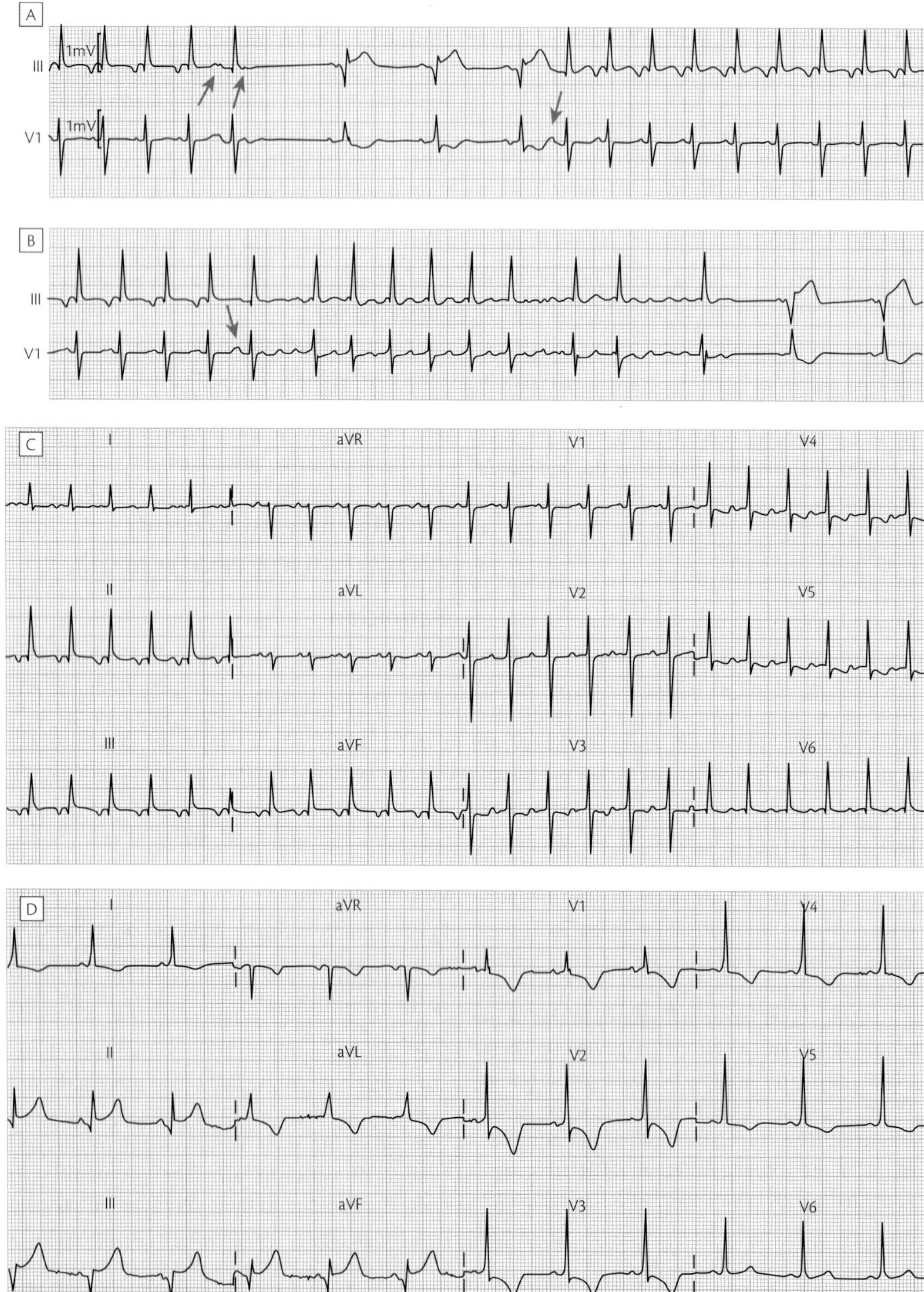

Figure 28.40 Continuously recurring PJRT using a slow, decrementally conducting left inferior VA AP, having its atrial insertion some 15mm from the ostium of the CS. (A) PJRT terminates after two consecutive spontaneously occurring APBs (green arrows). After three sinus beats with pre-excitation, an APB (arrow) initiates PJRT. (B) PJRT terminates by an APB that is followed by an unsustained run of AF. (C, D) 12-lead ECG during PJRT and sinus rhythm, respectively. The same AP was also capable of AV conduction with much shorter conduction times giving rise to patent pre-excitation in the short periods in which the patient was in sinus rhythm. Ablation during PJRT resulted in abolition of tachycardia and in the disappearance of pre-excitation.

slow AP, thus excluding anterograde concealed conduction over the AP.

Diagnosis

Clinical consequences

At rest, despite being in tachycardia, most patients do not perceive palpitations or only notice the scanty normal sinus beats that from time to time are observed between bursts of the arrhythmia. Patients frequently offer a long history of palpitations on exertion or with psychological stress. A few patients have syncope, most likely of vasovagal origin. In the past, cardiomegaly and echocardiographic signs of mild-to-moderate systolic left ventricular dysfunction was seen in 50–60% of cases [18] and congestive heart failure occurs in ≈30% [301]. Some patients are referred to tertiary centres with the diagnosis of dilated cardiomyopathy [18]. Sudden death has been reported in patients with PJRT and left ventricular dysfunction without heart failure [301]. Spontaneous resolution of PJRT has also been described [301]. Today patients are diagnosed and usually ablated at an earlier stage. An electrocardiographically and electrophysiologically identical tachycardia can develop with a paroxysmal, rather than permanent presentation. Interestingly, although left ventricular dysfunction was more frequently observed in the permanent form, the paroxysmal variety can also be associated with a reduced ejection fraction [302].

Electrocardiographic diagnosis

PJRT usually has a narrow QRS complex, a PR <RP, and negative P waves in inferior leads and frequently in V6 (➲ Fig. 28.28, 28.40, and 28.41). There are instances in which RP and PR intervals during PJRT have similar durations. The rate of PJRT varies from 90–250bpm depending on the autonomic tone. During sleep, PJRT may slow down or even disappear. At rest, tachycardia may be incessantly present or runs of different duration alternate with a few sinus beats. During physical or psychological stress, PJRT becomes truly incessant and its rate accelerates [18].

Although an APB is not required for the initiation of PJRT that usually begins spontaneously, if APBs are present, they may also elicit PJRT (➲ Fig. 28.40). The first RP interval is frequently shorter than the subsequent ones, and in some patients transient oscillations of the RP/PR intervals and of the resulting cycle lengths of the tachycardia can be observed. A few patients show alternating long-to-short RR intervals during tachycardia with an almost constant PR interval and oscillating RP times. The QRS width ranges from 80–100ms and may occasionally show LBBB if the patient has developed a tachycardiomyopathy. Spontaneous tachycardia terminations can be observed, particularly at rest, usually in the form of a retrograde block over the AP. The VA conduction time is shortened by isoprenaline, atropine and exercise, is prolonged by verapamil, and is not affected by ajmaline [18, 86].

From the electrocardiographic point of view, PJRT is similar to AT and to the uncommon fast–slow AVNRT (➲ Fig. 28.7). The induction of AV block by vagal or pharmacological manoeuvres without interrupting the tachycardia at the atrial level indicates an atrial origin. Vagal manoeuvres may terminate PJRT temporarily, usually by inducing retrograde conduction block. The continuously recurring nature of PJRT is very seldom observed in fast–slow AVNRT but does not exclude it.

Electrophysiological diagnosis

The complexities of electrophysiological studies in PJRT have been reviewed elsewhere [18, 86, 229, 299, 300]. In most PJRTs, an inferior paraseptal AP with long conduction times and decremental conducting properties is demonstrated. Other cases have a left inferior or even posterior atrial insertion (➲ Figs. 28.40 and 28.41) [18]. Exceptionally, PJRT is based on a fast–slow AV nodal re-entry mechanism.

Treatment

Because of the incessant nature of the tachycardia, no acute treatment should be used in these patients. Due to the risk of developing a tachycardiomyopathy, RFCA is recommended in asymptomatic patients with and without signs of left ventricular dysfunction (➲ Fig. 28.41) [301–303].

Other non-paroxysmal SVT

Focal junctional tachycardia

This type of SVT is also termed 'congenital' when discovered during the first 6 months of life [18, 304] where it is incessant and has a poor prognosis, with systolic left ventricular dysfunction, heart failure, and early death [305]. The ECG shows narrow QRS-complex tachycardia at 140–300bpm with AV dissociation or intermittent VA conduction. Amiodarone is the drug of choice in these infants [18]—flecainide and propafenone slow the tachycardia rate, whereas verapamil may accelerate it [306]. There are anecdotal reports of successful RFCA of this tachycardia with

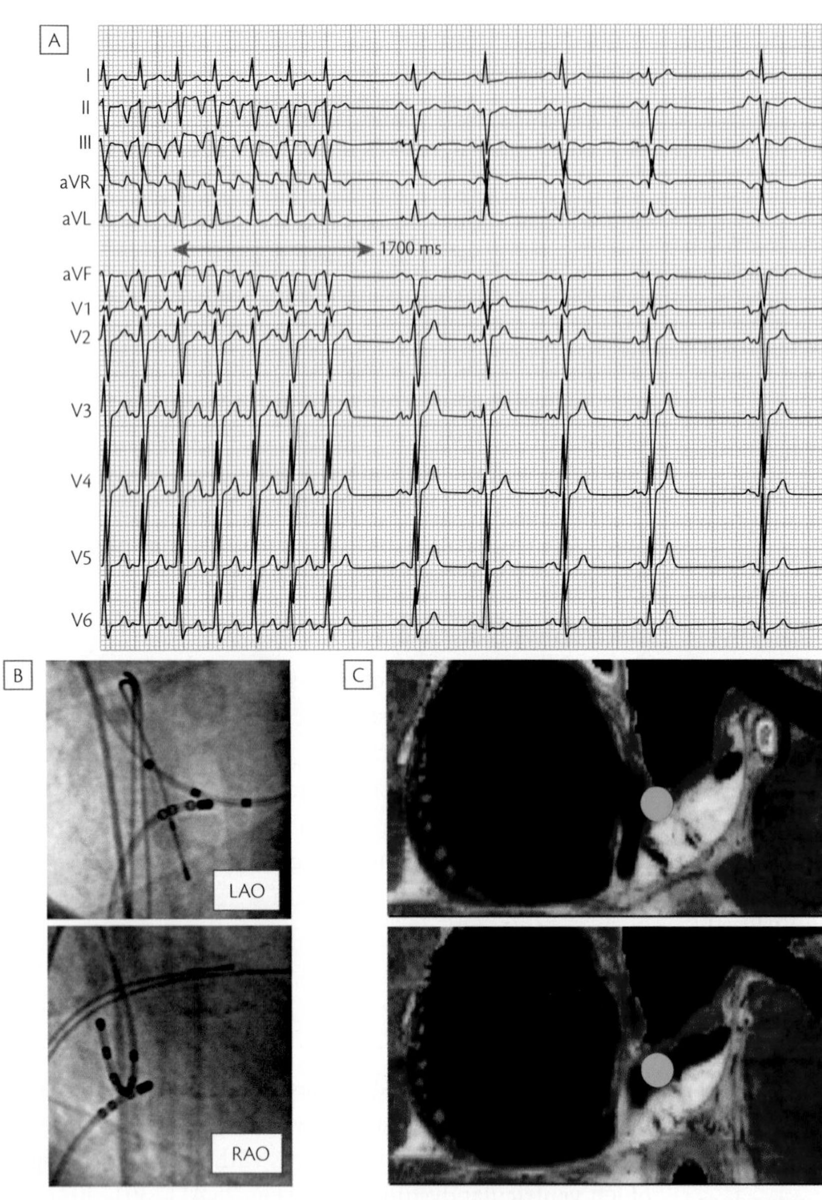

Figure 28.41 (A) PJRT in a 20-year-old male terminates 1700ms after the initiation of the application of RF current. (B) The atrial insertion of this slowly conducting AP was at 5mm from the mouth of the CS. (C) Anatomic sections of the heart at two levels in LAO projection illustrating the location of the ablation catheter at the site of block of the AP (blue circles).

preservation of AV nodal conduction [307, 308]. A more benign form of the arrhythmia, either paroxysmal or continuously recurring, may be rarely observed in adulthood becoming permanent during exercise or adrenergic stress [1].

Non-paroxysmal junctional tachycardia

NPJT is an accelerated AV junctional rhythm originating at the bundle of His or at the AV node. NPJT most of the time is secondary to ischaemia, digitalis intoxication, cardiac surgery, hyperthyroidism, percutaneous closure of an atrial septal defect with an implantable device, or application of radiofrequency current near the AV node (➲Fig. 28.18C). Although enhanced automaticity may be the underlying mechanism, other causes cannot be excluded [1]. Electrocardiographically, it is characterized by prolonged runs of an accelerated junctional rhythm, at 70–140bpm. During the arrhythmia there is AV dissociation with capture beats, or VA conduction. The QRS complex is narrow except for patients with organic bundle branch block. Focal NPJT is usually asymptomatic and does not require treatment.

Personal perspective

In the coming 10 years, various aspects of SVT will be explored from the viewpoint of molecular biology, genetics, and proteomics. CTI-dependent and atypical AFL will become more prevalent due to the longer life expectancy of the population and the escalating number of ablation procedures to treat AF.

The handling of new information will in itself be challenging. In the last decade of the 20th century an academic cardiologist could be well informed by following about ten journals, some of which were of a general medical orientation. Today, the number of periodical publications dealing with arrhythmias is on the rise and in spite of easier access through the Internet, time and economic constraints may impair the continuous education of cardiologists.

Internet-based portals devoted to cardiovascular medicine in general and arrhythmology in particular, can not only filter the overwhelming number of papers on offer, but will also make information available to physicians working in environments that simply cannot afford to pay the access to electronic journals. Open-access journals will, hopefully, become the norm although this may also make it more difficult keeping abreast with new relevant advances. In this scenario, the development of timely, independent, comprehensive, well referenced, profusely illustrated, and evidence-balanced guidelines will become badly needed. For the diffusion and consultation of such guidelines Gutenberg's press has to give way to 'e-publication' free-access technologies.

The strong diagnostic power of the 12-lead ECG needs to be maintained and enhanced with future investigations. Good teachers stimulating the interest of the coming generations of cardiologists on this 100-year-old diagnostic tool will also be needed. Industry will provide computer-based platforms enabling the storage of continuous recording of the 12-lead ECG for the subsequent editing of the relevant fragments to be sent to the hospital information system.

The fine art of thoughtful electrophysiological diagnosis, a blend of catheter mapping and stimulation criteria, currently threatened by a 'burning without learning' temptation, must be reinforced today so that it is not lost tomorrow.

Further reading

Blomström-Lundqvist C, Scheinman MM, Aliot EM, Alpert JS, Calkins H, Camm AJ, *et al.* ACC/AHA/ESC guidelines for the management of patients with supraventricular arrhythmias-executive summary: a report of the American College of Cardiology/American Heart Association Task Force on Practice Guidelines and the European Society of Cardiology Committee for Practice Guidelines. (Writing Committee to Develop Guidelines for the Management of Patients with Supraventricular Arrhythmias.) Developed in collaboration with NASPE–Heart Rhythm Society. *Eur Heart J* 2003; **24**: 1857–97.

Delacrétaz E. Supraventricular tachycardia. *N Engl J Med* 2006; **354**: 1039–51.

Huang SKS, Wood MA. *Catheter ablation of cardiac arrhythmia* 2006. Philadelphia, PA: Saunders-Elsevier.

Josephson ME. *Clinical cardiac electrophysiology. Techniques and interpretations*, 4th edn, 2008. Philadelphia, PA: Wolters Kluwer–Lippincott Williams & Wilkins.

Marine JE. Catheter ablation therapy for supraventricular arrhythmias. *JAMA* 2007; **298**: 2768–78.

➲ **For full references and multimedia materials please visit the online version of the book (http://esctextbook.oxfordonline.com).**

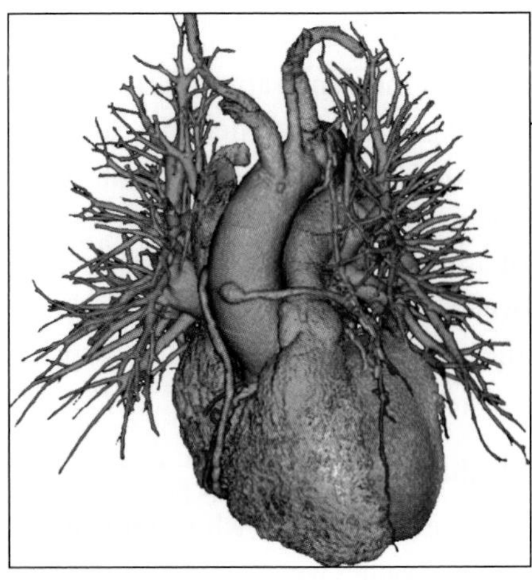

CHAPTER 29

Atrial Fibrillation

A. John Camm, Paulus Kirchhof, Gregory Y.H. Lip, Irina Savelieva, and Sabine Ernst

Contents

Summary

Atrial fibrillation (AF) is such a common arrhythmia that it is often wrongly regarded as an acceptable alternative to normal sinus rhythm. Its first onset may present with rapid and uncomfortable palpitations, breathlessness, dyspnoea, chest pain, and anxiety. Often it is entirely asymptomatic and discovered quite by chance. Paroxysmal and persistent recurrences may eventually lapse into permanent AF.

The causes of AF are legion and should be identified since many can be corrected and the management of the arrhythmia can be simplified. The consequences of AF may be dire: heart failure, stroke, sudden death, markedly reduced exercise capacity, and degraded quality of life. Appropriate thromboprophylaxis, adequate rate control, and sucessful rhythm control in suitable patients are essential.

Stroke risk can be diminished by appropriate thromboprophylaxis with aspirin or vitamin K antagonists as indicated by systematic risk stratification; heart failure can be improved by competent management of underlying comorbid disease and proper rate control. Rhythm control with antiarrhythmic drugs, including beta-blockers, and left atrial ablation techniques may be needed to ameliorate symptoms and alleviate anxiety.

Epidemiology

Atrial fibrillation in the general population

Detection of atrial fibrillation

AF can be recognized on the electrocardiogram (ECG) by an irregular ventricular rhythm without consistent P waves (➲Fig. 29.1) [1]. Epidemiological studies using short-term (often one single) ECG recording and symptoms have estimated the prevalence of AF in the population at 0.5–1% [2–5]. Continuous ECG monitoring of AF patients suggests that more than half of AF episodes are not detected by standard ECG recordings, even in symptomatic AF patients [6–8]. Hence, the 'true' prevalence of AF may be closer to 2% of the population [8]. As the population ages, it is expected that the number of patients with AF will double or triple in the next few decades (➲Fig. 29.2).

Prevalence of atrial fibrillation

The prevalence of AF increases with age. Less than 0.5% of 40–50-year-olds suffer from AF, while an estimated 5–15% of the population present with AF at the age of 80 years [3, 9–11] (➲Fig. 29.3). Men are more often affected than women, and the age of diagnosis is later in women, but women with AF appear to be more prone to AF-related complications [4, 12]. The recurrent, initially often self-terminating nature of the arrhythmia [13] translates to a lifetime risk of AF around 25% in current 40-year-olds [14, 15]. Furthermore, in the Western world the age-adjusted prevalence of AF has increased over the past decades [2, 3, 10].

Incidence of atrial fibrillation

Similar to AF prevalence, its incidence appears to increase with age, is higher in men than in women [2], and has risen in the last two decades [10], varying from 1.6–1.0% per annum [11] to 0.54 cases per 1000 person years [2]. A high proportion of undiagnosed AF suggests a large potential overlap between newly detected 'prevalent' and truly 'incident' AF in the context of scheduled surveys using ECG recordings.

Ethnicity and atrial fibrillation

The prevalence and incidence of AF in non-white populations are less well studied, but lower values were reported for Asians and African Americans [16]. In the health survey of 664,754 US veterans, white men were significantly more likely to have AF compared to all races but Pacific Islanders (odds ratios vs. blacks, 1.84; vs. Hispanics, 1.77; vs. Asians, 1.41; vs. Native Americans, 1.15; $p < 0.001$) [17]. Whites were more likely to have valvular heart disease, coronary artery disease, and congestive heart failure; blacks had the highest hypertension prevalence; Hispanics had the highest diabetes prevalence associated with AF. Racial differences remained after adjustment for age, body mass index, and other comorbidities.

Types of atrial fibrillation

Clinically, four types of AF are distinguished based on the presentation and duration of the arrhythmia: first diagnosed AF, paroxysmal AF, persistent AF, and permanent (accepted) AF (➲Fig. 29.4).

- **First diagnosed AF** is AF presenting for the first time, irrespective of the duration of the arrhythmia or of

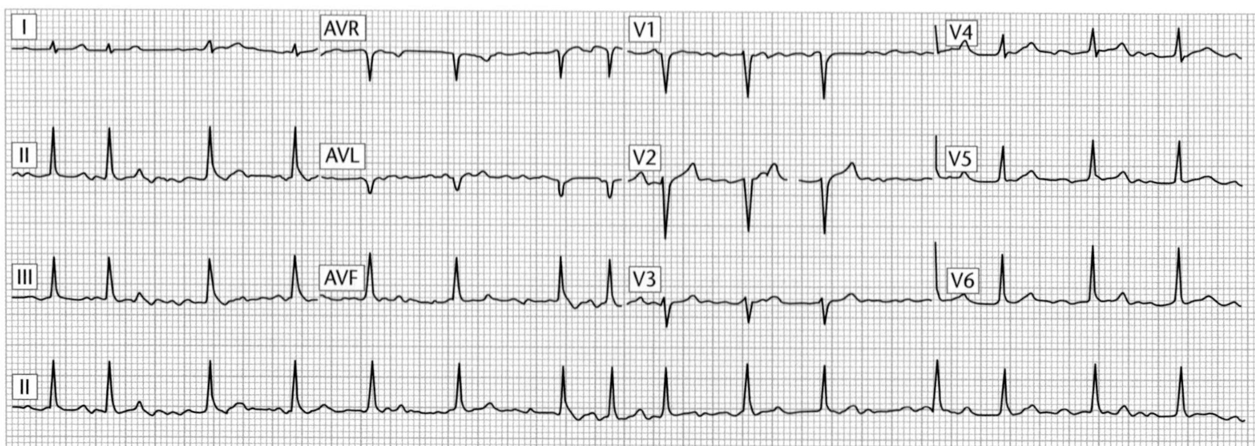

Figure 29.1 12-lead electrocardiogram demonstrating atrial fibrillation. Note the irregular ventricular response rate and the fine baseline oscillations due to 'f' waves. No consistent P-wave activity can be seen.

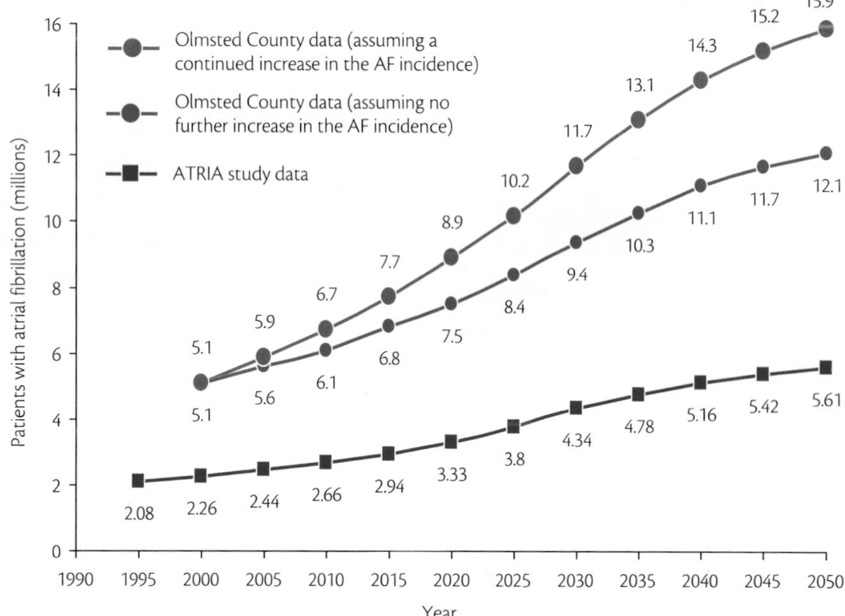

Figure 29.2 Projected number of adults with atrial fibrillation in the United States by 2050. ATRIA, AnTicoagulation and Risk Factors In Atrial Fibrillation. Data from Go AS, Hylek EM, Phillips KA, *et al.* Prevalence of diagnosed atrial fibrillation in adults: national implications for rhythm management and stroke prevention: the AnTicoagulation and Risk Factors in Atrial Fibrillation (ATRIA) Study. *JAMA* 2001; **285**: 2370–5 and Miyasaka Y, Barnes ME, Gersh BJ, *et al.* Secular trends in incidence of atrial fibrillation in Olmsted County, Minnesota, 1980 to 2000, and implications on the projections for future prevalence. *Circulation* 2006; **114**: 119–25.

the presence or severity of AF-related symptoms or complications.

- **Paroxysmal AF** is recurrent and self-terminating. Many of these patients present with frequent symptomatic paroxysms of AF, usually lasting 48 hours or less, and definitely <7 days. In clinical trials, AF is defined as any episode lasting >30s.
- **Persistent AF** lasts >7 days (by convention) or is terminated by cardioversion (either with drugs or electrical shocks). Persistent AF also implies that a rhythm-control therapy strategy is pursued. Long-term persistent forms of AF may last >12 months but assignment of AF as persistent rather than permanent implies that a rhythm-control strategy is pursued.
- **Permanent AF** is longstanding and by definition occurs when a rate control therapy is pursued, i.e. the presence of AF is 'accepted'. Hence, rhythm-control interventions (e.g. antiarrhythmic drugs, cardioversions, catheter ablation, or surgical interventions) are abandoned in patients with permanent AF.

This classification is useful for clinical management of AF patients, especially when AF-related symptoms are also considered. A symptoms score ('EHRA score'; ➲Table 29.1) [8] provides a simple clinical tool to assess symptoms during AF. Combined with a stroke risk estimation, the symptom score and AF classification guide clinical decisions in AF patients.

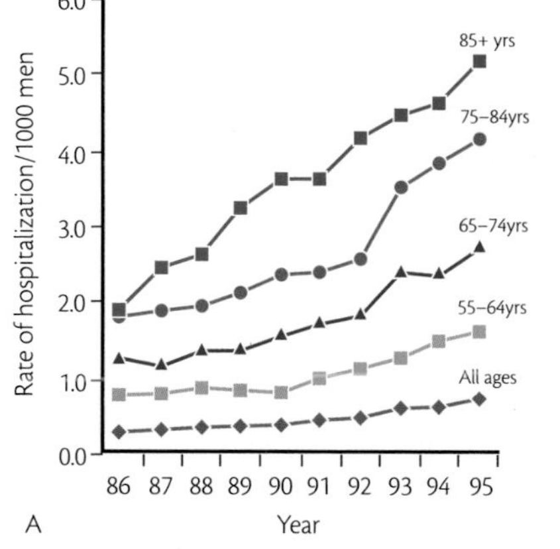

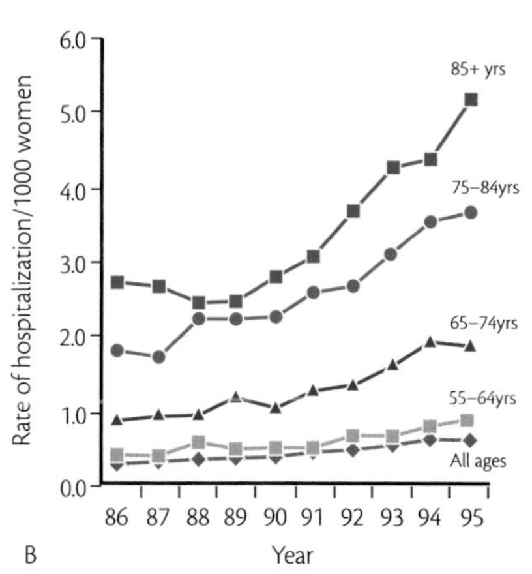

Figure 29.3 Increasing prevalence of atrial fibrillation among first-ever hospital admissions between 1986 and 1995. The greatest increase is seen among the elderly. (A) Men; (B) women. Reproduced with permission from Stewart S, Hart CL, Hole DJ, *et al.* Population prevalence, incidence, and predictors of atrial fibrillation in the Renfrew/Paisley study. *Heart* 2001; **86**: 516–21.

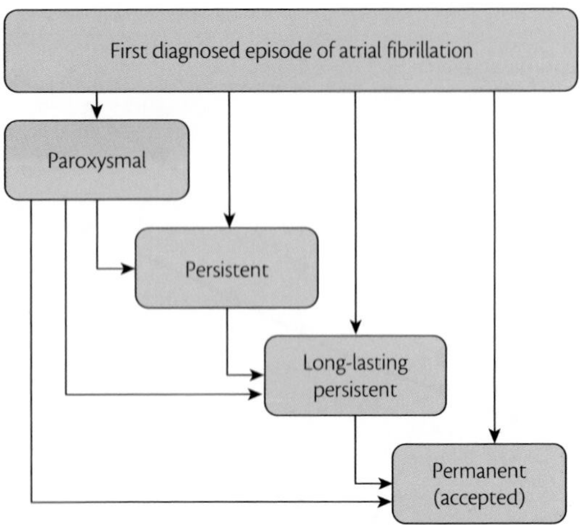

Figure 29.4 Temporal patterns of atrial fibrillation. The first detected episode of atrial fibrillation may not have begun recently or may have been preceded by other episodes which have been asymptomatic. The usual progression of this arrhythmia is through paroxysmal (self-terminating) forms to persistent (not-self terminating atrial fibrillation), implying attempts are made to restore and maintain sinus rhythm. Eventually the physician or the patient may not wish to attempt to restore sinus rhythm and accepts permanent atrial fibrillation. Recent advances in the maintenance of sinus rhythm in patients with long-standing atrial fibrillation suggest that a differentiation between 'persistent' and 'long-standing persistent' (e.g. duration of the present atrial fibrillation episode > 12 months) can be reasonable.

Development of atrial fibrillation over time in an individual patient

In the majority of patients, AF is a progressive arrhythmia. An AF patient may experience asymptomatic, self-terminating episodes of the arrhythmia before AF is first diagnosed. The rate of recurrent AF is 10% in the first year after the initial diagnosis, and approximately 5% per annum thereafter. Comorbidities and age significantly influence the progression and complications of AF [4]. In a small group of highly selected patients with 'lone AF' without concomitant conditions that contribute to progression of the arrhythmia, AF remains paroxysmal over several decades [18].

When persistent AF is cardioverted, the recurrence rate is between 30–70% in the first month. Most recurrences occur in the first few weeks after termination of AF [6, 19]. The frequency and duration of arrhythmia recurrence tends to increase over time, and the distribution and duration of arrhythmia episodes is not random [20], but clustered (➲Fig. 29.5) [8, 21, 22]. Hence, 'total AF burden' can vary markedly over months or even years in individual patients [22, 23]. Therefore reliable and valid assessment of AF

Table 29.1 Clinical classification of atrial fibrillation according to duration, therapeutic strategy, symptoms, and risk for thromboembolic events

Types of AF		
First episode	Any duration of AF	
Paroxysmal AF	Self-terminating AF of <7 days duration, but typically ≤48 hours	
Persistent AF	AF that terminates after >7 days or that is intentionally terminated by an intervention (cardioversion)	Implies the decision to pursue a rhythm-control therapy strategy
Permanent AF	AF without an intention to terminate the arrhythmia	Implies the decision to pursue a rate-control therapy strategy
Classification of AF-related symptoms (EHRA symptoms score)		
EHRA class	**Explanation**	
EHRA I	'No symptoms'	
EHRA II	'Mild symptoms'; normal daily activity not affected	
EHRA III	'Severe symptoms'; normal daily activity affected	
EHRA IV	'Disabling symptoms'; normal daily activity discontinued	
Risk factors in the $CHADS_2$ score for estimation of stroke risk in AF patients		
Risk factor	**Comments**	**Contribution to score**
Age >75 years	Patients aged 65–75 years carry an 'intermediate' stroke risk elevation	1 point
Hypertension	Irrespective of current blood pressure control	1 point
Diabetes mellitus	Managed by drugs (PO or insulin)	1 point
Heart failure	As a clinical diagnosis—possibly also as a diagnosis of poor left ventricular function	1 point
Prior stroke or TIA	Irrespective of persistence of neurological deficit	2 points

AF, atrial fibrillation; EHRA, European Heart Rhythm Association; TIA, transient ischaemic attack.

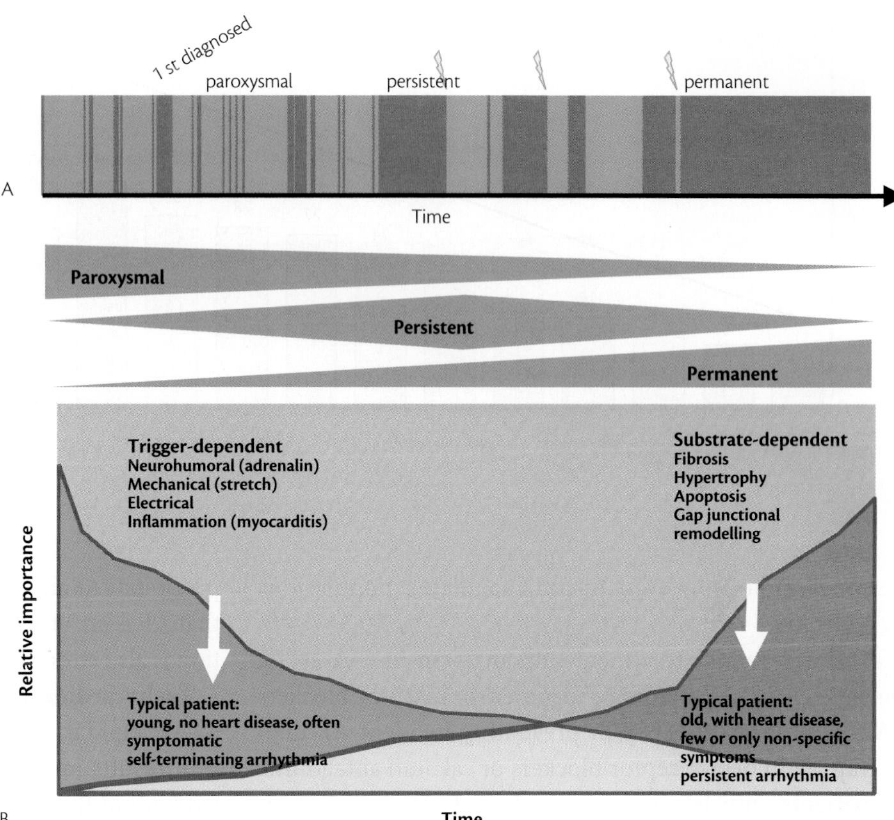

Figure 29.5 Progression of atrial fibrillation from paroxysmal to permanent and the importance of specific triggers and substrate formation. In the majority of patients, atrial fibrillation is a chronically progressive arrhythmia; patients may experience asymptomatic, self-terminating episodes of the arrhythmia before atrial fibrillation is first diagnosed. Recurrences of the arrhythmia are clustered, and periods with frequent paroxysms are often alternating with longer periods without any recurrences (A). Modified with permission from Kirchhof P, Auricchio A, Bax J, *et al.* Outcome parameters for trials in atrial fibrillation: executive summary. *Eur Heart J* 2007; **28**: 2803–17. Initially, atrial fibrillation can be a primary electrical disorder in response to specific triggers such as atrial premature beats, pulmonary vein tachycardia, or neurohumoral stimuli, followed by electrical, structural, and functional remodelling (B). Progression of atrial fibrillation relates to progression of the underlying disease and to continuous structural remodelling of the atria, including changes associated with ageing (e.g. fatty metamorphosis, myocyte degeneration, and fibrosis).

recurrences is difficult in clinical practice, and especially in clinical trials. Asymptomatic AF is common even in symptomatic patients, irrespective of whether the initial presentation was persistent or paroxysmal AF, and has important implications for therapy (dis)continuation.

Predisposing clinical conditions

AF is associated with a variety of cardiovascular conditions that may perpetuate the arrhythmia [4, 12, 24, 25]. These conditions may also be markers for global cardiovascular risk [26] and/or cardiac damage rather than causative factors.

Hypertension (➲Chapter 13) is the most common underlying condition in AF patients, found in approximately 2/3 of all AF patients in different surveys (➲Fig. 29.6) [4]. Inadequate control of blood pressure is a risk factor for incident (first diagnosed) AF in hypertensive patients and for AF-related complications such as stroke and systemic

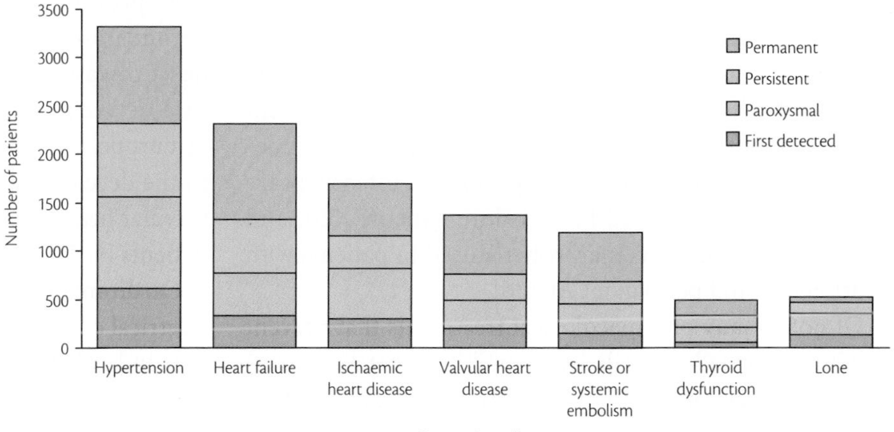

Figure 29.6 Types of atrial fibrillation by concomitant pathology in the Euro Heart Survey. Modified with permission from Nieuwlaat R, Capucci A, Camm AJ, *et al.* Atrial fibrillation management: a prospective survey in ESC member countries: the Euro Heart Survey on Atrial Fibrillation. *Eur Heart J* 2005; **26**: 2422–34.

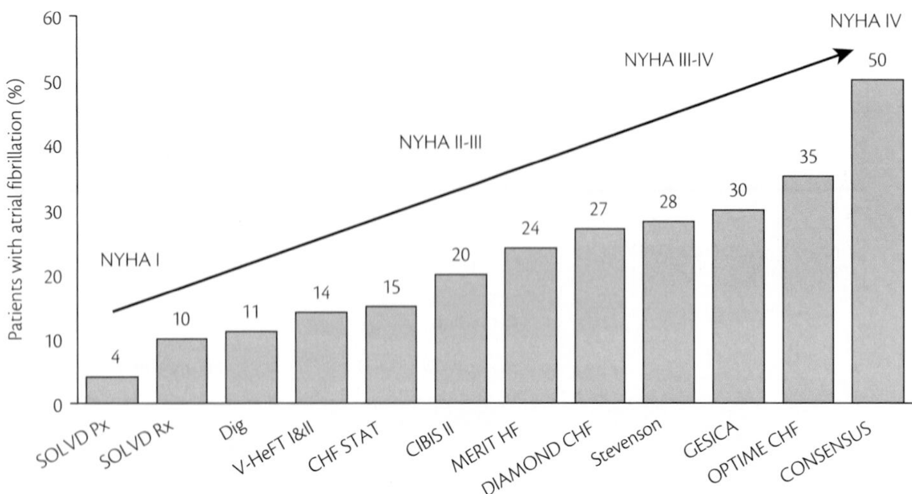

Figure 29.7 Prevalence of atrial fibrillation in studies of heart failure. Reproduced with permission from Savelieva I, Camm AJ. Atrial fibrillation and heart failure: natural history and pharmacological treatment. *Europace* 2004; **5** (Suppl.1): S5–19.

thromboembolism, even in anticoagulated populations [27–29].

Antihypertensive treatment with angiotensin-converting enzyme (ACE) inhibitors or angiotensin receptor blockers (ARBs) is more effective in preventing incident AF than therapy with beta-receptor blockers or calcium antagonists in patients with left ventricular (LV) dysfunction or LV hypertrophy, despite similar reductions in blood pressure [30, 31] but less so in patients with well-controlled hypertension and without structural heart disease [32]. This is because the former may prevent atrial remodelling (cellular hypertrophy and atrial fibrosis) in patients prone to such changes (see ➲'Upstream' therapy, p.1113).

Heart failure (➲Chapter 23), defined as heart failure with dyspnoea on exertion (New York Heart Association (NYHA) classes II–IV) is found in 30% of AF patients [4, 12], and AF is found in 5–50% of heart failure patients [33]. The prevalence of AF clearly increases with the clinical severity of heart failure, with an AF prevalence of almost 50% in patients with NYHA IV heart failure (➲Fig. 29.7) [34].

Heart failure can be either a consequence of AF (tachycardiomyopathy or decompensation in acute-onset AF) or a cause for the arrhythmia (by atrial pressure and volume overload, or chronic neurohumoral stimulation). In most patients, both conditions sustain each other to different degrees. Importantly, new-onset AF appears to be an independent predictor of death and prolonged intensive care unit stay in non-selected heart failure patients [35], and exercise performance is markedly reduced in patients with heart failure and permanent AF [36].

Of note, many pharmacological treatments that prevent death in heart failure trials (ACE inhibitors, beta-blockers) also prevent new-onset AF (see ➲'Upstream' Therapy, p.1113) [34]. The common myocardial damage mechanisms that precipitate AF and heart failure (see ➲Chapter 23) may suggest that AF is an 'atrial cardiomyopathy'. Diastolic LV dysfunction is also strongly correlated with the incidence of AF.

Tachycardiomyopathy is a form of LV dysfunction caused by AF: rapid irregular rate and loss of atrial contractile function results in severe LV dysfunction in selected patients with AF in the absence of structural heart disease. Similar effects have been described for other incessant tachycardias, including atrial and atrioventricular (AV) nodal tachycardia [37], and right ventricular outflow tract tachycardia [38]. Tachycardiomyopathy should be suspected when there is a fast ventricular rate and LV dysfunction but no signs for structural heart disease. Tachycardiomyopathy is confirmed when LV function is restored with adequate rate control or maintenance of sinus rhythm (➲Fig. 29.8). Recovery of LV function may require several weeks. In some patients, only repeated measurements of LV function over time can distinguish between mild forms of ventricular cardiomyopathy complicated by AF and tachycardiomyopathy.

Valvular heart disease (➲Chapter 21), especially mitral valve stenosis and regurgitation, induces left atrial (LA) pressure or volume overload that can provoke AF. Secondary to the improved earlier treatment of valvular heart disease and the prevention of rheumatic heart disease, severe mitral valve disease has become less common in Europe. The contribution of mild valvular heart disease to the development of AF is less clear, but some degree of valvular heart disease is found in approximately 30% of AF patients [4, 12].

Cardiomyopathies (➲Chapter 18) including the primary electrical cardiac diseases (➲Chapter 9 and 30) [39] carry a high individual risk for AF. In fact, sudden death and AF are clearly associated in epidemiological studies, suggesting the possibility of a common mechanism for both arrhythmias.

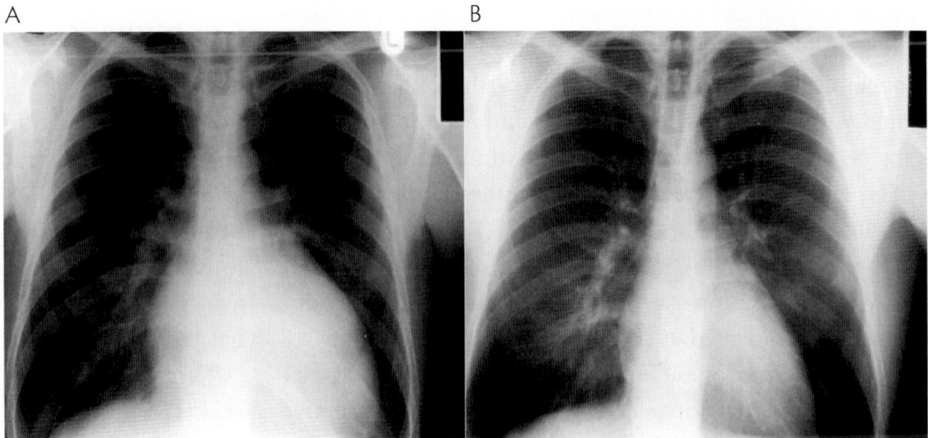

Figure 29.8 Resolving atrial fibrillation rate-related cardiomyopathy. This young man presented with atrial fibrillation and an average heart rate of 125bpm. He had been unwell for several months but was not aware of his heart rate during this time (A). Four weeks after cardioversion to sinus rhythm his heart size had reduced to normal (B).

The genetically determined cardiomyopathies comprise hypertrophic, dilated, and right ventricular cardiomyopathy. In addition 'electrical cardiomyopathies' such as long QT syndrome, short QT syndrome, Brugada syndrome, and catecholaminergic VT should be considered.

The high individual risk for AF at younger ages [40–43] probably explains why relatively rare cardiomyopathies are found in 10% of AF patients [4, 12]. Genetic studies suggest that a small proportion of patients with 'lone AF' are actually mutation carriers for 'primary electrical' cardiomyopathies [44].

With the possible exception of catecholaminergic ventricular tachycardia (VT), all genetically determined cardiomyopathies carry a risk for AF [41, 45]. In the long QT syndromes, 'AF' appears to be caused by after-depolarizations and prolongation [46, 47], rather than shortening of the action potential [48] (atrial 'torsade'). Occasionally, 'twisting' of the P waves during atrial arrhythmias has been reported in long QT syndrome (29.1). In short QT syndrome, AF appears to be even more prevalent than ventricular arrhythmias [49, 50].

There is a high prevalence AF in Brugada syndrome (➲Chapter 9) [42] but the mechanism is not delineated. It may be linked in some patients to mutations in the sodium channel (*SCN5A*) gene, and conduction slowing. In hypertrophic cardiomyopathy and arrhythmogenic right ventricular cardiomyopathy (ARVC) (➲Chapter 18), a mixture of altered myocardial structure, changes in haemodynamic function, and primary electrical changes appear to cause AF [51, 52]. The reported association between ventricular pre-excitation or Wolff–Parkinson–White syndrome and AF (29.2) may be either due to the more severe symptoms of AF in patients with rapid conduction of atrial activity via the bypass tract, or due to a common genetic cause (➲Table 29.4).

Atrial septal defects (➲Chapter 10) are associated with AF in 10–15% of patients according to earlier surveys [40]. This association has important clinical implications in the antithrombotic management of stroke or transient ischaemic attack (TIA) survivors with an atrial septal defect. In patients with large shunt volumes and/or a high atrial load due to the septal defect, AF may be secondary to pressure and volume overload. In others, the association between AF and septal defects points to a common abnormality (e.g. a genetic predisposition) that predisposes to both ASD and AF.

Other congenital heart defects (➲Chapter 10) are often associated with AF. Patients with single ventricles, atrial repair (Mustard operation) of a transposition of the great arteries, or after a Fontan procedure are at especially high risk for AF. Altered atrial anatomy, either due to the primary defect or secondary to repair surgery, and the ensuing altered atrial haemodynamics, may be one of the main predisposing factors for AF. AF can be highly symptomatic in these patients, and is often difficult to treat.

Coronary artery disease (CAD) (➲Chapters 16 and 17) is present in 20% of the AF population. Studies that recruited patients in hospital usually have higher prevalence of coronary heart disease than when outpatients are enrolled, most likely secondary to the relatively high likelihood of in-hospital treatment of coronary heart disease [53]. Whether CAD per se predisposes to AF is not known, given that the association between AF and CAD may be mediated via heart failure in survivors of a myocardial infarction, or by shared risk factors, such as hypertension. AF is rare in patients with stable CAD and preserved LV function, but indicates those with a poor prognosis after a myocardial infarction [54].

Thyroid dysfunction is an important cause of AF. In recent surveys, only a relatively small percentage of the AF population (10% in Germany, a country with a high prevalence of goitre due to iodine deficiency) presents with apparent hyper- or hypothyroidism [4, 12]. In a population-based study of 5860 subjects aged 65 years and older, the biochemical finding of subclinical hyperthyroidism is associated with AF on the resting ECG, and even in euthyroid subjects with normal serum thyroid-stimulating hormone (TSH) levels, serum free T4 concentration is independently associated with AF [55].

Obesity is found in 25% of AF patients [4]. In meta-analysis of the population-based cohort studies, obese individuals have an associated 49% increased risk of developing AF compared to non-obese individuals [56]. Obesity is associated with hypertension, sleep apnoea, chronic obstructive airways disease, and diabetes mellitus, among others, and most likely is a marker for cardiovascular risk that associates, among other events, with AF.

A proportion of patients with **metabolic syndrome** (see ➲Chapter 15) develop AF. An apparent correlation between the presence of metabolic syndrome and increased susceptibility to AF during a mean follow-up of 4.5 years has recently been demonstrated in a large (>28,000 subjects) community-based cohort in Japan [57]. Again, this association may reflect that metabolic syndrome summarizes several of the known conditions that predispose to AF.

Sleep apnoea is associated with an atrial pressure rise and dilatation and may predispose to AF [58]. The retrospective cohort study of 3542 Olmsted County adults who were referred for a diagnostic polysomnogram, has found that obesity and the magnitude of nocturnal oxygen desaturation, which is an important pathophysiological consequence of sleep apnoea, were independent risk factors for new incident AF in individuals <65 years of age [59].

Tall stature is associated with AF [60]. The mechanisms are unclear, but mechanical distension of pulmonary veins (PVs) and LA dilatation are possible.

Diabetes mellitus, when defined as a medical condition that requires treatment, is found in 20% of AF patients. It is conceivable that badly controlled diabetes mellitus may contribute to atrial cell death and 'structural remodelling', and thereby contribute to the perpetuation of AF [61].

Chronic obstructive pulmonary disease is found in 10–15% of AF patients [62]. In some patients, pulmonary disease may rather be a marker for cardiovascular risk in general than a specific predisposing factor for AF. Cancer of the bronchus may also present with AF.

Chronic renal disease (see ➲Chapter 15), measured as renal dysfunction, is present in 10–15% of AF patients. Renal failure appears to increase the risk for AF-related complications, especially cardiovascular complications. Renal failure, diabetes mellitus, and chronic obstructive pulmonary disease are more prevalent in patients with permanent AF.

Consequences of atrial fibrillation and its complications

During AF, regulation of heart rate by the sinus node is lost, and the ventricular rate is regulated by the conduction properties of the AV node ('arrhythmia absoluta'). The reduction of cardiac output is aggravated by loss of atrial contractile function. The latter leads to abnormal atrial stasis which, in association with abnormal blood constituents and endothelial alterations, fulfils Virchow's triad for thrombogenesis.

Through these main mechanisms, AF has important effects on health by causing or associating with death, stroke and other thromboembolic events, reduced quality of life and exercise capacity, and LV dysfunction. Due to these severe complications and its high prevalence, AF causes substantial cardiovascular morbidity on a population level. ➲Table 29.2 lists rates of relevant outcome events reported in recent large AF trials.

Death rates are doubled in association with AF in epidemiological studies. This is independent of other, known predictors of death (➲Table 29.3) [63–66]. Hence, the prevention of AF-related death is important, although difficult. The biological processes that cause AF-related deaths are not fully understood. So far, only antithrombotic therapy and treatment with dronedarone (see ➲Dronedarone, p.1107) has been shown to affect AF-related deaths and reduce thromboembolic strokes [67]. Patients without structural heart disease (lone AF), particularly who were <60 years at the time of AF diagnosis, appear to have a risk of death similar to that in a general population after 20–30 years [18].

Stroke is the most devastating consequence of AF (➲Fig. 29.9) [68–72]. Approximately every fifth to sixth stroke is due to AF [71, 73]. Strokes in AF patients are markedly more severe, more often result in death or permanent disability than strokes of other origin, and recur more commonly [68, 74, 75]. Paroxysmal AF carries the same stroke risk as permanent or persistent AF [76, 77]. Because much AF is asymptomatic, a number of so-called 'cryptogenic strokes' may be due to undetected (often paroxysmal) AF [78]. Cerebral microemboli may cause cognitive dysfunction in patients with AF in the absence of clinically overt stroke [79] and may contribute to the degraded quality of life in AF patients.

Quality of life and exercise capacity are impaired by AF in patients with AF-related symptoms. Patients with AF have significantly poorer quality of life than healthy controls, the general population, or patients with CAD in sinus rhythm [80]. Although many patients present with 'accidentally diagnosed' and/or asymptomatic AF, AF is one of the most common reasons for hospitalizations [81].

Table 29.2 Yearly rates of outcome events in recent large trials in atrial fibrillation. Outcome events have been classified following the classification given in ➲Table 29.1 [8]. All rates have been estimated based on the published reports of these studies and are expressed as per cent per year. Estimates for atrial fibrillation recurrence rates clearly depend on the intensity of ECG monitoring and will be higher when considering asymptomatic atrial fibrillation [8].

Trial acronym	Number of patients	Stroke	Death	Myocardial infarction	Heart failure	Proarrhythmia (VT, VF, TdP)	Persistent AF recurrence	Paroxysmal AF recurrence
ACTIVE W	6700	2.4/1.4	4	0.88/0.55				
AFFIRM	4060	1.2	5	1.1		1.7	66 at 5 years/18	
RACE	522	3.3	3.4		2	2.8	61 at 2 years/90 at 2 years	
SPORTIF III	3410	1.6/2.3	3.2	1.1/0.6				
SPORTIF V	3922	1.6/1.2	3.6/3.8	1.0/1.4				
AMADEUS	4576	0.9/1.3	3.2/2.9	0.8/0.6				
EURIDIS/ADONIS	1237	0.5/0.7	1.0/0.7		2.4/1.0	0.7/0.5		64/75
PAFAC	848		1.3			2.4	45/77	67/83
SOPAT	1012		1			0.1 –0.3		70/80
SAFE-T	665	2	4.36/2.84					30/60/80
AF-CHF	1376	1.5	9.5				*in AF 60/20*	
ANDROMEDA*	627		50/24 (?)					
ATHENA	4628	1.8/1.2	2.8/3.4	1.5	2.5–3			
Estimated event rate		**1.5**	**4**	**1**	**2**	**1**	**45/75**	**55/80**

* ANDROMEDA was terminated too early to adequately estimate yearly event rates; AF, atrial fibrillation; EPHESUS, Eplerenone Post-Acute Myocardial Infarction Heart Failure Efficacy and Survival Study AMADEUS, Atrial fibrillation trial of Monitored, Adjusted Dose vitamin K antagonist, comparing Efficacy and safety with Unadjusted SanOrg 34006/idraparinux; TdP, torsade de pointes; VF, ventricular fibrillation; VT, ventricular tachycardia. (See text for explanation of other trial acronyms.)

Even patients with otherwise asymptomatic AF report lower quality of life compared with subjects in sinus rhythm [82]. Adequate control of ventricular rate and successful maintenance of sinus rhythm can improve quality of life and exercise capacity in AF patients [83, 84].

LV function is often impaired by the irregular, fast ventricular rate and by loss of atrial contractile function and reduced end-diastolic LV filling in patients with AF [8, 36, 85–87]. Either adequate rate-control therapy or maintenance of sinus rhythm [87–90] can improve LV function

Table 29.3 Mortality after diagnosis of atrial fibrillation in epidemiological studies

Study	Number of patients	Follow-up	Mortality risk
Framingam, 1998	5202, age 55–94 years, 612 (11.9%) AF	40 years	All subjects, ACM: 1.5 (1.2–1,8) men 1.9 (1.5–2.2) women No heart disease, ACM: 2.4 (1.8–3.3) men 2.2 (1.6–3.1) women
Manitoba, 1995	3983 male aircrew recruits, age 18–62 years, 299 (7.5%) AF	154,131 person-years	ACM: 1.31; CVM: 1.41
Marshfield Epidemiologic Study Area, 2002	58,820 residents, 577 with AF, age 71 years	4775 person-years	All subjects, ACM: 2.4 (1.9–3.1) Lone AF, ACM: 2.1 (0.96–4.5)
Paris Prospective Study,1999	7746 male civil servants age 43–52 years	27 years	Lone AF, ACM: 1.95 (1.13–3.37) Lone AF, CVM: 4.31 (2.14–8.68)
UK cohort, 2002	1035 AF, 5000 general population controls, 40–89 years	AF; 1898 person-years; controls; 9261 person-years	ACM: 2.5 (2.1–3.0)
Olmsted County, 2007	4618 with AF, age 73 years	5.3 years	All subjects, ACM: 2.08 (2.01–2.16) Excluding first 4 months after diagnosis 1.66 (1.59–1.73)

ACM, all-cause mortality; AF, atrial fibrillation; CVM, cardiovascular mortality.

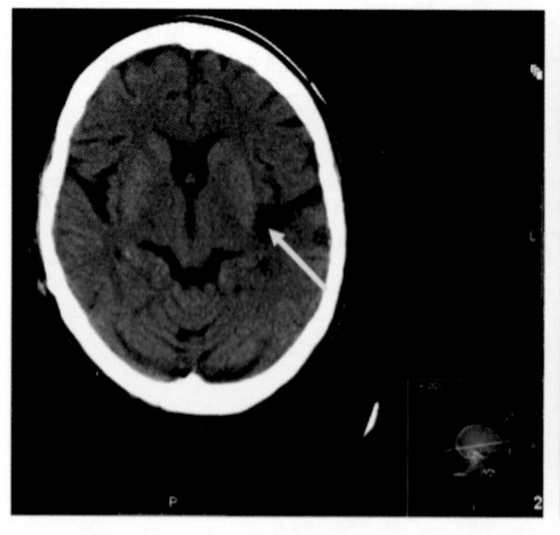

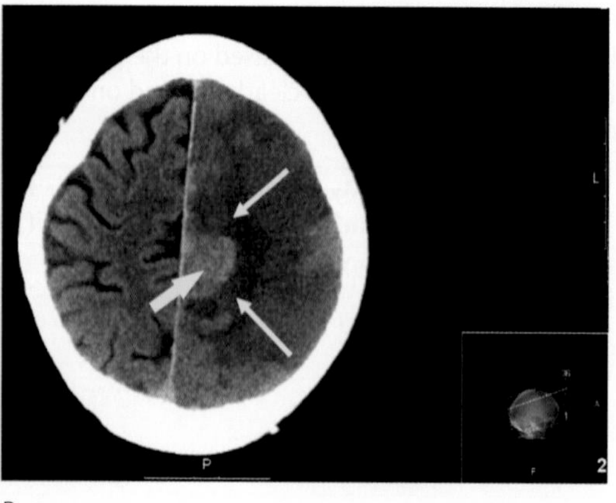

A B

Figure 29.9 A computer tomography image of cerebral infarct (arrow) in a patient with permanent atrial fibrillation and no neurological symptoms (silent infarct) (A). A computer tomography image of acute ischaemic stroke (thin arrows) with subsequent haemorrhagic transformation (thick arrow) (B).

in AF patients. This effect is most visible in patients with a first episode or recent-onset AF. Drugs that prevent progression of LV dysfunction and heart failure can prevent AF (see ➲'Upstream' therapy, p.1113) [34].

Pathophysiological changes that can cause atrial fibrillation

The genesis of AF is complex and multifactorial, unlike many other supraventricular arrhythmias, and is comparable only to the genesis of ventricular fibrillation and sudden death.

Electrical activation of the atria in atrial fibrillation and maintenance of the arrhythmia

The diagnosis of AF is based on irregular ventricular rate and the loss of discernible P waves in the surface ECG (➲Fig. 29.1) [91]. This apparently simple yet often missed ECG-based diagnosis [92] lumps together arrhythmias with completely or partially different mechanisms of initiation and/or maintenance. The ECG pattern of AF can be created by multiple, rapid repetitive atrial foci, single, rapid atrial foci with fibrillatory conduction [93], or re-entrant activity maintained via several simultaneous electrical wave fronts [94].

The simultaneous existence of multiple foci or a single wandering re-entrant electrical wave ('mother rotor') is possible, although less likely in clinical and experimental studies (➲Fig. 29.10). It has been assumed that multiple re-entrant wave fronts maintain AF in the majority of patients [95], but several 'drivers' may be present. Multiple wavelet re-entry requires several (at least two, but in most measurements four to eight) simultaneous meandering wavelets which maintain each other by creating areas of functional conduction block and slow conduction.

One condition that facilitates functional re-entry is a short 'wavelength' of the electrical activation waves, i.e. a short product of its atrial conduction velocity and refractory period. In normal atria activated during sinus rhythm, the wavelength is longer than the size of the atria, thereby precluding re-entrant activation. During AF, the conduction velocity of activation waves is markedly slowed and the action potential duration and refractory period are shortened. These factors shorten atrial wavelength to an extent that allows multiple areas of functional re-entry.

In concordance with the 'wavelength' concept, factors that either shorten the atrial refractory period or slow conduction (i.e. parameters that reduce atrial wavelength) contribute to the maintenance of AF. In long-standing AF or in atria with marked structural changes and conduction inhomogeneities, the number of simultaneous wavelets may be higher and their three-dimensional distribution can be complex [96], possibly secondary to increased 'electrical isolation' between cardiomyocytes and separation of atrial cardiac tissue by fibrotic tissue. Although not proven so far, the available experimental data and many aspects in the epidemiology and treatment of AF can be readily explained by the multiple wavelet hypothesis (➲Fig. 29.10).

Pathophysiological changes in the fibrillating atria

Initiation and maintenance of atrial fibrillation

The aetiology of AF is complex, and several different factors contribute to changes that promote focal atrial activity or one of the different forms of re-entry in the atria.

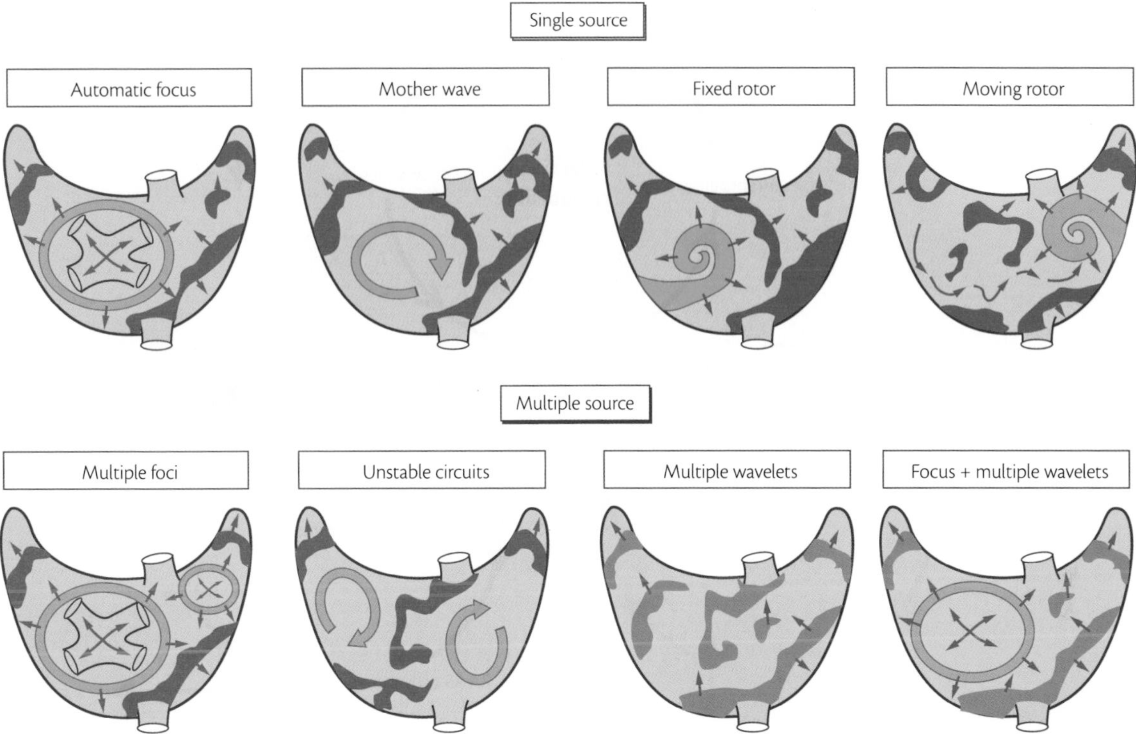

Figure 29.10 Mechanisms of atrial fibrillation.

Several experimental models have helped to dissect AF-induced pathophysiological changes that contribute to the perpetuation of AF. ➲Fig. 29.11 summarizes several of the known vicious circles that contribute to the initiation and perpetuation of AF. In a given patient (or a given experimental model), different pathophysiological changes may have more or less impact. These vicious circles are important because their interruption by therapeutic interventions (drugs, lifestyle changes, or catheter ablation) is probably the main determinant of treatment success for rhythm-control therapies.

Focal activity in the pulmonary veins

Focal ectopic activity in the PVs was first described in patients with AF [93]. Especially in the early phases of AF and in patients with so-called 'lone AF' (i.e. AF without concomitant conditions that might explain the arrhythmia), AF episodes are often initiated by rapid focal electrical activity originating from within the PV, the junction between PVs and posterior LA, and to a lesser extent in other regions of the venous parts of the atria [93]. Abnormal calcium release may be driving these focal discharges [97], although re-entry within the PV myocardium may also contribute to the initiation of 'focal activity' in the PVs [98]. Ablation therapy of AF which targets these focal sources has proven effective in its prevention (see ➲Catheter ablation strategies, p.1121) [99].

Electrical remodelling

The process of AF-induced 'electrical remodelling' was first described in goats with pacing-induced AF (➲Fig. 29.12) [100]. In essence, the atrial myocardium responds to the high atrial rate in the fibrillating atria by shortening of atrial refractoriness and atrial action potential duration. This is most likely a 'cellular survival mechanism' that helps to extrude excess intracellular calcium from the rapidly activated atrial myocardial cells [101]. On the molecular level, an altered expression and regulation of proteins involved in potassium and calcium channels reduces calcium currents and increases potassium currents (➲Fig. 29.13) [102, 103].

In addition to acceleration of repolarization (action-potential shortening), the resting membrane potential is more positive in chronic AF, most likely secondary to a constitutive activation of I_{KACh} [104]. However, shortening of the atrial action potential not only preserves viability during AF, but also renders the atria prone to recurrent AF. The atrial action potential normalizes in the first few weeks, and possibly even in the first few days, after restoration of sinus rhythm.

The concept of electrical remodelling provides a pathophysiological rationale for the use of drugs that prolong the atrial action potential to prevent recurrences of AF after cardioversion, i.e. in atria that underwent the process of electrical remodelling [105–108]. Time-dependent recovery from electrical remodelling in sinus rhythm suggests that

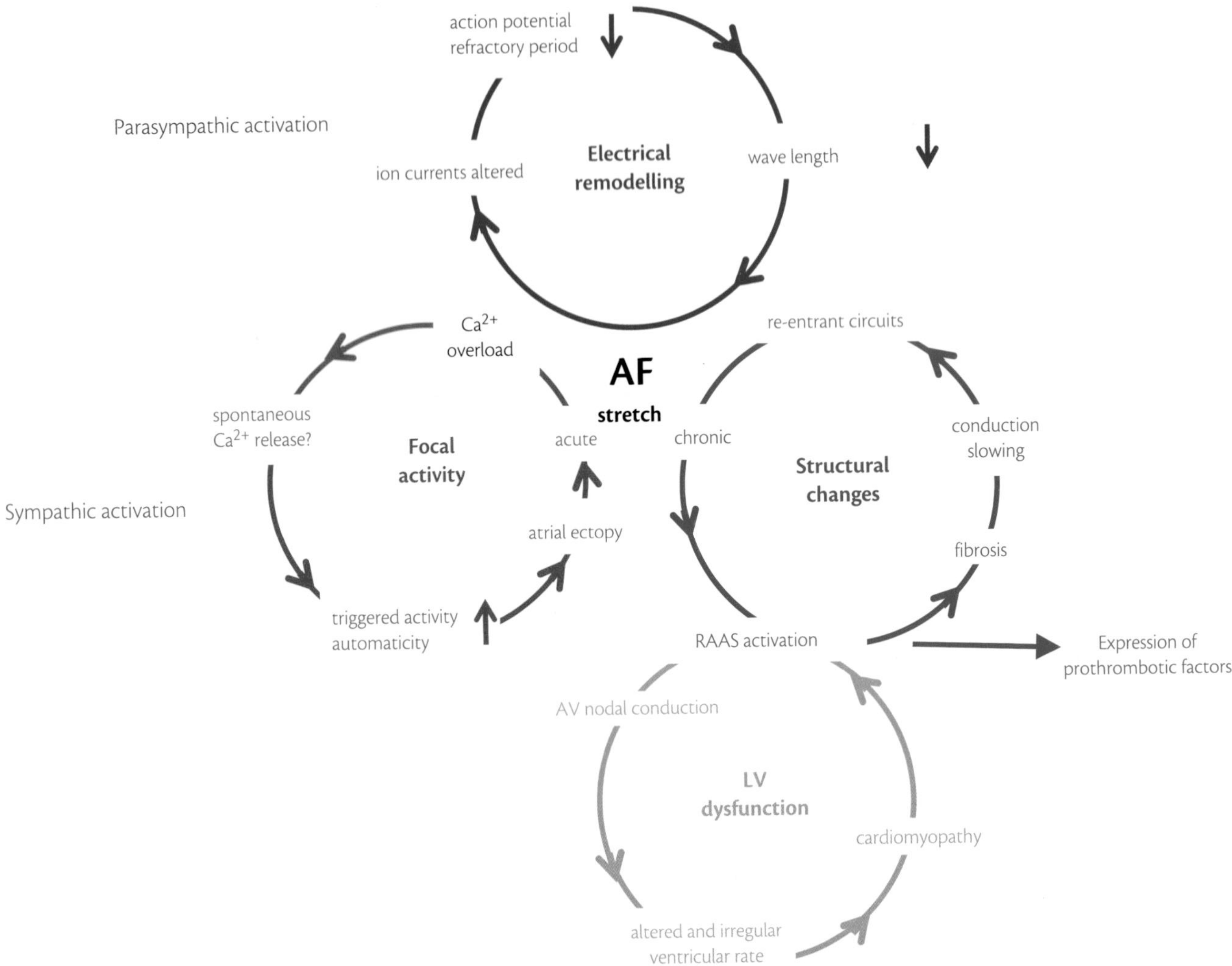

Figure 29.11 Vicious circles that contribute to the genesis of atrial fibrillation. Initiation and perpetuation of atrial fibrillation is caused by multiple factors in the vast majority of patients. Many of these are self-sustaining, i.e. they are part of 'vicious circles' that accelerate the progression of atrial fibrillation with each episode. The figure illustrates four of these vicious circles. Rapid atrial rates, e.g. caused by atrial fibrillation, atrial flutter, or atrial tachycardias, cause intracellular calcium overload. To protect itself against calcium-induced cell death, cardiomyocytes activate a 'survival programme' to extrude as much calcium as possible. This is done by shortening atrial action potential duration and refractoriness ('electrical remodelling'). Although preventing cell death, this mechanism reduces wave length and contributes to atrial fibrillation recurrence after premature atrial activations. Focal activity within the pulmonary veins, a frequent trigger of 'lone' paroxysmal atrial fibrillation, can be caused by stretch within the atrial–atrial fibrillation junction or by calcium load in cardiomyocytes leading to spontaneous calcium release and afterdepolarizations, especially in the presence of sympathetic stimulation. Via calcium load, sympathetic activation, and increased stretch at the LA (left atrial)–PV (pulmonary vein) junction this mechanism is prone to a second vicious circle. Atrial fibrillation-induced structural changes occur already after several hours of atrial fibrillation. Many of these changes are mediated via activation of the renin–angiotensin system due to atrial stretch, atrial pressure increase, and peripheral hypovolemia. Activation of renin–angiotensin–aldosterone system (RAAS) will increase extracellular matrix formation, lead to cardiomyocyte isolation, create localized conduction barriers which will facilitate reentry within the atria, and thereby reduce atrial wave length. Rapid and irregular rate during atrial fibrillation, in conjunction with loss of atrial contractile function, reduce cardiac output and can cause left ventricular (LV) dysfunction. The systemic response to LV dysfunction is, again, RAAS activation, sympathetic activation (with in turn even more rapid ventricular rates), and thereby perpetuation of atrial fibrillation. Last but not least, activation of any of the cellular changes involved in these vicious circles can activate expression of prothrombotic factors in atrial endothelium. As delineated later in the text, therapeutic approaches to disrupt each of these vicious circles exist: electrical remodelling: antiarrhythmic drugs; focal activity: pulmonary vein isolation, structural changes: upstream therapy; LV dysfunction: rate control therapy (and, to some extent, successful rhythm control therapy). Modified with permission from Koebe J, Kirchhof P. Novel non-pharmacological approaches for antiarrhythmic therapy of atrial fibrillation. *Europace* 2008; **10**: 433–7.

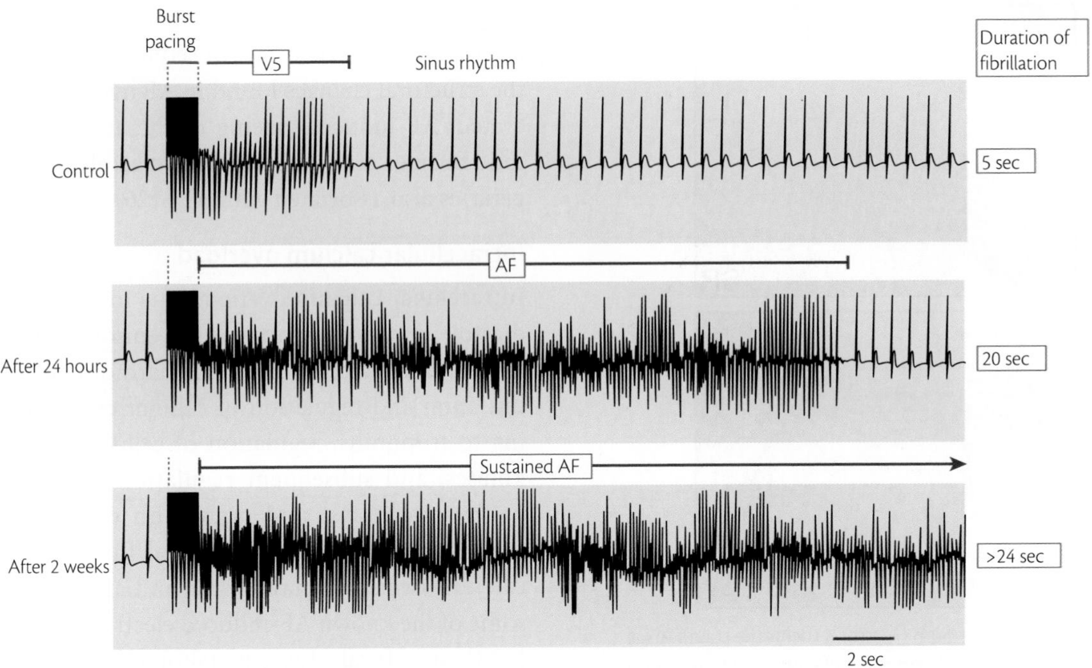

Figure 29.12 Atrial fibrillation 'begets' atrial fibrillation. In the control state a short burst of atrial pacing in this goat model induces a brief episode of rapid atrial fibrillation. Repeated re-induction of atrial fibrillation leads to progressive acceleration of the fibrillatory impulses and longer duration of the arrhythmia. After 2 weeks atrial fibrillation which is induced does not terminate spontaneously. Reproduced with permission from Wijffels MC, Kirchhof CJ, Dorland R, *et al.* Atrial fibrillation begets atrial fibrillation. A study in awake chronically instrumented goats. *Circulation* 1995; **92**: 1954–68.

therapy with ion channel-blocking agents may be stopped once electrical remodelling has been reversed [108].

Atrial fibrillation-induced contractile dysfunction

Continuous electrical reactivation of atrial cardiomyocytes results in reduced duration of electrical diastole, increased calcium influx through the sarcolemmal membrane, increased calcium release from the sarcoplasmic reticulum, and consequently a rapid intracellular calcium overload in the atrial myocardium [109]. The resulting altered expression and function of calcium-handling proteins and the ensuing altered regulation of the contractile apparatus reduces atrial contractile function and increases atrial size [110]. These changes persist for several weeks after restoration of sinus rhythm (atrial stunning)[111]. Contractile dysfunction suggests an important role for intracellular calcium overload in the maintenance of AF [112] and has also been regarded as a reason for anticoagulation in the first weeks after cardioversion [1].

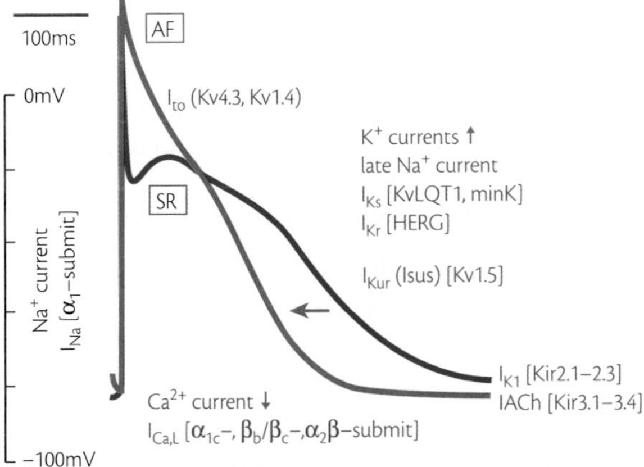

Figure 29.13 Atrial action potential recorded in cardiomyocytes isolated from two patients undergoing open-heart surgery. Patient 1 (blue) had no history of atrial fibrillation. Patient 2 (red) was in atrial fibrillation at the time of the operation. Atrial fibrillation-induced 'electrical remodelling' can be seen as shortening of the action potential and as the less negative resting membrane potential. Abbreviations indicate the main currents that contribute to action potential shortening. Modified with permission from Ravens U, Cerbai E. Role of potassium currents in cardiac arrhythmias. *Europace* 2008; **10**: 1133–7.

Atrial fibrillation-induced structural changes

The relatively high AF recurrence rate in the active-treatment arms of ion channel-blocking drug trials already suggests that electrical remodelling is not the only factor that maintains AF and/or provokes its recurrence. AF induces an increased expression of extracellular matrix proteins and increased atrial fibrosis (➲Fig. 29.14) [113]. These changes result in conduction slowing in the atria, and in electrical isolation of atrial cardiomyocytes, even prior to development of AF [114]. The molecular signalling pathways that mediate these structural changes are not fully understood, but the angiotensin system is activated, sympathetic stimulation is increased, a 'fetal' gene expression programme is activated, and thrombogenic molecules

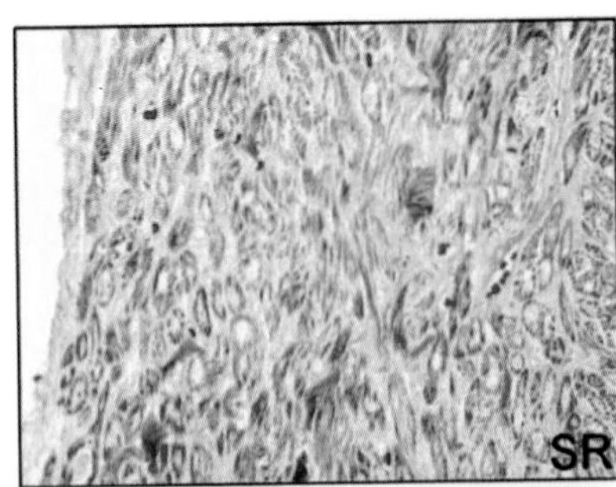

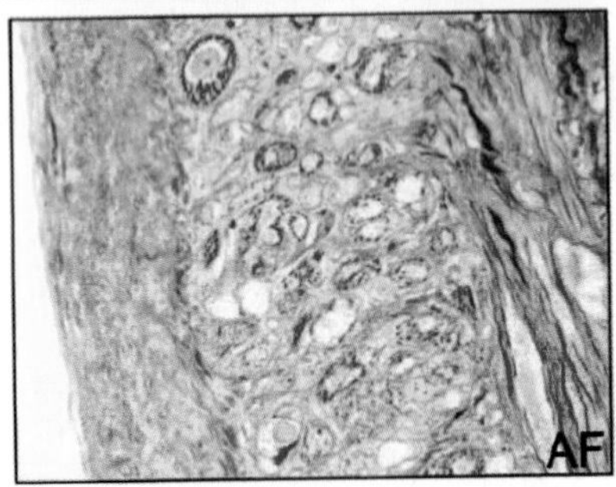

Figure 29.14 Atrial myocardium (Masson's trichrome stain). Atrial fibrillation induces an increased expression of extracellular matrix proteins and increased atrial fibrosis. AF, atrial fibrillation; SR, sinus rhythm. (Courtesy of Andreas Göette, University hospital Magdeburg, Germany.)

are expressed in the endothelium in AF [115]. Inhibition of either the ACE or the angiotensin II receptor in the heart can prevent some of these AF-induced changes [116].

The lack of intracellular ATP donators, possibly due to mitochondrial dysfunction, may contribute to extracellular matrix formation, cellular dysfunction, and potentially to cell death, and de-differentiation of atrial myocardium [115, 117]. This is one cause of major metabolomic changes in atrial tissue from AF patients [118] and animal models of AF [119]. The antifibrillatory effect of ACE inhibitors, ARBs, and statins is most likely explained by the effects of these drugs on AF-induced structural changes. Whether inflammation of the atrial myocardium [120, 121], identifiable by increased content of inflammatory cells in atrial tissue, and in part by increased C-reactive protein (CRP) levels in the blood of patients with AF [122, 123], is an independent process or not, is unknown.

Ageing and atrial fibrillation

The prevalence of AF is clearly age-dependent (see ➲Prevalence of atrial fibrillation, p.1070). Ageing is associated with an increased isolation of cardiomyocytes through altered expression of connexins and increased development of fibrous septa between atrial muscle fibres [124]. Denatured atrial natriuretic peptide creates amyloid-like deposits that also lead to fibre separation. AF-induced mitochondrial DNA deletions which are associated with altered mitochondrial energy production are comparable to the DNA alterations found in ageing myocardium [125]. In this regard, ageing is associated with some of the changes that are found as a structural consequence of AF. Conversely, the structural changes found in AF may be a form of accelerated 'AF-induced' ageing of the atrial myocardium. A mild form of genetically conferred accelerated ageing (progeria) is also associated with AF [126].

Intracellular calcium overload

Intracellular calcium overload due to the loss of electrical diastole occurs even after short episodes of AF. Calcium has several major roles in the cardiomyocyte, including initiation and regulation of cellular contraction by binding to troponins, regulation of cellular proteins, protein kinases, and subsequent regulation of intracellular signalling pathways, and regulation of sarcolemmal and sarcoplasmic reticulum electrical function. Intracellular calcium overload may be the initial event that triggers some of the known AF-induced electrical [127], contractile [128], structural [129], metabolomic, and inflammatory changes [130].

What causes the first atrial fibrillation episode?

In some patients, especially in patients without concomitant conditions, focal sources of electrical activity (often in the PVs) are the most likely cause of the first AF episode. Some of these patients, however, never develop sustained AF [18], while others present with sustained AF from the start. The likelihood of sustained forms of AF is almost linearly related to the number of predisposing conditions in the majority of (often elderly) patients with AF. Many of these factors, e.g. hypertension, diabetes and obesity, or heart failure, are present prior to the initial diagnosis of AF. The factors that precede AF may provide attractive therapeutic targets for the preventative treatment of the arrhythmias [131].

Atrial stressors that predispose to atrial fibrillation

Some of the pathophysiological responses to 'atrial stressors' that predispose to AF have been delineated in experimental studies: dogs in which ventricular pacing induces heart failure are prone to conduction slowing and inducible AF [132, 133]. In a sheep model of early-onset arterial hypertension, inducible AF was associated with electrical isolation of atrial cardiomyocytes, increased formation of extracellular matrix, and conduction disturbances without evidence for action-potential shortening [114]. Chronic dilatation of the atria secondary to chronic pressure and/or volume overload of the atria may induce these structural changes that appear to precede AF, possibly related to AF in the setting of severe valvular heart disease or heart failure [12, 134, 135].

Table 29.4 Genetic causes of atrial fibrillation—see text for details

Inherited cardiomyopathies associated with AF			
Cardiac abnormality	Genetic defect	… found in	AF prevalence (rough estimate)
Brugada syndrome	Loss-of-function *SCN5A* mutations (10–15% of patients)	Familial clusters	10–20%
Long QT syndrome	Late gain-of-function *SCN5A* and loss-of-function K channel mutations, among others	Familial clusters	5–10%
Short QT syndrome	Gain-of-function K channel mutations	Familial clusters	70%
Catecholaminergic VT	Loss-of-function ryanodine receptor mutation	Rare families	
Hypertrophic cardiomyopathy	Sarcomeric proteins	Unselected patient cohorts	5–15%
Wolff–Parkinson–White syndrome and abnormally LVH	*PRKAG* mutations	Family clusters	
Holt–Oram syndrome with AF	*TBX5* mutations (regulatory gene)	Family clusters	
Gene defects associated with AF			
Type of AF	Genetic defect identified	… found in	Associated with AF in
'Lone' AF	Loss-of-function *SCN5A* mutations	'Lone' AF cohorts	5% of 'lone' AF patients
AF and heart failure	*SCN5A* mutation	One large family	Rare forms
'Lone' AF	Gain-of-function K channel mutations	Single families	Rare families, associated with short QT syndrome
'Lone' AF	Loss-of-function K channel polymorphisms	Large association study	Rare families, associated with long QT syndrome
'Lone' AF	Loss-of-function Kv1.5 mutation (I_{Kur})	Selected patients	Rare patients
'Lone' AF	Somatic connexion 40 mutations	Unrelated patients	Not known (requires atrial tissue for testing)s
'Lone' AF	Frameshift (loss-of-function) ANP mutation	Familial clustering	Not known
All types of AF	*PITX2* polymorphism (involved in pulmonary and cardiac development)	Genome-wide association	Populations (Iceland and elsewhere)

ANP, atrial natriuretic peptide; LVH, left ventricular hypertrophy.

High-level endurance sports may be sufficient to predispose to AF, most likely via chronic atrial dilatation [58, 136]. Atrial ischaemia may also contribute to the initiation of AF. In another study in dogs with 'spontaneous' sustained AF, action-potential shortening was found prior to AF, suggesting that these electrical changes can also form prior to AF [109]. It is conceivable that many of the vicious circles mentioned earlier (➲Fig. 29.11) are activated prior to AF and contribute to its initiation. Retrospective analyses from randomized studies [34] suggest that structural changes that precede AF may be a reasonable target for primary prevention of AF.

Genetic factors associated with atrial fibrillation

AF, especially early-onset AF, can be clustered in families, and associations between familial AF and the first gene loci were described over a decade ago [137]. The past few years have brought about many reports of different genetic alterations in atrial fibrillation (➲Table 29.4).

Genetic alterations found in inherited cardiomyopathies (see ➲Chapter 9)

Sudden death and ventricular fibrillation in the young are often caused by inherited cardiomyopathies [138]. Many of the proteins that are mutated in these diseases are also expressed in the atria, and the same electrical abnormalities which are arrhythmogenic in the ventricles can cause AF. Patients with short QT syndrome, i.e. a genetic cause for short cardiac action potentials and a QT interval <0.33s, are at high risk for AF, e.g. detected by inappropriate defibrillator discharges [49, 50]. The first identified mutation found in a family with AF affects a gene that is also altered in the short QT syndrome (*KCNQ1*) [48]. Short QT syndrome can probably be considered a 'genetic' cause of atrial action potential shortening (see ➲Electrical remodelling, p.1079).

More recently, several groups have found an increased risk of AF in patients with long QT syndrome [41, 43, 46], polymorphisms associated with QT prolongation co-associate with AF [139], and mutations in long QT syndrome-causing genes are found in approximately 5% of patients with 'idiopathic' AF [44]. The limited available data suggest that prolongation of the atrial action potential and after-depolarizations cause AF in these patients [46] (29.1). Similar mechanisms may be present in patients with a nonsense mutation in the Kv1.5 gene responsible for the 'atrial-specific' potassium current I_{Kur} [135].

The pathophysiological factors that cause AF and other supraventricular arrhythmias in Brugada syndrome are less well established, but the prevalence of AF is high [42]. It is conceivable that the combination of a 'Brugada-type' ECG with AF is indicative of patients with a sodium channel mutation [44, 140], and that either conduction slowing in the atria [141–143] and/or prolongation of the atrial action potential and after-depolarizations ('atrial torsade de pointes') [46, 144] cause AF in such patients.

Sodium channel mutations have also been identified in patients with 'lone' AF [44, 145] and in a large family suffering from heart failure and atrial fibrillation [146]. Mutations in the cardiac ryanodine receptor, the calcium release channel in the sarcoplasmic reticulum, have been associated with AF and catecholaminergic VT [147]. Whether AF in hypertrophic cardiomyopathy is mediated via electrical changes, e.g. secondary to altered calcium handling by the mutated sarcomeric proteins, or a consequence of the increased atrial pressure and volume load in obstructive forms of the disease, has not been convincingly studied. A small group of patients suffer from a genetic abnormality in the *PRKAG* protein. Clinically, these patients carry a combination of AF, ventricular pre-excitation, and atypical LV hypertrophy [148, 149].

Other genetic abnormalities associated with atrial fibrillation

Somatic, i.e. 'heart-restricted' mutations in connexin 40 have been identified in a small series of patients in whom atrial tissue could be genetically studied [150], and a frameshift mutation in the gene coding for the atrial natriuretic peptide (ANP) [151] has recently been identified in patients with 'lone' AF. Hence, either genetically conferred conduction disturbances or genetically-conferred altered ANP signalling and/or hypertension may cause AF.

In addition to these genetic alterations with more or less known functional consequences, a population-wide study has associated a common variant in the *PITX2* gene with AF [152]. This finding was replicated in other cohorts.

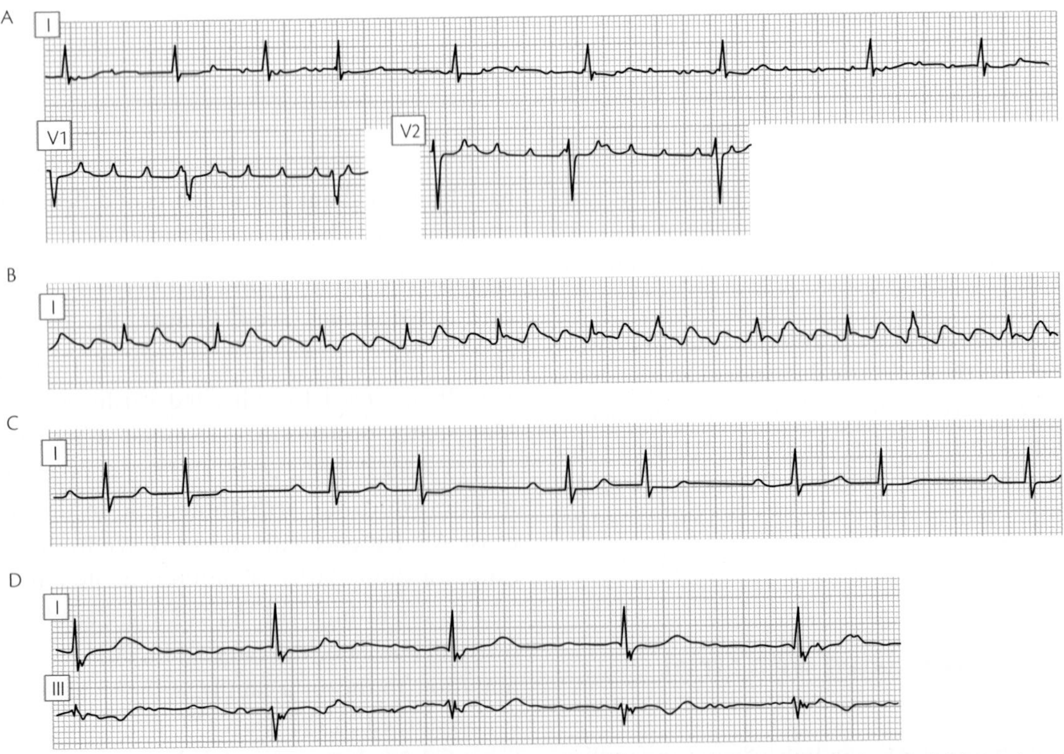

Figure 29.15 Atrial tachycardia (A), atrial flutter (B), and frequent atrial premature beats (C) that may mimic the irregular RR intervals typical for atrial fibrillation. Note first-degree atrioventricular block in (C). Atrial fibrillation may coexist with complete heart block, particularly, in elderly, and result in a regular slow rhythm (D).

PITX2 is an important regulator of cardiac development including formation of the LA and pulmonary tissue, and a part of the PVs [153, 154]. Another study found an association with TBX5, another regulator of cardiac development, and AF in patients with the Holt–Oram syndrome [155], and a transgenic model with enhanced atrial activity of TGFβ1 predisposes to AF, atrial fibrosis and conduction slowing [156–159].

Initial evaluation of patients with atrial fibrillation

Detection of atrial fibrillation

An irregular pulse should always raise suspicion of AF. The ECG diagnosis of AF follows simple criteria: AF is characterized by complete irregularity of RR intervals ('arrhythmia absoluta') and loss of discernible P waves (➲Fig. 29.1). As the anterior right atrium and the right atrial appendage often show organized atrial activation during AF, small atrial waves may be present in the right precordial leads in AF. Any arrhythmia that has the ECG characteristics of AF and lasts for 30s or longer should be considered AF [8], and episodes of at least 5-min duration are associated with an increased mortality in retrospective analyses [160]. The risk of AF-related thromboembolic complications (e.g. stroke) is not different between short AF episodes and sustained forms of the arrhythmia [76].

Differential diagnosis

Several supraventricular arrhythmias, most notably atrial tachycardias and atrial flutter, but also forms of frequent atrial ectopy, may conduct to the ventricles producing rapid irregular RR intervals, thereby mimicking AF (➲Fig. 29.15A–C). Usually, AF has an atrial cycle length of <200ms [46, 161, 162], while most atrial tachycardias and flutters are slower. This may be helpful for the differentiation of AF from atrial flutter or atrial tachycardia. Atrial cycle length during AF may be longer in patients receiving conduction-slowing or action potential-prolonging drugs, e.g. sodium channel blockers, sotalol, or amiodarone.

The differential diagnosis of slow AF includes severe sinus node dysfunction with changing ectopic pacemakers and unusual forms of higher degree AV block. AF may coexist with complete heart block, particularly in elderly patients, when the ventricular escape rhythm is often regular (➲Fig. 29.15D). These conditions can usually be discerned from the 12-lead ECG by a careful search for occasional, but definite, P waves which excludes the presence of AF.

To differentiate the common diagnosis of AF from the rare other rhythms with irregular RR intervals, a 12-lead ECG during the arrhythmia is usually needed. Therefore, any episode of suspected AF should be recorded by a 12-lead ECG of sufficient duration and quality to evaluate P waves. Occasionally, especially when the ventricular rate is high, AV nodal blocking techniques such as a Valsalva manoeuvre, carotid massage, or intravenous adenosine administration during the ECG recording can help to unmask P waves.

Silent atrial fibrillation

Silent AF may be found incidentally during routine physical examinations, pre-operative assessments, occupation assessments, or population surveys. The prevalence of sustained silent AF in epidemiology studies is believed to be about 25–30% of AF patients [163].

In some cases, silent AF is diagnosed only after a complication such as stroke or heart failure has occurred. Thus, in the Framingham Study database, AF was found incidentally in about 18% of admissions for stroke and subsequently diagnosed within 2 weeks in another 4.4% [164]. Therefore, a thorough screening for AF is needed in patients with such complications. Given that detection of AF has therapeutic consequences (e.g. anticoagulation), prolonged Holter ECG monitoring is recommended in such patients with suspected asymptomatic AF.

Wider use of implantable rhythm-control devices, such as pacemakers and cardioverter defibrillators, has shown that a significantly greater proportion of patients has silent AF than was previously thought. About 50–60% of patients may have unsuspected episodes of the arrhythmia, almost half of which last >48 hours [165]. The use of implanted monitors, ECG garments, or patient-operated ECG systems may allow expansion of the monitoring period for suspected AF [8].

Initial management of patients with atrial fibrillation

The acute management of AF patients aims to ameliorate symptoms and to estimate AF-associated risk. This can be remembered by the acronym SHS (Symptoms, Heart rate, Stroke risk assessment). Asymptomatic or mildly symptomatic AF does not require urgent diagnostic or therapeutic steps, but should result in a thorough risk evaluation. The EHRA symptom score and $CHADS_2$ stroke risk score should be estimated (➲Table 29.1). A thorough clinical evaluation is recommended to exclude other causes of acute dyspnoea. Symptomatic patients may require urgent rate control or cardioversion.

Clinical history

A complete diagnosis of AF includes analysis of associated medical conditions (see ➲ Predisposing clinical conditions, p.1073) and stroke risk factors. This will guide arrhythmia therapy as well as antithrombotic treatment. In addition, the clinician should assess bleeding risk if antithrombotic treatment is indicated. In symptomatic patients, vagal, adrenergic, and other potential trigger mechanisms should be considered. AF should be classified as first onset, paroxysmal, persistent, or permanent (➲ Fig. 29.4). AF may be symptomatic and asymptomatic in the same patient at different imes [163]. Symptoms may relate to the arrhythmia itself, or to the complications of AF, or the associated medical condition.

Vagal AF [166] is a paroxysmal arrhythmia that usually occurs in the evening, at night, or during weekends, particularly after heavy meals and possibly alcohol consumption. Usually sinus bradycardia or sinus pauses precede the development of the AF and during the AF the heart rate is relatively slow.

Adrenergic AF, on the other hand, is less common, occurs during the day and is provoked by physical or mental stress, and may sometimes be triggered by a stress test. An acceleration of sinus rhythm usually anticipates the arrhythmia and the ventricular rate during the AF tends to be rapid. Some patients have both autonomic forms of AF and many paroxysms are not classically one or the other.

Physical examination

AF presents with an irregular pulse, irregular jugular venous pulsations, and variations in the loudness of the first heart sound and in systolic blood pressure. There may be a deficit between number of heart beats and number of peripheral pulsations, especially when the ventricular rate is rapid. Signs of valvular heart disease, ventricular dilatation, and heart failure may be found.

Investigations

The **12-lead ECG** (➲ Chapter 2) should, in addition to the detection of AF, also be screened for signs of acute myocardial infarction and other signs for structural heart disease (e.g. prior myocardial infarction, LV hypertrophy, bundle branch block or ventricular pre-excitation, signs of cardiomyopathy or ischaemia). In sinus rhythm LA conduction delay is often present , and rare cardiac abnormalities may occasionally be found (🎥 29.4).

The ECG may also show other abnormal sinus node function, atrial arrhythmias (➲ Fig. 29.15A–C) that may trigger AF, or ventricular arrhythmias that may be a sign of heart disease. It is always important to distinguish aberrant conduction from VTs, especially when using antiarrhythmic drugs (➲ Fig. 29.16).

The **chest radiograph** may help to reveal cardiac enlargement (➲ Fig. 29.8) but is most helpful in detecting intrinsic pulmonary disease and abnormalities of the pulmonary vasculature as in heart failure and pulmonary hypertension.

Echocardiography should be performed at least once in all AF patients. It is indispensable for the management of AF-associated medical conditions. In addition, markers of thrombosis (spontaneous echo contrast) or even a thrombus may be found. Risk markers for stroke include LV hypertrophy or dysfunction, LA enlargement, and low-flow velocities in the LA appendage (LAA). Also, aortic plaques are associated with a high stroke risk. New technical developments have improved the performance of transthoracic echocardiography but for detection of thrombi (e.g. for echo-guided cardioversion) transoesophageal echocardiography is the current standard [1] (➲ Fig. 29.17; 🎥 29.5).

Laboratory evaluation may be limited to thyroid function tests, serum electrolytes, haemoglobin levels, a serum creatinine measurement, analysis for proteinuria, and a test for diabetes mellitus (usually a fasting glucose measurement). Markers of heart failure (BNP) or inflammation (CRP)

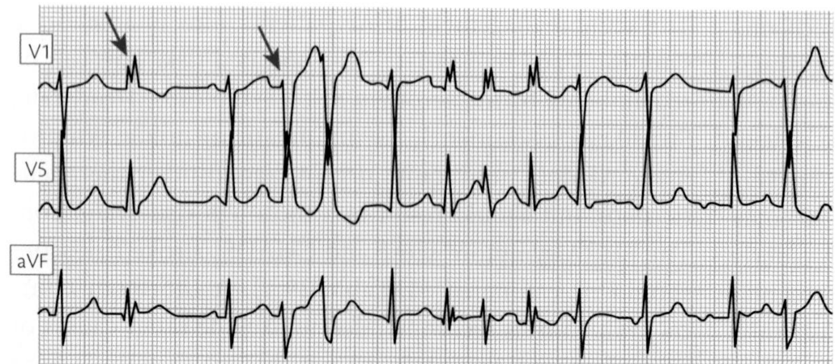

Figure 29.16 Holter strip of modified leads V1, V5, and aVF showing atrial fibrillation initiated by the second atrial premature beat (arrows) with left and right aberrant conduction in a patient treated with sotalol for paroxysmal atrial fibrillation. Note the long–short RR sequence at initiation of aberrant conduction. Sotalol may have enhanced onset of aberrancy in this case due to prolongation of refractoriness in the Purkinje system.

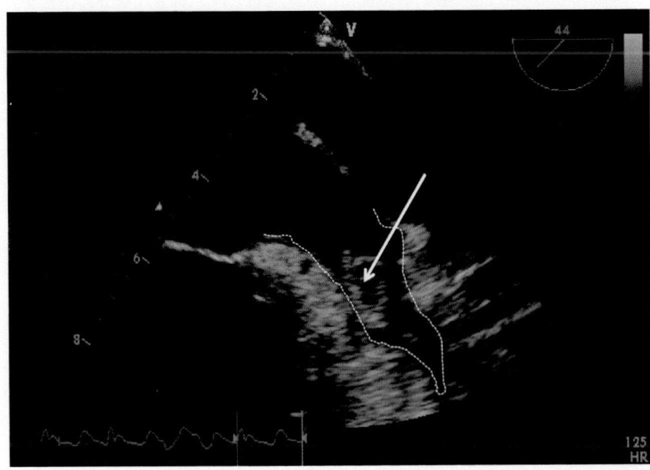

Figure 29.17 Transoesophageal echocardiogram. This demonstrates a ball thrombus (arrow) in the mouth of the left atrial appendage (dotted line). (Courtesy of Dr Andreas Göette, University Hospital Magdeburg, Germany.)

or infection may be useful. Thyroid and hepatic function should be assessed when treating patients with amiodarone.

Holter monitoring or event recorders may be used in order to establish the diagnosis of AF. In patients with an implanted device (pacemaker, implantable cardioverter defibrillator, or implantable loop recorder) the logging functions in the device may be very helpful. If patients remain symptomatic with palpitations or reduced exercise tolerance despite normal resting heart rate, the adequacy of rate control may be checked with Holter (or exercise testing in fit patients). AF may start during sinus bradycardia or tachycardia, with single or bouts of atrial ectopic beats, while the start of AF with a supraventricular tachycardia or transitions between AF and atrial flutter may also be seen. Identification of these initiating mechanisms may guide treatment, e.g. vagolytic or beta-blocking agents, atrial pacing or catheter ablation of focal AF or other initiating arrhythmias (see ➲Pacemaker and defibrillator therapy, p.1115). Although the AF burden (total duration or percentage of time in AF) can be measured, its clinical relevance is uncertain.

Exercise testing is useful in patients with permanent AF who remain symptomatic despite adequate rate control at rest. The test may reveal an excessive heart rate rise during the lower stages of exercise, thereby limiting exercise tolerance due to dyspnoea, fatigue, or palpitations. In these cases, rate-control drugs may be targeted to the heart rate during a lower level of exercise. Exercise testing may be useful in detecting ischaemic heart disease, which has consequences for antiarrhythmic treatment of AF. Finally, exercise testing may be used to evaluate the safety of antiarrhythmic drug treatment, e.g. for detecting excessive QRS widening on class IC drugs.

Electrophysiological evaluation may be needed in selected cases, especially in patients in whom other arrhythmias, sick sinus syndrome, or a focal origin is suspected. Many of these patients may receive catheter ablation or a pacemaker.

Antithrombotic therapy for atrial fibrillation

The risk of stroke- and thromboembolism-related AF has long been recognized. Independent studies, performed before the time when anticoagulation became recommended for these patients, verify a relative risk increase of 2.3–6.9 for patients in AF without signs of rheumatic mitral valve disease (so-called non-valvular AF) compared with arrhythmia-free controls [167]. In valvular AF, for example when AF is related to rheumatic mitral valvular disease, this risk of thromboembolism is increased 17-fold [168]. The risks of thromboembolism in non-valvular AF are not homogeneous, being related to the presence of other clinical risk factors.

Risk factors for stroke

Cohort data from one epidemiological study (Framingham) and non-warfarin arms of clinical trials have identified clinical and echocardiographic risk factors that can be related to an increased risk of stroke [167]. However, these risk factors represent what was prospectively documented in these studies, as (for example) peripheral artery disease was not systematically documented in the clinical trials.

The systematic review conducted as part of the United Kingdom National Institute for Health and Clinical Excellence (NICE) national clinical guidelines for AF management, identified a history of stroke or TIA (or thromboembolism), older age, hypertension, and structural heart disease (LV dysfunction or hypertrophy) as good predictors of stroke risk in AF patients [169]. In this overview, the evidence regarding diabetes mellitus, female gender, and other characteristics were less consistent in the AF population per se, although diabetes is regarded as an important risk for stroke generally.

In a systematic review of stroke risk factors in AF by the Stroke Risk in Atrial Fibrillation Working Group, prior stroke/TIA/thromboembolism (relative risk (RR) 2.5, averaging 10% per year), increasing age (RR 1.5 per decade), a history of hypertension (RR 2.0), and diabetes mellitus (RR 1.7) were found to be the most consistent independent risk factors [170]. Again, female sex was inconsistently associated with stroke risk, whereas the relevance of heart failure or CAD was considered 'inconclusive'.

Patients with paroxysmal AF should be regarded as having a similar stroke risk compared to persistent and permanent AF, in the presence of risk factors [171]. Patients with 'lone AF', that is, those with non-valvular AF aged <60 years and who have no clinical history or echocardiographic evidence of cardiovascular disease carry a very low cumulative stroke risk, estimated to be 1.3% over 15 years [18, 172]. In this group, cerebrovascular events occurred at the same rate in patients with a paroxysmal form of AF and in patients who progressed to permanent AF. All patients with lone AF who had a cerebrovascular event had developed at least 1 risk factor for thromboembolism (hypertension, heart failure, or diabetes) and the majority were not taking antiplatelet agents or anticoagulants at the time of stroke. Thus, the probability of stroke in young patients with lone AF appears to increase only after many years of disease (at least 25 years), with advancing age or development of hypertension. These observations emphasize the importance of re-assessment of risk factors for stroke over time.

The presence of moderate–severe LV systolic dysfunction on transthoracic echocardiography is the only independent echocardiographic risk factor for stroke on multivariate analysis [173]. On transoesophageal echocardiography, the presence of LA thrombus (➲Fig. 29.17), complex aortic plaques, spontaneous echo-contrast, and low LAA velocity on transoesophageal echocardiography have been suggested as predictors of stroke and thromboembolism [168].

➲Table 29.5 presents the risk categories for stroke or systemic embolism for the patient with non-valvular AF and additional risk factors.

'Definitive' risk factors (previously referred to as 'high risk' risk factors) are those that have been associated with an increased risk of stroke and thromboembolism, such as previous stroke, or TIA, or thromboembolism, the elderly (aged ≥75), or valvular heart disease (mitral stenosis or prosthetic heart valves).

'Combination' risk factors (previously referred to as 'moderate risk' risk factors) are heart failure (especially moderate–severe LV dysfunction, defined arbitrarily as ejection fraction ≤40%), hypertension, or diabetes. Note that risk factors are cumulative, and the simultaneous presence of two or more 'combination' risk factors would justify a high enough stroke risk to require anticoagulation.

Less validated **'combination' risk factors** (previously referred to as 'less validated risk factors') have a less robust evidence-base link for stroke and thromboembolism risk, and include female gender, age 65–74 years and vascular disease (specifically, myocardial infarction, as well as complex aortic plaque and peripheral artery disease). The available evidence is controversial as to whether thyrotoxic AF is an independent risk factor for stroke compared to other causes of AF. Thus, antithrombotic therapies should be chosen based on the presence of validated stroke risk factors.

The identification of stroke clinical risk factors has led to the publication of various stroke risk schemes. The simplest and most validated is the $CHADS_2$ (Cardiac failure, Hypertension, Age, Diabetes, Stroke doubled) score, as shown in ➲Table 29.1. The $CHADS_2$ risk index is based on a point system in which 2 points are assigned for a history of stroke or TIA and 1 point each is assigned for age >75 years, a history of hypertension, diabetes, or recent cardiac failure. As shown in ➲Table 29.6, there is a clear relation between $CHADS_2$ score and stroke rate [174]. The original validation of this schema classified a $CHADS_2$ score of 0 as low risk, 1–2 as moderate risk, and >2 as high risk.

The Stroke in AF Working Group [175] performed a comparison of 12 published risk stratification schemes to predict stroke in patients with non-valvular AF and concluded that there were substantial, clinically relevant differences among published schemes designed to stratify stroke

Table 29.5 Risk factors for stroke and thromboembolism in atrial fibrillation

'Definitive' risk factors	'Combination' risk factors	
Previous stroke, TIA, or systemic embolus	Heart failure or moderate–severe LV dysfunction (e.g. LVEF ≤40%)	Female gender
Age ≥75 years	Hypertension	Age 65–74 years
Mitral stenosis	Diabetes mellitus	Vascular disease*
Prosthetic heart valve**		

LV, left ventricular; LVEF, left ventricular ejection fraction (as documented by echocardiography, radionuclide ventriculography, cardiac catheterization, cardiac MRI, etc.); TIA, transient ischaemic attack. In patients with thyrotoxicosis, antithrombotic therapy should be chosen based on the presence of other stroke risk factors, as listed earlier.

* 'Vascular disease' refers to myocardial infarction, complex aortic plaque, carotid disease, peripheral artery disease, etc. ** If mechanical valve, target VKA therapy to international normalized ratio (INR) >2.5.

Table 29.6 CHADS$_2$ score and stroke rate

Patients (N = 1733)	Adjusted stroke rate (%/year)* (95% CI)	CHADS$_2$ score
120	1.9 (1.2–3.0)	0
463	2.8 (2.0–3.8)	1
523	4.0 (3.1–5.1)	2
337	5.9 (4.6–7.3)	3
220	8.5 (6.3–11.1)	4
65	12.5 (8.2–17.5)	5
5	18.2 (10.5–27.4)	6

* The adjusted stroke rate was derived from the multivariate analysis assuming no aspirin usage. Adapted with permission from Gage BF, Waterman AD, Shannon W, *et al.* Validation of clinical classification schemes for predicting stroke; results from the National Registry of Atrial Fibrillation. *JAMA* 2001; **285**: 2864–70.

risk in patients with AF. Most had modest predictive value in predicting stroke (c-statistic of approximately 0.6).

Similarly, it has been reported that the published stroke risk schemes had only fair discriminating ability, with c-statistics ranging from 0.56–0.62 [176]; also, the proportion of patients assigned to individual risk categories varied widely across the schemes, where the proportion considered high risk ranged from 16.4–80.4%. The CHADS$_2$ score categorized most subjects as 'moderate risk' and had a c-statistic of 0.58 to predict stroke in the whole cohort.

Nonetheless, especially given the observed rates of inadequate oral anticoagulation in AF patients, the CHADS$_2$ score is currently the most validated, simple system to give some initial estimate of stroke risk in AF patients. Other, as of now, less validated, risk factors for stroke, and estimators for bleeding risk, need to be applied with clinical judgement to decide optimal antithrombotic therapy in patients at 'intermediate risk' for stroke.

Thrombogenesis in atrial fibrillation

The risk of stroke or systemic embolism in patients with non-valvular AF is linked to a number of underlying pathophysiological mechanisms [177].

'Flow abnormalities' in AF are evident by stasis within the LA, with reduced LAA flow velocities and visualized as spontaneous echo-contrast on transoesophageal echocardiography. The LAA is a blind pocket, and inside, it is markedly trabeculated (➲Fig. 29.18A). The more the outflow velocity from the LAA decreases, the higher the risk for development of thrombi within its cavity [178]. The LAA volume has been measured by a cast technique in a necropsy study and found to vary between individuals, ranging between 0.7–19.2ml (➲Fig. 29.18B) [179]. There is also marked variability in the size of the LAA orifice (5–27mm) and the maximal diameter (10–40mm). The LAA of subjects with verified AF had generally larger dimensions than in those known to have been free from the arrhythmia. Persistence and permanence of AF is followed by structural remodelling [180], further depressing the function of the LAA.

'Vessel wall abnormalities'—essentially, anatomical and structural abnormalities—in AF include progressive atrial dilatation, endocardial denudation, and oedematous/fibroelastic infiltration of the extracellular matrix. Indeed, the LAA is the dominant source of embolism in AF patients [181] being the embolic source in 91% when AF is of non-valvular origin. ➲Fig. 29.17 illustrates a transoesophageal view of an LAA hosting a thrombus.

Finally, 'abnormalities of blood constituents' are well described in AF, and include haemostatic and platelet activation, as well as inflammation and growth factor abnormalities [177]. The presence of this 'triad' of abnormalities of blood flow, vessel wall abnormalities, and abnormalities of blood constituents, results in the fulfilment of Virchow's triad for thrombogenesis, and are in keeping with a

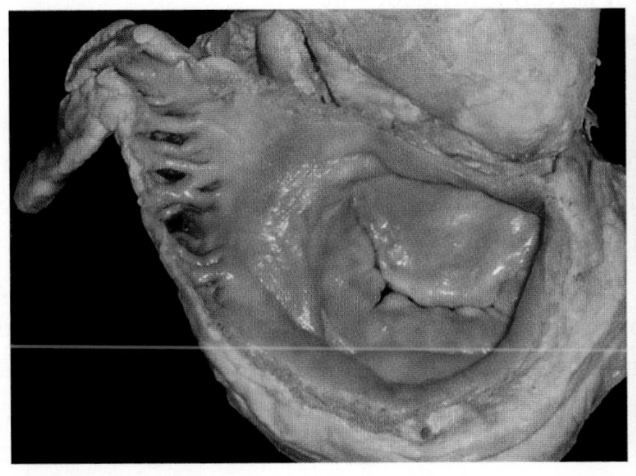
A

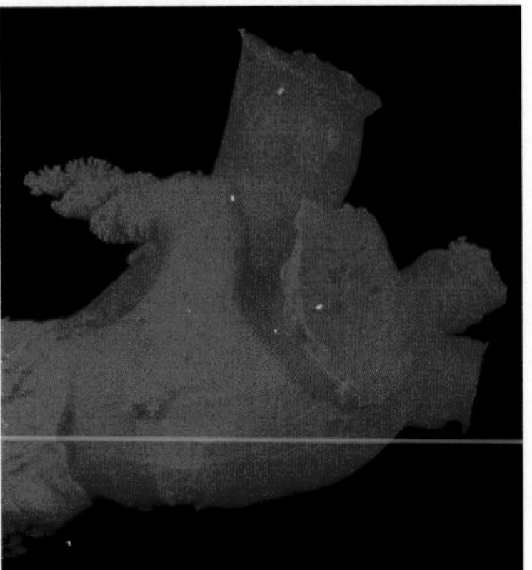
B

Figure 29.18 Left atrium cut open (A). Exposed are the mitral valve and the trabeculated atrial portion of the left atrial wall. The left atrial appendage volume has been measured by a cast technique in a necropsy study (B). It is found to vary between individuals, ranging between 0.7–19.2mL. (Courtesy of Prof. SY Ho, Royal Brompton Hospital, UK.)

prothrombotic or hypercoagulable state in AF, as first proposed in 1995 [182].

Embolic targets

An embolus originating from a fibrillating LA may follow the bloodstream to any part of the body. However, the incidence of stroke and of a clinically evident systemic embolism in non-valvular AF differs markedly from the proportion of blood flowing to the brain and to the rest of the body. Thus, the stroke rate is ten times higher than the rate of systemic embolism in patients with non-valvular AF who have not received any anti-thrombotic treatment. In one study of patients with non-valvular AF with incident peripheral embolism, small emboli are more likely to lodge in the cerebral circulation as a result of hydrodynamic, anatomic, and physical factors related to AF [183]. However, advanced age, atrial enlargement and other comorbidities may result in the formation of 'larger thrombi' per se which may bypass the carotid orifice merely as a function of size. Of note, 'silent' embolism is likely to be more common in the systemic circulation, although this may also occur in cerebral vessels [79, 184].

Antithrombotic therapy for atrial fibrillation

Numerous clinical trials have provided an extensive evidence base for the use of antithrombotic therapy in AF [168, 185].

The $CHADS_2$ score should be used as an initial, rapid, and easily memorable means of assessing stroke risk, particularly suited to primary care and non-specialists. In patients with a $CHADS_2$ score of ≥2, chronic oral anticoagulant therapy with a vitamin K antagonist (VKA) is recommended in a dose adjusted to achieve the target intensity INR of 2–3, unless contraindicated.

For a more detailed stroke risk assessment, a comprehensive risk factor-based approach is recommended. The presence of one 'definitive' risk factor merits anticoagulation with an oral VKA (to a target INR 2–3) (➲Table 29.7). Patients with two or more 'combination' risk factors should all be considered for anticoagulation. Where less validated 'combination' risk factors are being included, the decision should be individualized, after discussion of the pros and cons with the patient.

Patients with one 'combination' risk factor should be managed with antithrombotic therapy, either oral VKA or aspirin 75–325mg daily. Where possible, such patients at intermediate risk should be considered for a VKA rather than aspirin (➲Table 29.7). Where there is one less validated 'combination' risk factor patients should similarly be considered for antithrombotic therapy, either VKA or aspirin 75–325mg daily.

Table 29.7 Guidelines for antithrombotic therapy in atrial fibrillation

Risk category	Recommended antithrombotic therapy
One 'definitive' risk factor or two or more 'combination' risk factors	OAC (Class 1A)
One 'combination' risk factor	Antithrombotic therapy, either as OAC (Class 1A) or aspirin 75–325mg daily (Class 1B). Probably OAC rather than aspirin (Class 2A)
No risk factors	Aspirin 75–325 mg daily (Class 1B) or no antithrombotic therapy (Class 2A)

OAC, oral anticoagulation therapy, such as a VKA adjusted to an intensity range of INR 2–3 (target 2.5).

Full discussion with the patient would enable agreement to use VKA instead of aspirin to allow greater protection against ischaemic stroke, especially if these patients value stroke prevention much more than the (theoretical) lower risk of haemorrhage with aspirin and the inconvenience of anticoagulation monitoring. Of note, the Birmingham Atrial Fibrillation Treatment of the Aged Study (BAFTA) found no difference in major bleeding between warfarin (INR 2–3) and aspirin 75mg in an elderly AF population in primary care [186].

Patients with no risk factors are at low risk (essentially patients aged <65 years with lone AF, with none of the risk factors, whether definitive or combination risk factors can be managed with aspirin 75–325mg daily or no antithrombotic therapy, given the limited data on the benefits of aspirin in this patient group (that is, lone AF) and the potential for adverse effects [187].

➲Table 29.7 summarizes the guidelines for antithrombotic therapy in AF.

Anticoagulation therapy versus control

The possible benefit of prophylactic VKA therapy in non-valvular AF has been explored in several randomized controlled studies. The first to be published was the Danish Atrial Fibrillation, ASpirin, AntiKoagulation (AFASAK) study, illustrating a 54% relative risk reduction of stroke associated with a VKA regimen [188]. Since then, other randomized controlled studies exploring the role of VKA as stroke prevention in non-valvular AF have been published.

When pooled together in a meta-analysis, the relative risk reduction was highly significant and amounted to 64%, corresponding to an absolute annual risk reduction

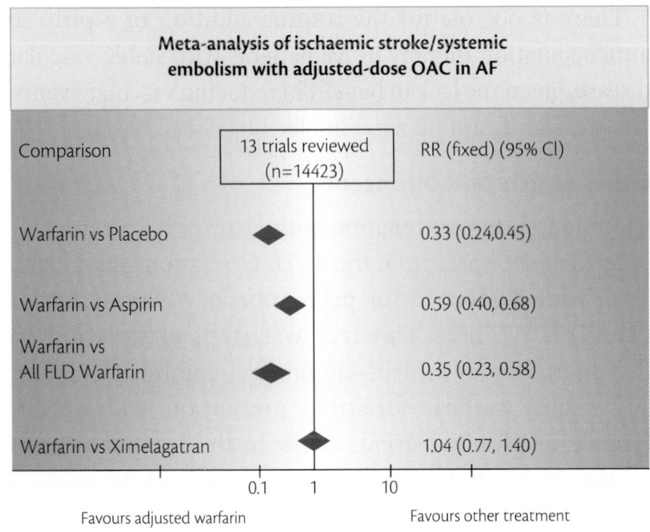

Figure 29.19 Meta-analysis of ischaemic stroke/systemic embolism with adjusted-dose oral anticoagulation in atrial fibrillation. Reproduced from Lip GYH, Edwards SJ. Stroke prevention with aspirin, warfarin and xilmelagatran in patients with non-valvular atrial fibrillation: a systematic review and meta-analysis. *Thromb Res* 2006; **118**: 321–33.

in all strokes of 2.7% [189]. When only ischaemic strokes were considered, adjusted-dose warfarin was associated with a 67% relative risk reduction (➲Fig. 29.19). Notably, this was the risk reduction in those patients who were *intended to take* oral anticoagulants in the trials. The relative risk reduction for the patients who did indeed use the medication was strikingly high at 85%. All-cause mortality was substantially reduced (26%) by adjusted-dose warfarin versus control. The risk of intracranial haemorrhage was small.

It is important to note that these studies generally excluded patients with low risk of embolism or markedly increased bleeding risk as well as those with the highest risk of embolism. The latter category, in which VKA treatment is strongly advised (although its benefit has not been illustrated in randomized clinical trials), includes patients who in addition to AF have a prosthetic valve, or suffer from rheumatic mitral valve disease or hypertrophic cardiomyopathy. In addition, AF in the setting of hyperthyroidism is often placed in this category, although the evidence for high stroke risk is weak.

Supported by the results of the trials cited above, VKA treatment is strongly recommended for patients with AF with 'definitive' or two or more 'combination' stroke risk indicators provided there are no contraindications.

Antiplatelet therapy versus control

Eight independent randomized controlled studies, together including 4876 patients, have explored the prophylactic effects of antiplatelet therapy, most commonly acetylsalicylic acid (ASA), compared with placebo on the risk of thromboembolism in patients with AF [189]. When aspirin alone was compared to placebo or no treatment in seven trials, meta-analysis showed that aspirin was associated with a non-significant 19% (CI, −1% to 35%) reduced incidence of stroke. There was an absolute risk reduction of 0.8% per year for primary prevention trials and 2.5% per year for secondary prevention [189]. When all randomized data from all comparisons of antiplatelet agents and placebo or control groups were included in the meta-analysis, antiplatelet therapy reduced stroke by 22%.

Of note, the dose of aspirin differed markedly between the studies, ranging from 50–1300mg daily. Furthermore, much of the beneficial effect of aspirin was driven by the results of the SPAF-I clinical trial, which suggested a 42% stroke risk reduction with aspirin versus placebo [190]. In this trial, there were inconsistencies for the aspirin effect in this trial between the results for the warfarin-eligible (relative risk reduction, 94%) and warfarin-ineligible (relative risk reduction, 8%) arms. Also, aspirin has less effect in people older than 75 years and did not prevent severe or recurrent strokes. The magnitude of stroke reduction of aspirin versus placebo is comparable to that seen if aspirin were given for vascular disease subjects—given that AF commonly coexists with vascular disease, the modest benefit seen for aspirin in AF is likely to be related to the effects on vascular disease.

Anticoagulant therapy versus antiplatelet therapy

Direct comparison between the effects of VKA and ASA has been undertaken in nine studies, illustrating that VKA was significantly superior with a relative risk reduction of 39% [189]. The latter relative risk reduction has largely been driven by the BAFTA trial, which showed that warfarin (target INR 2–3) was superior to aspirin 75mg in reducing the primary endpoint of fatal or disabling stroke (ischaemic or haemorrhagic), intracranial haemorrhage, or clinically significant arterial embolism by 52%, with no difference in risk of major haemorrhage between warfarin and aspirin (➲Fig. 29.20) [186].

When the trials prior to BAFTA were considered, the risk for intracranial haemorrhage was doubled with adjusted-dose warfarin compared with aspirin, although the absolute risk increase was small (0.2% per year) [189].

Combination therapies

Several attempts have been made to combine drugs with different antithromboembolic mechanisms, mostly low-dose VKA treatment with an antiplatelet drug. No study

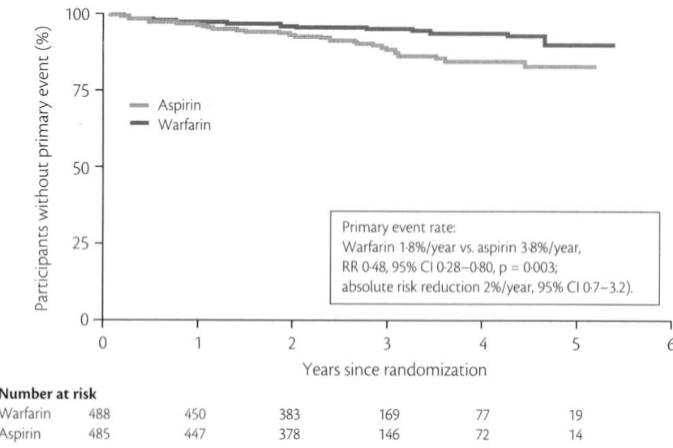

Figure 29.20 Warfarin versus aspirin for stroke prevention in an elderly community population with AF: the Birmingham Atrial Fibrillation Treatment of the Aged Study (BAFTA). Modified from Mant J, Hobbs FD, Fletcher K, *et al.*; BAFTA investigators; Midland Research Practices Network (MidReC). Warfarin versus aspirin for stroke prevention in an elderly community population with atrial fibrillation (the Birmingham Atrial Fibrillation Treatment of the Aged Study, BAFTA): a randomised controlled trial. *Lancet* 2007; **370**: 493–503.

has shown any superior outcome for such a drug combination compared with dose-adjusted VKA only in preventing stroke or embolism in non-valvular AF.

Antiplatelet therapy has also been combined with therapeutic anticoagulation in AF cohorts, and these have shown a high rate of bleeding in the combination treatment arm [191, 192]. An ancillary analysis from the SPORTIF (Stroke Prevention using an Oral Thrombin Inhibitor in Atrial Fibrillation) trials, which compared aspirin users with non-users [192] found no additive effect of taking aspirin for stroke prevention or a reduction in vascular events (including death or myocardial infarction) in patients who were given anticoagulation (warfarin or ximelagatran); instead, aspirin use resulted in a substantial increase in risk of bleeding.

There is no role for the routine addition of aspirin to anticoagulation therapy in AF patients with stable vascular disease, given the lack of benefit in reducing vascular events, and the significant increase in bleeding risks [193].

Other antithrombotic agents

Clopidogrel, in combination with aspirin, has been compared against warfarin in the Atrial fibrillation Clopidogrel Trial with Irbesartan for prevention of Vascular Events (ACTIVE W) trial. This trial was stopped early due to the inferiority of aspirin–clopidogrel combination therapy against warfarin for stroke prevention, with no difference in bleeding events between the treatment arms (➲ Fig. 29.21) [194]. An ancillary analysis of AF subjects participating in the Clopidogrel for High Atherothrombotic Risk and Ischemic Stabilization, Management, and Avoidance (CHARISMA) trial of patients with stable cardiovascular disease or multiple cardiovascular risk factors, which compared combination aspirin–clopidogrel therapy to aspirin alone, found no benefit of combination therapy but an excess of severe or fatal extra-cranial haemorrhage with combination therapy [195].

The recent ACTIVE-A trial tested the hypothesis that the addition of clopidogrel 75mg to aspirin would reduce the risk of vascular events in 7554 patients with AF [196]. At a median of 3.6 years of follow-up, major vascular events were reduced in patients receiving aspirin–clopidogrel (6.8%/year vs. aspirin alone, 7.6%/year: RR 0.89; 95% CI 0.81–0.98; P = 0.01). This difference was primarily due to a reduction in the rate of stroke with combination therapy (2.4%/year vs. 3.3%/year: RR 0.72; 95% CI, 0.62–0.83; P <0.001). However, major bleeding increased with combination therapy (2.0%/year vs. 1.3%/year. RR 1.57; 95% CI, 1.29–1.92; P<0.001). Thus, in AF patients for whom VKA

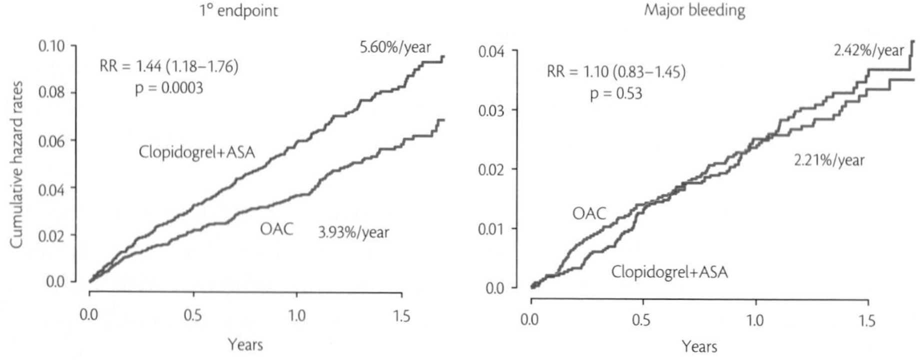

Figure 29.21 Primary endpoint (stroke, systemic embolus, myocardial infarction and vascular death in the ACTIVE W Study comparing oral anticoagulation with warfarin against a fixed dose of clopidogrel and aspirin (A). The occurrence of major bleeding (B). ASA, aspirin; OAC, oral anticoagulation. Modified with permission from Connolly S, Pogue J, Hart R, *et al.*; ACTIVE Writing Group on behalf of the ACTIVE Investigators. Clopidogrel plus aspirin versus oral anticoagulation for atrial fibrillation in the Atrial fibrillation Clopidogrel Trial with Irbesartan for prevention of Vascular Events (ACTIVE W): a randomised controlled trial. *Lancet* 2006; **367**: 1903–12.

therapy was unsuitable, the addition of aspirin–clopidogrel reduced the risk of major vascular events, especially stroke, but increased the risk of major haemorrhage. Nonetheless, 50% of subjects entered the trial due to 'physician perception of being unsuitable for VKA therapy' and 23% had a relative risk factor for bleeding at trial entry. However, of patients perceived not to be candidates for VKA therapy, only a small proportion still have the same relative contraindication to VKA a year later. Hence aspirin–clopidogrel therapy could be considered as an interim measure pending use of more effective thromboproplylaxis with VKA. Other antiplatelet agents such as indobufen and triflusal have been investigated in AF, with the suggestion of some benefit, but more data are required before definitive conclusions can be made [167].

Investigational drugs

Several new anticoagulant drugs—broadly in two classes, the oral direct thrombin inhibitors (DTI) and the oral factor Xa inhibitors (FXaI)—have been developed as possible alternatives to VKA (➲Fig. 29.22) [197]. The first oral DTI, ximelagatran was tested in two large-scale clinical studies, and was found to be as effective as adjusted-dose warfarin in the prevention of ischaemic strokes or systemic emboli (RR 1.04; 95% CI: 0.77–1.40) (➲Fig. 29.19) with less risk of major bleeding (RR, 0.74; 95% CI, 0.56–0.96) [198]. Further development of ximelagatran has been discontinued due to liver toxicity.

Other DTIs (e.g. dabigatran and AZD0837), as well as Factor Xa inhibitors (rivaroxaban, apixaban, edoxaban, YM150, etc.) and non-warfarin vitamin K antagonists (ATI-5923) are being developed for stroke prevention in AF [199]. The possible benefit of these drugs awaits the outcomes of clinical studies.

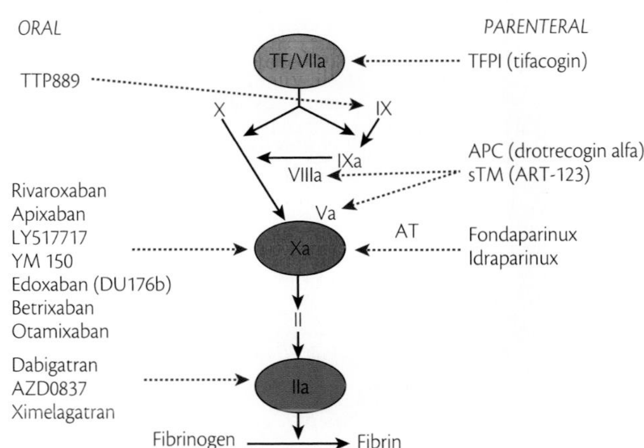

Figure 29.22 Simplified coagulation cascade and sites of action of new anticoagulant agents. Modified with permission from Turpie AG. New oral anticoagulants in atrial fibrillation. *Eur Heart J* 2008; **29**: 155–65.

One indirect FXaI, idraparinux, which requires once-weekly administration, was tested against warfarin in one trial [200]. This found that idraparinux was non-inferior to warfarin for stroke prevention, but there was a marked excess of bleeding with idraparinux compared to warfarin. A biotinylated version of idraparinux is undergoing a clinical trial in AF, with the potential of anticoagulant reversal should bleeding occur.

Optimal INR

Currently, the level of anticoagulation in a serum sample is expressed as the INR, which is the ratio between the actual prothrombin time and that of a standardized control serum. Although arguments have been raised against the accuracy of this comparative technique [201], it has become widely accepted.

Based on the pooled information from achieving a balance between stroke risk with low INRs and an increasing bleeding risk with high INRs [202, 203], a consensus has been reached that an INR of 2.0–3.0 is the likely optimal range for prevention of stroke and systemic embolism in patients with non-valvular AF. A mortality risk analysis in a VKA-treated population comprising >40,000 patients suggests that the target INR window should be narrower, with a target value close to 2.2–2.3 [204]. ➲Fig. 29.23 illustrates the risk of ischaemic stroke and intracranial bleeding relative to the INR level as well as the 1-month mortality risk in relation to INR in patients with AF.

Keeping within a target INR of 2–3 is difficult. One of the many problems with anticoagulation with VKA is the high inter- and intra-individual variation in INRs. VKAs also have significant drug, food, and alcohol interactions. Patients stay within target INR range (2–3) for 60–65% of the time [205], but many 'real life' studies even suggest that this figure may be <50%.

The elderly may pose a particular problem. One hospital-based cohort suggested a high bleeding rate in elderly subjects (>80 years old) initiated on warfarin, especially in the first 3 months following the start of warfarin [206]. In this study, increasing stroke risk was associated with an increasing risk of bleeding, which in turn led to more discontinuations. Whilst a lower target INR range (1.8–2.5) has been proposed for the elderly, this is not based on any trial evidence, and cohort studies even suggest a twofold increase in stroke risk at INR 1.5–2.0 [207], and is therefore not recommended. Also, the BAFTA trial shows the benefit of conventional dose warfarin over aspirin in the elderly (aged ≥75 years), irrespective of age categories [186].

In addition to the fear of drug-induced bleeding complications, VKA treatment is associated with several other

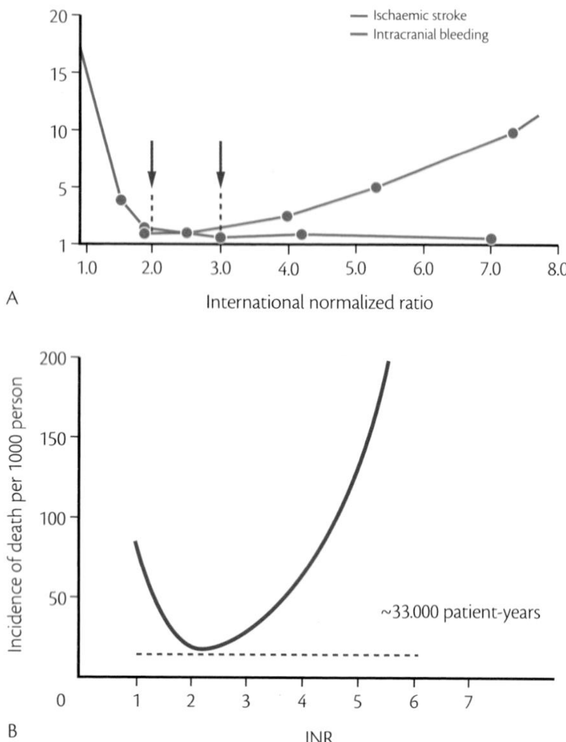

Figure 29.23 (A) Adjusted odds ratio for ischaemic stroke and intracranial bleeding in relation to international normalized ratio (INR). Reproduced with permission from Odén A, Fahlén M. Oral anticoagulation and risk of death: medical record linkage study. *Br Med J* 2002; **325**: 1073–5. (B) Risk of death during the month following an INR test in relation to the INR value. The blue line represents the mortality risk for a 71-year-old woman. The horizontal dotted red line represents the mortality risk for the entire population of 71-year-old females.

reasons that contribute to its underuse in patients with non-valvular AF [208]. In short, the barriers to the use of VKA treatment in non-valvular AF patients may relate to the doctor as well as the patient and the healthcare system. In addition, many patients with AF have limited understanding of the disease process as well as the need for anticoagulation therapy to prevent thromboembolism [209].

The maintenance, safety, and effectiveness of INR within range can be influenced by pharmacogenetics of VKA therapy, particularly the cytochrome P450 2C9 gene (*CYP2C9*) and the vitamin K epoxide reductase complex 1 gene (*VKORC1*). *CYP2C9* and *VKORC1* genotypes can influence warfarin dose requirements, whilst *CYP2C9* variant genotypes are associated with bleeding events [210]. The ability to determine mutations in the genes coding for these two proteins could influence future VKA dosing patterns (i.e. genotype-guided therapy), but just how much would these would really add to regular, conscientious monitoring of the INR and dose adjustment is undetermined. Ongoing trials are addressing this question.

Anticoagulation near-patient testing and self-monitoring

The need for regular monitoring of oral anticoagulation therapy has led to a substantial increased use of 'point of care' or 'near patient' testing schemes, as well as patient self-monitoring approaches (➲Fig. 29.24).

Thus, patients may have anticoagulation-monitoring testing at a local clinic (e.g. general practitioner clinic using an INR testing machine, or blood sample taken at a local clinic which is batched and sent to a central laboratory) and the INR result phoned to the patient, with VKA dose change, if necessary. Alternatively home monitoring can be performed using a personal INR testing machine allowing patients to alter the warfarin dose themselves [211].

Self-monitoring could be considered if the patient is physically and cognitively able to perform the self-monitoring test [212, 213] or a designated carer may be used. Appropriate training by a competent healthcare professional is needed and the patient must remain in contact with a named clinician.

Special situations

Paroxysmal atrial fibrillation

The stroke and thromboembolic risk in paroxysmal AF is less well defined, and such patients have represented the

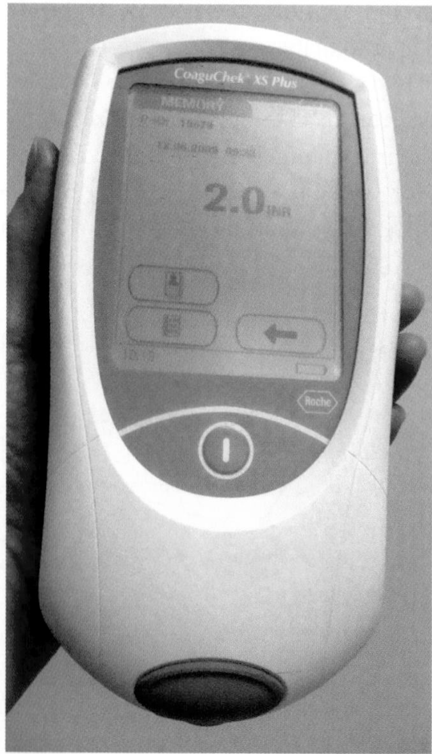

Figure 29.24 Self-testing device for assessment of international normalized ratio (INR) (CoaguChek XS® Plus system—PT/INR monitoring).

minority (usually <30%) in the clinical trials of thromboprophylaxis. A recent large trial programme did not identify a difference in stroke risk between paroxysmal or chronic forms of AF [77].

A retrospective hospital record study followed >400 individuals with paroxysmal AF for >25 years [214]. In these non-VKA taking patients, there was a clustering of thromboembolism at the time of onset of paroxysmal AF, namely 6.8% during 1 month. Later, the annual embolic rate varied from 0.6–2.6%. Following transition to permanent AF, which occurred in every third patient, the rate of embolism rose to a significantly higher level. Some of the observed differences in thromboembolic rates are clearly attributable to the presence or absence of stroke risk factors.

Another study, exploring the embolic risk factors in >700 patients with paroxysmal AF, verified a 2.2% annual rate of embolism, typically occurring in males above the age of 65 [77]. Importantly, individuals without any underlying disorder had a low embolic event rate (0.7% per year). Data from the non-VKA arms of clinical trials show that stroke risk in paroxysmal AF was comparable to that seen in permanent AF, and is dependent upon the presence of stroke risk factors [171, 215]. Thus, current guidelines suggest that prevention of thromboembolism is appropriate in patients with paroxysmal AF [1].

Perioperative anticoagulation

Patients with AF who are anticoagulated will require temporary interruption of a VKA before surgery or an invasive procedure. Many surgeons require an INR of <1.5 or even INR normalization before undertaking surgery. Thus, VKAs should be stopped approximately 5 days before surgery, to allow the INR to fall appropriately. VKA should be resumed at the 'usual' maintenance dose (without a loading dose) on the evening of (or the next morning) after surgery assuming there is adequate haemostasis. If surgery is urgent but the INR is still elevated (>1.5), the administration of low-dose oral vitamin K (1–2mg) to normalize the INR may be considered.

In patients with a mechanical heart valve or AF at high risk for thromboembolism, management can be problematic. Such patients should be considered for 'bridging' anticoagulation with therapeutic doses of heparin (either low-molecular-weight heparin (LMWH) or unfractionated heparin (UFH)) during the temporary interruption of VKA therapy [216].

Atrial fibrillation presenting with acute coronary syndrome and/or percutaneous coronary intervention with stenting

Increasing numbers of patients with AF may present with an acute coronary syndrome (ACS). Given that AF is also associated with CAD, some AF patients would require percutaneous coronary intervention, with the possibility of stent implantation. Current guidelines for ACS and/or PCI recommend the use of aspirin–clopidogrel combination therapy after ACS (9–12 months), and after a stent (4 weeks for a bare metal stent, 6 or more months for a drug-eluting stent).

However, there are limited data to guide the optimal antithrombotic regimen to use in anticoagulated patients with AF, given that bleeding with triple therapy (VKA, aspirin, and clopidogrel) may be substantial. The largest published cohort [217] suggests that non-VKA use was associated with an increase in mortality and major adverse cardiac events, with no significant difference in bleeding rates between VKA and non-VKA users.

Current consensus guidelines suggest that drug-eluting stents should be avoided and triple therapy (VKA, aspirin, clopidogrel) used in the short term, followed by more long-term therapy with VKA plus a single antiplatelet drug [218, 219].

Atrial fibrillation patients presenting with an acute stroke

Acute stroke is a common first presentation of a patient with AF, given that the arrhythmia often develops asymptomatically. There are limited trial data to guide our management, and there is concern that patients within the first 2 weeks of having had a cardioembolic stroke are at greatest risk of having stroke recurrence because of further thromboembolism. However, anticoagulation in the acute phase may result in intracranial haemorrhage or haemorrhagic transformation of the infarct. In most stroke survivors with AF it is reasonable to initiate anticoagulation at approximately 2 weeks after the stroke in patients with minor strokes or TIA, anticoagulation could be initiated earlier, after cerebral imaging as excluded any intracranial bleeding.

Atrial flutter

Large-scale prospective observational or interventional studies on the stroke rate in atrial flutter per se are lacking. However, the risk of stroke linked to atrial flutter has been studied retrospectively in a large number of older patients, and was similar to that seen in AF [219]. Thus, thromboprophylaxis in a patient with atrial flutter should follow the same guidelines as if the patient had AF [185].

Pregnancy

On occasion, AF may occur in pregnant women, especially in relation to valvular heart disease, prosthetic heart valves, or venous thromboembolism. A thorough discussion of the potential risks and benefits of any anticoagulation regimen is needed with the patient, and a close liaison on management between the cardiologist and obstetrician is mandatory.

VKAs can be teratogenic and in many cases should be substituted with UFH or LMWH for the first trimester of the pregnancy [221]. Pregnant patients with AF and mechanical prosthetic valves who elect to stop warfarin between weeks 6 and 12 of gestation should receive continuous intravenous UFH, dose-adjusted UFH, or dose-adjusted subcutaneous LMWH [222] and may start VKA in the second trimester at an only slightly elevated teratogenic risk. For pregnant women with acute venous thromboembolism, subcutaneous LMWH or UFH should be continued throughout pregnancy and anticoagulant prophylaxis continued for at least 6 weeks postpartum [221].

Cardioversion

The increased risk of embolism following cardioversion is well recognized. Therefore, full antithromboembolic treatment is considered mandatory before elective cardioversion in cases where AF duration exceeds 48 hours [185]. Despite these precautions, embolism has been reported to occur in up to 2% of all electrical cardioversions [223]. These occur typically during the initial few days following reappearance of sinus rhythm (➲Fig. 29.25).

The mechanism of post-cardioversion embolism is complex. Pre-existing thrombi may dislodge from the endocardial wall when the atria resume a slower and regular rhythm. However, following conversion from AF to sinus rhythm, the mechanical function of the atrial myocardium is not immediately restored ('atrial stunning'), presenting

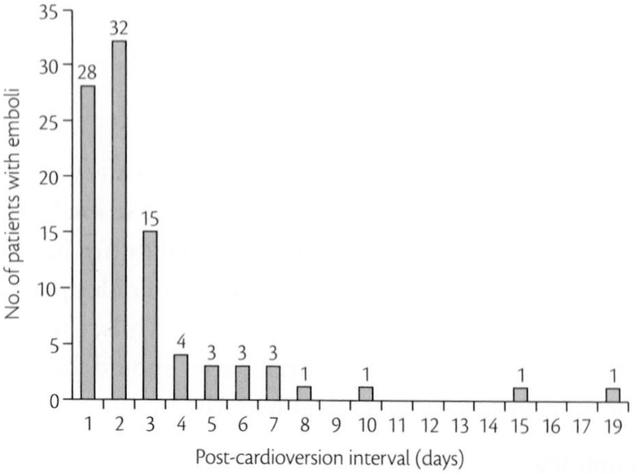

Figure 29.25 Interval between cardioversion and thrombotic events in 92 patients. Reproduced with permission from Berger M, Schweitzer P. Timing of thromboembolic events after electrical cardioversion of atrial fibrillation or flutter: a retrospective analysis. *Am J Cardiol* 1998; **82**: 1545–6.

an opportunity for thrombus formation. Furthermore, there is activation of coagulation and platelets, leading to a propensity to thrombogenesis in the immediate post-cardioversion period.

The importance of an adequate anticoagulation level at the time of cardioversion must be stressed. In a study of >2500 elective direct-current cardioversion attempts in almost 2000 patients, no post-cardioversion embolism could be confirmed when the INR exceeded 2.4 on the day of the procedure [224]. In contrast, embolism was increasingly more common at a lower INR and appeared to increase with decreasing INR.

Current guidelines state that VKA treatment (INR 2–3) should be given for at least 3 weeks before cardioversion of a patient in whom AF has been maintained for >48 hours or which is of unknown duration [185]. Thromboprophylaxis is recommended irrespective of whether the cardioversion is performed using a pharmacological or an electrical method. Anticoagulation treatment should be continued for a minimum of 4 weeks post-cardioversion. However, in patients with stroke risk factors, or those at high risk of AF recurrence, long-term VKA treatment is usually required.

Transoesophageal echocardiography-guided cardioversion

The 3–4-week period of adequate anticoagulation prior to cardioversion can be shortened with the use of transoesophageal echocardiography. This technique may not only show thrombi within the LAA or the LA proper but also identify indicators for thrombus formation, such as spontaneous echo-contrast or complex aortic plaque. The safety and applicability of transoesophageal echocardiography-guided cardioversion has been repeatedly verified [225, 226]. Following exclusion of any thrombus, anticoagulation can commence with LMWH [226, 227], the cardioversion performed, and anticoagulation post-cardioversion continued, as highlighted earlier. Oral anticoagulation is started and LMWH discontinued when the INR is therapeutic.

Silent stroke

A history of previous stroke or TIA is the most powerful risk factor for a recurrent cerebrovascular event. As stroke in patients with AF is primarily embolic, the detection of asymptomatic cerebral emboli may identify high-risk patients. The prevalence of silent cerebral infarct on computer tomography images of the brain in AF patients without neurological deficit ranged from 15–26% in the SPINAF and SPAF (Stroke Prevention Atrial Fibrillation) studies [228, 229]. These silent strokes may contribute to impaired cognitive function in AF patients.

Transcranial Doppler ultrasound may identify asymptomatic patients with an active embolic source or patients with prior stroke who are at high risk of recurrent stroke. During 1-hour bilateral Doppler monitoring from the middle cerebral arteries, the frequency of embolization was 13% in patients with previous AF-related stroke or TIA and 16% in those individuals without a history of a cerebrovascular event [230]. The incidence of embolic signals was higher in untreated patients compared with those receiving warfarin (11.9% vs. 1.5%) [231].

Non-pharmacological methods to prevent stroke in atrial fibrillation

Since the majority of all LA thrombi form in the LAA [181], different techniques have been developed that aim to eliminate the LAA as a possible source of thromboembolism. The result of LAA resection in patients who undergo cardiac surgery for other reasons has been tested in a series of >400 patients [231]. No strokes were reported following surgery and it has been suggested that the LAA should be resected 'whenever the chest is open'.

Other non-pharmacological techniques for elimination of the LAA as a possible thrombotic location are currently undergoing clinical evaluation, including thoracoscopic obliteration of the LAA as well as endocardial occlusion of the LAA with different devices [199, 232]. ➲Fig. 29.26 illustrates two different devices that can be inserted in the LAA to prevent thrombus formation and subsequent stroke. At the American College of Cardiology meeting in 2009, the PROTECT AF Trial, a Randomized Prospective Trial of Percutaneous LAA Closure vs Warfarin for Stroke Prevention in AF found that all cause stroke and all cause mortality risk using the WATCHMAN device was non-inferior to warfarin, with a lower haemorrhagic stroke risk. However, there were early safety events, specifically pericardial effusion.

Pharmacological therapy

The fundamental principles of pharmacological therapy for AF, apart from anticoagulation and treatment of underlying conditions associated with AF, include specific termination of the arrhythmia and maintenance of sinus rhythm, prevention of AF recurrence (secondary prevention), and control of ventricular rates during AF. Antiarrhythmic drugs can be used for rhythm control as sole agents or as an adjunct to catheter ablation or electrical cardioversion. Prevention and effective treatment of conditions that are commonly associated with the development of AF, such as hypertension and congestive heart failure, may prevent the occurrence of new AF (primary prevention) or reduce the recurrence rate, and delay the progression to permanent AF (secondary prevention) [233]. Treatment of the underlying heart disease to prevent atrial remodelling and formation of the substrate for AF is often termed 'upstream' therapy [34].

Rhythm versus rate control management

Symptomatic AF can be managed by therapy aimed either at restoring and maintaining sinus rhythm ('rhythm control')

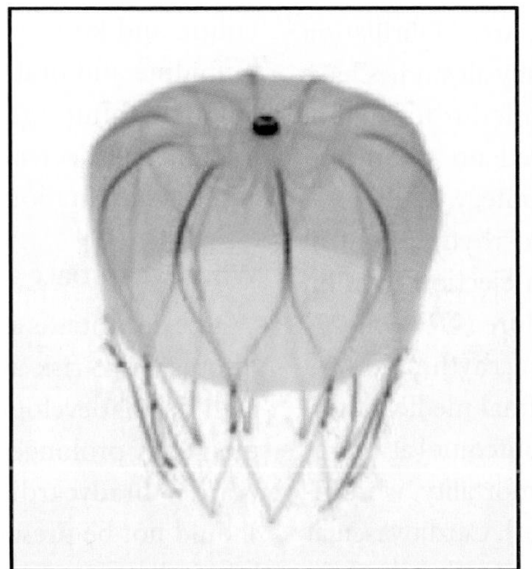
A

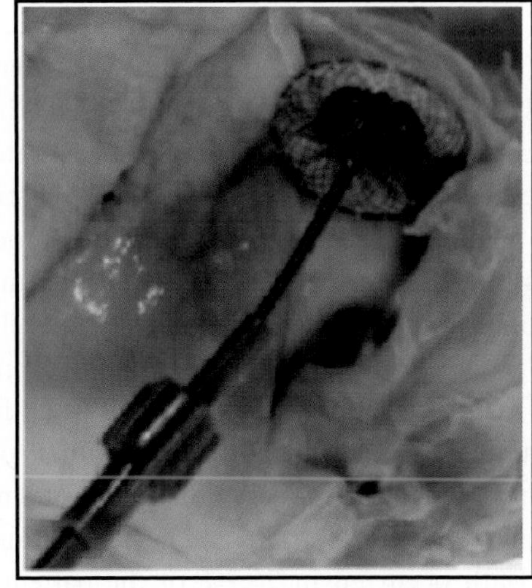
B

Figure 29.26 Two examples of left atrial occluder devices: Watchman (A) and Amplatz (B).

or therapy that controls ventricular rate ('rate control'). Sinus rhythm offers physiological control of heart rate and regularity, normal atrial activation and contraction, the correct sequence of AV activation, and normal valve function. Rhythm control might be an ideal approach for both stroke prevention and symptom alleviation and it might improve survival. However, the long-term maintenance of sinus rhythm has proven difficult to achieve, the recurrence rate is high, and rhythm-control management is time consuming, expensive (due to the cost of the antiarrhythmic drugs and the increased need for hospitalization, e.g. for cardioversion), and is not completely free from complications. A well-appreciated limitation of current rhythm-control management is poor long-term efficacy and the adverse effects of antiarrhythmic drugs (e.g. proarrhythmia and organ toxicity) that may negate the inherent advantage of sinus rhythm over AF [234].

The advantages of rate control are simplicity, availability, and low cost, although in some patients, adequate rate control may be difficult to achieve and may not result in symptom relief, or may be associated with adverse effects (e.g. bradycardia or worsening heart failure) and increased mortality [234, 235].

Rhythm- versus rate-control studies

Several randomized studies directly and prospectively compared the effect of rate and rhythm control on patient outcomes (➲Table 29.8). The major studies were the Atrial Fibrillation Follow up Investigation of Rhythm Management (AFFIRM) trial [237], the RAte Control versus Electrical Cardioversion (RACE) trial [238], and the Atrial Fibrillation Congestive Heart Failure (AF-CHF) trial [239]. There were also a series of pilot studies performed, including the Pharmacological Intervention in Atrial Fibrillation (PIAF) [240], Strategies of Treatment of Atrial Fibrillation (STAF) [241], and How to Treat Chronic Atrial Fibrillation (HOT CAFÉ) [242] among others. Virtually all studies have shown that primary rate control is not inferior to rhythm control. Meta-analysis has demonstrated no significant excess or reduced mortality with either strategy [243].

The AF-CHF trial compared rate- and rhythm-control strategies specifically in patients with an ejection fraction of 35% or less and NYHA II–IV heart failure (➲Fig. 29.27) [239]. The study showed no benefit from rhythm control (mainly with amiodarone) on top of optimal medical therapy on cardiovascular death (the primary outcome) as well as pre-specified secondary outcomes (total mortality, worsening heart failure, stroke, and hospitalization). Cardiovascular death occurred in 26.7% of the patients in the rhythm-control group compared with 25.2% in the rate-control arm.

Indications for rhythm versus rate control

Rate control as a primary strategy is now accepted in older, sedentary, and asymptomatic (or only mildly symptomatic) patients (EHRA I–II) who have had their arrhythmia for many years, without significant impairment of ventricular function and exercise tolerance. Following the AF-CHF study, rate control is a legitimate primary treatment option for patients with heart failure who can tolerate AF without worsening NYHA functional class. Rhythm control with antiarrhythmic drugs, cardioversion, or ablation remains treatment of choice in patients who are symptomatic, in patients with recent onset AF, or in young and active individuals.

On-treatment analysis of outcomes in the AFFIRM trial has shown a 47% reduction in the risk of all-cause death if sinus rhythm was maintained irrespective of the treatment strategy [244]. If safer and more effective antiarrhythmic agents were available, sinus rhythm might confer a favourable outcome and many new antiarrhythmic agents are under investigation (➲Fig. 29.28) [107].

Choice of antiarrhythmic drugs

The choice of an antiarrhythmic drug for cardioversion as well as for long-term management of AF depends on underlying heart disease (➲Fig. 29.29) [1]. Class IC antiarrhythmic agents (propafenone and flecainide), and class III agents (sotalol and ibutilide) are recommended for cardioversion of AF in patients with moderate structural heart disease or hypertension without LV hypertrophy. These agents are not recommended in patients with a history of heart failure, myocardial infarction with LV dysfunction, and significant LV hypertrophy. Amiodarone and dofetilide (dofetilide is not available outside the USA) can be used in patients presenting with symptoms of heart failure and known advanced heart disease. Although oral quinidine and oral or intravenous procainamide (class IA antiarrhythmic agents) are still available, there has been a significant decrease in their use worldwide. Quinidine as a fixed combination with verapamil has a limited use.

Where to initiate antiarrhythmic drug therapy

Where to initiate antiarrhythmic drug therapy must take into account risk and practicality. Patients at anticipated high risk of developing adverse effects (e.g. patients with an inherently prolonged QT interval, or patients at risk of tachycardia–bradycardia syndrome upon termination of AF), should not be prescribed antiarrhythmic drugs outside the hospital setting. For some antiarrhythmic agents, e.g. dofetilide, there is formal requirement for in-hospital initiation.

Table 29.8 Studies of rate versus rhythm control in atrial fibrillation

Study	PIAF	STAF	HOT CAFÉ	RACE	AFFIRM	AF-CHF	Metaanalysis‡
No. of patients	252	200	205	522	4060	1376	5239
Follow-up, years	1	1.6	1.7	2.3	3.5	3.1	–
Primary endpoint	Symptom improvement	Composite of ACM, cardiovascular events, CPR, TE	Composite of ACM, TE, bleeding	Composite of CVD, hospitalizations for CHF, TE, bleeding, pacemaker, AAD adverse effects	All-cause mortality	Cardiovascular mortality	–
Difference in primary endpoint	Symptoms improved in 70 RhyC vs. 76 RC patients (p = 0.317)	5.54%/year vs. 6.09%/year RhyC vs. RC (p = 0.99)	No difference (OR, 1.98, 95% CI, 0.28–22.3; p > 0.71)	22.6% vs. 17.2% RhyC vs. RC (HR, 0.73; 90% CI, 0.53–1.01; p = 0.11)	23.8% vs. 21.3% RhyC vs. RC (HR, 1.15; 95% CI, 0.99–1.34; p = 0.08)	27% vs. 25% RhyC vs. RC (HR, 1.06; 95% CI, 0.86–1.3; p = 0.59)	–
Mortality	Not assessed	2.5%/year vs. 4.9%/year RhyC vs. RC	3 (2.9%) vs. 1 (1%) RhyC vs. RC	6.8% vs. 7% RhyC vs. RC (for CVD)	As above	32% vs. 33% RhyC vs. RC (p = 0.68)	14.6% vs. 13% RhyC vs. RC (OR 0.87; 95% CI, 0.74–1.02; p= 0.09)
Thrombo-embolic event	Not assessed	3.1%/year vs. 0.6%/year RhyC vs. RC	3 (2.9%) vs. 1 (1%) RhyC vs. RC	7.9% vs. 5.5% RhyC vs. RC	Stroke: 7.1% vs. 5.5% RhyC vs. RC (p = 0.79); SE: 0.4% vs. 0.5% RhyC vs. RC (p = 0.62)	3% vs. 4% RhyC vs. RC (p = 0.32)	3.9% vs. 3.5% RhyC vs. RC (OR 0.50; 95% CI, 0.14–1.83; p = 0.3)
Heart failure	Not assessed	Improved: 16 vs. 26; worsened: 39 vs. 29 RhyC vs. RC patients (p = 0.18)	No difference	4.5% vs. 3.5% RhyC vs. RC	2.7% vs. 2.1% RhyC vs. RC (p = 0.58)†	28% vs. 31% RhyC vs. RC (p = 0.17)	–
Hospitalizations	69% vs. 24% RhyC vs. RC (p = 0.001)*	54% vs. 26% RhyC vs. RC (p < 0.001)	1.03 vs. 0.05 per pt RhyC vs. RC (p < 0.001)	More in RhyC (for DCC)	80% vs. 73% RhyC vs. RC (p < 0.001)	During the first year, 46% vs. 39% RhyC vs. RC (p = 0.0063)	–
Quality of life	No difference	No difference	Not assessed, but better functional capacity in RhyC	No difference	No difference, but trend towards better functional capacity in RhyC	Not yet available	–
Other findings	Better exercise tolerance but more adverse effects of AAD in RhyC (25% vs. 14%; p = 0.036)	18 out of total 19 primary endpoints occurred when patients were in AF	In RhyC, better exercise tolerance (p < 0.001), smaller LA and LV sizes, better LV systolic function	On-treatment analysis: more CHF in RC; smaller LA and LV sizes, better LV systolic function in RhyC	On-treatment analysis: maintenance of sinus rhythm was associated with lower mortality (HR, 0.53; 95% CI, 0.39–0.72; p <0 .0001)	On-treatment analysis: no survival benefit from maintenance of sinus rhythm (HR, 1.11; 95% CI, 0.78–1.58; p = 0.568)	–

AAD, antiarrhythmic drugs; ACM, all-cause mortality; AF, atrial fibrillation; AF-CHF, Atrial Fibrillation and Congestive Heart Failure; AFFIRM, Atrial Fibrillation Follow-up Investigation of Rhythm Management; CHF, congestive heart failure; CI, confidence intervals; CPR, cardiopulmonary resuscitation; CVD, cardiovascular death; DCC, direct current cardioversion; HR, hazard ratio; HOT CAFÉ, How to Treat Chronic Atrial Fibrillation; HR, hazard ratio; LA, left atrium; LV, left ventricle; OR, odds ratio; PIAF, Pharmacological Intervention in Atrial Fibrillation; RACE, Rate Control versus Electrical Cardioversion; RC, rate control; RhyC, rhythm control; STAF, Strategies of Treatment of Atrial Fibrillation; TE, thromboembolic event.

* including cardioversion; †reported as an adverse event; ‡mortality analysis: AFFIRM, HOT CAFÉ, PIAF, RACE, STAF; ischaemic stroke analysis: AFFIRM, HOT CAFÉ, STAF.

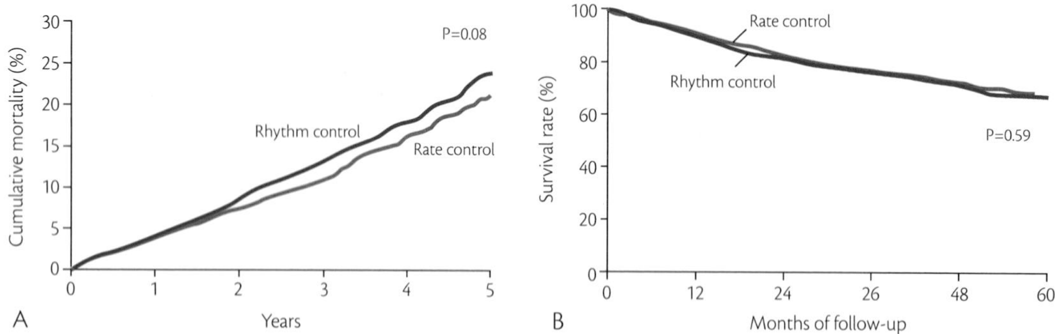

Figure 29.27 All-cause mortality in the rate control and rhythm control arms of the AFFIRM study (A). Cardiovascular mortality in the rate-control and rhythm-control arms of the AF-CHF study (B). In the AFFIRM study, more deaths occurred in the rhythm-control arm (356/2027 (26.7%)) than in the rate-control arm (310/2027 (25.9%)), but the difference was not statistically significant (hazard ratio, 1.15 (95% CI, 0.99–1.34); p = 0.08). In the AF-CHF study, 182 of 682 patients (27%) in the rhythm-control group died from cardiovascular causes compared with 175 of 694 patients (25%) in the rate-control group (hazard ratio, 1.06; 95% CI, 0.86–1.30). AFFIRM, Atrial Fibrillation Follow-up Investigation of Rhythm Management; AF CHF, Atrial Fibrillation in Congestive Heart Failure. Reproduced with permission from Wyse DG, Waldo AL, DiMarco JP, *et al.* A comparison of rate control and rhythm control in patients with atrial fibrillation. *N Engl J Med* 2002; **347**: 1825–33; and Roy D, Talajic M, Nattel S, *et al.* for the Atrial Fibrillation and Congestive Heart Failure Investigators. Rhythm control versus rate control for atrial fibrillation and heart failure. *N Engl J Med* 2008; **358**: 2667–77.

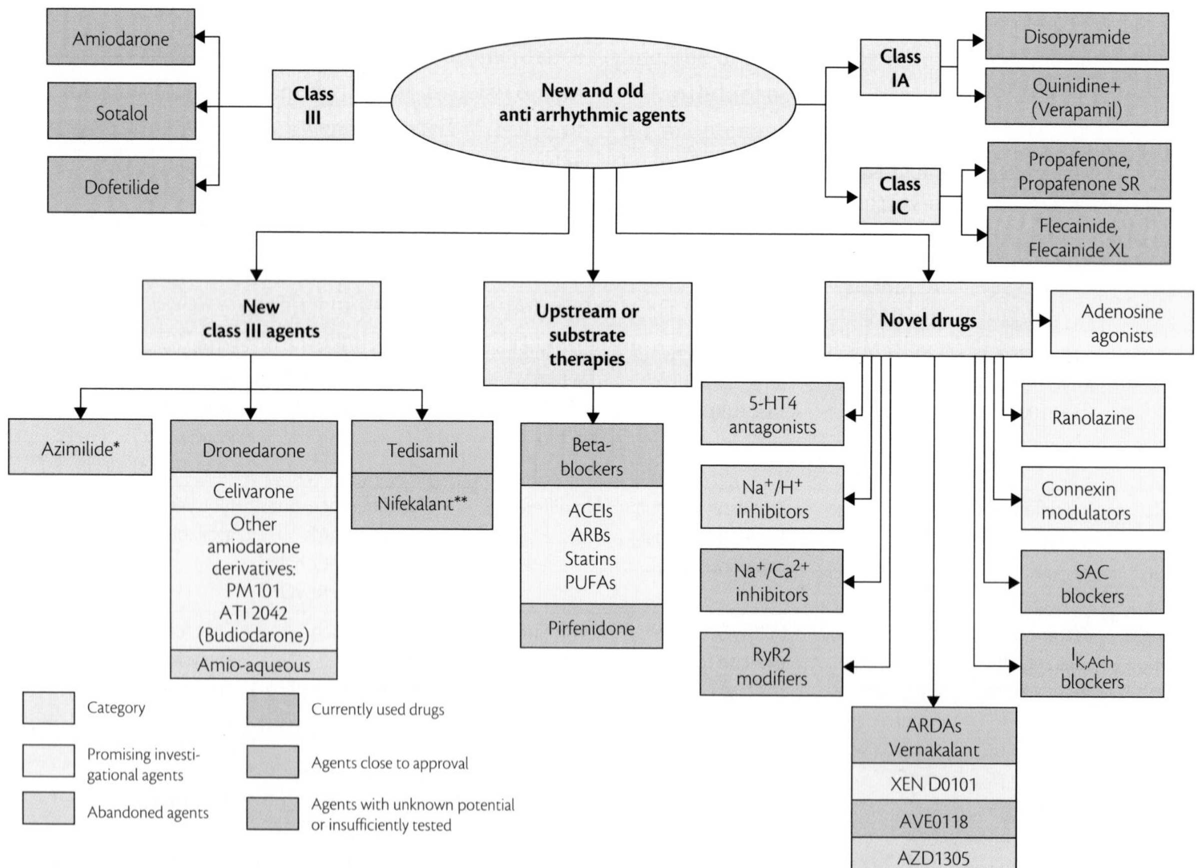

Figure 29.28 Antiarrhythmic agents for atrial fibrillation. *Azimilide is not used for treatment of atrial fibrillation; its use in patients with implantable defibrillators is under consideration. **Nifekalant is used in Japan, mainly for termination of ventricular tachycardia. ACEIs, angiotensin converting enzyme inhibitors; ARBs angiotensin type I receptor blockers; ARDAs, atrial repolarization delaying agents; HT, hydroxytryptamine; PUFA, polyunsaturated fatty acids; RyR, ryanodine receptors; SAC, stretch-activated channels. Reproduced with permission from Savelieva I, Camm J. Anti-arrhythmic drug therapy for atrial fibrillation: current anti-arrhythmic drugs, investigational agents, and innovative approaches. *Europace* 2008; **10**: 647–65.

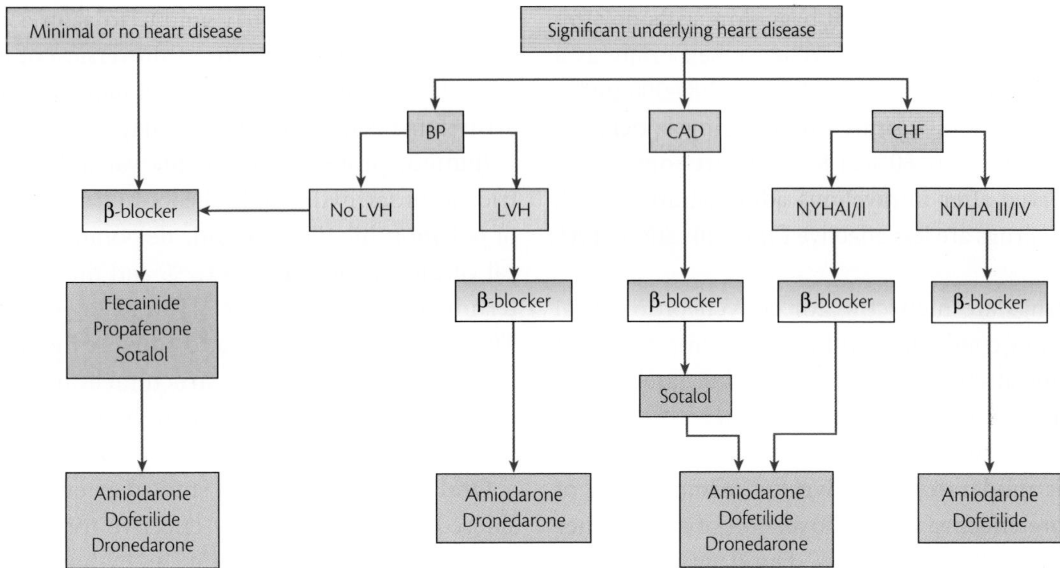

Figure 29.29 Selection of antiarrhythmic drugs for prevention of atrial fibrillation by underlying heart disease.

In the absence of proarrhythmia concerns and formal labelling, convenience and cost effectiveness favour out-of-hospital initiation, e.g. oral propafenone and flecainide (usually in combination with AV blocking drugs to prevent fast ventricular rates if atrial flutter occurs) in patients with lone AF or AF associated with hypertension without significant LV hypertrophy. Amiodarone can be safely started on an outpatient basis, given its long elimination half-life period and low probability of developing torsade de pointes. An ECG control and/or trans-telephonic ECG monitoring should be arranged to provide surveillance of heart rate, PR and QT interval durations (sotalol, amiodarone, dofetilide), QRS width (flecainide, propafenone), and assessment of the efficacy of treatment. When sotalol therapy is initiated outside hospital, the initial dose should be low and up-titration should depend on the heart rate and QT interval.

Pharmacological cardioversion

Cardioversion with antiarrhythmic drugs is usually effective if initiated early, i.e. within a week, probably even 3 days, after onset of AF. Within 24–72 hours, about 45% of patients with AF may convert spontaneously [245] and drug-assisted conversion will occur in approximately 70% [245–247].

Systematic analysis of placebo-controlled studies of pharmacological cardioversion for AF has shown that among patients with AF of <24 hours, 66% spontaneously converted to sinus rhythm compared with only 17% of those with AF of longer duration (odds ratio 1.8) [246].

'Pill in the pocket' approach

In patients with no or minimal structural heart disease and relatively infrequent (less than monthly), symptomatic paroxysms of AF of distinct onset which do not cause significant haemodynamic compromise (e.g. hypotension), a single loading dose of propafenone or flecainide can be used for expedient cardioversion [248]. In a proof of concept study, patients with paroxysmal AF, who had been successfully treated in hospital with either oral flecainide or propafenone, were instructed to take a single oral dose of the relevant drug within 5min of noticing palpitations. This 'pill in the pocket' strategy resulted in the reduction in the number of visits and hospitalizations, despite the same frequency of arrhythmia episodes [249].

The experience with this approach is limited and neither drug is licensed for patients to use for self-treating single attacks. As there is a danger of developing atrial flutter with 1:1 AV conduction, QRS widening, and rarely LV dysfunction, it is mandatory that the efficacy and safety of this strategy is first tested in-hospital. Furthermore, it is advisable to combine these agents with an AV-nodal slowing drug, e.g. a beta-receptor blocker, verapamil, or diltiazem. Atrial flutter was reported in 5–7% of patients who received oral loading doses of propafenone or flecainide for conversion of AF [250].

Drugs for cardioversion of atrial fibrillation

Intravenous **propafenone and flecainide** are very effective in cardioversion of AF of <72 hours' duration, with conversion rates as high as 80–90% within an hour after the start of infusion [251–253]. When taken orally as a loading dose (450–600mg for propafenone, 200–300mg for flecainide), restoration of sinus rhythm is more delayed, but conversion rates (70–80% at 8 hours) are comparable to those observed after intravenous administration [250, 254–259]. The drugs are less effective for termination of AF lasting >7 days.

Class IC drugs are ineffective for conversion of atrial flutter. They slow conduction within the re-entrant circuit and prolong the atrial flutter cycle length, but rarely interrupt the circuit. The efficacy rates have been reported to be as low as 13–40% [260].

Ibutilide is moderately effective for cardioversion of AF and is more effective for cardioversion of atrial flutter (31–44% vs. 56–70%) [261, 262]. The drug is available only as an intravenous formulation and is usually administered as a 1-mg bolus over 10min. Higher doses of ibutilide such as a single bolus of 2mg or two successive infusions of 1mg may be required for cardioversion of AF [261, 263, 264]. The antiarrhythmic effect of ibutilide decreases if the arrhythmia had persisted for >7 days.

Ibutilide prolongs the QT interval and may induce ventricular proarrhythmia. In the ibutilide trials, the incidence of polymorphic VT or torsade de pointes requiring electrical cardioversion was 0.5–1.7% and the incidence of self-terminating polymorphic VT was 2.6–6.7% [262, 265]. There are insufficient data to support the use of ibutilide in patients with significant structural heart disease as many controlled studies of ibutilide have only enrolled patients with mild or moderate underlying heart disease.

Oral dofetilide has been studied extensively and is considered safe and relatively effective for pharmacological cardioversion of AF including arrhythmia duration of >7 days. Two medium-size prospective studies, SAFIRE-D (Symptomatic Atrial Fibrillation Investigative Research

Table 29.9 Antiarrhythmic drugs for pharmacological cardioversion of atrial fibrillation

Drug	Route	Dose					Potential adverse effects
			Class	LOE	Class	LOE	
Flecainide	Oral or intravenous	Loading dose 200–300mg or 1.5–3.0mg/kg over 10–20min	I	A	IIb	B	Rapidly conducted atrial flutter; ventricular proarrhythmia in patients with myocardial ischaemia; possible deterioration of ventricular function in the presence of organic heart disease
Propafenone	Oral or intravenous	Loading dose 450–600mg or 1.5–2.0mg/kg over 10–20min	I	A	IIb	B	
Ibutilide	Intravenous	1mg over 10min; repeat 1mg if necessary	IIa	A	IIa	A	QT prolongation; torsade de pointes; hypotension
Sotalol	Intravenous	1–1.5mg/kg	III	A	III	B	QT prolongation; torsade de pointes; bradycardia; hypotension
	Oral	80mg initial dose; then 160–320mg in divided doses	IIb	B	III	B	
Dofetilide	Oral	125–500mg twice daily*	I	A	I	I	QT prolongation; torsade de pointes; contraindicated if creatinine clearance <2 ml/min
Amiodarone	Oral or intravenous	In-patient: 1200–1800mg daily in divided doses until 10g total; then 200–400mg daily Out-patient: 600–800mg daily until 10g total; then 200–400mg daily 5–7mg/kg over 30–60min intravenously; then 1200–1800mg daily oral until 10g total; then 200–400mg daily	IIa	A	IIa	A	Hypotension; bradycardia; QT prolongation; torsade de pointes (risk <1%); phlebitis (intravenous) gastrointestinal upset; constipation (oral); multiorgan toxicity in the long-term
Procainamide†	Intravenous	1000mg over 30min (33mg/min) followed by 2mg/min infusion	IIb	B	IIb	C	QRS widening; torsade de pointes; rapid atrial flutter

AF, atrial fibrillation; LOE, level of evidence; *dose depends on creatinine clearance: >60mL/min—500mg; 40–60mL/min—250mg; 20–40mL/min—125mg twice daily; contraindicated if creatinine clearance <20mL/min; † limited use or withdrawn agents.

on Dofetilide) and EMERALD (European and Australian Multicenter Evaluative Research on Dofetilide) reported a modest 30% cardioversion rate of persistent AF with high-dose (1000mcg twice daily) oral dofetilide compared with 1.2% of spontaneous conversion on placebo [266] and 5% on sotalol [267].

In the pooled analysis from the DIAMOND (Danish Investigations of Arrhythmia and Mortality ON Dofetilide) studies in patients with symptomatic heart failure (DIAMOND-CHF) or myocardial infarction with LV dysfunction (DIAMOND-MI), oral dofetilide had a neutral effect on mortality and also demonstrated a greater rate of conversion to sinus rhythm (44% vs. 14%) [236].

Dofetilide causes QT interval prolongation and a non-negligent risk of torsade de pointes. The effect on the QT interval is dose-related and proarrhythmia typically occurs within the first 2–3 days after initiation of therapy. Therefore, it is mandatory that dofetilide be initiated in-hospital and that patients should be monitored for at least 3 days. In addition, the dose of dofetilide requires adjustment to creatinine clearance (➲Table 29.9).

Intravenous **sotalol** (1–1.5mg/kg) is ineffective for acute pharmacological cardioversion of AF: the conversion rates at 10–20% were not different from placebo [261, 262, 268, 269]. The antifibrillatory effect of sotalol is limited by reverse use dependency of its effect on atrial refractoriness: sotalol prolongs the atrial effective refractory period at normal and slow atrial rates, but not during rapid AF.

There is evidence that oral sotalol may offer a modest benefit of facilitating conversion to sinus rhythm and, in addition, can ensure ventricular rate control in patients awaiting electrical cardioversion. In the Sotalol Amiodarone Atrial Fibrillation Efficacy Trial (SAFE-T), 24.2% of patients with persistent AF treated with sotalol converted to sinus rhythm within 28 days, compared with 27.1% on amiodarone and only 0.8% on placebo [19].

The adverse effects of sotalol include hypotension, bradycardia, QT interval prolongation, and associated ventricular proarrhythmia (torsade de pointes). Bradycardia and hypotension were the commonest with intravenous sotalol [19]. The risk of proarrhythmia is increased in the presence of LV hypertrophy and in renal failure and the drug is contraindicated in these conditions.

Amiodarone is considered a relatively safe drug for acute pharmacological cardioversion and is the drug of choice in patients with advanced underlying heart disease. Amiodarone does not have any negative inotropic effect, controls the ventricular rate, and is associated with a low incidence of torsade de pointes. In meta-analysis of 13 randomized controlled studies in 1174 patients, the placebo-subtracted efficacy of amiodarone was 44%, but its effect was delayed up to 24 hours [270]. Intravenous amiodarone followed by an oral maintenance dose increases the likelihood of conversion to sinus rhythm [271].

The mortality and morbidity study CHF-STAT (Congestive Heart Failure Survival Trial of Antiarrhythmic Therapy) in patients with a mean ejection fraction of 25% has shown that long-term treatment with oral amiodarone 400mg daily for the first year and 300mg daily for the remainder of the 4.5-year trial was associated with greater rates of conversion to sinus rhythm compared with placebo (31% vs. 7.7%) [272].

Unlike propafenone and flecainide, amiodarone preserves its efficacy in patients with long-standing AF. Thus, in patients with a mean AF of almost 2 years, amiodarone 600mg daily for 4 weeks restored sinus rhythm in 34% of patients compared with 0% in the placebo group [273].

Amiodarone prolongs the QT interval, but, unlike pure class III agents, exhibits a low arrhythmogenic potential (<1%) [274]. The most common adverse effects of intravenous amiodarone are hypotension and relative bradycardia.

Class IA drugs **procainamide** (oral and intravenous) and **quinidine** (oral) have been widely used for cardioversion of AF. In direct comparisons, the efficacy of intravenous procainamide 1000–1200mg was comparable to that of propafenone (69.5% vs. 48.7%) [275], flecainide (65% vs. 92%) [276], or amiodarone (68.5% vs. 89.1%) [277] for conversion of AF of <48 hours. Quinidine given orally in a cumulative dose of up to 1200–2400mg over 24 hours has been shown to cardiovert 60–80% of recent onset AF [278, 279].

Because of the non-target effects (vasodilatation, hypotension, anticholinergic action, AV node blockade, worsening heart failure, and in addition to these, gastrointestinal discomfort and a 6% increased risk of torsade associated with quinidine), the drugs are less commonly used for cardioversion of AF.

There is limited evidence for the efficacy of intravenous **disopyramide** for acute pharmacological cardioversion in patients with AF. In one study, disopyramide administered as a bolus of 2mg/kg over 5min restored sinus rhythm in (71%) patients with self-limiting lone AF and three of seven (43%) patients with atrial flutter [280]. There are concerns, however, that the adverse effects such as proarrhythmia, hypotension, asystole, and non-target effects resulting from anticholinergic activity of disopyramide, may offset its modest antiarrhythmic potential.

Vernakalant is a new antiarrhythmic drug agent [281] with an affinity to ion channels specifically involved in the repolarization processes in atrial tissue, in particular, the ultrarapid potassium repolarization current I_{Kur}, but has little impact on major currents responsible for ventricular repolarization. It does, however, inhibit the inward sodium current (I_{Na}) and slows myocardial conduction, especially at high rates.

In the randomized, double-blind, placebo controlled Atrial arrhythmia Conversion Trials (ACT), vernakalant administered as a 10-min infusion of 3mg/kg (followed by a second infusion of 2mg/kg if AF persisted after 15min) was significantly more effective than placebo in converting AF of <7 days (52% compared with 3.6–4%, respectively) [282, 283]. The highest efficacy was observed for AF of up to 72 hours (70–80%). Vernakalant was ineffective in converting AF of >7 days duration and did not convert atrial flutter.

The drug was well tolerated; the most common (>5%) side effects of vernakalant were dysgeusia, sneezing, and nausea. Minor QTc prolongation was reported but there has been little or no proarrhythmia [282, 284].

Magnesium sulphate Meta-analysis of eight studies in 476 patients showed that magnesium sulphate, administered intravenously at an initial dose of 1200–5000mg over 1–30min (in some studies followed by the second dose or continuous infusion for 2–6 hours), was superior to placebo or the active comparator in cardioverting AF with an odds ratio of 1.6 (95% CI, 1.07–2.39) [285]. The most common side effects were sensation of warmth and flushing. Magnesium prolongs the atrial and AV node refractory periods and therefore in addition to its antifibrillatory effect, it may slow the ventricular rate. Magnesium is not routinely used for pharmacological cardioversion of AF, but it may potentiate the effect of other antiarrhythmic agents.

Digitalis, **beta-blockers**, and **calcium antagonists** usually are ineffective for acute conversion of AF [286, 287]. Digoxin may even be profibrillatory due to its cholinergic effects which may cause a non-uniform reduction in conduction velocity and effective refractory periods of the atria [288]. Short-acting intravenous beta-blockers (e.g. esmolol) and non-dihydropyridine calcium antagonists (verapamil and diltiazem) are more commonly used for rate control than for restoration of sinus rhythm.

Prevention of atrial fibrillation

Prophylactic antiarrhythmic drug therapy is recommended for patients with paroxysmal AF when paroxysms occur frequently and are associated with significant symptoms or lead to worsening LV function, and for patients with persistent AF when the likelihood of maintenance of sinus rhythm is uncertain, especially in patients with structural heart disease and a remodelled LA. After cardioversion, approximately 25–50% patients will have the recurrence of persistent AF within the first 1–2 months (early recurrence). Thereafter, the recurrence rate is about 10% per year (➲Fig. 29.30).

A systematic review of 44 studies in 11,322 patients has shown that antiarrhythmic drugs significantly reduced AF recurrence after cardioversion; the number of patients needed to treat to prevent a recurrence ranged from two to nine, depending on the agent used (➲Fig. 29.31) [289]. The majority of large-size, high-quality studies were conducted in patients with persistent AF, mainly because the recurrence of a persistent episode is more 'predictable', is likely to occur during the first year, and is easier to recognize and document, especially when the time to first symptomatic recurrence is used as an outcome parameter. Hence, the efficacy of an antiarrhythmic drug to control paroxysmal AF is usually derived from the results of studies in persistent AF.

Beta-blockers are modestly effective in preventing AF and are mainly used for rate control. In anecdotal reports, the annual recurrence rate after cardioversion for persistent AF was slightly lower on beta-blockers (metoprolol 100mg or bisoprolol 5mg) than on placebo (48% vs. 60%) [290] or comparable to that on sotalol (42% vs. 41%) [291]. There is no evidence of superiority of one type of beta-blocker over the other for prevention of AF [292]. However, because of their safety and the effect on AV node conduction during rapid AF, beta-blockers are often used as initial therapy in patients with new onset AF.

In addition, beta-blockers may contribute to upstream therapy in AF associated with congestive heart failure: a meta-analysis of seven studies in 11,952 patients has

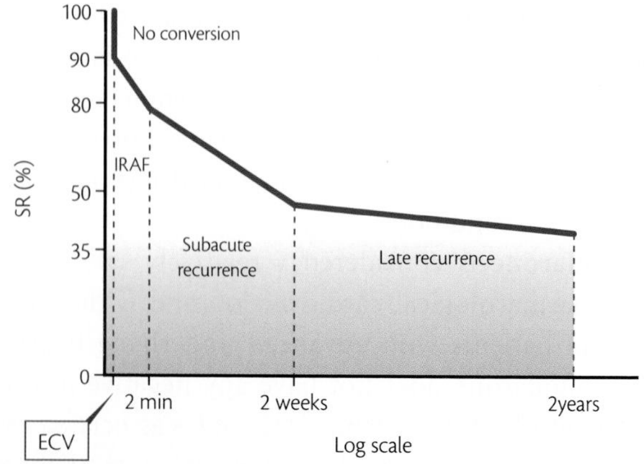

Figure 29.30 Recurrence of atrial fibrillation after cardioversion.

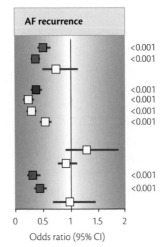

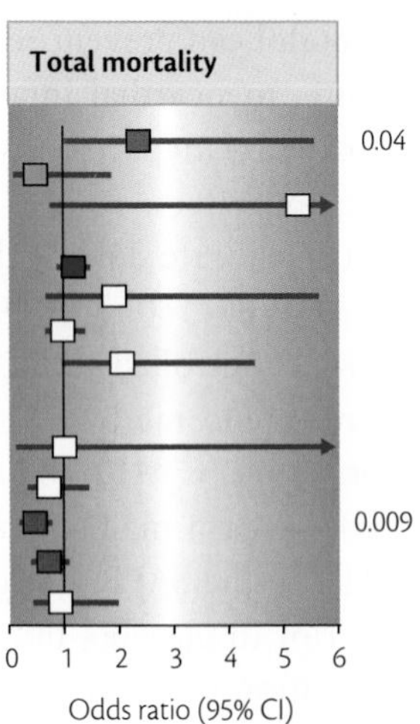

Figure 29.31 Antiarrhythmic drugs for prevention of atrial fibrillation after cardioversion. Modified with permission from Lafuente-Lafuente C, Mouly S, Longas-Tejero MA, *et al.* Antiarrhythmic drugs for maintaining sinus rhythm after cardioversion of atrial fibrillation: a systematic review of randomized controlled trials. *Arch Intern Med* 2006; **166**: 719–28.

shown that therapy with beta-blockers was associated with a statistically significant reduction in the incidence of new onset AF by 27% during mean follow-up of 1.35 years [295]. Beta-blockers are first-line therapy in patients with thyrotoxicosis or, rarely, adrenergically-mediated AF [293, 294].

Propafenone and **flecainide** are recommended as first-line therapy for AF in patients without significant structural heart disease, i.e. patients without congestive heart failure, LV dysfunction, marked hypertrophy, previous myocardial infarction, or CAD. Both propafenone (300–900mg daily in 2–3 divided doses) and flecainide (50–150mg twice daily) reduced the recurrence rate by approximately two-thirds [254, 289, 296–300], with no advantage of one drug over the other. In a meta-analysis of propafenone, the incidence of recurrent AF at 1 year was 56.8% (52.3–61.3%) [254]. All-cause mortality associated with propafenone was 0.3%. Several placebo-controlled and comparator trials of flecainide at 200–300mg daily have consistently reported a 60–70% likelihood of maintaining sinus rhythm after 1 year with an acceptable risk:benefit ratio [296, 299, 300].

Propafenone is available as a sustained-release (SR) formulation at 225, 325, or 425mg twice daily. In the North American Recurrence of Atrial Fibrillation Trial (RAFT) [301] and its European equivalent, ERAFT [302], propafenone SR was superior to placebo in prolonging time to first symptomatic recurrence of paroxysmal AF in patients with minor structural heart disease. Flecainide is also available as a long-acting formulation in some parts of Europe, but no formal studies of its safety and efficacy have been reported.

Drugs with class IC mode of action, other than flecainide and propafenone, are available in some countries, e.g. **pilsicainide** is available in Japan and **cibenzoline** is used in Japan and France. Both drugs are modestly effective in cardioversion (45% for pilsicainide) and/or prevention of AF (maximum 41% reported for pilsicainide and 50% for cibenzoline at 1 year) and exhibit a similar adverse event profile to other class IC agents [303, 304].

Quinidine has been used for treatment of AF since the discovery of its antiarrhythmic properties in the early 1920s. In a meta-analysis of six randomized controlled trials in 808 patients, published in 1990, 50% of patients treated with quinidine were in sinus rhythm after 1 year compared with 25% among controls [305]. The antiarrhythmic effect of quinidine was offset by high all-cause mortality and sudden death in the quinidine-treated patients compared with controls (2.9% vs. 0.8%; odds ratio 2.98) [305]. In a 2006 analysis which included two recent large-scale studies of quinidine, PAFAC (Prevention of Atrial Fibrillation After Cardioversion) and SOPAT (Suppression Of Paroxysmal Atrial Tachyarrhythmias), quinidine reduced recurrent AF by 49% [289]. In PAFAC [6] and SOPAT [7], quinidine was not associated with increased risk of death, probably because it was used at lower doses (320–480mg as opposed to 1000–1800mg daily in the previous trials [305]), in a fixed combination with verapamil (single combination tablet), and in patients with overall less significant structural heart disease. However, the foremost safety issue for quinidine remains its propensity to cause ventricular proarrhythmia including torsade de pointes even at low or sub-therapeutic doses [234].

Disopyramide is rarely used for treatment of AF because of its negative inotropic effect, the torsadogenic potential, and poor tolerance due to antimuscarinic properties. However, the use of disopyramide is advocated in patients with lone, vagally-mediated AF. Data on the efficacy of disopyramide in AF are sparse [305, 306].

Sotalol can prevent recurrent AF in the absence of heart failure, myocardial infarction, or hypertension with significant LV hypertrophy [308–310]. Because of its beta-blocking effect, sotalol offers the additional benefit of ventricular rate slowing during recurrences. The usual dose for AF is 80–160mg BID. In a meta-analysis of nine randomized controlled studies in 1538 patients, sotalol reduced the recurrence rate by 47% [289]. In the Canadian Trial of Atrial Fibrillation (CTAF), sotalol was inferior to amiodarone for the long-term maintenance of sinus rhythm (➲Fig. 29.32) [311]. In the SAFE-T study, sotalol 160mg twice daily was superior to placebo, but less effective than amiodarone in prevention of AF recurrence after electrical cardioversion [19]. At 2 years, approximately 30% of patients treated with sotalol remained in sinus rhythm compared with 60% of patients on amiodarone and 10% of patients on placebo. The efficacy of sotalol was similar to that of class I antiarrhythmic drugs and inferior to that of amiodarone in the AFFIRM sub-study (48%, 45%, and 66%, respectively) [312].

Hypotension and bradycardia were the most common cardiovascular adverse effects of sotalol with an incidence of 6–10%, while ventricular proarrhythmias associated with prolongation of the QT interval were reported in 1–4% of patients and were dose related [308, 310]. Ventricular proarrhythmia is a relevant concern and is often related to QT prolongation.

Dofetilide is relatively safe to use in patients with previous myocardial infarction and/or congestive heart failure. In the DIAMOND AF sub-study of DIAMOND-CHF and DIAMOND-MI trials, 506 patients with AF at baseline were more likely to remain in sinus rhythm on treatment with dofetilide 500mcg twice daily compared with placebo (79% vs. 42%) [236]. Patients treated with dofetilide had a lower incidence of new onset AF than those on placebo (1.23% vs. 3.78%) [311, 312]; this effect was more pronounced in patients with NYHA class III and IV heart failure enrolled in DIAMOND-CHF (1.98% vs. 6.55%) [313]. Dofetilide was almost twice as effective for the long-term prevention of atrial flutter than of AF (73% vs. 40%) [266].

The major safety concern about dofetilide is its torsadogenic potential which is dose related. For instance, the incidence of torsade de pointes with dofetilide ranges from almost 'zero' at doses below 250mcg BID to 10% or greater at doses higher than 500mcg BID, with more than three-quarters of episodes occurring during the first 3–4 days of drug initiation [234]. Dofetilide is excreted predominantly via kidneys and its dose should be adjusted for creatinine clearance (see ➲Table 29.9); the drug should not be prescribed in patients with significantly impaired renal function (creatinine clearance <20), hypokalaemia, hypomagnaesemia, or a QT interval of >500ms. If the QT interval is prolonged to >500ms or by >15% versus baseline, the dose should be reduced.

Amiodarone is the best available antiarrhythmic drug for maintenance of sinus rhythm in patients with advanced heart disease or in patients in whom class IC agents or sotalol were ineffective. Because of its neutral effect on all-cause mortality [274, 315, 316], amiodarone is considered a drug of choice for management of AF in patients with congestive heart failure, hypertrophic cardiomyopathy, and hypertension with significant LV hypertrophy.

In the CTAF trial of 403 patients with paroxysmal and persistent AF, amiodarone administered at 10mg/kg for 2 weeks, followed by 300mg per day for 4 weeks and

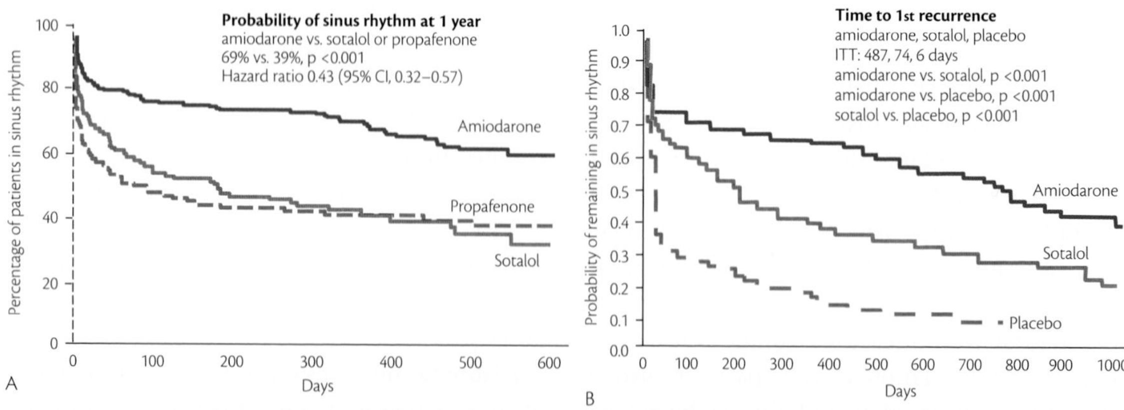

Figure 29.32 Probability of remaining free from recurrent atrial fibrillation with amiodarone and sotalol in the Canadian Trial of Atrial Fibrillation (CTAF) (A) and in the Sotalol Amiodarone atrial Fibrillation Efficacy Trial (SAFE-T) (B). ITT, intention to treat. Modified from Roy D, Talajic M, Dorian P, *et al.*; for the Canadian Trial of Atrial Fibrillation Investigators. Amiodarone to prevent recurrence of atrial fibrillation. *N Engl J Med* 2000; **342**: 913–20; and Singh BN, Singh SN, Reda DJ, *et al.*; Sotalol Amiodarone Atrial Fibrillation Efficacy Trial (SAFE-T) Investigators. Amiodarone versus sotalol for atrial fibrillation. *N Engl J Med* 2005; **352**: 1861–72.

a maintenance dose of 200mg reduced the incidence of recurrent AF by 57% compared with sotalol 160–320mg per day or propafenone 450–600mg (➲ Fig. 29.32) [309]. Patients who received amiodarone at a maintenance dose of 300mg per day in the CHF-STAT study had fewer recurrences, and were half as less likely to develop new AF compared with placebo [272].

Despite prolonging cardiac repolarization, amiodarone has a low (<1%) torsadogenic potential [234, 274]. The residual risk of torsade de pointes with amiodarone occurs mainly in patients with other risk factors, such as bradycardia or hypokalaemia. The reason for the low propensity of amiodarone to cause torsade de pointes is not clear, but is presumably related to its complex mode of action which involves class I, II, and IV effects alongside its class III properties and a low propensity to increase the heterogeneity of refractoriness across the myocardial layers.

A significant downside of amiodarone is multiple non-target effects, which range from transient and relatively trivial (e.g. gastrointestinal disturbances), to partially preventable (e.g. skin toxicity) and medically correctable (e.g. underactive thyroid), to serious such as pulmonary toxicity, liver damage, hyperthyroidism, bradycardia, significant or irreversible neurological symptoms (e.g. peripheral neuropathy), and visual disturbances (e.g. optic neuritis). Amiodarone is therefore not recommended as first-line therapy in patients with little or no structural heart disease for whom therapy with class IC drugs or sotalol is more appropriate. As many serious adverse effects of amiodarone develop after prolonged therapy (years), amiodarone therapy is less appropriate for younger patients.

Dronedarone is a structural analogue of amiodarone which is devoid of iodine atoms and is believed to have a better side-effect profile with lower risk of pulmonary fibrosis, ocular adverse effects, and skin photosensitivity. Dronedarone 400mg BID is moderately effective in preventing AF recurrences after electrical cardioversion [317, 318]. In the EURIDIS (EURopean trial In atrial fibrillation or flutter patients receiving Dronedarone for the maintenance of Sinus rhythm), the median time to the recurrence of AF was 41 days in the placebo group and 96 days in the dronedarone group (➲ Fig. 29.33) [318]. In the American–Australian–African equivalent of the European trial (ADONIS), the median time to recurrence was 59 on placebo and 158 days on dronedarone.

The post hoc analysis of the EURIDIS and ADONIS studies has shown that patients treated with dronedarone had a 27% reduction in relative risk of hospitalization for cardiovascular causes and death [318]. The beneficial effect of dronedarone on survival has been confirmed in a further study called ATHENA (A placebo controlled, double blind Trial to assess the efficacy of dronedarone for the prevention of cardiovascular Hospitalization or death from any cause in patiENts with Atrial fibrillation and flutter) in >4000 high-risk patients with AF (➲ Fig. 29.33) [319]. In ATHENA, dronedarone reduced cardiovascular hospitalizations or all-cause death by 24% compared with placebo. This effect was driven by the reduction in cardiovascular

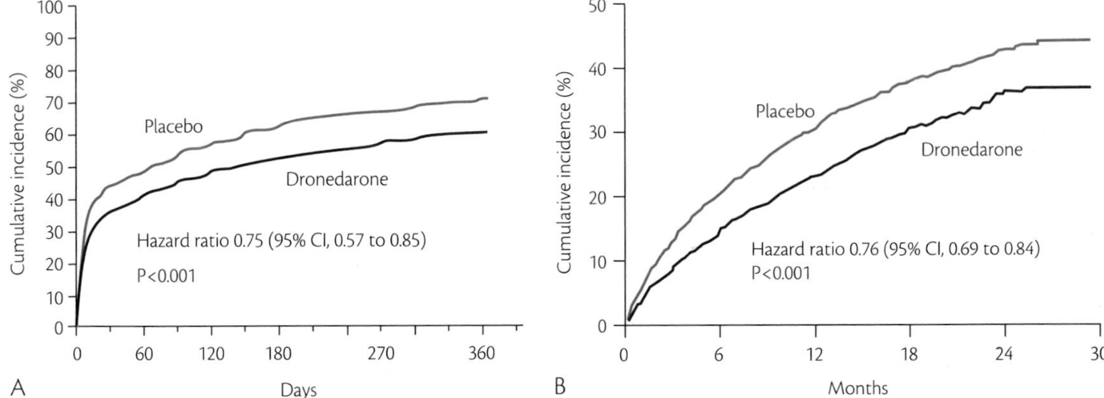

Figure 29.33 EURIDIS and ADONIS pooled analysis (A). Times to first recurrence of atrial fibrillation or flutter. Modified with permission from Singh BN, Connolly SJ, Crijns HJ, *et al.*; EURIDIS and ADONIS Investigators. Dronedarone for maintenance of sinus rhythm in atrial fibrillation or flutter. *N Engl J Med* 2007; **357**: 987–99. (B) Time to first cardiovascular hospitalization or death in the ATHENA trial of dronedarone versus placebo. Data from Hohnloser SH , Crijns HJ, van Eickels M, *et al.* Effect of dronedarone on cardiovascular events in atrial fibrillation. *N Engl J Med* 2009; **360**: 668–78. ADONIS, American-Australian-African trial In atrial fibrillation or flutter patients receiving DronedarONe for the maIntenance of Sinus rhythm; ATHENA, A placebo controlled, double blind Trial to assess the efficacy of dronedarone for the prevention of cardiovascular Hospitalization or death from any cause in patiENts with Atrial fibrillation and flutter. EURIDIS, EURopean trial In atrial fibrillation or flutter patients receiving Dronedarone for the maIntenance of Sinus rhythm.

hospitalizations (by 25%), particularly hospitalizations for AF (by 37%). The beneficial effect of dronedarone on cardiovascular hospitalizations and death was consistent across all subgroups of patients, including those who remained in AF throughout the study. In addition, dronedarone reduced the ventricular rate response during AF by 10–15bpm. All-cause mortality was similar in the dronedarone and placebo groups (5% and 6%, respectively); however, dronedarone significantly reduced deaths from cardiovascular causes.

Unlike the trials which reported a beneficial effect of dronedarone on cardiovascular mortality, the ANDROMEDA (ANtiarrhythmic trial with DROnedarone in Moderate to severe heart failure Evaluating morbidity DecreAse) study specifically enrolled patients with NYHA functional class III or IV heart failure and recent heart failure decompensation. The trial was stopped prematurely after 627 patients out of the 1000 planned were enrolled, because an interim safety analysis revealed an excess of deaths in the dronedarone arm compared with placebo (8% vs. 13.8%; hazard ratio 2.13) [320]. The risk of death was the greatest in patients with severely depressed ventricular function and there were more hospitalizations for heart failure in the dronedarone arm.

The adverse outcome in ANDROMEDA is in part thought to be associated with more frequent discontinuation of ACE inhibitors or angiotensin receptor blockers in patients who received dronedarone because of increases in creatinine levels which were misinterpreted as progressive renal failure. These increases were secondary to the now known inhibitory effect of dronedarone on renal tubular excretion of creatinine. Consequently, excess mortality in the dronedarone group was related to worsening heart failure. In the subsequent analysis of a small proportion of patients (n = 200) with NYHA class III heart failure, many of who had an ejection fraction of <35%, therapy with dronedarone was, in fact, associated with a lower likelihood of hospitalizations or death from cardiovascular causes as well as lower all-cause mortality compared with placebo. However, withdrawal of potentially life-saving therapy does not explain all fatalities in ANDROMEDA, and dronedarone is therefore contraindicated in patients with NYHA class IV heart failure.

Investigational antiarrhythmic agents

A raft of other amiodarone analogues (e.g. celivarone) and amiodarone-derivative with modified bonds within the molecule is currently at various stages of development (➲Fig. 29.28) [107]. An oral formulation of vernakalant 600mg BID has been reported to be useful for prevention of AF recurrence after electrical cardioversion, with a modest superiority to placebo (51% vs. 37%) [107]. There is evidence that an antianginal drug, ranolazine, may also produce an antiarrhythmic effect due to multiple channel blockade, particularly late sodium current blockade.

Antiarrhythmic drugs and direct current cardioversion

Antiarrhythmic drugs can be used to facilitate electrical cardioversion and to prevent immediate or early recurrence of AF. Synergistic action of antiarrhythmic drugs may be due to prolongation of atrial refractoriness, conversion of AF to a more organized atrial rhythm (e.g. flutter) which may be cardioverted with less energy, the suppression of atrial premature beats that may re-initiate AF, and prevention of atrial remodelling. The disadvantages are increased risk of ventricular proarrhythmia and bradycardia [321].

Pre-treatment with intravenous ibutilide, flecainide, or sotalol lowered the energy requirement by around 30% and improved the success rate of cardioversion, including previously failed electrical cardioversion [321–324]. Slightly higher rates of restoration and maintenance of sinus rhythm were reported in patients pre-treated with oral amiodarone, propafenone, verapamil, and diltiazem, but the evidence is inconsistent [325–327].

Risk of recurrence is increased (25–50%) during the first 1–2 months after electrical cardioversion. It is therefore important to continue antiarrhythmic drug therapy if risk of recurrence is deemed to be high (e.g. in patients who had previously reverted to AF). The CONVERT (CONtinuous Vs Episodic pRophylactic Treatment with amiodarone) study reported that patients who stopped amiodarone after 1 month of sinus rhythm following cardioversion had a higher incidence of recurrent AF (80% vs. 54%), as well as all-cause mortality and cardiovascular hospitalizations (53% and 35%) during a median follow-up of 2.1 years compared with those who continued amiodarone treatment [328].

Antiarrhythmic drug use after left atrial ablation

After LA ablation therapies, the incidence of AF or atrial tachycardia has been reported to be 45% during the first 3 months despite antiarrhythmic drugs [99]. In many cases, early recurrence of AF after ablation is transient and is thought to be secondary to inflammation after radiofrequency injury, nerve ending damage and resulting

Table 29.10 Drugs for acute rate control in atrial fibrillation

Drug	Route of administration	Dose	Onset	Recommendation (class)	Level of evidence
Esmolol	Intravenous	0.5mg/kg over 1min followed by 0.05–0.2mg/kg/min infusion	5min	I	C*
Metoprolol	Intravenous	2.5–5mg over 2min followed by repeat doses if necessary	5min	I	C*
Propranolol	Intravenous	0.15mg/kg	5min	I	C*
Diltiazem	Intravenous	0.25mg/kg over 2min followed by 5–15mg/hour infusion	2–7min	I	B
Verapamil	Intravenous	0.075–0.15mg/kg over 2min	3–5	I	B
Digoxin	Intravenous	0.25mg every 2 hours, max. 1.5mg	2 hours	IIb†	B
Amiodarone	Intravenous	As for cardioversion‡	6–8 hours	IIb‡	C
Sotalol	Intravenous	1–1.5mg/kg over 5–10min	15–30min	III	B

* For all beta-blockers; † a class I indication in patients with poor ventricular function and moderately fast ventricular rates, level of evidence B; ‡see ➲ Table 29.9, a class IIa indication in patients with poor ventricular function and moderately fast ventricular rates, level of evidence C.

imbalance of the cardiac autonomic nervous system, and a delayed effect of ablation associated with 'maturation' of lesions.

Early AF often subsides after 3 months upon the resolution of inflammation and restoration of autonomic regulation, without the need for re-ablation. Therefore antiarrhythmic drug therapy to suppress early recurrence of AF is commonly employed for the first 1–3 months after ablation or if the arrhythmia recurs after discontinuation of the antiarrhythmic drug. These are usually the same agents that have been previously ineffective, but may now be efficacious because of a synergistic effect with ablation. Amiodarone has been reported to be most commonly prescribed because of its antifibrillatory as well as AV conduction slowing properties. The synergistic effect of propafenone, flecainide, or sotalol has been demonstrated in the 5A (AntiArrhythmics After Ablation of Atrial fibrillation) study. The use of antiarrhythmic drugs increases the likelihood of staying in sinus rhythm by about 30% [329].

Pharmacological rate control

Acute rate control

The target heart rate for acute rate control is 80–100 beats per minute (bpm) during AF. In patients with rapid ventricular rate, intravenous **verapamil**, **diltiazem**, and **beta-blockers** (usually metoprolol or the rapidly-eliminated **esmolol**) are commonly used for rapid ventricular rate control (➲ Table 29.10) [330]. All drugs are equally effective in reducing the ventricular response rate by approximately 20–30% in 20–30min and have a similar risk of adverse effects (usually hypotension and bradycardia; although LV dysfunction and high-degree heart block may occur). Beta-blockers are preferable in patients with a history of myocardial infarction or if thyrotoxicosis is suspected as a cause of the arrhythmia, whereas verapamil and diltiazem are preferred in patients with acutely exacerbated chronic obstructive airways disease.

Intravenous **digoxin** is no longer the treatment of choice for acute rate control because of delayed onset of its therapeutic effect (>60min). However, because digoxin has a positive inotropic effect, it is a reasonable adjunct to beta-blockers in patients with impaired LV function and moderately fast ventricular rates.

Agents with the primary effect on the AV node should not be used for rate control in patients with known or suspected pre-excitation syndrome: these agents will only affect AV nodal conduction and will have no effect on rapid conduction via the accessory pathway. In patients with accessory pathways, sodium-channel blockers (e.g. intravenous ajmaline or flecainide) can slow anterograde conduction via the accessory pathway.

Intravenous **amiodarone** can be used for acute ventricular rate control when other agents have no effect on ventricular response or are contraindicated, for example, in haemodynamically unstable AF refractory to electrical cardioversion [331]. The AV blocking effect of amiodarone is complemented by its antifibrillatory action. The disadvantages of intravenous amiodarone are slow onset of action and increased risk of phlebitis. **Sotalol** can also slow down the ventricular rate due to its beta-blocking properties [332], but its negative inotropic effect in patients with LV dysfunction and risk of torsades due to QT interval prolongation reduce its value as a rate controlling agent.

There is limited evidence of the use of **clonidine** (due to its central sympatholytic activity) [333] and **magnesium** [285] for ventricular rate control. In a meta-analysis, intravenous magnesium reduced the ventricular rate to <90–100 within 5–15 min of infusion. **Adenosine** derivatives with a high specificity for adenosine A1 receptors and longer half-life periods (e.g. tecadenoson, selodenoson, and capadenoson) are currently under investigation [107, 334].

Rate control in paroxysmal and persistent atrial fibrillation

Rate control is an essential constituent of management of AF and is pertinent to all types of the arrhythmia. In paroxysmal and persistent AF, rate control is important during the recurrence or prior to electrical cardioversion. **Verapamil**, **diltiazem**, and **beta-blockers** (**metoprolol**, **atenolol**, **bisoprolol**, **carvedilol**, and **nadolol**) are drugs of choice. They are also commonly prescribed in combination with the class IC agents, propafenone and flecainide, to prevent fast ventricular rates due to 1:1 AV conduction when recurrent AF evolves to flutter.

Digoxin has been shown to reduce the ventricular rate during symptomatic paroxysms of AF by approximately 15bpm and has probably rendered some episodes asymptomatic [335], but because of its profibrillatory effect, digoxin usually should be avoided if the arrhythmia is self-terminating or electrical cardioversion is planned and rhythm control is pursued.

Some antiarrhythmic drugs, such as **sotalol**, **amiodarone**, and **dronedarone**, slow AV conduction and thus offer an additional benefit of ventricular rate control during recurrences of AF without significantly affecting the overall exercise capacity [19, 272, 336–338]. However, antiarrhythmic drugs are not likely to be routinely employed for long-term rate control, e.g. in permanent or accepted AF, because of potential proarrhythmic and non-target side effects.

Rate control in permanent atrial fibrillation

Current guidelines define adequate rate control as maintenance of the ventricular rate response between 60–80bpm at rest and 90–115bpm during moderate exercise, but few systematic studies explored the effect of rate slowing drugs on chronotropic competence in AF or defined upper limits of the appropriate ventricular rate response during exercise [339] and no controlled clinical trials have validated these values with regard to their effects on morbidity or mortality. In post hoc pooled analysis of the AFFIRM and RACE studies, patients with mean ventricular rates during AF within the AFFIRM (≤80bpm) or RACE (<100bpm) criteria had a better outcome than patients with ventricular rates ≥100bpm (hazard ratio 0.69 and 0.58, respectively for ≤80 and <100 compared with ≥100bpm) [340].

Although rapid ventricular rates can be detrimental, too slow heart rate can be problematic, particularly in patients with impaired diastolic filling, hypertension, and LV hypertrophy when loss of atrial contraction may cause a marked decrease in cardiac output. Furthermore, rhythm irregularity per se may contribute to ventricular dysfunction [341].

Ventricular rate control at rest does not always translate into effective control during exercise. Ambulatory 24-hour ECG monitoring is considered sufficient for assessment of rate control in elderly and sedentary individuals, whereas in younger individuals, an exercise stress test may be necessary (➲Figs. 29.34 and 29.35). RACE II was instigated to assess whether maintaining strict rate control, i.e. mean resting heart rate <80bpm and heart rate during mild exercise <110bpm, can offer any additional benefit to standard practice [342].

Drugs for rate control. Digoxin, beta-blockers, verapamil, and diltiazem, are commonly employed (➲Table 29.11). Digoxin is effective in controlling ventricular rates at rest as it prolongs AV node conduction and refractoriness through

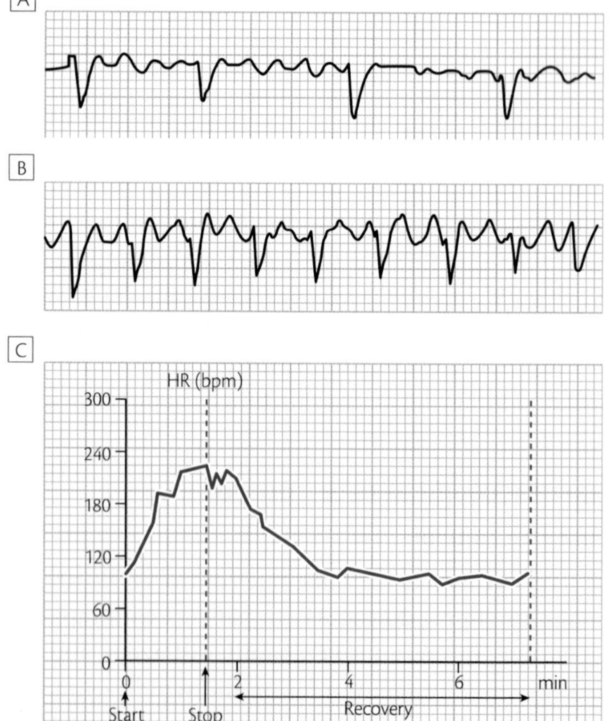

Figure 29.34 ECG strips recorded before (A) and after (B) exercise stress test in a young patient with atrial fibrillation and controlled ventricular rates at rest. Note a sharp increase in ventricular rates showing inadequate ventricular rate control after just 1.5min of exercise prompting early termination of the test (C).

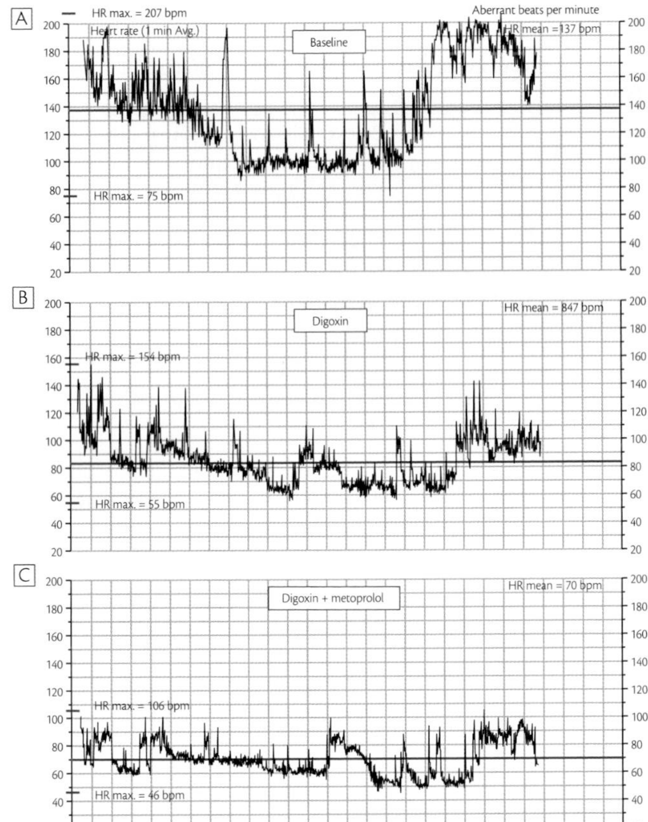

Figure 29.35 24-hour Holter ECG histograms show fast ventricular rates during untreated atrial fibrillation (A), during monotherapy with digoxin (B), and after digoxin in combination with a beta-blocker (C).

vagal stimulation, by direct effects on the AV node, and by increasing the amount of concealed conduction. However, the effect of digoxin is negated during exercise when most vagal tone is lost and AV conduction is further enhanced by the increased sympathetic tone. Digoxin alone was effective in only 58% of patients [343]. Therefore, digoxin as monotherapy can be used in older, sedentary patients, but a combination with beta-blockers or calcium antagonists is often necessary to achieve rate control in the majority of patients (➲Fig. 29.35).

Non-dihydropyridine calcium antagonists and beta-blockers are effective as primary pharmacological therapy for rate control, but multiple adjustments of drug type and dosage may be needed to achieve the desired effect [343–345]. For example, in the AFFIRM trial, only 58% of patients in the rate-control group achieved adequate rate control with the first drug or combination; drug switches occurred in 37% of the patients and drug combinations were commonly used [343]. Overall, adequate rate control was ascertained in 80% of patients at 5 years (most frequently on a beta-blocker with or without digoxin).

Atrial fibrillation in congestive heart failure

Patients with congestive heart failure are particularly prone to the adverse effects of antiarrhythmic drugs. Electrical cardioversion may be considered in younger patients with short arrhythmia duration who have compensated heart failure. **Amiodarone** or **dofetilide** are the drugs of choice to prevent recurrences as they have been shown to be safe and effective in this context [236, 272, 313–315]. Neither drug is associated with deterioration of LV function nor predisposes to proarrhythmic effects as long as they have been initiated and followed carefully. ECG monitoring of the QT interval is of special importance in this setting.

All patients with LV dysfunction should also be treated with **beta-blockers** and **ACE inhibitors** or **angiotensin receptor blockers** because, in addition to their proven beneficial effect on survival, they may delay atrial remodelling and deter onset of new AF and possibly prevent recurrent AF (see ➲'Upstream' therapy, p.1113) [34]. The magnitude of their effect may be modest but if applied to a very large population, the outcome could be significant.

Prevention of atrial fibrillation after cardiac surgery

Postoperative AF occurs predominantly during the first 4 days. More than 90% of patients present with a paroxysmal or first-onset form of the arrhythmia. Atrial flutter and atrial tachycardias, including multifocal atrial tachycardia, are also common. Electrical or pharmacological restoration of sinus rhythm with subsequent prophylactic antiarrhythmic therapy should be considered in haemodynamically unstable or highly symptomatic patients with postoperative AF. If AF is well tolerated, rate control may be sufficient as AF after isolated coronary bypass surgery is often self-limiting and there is a high likelihood of spontaneous conversion to sinus rhythm, usually within 6 weeks [346].

Beta-blockers should be considered the first-line treatment because of their beneficial effects on the hyperadrenergic postoperative state. The best evidence of the efficacy in prevention of postoperative AF has been accumulated for beta-blockers, sotalol, and amiodarone (➲Fig. 29.36) [346]. Two earlier meta-analyses of randomized controlled studies have shown that treatment with beta-blockers may reduce the incidence of postoperative AF by approximately 50% [347, 348]. In the recent meta-analysis of 27 trials in 3840 patients, therapy with beta-blockers reduced risk of postoperative AF by 61%; there was also a trend towards shorter length of stay [346]. The downside of

Table 29.11 Drugs for long-term rate control in atrial fibrillation

Drug	Dose	Type of recommendation	Level of evidence	Potential adverse effects
Digoxin	Loading dose: 250mcg every 2 hours; up to 1500mcg; maintenance dose 125–250mcg daily	I	B	Bradycardia; AV block; atrial arrhythmias; ventricular tachycardia
Diltiazem	120–360mg daily	I	B	Hypotension; AV block; heart failure
Verapamil	120–360mg daily	I	B	Hypotension; AV block; heart failure
Atenolol	50–100mg daily	I	C*	Hypotension; bradycardia; heart failure; deterioration of chronic obstructive pulmonary disease or asthma
Metoprolol	50–200mg daily	I	C*	
Propranolol	80–240mg daily	I	C*	
Bisoprolol	5–10mg daily	I	C*	
Carvedilol	25–100mg daily	I	C*	
Sotalol	80–320mg	IIb†	C	Bradycardia; QT prolongation; torsade de pointes (risk <1%); photosensitivity; pulmonary toxicity; polyneuropathy; hepatic toxicity; thyroid dysfunction; gastrointestinal upset
Amiodarone	800mg daily for 1 week, then 600mg daily for 1 week, then 400mg daily for 4–6 weeks; maintenance dose 200mg daily	IIb†	C	Bradycardia; QT prolongation; torsade de pointes (risk <1%); photosensitivity; pulmonary toxicity; polyneuropathy; hepatic toxicity; thyroid dysfunction; gastrointestinal upset

AV, atrioventricular.

* For all beta-blockers; †useful during the recurrence of atrial fibrillation.

beta-blockers is that they may increase risk of bradycardia (5–10%) and risk of longer ventilation (1–2%).

Magnesium (20 studies, 2490 patients), **amiodarone** (19 studies, 3295 patients), and **sotalol** (eight studies, 1294 patients) reduced the incidence of postoperative AF by 46%, 50%, and 65%, respectively, compared with placebo [346]. In the Prevention of Arrhythmias that Begin Early After Revascularization (PAPABEAR) trial of 601 patients undergoing isolated coronary artery bypass surgery, treatment with amiodarone 10mg/kg per day starting 7 days before surgery, was associated with a significant decrease in the incidence of postoperative AF compared with placebo (30% vs. 16%) reflecting a 52% reduction in relative risk [349]. The use of sotalol risks bradycardia and torsade

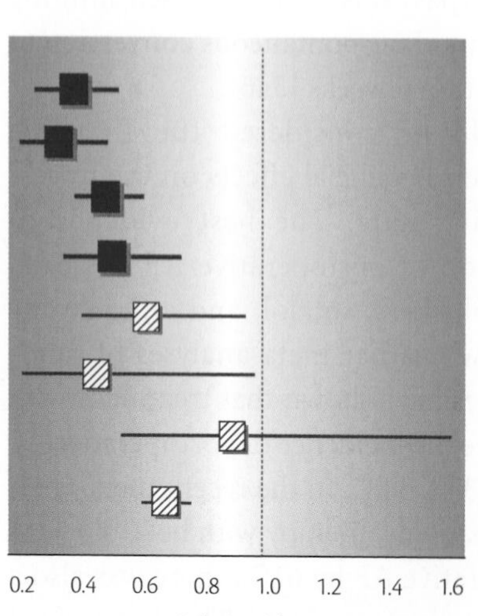

Drug	Studies N	Pts, N	RR	(95% CI)
Beta-blockers	27	3840	0.39	(0.28–0.52)
Sotalol	8	1294	0.35	(0.26–0.49)
Amiodarone	17	3007	0.50	(0.42–0.59)
Magnesium	20	2490	0.54	(0.38–0.75)
Propafenone	1	293	0.62	(0.43–0.91)
Procainamide	2	146	0.47	(0.22–0.99)
Verapamil	3	432	0.94	(0.56–1.58)
Diltiazem	5	638	0.64	(0.53–0.76)

Figure 29.36 Meta-analysis of pharmacological prevention of atrial fibrillation after heart surgery. Hatched boxes indicate agents that have not been rigorously tested. Data from Mitchell LB, Crystal E, Heilbron B, *et al.* Atrial fibrillation following cardiac surgery. *Can J Cardiol* 2005; **21**(Suppl. B): 45B–50B.

de pointes, especially in patients with electrolyte disturbances. Amiodarone may cause hypotension and bradycardia necessitating inotropic and chronotropic support or pacing.

The proarrhythmic potential and the negative inotropic effect of class I agents, ibutilide, and dofetilide offset their modest efficacy in prevention and/or conversion of AF after cardiac surgery.

Several randomized controlled studies have suggested the beneficial role of agents with anti-inflammatory properties, such as statins, or specific anti-inflammatory drugs such as corticosteroids [350, 351]. In the randomized prospective, double-blind, placebo-controlled study, ARMYDA-3 (Atorvastatin for Reduction of MYocardial Dysrhythmia After cardiac surgery), in 200 patients undergoing elective coronary bypass grafting surgery pre-treatment with atorvastatin starting 7 days before surgery was associated with a 61% reduction in the incidence of in-hospital AF [350]. Pre-treatment of patients with poly-unsaturated fatty acids for 5 days before coronary bypass grafting surgery reduced the occurrence of postoperative AF by 65% [352].

'Upstream' therapy

It has been recently appreciated that primary and secondary prevention of AF with 'upstream' therapy and risk factor modification is likely to produce a larger effect in the general population than will specific interventions [34, 233]. Angiotensin II, whose local synthesis is increased in AF, has been recognized as a key element in atrial remodelling. Angiotensin II produces a variety of direct and indirect effects on atrial structure and electrophysiology by stimulating atrial fibrosis and hypertrophy, promoting inflammation, modifying ion channels, uncoupling gap junctions, and disrupting calcium handling. Aldosterone, which can also be produced locally in the heart, may stimulate mediators of inflammation, activate fibroblasts and matrix metalloproteinases (MMPs), and probably, has direct electrophysiological effects.

There is accumulating evidence that, beyond its therapeutic effects on underlying heart disease, such as hypertension and heart failure, inhibition of the renin–angiotensin–aldosterone system may offer some protection against atrial structural and possibly electrical remodelling associated with AF (➲Fig. 29.37) [34, 233].

Meta-analysis of several retrospective reports as well as prospective studies in patients with congestive heart failure and hypertension has reported that therapy with ACE inhibitors and angiotensin receptor blockers reduced risk of new-onset AF by approximately 20–30% [116]. Furthermore, the results of small prospective studies of secondary prevention of AF have uniformly demonstrated a significant reduction in AF recurrence associated with ACE inhibitor or angiotensin receptor blocker plus amiodarone therapy compared with amiodarone alone before and after electrical cardioversion [34, 233]. However, the results of the GISSI-AF study which enrolled 1442 AF patients with typical risk factors (heart failure, hypertension, diabetes, CAD or peripheral artery disease) as well as patients with lone AF but with risk factors for AF such as a dilated LA, were disappointing [352]. Patients, the majority of whom had hypertension as a primary diagnosis, were randomized to receive valsartan 320mg daily or warfarin. There was no difference in the primary endpoint of time to first AF recurrence of AF (hazard ratio, 099, 95% CI, 0.85–1.15; p = 0.84) as well as no difference in secondary point of all-cause hospitalizations and hospitalizations for cardiovascular causes in the overall patient population or pre-specified groups. Several large prospective trials will assess the antiarrhythmic value of renin–angiotensin–aldosterone blockade in

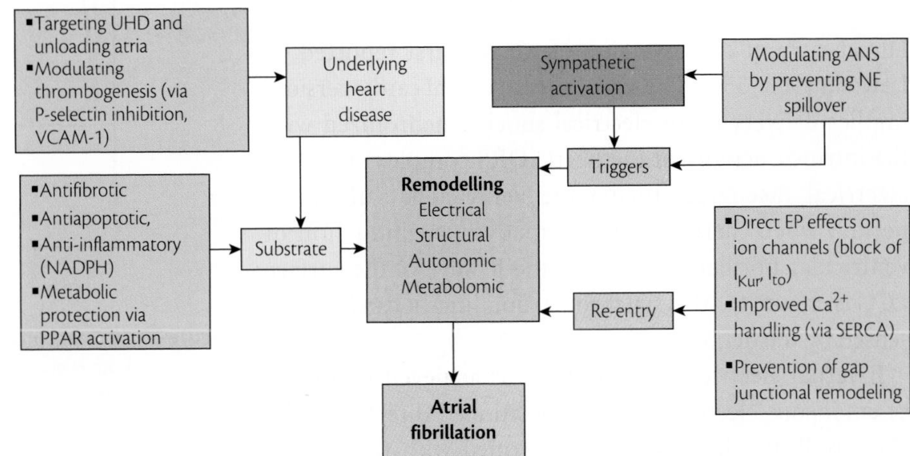

Figure 29.37 Angiotensin-converting enzyme inhibitors (ACEI) and angiotensin receptor blockers (ARB) for prevention of atrial fibrillation. ANS, autonomic nervous system; EP, electrophysiological effects; NADPH, nicotinamide adenine dinucleotide phosphate; NE, norepinephrine; PPAR, peroxisome proliferator-activated receptor; RCT, randomized clinical trials ; SERCA, sarco/endoplasmic reticulum C^{2+}-ATP-ase; UHD, underlying heart disease ; VCAM-1, vascular cell adhesion molecule-1. Modified from Savelieva I, Camm J. Is there any hope for angiotensin-converting enzyme inhibitors in atrial fibrillation? *Am Heart J* 2007; **154**: 403–6.

the absence of formal indications, e.g. myocardial infarction, heart failure, or severe hypertension.

Increased levels of CRP and pro-inflammatory cytokines (e.g. interleukin-1b, interleukin-6, and tumour necrosis factor-α) in AF have been reported in epidemiological and observational studies [35]. Higher CRP levels have been shown to be associated with a greater incidence of AF in the general population [123]. Recent meta-analysis of seven prospective observational studies has demonstrated that baseline CRP levels determine freedom from AF recurrence after electrical cardioversion [122].

Statins have strong anti-inflammatory and antioxidant effect and may, therefore, abolish AF mediated through these mechanisms [353]. By reducing oxidative stress and oxidized low-density lipoproteins which can up-regulate angiotensin II type 1 receptors, statins may counteract the arrhythmogenic effects of angiotensin II. In addition, statins may change ion channel conductance by altering the lipid content of the membrane. By increasing the synthesis of nitric oxide in the endothelium, statins protect atrial myocytes during ischaemia associated with rapid atrial rates and they may regulate the variety of MMPs which play a role in extracellular matrix remodelling in AF.

Meta-analysis of six randomized controlled studies in 3557 patients has shown that the use of statins was associated with a 61% reduction in the incidence of recurrent AF, but the effect was driven by the decrease in postoperative AF [355]. Several well-designed prospective trials were initiated to assess the antiarrhythmic value of statins. The role of polyunsaturated fatty acids in AF is controversial, but prospective studies are under way.

There is insufficient evidence to warrant a recommendation to expand the indications in wider patient populations at risk of AF.

Electrical cardioversion

Direct-current cardioversion of AF was first reported by Lown in 1963 [354]. The term 'direct-current cardioversion' implies delivery of an electrical shock synchronized with the intrinsic activity of the heart (QRS complex) to avoid electrical discharge during the ventricular vulnerable period, when there is a risk of inadvertent induction of ventricular fibrillation. Usually, the R wave of the surface ECG is chosen for this synchronization since it can be easily sensed by the defibrillator.

External electrical cardioversion is achieved by means of cutaneous electrode paddles positioned directly on the chest wall. Cardioversion is performed with the patient having fasted and under adequate general anaesthesia (or sedation) in order to avoid pain related to the delivery of the electrical shock. Success of cardioversion is determined by density of the current that traverses the muscle of the chamber to be defibrillated. The intensity of current that flows depends on the output waveform, selected energy level, and the transthoracic impedance. The higher the impedance, the lower the current delivered. The determinants of transthoracic impedance mainly include body habitus, the interface between the electrode and skin, and the size and position of the electrode paddles. For successful cardioversion, a critical mass of atrial muscle has to be encompassed by the electrical field. This is the rationale for using the anteroposterior paddle position rather than the anteroapical paddle position. Some randomized studies have shown greater success with anteroposterior configuration [357–359]. Since the anteroposterior paddle position has never been shown to be less effective than the anteroapical, this configuration is the first choice in clinical practice (29.6). Because the optimum paddle configuration for a given patient is not known before cardioversion, the clinician should consider an alternative arrangement if the initial position is unsuccessful.

Most devices used for external cardioversion deliver current with a monophasic waveform (Fig. 29.38) with a maximum energy output limited to 360J. The success rate for cardioversion of persistent AF is usually around 80% and is related to several clinical parameters such as long arrhythmia duration, patient age, LA enlargement, the presence of underlying heart disease, cardiomegaly, and obesity [360, 361].

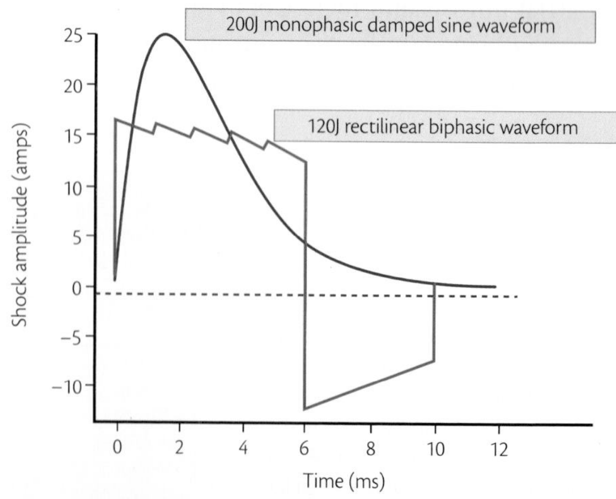

Figure 29.38 Monophasic versus biphasic waveforms. Reproduced with permission from Niebauer MK, Brewer JE, Chung MK, *et al.* Comparison of the rectilinear biphasic waveform with the monophasic damped sine waveform for external cardioversion of atrial fibrillation and flutter. *Am J Cardiol* 2004; **93**: 1495–9.

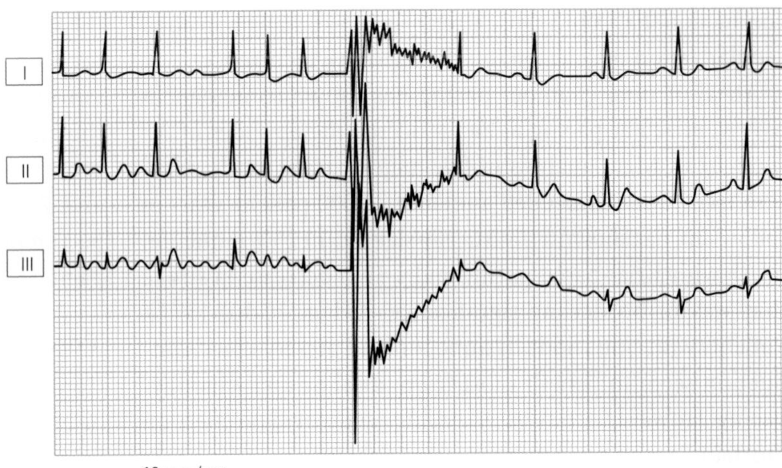

Figure 29.39 The 3-lead ECG of atrial fibrillation and successful cardioversion to sinus rhythm. Note the irregularity of the RR intervals and the fibrillation waves in leads V1 and V2. The artefact in the middle of the tracing represents the moment of DC electrical countershock.

The most modern type of external defibrillator delivers current with a biphasic waveform (➲Fig. 29.38). The maximum energy output is limited to 200J. Randomized studies have shown that biphasic defibrillators have a greater efficacy, require fewer shocks and lower delivered energy, and result in less skin burns than monophasic defibrillators [362–364]. The efficacy of transthoracic cardioversion was >90% with a biphasic shock waveform. Starting with higher energies may reduce the number of shocks (and thus total energy) delivered.

After one or two failed cardioversion attempts with maximum energy output with both paddle positions, antiarrhythmic drugs before further shock delivery, double shocks (delivery of energy with the use of two defibrillators) or internal cardioversion may be considered. Internal cardioversion of AF using high-energy (200–300J) direct current delivered between a catheter positioned in the right atrium and a backplate has been shown in a randomized trial to achieve higher conversion rates using a monophasic defibrillator for external cardioversion in the control group [365]. This can be useful in obese patients and patients with chronic obstructive lung disease, particularly if an electrophysiology study is planned for other purposes.

Other techniques for internal cardioversion apply low-energy (<20J) shocks via a large-surface electrode catheter (cathode) in the right atrium and another catheter (anode) positioned in the coronary sinus or the left pulmonary artery [366, 367]. Transoesophageal cardioversion has also been studied as an alternative approach for external cardioversion. With this technique, intermediate-level energy (20–50J) is delivered between oesophageal electrodes and a mid-sternum patch. It has been proved to be safe and efficacious [368] and can be combined with transoesophageal echocardiography to ensure that no atrial thrombus is present prior to cardioversion.

Transient ST-segment elevation may appear on the ECG after cardioversion and serum levels of creatine kinase may be increased whereas troponin-T and troponin-I levels are not. Myocardial damage related to electrical cardioversion is not observed at a microscopic level.

Cardioversion is contraindicated in patients with digitalis toxicity because a malignant ventricular arrhythmia may be triggered by the direct-current shock. However, at therapeutical levels, digoxin is not associated with the induction of malignant ventricular arrhythmias during cardioversion. Because hypokalaemia may precipitate a malignant ventricular arrhythmia after cardioversion, serum potassium levels should be in the normal range before direct-current shock delivery. Appropriate anticoagulation prior to cardioversion is mandatory.

Implantable pacemakers and defibrillators

Pacemaker and defibrillator therapy

Device-based therapy has been evaluated to treat AF with regards to two major concepts: the first concept seeks to avoid AF initiation by alleviation of bradycardia-induced dispersion of atrial activation and repolarization, and atrial overdrive suppression of premature atrial beats ('preventive pacing'). The second concept is to terminate AF episodes by high-rate pacing once the arrhythmia has started ('anti-tachycardia' pacing).

Physiological pacing (also see ➲Chapter 27)

The potential to maintain AV synchrony and prevent the development of mitral regurgitation and/or ventriculoatrial conduction that could cause stretch-induced changes in atrial repolarization may lessen the chance of AF recurrence.

Atrial or dual-chamber pacing has shown some benefit over ventricular pacing alone in decreasing episodes of AF [369–372]. Meta-analysis of five major pacing mode selection trials, which included a total of 35,000 patient-years of follow-up, has shown a statistically significant 20% reduction in AF with atrial-based pacing and a 19% decrease in stroke that was of borderline significance (➲Fig. 29.40) [373]. Patients with sinus node dysfunction and preserved AV conduction seem to benefit most from atrial or dual-chamber pacing. However, atrial-based pacing modes had no effect on mortality or the development of heart failure.

Minimizing ventricular pacing

It has been hypothesized that excessive right ventricular stimulation during dual-chamber pacing may worsen LV function and thus may negate the physiological advantage of AV synchrony and preservation of sinus node control over heart rate [374]. Thus, in patients with sinus syndrome and preserved native AV conduction enrolled in the MOST (Mode Selection Trial), the incidence of AF at 33.1 months (≈2.7 years) was 26.7% in the group assigned to ventricular-based pacing and 15.2% in the group assigned to physiological pacing [371].

The use of specific algorithms to minimize unnecessary ventricular stimulation in dual-chamber pacemakers has had no significant beneficial effect on mortality or heart failure, but has further reduced the risk of AF, in particular persistent AF, by 40% compared with conventional dual-chamber pacing [375]. In the SAVE PACe (Search AV Extension and Managed Ventricular Pacing for Promoting Atrioventricular Conduction) trial, which enrolled patients similar to those in the MOST study, the incidence of AF after 1.7 years was 12.7% in the group treated with conventional dual-chamber pacing and 7.9% in the group who treated with dual chamber-pacing plus an algorithm reducing unnecessary ventricular pacing [375].

'Preventative' pacing

Continuous pacing at selected sites (alternative, dual or bi-atrial) may change atrial activation patterns, increases homogeneity of left and right atrial electrical properties in conduction and refractoriness, reduce dispersion of refractoriness that occurs with premature atrial contractions (PACs) or with abrupt changes in atrial rate and thus prevent the development of atrial re-entry.

Alternative pacing sites: experimental and clinical studies have demonstrated that septal pacing, dual-site, or bi-atrial-site pacing shortens total atrial activation time [376, 377]. A number of clinical trials have evaluated the effects of selective atrial pacing sites on the prevention of AF in patients that required a pacemaker for other indications than AF, mainly with bradycardia as an indication (Bachmann bundle, inter-atrial septum) [377]. However, the largest randomized trial of right atrial pacing versus septal pacing ASPECT (Atrial Septal Pacing Efficacy Clinical Trial) failed to demonstrate a reduction in AF frequency and burden over a short follow-up [378].

Several techniques for bi-atrial stimulation have been proposed (right atrial and coronary sinus pacing) in

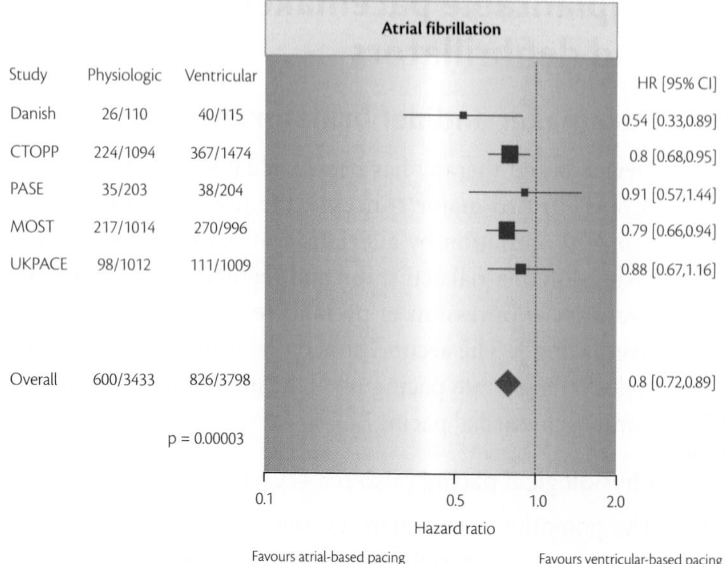

Figure 29.40 Effect of pacing mode on the incidence of atrial fibrillation in a meta-analysis of five major trials: CTOPP, Canadian Trial Of Physiologic Pacing; MOST, MOde Selection Trial; PASE, PAcemaker Selection in the Elderly; UKPACE, United Kingdom Pacing and Cardiovascular Events. Modified from Healey JS, Toff WD, Lamas GA, *et al.* Cardiovascular outcomes with atrial-based pacing compared with ventricular pacing: meta-analysis of randomized trials, using individual patient data. *Circulation* 2006; **114**: 11–17.

patients with sinus node dysfunction. In the DAPPAF (Dual site Atrial Pacing to Prevent Atrial Fibrillation) trial in antiarrhythmic drug-treated patients, dual right atrial pacing increased symptomatic AF-free survival compared with support pacing or high right atrial pacing, supporting the use of a hybrid approach to rhythm management [379].

Preventative pacing algorithms: the Atrial Fibrillation Therapy (AFT) trial, which investigated modes of onset of AF to determine potential arrhythmogenic triggers, has shown that AF is most commonly caused by premature atrial complexes (PACs) (48%) and sinus bradycardia (33%), whereas sudden onset was less common (17%) (➲Fig. 29.41) [380].

Specific algorithms are designed to prevent bradycardia and to avoid significant atrial rate variations associated with PACs. These include rate-adaptive pacing that monitors the underlying intrinsic rate to pace just above it, elevation of the pacing rate after spontaneous PACs, transient overdrive pacing after mode switch episodes, and increased post-exercise pacing to prevent an abrupt drop in heart rate.

The results of randomized clinical trials completed to date are not conclusive with respect to the beneficial effects of atrial pacing for AF and to the definition of an AF population (with except probably of patients with sinus node disease) that would obtain the most advantage from pacing strategies and which of these strategies are the best [380–384].

Atrial pacing prevention algorithms have modest to minimal incremental benefit for the prevention of AF and are not warranted in the absence of bradycardia indications for pacing [385]. At present, AF alone should not be an indication for preventative pacing, except for documented vagally-mediated AF.

'Antitachycardia' pacing

In some episodes, AF can be controlled with antitachycardia devices through the use of antitachycardia pacing or high-frequency atrial burst pacing. This approach is based on the concept that even AF may be sufficiently organized at its onset to allow pacing intervention, tissue capture, and arrhythmia termination [380]. Pace termination of atrial tachycardias or atrial flutter may prevent the development of AF and reduce the overall AF burden. However, when added to a pacing prevention algorithm, no further reduction of AF burden was demonstrated in a prospective randomized trial [381, 386]. In addition, there is so far no trial that demonstrates any long-term efficacy of device algorithms for both prevention or termination of AF.

Atrial defibrillator (within an implantable cardioverter defibrillator)

Initial short-term clinical experience with the 'stand-alone' atrial defibrillator suggested that atrial defibrillation was safe and effective. The first generation of atrial defibrillator was followed by a commercially available dual-chamber AV defibrillator. However, in a long-term analysis of 106 patients, only 39 were still actively using their device after a median of 40 months. In half, the device had been turned off or even explanted and in 14 patients it was solely used to monitor AF episodes [387]. The major drawback of internal cardioversion devices is that even a relatively low energy shock (<1J) is intolerably painful for the patient, making repetitive shocks in patients with frequent AF episodes a very unattractive treatment strategy [388].

For very selected patients who already have indications for implantable devices, device-based atrial defibrillation may be an option as a 'backup' option for managing AF

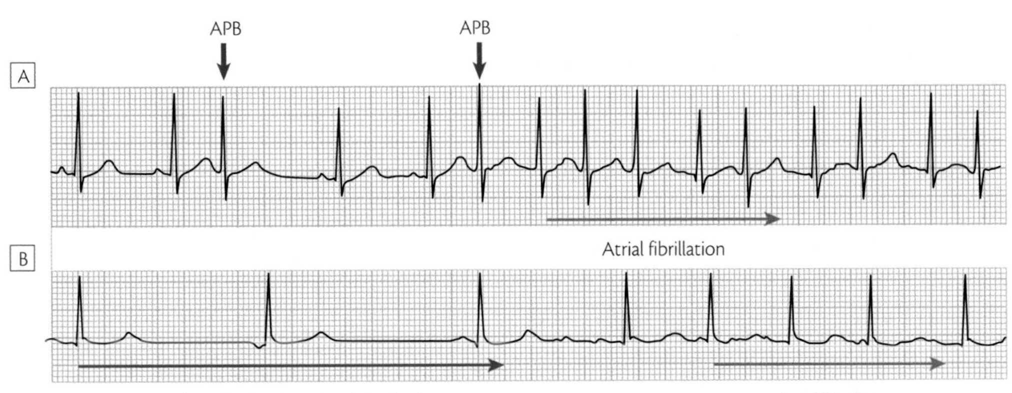

Figure 29.41 Patterns of initiation of atrial fibrillation which can be modified by pacing algorithms. Atrial premature beats (APB) that trigger atrial fibrillation (A) and bradycardia preceding atrial fibrillation in vagally-mediated AF (B).

A

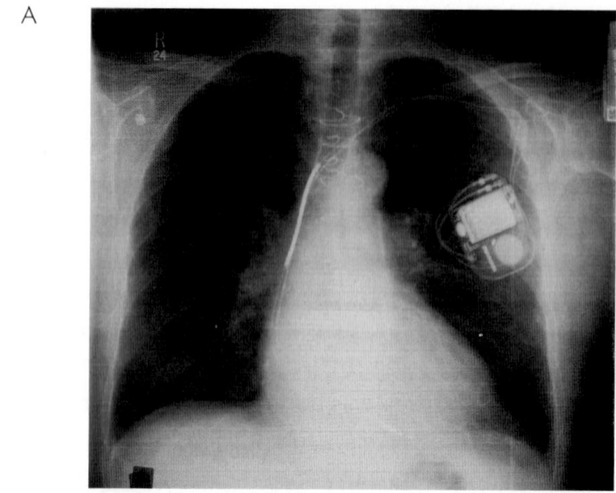

B

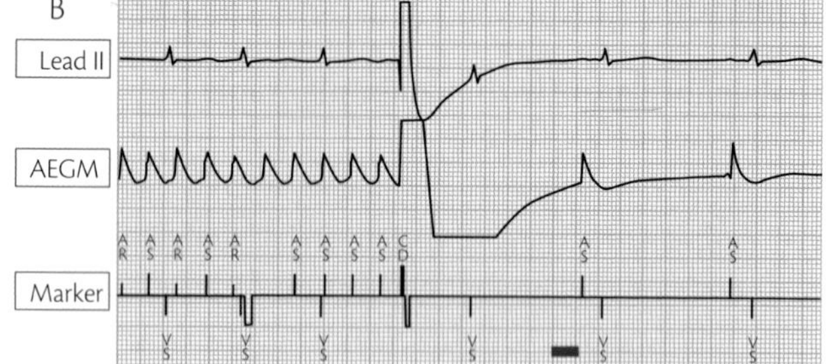

Figure 29.42 Chest X-rays showing a dual-chamber cardioverter defibrillator with atrial-tiered therapies (A). Internal cardioversion of atrial flutter/fibrillation with a 1J shock via the device (B).

when preventive pharmacological/electrical measures fail (➲Fig. 29.42). There is limited evidence that the combination of antitachycardia pacing, atrial shock, and preventative pacing is effective in reducing AF burden [389, 390].

Hybrid therapy for atrial fibrillation

Hybrid therapy involves the use of different types of treatment which together provide some form of synergism [389]. The three available rhythm management therapies are antiarrhythmic drugs, ablation, and devices. Antiarrhythmic drugs are often used in combination with ablation or device therapy. Increasingly, ablation and device therapy is combined. Although efficacy may be improved, side effects from both therapies may occur. Hybrid therapy does not refer, however, to the concomitant use of anticoagulation or upstream therapies. This remains largely a theoretical concept that has only been strictly evaluated in a small number of studies. Principles of hybrid therapy are listed in ➲Table 29.12.

Drug-induced atrial flutter: although atrial flutter and AF have different electrophysiological mechanisms, the two arrhythmias often coexist. Atrial flutter may initiate the first re-entrant circuit and may transform into AF as multiple wavelets develop [392]. The usual flutter pathway

Table 29.12 Principles of patient selection for hybrid therapy

General policy of combining treatments to reduce adverse effects whilst maintaining efficacy
Inadequate efficacy from single therapy
Rescue strategy when interventional approach is not fully effective
Management of proarrhythmia from single therapy which is otherwise effective
Arrhythmia mechanism suggests combined therapy will be more successful than single therapy
Need for monitoring as well as therapy

may continue to perpetuate AF whenever engaged. Typical atrial flutter is a relatively common finding in patients with AF treated with class IC and IA drugs and amiodarone (➲Fig. 29.43). These agents may modify wavefront activation by creating lines of functional block that interrupt multiple wavelets and promote conduction preferentially through a large single re-entrant circuit such as the isthmus-dependent flutter circuit. In these patients, ablation of the cavo-tricuspid isthmus can be considered first-line therapy before proceeding to LA ablation.

A less appreciated example of hybrid therapy is pacing for **drug-induced bradycardia** which allows dose up-titration

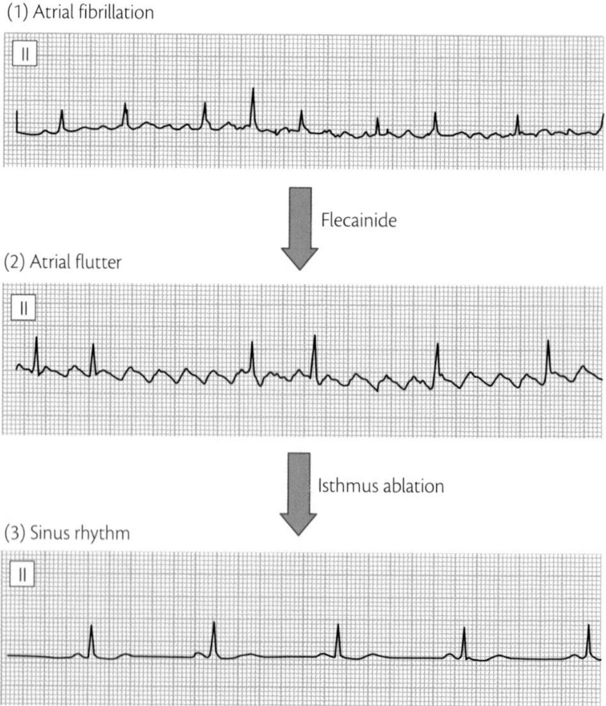

Figure 29.43 An example of hybrid therapy. A sodium-channel blocker flecainide converted atrial fibrillation into atrial flutter which was subsequently treated with isthmus ablation. Note that therapy with a sodium-channel blocker should continue after ablation to maintain sinus rhythm.

to achieve the best efficacy of antiarrhythmic drugs, although the intentional use of such combination therapy is limited [393].

Other examples of hybrid therapy include pacing-induced reduction of PACs and antiarrhythmic drug modification of substrate; device-based monitoring of rate/rhythm control in AF treated by pacing or antiarrhythmic drugs; biventricular pacing and ablation of the AV node in patients with AF and heart failure.

Catheter ablation of the atrioventricular node

Atrioventricular node ablation and modification

AF patients may benefit from control of both the ventricular rate and its regularity. Therefore, ventricular pacing after AV junction ablation to induce heart block ('ablate and pace') is a useful strategy for patients with permanent AF in whom rate control is difficult to accomplish by drugs (➲Fig. 29.44). The benefits of this procedure have been demonstrated in many controlled and non-controlled trials [394]. AV nodal ablation is especially useful when an excessive ventricular rate induces a tachycardia-mediated decline in ventricular systolic function despite appropriate medical therapy.

The 'ablate and pace' strategy improves exercise tolerance, cardiac function, healthcare utilization, and quality of life. Its safety has been established, and in a meta-analysis the risk of sudden death and total mortality was 2% and 6% respectively at 1 year [395], figures similar to the mortality observed with medical therapy of AF [396]. After total AV nodal block, ventricular pacing is performed from the apex of the right ventricle. This 'non-physiologic' activation from apex to base enhances cardiac dyssynchrony and can result in worsening of ventricular function, an effect which explains the deterioration of some patients [397].

By only modifying the AV node conduction properties to decrease the ventricular rate during AF ('AV node modulation or modification'), complete AV block and lifetime pacemaker therapy could be avoided. However, this technique is less widely performed because of lower success rates, the risk of inadvertent AV block, and the persistence of symptoms due to irregular beats during AF [398, 399].

Atrioventricular node ablation plus resynchronization therapy (also see ➲Chapter 27)

In the presence of congestive heart failure and AF, a significant benefit has been demonstrated for improvement of LV ejection fraction when a cardiac resynchronization therapy (CRT) device is implanted. Meta-analysis of five studies which compared the effect of CRT on outcomes in 1164 patients with sinus rhythm or AF, has shown that patients with AF have significant improvement after CRT, with similar improvement in ejection fraction as patients in sinus rhythm [400]. However, patients with AF seemed to gain smaller benefits in functional outcomes (NYHA functional class, 6-min walk, and quality of life).

The effect of CRT on outcome is significantly enhanced if the AV node is ablated [401, 402]. Recently, a large

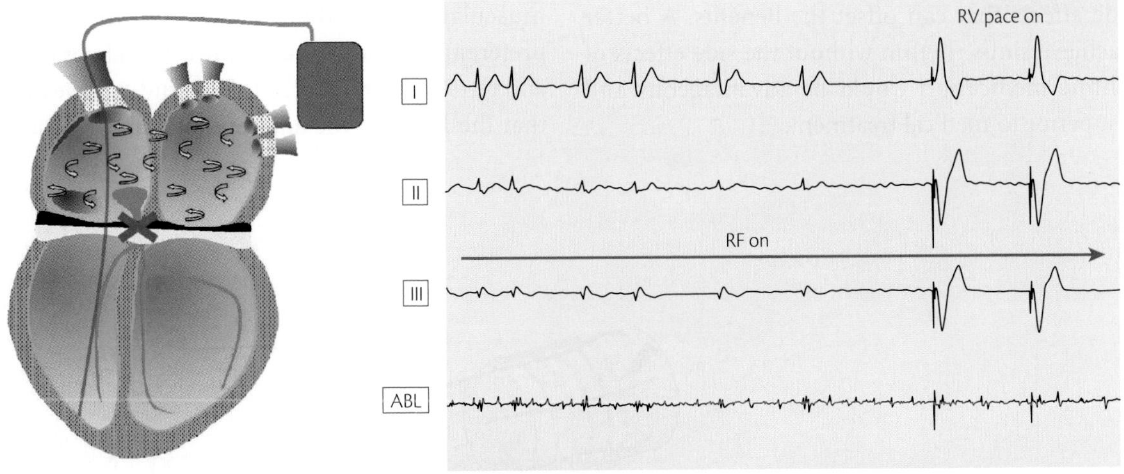

Figure 29.44 Schematic of atrioventricular node (AVN) ablation concept and pacemaker (grey box) implantation with single ventricular lead (VVI). Small arrows depict AF activation of the atria, which continues unaffected.

Table 29.13 Balloon isolation systems

Energy	Applied energy details	Sheath diameter	Balloon diameter	Single shot possible
Radiofrequency	Capacitive heating via coil inside the balloon: 200W, target temp. 55–60°C for up to 3min	12Fr	20–35mm	Yes
Cryo energy	Double balloon system with nitrous oxide as the refrigerant vaporizing inside the inner balloon lowering the temperature to ≤–30°C for up to 5min	1Fr	23 and 28mm	Yes
Ultrasound	Non-focused acoustic ultrasound	12Fr	22mm	Yes
Highly-focused ultrasound	Highly-focused ultrasound using a double balloon concept (acoustic power 45W)	14Fr	20, 25, and 30mm	Yes
Laser	Laser energy at 980nm, transmitted via the optical fibre to the tissue for 60s, achieving 6W/cm of arc length	15Fr	20, 25, and 30mm	No (arc-shape lesion)

registry suggested that AF patients who received a CRT device ('biventricular pacemaker') may have a better outcome with an 'ablate and pace' therapy than with pharmacological rate control [403].

On the other hand, AV node ablation and pacing preempts the later use of potentially newer and more effective non-pharmacological or pharmacological treatments, and should generally be reserved for patients refractory to other therapies. A specific atrial preventative pacing algorithm has been tested as adjunct to CRT, but although proven safe, it has had no effect on the 1-year incidence of AF [404].

Ablation of atrial fibrillation

In principle, the maintenance of sinus rhythm is of significant benefit for patients with AF [244]. The means to achieve stable sinus rhythm by antiarrhythmic medication however, are limited in their efficacy and have potential adverse side effects that can offset the benefits. A better means to achieve sinus rhythm without the side effects of antiarrhythmic medication would be advantageous and should be superior to medical treatment.

The first reports on catheter ablation of AF date back to 1994 [405]. Since then, multiple different strategies and technologies have been investigated (➲Table 29.13) with variable success. These developments have moved AF ablation from an experimental option in highly selected patients, to a reproducibly effective treatment option (PV isolation) for symptomatic patients with paroxysmal AF. However, ablation of persistent AF is still a challenge, with inconsistent results and unresolved acute ablation endpoints.

Role of the pulmonary veins in atrial fibrillation

Clinical AF results from the complex interaction of triggers with the perpetuators and substrate that then maintain fibrillation [406]. While theoretically all myocardial cells could act as a 'self-depolarizing' source of AF triggers, the PVs are clearly the dominant source, in up to 60–94% of paroxysms of AF (➲Fig. 29.45) [93, 407, 408]. Anatomical studies have demonstrated extension of a sleeve of atrial musculature into the PVs, thus creating the milieu for preferential conduction, unidirectional conduction block, and re-entry [409, 410]. Clinical studies have demonstrated that the PVs and the adjacent antrum of patients with AF

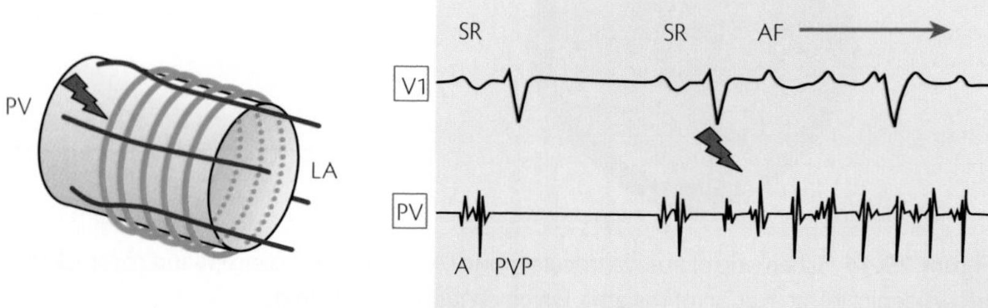

Figure 29.45 Atrial fibrillation initiation: concept and intracardiac recording from within the pulmonary vein.

have distinctive electrophysiological properties characterized by shorter refractory periods and greater anisotropy compared with patients without AF [411, 412]. These properties are capable of sustaining high-frequency activity [413, 414], especially when exposed to pulsatile stretch with every atrial contraction. Ablation of these arrhythmogenic structures forms an essential part of the ablation strategy for AF.

Catheter ablation strategies

Trigger elimination by direct focal ablation

The initial aim of AF ablation procedures was to eliminate focal triggers from within the PVs by direct localized ablation [93]. However, a trigger could only be localized when it was actually 'firing', a condition that was not necessary present during the procedure and was not easily provoked (pacing, pharmacological stress, etc.) [415]. In addition, multiple sites within a PV and multiple PVs could be arrhythmogenic and intra-PV ablation led to scarring of the ablated tissue and PV stenosis and/or occlusion.

Trigger elimination by pulmonary vein isolation

The initial experience led to the strategy of electrically isolating all PVs to prevent any interaction of these triggers with the atrial substrate [416, 417]. This approach was facilitated by circumferential mapping catheters that were positioned within the PV ostia to guide ablation targeting the 'connecting' fibres by 'segmental' ablation [416]. Ablation lesions were deployed relatively close to the PV ostia or just within (➲Fig. 29.46), risking ostial stenosis and/or occlusion. In addition, high AF recurrence rates were reported mostly due to electrical re-conduction of the PVs, but also to some extend due to 'ostial' triggers in the presence of more distally isolated PVs [418–421].

Linear pulmonary vein isolation and circumferential pulmonary vein ablation

In order to facilitate the ablation procedure and to reduce the risk of PV stenosis, the ablation sites have moved more into the atrium forming a long linear lesion around one PV or even both ipsilateral PVs together (➲Fig. 29.46) [414, 422, 423], the latter having the advantage that the small space between the PV ostia (ranging from as little a several mm to cm) is spared, reducing further risk of complications [424, 425] (29.7).

There is now strong evidence suggesting that the veins and the antrum are in fact critical for maintenance of AF, rendering the classification of 'trigger' versus 'substrate modification' inadequate to fully explain the role to the PVs. In patients with paroxysmal AF, who are undergoing PVI during AF, the AF cycle length slows during ablation and AF may finally terminate in up to 75% of cases [426]. Following PV isolation of all veins, about half of patients

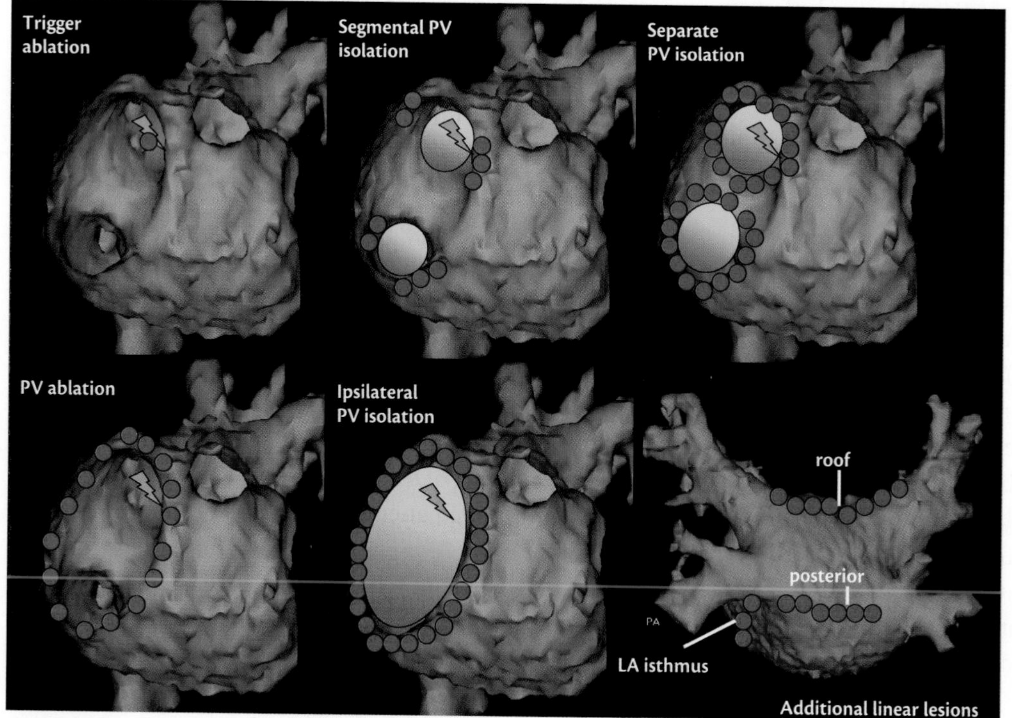

Figure 29.46 Different approaches for ablation of atrial fibrillation. The orange bolt depicts the trigger inside the left superior pulmonary vein (LSPV); red dots mark ablation sites and the shadowed yellow area demonstrates the area of isolation.

can no longer sustain AF, suggesting that in significant proportions of patients with paroxysmal AF the PVs form the substrate maintaining AF [427].

Circumferential pulmonary vein ablation

This is a purely anatomical approach that does not require the endpoint of electrical disconnection of the encircled area (➲Fig. 29.46) [428]. Since no simultaneous mapping within the PVs is performed, only a single trans-septal puncture is required. In addition, no waiting time after successful isolation is required, thereby shortening the procedure time dramatically. Using this technique up to 45% of PVs are not isolated, with persistent PV–LA conduction, which is potentially arrhythmogenic [429]. Reports from groups that have advocated the use of a purely anatomical approach have reported a significant incidence of organized arrhythmias occurring after such ablation. Indeed, a recent study reports that incomplete encircling lesions ('gaps') were the most predictive factor for the subsequent development of organized arrhythmias [430]. This finding argues further in favour of achieving complete lesions, with complete lesions being crucial for the prevention of macro re-entry; conversely, incomplete lesions promote the occurrence of atrial arrhythmias.

Is it really necessary to electrically disconnect the pulmonary veins? (29.10)

A recent expert consensus has recommended that complete electrical PV isolation should be achieved when treating patients with paroxysmal AF [99]. However, results from prospective trials investigating the need of permanently isolated ablation lines are still pending (e.g. GAP-AF trial).

Further evidence of the need for PVI is provided by studies that have evaluated the recurrence of AF after ablation. These studies have observed that the vast majority of patients with recurrence of AF demonstrate PV re-conduction. Repeat PVI in these patients has been associated with the elimination of AF in 90% of patients [424, 431]. In fact, patients with complete PV isolation fared best (SR in the absence of antiarrhythmic medication). Patients with re-conducting PVs with long conduction times were similar to patients with complete isolation, while patients with rapid conduction times required antiarrhythmic therapy and experienced AF recurrences [432]. These data implicate residual PV–LA connections in the development of clinical arrhythmia and serve to further accentuate the importance of achieving complete isolation. The rate of re-conduction of PVs in patients without symptomatic AF recurrences, however, is not known.

Additional lines for substrate modification

Despite exclusion of triggers, most patients with persistent or longstanding persistent AF may need additional substrate modification. The conceptual basis for substrate modification by compartmentalization of the atria is based on the multiple-wavelet hypothesis, which suggested that AF is maintained by multiple re-entrant wavelets propagating simultaneously in the atria and that a minimum mass of electrically continuous myocardium must be present to sustain the wavelets on re-entry.

Linear ablation is performed between anatomical or functional electrical obstacles in order to transect these regions and thereby preventing re-entry. A variety of different linear configurations has been investigated; however, prediction of which line is more suitable in a given patient has been elusive [433–436]. Typical applied lines are a *roof line* (connecting the upper PVs) or a so-called 'mitral' or 'left isthmus' line (connecting the inferior left PV to the mitral annulus (MA) (➲Fig. 29.46). Ablation of the *LA isthmus* offers several theoretical benefits over the other LA lesions [436]. This line is short but creates a contiguous long lesion with the ablated PVs and does not interfere with normal sinus activation of the atria. In addition, its proximity to the coronary sinus allows positioning of catheters on either side of the line to evaluate the integrity of the line. However, despite these features, ablation at this site requires 20–25min of radiofrequency energy application, with 68% requiring ablation within the coronary sinus. Due to the close proximity to the circumflex artery, substantial harm may result including acute coronary stenosis requiring immediate intervention [437].

An *anterior line* (from the roof line to the MA) would need to cross the LA insertion of Bachmann's bundle. This thick muscular connection between the right and LA is in fact the fastest connection between the atria and conduction block is difficult to achieve (due to the thickness of the tissue). However, complete anterior line deployment would result in a splitting of the P wave in sinus rhythm and in the presence of both a complete roof and LA isthmus line a completely isolated LAA [438].

A *posterior line* (between the septal and lateral PVs across the posterior wall of the LA) has been performed utilizing high power as part of the anatomical ablation strategy, leading in a number of patients to developed atrio-oesophageal fistulae [439].

Critical to the concept of linear lesions is that ablation has to be coalescent and transmural in order to achieve complete lesions. In some cases this can be challenging, with an increased procedural risk (particularly of tamponade, stroke and fistula formation). Incomplete linear lesions however may be pro-arrhythmic, resulting in rapid AV conduction of gap-related atrial tachycardia (➲Fig. 29.47) [440–442]. The completeness of the line should be validated in order to avoid iatrogenic complications even though an initially 'complete' linear lesion may exhibit conduction gaps in the long term. In addition, thoughtful placement of lesions can help to prevent formation of macro-reentrant circuits which will result in LA flutters. Their incidence varies widely between studies (and centres), in part due to slightly different anatomical positions of ablation lines and lesions.

After PV isolation alone, approximately 12% of patients have inducible macro re-entry and 5% present with spontaneous macro re-entry. Mapping and ablation have demonstrated that the vast majority of these use the ablated zone as a central obstacle, resulting in either peri-mitral or peri-PV re-entry being more prevalent in patients with larger atria [429].

When an anatomical approach of PV encircling has been utilized or no line validation has been performed, the reported incidence of re-entrant arrhythmias has been much higher, with some groups reporting spontaneous arrhythmias in up to 27%, presumably due to the greater but incomplete atrial ablation [441, 443, 444].

Alternative techniques for substrate modification

More recently, other techniques of substrate modification have been evaluated. The ablation of complex fractionated electrograms, without any isolation attempt of PVs has been proposed [445]. It is not clear why ablation of these points should be helpful, but reports from single centres are favourable. Interestingly, arrhythmia recurrences after such procedures seem to be dominated by arrhythmias arising from the PVs [446–450].

Several groups have described the results from ablating ganglionic plexuses (at atrial sites where a vagal response is observed after local stimulation), in addition to PV isolation [451–453]. However, long-term results of a procedure limited to these ganglia are not yet available.

Imaging tools to avoid intrapulmonary vein ablation (29.8)

Lesions performed to isolate the PVs should be placed within the atria or as proximally as possible rather than within the distal PVs [454]. This strategy not only reduces the incidence of PV stenosis, but may also improve efficacy by excluding proximal foci of activity from the arrhythmogenic substrate. When ablating along the anterior aspects of the left PVs, the catheter needs to be positioned along the 'ridge' between the PVs and the LAA. Catheter stability and lesion formation can be difficult, but avoidance of intra-PV ablation is key.

The use of a circular mapping catheter does not imply that the ablation lesions are being performed at the PV ostia. A distance >1 or 1.5cm between both catheters is commonly observed when ablation is performed atrially and careful identification of the respective PV ostia (e.g. by angiography, intracardiac echocardiography, etc.) is strongly recommended [99, 422]. The use of a circular mapping catheter also provides a very clear endpoint of complete isolation, which is achieved by wide encircling lesions around the PVs from within the atrium itself.

The use of pre-acquired three-dimensional imaging facilitates the understanding of the individual anatomy (which may vary substantially; ➲Fig. 29.48; 29.9), however careful registration is necessary to implement the three-dimensional volume of the LA correctly, so that the operator is not misled by an wrongly positioned image.

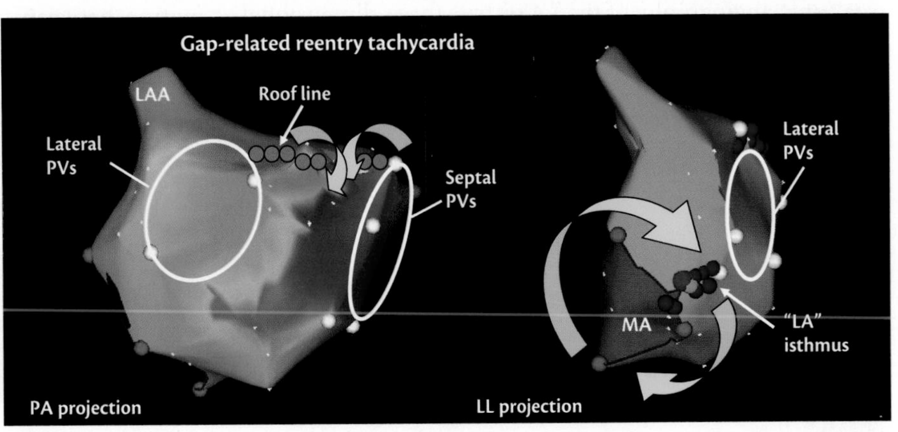

Figure 29.47 Iatrogenic 'gap-related' atrial tachycardia post-incomplete 'roof' line deployment (left panel). Reentry around mitral annulus (MA) caused by incomplete 'left atrial isthmus' line. The white lines depict the ostia of the pulmonary veins.

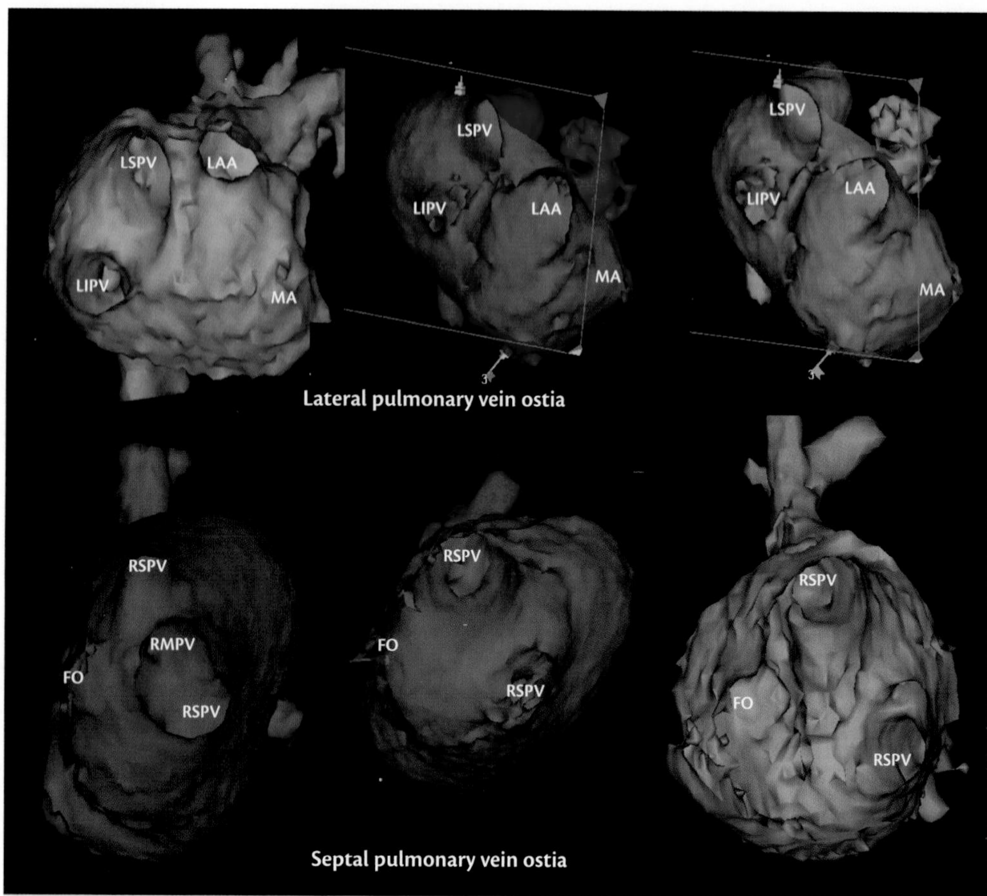

Figure 29.48 Variable anatomy of the pulmonary vein (PV) ostia depicted by three-dimensional imaging (cardiac magnetic resonance). Upper panel: lateral PVs, lower panel: septal PVs. LAA, left atrial appendage; MA, mitral annulus; FO, fossa ovalis; PV, pulmonary vein; RMPV, right middle pulmonary vein.

Accuracy of image fusion techniques vary and are reported to reach about 2mm, depending on the registration method [453–455].

While cardiac magnetic resonance (CMR) imaging does not add any radiation exposure to the patient, three-dimensional imaging by cardiac computer tomography (CT) exposes the patient to substantial radiation (about 20mSv) [458, 459]. Image quality, with properly applied imaging sequences are definitely comparable, therefore CMR is preferred whenever possible [460]. Intraprocedural rotational angiography of the LA or true three-dimensional intracardiac ultrasound may supplement these imaging modalities.

Complications

Despite significant improvements, catheter ablation of AF is still associated with major complications (➲ Fig. 29.49; Table 29.14) [99, 329].

Atrio-oesophageal fistula

An acutely life-threatening complication is a fistula formation between the LA and the oesophagus [439, 461].

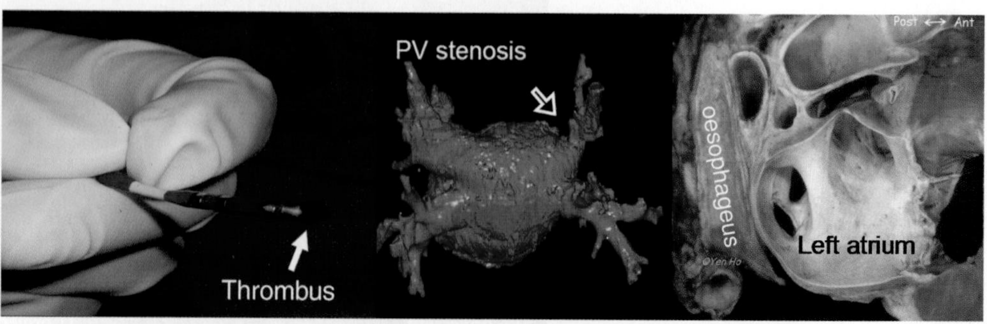

Figure 29.49 Complication of atrial fibrillation ablation. Thrombus at catheter tip (A); pulmonary vein stenosis (B); atrio-oesophageal fistula (C).

Table 29.14 Complications of left atrial ablation

Type of complication	Typical symptoms	Acute onset	Late onset	Reported incidence	Required action
Thromboembolic events	Stroke TIA PRIND (with symptoms related to infracted area)	Yes	With AF recurrence postablation	0.94% in WW survey	Periprocedural anticoagulation Exclusion of pre-existing intracardiac thrombi Continuous flush of trans-septal sheaths Use of irrigated tip catheters
PV stenosis/occlusion	Cough Pneumonia Dyspnoea Haemoptysis	Yes	Yes	1.6% in WW survey	Avoid intra PV ablation Imaging of PV ostium 3D imaging when typical symptoms Dilatation of symptomatic PV stenosis/recanalization if needed
Atrio-oesophageal fistula formation	High fever Dysphagia Neurologic signs (seizures)	Typically within 48 hours	Possible after penetration of an oesophageal ulceration	Only single case reports	Immediate 3D imaging Avoid endoscopy Emergency surgery
Air embolism	ST elevation Pressure drop and bradycardia Cardiac arrest	Within seconds	Only with fistula formation	Transient event, most likely underreported	Check sheaths for air leak Continuous flush of all trans-septal sheaths Perform CPR if necessary Wait!
Tamponade	Pressure drop and bradycardia Cardiac arrest	Within minutes	Rare	1.2% in WW survey	Pericardiocentesis Surgical intervention if percutaneous approach can't control the situation
Phrenic nerve injury	Diaphragm palsy with subsequent dyspnoea	Within seconds to minutes		0.48% [476]. Mostly transient event Incidence higher in balloon devices	Avoid ablation in vicinity of phrenic nerve (especially at RSPV)
Gastropathy	Dysphagia pyloric spasm gastric hypomotility	No	Yes	4/367 pts Likely to be underreported	Avoid excessive energy deployment
Vascular complication (AV fistula formation, groin haematomas, aneurysms)	Local pain Swelling Bruising	Yes	Yes	~1% in WW survey	Careful puncture technique Sheath removal after restored haemostasis

3D, three-dimensional; CPR, cardiopulmonary resuscitation; PRIND, prolonged reversible ischaemic neurological deficit; RSPV, right superior pulmonary vein; TIA, transitoric ischaemic attack; WW, world-wide.

Fortunately, this fatal complication is exceedingly rare [462] and may be avoided by careful lesion deployment along the posterior wall and energy reduction if ablation in this area is unavoidable (e.g. 30W). Static imaging of the moving oesophagus is a useless exercise that might even mislead the operator to falsely assume a 'safe' ablation position [463–465]. Similarly, the measurement of oesophageal temperatures can prevent some, but not all damage to the oesophagus, and might not always allow 'safe' ablation sites to be identified [466–468].

Pulmonary vein stenosis (29.11)

Using irrigated tip catheters, the current incidence of angiographic PV stenosis (>50% reduction in PV diameter) is <2%, with most patients being asymptomatic. This incidence is reduced significantly with lower-power ostial ablation and operator experience. Typical symptoms of significant PV stenosis or occlusion are persistent cough, pneumonia, and eventually haemoptysis [469–472]. The occurrence of such symptoms in a patient after AF ablation (even months later) should raise the suspicion of

PV stenosis. Imaging studies such as three-dimensional MRI (or CT in patients with devices) or functional assessment of PV flow velocities using transoesophageal echocardiography should be done immediately [473, 474].

Phrenic nerve injury

This complication has been recently recognized as a consequence of catheter ablation techniques for AF. There is a close relationship between the right phrenic nerve and the superior vena cava (SVC), and the anteroinferior part of the right superior pulmonary vein (RSPV) [475]. In addition, the left phrenic nerve is close to the LAA. Phrenic nerve injury can occur independently of the type of ablation catheter (4mm, 8mm, irrigated tip, balloon) or energy source used (radiofrequency, ultrasound, cryotherapy, or laser), however it has been more often reported when using balloon-based devices [476].

Although some patients with phrenic nerve injury after AF ablation remain asymptomatic, dyspnoea is the usual presentation. While causing adverse effects on functional status and quality of life, it is reversible in the most patients. However, recovery of PNI may take up to 1 year. High output pacing can be used to identify the PN and allows an exact three-dimensional localization to avoid ablation in immediately adjacent area [476].

Tamponade

Cardiac tamponade occurs either during the trans-septal puncture, mechanically during the mapping process, or during the ablation itself by steam-pop formation [477]. The incidence varies in reports from as low as 0.6% to up to 2.9% and is clearly associated with the experience of the operators [478, 479]. Most tamponade can be handled successfully by immediate pericardiocentesis; a small minority of patients however, require surgical drainage.

Thromboembolic events during and after ablation

Clot formation at the LA catheters is thought to be the cause of thromboembolic events during AF ablation (➲Fig. 29.49). While transoesophageal echocardiography is recommended prior to LA access to rule out any pre-existing LAA thrombus, small existing thrombi may be overlooked and dislocated mechanically during the mapping procedure [99]. The Worldwide Survey I quotes a 0.93% incidence for all events, ranging from TIAs with 0.66% to stroke with 0.28% [329]. To avoid intraprocedural events, close observation of activated clotting time (ACT) at regular intervals (e.g. every 30min) is recommended to allow individual adjustment of the anticoagulation parameters by intravenous heparin. As stated by expert consensus, oral anticoagulation should be continued for a minimum of 2 months after catheter ablation and thereafter according to the individual $CHADS_2$ score [98].

Death

Death is a relatively rare complication, occurring in approximately one of 1000 patients undergoing ablation for AF. In the Worldwide Survey II which reported on >45,000 procedures in >32,000 patients, causes of death included tamponade in eight patients, stroke in five, atrio-oesophageal fistula in five, and massive pneumonia in two patients [480]. Other causes of death included myocardial infarction, sudden respiratory arrest and asphyxia, torsade de pontes, pulmonary vein occlusion and perforation (extrapericardial), septicaemia, and intracranial bleeding.

Indications for left atrial catheter ablation

For paroxysmal AF, there must be sufficient potential benefit to justify a complex ablation procedure associated with potentially severe complications. In most centres and as per AF guidelines from 2006, patients are considered for ablation on the basis of frequent symptomatic episodes of AF that are resistant to at least one antiarrhythmic drug (class I or III) [481]. Ablation is only considered in patients with symptoms, as the benefit of AF ablation has not been demonstrated in asymptomatic patients. Success rates of 70–90% are frequently reported (➲Table 29.15) [482].

In a recent meta-analysis of four smaller randomized trials comparing catheter ablation versus antiarrhythmic medication, 162 of 214 patients (75.7%) in the ablation group had AT recurrence-free survival vs. 41 of 218 patients (18.8%) in the medication group [481]. In addition, there were fewer adverse events in the ablation group. However, there was much heterogeneity among the trials owing to differences in the subject populations, differences in the inclusion and exclusion criteria, disparity in the interventions and the control treatments, and variation in expertise of the physicians (➲Table 29.15) [482–489].

Several large prospective, multicentre randomized trials are currently underway, for example the Radiofrequency Ablation versus Antiarrhythmic Drugs for Atrial Fibrillation Treatment (RAAFT) study and the Catheter Ablation for the Cure of Atrial Fibrillation–2 (CACAF 2) study, investigating the value of AF ablation as first-line treatment. Several other large ongoing randomized trials are also exploring the place of catheter ablation in relation to other antiarrhythmic strategies, rate control, and anticoagulation e.g. Catheter Ablation versus Standard conventional Treatment in patients with LEft ventricular dysfunction

Table 29.15 Randomized controlled trials of radiofrequency ablation versus antiarrhythmic drugs or no treatment for atrial fibrillation

Study [reference]	No. of patients	Type of AF	Previous use of AAD	Ablation technique	Patients without AF, %—Ablation vs. AAD or no AAD
Krittayaphong *et al.* 2003 [483]	30	Paroxysmal or persistent	≥1 AAD failure[d]	PVI + LA lines + CTI ablation + RA lines	79 vs. 40
Wazni *et al.* 2005(RAAFT) [484]	70	Mainly paroxysmal	No	PVI	87 vs. 37
Stabile *et al.* 2006 (CACAF) [485]	137	Paroxysmal or persistent	≥2 AAD failure	PVI + LA lines ± CTI ablation	56 vs. 9
Oral *et al.* 2006 [486]	146	Persistent	≥1 AAD failure (mean 2.1 ± 1.2)	CPVA	74 vs. 4
Pappone *et al.* 2006 (APAF) [487]	198	Paroxysmal	≥2 AAD failure (mean 2 ± 1)	CPVA + CTI ablation	86 vs. 22
Jais *et al.* 2008 (A4 study) [488]	112	Paroxysmal	≥1 AAD failure	PVI ± LA lines ± CTI ablation	89 vs. 23
Forleo *et al.* 2009 [489]	70	Paroxysmal or persistent	≥1 AAD failure	PVI + CTI ablation ± LA lines	80 vs. 43
Thermocool 2008[f]	159	Paroxysmal	≥1 AAD failure[g]	PVI + CTI ablation ± LA lines ± RA focal ablation	66 vs. 17

[a]All patients in the ablation arm were treated with antiarrhythmic drugs; [b]patients in the control group received amiodarone and had up to two electrical cardioversions if required during the first 3 months; amiodarone was discontinued if patients were in sinus rhythm after 3 months; [c]with type 2 diabetes mellitus; [d]no previous use of amiodarone, but 'failed' drugs included beta-blockers, calcium-channel blockers, and digitalis in addition to class IA and IC agents; [e]after 1 year; not allowed during 1 year-follow-up; [f]presented at the Heart Rhythm Society meeting in May 2009; [g]including beta-blockers and calcium antagonists. All studies had a follow-up period of 1 year.

AAD, antiarrhythmic drugs; AF, atrial fibrillation; APAF, Ablation for Paroxysmal Atrial Fibrillation study; A4, Atrial fibrillation Ablation versus AntiArrhythmic drugs; CACAF, Catheter Ablation for the Cure of Atrial Fibrillation study; CPVA, circumferential pulmonary vein ablation; CTI, cavotricuspid isthmus; LA, left atrial; PVI, pulmonary vein isolation; RAAFT, Radiofrequency Ablation Atrial Fibrillation Trial; RA, right atrial.

and Atrial Fibrillation (CASTLE AF) and Catheter ABlation Versus ANtiarhythmic Drug Therapy for Atrial Fibrillation (CABANA).

In persistent or permanent AF, ablation is more difficult [490, 491]. Consequently, major symptoms should be associated with the arrhythmia to justify the procedure. However, there is emerging evidence to suggest that patients with complications related to AF may benefit from a primary ablation strategy; e.g. patients with heart failure, even in the absence of obvious symptoms, benefit from ablation as the ejection fraction may improve by about 20% with the maintenance of sinus rhythm (a much greater benefit than that reported with an 'ablate and pace' strategy) (➲Table 29.16, Fig. 29.50) [90, 492–496]. Ablation of persistent and permanent AF is associated with variable but encouraging success, but often requires several ablation attempts [425, 491]. However, these ablation procedures are long, difficult, technically challenging and associated with greater risk than PVI alone.

Surgical ablation

The curative approach for AF was pioneered by the cardiac surgeons who developed the Maze procedure and the Corridor procedure [497, 498]. Their idea was to 'compartmentalize' the atria in segments too small to sustain AF. Initially, these operations were performed using a 'cut-and-sew' technique requiring substantial bypass time and therefore prolonging the overall operation. Other tools, such as radiofrequency ablation, ultrasound, and microwave probes or cryoablation, have now been developed which allow the surgeon to perform AF ablation in less time [499].

Interestingly, most of the currently used intraoperative treatment strategies consist of a PV isolation (ranging from a box around all four PVs to '1 by 1'). In some instances, these PV isolations are combined with further line deployments. Since most of the operations are performed from the endocardial site, these procedures require total cardiac arrest, eliminating the opportunity to test for conduction block during line deployment. However, the visual assessment of the lesion formation is a clear advantage of the surgical procedure. Some techniques now allow an epicardial deployment of the PV isolation line, which in turn allows recording the endpoint of complete electrical isolation. In addition, minimally invasive operations can be performed, further reducing the patients' burden of these operations [500].

Table 29.16 Results of left atrial ablation procedures for patients with congestive heart failure, left ventricular dysfunction, and structural heart disease. Significant improvement of left ventricular ejection fraction is noted

Study/year	Number of patients	EF (%)	Paroxysmal AF	Intervention	Follow-up (months)	Outcome	Probable TCMP (%)
Chen *et al.* 2004 [492]	94	36 ± 8	43%	PVI	14 ± 6	Improvement in EF (by 4.6%, NS), quality of life	11
Hsu *et al.* 2004 [90]	58	35 ± 7	9%	PVI, LAA (91%)	12 ± 7	Significant improvement in EF (by 21 ± 13%), LV size, exercise tolerance, NYHA class	25
Tondo *et al.* 2006 [493]	40	33 ± 2	25%	PVI, LAA	14 ± 2	Significant improvement in EF (to 47 ± 3%), exercise tolerance, quality of life	Excluded
Gentlesk *et al.* 2007 [494]	67	42 ± 9	70%	PVI, non-PVI triggers	20 ± 9	Significant improvement in EF (to 56 ± 8%), LV and LA size	22
Efremidis *et al.* 2008 [495]	13	35 ± 5	0%	PVI, LAA	12	Significant improvement in EF (to 60 ± 4%), LV and LA size	Not stated
Lutomsky *et al.* 2008 [496]	18	41 ± 6	100%	PVI	6	Significant improvement in EF (to 51 ± 12%)	Not stated

AF, atrial fibrillation; EF, ejection fraction; LA, left atrial; LAA, left atrial ablation; LV, left ventricular; NS, not significant; PVI, pulmonary vein isolation; TCMP, tachycardia-induced cardiomyopathy

As with percutaneous ablation strategies, the best surgical strategy and technology is still being evaluated. Similar to the transcutaneous experience, incomplete linear lesions lead to re-conduction and iatrogenic arrhythmia. Most of these gap-related atrial tachycardias can be managed successfully by three-dimensional mapping and subsequent ablation by the interventional electrophysiologist [501, 502]. Good cooperation between the surgical and interventional groups is the key factor to ascertain optimal care for patients with arrhythmia recurrences after intraoperative AF ablation.

Currently, intraoperative AF ablation is predominantly advocated in patients with AF who need cardiac surgery for an additional reason (e.g. valvular or bypass surgery). It is generally agreed that in the absence of an indication for cardiac surgery, surgical therapy of AF should not be the first-line approach.

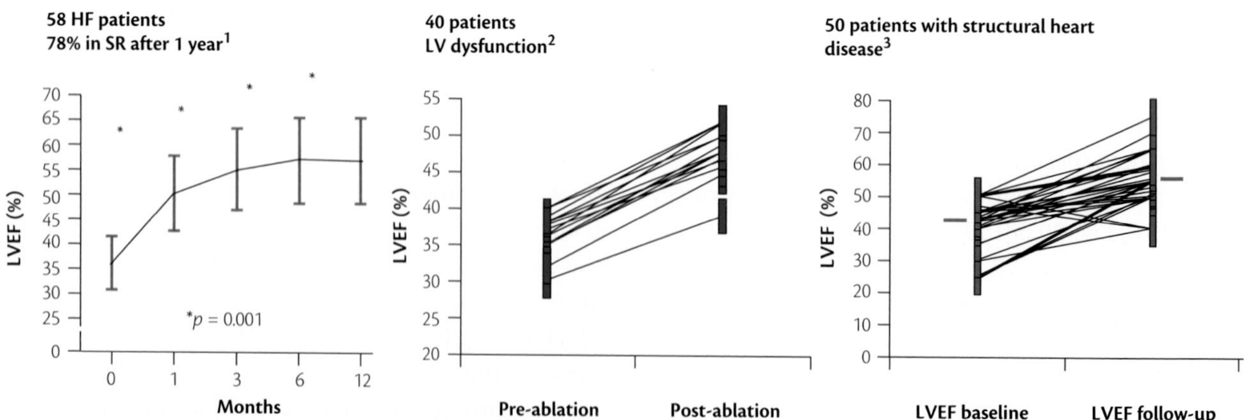

Figure 29.50 Improvement in left ventricular function after successful ablation for atrial fibrillation in patients with heart failure and structural heart disease. HF, heart failure; LVEF, left ventricular ejection fraction; SR, sinus rhythm. Modified with permission from Hsu LF, Jaïs P, Sanders P, *et al.* Catheter ablation for atrial fibrillation in congestive heart failure. *N Engl J Med* 2004; **351**: 2373–83; Tondo C, Mantica M, Russo G, *et al.* Pulmonary vein vestibule ablation for the control of atrial fibrillation in patients with impaired left ventricular function. *Pacing Clin Electrophysiol* 2006; **29**: 962–70; and Gentlesk PJ, Sauer WH, Gerstenfeld EP, *et al.* Reversal of left ventricular dysfunction following ablation of atrial fibrillation. *J Cardiovasc Electrophysiol* 2007; **18**: 9–14.

Follow-up considerations

Anticoagulation

Initially post-ablation, LMWH or intravenous heparin should be used as a bridge to resumption of systemic anticoagulation for a minimum of 2 months. Thereafter, the individual $CHADS_2$ score of the patient should determine if oral anticoagulation should be continued. Discontinuation of warfarin therapy postablation is generally not recommended in patients who have a $CHADS_2$ score of 2 or more [99].

Monitoring for atrial fibrillation recurrences

The most appropriate assessment of the clinical mid- and long-term outcome after AF ablation still remains a subject of discussion. Currently evaluation is usually based on Holter ECG, tele-ECG, or on patients' symptoms. A high prevalence of asymptomatic episodes of AF has been revealed indicating that patient interrogation alone may not be suitable for an accurate follow-up due to an overestimation of freedom from AF. Although antiarrhythmic medication is continued for some time (up to several months) in most studies, results should be reported off drugs with all atrial arrhythmias (including atrial tachycardia or frequent atrial premature beats) counting as failure [8, 99].

While 7-day Holter ECG has demonstrated that many AF episodes may not be recognized by the patient post-AF-ablation [503], a recent study in patients with pacemakers demonstrated a clear correlation between symptoms and AF recurrence [504]. The expert consensus recommends following AF ablation patients in 6-month intervals for at least 2 years, after an initial follow-up visit at 3 months [99]. However, as the indication for ablation is relief of symptomatic AF episodes, the therapeutic outcome can be monitored by symptom-driven ECGs in many routine clinical settings.

Personal perspective

The increased longevity of post-war 'baby boomers' who have survived despite underlying cardiovascular disease will give rise to a burgeoning number of elderly patients with AF associated with concomitant cardiac and extra-cardiac disease. Although definitive proof is not yet available, there is an expectation that early and aggressive treatment of patients prone to this arrhythmia may prevent the disease and its complications. Effective 'upstream' treatment of hypertension and congestive heart failure may reduce the occurrence of new-onset arrhythmia by alleviating and delaying underlying damage to the atria (primary prevention of AF).

Especially in patients with structural heart disease, AF represents a risk factor for serious cardiovascular complications such as stroke, heart failure, sudden cardiac death, and overall mortality. Unfortunately, AF is often 'silent' until these devastating complications occur, but chance or intended ECG monitoring may detect asymptomatic AF. The management of the disease involves risk stratification for these eventualities, appropriate anticoagulation, and comprehensive treatment of hypertension and ventricular dysfunction, including effective rate and/or rhythm control.

Paroxysmal AF in younger patients may occur independently of identifiable heart disease. The pathophysiological and genetic background of this disorder is currently being unravelled. This arrhythmia is often symptomatic with fast and irregular palpitations and associated anxiety. In the absence of risk factors for stroke, these patients do not need to be anticoagulated. Beta-blockers and/or antiarrhythmic drugs can often control the rhythm, and these are indicated to relieve symptoms (secondary prevention). Recurrences of this arrhythmia despite medical therapy should prompt consideration for interventional treatments such as LA ablation. Technological advances will render these procedures more effective and less harmful in the foreseeable future.

Atrial remodelling in response to paroxysms of the arrhythmia and secondary to underlying heart disease such as hypertension and LV dysfunction, may lead to progression of a self-limiting form to a more persistent variety that eventually resists cardioversion. It may prove possible to slow this progressive deterioration using 'upstream' pharmacological therapy, such as ACE inhibition or angiotensin receptor blockade, or statins, to counter the deterioration induced by the arrhythmia itself. Determined treatment of underlying heart disease (e.g. stringent blood pressure control in hypertension) may also prevent or delay the formation and maturation of the substrate for self-perpetuating AF.

The last decade has seen significant developments in our understanding of AF and has led to catheter ablation and surgical techniques that have demonstrated the feasibility of achieving cure of AF. While complete electrical PV isolation is recommended to treat paroxysmal AF, strategies for persistent and longstanding persistent AF are less clear. Additional substrate modifications using linear lesions or ablation of complex fractionated signals are still under investigation. Further technological improvements will broaden the use of curative AF techniques in the future, making catheter ablation a viable option for many AF patients.

AF and its complications present a substantial cost burden to healthcare providers. In the next several years, new antithrombotic medications, better antiarrhythmic agents, improved ablation techniques, strategies for the treatment and prevention of precursors of the arrhythmia and arrhythmia-induced cardiac damage, and better choice and implementation of adequate rate- and rhythm-control strategies will emerge. Together these developments will lead to more cost-effective management of this increasingly prevalent condition, be it a disease in itself or simply a marker of increased cardiovascular jeopardy.

Further reading

Blanc JJ, Almendral J, Brignole M, *et al.* Scientific Initiatives Committee of the European Heart Rhythm Association. Consensus document on antithrombotic therapy in the setting of electrophysiological procedures. *Europace* 2008; **10**: 513–27.

Calkins H, Brugada B, Packer DL, *et al.* HRS/EHRA/ECAS expert consensus statement on catheter and surgical ablation of atrial fibrillation: recommendations for personnel, policy, procedures and follow-up. A report of the Heart Rhythm Society (HRS) Task Force on Catheter and Surgical Ablation of Atrial Fibrillation developed in partnership with the European Heart Rhythm Association (EHRA) and the European Cardiac Arrhythmia Society (ECAS); in collaboration with the American College of Cardiology (ACC), American Heart Association (AHA), and the Society of Thoracic Surgeons (STS). Endorsed and approved by the governing bodies of the American College of Cardiology, the American Heart Association, the European Cardiac Arrhythmia Society, the European Heart Rhythm Association, the Society of Thoracic Surgeons, and the Heart Rhythm Society. *Europace* 2007; **9**: 335–79.

Cappato R. Calkins H, Chen SA, *et al.* Worldwide survey on the methods, efficacy, and safety of catheter ablation for human atrial fibrillation. *Circulation* 2005; **111**: 1100–5.

Cappato R, Calkins H, Chen SA, *et al.* Prevalence and causes of fatal outcome in catheter ablation of atrial fibrillation. *J Am Coll Cardiol* 2009; **53**: 1798–803.

Cosio FG, Aliot E, Botto GL, *et al.* Delayed rhythm control of atrial fibrillation may be a cause of failure to prevent recurrences: reasons for change to active antiarrhythmic treatment at the time of the first detected episode. *Europace* 2008; **10**: 21–7.

Fuster V, Rydén LE, Cannom DS, *et al.* ACC/AHA/ESC 2006 guidelines for the management of patients with atrial fibrillation-executive summary: A report of the American College of Cardiology/American Heart Association Task Force on practice guidelines and the European Society of Cardiology Committee for Practice Guidelines (Writing Committee to Revise the 2001 Guidelines for the Management of Patients with Atrial Fibrillation) Developed in collaboration with the European Heart Rhythm Association and the Heart Rhythm Society. *Eur Heart J* 2006; **27**: 1979–2030.

Kirchhof P, Auricchio A, Bax J, *et al.* Outcome parameters for trials in atrial fibrillation: executive summary: Recommendations from a consensus conference organized by the German Atrial Fibrillation Competence NETwork (AFNET) and the European Heart Rhythm Association (EHRA). *Eur Heart J* 2007; **28**: 2803–17.

Knight BP, Gersh BJ, Carlson MD, *et al*, Role of permanent pacing to prevent atrial fibrillation: science advisory from the American Heart Association Council on Clinical Cardiology (Subcommittee on Electrocardiography and Arrhythmias) and the Quality of Care and Outcomes Research Interdisciplinary Working Group, in collaboration with the Heart Rhythm Society. *Circulation* 2005; **111**: 240–3.

Kourliouros A, Savelieva I, Jahangiri M, *et al.* Current concepts in the pathogenesis of atrial fibrillation. *Am Heart J* 2009; **157**: 243–52.

Natale A, Raviele A, Arentz T, *et al*, Venice Chart international consensus document on atrial fibrillation ablation. *J Cardiovasc Electrophysiol* 2007; **18**: 560–80.

National Collaborating Centre for Chronic Conditions. *Atrial Fibrillation: National Clinical Guideline for Management in Primary and Secondary Care*, 2006. London: Royal College of Physicians. Available at http://rcplondon.ac.uk/pubs/books/af/index.asp

Fisher JD, Spinelli MA, Mookherjee D, *et al.* Atrial fibrillation ablation: reaching the mainstream. *Pacing Clin Electrophysiol* 2006; **29**: 523–37.

Hart RG, Pearce LA, Aguilar MI. Meta-analysis: antithrombotic therapy to prevent stroke in patients who have nonvalvular atrial fibrillation. *Ann Intern Med* 2007; **146**: 857–67.

Hughes M, Lip GYH. Guideline Development Group, National Clinical Guideline for Management of Atrial Fibrillation in Primary and Secondary Care, National Institute for Health and Clinical Excellence. Stroke and thromboembolism in atrial fibrillation; a systematic review of stroke risk factors, risk stratification schema and cost effectiveness data. *Thromb Haemost* 2008; **99**: 295–304.

Lafuente-Lafuente C, Mouly S, Longás-Tejero MA, *et al.* Antiarrhythmic drugs for maintaining sinus rhythm after cardioversion of atrial fibrillation: a systematic review of randomized controlled trials. *Arch Intern Med* 2006; **166**: 719–28.

Lip GY, Lim HS. Atrial fibrillation and stroke prevention. *Lancet Neurol* 2007; **6**: 981–93.

Lip GY, Tse HF. Management of atrial fibrillation. *Lancet* 2007; **18**; **370**: 604–18.

Rubboli A, Halperin JL, Airaksinen KE, *et al.* Antithrombotic therapy in patients treated with oral anticoagulation undergoing coronary artery stenting. An expert consensus document with focus on atrial fibrillation. *Ann Med* 2008; **40**: 428–36.

Savelieva I, Camm J. Statins and polyunsaturated fatty acids for treatment of atrial fibrillation. *Nat Clin Pract Cardiovasc Med* 2008; **5**: 30–41.

Savelieva I, Camm J. Anti-arrhythmic drug therapy for atrial fibrillation: current anti-arrhythmic drugs, investigational agents, and innovative approaches. *Europace* 2008; **10**: 647–65.

Singer DE, Albers GW, Dalen JE, *et al.* Antithrombotic therapy in atrial fibrillation: American College of Chest Physicians Evidence-Based Clinical Practice Guidelines (8th Edition). *Chest* 2008; **133**: 546S–592S.

Stroke Risk in Atrial Fibrillation Working Group. Independent predictors of stroke in patients with atrial fibrillation: a systematic review. *Neurology* 2007; **69**: 546–54.

Stroke Risk in Atrial Fibrillation Working Group. Comparison of 12 risk stratification schemes to predict stroke in patients with non-valvular atrial fibrillation. *Stroke* 2008; **39**: 1901–10.

Online resources

- National Collaborating Centre for Chronic Conditions. *Atrial Fibrillation: National Clinical Guideline for Management in Primary and Secondary Care*, 2006. London: Royal College of Physicians. http://rcplondon.ac.uk/pubs/books/af/index.asp
- German atrial Fibrillation competence NETwork (AFNET). An English version of this publicly funded scientific network is available. The site provides information for healthcare professionals and patients: http://www.kompetenznetz-vorhofflimmern.de

Additional online material

- 29.1 Atrial fibrillation with twisting of the P waves, suggestive of an 'atrial torsade de pointes', in a patient with long QT syndrome.
- 29.2 Wolff–Parkinson–White and atrial fibrillation with rapid conduction to the ventricles. ECG provided by G. Breithardt.
- 29.3 (A) Echocardiogram movie and (B) MRI from a patient with right atrial lipoma (not a thrombus). MRI provided by D. Maintz.
- 29.4 (A) Echocardiogram and (B) MRI movies from a patient with paroxysmal atrial fibrillation who had several cardiac abnormalities: Chiari's net, cor triatriatum, and a hypermobile septum. Echocardiogram provided by M. Stenzel, MRI by D. Maintz.
- 29.5 (A) Three-dimensional transoesophageal echocardiogram (TOE) and (B) two-dimensional 'sliced' TOE of a large thrombus in the left atrial appendage in a patient with atrial fibrillation. Echocardiogram provided by K. Tiemann.
- 29.6 Strictly anteroposterior electrode position for external cardioversion of atrial fibrillation.
- 29.7 Three-dimensional merge of three-dimensional magnetic resonance image with three-dimensional electroanatomical mapping.
- 29.8 Three-dimensional image of the whole heart of a patient undergoing atrial fibrillation catheter ablation.
- 29.9 Three-dimensional reconstruction of a cardiac magnetic resonance image of a patient with a common ostium of the lateral pulmonary veins.
- 29.10 Clipping plane view of the septal pulmonary veins (PV) of a patient undergoing PV isolation.
- 29.11 Stenosis of the right superior pulmonary vein as displayed in contrast computer tomography in a patient post atrial fibrillation ablation.

For full references and multimedia materials please visit the online version of the book (http://esctextbook.oxfordonline.com).

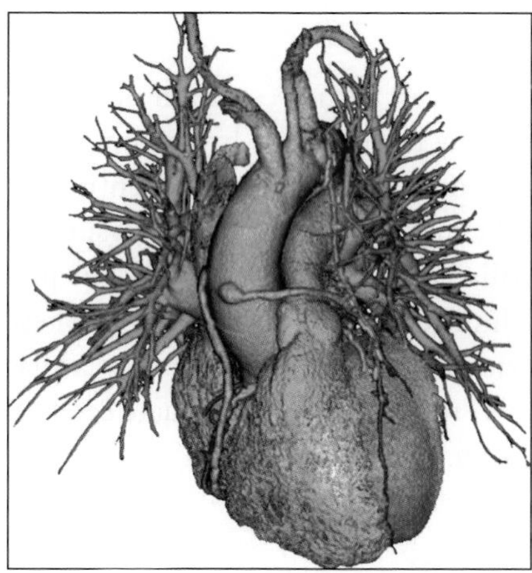

CHAPTER 30

Ventricular Tachycardia and Sudden Cardiac Death

Lars Eckardt, Günter Breithardt, and Stefan Hohnloser

Contents

Summary

Sudden cardiac death (SCD) continues to be a leading cause of death in Western countries, most often caused by ventricular tachyarrhythmias, such as ventricular tachycardia (VT) or fibrillation (VF), in the setting of structural heart disease. Ventricular arrhythmias can also be a mechanism of sudden death in patients with structurally normal hearts (e.g. ion channel disorders such as long or short QT syndrome, Brugada syndrome). Risk stratification for SCD remains a major challenge despite the development of numerous non-invasive risk factors. In contrast to VF, VTs are relatively organized tachyarrhythmias with discrete QRS complexes. They can be either sustained or non-sustained, and can be monomorphic or polymorphic. Polymorphic ventricular tachyarrhythmias tend to be faster and less stable than monomorphic. The correct diagnosis of a VT remains a challenge despite established criteria for the differentiation of ventricular from supraventricular tachycardia (SVT) with aberrant conduction. A re-entry mechanism accounts for the majority of ventricular tachyarrhythmias in patients with structural heart disease. The spectrum of therapies for VTs includes drug therapy, device implantation, and ablation techniques. The implantable defibrillator is an effective treatment modality not only for secondary, but also for primary prevention of SCD in selected patient populations. The management challenge is to deal both with the VT as the presenting symptom, and the SCD risk that may be the consequence of the arrhythmogenic substrate. As only a minority of victims of cardiac arrest survive to receive secondary preventive therapy, recent years have seen strong efforts to improve cardiopulmonary resuscitation. Probably the most important aspect in this regard is the development of the automatic external defibrillator, which effectively improves the outcome of victims of cardiac arrest.

Introduction

SCD remains one of the major challenges in cardiovascular medicine today. Ventricular tachyarrhythmias are the major cause of SCD in patients with structural heart disease, but can also be a mechanism of sudden death in patients with structurally normal hearts. This chapter summarizes the present state of knowledge regarding the pathophysiology and therapeutic approaches to patients with ventricular tachyarrhythmias. In large parts, this chapter is based on the published American College of Cardiology (ACC)/American Heart Association (AHA)/European Society of Cardiology (ESC) guidelines for management of patients with ventricular arrhythmias and the prevention of SCD [1] and the recent handbook *Sudden Cardiac Death* of the European Society of Cardiology (see ➲Further reading, p.1170 for more details).

Definitions

Ventricular tachycardia

VT is a relatively organized tachyarrhythmia with discrete QRS complexes. It can be either sustained (lasting >30s or requiring cardioversion in <30s) or non-sustained (defined as three or more beats but <30s), and can be monomorphic or polymorphic. If the same patient has monomorphic VTs with different morphologies, these are termed pleomorphic. Polymorphic VTs (i.e. markedly changing QRS complexes within the same episode) tend to be faster and less stable than monomorphic. Torsade de pointes (TdP) is a rapid, irregular non-sustained polymorphic VT that appears to twist around the isoelectric line, is associated with a long QT, and may degenerate into VF. Haemodynamically stable VT lasting hours has been termed 'incessant' [1]. A cluster of VT is defined as three or more episodes per 24 hours. The syndrome of very frequent episodes of VT requiring cardioversion has been termed 'VT storm'.

The rate of VT can range from 100 beats per minute (bpm) to >300bpm. At faster rates (usually 220bpm or faster), VT is so rapid that it may be impossible to distinguish the QRS complex from the T wave. This type of VT is referred to as ventricular flutter. VF is a completely disorganized (chaotic) tachyarrhythmia without discrete QRS complexes. When it begins, it is associated with a coarse electrical pattern. As the heart becomes less viable, the fibrillation becomes fine, and then, as an agonal event, all electrical activity ceases.

Cardiac arrest

Cardiac arrest is defined as an abrupt cessation of cardiac pump function, which may be reversible by prompt intervention but will lead to death in its absence. Ventricular tachyarrhythmias are the most common electrophysiological mechanism of cardiac arrest leading to SCD but primary non-tachyarrhythmic events are also common. These include pulseless electrical activity, asystole, or bradycardias that are severe enough to result in loss of adequate cerebral and other organ perfusion.

Sudden cardiac death

SCD is defined as 'natural death due to cardiac causes, heralded by abrupt loss of consciousness within one hour of the onset of acute symptoms; pre-existing heart disease may have been known to be present but the time and mode of death are unexpected' [2]. The key features that are central in the definition of SCD are the non-traumatic nature of the event and the fact that SCD should be unexpected and instantaneous. In order to limit sudden death to heart diseases, the word 'cardiac' has been added to forge the term SCD. The classification of deaths that occur unwitnessed, such as being found dead in bed, has been a difficult issue to deal with. Most investigators have elected to classify such events as SCD, even though it is often impossible to define when the patient was last alive or for what duration they suffered any symptoms prior to death.

Epidemiology of sudden cardiac death

Annual incidence rates of SCD range between 0.36–1.28 per 1000 inhabitants [2–4]. The incidence of SCD occurring out-of-hospital varies with age, gender, and presence or absence of a history of cardiovascular disease. For instance, a population-based study undertaken in Maastricht [5] monitored all cases of out-of-hospital cardiac arrest occurring in individuals aged 20–75 years. An overall yearly incidence of SCD of 1 per 1000 was observed. Overall, 21% of all deaths were sudden and unexpected in men and 14.5% in women. Most deaths occurred at home (80%) and only about 15% in public places; 40% of deaths were unwitnessed. Of note, a parental history of SCD was found to be an independent risk factor for SCD in >7000 men followed up for 23 years in the Paris Prospective Study I [6].

In the USA, there is an estimate of 300,000 cases of SCD per year. Myerburg and colleagues [7] reviewed the issue of risk of SCD in population subgroups. The population incidence of SCD was just over 1 in 1000 per year, implying that any intervention applied to the general population to reduce the risk of SCD would therefore be given to 999 out of 1000 individuals who will not die suddenly in 1 year in order to prevent one instance of SCD. Subgroups with progressively greater annual SCD risk comprise a progressively smaller proportion of the total numbers of SCDs in the population. Thus, the logical conclusion of these figures is that the greatest opportunity to reduce the population burden of SCD lies in the reduction of coronary artery disease in the population at large (see ➲Chapter 12, Prevention of Cardiovascular Disease).

Causes of sudden cardiac death

The single most important cause of death in the adult population of the industrialized world is SCD due to coronary artery disease (see ➲Chapter 17, Chronic Ischaemic Heart Disease). Although estimates vary, approximately 75–80% of SCD are due to this one underlying aetiology [7]. Accordingly, population studies in many industrialized countries have demonstrated that the risk factors for SCD are predominantly the same as those for atherosclerotic coronary disease, such as increasing age, male gender, family history of coronary artery disease, increased low-density lipoprotein cholesterol (LDL-C), hypertension (see ➲Chapter 13, Hypertension), smoking, and diabetes mellitus [6, 8, 9].

Idiopathic dilated cardiomyopathy (DCM) (➲Chapter 18), a chronic heart muscle disease characterized by left ventricular dilatation, impairment of systolic function, and congestive heart failure in the absence of coronary heart disease, is the second largest cause of SCD. DCM accounts for approximately 10–15% of all SCDs [10]. Despite a gradual decline in 5-year mortality from 70% in the early 1980s to approximately 20% nowadays, SCD accounts for at least 30% of all deaths in DCM.

In about 5–10% of cases, SCD occurs in the absence of coronary artery disease and congestive heart failure; ➲Table 30.1 provides a summary of the clinical syndromes that constitute this proportion of SCD cases. Despite the relatively low absolute number of SCDs due to these clinical entities, identification of individuals at risk is of paramount importance, as many of the afflicted individuals are destined to die at a young age.

Table 30.1 Cardiovascular diseases and SCD

Coronary artery disease
Dilated cardiomyopathy
Together, these two disease account for >90% of all SCDs
Other cardiomyopathies
Hypertrophic cardiomyopathy
Arrhythmogenic right ventricular cardiomyopathy
Primary 'electrical' disorders
Long QT syndrome
Brugada syndrome
Catecholaminergic right ventricular cardiomyopathy
Wolff–Parkinson–White syndrome
Sinus node AV node conduction disturbances
Mechanical cardiovascular disease
Aortic stenosis
Mitral valve prolapse
Myocardial bridging
Anomalous origin of coronary arteries
Miscellaneous disorders
Myocarditis
Chest trauma
Drug-induced torsade de pointes and SCD
Trained heart
SCD in the normal heart

Pathological anatomy in sudden cardiac death

Extensive coronary atherosclerosis is the primary anatomic hallmark of SCD in patients with coronary heart disease. In addition, the presence of plaque fissuring and/or erosion, platelet aggregation, and acute thrombosis within the matrix of coronary atherosclerosis is associated with SCD [11, 12]. This feature of coronary artery anatomy, superimposed upon chronic lesions, does not differ among the three primary expressions of acute coronary syndromes: namely SCD, acute myocardial infarction, and unstable angina pectoris (see ➲Chapter 16, Acute Coronary Syndromes). Myocardial pathology reflects the presence and extent of chronic coronary atherosclerosis, which is characterized by myocardial scars as a result of healed myocardial infarction. The association between extensive coronary disease and left ventricular hypertrophy is mainly a reflection of the presence of longstanding arterial hypertension as a risk factor in coronary heart disease patients. Both myocardial scars and left ventricular hypertrophy are considered important factors in arrhythmogenesis during transient ischaemia.

Among the less prevalent causes of SCD, anatomy depends upon the underlying aetiology. In DCM, pathological findings are non-specific, characterized by interstitial fibrosis and myocyte degeneration. In hypertrophic cardiomyopathy, there are obstructive and non-obstructive forms with apical versus concentric hypertrophy patterns (see ➲Chapter 18, Myocardial Disease).

In the small fraction of SCDs that is due to rare genetically determined disorders such as the long QT syndrome or Brugada syndrome, there may be no or only minimal myocardial pathology. A number of cases of SCD in infancy (often labelled as sudden infant death syndrome), and even of stillbirths, are actually due to the long QT syndrome [13–15].

Electrocardiographic diagnosis of ventricular tachycardia

The correct diagnosis of a wide complex tachycardia (QRS duration >120ms) remains a challenge despite numerous established criteria for the differentiation of ventricular from SVT with aberrant conduction. However, the correct diagnosis is important for the acute as well as long-term management of patients with broad QRS complex tachycardia. VT is the most common cause of wide QRS complex tachycardia, accounting for up to 80% of all cases [16]. Thus, all wide QRS complex tachycardia should be treated as if the rhythm was VT until proven otherwise!

A history of heart disease (prior myocardial infarction or heart failure) has a positive predictive accuracy of 95% for VT [17]. A history of heart disease (prior myocardial infarction, angina, or congestive heart failure) can serve as a good discriminator between a SVT and a VT as the cause of a wide QRS complex tachycardia!

On the other hand, if a patient has had similar episodes during previous years, a supraventricular origin is more likely than a VT. Termination of a tachycardia by manoeuvres, such as the Valsalva manoeuvre or adenosine injection, strongly suggests a supraventricular origin (see ➲Chapter 28, Supraventricular Tachycardia), although some VTs can also terminate with these manoeuvres (e.g. fascicular VT).

It is important to recognize that a wide QRS complex tachycardia in a patient who is alert and haemodynamically stable is not necessarily of supraventricular origin. If it is a VT in a patient with reduced systolic function, an intravenous injection of, for example, verapamil may result in severe hypotension and haemodynamic instability. Thus, calcium-channel blockers should not be used in patients to terminate wide QRS complex tachycardia of unknown origin (Class III Recommendation; Level of Evidence: C). Causes of VT in patients without structural heart disease are listed in ➲Table 30.2.

Table 30.2 Causes of wide complex tachycardias in patients without structural heart disease

Monomorphic configuration
SVT
◆ Bundle branch block: • Functional (RBBB more often than LBBB) • Pre-excitation • Rate related (RBBB more often than LBBB) ◆ Antidromic (i.e. retrograde conduction over AV node) • LBBB, superior axis (consider Mahaim, see text) ◆ Non-specific conduction delay • Class I or class III antiarrhythmic drugs • Electrolyte imbalance
VT
◆ LBBB, inferior axis: idiopathic right ventricular VT ◆ RBBB, superior axis: idiopathic left ventricular VT ◆ Pacemaker-mediated VT
Polymorphic configuration
SVT
◆ Atrial fibrillation with pre-excitation
VT
◆ TdP (long QT syndrome) ◆ Brugada syndrome ◆ Catecholaminergic polymorphic VT ◆ Short QT syndrome ◆ Early repolarization syndrome

AV, atrioventricular; LBBB, left bundle branch block; RBBB, right bundle branch block; SVT, supraventricular tachycardia; TdP, torsade de pointes.; VT, ventricular tachycardia.

Note: all wide complex tachycardias should be treated as if the rhythm was VT until proven otherwise.

How to distinguish between a supraventricular and a ventricular tachycardia?

In general, if an electrocardiogram (ECG) showing a wide QRS complex tachycardia does not look like aberration, it is most likely a VT (➲Fig. 30.1). The following ECG criteria distinguish between a VT and a SVT with aberration [18].

- *QRS morphologies in V1 and V6* (➲Fig. 30.1) [19]. Differential diagnosis of SVT and VT. In right bundle branch block (RBBB) pattern, a monophasic R wave, a broad (>30ms) R or a QR in V1 strongly suggests VT, while a three-phasic (RSR) pattern suggests a supraventricular origin. A monophasic R wave or an S greater than an R in V6 also suggests VT. In the presence of a left bundle branch block (LBBB) pattern, a broad R wave (usually >30ms) [20]

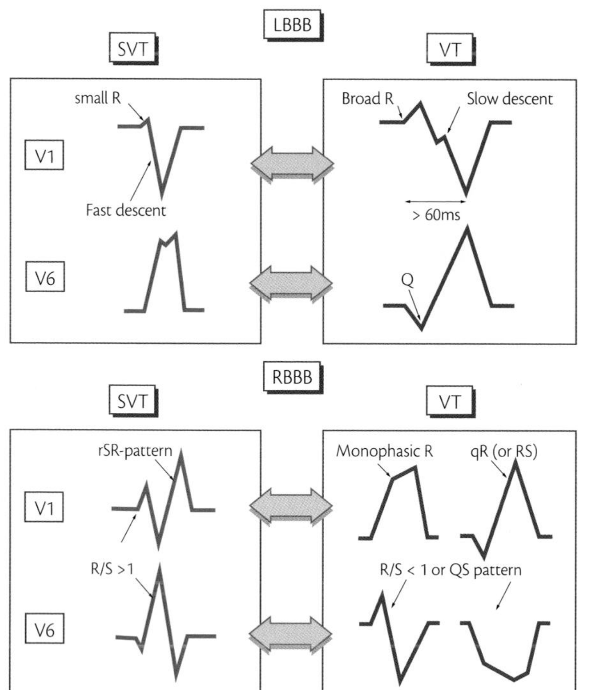

Figure 30.1 QRS criteria for differential diagnosis in broad complex tachycardia: ventricular tachycardia (VT) vs. supraventricular tachycardia (SVT) with left (LBBB) or right (RBBB) bundle branch block.

and/or a slow descent to the S wave nadir in V1 and a Q in V6 point towards a VT.

- *Atrioventricular (AV) dissociation.* This is one of the most useful criteria for distinguishing VT from SVT. It occurs in 20–50% of VT and almost never in SVT [16, 21, 22]. AV dissociation may be diagnosed by a changing pulse pressure, irregular canon A waves in the jugular veins, and a variable first heart sound. It is often very difficult to ascertain, particularly in rapid tachycardias. It often demands long 12-lead ECG recordings and careful ECG analysis. In addition, about 30% of VT has 1:1 retrograde conduction.
- *QRS complex duration.* VT is the probable diagnosis when the QRS duration with RBBB is >140ms, and >160ms with LBBB morphology [16]. However, a SVT can have a QRS width >140ms (RBBB) or 160ms (LBBB) in the presence of pre-existent bundle branch block (BBB) in the elderly with fibrosis in the bundle branch system and ventricular myocardium, when during SVT, AV conduction occurs over an accessory AV pathway or when class IC drugs (especially flecainide) are present during SVT (➲Fig. 30.2). On the other hand, a QRS width below the above named values may occur in VT having their origin in or close to the interventricular septum or within the fascicular system.
- *QRS axis.* A frontal axis of between 90° and ± 180° cannot be achieved by any combination of BBB and therefore suggests VT. Thus, predominantly negative QRS complexes in leads I, II, and III are useful criteria for identifying a VT (➲Fig. 30.3). Left axis deviation (to the left of −30°) suggests VT, but is not helpful in LBBB-shaped QRS complexes, in a SVT with conduction over a right-sided or posteroseptal accessory pathway or in the presence of SVT during use of class IC drugs. Right axis deviation (to the right of +90°) suggests VT in LBBB-shaped QRS [23].
- *Concordant negative ECG patterns in the precordial leads.* If all precordial leads are predominantly negative, a VT is the diagnosis (➲Fig. 30.4). If all precordial leads are predominantly positive, the differential diagnosis is an antidromic tachycardia using a left-sided accessory

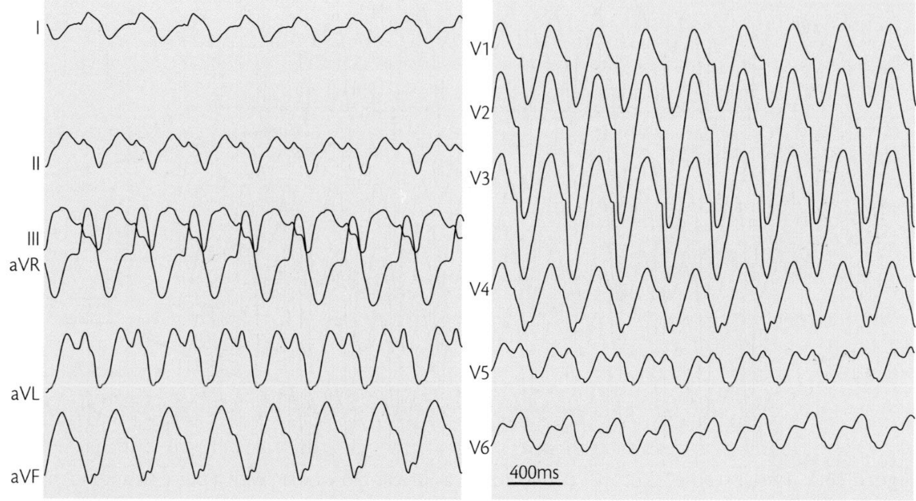

Figure 30.2 Atrial flutter with 2:1 conduction (CL 400ms) in patient with paroxysmal atrial fibrillation. The patient was advised to take 200mg flecainide in combination with a beta-blocker as a 'pill in the pocket' strategy to treat his symptomatic episodes of recurrent atrial fibrillation, but took 400mg instead. Note the broad LBBB morphology with a QRS duration of 0.22s.

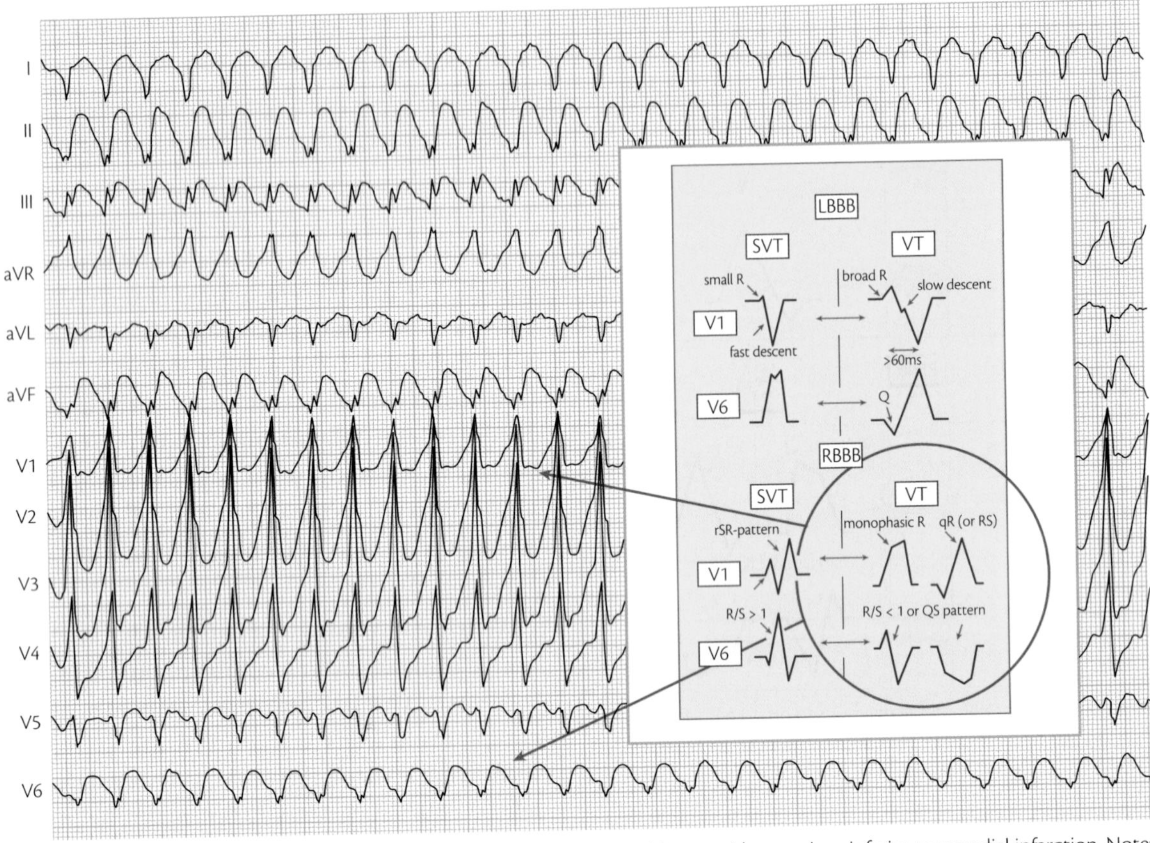

Figure 30.3 Twelve-lead-ECG of a ventricular tachycardia (CL 320ms) in a 73-year-old man with a previous inferior myocardial infarction. Note: the monophasic broad R wave V1 and the S greater than R in V6 suggest VT.

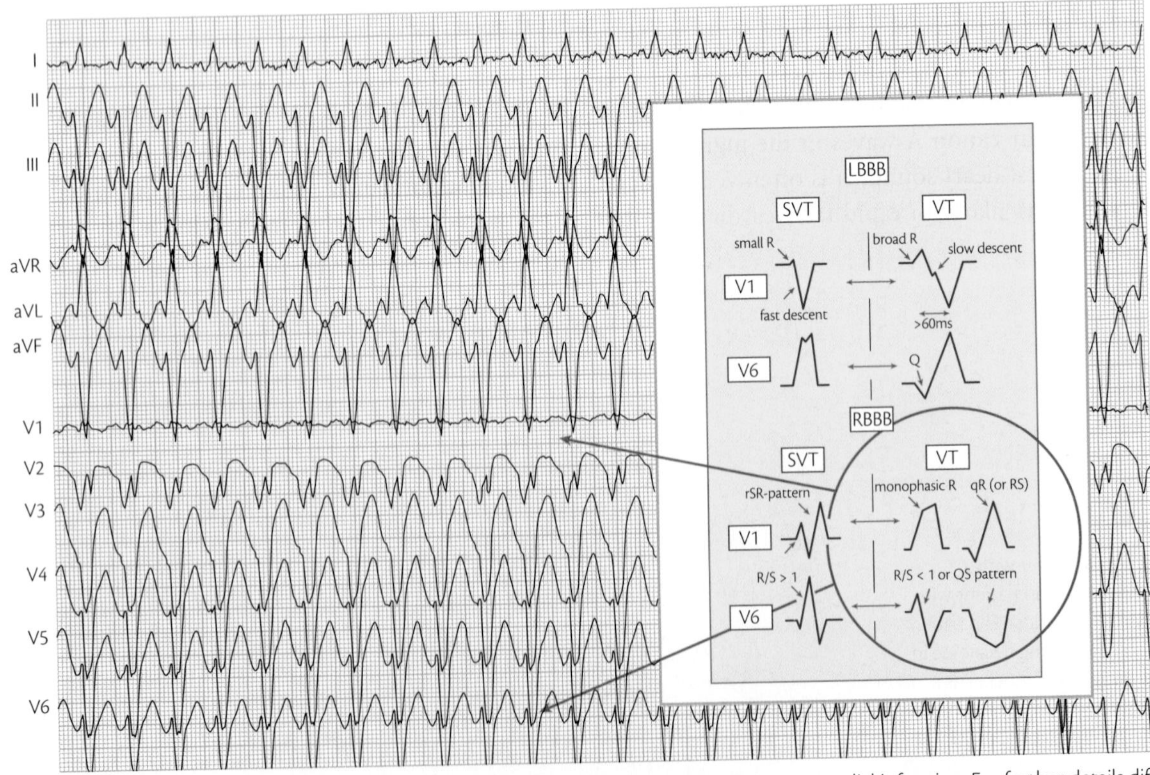

Figure 30.4 Twelve-lead-ECG of a VT (CL 400ms) in a 60-year-old woman with a previous anterior myocardial infarction. For further details differentiating SVT vs. VT see text.

pathway or a VT. An initial R wave in lead aVR rules out pre-excitation since activation of the ventricles over an accessory pathway proceeds from the base towards the apex of the heart yielding a negative QRS complex in lead aVR. It serves as a useful additional marker for a VT (➲Figs. 30.3 and 30.4) but may be negative in VT due to anteroseptal myocardial infarction, scar at a late activated ventricular site, fascicular VT, and VT exit sites close to the His–Purkinje system [24].

- *QR complexes.* A QR (but not a QS) complex during a broad QRS tachycardia indicates a scar in the myocardium usually caused by myocardial infarction (➲Fig. 30.5). QR complexes during VT are present in approximately 40% of VT after myocardial infarction [25].
- *Capture or fusion beats.* These result from AV conduction of dissociated atrial complexes during VT and may occur in patients with slow VT (e.g. in the presence of amiodarone) (➲Fig. 30.5). They are a specific finding for VT but are only found in a limited number of patients [21].

The ECG and site of ventricular tachycardia origin

The 12-lead ECG during VT can be helpful in providing an approximation of the site of origin, which may be useful for guiding diagnostic management and catheter ablation (➲Fig. 30.6). In general, VTs that have a LBBB-like morphology in V1 have an exit in the right ventricle or the interventricular septum. A QRS axis that is directed superiorly generally indicates an exit in the inferior wall; an axis directed inferiorly indicates an exit in the anterior (superior) wall. In V2–V4, dominant R waves usually indicate an exit near the base of the ventricle. In idiopathic right ventricular outflow tract (RVOT) tachycardia (see ➲Idiopathic outflow-tract ventricular tachycardia, p.1163), the QRS duration during VT is usually >140ms if it originates from the free wall of the RVOT, and <140ms if the arrhythmia originates from the septal site of the RVOT. The precordial R-wave transition in RVOT VT usually occurs in leads V2–V4 and becomes earlier as the site of origin advances more superiorly along the septum. An R-wave transition in lead V2 points to a site of origin immediately inferior to the pulmonic valve or the left ventricular outflow tract [26] (➲Fig. 30.7).

In wide QRS complex tachycardia with LBBB morphology and a left superior axis (➲Fig. 30.8), one should always consider an atriofascicular (Mahaim) accessory pathway (see ➲Chapter 28, Supraventricular Tachycardia). Patients with these pathways may have episodes of pre-excited tachycardia without exhibiting pre-excitation during sinus rhythm. Narrow QRS complex tachycardias almost never

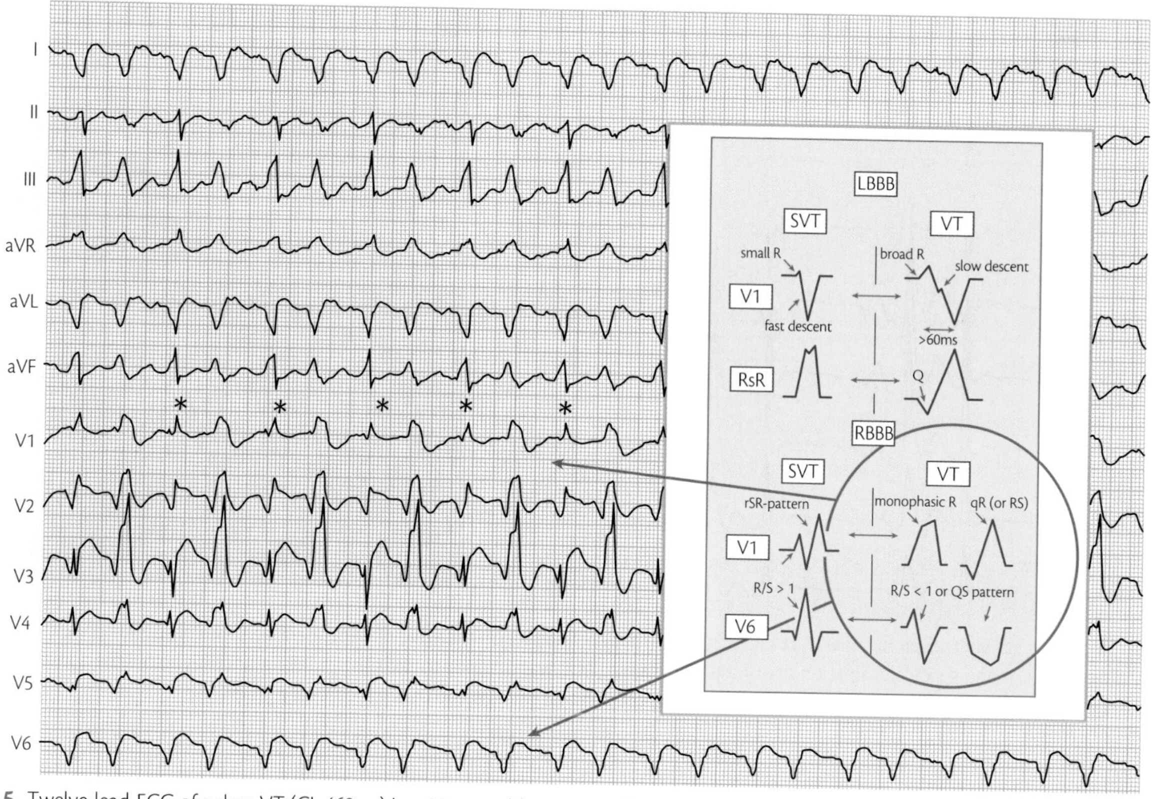

Figure 30.5 Twelve-lead-ECG of a slow VT (CL 460ms) in a 83-year-old woman with a previous anterior myocardial infarction and a large anteroseptal aneurysm. Due to the slow VT rate every second beat is a capture/fusion beat (*). Note the deep right precordial Q waves.

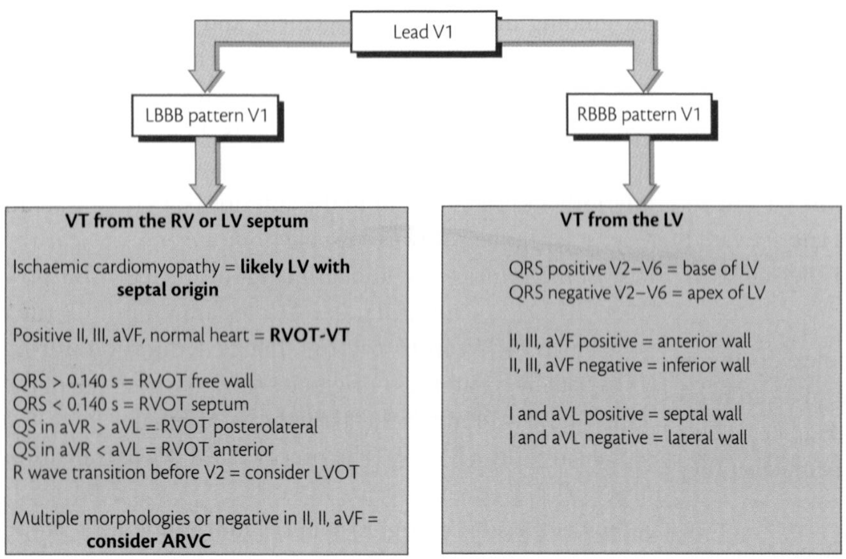

Figure 30.6 Algorithm for localization of the exit site of VT.

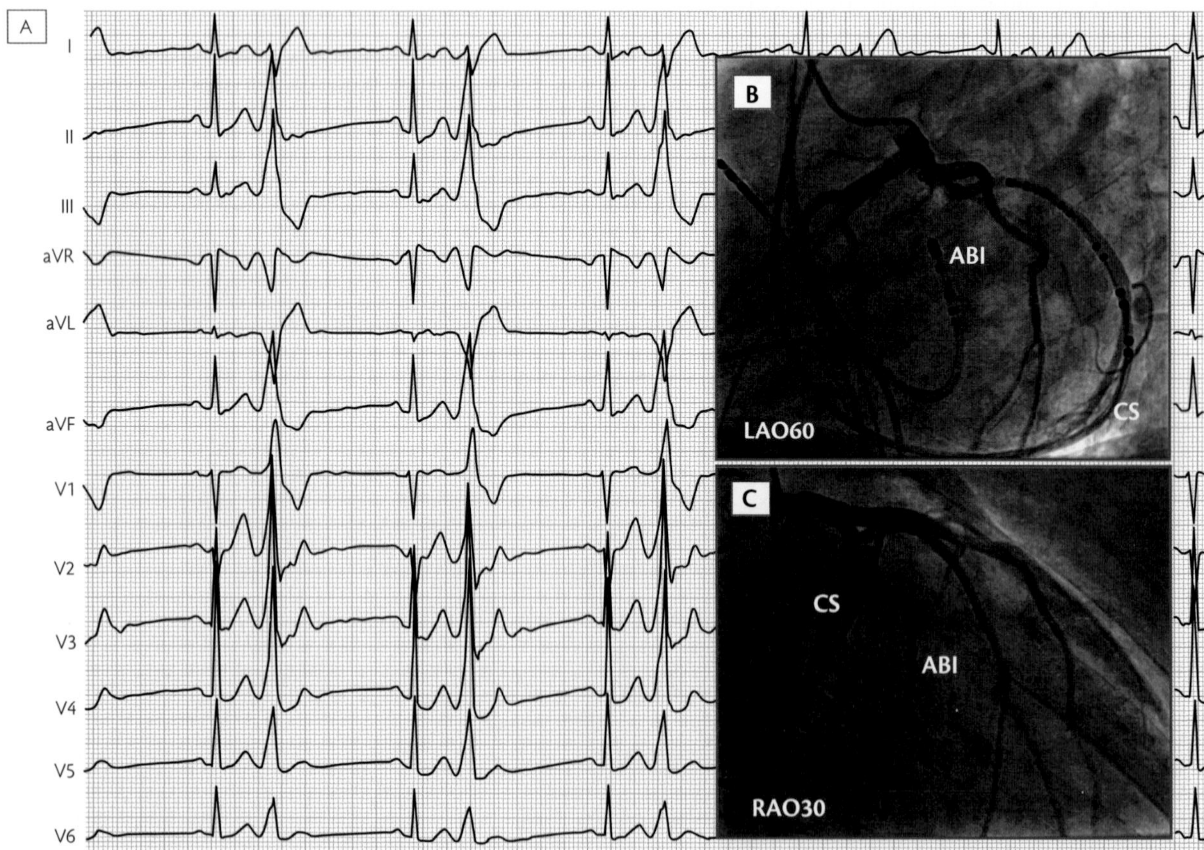

Figure 30.7 Idiopathic left ventricular outflow tract bigeminus. The patients had recurrent exercise-dependent episodes of sustained tachycardia of the same morphology. The exit and successful ablation site of the tachycardia (Abl) was mapped to the superior mitral annulus below the aortic valve. The angiogram of the left coronary artery illustrates the relation between the ablation site and the LCA. CS, coronary sinus.

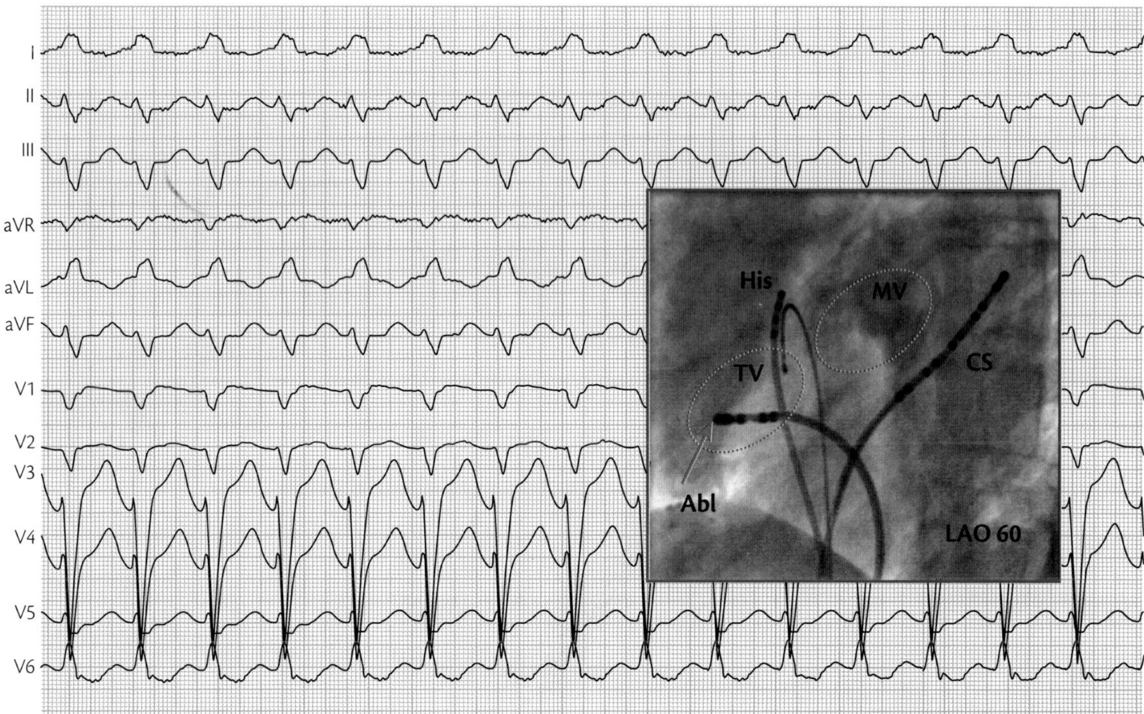

Figure 30.8 Typical ECG of an antidromic AV re-entrant tachycardia via an atriofascicular bypass tract (Mahaim fibre). Note the LBBB morphology with the superior axis. The differential diagnosis would be a right VT in ARVC. Abl: successful ablation site at the tricuspid annulus, CS: coronary sinus; His: His bundle catheter; MV and TV: mitral and tricuspid annulus.

occur due to the absence of retrograde conduction over the accessory pathway. The QRS morphology during tachycardia typically shows a small, short, initial R wave followed by a steep downstroke in the precordial ECG leads.

Electrophysiological mechanisms of ventricular tachycardia

Re-entrant ventricular arrhythmias

A re-entry mechanism accounts for the majority of monomorphic VT. In contrast with automatic arrhythmias, the conditions for re-entry tend to be associated with chronic rather than acute disease (see ➲Chapter 17, Chronic Ischaemic Heart Disease). Endocardial catheter mapping and intraoperative mapping have shown that these arrhythmias originate within or at the border zone of the diseased myocardium. The size of the re-entrant circuit may be large, especially in patients with a left ventricular aneurysm, or may be confined to a small area.

Re-entry requires a series of conditions to be satisfied for its occurrence:

1) two potentially conducting pathways or more;
2) unidirectional block occurring in one pathway;
3) an activation wavefront travelling around that zone of unidirectional block over the alternative pathway;
4) then activation of myocardium distal to the zone of unidirectional block with delay (i.e. with slow conduction); so allowing
5) the activation wavefront to invade the zone of block retrogradely and re-excite the tissue where the activation wavefront originated.

Zones of slowly conducting myocardium may be identified during endocardial catheter mapping by fractionated and/or mid-diastolic electrograms (➲Fig. 30.9), continuous electrical activity, or a long delay between a stimulus artefact and the resulting QRS complex. However, not all areas of slow conduction participate in the re-entry circuit, i.e. 'dead end' or 'bystander' pathways may exist. Therefore, for successful ablation, localization procedures have to provide evidence that a mapping site is actually within the re-entry circuit and is critically linked to the perpetuation of the arrhythmia. If a VT is not inducible or haemodynamically not tolerated during an ablation procedure, electro-anatomical mapping systems can be used to locate critical isthmus regions, such as the mitral isthmus (➲Fig. 30.10) and to guide successful ablation.

Of note, in the presence of heart failure, re-entry in the His–Purkinje system (bundle branch re-entry; ➲Fig. 30.11)

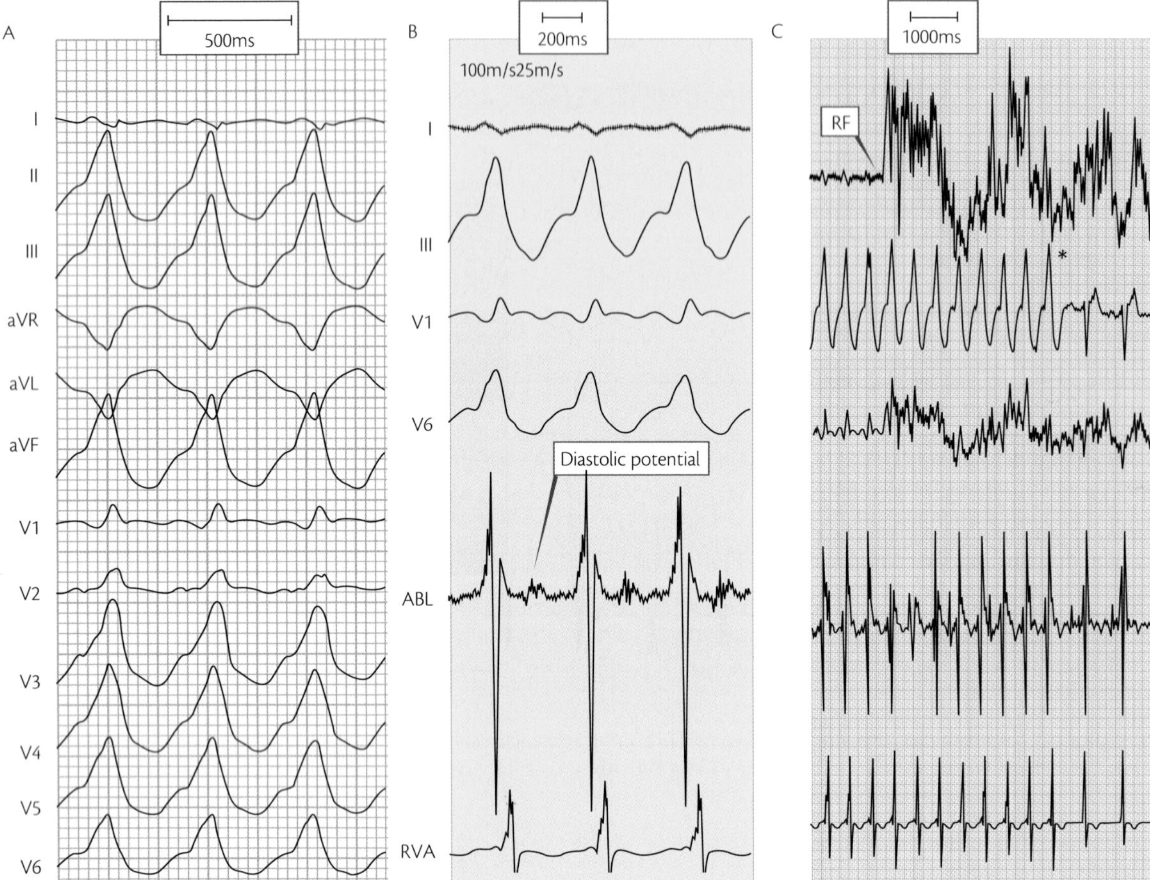

Figure 30.9 ECG recording in a patient with previous anterior myocardial infarction and recurrent sustained VT. (A) Catheter mapping and subsequent catheter ablation were performed. (B) Leads I, III, V1 and V6, as well as intracardiac signals from the right ventricular apex (RVA) and the ablation catheter at the successful ablation site (ABL) anteroseptal at the left-ventricular base are displayed. Note: the fragmented diastolic potential at the successful ablation site (for further details, see text), where the VT terminated a few seconds after starting radiofrequency (RF) ablation (C).

accounts for a substantial number of monomorphic VTs. The re-entry wavefront proceeds down one bundle branch (mostly the right bundle branch), and up the contralateral bundle. This creates a QRS complex that has a LBBB contour and a normal or leftward frontal plane axis. Its significance lies in the fact that it can be easily cured by catheter ablation of the right bundle branch.

Automatic ventricular arrhythmias

Abnormal automaticity accounts for a minority of VT. Automatic VT tends to be associated with conditions such as acute myocardial infarction, hypoxaemia, electrolyte abnormalities, and a high adrenergic tone. Automatic VTs that occurs during the first 24–48 hours after an acute myocardial infarction are a major cause of SCD. They are probably related to the residual ischaemia seen acutely in the zone of infarction. Once the infarction heals, the substrate for these arrhythmias disappears (but the one for re-entry evolves). Because automatic arrhythmias generally occur secondarily to metabolic abnormalities, treatment should be aimed at identifying and reversing the underlying cause whenever possible.

Triggered activity

Although VTs based on triggered activity are uncommon, two distinct clinical syndromes involving triggered activity have been identified: pause- and catecholamine-dependent arrhythmias. In each syndrome, patients develop polymorphic VT. These arrhythmias tend to occur in relatively short bursts that may be accompanied by light-headedness or syncope, but may also degenerate into VF and SCD.

Pause-dependent triggered activity is caused by afterdepolarizations that occur during phase 3 of the action potential (early afterdepolarizations). If these afterdepolarizations reach the threshold potential of the cardiac cell, another action potential is generated. Pause-dependent triggered activity may be related to congenital ion-channel abnormalities (see ➲Long QT syndrome, p.1163, and ➲Chapter 9), and/or to specific conditions (hypokalaemia and

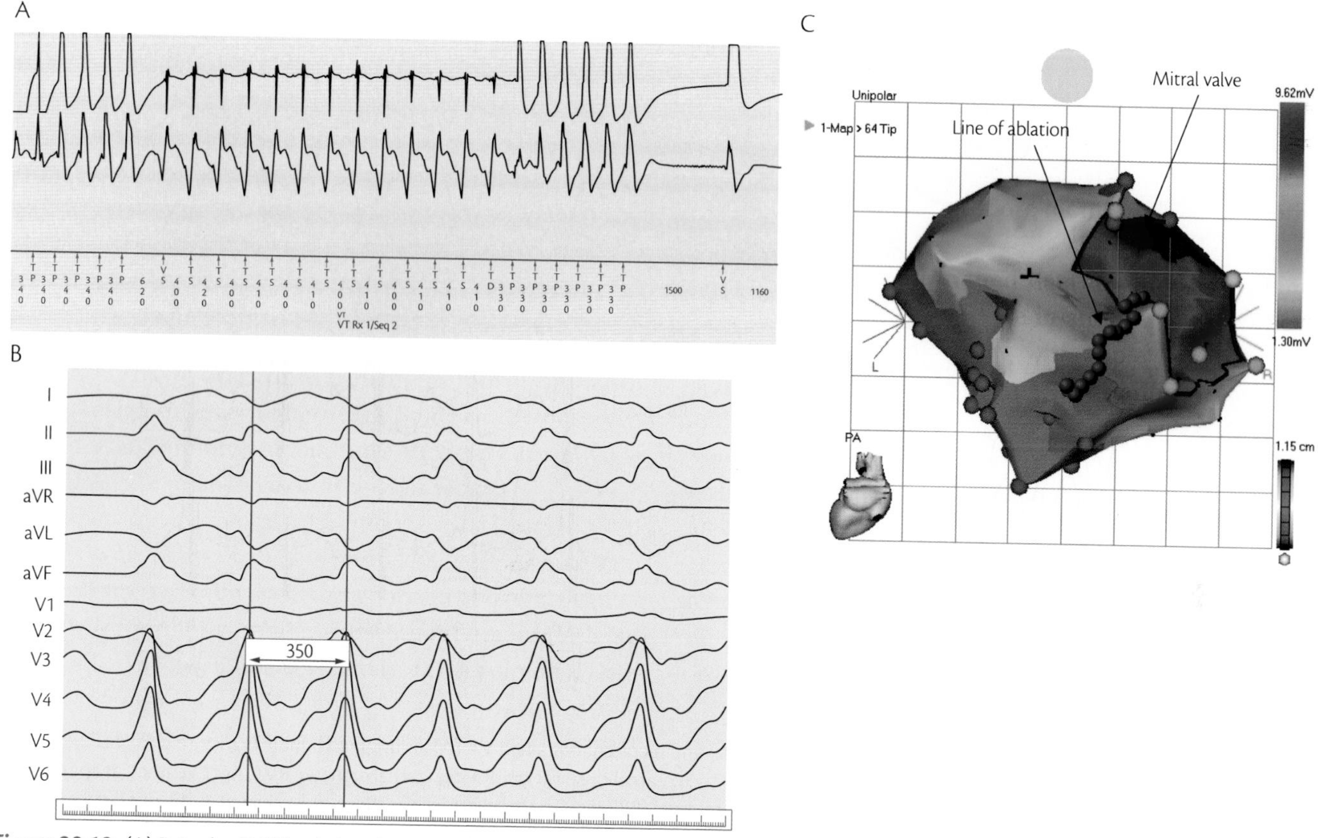

Figure 30.10 (A) Episode of VT (cycle length ~ 400ms) detected and terminated by an implantable cardioverter-defibrillator in a patient with a remote inferior myocardial infarction who experienced recurrent VT episodes. (B) Twelve-lead ECG of the VT in the same patient. (C) Posterior view of an electroanatomic voltage map (Carto) of the left ventricle. Electroanatomic mapping can be used to define isthmus boundaries and thus guide successful ablation. Colour range represents voltage amplitude. Grey denotes dense scar tissue. A linear ablation lesion was placed from the mitral annulus to the edge of the scar tissue to prohibit mitral 'isthmus' re-entrant tachycardias (around the mitral valve and/or around the posterior scar).

hypomagnesaemia), and/or the use of non-cardiovascular or cardiovascular drugs that prolong repolarization (i.e. acquired QT syndrome). Individuals who develop ventricular tachyarrhythmias (i.e. torsade de pointes (➲Fig. 30.12) see ➲Risk factors for torsade de pointes, p.1166) in the presence of these conditions have a reduced repolarization reserve [27].

Catecholamine-dependent triggered activity is caused by afterdepolarizations that occur during phase 4 of the cardiac action potential (delayed afterdepolarizations). They occur in the setting of congenital ion-channel abnormalities (see ➲Catecholaminergic polymorphic ventricular tachycardia, p.1164 and ➲Chapter 9), digitalis toxicity, or cardiac ischaemia and may present as a bidirectional VT (➲Fig. 30.13). Catecholamine-dependent triggered activity generally is not dependent on pauses. Instead, these arrhythmias may arise in conditions of high sympathetic tone and underlying sinus tachycardia. Thus, patients experience VT (manifested by syncope or cardiac arrest) during times of exercise or of emotional stress.

Ventricular tachycardia: clinical presentation

The clinical presentation of VT depends on the haemodynamic consequences it produces. These depend partly on VT rate, the degree of myocardial dysfunction, and autonomic factors. Physical examination in a patient presenting with VT often indicates haemodynamic distress (low blood pressure, heart failure, or cardiogenic shock). When cardiac output and blood pressure are maintained and/or when the VT is short-lived, the arrhythmia may present as palpitations, breathlessness, or chest pain. Sometimes, especially in patients without structural heart disease (➲Table 30.2), no symptoms are reported during VT. Persistent, slow (<150bpm) VT may lead to dyspnoea, pulmonary congestion, and oedema.

Syncope (➲Chapter 26) is the single most important clinical event for grading SCD risk in heart failure [28]. VT was found to be the cause of syncope in 35% of these

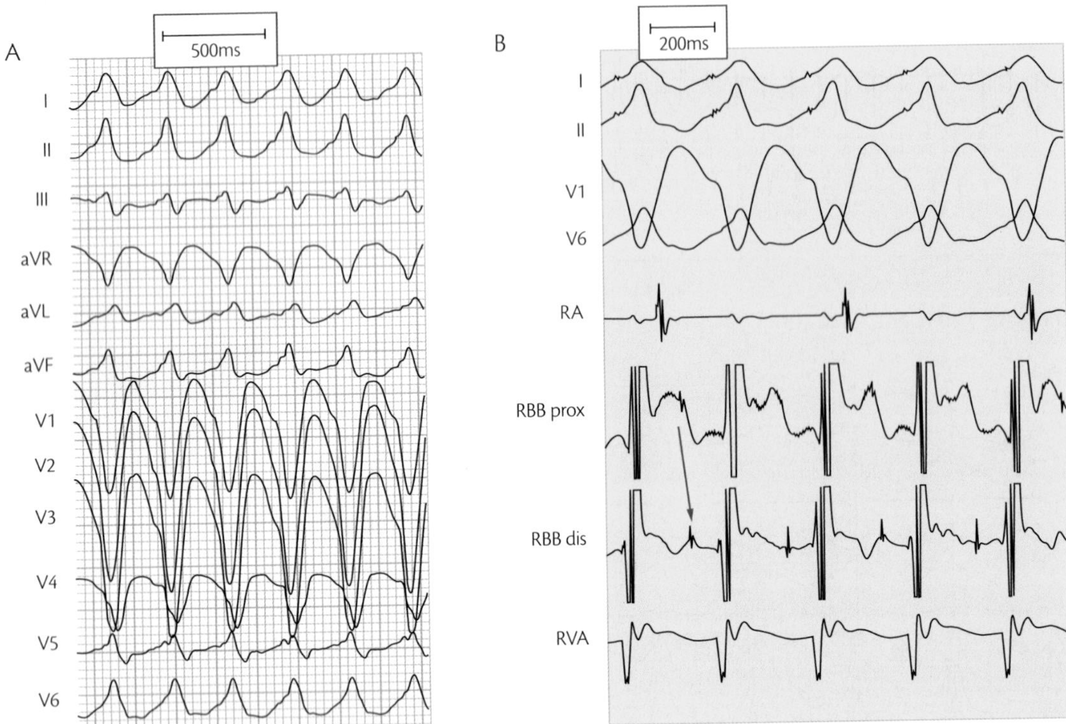

Figure 30.11 ECG recording in a patient with dilated cardiomyopathy and recurrent sustained VT. (A) A sustained bundle branch re-entry tachycardia with a LBBB morphology is displayed. Intracardiac signals (B) reveal ventriculo-atrial dissociation (RA, right atrial catheter; RVA, right ventricular apex) and activation of the right bundle branch (RBB) from proximal (RBB prox) to distal (RBB dis). The tachycardia was successfully ablated at the distal right bundle branch using radiofrequency current.

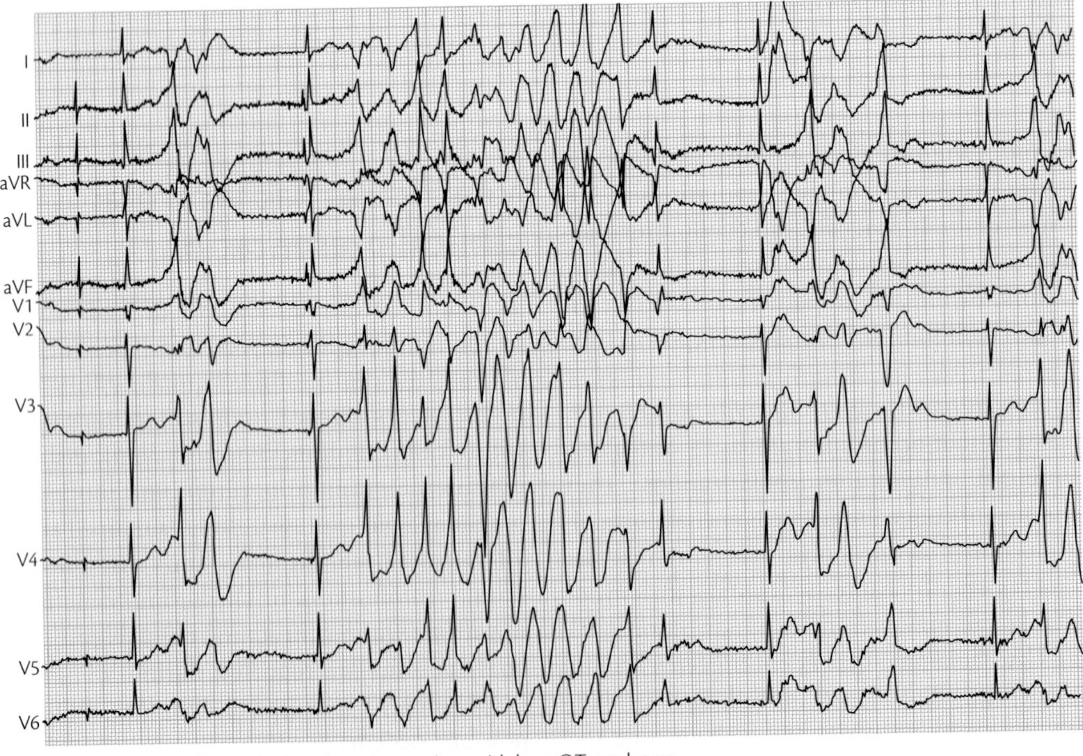

Figure 30.12 Recurrent episodes of torsade de pointes in a patient with long QT syndrome.

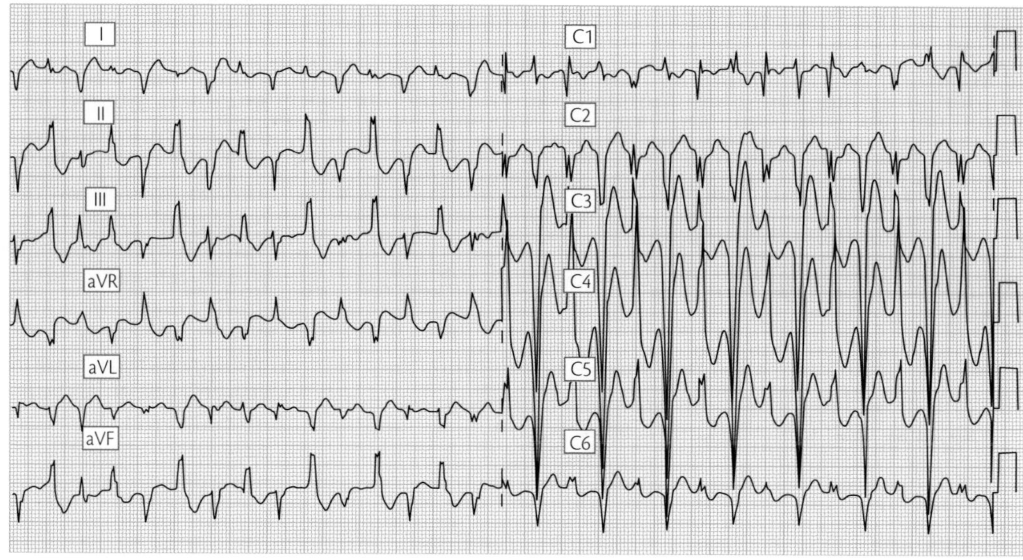

Figure 30.13 Bidirectional tachycardia after exercise in a patient with catecholaminergic polymorphic VT.

patients [29]. Patients with heart failure and unexplained syncope have a 1-year sudden death rate of up to 45% [29]. The frequency and complexity of VT parallel the severity of ventricular dysfunction. In total, 15–20% of patients with New York Heart Association (NYHA) class I–II heart failure have non-sustained VT compared with 50–70% of patients with class IV heart failure. *Sustained polymorphic VT* is less stable than monomorphic VT. It is usually rapid and often degenerates into VF. *Sustained monomorphic VT* may be haemodynamically tolerated, but may also precipitate VF or may cause syncope before terminating spontaneously. Patients presenting with haemodynamically tolerated VT have a lower risk of SCD than patients whose initial episode causes cardiac arrest, but the risk is still substantial.

Broad QRS complex tachycardia: clinical approach

The clinical approach to a broad QRS complex tachycardia depends on the patient's history and the electrocardiographic documentation. If the documented tachycardia is most likely a SVT with aberrant conduction only very few clinical tests are required (see ➲Chapter 28, Supraventricular Tachycardia).

Intraventricular conduction delay can result from heart rate changes, as well as from fixed pathological lesions in the conduction system. In patients with pre-existing or 'fixed' (present during the normal baseline rhythm) BBB, any SVT results in a broad complex tachycardia. However, rate related and/or 'functional' (present only during tachycardia) BBB may also result in a broad complex tachycardia.

Functional aberration results from sudden increases in cycle length when parts of the His–Purkinje system are partially or wholly inexcitable. Functional RBBB occurs more frequently than functional LBBB because of the longer refractoriness of the former [30]. Functional BBB may persist for several successive impulses because the bundle branch that is blocked antegradely may be activated transseptally via its contralateral counterpart, a process known as linking phenomenon [31]. As the duration of the refractory period is a function of the immediately preceding cycle length (the longer this cycle length, the longer the subsequent refractory period), abrupt cycle length variations (i.e. long-to-short or short-to-long) predispose to the occurrence of functional BBB. This is known as the Ashman phenomenon [32] (➲Fig. 30.14). It can often be observed in patients with atrial fibrillation and should not be interpreted as a non-sustained VT.

Non-invasive work-up

Apart from a detailed history and physical investigation the non-invasive work-up has to include a 12-lead ECG and an echocardiogram.

The ECG may reveal the diagnosis of Wolff–Parkinson–White (WPW) syndrome (➲Chapters 21 and 28). Pre-excited tachycardias in WPW syndrome account for a minority of wide QRS complex tachycardias. In these tachycardias, ventricular activation occurs predominately or exclusively via an accessory pathway. Variations in pre-excitation (➲Fig. 30.15) along with cycle lengths changes are seen when atrial fibrillation conducts over the pathway, whereas a monomorphic picture of pre-excitation is almost always due to a re-entrant tachycardia (with the exception

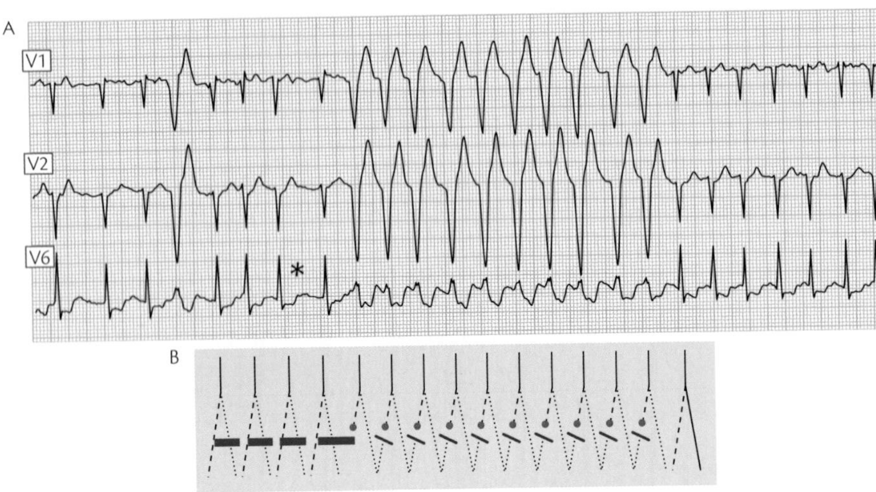

Figure 30.14 Atrial fibrillation with ventricular aberration resulting from the Ashman phenomenon, and concealed trans-septal conduction. (A) After a long pause (*) the refractory period of the left bundle branch is prolonged which results in ten RS complexes with LBBB morphology. The aberration is probably perpetuated by concealed trans-septal conduction ('linking phenomenon') from the right into the left bundle with block of antegrade conduction of the subsequent impulses in the left bundle. (B) The solid line represents the His bundle; the dashes (dots) represent the left (right) bundle. The solid horizontal bars represent the refractory period.

of an atrial tachycardia and/or atrial flutter conducted over the accessory pathway). In the presence of atrial fibrillation, rapid ventricular rates due to AV conduction over an accessory pathway (➲Fig. 30.16) may cause VF and SCD. The incidence of SCD in patients with WPW syndrome is estimated to be <1 per 100 patient-years follow-up; 70% of patients who experience ventricular tachyarrhythmias have a previous history of symptoms [33]. The ECG of a pre-excited SVT can be indistinguishable from a VT originating at the base of the ventricles (see ➲Chapter 28, Supraventricular Tachycardia).

In patients with monomorphic VT, an exercise test should be performed after excluding acute coronary syndrome. It is of particular value in patients with idiopathic exercise-dependent VT (e.g. idiopathic RVOT VT and fascicular tachycardia) and catecholaminergic polymorphic VT (Class I indication, Level of Evidence B) [1], but may also just unmask ischaemic heart disease or even induce a polymorphic ischaemia-related VT (➲Fig. 30.17). Of note, sustained monomorphic VT only very rarely indicates acute ischaemia and is unlikely to be affected by revascularization.

An echocardiogram is helpful in ruling out structural heart disease (e.g. old myocardial infarction, reduced left ventricular function) and congenital abnormalities (➲Chapter 10). Some rare congenital disorders such as Ebstein's anomaly are often associated with right-sided accessory pathways. In LBBB tachycardia, echocardiographic signs for arrhythmogenic right

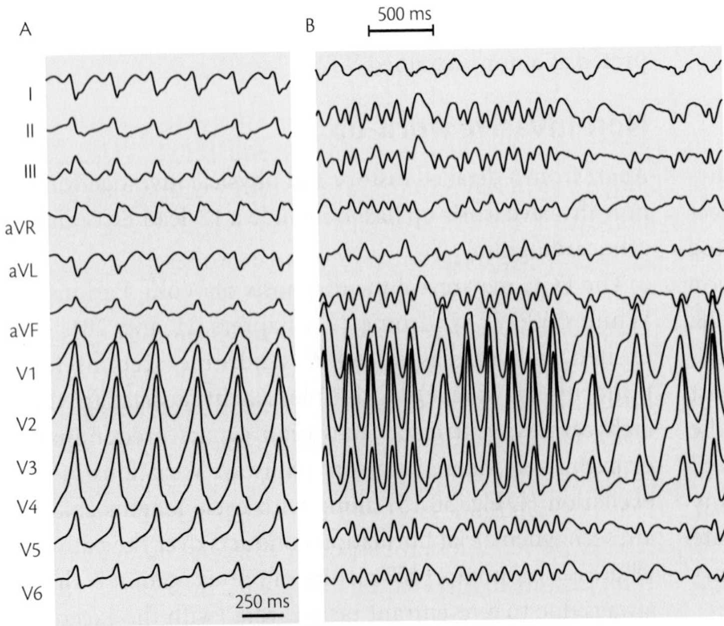

Figure 30.15 Antidromic tachycardia (A) over a left-sided accessory pathway in a patient with WPW syndrome. (B) Atrial fibrillation with rapid conduction over the pathway in the same patient (shortest RR interval 200ms).

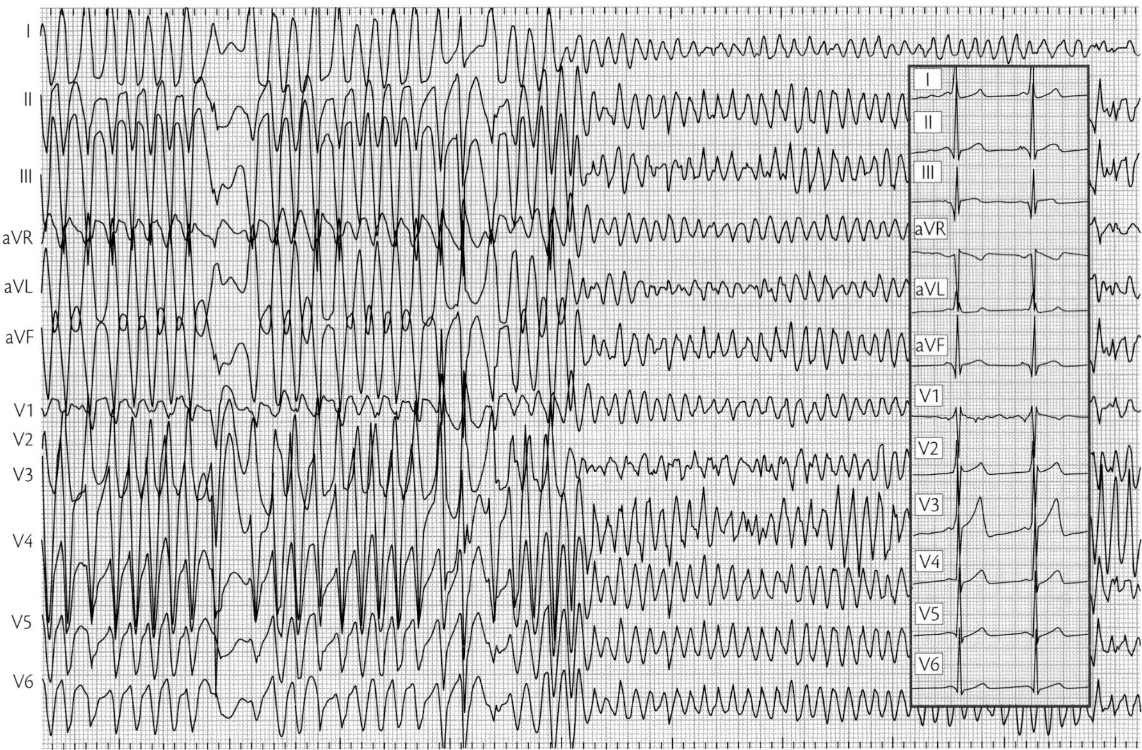

Figure 30.16 Atrial fibrillation with rapid conduction over the accessory pathway degenerating into VF. The inlet shows the 12-lead ECG after defibrillation showing only minimal pre-excitation.

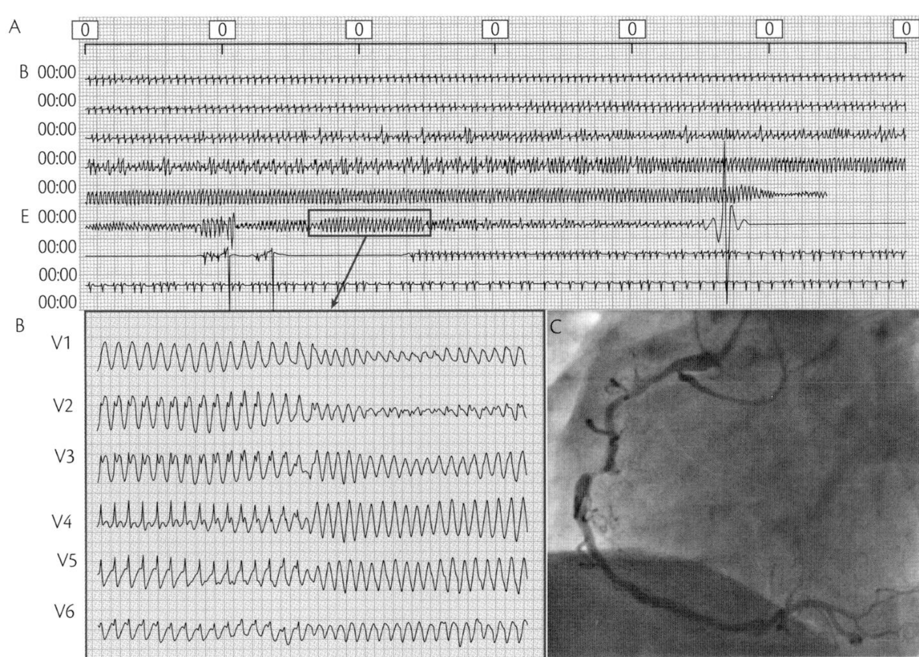

Figure 30.17 Exercise test (A) in a patient with a previous syncope showing the occurrence of a sustained polymorphic VT (B) during exercise that spontaneously terminated. The angiogram (C) of the right coronary artery showed a severe stenosis.

Table 30.3 Differences between idiopathic RVOT VT and ARVC

Features	Idiopathic RVOT VT	ARVC
Clinical presentation		
Arrhythmias	LBBB inferior axis (+II, III, aVF; −aVL)	May be the same Frequently different: LBBB −II, III, aVF, + aVL
SCD	Not increased	About 1% per year
Family history of SCD	No	Often yes
ECG		
Wave morphology	Upright V2–V5	Inverted beyond V1
QRS duration	<0.12s in V1–V3	QRS duration >0.11s
Epsilon wave	Absent	Present in 30%
Prolonged S-wave upstroke	Absent	Present in 95%
Signal averaged ECG	Normal	Usually abnormal
Imaging features		
RV ventriculogram	Normal	Usually abnormal
Echocardiogram	Normal	Usually abnormal
MRI	Normal	Usually abnormal

ARVC, arrhythmogenic right ventricular cardiomyopathy; LBBB, left bundle branch block; MRI, magnetic resonance imaging; RV, right ventricle; RVOT, right ventricular outflow tract; SCD, sudden cardiac death.

ventricular cardiomyopathy (ARVC) (e.g. prominent trabeculation, aneurysmatic out-pouchings) may be detected (see ➲Chapter 18, Myocardial Disease) (➲Table 30.3). In selected cases, cardiac magnetic resonance imaging, cardiac computed tomography, or radionuclide angiography (see ➲Chapters 5–7 respectively) can be useful when echocardiography does not provide accurate assessment of LV and RV function. MRI with delayed contrast enhancement may also identify abnormalities such as myocarditis, sarcoidosis, or amyloidosis, but this is not part of a routine work-up.

Invasive work-up

If the documented tachycardia and the history of the patient clearly indicate a supraventricular origin, an invasive approach to rule out structural heart disease is not necessary. On the other hand, urgent angiography with a view to revascularization is indicated in patients with polymorphic VT when myocardial ischaemia cannot be excluded (Class I Recommendation, Level of Evidence: C [1]). Besides, the majority of patients presenting with a sustained monomorphic VT should undergo invasive imaging to exclude coronary artery disease (see ➲Chapter 8, Invasive Imaging and Haemodynamics). The only exception is idiopathic left or right VT e.g. LBBB tachycardia with an inferior axis (originating in the RVOT with no echocardiographic evidence for ARVC (see ➲Chapter 18, Myocardial Disease) or ion channel disorders such as long QT syndrome. If there is doubt, a right ventricular angiogram is helpful to rule out ARVC. Nevertheless, differentiating idiopathic RVOT VT from an outflow tract tachycardia in ARVC may be difficult (➲Table 30.3).

Invasive electrophysiological testing is of limited value in patients with sustained VT and structural heart disease as these patients have an increased risk of SCD and require an implantable cardioverter defibrillator (ICD; see ➲Prevention of sudden cardiac death, p.1150). However, in patients with non-sustained VT and moderate left ventricular function (left ventricular ejection fraction (LVEF) between 35–40%) an electrophysiological study may be considered (see ➲Risk stratification, p.1148). Besides, in a patient with a previous myocardial infarction presenting with a syncope one should always assume that a VT caused the syncope and perform an electrophysiological study.

Risk stratification

Depressed left ventricular function

Risk stratification has always been important in cardiology but its interest has taken a sudden twist in recent years, largely as a consequence of the results of the major ICD trials (MADIT I, II, SCD-HeFT) [34, 35]. Indeed, the emerging indication of considering ICD implants in all post-myocardial infarction patients with a LVEF ≤30% [1] is causing havoc in the national health services of European countries. Accordingly, this section will focus primarily on this issue. For more general and traditional risk stratification, the reader is referred to recent guidelines [36].

Owing to space limitations, only those risk markers that, other than LVEF, have received a class IA recommendation by the Task Force Report of the ESC are discussed here. These markers are the demographic variables, heart rate variability (HRV)/turbulence or baroreflex sensitivity (BRS), and microvolt T-wave alternans (MTWA). Other markers that could contribute to better risk stratification, in association with low LVEF, include the following: ECG variables such as QRS duration, late potentials, and electrophysiological testing. For example, a publication from the Multicenter Unsustained Tachycardia Trial (MUSTT) trial indicated that the presence of LBBB or intraventricular conduction defect assessed from the surface in 1638 coronary patients with depressed left ventricular function carried a 50% increased risk of total and arrhythmic mortality [37]. This prognostic information was independent of other risk markers such as

LVEF or results of electrophysiological evaluation. In addition, ECG signs of left ventricular hypertrophy were also a significant predictor of arrhythmic mortality (hazard ratio 1.35; 95% confidence interval (CI) 1.08–1.69).

Ventricular ectopy and non-sustained ventricular tachycardia

Ventricular premature beats (VPBs) and non-sustained VT (NSVT) are common findings in patients with structural heart disease. Most studies cite a frequency of 10 VPBs per hour and the occurrence of repetitive forms of ventricular ectopy as thresholds for increased risk. The positive predictive value of VPBs after myocardial infarction ranges from 5–15%, with a negative predictive value of 90% or more [38]. When combined with reduced left ventricular function, ectopy becomes a stronger marker for mortality [36]. Nevertheless, prophylactic antiarrhythmic drug therapy is not indicated to reduce mortality in patients with asymptomatic non-sustained ventricular arrhythmias [1]. The Cardiac Arrhythmia Suppression Trial (CAST) [39] demonstrated that markers of risk are not necessarily appropriate targets for therapy. Suppression of ectopy after myocardial infarction with type IC antiarrhythmic drug therapy increased mortality [1].

In post-myocardial infarction patients with LVEF <35%, the incremental risk stratification with ventricular ectopy/non-sustained VT remains unclear [36] but in patients with moderate LV dysfunction (LVEF between 35–40%) patients with documented ectopy and induced VT at electrophysiological study have been shown to benefit from ICD therapy [1, 40]. The relationship of ventricular ectopy and cardiac arrest in patients with non-ischaemic cardiomyopathy is unclear. The positive predictive value is low, ranging from 20–50% [36]. Thus, according to the current practice guidelines there is no indication to treat NSVT in post-myocardial infarction or non-ischaemic cardiomyopathy subgroups, except in the relatively uncommon circumstances of frequent or very rapid episodes compromising haemodynamic stability [36]. In these cases, initial pharmacological therapy of symptomatic NSVTs should consist of beta-blocking agents. If symptomatic NSVTs are unresponsive to these drugs, amiodarone or sotalol remain pharmacological options [1].

Microvolt T-wave alternans (also see ➲Chapter 2)

The presence of subtle changes in the repolarization phase of the ECG, termed microvolt T-wave alternans (MTWA), is associated with an increased risk of SCD or other serious ventricular tachyarrhythmic events. MTWA refers to the presence of changes in T-wave amplitude on an every-other-beat basis, which are not detectable on the surface ECG. Utilizing contemporary signal processing techniques, however, these changes can be detected upon an increase in heart rate. This heart rate increase is produced either by atrial pacing or, preferably, non-invasively by means of exercise testing. In ➲Fig. 30.18, examples of a positive, negative, and indeterminate MTWA testing are shown.

Several clinical studies have demonstrated that assessment of MTWA in patients with structural heart disease may yield prognostic information. Particularly in patients with ischaemic and non-ischaemic cardiomyopathy, assessment of MTWA is useful for prediction of arrhythmic complications during the subsequent course of these patients [36]. For instance, a recent report on 129 patients with ischaemic cardiomyopathy found that over 24-month follow-up no major arrhythmic event or SCD occurred in those patients who were negative; on the other hand, in MTWA-positive patients or in those with an indeterminate test result, the event rate was 15.6% [41]. This indicates that analysis of MTWA may be helpful to avoid unnecessary ICD implantations in patients with depressed left ventricular function who test negative for MTWA.

Heart rate variability, baroreflex sensitivity, and heart rate turbulence (also see ➲Chapter 2)

HRV provides a means of assessing autonomic nervous system modulation of cardiac rate. HRV is almost completely due to autonomic input to the sinus node. Both HRV and BRS have been assessed prospectively. They provide a surrogate for the autonomic effects in the ventricle that are postulated to be important in the pathophysiology of VT and SCD. In most population studies using multivariate analysis, HRV provides significant independent prognostic information. The Autonomic Tone and Reflexes After Myocardial Infarction (ATRAMI) study [42, 43] showed that after myocardial infarction, patients with low HRV had a relative mortality risk of 3.2. Specifically, within the patients with LVEF of <35%, those with preserved BRS had a significantly better 2-year survival than patients with depressed BRS (7% vs. 18%). This was even more evident for major arrhythmic events (3% vs. 16%) (➲Fig. 30.19). Camm *et al.* [44] studied 3717 post-myocardial infarction patients with left ventricular dysfunction and reported data on the prognostic importance of HRV. By multivariate

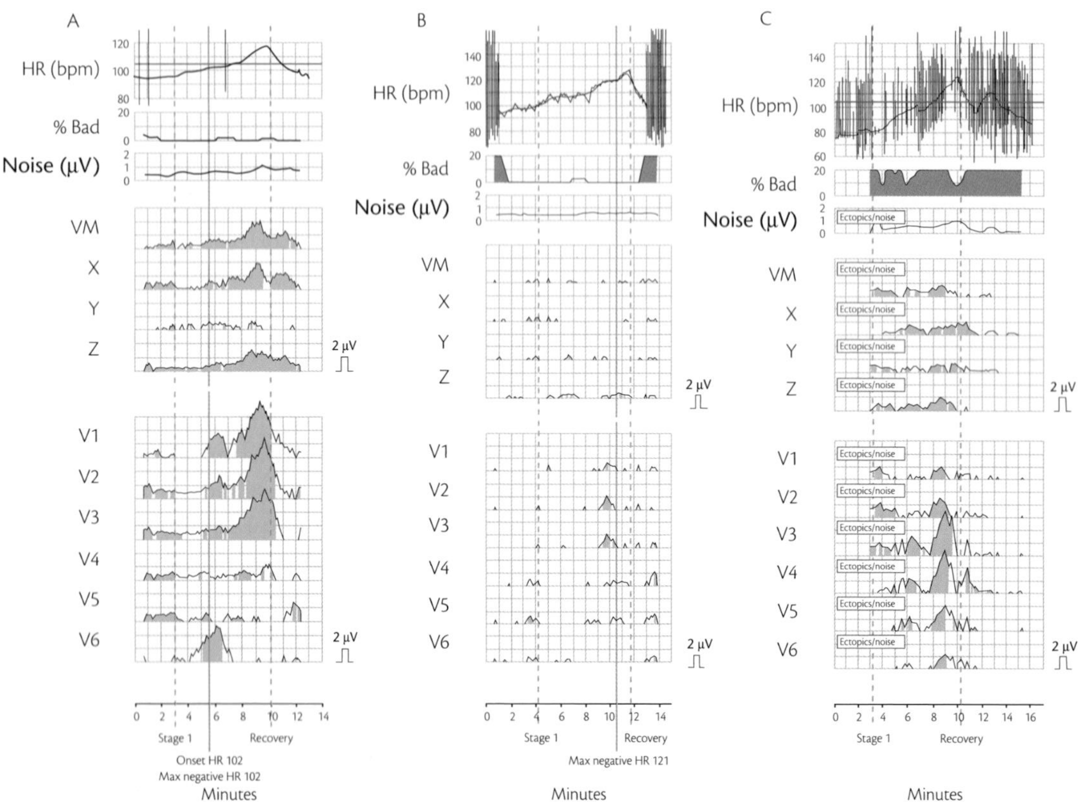

Figure 30.18 Examples of MTWA-positive, -negative, and indeterminate test results. Shown from top to bottom: heart rate trend, percentage of bad beats, noise level, MTWA amplitudes in vector magnitude lead VM, orthogonal leads X, Y, and Z and from ECG leads V1–V6. (A) Example of bicycle exercise-induced sustained MTWA (grey shaded area), which starts at an onset rate of 102 bpm (B) Absence of MTWA during exercise-induced elevation of heart rate to a maximum rate of 121 bpm (C) Indeterminate MTWA test due to the presence of frequent ectopic beats that are indicated by the vertical lines in the heart rate trend pictogram.

analysis, a low HRV increased risk of all-cause mortality with a hazard ration of 1.46 (95% CI 1.1–1.94), but low HRV did not predict arrhythmic mortality. Thus, low HRV may be a better marker for non-arrhythmic mortality than for SCD.

Heart rate turbulence describes the short-term fluctuation in sinus cycle length that follows a VPB [45]. It has been postulated that it measures vagal responsiveness similar to BRS. It is a potentially attractive risk factor as it can be performed with a relative small number of premature beats from 24-hour Holter ECG. Further studies are needed to establish whether there is clinical utility for risk stratification.

Therapy of ventricular tachycardias in patients with structural heart disease

The spectrum of therapies for VTs includes drug therapy, device implantation, and surgical or catheter ablation techniques. The indication for therapy is either based on VT as the presenting symptom or the potential risk of sudden (arrhythmic) death as the consequence of the arrhythmogenic substrate.

Acute treatment of sustained ventricular tachycardia

In patients with sustained monomorphic VT and haemodynamic compromise immediate cardioversion with appropriate sedation is recommended [1]. If the VT is refractory to cardioversion or resumes shortly afterwards, intravenous amiodarone should be given [1]. If the patient is haemodynamically stable, intravenous procainamide or ajmaline (only available in some European countries) can be administered [1]. Amiodarone is only poorly effective in this situation [46].

Prevention of sudden cardiac death

As SCD has a multifactorial aetiology, a variety of therapeutic targets may be considered. For instance, in the case of

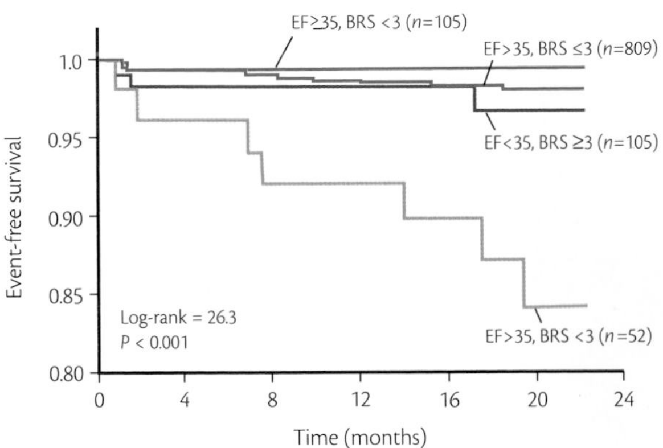

Figure 30.19 Risk prediction for major arrhythmic events according to determination of LVEF and assessment of BRS.

coronary artery disease such therapeutic interventions may range from limitation of infarct size and prevention of new ischaemic events, resulting from progression of disease and plaque instability, to modulation of neuroendocrine activation, and antiarrhythmic and antifibrillatory actions. All of these treatment modalities are designed to either prevent or terminate ventricular tachyarrhythmias.

The terms 'primary' and 'secondary' prophylaxis of SCD usually refer to whether or not a patient has a history of sustained (hypotensive) VT or aborted SCD due to VF. In patients without prior sustained ventricular tachyarrhythmias who are nevertheless deemed to be at high risk for SCD, therapy is usually described as 'primary' prophylaxis. Similar prophylactic therapy, recommended for patients who have already suffered a cardiac arrest or sustained VT, is termed 'secondary' prophylaxis.

Device and drug therapy of ventricular tachyarrhythmias in patients with structural heart disease

When VT is the consequence of structural cardiac disease, persistence or evolution of an arrhythmogenic substrate, even after successful treatment of a presenting VT, militates against any *curative* therapy. For a long time, management of VT was dominated by drug therapy or antitachycardic surgery. However, nowadays the ICD is the best available therapy to prevent sudden cardiac death from VT (Class I indication, Level of Evidence B [47]) (➲Figs. 30.20 and 30.21). In clinical use since 1980, the ICD is a self-contained device that is capable of identifying VT and VF and automatically terminating these arrhythmias by antitachycardia pacing or delivering a shock, usually about 35J or less, directly to the heart. According to current practice guidelines, Class I and II criteria for ICD implantation are listed in ➲Table 30.4.

Secondary prevention of sudden cardiac death

Patients with documented sustained VT or resuscitated cardiac arrest have been traditionally treated with drugs with electrophysiological properties to prevent recurrent ventricular tachyarrhythmic events. With the advent of the ICD, device therapy has progressively become the cornerstone of treatment of these patients (➲Figs. 30.22 and 30.23). Three randomized clinical trials have compared the efficacy of the device to the efficacy of amiodarone in prolonging life in such high-risk patients [48, 49].

The Antiarrhythmics Versus Implantable Defibrillator trial

The Antiarrhythmics Versus Implantable Defibrillator (AVID) trial [50] was the first large-scale randomized trial that compared ICD therapy with antiarrhythmic drug treatment in patients with documented symptomatic VT (55%) or VF (45%). Patients with VT also had either syncope or other serious cardiac symptoms, along with a LVEF of <40%; 81% of these patients had coronary artery disease. In total, 1016 patients with documented VT were randomized to ICD or antiarrhythmic drug therapy, almost exclusively with amiodarone. Mortality in the group treated with antiarrhythmic drugs was 17.7%, 25.3%, and 35.9% after 1, 2, and 3 years respectively. It was significantly reduced by 39% in the ICD group after 1 year and by 27% and 31% after 2 and 3 years respectively. The results of AVID were consistent among all pre-specified subgroups: coronary artery disease versus other diseases, VF versus VT, all age groups, and all ejection fractions. There was a trend towards less benefit in patients with an ejection fraction >35%.

The Canadian Implantable Defibrillator Study and the Cardiac Arrest Study Hamburg

The Canadian Implantable Defibrillator Study (CIDS) [48] and the Cardiac Arrest Study Hamburg (CASH) [49] recruited similar patient cohorts as AVID. CIDS [48] randomized 659 patients with symptomatic VT, aborted sudden death, or syncope in the presence of inducible VT to ICD treatment or empirical amiodarone. Two-year mortality in the drug arm was about 22%. There was a reduction of total death rate by ICD implantation (risk reduction 19.6% at 3 years) but this did not reach statistical significance. A recent study, however, compared the long-term outcome of 120 patients who were enrolled in the CIDS and who were

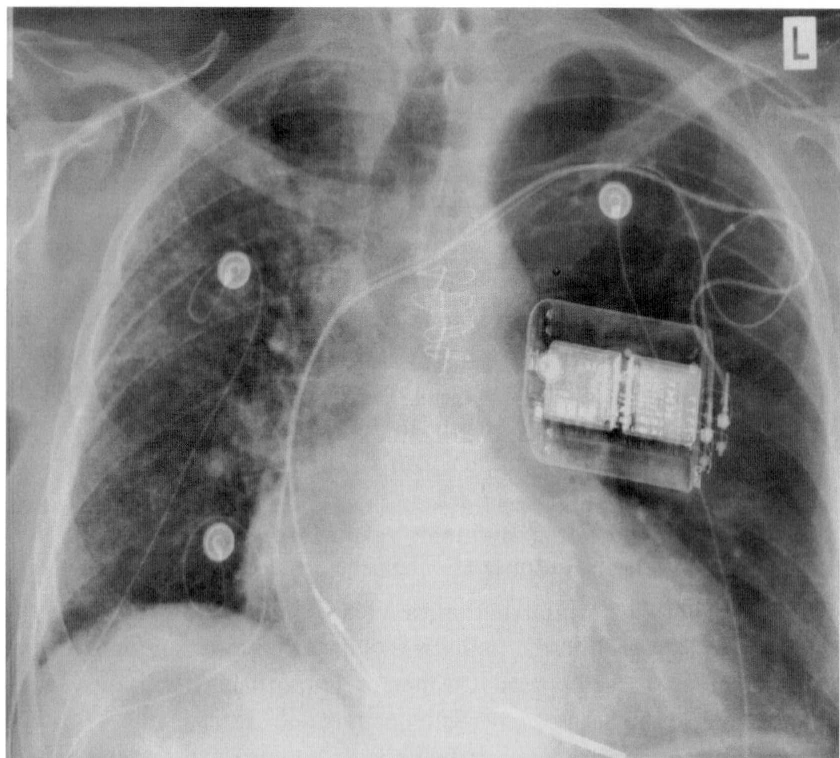

Figure 30.20 Example of a dual-chamber ICD implanted in a patient with ischaemic cardiomyopathy and prior coronary artery bypass grafting.

followed for 11 years [51]. One-half of these patients had been implanted with the device; the other half had been randomized to receive amiodarone and were kept on the drug after the official end of the trial. After a mean follow-up of 5.6 years, 28 deaths occurred in the amiodarone group (47%) compared with 16 deaths (23%) in the ICD group ($p = 0.021$).

Over the observation time, 49 patients (82%) developed side effects related to amiodarone, which required drug discontinuation. Although this study has limitations owing to the small patient population, it suggests that the strategy of using amiodarone as first-line monotherapy for secondary prevention of SCD results in a substantial arrhythmogenic risk and a high incidence of side effects (➲Table 30.5) necessitating drug discontinuation. In this small study, the benefit from the ICD in reducing all-cause mortality extends to more than 10 years of follow-up. This may be particularly relevant to patients after a survived cardiac arrest with only moderately impaired LV function in whom the benefit of ICD therapy may only accrue after a prolonged time period.

In CASH [49], a total of 346 patients with a history of cardiac arrest were randomized to ICD, or treatment with metoprolol, amiodarone, or propafenone. After inclusion of 230 patients that were randomly assigned to propafenone, amiodarone, metoprolol, or the implantable defibrillator, the propafenone arm was stopped based on a per-protocol analysis because of excess mortality compared with the ICD

Counter

Last test: 24 Sept 2004 10:26;08

	Since last test	Since last clearance	Since implantation
Episodes	01, Apr 2004	09, Oct 2002	
VF	0	3	3
FVT	0	0	0
VT	1	3	3
SVT/NST	3	582	582
% Stimulation			
Sensed	98%	99%	99%
Paced	1%	0%	0%
Additional counters			
Single	313667	430195	430195
VES salvos	7958	17542	17542
V. freq stabilizing stimuli	0	0	0
Salvos of V freq. stab. stimuli	0	0	0

Episode report

Last test: 24 Sep 2004 10:26:08

VT/VF-episodes

ID	Date/time	Art	V. cycle	Last Rx	Success	Duration
6	27 Aug 23:51:09	VT	300 ms	VT Rx 1	Yes	27 Sec

SVT/NST-episodes

ID	Date/time	V. cycle	Duration	Reason
582	06 Aug 20:41:58	360 ms	5 strikes	Non-sustained
581	12 Jul 21:38:37	340 ms	5 strikes	Non-sustained
580	28 Jun 16:55:09	370 ms	7 strikes	Non-sustained

Figure 30.21 Read-out of a single chamber ICD device memory including number and timing of device-delivered therapy for VT and VF.

Table 30.4 Class I and II indications for an ICD according to the ACC/AHA/HRS 2008 guidelines

Class I
◆ ICD is indicated in survivors of cardiac arrest due to VF/VT after evaluation to define the cause of the event and to exclude any completely reversible causes (Level of Evidence: A)
◆ ICD is indicated in patients with structural heart disease and spontaneous sustained VT (Level of Evidence: B)
◆ ICD is indicated in patients with syncope of undetermined origin with clinically relevant, haemodynamically significant sustained VT or VF induced at electrophysiological study (Level of Evidence: B)
◆ ICD is indicated on patients with LVEF <35% due to prior MI who are at least 40 days post-MI and are in NYHA functional class II or III (Level of Evidence: A)
◆ ICD is indicated in patients with dilated cardiomyopathy who have an LVEF ≤35% and who are in NYHA functional class II or III (Level of Evidence: B)
◆ ICD is indicated on patients with LV dysfunction due to prior MI who are at least 40 days post-MI, have an LVEF <30%, and are in NYHA functional class I (Level of Evidence: A)
◆ ICD is indicated in patients with non-sustained VT due to prior MI, LVEF <40%, and inducible VF or sustained VT at electrophysiological study (Level of Evidence: B)
Class IIa
◆ ICD is reasonable for patients with unexplained syncope, significant LV dysfunction, and dilated cardiomyopathy (Level of Evidence: C)
◆ ICD is reasonable for patients with HCM who have one or more risk factors for SCD (Level of Evidence: C)
◆ ICD is reasonable for the prevention of SCD in patients with ARVC who have one or more risk factors for SCD (Level of Evidence: C)
◆ ICD is reasonable for patients with long QT syndrome who are experiencing syncope and/or VT while receiving beta-blockers (Level of Evidence: B)
◆ ICD is reasonable for patients with Brugada syndrome who have had a syncope or a documented VT that has not resulted in cardiac arrest (Level of Evidence: C)
◆ ICD is reasonable for patients with catecholaminergic polymorphic VT who have had a syncope and/or documented VT while receiving beta-blockers (Level of Evidence: C)
◆ ICD is reasonable for patients with cardiac sarcoidosis, giant cell myocarditis, or Chagas diseases (Level of Evidence: C)
Class IIb
◆ ICD may be considered in patients with non-ischaemic heart disease who have a LVEF of ≤35% and who are in NYHA functional class I (Level of Evidence: C)
◆ ICD may be considered in patients with long QT syndrome and risk factors for SCD (Level of Evidence: C)
◆ ICD may be considered in patients with syncope and advanced structural heart disease in whom thorough invasive and non-invasive investigation have failed to define a cause (Level of Evidence: C)
◆ ICD therapy may be considered in patients with familial cardiomyopathy associated with sudden death (Level of Evidence: C)
◆ ICD therapy may be considered in patients with LV non-compaction (Level of Evidence: C)

AVRC, arrhythmogenic right ventricular cardiomyopathy.

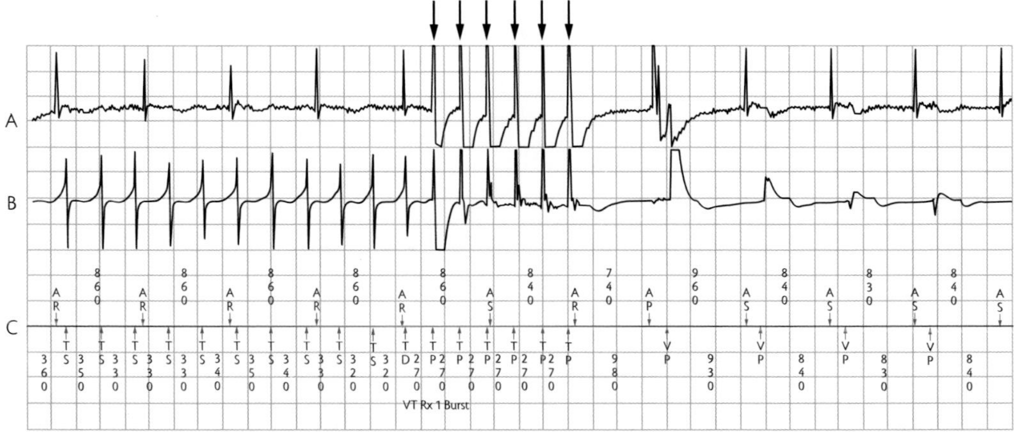

Figure 30.22 Example of an electrogram read-out of a dual-chamber ICD. (A) Atrial electrograms; (B) ventricular electrograms; (C) marker annotations. Note the VT on the left-hand side of the tracing (AV dissociation), which is terminated by antitachycardia pacing (arrows).

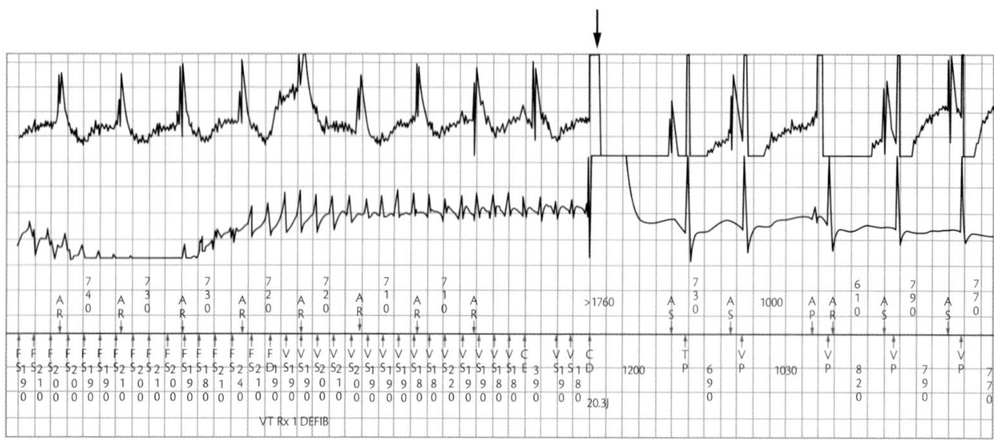

Figure 30.23 Example of an electrogram readout of a dual-chamber ICD. Note the presence of VF on the left-hand side of the tracing which is terminated by the ICD delivering a high-voltage shock (arrow).

group [49]. This study demonstrated a 37% survival benefit of patients receiving ICDs in comparison with metoprolol or amiodarone at 2 years. Two-year mortality in these arms was 19.6%. Of note, the ejection fraction of the patients in CASH (0.46) was much higher than in AVID (0.32) or CIDS (0.34). In CASH, primary VF patients had also been included.

Data from AVID, CIDS, and CASH (only amiodarone and ICD arms) were merged into a meta-analysis [52]. This analysis showed a significant reduction in death from any cause, with the ICD having a mean hazard ratio of 0.72. This 28% reduction in the relative risk of death with the ICD was largely the result of the reduction in arrhythmic death. Survival was extended by a mean of 4.4 months by the ICD over a follow-up period of 6 years. Patients with LVEF of ≤35% had a significantly higher benefit from ICD therapy than those with better-preserved left ventricular function. This was also found in a post hoc analysis of CIDS [53]. This analysis showed that three clinical risk factors were predictors of death and benefited from the ICD: age ≥70 years, LVEF ≤35%, and NYHA class III or IV.

Table 30.5 Summary of reported side effects related to amiodarone in large amiodarone trials

Study	GESICA	CHF-STAT	MADIT	EMIAT	CAMIAT *	AVID	CIDS	CASH	AMIOVIRT	CIDS	SCD-HeFT
Pulmonary toxicity		3.0	3.0	4.0	3.8	5.0	5.7	0		10.0	
Visual symptoms				0.7	0.8		14.5			10.0	
Photosensitivity							10.3				
Bradycardia	3.8	1.8	3.0	0.1	1.3		3.0			20.0	
Proarrhythmia				0.0	0.3	0.2					
Skin discolouration		0.3		0.0	1.9		6.3			18.3	
Gastrointestinal	0.8	6.0		2.0	2.1					16.7	
Liver disorders		1.2		0.8	1.0					15.0	
Neurotoxicity		4.8		1.1	3.1		17.2			48.3	
Tremor							15.4				4.0
Sleep disturbance					1.7		19.3				
Thyroid										20.0	
Hyperthyroidism		0.6		0.5	0.6			3.3			
Hypothyroidism		0.6	1.0#	0.0	3.3	16.0					6.0
Poor compliance				9.4	7.3						

*= reasons for stopping amiodarone;

#= data of all conventionally treated pts (n = 101, including n= 74 patients treated with amiodarone).

Secondary prophylaxis in dilated cardiomyopathy

In contrast to patients with coronary artery disease, risk stratification in patients with *idiopathic DCM* is much more difficult. These patients are under-represented in all ICD studies. In AVID, CASH, and CIDS, only 15%, 11%, and 10%, respectively, of all patients had idiopathic DCM. All of these studies showed a reduction of total mortality in patients with non-ischaemic DCM of 20–40% compared with conventional therapy [48–50]. However, the confidence intervals for patients with non-ischaemic DCM were much wider than for patients with coronary artery disease. In the meta-analysis of these three studies, only 225 out of 1832 patients had non-ischaemic cardiomyopathy [52]. These patients had a hazard ratio for reduction of total mortality of 0.78, which was very similar to the total cohort (0.72). However, the 95% CIs for these patients ranged from 0.45–1.37.

The significance of syncope in DCM without documented VT is still unclear. A non-randomized study showed similar event rates of appropriate ICD discharges in patients who received an ICD because of syncope, and patients who received a defibrillator after aborted sudden death, or episodes of VT, or VF [54]. Another study showed significantly lower event rates in a series of consecutive patients treated with an ICD than in conventionally treated patients [55]. Hence, it seems reasonable to treat patients with non-ischaemic DCM and syncope similar to those after aborted SCD if other causes of syncope are excluded.

Primary prophylaxis

There are three different therapeutic modalities by which primary prevention of SCD in patients with structural heart disease is pursued: therapy using drugs that have no electrophysiological properties, therapy using drugs with distinct electrophysiological properties, and ICD therapy.

Drugs without distinct electrophysiological properties

According to the Task Force on Sudden Cardiac Death of the ESC, there are at least three different drug classes that do not have electrophysiological properties but have been shown to reduce not only all-cause mortality, but also SCD. Treatment with angiotensin-converting enzyme (ACE) inhibitors in patients after myocardial infarction and/or congestive heart failure has resulted in a reduction in SCD in the range of 30–54% [56, 57]. The second class of drugs, which have been shown to reduce SCD are aldosterone receptor blockers; the RALES study [58] has demonstrated a 30% reduction in the relative risk of SCD. The mechanism of this protection is not entirely clear but may include prevention of hypokalaemia and regression of aldosterone-related interstitial fibrosis, but at the expense of an increased risk of hyperkalaemia. These results were substantiated in a much larger study comprising 6632 survivors of acute myocardial infarction with left ventricular dysfunction [59]. In this large-scale randomized trial, the aldosterone blocker eplerenone reduced all-cause mortality, which was the primary end-point of the trial (relative risk 0.85, 95% CI 0.75–0.96, p = 0.008). Mortality from SCD was also significantly reduced by eplerenone (relative risk 0.79, 95% CI 0.64–0.97, p = 0.03). Finally, there is evidence from several randomized controlled clinical trials that lipid-lowering agents may not only reduce overall mortality but also SCD mortality in coronary patients [60, 61].

Drugs with distinct electrophysiological properties

With respect to drugs with distinct electrophysiological properties, there is ample evidence that treatment with beta-blockers is associated with an improved outcome in several patient groups. A recent analysis of 31 beta-blocker trials showed that only 13 trials reported data on reduction of SCD [62, 63]. These 13 trials indicated a reduction in SCD from 51% in the control patients to 43% in patients receiving anti-adrenergic therapy. The greatest beneficial effect in terms of mortality reduction was shown in patients with congestive heart failure or depressed left ventricular function. Importantly, concomitant therapy with important other categories of drugs such as ACE inhibitors, aldosterone receptor blockers, or aspirin does not appear to limit the independent benefit on clinical outcome provided by beta-blockers, as suggested by the evidence of residual risk reductions of between 30–50% [64]. Accordingly, beta-blocking drugs are to be regarded as a fundamental prophylactic treatment for survivors of myocardial infarction and in patients suffering from congestive heart failure (➲Table 30.6).

Amiodarone, which is predominantly a class III anti-arrhythmic compound but also possesses anti-adrenergic, sodium-channel and calcium-channel blocking properties, has been subjected to a number of randomized controlled trials evaluating the primary preventive efficacy of this drug in various patient subsets. Although early studies showed a reduction in SCD in patients receiving amiodarone [65], more recent trials demonstrated that amiodarone has little or no effect on all-cause mortality. A meta-analysis comprising data from 13 randomized controlled trials in 6553 patients with various forms of heart disease reported a small albeit significant reduction in all-cause mortality in

Table 30.6 Primary prevention antiarrhythmic trials: relative risk for all-cause mortality

Antiarrthythmic compound	No. of patients	Relative risk of death (95% CI)	*p*- value
Sodium channel blockers post-myocardial infraction			
Class 1A	6582	1.19 (0.99–1.44)	0.07
Class 1B	14033	1.06 (0.89–1.26)	0.50
Class 1C	2538	1.31 (0.95–1.79)	0.0006
Flecainide and encainide	1455	**3.6 (1.7–8.5)**	**0.0006**
Beta-blocker			
During myocardial infraction	28970	0.87 (0.77–0.98)	0.02
After myocardial infraction	24298	0.77 (0.70–0.84)	<0.0001
Carvedilol	1959	0.77 (0.60–0.98)	0.03
		0.74 (0.51–1.06)	**0.098**
Beta-blocker in CHF			
Carvedilol	1094	0.44 (0.28–0.69)	<0.0001
		0.51 (0.28–0.92)	NA
Bisoprolol	2647	0.66 (0.54–0.80)	<0.0001
		0.56 (0.39–0.80)	**<0.01**
Metoprolol	3991	0.66 (0.53–0.81)	0.0009
		0.59 (0045–0.78)	**0.0002**
Class III antiarrthythmic drugs			
Amiodarone	6500	0.87 (0.78–0.99)	0.03
		0.71 (0.59–0.85)	**0.0003**
d-Sotalol	3121	1065 (1.15–2.36)	<0.006
		1.77 (1.15–2.74)	**0.0008**
Dofetilide	1518	0.95 (0.81–1.11)	>0.05

Figures relating to sudden death appear in bold text.

CHF, congestive heart failure; NA, not applicable.

Adapted with permission from Priori SG, Aliot E, Blømstrom-Lundqvist C, *et al.* Task Force on Sudden Cardiac Death, European Society of Cardiology. *Eur Heart J* 2001; **22**: 1374–450.

favour of amiodarone over placebo (hazard ratio 0.87; 95% CI 0.78–0.99, $p = 0.03$) (➲Fig. 30.24) [66].

SCD-HeFT, in which patients with congestive heart failure were randomized to best medical therapy alone, or in addition to amiodarone or the ICD demonstrated that amiodarone was not different from placebo [67]. However, the neutral effect on mortality and the good cardiovascular safety profile indicate that amiodarone can be safely administered to treat non-sustained ventricular arrhythmias or atrial fibrillation in patients after myocardial infarction or congestive heart failure [68]. Side effects (➲Table 30.5) are a major problem with 14% more patients discontinuing amiodarone than placebo by 2 years of follow-up [66].

Implantable cardioverter defibrillator trials for primary prevention of sudden cardiac death

ICD therapy (➲Figs. 30.20 and 30.21) in primary prevention of SCD has been evaluated in patients deemed to be at high risk of serious ventricular tachyarrhythmias (➲Fig. 30.25). The MADIT I [34] and the MUSTT [69] trials used invasive electrophysiological testing to identify coronary patients at risk for SCD. In both trials, the ICD was clearly superior to conventional antiarrhythmic therapy (mostly amiodarone) in reducing not only sudden death but more importantly all-cause mortality. A similar effect was demonstrated in MADIT II, a trial which randomized coronary patients only on the basis of a reduced left ventricular function (LVEF ≤30%) without using other risk stratifiers [35] (➲Fig. 30.26). After inclusion of 1232 patients, the trial was terminated because of a significant (31%) reduction in all-cause death in patients assigned to ICD therapy.

In a post hoc analysis, Moss and colleagues [34] found that patients with an ejection fraction of <26% had a far greater benefit from ICD implantation than patients with an ejection fraction between 26–35% [70]. Later they

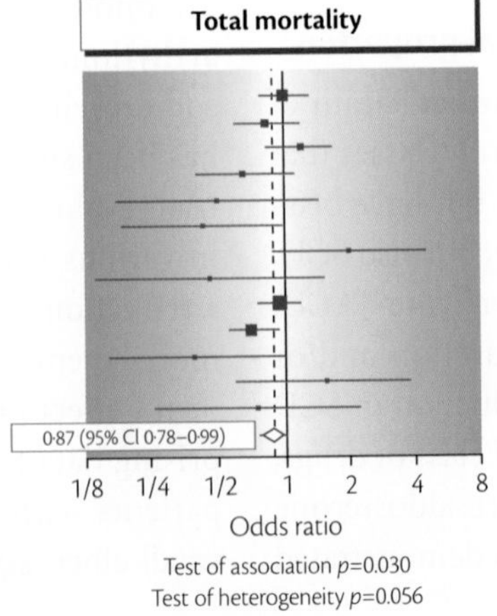

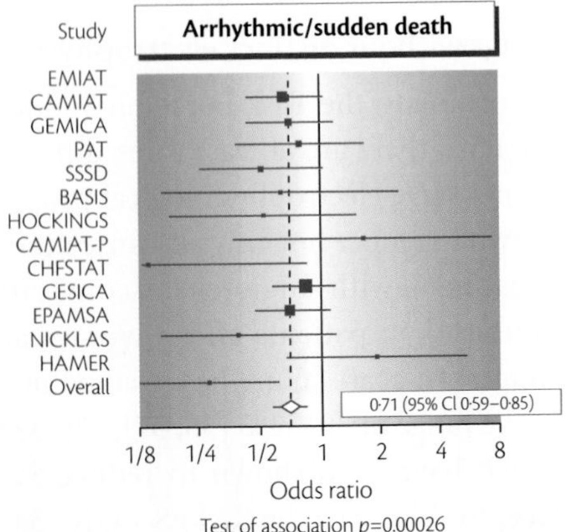

Figure 30.24 Meta-analysis of 13 studies comparing the effects of amiodarone to placebo on all-cause mortality (left) and arrhythmic mortality (right). Overall mortality showed a 13% decrease for patients who received amiodarone compared with control subjects. Adapted with permission from Amiodarone Trials Meta-Analysis Investigators. Effect of prophylactic amiodarone on mortality after acute myocardial infarction and in congestive heart failure: meta-analysis of individual data from 6500 patients in randomised trials. *Lancet* 1997; **350**: 1417–24.

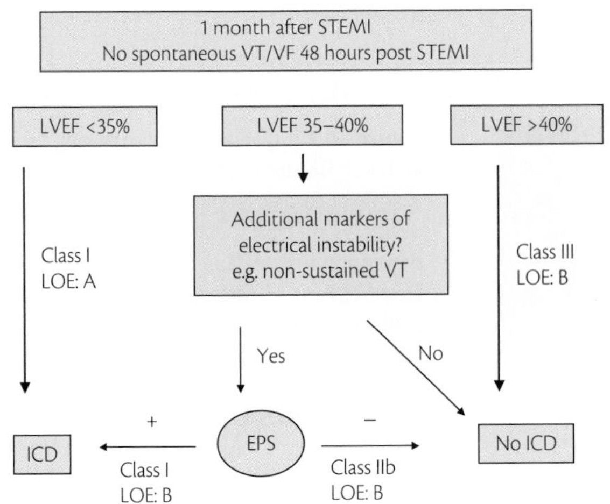

Figure 30.25 Algorithm for primary prevention of SCD in post-STEMI patients without spontenous VT/VF at least 1 month post STEMI and diminished ejection fraction. LVEF left ventricular ejection fraction; STEMI ST-elevation myocardial infarction; EPS electrophysiological study; LOE Level of Evidence.

identified three independent risk factors: ejection fraction ≤25%, QRS duration ≤120ms, and a history of heart failure treatment [71]. The benefit from ICD treatment increased with the number of risk predictors. Thus, in patients with chronic coronary heart disease, the magnitude of the survival benefit from the ICD is directly related to the severity of cardiac dysfunction and its associated mortality risk.

The DEFINITE (Defibrillators in Non-Ischemic Cardiomyopathy Treatment Evaluation) trial showed in patients with non-ischaemic cardiomyopathy a strong trend towards a reduction in all-cause mortality in patients randomized to ICD therapy compared with medically treated patients [72]. It was the first large-scale trial investigating the use of ICD for the primary prevention of SCD in patients with non-ischaemic DCM. It enrolled a total of 458 patients with non-ischaemic DCM, left ventricular dysfunction (ejection fraction <35%), NYHA class I–III heart failure, and spontaneous premature ventricular complexes or non-sustained VT. In a subset of patients with NYHA class III heart failure, the ICD caused a significant reduction in all-cause mortality (67% relative risk reduction in all-cause mortality compared with those who received drug therapy alone ($p = 0.009$)). Desai *et al.* [73] performed a meta-analysis of five randomized trials that evaluated the benefits of prophylactic ICD therapy in 1854 patients with non-ischaemic cardiomyopathy. There was a 39% reduction in all-cause mortality in patients with an ICD (hazard ratio 0.61, 95% CI 0.55–0.87, $p = 0.002$) (➲Fig. 30.27).

The majority of ICD trials reporting benefits of ICD therapy is contrasted by two trials that could not demonstrate a survival advantage of ICD-treated patients compared with control subjects. The CABG-Patch (prophylactic use of ICDs in patients at high risk for ventricular arrhythmias after coronary-artery bypass surgery) trial used the presence of late potentials on the signal-averaged ECG and reduced LVEF to randomize patients who were scheduled for elective coronary artery bypass grafting [74]. The study was terminated prematurely because an interim analysis showed no benefit of device therapy. The Defibrillator in Acute Myocardial Infraction Trial (DINAMIT) (prophylactic use of an ICD after acute myocardial infarction) [75] randomized patients who had survived a recent myocardial infarction (6–40 days enrolment window) with a LVEF of <36% and signs of autonomic imbalance to best medical therapy with or without ICD implantation. A total of 674 patients were followed for a mean of 2.5 years. Whereas the ICD was associated with a significant reduction in arrhythmic mortality, there was no effect on all-cause mortality (➲Fig. 30.28). This neutral effect was due to an unexpected increase in non-arrhythmic mortality in patients randomized to receive the ICD.

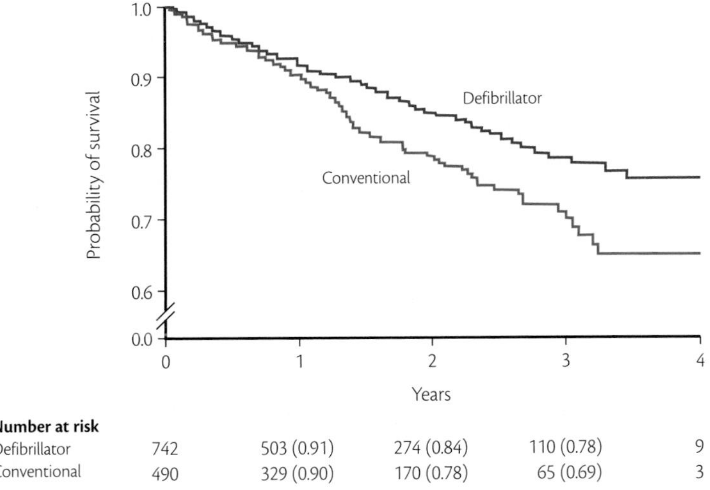

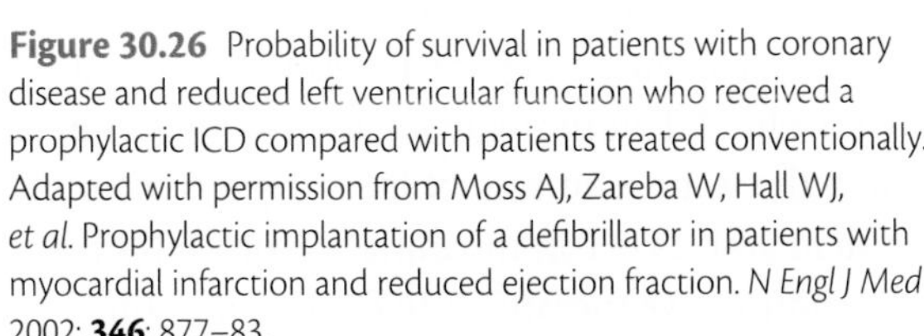

Figure 30.26 Probability of survival in patients with coronary disease and reduced left ventricular function who received a prophylactic ICD compared with patients treated conventionally. Adapted with permission from Moss AJ, Zareba W, Hall WJ, *et al.* Prophylactic implantation of a defibrillator in patients with myocardial infarction and reduced ejection fraction. *N Engl J Med* 2002; **346**: 877–83.

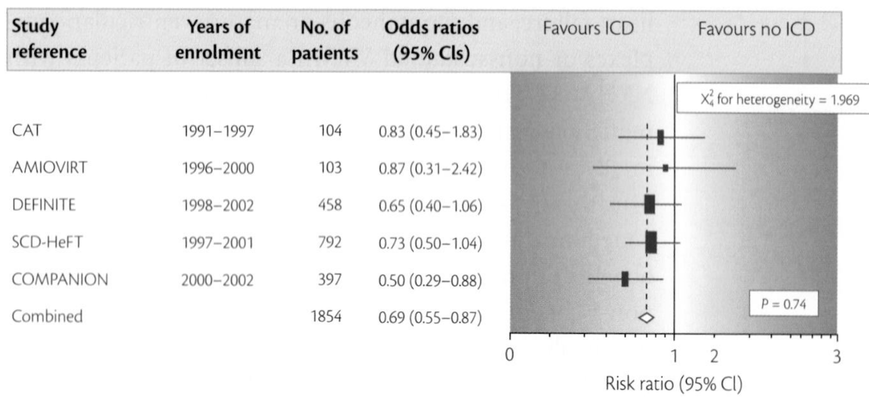

Study reference
Years of enrolment
No. of patients
Odds ratios (95% CIs)
Favours ICD
Favours no ICD
χ²₄ for heterogeneity = 1.969
CAT 1991–1997 104 0.83 (0.45–1.83)
AMIOVIRT 1996–2000 103 0.87 (0.31–2.42)
DEFINITE 1998–2002 458 0.65 (0.40–1.06)
SCD-HeFT 1997–2001 792 0.73 (0.50–1.04)
COMPANION 2000–2002 397 0.50 (0.29–0.88)
Combined 1854 0.69 (0.55–0.87)
P = 0.74
0
1
2
3
Risk ratio (95% CI)

Figure 30.27 Overall mortality among patients with non-ischaemic cardiomyopathy rendomized to ICD (or cardiac resynchronization therapy device) vs. medical therapy in five primary prevention trials. Adapted with permission from Desai AS, Fang JC, Maisel WH, *et al.* Implantable defibrillators for the prevention of mortality in patients with nonischemic cardiomyopathy: a meta-analysis of randomized controlled trials. *JAMA* 2004; **292**: 2874–9.

DINAMIT contrasts all other primary preventive ICD trials in coronary patients by the fact that it included patients early after a myocardial infarction, whereas patients entering the other trials were for the most part years after their last infarct. It appears therefore that survival benefit of the ICD in infarct survivors accrues after a considerable time having elapsed from the most recent myocardial infarction, presumably 6 months or perhaps more. Importantly, this notion is supported by evidence stemming from the Multicenter Automatic Defibrillator Implantation Trial (MADIT II). Wilber *et al.* [76] examined the relationship between ICD-associated survival benefit and the time interval from the most recent myocardial infarction to study enrolment in MADIT II. They found that patients who entered the trial within 18 months of their last infarction had no benefit from device therapy as opposed to those who entered the study years after their last myocardial infarction.

In summary, therefore, there is a comprehensive database on the efficacy of ICD therapy for primary prevention of SCD in various patient populations. This database can and must be used to tailor ICD therapy to those patient groups in which the benefit is greatest. As all positive trials reported relatively small absolute reductions in all-cause mortality, it is of paramount importance to tailor device therapy to individuals who are most likely to receive the largest benefit. Even then, the cost associated with device therapy is high and all societies will face enormous problems in translating trial results to everyday clinical practice. The most reasonable approach to reduce costs without affecting benefit lies in the improvement in risk stratification, with the goal of reducing the number of 'false-positives'.

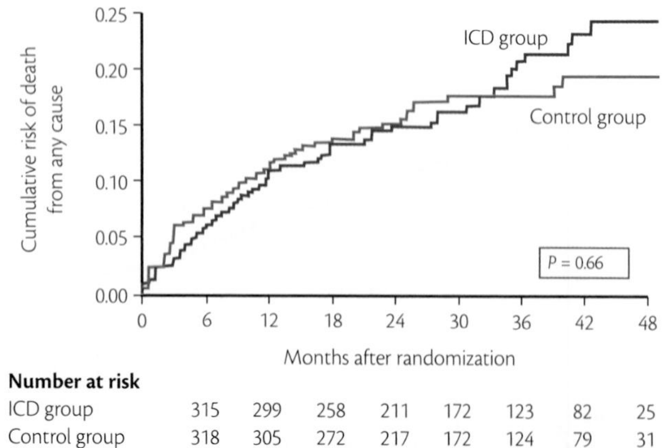

Figure 30.28 Cumulative risk of death from any cause according to treatment assignment in the DINAMIT trial. Adapted with permission from Hohnloser SH, Kuck KH, Dorian P, *et al.* Prophylactic use of an implantable cardioverter-defibrillator after acute myocardial infarction. *N Engl J Med* 2004; **351**: 2481–8.

Catheter ablation or surgical treatment of ventricular tachyarrhythmias

Approximately 20% of patients with an ICD implanted for primary prevention of SCD will experience one or more episodes of spontaneous VT within 3–5 years after ICD implantation [77–79]. In addition, ICD shocks can be painful and traumatic, and some patients consequently require therapy to reduce or prevent even infrequent episodes [78, 79]. Catheter ablation might be an adjunctive but rarely curative option for a selected group of patients with refractory or incessant VT (see ➲Figs. 30.9 and 30.10). Catheter ablation has been successfully applied in VT that is caused by ischaemic heart disease. Results with computerized mapping systems and mapping techniques using non-contact mapping systems that do not require sustained VT during the ablation procedure have demonstrated promising results in VT ablation. There are strategies to ablate VF or polymorphic VT in individual patients. Studies have demonstrated the important role of focal triggers from the Purkinje system and RVOT in the initiation of VF [80], but it remains an adjunctive therapy to ICD implantation.

Surgical techniques for treatment of VT may be effective in ICD carriers with sustained monomorphic VT resulting from coronary artery disease, especially when a discrete left ventricular aneurysm and inducible monomorphic VT are present. In selected patients, antitachycardia operations can be carried out with an acceptable mortality and a relatively high long-term survival rate. However, these procedures cannot be expected to alter the natural history of the underlying heart disease. Bundle branch re-entrant VT, which may occur in idiopathic DCM, is particularly amenable to catheter ablation (see ➲Electrophysiological mechanisms of ventricular tachycardia, p.1141).

Recurrent ventricular tachycardia/ ventricular fibrillation in patients with implantable cardioverter defibrillator

Recurrent appropriate ICD discharges or electrical storm (three or more appropriate ICD discharges in a 24-hour period) require an urgent search for reversible causes such as ischaemia, decompensated heart failure, electrolyte imbalance, or proarrhythmic side effect of drugs. Electrical storm occurs in up to 20% of patients with incessant VT [81–84]. After the initial assessment the patient should be treated with intravenous amiodarone and as much beta-blockade as blood pressure can tolerate. Sotalol may be an alternative to amiodarone [85] in suppressing ventricular arrhythmias, but due to the low ejection fraction in most of these patients and/or a depressed renal function amiodarone is usually first choice. Sedation and intubation may be necessary to blunt the adrenergic drive that ICD discharges provoke, which may perpetuate recurrent tachycardia. Animal studies [86, 87] have shown the benefits of neural modulation via spinal cord approaches. In addition, catheter ablation (see ➲Catheter ablation or surgical treatment of ventricular tachyarrhythmias, p.1158) is often required for control of the recurrent VT and associated ICD shocks.

Other cardiomyopathic conditions

Arrhythmogenic right ventricular cardiomyopathy

Arrhythmogenic right ventricular cardiomyopathy (ARVC) was first described in 1982 [88] and since then has been diagnosed with increasing frequency. ARVC is a primary myocardial disorder with a genetic background. The disease is a major cause of ventricular arrhythmias and SCD, particularly in young patients and athletes with apparently normal hearts. ARVC is characterized by localized or diffuse atrophy of predominantly right ventricular myocardium, with subsequent replacement with fatty and fibrous tissue, and usually manifests with VT and/or sudden death, frequently before structural abnormalities become apparent [88–90]. Diagnostic criteria of ARVC were proposed by an international study group [91] and include major and minor criteria in different categories (see ➲Chapter 18, Myocardial Disease). Twelve chromosomal loci for autosomal dominant forms of ARVC and two loci for autosomal recessive inheritance (one of which is Naxos disease) have been reported. In Naxos disease, a syndromic variant of ARVC with palmoplantar keratosis and woolly hair, a mutation in the gene encoding the cytoskeletal protein plakoglobin was identified. Mutations in the desmosomal protein plakophilin-2 are common in arrhythmogenic right ventricular cardiomyopathy [92]. In addition, a mutation in the desmoplakin gene, another protein involved in cell-to-cell junctions (adherens junctions and desmosomes), was identified in a classical form of ARVC (ARVC-8), with frequent left ventricular involvement. In a rare and rather atypical subgroup of ARVC (ARVC-2) with minor right ventricular abnormalities and polymorphic ventricular arrhythmias, a mutation in the gene encoding the cardiac ryanodine receptor (RyR2) was identified.

In ARVC, episodes of VT are frequently well tolerated, mainly due to the preserved left ventricular function. The main differential diagnosis is idiopathic RVOT tachycardia (➲Table 30.3). Antiarrhythmic treatment of ARVC includes drug therapy, catheter ablation (➲Fig. 30.29), and ICD implantation. There are no prospective randomized trials of pharmacological therapy versus ICD therapy in patients with ARVC. The available but limited data on risk stratification indicate that patients with severe right ventricular dysfunction, left ventricular involvement, a history of syncope or cardiac arrest, family history of SCD, inducible VT/VF, and ECG abnormalities (e.g. epsilon potentials, late potentials) are more prone to life-threatening VT and SCD. In patients with ARVC and low risk of SCD, antiarrhythmic drug therapy is an alternative option. Low-risk cohorts include patients with localized right ventricular disease and monomorphic VT suppressed by antiarrhythmic drugs.

Despite high efficacy rates of radiofrequency catheter ablation in abolishing regional sites of VT, there is a high recurrence rate due to new VT morphologies and origins as a consequence of disease progression. Main indications for catheter ablation in ARVC include monomorphic VT in localized right ventricular abnormalities and incessant or frequent VT not suppressed by antiarrhythmic treatment.

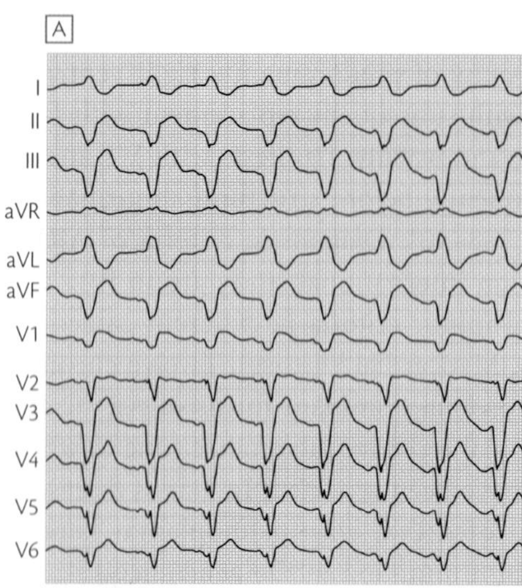

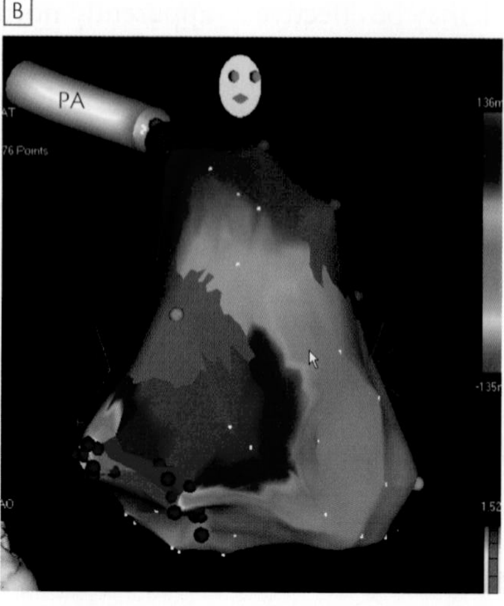

Figure 30.29 (A) Slow right VT with LBBB/superior axis (CL 660ms) in a patient with severe arrhythmogenic right VT with chronic amiodarone treatment. (B) Right anterior oblique view of an electroanatomic activation map of the VT (CARTO). Red colour represents earliest depolarization. A zone of slow conduction was mapped close to the exit of the VT where a short line of ablation terminated the VT.

Recent studies [93, 94] in high-risk patients with ARVC after resuscitated cardiac arrest, life-threatening VT, or drug-refractory VT demonstrated the high efficacy of ICD implantation in the prevention of SCD. The estimated survival benefit of ICD therapy was 21%, 32%, and 36% after 1, 3, and 5 years of follow up, respectively. The role of ICD therapy for primary prevention of SCD in ARVC remains unclear to date because only limited data are available. Patients with well-tolerated and non-life-threatening VT are usually treated empirically with antiarrhythmic drugs, including amiodarone, sotalol, beta-blockers, flecainide, and propafenone, alone or in combination. Wichter *et al.* [41] found that, in a series of 60 patients in a single centre during a mean follow-up of 80 ± 43 months, the event-free rate after 5 years was only 26% for VT and 59% for potentially fatal VT with a rate >240bpm Extensive right ventricular dysfunction was identified as a predictor for appropriate ICD discharges.

Hypertrophic cardiomyopathy

Hypertrophic cardiomyopathy (HCM) is an inherited myocardial disorder with an autosomal dominant trait, which is caused by mutations in one of ten genes known so far, each encoding for protein components of the cardiac sarcomer. It affects approximately one of every 500 persons in the general population and is the most common cause of SCD in individuals younger than 40 years of age [36, 47]. There is broad heterogeneity not only concerning disease-causing genetic mutations, but also in terms of phenotypic expression, treatment, and prognosis. Patients with HCM often present with ventricular ectopy or non-sustained VT. Symptoms of HCM range from dyspnoea and angina pectoris to palpitations, dizziness, and syncope [95]. Treatment of symptomatic HCM patients includes drugs (verapamil, beta-blockers, or disopyramide) or non-pharmacological options (septal myectomy, DDD pacing, alcohol septal ablation) in those with obstructive HCM [96] (see ➲Chapter 28, Myocardial Disease). These treatment options are targeted to reduce symptoms and improve quality of life, but have not been shown to have an impact on survival.

SCD may occur without warning signs or symptoms as the initial disease manifestation, and may be triggered by vigorous exercise or competitive sports activity. The highest risk for SCD has been associated with prior cardiac arrest or spontaneous sustained VT/VF. In such patients, the implantation of an ICD is strongly recommended for secondary prevention of sudden death (➲Table 30.4). In a multicentre retrospective study in high-risk HCM patients, appropriate ICD interventions occurred in 25% of patients after a follow-up period of only 3 years. Potentially life-saving ICD therapies were reported at a rate of 11% per year in patients receiving the ICD for secondary prevention (aborted sudden death or sustained VT/VF), compared with a rate of 5% per year in the primary prevention cohort (based solely on non-invasive risk factors) [97].

A consensus document on HCM from the ESC and the ACC categorized known risk factors for SCD as 'major' and 'possible' in individual patients [86] (➲Table 30.7). The severity of other symptoms, such as dyspnoea, chest pain, and effort intolerance, has not been correlated with increased risk of SCD. ICD implantation is considered the most effective and reliable treatment option and has been recommended in HCM patients at high risk of sudden death [97–99]. Of note, an important proportion of ICD discharges occur in primary prevention patients who undergo ICD implantation for a single risk factor. Thus, a single risk marker of high risk for SCD may be sufficient to justify consideration for prophylactic ICD implantation

Table 30.7 Risk factors for sudden cardiac death in hypertrophic cardiomyopathy

Major risk factors
Previous VF arrest
Spontaneous sustained VT
Family history of SCD
Syncope
Left ventricular thickness >30mm
Abnormal blood pressure response to exercise
Non-sustained ventricular tachycardia
Possible in individual patients
Atrial fibrillation
Left ventricular outflow obstruction
High-risk mutation
Intense competitive sports

Modified with permission from Maron BJ, McKenna WJ, Gordon K, *et al.* American College of Cardiology/European Society of Cardiology Clinical Expert Consensus Document on Hypertrophic Cardiomyopathy. *Eur Heart J* 2003 **24**:1965–91.

in selected patients [100]. HCM patients without risk factors are at low risk of SCD and should be reassured and followed clinically. Little or no restriction is necessary with regard to employment and recreational activities but patients should be excluded from strenuous exercise and competitive sports.

Sudden cardiac death and valvular heart disease (also see ➲Chapter 21)

According to a pathological registry of 1000 adults <65 years of age with no previous history of SCD, valvular heart disease was the fourth largest cause of SCD after coronary heart disease, left and right ventricular cardiomyopathies, and tissue conduction abnormalities [101]. The development of symptoms and signs of left ventricular dysfunction are major predictors of SCD. Currently, the only documented indication for an ICD in patients with valvular heart disease is a history of cardiac arrest or symptomatic sustained ventricular arrhythmias. For primary prevention of SCD there is lack of data. The effectiveness of mitral valve repair or replacement to reduce the risk of SCD in patients with mitral valve prolapse, severe mitral regurgitation, and serious ventricular arrhythmias is not well established.

Ventricular tachycardia in patients without structural heart disease:'idiopathic ventricular tachycardia'

'Idiopathic VT' is a non-specific term that represents a heterogeneous group of arrhythmias. Awareness of this entity has existed since it was first described by Gallavardin [102] in 1922. Patients can be completely asymptomatic or have transient symptoms including palpitations, dizziness, or presyncope, but these arrhythmias, with the exception of rapid polymorphic VT or idiopathic VF occurring in the setting of inherited arrhythmic syndromes, are very rarely life threatening. The underlying mechanisms include reentry, triggered activity, and catecholamine-mediated automaticity. Idiopathic VT can be categorized according to the clinical presentation (non-sustained vs. sustained), precipitating factors (e.g. exercise), site of origin (i.e. left or right ventricle), by response to antiarrhythmic drugs (e.g. adenosine or verapamil), or on the basis of an underlying organic heart disease (primary electrical disorder vs. inherited myocardial disease).

Ventricular tachycardia in patients without structural heart disease amenable to curative therapies

Idiopathic outflow tract ventricular tachycardia

This arrhythmia, which has also been termed *repetitive monomorphic VT*, usually originates in the right ventricular outflow tract (RVOT VT), but approximately 10–15% arise from the left ventricular outflow tract (LVOT VT), or various other basal left ventricular sites (e.g. aortomitral continuity and the mitral annulus) [103–105]. It is usually seen in female patients without structural heart disease and accounts for up to 70% of idiopathic VT. Although the majority of cases appear to occur sporadically rather than on a familial basis, the condition is generally considered as a 'primary electrical disease'. It is important in the differential diagnosis of various entities, in particular mild or subclinical forms of ARVC (➲Table 30.3). Most data suggest that the mechanism of idiopathic outflow tract VT is triggered activity by adenylcyclase-mediated delayed afterdepolarizations [106]. They are usually exertion- or stress-related arrhythmias. They can also present as recurrent extrasystoles (➲Fig. 30.30) or non-sustained arrhythmias tending to occur at rest ('repetitive monomorphic VT') (➲Fig. 30.31), or provoked only with exercise (Gallavardin's tachycardias [102]). However, these forms just represent different spectra of the same arrhythmia. Idiopathic outflow tract tachycardia is usually well tolerated, probably owing to the preserved ventricular function. Hence, RVOT VT has a favourable long-term prognosis compared with VT in structural heart disease. It manifests as a LBBB VT with an inferior axis (➲Fig. 30.30). The arrhythmia is often responsive to therapy with beta-blockers [107], sotalol [107, 108] or calcium-channel

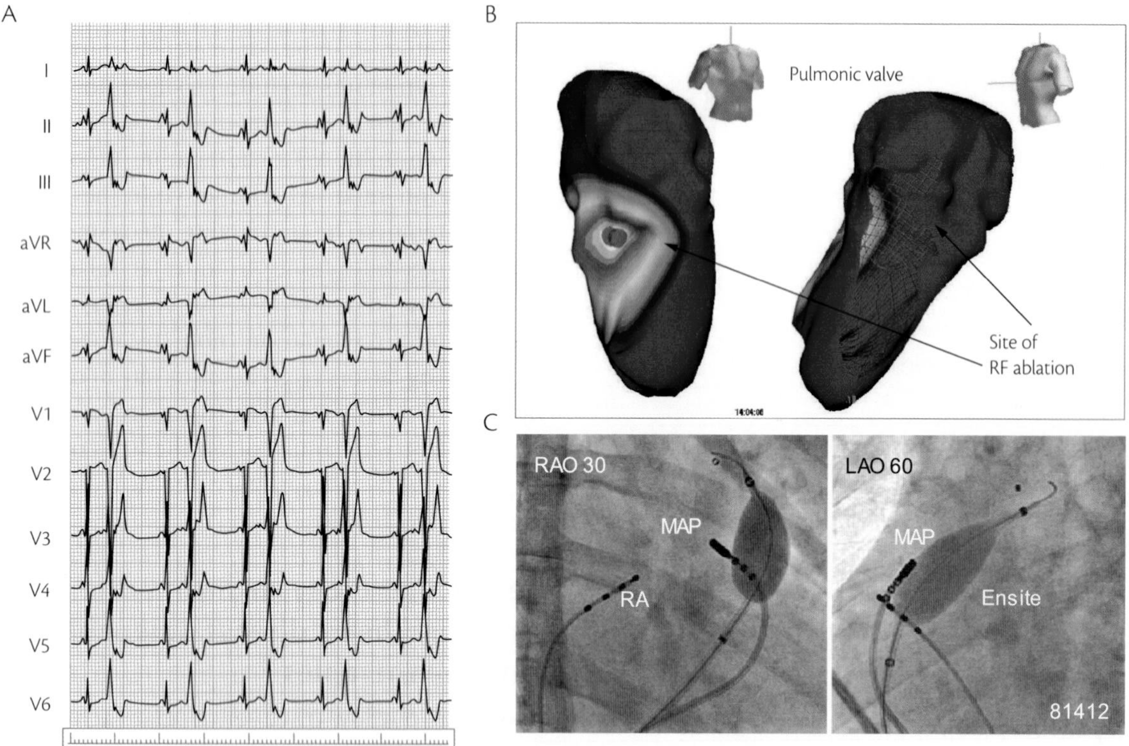

Figure 30.30 Non-contact mapping of a ventricular bigeminus with LBBB inferior axis morphology originating from the right ventricular outflow tract in a highly symptomatic patient (A). The multielectrode array catheter (MEA) is part of the non-contact mapping system (EnSite 3000; Endocardial Solutions). The system permits mapping of a single complex. The MEA, which is filled with a contrast saline medium, is positioned in the right ventricular outflow tract (RAO/LAO, right/left anterior oblique views). The system calculates electrograms from 3000 endocardial points simultaneously by reconstructing far-field signals. Non-depolarized myocardium is shown in purple in this three-dimensional isopotential map (B). The map also shows the site of earliest depolarization (white circle). At this site the extrasystoles were successfully ablated using radiofrequency ablation. The ablation catheter is located at the successful ablation site. RA, diagnostic catheter in the right atrium (C).

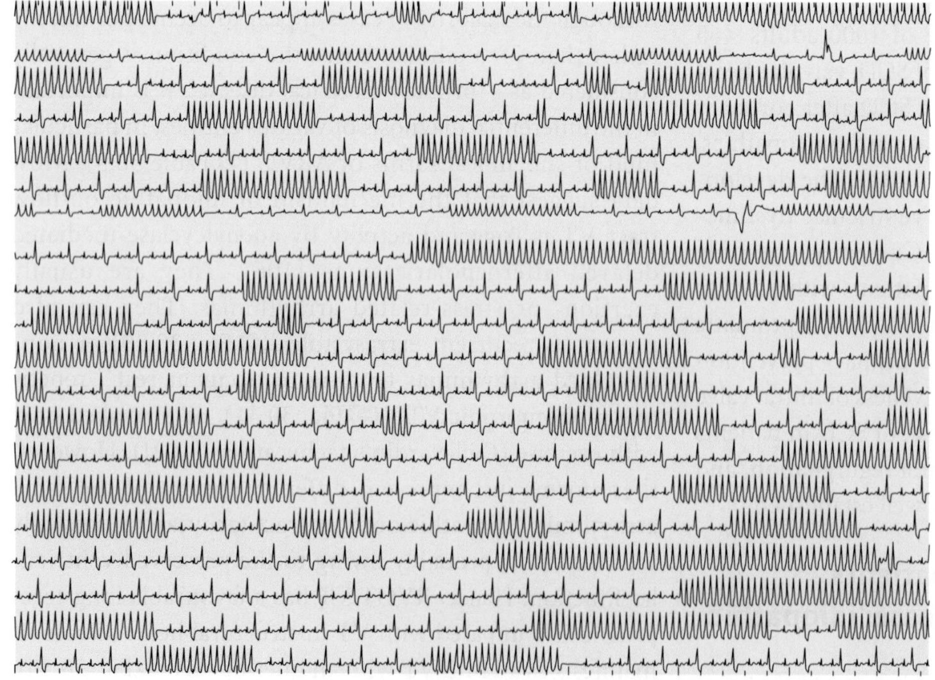

Figure 30.31 Repetitive monomorphic ventricular tachycardia in a 34-year-old female with idiopathic outflow tract tachycardia.

blockers [93], and can also be amenable to catheter ablation (➲Fig. 30.30) [1, 109, 110].

Idiopathic left fascicular ventricular tachycardia

This arrhythmia tends to occur in younger, predominantly male patients, without structural heart disease [111, 112]. The arrhythmia has a relatively narrow (0.10–0.14s) RBBB morphology with a rapid downstroke of S waves in the precordial leads and a left superior axis (➲Fig. 30.32). It is mostly inducible with programmed stimulation or isoproterenol infusion. ILVT is thought to have a re-entrant basis or derives from triggered activity secondary to delayed afterdepolarizations [113]. It arises on or near to the septum near the left posterior fascicle [114–117]. Rarely, VT can arise from the left anterior fascicle [111] and thus produce an RBBB pattern with right-axis deviation. Catheter ablation (➲Fig. 30.32) [118] offers curative therapy and is recommended early in the management of symptomatic patients. It can be performed using pace mapping [114, 119], presystolic Purkinje potential [119, 120] or diastolic potential during VT [116]. Alternatively, ILVT tends to respond to therapy with beta-blockers and calcium-channel blockers [111, 121].

Ventricular tachycardia in patients without structural heart disease but not currently amenable to curative therapies

Long QT syndrome

Long QT syndrome (LQTS) is characterized by a prolonged QT interval in the surface ECG, recurrent syncope, or sudden death resulting from TdP (➲Fig. 30.12) [122–125] (➲Chapter 9). The ECG, while in sinus rhythm, usually shows prolongation of the QT interval. In addition, distortion of the T wave and often distinct U waves may occur. The longer the previous cycle length, the more exaggerated the TU wave aberration of the following complex; hence the condition is'pause-dependent'. The treatment of pause-dependent triggered activity is aimed at reducing the prolonged repolarization. Drugs that prolong the QT interval must be discontinued and avoided. Electrolyte abnormalities should be rapidly corrected. Intravenous magnesium

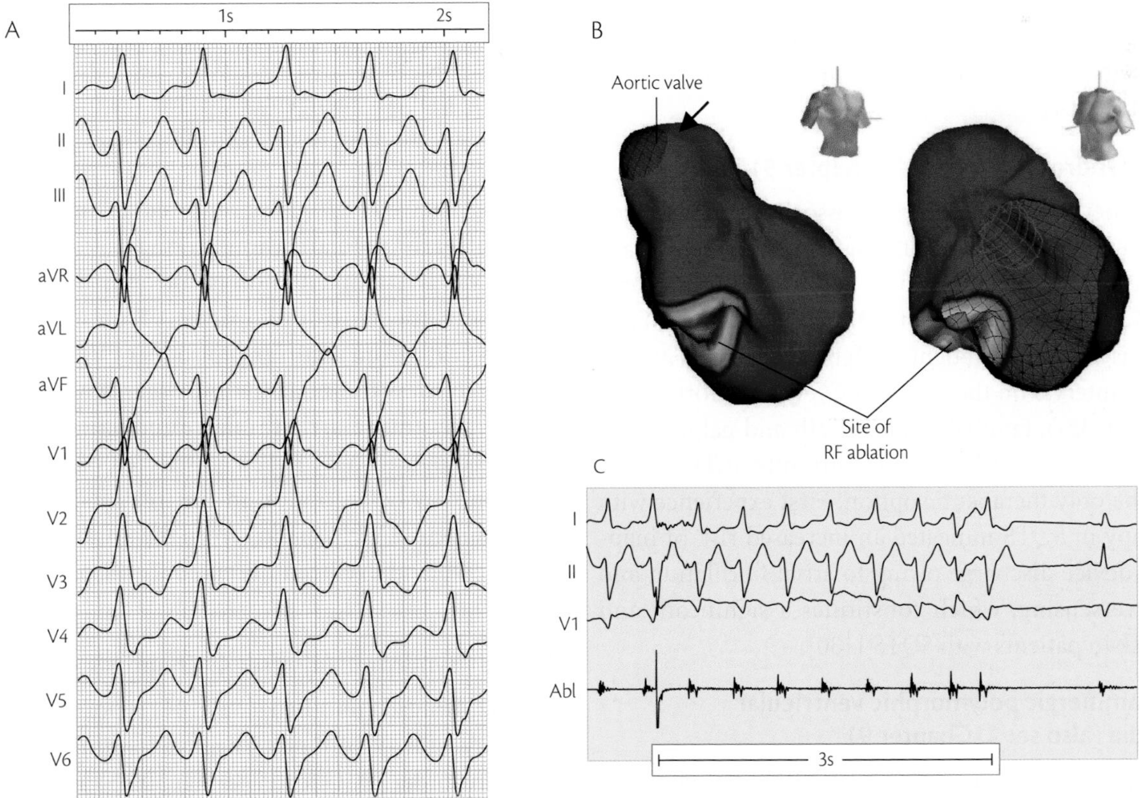

Figure 30.32 Non-contact mapping of an idiopathic left ventricular tachycardia with RBBB left axis deviation (A). The multiple electrode array (Ensite 3000, Endocardial Solutions) was placed in the left ventricle (for details, see legend to ➲Fig. 30.30). At the distal part of the left posterior fascicle, radiofrequency ablation almost immediately terminated the ventricular tachycardia (C), which, thereafter, was no longer inducible.

sulphate ameliorates these arrhythmias. In addition, pauses can be eliminated by either atrial or ventricular pacing, or by isoproterenol infusion.

The incidence of LQTS has been estimated as 1 in 7000 to 1 in 10,000 live births. Mutations involve genes encoding potassium channels (LQT1, 2, 5, and 6, Jervell Lange–Nielsen (JLN) 1 and 2), sodium channels (LQT3), and ankyrin B (LQT4), which acts as a targeting and anchoring molecule for the sodium channel. In 30–40% of all patients with LQTS, no gene defect can be found, pointing towards a large heterogeneity of gene loci. For long QT syndrome, Priori *et al.* [126] presented a scheme for risk stratification, based on analysis of 647 patients. High risk was considered in patients with LQT1 and QT_c >500ms$^{1/2}$ and in male patients with LQT2 or LQT3 and QT_c >500ms$^{1/2}$. In a recent report on LQT after the age of 40 years a recent syncope (<2 years ago) was the predominant risk factor in affected subjects, and the LQT3 genotype was identified as the most powerful predictor of outcome [127].

According to the current guidelines [1] patients with LQTS should be treated prophylactically using beta-blockers, although the effect is less beneficial in patients with LQT3. Beta-blocker therapy is associated with a significant reduction in the rate of cardiac events. There is only limited information available on the role of ICD therapy in patients with LQTS but ICD implantation is reasonable for patients with recurrent syncope despite drug therapy [36, 47] (➲Table 30.4).

Short QT syndrome (also see ➲Chapter 9)

Recently, a new inherited syndrome associated with sudden cardiac death in otherwise healthy patients with structurally normal hearts has been described, the short QT syndrome (SQTS) [128, 129] (see ➲Chapter 9). The prevalence of this syndrome is unknown. Patients with the SQTS present with a short QT interval on the 12-lead ECG (QT_c shorter than about 0.32–0.35s), familial sudden death and palpitations, syncope, or sudden cardiac arrest. Currently, ICD implantation is the only therapeutic option. First experience with ICD therapy in SQTS indicated an increased risk of inappropriate device discharge owing to atrial fibrillation and T-wave oversensing, which constitutes a significant and specific risk in patients with SQTS [130].

Catecholaminergic polymorphic ventricular tachycardia (also see ➲Chapter 9)

Catecholaminergic polymorphic VT (CPVT) is a clinically and genetically heterogeneous disease. It is characterized by episodes of syncope or SCD in response to physiological or emotional stress occurring in structurally normal hearts [131–136]. Documented arrhythmias include bidirectional VT (➲Fig. 30.13), polymorphic VT, and, in rare patients, catecholaminergic idiopathic VF. Mortality is high and reaches up to 30–50% by the age of 30 years [137]. Current treatment of CPVT consists of beta-adrenergic blockers [133, 138], antiarrhythmic drugs, and/or ICD implantation, mainly based on empirical grounds or the results of serial exercise/pharmacological testing [137]. The current guidelines (➲Table 30.4) recommend ICD therapy in patients who have syncope and/or documented VT while receiving beta-blockers.

Idiopathic ventricular fibrillation

In 5–10% of survivors of cardiac arrest due to ventricular arrhythmias, no structural abnormality of the heart as the underlying cause is found. In the absence of demonstrable structural heart disease, myocardial ischaemia, drug effects, electrolyte or metabolic abnormalities and toxicity, and VF, and unexplained cardiac arrest is rare [139–142]. However, it appears to be more frequent than previously thought and accounts for approximately 6–12% of all sudden deaths (lifetime prevalence <0.5 in 10,000), with a higher percentage in the young population below the age of 40 years. VF in patients with apparently normal hearts may represent a true 'primary electrical disease', but it may also be the first manifestation of a cardiomyopathy. The diagnosis of idiopathic VF must therefore be made by exclusion, implying that adequate and extensive diagnostic evaluation is necessary in order to rule out subclinical structural heart disease [143].

Haissaguerre *et al.* [143] reported an increased prevalence of early repolarization among patients with idiopathic VF. ICD implantation is currently the treatment of choice in patients with idiopathic VF in order to prevent sudden death from recurrent episodes of VF. In one report, quinidine (class IA antiarrhythmic agent) was highly effective in preventing arrhythmia re-induction during electrophysiological study [142]. In selected patients, catheter ablation may be an option in the treatment of idiopathic VF by targeting VPBs arising from the Purkinje conducting system, which have been observed to trigger polymorphic VT [80].

Brugada syndrome (also see ➲Chapter 9)

In 1992, Brugada and Brugada [144] reported a new clinical entity with a RBBB pattern and ST segment elevation in right precordial ECG leads (➲Fig. 30.33) and a high incidence of SCD in patients with structurally normal hearts, later referred to as Brugada syndrome (see ➲Chapter 2). It manifests with episodes of polymorphic VT, syncope,

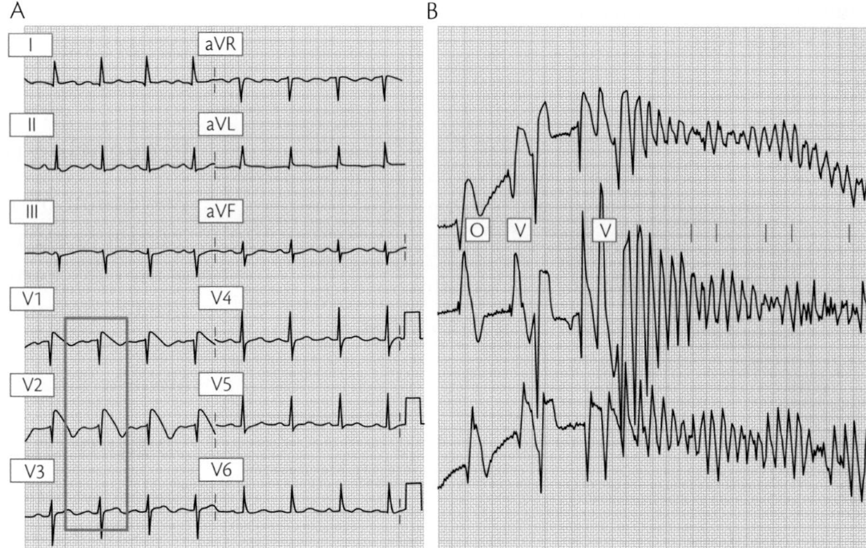

Figure 30.33 Twelve-lead ECG of a resuscitated patient with Brugada syndrome. The ECG is characterized by a prominent coved ST segment elevation displaying a J wave amplitude or ST segment amplitude elevation of ~0.2mV at its peak, followed by a negative T wave, with little or no isoelectric separation (A). Patients with such an ECG may develop syncope or sudden cardiac death due to fast polymorphic VT (B: for details, see text).

and cardiac arrest. Diagnostic criteria were proposed and reported in a consensus document [145] and mainly rely on electrocardiographic abnormalities after exclusion of structural heart disease by detailed cardiac investigation. The electrocardiographic manifestations of Brugada syndrome may be transient or concealed but can be unmasked with sodium-channel blockers (i.e. ajmaline, flecainide, and others) [146, 147], vagotonic stimulation [148], or fever [149] (so-called acquired Brugada syndrome).

The diagnostic and prognostic impact of an incidental finding of Brugada-type ECG signs in asymptomatic individuals without a family history represents a controversial and currently unresolved yet growing problem in clinical decision-making [150]. The role of programmed electrical stimulation for risk stratification has been a matter of controversial discussion. Recent meta-analysis [151, 152] did not find a correlation between VT/VF recurrence and inducibility of ventricular tachyarrhythmias. Hence, patient management and therapeutic strategies are controversial and under constant debate and refinement. Currently, ICD implantation is the treatment of choice in secondary and primary prevention of sudden death in high-risk patients with Brugada syndrome [153, 154].

Drug-induced ventricular tachyarrhythmias

Drug-induced ventricular tachyarrhythmias may be caused by cardiovascular drugs, non-cardiovascular drugs, and even non-prescription agents. They may result in SCD. If a new arrhythmia or aggravation of an existing arrhythmia develops during therapy with a drug at a concentration usually considered not to be toxic, the situation is defined as proarrhythmia. It may occur in individuals with or without structural heart disease. The major causes of proarrhythmia include drugs that affect ion channels of the heart directly such as cardiac glycosides, QT prolonging agents, or sodium-channel blocking drugs. The proportion of patients with proarrhythmia who present with sudden death, and the extent to which proarrhythmia contributes to the overall problem of sudden death are unknown. General treatment guidelines focus on avoiding drug treatment in high-risk patients, recognizing the syndromes of drug-induced proarrhythmia, and withdrawal of the culprit agent(s).

Drug-induced long QT syndrome

Drug effects are the most common cause of LQTS (see ➲Long QT syndrome, p.1163). It has become apparent that in addition to antiarrhythmic drugs, a large spectrum of non-cardiac drugs (➲Table 30.8) can cause QT prolongation and TdP (see ➲Fig. 30.12). TdP is characterized by a polymorphic, usually non-sustained, pause-dependent VT that may develop in association with an excessively prolonged QT interval [27]. It may be associated with syncope or may degenerate into VF. The ECG recorded just prior to or after termination of a polymorphic VT help to distinguish TdP from other polymorphic VT mainly occurring in patients with structural heart disease. Features diagnostic for TdP include a prolonged QT interval, the presence of U waves before the onset or after the termination of the arrhythmia, relatively long coupling intervals, or a typical initiating sequence.

Table 30.8 Risk factors that favour the genesis of drug-induced torsade de pointes

Female gender
Bradycardia
Prolonged baseline QT
Abnormally prolonged QT interval and QTc during drug treatment
T-wave lability
T-wave morphology changes during drug treatment
Electrolyte disturbances (hypokalaemia, hypomagnesaemia)
High drug doses or concentrations
Rapid intravenous injection/infusion
Use of drugs interfering with the metabolism of drugs known to cause TdP (e.g. inhibitors of cytochrome P450 enzymes such as erythromycin, ketoconazole, and grapefruit juice)
Cardiac hypertrophy
Diuretic use
Recent cardioversion from atrial fibrillation
Genetic risk factors, i.e. asymptomatic/symptomatic carriers of mutations encoding for potassium or sodium channels

In acquired LQTS, short–long–short cycle length changes constitute the typical pattern of initiation of TdP and may be regarded as a warning sign of an impending TdP. VPBs are often found to arise from exaggerated T/U waves after longer intervals, e.g. post extrasystolic pauses (see ➲Fig. 30.12). The torsadogenic potential of drugs is extremely variable, even within the same class of drugs [155]. Some drugs may only provoke TdP in the setting of overdose, concomitant administration of other QT-prolonging drugs, or in the presence of risk factors such as hypokalaemia, whereas others may induce TdP alone, even at therapeutic level, and in the absence of additional risk factors.

Risk factors for torsade de pointes

Several risk factors for the development of drug-related TdP are known. Patients who developed drug-related TdP were found to have a borderline or prolonged (>0.44s) QTc intervals before drug administration. The fact that the QT interval is longer in women compared with men accounts for the two- to threefold higher incidence of abnormal QT prolongation and TdP in females. Patients who had a previous history of drug-related TdP are very likely to develop further episodes when exposed to any other QT-prolonging drug. Acquired abnormal QT prolongation and TdP has been observed in patients with various types of heart diseases as well as in patients without detectable heart disease. Other risk factors that can affect repolarization and reduce the repolarization reserve apart from the congenital LQTS and drugs are listed in ➲Table 30.9. Drugs that prolong the QT interval, and thereby predispose to torsade de pointes, are listed on websites such as http://www.qtdrugs.org.

Prevention of acquired torsade de pointes

Prevention of a potentially adverse response of the QT interval to a drug requires careful and regular observation of the ECG. Particular attention should be directed to excessive QT prolongation, QT dispersion [156], and emerging evidence of T/U abnormalities such as negative or notched/biphasic T waves and appearance of prominent U waves.

Sodium-channel blocker related toxicity

Antiarrhythmic drugs are the most common precipitants of sodium-channel blocker-related toxicity, although other agents (e.g. antidepressants and cocaine) may produce some of their toxicities through their sodium-channel blocking properties. Sodium channel-blocking drugs with slower rates of dissociation from the sodium channel (e.g. flecainide, propafenone, and quinidine) tend to generate these adverse effects more commonly. These drugs tend to prolong QRS duration even at normal heart rates because of the slow dissociation rate. In contrast to the occurrence of TdP, which is promoted by a slow heart rate, induction of a VT by a class IC drug is promoted by a fast heart rate. In CAST [39], patients with frequent ventricular ectopy following a myocardial infarction who were treated with flecainide had a higher mortality rate than patients treated with placebo. Sodium-channel blockers may also 'convert' atrial fibrillation to atrial flutter with 1:1 AV conduction with wide QRS complexes. This drug-induced arrhythmia can mistakenly been regarded as VT (see ➲Fig. 30.2). Thus, when used in atrial fibrillation, an AV nodal-blocking drug should be co-administered to prevent rapid ventricular rates in case of atrial flutter.

Some patients treated with sodium-channel blocking drugs (particularly flecainide and propafenone) may develop slow, incessant VT, which occasionally may be resistant to cardioversion [1]. Those VTs may be haemodynamically tolerated due to the slow heart rate, but may also degenerate into a haemodynamically significant VT or fibrillation and be lethal. In such a situation, the antiarrhythmic drug should be immediately discontinued. Hypertonic saline or sodium bicarbonate may reverse the conduction slowing and terminate or accelerate the arrhythmia [157].

Acquired Brugada syndrome

A number of drugs and conditions, which cause an outward shift in current active at the end of phase 1 of the action potential, have been reported to induce transient Brugada-like ST segment elevation (see ➲Brugada syndrome, p.1164). Whether this 'acquired' form of the Brugada syndrome unmasks individuals with clinically inapparent Brugada syndrome ('forme fruste') or just one end of a broad spectrum of responses to sodium-channel blocking drugs is not known. However, in the majority of reported cases of acquired Brugada syndrome, the characteristic type-1 Brugada ECG pattern disappeared after the withdrawal of the drugs and could not be reproduced with the subsequent flecainide tests on these patients.

Among antiarrhythmic drugs, class IC drugs most effectively amplify or unmask ST segment elevation due to their strong effect to block I_{Na}, and are therefore used as a diagnostic tool in Brugada patients with transient ECG abnormalities. Class IA antiarrhythmic drugs (e.g. ajmaline, procainamide, disopyramide) which exhibit less use-dependent blocking of I_{Na} due to faster dissociation of the drug from the sodium channels, show weaker ST segment elevation than class IC drugs [147]. Of note, quinidine, another class IA drug generally normalizes ST segment elevation owing to its relatively strong I_{to} blocking effect, and is proposed as a pharmacologic treatment of Brugada syndrome (see ➲Chapter 9). Several psychotropic drugs including tricyclic antidepressants (e.g. amitriptyline, nortriptyline, desipramine, clomipramine), tetracyclic antidepressants (e.g. maprotiline), phenothiazine (e.g. cyamemazine), and selective serotonin re-uptake inhibitors (e.g. fluoxetine) have been reported to unmask Brugada like ST segment elevation, secondary to block of fast I_{Na} associated with overdoses of these drugs. It has been postulated that this could be an important mechanism for drug-related SCD in patients on chronic treatment with antidepressants and neuroleptics.

Resuscitation

Out-of-hospital resuscitation

Survival of cardiac arrest outside the hospital continues to be very poor. In general, survival is critically depending on the characteristics of the cardiac arrest (i.e. cardiac aetiology or not, VF vs. pulseless electrical activity, witnessed or not, etc.) and on the patient's condition prior to cardiac arrest. Before the introduction of the automated external defibrillator (AED), only approximately 15% of all out-of-hospital cardiac arrest victims had restoration of spontaneous circulation and reached the hospital alive. However, only one-half of these survived to discharge (5–7%). Survival rates were somewhat better if only patients with documented VF as the cause of their cardiac arrest are considered. In areas with early defibrillation programmes in place, more patients are found in VF owing to shorter arrival times or use of the automated defibrillator; in such areas, higher hospital discharge rates reaching 20–25% have been reported [158, 159].

Most instances of cardiac arrest occur at home, in men aged >50 years, and during daytime. As recently pointed out, this profile of the cardiac arrest victim is useful to identify the profile of the potential bystander of such an event. These persons constitute the primary target group for teaching cardiopulmonary resuscitation (CPR) to laypersons.

The European 2005 guidelines for basic life support [160, 161] are basically a step moving towards simplicity and thus making public CPR education more feasible. The main principles are shown in ➲Figs. 30.34 and 30.35. Basic life support has to be followed by advanced cardiac life support (ACLS). Such guidelines have been established by the European Resuscitation Council, the AHA, and other societies [160, 162] and are regularly updated.

Electrical means of resuscitation

Cardiac arrest is most often due to VF that does not end spontaneously in the human heart. When VF continues for more than 3–4min, there is irreversible damage to the central nervous system and other organ systems, which affects survival even in the case of successful defibrillation. Accordingly, the most important therapeutic means to prevent death from cardiac arrest is to accomplish

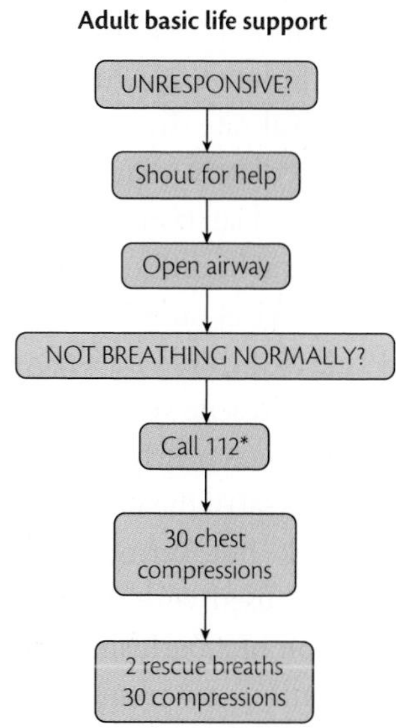

Figure 30.34 Main principles of basic life support according to European Resuscitation Council Guidelines for Resuscitation 2005.

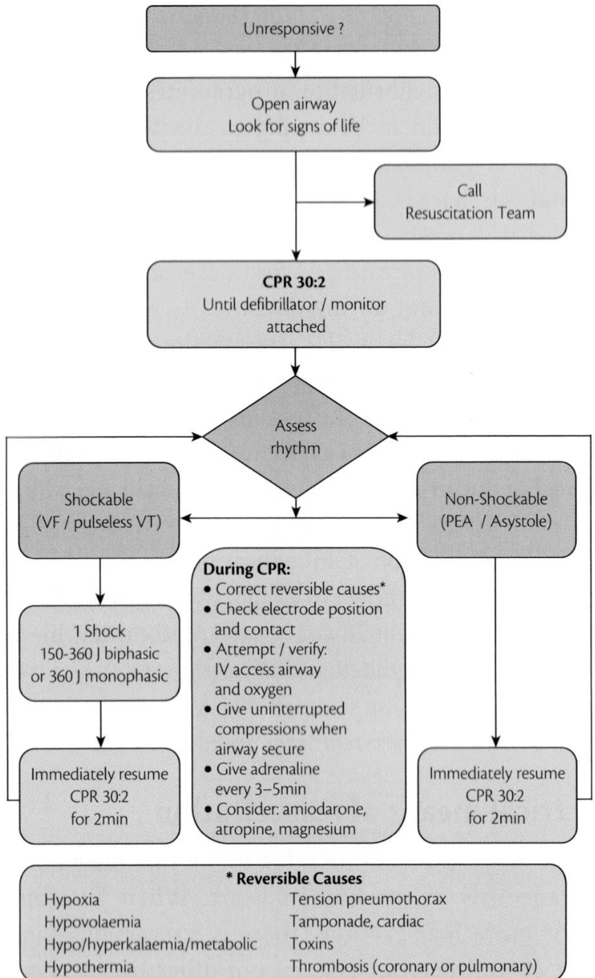

Figure 30.35 Main principles of advanced life support life support according to European Resuscitation Council Guidelines for Resuscitation 2005.

successful and early termination of VF by prompt defibrillation [163]. It has been estimated that for each minute of delay of defibrillation, survival rate drops by about 7–10%, even if CPR is started immediately. The relation between delay time to defibrillation and survival explains, to a large extent, the variation in survival in different published studies. The regions with high survival rates have a shorter delay time to defibrillation. Prior to the initial development of the community-based emergency rescue system in Seattle [163], out-of-hospital cardiac arrest was nearly uniformly fatal.

'Defibrillation' means 'reversal of the fibrillation'. Defibrillation does not mean 'shock' but 'termination of fibrillation' and should not be confused with other resuscitation outcomes, such as restoration of a perfusing rhythm, recovery of spontaneous circulation, or admission to hospital and discharge survival [164]. These endpoints may occur during resuscitation as a consequence of many other variables such as collapse to shock time and drug therapy during resuscitation attempt. These different endpoints should be taken into account when considering clinical research results.

Defibrillation consists of the passage of sufficient electric current (amperes) through the heart. The energy chosen (joules) and the transthoracic impedance (ohms) or resistance to current flow determine effective current flow. Factors that determine transthoracic impedance include energy selected, electrode size, paddle skin coupling material, number and interval of previous shocks, size of the chest, phase of ventilation, and paddle electrode pressure [165].

New defibrillators, including AEDs, may provide monophasic and biphasic energy waveforms. Monophasic waveforms deliver current that is primarily of one polarity: the direction of current flow is one-way. The recommended energy for monophasic waveforms is 360J. Biphasic waveform is a sequence of two current pulses of two different polarities (the current flows in a positive direction for a specific duration, then reverses and flows in a negative direction for the remaining time of the electrical discharge): the polarity of the second flow is opposite to that of the first. The first successful experience with biphasic waveforms stems from implantable defibrillators [166]. Subsequently, many studies using implantable but also external biphasic defibrillators have clearly demonstrated the superiority of this particular waveform over monophasic shocks in terminating VF [167].

Wearable automatic defibrillator

The wearable automatic defibrillator is a vest-like device worn under the clothing that continuously monitors the rhythm and automatically delivers electric shock when a VT is detected. It is mainly used for patients with transient high risk for VF (e.g. patients awaiting cardiac transplantation; patients requiring temporal removal of an infected implanted defibrillator).

Adjunctive drug therapy during resuscitation

Although various pharmacological interventions have been recommended in older versions of resuscitation guidelines, most of these do not have sufficient evidence to support their routine use. From the various interventions, only the administration of adrenaline is recommended in the most recent guidelines for ACLS. Routine administration of sodium bicarbonate is not advised, as one prospective randomized trial failed to demonstrate improved survival by using buffering agents during CPR [168, 169]. Probably the longest controversy in this regard exists with respect to the use of antiarrhythmic drugs to improve outcome of cardiac arrest victims. From the published literature, however, there is no evidence that administration of lidocaine (lignocaine), bretylium, or procainamide has any beneficial effect during resuscitation.

Two prospective randomized controlled trials, however, strongly indicate that the administration of intravenous amiodarone may improve chances of survival to hospital admission [170]. Accordingly, administration of amiodarone has been incorporated in the latest recommendations of European Resuscitation Council Guidelines [170].

Automatic external defibrillator

AEDs are considered to be one of the key links in the chain of survival. AEDs were first developed in the 1970s and pre-hospital care systems in various locations in the USA and the UK began to use them in the early 1980s. Since that time, research has established that AEDs are among the most successful technological innovations in emergency cardiac care. AED devices include an automated rhythm analysis system and a shock delivery system. The AED automatically 'analyses' the rhythm of a patient and 'advises' a shock. Fully automated external defibrillators do not require pressing the shock button, but are available only for specific situations. The commonly used AED is better defined as 'semi-automatic' as the operator needs to press the 'shock' button to deliver electric shock. AEDs are programmed to detect and analyse multiple features of surface ECG signal through a highly sophisticated microprocessor-based system. Frequency, amplitude, and slope or wave morphology are the ECG features analysed in order to classify the rhythm as 'shockable' or 'non-shockable'. When a shockable rhythm is recognized, the AED charges and shock delivery is permitted.

Some devices are programmed to recognize patients' movements (spontaneous or by others) and to filter them out from ECG analysis. The diagnostic accuracy of AEDs is high, with a specificity of the diagnostic algorithm for VF of about 100%, along with a sensitivity of about 90–92%. If it fails, it fails only to shock fine VF, which is more properly termed *coarse asystole* [171]. Rarely, when used improperly in patients who are not in cardiac arrest, AEDs have been reported to deliver shocks to non-VF/VT rhythm. However, these events are rare and represent an improper use of the device by the operator rather than a low diagnostic accuracy of the AED. The AED should be operated only on patients who are unresponsive, not breathing, and who have no signs of circulation.

The incremental survival benefit associated with early defibrillation using the AED was recently demonstrated in a large randomized multicentre trial [172]. The Public Access Defibrillation (PAD) trial involved >19,000 volunteer responders from 993 community places in the USA. One-half of these responders were trained in CPR alone and the other half were trained in CPR plus the use of the AED. There were more survivors to hospital discharge in the units assigned to have volunteers trained in CPR plus the use of the AED (30 survivors among 128 cardiac arrests) than there were in the units assigned to have volunteers trained only in CPR (15 out of 107; relative risk 2.0, 95% CI 1.07–3.77, $p = 0.03$). No inappropriate shocks were delivered in the entire study. Thus, this trial proves the concept of trained laypersons being able to safely and effectively use the AED.

Based on results from controlled studies [163, 166, 171–178], first responders to cardiac arrest, who should undergo training in the use of the AED according to the recent ESC guidelines, may be subdivided into the following categories:

- traditional first responders: ambulance personnel;
- non-traditional first responders: firefighters, police, security personnel, airline cabin crew, first-aiders;
- targeted lay first responders: trained citizens at work sites or public places, family of high-risk patients.

The same guidelines recommend that:

- every ambulance must carry a defibrillator on board, with personnel who are trained in its use;
- defibrillation should be one of the core competencies of doctors, nurses, and other healthcare professionals;
- defibrillators should be widely placed on general hospital wards;
- the feasibility and efficacy of allowing lay rescuers in the community to be trained and permitted to defibrillate should be investigated.

Conclusion

During the recent decades, our understanding of the clinical problem of VT and SCD has markedly changed. When, about 40 years ago, intracardiac stimulation studies were started nobody could have predicted the advances that were going to be made in the years thereafter. The field of experimental and clinical research on VT and SCD remains one of the almost ideal examples of translational research 'from bench to bedside' and vice versa. Understanding and managing VT and SCD has dramatically changed. The importance of ICD therapy for primary prevention of SCD is continuously rising. Nevertheless, SCD continues to present an important challenge in Europe, the USA, and other developed countries. The major challenge still is to identify individuals being at risk of life-threatening VT and SCD.

Personal perspective

Basic and clinical research efforts over the last 40 years have led to a tremendous increase in our knowledge on the pathophysiology of VT and SCD, on identification of patients at risk for this event, and on secondary and primary preventive therapeutic modalities. This awareness of the problem of SCD, not only among patients with cardiovascular diseases, but also among the general population, has resulted in better ways of delivering basic and advanced cardiac life support to the victim of cardiac arrest. The development of the AED has clearly been a milestone in that respect.

Continued experimental and clinical research is likely to result in an even better understanding of the molecular and genetically determined factors predisposing individuals to SCD. Based on such pathophysiological considerations, better methods to risk-stratify patients might be developed, allowing the targeting of preventive therapy to those individuals who are at highest risk for life-threatening ventricular tachyarrhythmias. In concert with clinicians, industry will continue to play a major role in refining technology, particularly with respect to ICD therapy. One of the biggest challenges here will be the development of leadless devices since lead problems can be regarded as the 'Achilles heel' of ICD therapy.

Finally, perhaps the most significant advances in the fight against SCD will be derived from better 'upstream therapy' of coronary artery disease. Preventing this disease in a sizable number of individuals will undoubtedly have the largest impact on the prevalence of out-of-hospital cardiac arrest and SCD. The theme for these activities has perhaps been best expressed by a citation of Michel Mirowski, the inventor of the implantable defibrillator, who used to say: 'The bumps in the road are not bumps, they are the road!'

Further reading

Epstein AE, Dimarco JP, Ellenbogen KA, *et al.* ACC/AHA/HRS 2008 Guidelines for Device-Based Therapy of Cardiac Rhythm Abnormalities: a report of the American College of Cardiology/American Heart Association Task Force on Practice Guidelines. Developed in collaboration with the American Association for Thoracic Surgery and Society of Thoracic Surgeons. *Circulation* 2008; **117**: e350–e408.

Goldberger JJ, Cain ME, Hohnloser SH, *et al.* American Heart Association/American College of Cardiology Foundation/Heart Rhythm Society scientific statement on noninvasive risk stratification techniques for identifying patients at risk for sudden cardiac death: a scientific statement from the American Heart Association Council on Clinical Cardiology Committee on Electrocardiography and Arrhythmias and Council on Epidemiology and Prevention. *Circulation* 2008; **118**: 1497–518.

Handley AJ, Koster R, Monsieurs K, *et al.* European Resuscitation Council guidelines for resuscitation 2005. Section 2. Adult basic life support and use of automated external defibrillators. *Resuscitation* 2005; **67**(Suppl.1): S7–S23.

Haverkamp W, Breithardt G, Camm AJ, *et al.* The potential for QT prolongation and pro-arrhythmia by non-anti-arrhythmic drugs: clinical and regulatory implications. Report on a Policy Conference of the European Society of Cardiology. *Cardiovasc Res* 2000; **47**: 219–33.

Maron BJ, McKenna WJ, Danielson GK, *et al.* American College of Cardiology/European Society of Cardiology Clinical Expert Consensus Document on Hypertrophic Cardiomyopathy. A report of the American College of Cardiology Foundation Task Force on Clinical Expert Consensus Documents and the European Society of Cardiology Committee for Practice Guidelines. *Eur Heart J* 2003; **24**: 1965–91.

Nolan JP, Deakin CD, Soar J, *et al.* European Resuscitation Council guidelines for resuscitation 2005. Section 4. Adult advanced life support. *Resuscitation* 2005; **67**(Suppl.1): S39–S86.

Priori SG, Aliot E, Blomstrom-Lundqvist C, *et al.* Task Force on Sudden Cardiac Death, European Society of Cardiology. *Europace* 2002; **4**: 3–18.

Priori SG and Zipes DP (eds.). *Sudden Cardiac Death*, 2006. Malden, MA: Blackwell Publishing.

Soar J, Deakin CD, Nolan JP, *et al.* European Resuscitation Council guidelines for resuscitation 2005. Section 7. Cardiac arrest in special circumstances. *Resuscitation* 2005; **67**(Suppl.1): S135–S170.

Task Force for cardiac pacing and resynchronization therapy of the European Society of Cardiology. Developed in collaboration with the European Heart Rhythm Association. Guidelines for cardiac pacing and cardiac resynchronization therapy. *Eur Heart J* 2007; **28**: 2256–95.

Zipes DP, Camm AJ, Borggrefe M, *et al.* ACC/AHA/ESC 2006 guidelines for management of patients with ventricular arrhythmias and the prevention of sudden cardiac death – executive summary: A report of the American College of Cardiology/American Heart Association Task Force and the European Society of Cardiology Committee for Practice Guidelines (Writing Committee to Develop Guidelines for Management of Patients with Ventricular Arrhythmias and the Prevention of Sudden Cardiac Death). Developed in collaboration with the European Heart Rhythm Association and the Heart Rhythm Society. *Eur Heart J* 2006; **27**: 2099–140.

Online resources

- QT Drug Lists by Risk Groups. Available at Arizona CERT: Center for Education and Research on Therapeutics: http://www.qtdrugs.org.

For full references and multimedia materials please visit the online version of the book (http://esctextbook.oxfordonline.com).

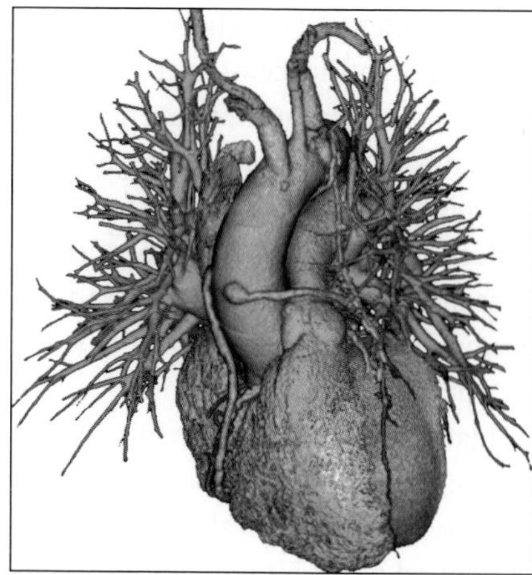

CHAPTER 31

Diseases of the Aorta and Trauma to the Aorta and the Heart

Christoph A. Nienaber, Ibrahim Akin, Holger Eggebrecht, Raimund Erbel, and Axel Haverich

Contents

Summary

Both chronic and acute diseases of the aorta, including trauma, are attracting increasing attention both in the light of an ageing Western population and with the advent of modern diagnostic modalities and therapeutic options to manage aortic pathology. For aortic aneurysm, an individual rate of expansion and the risk of rupture may be assessed from co-morbidities, hypertensive state, or connective tissue disease, and may be quantified regardless of anatomic location for timely selection and treatment. Acute aortic syndrome, a new term comprising acute dissection, intramural haematoma, and penetrating aortic ulcers, may share common ground by the observation of microapoplexy of the aortic wall, eventually leading to higher wall stress, facilitating progressive dilatation, intramural haemorrhage, dissection, and rupture; chronic hypertension and connective tissue disorders are likely to promote this mechanism as well.

While classical surgical strategies still dominate care for acute and chronic pathology of the ascending aorta and the proximal arch region, new endovascular concepts are emerging and are likely to evolve as primary treatment for descending and abdominal aortic pathology in selected and suitable patients. Additionally, aortic arch pathologies are treated in a hybrid approach combining surgical head-vessel debranching and interventional stent-graft implantation in the attempt to improve outcome. Life-threatening aortic emergencies, including aortic trauma involving the descending aorta, are accepted indications for endovascular stent-grafts.

In summary, the newly discovered field of clinical aortic pathology is unfolding; optimized multimodality diagnostic and therapeutic strategies require the collaborative effort of a multidisciplinary approach probably organized best in association with an emergency unit which includes a chest pain unit.

Aneurysms of the thoracic aorta

Definition

Aneurysmal degeneration can involve every part of the aortic vessel. The segment above the cusp of the aortic valve extending to the sinotubular ridge is known as the sinus of Valsalva. The proper ascending aorta extends from the sinotubular ridge to a line drawn at a right angle to the origin on the innominate artery, while the aortic arch is defined from the line drawn at a right angle proximal to the innominate artery origin to a line drawn in a right angle distal to the origin of the left subclavian artery. The descending thoracic aorta is the part from the left subclavian artery to the aortic hiatus in the diaphragm, followed by the abdominal aorta extending to the bifurcation of the aorta, where it is further divided into its sub segments (➲Fig. 31.1) [1, 2]. The aortic wall consists of the intima, media, and adventitia, with a thickness of about 4mm. The intima is thin, the media contains elastic fibres and smooth muscle cells forming a spiral layer of tissue that provides the strength of the aortic wall, and the adventitia provides the nutrition with arterial and venous vasa vasorum. The normal diameter of the ascending aorta can be calculated [3, 4] and has been defined as 2.1cm/m^2; the value for the descending aorta is 1.6cm/m^2 [5]. The normal diameter of the abdominal aorta is regarded to be <3.0cm. Any influence of anthropometric data on the aortic diameters was not apparent in the study of Hager and associates [4]. The analyses of variance revealed no influence of weight, height, or body surface area, but it did reveal influence of sex and age [4]. Concerning the influence of age, this study matches with the study of Aronberg and associates, who showed that aortic diameters increase about 1mm per decade during adulthood [3]. On the basis of these data, dilatation of aortic segments should be defined as a deviation of more than two standard deviations from the normal value. Therefore, localized aneurysm should continue to be defined as a >50% dilatation compared to the diameter of the adhering normal vessel [2]. Aneurysms below the origin of the left subclavian artery are classified according to the Crawford classification (thoracic aortic aneurysm (TAA) type I to type IV), recently adapted by Safi (TAA type V) (➲Fig. 31.2) [6, 7].

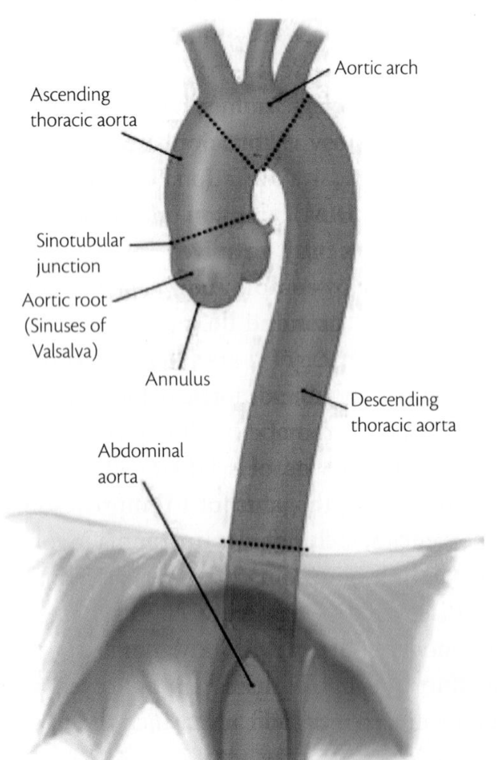

Figure 31.1 Anatomy of the aorta. ©Massachusetts General Hospital Thoracic Aortic Center, reproduced with permission.

Various forms of aneurysm can be defined: 'true aneurysm' denotes enlargement of the inner lumen due to vessel wall expansion, whereas 'false aneurysm' (also called pseudo-aneurysm) denotes lumen enlargement due to perforation (penetration) of all parts of the vessel wall, forming an outer sac in communication with the inner lumen of the aorta. The term 'dissecting aneurysm' should be replaced:

- 'circumscript (localized) aneurysm' denotes involvement of only segments of the entire aorta;
- 'diffuse aneurysm' denotes enlargement of the ascending aorta, aortic arch, descending thoracic, or abdominal aorta, or even the whole aorta.

Epidemiology

Over the past 30 years, reported incidence of TAAs has increased with better diagnostics and with more patients living to advanced age. Little is known, however, about the true prevalence and mortality rate of TAAs in a particular population. TAAs and thoracoabdominal aortic aneurysms (TAAAs) are less common than infrarenal abdominal aortic aneurysms (AAAs), comprising not more than 2–5% of the spectrum of degenerative aortic aneurysms. The incidence of death in white males with TAA was reported to be 0.7/100,000 per year and for dissecting aneurysms 1.5/100,000 per year [8, 9]. Accordingly, a population-based study reported an age- and gender-adjusted incidence of 5.9 new aneurysms per 100,000 person-years in a Midwestern community over a 30-year period with median ages of 65 years for men and 77 years for women,

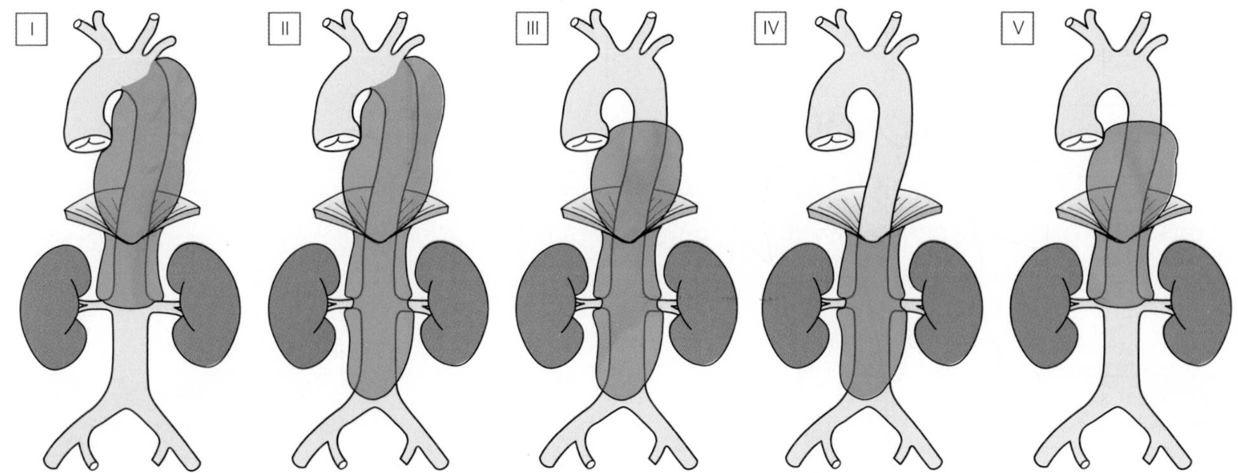

Figure 31.2 Thoracoabdominal aortic aneurysm (TAA) classification. Type I, from below the left subclavian artery to above the celiac axis, or opposite the superior mesenteric and aove the renal arteries. Type II, from below the left subclavian and including the infrarenal abdominal aorta to the level of the aortic bifurcation. Type III, from the 6th intercostals space tapering to just above the infrarenal abdominal aorta to the iliac bifurcation. Type IV, from the 12th intercostals space, tapering to above the iliac bifurcation. Type V, from the 6th intercostals space, tapering to just above the renal arteries. Modified with permission from Safi HJ, Miller CC. Spinal cord protection in descending thoracic and thoracoabdominal aortic repair. *Ann Thorac Surg* 1999; **67**:1937–39.

and a distribution to the ascending aorta in 51%, to the arch in 11%, and to the descending thoracic aorta in 38% [10]. In contrast to abdominal aneurysms with male predominance, up to one-half of the TAAs were identified in women [9, 10]. Moreover, a quarter of the patients had concomitant infrarenal aneurysmal aortic disease and up to 13% had multiple aneurysms, whereas the risk of having a TAA, when AAA was diagnosed, is 3.5–12% [11]. Of the patients with aortic aneurysm and dissection, 22% did not reached the hospital alive (with the diagnosis made at autopsy) and aortic rupture occurred in 74% of all TAAs with a mortality rate of 94.3% [12].

Aetiology

The aorta ages during its lifetime [4, 5, 13]. Ageing involves all segments, with an increase in the luminal diameter of the entire aorta during childhood and young adulthood (➲ Fig. 31.3) Ageing processes are gender specific (➲ Fig. 31.4). In adulthood, aortic size is related to exercise and workload. During further ageing, vessel wall stiffness increases due to

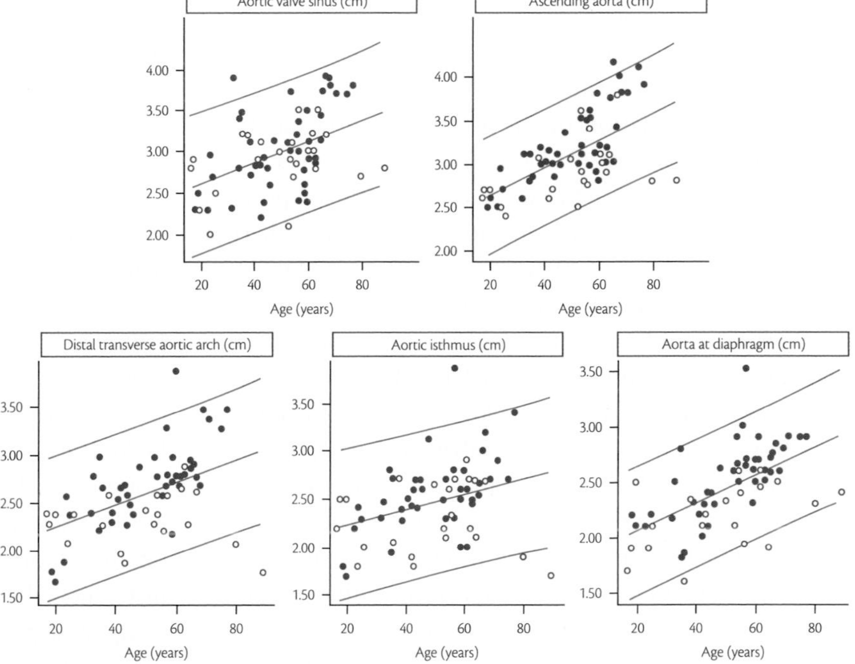

Figure 31.3 Changes in aortic size during life illustrated for the following aortic segments: aortic root, ascending aorta, transverse descending aorta, aortic isthmus, diaphragm. Reproduced with permission from Hager A, Kaemmerer H, Rapp-Bernhardt U, *et al.* Diameters of the thoracic aorta throughout life as measured with helical computed tomography. *J Thorac Cardiovasc Surg* 2002; **123**: 1060–6.

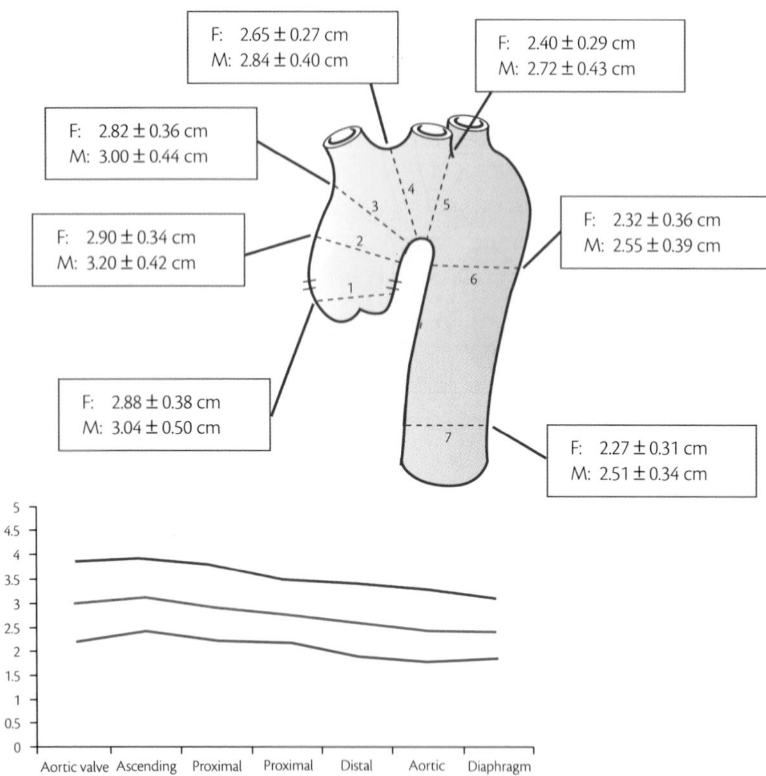

Figure 31.4 Gender related normal values for the diameter at seven aortic segments. Mean values ± standard deviation. Reproduced with permission from Hager A, Kaemmerer H, Rapp-Bernhardt U, *et al*. Diameters of the thoracic aorta throughout life as measured with helical computed tomography. *J Thorac Cardiovasc Surg* 2002; **123**: 1060–6.

structural changes induced by aortic sclerosis [4]. Risk factors include hypertension, hyperlipidaemia, diabetes mellitus, and smoking. Aortic wall components demonstrate increasing amounts of collagen and lipids as well as calcium deposits. Aortic wall thickness increases with up to 7mm as the upper normal limit [5]. As a result, pulse pressure is enhanced and pulse wave velocity elevated, decreasing the resulting organ perfusion, particularly diastolic myocardial perfusion. Further development of aortic sclerosis is characterized by intimal thickening, plaque formation, ulceration, and thrombus formation.

Aneurysm formation of the ascending aorta has been regarded as a forme fruste of Marfan syndrome, but actually represents a specific genetically determined disease process, where the aortic arch is usually not involved [14]; there is also a 1% prevalence of bicuspid aortic valve (BAV) [15]. In a review of 21,417 cases with 161 patients suffering from aortic dissection, BAV was tenfold more prevalent than in controls [16] and found in 6–10% of all dissections [17]. Patients with BAV have a ninefold higher risk of dissection than those with tricuspid aortic valves [14]. There is also a high incidence of BAV in patients with aortic coarctation. In patients with BAV, enlarged ascending aortic diameters are reported [18]. It was once thought that such aneurysms were due to 'poststenotic dilatation' of the ascending aorta. Yet even young patients with normally functioning BAVs were found with aortic dilatation [19]. Cystic medial degeneration has been identified as a common denominator of aortic dilatation in a variety of conditions including a BAV; 75% of patients with a BAV undergoing aortic valve replacement had biopsy-proven cystic medial necrosis of the ascending aorta, compared to 14% of those with tricuspid aortic valves undergoing similar surgery [20]. Inadequate fibrillin-1 during embryogenesis is one suggestion to explain both the BAV and a weakened aortic wall [21]. Additionally, compared with tricuspid aortic valve controls, the aortic wall tissue of those with a BAV demonstrated more lymphocyte infiltration and smooth muscle cell apoptosis suggesting that the walls of aneurysms associated with BAVs may be weaker than in typical aneurysms [22].

The medial layer of the aorta is composed of both vascular smooth muscle cells and extracellular matrix (ECM) proteins, primarily elastin and collagen; a balanced composition of vascular smooth muscle cells and ECM proteins appears critical for preserving functional properties of the aorta, and especially its mechanical compliance with pulsatile flow. Disturbance of metabolic balance resulting in excessive ECM degradation may be key to progressive aortic wall deterioration with subsequent expansion or rupture. Another mechanism relates to matrix metalloproteinases (MMP-family of more than 20 zinc-dependent proteolytic enzymes) instrumental for ECM metabolism and aortic wall remodelling, and potentially relevant for development of aneurysms or dissection [23]. Increased MMP-9 expression has

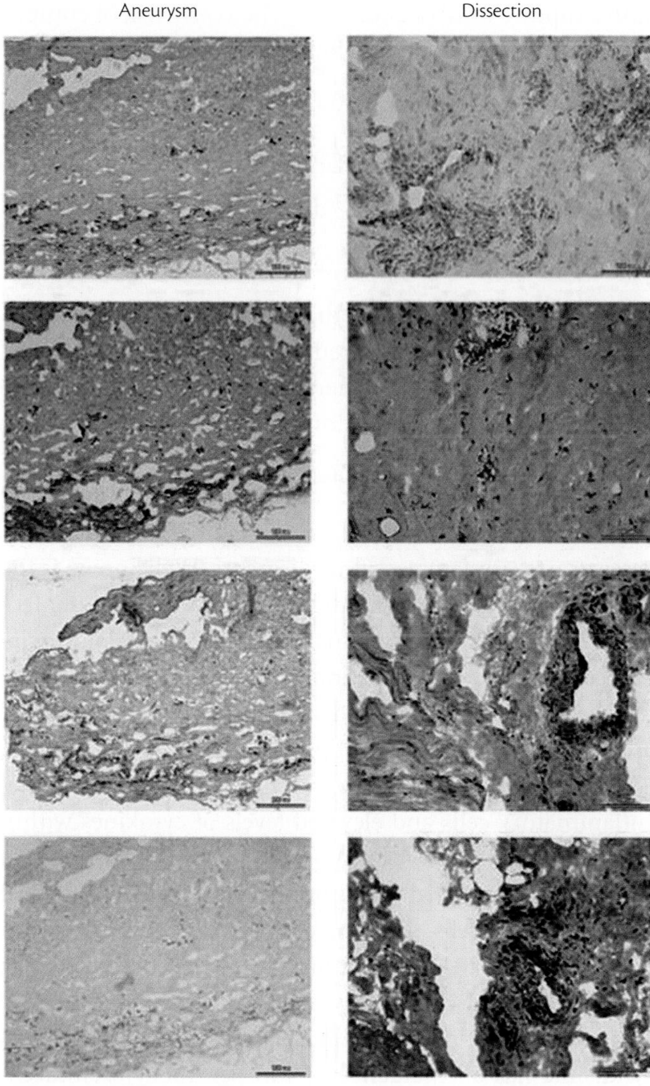

Figure 31.5 Immunohistology and staining of increased expression of both MMP-2 and MMP-9, as well as low TIMP-1 and TIMP-4 especially in the vascular tissue of a patient with thoracic aortic aneurysm as compared to another case with aortic dissection. (Original magnification × 200.) Reproduced with permission from Ince H, Nienaber CA. Etiology, pathogenesis and management of thoracic aortic aneurysm. *Nat Clin Pract Cardiovasc Med* 2007; **4**: 418–27.

also been observed in patients with thoracic aortic disease (➲Fig. 31.5) [24, 25]. Thus, it is not surprising that the MMP-9 gene (*MMP9*) has emerged as target for investigation and MMP-9 –8202A/G polymorphism has been reported to be associated with TAAs although the functional role of the -8202A/G variant in matrix MMP9 expression still needs to be determined [26].

Genetic defects are usually involved in thoracic aneurysm formation. Three major inherited disorders are known to cause aortic diseases: Marfan syndrome, Ehlers–Danlos syndrome, and other familial forms of connective tissue diseases. Most cases, however, represent so called 'overlap' syndromes reflecting the currently incomplete knowledge of genetic defects associated with aortic diseases. The classic phenotype of Marfan syndrome reveals aortic root dilatation and cystic medial degeneration prior to aneurysm formation; more than 125 spot mutations have been identified on the fibrillin-1 (*FBN1*) gene to date [27]. Prevalence is about 1 in 5000 [28] and it accounts for 6–9% of all dissections [29]. Dilatation of the aorta is found in 50% of childhood Marfan syndrome and will progress over time. In one study of 76 patients at an average age of 30 years, the greatest progression of aortic dilatation occurred in the aortic root at 0.2cm/year [29, 30]. Complications are aortic aneurysms, aortic regurgitation due to aortic ring dilatation, and aortic dissection. Other familial clusters of TAA have also been identified in about 20% of 1600 patients [30]. Also see ➲Chapter 9.

Annulo-aortic ectasia affects 5–10% of patients undergoing valve replacement and has been described in association with a familial sex-linked aggregation with the probable existence of genetic heterogeneity [31, 32]. AAA formation is uncommon before the sixth decade. The process is often combined with more proximal disease [33]. The prevalence in men over the age of 50 years is 5% [34, 35]. A familial aggregation is suggested that predominantly affects women, whereas men who are affected tend to be younger [36]. A genetic mutation has been described [37].

TAA and/or thoracic aortic dissection (TAD) may occur in the context of inherited connective tissue disorders such as the above mentioned fibrillinopathies, Marfan syndrome and Ehlers–Danlos syndrome. Familial clustering of common TAD is, however, more complex and heterogeneous and at least three causal loci have been mapped to chromosomes 11q23.2–q24 (AAT1), 5q13–14 (AAT2) and 3p24–25 (AAT3) [38, 39].

Pathological–anatomical studies demonstrate typical cystic degeneration of the aortic media, mucoid material, and loss of elastic fibres (➲Fig. 31.6). The loss of elastic fibres, deposits of mucopolysaccharide-like material and cystic anomalies are found in Marfan syndrome as well as annulo-aortic ectasia [40]. This leads to a weakening of wall strength and consequent vessel dilatation. The circumferential wall stress (W) can be calculated according to Laplace's law for thin-walled structures:

$$W = Pr/2h$$

where P represents pressure, r radius, and h wall thickness.

Hypertension, wall thinning, and aortic enlargement are the most important factors increasing wall stress leading to aortic rupture or dissection [41, 42]. Aortic diameter is a marker of risk but is not always enlarged. In connective tissue disease up to 40% of cases show aortic enlargement

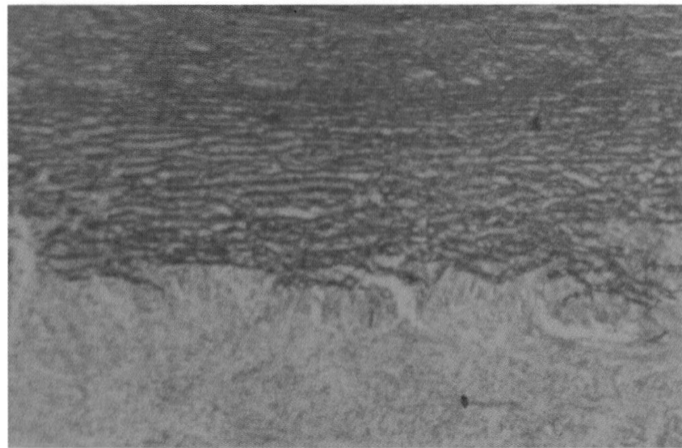

Figure 31.6 Aortic aneurysm specimen: histological view of aortic wall structure with mucoid medial degeneration and fibre rupture.

of more than the normal range, although in other forms this degree of enlargement is found in only 10%. The critical point of rupture (➲Fig. 31.7) is at 6cm for the ascending aorta and 7cm for the descending aorta [30]. When this point is reached, up to 30% with enlargement of the ascending aorta and 40% with enlargement of the descending aorta suffer rupture or dissection [30]. The yearly risk of complications can be calculated as follows [43]:

$$\text{Ln} = -21.055 + 0.0093\,(\text{age}) + 0.842\,(\text{pain}) + 1.282\,(\text{COPD}) + 0.643\,(\text{descending aortic diameter}) + 0.405\,(\text{abdominal aortic diameter})$$

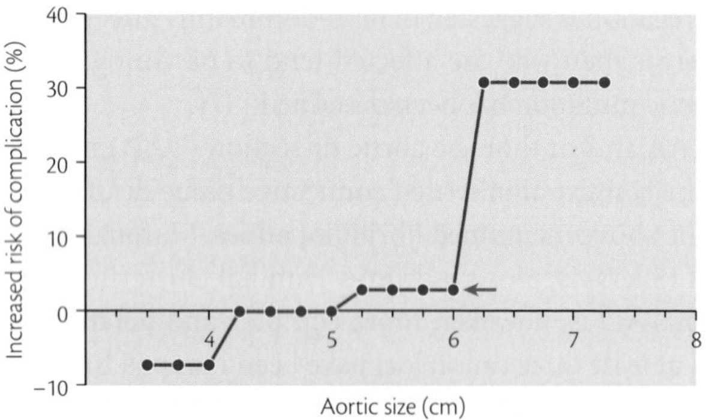

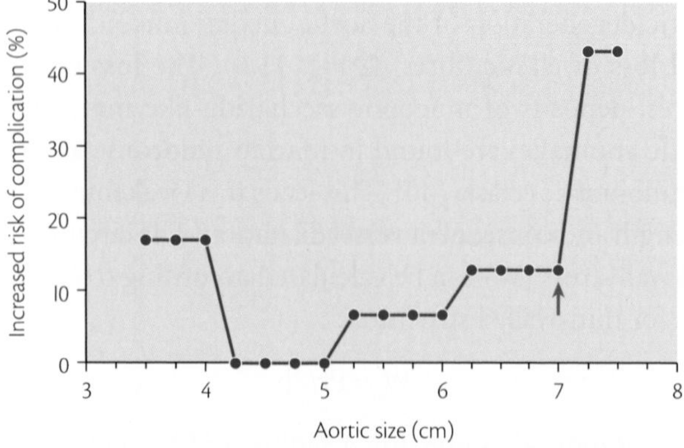

Figure 31.7 Influence of aortic size on cumulative lifetime incidence of natural complications of aortic aneurysm: y-axis, incidence of natural complications (rupture/dissection); x-axis, aortic size. (A) Ascending aorta, hinge point at 6cm. (B) descending aorta, hinge point at 7cm. Reproduced with permission from Elefteriades JA. Natural history of thoracic aortic aneurysms: indications for surgery, and surgical versus nonsurgical risks. *Ann Thorac Surg* 2002; **74**: S1877–S80.

Aortic sclerosis of both, the thoracic and the abdominal aorta, is only a weak predictor of expansion [44, 45]. Patients with the most atherosclerotic burden have the slowest growth of the abdominal aorta [45]. Smoking increases growth rate by 15–20%.

Weakening of the aortic wall can also be induced by inflammation. This can be the result of microbiological diseases or multisystem vasculitic disorders. Well known is the aortitis induced by syphilis and *Staphylococcus aureus* infection. Kawasaki's syndrome is characterized by more circumscript aneurysm formation, whereas syphilis can induce diffuse wall thickening and aneurysm formation of the ascending aorta, but penetrating ulcers can also be observed. The risk of rupture increases with the diameter of the aorta. Inflammatory cells and elevated levels of cytokines within the aneurysm wall have been observed [46]. Cytokines may trigger increased production of MMP by macrophages and smooth muscle cells [47]. There is a strong relation between infiltration and MMP activation [46]. Behçet's disease, like other forms of vasculitis, may lead to local aneurysm formation and perforation rather than dissection [48]. Kawasaki's syndrome has an incidence of 135 per 100,000 children, with 8–17 cases in 100,000 children under the age of 5 years [49]. Coronary aneurysm is the leading sign, but other arterial segments can also be involved. In giant-cell arteritis, thoracic and abdominal aneurysm may develop [50]. The use of cocaine and amphetamines can also lead to aortic wall thinning and aneurysm formation.

In aortic stenosis, poststenotic aneurysm formation can occur, which may even be enhanced after aortic valve prosthesis implantation [51]. Previous surgery accounts for 2–4% of patients receiving aortic root surgery [45]. An important cause of aneurysm formation is related to trauma, particularly high-speed deceleration trauma involving the aortic isthmus in 95% [52] and about 15–20% of deaths are related to aortic trauma in these patients.

Natural history

The natural history of TAAs has not been sufficiently defined. One reason for this is that both the aetiology and location of an aneurysm may affect its rate of growth and propensity for dissection or rupture. The Yale group showed in their longitudinal data that the mean rate of growth for all thoracic aneurysms was significantly lower (0.1cm/year) than of abdominal aneurysms (0.2–0.5cm/year). The rate of growth, however, was greater for aneurysms of the descending aorta versus ascending aorta, and was greater for dissected versus non-dissected aneurysms, and eventually most pronounced in Marfan syndrome [9]. Initial size can also be an important predictor of the rate growth; a study based on 721 patients supported the fact that TAA size had a profound impact on risk for rupture with an annual rate of 2% in aneurysms <5cm, 3% in aneurysms 5–5.9cm, and 7% for aneurysms >6cm in diameter. Therefore, the risk appears to rise abruptly as thoracic aneurysms reach a size of 6cm [53]. Similar results were reported over 5 years of follow-up in 133 patients with a rupture risk of 0% for ectasia <40mm, compared to 16% and 31% for aneurysms of 40–59 and ≥65mm, respectively (➲Fig. 31.7; ➲Table 31.1) [30, 31]. In several series, aneurysm rupture occurred in 32–68% of medically treated patients and rupture accounted for 32–47% of deaths; thus the 1-, 3-, and 5-year survival rate of thoracic aneurysms left without repair was 65%, 36%, and 20%, respectively [41]. Beyond this dimensional view, non-dimensional variables with impact on expansion rate and risk of rupture should also be evaluated. The Mount Sinai group identified older age, the sensation of even uncharacteristic pain, and the history of COPD as independent risk factors for rupture of TAA in a multivariate regression analysis; in this context, symptomatic TAAs have a 27% 5-year survival, compared to 58% in asymptomatic patients [54]. For TAAs who are unfit for or who refused surgery, a survival rate of only 24% at 2 years was reported [8]. According to the natural history in 76 patients with arteriosclerotic aneurysms of the thoracic aorta, of whom 63 did not undergo surgery for aneurysms, 25 (40%) eventually died of rupture and 27% of unrelated cardiovascular conditions [55].

Clinical features

Patients with TAAs are often asymptomatic at the time of diagnosis. However, depending upon size and location, chest, back, flank, or abdominal pain can result. Symptoms are usually attributed to unilateral compression, erosion, or distortion either of adjacent vessels, with vascular consequences such as superior vena cava compression syndrome, aortic regurgitation, or thromboembolic sequelae, or neighbouring structures leading to phrenic nerve dysfunction or hoarseness. Ascending aortic aneurysms may present first with clinical signs of aortic valve regurgitation or heart failure from aortic regurgitation or from aortic root dilatation and annular distortion. More importantly, aneurysm involving a sinus of Valsalva can rupture into right-sided cardiac chambers, leading to continuous shunting of blood and eventually to heart failure. Moreover, ascending and arch aneurysms can erode into the mediastinum, producing hoarseness from compression of vagus or recurrent laryngeal nerve, or from hemidiaphragmatic paralysis due to compression of the phrenic nerve; wheezing, cough, haemoptysis, dyspnoea, or pneumonitis in case of compression of the tracheobronchial tree, and dysphagia from oesophageal compression or from superior vena cava syndrome; at advanced stage, compression of other intrathoracic structures or erosion of adjacent bony structures may even cause continuous chest or back pain. Occasionally, emboli from layered thrombus within the aneurysm may cause cerebral, renal, and mesenteric ischaemia or claudication.

Diagnostic procedures

Various tomographic imaging techniques can be used to diagnose aortic aneurysm formation, which in many instances is an accidental finding. Chest radiography may reveal widening of the mediastinum, left-sided visible enlargement of the ascending aorta, changes in the aortic knob, or an enlarged and often elongated descending aorta. Circumscript aneurysm formation may result in multiform chest radiographic abnormalities. However, chest x-ray is likely to fail to distinguish aneurysm from a tortuous aorta and, thus, some aneurysms are subsequently missed (➲Fig. 31.8). On plain chest film, abnormalities were detected in only 22 of 36 patients (61%) even in presence of recent chest or back pain [56].

Table 31.1 Annual risk (%) of complications based on aortic size

	Aortic size (cm)			
Risk/year	>3.5	>4	>5	>6
Rupture risk	0	0.3	1.7	3.6
Dissection	2.2	1.5	2.5	3.7
Mortality	5.9	4.6	4.8	10.8
Any event	7.2	5.3	6.5	14.1

Reproduced with permission from Ellis PR, Cooley DA, Bakey ME. Clinical consideration and surgical treatment of annuloaortic ectasia. *J Thorac Cardiovasc Surg* 1961; **42**: 363–70.

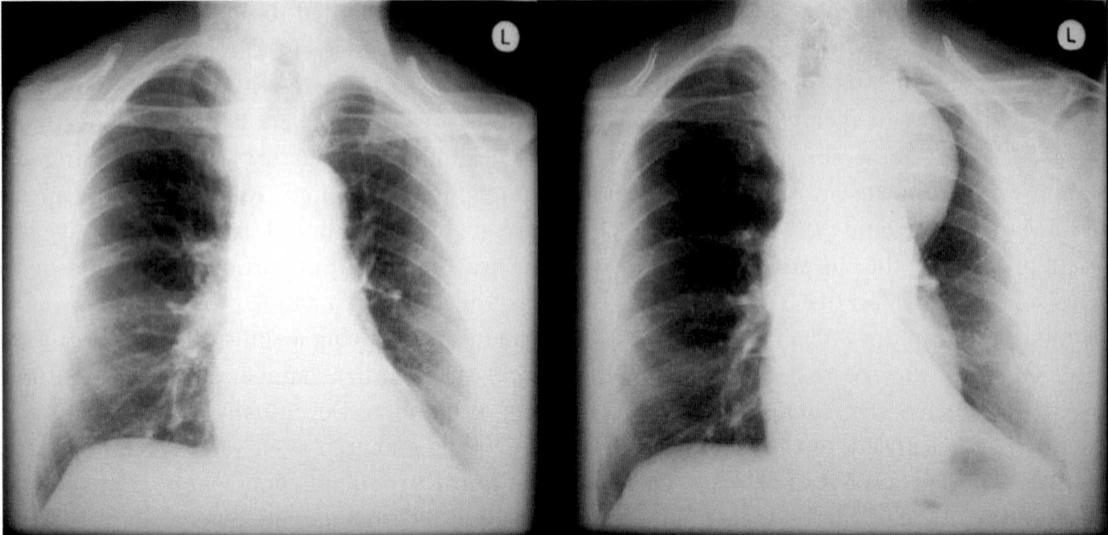

Figure 31.8 Serial chest radiograph of a patient with a true aortic aneurysm. (A) Baseline study demonstrates a normal anteroposterior chest film despite an enlarged aortic diameter. (B) Follow-up chest radiograph upon admission reveals a remarkable enlargement of the aortic knob and the descending thoracic aorta with an aortic diameter of 9cm.

Computed tomography (CT), especially with contrast image enhancement, is instrumental in determining location, size, and/or any complications. Aortic wall thickness, calcium deposits in the area of the coronary arteries and aortic wall, and side-branch anatomy can be visualized (➲ Fig. 31.9). The use of standardized techniques yields high reproducibility for follow-up studies to estimate changes over time. Complications such as perforation with mediastinal haematoma, pleural effusion, pericardial effusion, and signs of aortic syndrome are detected [13, 57–59]. Disadvantages are the use of potentially toxic contrast agents and the inability to visualize aortic regurgitation and left ventricular wall motion abnormalities (➲ Chapter 6).

Magnetic resonance imaging (MRI) produces unrestricted high-resolution views of the aorta in transverse, sagittal, and coronal planes. Because of its higher quality images, MRI provides optimal delineation of the origin and extent of aneurysm formation (➲ Fig. 31.10). Left ventricular wall thickness and function can be studied, but visualization of coronary stenoses or aortic sclerosis is less accurate. The size of an aortic aneurysm, its location, and extent is easily measured [60–62]. A big advantage is the lack of radiation burden, which allows multiple follow-up studies, particularly in young adults and women of childbearing age. Renal failure occurs to a lesser extent than with radiographic contrast material injection. MRI contrast studies are not allowed in renal failure due to the potential danger of the development of nephrogenic systemic fibrosis [63].

Ultrasound can visualize the whole aorta using transthoracic, suprasternal, subcostal, and abdominal interrogation, usually combined with colour duplex imaging. However, the ascending part of the aortic arch cannot be imaged even

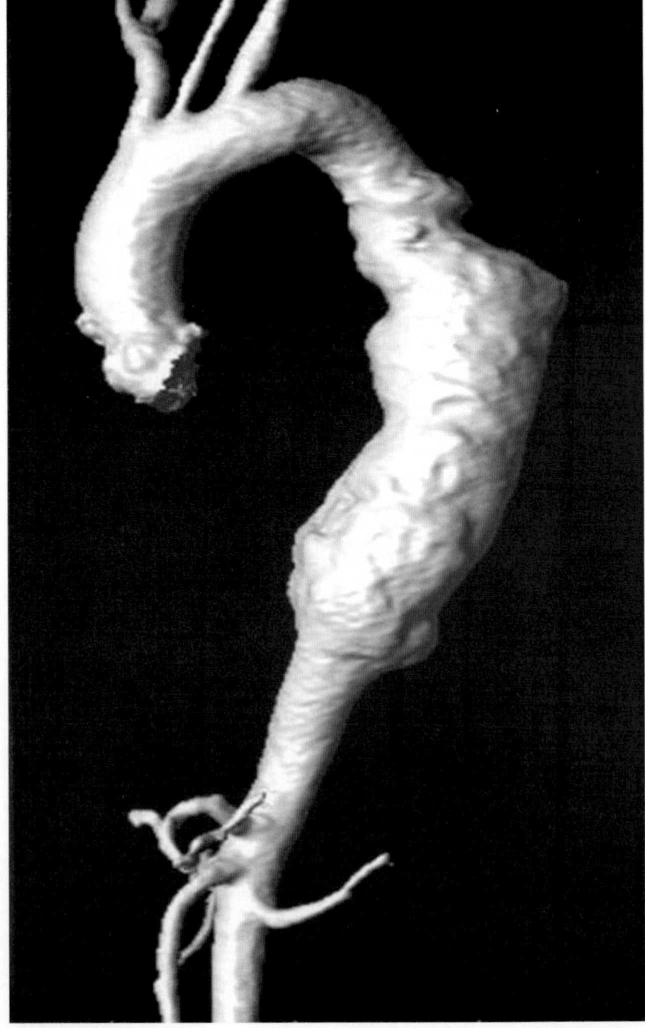

Figure 31.9 Contrast-enhanced CT of the thoracic aorta with surface rendering for 3D-reconstruction. 3D shaded-surface rendering image demonstrates a large true aneurysm of the thoracic descending aorta and the spatial relationship to side branches.

by

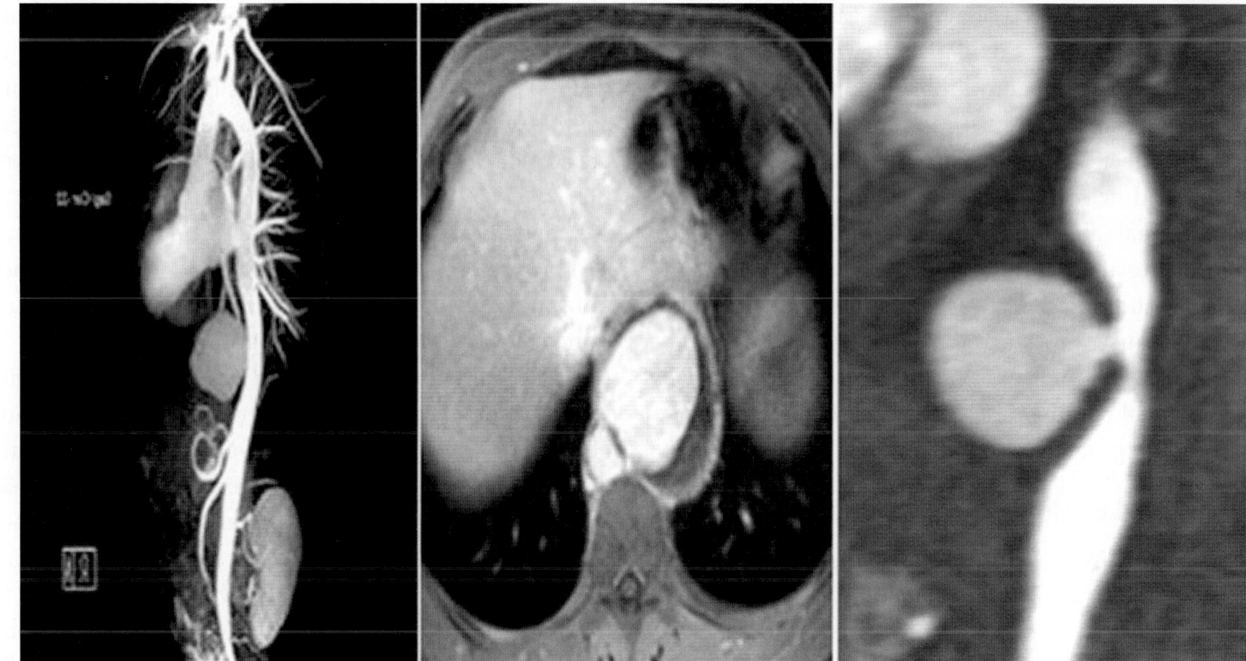

Figure 31.10 MRI of discrete false aneurysm of the descending aorta reconstruction.

transoesophageal echocardiography because of the interposition of the trachea and the right mainstem bronchus between the oesophagus and the aorta at this location [64, 65]. This technique has high resolution but spatial orientation is limited. Aneurysms can be detected but the full extent and size are difficult to assess. With endovascular interventions, however, intravascular ultrasound and transoesophageal echocardiography are of great importance [66, 67].

The invasive technique most widely used is aortography, which allows visualization of aortic regurgitation, ventricular function, coronary artery disease, side-branch involvement, and aneurysm location, size, and extent. The disadvantage is the exposure to radiation and the use of contrast agents. The technique is the basis for interventional procedures [68–71]. Moreover, intravascular ultrasound using transducers of 7–10MHz also has great diagnostic potential. Mechanical and electronic sector scanners are available which show cross-sectional images but without flow imaging. This disadvantage can be eliminated with the use of flexible, steerable, linear 8F ultrasound catheters, which have all the capabilities of other echocardiographic and sonographic machines.

Positron emission tomography (PET) is able to detect increased metabolic activity in thoracic and abdominal aneurysms [72]. ^{18}F-fluorodeoxyglucose uptake at the level of the aneurysm is a strong predictor of aneurysm expansion and rupture, and the combination of PET and CT may potentially offer new insights, especially with regards to ongoing local inflammation or aortitis (➲Chapter 7) [73].

Besides imaging techniques, laboratory tests may be helpful for identifying active inflammatory processes. Elevated levels of fibrinogen, α_1-antitrypsin, haptoglobin and ceruloplasmin C-reactive protein and d-dimers are frequently found [74, 47].

Medical management

Asymptomatic aneurysms are initially managed medically, while surgery is indicated for symptomatic and expanding aneurysms, or those beyond 55mm in diameter in the ascending aorta or 60mm in diameter regardless of site or symptoms. A novel predictor for rupture of TAA, the aortic size index, may be useful to predict increasing rates of rupture, dissection, or death. Individual body surface area information is utilized for the aortic size index (aortic diameter/m^2) enabling improved and individualized selection for surgical repair. With the aortic size index stratification is possible into ≥2.75cm/m^2 representing low risk (approximately 4%/year), 2.75–4.24cm/m^2 for moderate risk (approximately 8% per year), and >4.25cm/m^2 at high risk (approximately 20% per year) underlining the importance of relative aortic size for predicting complications [75]. In an asymptomatic patient, medical management includes aggressive blood-pressure lowering and particularly anti-impulse medication such as potent beta-adrenergic receptor blocking agents; the adjacent use of additional antihypertensive drugs may be necessary, but decreasing dP/dt is the mainstay of medical therapy besides surveillance and serial tomographic imaging by CT or MR to evaluate growth and structure of the aneurysm. Beta-adrenergic receptor blocking agents may be of some benefit for reducing the rate of aortic dilatation, particularly in children and adolescents with Marfan syndrome. Today, some early experimental evidence may suggest that oxidative stress is involved in the pathogenesis of atherosclerotic TAA and that perhaps statin therapy and angiotensin II receptor blockers may have a protective effect [76]. Moreover patients should be counselled to avoid heavy lifting or straining, because isometric exercise may abruptly increase intrathoracic pressure and blood pressure. As detailed earlier, several aetiologies of TAAs, including a BAV, may have some genetic components. Because TAAs are typically asymptomatic, the only way to detect their presence among other potentially affected familial members is with formal screening by non-invasive imaging.

Surgical and endovascular management

Important measures for preventing enlargement and progression of aneurysm include cessation of smoking and lowering of blood pressure. Beta-adrenergic blocking agents or other agents that lower blood pressure may be used in combination. For abdominal aneurysms, smoking and hypertension were predictors of late death after aortic surgery [77]. In addition to medical treatment with beta-blocking agents, surgical and/or endovascular management may become necessary. Aortic dissection and rupture are the most severe complication of aortic aneurysm formation, leading to high operative risk in urgent or emergency situations [5]. Operative mortality has been reported to be 1.5% for elective, 2.6% for emergency, and 11.7% for urgent surgery. Thus, elective surgery has been recommended for aneurysms of the ascending aorta >5.5cm diameter and for those >4.5cm in Marfan syndrome or other connective tissue disease [13, 30].

Composite mechanical valve conduits have been used since their introduction by Bentall and De Bono in 1968 [78]. Most often, modified procedures are used [77]. The open technique has replaced the inclusion wrap technique, with the Carrel button technique to reattach the coronary ostia [79]. In order to create an optimal sinutubular junction with a 1:1 relation to the valve cusp's free margin and annulus diameter, Dacron tubes of 26–30mm are chosen [77]. Valve-preserving procedures would be ideal because anticoagulation can be avoided, but often the valve apparatus itself contains connective tissue abnormalities [80, 81]. If the aortic root exceeds 6cm, most of the cusps demonstrate abnormalities [82]. Therefore, it is not surprising that in 203 patients operated in the Mayo Clinic, composite valve conduit reconstruction resulted in a more durable result during a follow-up period of 20 years [77]. After 5 years, 12% versus 40% were free from reoperation. Sarsam and Yacoub [83], as well as David and Feindel [84], have developed a valve-preserving reconstruction technique. The reoperation rate was reported to be 11% at 10 years [85] and only 3% at 10 and 8 years, respectively [86]. However, a high rate of residual aortic regurgitation developed in 25–45% at 8–10 years [82, 86].

Reoperation is necessary in 10–20% of the patients during a follow-up of 10–20 years, with a trend for more reoperations in those with valve-preserving aortic root reconstruction versus composite graft replacement (16% versus 5%) [87]. A predictor for reoperation was found to be an annulus diameter >2.5cm [88]. Other predictors were found to be Marfan syndrome, mitral valve prolapse, preoperative atrial fibrillation, aortic valve-preserving operation, and concomitant procedures performed, with a mean time to reoperation of 4.5 ± 5 years [77]. Recurrent aortic aneurysm was found in 3.5%, mitral valve disease in 2%.

Long-term problems can arise from anticoagulation in patients with mechanical valve prosthesis. Thromboembolism is reported in up to 0.42 per 100 patient-years [89], depending on whether patients with atherosclerotic aneurysms are included in the analysis [77]. Valve thrombosis was observed in 1% and life-threatening haemorrhage in 2% of 203 patients, with a time of 5.4 ± 4.9 years to the event. Endocarditis was found in only 1%, but usually within 1 year after surgery. Main predictors of late death are female sex, increased age, untreated with beta-blockers, mitral regurgitation III°–IV° at presentation, mitral ring calcification, postoperative dysrhythmia, and postoperative inotropes. The overall 20-year survival rate reaches 50% [77].

For the aortic arch, surgical intervention is most likely to be the method of choice, which nowadays is more frequently combined with stent-graft implantation in order to seal the distal aortic arch to the descending aorta. Special systems have been designed so that implantation can be performed via an antegrade strategy [90].

For thoracic descending or TAAAs, the current surgical strategy has been developed over the last 15 years in order to prevent ischaemic complications and includes: permissive mild hypothermia (32–34°C nasopharyngeal); moderate heparinization with 1mg/kg; renal artery perfusion with 4°C crystalloid solution; aggressive reattachment of segmental arteries (especially between T8 and L1); sequential aortic clamping as well as cerebrospinal fluid drainage; stent graft implantation into the proximal descending aorta; left heart bypass during proximal anastomosis; and selective perfusion of coeliac and superior mesenteric arteries during intercostal, visceral, and renal anastomosis [90, 91, 92]. The technique for spinal cord protection can reduce the rate of

Table 31.2 Current possible indications for endovascular treatment of symptomatic thoracic aortic disease

Disease aetiology
Aortic aneurysms
Atherosclerotic/degenerative
Post-traumatic
Anastomotic
Cystic medial necrosis
Stanford type B aortic dissection
Acute
Chronic
Giant penetrating ulcer
Traumatic aortic tear
Aortopulmonary fistula
Aneurysm morphology
Aneurysm of the descending aorta
Proximal neck length = 2cm
<2cm if supra-aortic vessels have been transposed prior stent-graft placement
Distal neck length = 2cm
Diameter ≥ 6 cm
Patient's condition
Preferentially older age
Unfit for open surgical repair or high-risk patients
Chronic obstructive pulmonary disease
Severe coronary heart disease
Severe carotid artery disease
Renal insufficiency
Suitable vascular access site
Life expectancy of >6 months

paraplegia from about 15 to <5% [93]. Also, renal failure (serum creatinine elevation >50% above baseline value) could be reduced from about 60% to 20% [94]. The 5-year survival of 1773 patients reached nearly 75% compared with only 20% [8, 90].

For circumscript localized aortic pathologies, regardless of true or false aneurysms, percutaneous stent-graft implantation has become an alternative treatment option. Currently, there is ongoing controversy regarding which patients should be treated by endovascular means (➲Table 31.2). The long-term durability of aortic stent-grafts is promising, but not yet fully proven, and cautious patient selection is still recommended [95]. The suitability of a given patient for endovascular repair is based on both clinical and anatomical considerations. At present, stent-grafts are routinely used to treat patients with thoracic aneurysms distal to the aortic arch, and infrarenal abdominal aorta (➲Fig. 31.11). Endovascular treatment of TAAs is achieved by transluminal placement of one or more stent-graft devices across the longitudinal extent of the lesion. The prosthesis bridges the aneurysmal sac to exclude it from high-pressure aortic blood flow, thereby allowing for sac thrombosis around the endograft and possible remodelling of the aortic wall. Thoracotomy, aortic cross-clamping, left-heart bypass, and single-lung ventilation are all avoided with an endovascular aortic procedure. The use of stent-grafts in TAAs was first reported by Volodos *et al.* in 1988 in a patient with post-traumatic pseudoaneurysm of the thoracic aorta [96, 97].

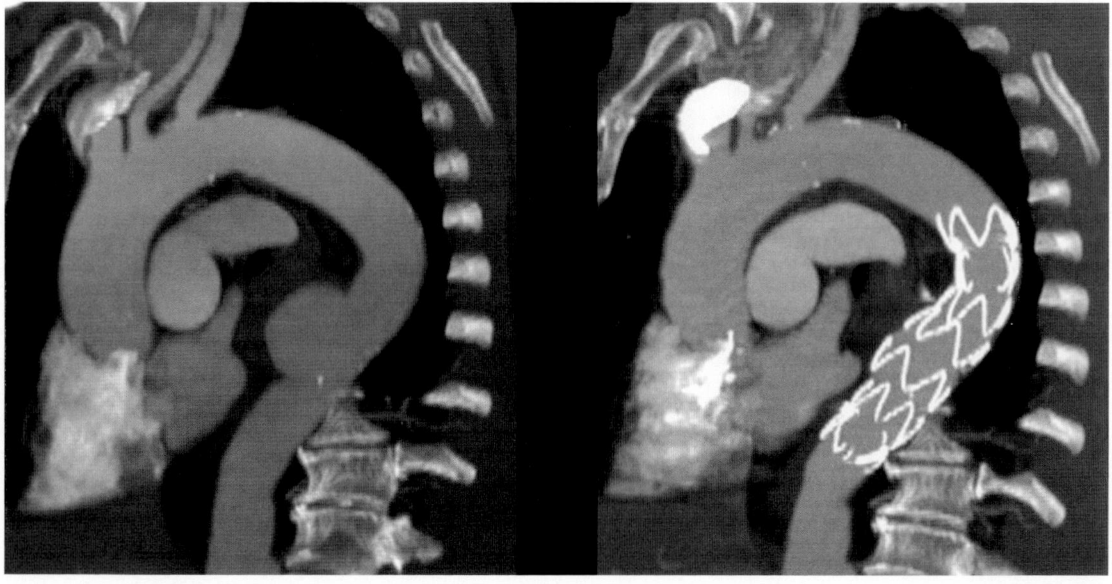

Figure 31.11 (A) CT-angiogram showing a circumscript aneurysm of the descending thoracic aorta in a middle-aged male patient selected for endografting. (B) 1-year follow-up after successful endovascular exclusion of the aneurysm by stent-graft placement demonstrates marked shrinkage of periprothetic aneurysm and optimal wall apposition of the stent-graft.

The initial experience with endovascular repair of TAAs was gained by using home-made devices. With technology proceeding at fast pace, both custom-designed and commercially produced stent-grafts are available for treating thoracic aortic disease and various institutions have substantiated both safety and effectiveness of stent-grafts for the repair of TAAs (➲Table 31.3) [97–117].

Despite limited follow-up, endovascular techniques appear attractive in emergency situations, with high procedural and clinical success rates. The teamwork of cardiologists, radiologists, anaesthesiologists, and cardiovascular surgeons is necessary for optimal results. The intervention is mostly performed under general anaesthesia, but local anaesthesia has also been used [118]. Access to the peripheral artery requires surgical cut-down for the 22–24F sheaths. The preferred and most common site (41–58%) of vascular access is the common femoral artery. Less frequently, access to the iliac artery (9–44%) via an extraperitoneal approach is required. Retroperitoneal exposure to the abdominal aorta is necessary in 14–30% of cases, especially in tiny elderly women [119]. In patients with multiple aortic aneurysms involving both the thoracic and abdominal aorta, a combination of conventional abdominal aortic replacement with endovascular stent-graft placement into the thoracic aorta under fluoroscopic guidance is feasible. Under fluoroscopic guidance the stent-graft is advanced using a stiff wire in order to overcome the elongation of the iliac arteries and the aorta, which can be difficult [71]. Positioning of the customized stent-graft is regarded as crucial and can be aided by transoesophageal ultrasound, whereas for surgery of the abdominal aorta it is helpful to have the intravascular ultrasound probe located in the inferior vena cava. Lowering the blood pressure by rapid right ventricular pacing is essential

Table 31.3 Overview of the published data regarding endovascular treatment of thoracic aortic aneurysms

Author, year [reference]	N	Follow-up (month)	Technical success (%)	30-day mortality (%)	Paraplegia (%)	Endoleak (%)	Long-term survival (%)	Devices
Dake, 1998 [95]	103	22	83	9	3	24	73 (2 years)	Home-made
Ehrlich, 1998 [96]	10	NA	80	10	0	20	NA	Talent
Cartes-Zumelzu, 2000 [97]	32	16	90.6	9.4	3.1	15.4	90.2 (32 months)	Excluder, Talent
Grabenwoger, 2000 [98]	21	NA	100	9.5	0	14.3	NA	Talent, Prograft
Najibi, 2002 [99]	24	12	94.7	5.3	0	0	89.5 (1 year)	Excluder, Talent
Heijmen, 2002 [100]	28	21	96.4	0	0	28.6	96.4 (21 months)	Talent, Excluder
Schoder, 2003 [101]	28	22.7	100	0	0	25	80.2 (3 years)	Excluder
Bell, 2003 [102]	67	17	NA	2	4	4.8	89 (1 year)	Gore, Talent
Lepore, 2003 [103]	21	12	100	9.5	4.8	19	76.2 (1 year)	Excluder, Talent
Ouriel, 2003 [104]	31	6	NA	12.9	6.5	32.3	81.6	Excluder, Talent
Czerny, 2004 [105]	54	38	94.4	9.3	0	27.8	63 (3 years)	Excluder, Talent
Makaroun, 2004 [106]	142	29.6	97.9	1.5	3.5	8.8	75 (2 years)	TAG
Leurs, 2004 [107]	249	1–60	87	10.4	4	4.2	80.1 (1 year)	Excluder, Talent, Zenith, Endofit
Glade, 2005 [108]	42	15	NA	NA	2	NA	NA	Gore, Talent
Greenberg, 2005 [109]	100	14	NA	NA	1	6	83 (1 year)	Zenith
Riesenmann, 2005 [110]	50	9	96	NA	0	10	79.4 (1 year)	Talent
Ricco, 2006 [111]	166	NA	NA	5	3.6	16.2	NA	Gore, Talent
Wheatley, 2006 [112]	156	21.5	98.7	3.8	0.6	11.5	76.6 (1 year)	Gore
Bavaria, 2007 [113]	140	24	98	2.1	2.9	10	NA	Gore

before deploying a stent-graft in order to avoid a stent shift [120]. Angiography after implantation will reveal satisfying wall apposition of the stent. If endoleaks are found, additional balloon inflations may be necessary to obtain good strut apposition to the wall. After stenting, patients can usually be rapidly extubated and discharged after a few days. In some patients inflammation is seen, described as graft disease with high levels of C-reactive protein but negative values for procalcitonin, leading to some chest discomfort that responds to indometacin. The aortic arch morphology is challenging because of angulation and the proximity of the supra-aortic branches that need to be preserved.

Traditional open arch reconstruction using hypothermic cardiac arrest, extracorporeal circulation, and selective cerebral perfusion has been demonstrated to effectively manage aortic arch pathologies. However, this current standard procedure for any arch pathology carries significant mortality (2–9%) and risk of paraplegia and cerebral stroke in 4–13% of cases [121, 122]. Therefore, open repair is often reserved for low-risk patients. Hybrid arch procedures (HAP) are a combination of debranching bypass (supra-aortic vessel transposition) to establish cerebral perfusion and subsequent thoracic endografting to provide patient-centred solutions for complex aortic arch lesions. HAP is performed without hypothermic circulatory arrest and extracorporeal circulation and could expand the treatment group to older patients with severe co-morbidities and redo-surgery currently ineligible for open surgical intervention. To treat distal arch aneurysms involving both the left subclavian and the left common carotid artery, those vessels can be translocated upstream to the right common carotid artery approached via cervical access (hemi-arch debranching). For arch aneurysms extending to the innominate artery the ascending aorta can be used, via sternotomy, as a donor site to revascularize all three supra-aortic arteries (total arch debranching) [123–129]. The key to success is the quality of the unimpaired ascending aorta as a donor site for the debranching bypass and proximal landing zone for the endografts (➲Fig. 31.12). Primary technical success was generally defined as complete exclusion of the TAA, endograft patency, and restoration of normal blood flow immediately after EVR. Secondary technical success was defined as complete TAA exclusion, graft patency, and restoration of blood flow within 30 days of endograft placement. Endoleak was defined as perigraft leakage of contrast medium into TAA sac as demonstrated by imaging either postinterventionally or during follow-up examinations. Endoleaks result from incomplete exclusion of the aneurysm. Type I endoleaks are defined as those occurring around the stent-graft, while type II endoleaks are those occurring through collateral arteries. Type III endoleaks are those resulting

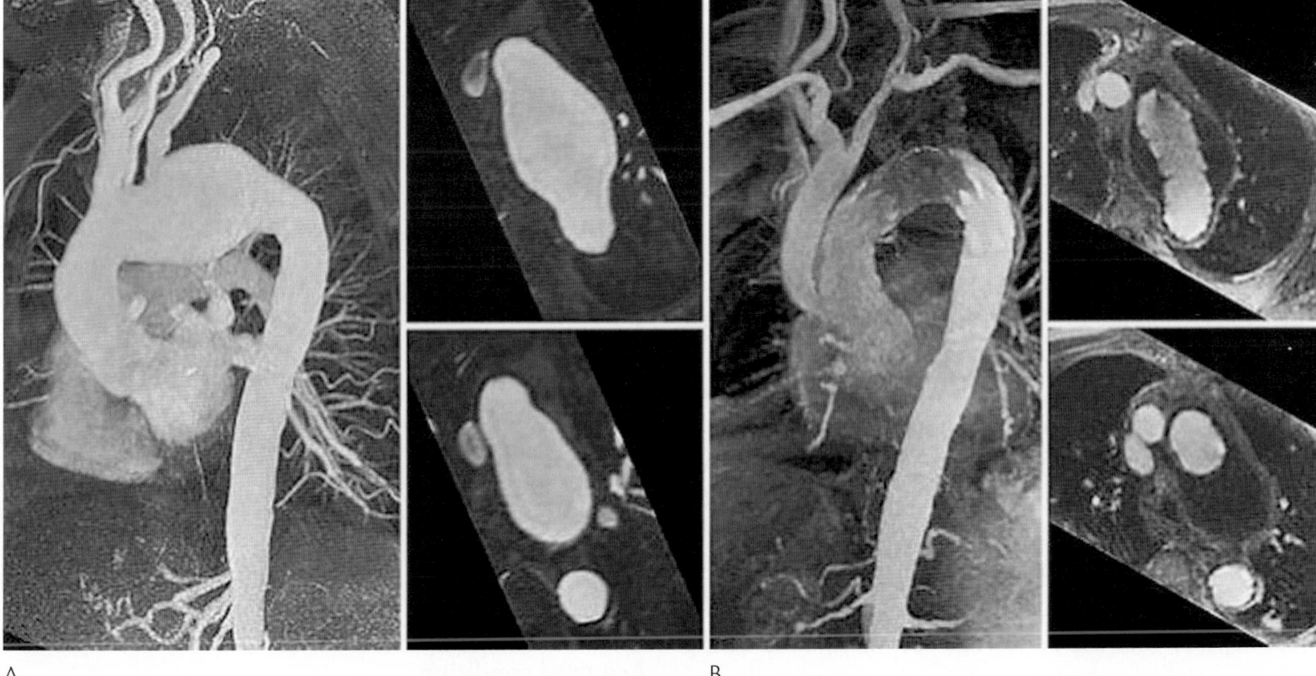

Figure 31.12 Contrast-medium enhanced MR-angiography of the aorta in a case of an aortic arch aneurysm. (A) Aneurysm of the aortic arch involving the supra-aortic branches. (B) Postinterventional-surgical result after hybrid procedure with debranching of the supraaortic vessels and stent-graft implanatation in the aortic arch.

from small holes in the graft, and type IV endoleaks are due to large holes. Several studies reported high success rates with 85–100% of procedures in successful deployment and functional exclusion of the aneurysm. Major complications occurred in 14–18% of patients depending upon the acuity at presentation with very low incidence of paraplegia. Early and late mortality rate ranged from 0–14% and is usually attributable to the preoperative status of the patients. Most studies showed a patient survival rate of 70–80% at 1, 3, and 5 years. Data from 457 patients treated with stent-grafts and collected in a registry (113 emergency and 344 elective cases) revealed that among 422 patients who survived the interventional procedure (in-hospital mortality 5%), mortality during follow-up was 8.5% (36 patients), of which 11 patients had died from the aortic disease; persistent endoleak was reported in 64 cases, and Kaplan–Meier overall survival estimates at 1, 3, and 5 years were 90.9%, 85.4%, and 77.5%. At the same intervals, freedom from a second procedure (either open conversion or endovascular) was 92.5%, 81.3%, and 70.0%, respectively [130]. A 6-year prospective case series involving 84 patients was completed by Ellozy *et al.* Primary technical success was achieved in 90%, and successful exclusion of the aneurysm was achieved in 82%. However, major procedure-related or device-related complications occurred in 38%, including proximal attachment failure (8%), distal attachment failure (6%), mechanical device failure (3%), periprocedural death (6%), and late aneurysm rupture (6%). More encouraging was the fact that only 3% suffered persistent neurological complications [131–133].

Dissection of the thoracic aorta

Aortic dissection results from separation of aortic wall layers in the setting of elevated blood pressure and concomitant degenerative changes in the aortic media. As the proximal aorta is subject to the steepest fluctuations in pressure, it has the highest risk of dissection. Degeneration of the aortic media is part of the normal ageing process, but is accelerated in the setting of BAV, Turner's syndrome, inflammatory arteritis, or inherited diseases of collagen formation (➲Table 31.4). Propagation of the dissection causes much of the morbidity associated with aortic dissection by disrupting blood flow across branch vessels, by direct rupture into the pericardial sac, or by obstructing aortic flow (Lériche syndrome). Over time, the false lumen of the dissection may expand critically with aortic rupture and exsanguination [134–156].

Table 31.4 Risk conditions for aortic dissection

Long-standing arterial hypertension		
	Smoking, dyslipidaemia, cocaine/crack	
Connective tissue disorders		
	Hereditary fibrillinopathies	
		Marfan syndrome
		Ehlers–Danlos syndrome
	Hereditary vascular disease	
		Bicuspid aortic disease
		Coarctiation
Vascular inflammation		
	Giant cell arteritis	
	Takayasu's arteritis	
	Behçet's disease	
	Syphilis	
	Ormond's disease	
Deceleration trauma		
	Car accident	
	Fall from height	
Iatrogenic factors		
	Catheter/instrument intervention	
	Valvular/aortic surgery	
		Side- or cross-clamping/aortotomy
		Graft anastomosis
		Patch aortoplasty
		Aortic wall fragility

Epidemiology

Aortic dissection is a rare disease, with an estimated incidence of approximately 2.6–3.5 cases per 100,000 person/year with high prevalence in Italy (4.04/100,000/year) [134, 157]. Around 0.5% of patients presenting to an emergency department with chest or back pain suffer from aortic dissection [139]. Two-thirds of patients are male, with an average age at presentation of approximately 65 years. A history of systemic hypertension, found in up to 72% of patients, is by far the most common risk factor [15, 134]. Atherosclerosis, a history of prior cardiac surgery, and known aortic aneurysm are other major risk factors [134]. The epidemiology of aortic dissection is substantially different in young patients (<40 years of age) where risk factors such as Marfan syndrome take precedence. Conditions for aortic dissection can be distributed in (➲Table 31.5):

Acquired conditions

Chronic hypertension affects arterial wall composition, causing intimal thickening, fibrosis and calcification, and

Table 31.5 Demographics and history of patients with acute aortic dissection

Variable	n* (%)	Type A, n (%) (N=289)	Type B, n (%) (N=175)	P Type A vs. B
Demographics				
Age, mean (SD), years	63.1 (14.0)	61.2 (14.1)	66.3 (13.2)	<0.001
Male	303 (65.3)	182 (63.0)	121 (69.1)	0.18
Patient history				
Marfan syndrome	22/449 (4.9)	19 (6.7)	3 (1.8)	0.02
Hypertension	326/452 (72.1)	194 (69.3)	132 (76.7)	0.08
Atherosclerosis	140/452 (31.0)	69 (24.4)	71 (42)	<0.001
Prior aortic dissection	29/453 (6.4)	11 (3.9)	18 (10.6)	0.005
Prior aortic aneurysm	73/453 (16.1)	35 (12.4)	4 (2.3)	0.006
Diabetes	23/451 (5.1)	12 (4.3)	11 (6.6)	0.29
Prior cardiac surgery	83 (17.9)	46 (15.9)	37 (21.1)	0.16

N=464.

* Denominator of reported responses is given if different than stated in the column heading.

Reproduced with permission from Hagan PG, Nienaber CA, Isselbacher EM *et al.* The international registry of acute aortic dissection (IRAD): new insights into an old disease. *JAMA* 2000; **283**: 897–903.

extracellular fatty acid deposition. In parallel the extracellular matrix undergoes accelerated degradation, apoptosis and elastolysis with hyalinization of collagen. Both mechanisms may eventually lead to intimal disruption. Moreover, adventitial fibrosis may obstruct nutrient vessels feeding the arterial wall as well as small intramural vasa vasorum. Both result in necrosis of smooth muscle cells and fibrosis of elastic structures, rendering the vessel wall vulnerable to pulsatile forces and creating a substrate for aneurysms and dissections [15, 144–147]. In addition to chronic hypertension, smoking, dyslipidaemia and, potentially, the use of crack cocaine are modulating risk factors. On rare occasions, inflammatory diseases destroy the media layers and cause weakening, expansion, and dissection of the aortic wall. Iatrogenic aortic dissection may occur in association with invasive retrograde catheter interventions, during or after valve aortic surgery [15, 148–150]. Given the morbidity and mortality of iatrogenic aortic dissection, careful assessment is strongly encouraged in patients with unexplained haemodynamic instability or malperfusion syndromes following invasive vascular procedures or aortic surgery (➲Table 31.6).

Finally, pregnancy-related dissection, although a dramatic scenario, is a rare event as long as the patient is not affected by any form of connective tissue disease. The putative association of pregnancy in otherwise healthy women and acute dissection may largely be an artefact of selective reporting. Pregnancy is a common condition and may coincidentally occur only with concomitant existence of other risk factors, such as long-standing or pregnancy-associated hypertension, or Marfan syndrome. Preliminary data from the International Registry of Aortic Dissection (IRAD) show that pregnancy in Marfan syndrome is not associated with aortic tears unless root size exceeds 40mm.

Marfan syndrome

Among hereditary diseases, Marfan syndrome is the most prevalent connective tissue disorder, with an estimated incidence of 1 in 7000 and autosomal dominant inheritance with variable penetrance. More than 150 mutations on the fibrillin-1 (*FBN-1*) gene have been identified encoding for a defective fibrillin in the ECM, which may affect the ocular, cardiovascular, skeletal, and pulmonary systems, as well as skin and dura mater. The diagnosis of Marfan syndrome is currently based on the revised clinical criteria of the 'Gent nosology' [151]. The Gent criteria pay particular attention to genetic information, e.g. the appearance of Marfan syndrome in kindreds of an unequivocally affected individual. Moreover, both skeletal and cardiovascular features are major (i.e. diagnostic) criteria if four of eight typical manifestations are present. However, borderline manifestations such as the MASS phenotype or subtle phenotypic features

Table 31.6 Aetiology of iatrogenic aortic dissection in International Registry of Aortic Dissection (IRAD)

Cause	Type A	Type B
Cardiac surgery	18 (69%)	1 (12%)
Coronarography/intervention	7 (27%)	7 (87%)
Renal angioplasty	1 (4%)	–
Complication	**Iatrogenic**	**Spontaneous**
Myocardial ischaemia	36%*	5%
Myocardial infarction	15%*	3%
Limb ischaemia	14%	8%
Mortality (30 days)	35%	24%

* $p \leq 0.001$.

Reproduced with permission from Hagan PG, Nienaber CA, Isselbacher EM *et al.* The international registry of acute aortic dissection (IRAD): new insights into an old disease. *JAMA* 2000; **283**: 897–903.

(forme fruste), the molecular analysis of suspected Marfan syndrome and the delineation of criteria for differentiating other inherited conditions (genotypes) from the Marfan phenotype are attracting interest [27, 152–155]. The clinical variety of Marfan syndrome is only partially explained by the number of mutations on the *FBN-1* gene. Genetic heterogeneity and the involvement of a second gene (*MFS2*, Marfan syndrome type 2) may further add to the broad spectrum of symptoms [156, 157].

A common denominator of all phenotypic forms of aortic wall disease is the dedifferentiation of vascular smooth muscle cells, not only with classic aneurysm formation but also from enhanced elastolysis of aortic wall components [158], as shown in a fibrillin-1-deficient animal model [159]. Moreover, enhanced expression of metalloproteinases in vascular smooth muscle cells of the Marfan aorta may promote both fragmentation of medial elastic layers and elastolysis, thus initiating an activated phenotype of smooth muscle cells [160]. In parallel, expression of peroxisome proliferator activated receptor (PPAR) is upregulated in smooth muscle cells of Marfan aorta and with cystic medial degeneration and correlates with clinical severity, while vascular smooth muscle cell apoptosis is likely to be related to progression of aortic dilatation. Thus, PPAR expression might reflect the pathogenesis of cystic medial degeneration and disease progression in the aorta of both Marfan syndrome and non-Marfan disease without any vascular inflammatory response [161].

Ehlers–Danlos syndrome

Ehlers–Danlos syndrome is a heterogeneous group of hereditable connective tissue disorders characterized by articular hypermobility, skin hyperextensibility, and tissue fragility. Eleven types of Ehlers–Danlos syndrome have been characterized; the true prevalence is unknown. An aggregate incidence of 1 in 5000 births is often cited, with no racial or ethnic predisposition. Aortic involvement is seen primarily in autosomal dominant Ehlers–Danlos syndrome type IV [162].

Annulo-aortic ectasia and familial aortic dissection

More than five mutations in the *FBN-1* gene have now been identified in patients presenting with either sporadic or familial forms of TAA and dissection [163, 164]. Histological examination of the aortic wall reveals elastolysis or loss of elastic fibres, deposits of mucopolysaccharide-like material, and cystic medial degeneration similar to that in Marfan syndrome. However, no abnormalities of types I and III collagen or any specific fibrillopathy have been found in fibroblast cultures.

AAA and dissection

Careful examination of family pedigrees often reveals both involvement of the abdominal aorta and disease in proximal aortic segments, or other features suggestive of Marfan or Ehlers–Danlos syndrome. Differentiation of familial forms of AAA/dissection from TAA/dissection with an abdominal component is difficult considering that only one mutation within the *COL3A1* gene is known [164]. In fact, many candidate genes encoding for collagens, fibrillins, fibrullins, microfibril-associated glycoproteins, and MMPs and their inhibitors have been investigated but no mutation has been identified. Similar pathogenetic processes have been described with coarctation and with the BAV architecture [144, 145].

Definition and classification

According to the acuity, aortic dissection diagnosed within 2 weeks of the onset of symptoms during the early phase of high mortality is an acute dissection. Patients who survive 2 weeks without treatment are considered subacute or even chronic cases after 8 weeks. About one-third of patients with aortic dissection fall into the chronic category [165]. Aortic dissections are further classified according to their anatomic location using the Stanford and DeBakey classification. The fundamental distinction is whether the dissection is proximal (involving the aortic root or ascending aorta) or distal (beyond the left subclavian artery). The Stanford classification of aortic dissection distinguishes between type A and type B (➲Fig. 31.13) [166, 167]. Type A involves the ascending aorta, while type B dissection does not. The De Bakey classification subdivides the dissection process into type I dissection involving the entire aorta, type II dissection involving only the ascending aorta, and type III dissection sparing the ascending aorta and the arch. Various attempts to further subdivide both classification systems have not been established [168, 169], although the arch region deserves integration into a modern classification system. Recent observations highlight the importance of precursors of typical aortic dissection such as intramural haematoma, penetrating aortic ulcers, or localized intimal tears as variants of a wall-dissecting process (➲Fig. 31.14) [170–173].

Classic aortic dissection

Acute aortic dissection is characterized by the rapid development of an intimal flap separating the true and false lumen [174–176]. In the majority of cases (approximately 90%) intimal tears are identified as sites of communication between true and false lumen. The dissection can spread in

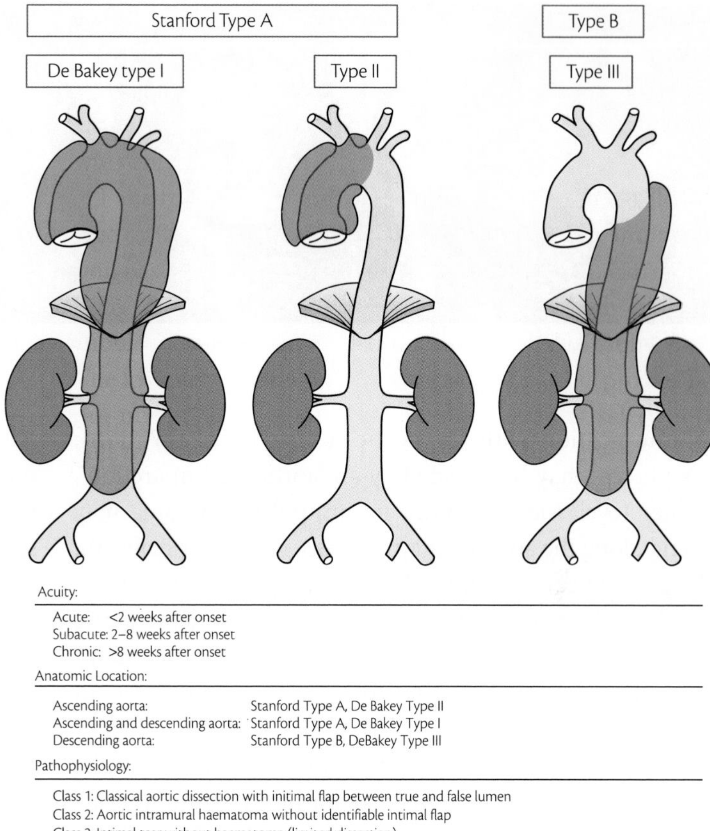

Stanford Type A
Type B
De Bakey type I
Type II
Type III
Acuity:
Acute: <2 weeks after onset
Subacute: 2–8 weeks after onset
Chronic: >8 weeks after onset
Anatomic Location:
Ascending aorta: Stanford Type A, De Bakey Type II
Ascending and descending aorta: Stanford Type A, De Bakey Type I
Descending aorta: Stanford Type B, DeBakey Type III
Pathophysiology:
Class 1: Classical aortic dissection with initimal flap between true and false lumen
Class 2: Aortic intramural haematoma without identifiable intimal flap
Class 3: Intimal tear without haematoma (limited dissection)
Class 4: Atherosclerotic plaque rupture with aortic penetrating ulcer
Class 5: Iatrogenic or traumatic aortic dissection (intra-aortic catheterization, high-speed deceleration injury, blunt chest trauma)

Figure 31.13 The most common classification systems of thoracic aortic dissection.

an antegrade or retrograde fashion, involving side branches and causing complications such as malperfusion syndrome by dynamic or static obstruction (from coronary to iliac arteries), tamponade, or aortic insufficiency. The arbitrary classification of acute, subacute, or chronic dissection appears helpful for neither didactic nor differential therapeutic considerations, but may rather be used to describe the individual situation and time span of survival of a given patient. From a pathophysiological point of view, progression of dissection is difficult to predict once a patient with dissection has survived the initial 2 weeks after its inception, although false lumen expansion is likely to develop over time. Several clinical features may be used to roughly estimate late risk, including evidence of persistent communication, patent false channel, and others [169, 174, 175].

Intramural haematoma

Aortic intramural haematoma is considered a precursor of classic dissection, and originates from ruptured vasa vasorum in medial wall layers, eventually provoking a secondary

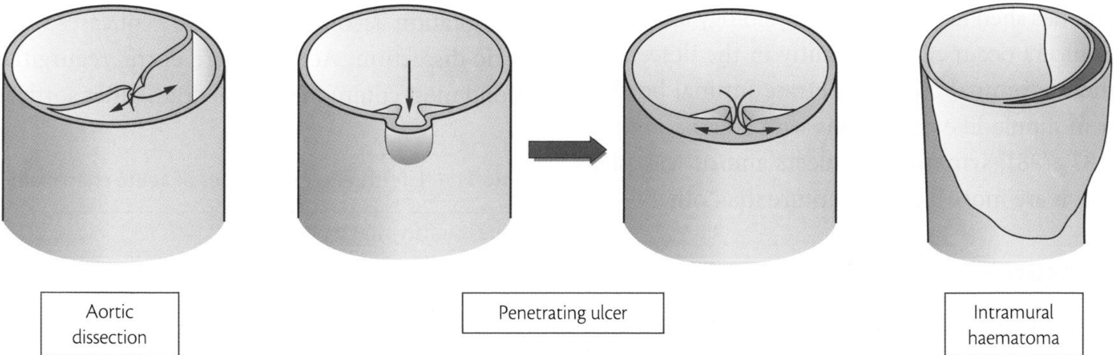

Figure 31.14 Schematic representation of AD (left), penetrating ulcer (middle) and IMH (right).

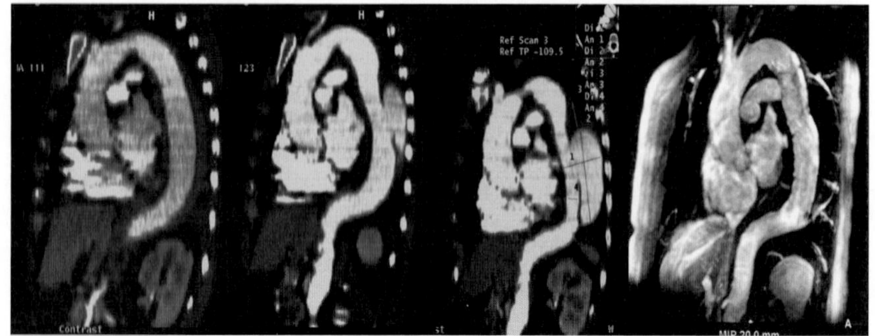

Figure 31.15 Evolutions of acute IMH of the descending aorta (left) to growing local dissection and formation of an aneurysm on spiral contrast-enhanced CAT scans within 4 months; reconstruction of the dissected aorta and exclusion of aneurysm after interventional stent-graft placement. F/U indicates follow-up.

communication with the aortic lumen [172, 177, 178]; this process may be initiated by an 'aortic wall infarction'. Similar to classic dissection, intramural haematoma may extend along the aorta or may progress, regress, or reabsorb. The prevalence of intramural haemorrhage is 10–30% [172, 178–180]. Intramural haematoma can lead to acute aortic dissection in 21–47% of patients or to regression in about 10%. Involvement of the ascending aorta is considered an indication for expeditious surgery due to the inherent risk of rupture, tamponade, or compression of coronary ostia. Distal intramural haematoma may warrant watchful waiting and, potentially, stent-graft placement (➲Fig. 31.15) [178, 180–183]. Studies in Asian patients from Japan and Korea have argued that wall haematoma reflects a more benign condition, in which aggressive medical therapy and serial imaging allow a watchful waiting strategy [181, 182]. The reasons for this disparity may relate either to a different gene pool of Asian and white patients or to semantic differences. However, at present the cardiological and surgical communities have generally concluded that acute intramural haematoma involving the ascending aorta should be managed surgically in the same way as type A dissection.

Plaque rupture/ulceration

Ulceration of atherosclerotic aortic plaques can lead to aortic dissection or perforation [184–186]. Non-invasive imaging of aortic ulceration has been improved by tomographic scanning and has shed light on pathophysiology and aetiology. Aortic ulcers occur predominantly in the descending thoracic and abdominal aorta, penetrate intimal borders, and appear in nipple-like projections with an adjacent haematoma [187, 188]; symptomatic ulcers and/or with signs of deep erosion are more likely to rupture than others.

Clinical features

The challenge in managing acute aortic syndrome, and especially dissection, is appropriate clinical suspicion and action in pursuing diagnosis and therapy [189, 190]. The differential diagnosis for acute aortic dissection includes acute coronary syndrome, pulmonary embolus, pneumothorax, pneumonia, musculoskeletal pain, acute cholecystitis, oesophageal spasm or rupture, acute pancreatitis, and acute pericarditis (➲Table 31.7). Typical features of dissection are the acute onset of chest and/or back pain of blunt, radiating, and migrating nature. The pain could be sharp, ripping, tearing, or knife-like in nature, but the abruptness is the most specific characteristic of the pain. According to a report on 464 patients from the IRAD, 95% of patients reported any pain, and 85% reported an abrupt onset [134]. Sharp pain was reported by 64% of patients, whereas the classic tearing or ripping type of pain was reported by 51% of patients. The most common site of pain was the chest (73%), with anterior location being more common than the posterior location (61% vs. 36%, respectively). Back pain was experienced in 53% of patients, and abdominal pain was experienced by 30% of patients. Extension of the pain down to the back, abdomen, hips, and legs indicates the extension of the dissection process distally. Chronic hypertension is common if obvious signs of connective tissue disorders are absent. Clinical manifestations of acute aortic dissection are often explained by specific malperfusion syndrome from dissection-related side-branch obstruction. More than one-third of the patients with aortic dissection demonstrate signs and symptoms secondary to the organ system involvement [134]. Aortic regurgitation accompanies 18–50% of cases with proximal aortic dissection. Acute, severe aortic regurgitation is the second most common cause of death (after aortic rupture) in

Table 31.7 Life-threatening causes of acute chest pain

Acute coronary syndromes
Aortic dissection
Pulmonary embolus
Tension pneumothorax
Oesophageal rupture

patients with aortic dissection. Patients with this condition usually present with acute cardiac decompensation and shock. The mechanism of aortic regurgitation in aortic dissection include dilatation of the aortic root and annulus, tearing of the annulus or valve cusps, downward displacement of one cusp below the line of the valve closure, loss of support of the cusp, and physical interference in the closure of the aortic valve by an intimal flap. Although most patients with aortic dissections have hypertension at time of presentation, an initial systolic BP <100mmHg has been reported in about 25% of patients with aortic dissection. Hypotension and shock in patients with aortic dissection are caused by acute severe aortic regurgitation, aortic rupture, cardiac tamponade, or left ventricular systolic dysfunction [134]. The presence of pulse differentials is the most specific physical sign of aortic dissection, and it has been reported in 38% of patients with aortic dissection [134]. Every fifth case of acute aortic dissection may present with syncope from tamponade, severe hypotension, or carotid obstruction [134–140]. Cerebrovascular manifestations, limb ischaemia, or pulse deficits are caused by involvement of a side-branch orifice into the dissection or obliteration of the true lumen by an expanding false lumen [141, 191]. Paraplegia may emerge if too many pairs of intercostal arteries are separated from the aortic lumen (➲Table 31.8).

Recurrent abdominal pain, elevation of acute-phase proteins, and increase of lactate dehydrogenase are indicators of involvement of either the coeliac trunk (observed in approximately 8%) or superior mesenteric artery (in 8–13%).

Table 31.8 Clinical findings in aortic dissection

Clinical findings
Hypotension or shock due to: a. Hemopericardium and pericardial tamponade b. Mediastinal bleeding c. Acute aortic insufficiency due to dilatation of the aortic annulus d. Aortic rupture e. Lactic acidosis f. Spinal shock
Acute myocardial ischaemia/infarction due to coronary ostial occlusion
Pericardial friction rub due to hemopericardium
Syncope
Pleural effusion or frank haemothorax
Pressure differences, pulse deficits, Leriche syndrome
Acute renal failure due to dissection across renal arteries
Mesenteric ischaemia due to dissection across intra-abdominal arteries
Neurologic deficits: a. Stroke due to occlusion of arch vessels b. Limb weakness c. Spinal cord deficits due to cord ischaemia d. Hoarseness due to compression of left recurrent laryngeal nerve

Involvement of renal arteries may result in oliguria or anuria and propagation of dissection is heralded by repetitive bouts of pain or a deteriorating clinical picture [21, 152].

Pulse deficits on physical examination occur in about 20% and are important clues heralding complications and bad outcome (➲Fig. 31.16). A diastolic murmur indicative of aortic regurgitation is seen in approximately 50% of patients with proximal dissection. Signs of pericardial effusion, jugular venous distension, or a paradoxical pulse should provoke confirmation of the diagnosis. Shock may be a presenting sign, resulting from tamponade, coronary compression, acute aortic valve incompetence, or loss of blood and imminent exsanguinations [134, 141, 143, 189].

Consequently, the differential diagnosis of acute aortic dissection should always be considered in patients presenting with chest pain, back pain, unexplained syncope, abdominal pain, stroke, acute onset of congestive heart failure, pulse differentials, or malperfusion syndrome of extremities or viscera. In the present absence of useful specific biomarkers for aortic dissection, interpretation of positive cardiac markers may be even more complex in the scenario of aortic dissection compromising coronary ostia.

Natural history

Despite major advances in the non-invasive diagnosis of aortic dissection and in therapy, up to 28–55% of patients die without a correct ante mortem diagnosis [165]. The risk of death is increased in patients with complications such as pericardial tamponade, involvement of coronary arteries, or malperfusion of the brain or intestine [175, 192, 193]. Other predictors of increased in-hospital death include age ≥70 years, hypotension, kidney failure, and pulse deficits (➲Table 31.9) [134, 192]. Less appreciated predisposing factors for type A dissection include prior cardiac and valvular

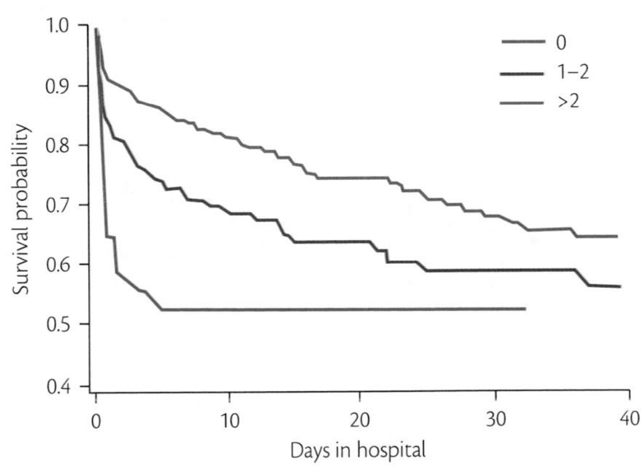

Figure 31.16 Kaplan–Meier survival curves from patients with and without pulse deficits; log-rank for curves of patients with 1, 2, or 3 or more pulse deficits differ from patients with no pulse deficits (*P* <0.03 and 0.004).

Table 31.9 Independent predictors of in-hospital death after aortic dissection

	Overall type A,%	Among survivors,%	Among deaths,%	Parameter coefficient	P	OR for death (95% CI)
Age >70 years	35.2	30.0	46.1	0.53	0.03	1.70 (1.05–2.77)
Female	34.5	30.7	42.7	0.32	0.20	1.38 (0.85–2.27)
Abrupt onset pain*	84.5	82.3	89.0	0.96	0.01	2.60 (1.22–5.54)
Abnormal ECG*	69.6	65.2	79.5	0.57	0.03	1.77 (1.06–2.95)
Any pulse deficit*	30.1	24.7	41.1	0.71	0.004	2.03 (1.25–3.29)
Kidney failure**	5.6	2.9	11.9	1.56	0.002	4.77 (1.80–12.6)
Hypotension/shock/ tamponade*	29.0	20.1	47.1	1.09	<0.0001	2.97 (1.83–4.81)

OR indicates odds ratio; CI, confidence interval.

* On presentation;

** On presentation and before surgery.

Reproduced with permission from Hagan PG, Nienaber CA, Isselbacher EM *et al.* The international registry of acute aortic dissection (IRAD): new insights into an old disease. *JAMA* 2000; **283**: 897–903.

surgery (15%) and iatrogenic dissection from cardiac surgery or catheterization (5%). Iatrogenic aortic dissection carries a mortality slightly higher than non-iatrogenic (35% versus 24%) [15, 134]. Data from the largest registry of acute aortic dissection showed that in the absence of immediate surgical repair, medical management is associated with a mortality of nearly 24% at day 1, 29% at 48 hours, 44% at day 7, and 50% after 2 weeks (➲Fig. 31.17) [5, 144]. Less than 10% of untreated patients with proximal aortic dissection live for 1 year, and almost all patients die within 10 years. Most of these deaths occur within the first 3 months. The risk of fatal aortic rupture in patients with untreated proximal aortic dissection is around 90%, and 75% of these ruptures take place in the pericardium, the left pleural cavity, and the mediastinum. Even with surgical repair, in-hospital mortality rates are 10% after 1 day, 12% at 2 days, and nearly 20% at 2 weeks with aortic rupture, stroke, visceral ischaemia, cardiac tamponade, and circulatory failure as the most common causes for death [5, 15, 134].

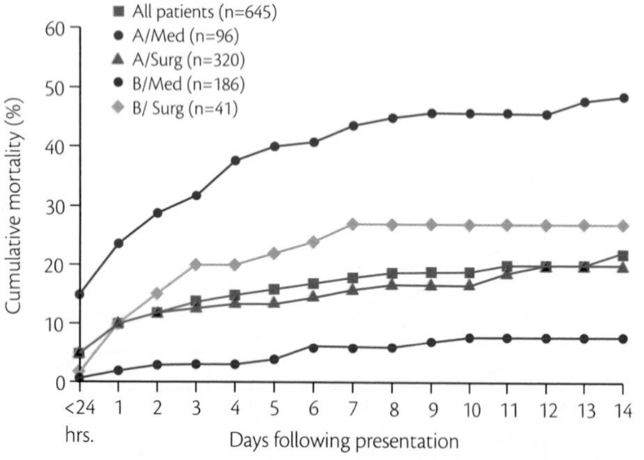

Figure 31.17 Fourteen-day mortality in 645 patients from the IRAD registry stratified by medical and surgical treatment in both type A and B aortic dissection. Reproduced with permission from Hagan PG, Nienaber CA, Isselbacher EM *et al.* The international registry of acute aortic dissection (IRAD): new insights into an old disease. *JAMA* 2000; **283**: 897–903.

Acute aortic dissection of the descending aorta is less frequently lethal. In the absence of treatment, survival rates are 89% at 1 month, 84% at 1 year, and 80% at 5 years [135]. However, patients with complications such as renal failure, visceral ischaemia, or contained rupture often require urgent repair, with a mortality of 20% at day 2 and 25% at 1 month. Similar to type A dissection, advanced age, rupture, shock, and malperfusion are important independent predictors of early mortality [134].

Proximal location of IMH is clearly considered an independent predictor of progression to dissection, contained rupture, or aneurysm formation independent of age, sex, hypertension, Marfan syndrome, BAV, or local extent and diameters of IMH [178]. Global experience suggests mortality at 30 days at around 20% with an early death rate of 16% [171, 194]. Proximal (type A) IMH is no longer related to early death when surgical repair is performed [195]. The high risk of 'wait and see' in type A IMH, though, is reflected in 55% early mortality with medical treatment compared to 8% with surgical repair ($p = 0.004$). Considering a 12% early mortality after surgery, and a 24% death rate with medical treatment, global experience from the IRAD confirmed a trend of improved outcome after surgery of proximal IMH ($p = 0.12$) [195]. Moreover, actuarial survival analysis showed better long term survival on oral beta-blocker treatment with 95% versus 67% without beta-blockers (p = 0.004). Beta-adrenergic blocking agents protect by reducing wall stress, systolic arterial pressure, and the rate of pressure changes and, presumably stabilize the extracellular vascular matrix of the aorta [171, 195]. The observation that older age (>55 years) at initial diagnosis of IMH has a better long-term prognosis may be explained by more focal microscars along the aortic wall inherently limiting the longitudinal progression of IMH [187]. Accordingly, favourable outcomes of IMH are consistently reported in patients beyond 65 years [187]. Thus, considering both advanced aortosclerosis with older age and the lower risk of progression, a conservative strategy (with beta-blockade and serial imaging) may be justified in elderly multimorbid patients and in distal IMH [187].

Ulcer-like projections in aortic segments of IMH identify a subset of patients at high risk. Penetrating atherosclerotic ulcers (PAU) are known to result from progressive erosion of mural plaque penetrating the elastic lamina and finally separating media layers, thus setting the stage for adjacent IMH. PAUs are preferentially (>90%) observed in IMH of the descending aorta, while IMH without PAU is more frequently present in the ascending aorta. Symptomatic PAU infers complications such as formation of aneurysm, pseudoaneurysm, and dissection, or unpredictable rupture. Careful imaging is vital to identify both diameter and depth of ulcers with IMH, since width >2cm and depth >1cm may herald the need for interventional or surgical repair to avoid rupture and death [141].

Diagnostic procedures

The diagnosis of aortic dissection begins with clinical suspicion, as the most crucial step in work-up of this catastrophic condition. The diagnostic modalities currently available include aortography, contrast-enhanced CT, MRI, and transthoracic (TTE) or transoesophageal echocardiography (TOE) (➲Table 31.10). Most importantly, any diagnostic study must confirm or refute the diagnosis of aortic dissection. Second, the diagnostic modality must discern whether the dissection involves the ascending aorta or is confined to the descending aorta or arch. Third, anatomic features of the dissection, including its extent, the sites of entry and re-entry, the presence of thrombus in the false lumen, branch vessel involvement by the dissection, presence or absence of pericardial effusion, and any coronary involvement need to be known. Unfortunately, no single imaging modality provides all details. The diagnosis should be confirmed rapidly and accurately, preferable with an easily available non-invasive modality.

Table 31.10 Comparative diagnostic utility of imaging techniques in aortic dissection

	TOE	CT	MRI	Aortography
Sensitivity	++	++	+++	++
Specificity	+++	++	+++	++
Classification	+++	++	++	+
Intimal flap	+++	–	++	+
Aortic regurgitation	+++	–	++	++
Pericardial effusion	+++	++	++	–
Branch vessel involvement	+	++	++	+++
Coronary artery involvement	++	+	+	+++

Reproduced from Erbel R, Alfonso F, Boileau C *et al.* Task Force on Aortic Dissection of the European Society of Cardiology. Diagnosis and management of aortic dissection. *Eur Heart J* 2001; **22**: 1642–81.

In laboratory analyses a mild-to-moderate leucocytosis occurs in two-thirds of patients, and anaemia may occur as a result of leakage of the dissection or from sequestration of blood in the false lumen. This is also the reason for extensive D-dimer elevation found particularly in acute dissection, which reaches the level of pulmonary embolism. Aortic dissection causes extensive damage to the smooth muscle cells of the media, leading to the release of structural proteins of the smooth muscle cells including smooth muscle myosin heavy chain into the circulation. The most common electrocardiographic abnormality is left ventricular hypertrophy from systemic hypertension. Acute electrocardiographic changes occur in up to 55% of patients and include ST segment depression, T-wave changes, and ST segment elevation. Myocardial infarction occurs in 1–2% of patients due to compromise of the coronary ostium by the haematoma or intimal flap [143].

In the emergency department, chest radiography is a mainstay of the evaluation of acute chest pain. Moreover, routine chest radiography is abnormal in 56% of cases of suspected aortic dissection [143]. The classic radiographic sign that is suggestive of aortic dissection is the widening of the mediastinal shadow. Other signs are altered configuration of the aorta, a localized hump on the aortic arch, a widening of the aortic knob past the origin of the left subclavian artery, aortic wall thickness indicated by the width of the aortic shadow beyond intimal calcification, displacement of the calcification in the aortic knob. TTE has a sensitivity of 60% and a specificity of 83% for type A dissection and also shows aortic regurgitation, pleural effusion, and pericardial effusion/tamponade [196]. TOE with colour Doppler interrogation overcomes the limitations of transthoracic echocardiography, with a sensitivity of 94–100%

for identifying an intimal flap and 77–87% for identifying the site of entry; specificity ranges from 77–97% [136]. In addition to providing excellent visualization of the thoracic aorta, TOE provides superb images of the pericardium and detailed assessment of aortic valve function. A significant advantage of TOE is its possibility, allowing rapid diagnosis at the bedside. For this reason, it is particularly useful for evaluation of patients who are haemodynamically unstable and are suspected to have an aortic dissection.

Multislice CT is available in many hospitals and is usually offered on an emergency basis [58]. It provides complete anatomical information of the aorta including branch vessel involvement and enables visualization of the ostium and proximal part of both coronary arteries. CT has a sensitivity of 83–100% and a specificity of 90–100% for aortic dissection [134–136]. In randomized trials, cardiac MRI was more precise than transoesophageal echocardiography and CT and nearly 100% specific for aortic dissection. For identifying the site of entry, sensitivity was 85% and specificity 100% [137, 139]. Aortography, an invasive procedure, is no longer required for diagnosing aortic dissection. The sensitivity and specificity of aortography are inferior to less invasive imaging modalities. False negatives may occur if both the true and false lumen opacify equally with contrast, or if the false lumen is sufficiently thrombosed to preclude any installation of contrast. Aortography cannot identify aortic intramural haematomas, is invasive and highly operator dependent, and requires nephrotoxic contrast. Coronary angiography adds little to the decision-making process and should generally be avoided in type A dissection [136]. In the large IRAD, the first diagnostic step was transthoracic echocardiography and transoesophageal echocardiography in 33%, CT in 61%, MRI in 2% and angiography in 4%. In 56% transthoracic echocardiography and transoesophageal echocardiography, in 18% CT, in 9% MRI, and in 17% angiography were used as secondary techniques. Therefore, an average of 1.8 methods were utilized to diagnose aortic dissection [197].

Medical management

Patients with suspected acute aortic dissection should be admitted to an intensive care or monitoring unit and undergo diagnostic evaluation immediately. Pain and blood pressure control to a target systolic pressure of 110mmHg can be achieved using morphine sulfate and intravenous beta-blockers (metoprolol, esmolol, or labetalol) or in combination with vasodilating drugs such as sodium nitroprusside or angiotensin-converting enzyme inhibitors. Intravenous verapamil or diltiazem may also be used if beta-blockers are contraindicated. Monotherapy with beta-blocking agents

Table 31.11 Management of patients with suspected aortic dissection

Recommendation	Class I, IIa, IIb, III
ECG: documentation of ischaemia	I
Heart rate and blood pressure monitoring	I
Pain relief (morphine sulfate)	I
Reduction of systolic blood pressure using beta-blockers (IV metoprolol, esmolol, or labetolol)	I
In patients with severe hypertension despite beta-blockers, additional vasodilator (IV sodium nitroprusside) to titrate blood pressure to 100–120 mmHg	I
In patients with obstructive pulmonary disease, blood pressure lowering with calcium-channel blockers	II
Imaging in patients with ECG signs of ischaemia before thrombolysis if aortic pathology is suspected	II
Chest X-ray	III
Diagnostic imaging (non-invasive)	I

Reproduced from Erbel R, Alfonso F, Boileau C *et al.* Task Force on Aortic Dissection of the European Society of Cardiology. Diagnosis and management of aortic dissection. *Eur Heart J* 2001; **22**: 1642–81.

may be adequate to control mild hypertension and, in concert with sodium nitroprusside at an initial dose of 0.3mcg/kg/min, is often effective in a severe hypertensive state (➲Tables 31.11 and 31.12). In normotensive or hypotensive patients, careful evaluation for loss of blood, pericardial effusion, or heart failure (by cardiac ultrasound) is mandatory before administering volume. Patients with profound haemodynamic instability often require intubation, mechanical ventilation, and urgent bedside transoesophageal echocardiography or rapid CT for confirmatory imaging. In rare cases, the external ultrasound diagnosis of cardiac tamponade may justify immediate sternotomy and surgical access to the ascending aorta to prevent circulatory arrest, shock and ischaemic brain damage. Percutaneous pericardiocentesis as a temporizing step has often failed, and can accelerate bleeding and shock [198].

Surgical management

The aim of surgical therapy in proximal type A (type I, II) aortic dissection is prevention of rupture or development of pericardial effusion, which may lead to cardiac tamponade and death. Similarly, sudden onset of aortic regurgitation and coronary flow obstruction require urgent surgical intervention, with the aim of resecting the region of intimal tear in dissection limited to the ascending aorta and replacement by a composite or interposition graft (if the aortic valves are intact or resuspendable). When the dissection extends to the aortic arch or the descending

Table 31.12 Initial medical treatment in patients with acute aortic dissection and hypertension

Name	Mechanism	Dose	Cautions/contraindications
Esmolol	Cardioselective beta-1 blocker	Load: 500mcg/kg IV Drip: 50mcg kg^{-1} min^{-1} IV Increase by increments of 50mcg/min	Asthma or bronchospasm Bradycardia 2nd- or 3rd-degree AV block Cocaine or methamphetamine abuse
Labetalol	Nonselective beta 1,2 blocker Selective alpha-1 blocker	Load: 20mg IV Drip: 2mg/min IV	Asthma or bronchospasm Bradycardia 2nd- or 3rd-degree AV block Cocaine or methamphetamine abuse
Enalaprilat	ACE inhibitor	0.625–1.25mg IV q 6 hours Max dose: 5mg q 6 hours	Angioedema Pregnancy Renal artery stenosis Severe renal insufficiency
Nitroprusside	Direct arterial vasodilator	Begin at 0.3mcg kg^{-1} min^{-1} IV Max dose 10mcg kg^{-1} min^{-1}	May cause reflex tachycardia Cyanide/thiocyanate toxicity especially in renal or hepatic insufficiency
Nitroglycerin	Vascular smooth muscle relaxation	5–200mcg/min IV	Decreases preload contraindicated in tamponade or other preload-dependent states Concomitant use of sildenafil or similar agents

aorta, resection of the entire intimal flap may not be possible or the patient may require partial or total arch replacement [199]. A recent report highlights the problem of either resecting or leaving unrecognized intimal tears in the arch or descending thoracic aorta, which is seen in 20–30% and predisposes to later distal aortic reoperation [200]. With an operative mortality of 15–35% even in centres of excellence, adjunctive measures such as profound hypothermic circulatory arrest and selective retrograde perfusion of head vessels have been used in the surgical management of arch repair or an open distal anastomosis [201]. Although the latter is gaining growing acceptance for improved outcome (5-year survival of 73 ± 6%), profound hypothermic circulatory arrest has failed to improve early complications, survival, and distal reoperation rates in patients with acute type A dissection; 30-day, 1-year, and 5-year survival estimates are 81 ± 2%, 74 ± 3%, and 63 ± 3%—no different from other techniques using propensity-matched retrospective analysis [199]. The key to success is rapid surgery prior to any haemodynamic instability or deterioration (➲Table 31.13).

Once the patient is on extracorporeal circulation and preferably antegrade cerebral perfusion, which is usually established after cannulation of one femoral artery and the right atrium, the aorta is mobilized to visualize the innominate artery and the aortic root. If the valve leaflets are intact, aortic valve reconstruction using David's or Yacoub's resuspension technique is gaining growing acceptance over valve replacement (➲Fig. 31.18) [83, 84].

The approach to an acute type A (type I, II) dissection in a previously ectatic proximal aorta requires a different approach. In such instances, mostly in patients with Marfan syndrome, a composite graft (aortic tube graft with integrated valve) is preferred, with coronary reimplantation [78, 79, 202]. Surgical allografts and xenografts are experimental since late postoperative degeneration may require reoperation on the aortic root. Valve-sparing operations are delicate endeavours in an emergency and require great surgical competence in centres with expertise in elective cases. If the dissection compromises the left or right ostium without disrupting the coronary vessel, the ostium can usually be preserved. An ostium completely surrounded by dissected

Table 31.13 Surgical therapy of acute type A (type I and II) aortic dissection

Recommendation	Class I, IIa, IIb, III
Emergency surgery to avoid tamponade/aortic rupture	I
Valve-preserving surgery tubular graft if normal sized aortic root and no pathological changes of valve cusps	I
Replacement of aorta and aortic valve (composite graft) if ecstatic proximal aorta and/or pathological changes of valve/aortic wall	I
Valve-sparing operations with aortic root remodelling for abnormal valves	IIa
Valve preservation and aortic root remodelling in Marfan patients	IIa

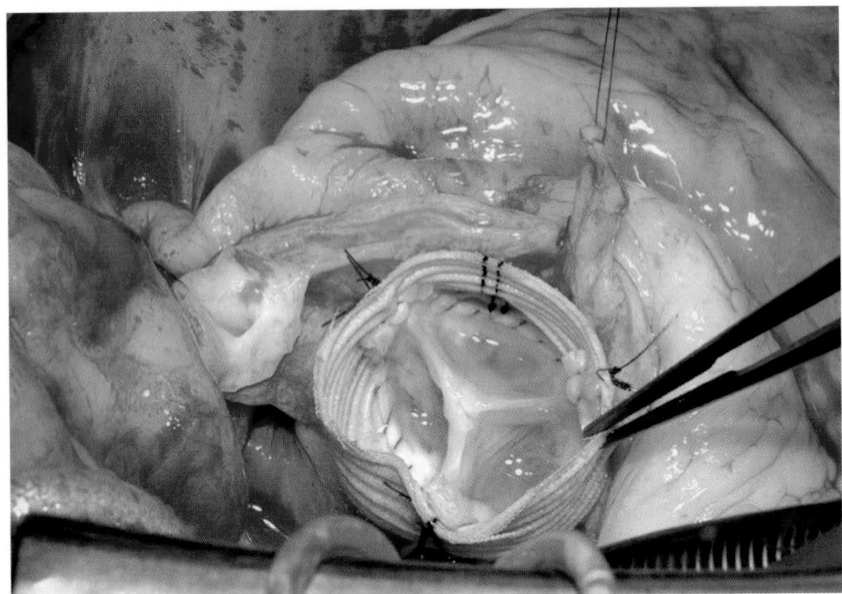

Figure 31.18 Intraoperative view of a reimplanted aortic valve (David technique).

aortic wall may be excised in button form. The dissected layers around the ostium are conjoined using tissue adhesive and over-and-over suturing before the anastomosis to a tube graft is accomplished. Bypass grafting of coronary arteries using saphenous vein segments is limited to those instances where a small torn ostium precludes reconstruction.

Aortic arch in acute type A (type I and II) dissection

Treatment of the acutely dissected aortic arch remains an unresolved issue. At present there is growing consensus that any dissected arch should be explored during hypothermic circulatory arrest [202, 203]. In the absence of an arch tear, an open distal anastomosis of the graft and the conjoined aortic wall layers at the junction of the ascending and arch portions is justified. Arch tears occur in up to 30% of patients with acute dissection [203, 204]. Whenever extensive tears are found that continue beyond the junction of the transverse and descending aortic segments, or with acute dissection of a previously aneurysmatic arch, subtotal or total arch replacement may be required, with reconnection of some or all supra-aortic vessels to the graft during hypothermic circulatory arrest and antegrade head perfusion [205].

In dissecting and non-dissecting aneurysms extending to the downstream aorta, an elephant trunk extension of the arch graft is an option described by Borst *et al.* [206]. This technique greatly facilitates later procedures on the downstream aorta. Instead of performing a conventional anastomosis between the end of the graft and the descending aorta, the graft is allowed to float freely in the aortic lumen. In a later procedure the elephant trunk section of the graft may be either connected surgically to the distal descending aorta directly or extended with another tubular prosthesis or interventionally by a customized endovascular stent-graft that may then be anastomosed at any desired downstream level of the aorta (➲Fig. 31.19).

In summary, surgery is advised without delay in acute type A (type I and II) dissection in order to prevent aortic rupture, pericardial tamponade and death, and to relieve aortic regurgitation. In selected cases with high anticipated surgical mortality, endovascular stent-graft placement has been successfully carried out by sealing a single proximal entry tear in the ascending aorta (➲Fig. 31.20) [207].

Surgery in type B (type III) aortic dissection

In the current era, the indications for operative treatment in patients with acute type B (type III) are limited to the prevention or relief of life-threatening complications such as intractable pain, a rapidly expanding aortic diameter, or signs of imminent aortic rupture, although these can also be managed by interventional stent-graft placement. The onset of complications such as malperfusion of vital aortic side branches warrants interventional therapy via stent-grafting to improve distal true lumen flow or, in rare instances, via catheter-guided fenestration of an occlusive lamella. When this approach does not lead to prompt relief of symptoms, surgical intervention may still be required. At present uncomplicated type B (type III) aortic dissections are usually treated conservatively, since surgical repair has no proven superiority over medical or interventional treatment in stable patients. In complicated cases, the concept of

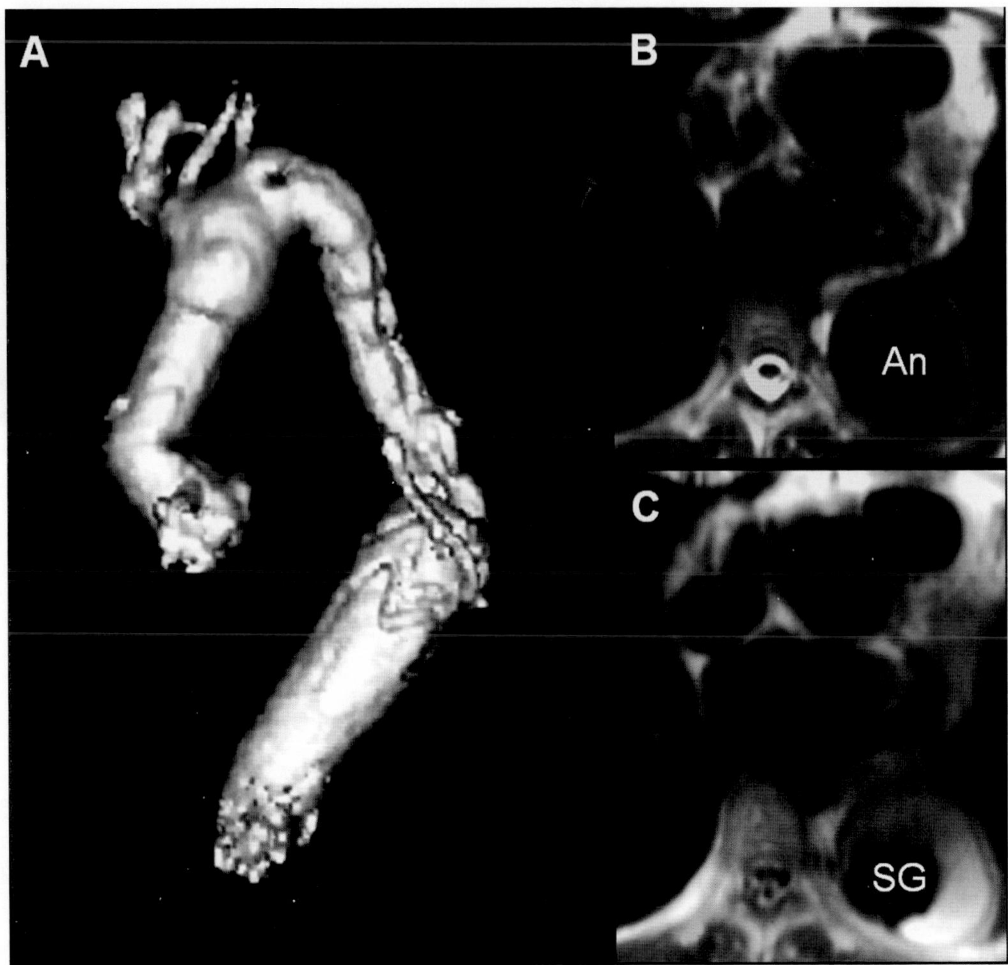

Figure 31.19 (A) Reconstructed 3D MRI after percutaneous use of a customized stent-graft to connect a surgically inserted elephant trunk with the upper abdominal aorta in order to exclude an aneurysm that had formed at the distal end of the elephant trunk (B); after placement of the customized stent-graft, the thoracic aneurysm was successfully excluded from circulation with thrombus formation around the stent-graft protheses (C).

interventional stent-graft placement seems to be associated with higher survival rates than the open surgical approach [208, 209].

Interventional endovascular strategy

Conventional treatment of Stanford type A (De Bakey type I, II) dissection consists of surgical reconstruction of the ascending aorta with complete or partial resection of the dissected aortic segment; endovascular strategies have no clinical application except for relief of critical malperfusion prior to surgery of the ascending aorta by distal fenestration in cases of thoracoabdominal extension (De Bakey type I) and peripheral ischaemic complications. However, endovascular stent-graft placement in addition to the conventional surgical treatment, has the potential to reconstruct the aorta by sealing one (or multiple) proximal entry tears with a Dacron-covered scaffold, thus initiating thrombosis of the false lumen [69, 91, 92, 208–210]. Reconstruction of a collapsed true lumen might result in re-establishment of side-branch flow (➲Fig. 31.21). Most scenarios of malperfusion syndrome are amenable to endovascular management, considering that surgical mortality rates in patients with acute peripheral vascular ischaemic complications are similar to those in patients with mesenteric ischaemia, reaching 89% in-hospital mortality [211, 212].

The interventional management of Stanford type B (De Bakey type III) dissection and the use of stent-grafts evolved to avoid the risk of paraplegia from spinal artery occlusion, as seen in up to 18% after open surgery [144, 145]. In the near future, combined surgical and interventional procedures even for proximal dissection are likely to emerge [213, 214] and even endovascular procedures have been applied successfully to the ascending aorta (➲Fig. 31.20).

Indications for stent-graft placement

There appears to be a role for interventional concepts in the treatment of static or dynamic obstruction of aortic branch arteries: static obstruction of a branch can be

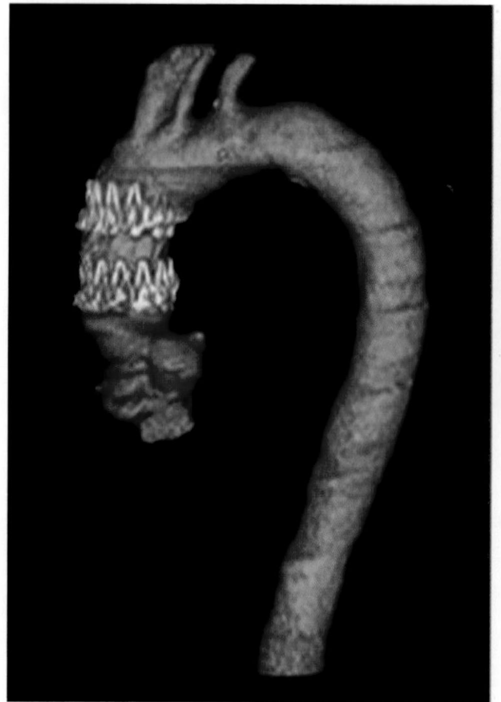

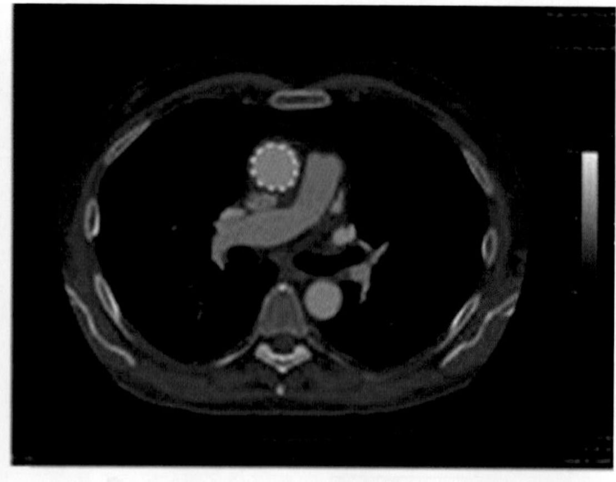

Figure 31.20 Stent-graft implantation in the ascending aorta.

overcome by placing endovascular stents in the ostium of the compromised side branch, and dynamic obstruction may benefit from stents in the aortic true lumen. In classic aortic dissection, successful fenestration leaves false lumen pressure unchanged. Sometimes bare stents deployed from the true lumen into side branches are useful for buttressing the flap in a stable position [215]. Conversely, fenestration may increase the long-term risk of aortic rupture because a large re-entry tear promotes flow in the false lumen and provides the basis for aneurysmal expansion of the false lumen; moreover, there is a risk of peripheral embolism from a perfused but partially thrombosed false lumen.

The most effective method for excluding an enlarging and aneurysmal dilated false lumen is the sealing of proximal entry tears with a customized stent-graft; the absence of a distal re-entry tear is desirable for optimal results but not a prerequisite. Adjunctive treatment by fenestration and/or ostial bare stents may help establish flow to compromised aortic branches. Compression of the true aortic lumen cranial to the main abdominal branches with distal malperfusion (so called pseudo-coarctation) may also be corrected by stent-grafts that enlarge the compressed true lumen and improve distal aortic blood flow [69, 208, 209, 212–215]. Depressurization and shrinking of the false lumen is the most beneficial result

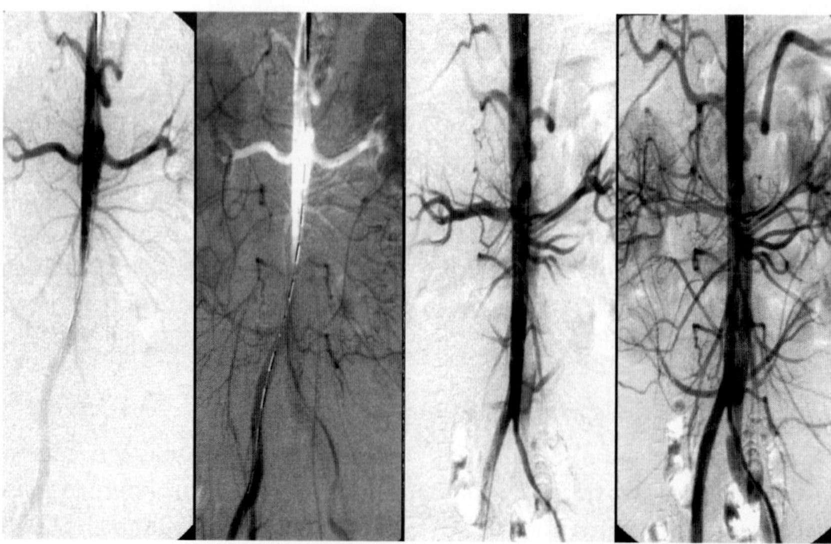

Figure 31.21 Malperfusion of distal aorta by occlusive type B dissection. Stent-graft placement in the true lumen of the proximal descending aorta re-established flow to the abdomen and legs.

to be gained, ideally followed by complete thrombosis of the false lumen and remodelling of the entire dissected aorta; on rare occasions, this even occurs in retrograde type A dissection [215]. Similar to previously accepted indications for surgical intervention in type B dissection, scenarios such as intractable pain with descending dissection, rapidly expanding false lumen diameter, extra-aortic blood collection as a sign of imminent rupture or distal malperfusion syndrome are accepted indications for emergency stent-graft placement [209, 215–218]. Moreover, late onset of complications such as malperfusion of vital aortic side branches may justify endovascular stent-grafting as a first option (➲Table 31.11).

Interventional therapy in an elective setting

Medical therapy, as the first-line approach to uncomplicated type B aortic dissections, is justified because of a relatively good short-term prognosis with 85% of patients surviving their initial hospital stay. The reported 30-day mortality of uncomplicated type B dissections is 11% versus 30% in complicated causes with extremity ischaemia, renal failure, visceral ischaemia, or contained rupture [134]. Unfortunately, the long-term outcome of medical therapy alone is suboptimal with reported 50% mortality at 5 years and delayed expansion of the false lumen in 25% patients at 4 years. This expansion of the false lumen predisposes patients to aortic rupture or retrograde migration of the dissection plane with involvement of the ascending aorta and a consequent increased mortality rate [219]. Initial experience for the treatment of chronic aortic dissection with stent-graft versus open surgery was reported by Nienaber *et al.* There were no mortality or morbidity for stent-grafts whereas conventional surgery was associated with four deaths and five serious adverse events in their series [220].

With both bare stents in side branches and sometimes fenestrating manoeuvres, compromised flow can be restored in >90% (range 92–100%) of vessels obstructed by aortic dissection (➲Table 31.14). The average 30-day mortality rate is 10% (range 0–25%) and additional surgical revascularization is rarely needed. Most patients remain asymptomatic over a mean follow-up time of about 4 years. Fatalities related to the interventional procedure may occur as a result of non-reversible ischaemic complications, progression of the dissection, or complications of additional reconstructive surgical procedures on the thoracic aorta. Potential problems may arise from unpredictable haemodynamic alterations in the true and false lumen after fenestration and side-branch stenting. These alterations can result in loss of previously well-perfused arteries or initially salvaged side branches.

Table 31.14 Interventional therapy in aortic dissection

Recommendation	Class I, IIa, IIb, III
Stenting of obstructed branch origin for static obstruction of branch artery	IIa
Balloon fenestration of dissecting membrane plus stenting of aortic true lumen for dynamic obstruction	IIa
Stenting to keep fenestration open	IIa
Fenestration to provide re-entry tear for dead-end false lumen	IIa
Stenting of true lumen:	
+ to seal entry (covered stent)	IIb
+ enlarge compressed true lumen	IIa

Reproduced from Erbel R, Alfonso F, Boileau C *et al.* Task Force on Aortic Dissection of the European Society of Cardiology. Diagnosis and management of aortic dissection. *Eur Heart J* 2001; **22**: 1642–81.

Paraplegia may occur after use of multiple stent-grafts but still appears to be a rare phenomenon, especially with stented segment of <16cm. Results of short-term follow-up are excellent, with a 1-year survival rate of >90%; tears can be re-adapted and aortic diameters generally decrease with complete thrombosis of the false lumen. This suggests that stent placement may facilitate healing of the dissection, sometimes of the entire aorta, including abdominal segments (➲Fig. 31.22). However, late reperfusion of the false lumen has been observed occasionally, underlining the need for stringent follow-up imaging.

Recent reports suggest that percutaneous stent-graft placement in the dissected aorta is safer and produces better results than surgery for type B dissection. Data from the IRAD registry on 571 patients with acute type B aortic dissection provided better survival rates after endovascular treatment versus open surgical repair in patients with complicated type B dissection. Of the 571 patients, 390 (68.3%) were treated medically, 59 (10.3%) with standard open surgery,and 66 (11.6%) with an endovascular approach. Indications for interventional and surgical treatment modality were recurrent pain (46.3% vs. 22.0%; p = 0.008), refractory pain (19.5% vs. 15.3%; p = n.s.), limb ischaemia (19.5% vs. 11.9%; p = n.s.), visceral ischaemia (22% vs. 18.6%; p = n.s.), and extension of dissection (26.8% vs. 47.5%; p = 0.003) with 217 hours versus 81.6hours from diagnosis to treatment (p<0.001). In-hospital complications occurred in 20% of patients subjected to endovascular technique and in 40% of patients after open surgical repair. In-hospital mortality was significantly higher after open surgery (33.9%) than after endovascular treatment (10.6%; p = 0.002). After propensity and multivariate adjustment, open surgical repair was associated with an increased risk

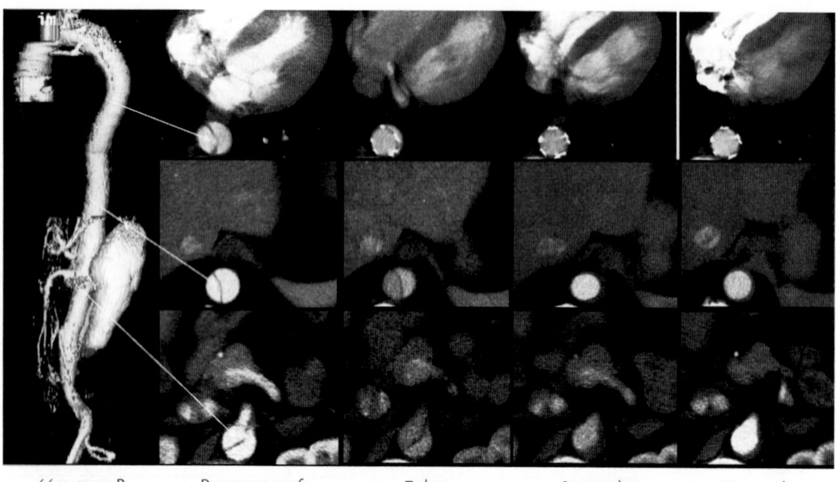

Figure 31.22 Acute type B aortic dissection in a 44-year-old man; note the communications between the true and false lumen at the thoracic and abdominal level. After stent-graft placement across the proximal thoracic entry, the entire aorta including the abdominal segment is reconstructed with time, with complete 'healing' of the dissected aortic wall and closure of distal communication.

of in-hospital mortality [OR: 3.41; 95% confidence interval: 1.00 to 11.67; p = 0.05) (➲Fig. 31.23) [221].

Interventional therapy in an emergency setting

The concept of emergency stent-graft placement for urgent endovascular aortic repair of dissection is attractive, and a growing number of acute type B aortic dissections undergo endovascular repair (with little evidence of periprocedural morbidity, aborted malperfusion, or leakage) and reconstruction of the dissected aorta; stent-graft placement in complicated distal aortic dissection is an emerging concept and is free from excessive peripheral or neurological complications in experienced hands [216, 217, 222, 226]. Even endovascular procedures to the ascending aorta have been performed.

In conclusion, current advances with stent-graft thoracic intervention must be viewed as exciting new developments that offer hope to many patients with type B dissection.

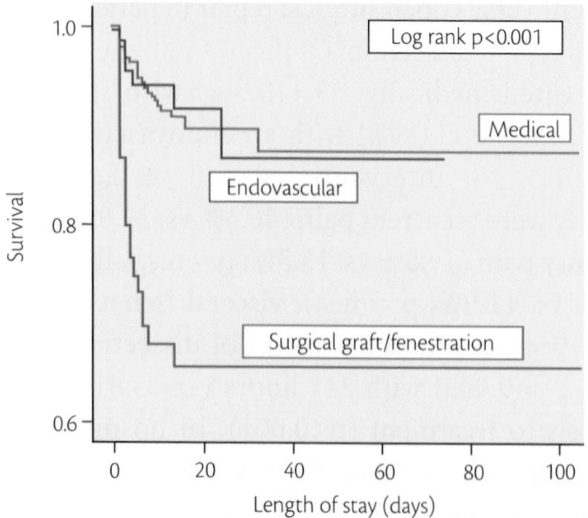

Figure 31.23 Comparison of medical, surgical and endovascular treatment of complicated type B aortic dissection. Reproduced from Fattori R, Tsai TT, Myrmel T, *et al.* Complicated acute type B dissection: is surgery the best option?. A report from the International Registry of Acute Aortic Dissection. *JACC Cardiovas Interv* 2008; **1**: 395–402.

Technical strategies and devices continue to evolve and it is likely that these techniques will soon become first-line therapy for most patients presenting with anatomically suitable thoracic and thoracoabdominal aortic lesions.

Long-term therapy and follow-up

The long-term approach to patients with successful initial treatment of acute aortic dissection begins with the appreciation of a systemic illness. Systemic hypertension, advanced age, aortic size, and presence of patent false lumen are all factors which identify higher risk, as does the entire spectrum of Marfan syndrome [221–225]. All patients merit aggressive medical therapy, follow-up visits, and serial imaging. It has been estimated that nearly one-third of patients surviving initial treatment for acute dissection will experience extension of dissection or aortic rupture, or require surgery for aortic aneurysm formation within 5 years of presentation. Treatment with effective beta-blockade is the cornerstone of medical therapy, but it has to be taken into account that 40% of the patients develop resistent hypertension and need up to 6 drugs [227]. By lowering both blood pressure and dP/dt, beta-blockers have been shown to retard aortic expansion in Marfan syndrome and that associated with chronic AAAs. Blood pressure should be titrated to <135/80mmHg in usual patients and to <130/80mmHg in those with Marfan syndrome [5, 228, 229]. Additionally, heart rate should controlled tight. A heart rate <60bpm significantly decreases the secondary adverse events (aortic expansion, recurrent aortic dissection, aortic rupture and/or need for aortic surgery) in type B aortic dissection compared to conventional control of >60 bpm [230].

Serial imaging of the aorta is an essential component of long-term management (before and after surgery or stent-graft placement) in Marfan disease and in all cases of chronic dissection. Choice of imaging modality is dependent on institutional availability and expertise. Previous recommendations suggest follow-up imaging at 1, 3, 6, 9, and 12 months following discharge, and annually thereafter [5]; this aggressive strategy underlines the observation that both hypertension and aortic expansion/dissection are common and not easily predicted in the first months following hospital discharge. Imaging should not be confined to the region of initial involvement since both dissection and aneurysm formation may occur anywhere along the entire length of the aorta.

Development of an ascending aortic diameter of 4.5–5.0cm is an indication for surgical repair in Marfan syndrome. In non-Marfan patients, an aortic diameter of 5.5–6cm warrants repair, as does distal aortic expansion to 6.0cm or more in all types of patients. As with non-dissecting aneurysms, rate of growth and size of the aorta are both important factors to consider when it comes to prophylactic vascular surgery. An ascending aortic aneurysm of 5.0cm may merit urgent repair in a young patient with Marfan syndrome [228]. Conversely, an aneurysm of 5.0cm present for 3 years in an elderly person with well-controlled blood pressure is unlikely to rupture. Patients who have been treated with surgery and/or endovascular stent-grafting warrant similar follow-up to those whose initial treatment was limited to medical therapy.

Aortitis

Definition

Aortitis is defined by inflammation of the aorta, categorized by the underlying aetiology into:

- infective syphilitic aortitis;
- infective non-syphilitic (bacterial or fungal) aortitis; or
- non-infective aortitis due to large-vessel vasculitis (e.g. Takayasu's arteritis, giant-cell arteritis (GCA)) or atherosclerosis.

Determining the individual aetiology of aortitis is of particular importance because immunosuppressive therapy can aggravate an active infectious process [231].

Epidemiology

Although data on the incidence of aortitis are not available, the epidemiology of the large-vessel vasculitides GCA and Takayasu's arteritis has been studied. The overall incidence of GCA has been estimated to be 18.8/100,000/year with a man to women ratio of 2:1 and a mean age of 75 years [232]. For the Takayasu arteritis an incidence of 0.4–1.0 case per million resident per year has been reported [233].

Pathogenesis

The most common causes of aortitis are the non-infectious large-vessel vasculitides GCA and Takayasu's arteritis. Furthermore, a variety of bacterial, mycobacterial, and fungal organisms may infect the walls of the aorta (➲Table 31.15). Microorganisms may gain a foothold through several mechanisms:

- seeding of the vasa vasorum during haematogenous spread;
- direct invasion of the wall from the aortic lumen in light of a pathologic aortic wall;
- spread of infection from contiguous structures;
- traumatic aortic injury with subsequent infection;
- septic emboli.

Table 31.15 Aetiology of aortitis

Non-infective:
Large-vessel vasculitis
Giant cell arteritis (GCA)
Takayasu's arteritis
Rheumatoid arteritis
Systemic lupus erythematodes
HLA-B27 associated spondyloarthropathies
ANCA-asscoiated vasculitides
Wegener's arteritis
Churg–Strauss syndrome
Kawasaki disease
Behçet's disease
Sarcoidosis
Cryoglobunemia
Henoch–Schönlein purpura
Goodpasture syndrome
Infective non-syphilitic:
Gram-positive (60%)
Staphylococcus aureus (30–50%)
Streptococcus (20%)
Gram-negative (20–40%)
Salmonella
Infective syphilitic

Bacterial or fungal infections may trigger non-infectious vasculitis by generating immune complexes or by cross-reactivity. By analogy with infective endocarditis, bacterial or fungal aortitis often develops following bacteraemia in the place of least resistance (e.g. existing atherosclerotic lesions or aneurysms) [231, 234, 235].

Aortitis is the principal cardiovascular manifestation of tertiary syphilis, found mainly in the ascending aorta [5]. Whereas cardiovascular syphilis was a relatively frequent disorder at the beginning of the last century, tertiary syphilis has been almost eradicated with the use of penicillin and is today a medical curiosity. However, tertiary syphilitic lesions may persist despite treatment in patients with compromised immune status [236].

Staphylococcus aureus accounts for the majority of Gram-positive infections; aortitis has also been observed in association with streptococci [237, 238]. Gram-negative bacilli such as *Salmonella* and *Proteus* species, and *Escherichia coli* have been described [235]. Less common causes include tuberculous infections and fungal agents such as *Candida*, *Cryptococcus*, and *Aspergillus* species [238–240].

Autoimmune disorders can severely affect the vasa vasorum, and decrease the blood supply of the media [5]. Diseases affecting the aorta are diverse and include serum sickness, cryoglobulinaemia, systemic lupus erythaematosus, rheumatoid arthritis, relapsing polychondritis, Behçet's disease, Henoch–Schönlein purpura, and postinfectious or drug-induced immune complex disease [48, 241–245]. Also, antineutrophil cytoplasmic auto-antibody (ANCA)-associated small-vessel vasculitides can affect the large vessels, as in Wegener's granulomatosis, microscopic polyangiitis, and Churg–Strauss syndrome [197]. Other antibodies, such as antiglomerular basement membrane (Goodpasture's syndrome) and anti-endothelial (Kawasaki's disease), can also be targets. Transplant rejection, inflammatory bowel diseases, and paraneoplastic vasculitis also may afflict the large vessels.

The causes of aortitis in Takayasu's arteritis and GCA (temporal arteritis, granulomatous arteritis) are unknown. Both are thought to be antigen-driven cell-mediated autoimmune processes. Takayasu's arteritis is a chronic inflammatory disease of the large vessels that mainly affects the thoracic aorta and its branches, but can also occur anywhere in the vascular system [246, 247]. GCA usually affects the medium-sized extracranial arteries but may also affect the aorta in 10–15% of patients [248, 249]. Both GCA and Takayasu's arteritis are associated with an inflammatory cellular infiltrate of the aortic media, adventitia, and vasa vasorum that contains a predominance of lymphocytes, macrophages, and multinucleated giant cells. Over time, scarring of the aortic wall media and destruction of the elastic lamina occur.

Histologically, aortitis is characterized by inflammatory lymphocytic infiltrates within the medial layers of the aortic wall and around the vasa vasorum, smooth muscle, and fibroblast necrosis, and fibrosis of the vessel wall [5]. In syphilitic aortitis, *Treponema pallidum* invades the vasa vasorum, initiating inflammatory changes consisting of lymphocytic and plasma cell perivascular infiltrates that lead to endarteritis obliterans, adventitia scarring, and patchy necrosis of the medial layer with elastic fibre destruction [250]. The inflammatory reactions within the aortic wall may cause local weakening resulting in aortic dilation up to aneurysm formation [5]. Clinically evident involvement of the cardiovascular system occurs in about 10% of patients with untreated tertiary syphilis of long duration. About half of patients with untreated syphilis for >10 years have autopsy evidence of cardiovascular involvement. 'Mycotic' aneurysms are often characterized by rapid expansion. Moreover, aortitis can cause fibrous thickening of the aortic wall and subsequent ostial stenosis of major branches up to chronic arterial occlusions [251].

Clinical features

Diagnosing aortitis is clinically challenging because symptoms are non-specific and present as fatigue, malaise, joint aches, and low-grade fever as well as raised serum markers of inflammation. Fever is the most constant sign (70%). Shoulder, dorsal, or thoracic pains are often present (60%). Abdominal pains may also be noticed (20%). Carotidynia due to vascular inflammation presenting as neck pain can be an important clue. These symptoms can be accompanied by more specific clinical symptoms due to inflammatory stenoses of major arterial branches, such as reduced or absent peripheral pulses, ocular disturbances, neurological deficits, claudication up to ischaemic gangrene, or angina pectoris up to myocardial infarction in cases of coronary ostial involvement [250]. Aortitis-related aneurysm of the ascending aorta may become clinically overt with the appearance of new-onset diastolic murmur and signs of heart failure in cases of severe aortic regurgitation. However, the combination of clinical signs of infection (fever, raised laboratory markers), new-onset murmur, and multiple ischaemias may mimic infective endocarditis. Syphilitic or mycotic aneurysms are often indolent and show rapid progression (➲Table 31.16) [250, 252].

Diagnostic procedures

On physical examination, patients appear chronically ill with mild fever. Reduced blood pressure or laterality (i.e. a difference >10mmHg between left and right arms) suggests

Table 31.16 Characteristics of aortitis

Data	Results
Sex ratio men:women:	
General case	3:1
Mean age:	
General case	65 years old
Clinical presentation	Fever (70%)
	Pains:
	Dorsal and thoracic (60%)
	Abdominal (20%)
	Compressive signs
	Aneurysmal disease
	Cardiac abnormalities
	Aortic thrombosis with distal embolization
	Aortic dissection

vascular obstruction. Arterial pulse intensity in any of the limbs may be diminished. Bruits may be audible at carotid arteries, abdominal aorta, and even the subclavian and brachial arteries. When the diagnosis of aortitis is suspected on the basis of clinical presentation, expending imaging of the entire aorta with an appropriate modality is critical to establish the diagnosis.

Blood cultures have cardinal importance in the assumption of responsibility of the infection. They are indeed the only means of microbiological diagnosis before surgical or interventional therapy and they help to find the best adapted antibiotic therapy. The blood cultures have a rate of positivity varying from 50–90%. This poor rate is probably partly related to the frequency of antibiotic prescription before realization of blood cultures. Although the diagnosis of aortitis generally is based on clinical presentation and aortic imaging, key laboratory tests are helpful. Laboratory examination may reveal elevated acute-phase proteins (CRP, fibrinogen) and erythrocyte sedimentation rate as evidence of inflammatory processes. Additional laboratory testing should be based on the clinical assessment of the patient and the differential diagnosis of the underlying cause.

Standard chest X-rays find aortic aneurysms, shown by opacities of different size in the mediastinum. Traditionally, angiography was used as the imaging 'gold standard' for diagnosing aortitis by detecting luminal abnormalities (aneurysms or ostial stenosis of major branches) but is not useful for detecting early mural findings. Nowadays, modern tomographic imaging techniques are considered the method of choice, as they allow evaluation of early changes within the vessel wall [253, 254]. Characteristic features on contrast-enhanced CT, MRI, or TOE include thickening of the aortic wall with or without stenosis of major adjacent aortic branches, irregular enhancement of peri-aortic tissue, aortic dilatation or (irregular) aortic aneurysms [255–257]. A peri-aortic collection of blood, fluid or gas or adjacent vertebral osteomyelitis may suggest infectious aortitis [235]. These modalities are also used in the follow-up of patients, because MRI and CT are able to show reduction of wall thickening after initiation of treatment [253]. Recently, ^{18}F-fluorodeoxyglucose PET has been shown sensitive in detecting inflammatory aortic changes (➲Fig. 31.24) [204].

Therapeutic management

The prognosis is related to the infectious attack and the specific complications which it can involve. The severity of this disease is particularly related to the risk of rupture of the aneurysm. Without any treatment, the aneurysm will progressively increase, leading to a fatal rupture without emergency surgery. Once the diagnosis of aortitis has been established, the approach to management depends on the underlying cause. The uncommon case of infectious aortitis requires rapid diagnosis, antibiotic therapy, and consultation with a vascular surgeon. The initial treatment of suspected infectious aortitis is intravenous antibiotics with broad antimicrobial coverage of the most likely pathological organisms. In syphilitic aortitis, antibiotic treatment with benzylpenicillin 10–20 million units is the widely accepted treatment, although no controlled trials have shown its efficacy [250]. The optimal management of infective non-syphilitic aortitis requires early surgical intervention in addition to prolonged antibiotic/antimycotic administration [235, 238, 258]. With mere antimicrobial therapy, the mortality rate of infective aneurysms approaches 90% due to continued aneurysm growth and subsequent rupture [238]. Early surgical intervention with resection of the infected aorta with wide débridement and extra-anatomical bypass grafting has greatly increased survival [259, 260]. After surgery, bactericidal antibiotic therapy is usually continued for at least 6 weeks [260]. The mainstay of therapy for patients with non-infective aortitis is corticosteroids; however, a substantial percentage of patients require additional immunosuppressive agents such as cyclophosphamide, methotrexate, or mycophenolate mofetil. Daily prednisone in doses of 1mg/kg, not to exceed 60mg/day, should be given for 1–3 months to patients with active arteritis. Long-term low-dose prednisone therapy may be necessary to prevent progression of arterial stenoses. Endovascular stent-graft placement has been suggested as a novel, less invasive alternative [261]. Balloon angioplasty, stenting, or bypass surgery may be necessary for revascularization of aortitis-related arterial stenosis [262–264].

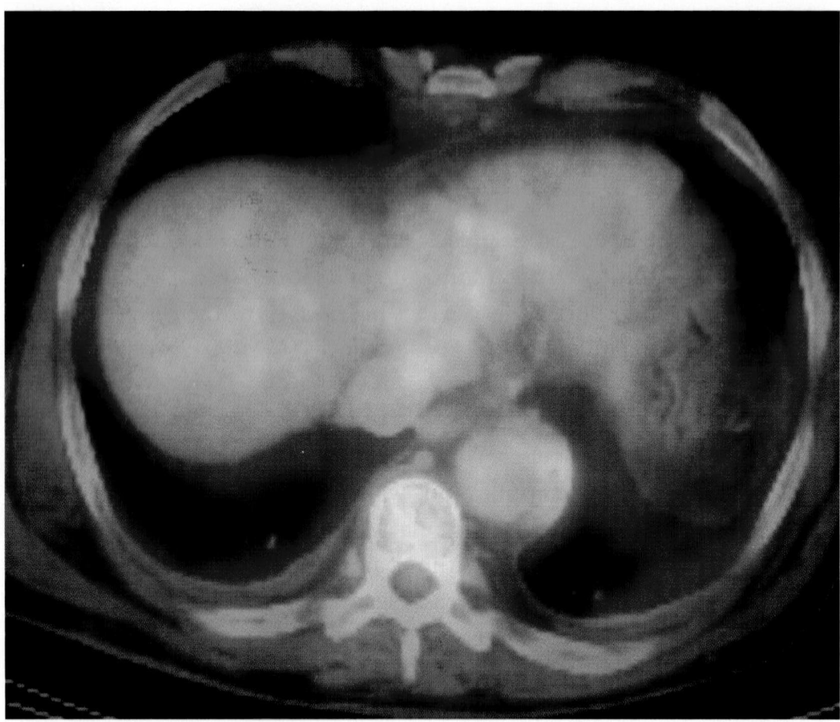

Figure 31.24 Demonstration of increased ^{18}F-desoxyglucose uptake within the wall of the descending thoracoabdominal aorta by PET-CT, indicating non-infective aortitis due to severe atherosclerosis.

In cases of enlarging aortic aneurysms due to non-infective aortitis, radical surgical resection is indicated [251].

Aortic atheromatous disease: thrombotic or cholesterol emboli

Thrombotic or cholesterol emboli of peripheral organs can arise from atheromatous disease of the aorta, with morphological or functional alterations of the aortic wall. Most frequently, atheromatous plaque or ulcers are encountered in the aortic arch and the descending aorta. Aortic intimal morphology is graded according to plaque characteristics [265].

- Grade I: normal intima.
- Grade II: increased intimal echo-density without lumen irregularity.
- Grade III: increased intimal echo-density with single or multiple well-defined atheromatous plaque of 3mm.
- Grade IV: atheroma > 3mm or mobile or ulcerated plaque.

Interestingly, reduced compliance of the aortic wall is considered an early expression of atheromatous disease and may promote atheromatous progression. Certainly, dissection membranes and aneurysmatic widenings will alter the laminar flow profile of the aorta and therefore cause mostly thrombotic emboli.

Spontaneous emboli frequently have their origin in ulcerated plaque or plaque with pedunculated or mobile parts [266]. These mobile parts consist of atheromatous material or adhesive thrombotic material; embolic events arise more from plaques without calcifications than from calcified lesions. In echocardiographic images the structures appear mostly echolucent. The incidence of aortic thrombus has been estimated as 2–5% [267–269].

Besides being spontaneous, emboli can be provoked by iatrogenic manipulations. Mechanical manipulation with wires or catheters, for instance during cardiac catheterization, can loosen mobile parts or even cause limited dissections, especially in diseased regions of the aortic wall [270]. Showering of cholesterol crystals occur especially during cardiac catheterization in 1–2%, often with cutaneous signs, renal insufficiency [271], and elevation of CRP [272]. Surgical manipulations during cardiovascular interventions and aortic cannulation or cross-clamping can likewise cause detachment of aortic debris.

Risk factors for such emboli include smoking, hypercholesterolaemia, hypertension, diabetes, elevated homocysteine levels, and increased fibrinogen levels. Furthermore, hormone therapy and procoagulative disease can increase aggregation of thrombocytes and promote thrombotic events. While embolic events into the lower limbs or the abdominal organs rarely cause significant clinical symptoms, embolic events to the brain and the retina are symptomatic. Amarenco *et al.* [273] have identified aortic plaque (measured as aortic wall thickness) of 4mm as a major risk factor for cerebral stroke besides the occurrence of atrial fibrillation and internal carotid stenosis. In patients with such atheromatous plaques, the annual risk of an embolic stroke is 12% [274].

The diagnosis of patients at risk for embolic events is often prompted when the first embolic event has already occurred. Transoesophageal echocardiography is the first modality to be employed and gives adequate image quality for assessment of the aortic valve, the ascending aorta, as well as the descending part to the level of the diaphragm. However, it should be noted that the TOE is unable to analyse the abdominal aorta or parts of the aortic arch as the left main bronchus is interposed between the oesophagus and the aortic arch [5]. The aorta can be further analysed by contrast-enhanced CT and by MRI using 1.5-T machines with good resolution especially for small pathological changes of the aortic wall. Experimental studies reveal that the diagnostic use of small iron oxide particles can improve plaque imaging of the aortic wall [275].

Intravascular ultrasound certainly has a higher risk of complications than non-invasive techniques but is clearly superior in imaging quality and is suited for differential diagnosis [280].

As there is no clear therapy for emboli, medical strategies should be clearly directed towards risk factor management and prevention. In this context, blood pressure control and cholesterol reduction using statins as well as optimization of blood glucose are considered important. Moreover, platelet inhibition is recommended as a preventive measure, while the use of antiaggregatory agents or anticoagulant drugs is controversial. Only few authors see a clear risk reduction in cerebral events with an INR value between 1.5 and 3 [277]. In general, a note of caution is raised on the use of anticoagulant drugs. Anecdotal reports have indeed suggested that in patients with cholesterol emboli, anticoagulation may favour further embolization (e.g. blue-toe syndrome). The hypothesis is that anticoagulation prevents thrombus formation on ulcerated plaques, allowing the release of atheromatous material contained in the plaques. Although the value of antithrombotic drugs is controversial, such patients are at high risk of vascular events [278]. In patients with atheromatous disease of the aorta or at risk for embolic events, statin therapy has shown superior outcome than warfarin or antiaggregation [279].

In summary, thrombotic or cholesterol emboli are a clearly underestimated clinical entity. In particular, cholesterol embolization is a rare but serious complication of cardiac catheterization. Our goal should be directed at the identification of risk groups and individual patients at risk for such events. Patients with suspected aortic disease should undergo a detailed analysis of the entire aorta using transoesophageal echocardiography and non-invasive tomographic imaging modalities. The therapy should be individualized and aimed at the reduction of risk factors and should include the use of statins.

Traumatic rupture of the aorta

Aetiology

Traumatic aortic rupture (TAR) is a lesion due to blunt trauma involving the aortic wall, from the intima to the adventitia. The first annotation of TAR was in 1557 by Vesalius, who described a patient with an aortic rupture after falling off a horse. In 1923 Dshanelidze in Russia reported the first successful repair of TAR in a penetrating lesion of the ascending aorta, followed by pioneering reports in the 1950s [280]. A pathological study, which is still the largest series of 296 cases, clearly defined the characteristics of aortic lesions and emphasized the time relationships between the trauma and subsequent death. The era of high-speed motor vehicles has brought an increased incidence of TAR [281]. Between 1936 and 1942 in a cohort of 7000 autopsies, Strassman [282] found only 51 patients with TAR secondary to vehicular collision, whereas several recent investigations have shown that TAR occurs in 10–30% of adults sustaining fatal blunt trauma. Richens *et al.* [283] reported 21% of mortality due to aortic rupture in a sample of 613 fatalities of road traffic accidents and accounts for 8000 victims per year in the USA [282, 284].

Pathogenesis

TAR can result from car and motorcycle collisions, falls from a height or blast injuries, airplane and train crashes, and skiing and equestrian accidents. In a demographic analysis of 144 patients with aortic rupture, Hunt *et al.* [285] reported motor vehicle crash in 83%, motorcycle in 4.9%, pedestrian in 7%, and falls in 2.1% of cases. Even lateral impact accounts for 20–40% of cases in recent studies [284]. The shearing forces in lateral collision seem to produce most frequently a partial laceration involving the lesser curvature of the distal part of the aortic arch, just above the isthmus [286, 287]. Airbags and seatbelts do not protect against this type of impact [284, 286]. The region subject to the greatest strain is the isthmus, where the relatively mobile thoracic aorta joins the fixed arch and the insertion of the ligamentum arteriosus. Aortic ruptures occur at this site in 80–95% [283, 285, 286]. Because of the high immediate mortality of traumatic rupture of the ascending aorta, this location has been reported in 10–20% of the autopsy series versus 5% of the surgical cases [286, 288]. Other less common locations are distal segments of the descending aorta (12%) or the infrarenal segment (4.7%). Multiple sites of aortic tears are found in some reports [52]. Different theories have been advanced to explain the mechanism of aortic injury. Considering different causes and types of impact that produce the aortic lesion, it is reasonable to claim not only one mechanism but a combination of many [289–293].

Mechanisms of rupture

A traumatic lesion may be classified as:

- intimal haemorrhage;
- intimal haemorrhage with laceration;
- medial laceration;
- complete laceration of the aorta;
- false aneurysm formation;
- peri-aortic haemorrhage [52].

Intimal haemorrhage may leave an intact endothelial layer or may be associated with circumscribed laceration of the endothelial and internal elastic lamina of the intima. When the lesion involves intimal and medial layers, false aneurysm formation can occur. The aneurysm is fusiform in the case of a circumferential lesion, involving the entire wall on the transversal plane, while in a partial lesion in which only a portion of the wall is lacerated, it appears as a localized diverticulum. Peri-aortic haemorrhage occurs independently of the type of lesion. While complete rupture of the aorta including adventitia and peri-adventitial connective tissue leads to immediate death, formation of an aneurysm or occlusion of the site of rupture may permit temporary survival.

Clinical presentation

Despite the severe nature of injury, clinical signs may not be impressive and thus it is imperative to maintain a high index of suspicion in victims of high-speed decelerating injuries, regardless of external evidence of thoracic injury.

The signs of aortic rupture are not specific, and the presence of coexisting head, facial, orthopaedic, and visceral lesions dominates the physician's attention. Dyspnoea and chest pain are prominent symptoms, localized in the back in 20–76% of cases. Loss of consciousness and hypotension are also frequent, as generally reported in polytraumatized patients, while generalized hypertension is reported in about 17% [294]. Systolic blood pressure <90mmHg despite adequate fluid resuscitation is considered to be a sign of haemodynamic instability and associated with higher mortality [283]. Less frequent symptoms include dysphagia and hoarseness. A small number of patients (6%) have paraplegia without obvious spinal malperfusion [295]. Difference in pulse amplitude between upper and lower extremities from compression of the aortic lumen by a peri-aortic haematoma is seen in 23–37% [294, 296]. If the intimal and media tear forms a flap which acts as a ball valve, partial aortic obstruction occurs, with upper extremity hypertension reported as 'acute coarctation syndrome' or 'pseudo-coarcation' [297]. Hypertension may be secondary to stretching or stimulation of the cardiac plexus. Hypotension <90mmHg despite adequate fluid volume resuscitation and free exsanguination into the pleural space, often worsening despite thoracotomy, are considered to be signs of forthcoming free aortic rupture [283, 298–301]. Likewise, vocal cord palsy, or tracheal and superior vena cava compression may herald severe expansion [296].

Associated lesions are present in almost all patients with TAR, ranging from fractures and head injuries to spleen, liver, and cardiac as well as lung contusion [294, 302, 303]. The latter can cause respiratory insufficiency, while cardiac contusion results from compression of the heart between the sternum and the vertebral column in 20% of cases, frequently if the ascending aorta is involved. Finally, normal physical findings are reported in 5–14% of cases [288, 294].

Diagnostic procedures

The common denominator of TAR is its unpredictable and unfavourable outcome. Therefore, early diagnosis and appropriate treatment are essential. The most important diagnostic imaging modalities are transoesophageal echocardiography, contrast-enhanced CT, MRI, and contrast angiography. There is growing interest in, and use of, three-dimensional MRI and CT due to the high sensitivity of reconstruction. Computer-enhanced three-dimensional reconstruction of the aorta can serve as a blueprint for surgical or interventional therapeutic procedures.

Therapeutic management

With improved resuscitation and transport logistics, almost all patients with TAR who reach the hospital alive are candidates for aortic repair. Until recently, emergency surgery was universally accepted for TAR [52]; however, immediate surgery has been characterized by high mortality and morbidity. Surgery within 6 hours of arrival had an intraoperative mortality of 10.2%, postoperative mortality of 18.4%, and major postoperative morbidity (e.g. paraplegia) of 10.5%

[285]. Because of these unsatisfactory results of surgery, alternative treatment protocols have been explored [302–306].

Maggisano *et al.* [307] showed that there are two populations of patients with TAR. The first group is represented by patients who reach the hospital in an unstable haemodynamic condition with signs of active bleeding; the survival rate of these patients is low at 17.7%. The second group includes haemodynamically stable patients in whom the diagnosis is obtained by chest radiography and aortography. Surgical repair can be delayed if coexisting injuries increase the risk of operative mortality and morbidity. The risk of fatal free rupture in these patients is low (4.5% within 72 hours) and justifies waiting.

If complete rupture of the aorta does not occur with the traumatic impact, the adventitia and the surrounding mediastinal structures guarantee continuity of the aortic wall. This first phase after the trauma is life-threatening and victims should be taken to hospital as quickly as possible. Prompt diagnosis of aortic wall injury is mandatory and therapeutic hypotension with vasodilators and beta-blocking drugs should reduce aortic wall stress and the risk of lethal aortic rupture. Pate *et al.* [308] analysed 15 years of data and their own experience of risk of free haemorrhage in patients affected by acute TAR in the interval between diagnosis and delayed surgical repair. Of the 492 patients in reports specifying the cause of death, 22 (4.5%) died of aortic rupture, mostly presenting with haemodynamic instability and active bleeding into the pleural space on arrival; in patients in whom the pseudo-aneurysm or haematoma was contained within the mediastinum and who did not present with signs of haemodynamic instability or exsanguination, rupture appeared to be uncommon.

On subsequent days after the trauma, a process of organization of the haematoma usually develops and with time it will turn into strong fibrous tissue, with the formation of a pseudo-aneurysm, which has the same risk of rupture as a true aneurysm of similar size. An arterial systolic pressure exceeding 90mmHg should be an indication to limit fluid replacement for haemodynamic support in hypotensive patients. Monitoring of respiratory function and eventual intubation and mechanical ventilation are fundamental in polytraumatized patients with respiratory insufficiency from injury to the central nervous system, pulmonary contusion, and pleural effusion [308, 309].

The strategy of delaying surgical repair of post-traumatic aortic aneurysms in selected patients offers clear advantages. The overall mortality and incidence of major complications are reduced in an elective scenario compared with an emergency operation. All the necessary procedures of distal aortic perfusion can be safely performed and the mortality is also reduced by prior treatment of potentially lethal associated lesions in polytraumatized patients [298, 310]. Therefore, the treatment of associated lesions is fundamental in these patients and is another incentive to delay surgical intervention in the aorta. However, delayed surgery cannot be applied in every case [311–313]. Even if the majority of traumatic aortic ruptures are stable lesions, in approximately 5% of them the risk of rupture may be high in the acute phase. Signs of impending rupture, such as peri-aortic haematoma, repeated haemothorax, contrast medium extravasation, and uncontrolled blood pressure, are considered signs of instability. Sometimes the aortic tear, acting as a valve mechanism, may cause a pseudo-coarctation syndrome, producing a reduction of flow in the descending aorta with lower extremity ischaemia. This complication, which represents a surgical emergency, accounts for 10% of victims.

Endovascular techniques offer a less invasive option for these patients in whom emergency treatment is necessary. By avoiding thoracotomy and heparin, this technique can be applied in the acute phase without the risk of destabilizing pulmonary, head or abdominal traumatic lesions. The correct timing of aortic repair in a polytraumatized patient should be balanced against other injuries, without a fixed priority.

Surgical and interventional procedures in typical TAR

For surgery the patient is positioned in the right lateral decubitus position with the left hip rolled back to expose the left groin sufficiently to allow access to the femoral vessels. The aortic isthmus is approached via a left posterolateral thoracotomy through the fourth or fifth intercostal space. After opening the pleural space and removing any clots that may be present, the aorta must be controlled above and below the adventitial haematoma. The damaged aortic wall is manipulated only after vascular clamping. The proximal clamp can be positioned below or above the left subclavian artery depending on its involvement within the rupture; various techniques can ensure perfusion of the distal aorta and are discussed below. Once the haematoma is opened, the margins of the rupture can be identified; if the aortic tear is sufficiently limited, a primary wall repair with stitches reinforced with Teflon pledgets should be considered. Frequently, an interposition of preclotted Dacron graft is required. The choice of surgical technique is based on the type of lesion and the time of execution: primary sutures (also with pledgets) (➲ Fig. 31.25A) and end-to-end anastomoses are suitable in patients with linear lesions without extensive dissection and in young patients with an

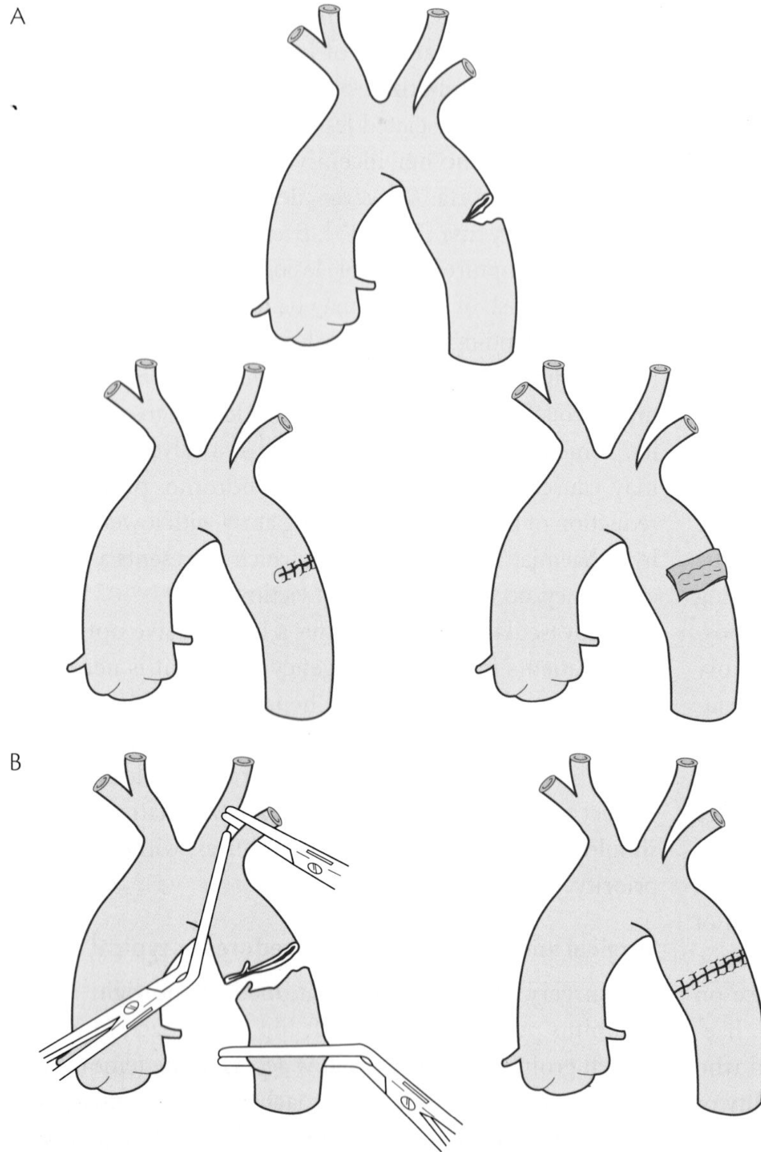

Figure 31.25 (A) Surgical patch repair after traumatic rupture of the descending aorta at the isthmus. (B) Clamping and end-to-end anastomosis after complete transsection of the aorta.

easily mobilized aorta (➲Fig. 31.25B). A tube prosthesis is recommended in lacerated or multiple lesions, with wide intimal dissection, and in elderly patients with atherosclerotic lesions (➲Fig. 31.26).

Rupture involving the anterior portion of the aortic arch is usually characterized by partial or complete avulsion of the brachiocephalic trunk. In these cases the surgical approach is via a median sternotomy and the operation is performed with the patient in cardiopulmonary bypass and deep hypothermia with complete circulatory arrest. The extracorporeal circulation can be right atrium–femoral artery or femoral vein–femoral artery to be implanted before sternotomy. The operation involves completely detaching the brachiocephalic trunk, repairing the aortic arch with a Dacron patch or replacing it with a Dacron tube prosthesis and re-implanting the brachiocephalic trunk on the ascending aorta with the interposition of a prosthesis. In the case of rupture of the ascending aorta, the involved segment needs to be replaced during heart cardioplegic arrest and extracorporeal circulation, either right atrium–femoral artery or femoral vein–femoral artery.

Spinal cord protection

All surgical techniques that use aortic clamping at the level of the descending aorta disrupt spinal cord perfusion and blood pressure; hypertension is extensive above the cross-clamp while hypotension may compromise the spinal cord, kidneys, and other abdominal organs below the clamp. The risk of paraplegia, common in operations on the thoracic descending aorta, is particularly elevated in patients with traumatic aortic rupture. Katz *et al.* [314] found a 24% incidence of ischaemic damage to the spinal cord with

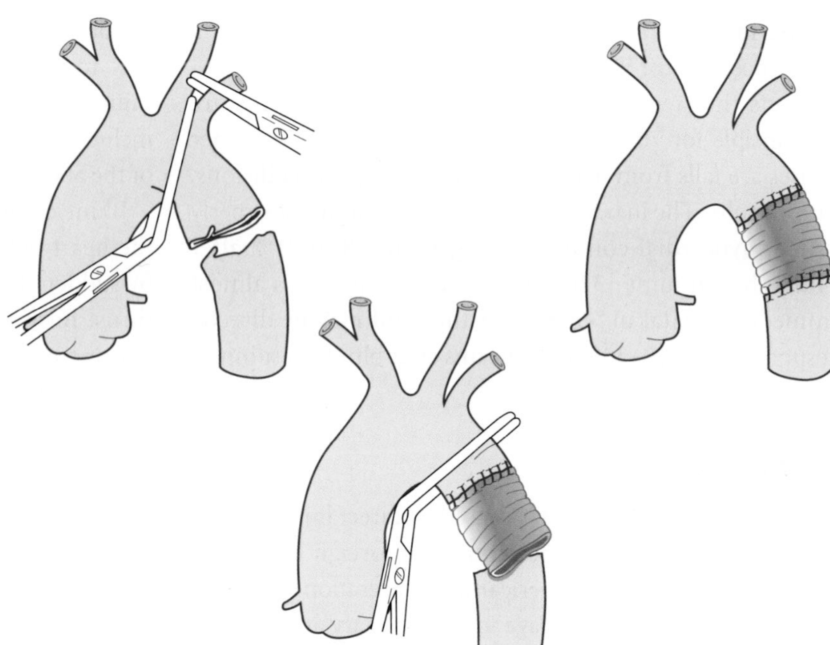

Figure 31.26 Surgical repair by clamping and insertion of an inter-position graft for complete traumatic transsection of the aorta.

postoperative paraplegia. This complication is directly correlated with the length of flow interruption and increases proportionally beyond 30min. Efforts to reduce the incidence of cordal ischaemia by whole-body surface hypothermia, localized cooling of the spinal cord, intrathecal administration of drugs, systemic administration of steroids, and perfusion of the distal aorta were not all convincing [315–317]. An extracorporeal circulation can be used with partial bypass between the femoral vein and artery; this procedure implies total heparinization of the patient and therefore carries a risk of haemorrhage. Left atrium–femoral artery bypass with partial or without heparinization performed with a centrifugal pump offers an adequate blood flow to the distal aorta and the abdominal organs, reduces blood volume overload and the overall pressure to the cardiocirculator system above the cross-clamp, and prevents possible haemorrhagic complications [318].

An overview by von Oppel *et al.* in 1994 [301] disclosed a 25% incidence of paraplegia when the surgical repair was performed by simple cross-clamping. By significantly increasing the distal perfusion the incidence of paraplegia was reduced to 5.2%. Moreover, the two types of distal perfusion differed significantly, because paraplegia developed in 15.6% of patients submitted to 'passive' perfusion and in 2.5% of patients submitted to 'active' perfusion. However, overall operative mortality is still 18.2% for cardiopulmonary bypass, 11.9% for perfusion without heparin, 12.5% for shunts and 16% for simple aortic cross-clamping.

Outcomes

After initial limited series and case reports, endovascular treatment is going to become the method of choice in the management of TAR [319–323]. By avoiding thoracotomy and the use of heparin, endovascular repair can be applied in the acute patient without the risk of threatening pulmonary, head or abdominal traumatic lesions. The risk of paraplegia seems to be very low in endovascular techniques. Therefore we may expect a very low rate or absence of paraplegia when using short stent-graft coverage of a post-traumatic aneurysm.

Trauma to the heart

Aetiology

Trauma is the most common cause of death for men <40 years of age, with 25% related to chest trauma. Isolated chest trauma is responsible for 10% of all fatal traumas [324] as a result of penetrating or non-penetrating injuries or blunt trauma to the heart. For penetrating injuries, the underlying cause may be stab wounds from knife, ice pick, stiletto, or screwdriver that has been violently driven into the chest. Other causes are missiles, shotgun wounds, or iatrogenic injury such as chest tubes or needle biopsy. While stab wounds most commonly injure the right ventricle, high-velocity missiles rupture the heart.

The most common cause of blunt cardiac injury is a high-speed motor vehicle crash in which the driver's chest impacts the steering wheel. Motor vehicle accidents are responsible for 70% of all chest wall injuries [325]. Other causes are falls from height, blast injuries, sports collisions, and assaults. The incidence of blunt cardiac injury, formerly called myocardial contusion, ranges from 8 to 71% after blunt chest trauma [326]. Blunt cardiac rupture is almost immediately fatal in >90% of victims and may be directly responsible for 10–30% of all deaths after blunt chest injury [324, 327].

Pathogenesis

Penetrating cardiac trauma is caused by direct injury of cardiac structures due to penetration of a foreign body. The result may be injury to the pericardium, laceration of the epicardium with possible damage to the coronary arteries, and penetration through the myocardial wall opening a connection between the chambers and the pericardium. All structures of the heart can be injured directly and may cause the specific pathophysiological patterns observed for myocardial infarction, acute valvular insufficiency, creation of intracardiac shunts, and injury to the conduction system (➲Fig. 31.27). However, most stab wounds result in acute pericardial tamponade, although rapidly exsanguinating haemorrhage into the pleural space is also possible. Therefore, the clinical presentation of patients with stab wounds is dominated by the typical signs of cardiac tamponade and/or haemorrhagic shock. Cardiac wounds caused by missiles usually result in acute haemorrhagic shock with frequently fatal outcome. The clinical status is typically profound hypotension with tachycardia and collapsed veins. On their way to the heart, penetrating foreign bodies frequently injure the pleural space, internal mammary vessels, lung including pulmonary vessels, and/or occasionally structures of the abdominal viscera.

Blunt cardiac injury may be caused by compression of the heart between the sternum and vertebral column, or by sudden deceleration of the chest causing the heart to be thrust forward against the sternum with consequent sudden increase in intracardiac pressure. The possible result may be rupture of the free cardiac wall, the ventricular septum, the tensor apparatus, or leaflets of the atrioventricular valves or the cusps of the aortic valve. Also described are coronary artery fistula to a cardiac chamber, injury with coronary artery thrombosis, and damage to the conduction system causing bundle branch block or arrhythmias with cardiac arrest or ventricular fibrillation. If the blunt chest impact is less violent, contusion of the myocardium may be the result. Myocardial contusion may result in subepicardial and myocardial haemorrhage and disruption, inflammatory cell infiltration, and interstitial oedema.

Clinical features

Penetrating cardiac injury

The diagnosis of cardiac injury must be considered any time the chest is penetrated by a missile or a knife. This is especially true when the entry is medial to the nipple anteriorly or medial to the scapula posteriorly. Careful inspection of the undressed chest is mandatory since stab wounds of stilettos may be missed. The clinical presentation of penetrating cardiac injuries ranges from complete haemodynamic stability

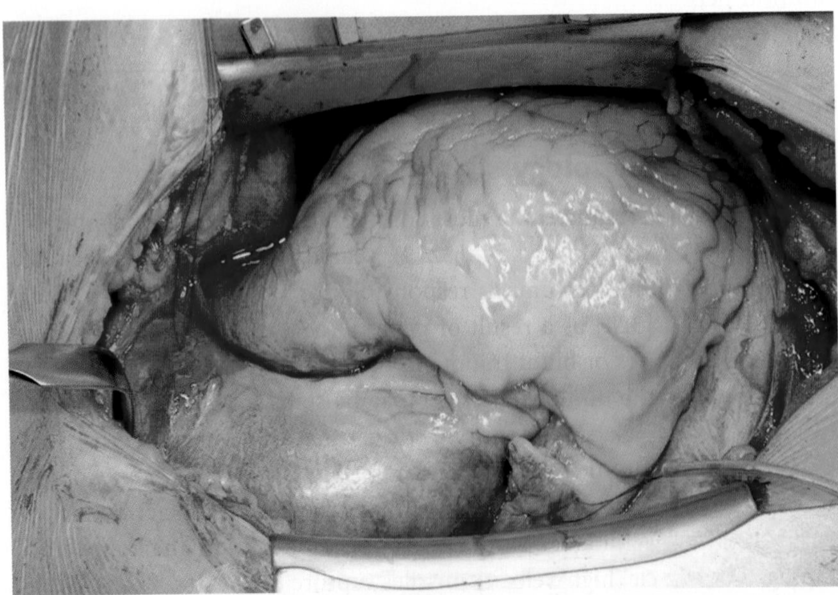

Figure 31.27 Intraoperative aspect of a 'blue aorta' after acute aortic dissection Stanford type A.

to acute cardiovascular collapse and frank cardiopulmonary arrest. Distended neck veins, muffled heart sounds, and hypertension represent the classical Beck's triad [328] of patients presenting with full-blown pericardial tamponade. Kussmaul's sign (paradoxical inspiratory distension of neck veins upon expiration) is another classic sign attributed to pericardial tamponade. When blood loss exceeds 40–50% of intravascular blood volume, cessation of cardiac function will occur. It has been controversially discussed that pericardial tamponade has protective as well as negative impacts on outcome after penetrating cardiac injury, i.e. avoidance of exsanguination versus compression of the heart leading to cardiopulmonary arrest [329–331]. However, medical staff of emergency departments should be aware that cardiac injuries can be extremely deceptive in their clinical presentation. If the patient's condition permits, chest radiography and techniques of cardiac investigation are helpful, such as transthoracic echocardiography, MRI, and/or CT. However, the majority of patients with penetrating cardiac injury will reach the emergency room in an unstable condition, often under resuscitation or presenting with pericardial tamponade [332]. Therefore, diagnostic procedures are restricted to the identification of the cause of haemodynamic instability or shock.

The established standard for diagnosis of pericardial tamponade remains subxiphoid access with transthoracic echocardiography [330–333]. Surgical inspection has been relegated to a second line of evaluation. Two-dimensional echocardiography is also the tool of choice for diagnosis of penetrating cardiac injuries, with 90% accuracy, 97% specificity, and 90% sensitivity in haemodynamically stable patients [334]. When a haemopneumothorax is associated, the usefulness and value of echocardiography declines significantly [326]; however, echocardiography should be employed both in stable and unstable patients with suspected penetrating cardiac injury, allowing the surgeon to proceed directly to median sternotomy. If diagnostic tools fail to show definite evidence of cardiac penetration in patients presenting with penetrating thoracic injury, diagnostic sternotomy or thoracotomy should be considered liberally.

Blunt cardiac trauma

Blunt cardiac trauma manifests as a variety of clinical conditions, usually in association with multiorgan injuries. The patient with blunt cardiac injury may exhibit severe (or no) symptoms of precordial pain, dysrhythmias, symptoms of acute valvular incompetence, myocardial infarction, intracardiac shunts, or the complete picture of cardiac tamponade or shock due to exsanguinating haemorrhage. The most important determinant for diagnostic management is haemodynamic stability. A normal ECG and blood pressure virtually excludes significant injury to the heart. Haemodynamic instability may be related to blood loss caused by additional injuries, but cardiac tamponade must be excluded. The classic 'bruit de Moulin' demonstrates the sound of the heart beating in a pericardium partially filled with air and blood and sounds like a splashing millwheel. Immediate objective assessment of unstable patients suspected of blunt cardiac injury is provided in the majority of cases by echocardiography in the emergency room. If echocardiography shows a mechanical cause for hypotension, rapid surgical intervention is warranted.

The significance of making the diagnosis in asymptomatic patients is not clear, nor is the best method. Probably only 1–20% of asymptomatic patients will develop complications that require treatment [326]; one scenario may be the development of an aneurysm of the left ventricle after cardiac contusion. Therefore, transthoracic ultrasound, ECG, measurement of cardiac enzymes, and use of echocardiography in selected cases are all useful for assessment of stable patients. A normal ECG helps to identify a very-low risk patient. ECG changes are neither specific nor sensitive for significant myocardial dysfunction but have a high negative predictive value for cardiac complications [338]. Routine measurement of cardiac enzymes such as cardiac troponin I in asymptomatic patients suspected of cardiac trauma is recommended [324, 326, 335, 336] but evidence for benefit in the accurate diagnosis of cardiac trauma in asymptomatic patients is lacking [327]. At present, an admission ECG should be performed on all patients in whom there is suspected blunt cardiac injury, and echocardiography should be obtained in haemodynamically unstable patients. If aortic rupture is a potential differential diagnosis, echocardiography and CT should be performed. A normal ECG should terminate the pursuit of diagnosis since the risk of having blunt cardiac injury that requires treatment is insignificant. No other imaging studies or measurement of cardiac enzymes are recommended for screening of cardiac injury or for predicting complications related to blunt cardiac injury [327].

Therapeutic management

Medical management

In this era of progressively earlier ambulation of patients with acute myocardial infarction, a similar approach appears to be reasonable after several days of close observation for myocardial contusion. Several groups have concluded that in trauma patients in stable condition, contusion neither increases the complication rate nor necessitates monitoring [337, 338]. In a study from the Boston City Hospital, Jimenez et al. [334] prospectively divided 336 patients admitted to the surgical intensive care unit with possible myocardial contusion into three groups: (1) those with a normal ECG; (2) those with an abnormal one; and (3) those with either normal or abnormal ECG but with many associated thoracic or extrathoracic injuries. Non-invasive studies were abnormal most often in the latter group, while cardiac complications were absent in groups 1 and 2. The authors concluded that young patients with minor blunt trauma and a normal or slightly abnormal ECG do not benefit from cardiac monitoring and should be subject to regular mobilization and rehabilitation. However, treatment with anticoagulants, and clearly with thrombolytics, is contraindicated because intramyocardial or intrapericardial haemorrhage may be precipitated or exacerbated. Atrial fibrillation, when present, usually reverts to sinus rhythm spontaneously; digitalis glycosides may be used to slow the ventricular rate and accelerate reversion to sinus rhythm. Chest pain is best treated with analgesics; non-steroidal anti-inflammatory agents are not advised because they might interfere with myocardial healing. Corticosteroids have proved helpful only in Dressler's syndrome [339].

As already noted, the prognosis for complete or partial recovery is generally excellent but careful follow-up to screen for late complications, ranging from ventricular arrhythmias to cardiac rupture, is recommended. Coronary occlusion [339–342], aorta–right atrial fistula [343], and ventricular aneurysms [330] are occasional sequelae.

Although many analogies can be drawn between cardiac necrosis caused by trauma and that caused by ischaemic heart disease, a number of crucial differences must be emphasized. Patients with acute myocardial infarction secondary to coronary artery disease generally have diffuse, obstructive, gradually progressive coronary atherosclerosis, are frequently middle-aged or elderly, and may have underlying heart disease. Patients with traumatic myocardial contusion generally have normal coronary vessels and only a discrete area of myocardial damage; most often, they are young and without underlying cardiovascular illness. Hence, the long-term prognosis in surviving patients with myocardial necrosis secondary to trauma tends to be far better than in patients with myocardial infarction and coronary disease.

Patients with external rupture of the heart obviously require emergency surgery if they reach a hospital. Pericardiocentesis and expansion of the intravascular volume can be carried out while the most rapid preparation possible for operation is undertaken [344–349]. In contrast, patients with rupture of the interventricular septum do not always require emergency operation. Indeed, many defects are small, with minimal left-to-right shunts, and may even heal spontaneously. If heart failure develops subsequently, as occurs in many patients, surgical correction should be carried out promptly and is often successful [347].

Surgical management

In the majority of patients with cardiac trauma, surgical intervention is aimed at preserving life in patients with a poor prognosis. Recently, the American Association for the Surgery of Trauma and its Organ Injury Scaling Committee have developed a cardiac injury scale for uniformly describing cardiac injuries [350]. It remains questionable if this complex but comprehensive scale will be usable for emergency situations in the emergency or operating room, but it defines the severity, mechanism, and location of both penetrating and blunt trauma in a scale from I to VI. Treatment strategies could be developed with regard to the heart injury scale, and prognosis of mortality becomes predictable to a certain degree [330].

In stable patients with evidence of penetrating cardiac injury, immediate transport to the operating room, general anaesthesia, and thoracotomy is mandatory. Median sternotomy is the incision of choice. This is especially true in stable patients with stab wound. If the stabbing device is still in place when the patient is admitted to the emergency room, it is not removed until the surgical approach has been made and ideally not until the pericardium has been opened [351]. In unstable patients who arrive in the emergency room in extremis, unconscious, with or without reduced vital signs but with evidence of cardiac or great vessel wound as the cause, immediate thoracotomy in the emergency unit is indicated. Left anterolateral thoracotomy remains the incision of choice, and can be extended across the sternum as bilateral anterolateral thoracotomies if the patient's injuries extend into the right hemithoracic cavity [329]. Evaluation of the extent of haemorrhage present within the left hemithoracic cavity is then carried out. If necessary, the descending aorta can be reached and cross-clamped, the location of penetrating injury found, and immediate digital control can be established. If the repair appears to be a simple one, repair is then performed. Otherwise, the patient is transferred to a prepared operating room while digital control of the haemorrhage is maintained. Atrial wounds can be controlled by partial occlusion with a Satinsky vascular clamp or Allis clamps followed by a closing suture line; total inflow occlusion by clamping of both venae cavae should be avoided since the acidotic and ischaemic heart will not tolerate the manoeuvre [329, 330]. Ventricular wounds are best controlled by digital occlusion while placing running or horizontal mattress sutures with 2-0 Prolene. If coronary arteries are injured, either ligation (of distal portion) or immediate establishment of cardiopulmonary bypass and coronary artery bypass grafting are indicated (➲Fig. 31.28). Since most septal injuries from penetrating trauma close spontaneously, no patient should be considered for operation acutely. Only if an intracardiac shunt greater than 2:1 is confirmed by cardiac catheterization should surgery be considered in a stable patient.

Cardiac contusion is no indication for surgery [339, 340]. Close follow-up management is indicated in order to detect delayed cardiac rupture, valvular dysfunction, or aneurysm formation. Rupture of atrioventricular and aortic valves requires surgical repair, but proper timing of the procedure may improve results. Stabilization of a traumatized patient prior to surgery is attempted, although left ventricular failure may require immediate operation. If possible, septal defects with a left-to-right shunt and a Q_p:Q_s ratio >2:1 should be repaired electively to improve long-term outcome. Immediate surgery for blunt cardiac trauma is mandatory in both cardiac rupture and injury or occlusion of a coronary artery. In contrast to penetrating cardiac injuries, pericardiocentesis should not be used to diagnose haemopericardium in a stable patient with suspected cardiac injury; instead, the patient should be transported to the operating room with cardiopulmonary bypass equipment available. The operative approach for repairing cardiac injury is a median sternotomy. Surgical techniques are similar to those used for penetrating cardiac injuries; use of cardiopulmonary bypass is required for coronary artery bypass grafting of valve repair but rarely for the repair of cardiac rupture [340].

Outcome after cardiac trauma

Survival after penetrating cardiac trauma is directly related to the patient's status on presenting to the emergency department. Of those who reach the emergency room alive, 80% of patients survive. Survival of patients with cardiac missile wounds is poor, with 40% of these reaching the emergency room. Generally, stab wounds have a better outcome than missile wounds [351]. In a prospective study, a total of 105 patients sustained penetrating injuries over a 2-year period, with 65% due to gunshots and 35% to stab wounds [330]. Survival of patients with gunshot wounds was 16% but was 65% in those with stab wounds. Emergency department thoracotomy was performed in 71 patients (68%), but only 10 patients survived. The site of injury and the presence of tamponade did not predict survival.

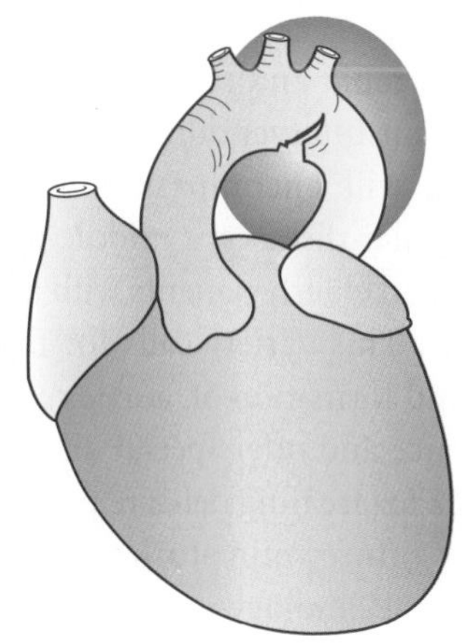

Figure 31.28 Schematic view of an aortic rupture 'loco typico'.

Outcome after blunt heart trauma depends on the severity of the injury. The prognosis after myocardial contusion is generally benign. A prospective study of 118 patients with blunt chest trauma revealed 14 patients (12%) with myocardial contusion. All but one patient survived the acute hospitalization and 1-year follow-up without new cardiac pathologies [352]. However, cardiac rupture may be a diagnostic challenge since institutional algorithms may not identify those patients with remarkably few symptoms before [342]. Cardiac rupture has a poor prognosis, with a mortality of >90% [327]; if patients showing vital signs at admission reach a surgical unit, prognosis increases significantly. Outcome of emergency thoracotomy after blunt chest trauma in the admission room is poor [353–355].

Personal perspective

Cardiovascular and aortic disease, in both acute syndromes and chronic stages, will constitute an increasing share of cardiology and vascular medicine. With improved awareness and easy access to non-invasive tomographic imaging, aortic pathology emerges as a major focus and will require more attention than before; cardiology in particular will shoulder the major burden of the multifaceted acute and chronic aortic pathology. Thus the cardiovascular community has to handle the complexity and the challenges with regard to screening patients at risk, rapid and reliable diagnosis, and, eventually, competent interventional or surgical treatment. The spectrum will encompass young patients with hereditary vascular diseases, a middle-aged cohort with hypertension, and elderly patients with advanced general atherosclerosis. This variety calls for multidisciplinary cooperation and formation of 'aortic centres' to concentrate competence and offer special diagnostic and interventional skills for treating delicate patients.

In the near future, miniaturization and refinement of endovascular technology will allow endo-aortic interventions to be performed percutaneously under local anaesthesia, and more physiological stent-grafts will even mimic the rotational three-dimensional systolic twist of both the ascending and descending thoracic aorta, while contemporary surgical techniques are less likely to improve. More importantly, even successful aortic surgery will not abolish any of the associated risk factors from comorbid conditions and therefore late outcome will remain dominated by the individual prognosis (comorbid state). As a consequence, in centres of excellence for aortic disease the endovascular treatment options are more likely to prevail even in highly comorbid subsets of patients, since at least the surgical risk will be eliminated with endovascular techniques. A definitive answer to the ethical justification for treatment in the very old patient is not established, because prospective data from randomized studies or registries are scarce in aortic diseases. However, when insisting on strict proof (or disproof) in empirical science, one will never benefit from experience. In a world of rapidly advancing technology, it is wise to remember the old principles of responsible use of clinical judgement and experience for the benefit of our patients. The growing segment of older patients with multiorgan comorbidities deserve an holistic approach, the intelligent use of prognosticating tools, and close interdisciplinary cooperation.

Further reading

Amarenco P, Cohen A, Tzourio C, *et al.* Atherosclerotic disease of the aortic arch and the risk of ischemic stroke. *N Engl J Med* 1994; **331**: 1474–9.

Erbel R, Alfonso F, Boileau C *et al.* Diagnosis and management of aortic dissection. Recommendations on the Task Force on Aortic Dissection, European Society of Cardiology. *Eur Heart J* 2001; **22**: 1642–81.

Fattori R, Tsai TT, Myrmel T, *et al.* Complicated acute type B dissection: is surgery still the best option? A report from the International Registry of Acute Aortic Dissection (IRAD). *J Am Coll Cardiol Intv* 2008; **1**: 395–402.

Gornik HL, Creager MA. Aortitis. *Circulation* 2008; **117**: 3049–51.

Greenberg RK, Lu Q, Roselli EE, *et al.* Contemporary analysis of descending thoracic and thoracoabdominal aneurysm repair. A comparison of endovascular and open techniques. *Circulation* 2008; **118**: 808–17.

Hunt JP, Baker CC, Lentz CW, *et al.* Thoracic aorta injuries: management and outcome of 144 patients. *J Trauma* 1996; **40**: 547–56.

Karmy-Jones R, Jurkovich GJ. Blunt chest trauma. *Curr Probl Surg* 2004; **41**: 211–21.

Nienaber CA, Fattori R, Lund G, *et al.* Nonsurgical reconstruction of thoracic aortic dissection by stent-graft placement. *N Engl J Med* 1999; **340**: 1539–45.

Nienaber CA, Zannetti S, Barbieri B, *et al.* Investigation of Stent grafts in patients with type B Aortic Dissection Design of the INSTEAD trial- a prospective, multicenter, European randomized trial. *Am Heart J* 2005; **149**: 592–9.

Patel HJ, Deeb M. Ascending and arch aorta: pathology, natural history, and treatment. *Circulation* 2008; **118**: 188–95.

Svensson LG, Kouchoukos NT, Miller DC, *et al.* Expert consensus document on the treatment of descending thoracic aortic disease using endovascular stent-grafts. *Ann Thorac Surg* 2008; **85**: S1–41.

Tsai TT, Nienaber CA, Eagle KA. Acute aortic syndromes. *Circulation* 2005; **112**: 3802–13.

➲ **For full references and multimedia materials please visit the online version of the book (http://esctextbook.oxfordonline.com).**

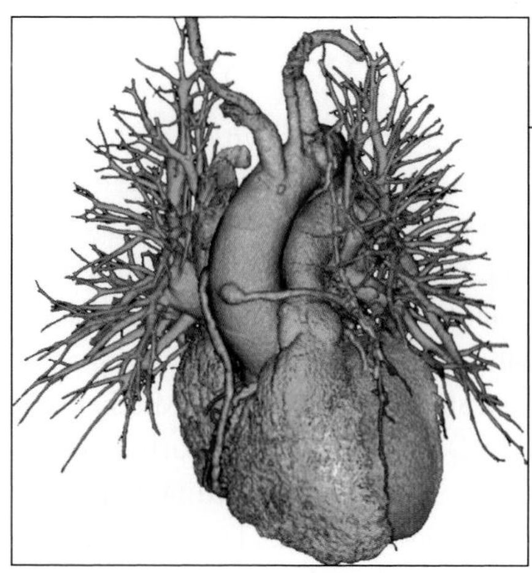

CHAPTER 32

Sports and Heart Disease

Domenico Corrado, Cristina Basso, Antonio Pelliccia, and Gaetano Thiene

Contents

Summary

Sports activity is recommended by the medical community because it improves fitness and reduces cardiovascular morbidity and mortality. However, physical exercise may precipitate acute fatalities in both adults and young competitive athletes with concealed heart diseases. The risk:benefit ratio of physical exercise differs among these two age groups. In adults, physical activity can be regarded as a 'two-edged sword': vigorous exertion increases the incidence of acute coronary events in individuals who did not exercise regularly, whereas habitual physical activity reduces the overall risk of myocardial infarction and sudden coronary death by preventing development and progression of coronary atherosclerotic lesions. In adolescents and young adults, competitive sport is associated with a significant increase of the risk of sudden death. Sports is not the 'per se' cause of the enhanced mortality in this age group; rather, it acts as a trigger of cardiac arrest in those athletes who are affected by silent cardiovascular conditions, mostly cardiomyopathy, premature coronary artery disease, and congenital coronary anomalies, which predispose to life-threatening ventricular arrhythmias during effort. This points to the need for a preparticipation screening aimed at early identification and disqualification of those subjects affected by at-risk cardiovascular diseases.

This chapter will focus on the physiologic adaptive changes of the cardiovascular system to sustained physical exercise ('athlete's heart'); the causes and mechanisms of the increased cardiovascular risk during sports activity; the prevention of sudden death by preparticipation screening; and the management strategies, including eligibility to competitive sports activity, of athletes diagnosed with a potentially lethal cardiovascular disease.

Introduction

Regular physical exercise is recommended by the medical community because it improves fitness and reduces cardiovascular morbidity and mortality [1]. Several epidemiological, clinical, and experimental studies have provided solid scientific evidence that habitual physical activity prevents the development of atherosclerosis and reduces the incidence of coronary events [2, 3]. In addition, physical exercise may confer protection against other diseases such as obesity, osteoporosis, diabetes, malignancies and depression. On the other hand, vigorous exertion may acutely and transiently increase the risk of acute myocardial infarction and sudden death in susceptible individuals [4–10]. For centuries it was a mystery why cardiac arrest should occur in competitive athletes, who had previously achieved extraordinary exercise performance without complaining of any symptoms. The cause was generally ascribed to myocardial infarction, even though evidence of ischaemic myocardial necrosis was rarely reported. It is now clear that the most common mechanism of sudden death during sports activity is an abrupt ventricular tachyarrhythmia as a consequence of a wide spectrum of cardiovascular diseases, either acquired or congenital [4, 9]. The culprit diseases are often clinically silent and unlikely to be suspected or diagnosed on the basis of spontaneous symptoms. Systematic preparticipation screening of all subjects embarking in sports activity has the potential to identify those athletes at risk and to reduce mortality. Guidelines for athletic participation have been developed based on the best available information regarding the risks of the underlying cardiovascular condition and the specific sport disciplines. The use of internal and external defibrillators for treatment of on-the-field arrhythmic cardiac arrest is an emerging clinical and legal issue.

There are four important areas of sports cardiology:

1) physiologic adaptive changes of the cardiovascular system to sustained physical exercise (athlete's heart);
2) causes and mechanisms of the increased cardiovascular risk during sports activity;
3) prevention of sudden death by preparticipation screening; and
4) disqualification from competitive sports activity and management strategies of athletes diagnosed with a potentially lethal cardiovascular disease.

Classification of sports

The cardiovascular impact of a sports activity is related to its specific workload on the heart, mostly in terms of increase of blood flow and pressure, which, in individuals with existing heart disorders, may induce life-threatening ventricular arrhythmias, acute coronary events, and disease progression. The classification for the assessment of specific sports-related cardiovascular risk proposed by Mitchell and colleagues is provided in ➲Table 32.1 [11]. Sports activities are classified into two main categories according to general types of exercise (i.e. dynamic and static). Dynamic exercise involves changes in the muscle length and joint movement with rhythmic contractions that develop a relatively small intramuscular force. Static exercise involves the development of a relatively large intramuscular force with little or no change in muscle length or joint movement. Each sport can be classified as low, moderate, and high based on the level

Table 32.1 Classification of sports

	A. Low dynamic	B. Moderate dynamic	C. High dynamic
I. Low static	Archering Bowling Cricket Golf Riflery	Baseball* Table tennis Tennis (doubles) Volleyball	Badminton Cross-country skiing (classic) Running (marathon) Walking
II. Moderate static	Auto racing*† Diving† Equestrian*† Gymnastics*† Karate/Judo*† Motorcycling*† Sailing	Fencing Field events (jumping) Figure skating* Lacrosse* Running (sprint)	Basketball* Biathlon Cross-country skiing (skating) Field hockey* Football* Ice hockey* Running (mid/long) Soccer* Squash* Swimming Team handball* Tennis (single)
III. High static	Bobsledding *† Field events (throwing) Luge*† Rock climbing*† Waterskiing*† Weight lifting*† Windsurfing*†	Body building*† Downhill skiing*† Wrestling*	Boxing* Canoeing, kayaking Cycling*† Decathlon Rowing Speed skating

* Danger of bodily collision.† Increased risk if syncope occurs. Also see ➲Table 12.5, p.421 and ➲Table 25.11, p.946.

Modified with permission from Mitchell J, Haskell WL, Raven PB. Classification of Sports. *J Am Coll Cardiol* 1994; **24**: 864–6.

of intensity of exercise (either dynamic or static) required to perform that sport during competition. This classification is intended to provide a schematic indication of the cardiovascular demand associated with different sports, with an additional notification of those disciplines associated with increased risk of bodily collision and those associated with an enhanced risk if syncope occurs. In terms of their dynamic and static demands, sports are classified as III C (high static and high dynamic), II B (moderate static and moderate dynamic), or IA (low static and low dynamic) (➲Table 32.1). For instance, an athlete with a cardiovascular disorder that contraindicates a sport that produces a high pressure load on the left ventricle may be advised to avoid sports classified as III A, III B, and III C. The Mitchell classification should be regarded as largely theoretical and limited because it does not take into account a number of additional significant factors such as the emotional involvement of the athlete during a competitive match, environmental exposure during athletic competition, and training programmes requiring a different type of exercise and more demanding physical activity than the competition itself. However, the classification provides a reasonable estimate of the risk associated with specific sports activity and is currently used in sports medical practice.

The athlete's heart

During intense aerobic exercise, the oxygen consumption of muscle tissue increases markedly, and cardiac output must rise to meet the demands. Participation in sports activity and regular physical training is associated with physiological structural and electrophysiological cardiac changes (athlete's heart) that enable sustained increases in cardiac output for prolonged periods [12]. First demonstrated in 1935, adaptive structural changes of the athlete's heart consist principally of left ventricular (LV) remodelling with increased LV wall thickness and chamber size, with preserved systolic and diastolic ventricular function [13–15] (➲Fig. 32.1). Moreover, physiologic adaptation of the cardiac autonomic nervous system (i.e. increased vagal tone and/or withdrawal of sympathetic activity) to athletic conditioning results in sinus bradycardia, atrioventricular (AV) conduction impairment, and early repolarization [16]. The extent of cardiac morphological and electrical changes in trained athletes varies with the athlete's gender, race, level of fitness, and type of sport [16–25]. Adaptive changes are more prevalent and significant in male athletes and athletes of African-Caribbean descent [19, 26, 27]. This most likely reflects the role of genetic/ethnic predisposing factors which account for a more prominent cardiovascular remodelling, either structural or neuro-autonomic, in response to physical training and competition. Genotype and different polymorphisms of the angiotensin-converting enzyme or angiotensinogen genes can result in different phenotypic expression of the athlete heart [28, 29].

Although short-term sports conditioning does not induce changes of cardiac dimensions, prolonged training is commonly associated with structural left ventricular remodelling. The morphological changes depend on the type of exercise undertaken [22, 23]. High dynamic (isotonic) forms of exercise found in endurance sports, such as long-distance running and cycling, are more likely to result in an increase in absolute ventricular chamber dimensions with a proportional increase in wall thickness (eccentric hypertrophy). Such a type of ventricular change is required to adapt to the volume overload associated with the exceptionally large increases in cardiac output during activity. In contrast, high static (isometric) exercise, such as weight lifting and wrestling, tends to increase LV mass without increasing chamber size (concentric hypertrophy), in response to the pure pressure overload produced by the very high systemic arterial pressures generated by this sporting activity. Athletes who participate in sports involving combined high dynamic and high static demands, such as rowing and canoeing, exhibit intermediate morpho-functional changes. Adaptive LV hypertrophy is typically symmetric (i.e. hypertrophy of the septum and left ventricular free wall is equal), occurs early in conditioning, and rapidly reverses to baseline within weeks of detraining. The electrocardiogram (ECG) of athletes characteristically shows sinus bradycardia/arrhythmia, increased QRS voltages, and early repolarization changes (➲Chapter 2) [16, 30]. Participation in an endurance sports discipline, such as cycling, cross-country skiing, and rowing/canoeing, provokes greater cardiac remodelling, and is significantly associated with a higher rate and greater extent of physiologic ECG changes such as sinus bradycardia and increase of QRS voltages.

Physiologic structural and electrical changes seen in the athlete's heart may partially overlap with pathologic features of cardiovascular conditions at risk of sudden death during sports, thus raising the need for an accurate diagnosis [15, 30]. Recognition of variations in physiologic adaptive ECG changes by race is mandatory for differentiating athlete's heart from cardiomyopathy. A recent study [27] showed that almost 20% of black athletes exhibit left ventricular hypertrophy compared with just 4% of white athletes and 3% of black athletes (but none of the white athletes) have

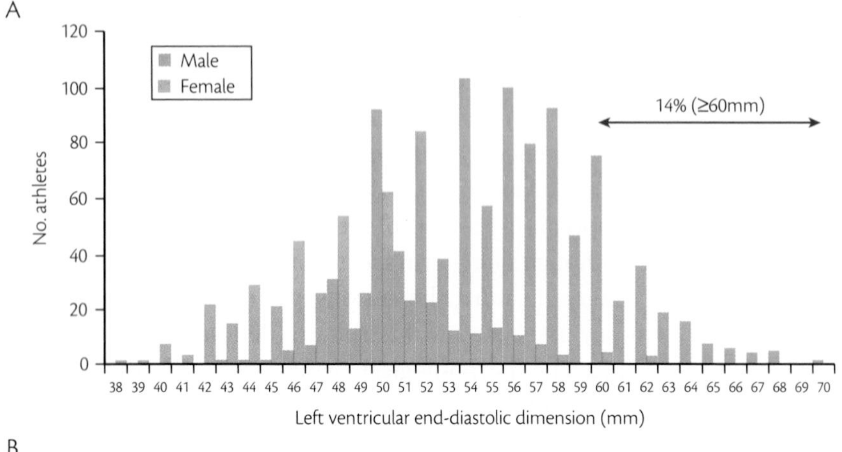

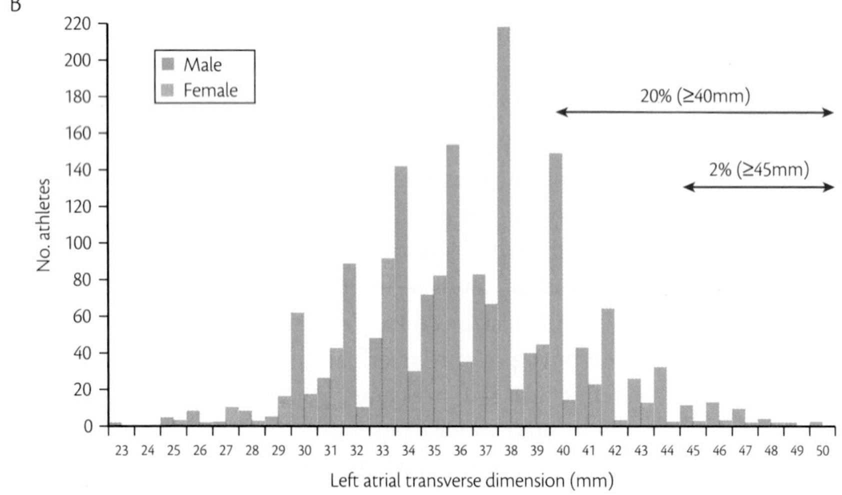

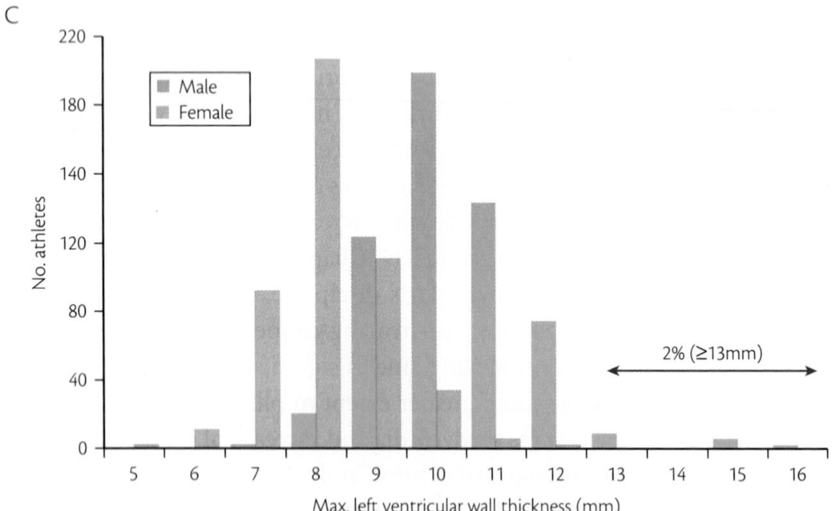

Figure 32.1 Distribution of cardiac dimensions in large populations of highly trained male and female athletes. (A) LV end-diastolic cavity dimension; 14% of athletes have enlargement of 60–70mm. (B) Transverse left atrial dimension; 20% of athletes have transverse left atrial dimension 40mm. (C) Maximum (Max.) LV wall thickness; 2% of men and 0% of women have wall thickness 13mm. Modified from Maron BJ, Pelliccia A. The heart of trained athletes: cardiac remodeling and the risks of sports, including sudden death. *Circulation* 2006; **114**: 1633–44.

substantial increase of LV thickness (>15mm), which may be consistent with morphologically mild HCM. Moreover, black athletes have more prevalent and pronounced ECG changes, including voltage criteria for left ventricular hypertrophy and early repolarization changes which reflect the race-related greater magnitude of left ventricular hypertrophy and/or increased vagal sensitivity [27, 28].

Epidemiology of sudden death in the athlete

The sudden and unexpected death of an athlete is always a powerful and tragic event, which devastates families, other competitors, institutions (high school, college, or professional organization), sports medicine teams, and the community [9, 31, 32]. The sudden demise of an athlete has a tremendous appeal to the media because it affects apparently healthy individuals who are regarded as heroes and the healthiest group in society. Instinctively, everyone wonders what intervention might have prevented the death.

Incidence of sudden death

The assessment of the precise frequency with which sudden death occurs in athletes is hampered by the retrospective nature of most analyses. The sudden death incidence is fortunately low and varies in the different athlete series reported in the literature. In apparently healthy adults (>35 years of age), joggers or marathon racers, the estimated rate of sports-related fatalities ranges from 1:15,000 to 1:50,000 [33]. In comparison a significantly lower incidence of fatal events have been reported in young competitive athletes (≤35 years of age). Van Camp *et al.* [34] in a nationally-based survey estimated the prevalence of sudden death in high school and college athletes in the USA to be 0.4 per 100,000 athletes per year. Maron *et al.* [35] showed the prevalence of cardiovascular sudden deaths in competitive high school athletes (age 13–19 years, mean 16 years) from Minnesota to be 0.35 per 100,000 sports participations, and 0.46 per 100,000 individual participants per year (0.77 per 100,000 male athletes). A prospective population-based study in the Veneto Region of Italy reported an incidence of sudden death of 2.3 (2.62 in males and 1.07 in females) per 100,000 athletes per year from all causes, and of 2.1 per 100,000 athletes per year from cardiovascular diseases [36].

The risk of sudden death in athletes increases with age and is greater in men [32, 33, 36]. This explains why the mortality rates found in the Italian investigation were significantly higher than those reported in the USA. Compared with US high school and college participants, the Italian athletic population included older athletes (age range 12–35 years vs. 12–24 years) and a significantly higher proportion of men (82% vs. 65%).

The striking male predominance (male:female ratio up to 10:1) of sudden death in athletes has been related to the higher participation rate of men compared with women in competitive sports, as well as the more intensive training load and level of athletic achievement of men. Furthermore, male gender was reported to be an independent predictor of sports-related sudden death, most likely as a consequence of the greater prevalence and/or phenotypic expression in young males of cardiac diseases at risk of arrhythmic cardiac arrest, such as cardiomyopathies and premature coronary artery disease [36–38].

Risk of sudden death (also see ➲Chapter 30)

Death usually occurs either during (80%) or immediately after (20%) athletic activity, suggesting that participation in competitive sports increases the likelihood of cardiac arrest [31]. The risk:benefit ratio of physical exercise differs between adults and young competitive athletes [4, 39]. This may be explained by the different nature of cardiovascular substrates underlying sport-related sudden death in the two age-groups (➲Table 32.2). Atherosclerotic coronary artery disease is the most common cause of sudden death in adults and elderly exercising subjects [40, 41]. Several epidemiologic studies have assessed the relationship between physical exercise and the risk of sudden coronary events in the middle-aged and older population, in which physical activity can be regarded as a 'two-edged sword' [4, 39, 42]. The available evidence indicates that vigorous exercise acutely increases the incidence of both cardiac arrest and acute myocardial infarction in those who do not exercise regularly. In comparison, epidemiologic studies support the concept that habitual sport activity may offer protection against cardiovascular events over the long-term [4, 43–46]. The relative risk of cardiac arrest or myocardial infarction is greater during exercise than at rest; however, the overall incidence of cardiac arrest, both at rest and during exercise, decreases with increasing exercise levels. Regular exercise prevents development and progression of atherosclerotic coronary artery disease by favourable effects on lipid metabolism and weight reduction and enhances

Table 32.2 Cardiovascular causes of sudden death associated with sports

Age ≥35 years
Coronary artery disease
Age <35 years
Hypertrophic cardiomyopathy
Arrhythmogenic right ventricular cardiomyopathy
Congenital anomalies of coronary arteries
Myocarditis
Aortic rupture
Valvular disease
Pre-excitation syndromes
Cardiac conduction diseases
Ion channel diseases
Congenital heart disease, operated or unoperated

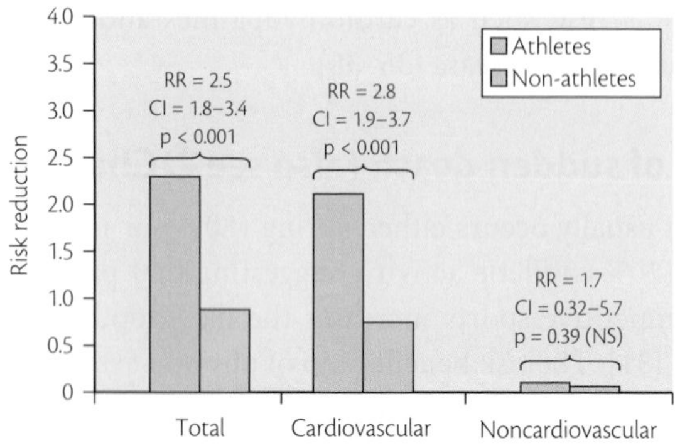

Figure 32.2 Incidence and relative risk (RR) of sudden death among young athletes and non-athletes from total (A), cardiovascular (B) and non-cardiovascular causes. Modified with permission from Corrado D, Migliore F, Basso C, *et al.* Exercise and the risk of sudden cardiac death. *Herz* 2006; **31**: 553–8.

both coronary artery plaque and myocardial electrical stability [4, 39].

Unlike older athletes, a broad spectrum of cardiovascular substrates (including congenital and inherited heart disorders) may underlie sudden death in young competitive athletes (age ≤35 years) [9, 10, 32, 47–55]. An Italian prospective study demonstrated that adolescent and young adults involved in sports activity have 2.8-fold greater risk of sudden cardiovascular death than their non-athletic counterparts [36] (➲Fig. 32.2). However, sports is not itself the cause of the enhanced mortality, since it triggers cardiac arrest in those athletes who are affected by cardiovascular conditions which predispose to life-threatening ventricular arrhythmias during physical exercise. This reinforces the need for systematic evaluation of adolescent and young individuals embarking on sporting activity in order to identify those with potentially lethal cardiovascular diseases and protect them from the increased risk of sudden death.

Causes of sudden death

The vast majority of athletes who die suddenly have underlying structural heart diseases, which provide a substrate for ventricular tachycardia/fibrillation leading to cardiac arrest. As reported in ➲Table 32.2, the causes of sudden death reflect the age of participants. Atherosclerotic coronary artery disease (see ➲Chapter 17) accounts for the vast majority of fatalities in adults (age >35 years) [40, 41, 56–59], while cardiomyopathies have been consistently implicated as the leading cause of sports-related cardiac arrest in younger athletes [32, 47–55]. Hypertrophic cardiomyopathy (HCM) (see ➲Chapter 18) has been reported to account for more than one-third of fatal cases in the USA [32, 52, 60–63] (➲Fig. 32.3), and arrhythmogenic

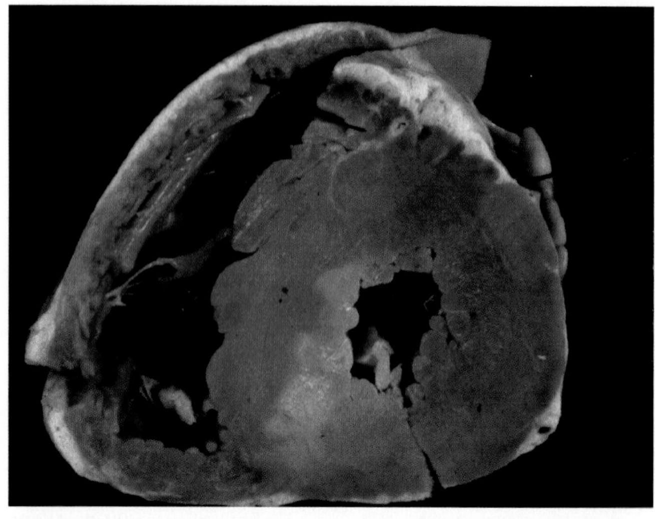
A

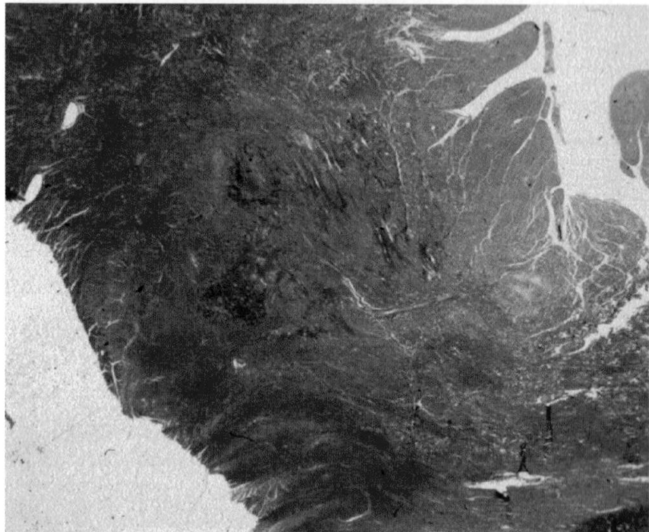
B

Figure 32.3 A 15-year-old basketball player who died suddenly. (A) Short-axis view of the heart showing massive left ventricular hypertrophy and a large scar in the posteroseptal region. (B) Corresponding panoramic histologic section showing intraseptal replacement-type fibrosis (Azan stain, original magnification × 3). Modified with permission from Basso C, Thiene G, Corrado D, *et al.* Hypertrophic cardiomyopathy: pathologic evidence of ischemic damage in young sudden death victims. *Hum Pathol* 2000; **31**: 988–98.

right ventricular cardiomyopathy (ARVC) (see ➲Chapters 9 and 18) for approximately one-fourth in the Veneto Region of Italy [10, 36, 38, 50, 64–68] (➲Fig. 32.4). Other cardiovascular substrates for sports-related sudden death in the young include premature atherosclerotic coronary artery disease [37, 59] (➲Fig. 32.5), congenital coronary anomalies [48, 49, 51] (➲Fig. 32.6), myocarditis [36, 55, 69], dilated cardiomyopathy, mitral valve prolapse, conduction system diseases, and Wolff–Parkinson–White (WPW) syndrome [10, 36, 49, 53] (see ➲Chapter 28).

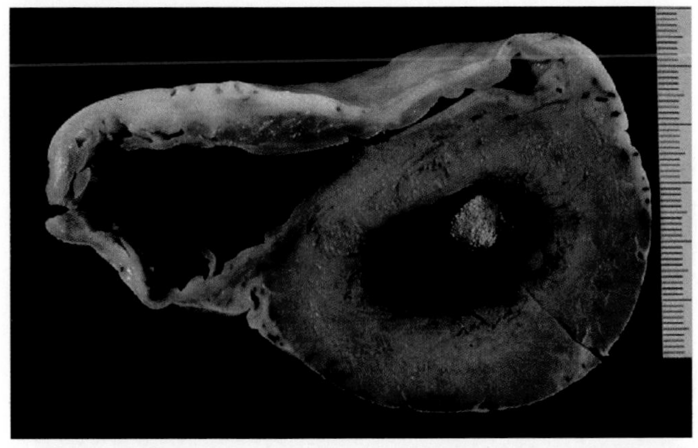

A

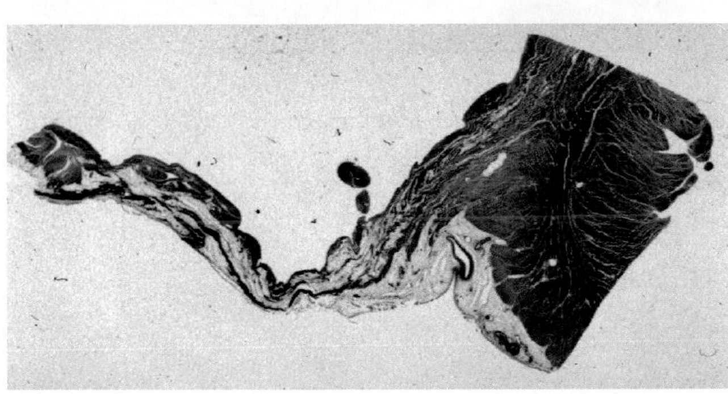

B

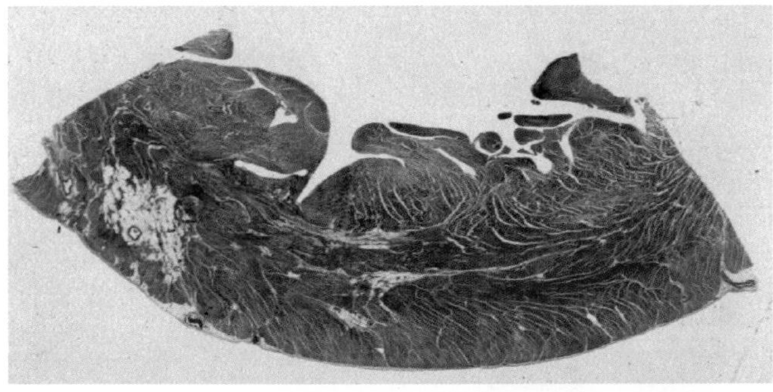

C

Figure 32.4 A 17-year-old soccer player who died suddenly. (A) Cross section of the heart specimen with infundibular and inferior sub-tricuspid aneurysms. (B) Panoramic histologic view of the aneurysm of the inferior region showing wall thinning with fibro-fatty replacement of the right ventricle (Azan stain, original magnification, × 2.5). (C) Panoramic histologic view of the left ventricle showing a spot of fibro-fatty myocardial replacement (Azan stain, original magnification, × 2.5). Modified from Basso C, Thiene G, Corrado D, *et al.* Arrhythmogenic right ventricular cardiomyopathy. Dysplasia, dystrophy, or myocarditis? *Circulation* 1996; **94**: 983–91.

Two to five per cent of young people and athletes who die suddenly have no evidence of structural heart diseases and the cause of their cardiac arrest is in all likelihood related to a primary electrical heart disorders such as inherited cardiac ion channel defects (channelopathies) [36, 55] (see ➲Chapters 9 and 30), including long and short QT syndromes [70], Brugada syndrome [54, 71, 72], and cathecholaminergic polymorphic ventricular tachycardia [73].

Sudden death may be also caused by either a non-arrhythmic mechanism e.g. spontaneous aortic rupture complicating Marfan syndrome (➲Chapter 31) or bicuspid aortic valve (➲Chapter 21) [49], or by diseases not related to the heart—e.g. bronchial asthma or rupture of a cerebral aneurysm [36].

Blunt, non-penetrating, and often innocent-appearing blows to the precordium may trigger ventricular fibrillation without structural injury to ribs, sternum, or heart itself (commotio cordis) [74–77] (see ➲Chapter 30).

Prevention of sudden death by preparticipation screening

Preparticipation medical evaluation of the athletic population allows identification of asymptomatic athletes who have potentially lethal cardiovascular abnormalities, and their protection from the risk of sudden death during sports activity [78–86].

The Italian screening protocol

Italy is the only country in the world where law mandates that every subject engaged in competitive sports activity must undergo a clinical evaluation to obtain eligibility before entering in competitive sports [83–85]. A nationwide mass preparticipation screening programme, essentially based on the 12-lead ECG, has been the practice for >25 years [47, 68, 84–86]. The preparticipation evaluation involves nearly 6 million athletes of all ages annually, representing about 10% of the overall Italian population. A flow chart illustrating the Italian screening protocol is reported in ➲Fig. 32.7. The initial cardiovascular evaluation consists of complete personal and family history, physical examination including blood pressure measurement, and 12-lead ECG. The athletic evaluation is performed by a physician with the specific training, medical skill, and cultural background to reliably identify clinical symptoms and signs associated with those cardiovascular diseases responsible for exercise-related sudden death. In Italy, physicians primarily responsible for preparticipation screening and eligibility for competitive sports attend postgraduate residency training programmes in sports medicine (and sports cardiology) full-time for 4 years. Such specialists work in sports medical centres specifically devoted to periodical evaluation of athletes. The screening starts at the beginning of competitive athletic activity that for the majority of sports disciplines corresponds to an athlete age of 12–14 years. Preparticipation evaluation is repeated on a regular basis (every 1 or 2 years) in order to timely identify time-dependent progression of some diseases.

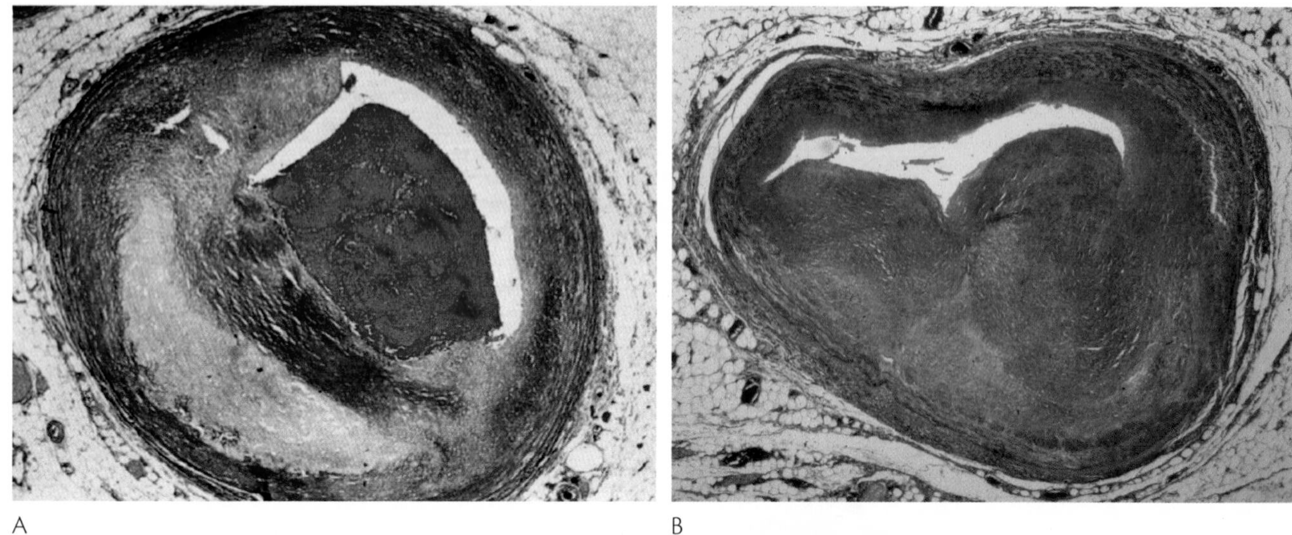

Figure 32.5 (A) A 33-year-old athlete who died suddenly. Fresh occlusive thrombosis of the proximal anterior descending coronary artery superimposed on an eccentric atheromatous plaque with a large lipid core (Azan stain, original magnification × 25). (B) A 30-year-old athlete who died suddenly. Cross section of the proximal left anterior descending coronary artery showing a severe obstructive fibro-cellular plaque (Azan stain, original magnification × 25). Modified from Corrado D, Basso C, Poletti A, *et al*. Sudden death in the young: is coronary thrombosis the major precipitating factor? *Circulation* 1994; **90**: 2315–23.

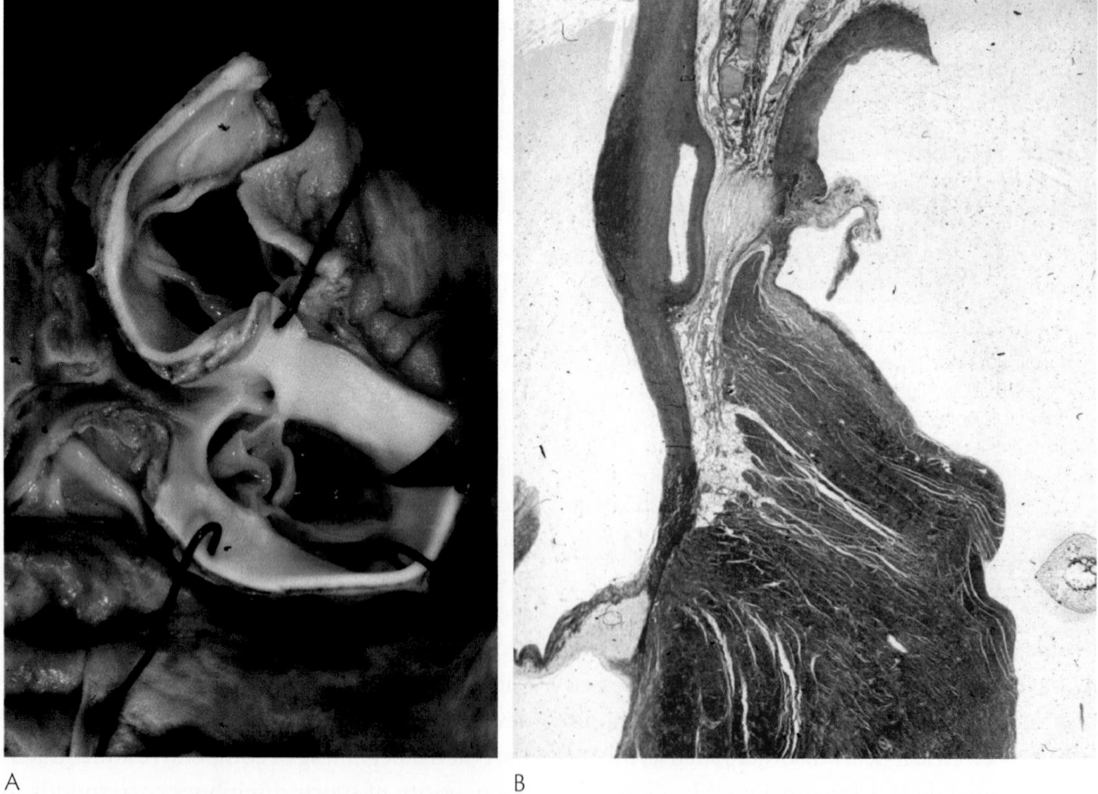

Figure 32.6 A 22-year-old soccer player who died suddenly. (A) View of the aortic root showing the right coronary artery ostium arising from the left (wrong) coronary sinus. (B) Histology of proximal right coronary artery, which appears to run within the aortic wall (intramural course), with a slit-like lumen (Azan stain, original stain × 10). Modified with permission from Corrado D, Thiene G, Nava A, *et al*. Sudden death in young competitive athletes: clinico-pathologic correlations in 22 cases. *Am J Med* 1990; **89**: 588–96.

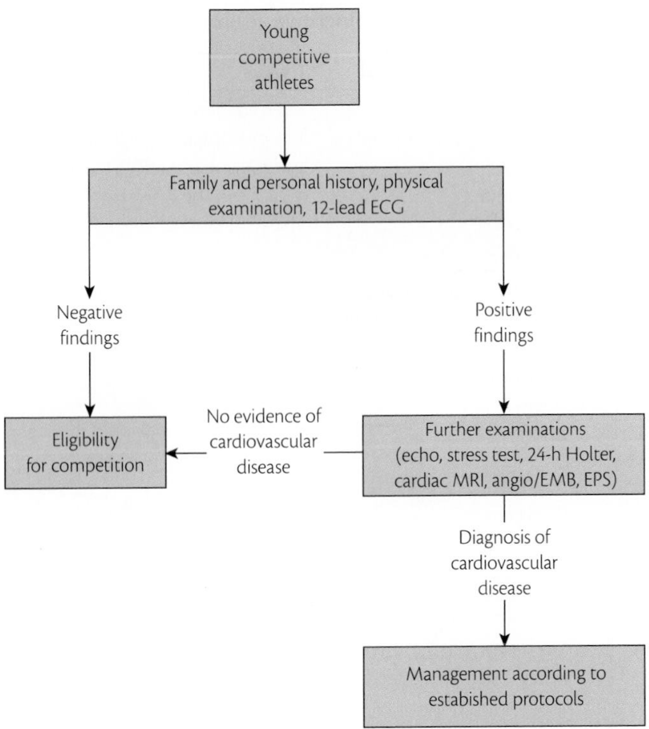

Figure 32.7 Flow chart of the Italian protocol of cardiovascular screening of young competitive athletes, see text for explanation. Angio/EMB, contrast angiography/endomyocardial biopsy; EPS, electrophysiologic study with programmed ventricular stimulation; MRI, magnetic resonance. Modified with permission from Corrado D, Pelliccia A, Bjornstad HH, *et al.* Cardiovascular pre-participation screening of young competitive athletes for prevention of sudden death: proposal for a common European protocol. Consensus Statement of the Study Group of Sport Cardiology of the Working Group of Cardiac Rehabilitation and Exercise Physiology and the Working Group of Myocardial and Pericardial Diseases of the European Society of Cardiology. *Eur Heart J* 2005; **26**: 516–24.

Medical history

The majority of conditions at risk of sudden death during sports are genetically determined diseases with an autosomal dominant pattern of inheritance; hence the importance of family history in identifying affected athletes. The family history is considered positive when a close relative has experienced a premature heart attack or sudden death (<55 years of age in males and <65 years in females), or in the presence of a family history of cardiomyopathy, Marfan syndrome, long QT syndrome, Brugada syndrome, severe arrhythmias, coronary artery disease, or other disabling cardiovascular diseases. The personal history is considered positive in case of exertional chest pain or discomfort, syncope or near-syncope, irregular heartbeat or palpitations, and in the presence of shortness of breath or fatigue, out of proportion to the degree of exertion.

Physical examination

Positive physical findings include musculoskeletal and ocular features suggestive of Marfan syndrome, diminished and delayed femoral artery pulses, mid-or end-systolic clicks, a second heart sound single or widely split and fixed with respiration, marked heart murmurs (any diastolic and systolic grade ≥2/6), irregular heart rhythm, and brachial blood pressure >140/90mmHg (on more than one readings).

ECG

The 12-lead ECG is considered positive in the presence of one or more of the findings reported in ➲Table 32.3. Subjects who have positive findings at basal evaluation are referred for additional testing, initially 'non-invasive' such as echocardiography, 24-hour ambulatory Holter monitoring, and exercise testing. Alternatively or in uncertain cases 'invasive' tests such as contrast ventriculography (both right and left), coronary angiography, endomyocardial biopsy, and electrophysiologic study may be necessary in order to confirm or rule out suspected heart disease. Finally, subjects recognized to be affected by cardiovascular conditions, potentially responsible for sudden death in association with exercise and sport participation, are managed according to the available recommendations for sports eligibility [87, 88].

The Italian protocol has been recommended as the most appropriate screening modality of young competitive athletes by the Working Group of Sports Cardiology of the European Society of Cardiology [85].

Efficacy of preparticipation ECG screening

HCM (➲Chapter 18) has been reported to be the leading cause of sudden death in young competitive athletes, accounting for up to 40% of athletic field deaths in the USA [32, 34, 58, 60, 61]. Although echocardiography is the main diagnostic tool for recognition of HCM, it is expensive and impractical for screening large athletic population [79]. The Italian experience demonstrated that a protocol utilizing the ECG in addition to history and physical examination successfully identified HCM in the general population of young competitive athletes. Among 33,735 athletes undergoing preparticipation screening at the Centre for Sport Medicine of Padua from 1979–1996, 22 (0.07%) showed definitive, clinical, and echocardiographic evidence of HCM [47]. An absolute value of screening sensitivity for HCM in young competitive athletes can not be derived from this study, because systematic echocardiographic data were not available. However, this 0.07% prevalence of HCM in the white athletic population of the Veneto Region of Italy, that was evaluated by history, physical examination, and ECG, is similar to that of 0.1% reported in young white individuals in the USA assessed by echocardiography [89]. This indicates that Italian screening essentially based on the 12-lead

Table 32.3 ECG features of cardiac diseases detectable at preparticipation screening in a young competitive athlete

Disease	QTc interval	P wave	PR interval	QRS complex	ST interval	T wave	Arrhythmias
Hypertrophic cardiomyopathy	Normal	(Left atrial enlargement)	Normal	Increased voltages in mid- left precordial leads; abnormal 'Q' waves in inferior and/ or lateral leads; (LAD, LBBB); (delta wave)	Down-sloping (up-sloping)	Inverted in mid- left- precordial leads; (giant and negative in the 'apical' variant)	(Atrial fibrillation); (PVB); (VT)
Arrhythmogenic right ventricular cardiomyopathy	Normal	Normal	Normal	Prolonged >110ms in right precordial leads; epsilon wave in right precordial leads; reduced voltages ≤0.5mV in frontal leads; (RBBB)	(Up-sloping in right precordial leads)	Inverted in right precordial leads	PVB with a LBBB pattern; (VT with a LBBB pattern)
Dilated cardiomyopathy	Normal	(Left atrial enlargement)	(Prolonged ≥0.21s)	LBBB	Down-sloping (up-sloping)	Inverted in inferior and/or lateral leads	PVB; (VT)
Myocarditis	(Prolonged)	Normal	Prolonged ≥0.21s	(Abnormal 'Q' waves)	Down- or up-sloping	Inverted in ≥2 leads	(Atrial arrhythmias); (PVB); (2nd or 3rd degree AV block); (VT)
Long QT syndrome	Prolonged >440ms in males; >460ms in females	Normal	Normal	Normal	Normal	Bifid or biphasic in all leads	(PVB); (torsade de pointes)
Brugada syndrome	Normal	Normal	Prolonged ≥0.21s	S1S2S3 pattern; (RBBB/LAD)	Up-sloping 'coved-type' in right precordial leads	Inverted in right precordial leads	(Polymorphic VT); (atrial fibrillation); (sinus bradycardia)
Lenègre disease	Normal	Normal	Prolonged ≥0.21s	RBBB; RBBB/LAD; LBBB	Normal	Secondary changes	(2nd or 3rd degree AV block)
Short QT syndrome	Shortened <300ms	Normal	Normal	Normal	Normal	Normal	Atrial fibrillation (polymorphic VT);
Pre-excitation syndrome (WPW)	Normal	Normal	Shortened <0.12s	Delta wave	Secondary changes	Secondary changes	Supraventricular tachycardia; (atrial fibrillation)
Coronary artery diseases§	(Prolonged)	Normal	Normal	(Abnormal 'Q' waves)‡	(Down- or up-sloping)	Inverted in ≥2 leads	PVB; (VT)

Less common or uncommon ECG findings are reported in brackets; §coronary artery diseases, either premature coronary atherosclerosis or congenital coronary anomalies; ‡abnormal 'Q' waves, (see ➲Table 32.3); LBBB, left bundle branch block; LAD, left axis deviation of −30° or more; PVB, either single or coupled premature ventricular beats; QTc, QT interval corrected for heart rate by Bazett's formula; RBBB, right bundle branch block; VT, either non-sustained or sustained ventricular tachycardia.

Modified with permission from Corrado D, Pelliccia A, Bjørnstad HH, *et al.* Cardiovascular pre-participation screening of young competitive athletes for prevention of sudden death: proposal for a common European protocol. Consensus Statement of the Study Group of Sport Cardiology of the Working Group of Cardiac Rehabilitation and Exercise Physiology and the Working Group of Myocardial and Pericardial Diseases of the European Society of Cardiology. *Eur Heart J* 2005; **26**: 516–24.

ECG may be as sensitive as screening by echocardiography in detecting HCM in the young athletic population.

The 12-lead ECG offers the potential to detect (or to raise clinical suspicion about) lethal conditions (other than HCM) manifesting with ECG abnormalities, such as ARVC, dilated cardiomyopathy, long QT syndromes, Lenègre disease, Brugada syndrome, short QT syndrome, and WPW syndrome (➲Table 32.3) (➲Chapter 9). Overall these conditions (including HCM) account for up to 60% of sudden deaths in young competitive athletes [32, 36, 47, 61, 68].

The possibility of detecting young competitive athletes with either premature coronary atherosclerosis or an anomalous coronary artery is limited by the scarcity of baseline ECG signs of myocardial ischaemia [37, 48, 51]. However, we reported that approximately one-fourth of young athletes who died from coronary artery diseases had warning symptoms and/or

ECG abnormalities at preparticipation screening that could raise the suspicion of a cardiac disease [47, 68].

Echocardiographic study in addition to the basal protocol does not seem to significantly improve efficacy of the preparticipation screening in identifying HCM. Pelliccia and colleagues. did not identify any HCM by routine echocardiographic examination in 4450 elite athletes previously cleared by ECG at preparticipation evaluation [63].

Mortality reduction by preparticipation ECG screening

A time-trend analysis of the incidence of sudden cardiovascular death in young competitive athletes in the Veneto region of Italy over 26 years (1979–2004) demonstrated a sharp decline of mortality rates after the introduction of the nationwide screening programme [68]. The annual incidence of sudden cardiovascular death in athletes decreased by 89%, from 3.6 per 100,000 athlete-years in the pre-screening period (1979–1981) to 0.4 per 100,000 athlete-years in the late-screening period (1993–2004) (➲Fig. 32.8). By comparison, the incidence of sudden cardiovascular death in the unscreened non-athletic population of the same age did not change significantly over that time. The decline in death rate started after mandatory screening was launched and persisted to the late screening period. Most of the reduced death rate was due to fewer cases of sudden cardiovascular death from cardiomyopathies. A parallel study of eligibility for competitive sports showed that the proportion of athletes identified and disqualified because of cardiomyopathies (mostly HCM and ARVC) doubled from the early to the late screening period. This substantiates the concept that the decrease of mortality from cardiomyopathy was the result of increasing identification over time of affected athletes at preparticipation screening.

Cost–benefit considerations

Screening of large athletic populations has a significant socio-economic impact. Strategies for implementing the screening programme depend on the particular socio-economic and cultural background as well as on the specific medical systems in place in different countries. In Italy, screening is made feasible thanks to the National Health System, which is developed in terms of healthcare and prevention services, and to the limited costs of cardiovascular evaluation in the setting of a mass-programme [85, 86]. The cost of performing a preparticipation cardiac history, physical examination, and ECG by qualified physicians has been estimated to be €30 (approximately US$40) per athlete. The screening cost is covered by the athlete or the team, except for athletes younger than 18 years, for whom the expense is supported by the National Health System. Moreover, the cost of further evaluation of athletes with positive findings at first-line examination is smaller than expected on the basis of the presumed low specificity of the 12-lead ECG. The percentage of athletes requiring additional testing, mainly echocardiography, did not exceed 9%, with a modest proportional impact on cost [47, 68] (➲Fig. 32.9).

Costs of infrastructure and training courses for preparticipation screening must also be taken into account in the calculation of the overall screening cost. Strategies for screening implementation should be in the hands of healthcare policy makers and services providers, with their programme development based on the specific national health and socio-economic systems [86].

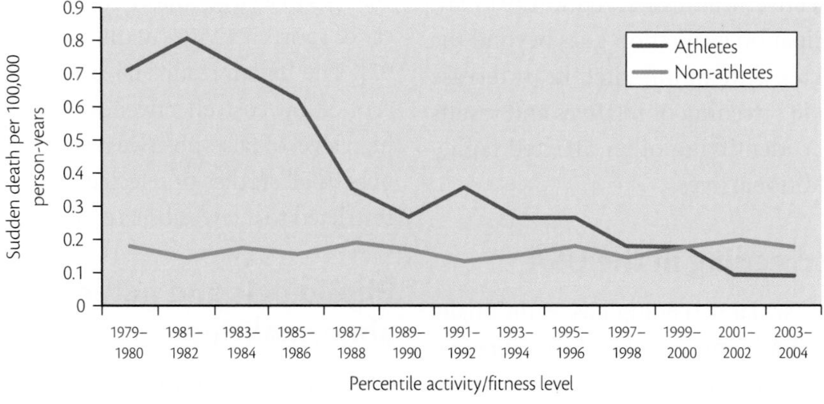

Figure 32.8 Annual incidence rates of SCD per 100,000 athlete-years, among screened competitive athletes and unscreened non-athletes 12–35 years of age in the Veneto Region of Italy, from 1979–2004. During the study period (the nationwide preparticipation screening programme was launched in 1982), the annual incidence of SCD declined by 89% in screened athletes (p for trend <0.001). In contrast, the incidence rate of SCD did not demonstrate consistent changes over time in unscreened non-athletes. Modified with permission from Corrado D, Basso C, Pavei A, *et al.* Trends in sudden cardiovascular death in young competitive athletes after implementation of a preparticipation screening program. *JAMA* 2006; **296**: 1593–601.

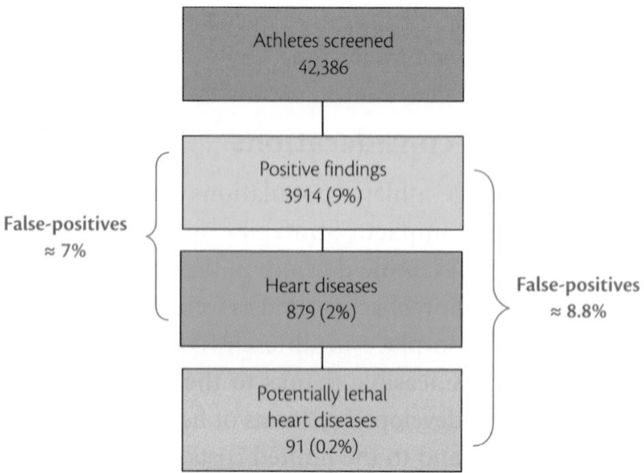

Figure 32.9 Results of preparticipation screening from 1982–2004 at the Centre for Sports Medicine of Padua, Italy. Among 42,386 athletes initially screened by history, physical examination, and 12-lead ECG, 3914 (9%) had positive findings as to require further examination, 879 (2%) were diagnosed with cardiovascular disorders, and 91 ultimately disqualified for potentially lethal heart diseases. The percentage of false-positive results, i.e. athletes with a normal heart but positive screening findings, was 7% for all cardiovascular disorders and 8.8% for heart diseases at high risk of sudden death during sports.

The young age of the screened athlete population and the genetic nature of the causes of sudden cardiac death in this age-group profoundly impact cost–benefit considerations. Unlike older patients with coronary artery diseases or heart failure, adolescents and young adults diagnosed with a genetic disease at risk of arrhythmic sudden cardiac death will survive for many decades with normal or nearly normal life expectancy, thanks to restriction from competition and prophylactic therapy against life-threatening arrhythmias [90]. This large saving of life-years influences cost-effectiveness analysis and explains why all reports on ECG screening of young individuals have provided cost estimates per year of life saved well below US$50,000, which is the traditional threshold for a cost-effective health intervention [91–94]. The benefit of preparticipation evaluation goes beyond the detection of index athletes with an inherited heart disease because it enables cascade screening of relatives and results in a multiplier effect for identifying other affected family members and saving additional lives.

Preparticipation screening in the USA

Preparticipation cardiovascular screening has traditionally been performed in the USA by means of history (personal and family) and physical examination, without 12-lead ECG [78–82]. This screening method is currently recommended by the American Heart Association on the assumption that the 12-lead ECG is not cost-effective for screening large population of young athletes due to its low specificity [79].

The US screening strategy, however, has a limited power to detect potentially lethal cardiovascular abnormalities in young athletes. One retrospective analysis in 134 high school and college athletes who died suddenly showed that cardiovascular abnormalities were suspected by standard history and physical examination screening in only 3% of the examined athletes and, eventually, <1% received an accurate diagnosis [61]. The Italian screening programme has shown that ECG makes the difference. Among 22 athletes with HCM who were detected by ECG screening at the Center for Sport Medicine in Padua and disqualified from competition, only five (23%) would had been identified on the basis of a positive family history, symptoms, or abnormal physical findings, in the absence of an ECG [85, 86]. These findings indicate that ECG screening has a 77% greater power for detecting HCM than the US protocol limited to history and physical examination.

Interpretation of the athlete's ECG

It is traditionally believed that ECG is a poor screening tool for cardiovascular disorders in athletes because its presumed low specificity [16, 79]. This presumption relies on (1) the knowledge that ECG abnormalities occur frequently in trained athletes as a consequence of electrical/structural adaptive changes of the heart to sustained physical exercise ('athlete's heart'); (2) the misconception that most athletes' ECG abnormalities overlap significantly with ECG findings of cardiovascular diseases at risk of sudden death during sports [16, 30, 79, 95, 96].

The long-term Italian experience with systematic ECG screening has offered the unique opportunity to extensively investigate prevalence, type, and determinants of ECG changes in a large cohort of athletes, engaged in a broad variety of sports activities at different levels of fitness [16, 47, 68, 97]. The Italian results have actually disproved the old concept of low cost-effectiveness of ECG screening because of a high level of false-positive results, which was based on previous, small studies of selected cases of highly trained athletes restricted to a few subsets of sports disciplines [95, 98].

Physiologic and pathologic ECG abnormalities

In ➲Table 32.4 the athlete ECG abnormalities are divided in two groups according to their prevalence, relation to exercise training, association with an increased cardiovascular risk, and need for further clinical investigation to confirm (or exclude) an underlying cardiovascular disease.

Table 32.4 Classification of abnormalities of the athlete ECG

Common and training-related ECG changes	Uncommon and training-unrelated ECG changes
Sinus bradycardia	T-wave inversion
First degree AV block	ST-segment depression
Incomplete RBBB	Pathological Q waves
Early repolarization	Left atrial enlargement
Isolated QRS voltage criteria for left ventricular hypertrophy	Left axis deviation/left anterior hemiblock
	Right axis deviation/left posterior hemiblock
	Right ventricular hypertrophy
	Complete LBBB or RBBB
	Ventricular pre-excitation
	Long or short QT interval
	Brugada-like pattern

Modified with permission from Corrado D, McKenna WJ. Appropriate interpretation of the athlete's electrocardiogram saves lives as well as money. *Eur Heart J* 2007; **28**: 1920–2.

Athlete's heart is commonly (up to 80%) associated with ECG changes such as sinus bradycardia, first-degree AV block (➲Chapter 27), and early repolarization (➲Chapter 2) (Group 1) resulting from physiologic adaptation of cardiac autonomic nervous system to training, i.e. increased vagal tone and/or withdrawal of sympathetic activity. Moreover, the ECG of trained athletes often exhibits pure voltage criteria for LV hypertrophy that reflect the physiological LV remodelling, consisting of increased LV wall thickness and chamber size. Although these ECG changes are abnormal in a strict statistical sense, they do not imply the presence of cardiovascular disorder or an increase of cardiovascular risk in the athlete. These ECG abnormalities should be clearly separated from uncommon ECG patterns (<5%) such as ST-segment and T-wave repolarization abnormalities, pathologic Q waves, intraventricular conduction defects, ventricular pre-excitation, long and short QT interval (➲Chapter 9), and ventricular arrhythmias (➲Chapter 30) (Group 2) which are unrelated to athlete training and may be an expression of cardiovascular disorders, notably cardiomyopathies and cardiac ion channel diseases, at risk of sudden arrhythmic death during sports.

The ECG should be evaluated in light of the athlete's gender, age and race, family history of cardiovascular disease and/or sudden death, clinical symptoms, and physical examination. In asymptomatic athletes with a negative family history, ECG changes due to cardiac adaptation to physical exertion (Group 1) do not cause alarm and allow eligibility to competitive sports without additional evaluation. Further diagnostic work-up is reserved to the limited subset of athletes with ECG changes potentially reflecting underlying heart disease (Group 2), and/or to those with a positive medical history or an abnormal physical examination (➲Figs. 32.7 and 32.9).

Appropriate interpretation of the athlete's ECG

HCM and ARVC (➲Chapter 18), which have been consistently implicated as leading causes of sports-related cardiac arrest in young competitive athletes, are often in the differential diagnosis of an asymptomatic athlete showing ECG abnormalities at preparticipation evaluation [9, 32, 34]. The Italian screening experience has demonstrated the crucial importance of appropriate interpretation of ECG abnormalities by qualified specialists in Sports Medicine for proper cardiovascular evaluation and management of young competitive athletes [85, 87]. Misinterpretation of ECG by non-experienced physicians may lead to serious consequences. Athletes may undergo expensive diagnostic work-up or may be unnecessarily disqualified from competition for abnormalities that fall within the normal range for athletes. ECG abnormalities in HCM are a good example since they overlap marginally with ECG findings in healthy trained athletes. Isolated QRS voltage criteria for LV hypertrophy (Sokolov–Lyon or Cornell criteria) are unusual in patients with HCM in whom pathologic hypertrophy is characteristically associated with additional non-voltage criteria such as left atrial involvement, left QRS axis deviation, a 'strain' pattern of repolarization, and delayed intrinsicoid deflection; T-wave inversion; and pathologic Q waves [60, 99, 100] (➲Fig. 32.10). Such ECG abnormalities of HCM need to be clearly distinguished from the ECG patterns of healthy trained athletes in whom physiologic hypertrophy manifests as an isolated increase of QRS amplitude, with right QRS axis deviation, normal atrial and ventricular activation patterns, and normal ST–T repolarization [16, 98, 101, 102]. A corollary is that further investigation by echocardiography is not recommended in athletes showing an isolated increase of QRS voltages at preparticipation screening, unless such subjects have other ECG changes suggesting pathologic LV hypertrophy, relevant symptoms, abnormal physical examination, or a positive family history for cardiovascular diseases and/or sudden cardiac death.

On the other hand, signs of potentially lethal organic heart disease may be misinterpreted as normal variants of the athlete ECG. For instance, there is a general misconception that inverted T-waves in precordial leads are frequently encountered in trained athletes, being part of the spectrum of cardiovascular adaptive changes to physical exercise [95]. Particularly, T-wave inversion in right precordial leads (beyond V1) is often dismissed in young competitive

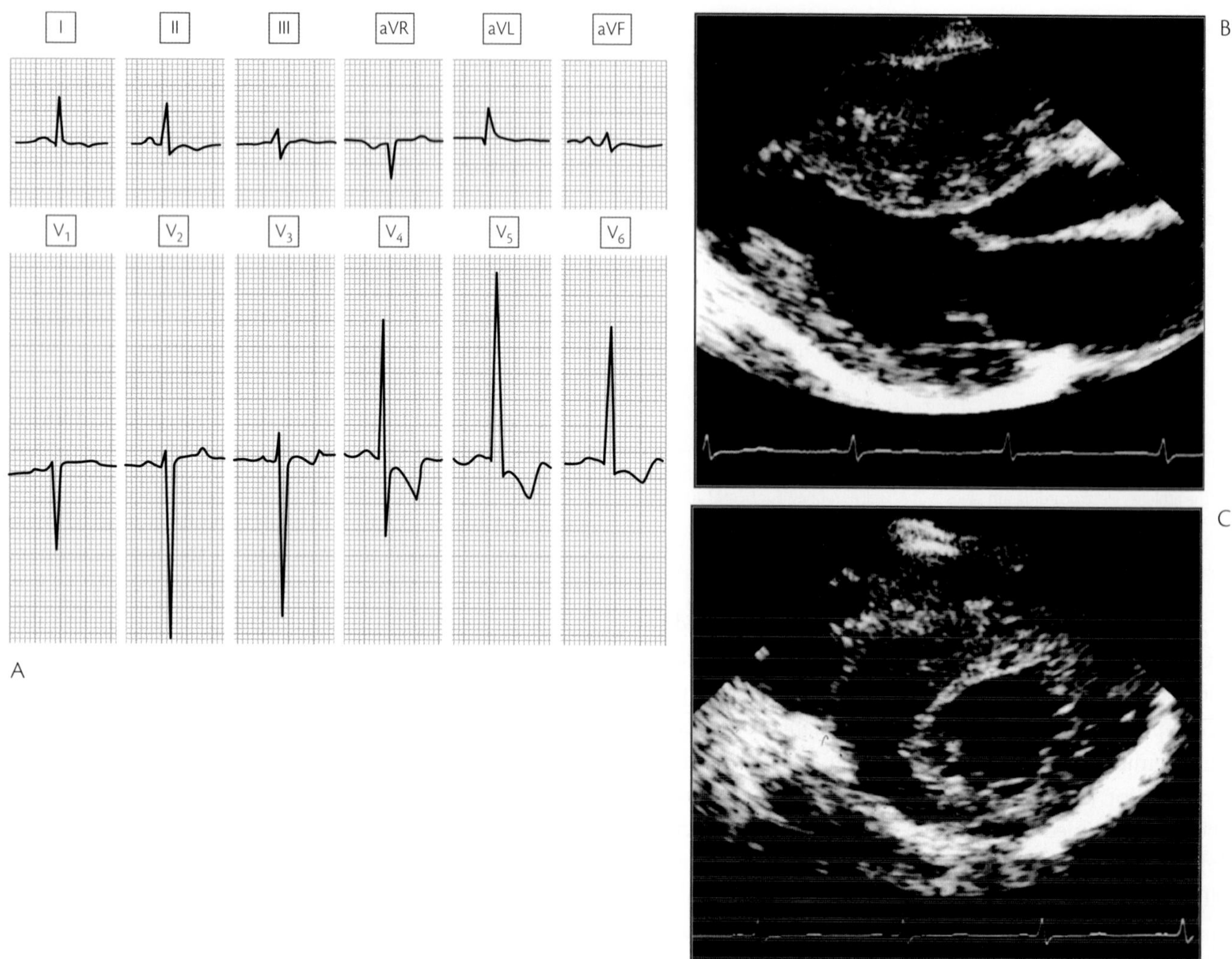

Figure 32.10 ECG and echocardiographic findings in an asymptomatic athlete diagnosed with HCM. The disease was suspected at preparticipation evaluation thanks to ECG abnormalities consisting of increased QRS voltages and flat/inverted T-waves in the inferolateral leads (A). HCM was diagnosed by echocardiography showing marked and asymmetric (predominantly septal) left ventricular hypertrophy; (B) long-axis view and (C) short-axis view.

athletes as non-specific or as persistence of the juvenile T-wave pattern. On the contrary, detailed analysis of available data, shows that the prevalence of T-wave inversion ≥2 precordial leads did not exceed 4% in large athlete populations (age ≥14 years), regardless of training intensity and duration; moreover, there does not seem to be a greater prevalence in trained athletes compared to sedentary people [97, 103]. On the other hand, T-wave inversion is an important ECG marker of cardiomyopathies, including HCM, ARVC, dilated cardiomyopathy, and cardiac ion channelopathies; ischaemic heart disease; and aortic valve disease [75, 95]. Of note, right precordial T-wave inversion is present in up to 87% of patients who have ARVC, a leading cause of sudden death on the athletics field [38, 53, 103] (➲Fig. 32.11). Such a finding raises suspicion of an underlying cardiovascular condition and the athlete should be thoroughly investigated by imaging techniques, electrophysiologic studies, and, when appropriate, by genetic testing to exclude a pathologic basis. Genotype–phenotype correlation studies in cardiomyopathy showed that ECG abnormalities can represent the only sign of disease expression in gene mutation carriers, even in the absence of any other features or before structural changes in the heart can be detected [104]. T-wave inversion in young and apparently healthy athletes may represent the initial clinical expression of a heart muscle disease that may not be evident until many years later and may ultimately be associated with adverse outcomes [105]. Accordingly, the perspective that T-wave inversion is due to cardiovascular adaptation in an athlete should only be accepted once inherited forms of cardiovascular disease have been definitively excluded by a comprehensive clinical work-up including investigation of family members. Moreover, continued clinical surveillance and follow-up by

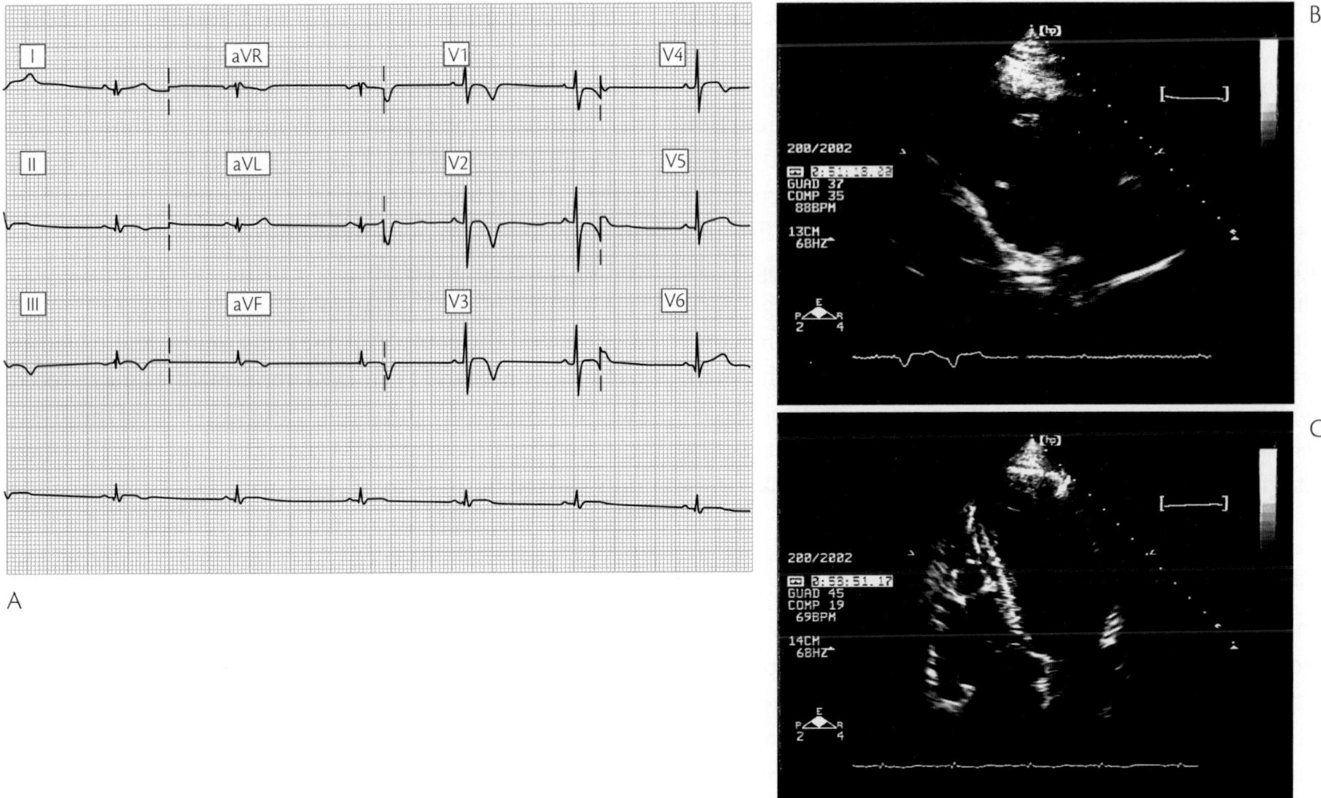

Figure 32.11 ECG and echocardiographic findings in an asymptomatic athlete diagnosed with ARVC. The athlete was referred for further evaluation because of ECG abnormalities found at preparticipation evaluation which consisted of inverted T-waves in the inferior and anteroseptal leads and low QRS voltages in the peripheral leads (A). ARVC was suspected at echocardiographic examination showing mild RV dilatation, basal and apical wall motion abnormalities with diastolic bulging of the RV inflow tract, and trabecular disarrangement; (B) RV long-axis view and (C) four-chamber view. Final diagnosis was achieved by CMR (not shown).

serial ECG and echocardiography is warranted in trained athletes with T-wave repolarization abnormalities, even in the absence of clinically demonstrable heart disease.

Management of athletes with cardiovascular diseases

Since 1985 the 16th, 26th, and 36th Bethesda Conferences (sponsored by the American College of Cardiology) have offered recommendations for eligibility of competitive athletes with cardiovascular abnormalities [87, 106, 107]. European guidelines have been recently elaborated by the Study Group of Sports Cardiology of the European Society of Cardiology [88]. These expert consensus recommendations provide a framework on which to base eligibility decisions in a competitive athlete once a cardiovascular abnormality is identified, by taking into account the nature and severity of the disease as well as the type and level of sports training and competition. Both US and European recommendations are based on the concept that intense physical activity (both training and competition) in subjects with a predisposing cardiovascular disorder will increase the risk of sudden cardiac death and/or disease progression.

Early identification and proper management of athletes with clinically significant cardiovascular disorders offers the possibility of prolonging life and prevention of disease progression by lifestyle modification, including restriction of competitive sports activity, and concomitant clinical interventions such as antiarrhythmic drugs, beta-blockers, and implantable cardioverter defibrillator (ICD) therapy [68, 86].

Athlete disqualification may be associated with an important individual cost in terms of health, contentment, and even future opportunity for professional sports. However, the risk of sudden cardiac death associated with competitive sports in the setting of life-threatening cardiovascular disease is a controllable factor, and the devastating impact of even infrequent fatal events in the young athlete population justifies appropriate restriction from competition [87].

The prevalence of Italian athletes who were diagnosed and disqualified because of cardiovascular diseases was approximately 2%; however, true potentially lethal conditions such as cardiomyopathies, rhythm and conduction disturbances, long QT syndrome, valvular heart disease (predominantly aortic valve stenosis), premature coronary artery disease, and Marfan syndrome were identified in a smaller subgroup not exceeding 0.2% [68, 86] (➲Fig. 32.9). This has significant implications for optimizing sports eligibility guidelines and the management of young competitive athletes with cardiovascular diseases. The main objective should be to reduce the number of unnecessary disqualifications and to adapt (rather than restrict) sports activity in relation to the specific cardiovascular risk.

Cardiomyopathies

The ultimate diagnosis of heart muscle diseases may be problematic in highly trained athletes due to the presence of physiologic adaptive changes of cardiac morphology to physical exercise, such as an increase of ventricular cavity dimension and/or wall thickness, which may show some similarities with structural abnormalities seen in cardiomyopathy (➲Chapter 18) [15]. Accurate differential diagnosis is crucial because of the potentially adverse outcome associated with cardiomyopathy in an athlete and, on the other hand, the possibility of misdiagnosis of pathologic conditions requiring unnecessary disqualifications from sport with financial and psychological consequences.

The majority (up to 95%) of HCM patients (➲Chapter 18) show ECG abnormalities, including increased QRS voltages, pathologic Q-waves, and deeply inverted T-waves. HCM is diagnosed by echocardiography in the presence of an otherwise unexplained increase of the LV wall thickness ≥13mm, although more substantial LV hypertrophy is usually found, with asymmetric distribution and sharp transition between contiguous segments [60]. Diastolic LV filling (by Doppler echocardiography) and tissue Doppler imaging (TDI) are abnormal in the majority of HCM patients and may precede the development of LV hypertrophy [108]. Other alterations include malformation of the mitral valve and anomalous insertion of papillary muscles. In contrast, distribution of LV hypertrophy is symmetric in athletes and maximum LV wall thickness does not exceed 15–16mm [17]. The LV cavity is enlarged (i.e. end-diastolic diameter ≥55mm) with a normal shape, a normally positioned mitral valve, and no outflow tract obstruction. LV filling (by Doppler echocardiography) and relaxation (by TDI) are normal. Most importantly, serial echocardiographic studies demonstrate reduction in LV wall thickness after complete deconditioning [109]. Additional criteria include peak oxygen consumption (with VO_2max >50mL/kg/min being more consistent with athlete's heart) [110] and gender, because female athletes do not usually show LV wall thickening >12mm [19]. Cardiac MR (➲Chapter 5) is indicated, when echocardiography is inadequate, in identifying an atypical pattern of hypertrophy or apical HCM. Genetic testing is still not widely available in the current clinical practice because of the substantial genetic heterogeneity of the disease, and the complex, time consuming, and expensive techniques needed [111]. ECG abnormalities may precede the LV hypertrophy and should raise suspicion of the disease in family members of HCM patients [104]. Special attention should be paid to athletes with ECG abnormalities (such as markedly increased QRS voltage, widespread T-wave inversion, deep Q-waves in precordial leads) suggestive for HCM, in the absence of LV hypertrophy [105]. Evaluation of these athletes should include complete family screening, personal history, echocardiography, and 24-hour Holter ECG monitoring. When sudden death or HCM in the family are excluded, and in the absence of symptoms, arrhythmias, and LV hypertrophy, and with a normal diastolic filling/relaxation, there is no reason to restrict athletes from competitive sports, but periodical clinical and diagnostic follow-up is recommended [87, 88].

Diagnosis of ARVC (➲Chapter 18) is based on the criteria previously proposed by an International Task Force [65, 112]. The ECG is of particular value in raising suspicion for ARVC, in consideration that ECG abnormalities are present in the majority of patients [66]. The most common abnormalities include prolonged QRS duration ≥110ms, epsilon waves (low amplitude potentials at the end of QRS complex), and inverted T-waves in the right precordial leads, as well as ventricular arrhythmias with left bundle branch block pattern suggesting their RV origin [113]. Echocardiography, RV angiography, and cardiac magnetic resonance (CMR) show an enlarged RV cavity, segmental morphologic abnormalities (with thinning, bulging, and aneurysms in the RV wall), and wall motion abnormalities [66]. Cardiac MR may also identify areas of altered signal intensity consistent with fatty replacement and ventricular late-enhancement by gadolinium corresponding to fibro-fatty scars into the RV and/or the LV [114, 115]. An enlarged RV, in association with an enlarged LV, may also be found in healthy elite athletes (mostly engaged in endurance disciplines, such as cycling, rowing/canoeing); however, in these instances RV wall thickness is normal and no segmental wall motion abnormalities are present [115]. Genetic diagnosis of ARVC is still limited to selected individuals [67].

Given the frequency of sudden death in young athletes with HCM and ARVC, the increased incidence of sudden death in affected athletes versus non-athletes, and the difficulty to accurately predict sudden death risk in a given individual, the available guidelines recommend that all athletes with probable or unequivocal clinical diagnosis of inherited cardiomyopathies (including cardiac ion channel diseases) should be excluded from most competitive sports, except possibly low-intensity activities such a bowling or golfing [87, 88] (➲Table 32.5). This recommendation applies regardless of an ICD back up.

Myocarditis (also see ➲Chapter 18)

The clinical picture of myocarditis (➲Chapter 18) usually starts with upper respiratory or gastrointestinal symptoms, but palpitations, fatigability, exertional dyspnoea, or syncope may also be the clinical onset. Evidence of flu-like illness, or epidemiological circumstances supporting viral infection should be assessed. The ECG abnormalities include frequent and/or complex ventricular and/or supraventricular arrhythmia, ST-segment changes (either ST-segment depression or elevation), T-wave inversion and, occasionally, left bundle branch block or AV block [116]. Global LV dilatation/dysfunction can be evident in certain cases; however, localized wall motion abnormalities, slightly enlarged LV cavity, and borderline systolic dysfunction are common [117]. Endomyocardial biopsy is not routinely performed and is reserved to selected circumstances, for therapeutic or medico-legal purposes. Myocarditis may evolve into a chronic inflammation, often with a subclinical course and may progress into dilated cardiomyopathy. Sudden death may occur in the active or healed phases of myocarditis as a consequence of life-threatening ventricular arrhythmias, which develop in the setting of an unstable myocardial substrate, namely inflammatory infiltrate, interstitial oedema, myocyte necrosis, and fibrosis [69]. It is of utmost importance to respect an adequate period of athletic rest until the disease has completely resolved.

Table 32.5 Recommendation for competitive sport participation in athletes with inherited cardiomyopathies (including channelopathies)

Lesion	Evaluation	Criteria for eligibility	Recommendations	Follow-up
HCM	History, PE, ECG, Echo	Definite diagnosis of HCM	No competitive sports	—
HCM with low risk profile	History, PE, ECG, Echo, ET, 24-hour Holter	No SD in the relatives, no symptoms; mild LVH, Normal BP response to exercise; no ventricular arrhythmias	Low dynamic, low static sports (IA)	Yearly
ARVC	History, PE, ECG, Echo (CE-CMR)	Definite diagnosis of ARVC	No competitive sports	—
DCM	History, PE, ECG, Echo	Definite diagnosis of DCM	No competitive sports	—
DCM with low risk profile	History, PE, ECG, Echo, ET, Holter	No SD in the relatives, no symptoms; mildly depressed EF (≥40%), normal BP response to exercise; no complex ventricular arrhythmias	Low–moderate dynamic and low static sports (IA, IB)	Yearly
Long QT syndrome	History, ECG, (ET, Holter, genetic testing)	Definite diagnosis of long QT syndrome	No competitive sports	—
Short QT syndrome	History, ECG, (Holter, genetic testing)	Definite diagnosis of short QT syndrome	No competitive sports	—
Brugada syndrome	History, ECG, Echo, provocative test	Definite diagnosis of Brugada syndrome	No competitive sports	—
Catecholaminergic Polymorphic VT	History, ECG, ET (genetic testing)	Definite diagnosis of Catecholaminergic polymorphic VT	No competitive sports	—
Lenègre disease	History, ECG, ET (genetic testing)	Definite diagnosis of Lenègre disease	No competitive sports	—
Healthy gene carriers	Disease-specific clinical assessment	No symptoms, no phenotype, no ventricular arrhythmias	Only recreational, non-competitive sport activities	Yearly

ARVC, arrhythmogenic right ventricular cardiomyopathy; BP, blood pressure; DCM, dilated cardiomyopathy; HCM, hypertrophic cardiomyopathy; Echo, echocardiography; EF, ejection fraction; ET, exercise testing; Holter, 24-hour ECG monitoring; LV, left ventricular; LVH, left ventricular hypertrophy; PE physical examination; SD, sudden death; Sport type (see ➲Table 32.1); VT, ventricular tachycardia.

Modified with permission from Pelliccia A, Fagard R, Bjørnstad HH, *et al.* Recommendations for competitive sports participation in athletes with cardiovascular disease: a consensus document from the Study Group of Sports Cardiology of the Working Group of Cardiac Rehabilitation and Exercise Physiology and the Working Group of Myocardial and Pericardial Diseases of the European Society of Cardiology. *Eur Heart J* 2005; **26**: 1422–45.

Athletes with a clinical diagnosis of myocarditis should be temporarily excluded from competitive and amateur-leisure time sport activity [87, 88]. This recommendation is independent of age and gender and does not differ for athletes with only mild symptoms and under treatment with drugs. After resolution of the disease signs (at least 6 months after the onset of the disease), clinical reassessment is indicated before the athlete re-enters competitive sporting activity. Moreover, clinical evaluation should be repeated every 6 months during the follow-up [88].

Rhythm and conduction abnormalities

Clinical evaluation and recommendations for sports eligibility of athletes with rhythm and conduction abnormalities are summarized in ➲Tables 32.6 and 32.7. Athletes with WPW syndrome and ventricular arrhythmias deserve particular consideration.

Wolff–Parkinson–White syndrome (also see ➲Chapter 28)

This condition carries a small but definite risk of sudden cardiac death [118]. Symptomatic individuals with WPW syndrome (➲Chapter 28) should not participate in sports until they have been cured with radiofrequency ablation. Sudden death may be the first clinical manifestation of the WPW syndrome and it may be triggered by physical exercise. Although there is no universal consensus on how to manage asymptomatic individuals, competitive athletes with asymptomatic ventricular pre-excitation should undergo

Table 32.6 Recommendation for competitive sport participation in athletes with rhythm and conduction abnormalities (I—bradyarrhythmias and supraventricular tachyarrhythmias)

Lesion	Evaluation	Criteria for eligibility	Recommendations	Follow-up
Marked sinus bradycardia (≤40bpm) and/or sinus pauses ≥3s with symptoms	History, ECG, ET, Holter, Echo	(a) If symptoms# are present (b) After >3 months from resolution of symptoms#; off therapy	(a) Temporary interruption of sport (b) All sports	Yearly
AV block 1st and 2nd degree, type 1	History, ECG, ET, Holter, Echo	If no symptoms, no cardiac disease, with resolution during exercise	All sports	Yearly
AV block 2nd degree, type 2 or advanced	History, ECG, ET, Holter, Echo	In the absence of symptoms, cardiac disease, ventricular arrhythmias during exercise, and if resting heart rate is >40bpm	Low-moderate dynamic, low-moderate static sports (I, II A, B)	Yearly
Supraventricular premature beats	History, ECG, thyroid function	No symptoms, no cardiac disease	All sports	Not required
Paroxysmal supraventricular tachycardia (AVNRT or AVRT over a concealed accessory pathway)	History, ECG, Echo, EP study	Ablation is recommended: (a) After catheter ablation: if no recurrences for >1 month, and no cardiac disease (b) If ablation is not performed and AVNRT is sporadic, without cardiac disease, without haemodynamic consequences and without relation with exercise	(a) All sports (b) All sports, except those with increased risk	Yearly
Ventricular pre-excitation and: (a) Paroxysmal AV reentry tachycardia (b) Atrial fibrillation or flutter (c) Asymptomatic pre-excitation pattern	(a), (b), (c) History, ECG, Echo, EP study	Ablation is mandatory in cases (a), (b). After catheter ablation: if no recurrences, no cardiac disease Ablation is recommended but not mandatory in case (c)	(a) (b) All sports (c) Asymptomatic athletes at low risk and not ablated: all sports, except those with increased risk*	Yearly
Atrial fibrillation (paroxysmal, permanent)	History, ECG, Echo, ET, Holter	(a) After paroxysmal AF: if no cardiac disease, no WPW, and stable sinus rhythm >3 months (b) Permanent AF in the absence of cardiac disease, and WPW: assess heart rate and LV function response to exercise	(a) All sports (b) Assessed on individual basis	(a) Yearly (b) Every 6 months
Atrial flutter	History, ECG, Echo, EP study	Ablation mandatory: after ablation: if no symptoms for >3 months, no cardiac disease or WPW, without therapy;	All sports	Yearly

AF, atrial fibrillation; AVNRT, atrioventricular nodal re-entrant tachycardia; AVRT, atrioventricular re-entrant tachycardia; ECG, 12-lead electrocardiogram; Echo, echocardiography; ET, Exercise testing; Holter, 24-hour ECG monitoring; EP, electrophysiologic; WPW, Wolff–Parkinson–White syndrome. *Increased risk if syncope occurs (see ➲Table 32.1); # symptoms include presyncope, lightheadedness, exertional fatigue.

Modified with permission from Pelliccia A, Fagard R, Bjørnstad HH, *et al.* Recommendations for competitive sports participation in athletes with cardiovascular disease: a consensus document from the Study Group of Sports Cardiology of the Working Group of Cardiac Rehabilitation and Exercise Physiology and the Working Group of Myocardial and Pericardial Diseases of the European Society of Cardiology. *Eur Heart J* 2005; **26**: 1422–45.

Table 32.7 Recommendation for competitive sport participation in athletes with rhythm and conduction abnormalities (II—ventricular tachyarrhythmias and electrical devices)

Lesion	Evaluation	Criteria for eligibility	Recommendations	Follow-up
Premature ventricular beats	History, ECG, Echo (ET, Holter, in selected cases invasive tests)	In the absence of: cardiac disease or arrhythmogenic condition†, family history of SD, symptoms (syncope), relation with exercise, frequent and/or polymorphic PVBs and/or frequent couplets with short RR interval	All sports	Yearly
Non-sustained VT	History, ECG, Echo (ET, Holter, in selected cases invasive tests)	In the absence of: cardiac disease or arrhythmogenic† condition, family history of SD, relation with exercise, multiple episodes of NSVT with short RR interval	All sports	Every 3 months
Slow VT, fascicular VT, RVOT VT	History, ECG, Echo, ET, Holter (in selected cases EP study)	In the absence of: cardiac disease or arrhythmogenic† condition, family history of SD, symptoms (syncope)	All sports, except those with increased risk*	Every 3 months
Syncope	History, ECG, Echo, ET, Holter; Tilt Test	(a) Neurocardiogenic (b) Arrhythmic or primary cardiac	(a) All sports (except those with increased risk*) (b) See specific cause	Yearly
Pacemaker	ECG, Echo, ET, Holter	Normal heart rate increase during exercise, no significant arrhythmias, normal cardiac function	Low–moderate dynamic and low static sports (I, II A), except those with risk of bodily collision	Yearly
ICD	ECG, Echo, ET, Holter	No malignant VTs; normal cardiac function; at least 6 months after the implantation or the last appropriate intervention	Low–moderate dynamic and low static sports (I, II A), except those with risk of bodily collision	Yearly

ECG, 12-lead electrocardiogram; Echo, echocardiography; ET, Exercise testing; Holter, 24-hour ECG monitoring; EP, electrophysiologic; PVBs, premature ventricular beats; RVOT, right ventricular outflow tract; VT, ventricular tachycardia; Sport types (see ➲Table 32.1). * Increased risk if syncope occurs (see ➲Table 32.1); symptoms include presyncope, lightheadedness, exertional fatigue; †arrhythmogenic conditions include cardiomyopathies, ischaemic heart disease and channelopathies. NB. For athletes with structural heart disease, see the recommendations of the disease.

Modified with permission from Pelliccia A, Fagard R, Bjørnstad HH, *et al.* Recommendations for competitive sports participation in athletes with cardiovascular disease: a consensus document from the Study Group of Sports Cardiology of the Working Group of Cardiac Rehabilitation and Exercise Physiology and the Working Group of Myocardial and Pericardial Diseases of the European Society of Cardiology. *Eur Heart J* 2005; **26**: 1422–45.

an electrophysiological study, either transoesophageal or intracardiac, for evaluation of eligibility to athletic competition, risk stratification, and therapy, including catheter ablation [119]. Electrophysiological findings considered to be associated with an increased risk of sudden death include an antegrade refractory period <250ms at baseline, a pre-excited R–R interval <240ms at baseline or <220ms during isoproterenol infusion, inducibility of AV reciprocating tachycardia, or atrial fibrillation, and the presence of multiple or septal (mainly posteroseptal and mid-septal) accessory pathways [88]. In athletes with at-risk AV accessory pathways, catheter ablation is recommended given its high success rate and low incidence of complications. For athletes who refuse ablation, or in case the procedure is associated with high risk (i.e. anteroseptal AV accessory pathways), competitive sport activity is allowed when the electrophysiological study demonstrates the absence of at-risk parameters and the specific sport is not associated with an increased risk of loss of consciousness (➲Table 32.1).

Atrial fibrillation

The prevalence of atrial fibrillation in competitive athletes is not well known, although is supposed to be higher than in the general population [120–123]. Increased sympathetic activity may trigger atrial fibrillation during physical exercise, particularly in those athletes with predisposing factors (such as hypertension), whereas athlete hypervagotonia may favour the development of bradycardia-related events. Morphofunctional heart remodelling in response to endurance training may also act as a structural substrate for atrial fibrillation [123]. In ≈40% of athletes with atrial fibrillation, a possible substrate, such as WPW syndrome, cardiomyopathy, or silent myocarditis can be found [124]. Use of doping substances, such as anabolic steroids, can also possibly cause atrial fibrillation in athletes [125]. Pulmonary vein catheter ablation is not yet established as a routine therapeutic strategy for atrial fibrillation, due to its limited acute and long-term success rates [≈50] and the occurrence of rare but potentially life-threatening complications such as pulmonary vein stenosis, tamponade, and periprocedural stroke [126–128]. In athletes with unsuccessful rhythm control or in athletes under rate-control therapy, anticoagulation may be necessary, depending also on the presence of risk factor for thromboembolic events [129]. Recommendations for sports eligibility are summarized in ➲Table 32.6. Anticoagulant therapy excludes individuals from sports with a risk of bodily collision or trauma (see ➲Table 32.1).

Ventricular arrhythmias

Ventricular arrhythmias (➲Chapter 30) confer adverse prognosis when underlying heart disease is present [31, 130]. Systematic investigation of sudden cardiac death victims in the Veneto region of Italy demonstrated that the presence of even isolated premature ventricular beats on basal ECG at preparticipation screening may be the only clinical warning sign of heart disease at high risk of arrhythmic cardiac arrest in otherwise asymptomatic athletes [10, 47, 68]. The first objective of cardiovascular evaluation of an athlete with ventricular arrhythmias is to search for underlying cardiovascular disease at risk of sudden death. First-line examination includes echocardiogram, 24-hour Holter monitoring, exercise testing, and signal averaged-ECG. A careful echocardiographic evaluation of even subtle morphofunctional ventricular abnormalities is required. Twenty-four-hour Holter recordings (➲Chapter 2) have to be performed during periods of intense physical activity and preferably whenever the athlete is performing specific sport activity. The likelihood of underlying cardiovascular abnormalities and the arrhythmic risk increases with frequent and complex premature ventricular beats (>2000/24 hours), different morphologies, and couplets/non-sustained ventricular tachycardia [130]. Exercise tests (➲Chapter 25) should be adapted to the specific type of exercise/sport responsible for the arrhythmic events, because a conventional exercise test may not replicate the specific clinical situation and the arrhythmogenic mechanisms produced by actively participating in the sport. Increase in the arrhythmia frequency at the beginning of exercise, disappearance at peak-exercise, and re-appearance during recovery usually suggest the benign nature of the ectopic ventricular rhythm. Instead, triggering or worsening of ventricular arrhythmia during exercise may point to underlying inherited cardiomyopathies or ion channel diseases and may predict malignant arrhythmic events at risk of sudden death during sports. A possible exception is the right ventricular outflow tract (RVOT) ventricular tachycardia (➲Chapter 30), which is characterized by repetitive monomorphic bouts of premature ventricular beats or paroxysmal sustained episodes, with the typical left bundle branch block/inferior axis pattern [131, 132]. RVOT tachycardia (➲Chapter 30) is usually triggered by exercise and can be interrupted by adenosine. It is an idiopathic and benign arrhythmic condition, provided that an underlying ARVC is carefully excluded. The induction of polymorphic ventricular tachycardia during exercise always carries a bad prognosis. Polymorphic ventricular tachycardia with alternating complexes ('bi-directional' pattern), induced during exercise suggests a specific inherited ion channel disorder, i.e. 'catecholaminergic polymorphic ventricular tachycardia' (➲Chapter 9), which predisposes to exercise-induced arrhythmic cardiac arrest in absence of structural heart disease [73].

Registration of late potentials by the signal averaged-ECG (SAECG) (➲Chapters 2 and 30) may be a sign of delayed ventricular activation and a pro-arrhythmogenic substrate. A positive SAECG has been found to be a criterion for detecting early or minor forms of ARVC (➲Chapter 18), and may help in the differential diagnosis with idiopathic RVOT ventricular arrhythmia [132].

There should be attempts to document a 12-lead ECG of the ventricular arrhythmias (➲Chapter 30) by exercise testing or 12-lead Holter monitoring. Careful assessment of the morphology of the arrhythmic QRS complex and the coexistent ECG abnormalities may help to characterize the anatomic origin and the cause/mechanism of the arrhythmia. A left bundle branch morphology and inferior QRS axis (with negative QRS-complexes in V1 and electrical transition between V2–V3 or V3–V4) is a hallmark of idiopathic RVOT ventricular arrhythmias [131]. Similar morphology but with earlier precordial transition may indicate origin in the LV outflow tract.

A rare clinical entity is ventricular arrhythmia with a borderline width QRS (≤0.12s) and a right bundle branch block/superior axis pattern, which is pathognomonic for origin in the left posterior fascicle (so called 'fascicular ventricular tachycardia') (➲Chapter 30) [133]. It carries no adverse prognosis unless associated with syncope during exercise or heart disease. Finally, a polymorphic bi-directional pattern indicates a catecholaminergic polymorphic ventricular tachycardia (➲Chapter 9) [73].

The analysis of concomitant repolarization/depolarization ECG abnormalities may provide relevant information to interpret the clinical significance of a documented ventricular arrhythmia. The association between a premature ventricular beat with a left bundle branch block pattern and repolarization abnormalities, such as T-wave inversion in right precordial leads is highly suggestive for ARVC

(➲Chapter 18) [10, 47]. The coexistence of a RV conduction defect in the form of a prolonged QRS duration or a delayed S-wave upstroke in V1 to V3, further increases the likelihood of an ARVC. On the other hand, premature ventricular beats originating from the LV, associated with negative T-waves in the left precordial leads, must raise the suspicion of a LV heart muscle disease such as a dilated/inflammatory cardiomyopathy, HCM, LV non-compaction, or a predominantly left-sided ARVC [134].

In selected athletes in whom previous clinical and instrumental findings are inconclusive, contrast-enhanced CMR, nuclear scintigraphy, or other invasive tests such as electrophysiological study, ventriculo-coronary angiography, and endomyocardial biopsy may be required to achieve a definite diagnosis. Molecular genetic studies are increasingly available for preclinical diagnosis of inherited arrhythmogenic heart muscle diseases, including channelopathies (➲Chapter 9) [111, 135].

Work up should also include a search for agents that may enhance electrical ventricular irritability, such as use of excessive amount of alcohol, illicit drugs, or stimulants, particularly ephedrine and caffeine [136].

Atherosclerotic coronary artery disease

Athletes with a definitive diagnosis of ischaemic heart disease (➲Chapter 16 and 17) have an high probability for exercise-induced adverse cardiac events and should be disqualified from all competitive sports (or restricted to low-intensity sports activity) in the presence of one or more of the following criteria [88, 137]:

- exercise-induced myocardial ischaemia;
- exercise-induced pathological dyspnoea (angina equivalent), or syncope;
- left ventricular ejection fraction <50%;
- frequent, complex ventricular tachyarrhythmias at rest and/or during stress testing;
- significant coronary stenosis of major coronary arteries (i.e. >70%) or left main stem (>50%) on coronary angiography.

In athletes with ischaemic heart disease and no symptoms, exercise-induced myocardial ischaemia, major arrhythmias, or significant coronary stenosis/left ventricular dysfunction the probability of adverse cardiac events is low and participation in low-moderate dynamic and low static sports (IA, B) is allowed.

In athletes without evidence of ischaemic heart disease but with one or more risk factors, the eligibility decisions may vary on the basis of the estimated risk of coronary events according to available scoring systems [138].

Congenital coronary anomalies

In athletes, the diagnosis of anomalous origin and course of a coronary artery is challenging and requires a high index of suspicious. Because >50% of sudden death victims with post-mortem diagnosis of a coronary anomaly have experienced chest pain or syncope, the condition should be suspected in the presence of such symptoms [51]. The 12-lead ECG, either basal or during effort, shows a low diagnostic sensitivity. False-negative results of exercise testing in subjects who have subsequently died suddenly from coronary anomalies has been explained by the difficulty of reproducing in the clinical setting the particular mechanisms of myocardial ischaemia due to the aberrant coronary origin and course [48]. Definitive diagnosis relies on demonstration of the anomalous coronary artery by either conventional coronary angiography (➲Chapter 8) or by modern imaging techniques such as coronary artery computed tomography or CMR (➲Chapter 5) [139, 140]. All individuals with anomalous origin of a coronary artery from the wrong coronary sinus and a course between the great arteries should be excluded from competitive sports until the anomaly is surgically corrected. After surgical repair, athletes should undergo a new evaluation for ischaemia, arrhythmia, and LV dysfunction at 3–6 months [87, 88]. If no abnormalities are detected, there are no prohibitions to participation in competitive athletics.

Valve diseases

Clinical evaluation and recommendations for sports eligibility of athletes with valve diseases are summarized in ➲Table 32.8. Postoperative patients with mechanical valves (or bioprosthetic valves in selected cases) need systematic anticoagulation treatment, which further limits their potential for participation in competitive sports, notably those at risk of bodily collision (see ➲Table 32.1) [88].

Implantable defibrillator

Patients with an ICD (➲Chapter 30) usually have a cardiac disease which represents per se a contraindication for competitive sports. Individuals with ICD and no evidence of structural heart disease and preserved cardiac function can be allowed to participate in sports with only low dynamic or static demand, which do not pose a risk of trauma to

Table 32.8 Recommendations for competitive sport participation in athletes with valvular diseases

Lesion	Evaluation	Criteria for eligibility	Recommendations	Follow-up
Mitral valve stenosis	History, PE, ECG, ET, TTE	Mild stenosis, stable sinus rhythm	All sports, with exception of high dynamic and high static (III C)	Yearly
		Mild stenosis in atrial fibrillation, and anticoagulation	Low-moderate dynamic, low-moderate static (I–I, A–B), No contact sport	Yearly
		Moderate and severe stenosis (atrial fibrillation or sinus rhythm)	Low dynamic and low static (IA) No contact sport	Yearly
Mitral valve regurgitation	History, PE, ECG, ET, TTE	Mild to moderate regurgitation, stable sinus rhythm, normal LV size/function, normal exercise testing	All sports	Yearly
		Mild to moderate regurgitation, normal LV size and function, normal exercise testing, if atrial fibrillation, in anticoagulation	All sports, with exception of contact sport	Yearly
		Mild to moderate regurgitation, mild LV dilatation, normal resting LV function, in sinus rhythm	Low-moderate dynamic, low-moderate static (I–II, A–B)	Yearly
		Mild to moderate regurgitation, LV enlargement (LVEDDI > 3.0 mm/m^2) or LV dysfunction	No competitive sports	
		Severe regurgitation	No competitive sports	
Aortic valve stenosis	History, PE, ECG, ET, TEE	Mild stenosis, normal LV size and function at rest and under stress, no symptoms, no significant arrhythmia	Low-moderate dynamic, low-moderate static (I–II, A–B)	Yearly
		Moderate stenosis, normal LV function at rest and under stress, frequent/complex arrhythmias	Low dynamic and low static (IA)	Yearly

the device, and do not specifically trigger malignant ventricular tachycardias (such as torsade de pointes in congenital long QT syndrome (➲Chapter 9) and polymorphic catecholaminergic ventricular tachycardia) (➲Table 32.7). Sports participation can be allowed at least 6 months after the ICD implantation, or after the most recent arrhythmic episode requiring defibrillator intervention (including pacing, antitachycardia pacing, or shock). To reduce the risk of inappropriate shocks related to sinus tachycardia induced by exercise, the cut-off heart rate for the ICD needs to be appropriately set by exercise testing and 24-hour Holter monitoring [142].

Automatic external defibrillator programme

The presence of a free-standing automated external defibrillator (➲Chapter 30) at sporting events may be a valuable back up for conditions unrecognized by ECG screening such as coronary artery diseases—either atherosclerotic or congenital—but should not be considered either a substitute of preparticipation evaluation or a justification for participation in competitive sports of athletes with at risk-heart diseases. Chances for on-field successful resuscitation are remote, even if cardiopulmonary resuscitation is started immediately and defibrillation equipment is readily available. Drezner *et al.* showed significant limitations of this strategy in the young athletic population, in which cardiovascular conditions other than coronary artery disease are the leading causes of cardiac arrest [142]. Only one of nine athletes (11%) survived, although most cases had a witnessed collapse, timely cardiopulmonary resuscitation, and prompt defibrillation (average time from cardiac arrest to defibrillation of 3.1min). On the other hand, Maron *et al.*[143] analyzed 128 cases from the United States Commotio Cordis Registry and found an overall survival rate of 46% (19 of 41) in the individuals who received early defibrillation. A plausible explanation for the discrepancy between the two studies is that the majority of athletes in the Drezner study had an underlying structural heart disease and that ventricular tachycardia/fibrillation in the presence of cardiac structural abnormalities may be more resistant to defibrillation (specially if non-immediate) than arrhythmic cardiac arrest in a structurally normal heart, such as in commotio cordis. Other factors that may decrease the efficacy of defibrillation in athletes include the high catecholamine levels and metabolic changes occurring during strenuous physical exercise and interacting unfavourably with the underlying cardiomyopathic substrate. In conclusion, the concept of prevention of athletic-field sudden death by using early automated external defibrillators programmes, although promising, is still evolving and further studies are needed [31].

Personal perspective

The future for prevention of sports-related fatalities lies in continuing efforts to better understand the substrates and mechanisms underlying sudden death in the athlete and to design more specific and efficient screening strategies. An international registry collecting all fatal events in young competitive athletes is warranted to evaluate whether genetic and/or environmental factors may influence the distribution of cardiovascular causes of sudden death in the different European countries.

The 25-year Italian experience with preparticipation screening of millions of athletes demonstrated that such a population-based prevention strategy allows successful identification of athletes affected by potentially malignant cardiovascular diseases and to substantial reduction of mortality. Until other studies, either observational or randomized, on athletic populations of comparable size and follow-up are conducted, the existing data provide good evidence that ECG screening decreases the risk of sudden cardiac death in athletes. Accordingly, preparticipation ECG screening is currently recommended by the International Olympic Committee ('Lausanne Recommendations') [144] as well as by most European Cardiology Societies and Sports Medical Federations [86]. However, major obstacles for the launch of definitive screening still exist because of the lack of national legislation. Continued cooperative efforts between medical societies and sports organizations, may persuade healthcare policy makers to seriously consider implementation of such screening programmes in the near future.

The extraordinary advances in molecular genetics during the last two decades have allowed identification of a growing number of defective genes involved in the pathogenesis of inherited cardiomyopathies, including cardiac ion channel disorders [145, 146]. It is hoped that in the near future genetic molecular tests will be clinically available for definitive differential diagnosis between cardiomyopathies and athletic training-related physiologic changes of the cardiovascular system.

Further reading

Corrado D, Pelliccia A, Bjornstad HH, *et al.* Cardiovascular pre-participation screening of young competitive athletes for prevention of sudden death: proposal for a common European protocol. Consensus Statement of the Study Group of Sport Cardiology of the Working Group of Cardiac Rehabilitation and Exercise Physiology and the Working Group of Myocardial and Pericardial Diseases of the European Society of Cardiology. *Eur Heart J* 2005; **26**: 516–24.

Corrado D, Basso C, Link MS, *et al.* Sudden death in athletes. In Priori SG, Zipes D (eds.) *Sudden Cardiac Death: A Handbook For Clinical Practice*, 2006. The ESC educational series. Oxford: Blackwell Publishing, pp. 189–202.

Maron BJ, Zipes DP. 36th Bethesda Conference: recommendations for determining eligibility for competition in athletes with cardiovascular abnormalities: *J Am Coll Cardiol* 2005; **45**: 1373–5.

Pelliccia A, Fagard R, Bjornstad HH, *et al.* Recommendations for competitive sports participation in athletes with cardiovascular disease: a consensus document from the Study Group of Sports Cardiology of the Working Group of Cardiac Rehabilitation and Exercise Physiology and the Working Group of Myocardial and Pericardial Diseases of the European Society of Cardiology. *Eur Heart J* 2005; **26**: 1422–45

Pelliccia A, Zipes DP, Maron BJ. Bethesda Conference #36 and the European Society of Cardiology Consensus Recommendations revisited. A comparison of U.S. and European criteria for eligibility and disqualification of competitive athletes with cardiovascular abnormalities. *J Am Coll Cardiol* 2008; **52**: 1990–6.

➲ For full references and multimedia materials please visit the online version of the book (http://esctextbook.oxfordonline.com).

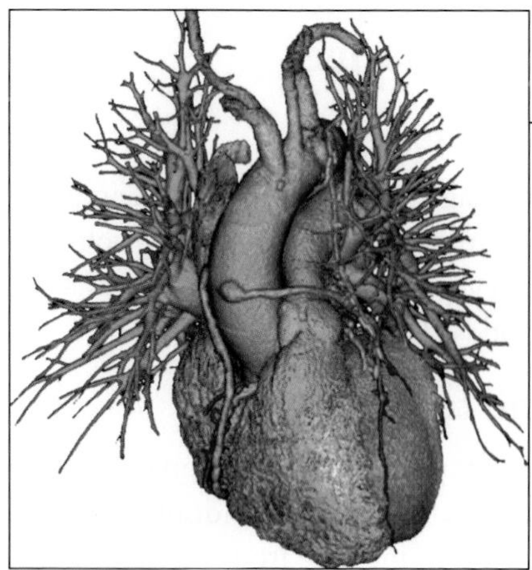

CHAPTER 33

Pregnancy and Heart Disease

Patrizia Presbitero, Giacomo G. Boccuzzi, Christianne J. M. Groot, and Jolien W. Roos-Hesselink

Contents

Summary

Heart disease, though rare, is in Western countries a major cause of maternal mortality. Heart disease can be present or discovered during pregnancy because of haemodynamic overload of the heart, particularly during the third trimester when cardiac output doubles.

Most of the knowledge in recognition and treatment of cardiac disease during pregnancy is not based on evidence from randomized trials, but is derived from clinical experience, few case reports, and small consecutive series. These are summarized in the guidelines on 'Management of Cardiovascular Diseases During Pregnancy' from the European Society of Cardiology, the basis for this chapter. The physiological changes that occur during pregnancy have a different impact depending on the type and severity of cardiac anomalies. Differential diagnosis with normal pregnancy related physiological changes is also discussed.

Particular emphasis is placed on early and accurate diagnosis of congenital or acquired cardiac anomalies because often early intervention is essential for a safe pregnancy and delivery.

Women at low risk are those in New York Heart Association (NYHA) class I or II with good ventricular function, without severe left ventricular inflow or outflow obstruction or pulmonary hypertension, and who do not need to take anticoagulants. Women at high risk are those showing symptoms of severe mitral or aortic stenosis, the ones with cyanotic congenital heart disease with or without pulmonary hypertension, the ones with significantly impaired systemic ventricular function and/or life-threatening arrhythmias, the ones with wide aorta in Marfan syndrome, and finally the ones with mechanical valves. The same conditions that endanger the mother also affect fetal morbidity and mortality.

Multiple therapeutic options including percutaneous or surgical intervention are now available to allow for a safe completion of the pregnancy. Management of these patients requires teamwork from cardiologists, obstetricians, anaesthetists, neonatologists, and, sometimes, cardiac surgeons.

Cardiovascular adaptations during normal pregnancy

Pregnancy physiology is characterized by significant haemodynamic changes that allow the uterus and developing fetus to receive an adequate blood supply. These adaptations are well tolerated by the normal heart but may result in haemodynamic problems for the diseased heart. This implies that pregnancy may unmask previously silent heart disease.

Heart disease is present in 0.5–1% [1, 2] of all pregnant women and accounts for about 10–15% of all maternal mortality [3]. Although the incidence of acquired disease has fallen (to <0.2%) in Western countries due to the reduction in the incidence of rheumatic fever following the introduction of penicillin [1, 2], rheumatic heart disease is still the prevalent cause. Congenital heart disease is becoming an increasing problem during pregnancy as a result of the success of neonatal corrective or palliative cardiac surgery [4](➲Chapter 10). Because of the increased delay to first pregnancy, maternal older age, and the increase in women's smoking habits, symptomatic coronary disease, although rare, can occur and is likely to increase.

Haemodynamic changes during pregnancy

The evaluation and management of heart disease in pregnant women require knowledge of the normal physiological changes associated with gestation, labour, delivery, and the early postpartum period (➲Fig. 33.1).

Blood volume and cardiac output

The most remarkable change related to pregnancy is the increase in blood volume, which almost doubles by the end of pregnancy. It starts to increase from the sixth week, rising rapidly in the second trimester and becoming stable in the last 8 weeks [5]. Red cell mass increases later in pregnancy but to a lesser extent than the plasma volume, leading to slight haemodilution and the physiological anaemia of pregnancy, with haematocrit at about 33–34% and haemoglobin around 11–12g/dL [6]. These changes are more marked in twin or multiple pregnancies. In the last trimester, peripheral arterial vasodilatation may reduce arterial vascular filling and thereby induce sodium and water retention mediated by aldosterone. In an average

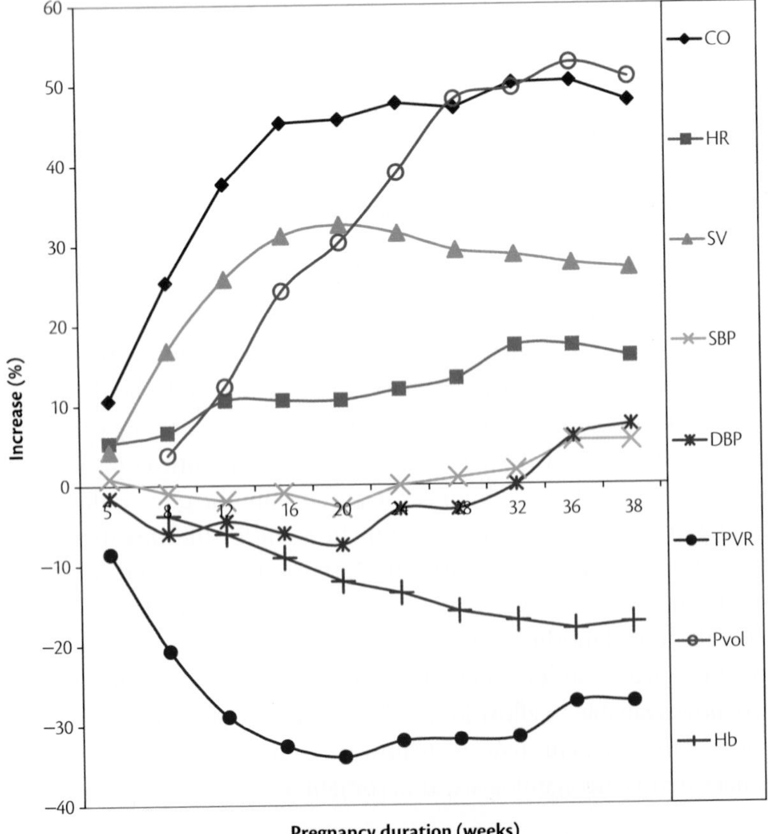

Figure 33.1 Changes in cardiac output (CO), stroke volume (SV), plasma volume (PV), total peripheral vascular resistance (TPVR), heart rate (HR), blood pressure (SBP, systolic blood pressure; DBP, diastolic blood pressure) and haemoglobin concentration (Hb) during pregnancy. Reproduced from Karamermer Y, Roos-Hesselink JW. Pregnancy and adult congenital heart disease. *Expert Rev Cardiovasc Ther* 2007; **5**: 859–69 with permission from Expert Reviews Ltd.

pregnancy, there is a gradual accumulation of 500–900mEq of sodium and total body water increases by 6–8L, mostly extracellular. All these haemodynamic changes, which evolved to protect the mother from blood loss at delivery, could play a role in the pathogenesis of heart failure.

Cardiac output also increases to about 40% above the non-pregnant value. Most of this increment is achieved early in pregnancy, with peak values at 20–24 weeks [7]. This is achieved by an increase in stroke volume and heart rate. In late pregnancy the increase in venous return is sensitive to posture: a sharp drop in preload due to inferior vena cava compression by the gravid uterus in the supine position may cause hypotension, with weakness and light-headedness or syncope and even (short) fetal distress. These symptoms are easily resolved by turning the woman from the supine to the lateral decubitus position.

Heart rate

Heart rate starts to increase in the first weeks of pregnancy and peaks in the first half of the third trimester. The increase in resting heart rate averages 10–20 beats per minute (bpm). Atrial tachyarrhythmias can be present in normal pregnancy due to increased plasma catecholamine concentrations and/or adrenoreceptor sensitivity, and to the stretched atrial wall because of increased heart volumes [8].

Peripheral vascular resistance

Maternal peripheral and pulmonary vascular resistance fall as a result of the low-resistance uteroplacental circulation, decreased mean aortic pressure, and endogenous hormones. Some reports focused on the role of nitric oxide in the pathogenesis of vasodilatation [9]. Venous return increases, with a consequent rise in left ventricular end-diastolic volume, although the filling pressure does not rise because of ventricular structural changes (increased compliance). In the first two trimesters, the fall in systemic vascular resistance, which exceeds the increase in cardiac output, leads to a drop in both systolic and, especially, diastolic blood pressure, resulting in a wide pulse pressure.

Haemostasis

Pregnancy induces complex changes in the physiological systems concerned with haemostasis. The hypercoagulable state of pregnancy is due to alterations in the coagulation and fibrinolytic systems, which include a decreased releasable tissue plasminogen activator (tPA), increased fast-acting tPA inhibitor, change in the level of coagulation factors, and reduction in functional protein S levels [10]. These alterations, together with the increased blood volume and unique phenomenon of myometrial contraction, help to combat the hazard of haemorrhage during and after placental separation; however, they carry the risk of more rapid and increased response to any coagulant stimuli [10].

Labour, delivery, and early postpartum period

The most dramatic swings in haemodynamic parameters occur during labour, delivery, and the immediate postpartum period. Uterine contractions significantly increase venous return, and during a contraction cardiac output may rise by a further 25%. Pain and anxiety cause an increase in sympathetic tone during the second stage of labour, which in turn enhances cardiac output and blood pressure. These changes may be influenced by the type of anaesthesia and analgesia used in labour and by the mode of delivery [11]. Reduction of pain and apprehension can be achieved by local and caudal anaesthesia. The patient should be lying in the left lateral position during labour.

During the early postpartum period, cardiac output increases as a result of a blood shift from the contracting uterus to the systemic circulation and because of inferior vena cava decompression (autotransfusion) [12]. There are no haemodynamic differences between lactating and non-lactating mothers. The cardiovascular adaptations associated with pregnancy regress by approximately 6 weeks after delivery.

Cardiac evaluation in normal pregnancy

During pregnancy, cardiovascular disease or worsening of a previous cardiac disease is difficult to detect: cardiopulmonary signs and symptoms typically reported during normal pregnancy may mimic heart disease. Fatigue and decreased exercise capacity are common, along with chest pain at rest that may be caused by oesophageal reflux. As many as 75% of women may complain of mild dyspnoea, whereas progressive orthopnoea or paroxysmal nocturnal dyspnoea are rare. Palpitations are very common and are due to either a physiological increase in the resting heart rate or atrial or ventricular ectopic beats [13] (➲Table 33.1).

Physical examination

The physical examination of a healthy pregnant woman shows a slightly fast resting heart, a bounding pulse, a widened

Table 33.1 Symptoms and signs during pregnancy

	Normal pregnancy	Indicators of heart disease
Symptoms	Mild dyspnoea	Severe or progressive dyspnoea
	Fatigability	Paroxysmal nocturnal dyspnoea
	Decreased exercise tolerance	Syncope with exertion
	Rest chest pain	Effort or emotion chest pain
	Palpitations	
Signs	Pedal oedema	Severe peripheral oedema
	Warm extremities	Clubbing and cyanosis
	Full, sharp, and collapsing pulse	Persistent neck vein distension
	Prominent left ventricular impulse	Cardiomegaly
	Third heart sound (S_3)	Fourth heart sound (S_4)
	Grade 1–2 systolic ejection murmurs	Grade ≥3 systolic ejection murmurs
	Premature beats	Sustained arrhythmias
	Continuous murmurs	Diastolic murmurs

pulse pressure, and warm flushed peripheries. In addition, a slight elevation of venous pressure, the presence of 'tense' soft tissues, and peripheral oedema (pedal oedema) are common. The thyroid gland may be enlarged in the absence of clinical hyperthyroidism.

The precordial impulse is hyperkinetic and the first heart sound (S_1) is increased, with prominent splitting that may be misinterpreted as a fourth heart sound (S_4) or as a systolic click. During the later stages of pregnancy, the physiological splitting of the second heart sound (S_2) may seem fixed. Third sound gallop (S_3) is frequently present by week 20 of gestation, whereas S_4 is uncommon and requires further evaluation.

Murmurs develop in nearly all women during pregnancy. They are usually soft, mid-systolic, and heard at the mid to upper left sternal border, and are secondary to increased pulmonary blood flow. Benign murmurs include the continuous bruit resulting from increased blood flow to the breasts, the 'mammary soufflé', and the suprasternal venous hums, which can be obliterated through ipsilateral jugular digital compression or by firm pressure of the stethoscope. Diastolic murmurs are unusual and therefore call for further evaluation. The murmurs of stenotic heart valves (aortic stenosis, pulmonary stenosis, mitral stenosis) may increase in intensity because of the physiological increase in cardiac output and fall in systemic vascular resistance. On the other hand, the murmurs of incompetent heart valves (aortic insufficiency, mitral insufficiency) may decrease. Detection of murmurs as diastolic murmurs, continuous murmurs, and loud systolic murmurs equal or greater than grade III in intensity cannot be considered physiological and hence need further careful examination, starting with transthoracic echocardiography (➲Table 33.1) [14].

Additional diagnostic tools

Electrocardiogram

In normal pregnancy, there are no characteristic electrocardiographic changes except for a slight leftward shift of the electrical axis, which can give rise to a small Q wave in lead III [15]. Severe left-axis deviation is not a normal pregnancy variant and needs further evaluation (➲Chapter 2).

Doppler echocardiography

Because of its safety and diagnostic power, transthoracic Doppler echocardiography is the first advisable diagnostic tool. In a normal pregnancy, serial echocardiography usually shows a significant increase in cardiac output, cardiac index, left ventricular end-diastolic volume, and left ventricular wall thickness. An increase in left (up to 6%) and right (up to 12%) ventricular diastolic dimensions is present [16]. A mild increase in left and right atrial size (up to 20%) and transvalvular flow velocities and the presence of mild atrioventricular valve regurgitation are normal echocardiographic findings during pregnancy [17] (➲Fig. 33.2). Transoesophageal echocardiography is used to confirm a diagnostic hypothesis or to minimize the radiating dose during percutaneous procedures (such as aortic and mitral valvuloplasty)(➲Chapter 4).

Chest radiography

Exposure to ionizing radiation should be avoided whenever possible, especially during early pregnancy since malignancies and congenital abnormalities in offspring have been described. Routine chest radiography (1.5mGy) exposes the uterus to a minimal (0.05mGy) radiation dose. Chest radiography should therefore be used only if clinically indicated and performed with the minimum amount of radiation, shielding the pelvic area. In addition, whenever possible it should be delayed until at least the completion of the first trimester. In normal pregnancy, the heart may appear enlarged due to the horizontal position, and increased lung markings and small pleural effusions can be detected [18].

Magnetic resonance imaging

Indications for magnetic resonance imaging (MRI) during pregnancy for cardiovascular disease are very rare

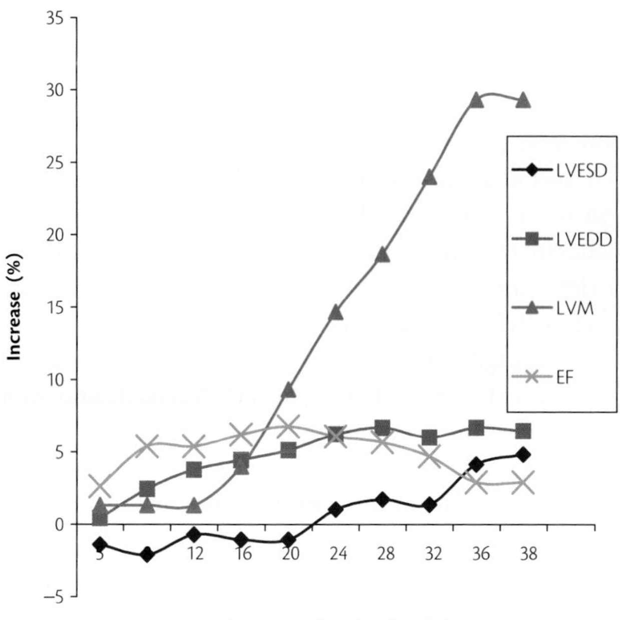

Figure 33.2 Changes in left ventricular end-diastolic and end-systolic dimension (LVEDD/LVESD), left ventricular ejection fraction (EF), and left ventricular mass indexed for body surface area (LVM) during pregnancy. Reproduced from Karamermer Y, Roos-Hesselink JW. Pregnancy and adult congenital heart disease. *Expert Rev Cardiovasc Ther* 2007; **5**: 859–69 with permission from Expert Reviews Ltd.

(for example, when aortic dissection diagnosis is doubtful even after transoesophageal echocardiography). Most of the time MRI can be performed with good diagnostic accuracy without contrast agent. The emergence of an association between gadolinium-based contrast agents and nephrogenic syndrome has led to a reassessment of contrast-enhanced MR imaging. Following intravenous administration, small amounts of gadolinium-based contrast agents cross the placenta and enter fetal circulation. Subsequently, they are excreted by the fetus into amniotic fluid, where they may remain or can be swallowed by the fetus. Although no teratogenic or mutagenic effects secondary to gadolinium-based contrast exposure have been demonstrated in humans, current radiology practices and recommendations discourage the use of gadolinium during pregnancy [19] (➲Chapter 5).

Computed tomography

The main indications for computed tomography (CT) scan during pregnancy is suspected pulmonary embolism. Based on the fact that a threshold dose of 50mGy is required for induction of deterministic effects, none of the potential hazards such as fetal death, malformation, or mental retardation are a specific risk with the low exposures of ionizing radiation used in diagnostic imaging. However, some recent studies revealed that there may be an increased risk of cancer induction after radiation exposure during CT to radiosensitive organs in pregnant patients, particularly in breast tissue. Therefore avoiding or reducing the radiation dose exposure is mandatory. There are a number of ways of minimizing the radiation dose to mother and fetus: reduce milliampere-second (mAs), reduce kilo voltage (kVp), increase pitch, increase detector and beam collimation, reduce field of view, reduce z-axis scan volume (caudal extent limited to top of diaphragm), eliminate frontal and lateral scout views, and circumferential shielding of the abdomen and pelvis. The iodine component of the contrast media given to a pregnant patient has the potential to produce neonatal hypothyroidism and cretinism, so screening for hypothyroidism in infants is mandatory. The risk:benefit ratio has to drive the use of such imaging techniques [19–20] (➲Chapter 6).

Assessment of heart disease in pregnancy

The assessment of women with heart disease should take place before conception in order to counsel them adequately and to minimize maternal and fetal morbidity and mortality. Preconception counselling has to address: the risk for the mother; the risk to the fetus; the risk of recurrence in the offspring; and maternal life expectancy. The type and severity of cardiac disease, general conditions, previous cardiovascular and cerebral events, NYHA class, medications, and obstetric and family history should be taken into account in evaluating the risks and possibility of successful pregnancy. For example, aortic insufficiency is normally well tolerated during pregnancy because of the low peripheral resistance; however, if systemic hypertension, NYHA class III–IV, an ejection fraction around 40%, or ventricular arrhythmias are present, it becomes a high-risk condition. The risk of recurrence in the offspring should be discussed.

All patients with congenital heart diseases should have informed genetic counselling before conception, the risk of recurrence varies between about 3–12% (for lesions with autosomal dominant inheritance the risk for recurrence of congenital heart disease can be as high as 50%) compared with a background risk of 0.8% for the general population (➲Table 33.2). Referral of the woman to a geneticist is indicated due to the increasing possibilities for identifying genetic underlying causes in many congenital diseases. An exercise test before pregnancy is very important for evaluating functional capacity; the physiological changes of pregnancy are similar to the ones that occur during exercise but over an extended period, so a good exercise test will predict

Table 33.2 Recurrence risks of congenital heart disease in offspring*

Type of heart disease	Total risk (%)	Mother affected (%)	Father affected (%)
Acyanotic congenital heart disease			
Atrial septal defect	3–5	4.5–6	1.5–3.5
Ventricular septal defect	4–8	6–9.5	2–3.6
Atrioventricular septal defect	10–15	7.5–15	1–7
Patent ductus arteriosus	3–4	4	2
Pulmonary stenosis	4	5.3–6.5	2–3.5
Left ventricular obstruction	11–15	10–11	3
Coarctation of aorta	6	4–6.3	2.5–3
Cyanotic congenital heart disease			
Tetralogy of Fallot	2.2–3.1	2–2.5	1.5–2.2
Transposition of great vessels	0.5		
Mendelian disorders			
Holt–Oram syndrome	50	50	50
Noonan syndrome	50	50	50
Marfan syndrome	50	50	50

* Based on multiple studies [36, 38, 41, 51, 53].

a well-tolerated pregnancy. Echocardiography is required to assess cardiac haemodynamics, particularly pulmonary pressure, left ventricular systolic function, and severity of valve obstructions. When the heart disease is severe (e.g. severe mitral stenosis), balloon valvuloplasty or mitral valve surgery should be considered before pregnancy.

If a woman with heart disease presents and is already pregnant, her cardiac status and medication should be evaluated and should be treated by a specialized team of cardiologists, obstetricians, and anaesthesiologists. A detailed plan for her pregnancy and delivery should be made early in pregnancy and changed if cardiac deterioration occurs. Our recommendation for follow-up visits is a visit at the end of each trimester and in case of deterioration the patient has to be re-evaluated immediately.

There are other conditions outside heart diseases that can affect the maternal and fetal morbidity and mortality: an increase in childbearing age, smoking habits, multiple pregnancies due to advances in reproductive technology, comorbidities like diabetes and collagenopathies. To assess the global (maternal and neonatal) risk associated with pregnancy these conditions have to be recognized before conception because they can complicate mild heart disease and add further risk to severe heart disease.

Maternal low-risk conditions

All the conditions which benefit from the decrease in systemic vascular resistance that occurs during pregnancy are well tolerated, provided that left and right ventricular function is not impaired. These conditions include mild and moderate valve regurgitation [21] and small–moderate left-to-right shunts without pulmonary hypertension. Though much better tolerated than severe stenosis, severe mitral or aortic regurgitation can worsen during pregnancy due to the increased overload leading to NYHA class deterioration, arrhythmias, and heart failure [22].

Also, the mild forms of cardiac disease are well tolerated even if some of them can worsen during pregnancy (mild valve stenosis, mild cardiomyopathies with left ventricle ejection fraction around 45%, Ebstein's anomaly). Some of them can never go back to the previous status after delivery and can continue to worse [21–24].

In patients who have undergone previous successful surgical repair without mechanical heart valve implantation, pregnancy is well tolerated if normal exercise tolerance, good functional status, and normal ventricular function are present. The exercise test is a very tool to predict an uneventful pregnancy: the patient should accomplish the Bruce stage 2 without symptoms, with no drop in arterial pressure or oxygen saturation [21–25].

Even if close follow-up is recommended (cardiac assessment every trimester), these patients need only to be reassured and vaginal delivery should be planned; Caesarean section should be performed only in case of obstetrics indications. However, patients need to be informed about the additional risk (though often small) compared to healthy women.

Maternal high-risk conditions

Previous studies have recognized that prior cardiac events or arrhythmias, poor functional class, cyanosis, left heart obstruction, and left ventricular systolic dysfunction independently predict maternal cardiac complications. The expected cardiac event (congestive heart failure, arrhythmias, stroke, or death) rate in pregnancies with 0, 1, or >1 of these risk factors is 5%, 27%, and 75% respectively [26, 27]. There are some specific conditions at particular risk during pregnancy.

Pulmonary hypertension

A 30–50% maternal mortality risk is still reported in patients with severe pulmonary vascular disease (➲Chapter 24), either with septal defects (Eisenmenger's syndrome) (➲Chapter 10) or without [28, 29], and fetal loss is of a similar magnitude. Systemic vasodilatation increases the right-to-left shunt and decreases pulmonary output, leading to a low-output status. Death occurs in the last months of pregnancy or in the first few days after delivery because of pulmonary hypertensive crises, mostly due to fibrinoid necrosis, rarely to pulmonary thrombosis. It can happen even in patients with little or no disability before or during pregnancy. The level of pulmonary hypertension that should be considered at risk is around 70mmHg systolic or >30mmHg mean pulmonary pressure. Even moderate forms of pulmonary vascular disease can worsen during pregnancy as a result of the decrease in systemic resistance and of overload of the right ventricle. Termination of pregnancy is advisable. If pregnancy continues, patients should restrict their physical activity, avoid the supine position, and take subcutaneous heparin as prophylaxis against thromboembolism [23]. Intravenous or pulmonary infusion of prostacyclin (epoprostenol) has been occasionally used to decrease pulmonary pressure during delivery and postpartum in order to manage pulmonary hypertensive crises [30, 31]. Further evaluation is needed before using new drugs such as the oral phosphodiesterase inhibitor sildenafil and the endothelin receptor antagonist bosentan during pregnancy [32, 33]. Invasive monitoring during labour and delivery is recommended.

Severe left ventricular tract obstruction

Congenital, most often bicuspid, aortic valve stenosis is rare during pregnancy because it is more frequently encountered in males and patients have usually had percutaneous or surgical valvuloplasty in childhood or before conception. Occasionally severe rheumatic aortic valve stenosis can occur rarely isolated, most often together with mitral stenosis. In severe aortic stenosis (aortic valve area ≤1.0cm^2 or V_{max} >4m/sec or echo mean gradient >50mmHg or haemodynamic peak gradient >64mmHg) the fixed resistance may not be able to accommodate the increased cardiac output that occurs during pregnancy. An increase in both gradient and left ventricular end-diastolic pressure is induced and can cause heart failure, low output, and reduction in uteroplacental perfusion. Important electrocardiogram (ECG) changes of left ventricular overload in a previously normal ECG, signs of heart failure, and low systemic blood pressure can appear. Serial echocardiography during pre-pregnancy and pregnancy period show a significant increase in the transvalvular aortic mean and peak gradients, a higher left ventricular mass and significant increase in left ventricular twist (defined as a wringing-like systolic motion of the heart around the long axis with the apex rotating counterclockwise and the base clockwise) [34]. The clinical symptoms occur typically at 20–24 weeks of gestation. Women with an aortic valve area <1.0cm^2 should be discouraged from conceiving before treatment especially when they are symptomatic, even if recent pregnancy reports in aortic stenosis patient are encouraging, showing a favourable pregnancy outcome with low major cardiovascular complications [35, 36], but with high rate of interventions in severe cases.

The recent study of Yap and colleagues found important cardiovascular events (i.e. heart failure, transient ischaemic attack, and arrhythmias) in only 5 of 53 pregnancies (9.4%) in a cohort of women with aortic stenosis and one or more completed pregnancy [35]. High mortality in previous series [37] was probably due to: the underestimation of clinical signs during pregnancy; the lack of immediate intervention when the symptoms occurred; and the worse NYHA functional class of the population. Risk assessment has to be based on: symptomatic status (high risk when NYHA >II); left ventricular function (high risk when ejection fraction <40%); occurrence of pulmonary hypertension; and poor exercise tolerance. If the fetus is viable (>34 weeks) delivery is advised, thus restoring the pre-pregnancy haemodynamic status. If the valve is not heavily calcified and no regurgitation is present, percutaneous balloon valvotomy can be successfully performed. Many cases have been reported, with significant reduction of valve gradient, enabling the pregnancy to continue [38–40]. Surgery can be an alternative in a small subset of patients in the presence of a heavily calcified valve or significant aortic valve regurgitation [41]. The majority of patients required elective aortic valve replacement after pregnancy, and balloon valvuloplasty should therefore be regarded as a palliative procedure, enabling the pregnancy to continue safely and deferring definitive treatment to a later date.

Focusing on maternal cardiac complications we should not forget the obstetric and perinatal complications. Non-cardiac complications are not infrequent, including premature deliveries (varies from 8–13.2%), small-for-gestational-age births (varies from 2–13.2%), and a slight rise of hypertension-related disorders (11.3% vs. 8% in the general population) [34].

Impaired systemic ventricular ejection function

Besides basic cardiac disease, systemic ventricular function is one of the main determinants of maternal and neonatal outcome. As far the left ventricle is concerned, no reviews are available that indicate a cut-off value for left ventricular ejection fraction below which pregnancy is contraindicated. An echocardiographic ejection fraction >40% with a good rise in systemic arterial pressure on exercise testing allows the continuation of pregnancy, although complications can still occur. Pregnancy termination should be advised if ejection fraction is <40% with increased left ventricular dimensions and the patient is markedly symptomatic. After peripartum cardiomyopathy (see ➲Chapter 18, Myocardial Disease), even if a complete recovery is achieved in 30-40% of the cases, left ventricle dysfunction and clinical deterioration can occur in subsequent pregnancies. However, when incomplete recovery of ventricular function is achieved after the first pregnancy, complications are around 50%; discourage of further pregnancies is indicated.

When the right ventricle is sustaining the systemic circulation, as in women with complete transposition of the great arteries (TGA) corrected with Mustard or Senning repair or in single ventricle right ventricle type, no cut-off value for ejection fraction which would predict adverse outcome is available. However, if a moderate impairment of systemic ventricle is present, pregnancy should be discouraged.

During pregnancy, restriction of physical activity and serial echocardiogram evaluation should be performed. Particular attention should be focused on the recognition of ventricular arrhythmias during pregnancy and after delivery, in which case telemetric monitoring is indicated. Particular attention should be paid when valvular disease with impaired ventricular function is present because the prognosis can be worse.

A planned delivery has to be discussed in every high-risk patient because normal labour involves intermittent deep haemodynamic changes during uterine contractions which may be potentially dangerous. Vaginal delivery with epidural analgesia, shortening the second stage of labour, may be suitable for selected patients. Most of the high-risk patients (and always if there is obstetric concern that labour may be prolonged), will undergo an elective Caesarean section under either epidural or general anaesthesia. This strategy prevents swings in blood pressure and minimizes maternal metabolic need, reducing the cardiovascular stress. Nowadays, blood loss during Caesarean section is reduced to 200Ml by the improved technique. The vasodilatation and hypotension secondary to anaesthesia (also epidural) can, in some conditions, cause a fall in cardiac output that has to be managed very carefully with liquids infusion or vasoconstrictors such as phenylephrine.

The immediate postpartum period represents a high-risk stage mainly because of the autotransfusion (500mlL or more of blood returned into the circulation from the uterus and placenta) and requires as close haemodynamic monitoring as the delivery period.

Other conditions

Mechanical valve prosthesis particularly in mitral position and when atrial fibrillation is present, Marfan syndrome with aortic root >40–45mm, severe mitral stenosis, and cyanotic congenital heart diseases are also maternal high-risk conditions and are discussed in ➲Specific conditions, p.1252.

Congenital heart disease and pregnancy

As a consequence of early surgical intervention, many patients with congenital cardiac malformations will reach child-bearing age and may become pregnant. Many of these patients have major or minor residua (abnormalities left behind) or sequelae (abnormalities caused by surgery but not technically considered complications) and have to be evaluated before pregnancy. As shown in a peer-reviewed literature which describes the outcome of 2491 pregnancies in patients with congenital heart disease, most pregnancies are successful, with an offspring mortality higher than the one in the general population (4% vs. 1%), but the rate of miscarriages become higher as the disease become more complex, as in pulmonary atresia with ventricular septal defect, diseases repaired with Fontan procedure, or cyanotic patients (➲Fig. 33.3) [42]. Similarly, maternal complications such as arrhythmias, heart failure, cardiovascular events, were present in 11% of completed pregnancies but again were higher as the disease becomes more complex. (➲Fig. 33.4)

Mild, moderate, and moderately severe right ventricular outflow tract obstruction are very well tolerated during pregnancy, as shown by previous series in which no deaths and a low incidence of complications have been reported [23]. However, the severe form of pulmonary valve stenosis and moderate stenosis with impaired right ventricular function should be treated before conception. Percutaneous pulmonary balloon valvuloplasty during pregnancy may be indicated in very severe (gradient suprasystemic) and/or symptomatic cases. A few successful cases have been reported [40] (➲Fig. 33.5). Stenting of pulmonary arteries can also be performed successfully during pregnancy. Mild left ventricular outflow tract obstruction is well tolerated during pregnancy even if pressure gradient doubles due to the increased cardiac output (➲Fig. 33.6) [23], whereas the moderate form must be followed carefully due to the possibility of rapid clinical deterioration.

Aortic coarctation carries a small risk of dissection [43] and should be corrected before pregnancy. Retrospective

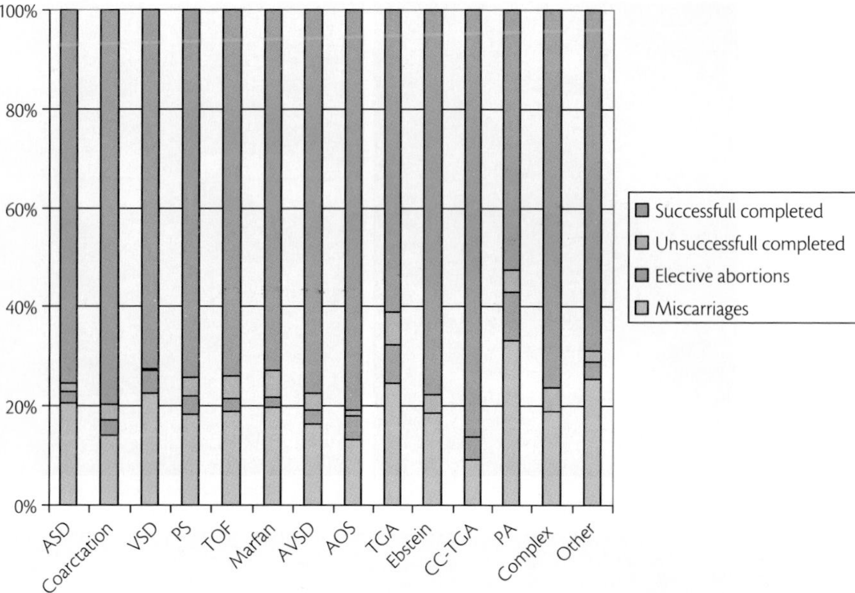

Figure 33.3 Pregnancy outcome in women with congenital heart disease. Distribution of successful/unsuccessful (fetal and neonatal mortality) completed pregnancies, elective abortions, and miscarriage for each congenital heart disease are shown separately. AOS, aortic stenosis; ASD, atrial septal defect; AVSD, atrioventricular septal defects; CC-TGA, congenital corrected transposition of the great arteries; Coarctation, aortic coarctation; Complex, other complex cyanotic heart disease according to Task Force; Ebstein, Ebstein's anomaly; Marfan, Marfan syndrome; PA, pulmonary atresia; PS, pulmonary valve stenosis; TGA, complete transposition of the great arteries; TOF, tetralogy of Fallot; VSD, ventricular septal defect. Data from Dutch ZAHARA study (1796 pregnancies). Drenthen W, Pieper PG.

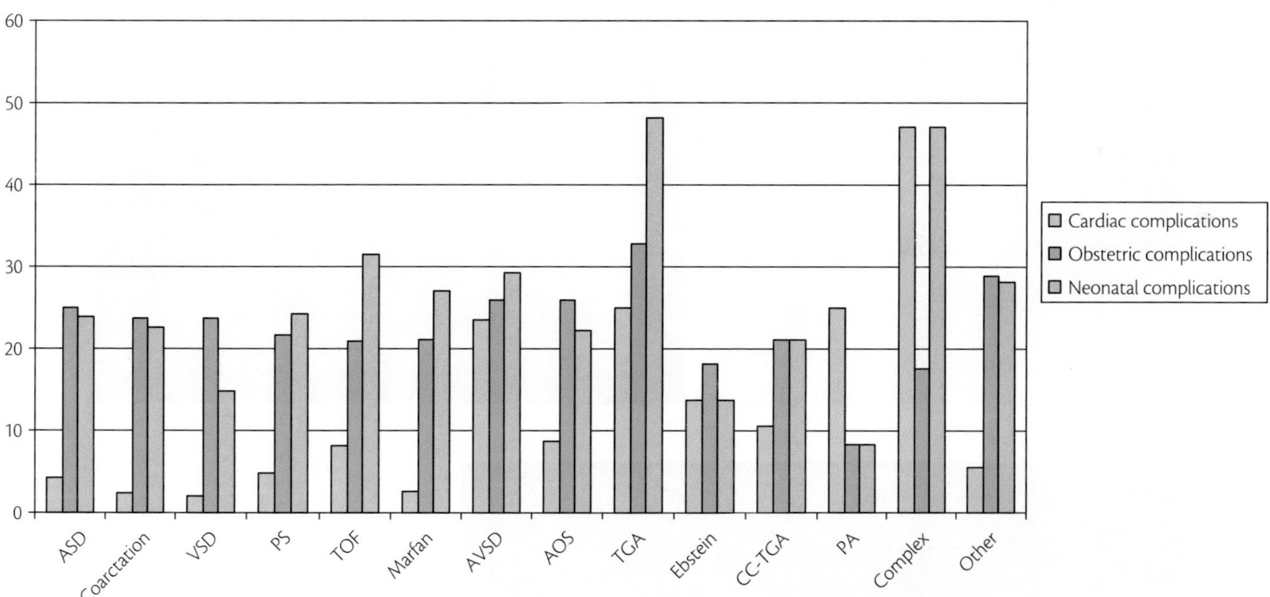

Figure 33.4 Distribution of complications in completed pregnancies in women with congenital heart disease. Overview of the most important complications encountered during pregnancy in women with structural congenital heart disease for each congenital heart disease separately. AOS, aortic stenosis; ASD, atrial septal defect; AVSD, atrioventricular septal defects; CC-TGA, congenital corrected transposition of the great arteries; Coarctation, aortic coarctation; Complex, other complex cyanotic heart disease according to Task Force; Ebstein, Ebstein's anomaly; Marfan, Marfan syndrome; PA, pulmonary atresia with; PS, pulmonary valve stenosis; TGA, complete transposition of the great arteries; TOF, tetralogy of Fallot; VSD, ventricular septal defect.
Composite cardiac complications: clinically significant ('requiring treatment') episodes of arrhythmia or heart failure; cardiovascular events (thromboembolic complications, myocardial infarction, cardiovascular mortality, and/or cerebrovascular accidents), endocarditis (including first 6 months' postpartum).
Composite obstetric complications: pregnancy-induced hypertension (PIH, new onset hypertension: blood pressure >140mmHg systolic or >90mmHg diastolic without proteinuria after 20 weeks of gestation); pre-eclampsia (PIH with >0.3g proteinuria in 24-hour urine sample); eclampsia (pre-eclampsia with grand mal seizures); haemolysis elevated liver enzymes low platelets (HELLP) syndrome according to the guideline of the European society of Gynaecology and Obstetrics; premature labour (<37 weeks' gestation); postpartum haemorrhage (vaginal delivery >500mL, Caesarean section >1000mL).
Composite neonatal complications: premature delivery (delivery <37 weeks); small-for-gestational-age birth weight (<10th percentile); offspring mortality (demise: in utero (>20 weeks' gestation)—the first year postpartum). Data from Dutch ZAHARA study (1302 pregnancies >20 weeks' gestation). Drenthen W, Pieper PG.

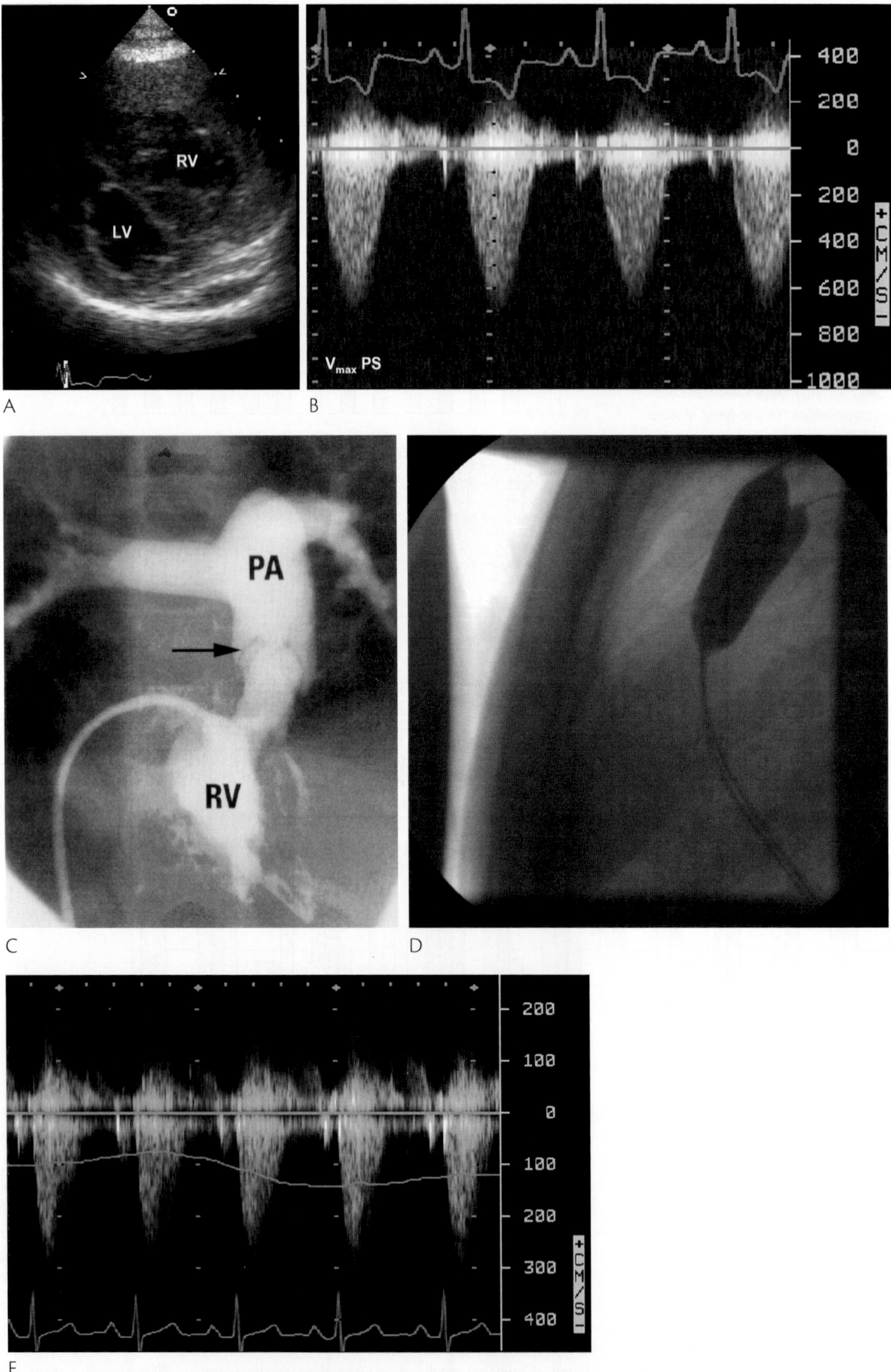

Figure 33.5 (A,B) Echocardiographic (A, parasternal short-axis view; B, continous-wave Doppler) and (C) angiographic image of a pregnant woman with severe pulmonic stenosis. Peak gradient was 144mmHg. She was treated with balloon dilatation during pregnancy (D), the peak gradient decreasing to 40mmHg after dilatation (E). RV, right ventricle; LV, left ventricle; PA, pulmonary artery; V_{max}, maximal velocity (m/s) measured over the pulmonic valve.

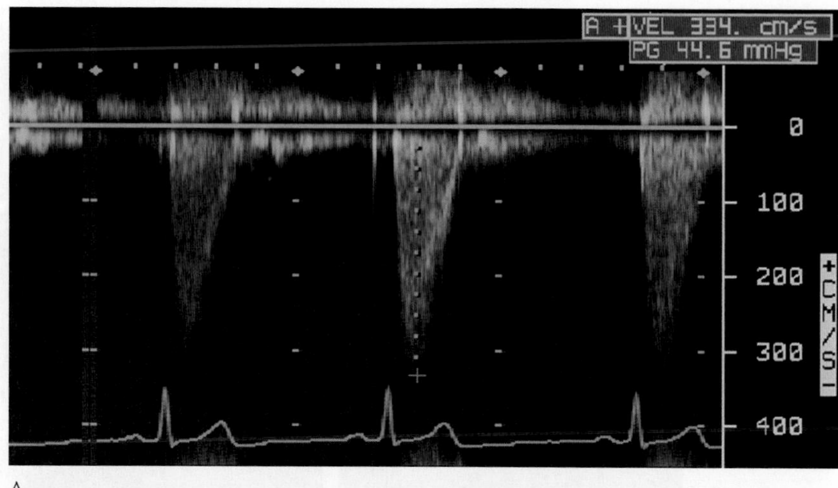

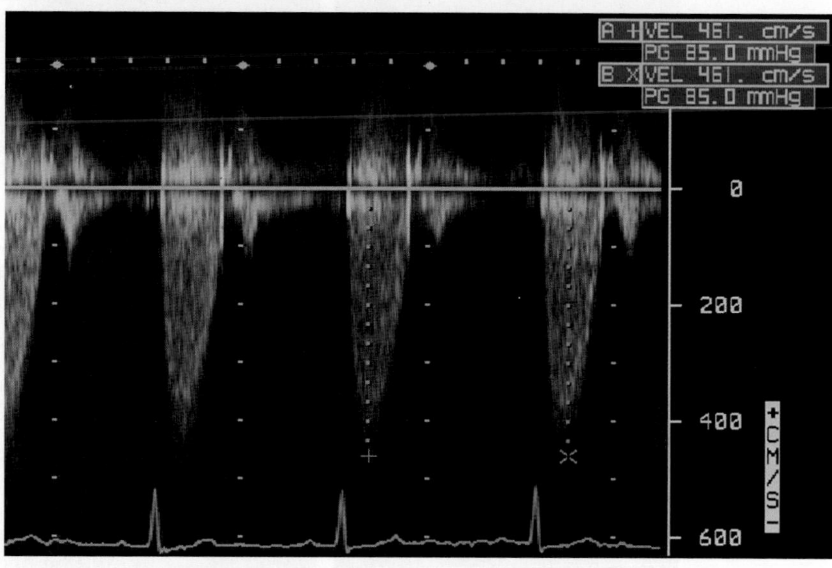

Figure 33.6 Echocardiographic continous-wave Doppler images of a severe aortic stenosis in a pregnant woman. The peak gradient changed from 45mmHg before pregnancy (A) to 85mmHg after 18 weeks of pregnancy (B).

studies on outcome of pregnancy in patients with repaired aortic coarctation show that pregnancy is in general well tolerated [44-45]. However, hypertension and pre-eclampsia are, along with a high number of miscarriages, common problems in patients with repaired aortic coarctation. This may be explained by shared aetiological factors such as endothelial dysfunction [46]. During pregnancy, women with mild coarctation should undergo close monitoring of blood pressure and treatment with a beta-blocking agent will be indicated if hypertension develops [44]. Percutaneous balloon angioplasty should be avoided in coarctation during pregnancy because of the risk of aortic dissection or rupture [47]. Stenting of the aorta for native or recoarctation with an uncovered or covered stent is the treatment of choice outside pregnancy and can be performed also during pregnancy in cases of severe disease. We report a unpublished case of a 19-year-old primigravida, diagnosed at 9 weeks, to have severe, native coarctation with very high blood pressure in the upper extremities. She underwent a staged percutaneous treatment consisting of the implantation of a covered stent at 12 weeks followed by additional dilatation 6 months after uneventful delivery (➲ Fig. 33.7). Because of the risk of restenosis after repair of coarctation in childhood, all women with a history of operated coarctation who consider pregnancy should be assessed.

The assessment of patients with congenital heart disease imply not only the evaluation of the underlying defects, but also the type and patency of surgically implanted conduits, valves, or baffles, the presence of postoperative sequelae such as arrhythmias, ventricular dysfunction, and the presence of devices such as pacemaker or defibrillators and/or prosthetic material (as patches), all of which are more common in the complex disorders. Furthermore, we don't know the effect of pregnancy on long-term survival

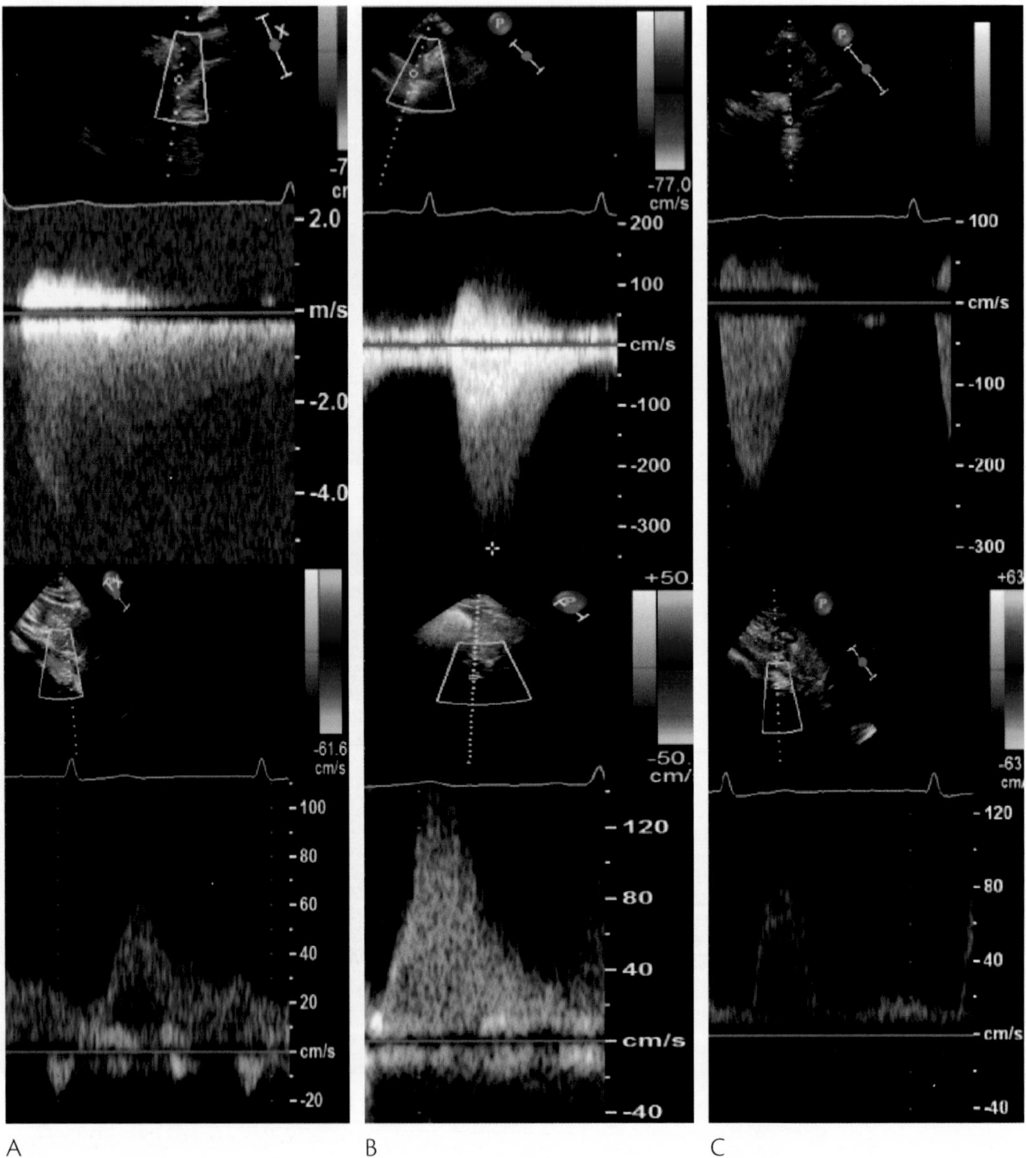

Figure 33.7 Flow patterns of the descending and abdominal aorta at three different stages: (A) Flow pattern native coarctation. (B) Flow pattern after stenting. (C) Flow pattern after repeat dilatation. With permission of Karamermer Y and Ross-Hesselink JW.

in patients with complex heart disease. We known now for example, that 25% of women with intra-atrial repair of TGA experience deterioration of their right (systemic) ventricular function during pregnancy and most of them do not recover to the baseline level [48]. Many patients who are left after the operation with overloaded right ventricles (pulmonary regurgitation in tetralogy of Fallot; pulmonary stenosis or atresia; tricuspid regurgitation in Ebstein's anomaly or long lasting left-to-right shunts) can develop heart failure during pregnancy and can deteriorate their right ventricular function. Not only right ventricular failure but also left heart failure (pulmonary congestion) has been reported in patients with severe pulmonary regurgitation and/or impaired subpulmonary ventricular dysfunction due to right-to-left ventricular interaction [49].

When percutaneous pulmonary valve implantation becomes the standard therapy it should be considered early before pregnancy in case of important residual pulmonary insufficiency and before right ventricular deterioration.

When the right ventricle is sustaining the systemic circulation as in women with complete TGA corrected with Mustard or Senning repair or in single ventricle right ventricle type, the assessment of ventricular function is mandatory: decreased ventricular contractility before pregnancy is associated with high rate of complications during pregnancy [50].

Due to the atrial scar tissue secondary to the extensive atrial surgery performed for congenital heart defects, supraventricular arrhythmias are often present in these adult patients and can be exacerbated during pregnancy due to the overloaded right atrium and to the enhanced adrenergic receptor excitability caused by hormones. Particularly at risk are patients with Fontan repair (atriopulmonary anastomosis) and with atrial repair (Mustard or Senning) with baffle for TGA [22]. These patients can develop 1:1 atrioventricular conduction flutter which can degenerate in ventricular fibrillation. If bradyarrhythmias are not present beta-blockers prophylactic treatment should be considered.

Some authors suggest that thromboembolic complications can be seen more often in pregnant women with congenital heart disease compared to the general population [47], either for chronic or recurrent arrhythmia, sluggish blood flow, or heart valve prostheses. Patients with a Fontan procedure and dilated right atrium are at high risk for thromboembolic events, even outside pregnancy. The risk is increased sixfold during pregnancy and 11-fold in the puerperium; thus anticoagulation therapy is mandatory.

Cyanotic heart disease without pulmonary hypertension

Cyanotic congenital heart diseases are usually corrected before pregnancy, but some inoperable or palliated cases can reach child-bearing age. The degree of maternal hypoxaemia is the most important predictor of maternal and fetal outcome (➲Fig. 33.8). With resting maternal blood saturation below 85%, maternal mortality is 2–5%, fetal loss is 85% and premature delivery or a low-birth-weight neonate is around 50%; pregnancy should therefore be discouraged [51]. Maternal complications (heart failure, pulmonary or systemic thrombosis, supraventricular arrhythmias) occur in 30% of cases. Low-dose heparin prophylaxis is widely used and recommended, although its value has not been proved. If oxygen saturation is 85–92%, it is advisable to measure it during exercise. If there is a sudden and important drop in oxygen saturation during exercise, the pregnancy has a poor prognosis and should be discouraged.

Tetralogy of Fallot is the most common cyanotic congenital heart defect. Comparing fetal and maternal outcome in uncorrected (i.e. cyanotic) and corrected tetralogy of Fallot, it is evident that persistent cyanosis is the most important determinant of maternal and fetal outcome (➲Fig. 33.9) [51, 52]. Offspring of mothers with tetralogy of Fallot, regardless of correction, carry a 3–10% risk of having congenital heart disease (➲Table 33.2).

Fetal high-risk conditions

The fetal risks are as follows:

- The recurrence risk of congenital malformations in the offspring of patients with major heart defects (➲Table 33.2) ranges from 2–50% depending on the type of parental disease, with an excess in the offspring of affected women [53–57]. A fetal nuchal translucency measurement at 12–13 weeks' gestation is a useful first screening test. Fetal echocardiography can detect the presence of congenital heart disease and should be performed at 18–20 weeks' gestation if the mother or father has congenital heart disease. Fetal echocardiography in weeks 18–20 can reliably exclude major forms of congenital heart disease, less complex lesions can be missed. These minor forms of congenital heart disease can be diagnosed with a careful postnatal paediatric cardiac assessment [58].
- Abortion.

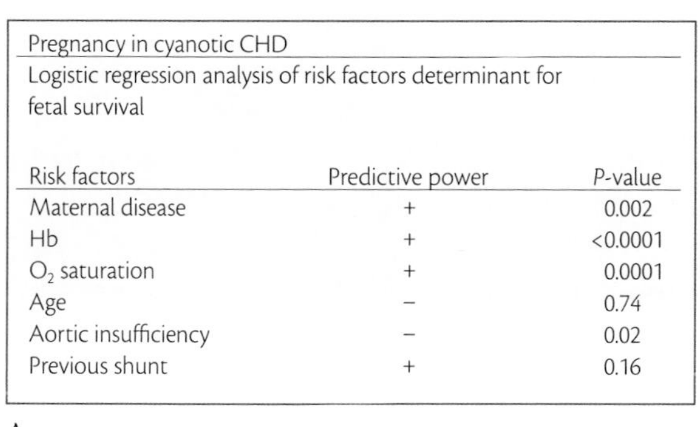

Pregnancy in cyanotic CHD

Logistic regression analysis of risk factors determinant for fetal survival

Risk factors	Predictive power	*P*-value
Maternal disease	+	0.002
Hb	+	<0.0001
O_2 saturation	+	0.0001
Age	–	0.74
Aortic insufficiency	–	0.02
Previous shunt	+	0.16

A

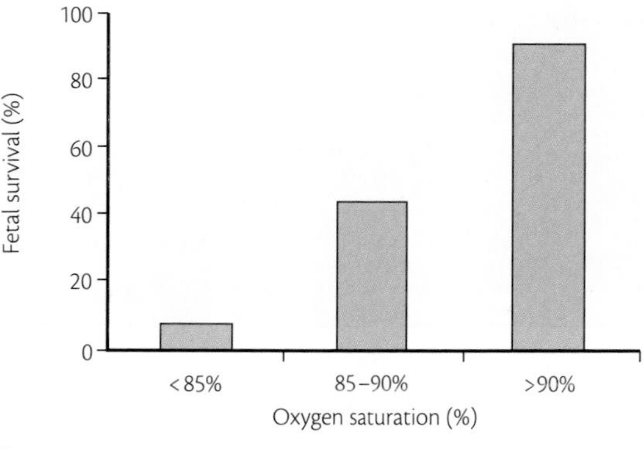

B

Figure 33.8 Risk factors affecting fetal survival: (A) multiple regression analysis shows that maternal disease, haemoglobin and oxygen saturation are significantly related to fetal survival; (B) fetal survival declines with the decrease in maternal oxygen saturation.

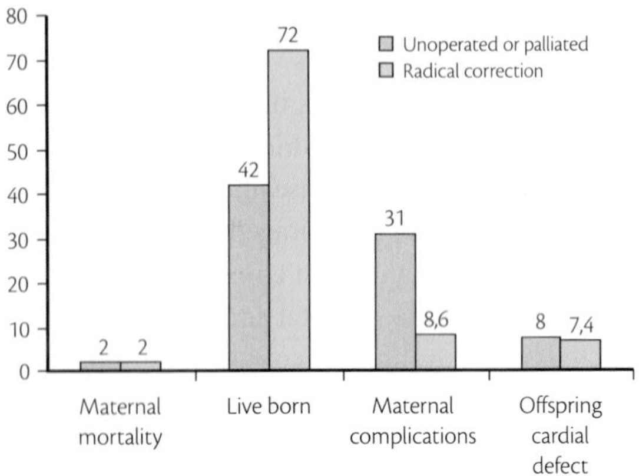

Figure 33.9 Maternal and fetal complications in cyanotic patients (mostly tetralogy of Fallot) selected to receive either no operation/palliation or radical correction. Maternal complications decreased and live births increased substantially with radical correction.

- Intrauterine growth retardation.
- Prematurity (➲Fig. 33.10).
- Perinatal mortality.

The last four complications depend on type and severity of maternal disease and poor maternal functional class (NYHA >II). Additional risk factors for adverse fetal/neonatal events, besides the conventional obstetric ones (history of premature delivery or rupture of membranes, incompetent cervix, or Caesarean section; intrauterine growth retardation, antepartum bleeding >12 weeks' gestation, febrile illness, or uterine/placental abnormalities during present pregnancy), include maternal age >35, multiple gestation, smoking during pregnancy, and anticoagulation therapy [59]. Besides cyanotic heart disease, another condition that carries an adverse fetal outcome (45% fetal survival) is the Fontan repair for tricuspid atresia or single ventricle. In this condition the venous congestion that occurs during pregnancy leads to congestion of the intrauterine veins, with a very high incidence of spontaneous abortion. Nowadays conversion from classic Fontan to total cavopulmonary connection should be considered before pregnancy. We have to emphasize that the prematurity associated with poor maternal condition carries a high risk of newborn disabilities: 30% when the fetus is delivered at 27 weeks, 60% at 24 weeks. Prematurity is also associated with high neonatal mortality.

Specific conditions

Mitral valve stenosis

Although its incidence is decreasing in Europe, rheumatic heart disease is still responsible for most of the cardiac complications during pregnancy. Mitral valve stenosis, nearly always of rheumatic origin, is the most common (90%) and important cardiac valvular problem during pregnancy. Mortality among pregnant women with minimal symptoms is <1% but in severe disease can reach 5%. Labour, delivery, and the immediate puerperium appear to be the periods most at risk [60–62].

The pressure gradient across the narrowed mitral valve may increase greatly during pregnancy because of the physiological increase in heart rate (decreasing left ventricular

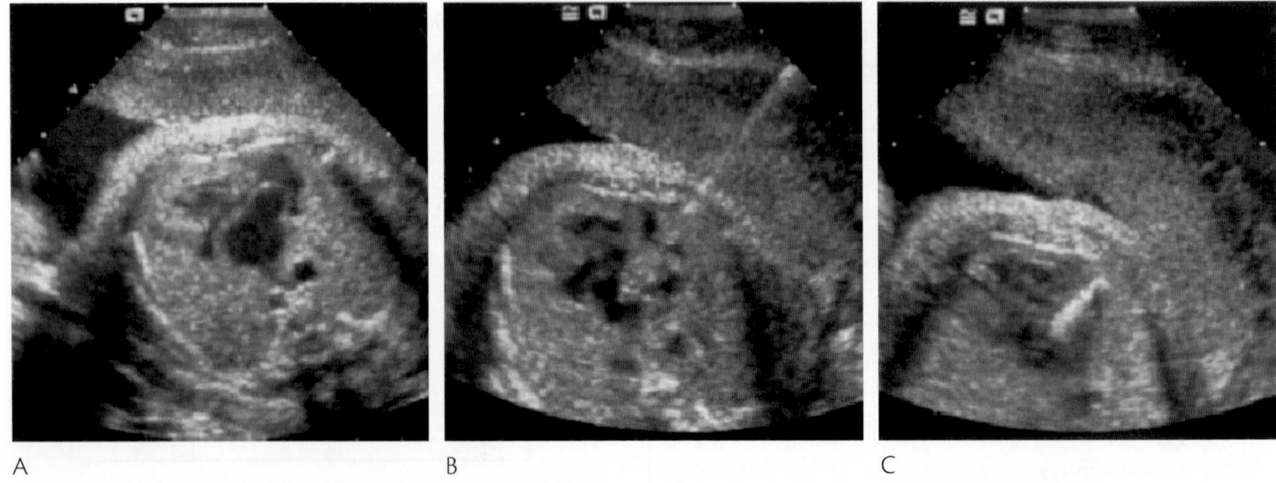

Figure 33.10 Creation of an atrial septal defect *in utero* for fetus with hypoplastic left heart syndrome and intact atrial septum. Transabdominal ultrasound image of the heart in a fetus with dilated left atrium and thin bulging atrial septum before atrial septal puncture (A), during septal puncture with Chuba needle (B) and during dilatation with 3-mm coronary angloplasty balloon (C). Reproduced with permission from Marshall AC, van der Velde ME, Tworetzky W, *et al.* Creation of an atrial septal defect in utero for fetuses with hypoplastic left heart syndrome and intact or highly restrictive atrial septum. *Circulation* 2004; **110**: 253–8.

diastolic filling time) and cardiac output. This can lead to a rise in left atrial and pulmonary wedge pressures and inability of cardiac output to increase appropriately with exercise. The onset of clinical symptoms (excessive fatigue, breathlessness on exertion, orthopnoea, and nocturnal dyspnoea) may occur even in women with moderate valve stenosis or who were previously symptom-free, usually in the middle trimester. Development of atrial fibrillation could further aggravate the clinical status, leading to acute pulmonary oedema.

Predictors of adverse maternal outcomes include degree of mitral valve stenosis (valve area <1.5cm^2), NYHA functional class II or more before pregnancy, and history of cardiac events [59]. Patients with mild valve stenosis (valve area >1.5cm^2) who are either asymptomatic or have minor symptoms can almost always be managed with behavioural advice (restriction of salt intake, reduction of physical activity up to complete bed rest) and judicious medical therapy (diuretics to reduce pulmonary and venous congestion; beta-blockers to reduce heart rate and increase diastolic filling period). The onset of tachyarrhythmias such as atrial fibrillation or supraventricular tachycardia requires immediate treatment with cardioversion. Anticoagulation therapy is indicated in patients with atrial fibrillation. In patients with moderate mitral valve stenosis (valve area 1.1–1.5cm^2), the different therapeutic strategies depend on the severity of symptoms before and during pregnancy and the rise in pulmonary pressure: patients who are either asymptomatic or mildly symptomatic (NYHA I–II) should undergo close follow-up with serial echocardiographic assessment (measurement of mean transmitral gradient and pulmonary artery pressure) and clinical evaluation; percutaneous balloon valvuloplasty or valve repair/replacement during pregnancy should be considered in cases with persistent symptoms despite optimal medical therapy. In patients with severe mitral valve stenosis (valve area <1cm^2), percutaneous balloon valvuloplasty or surgical intervention before conception is indicated. In pregnant women, careful monitoring and performance of these procedures at the right time have to be planned.

Percutaneous balloon valvuloplasty has been shown to be a successful and safe procedure during pregnancy in experienced centres, and has become the first-choice interventional treatment in anatomically suitable valves (young patients with non-calcified pliable valves without too much subvalvular thickening or significant mitral regurgitation) are present as a result of the significant reduction in fetal and neonatal mortality [40, 46, 63].

Labour and delivery should be planned carefully. Effective analgesia to minimize pain and anxiety, in addition to shortening of the second stage of labour, will decrease the haemodynamic demand on the maternal heart. Bedside ECG monitoring should be used to document rhythm disturbances. Swan–Ganz catheters are frequently used in moderate and severe mitral stenosis to monitor fluid balance. The safety of breastfeeding depends on the mother's medication in the postpartum period.

Hypertrophic cardiomyopathy

Although symptoms, particularly chest pain or dyspnoea, may increase, pregnancy is generally well tolerated and absolute maternal mortality is very low and mostly limited to very high-risk patients [64–66]. The only two reported maternal deaths in the Italian series were one in a patient in NYHA functional class IV with severe left ventricular hypertrophy (wall thickness 30mm) and left ventricular outflow obstruction (basal gradient 115mmHg at cardiac catheterization) and the second in a patient with a particularly malignant family history of sudden death due to hypertrophic cardiomyopathy. It has to be outlined that the two patients died of arrhythmias and none of them had an implantable cardioverter defibrillator (ICD). In a recent reported series of 400 patients no maternal deaths occurred. If symptoms are not present before pregnancy we can expect no clinical deterioration during pregnancy will occur (<5% of the patients). Management of hypertrophic cardiomyopathy during pregnancy should not differ from that outside pregnancy. No treatment other than reassurance is indicated in asymptomatic or mild symptomatic women, whereas in symptomatic patients beta-blockers and low-dose diuretic therapy may be indicated. Normal vaginal delivery is safe but careful monitoring of blood loss is needed [64–66].

Prosthetic heart valves

In women of child-bearing age, surgical valve repair is always preferable to replacement and must be performed whenever possible. If valve replacement is needed, the decision about the best type of valve prosthesis to use should take into account the woman's age (in very young women rapid tissue valve degeneration is common), the presence of other conditions such as atrial fibrillation requiring anticoagulant therapy, and the risk of reoperation (complex anatomy, re-repeat). Bioprosthetic valves appear to be the best choice provided that the woman is informed about the structural valve deterioration associated with pregnancy and the inevitability and risk of reoperation. Previous studies have shown that pregnancy is associated with an accelerated rate of structural valve deterioration (12–60%) [67–70]. In previous published studies the incidence of prosthetic valve reoperation was 60–80% at 5–10 years' follow-up, and the mortality of reoperation was 2–3.8% [67–70]. Due to the longer life expectancy of some currently available bovine valves, to the lower mortality rate at reoperation, biological valve replacement is probably the best option in women in childbearing age. The management of women with bioprosthetic valves should include serial clinical evaluation and two-dimensional echocardiography for early detection of valve structural deterioration; antibiotic prophylaxis at delivery is recommended particularly in high risk patients. In women with mechanical valves, pregnancy is associated with a 10% risk of prosthetic valve thrombosis and/or systemic embolization, necessitating the use of some form of anticoagulation during pregnancy throughout pregnancy. In a systematic review of the literature the overall pooled of maternal mortality rate was 2.9%, while major bleeding occurred in 2.5% of all pregnancies, mostly at the time of delivery [70]. The use of warfarin, particularly between weeks 6–12 of pregnancy, is associated with fetal embryopathy (nasal hypoplasia, bone, and optic atrophy) that occurs in approximately 6% of cases and an increased risk of miscarriage or stillbirth (cerebral fetal haemorrhage). Because of this maternal and fetal 'double jeopardy', women with mechanical valves should be informed about the risks of pregnancy and the necessity for immediate pregnancy testing if menstrual periods are missed.

The most appropriate anticoagulation regimen will be based on several factors: type of valve prosthesis (e.g. old generation caged-ball prosthesis vs. new bileaflet tilting disc), valve position (mitral vs. aortic), history of previous thromboembolism, warfarin dose, presence of atrial fibrillation, and the desires of prospective parents. The risks of anticoagulant treatment (➲Table 33.3) always have to be discussed with parents.

Due to the lack of trials and limited data the management of anticoagulant treatment in pregnant women remains controversial [71–77]. Although the widespread use of low-molecular-weight-heparin (LMWH) utilization outside and during pregnancy, doubt has been raised about their effectiveness for the prevention of thromboembolism during pregnancy [75, 76]. In the recently published evidence-based clinical practice guidelines (8th edition) for antithrombotic therapy and pregnancy from the American College of Chest Physicians, a warning from a LMWH manufacturer about the safety of LMWH use during pregnancy has been reported. This warning was based on post-marketing reports of valve thrombosis in an undisclosed number of patients receiving this LMWH, as well as by clinical outcomes in a open randomized study comparing LMWH (enoxaparin) with warfarin and unfractionated heparin (UFH) in pregnant women with prosthetic heart valves [75, 77]. The study was terminated after 12 of the planned 110 patients were enrolled because of two deaths in the enoxaparin arm. The published review of Oran and colleagues underlined the importance of a close monitoring and dose-adjusting to maintain target anti-Xa levels. The thromboembolic rate in pregnant women with mechanical heart valves treated with LMWH varies from 12% (ten of 81 cases) in the overall population to 2% (one of 51 cases) among pregnancies in which anti-factor Xa LMWH levels were closely monitored [78].

On the basis of the current knowledge and practice our recommendations are:

- *UFH and warfarin combination*: stop warfarin treatment as soon as the pregnancy test is positive. UFH in the first 13 weeks of pregnancy, switching to warfarin in the second trimester, continuing it until week 36 of gestation or 2 days before the planned delivery and then changing again to heparin until 4–5 days after delivery. Heparin should be terminated at the onset of labour and re-instituted shortly (12–24 hours) after delivery. During pregnancy heparin should be given subcutaneously two or three times daily and the dose adjusted to maintain the partial thromboplastin time at greater than twice control levels at all times; the monitoring should be performed at least twice weekly.

Table 33.3 Anticoagulant treatment during pregnancy*

		Warfarin	Heparin (in the first trimester)	Heparin throughout pregnancy	LMWH
Fetal risk	Death	30%	24%	–	12%
	Embryopathy	4–10%	2%	–	?
Maternal risk	Death	1.8%	4.2%	7%	?–16%
	Thromboembolism	3.9%	9–24%	25–33.3%	1.9–12.3%

* Based on multiple studies. LMWH, low-molecular-weight-heparin.

- *LMWH and warfarin combination*: stop warfarin treatment as soon as the pregnancy test is positive. LMWH in the first 13 weeks of pregnancy, switching to warfarin in the second trimester, continuing it until week 36 of gestation or 2 days before the planned delivery and then changing to heparin. LMWH should be given subcutaneously twice daily and the dose adjusted to body weight to maintain anti-Xa between 0.7–1.2U/mL 4–6 hours after injection. The checking of anti Xa levels should be performed weekly because dose requirements are likely to increase during pregnancy [79]. LMWH does not cross the placenta. Meticulous attention should be paid when shifting from one regimen to the other because most of the complications reported occur during these periods. These therapy changes are best followed with a hospitalized regimen.
- LMWH throughout the whole of pregnancy, administered twice daily with dose adjusted to body weight (to achieve the anti-Xa levels between 0.7–1.2U/mL 4–6 hours after subcutaneous injection). The checking of anti Xa levels should be performed weekly because dose requirements are likely to increase during pregnancy. This regimen is probably indicated in the low-risk conditions.
- Women judged to be at very high risk of thromboembolism (e.g. older-generation prosthesis in the mitral position or history of thromboembolism) particularly those in whom a low-daily dose of warfarin or acenocoumarol (warfarin dose <5mg and acenocoumarol dose <2mg) is necessary to achieve a proper INR value, can be treated with warfarin throughout the whole of pregnancy with replacement by UFH or LMWH (as described earlier) close to delivery [80]. Cotrufo found no cases of embryopathy in a small series of 20 women requiring <5mg of warfarin per day treated throughout pregnancy [81]. A thorough discussion of the potential risks and benefits of this approach with the patient are required before choosing this option.
- For pregnant women with prosthetic valves at high risk of thromboembolism, we recommend the addition of low-dose aspirin, 75–100mg/day [82].

In patients on anticoagulation therapy, elective Caesarean section at 38 weeks is indicated because it provides a safer birth route but it also minimizes the length of time that the mother is unprotected by anticoagulation therapy.

Marfan syndrome

With a population incidence of 1 in 5000, Marfan syndrome (➲Chapter 31) is the most frequently encountered fibrillin-1 deficiency disorder. It is transmitted as an autosomal dominant trait and is characterized by multiorgan dysfunction, predominantly affecting the eyes, skeleton, and cardiovascular system. There are three main problems in a woman with Marfan syndrome who is contemplating pregnancy:

1) the risk of serious maternal complications during or shortly after pregnancy;
2) the risk of obstetric and/or neonatal complications;
3) the risk of recurrence in offspring.

The predisposition to aortic dissection is due to: the hyperdynamic and hypervolaemic status of pregnancy. Furthermore, oestrogen has been reported to inhibit the deposition of collagen and elastin leading to fragmentation of reticular fibres. Whenever possible before starting pregnancy, any woman with Marfan syndrome should undergo a full clinical assessment (family history, ultrasound examination of the entire aorta, echocardiography, MRI) and a careful counselling of maternal and fetal risk. The risk of aortic dissection or other serious cardiovascular complication (endocarditis or congestive heart failure) during pregnancy is 1% even in the absence of aortic root dilatation, and may further increase, reaching 10%, in the presence of poor family history, rapid dilatation during pregnancy, aortic root diameter >45mm at the start of the pregnancy, and significant mitral or aortic valve regurgitation [83]. In addition to the increased risk of maternal complications, a recent study showed an increase of obstetric and/or neonatal complications such as premature deliveries (15%) and an increased combined fetal and neonatal mortality of 7% (2% and 5% respectively). Due to the high rate of pelvic instability, Caesarean section is more indicated than vaginal delivery. In a prospective long-term follow-up study Rossiter and colleagues demonstrated that pregnancy in patients with Marfan syndrome in whom cardiovascular involvement is minor and aortic root diameter is <40mm is usually well tolerated without subsequent evidence of aggravated aortic root dilatation over time [84].

Besides the risk of cardiovascular involvement, women with Marfan syndrome must know and accept that due to the autosomal-dominant nature of the disorder, each offspring of an affected Marfan's parent has a 50% chance of inheriting the genetic mutation and that the degree of severity of the disease could be worse than that of the parent. Genetic counselling should be encouraged for all patients with Marfan syndrome [84-85].

The recommendations are as follows.

- Patients with aortic root enlargement >4.5–5cm should undergo elective surgery before pregnancy; otherwise they will be advised against pregnancy.
- In patients with aortic root enlargement of 4–4.5cm, aortic root dimension assessment with serial echocardiography (each trimester until 6 months after delivery) should be recommended. During pregnancy, physical activity should be limited and the use of beta-blocker therapy is recommended.
- Even in patients without cardiovascular involvement, the relatively 'small' risk of complications (1%) should be discussed, as these can occur outside pregnancy. Clinical and echocardiographic monitoring should be performed during pregnancy and normal vaginal delivery should be conducted. Postpartum uterine haemorrhage should be anticipated as a complication and has been reported in nearly 40% of women.

Since the rate of aortic root dilatation is 0.2cm per year and only 30% of Marfan's patients will reach the age of 25–30 years without aortic root dilatation, pregnancy should be planned at a younger age.

Turner syndrome

Turner syndrome affects approximately one in 2500 liveborn females (➲Chapter 9). The diagnosis requires the presence of characteristic physical features in phenotypic females coupled with complete or partial absence of the second sex chromosome, with or without cell line mosaicism. Several recent imaging studies have investigated the prevalence of aortic coarctation and bicuspid aortic valve (BAV) in large groups of girls and women with Turner syndrome. These studies suggest that on average, approximately 11% have coarctation and approximately 16% have BAV. Spontaneous or assisted pregnancy (assisted reproductive technology, ART) should be undertaken only after thorough cardiac evaluation by a cardiologist familiar with the spectrum of cardiovascular issues encountered in this syndrome. Alarming reports of fatal aortic dissection during pregnancy and the postpartum period have raised concern about the safety of pregnancy in Turner syndrome. The evaluation should include: two-dimensional and colour Doppler echocardiography, a baseline ECG, and cardiac MRI of the aorta. A history of surgically repaired cardiovascular defect, the presence of BAV or current evidence of aortic dilatation or systemic hypertension should probably be viewed as relative contraindications to pregnancy. Due to the high rate of cardiac complications in patients during ART, a meticulous screening is mandatory in these patients. For those who become pregnant, close cardiology involvement throughout pregnancy and the postpartum period is essential [86].

Coronary heart disease

Acute myocardial infarction (➲Chapter 16) rarely occurs in women of child-bearing age and has been estimated to occur in only 1 in 10,000 women during pregnancy [87]. However, with the current trend of child-bearing at an older age and the ongoing effects of cigarette smoking, diabetes, and stress, the occurrence of acute myocardial infarction during pregnancy can be expected to increase [87, 88]. Myocardial infarction occurs at all stages of pregnancy and mostly in multiple pregnancies. Myocardial infarction location is mainly in the anterior wall. The reported maternal mortality rate, before the current practice of primary percutaneous coronary angioplasty, varied from 21–48%, either at the time of infarction (mostly in the third trimester) or within 2 weeks of the infarction. The maternal mortality rate decreased to 11% with an associated incidence fetal mortality of 9% in the recent reports [87].

The differential diagnosis of ischaemic chest pain includes haemorrhage, sickle crises, pre-eclampsia, acute pulmonary embolism, and aortic dissection [88]. It is confirmed by ECG changes and increase in enzyme levels. Due to the physiological increase in the concentration of creatine kinase and its MB fraction in the postpartum period, assessment of the troponin I or T levels is recommended. Echocardiography is safe during pregnancy and can be used to evaluate the presence of wall-motion abnormalities. Management includes coronary angiography with abdominal shielding. Intracoronary thrombus with or without an underlying atherosclerotic plaque can be present. Spontaneous coronary dissection of the proximal left anterior coronary artery is a common cause of myocardial infarction in the peripartum period and especially in the postpartum period. Physiopathological hypotheses are: the excess of progesterone leading to biochemical and structural changes to the vessel wall and the association among oeosinophils and a lack of prostacyclin synthesis-stimulating plasma factor and elevated lipoprotein (a).

Successful treatment includes mostly coronary stenting (bare metal stenting); few data are available on emergency coronary artery bypass grafting. The use of radiation should be kept a minimum but cardiac catheterization and interventional procedures are expected to yield <0.01Gy of radiation. In the assessment of adverse effects and fetus protection it is necessary to know the absorbed dose. Although termination of pregnancy is not generally recommended for fetal doses of radiation <0.05Gy, it may be considered when the dose exceeds 0.1Gy. Thrombolytic therapy should be considered a second choice to primary percutaneous coronary intervention in patients with ST-segment elevation acute myocardial infarction during pregnancy [89–91]. Pharmacological treatment should in general follow the usual standard of care and will be discuss in the next subsection.

If possible, the delivery should be postponed for at least 2 or 3 weeks after the myocardial infarction to allow adequate healing. The mode of delivery should be determined by obstetric reasons and the clinical status of the mother.

Cardiac transplantation

According to the actual recommendations individual factors should be considered when offering advice for timing of pregnancy. These considerations include: risk of acute rejection and infection; concomitant therapy with potentially toxic and teratogenic medications; and adequacy of graft function [92]. If ventricular function is normal and there are no signs of rejection, pregnancy is usually successful. The absence of rejection should be established before conception and needs to be assessed during pregnancy. Levels of immunosuppressants can decline during pregnancy; they should be monitored frequently and doses adjusted accordingly. Preconceptional genetic counselling is necessary depending on the indication for transplantation, such as mitochondrial myopathy or familial dilated cardiomyopathy. Management during pregnancy includes monitoring left ventricular function and preventing complications such as hypertension, infection, preterm labour, intrauterine growth restriction, and pre-eclampsia [93, 94]. Most patients on cyclosporine and tacrolimus require dosage adjustments during pregnancy. Teratogenicity and mutagenicity have not been documented with the currently used dosages. In addition, the rates of fetal malformations do not appear to be higher than expected. However, both cyclosporine and tacrolimus have been associated with intrauterine growth retardation, low birthweight, and small size for gestational age [95–97]. The choice of delivery mode is based on obstetric indications [93, 94].

Hypertension and pre-eclampsia

As the most common medical disorder of pregnancy, hypertension affects 10% of all pregnant women and contributes significantly to stillbirths and neonatal morbidity and mortality. Hypertensive disorders (➲Chapter 13) during pregnancy are one of the leading causes of maternal mortality, accounting for almost 15% of such deaths. In normal patients the blood pressure tends to fall in the first half of pregnancy, rising to pre-pregnancy levels or higher from about 30 weeks' gestation. Hypertension occurring during pregnancy, the so-called pregnancy-induced hypertension, has to be distinguished from pre-existing hypertension (chronic hypertension). As might be expected, the impacts of the different conditions on the mother and fetus are different as are the management strategies. Both hypertensive forms can lead to pre-eclampsia when proteinuria occurs. Pre-eclampsia is responsible for about half of induced pre-term deliveries and the need to detect pre-eclampsia as early as possible is a major reason for antenatal care.

Due to the physiopathology, in pregnancy there are specific problems relating to the position of the patient. Blood pressure should be measured in the left lateral or sitting positing (preferred position). Blood pressure levels are classified as mild (systolic blood pressure 140–159mmHg and diastolic pressure 90–109mmHg) or severe hypertension (systolic blood pressure >160mmHg and diastolic pressure >110mmHg). Laboratory tests recommended to follow hypertensive patients during pregnancy in order to detect as soon as possible pre-eclampsia include haemoglobin and haematocrit, platelet count, serum creatinine level, serum uric acid level, serum transaminase levels, serum albumin, lactic acid dehydrogenase, coagulation profile, and quantification of protein excretion.

As previously reported, the hypertensive disorders of pregnancy can be classified as chronic hypertension, gestational hypertension, pre-eclampsia, and pre-eclampsia superimposed on chronic hypertension [98].

Chronic hypertension is defined as blood pressure >140mmHg systolic or >90mmHg diastolic either predating pregnancy or developing before 20 weeks' gestation.

The woman who has blood pressure elevation (blood pressure >140mmHg systolic or >90mmHg diastolic) detected for the first time in the latter half of pregnancy (after 20 weeks' gestation) without proteinuria is classified as having gestational hypertension. Pregnancy-induced hypertension when sustained can lead to pre-eclampsia, a syndrome that manifests clinically as new-onset hypertension in later pregnancy with associated proteinuria: 1+ on dipstick and >0.3g per 24-hour urine collection. Hypertension is only one aspect of pre-eclampsia, it is variable in its expression and may even be absent in patients who otherwise have severe manifestations of the condition. Pre-eclampsia has to be suspected even if there is not proteinuria when a hypertensive pregnant woman manifests symptoms such as epigastric pain, neurological symptoms, thrombocytopaenia, and small fetus [99]. Pre-eclampsia occurs in 3–8%

of all pregnancies and is thought to be a consequence of abnormalities in the maternal blood vessels that supply blood to the placenta. Pre-eclampsia is a multisystem disease, affecting the endothelium of all blood vessels and characterized by vasospasm, activation of the coagulation system, and perturbations in many humoral and autacoid systems related to volume and pressure control. Risk factors for developing pre-eclampsia include dyslipidaemia, insulin resistance or diabetes, hypercoagulability inflammation disorders, and multiparity. A previously published epidemiological study showed an increased risk of cardiovascular disease in women with a history of preterm pre-eclampsia is not yet confirmed by prospective studies. Based on the current knowledge, in women with hypertensive disorders during pregnancy (particularly in case of pre-eclampsia) an aggressive treatment of cardiovascular risk factors is to be indicated.

The diagnosis of superimposed pre-eclampsia is made when a new-onset proteinuria is seen in a women with hypertension and no proteinuria early in pregnancy or when a sudden increase in proteinuria or blood pressure are seen in a woman with hypertension and proteinuria before 20 weeks' gestation. The definitive treatment for pregnancy-induced hypertension is delivery. Because this kind of hypertension occurs late in pregnancy, a proper planned delivery most often with Caesarean section should be organized. If severe hypertension is present early during pregnancy, interruption is the best option because the evolution toward pre-eclampsia and eclampsia is almost always the rule. When to use antihypertensive medications and what level of blood pressure to target is a matter for discussion. Although the goal of treatment of hypertensive disorders is to reduce maternal risk, the agents selected must be efficacious and safe for the fetus. Pregnancy and pre-eclampsia do not last for long enough to justify or need treatment of hypertension to prevent long-term complications, long-term risks do not exist, the target is to arrive to a proper time for a safe delivery. The benefit of antihypertensive therapy for mild hypertension, either chronic or pregnancy induced, have not been demonstrated in clinical trials. If clinically indicated (presence of underlying renal dysfunction), antihypertensive therapy can be started. First-line agents for non-severe hypertension are methyldopa and labetalol, with nifedipine as second line. Due to the physiopathology of pre-eclampsia (characterized by poor organ perfusion) diuretics are not recommended.

There is consensus that severe hypertension in pregnancy requires treatment, because these women are at an increased risk of intracerebral haemorrhage, and that treatment decreases the risk of maternal death. First-line agents are intravenous labetalol (start with 20mg IV as a bolus; if ineffective repeat bolus at increasing dosage every 10min, maximum dosage 220mg) and hydralazine (start with 5mg IV to be repeated every 20min until blood pressure control is achieved). Oral nifedipine is indicated in case of no parenteral treatment [98–100].

A complete remission of hypertension and symptoms and signs of pre-eclampsia is to be expected by 6 weeks' postpartum; if not, the patient has to be revaluated 6 weeks later. Few cases, particularly when risk factors are present, can evolve toward essential hypertension.

The recurrence rate in future pregnancies is related to the severity of disease in the first pregnancy: if the pre-eclampsia occurred very late and in a mild form the recurrence rate is around 10%, while if pre-eclampsia occurred early and in a severe form the recurrence rate can reach 40%.

Arrhythmogenic right ventricular cardiomyopathy

Arrhythmogenic right ventricular cardiomyopathy (ARVC) (➲Chapters 9 and 30) is characterized by progressive fibrous or fibrofatty tissue replacement of the right ventricular myocardium. The clinical spectrum of ARVC includes asymptomatic premature ventricular complexes, but also ventricular tachycardia and sudden death. Many cases of patients with an implantable defibrillator and uneventful pregnancy have been reported. Patients with ARVC should be managed with close monitoring during pregnancy for signs and symptoms of arrhythmia and preventive obstetric care appropriate to their clinical profile to optimize normal deliveries [101].

The long QT syndrome

Previous studies have pointed out that among women with long QT syndrome (LQTS) (➲Chapters 9 and 30) the postpartum period (9-month postpartum time) is associated with a 2.7-fold increased risk of experiencing a cardiac event (mostly syncope) and 4.1-fold increased risk of experiencing a life-threatening event (aborted cardiac arrest and LQTS-related sudden death) when compared with the preconception time period [102]. This is recognized especially for women with an LQTS type 2 [102, 103]. The risk of any cardiac events returns to the baseline after this high-risk period. The pregnancy period is associated with a reduced risk for cardiac events. Treatment with beta-blockers, which has proven to significantly reduce the number of cardiac events in congenital LQTS patients, also during the postpartum period, should be continued [102]. A close cardiac follow-up after pregnancy in LQTS2 is recommended. Serial ECG (every 1–2 weeks after delivery) could be useful to recognize patients with a QT duration significantly prolonged in comparison with prepregnancy values or when QTc exceeds 500msec.

The pregnant patient with a pacemaker or ICD

Patients with a pacemaker tolerate pregnancy well. Serious complications are rare, the most common being irritation or ulceration at the implantation site, particularly with old type pacemaker generators. For patients with an ICD, given the proven safety of cardioversion during pregnancy, the problems are similar to those of having a pacemaker. However, caution has to be used when many leads are implanted in the right atrium or ventricle, particularly when intracardiac shunts are present. In fact due to the hypercoagulable state during pregnancy (secondary to relative decreases in protein S activity, stasis, and venous hypertension), thrombotic vegetations can develop around pacemaker leads leading to intracardiac thrombosis (➲Fig. 33.11) or peripheral embolization. Even if no consensus is present, anticoagulation therapy should be considered, particularly in high-risk conditions.

Cardiovascular treatment during pregnancy

Treatment in pregnancy is not based on randomized trials but on limited data from case reports (successes tend to be reported), observational studies, and clinical individual experience. The safety of both mother and fetus has to be taken into account because treatment for one can have adverse effects on the other. Pregnant patients with heart disease and their close relatives should receive general advice such as limitation of physical activity, with complete bed rest in severe cases, and salt and fluid restriction. Self-weighing should be encouraged and in the case of sudden unexpected weight gain the physician should be contacted. Other general advice includes stopping smoking and avoiding excessive alcohol intake and all unnecessary medications.

Pharmacological therapy

The use of any medication in pregnancy and during lactation has to consider the safety and tolerability for the fetus and infant, the physiological maternal changes, and the risk:benefit ratio. In patients who are already taking cardiovascular medications, discontinuation or the switch to a 'safer' drug should be discussed before conception. Because of the lack of randomized trials and the fear of tragedies such as the thalidomide disaster, there is an extreme reluctance to introduce any new drugs in pregnancy. Drugs with the longest record of safety should be used as the first-choice therapy. However, the fear of 'unpredictable' complications must not overcome the correct use of drug treatment in pregnancy, because most of the drugs used to treat heart disease can be prescribed safely during pregnancy.

The effective plasma concentration of drugs varies during pregnancy. For example, the progesterone-induced reduction in gastrointestinal motility and the oestrogen-induced increase in gastric secretion may result in altered drug absorption. Intravascular volume is increased during pregnancy, resulting in enhanced volume distribution and lower serum concentrations that may require an increase in the loading dose. Serum protein concentration falls during pregnancy, causing a reduction in protein binding and an increase in the non-protein-bound fraction. Increases in renal blood flow and glomerular filtration rate may augment drug clearance. The transplacental transfer of drugs depends on liposolubility or hydrosolubility and molecular weight of the drug, the pH of maternal and fetal fluids, the link with carrier protein, and the gradient between maternal and fetal concentration [90–93].

A useful tool for checking every drug before its use in pregnancy and lactation is found at the TOXNET: Databases on toxicology, hazardous chemicals, environmental health, and toxic releases website: http://toxnet.nlm.nih.gov.

➲Table 33.4 categorizes drugs according to the reliability of evidence of fetal risk and the potential risk:benefit ratio [12, 104, 105, 107–112, 117, 118, 121–124].

Therapy of heart failure

Diuretics are the first drugs to be employed in order to reduce hypervolaemia in patients with severe symptomatic congestive heart failure not responding to water and salt restriction. Diuretics are not recommended for management of pedal oedema or prophylaxis of eclampsia. In patients already receiving diuretics, the therapy should be continued during pregnancy and the peripartum period independently of the presence of mild hypotension. Although furosemide crosses the placental barrier, it is the drug of choice because no teratogenic or cardiovascular fetal effects have been described. Collateral effects to be controlled are hypovolaemia and hypokalaemia. Particular caution should be taken in cyanotic patients because haemoconcentration can cause thrombosis. No adverse events have been reported in

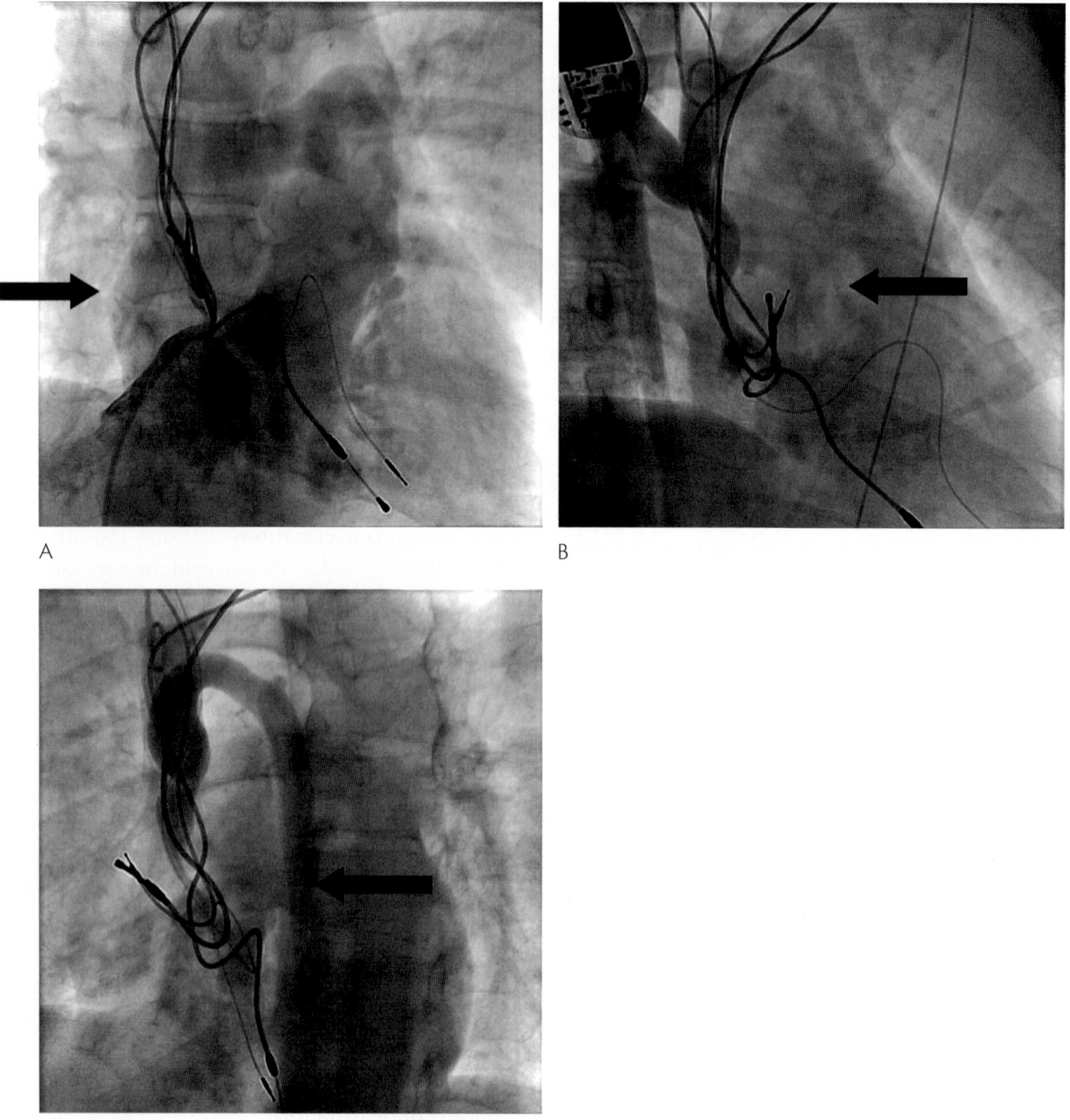

Figure 33.11 (A) Inferior vena cava venogram in the anterior posterior view demonstrates the presence of massive right atrial thrombosis (black arrow). The patient was treated after delivery with surgical removal of the atrial thrombus and pacemaker leads, and new implantation of single ventricular lead. (Courtesy of Dr M.Gasparini, Istituto Clinico Humanitas.) (B) Superior vena cava venogram in the right anterior oblique view. Massive right atrial thrombosis (black arrow). (C) Superior vena cava venogram in the left anterior oblique view. Massive right atrial thrombosis (black arrow).

patients treated with spironolactone, particularly indicated in cases of hypokalaemia. Thiazides are not recommended due to the reported neonatal thrombocytopaenia, jaundice, hyponatraemia and bradycardia [107].

Angiotensin-converting enzyme (ACE) inhibitors should be withdrawn during pregnancy because of teratogenic effects. Reported complications include fetal and neonatal renal failure, oligohydramnios, intrauterine growth retardation, and hypoplasia of skull bones especially in the second and third trimester, but also in the first trimester as recently published [108, 109]. There are not much data available about angiotensin II receptor antagonists in pregnancy, but because their actions are similar to those of ACE inhibitors their use is contraindicated.

Specific information on the safety of nitrates and sodium nitroprusside is lacking. Intravenous as well as oral nitrates have been used in a few patients for the treatment of hypertension, myocardial ischaemia, and heart failure,

Table 33.4 Cardiovascular drugs during pregnancy*

Drug	Use during pregnancy	Adverse fetal or neonatal effects	Breastfeeding
Antiarrhythmic agents			
Adenosine	First-line treatment: paroxysmal supraventricular tachycardia	No teratogenicity or other side effects	The short half-life makes it unlikely to be a problem
Amiodarone	Refractory maternal and fetal arrhythmias Maternal arrhythmias in presence of impaired left ventricular	Intrauterine growth retardation, premature birth, fetal hypothyroidism	Secreted in maternal milk Not recommended
Beta-blockers: atenol, propranolol, metoprolol	Control ventricular rate in atrial fibrillation Second-line treatment maternal supraventricular arrhythmias Prophylactic therapy for supraventricular and ventricular tachycardias	No teratogenicity Fetal bradycardia, hypoglycaemia, premature labour and metabolic abnormalities	Compatible
Digoxin (see heart failure)			
Flecainide	Second-line: maternal and fetal supraventricular arrhythmias	No reports of teratogenicity	Limited data
Lidocaine	Maternal ventricular arrhythmias Local anaesthesia	Fetal bradycardia Central nervous system toxicity	Limited data
Propafenone	Second-line: maternal supraventricular arrhythmias		Limited data
Sotalol	Second-line: maternal supraventricular arrhythmias Fetal tachycardia	Fetal bradycardia, intrauterine growth retardation	Limited data
Verapamil	Second-line: maternal supraventricular arrhythmias	Maternal hypotension an subsequent fetal hypoperfusion	Limited data
Heart failure therapy			
ACE inhibitors	Not recommended	Teratogenic effects	Compatible
Angiotensin II receptor antagonists	Not recommended	Limited data	Limited data
Digoxin	Prophylactic therapy for supraventricular tachycardias Control ventricular rate in atrial fibrillation Fetal tachycardia Heart failure	No reports of teratogenicity	Compatible
Loop diuretics: furosemide	Severe symptomatic congestive heart failure	No teratogenic or cardiovascular fetal effects	Compatible
Potassium sparing diuretics: spironolactone	Congestive heart failure and hypokalaemia	No teratogenic effects	Compatible
Nitrates	Myocardial ischaemia Heart failure Hypertension	Fetal heart deceleration Maternal hypotension and subsequent fetal hypoperfusion	Limited data
Hypertensive disease therapy			
Prophylactic treatment in women with historical risk factors			
Aspirin	Reduces the risk of perinatal death and pre-eclampsia	Haemorrhage, prolongation of labour	
Calcium supplementation	Positive impact on maternal and fetal morbidity need to be confirmed		Limited data
Magnesium sulphate	Reduces the risk of eclampsia in women with severe pre-eclampsia		Limited data
Severe hypertension			
Hydralazine	Second-line therapy	Neonatal bradycardia	Compatible
Labetalol	First-line therapy	Neonatal bradycardia	Limited data
Nifedipine	First-line therapy	Fetal distress	Limited data
Nitroprusside	Second-line therapy	Thiocyanate poising	Limited data

* Based on multiple studies [66–82].

although case reports of fetal heart decelerations have been reported.

Dopamine and dobutamine can be used in low-output congestive heart failure. A few cases have been reported with no adverse effect [104, 105]. However, during pregnancy with a viable fetus, fetal monitoring is advisable.

The experience with digoxin is extensive and there are no reports of teratogenicity associated with its use. It is considered a preferred choice for treatment of congestive heart failure, especially when supraventricular arrhythmias and systolic dysfunction are present. Furthermore, digoxin is the first-line drug for maternal and fetal rate control in atrial fibrillation/flutter and for the treatment of fetal supraventricular tachycardias [12, 106]. Because of increased renal clearance, the serum digoxin concentration may be lower and so maternal dose should be increased. In the presence of decreased renal function or concomitant administration of amiodarone, maintenance doses may require reduction. Even if higher doses are required during pregnancy, caution in changing the amount of digitalis is advised because digitalis toxicity has been associated with miscarriage and fetal death. In the third trimester, serum digoxin levels may appear falsely elevated because of the presence of digoxin-like substances interfering with radioimmunoassays. Hence, the monitoring of digoxin levels would not be helpful in guiding treatment [110–112].

Management of arrhythmias

Pregnancy may increase the incidence of arrhythmias. Knowledge of the underlying heart disease is important for the correct treatment. Most of the antiarrhythmic drugs can be prescribed safely in pregnancy but an attempt to recognize a correctable cause should be undertaken before starting therapy. All antiarrhythmic drugs cross the placental barrier and their potentially toxic effect on the fetus should be taken into consideration, particularly during the first weeks of pregnancy [111].

Maternal tachyarrhythmias

Ectopic beats are present in one-third of pregnant women but are generally benign and well tolerated. No treatment other than reassurance and correction/elimination of potential stimulants are indicated. An increased risk of new-onset, and exacerbation of, supraventricular tachycardia during pregnancy has been reported (3%), while ventricular tachycardia is rare. Recurrence of arrhythmia during the antepartum period increases the risk of adverse fetal complications, independent of other maternal and fetal risk factors [113]. When dysrhythmias such as atrial fibrillation or flutter are present during pregnancy, an underlying cause should be considered.

Electrical cardioversion is the treatment of choice for all drug-refractory maternal arrhythmias or those causing haemodynamic compromise and can be performed safely at any time during pregnancy. Paroxysmal supraventricular tachycardias are usually well tolerated and require active therapy only if very frequent or long-lasting or with haemodynamic instability. Vagal manoeuvre should be tried first and, if ineffective, intravenous adenosine would be the first-choice drug. Maternal effects may include facial flushing, headache, dyspnoea, and nausea. Adenosine crosses the placenta but no adverse fetal effects have been described. Second-line drugs include beta-blocking agents or propafenone. Intravenous verapamil can be used but maternal hypotension, heart failure, and inhibition of labour have been reported. If prophylactic drug therapy is needed, then β_1 receptor blockers or digoxin are the first choice.

Atrial fibrillation and flutter are rare in pregnancy and often secondary to congenital or valvular heart disease. However, due to the increased maternal age any patient with atrial scar or atrial overload can develop arrhythmias during pregnancy. Therapy includes ventricular rate control using digoxin or beta-blocking agents and conversion to sinus rhythm using propafenone or amiodarone (termination of atrial episodes should be attempted in order to avoid anticoagulation therapy). Ventricular tachycardia during pregnancy is rare in healthy women without organic disease but it can occur when ventricular scars are present (e.g. tetralogy of Fallot). Beta-blockers are the first-line therapy when ventricular function is preserved. Some forms of non-sustained ventricular tachycardia in normal hearts respond well to verapamil. If ventricular function is impaired, amiodarone is the only option. Chronic administration of amiodarone can have adverse effects on the mother in 3–5% of cases, including thyroid malfunction, photosensitivity, and corneal deposition. In the fetus, long-term treatment with amiodarone can cause neonatal hypothyroidism, which is however reversible.

Although catheter ablation has been performed in a pregnant patient, it should be recommended only in patients with drug-refractory, poorly tolerated, or life-threatening arrhythmias [111, 114]. Catheter ablation in patients with CHD can be very complex due to the multiple sites of re-entry circuits secondary to the atrial scars; due the high radiation exposure time in these patients should be avoided. The presence of an ICD should not be considered a contraindication to pregnancy [115], but implantation during pregnancy has never been reported in the literature.

Maternal bradyarrhythmias

Compared with the tachyarrhythmias, bradyarrhythmias are uncommon, but when they do occur they are usually well tolerated. Management should not be influenced by pregnancy. A temporary or permanent pacemaker, if required, can be implanted at any stage of pregnancy, although treatment is generally not indicated unless the conduction abnormality causes symptoms. Women with congenital complete heart block, as previously reported, can accomplish an uneventful and successful pregnancy [116] with or without a pacemaker.

Fetal arrhythmias

Intermittent extrasystoles, which are frequently encountered in clinical practice, do not require treatment. Fetal tachycardia, defined as a heart rate >180bpm, is a condition that occurs in approximately 0.4–0.6% of all pregnancies, and may cause non-immune fetal hydrops and lead to fetal morbidity and mortality. Prompt treatment with either anti-arrhythmic drugs or delivery must be considered. Maternal full-dose digoxin is the first-line antiarrhythmic agent in non-hydropic fetuses, while verapamil and beta-blocking agents are second-line therapy. In drug-refractory fetal tachycardia, particularly if accompanied by hydrops fetalis or ventricular dysfunction, amiodarone represents a safe and effective option [117]. Sotalol should be considered a valuable treatment option for fetal atrial fibrillation, which is extremely rare [118].

Prophylaxis of endocarditis

As in the non-pregnant state, antibiotic prophylaxis is indicated before undergoing a procedure likely to cause bacteraemia. Since the incidence of bacteraemia following vaginal delivery has been reported to be low (0–5%), routine antibiotic prophylaxis for uncomplicated vaginal delivery or primary (or planned) Caesarean section in women with heart disease is not recommended. However, the high morbidity and mortality associated with cardiac infection, the risk of unpredictable complications and the relatively safety of antibiotic prophylaxis in patients who are already receiving it should lead to consideration of antibiotic prophylaxis in all high-risk cardiac conditions (patients with prosthetic heart valves, a previous history of endocarditis, complex congenital heart disease, or a surgically constructed systemic-pulmonary conduit). Antibiotic therapy should be administered 30min before Caesarean section or at the beginning of spontaneous delivery [119, 120].

Percutaneous therapy

Over the last 20 years, interventional cardiology has emerged as a new therapeutic tool and as an effective alternative to surgical therapy in several cardiac diseases, such as valve stenosis and coronary artery disease [40]. Cardiac catheterization in the pregnant patient carries the risk of fetal radiation exposure. The effects of radiation on the fetus depend on the radiation dose and the gestational age at which exposure occurs. As previously reported, the maximum permissible dose of radiation to the pregnant woman has been set at 5mGy. During cardiac catheterization the mean radiation exposure to the unshielded abdomen is 1.5mGy, and <20% of this reaches the fetus because of tissue attenuation. If the radiation fetal dose is in excess of 25rad, elective pregnancy termination should be recommended because the risk of an adverse outcome is high. The effect of radiation during pregnancy can be divided into three main phases: preimplantation period (0–9 days) tends to cause death rather than anomalies; active organogenesis period (9–42 days) radiation causes severe structural anomalies; and second- and third-trimester risks are primarily related to the development of childhood leukaemia and other malignancies. Shielding the gravid uterus from direct radiation, shortening fluoroscopic time and delaying the procedure until at least the completion of the period of major organogenesis (>12 weeks after menses) will minimize radiation exposure. The best time for performing percutaneous intervention procedures is considered to be the fourth month, during which period organogenesis has been completed, the fetal thyroid is still inactive, and the volume of the uterus is still small, so that there is a greater distance between the fetus and the chest than in the following months. With these provisions, cardiac catheterization and interventional procedures during pregnancy are safe for the fetus but should be considered only in patients not manageable with medical therapy or in whom drug therapy is more dangerous for the fetus than catheter based treatment (refractory arrhythmias).

➲Table 33.5 shows the most common percutaneous interventions during pregnancy, but many others are possible and some are occasionally reported in the literature: transcatheter embolization of bronchial artery in massive haemoptysis, ablation of recurrent supraventricular tachycardias, patent foramen ovale closure after transient ischaemic attack, and stenting of a Blalock–Taussig shunt.

Cardiac surgery

Open heart surgery can be performed during pregnancy, with the same risk to the mother as outside pregnancy but with a high incidence of fetal death (20–33%). The best period to perform surgery is early in the second trimester

Table 33.5 Interventional cardiology procedures in pregnancy

Procedure	Indication	Outcome
Mitral valvuloplasty	Severe mitral stenosis NYHA III–IV Echo score <8	Many reports Good results
Aortic valvuloplasty	Severe aortic stenosis Symptomatic No aortic regurgitation No calcification	Some reports Good results
Pulmonary valvuloplasty	Severe pulmonary stenosis Symptomatic	Few cases Excellent result
Percutaneous coronary intervention	Acute coronary syndrome STEMI NSTEMI	Few cases Mixed results
Aortic stenting	Coartation Re-coartation	Few cases Good results

because in the first trimester it may cause abortion and later in the third trimester premature labour. The poor fetal outcome is due to non-pulsatile blood flow and hypotension associated with cardiopulmonary bypass that can adversely affect placental blood flow. Cardiopulmonary bypass in pregnancy must be performed at high flow and high pressure, in normothermia, with the shortest possible cross-clamping time.

Personal perspective

The panorama of heart disease in women of child-bearing age has changed and will change further. Mild uncorrected or corrected diseases with few sequelae will represent the majority of the cases and pregnancy should be encouraged. The profile of the cases at risk has become different: pulmonary hypertension and cyanotic heart disease are rare because of early correction during infancy; palliated or corrected forms of congenital heart disease with residual defects, aorta pathology, valvular heart disease in immigrants, and cardiomyopathies with or without coronary artery disease in older women have become more frequent.

Multiple other factors can increase the risk during pregnancy in women with heart disease. Older age at pregnancy, smoking habits, diabetes, and twin or triple pregnancy secondary to frequent *in vitro* fertilization are much more common and have to be taken into consideration when assessing the risk. Heart failure secondary to impaired left or right ventricular function has become a common complication in this setting and its early recognition and treatment is mandatory. The risks of hormone therapy for infertility treatment in non-pregnant patients with heart disease are not well known, but heart failure may occur. Correction of residual defects or aortic or mitral valve disease, particularly stenotic valves even with moderate degrees of stenosis, should be considered before pregnancy. Percutaneous procedures or minimally invasive surgical repair can today be performed in these young women with low rates of complications, making it easier to accomplish pregnancy without problems.

Nowadays heart surgery, particularly during the second and third trimesters, can be done with acceptable risks for mother and fetus. From the surgical standpoint, short pump runs with high flow rates are essential criteria, ensuring lower levels of fetal loss.

Interventional cardiology is rapidly progressing. New interventional techniques and devices will offer a very important contribution to the treatment of women with cardiac disease outside and during pregnancy with a partial replacement of the surgical procedures. The feasibility of low-exposure or MRI-guided interventional procedures will further increase the possibilities of treatment during pregnancy.

The failing ventricles with congestive symptoms continues to be a main unresolved problem. Rest is the first step in all patients at risk. Heart failure should be managed according to conventional guidelines, except for the use of ACE inhibitors because of their known fetal toxicity. Particular attention should be paid to fluid retention in the immediate postpartum period.

Advances in ART will enable increasing numbers of women with cardiac disease to contemplate the possibility of pregnancy even in advanced age. Pre-pregnancy counselling and multidisciplinary care including cardiologists, gynaecologists, and general practitioners are essential to help these women to reduce risk.

Further reading

Oakley C, Warnes CA (eds.). *Heart Disease in Pregnancy*, 2nd edn., 2007. Oxford: Blackwell Publishing Group.

Perloff JK, Child JS, Aboulhosn J (eds.). *Congenital Heart Disease in Adults*, 3rd edn., 2008. Philadelphia, PA: Saunders.

Warnes CA (ed.). *Adult Congenital Heart Disease*, 2009. London: Wiley-Blackwell Publishing Group.

Online resources

TOXNET: Databases on toxicology, hazardous chemicals, environmental health, and toxic releases from the US Library of Medicine: http://toxnet.nlm.nih.gov

➲ For full references and multimedia materials please visit the online version of the book (http://esctextbook.oxfordonline.com).

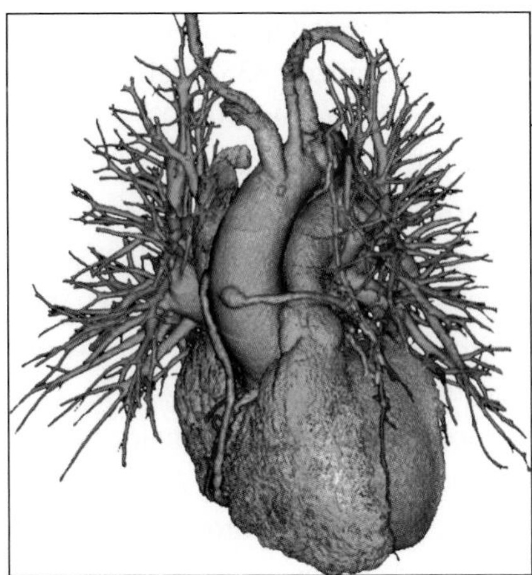

CHAPTER 34

Non-cardiac Surgery in Cardiac Patients

Sanne Hoeks and Don Poldermans

Contents

Summary

The number of cardiac patients undergoing non-cardiac surgery is steadily increasing. Some patients may be at substantial risk of perioperative morbidity and mortality. In this respect, vascular surgery is considered as high-risk surgery. Perioperative myocardial infarctions (PMIs) are the predominant cause of morbidity and mortality in patients undergoing non-cardiac surgery. The pathophysiology of PMI is complex. Prolonged myocardial ischaemia due to the stress of surgery, in the presence of a haemodynamically significant coronary lesion leading to subendocardial ischaemia, and acute coronary artery occlusion after plaque rupture and thrombus formation, contribute equally to these devastating events. Preoperative management aims at optimizing the patient's condition by identification and modification of underlying cardiac risk factors and diseases. Beta-blockers and statins are widely used in this setting. In contrast, the role of prophylactic coronary revascularization has been restricted to the same indications as the non-operative setting. This chapter will review the main aspects of perioperative care and management of cardiac patients undergoing non-cardiac surgery in line with the recent European Society of Cardiology guidelines on perioperative care.

Introduction

Patients undergoing non-cardiac surgery are at increased risk of cardiovascular morbidity and mortality. Hertzer's landmark study in 1000 consecutive patients undergoing operations for peripheral arterial disease (PAD) who underwent preoperative cardiac catheterizations reported that only 8% of their patients (who were roughly divided into thirds—aortic, infrainguinal, and carotid disease) had normal coronary arteries, and approximately one-third had severe-correctable or severe-inoperable coronary artery disease (CAD) [1]. More recent studies using functional tests for CAD, such as dobutamine stress echocardiography, confirmed these findings. In a study population of 1097 vascular surgical patients, the incidence of rest wall-motion abnormalities was nearly 50%, while one-fifth of patients had stress-induced myocardial ischaemia [2]. Careful management of patients undergoing surgery is therefore mandatory in the perioperative setting. In general, the risk of perioperative complications depends on the condition of the patient prior to surgery, the prevalence of comorbidities, and the severity and duration of the surgical procedure. Cardiac complications are especially suspected in patients with documented or hidden CAD undergoing procedures that are associated with prolonged haemodynamic and cardiac stress.

Although the perioperative event rate has declined over past decades as a result of achievements in anaesthesiologic and surgical techniques, perioperative complications remain a significant problem. Importantly, a large study showed that long-term prognosis of vascular surgery patients was significantly worse than for patients with CAD [3]. Estimations of cardiac outcome can be derived from the few large-scale clinical trials and registries that have been undertaken in patients undergoing non-cardiac surgery. Lee and colleagues studied 4315 patients undergoing elective major non-cardiac procedures in a tertiary-care teaching hospital during 1989–1994 [4]. Major cardiac complications, including cardiac death and myocardial infarction (MI), were observed in 2.1% of this patient cohort. In a cohort of 108,593 consecutive patients who underwent surgery during 1991–2000 in a university hospital in The Netherlands, perioperative mortality occurred in 1877 (1.7%) cases, of whom 543 (0.5%) were attributed to cardiovascular causes. The Dutch Echographic Cardiac Risk Evaluating Applying Stress Echo (DECREASE) -I, -II, and -IV trials enrolled 3893 surgical patients during 1996–2008, consisting of intermediate- and high-risk patients, and 136 (3.5%) had perioperative cardiac death or MI [5–7]. The recently published RCT PeriOperative ISchemic Evaluation trial (POISE) randomized 8351 patients who underwent non-cardiac surgery in the period 2002–2007 and perioperative mortality occurred in 226 patients (2.7%), of whom 133 (1.6%) had cardiovascular death, whereas non-fatal MI was observed in another 367 (4.4%) subjects [8]. Overall, major non-cardiac surgery is associated with an incidence of cardiac death between 0.5–1.5%, and an incidence of major cardiac complications in the range of 2–3.5%.

The global ageing phenomenon will have a major impact on perioperative management in future years. Ageing of the world's population can be seen as an indicator of improving global health but also enforces a change in healthcare toward the elderly population. Furthermore, the burden of cardiovascular disease (CVD) will further increase in the coming years. It is estimated from primary care data that in the 75–84 year age group 19% of men and 12% of women have some degree of CVD [9]. In contrast to the past, major surgical interventions are increasingly performed in the elderly. Demographics of patients undergoing surgery indeed show a trend toward an enlarged number of preoperative risk factors, including increasing age and more comorbidities [10].

With the growing elderly population, increased incidence of CVD, and the availability of advanced surgical techniques, preoperative cardiac risk assessment and perioperative cardiac management continues to be a major challenge.

Pathophysiology of myocardial infarction

Perioperative myocardial infarction (PMI) is one of the most important predictors of short- and long-term morbidity and mortality associated with non-cardiac surgery. The highest incidence of PMI is within the first 3 days after surgery (± 5%) [11–13].

The prevalence of acute coronary syndrome with symptomatic or asymptomatic perioperative myocardial ischaemia assessed by serum troponin I or T in major vascular surgery patients is high, even 15–25%. Hence, the prevention of a PMI is the cornerstone for improvement in overall postoperative outcome. To achieve this, knowledge about the pathophysiology of a PMI is essential.

Unfortunately the exact underlying mechanism of a PMI is still not clear, but seems to be the same as in other settings. Coronary plaque rupture, leading to thrombus formation and subsequent vessel occlusion, is considered to be an important cause of acute perioperative coronary syndromes. This is similar to MIs occurring in the non-operative setting (➲Chapter 3). Surgery itself is a significant stress factor leading to an increased risk of plaque rupture. The perioperative surgical stress response includes a catecholamine surge with associated haemodynamic stress, vasospasm, reduced fibrinolytic activity, platelet activation, and consequent hypercoagulability [11]. Two retrospective studies investigated the coronary pathology of fatal PMI. As demonstrated in the autopsy study by Dawood and colleagues, 55% of the fatal perioperative MIs have direct evidence of plaque disruption defined as fissure or rupture of plaque and haemorrhage into the plaque cavity [14]. Similar autopsy results were found in the study of Cohen and Aretz; a plaque rupture was found in 46% of patient with postoperative MI [15]. Time-to-death interval in patients with plaque rupture was significantly longer than in patients without plaque rupture.

In patients with significant CAD, PMI may also be caused by a sustained myocardial supply/demand imbalance due to tachycardia and increased myocardial contractility [11]. Episodes of perioperative ST-depression, indicating subendocardial myocardial ischaemia, has been described in up to 41% of vascular surgery patients, mostly occurring within the first 2 days after operation [16]. The association of PMI with myocardial ischaemia and non-transmural or circumferential subendocardial infarction supports this mechanism. Landesberg and colleagues demonstrated that 85% of postoperative cardiac complications were preceded by prolonged ST-segment depression [17]. Fleisher and colleagues found that 78% of patients with cardiac complications had at least one episode of prolonged myocardial ischaemia (i.e. >30min) either before or at the same time of the cardiac event [18]. In the majority of cases, it presents without Q waves. The hypothesis that ST-depression can lead to PMI is further supported by increased troponin T levels during or shortly after prolonged ST-depression ischaemia [19].

ST-elevation-type ischaemia is considered relative uncommon, confirmed by the incidence (12%) of intraoperative ST-elevation in a study by London and colleagues [14]. Few data exist on this topic. Using cardiac testing, one can identify the patient at risk; however, the location of the PMI is difficult to foresee due to the unpredictable progression of (asymptomatic) coronary artery lesions towards unstable plaques during the stress of surgery.

Risk stratification

The first question arising in perioperative care is which patients are at risk for perioperative cardiac events. This is an important issue as patients with a suspected low cardiac risk can be operated on safely without any delay while patients with an increased cardiac risk could benefit from preoperative risk reduction strategies (➲Fig. 34.1). In this context, adequate risk stratification of patients undergoing non-cardiac surgery is of utmost importance. Several risk indices have therefore been developed in the past decades for non-cardiac surgery patients. Goldman and colleagues were in 1977 the first to develop a multifactorial risk index specifically for perioperative cardiac complications. This risk index was developed in a non-cardiac surgical population and included nine independent risk factors correlated with major cardiac complications [20]. This index was subsequently modified by Detsky and colleagues in 1986, who added the presence of angina and a remote history of MI to

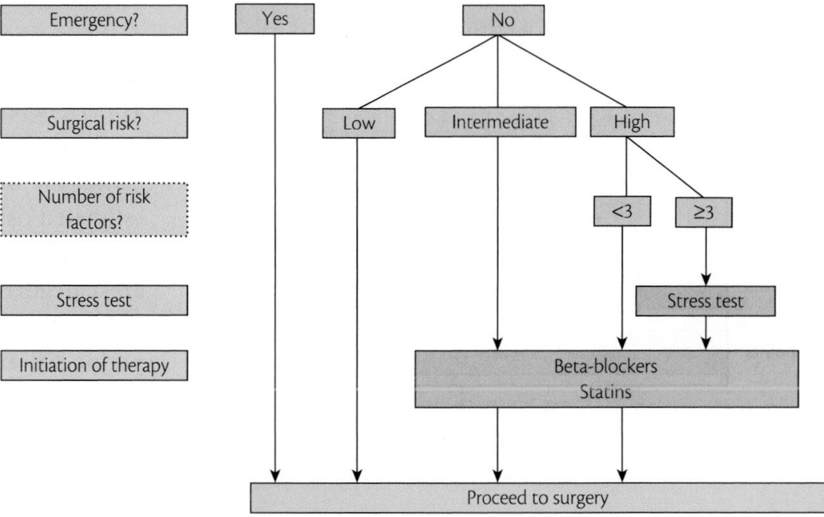

Figure 34.1 Decision tree for perioperative care.

the original model [21]. Nowadays, the Lee index is considered by many clinicians and researchers to be the best currently available cardiac risk prediction model in non-cardiac surgery [4]. This risk index was developed in 1999 on a cohort of 2893 consecutive patients who underwent a wide spectrum of procedures. The Lee index consists of six independent predictors of major cardiac complications: high-risk surgery, ischaemic heart disease, congestive heart failure, cerebrovascular disease, insulin-dependent diabetes mellitus, and renal failure (➲Fig. 34.2). All factors contribute equally to the index with each factor assigned to 1 point. The incidence of major cardiac complications in the validation cohort (n = 1422) was estimated at 0.4%, 0.9%, 7%, and 11% in patients with an index of 0, 1, 2, or ≥3 points, respectively. Evidence exists in 108,593 patients undergoing all types of non-cardiac surgery that this revised cardiac risk index was indeed predictive of cardiovascular mortality but could be substantially improved by adding age and an extensive description of the type of surgery (C-statistic improved from 0.63 to 0.85) [22]. The Lee index was also included in the algorithm of the 2007 American College of Cardiology (ACC)/American Heart Association (AHA) guidelines on perioperative cardiovascular evaluation. Furthermore, it was recently shown that the preoperative Lee index is not only an important prognostic factor for in-hospital outcome but also for late mortality and impaired health status in patients with PAD.

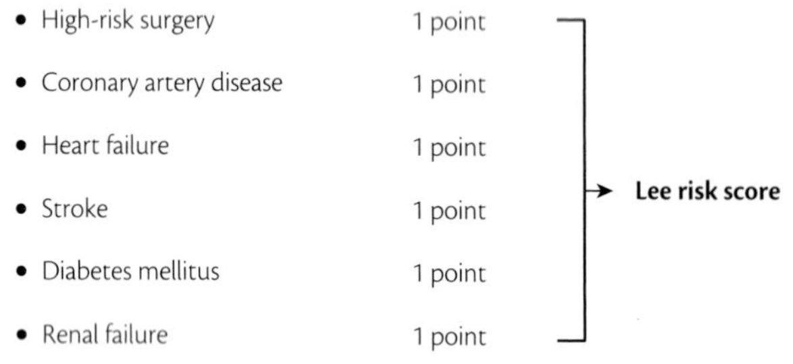

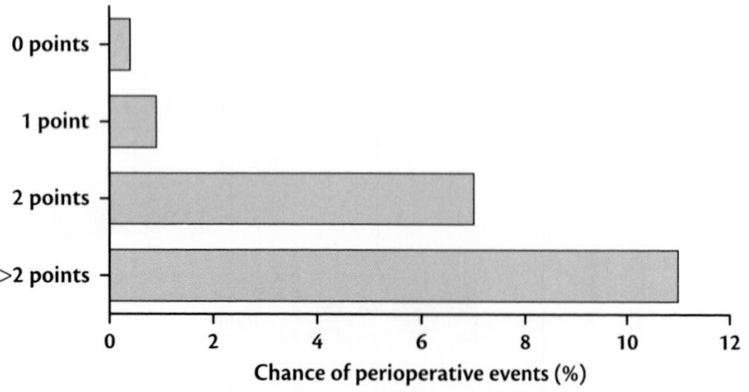

Figure 34.2 Risk factors according to the Lee risk index [4].

Surgery

The extent of preoperative cardiac evaluation will also depend on the type and urgency of the surgery in question [22–24]. Every operation will elicit a stress response to injury. This response is initiated by tissue injury and mediated by neuro-endocrine factors inducing tachycardia and hypertension. Fluid shifts in the postoperative period add to the surgical stress. This stress will influence the balance between myocardial oxygen supply and demand. Surgery will also cause alterations in the balance between prothrombotic and fibrinolytic factors resulting in hypercoagulability (elevation of fibrinogen and other coagulation factors, increased platelet aggregation and activation, reduced fibrinolysis). This is relative to the extent and duration of the intervention. Other factors that can influence cardiac stress are blood loss, perioperative fluid shifts, and body core temperature. These may cause haemodynamic changes and/or cardiac depression and are related to an increased cardiac risk.

Firstly, the urgency of the surgery determines the weight of cardiac evaluation. In case of true emergency and life-saving operations such as ruptured abdominal aortic aneurysm, or major trauma, cardiac evaluation will not change the course and result of the intervention. However, it can influence the management in the immediate postoperative period. With regard to cardiac risk, surgical interventions can be divided into a high-, intermediate-, and low-risk group with an estimated event rate of <1%, 1–5%, and >5%, respectively (➲Table 34.1). In cases of non-emergent but urgent surgical conditions, such as bypass for acute limb ischaemia or treatment of bowel obstruction, cardiac evaluation may influence the perioperative measures taken to reduce the cardiac risk but will not influence the decision to perform the intervention or allow for prophylactic coronary revascularization. When cardiac risk evaluation in patients scheduled for elective surgery demonstrates high cardiac risk, less invasive interventions such as peripheral angioplasty instead of infra-inguinal bypass can be considered. Moreover, it can be decided to delay or cancel the intended surgical intervention in case of high estimated risk.

Special attention is given to vascular procedures as they are categorized as high-risk procedures. Furthermore, although minimally invasive, the risk associated with peripheral angioplasties should not be neglected. Long-term survival does not seem to be influenced by the surgical technique that is used, but is determined by underlying cardiac disease [25].

Table 34.1 Cardiac risk from surgical interventions

Low risk: <1%
Breast
Dental
Endocrine
Eye
Gynaecologic
Orthopaedic—minor
Reconstructive
Urologic—minor
Intermediate risk: 1–5%
Abdominal
Carotid
Endovascular aneurysm repair
Head and neck surgery
Neurologic
Orthopaedic—major
Peripheral angioplasty
Pulmonary
Renal transplant
Urologic—major
High risk: >5%
Aortic and major vascular surgery
Peripheral vascular surgery

Chronic heart failure

The prevalence of chronic heart failure (CHF) is high in the overall population and still increasing (➲Chapter 23). Furthermore, it has been suggested that the prevalence of patients with symptomatic CHF is similar to the prevalence of patients with asymptomatic CHF, which may lead to an underestimation of the extent of heart failure in the general population [26]. CHF can be considered as a large health problem with major clinical impact. The prognosis of patients with diagnosed CHF is poor. Half of the patients will die within 4 years and of patients diagnosed with severe heart failure >50% will die within 1 year [27].

The effect of CHF on postoperative outcome was first described by Kazmers and colleagues who concluded that survival rates are reduced in patients with an impaired LV ejection fraction of ≤35% [28]. Historically, heart failure is also part of many different cardiac risk stratification models [4, 20–22, 29]. Although previous studies emphasize ischaemic heart disease as the most important risk factor for perioperative complications, heart failure has been suggested to be equally important [30]. Recently, Hammil and colleagues demonstrated that elderly patients with heart failure who undergo major non-cardiac surgery have an increased risk of operative mortality and hospital readmission compared to CAD patients [31]. They noted that improvements in perioperative care are needed for this growing population of heart failure patients undergoing surgery. Coupled to the growing prevalence of CHF and the elderly population, is the increase in surgical procedures. Therefore, adequate treatment of CHF in the perioperative setting is of pivotal importance to reduce morbidity and mortality after non-cardiac surgery. Perioperative management of these patients is aimed at optimizing haemodynamic status and providing intensive postoperative surveillance. In 2006, Feringa and colleagues concluded that the use of beta-blockers in patients with heart failure undergoing major vascular surgery was associated with a reduced incidence of in-hospital and long-term postoperative mortality [32]. Statins, angiotensin-converting enzyme (ACE)-inhibitors, and aspirin may also be of benefit in patients with LV dysfunction because these patients frequently have CAD comorbidity.

Recent studies showed that an increased plasma level of N-terminal pro-B-type natriuretic peptide (NT-proBNP) or B-type natriuretic peptide (BNP) is associated with adverse postoperative outcome. NT-proBNP is increased in patients with left ventricular (LV) dilatation caused by fluid overload (e.g. CHF and renal dysfunction), pressure overload (e.g. aortic valve stenosis), and myocardial ischaemia, which might explain the excellent correlation with adverse postoperative outcome. Feringa *et al.* reported on the prognostic value of NT-proBNP in 170 patients scheduled for major vascular surgery. Patients with NT-proBNP levels >533pg/mL had an independent 17-fold increased risk for postoperative cardiac events, even after adjustment for preoperative dobutamine stress echocardiography results (➲Fig. 34.3) [33]. The general assessment of postoperative patients with decompensated heart failure should be focused on evaluating asymptomatic and unstable myocardial ischaemia. The diagnosis of postoperative MI is often difficult to make since it often presents atypically and may have a different aetiology compared to non-postoperative MI. The evaluation of postoperative MI should include cardiac monitoring, electrocardiography, and serial cardiac enzyme measurements. Special attention should be given to perioperative volume infusion since excessive fluid administration is a common cause of decompensated heart failure. Once the aetiology of postoperative decompensated heart failure is diagnosed, treatment should

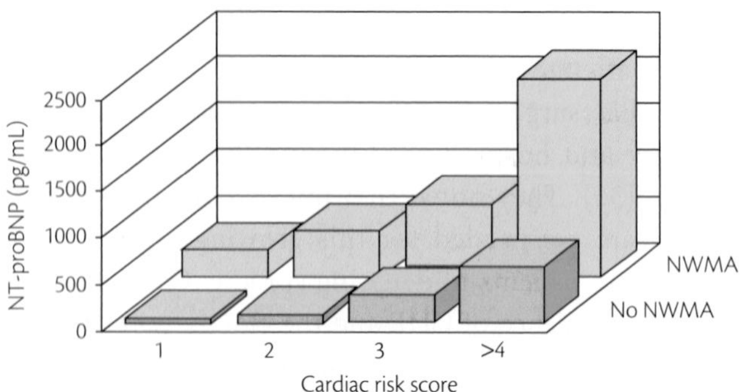

Figure 34.3 N-terminal pro-B-type natriuretic peptide (NT-pro-BNP) levels in relation to cardiac risk and DSE results. NWMA, new wall motion abnormalities. Reproduced from Feringa HH, Bax JJ, Elhendy A, *et al.* Association of plasma N-terminal pro-B-type natriuretic peptide with postoperative cardiac events in patients undergoing surgery for abdominal aortic aneurysm or leg bypass. *Am J Cardiol* 2006; **98:** 111–15. Copyright 2006, with permission from Elsevier.

be no different compared to the management of CHF during a general medical service admission [19].

Valvular disease

Valvular heart disease (VHD) (➲Chapter 21) is a common finding in patients presenting for non-cardiac surgery. These patients are known to be at increased risk for perioperative cardiovascular complications during non-cardiac surgery [34]. Aortic stenosis is the most common VHD in Europe, particularly among the elderly [35]. Severe aortic stenosis (defined as aortic valve area <1cm^2, <0.6cm^2/m^2 body surface area) constitutes a well-established risk factor for perioperative mortality and MI [36]. In symptomatic patients, aortic valve replacement should be considered before elective surgery. In patients who are not candidates for valve replacement due to either high risk associated with serious comorbidities or those who refuse, non-cardiac surgery should be performed only if strictly needed. In these patients, percutaneous balloon aortic valvuloplasty may be a reasonable therapeutic option before surgery [34].

Non-cardiac surgery can be performed at relatively low risk in patients with non-significant mitral stenosis (valve area >1.5cm^2) and in asymptomatic patients with significant mitral stenosis (valve area <1.5cm^2) and systolic pulmonary artery pressure <50mmHg.

Non-significant aortic regurgitation and mitral regurgitation do not independently increase risk of cardiovascular complications during non-cardiac surgery. Patients with severe mitral regurgitation and aortic regurgitation may benefit from optimization of pharmacological therapy to produce maximal haemodynamic stabilization before high risk surgery.

Renal

A decreased level of kidney function is an independent risk factor for adverse postoperative CVD outcomes including MI, stroke, and progression of heart failure (➲Chapter 15). Traditionally, this function is assessed by serum creatinine concentration. For example, the serum creatinine cut-off value of >2.0mg/dL (177mmol/L) is used in the Lee index [4]. However, creatinine clearance (mL/min) incorporating serum creatinine, age, and weight to provide a more accurate assessment of renal function than serum creatinine alone. Most commonly used is the Cockcroft–Gault formula [37]:

$$([140 - \text{age in years}] \times [\text{weight in kg}] \times 0.85\ [\text{if female}]) \,/\, (72 \times \text{serum creatinine in mg/dL})$$

Kertai *et al.* evaluated 852 subjects undergoing major vascular surgery and demonstrated an increase in mortality as serum creatinine was >2.0mg/dL, experiencing odds for perioperative mortality of 5.2 (95% confidence interval (CI) 2.9–10.8) [38]. However, it might be argued that patients with less pronounced renal insufficiency also do worse compared to patients with normal serum creatinine values. Using creatinine clearance among the entire strata of renal function a 10mL/min decrease in creatinine clearance was associated with a 40% increased risk of postoperative mortality (odds ratio (OR) 1.4; 95% CI 1.2–1.5; receiver operating characteristic (ROC) area: 0.70, 95% CI 0.63–0.76). ROC curve analysis showed that the cut-off value of 64mL/min for creatinine clearance yielded the highest sensitivity/specificity to predict postoperative mortality.

In addition to the preoperative renal function, changes in kidney function in the postoperative period frequently occur and are predictive for adverse outcome. Ellenberger and colleagues reported an elevated mortality within 30 days after elective abdominal aortic surgery in patients with a serum creatinine >0.5mg/dL within 3 days after surgery, compared with baseline value [39]. Furthermore, worsening of kidney function in the postoperative period has shown to be a prognostic factor for late outcome. In 1324 patients who underwent elective open abdominal aortic aneurysm surgery creatinine clearance was measured preoperatively and on days 1, 2, and 3 after surgery [40]. Patients were divided into three groups according to the change in renal function after surgery compared to baseline. Group 1 showed an improved or unchanged (change in creatinine clearance, ± 10% of function compared with baseline); group 2 showed a temporary worsening (worsening >10% at day 1 or 2, then complete recovery within 10% of baseline at day 3); and group 3 experienced a persistent worsening (>10% decrease compared with baseline). Mortality during

30 days after surgery was 1.3%, 5.0%, and 12.6% in groups 1 to 3, respectively. Adjusted for baseline characteristics and postoperative complications, 30-day mortality was the greatest in patients with persistent worsening of renal function (hazard ratio (HR) 7.3; 95% CI 2.7–19.8), followed by those with temporary worsening (HR 3.7; 95% CI 1.4–9.9). During 6.0 ± 3.4 years of follow-up, 348 patients (36.5%) died. Risk of late mortality was 1.7 (95% CI 1.3–2.3) in the persistent-worsening group followed by those with temporary worsening (HR 1.5; 95% CI 1.2–1.4). This study showed that although renal function may recover completely after aortic surgery, temporary worsening of renal function was associated with an increased long-term mortality.

Identification of patients who might experience perioperative worsening of renal function is important in order to initiate supportive measures as maintenance of adequate intravascular volume for renal perfusion and vasopressor use. In a large retrospective study, risk factors for postoperative acute renal failure within the first 7 days after major non-cardiac surgery among patients with previously normal renal function were evaluated. Thirty-day, 60-day, and 1-year all-cause mortality was also evaluated. A total of 65,043 cases between 2003–2006 were reviewed [41]. Of these, 15,102 patients met the inclusion criteria; 121 patients developed acute renal failure (0.8%), and 14 required renal replacement therapy (0.1%). Seven independent preoperative predictors were identified ($p < 0.05$): age, emergency surgery, liver disease, body mass index, high-risk surgery, peripheral arterial occlusive disease, and chronic obstructive pulmonary disease (COPD) necessitating chronic bronchodilator therapy.

Neurological

Stroke (➲ Chapter 15) is one of the leading causes of death in the Western world and an established risk factor in non-cardiac surgery. The risk of clinically apparent perioperative brain injury varies widely among different types of surgery and depends on the type and complexity of the surgical procedure. Whereas patients undergoing general surgery appear to be at low risk (0.08–0.7%), those undergoing heart valve surgery and aortic arch repair have a high incidence of perioperative stroke (8–10%) [42–44]. The increasing population of elderly patients undergoing surgery will draw even further attention to the risk of cerebrovascular diseases in this population. Importantly, the true incidence of cerebral complications is probably underestimated because of lack of major sensory-motor symptoms or the presence of only subtle neuropsychological deficits, which are more difficult to identify. Perioperative strokes are predominantly ischaemic and embolic instead of related to hypoperfusion. Risk factors for perioperative (a)symptomatic transient or permanent cerebrovascular events (transient ischaemic attack/stroke) are embolism or haemodynamic compromise in large (aorta, carotid, vertebral, and main cerebral arteries intracranially) or small vessels (perforating and penetrating arterioles and capillaries). The diagnosis of significant carotid stenosis itself is a major indicator of the atherosclerotic burden associated with an increased stroke risk. Although fatal and non-fatal stroke can be reduced significantly in symptomatic patients with moderate/severe carotid stenosis associated with ipsilateral symptoms in particular if treated early, the benefit of this interventional/surgical treatment might be smaller in neurologically asymptomatic subjects. Preoperative risk evaluation should carefully identify patients and procedure-related factors associated with an increased risk of perioperative stroke to evaluate the individual risk:benefit ratio and optimize care, including appropriate risk modification and timing of surgery. A history of recent stroke or transient ischaemic attack is a strong predictor for perioperative stroke. Therefore, physicians should inquire specifically about the history of cerebrovascular events and treat the patient accordingly.

Arrhythmias

Cardiac arrhythmias (➲ Chapters 28, 29, and 30) are frequent perioperative cardiovascular abnormalities in patients undergoing both cardiac and non-cardiac surgery. Their significance must be considered in association with many other factors, especially the presence and severity of underlying heart disease, since their presence alone is usually of little importance.

Chronic obstructive pulmonary disease

COPD is associated with CVD, increasing the risk by two to threefold for cardiovascular mortality. For every 10% reduction in forced expiratory volume at 1s (FEV_1) value, the risk of non-fatal coronary events increased with 20% and the risk of cardiovascular mortality with 28% [68]. Consequently, it might be suggested that the presence of COPD affects postoperative cardiac outcome in surgical patients. Although contradictory results have been reported on 30-day mortality in patients undergoing surgical repair of abdominal aortic aneurysm [69–71], there is no consistent evidence indicating that COPD is associated with higher risk of perioperative cardiac complications and death in patients undergoing non-cardiac vascular surgery. Preoperative identification of patients with COPD might encourage clinicians to start a more stringent pulmonary therapy and may reduce the perioperative cardiac morbidity and mortality. In contrast to the small postoperative cardiac risk, pulmonary complications frequently occur in surgical patients with COPD, especially after abdominal or thoracic surgery. Preoperative COPD management is therefore important in these surgical patients, including optimization of pulmonary function to prevent deterioration during or after surgery. Bronchodilators and/or corticosteroids are essential in the preoperative pulmonary management of patients with COPD.

Although beta-blockers are often recommended in patients undergoing non-cardiac surgery [24], beta-blockers are frequently withheld from patients with concomitant COPD because of fear of bronchoconstriction from blockade of beta-2-adrenoreceptors. Nevertheless, there is substantial evidence that cardioselective beta-blockers can be used in COPD patients without provoking bronchospasm and pulmonary deterioration [72, 73]. In addition, (cardioselective) beta-blockers are associated with reduced 30-day (and long-term) mortality in COPD patients after vascular surgery [74]. However, even cardioselective beta-blocking agents have slight effects on the beta-2-adrenoreceptors, and these medications still need to be used cautiously in patients with COPD. The drug should be initiated at a low dose and, if tolerated well, carefully increased to the target dose.

In addition to beta-blockers, statins are also associated with reduced 30-day mortality and long-term mortality in vascular surgery patients with concomitant COPD [75]. Besides of this, it is suggested that statins might have additional effects in patients with COPD because of the anti-inflammatory properties associated with a reduced number of hospitalizations [76], exacerbations, and intubations [77]. However, more research is needed before new therapeutic strategies can be made.

Non-invasive testing

When the preoperative risk assessment identifies a patient with an increased cardiac risk, or if there is a suspicion of CAD upon examination, further cardiac testing is warranted in this patient [24]. A Dutch survey showed poor agreement between ACC/AHA guideline recommendations and daily clinical practice [78]. Only one of every five patients underwent non-invasive testing when recommended. Furthermore, patients who had not undergone testing despite recommendations received as little cardiac management as the low-risk population. The goals of non-invasive risk stratification are:

- to identify patients at extremely high risk in whom surgery should be cancelled, or another less hazardous procedure should be considered;
- to identify those patients in whom the optimization of medical therapy or a coronary revascularization before surgery might reduce the risk of the surgical procedure;
- to identify those patients in whom an invasive and intensive monitoring might reduce the risk of perioperative events;
- to assess the long-term risk of a future cardiac event.

Several non-invasive and (non-) exercise stress tests are available for perioperative risk assessment. The most commonly used stress test for detecting myocardial ischaemia is treadmill or cycle ergometer test. These tests provide an estimate of the functional capacity, haemodynamic response, and detect myocardial ischaemia by ST-segment changes. The accuracy varies widely among studies [79]. However, an important limitation in patients undergoing non-cardiac surgery is the frequently limited exercise capacity in the elderly, the presence of claudication, arthrosis, or COPD. Consequently, non-physiological stress tests like dobutamine stress echocardiography (DSE) and dipyridamole myocardial perfusion scintigraphy (MPS) are recommended in patients with limited exercise capacity.

Stress agents

Exercise stress testing is more physiologic compared to pharmacologic stress, however, in many situations it is not generally feasible. Pharmacologic stress testing is performed during the infusion of a catecholamine, dobutamine, for increased contractility or oxygen consumption or agents with vasodilatory properties such as adenosine and dipyridamole.

Although vasodilators (i.e. dipyridamole or adenosine) may have advantages for assessment of myocardial perfusion, dobutamine is the preferred pharmacological stressor when the test is based on assessment of regional wall-motion abnormalities [80]. Dobutamine is a synthetic cathecholamine with predominantly β_1-receptor stimulating properties resulting in a strong positive inotropic and modest chonotropic effect on the heart. During the stress test dobutamine is intravenously administered, and during dobutamine infusion contractility and heart rate increase, leading to increased myocardial oxygen demand. Myocardial ischaemia leading to systolic contractile dysfunction occurs in regions supplied by haemodynamically significant stenotic coronary arteries. Performing stress-rest tests requires careful patient monitoring, access to antidotes to stress agents, and the presence of an experienced physician.

Stress echocardiography (➲ Chapter 4)

As most patients with peripheral vascular disease are not able to exercise maximally, stress echocardiography with pharmacological stressors such as dobutamine is a good alternative. A graded dobutamine infusion starting at 5mcg/kg/min and increasing at 3-min intervals to 10, 20, 30, and 40mcg/kg/min is the standard for DSE.

Tissue harmonic imaging is advised for stress echocardiography. This special imaging setting reduces near-field artefact, improves resolution, enhances myocardial signals, and is superior to fundamental imaging for endocardial border visualization. The improvement in endocardial visualization is further improved by the use of contrast agents for LV opacification. Contrast agents increase the number of interpretable LV wall segments. These recent developments have decreased interobserver variability and improved the sensitivity of stress echocardiography [81].

Many reports have demonstrated that DSE predict perioperative events in patients undergoing vascular surgery [82–85]. The negative predictive value of dobutamine stress tests is high but the positive predictive value is much lower.

Kertai and colleagues reported a weighted sensitivity of 85% (95% CI 74–97%) and a specificity of 70% (95% CI 62–69%) for DSE in 850 patients from eight studies [79]. A recent meta-analysis by Beattie and colleagues analyzed the predictive value of pharmacological stress testing compared to myocardial perfusion scintigraphy [86]. This report included 25 studies (3373 patients) of mainly dobutamine and several dipyridamole stress echocardiography. The likelihood ratio of a perioperative event with a positive stress echocardiogram was 4.09 (95% CI 3.21–6.56).

Myocardial perfusion scintigraphy

Since their introduction in the early 1970s, positron emission tomography (PET) and single photon emission computed tomography (SPECT) have been widely used as diagnostic tools in the detection of CAD. Both PET and SPECT scanners globally assess LV function by detecting gamma radiation emitted by radiotracers, which are administrated intravenously in a small quantity. In PET scanning, radiotracers with short half-lives are used; such as [^{15}O]water, [^{13}N]ammonia, and rubidium-82 (^{82}Rb). With half-lives of 2min and 10min respectively, an on-site cyclotron is needed for the clinical use of [^{15}O]water and [^{13}N]ammonia. ^{82}Rb, with an half-life of 78s can be readily produced with a ^{82}Rb generator without the need of a cyclotron (see ➲Chapter 7, Nuclear Cardiology). In SPECT scanning, thallium-201 (^{201}Tl) and technetium-99 labelled agents such as sestamibi (Cardiolite™), tetrofosmin (Myoview™), and teboroxime (Cardiotec™) are available. Due to difficulties in imaging, teboroxime (Cardiotec™) is not used for clinical practice (➲Chapter 7).

Nuclear imaging differs from other imaging techniques by focusing on physiologic processes in the LV myocardium instead of anatomy [7]. Myocardial uptake of radiotracers is the result of: 1) blood flow-dependent delivery of radiotracers to the cell surface and 2) subsequent extraction and retention of radiotracers into the cell, a process dependent on cell membrane integrity and viability [88]. The detection of CAD is based on a difference in blood-flow distribution through the LV myocardium. These perfusion abnormalities can be explained by insufficient coronary blood flow based on coronary stenosis. To assess the extent of abnormal myocardial tissue a distinction should be made between non-viable myocardium (scar tissue) and viable myocardium, which is dysfunctional. Viable myocardium is still alive, therefore a potential target for revascularization treatment, and can be subdivided in stunning and hibernating myocardium. Myocardial stunning is a temporary post-ischaemic myocardial dysfunction, characterized by a flow–contraction mismatch, which will persist for several hours to days following the ischaemic event and restoration of flow [89, 90] Myocardial hibernation is a chronic process of diminished myocardial contractile function, caused by a persistent reduction in coronary blood flow (flow-contraction match) and can be considered as a protective mechanism of the heart to prevent irreversible damage of myocytes [89, 91].

To evaluate myocardial viability, a MPS is performed during rest, exercise, or pharmacological-induced stress. Pharmacological agents such as adenosine, dipyridamole, and dobutamine are used to obtain maximal vasodilatation, needed to evaluate perfusion abnormalities during stress. To distinct viable and irreversible myocardial abnormalities, results derived from stress and rest MPS should be compared [92]. Different patterns of wall motion or perfusion responses can be assessed to a graded infusion of dobutamine, such as:

1) a normal wall motion or perfusion response;
2) a biphasic response, with initial improvement of wall motion or perfusion at low doses of dobutamine followed by worsening at higher infusion rates (ischaemic viable myocardium); and
3) lack of initial improvement in wall motion or perfusion response (non-viable myocardium).

A biphasic and ischaemic response to dobutamine signifies viable myocardium with possible improvement of LV dysfunction after revascularization [93, 94]. This might be an indication to delay surgery and perform a cardiac intervention first, based on the patient's individual profile.

PMI occurs in 2–15% of patients undergoing vascular surgery with great impact on postoperative cardiovascular outcome [11]. Many patients undergoing vascular surgery are unable to exercise, therefore a non-exercising test, such as MPS, is mandatory. MPS has been widely used for the evaluation of patients undergoing vascular surgery and serves as a valuable diagnostic tool in preoperative risk stratification. The major goal of non-invasive risk stratification with MPS is to identify patients at high risk for developing unrecognized MI or myocardial ischaemia perioperatively.

Previous studies indicate that MPS is highly sensitive in predicting cardiac complications; however, the positive predictive value of MPS remains less satisfactory. A meta-analysis conducted by Kertai and colleagues reported a sensitivity of 83% (95% CI 77–89%) and a much lower specificity of 47% (95% CI 41–57%) for ^{201}Tl MPS to predict perioperative cardiac events [79]. Although MPS demonstrated lower diagnostic accuracy compared to DSE they conclude MPS is a valuable test for cardiac risk assessment, especially in patients with contraindications to DSE. Using several specific analysis, Beattie and colleagues conclude that DSE has a superior negative predictive value in preoperative cardiac assessment compared to MPS [86]. This meta-analysis identified 75 studies of preoperative non-invasive testing, including 25 MPS and 50 DSE studies involving vascular surgery patients over a 20-year period. They demonstrated that the likelihood ratio of a postoperative cardiac event was higher for DSE (likelihood ration (LR) 4.09; 95% CI 3.21–6.56; $p = 0.001$) compared to MPS (LR 1.83; 1.59–2.1; $p = 0.001$). Prognostic variables which increase the positive predictive value of future cardiac events are:

- a large defect size (>20% of the LV);
- defects in >1 coronary vascular supply region (suggestive for multivessel CAD); and
- large numbers of non-reversible defects (even in the supply region of a single coronary artery) [95].

Although MPS is a diagnostic tool with low specificity, the negative predictive value derived from a normal scan is high in predicting future MI and cardiac death. A meta-analysis by Shaw and colleagues identified the results of ten articles describing the use of dipyridamole-^{201}Tl in vascular surgery patients in a time period of 10 years. They conclude that cardiac death and non-fatal MI was correlated with the positive predictive value of a reversible ^{201}Tl defect. Cardiac event rates were low in patients without a history of CAD compared with: 1) patients with CAD and a normal or fixed defect pattern and 2) patients with one or more ^{201}Tl redistribution abnormalities—1% ($n = 176$), 4.8% ($n = 83$), and 18.6% ($n = 97$), $p = 0.0001$, respectively [85]. Boucher and colleagues evaluated 49 patients scheduled for peripheral vascular surgery and performed dipyridamole-thallium imaging preoperatively. Half of the patients with thallium redistribution had cardiac events, whereas no events occurred in patients with a normal scan or with non-reversible defects only [96]. Husmann and colleagues evaluated the diagnostic accuracy of PET ([^{13}N] ammonia-PET) and SPECT (^{201}TICI-SPECT and MIBI-SPECT) imaging using coronary angiography as the standard of reference. PET imaging showed a higher sensitivity for locating coronary artery stenosis compared to SPECT (95% and 77% respectively); however, no difference in specificity was found (84% in both groups). In detecting ischaemia the specificity of PET was 91% compared to 74% for SPECT [97].

Preoperative risk assessment with non-invasive stress tests, such as MPS and DSE, is indicated only in high-risk patients without unnecessary delay for vascular surgery. The use of dipyridamole, in both MPS and stress echocardiography, is contraindicated in patients: 1) receiving theophylilline treatment; 2) with bronchospasms; 3) with unstable carotid disease; 4) with second- and third-degree atrioventricular block; and 5) asthmatic patients. DSE is contraindicated in patients with severe hypertension and relative hypotension [98, 99]. When choosing between MPS and DSE the following advantages are in favour of DSE: 1) higher specificity; 2) higher versatility; 3) greater convenience; and 4) lower costs. The advantages of stress perfusion imaging include: 1) higher sensitivity; 2) higher technical success rate; and 3) better accuracy when multiple resting left-wall abnormalities are present [99]. All these factors should be considered when deciding which non-invasive stress tests to use for preoperative risk stratification.

In the future, a combination of non-invasive coronary angiography and MPS could provide a new non-invasive strategy focusing on the physiologic processes in the LV myocardium as well as the anatomy.

Myocardial perfusion magnetic resonance imaging (➲Chapter 5)

As already noted, the identification of viable myocardium in patients undergoing non-cardiac surgery is of significant clinical relevance. Currently, stress echocardiography and MPS are the most established methods in the identification of viable myocardium. However, perfusion cardiac magnetic resonance imaging (CMR) has also shown to assess the extent of injury after MI including the ability to discriminate viable from non-viable zones. CMR protocols focus on wall motion analysis, wall thickness, tissue characteristics, and perfusion imaging [100]. Pharmacological protocols with stress perfusion MRI have been adapted from stress imaging with echocardiography, PET, or SPECT with the use of adenosine, dipyridamole, and dobutamine. During stress perfusion MRI the heart is analyzed after administration of gadolinium chelates, which serves as contrast. Gadolinium chelates are large molecules that rapidly diffuse from the intravascular space into the interstitium and remain in the extracellular space of the myocardium, provided that the tissue cell membranes are intact [101]. Gadolinium clearance from the normal myocardium is a process dependent by several factors such as: 1) the wash out rate of gadolinium contrast from the myocardium; 2) overall cardiac function; 3) renal function; and 4) the administrated dose of gadolinium [102]. Ischaemic areas show up as areas with delayed and diminished contrast enhancement [103], although acutely stunned or chronic hibernating myocardium with a decreased function but intact cell membranes do not show delayed enhancement on MRI [102].

Ishida and colleagues compared CMR with SPECT in patients without MI and evaluated which diagnostic tool correlated most closely to results obtained with quantitative coronary angiography. They note an overall sensitivity of cMRI of 90% for depicting at least one coronary artery with significant stenosis compared to a sensitivity of SPECT ranging from 76–86%. The specificity of CMR for the identification of patients with significant coronary artery stenosis was 85% [104]. Gutberlet and colleagues compared dobutamine cMRI with ^{201}Tl SPECT for viability assessment both before and after coronary artery bypass grafting (CABG). CMR performed best with a sensitivity of 99% and a specificity of 94% for viability compared to SPECT which showed a high sensitivity of 86% and a low specificity of 68% [105].

Nagel and colleagues compared cMRI with dobutamine stress MRI in patients referred for diagnostic coronary angiography and showed dobutamine stress MRI provided superior sensitivity and specificity, of 89% vs. 74% and 86% vs. 70% respectively, in detecting CAD [106]. As already noted, pharmacologic protocols with MRI have been adapted from other imaging methods, therefore contraindications towards stress agents are identical. Tomlinson and colleagues propose a pragmatic approach to the decision regarding which test to choose for additional diagnostic information in viability assessment. Recourse implications in terms of personnel and cost favour DSE. If resting echo shows adequate imaging quality and complete wall-motion scoring is possible, the proposed next step should be to perform DSE. Conversely, when image quality derived from resting echo is poor and complete wall-motion scoring is not possible, cMRI is the diagnostic tool of preference [107].

Little is known about the use of stress CMR to predict cardiac risk in patients undergoing non-cardiac surgery. However, dobutamine stress CMR has shown to be feasible in predicting myocardial recoverability in patients undergoing CABG [108]. Future studies will have to evaluate the role of stress cMRI in preoperative risk stratification in patients undergoing non-cardiac surgery.

Myocardial stress computed tomography

Myocardial perfusion imaging with pharmacologic stress computed tomography (CT) has been used to evaluate subendocardial ischaemia in patients with CAD [109]. Disadvantages of cardiac CT imaging compared to other non-invasive imaging modalities are: 1) the use of an iodine contrast medium which may cause an adverse reaction and 2) X-ray exposure [110]. However, acceptability of metal devices such as an infusion pump, pacemaker, and an intra-aortic balloon pump is an advantage compared to myocardial perfusion MRI. Kurata and colleagues evaluated the use of contrast-enhanced multislice CT to detect myocardial ischaemia as hypoperfusion areas using adenosine triphosphate as a coronary vasodilator. They conclude that myocardial stress CT is a potential alternative to stress MPS; however, they note that rest images were of higher quality and therefore more feasible for clinical use at present [109]. In animal models the use of myocardial perfusion CT during adenosine stress shows promising results. George and colleagues evaluated myocardial perfusion CT in a canine model of left anterior descending artery stenosis and conclude that differences in myocardial perfusion can be reliably assed using this diagnostic tool. In conclusion, myocardial stress CT to assess myocardial perfusion at rest and stress is currently being explored and is not clinically established yet (➲Chapter 6).

Invasive testing

Coronary angiography is a well-established invasive diagnostic procedure for the evaluation of cardiac patients. However, in patients scheduled for non-cardiac surgery there is paucity of information focusing on the efficacy of this procedure. Nevertheless, as already extensively discussed, the majority of the patients scheduled for non-cardiac surgery presents with underlying ischaemic heart disease. Invasive testing should only be performed if test results will alter preoperative or perioperative management. In patients with known CAD, indications for perioperative coronary angiography and revascularization should be similar to angiography indications for the non-operative setting [111–114].

Medical therapy

Pharmacological risk reduction is one of the most important elements of perioperative management. Data from observational studies and registries, however, observe a poor compliance with guidelines in pharmacological treatment [115–117]. In particular, it has been shown that the prescription rate of beta-blockers is low in patients undergoing non-cardiac surgery.

Beta-blockers

Randomized controlled trials investigating the effect of beta-blockers in the perioperative period have shown divergent results (➲Fig. 34.4). There are different explanations regarding this conflicting evidence for perioperative beta-blocker use. In particular, the initiation time and dose of beta-blocker therapy, dose adjustments for heart rate control, and patients' underlying cardiac risk are important factors that may relate to the effectiveness of therapy [118].

Evidence supporting the use of beta-blockers is based mainly on two small, prospectively randomized clinical trials and several observational studies. In the first study, Mangano and colleagues randomized 200 patients with either known or suspected CAD undergoing high-risk non-cardiac surgery to receive atenolol (50mg or 100mg) or placebo just before the induction of anaesthesia [119]. Atenolol therapy was not associated with an improved in-hospital outcome (cardiac death or MI); however, it was associated with a 50% reduction in electrocardiogram evidence of myocardial ischaemia detected with continuous 3-lead Holter monitoring during the first 48 hours after surgery. Furthermore, although the study of Mangano did not demonstrate a perioperative effect, atenolol use was associated with significantly lower mortality rates at 6 months after discharge (0% vs. 8%; p = 0.005), and after 2 years (10% vs. 21%; p = 0.019).

The other trial, the DECREASE-I trial, randomized 112 vascular surgery patients with evidence of myocardial ischaemia on preoperative DSE. The DECREASE-I trial started bisoprolol at an average of 37 (range 7–89) days before surgery and careful titration was performed. Poldermans and colleagues showed a tenfold reduction in the incidence of perioperative cardiac death and MI with perioperative bisoprolol use compared with placebo (3.4% vs. 34%; p <0.001) [7]. The high incidence of perioperative cardiac events was explained by the selection of high-risk patients for study. From a population of 1351 patients, only 112 met entrance criteria of inducible myocardial ischaemia.

Several trials also showed evidence not supporting the use of perioperative beta-blockade. The MAVS (Metoprolol After Vascular Surgery) trial randomized 496 patients to metoprolol or placebo starting 2 hours before surgery until hospital discharge or a maximum of 5 days after surgery [120]. The combined endpoint of death, MI, heart failure, arrhythmias, or stroke at 30 days did not differ between the metoprolol and the placebo groups (10.2% and 12%

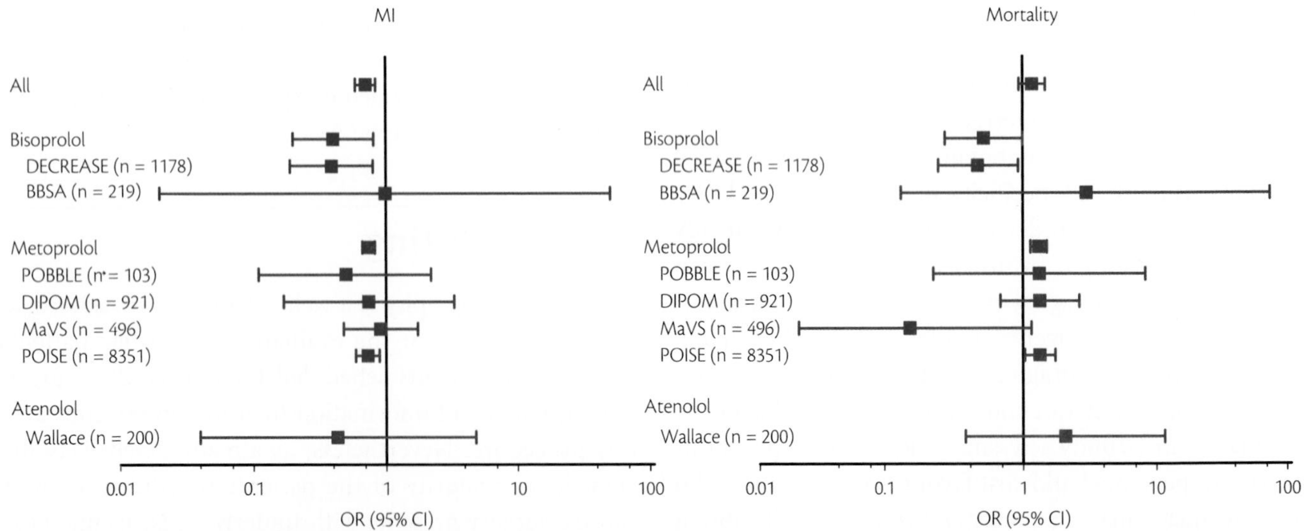

Figure 34.4 Effect of beta-blockers on 30-day rates of non-fatal MI and all-cause mortality.

respectively, p = 0.057). In the POBBLE (PeriOperative Beta-BLockadE) trial, only low-risk patients (history of ischaemic heart disease was an exclusion) scheduled for vascular surgery were studied [121]. In total, 103 patients were randomized to receive either metoprolol 25mg or 50mg, or placebo, starting the day before until 7 days after surgery. There was no difference in the incidence of perioperative cardiovascular events between the placebo and metoprolol groups (34% vs. 32%; relative risk (RR) 0.87, 95% CI 0.48–1.55). The duration of hospitalization though was shorter for those patients receiving metoprolol versus placebo (10 days vs. 12 days). The DIPOM (Diabetic Postoperative Mortality and Morbidity) trial also showed no differences in 30-day morbidity and mortality (21% vs. 20%; p = 0.66). In this study, 921 diabetic patients were randomized to 100mg metoprolol or placebo started the evening before major non-cardiac surgery [122].

Recently the results of the large randomized POISE trial were published. A total of 8351 patients were randomized to controlled-release oral metoprolol succinate, or placebo. Patients >45 years were included if they had known CVD, at least three out of seven clinical risk factors, or would undergo major vascular surgery. The POISE trial initiated randomized treatment of controlled-release metropolol just before surgery, and the maximum recommended therapeutical dose (400mg) could already be achieved within the first day of surgery (➲Fig. 34.5). The primary endpoint of cardiac death, MI, or cardiac arrest was reduced in the metoprolol group, compared to placebo (5.8% vs. 6.9%; HR 0.83; 95% CI 0.70–0.99; p = 0.04). However, the 30% decrease of non-fatal MI (3.6 vs. 5.1%: p = 0.0008) was accompanied by a 33% increase in total mortality (3.1% vs. 2.3%; p = 0.03) and a twofold increase risk in stroke (1.0 vs. 0.5%; p = 0.0005). Stroke was associated with perioperative bradycardia, hypotension, and bleeding in patients randomized to metoprolol with a diseased cerebrovascular tree. Post hoc analysis also showed that hypotension had the largest population-attributable risk for death and stroke. Importantly, hypotension can be related to the use of a high dose of metoprolol without dose titration.

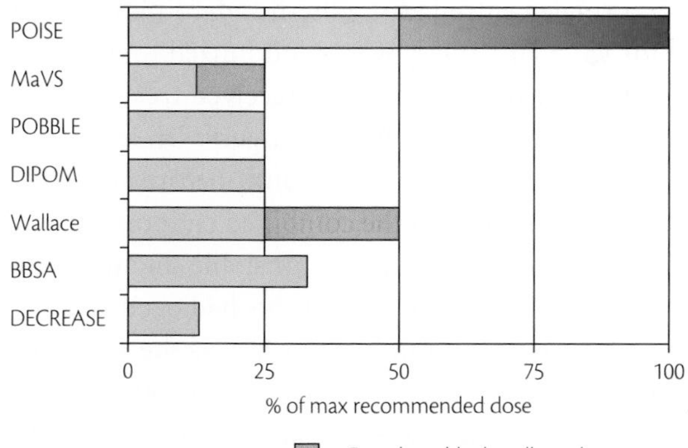

Figure 34.5 Beta-blocker trials and dosage used.

Importantly, the earlier mentioned randomized trials assessing the effect of beta-blocker use in the perioperative period differ in the population of surgical patients at risk. The MAVS trial and DIPOM trial both included many patients at low risk for complications. In the MAVS trial almost 60% had a Lee risk index of only 1. This is in contrast to the DECREASE study which randomized vascular surgery patients with a positive dobutamine echocardiography. In a large retrospective cohort study of 782,969 patients undergoing major non-cardiac surgery, a relationship between the effect of beta-blocker use and the patient risk profile was observed [123]. Beta-blocker use was associated with a significant beneficial effect in high-risk patients but showed no effect or possible harm in low-risk patients.

Other explanations regarding the divergent results of the perioperative beta-blocker studies are related to the beta-blocker treatment protocol. First, the use of a fixed versus individualized dose titrated to the patient's heart rate is of significant importance. In a study of 150 patients, Raby and colleagues assessed the heart rate threshold for myocardial ischaemia before surgery using Holter monitoring [124]. Patients with myocardial ischaemia (n = 26) were then randomized to receive intravenous esmolol titrated to aiming at tight heart rate 20% less than the ischaemic threshold but >60 beats per minute (bpm), or placebo. Of the 15 patients receiving esmolol, nine had mean heart rates below the ischaemic threshold and none experienced postoperative ischaemia. Four of 11 patients receiving placebo had a mean heart rate below the ischaemic threshold, and three of the four had no postoperative ischaemia. Together, of the 13 patients with heart rates below the ischaemic threshold, one (7.7%) had postoperative electrocardiogram myocardial ischaemia versus 12 of 13 (92%) patients with heart rates exceeding the ischaemic threshold. Feringa and colleagues found similar results in a study of 272 patients receiving beta-blocker therapy and undergoing vascular surgery [125]. In that study it was shown that higher doses of beta-blockers and lower heart rate were associated with reduced Holter monitoring-detected perioperative myocardial ischaemia (HR 2.49; 95% CI 1.79–3.48) and troponin T release (HR 1.53; 95% CI 1.16–2.03) (➲Fig. 34.6). These data suggest that monitoring of the heart rate and consequent beta-blocker dose adjustment is of critical importance for the likelihood that a patient will receive benefit

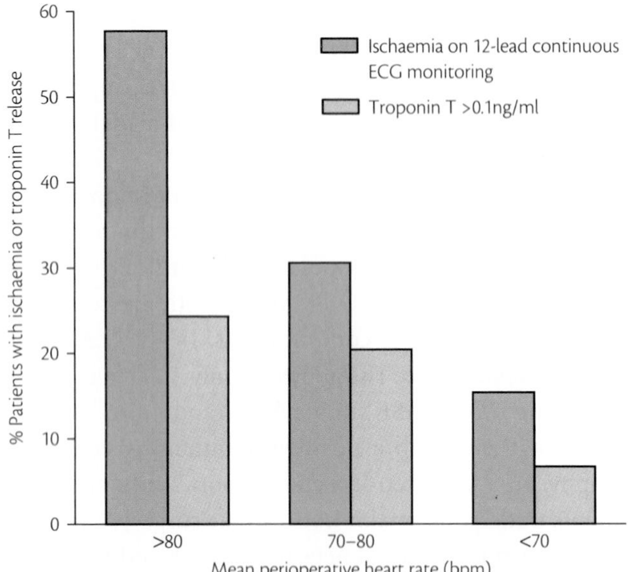

Figure 34.6 Mean heart rate in relation to myocardial ischaemia assessed by continuous electrocardiography and troponin T release. Based on data from Feringa HH, Bax JJ, Boersma E, *et al.* High-dose beta-blockers and tight heart rate control reduce myocardial ischemia and troponin T release in vascular surgery patients. *Circulation* 2006; **114** (Suppl.1): I344–I349.

of beta-blockade. Another important explanation is the variation in the starting time and duration of therapy. In contrast to the instant effect on heart rate control, the effect of beta-blockers on plaque stabilization may be achieved only after prolonged treatment. This can be argued by the pathophysiology of PMI. The DECREASE-I trial showed the largest effect of perioperative beta-blocker treatment [7]. In this trial the mean time between initiation and surgery was 37 days. In contrast, the DIPOM, POBBLE, and POISE trials started beta-blocker therapy only the day before surgery. As mentioned earlier, in the Mangano *et al.* study the benefits of atenolol were observed in the months after surgery [119]. These supposed long-term beneficial effects of beta-blockers were recently confirmed by a pooled analysis of four intravascular ultrasonography trials showing a decreased progression of coronary atherosclerosis [126].

Further, withdrawal of beta-blocker therapy shortly before surgery, or in the immediate postoperative period, might contribute to adverse myocardial effects resulting from a 'rebound' effect resulting in increased arterial blood pressure, heart rate, and plasma noradrenalin concentrations [127]. Redelmeier and colleagues have recently shown that the long-acting agent atenolol was superior to the short-acting drug, metoprolol, when given perioperatively, probably as the result of acute withdrawal effects from missed doses of short-acting beta-blockers [128].

On the other hand, care should be taken not to overtreat the patient. In the POISE study, for metoprolol succinate, a long-acting beta-blocker, the starting dose was 100mg, 2–4 hours prior to surgery, again 100mg 0–6 hours after surgery, and a dose of 200mg 12 hours after the first postoperative dose. Thereafter the daily maintenance dose was started at 200mg. Medication was withheld if blood pressure dipped below 100mmHg or heart rate was <50bpm. So, on the first day of surgery, metoprolol succinate could have been administered at a dose up to 400mg on the day of surgery, 100% of the maximum daily therapeutic dose (MDTD). In the non-surgical setting, much lower starting doses are recommended, for instance in patients with NYHA class II heart failure 12.5–25mg daily is started for 2 weeks and for hypertension the initial dose is 25–100mg, usually increased at weekly intervals.

Statins

Statins are widely prescribed in patients with or at risk for CAD because of their effectiveness in lowering serum cholesterol concentrations through 3-hydroxy-3-methylglutaryl coenzyme A reductase inhibition. Reduction of low-density lipoprotein cholesterol is one of the primary objectives of CVD prevention. Beyond the lipid-lowering effect of statins alone, evidence suggests that the more immediate benefits are related to the so-called pleiotropic effects of statins. These pleiotropic effects are thought to include improved endothelial function, enhanced stability of atherosclerotic plaques, decreased oxidative stress, and decreased vascular inflammation [129]. These effects of statins may consequently prevent plaque rupture and subsequent MI in the proinflammatory and prothrombotic environment of the perioperative period.

Two randomized controlled clinical trials have been performed to date evaluating the effect of statins in patients undergoing non-cardiac surgery, i.e. vascular surgery. Durazzo and colleagues performed the first prospective randomized controlled trial in a small population carried out at a single centre [130]. One-hundred patients scheduled for vascular surgery were randomized to either 20mg atorvastatin or placebo. Patients received treatment for 45 days and at least 2 weeks before surgery. On average, statins were prescribed around 1 month before surgery. The outcome of this trial was the combined endpoint of cardiac death, non-fatal MI, stroke, or unstable angina pectoris. After 6 months cardiovascular events had occurred in 26% of the placebo group but only in 8% of the statin group ($p = 0.03$). Though not powered to assess 30-day postoperative outcome, there was a clear trend for the beneficial effect of statins (OR 0.23; 95%CI 0.09–1.30). Lindenauer performed a large retrospective cohort study of 780,591

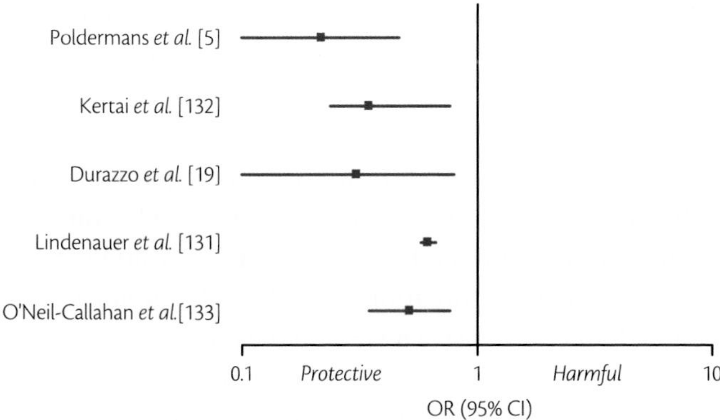

Figure 34.7 Perioperative statin therapy. Results of the effect of perioperative statin therapy in different studies.

patients undergoing major non-cardiac surgery at 329 hospitals (➲Fig. 34.7) [131]. The authors concluded that the 70,159 statin users had a 1.4-fold reduced risk of in-hospital mortality (adjusted OR 0.62; 95% CI 0.58–0.67). The meta-analysis by Hindler and colleagues including the randomized trial of Durazzo *et al.* and 6 other observational studies (n = 5373) demonstrated in the vascular surgery subgroup that preoperative statin therapy reduced the risk of short-term mortality significantly by 59% (1.7% vs. 6.1%; p <0.001) [134]. Although this confirmed the observed beneficial effect of perioperative statin therapy in large systematic reviews [134, 135], the authors concluded that evidence was insufficient to recommend routine statin treatment. The recently reported DECREASE III study is the first adequately powered randomized controlled trial which could address the role of statins in the perioperative period. This trial randomized 497 vascular surgery patients to either fluvastatin extended-release 80mg once daily or placebo [136]. The incidence of the MI in fluvastatin and placebo allocated groups respectively was 10.8% vs. 19.0% (OR 0.55; 95% CI 0.34–0.88) (➲Fig. 34.8). The incidence of the secondary, composite endpoint of cardiac death or myocardial ischaemia was 4.8% vs. 10.2% (OR 0.47; 95% CI 0.24–0.94). With respect to intermediate-risk surgical patients, the DECREASE IV trial assessed the effectiveness and safety of beta-blockers, statins, and their combination, on the incidence of perioperative cardiac death and MI. Patients randomized to fluvastatin experienced a lower incidence of the primary endpoint than those randomized to fluvastatin-control therapy (3.2% vs. 4.9% events; HR 0.65; 95% CI 0.35–1.10), but statistical significance was not reached (p = 0.17). This study was, however, limited by its lack of power.

An important issue in the perioperative setting is the use of concomitant medical treatment. The risk of myopathy might increase with concomitant drugs that are myotoxic or

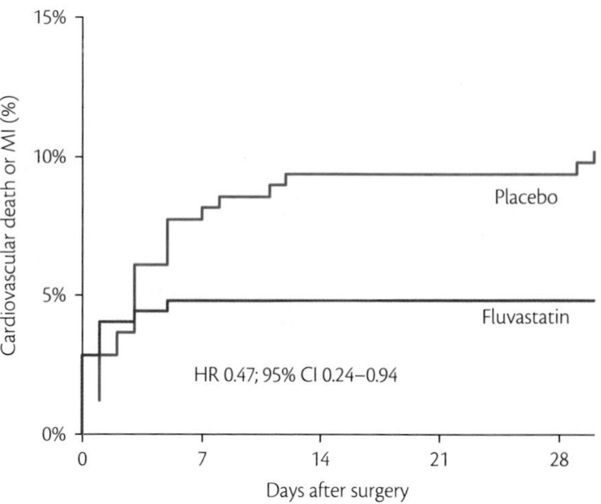

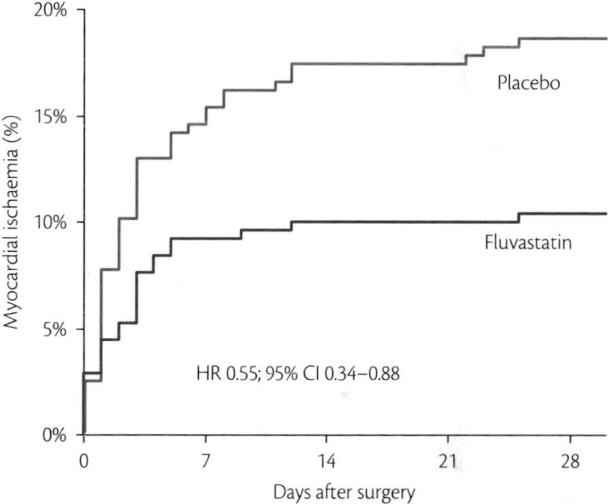

Figure 34.8 Results of the DECREASE III study. Kaplan–Meier curves of the cumulative probability of cardiovascular death or MI (top) and perioperative myocardial ischaemia (bottom). Reproduced from Schouten O, Boersma E, Hoeks S, *et al.* Fluvastatin XL use is associated with improved cardiac outcome after major vascular surgery. Results from a randomized placebo controlled trial: DECREASE III. *Eur Heart J* 2008; **29:** (Abstract suppl.) (Hotline session ESC).

increase serum statin levels. Besides concomitant medication use, numerous other factors like renal impairment in the perioperative setting might increase the risk of statin-induced myopathy. Importantly, the recent DECREASE III study also did not observe myopathy or rhabdomyolysis within 30 days after surgery (➲Table 34.2) [136]. Considering that the risk of cardiovascular complications is far greater than the risk of statin-induced myopathy and rhabdomyolysis in the perioperative period, the potential benefits of perioperative statin use seem to outweigh the potential hazards.

Another important concern is the continuation of statins in patients undergoing non-cardiac surgery. Because of the unavailability of an intravenous formula of statins and the not readily appreciated pleiotropic effects of statins, statin withdrawal is a well-known phenomenon in the immediate

Table 34.2 Safety measures of statin use (DECREASE-III study) [134]

	Placebo (n = 247)	Fluvastatin (n = 250)	p-value
Discontinuation: no. (%)	18 (7.3)	16 (6.4)	0.73
CK >10 × ULN: no. (%)	8 (3.2)	10 (4.0)	0.81
CK (U/L): median no.	113	141	0.24
ALAT >3 × ULN: no. (%)	13 (5.3)	8 (3.2)	0.27
ALAT (U/L): median no.	23	24	0.43
Myopathy: no. (%)	–	–	
Rhabdomyolysis: no. (%)	–	–	

ALAT, alanine aminotransferase; CK, creatine kinase; no., number of patients; ULN, upper limit of normal.

Reproduced from Schouten O, Boersma E, Hoeks S, *et al.* Fluvastatin XL use is associated with improved cardiac outcome after major vascular surgery. Results from a randomized placebo controlled trial: DECREASE III. *Eur Heart J* 2008; **29:** (Abstract suppl.) (Hotline session ESC).

postoperative period. From patients with CAD it is known that sudden withdrawal of statin therapy can be harmful [138, 139]. Recently, it has been demonstrated in vascular surgery patients that statin discontinuation was associated with an increased risk for postoperative troponin release (HR 4.6; 95% CI 2.2–9.6) and the combination of MI and cardiovascular death (HR 7.5; 95% CI 2.8–0.1) [140]. This increased postoperative risk associated with the withdrawal of statins was also observed by Le Manach and colleagues [13]. However, in one out of four patients included in the DECREASE III trial, statins had to be interrupted for a median of 2 days after surgery, but this did not result in a significant increase in adverse outcome (adjusted OR 1.1; 95% CI 0.48–2.52) [136]. These findings suggest that statins with a prolonged half-life time or with an extended-release formula should be preferred and that statins should be restarted after surgery as soon as possible.

Antiplatelet therapy

Acetylsalicylic acid (ASA) is one of the cornerstones in the primary and secondary prevention of CVDs. Furthermore, dual antiplatelet therapy, and the combination of ASA and clopidogrel, has proven to be effective for the prevention of stent thrombosis. The evidence of ASA in the perioperative period in patients undergoing non-cardiac surgery is less clear. Trials of patients undergoing carotid surgery showed some evidence in favour of ASA, although the evidence was inconclusive for all endpoints [141, 142]. The meta-analysis of Robless and colleagues in 2001 demonstrated a reduction of serious vascular events and vascular death in patients with peripheral vascular disease [143]. This study included ten trials of antiplatelet treatment in lower limb bypass surgery of which six involved ASA treatment. However, the benefit of antiplatelet therapy did not reach statistical significance for the combined endpoint of vascular events (OR 0.76; 95% CI 0.54–1.05) in this vascular surgery population.

An important issue is how to manage patients with antiplatelet therapy in the perioperative period. Concerns of promoting perioperative haemorrhagic complications often withheld continuation of ASA in the perioperative period. In their extensive review on the impact of antiplatelet therapy on perioperative bleeding complications, Harder and colleagues concluded that monotherapy with aspirin or clopidogrel alone usually does not have to be discontinued in the perioperative period [144]. This conclusion was confirmed in the meta-analysis of Burger and colleagues [145]. In 41 studies, including a total of 49,590 patients undergoing a variety of non-cardiac surgical procedures (14,981 on perioperative aspirin and 34,609 not on aspirin), they found that aspirin continuation led to a 1.5 times increased risk of bleeding complication, but not to a higher level of the severity of bleeding complications. They concluded that based on their meta-analysis aspirin should only be discontinued perioperatively if 'bleeding risks with increased mortality or sequels are comparable with the observed cardiovascular risks after aspirin withdrawal'.

Revascularization

Prophylactic coronary revascularization

Preoperative cardiac risk evaluation by means of risk factor assessment and non-invasive testing may often identify patients at increased cardiac risk. Importantly, the number of patients with CAD undergoing non-cardiac surgery is steadily increasing. These patients may either have documented symptomatic involvement or be fully asymptomatic. Furthermore, they may present with a life-threatening condition requiring immediate non-cardiac surgery or have a need for an elective intervention in which case a full cardiac work-up can be planned if indicated. Faced with a medical emergency, there is no other choice than to proceed with surgery and to postpone cardiac evaluation until afterwards. If not, the need for diagnostic evaluation and subsequent revascularization will have to be questioned, in particular in those patients requiring surgery within weeks or a few months. After the presence of severe CAD is confirmed by angiography, coronary revascularization via percutaneous coronary intervention (PCI) or CABG can be considered as prophylactic therapy in these patients prior to non-cardiac surgery.

The main goal of preoperative coronary revascularization is the prevention of the occurrence of PMI in patients with significant CAD scheduled for non-cardiac surgery. The cumulative risk of prophylactic coronary revascularization and non-cardiac surgery needs to be weighted against the risk of the surgical procedure performed without preoperative interventions.

In recent years two conducted randomized controlled trials have shed some light on the controversial role of prophylactic revascularization prior to non-cardiac surgery. Former evidence was based on small-scale observational studies and expert opinions [146–148]. The Coronary Artery Revascularization Prophylaxis (CARP) trial conducted by McFalls and colleagues was the first randomized trial that investigated the benefit of coronary revascularization before elective major vascular surgery [149]. Of 5859 screened patients at 18 Veterans Affairs US hospitals, 510 patients with significant artery stenosis were randomized to either revascularization or no revascularization before surgery. The main finding of this study was that there was no difference in the primary outcome of long-term mortality (median follow-up 2.7 years) in patients who underwent preoperative coronary revascularization compared to patients who received optimized medical therapy (22% vs. 23%; RR 0.98; 95% CI 0.70–1.37). The corresponding Kaplan–Meier curve is shown in ➲Fig. 34.9. Although the study was not powered to test the short-term benefit of prophylactic revascularization, no reduction in the number of MIs, deaths, or length of hospital stay was observed within 30 days after vascular surgery. The results of this trial suggest that prophylactic revascularization might not provide additional benefit in reducing the incidence of perioperative and long-term cardiac morbidity and mortality in cardiac stable, elective vascular surgery patients. The generalizability of this trial to patients with multivessel disease has, however, been questioned because the majority of the patients in the CARP trial had only one- or two-vessel disease. To address this issue, the CARP investigators recently studied the long-term outcome of all screened patients (randomized + registry) who underwent coronary angiography before vascular surgery from the original population [150]. Of the total 1048 patients who underwent a preoperative coronary angiography before their vascular operation, multivessel CAD without previous CABG was present in 382 (36.5%). In line with the results of the randomized CARP results, no long-term survival benefit was observed in patients with two- and three-vessel disease. In contrast, in the cohort of 48 patients (4.6%) with left main coronary artery stenosis, patients who had undergone preoperative revascularization did seem to have an improved 2.5-year survival (84% vs. 52%) (➲Fig. 34.10).

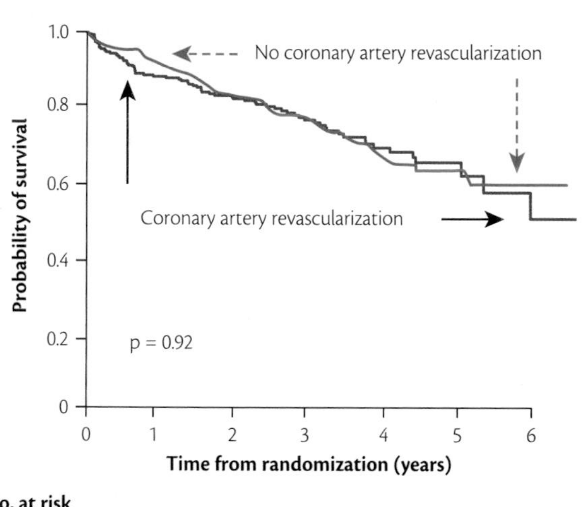

Figure 34.9 Results of the CARP study: long-term survival among patients assigned to undergo coronary-artery revascularization or no revascularization. Reproduced with permission from McFalls EO, Ward HB, Moritz TE, *et al.* Coronary-artery revascularization before elective major vascular surgery. *N Engl J Med* 2004; **351**: 2795–804.

In a recent study evaluating vascular surgery patients with predominantly three-vessel disease similar findings were obtained [151]. Cardiac-stable, elective vascular surgery patients were screened for risk factors, and those with three or more clinical risk factors (age >70 years, MI, angina pectoris, congestive heart failure, diabetes mellitus, renal failure, and cerebrovascular events) underwent cardiac stress testing. All patients with extensive stress-induced ischaemia were randomly assigned for additional revascularization. All patients received optimized medical therapy including beta-blockers aiming at a heart rate of 60–65bpm and continued antiplatelet therapy. Of 430 high-risk patients, 101 (23%) showed extensive ischaemia and were randomly assigned to revascularization (n = 49) or no-revascularization (n = 52). Coronary angiography showed two-vessel disease in 12 (24%), three-vessel disease in 33 (67%), and left main disease in four (8%). This study population reflects the patients at highest cardiac risk in the perioperative period. Revascularization did not improve perioperative outcome, the incidence of cardiac death and MI was 43 vs. 33% (OR 1.4; 95% CI 0.7–2.8; p = 0.30). Also no benefit during 1-year follow-up was observed after coronary revascularization, 49 vs. 44% (OR 1.2; 95% CI 0.7–2.3; p = 0.48) (➲Fig. 34.11).

To summarize, both randomized trials hint that prophylactic coronary revascularization of cardiac stable patients provides no benefit for postoperative outcome. Although limited by the small patient number and its observational nature, the CARP trial indicates that prophylactic coronary revascularization seems to be only beneficial in patients with left main coronary artery stenosis. No trials exist

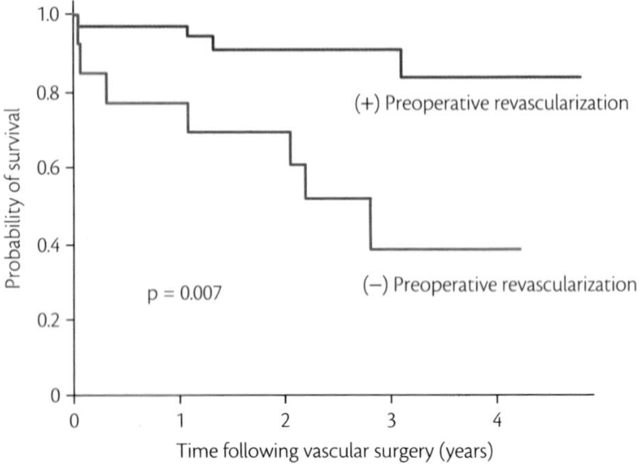

Figure 34.10 Kaplan–Meier survival curve according to preoperative coronary artery revascularization for patients with unprotected left main coronary artery stenoses. Reproduced from Garcia S, Moritz TE, Ward HB, *et al.* Usefulness of revascularization of patients with multivessel coronary artery disease before elective vascular surgery for abdominal aortic and peripheral occlusive disease. *Am J Cardiol* 2008; **102:** 809–13. Copyright 2008, with permission from Elsevier.

investigating the role of prophylactic revascularization in patients with unstable angina pectoris requiring non-cardiac surgery. If non-cardiac surgery can be postponed safely, diagnosis and treatment for these patients should be in line with the recent guidelines on unstable angina management [112].

The reasoning behind the apparent lack of benefit of prophylactic revascularization is not fully understood. It could likely be related to the fact that patients with stress-induced ischaemia not only suffer from a blood flow-limiting coronary lesion but also from (multiple) non-significant lesions which are vulnerable to rupture due to the stress of surgery. The perioperative stress response, which includes a cytokine response, catecholamine surge with associated haemodynamic stress, vasospasm, reduced fibrinolytic activity, platelet activation, and consequent hypercoagulability triggers coronary plaque rupture, leading to thrombus formation and subsequent vessel occlusion. Importantly, as discussed earlier, autopsy reports have shown that half of the cases of PMI have coronary plaque rupture as the underlying pathophysiologic mechanism. This also explains the lack of specificity of stress echocardiography or nuclear imaging techniques in predicting infarct-related coronary artery lesions [152, 153]. Surgical or percutaneous treatment of the culprit coronary lesion(s) apparently provides insufficient extra protection on top of medical treatment for rupture of these unstable lesions.

Previous coronary revascularization

Another important clinical situation is the management of patients with previous coronary stenting undergoing non-cardiac surgery [154]. The risk of perioperative stent thrombosis in these patients is increased by the non-cardiac surgical procedure, especially when surgery is performed early after stent implantation and particularly if dual antiplatelet therapy is discontinued. When possible, delaying surgery is advised until after the time window that requires dual antiplatelet therapy.

In the early days of angioplasty, it seemed that conventional percutaneous transluminal coronary angioplasty (PTCA) did not worsen outcomes after surgery even if performed as early as 11 days after PTCA [155]. However, the introduction of stenting accompanied with frequent occurrence of acute stent thrombosis directed physicians to postpone elective surgery up to 3 months after bare metal stent placement [156]. Thrombosis of a stent is associated with major morbidity and mortality. Dual antiplatelet therapy during the period of stent endothelization effectively reduces the risk of stent thrombosis to <1% and is therefore recommended. An important issue is the timing of the non-cardiac surgical procedure after PCI. A recent large study of

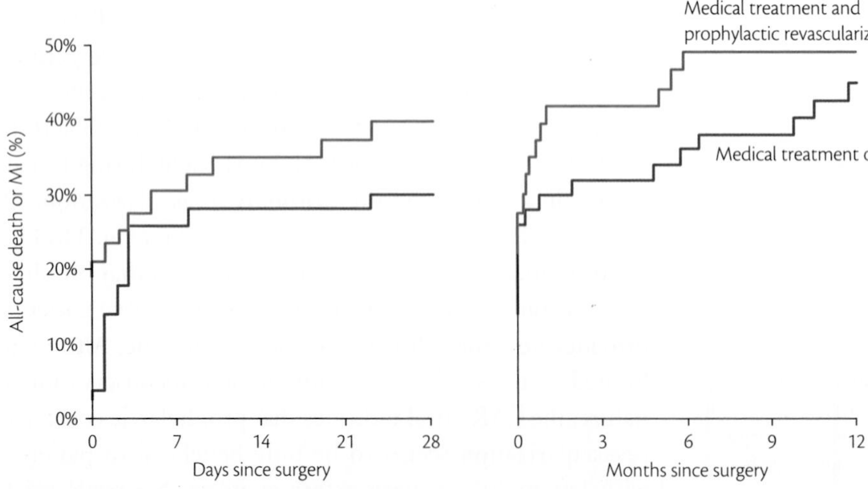

Figure 34.11 Results of the DECREASE V trial. Kaplan–Meier curves of the cumulative probability of all-cause death or MI during 1 year of follow-up according to the allocated strategy in patients with three or more cardiac risk factors with extensive stress-induced ischaemia. Reproduced from Poldermans D, Schouten O, Vidakovic R, *et al.* A clinical randomized trial to evaluate the safety of a non-invasive approach in high-risk patients undergoing major vascular surgery: the DECREASE-V Pilot Study. *J Am Coll* Cardiol 2007; **49:** 1763–9. Copyright 2007 with permission from the American College of Cardiology.

899 patients demonstrated a clear association between the duration of time between PCI and non-cardiac surgery and ischaemic cardiac events [157]. The incidence of major cardiovascular events was lowest (2.8%) if non-cardiac surgery was performed at least 90 days after PCI with bare metal stent. Bleeding events were not associated with duration of time between PCI and non-cardiac surgery.

In 2002, drug-eluting stents were introduced in Europe to further reduce in-stent restenosis. The use of these stents has grown exponentially over the last few years. However, their major drawback is the need for prolonged dual antiplatelet therapy by aspirin and clopidogrel from 3 up to 12 months. It is now generally accepted that after drug-eluting stent placement elective surgery should not take place before 12 months [158].

Conclusion

Patients undergoing non-cardiac surgery have an increased risk of cardiovascular perioperative morbidity and mortality. Preoperative management aims at optimizing the patient's condition by identification and modification of underlying cardiac risk factors and diseases. Systemic medical therapy with beta-blockers and statins is currently one of the cornerstones of individualized perioperative management.

Personal perspective

Preoperative cardiac risk evaluation currently aims to stratify patients into three main categories; patients at low risk in whom additional testing and medical therapy are redundant, and can be send for surgery safely without delay; patients in whom the risk of surgery clearly outweighs the potential benefit of the procedure; and patients in whom medical therapy and/or coronary revascularization reduces the potential risk significantly and can be send for surgery afterwards. Commonly, in the latter group, non-invasive cardiac testing is performed after an initial screening with common clinical cardiac risk markers and biomarkers such as high-sensitive C-reactive protein or NT-proBNP. Medical therapy has been shown to improve postoperative outcome in patients with CAD and heart failure, similar to the non-surgical setting. The question to be answered will be: is therapy safe to be initiated prior to surgery? Statin therapy seems to fulfil this criterion. It is safe and effective. However, a potential problem is the lack of intravenous formula. This might induce effects of statin withdrawal in those patients who cannot take oral medication after surgery. Long-acting statins or the development of statins for rectal administration might be alternatives. Beta-blockers are still controversial. Although proven to be effective in the non-surgical setting in patients with heart failure and CAD, safety issues such as hypotension and bradycardia leading to stroke are a potential problem. The use of low-dose regimens with careful up-titration and intraoperative use of ultra-short-acting beta-blockers are currently recommended. Additional randomized clinical trials including sufficient number of patients are warranted to prove the safety and efficacy of these treatment regimens.

The more widespread use of perioperative cardioprotective medication will reduce the indication for additional preoperative non-invasive cardiac testing, as outcome is improved and coronary revascularization as a consequence of test results is unlikely to improve postoperative outcome further. For instance, in patients in whom the risk can be reduced to <2%, coronary revascularization with its procedure-related morbidity and mortality, is unlikely to be of additional benefit. Moreover, the introduction of coronary stents in patients treated with a percutaneous coronary intervention necessitates use of antiplatelet therapy early after stent placement with the risk of perioperative surgical bleeding, while early interruption might lead to in-stent thrombosis.

Most of medical therapies and interventions have focused on restoration of the oxygen demand/supply mismatch in patients with CAD. However, coronary plaque instability due to the stress of surgery has become an important topic. Currently, non-specific anti-inflammatory medication such as aspirin and statins are considered. However, potentially interesting is the use of selective immunomodulation in patients at risk. The lessons we have learned from differences in outcome of perioperative beta-blocker trials highlight the importance of careful evaluation and understanding of the complex changes that occur during surgery with respect to haemodynamic changes by endogenous catecholamine surge and anaesthetic therapies. Although there seems to be a trend towards less non-invasive testing, it should be considered that testing also serves additional purposes such as patient counselling about postoperative outcome, choice of anaesthesia technique, and the consideration of alternative surgical procedures in high-risk patients.

Further reading

ESC guidelines on perioperative care. *Eur Heart J* 2009, in press.

Hertzer NR, Beven EG, Young JR, *et al.* Coronary artery disease in peripheral vascular patients. A classification of 1000 coronary angiograms and results of surgical management. *Ann Surg* 1984; **199**: 223–33.

Fleisher LA, Beckman JA, Brown KA, *et al.* ACC/AHA 2007 Guidelines on Perioperative Cardiovascular Evaluation and Care for Non-cardiac Surgery: Executive Summary: A Report of the American College of Cardiology/American Heart Association Task Force on Practice Guidelines (Writing Committee to Revise the 2002 Guidelines on Perioperative Cardiovascular Evaluation for Non-cardiac Surgery). Developed in Collaboration With the American Society of Echocardiography, American Society of Nuclear Cardiology, Heart Rhythm Society, Society of Cardiovascular Anesthesiologists, Society for Cardiovascular Angiography and Interventions, Society for Vascular Medicine and Biology, and Society for Vascular Surgery. *J Am Coll Cardiol* 2007; **50**: 1707–32.

McFalls EO, Ward HB, Moritz TE, *et al.* Coronary-artery revascularization before elective major vascular surgery. *N Engl J Med* 2004; **351**: 2795–804.

Poldermans D, Hoeks SE, Feringa HH. Pre-operative risk assessment and risk reduction before surgery. *J Am Coll Cardiol* 2008; **51**: 1913–24.

Rabbitts JA, Nuttall GA, Brown MJ, *et al.* Cardiac risk of non-cardiac surgery after percutaneous coronary intervention with drug-eluting stents. *Anesthesiology* 2008; **109**: 596–604.

Schouten O, Boersma E, Hoeks S, *et al.* Fluvastatin XL use is associated with improved cardiac outcome after major vascular surgery. Results from a randomized placebo controlled trial: DECREASE III. *Eur Heart J* 2008; **29:** (Abstract suppl.) (Hotline session ESC).

➲ For full references and multimedia materials please visit the online version of the book (http://esctextbook.oxfordonline.com).

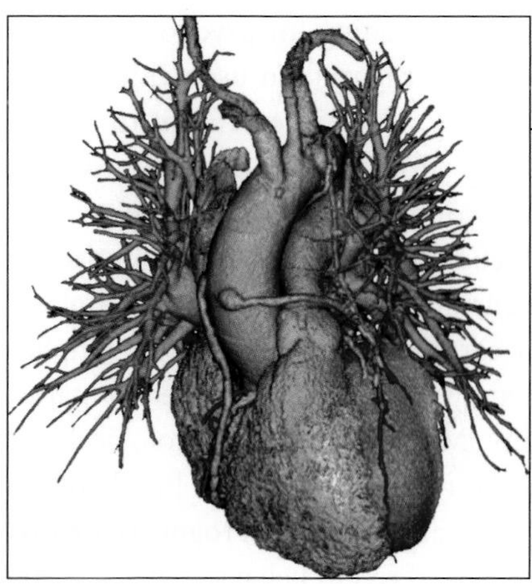

CHAPTER 35

Psychological Factors and Heart Disease

Susanne S. Pedersen, Nina Kupper, and Johan Denollet

Contents

Summary

Patients diagnosed with heart disease often experience emotional distress due to the life-threatening nature of their disease and are faced with functional impairments that may influence quality of life. In turn, these psychological manifestations interfere with adherence to treatment and increase the risk for mortality and morbidity. The risk incurred by psychological factors is of equal magnitude to that of standard risk factors, including somatic indicators of disease severity, such as left ventricular dysfunction.

This chapter focuses on the psychological impact of heart disease and consequences of psychological manifestations for prognosis, with emphasis on depression, anxiety, social isolation, health status, and Type D personality. Mechanisms, both biological and behavioural, that may be responsible for the link between psychological factors and cardiac prognosis are discussed. Results of recent behavioural and pharmacological intervention trials targeting psychological factors are also presented.

In order to enhance secondary prevention in patients with established heart disease, patients should be screened for psychological risk factors in clinical practice. When seeing patients, it is important that cardiologists take the time to listen carefully to patients, use clear and succinct communication, and make specific and simple recommendations. Time should also be allocated to follow-up patient adherence with medication and lifestyle changes. Patients with psychological comorbidity may need to be referred to healthcare professionals that are specialists in the area of psychological management, as they may require more intensive monitoring and treatment of a behavioural and psychological nature.

Introduction

In 2003, behavioural and psychological factors were introduced for the first time in the official European guidelines on cardiovascular disease (CVD) prevention [1, 2]. In 2004, the landmark case–control INTERHEART study, based on 15,152 myocardial infarction (MI) patients and 14,820 controls recruited from 52 countries, helped further cement their role in heart disease, as psychological factors were shown to incur a twofold increased risk of incident MI independent of standard risk factors [3]. The European guidelines on CVD prevention (➲Chapter 12) have since been updated, with psychological factors as potential risk factors in heart disease having earned a solid place in the guidelines [4].

Research into psychological factors in the context of heart disease has grown considerably in the last decades, with increasing recognition that a patient's psychological profile not only plays a major role in the adaptation to the disease, but also impacts on mortality, morbidity, and quality of life [4–6]. Psychological factors also impede adaptation of lifestyle changes, moderate treatment outcomes, and serve as obstacles for treatment adherence—including participation in cardiac rehabilitation (CR) (➲Chapter 25) [4]. Importantly, psychological risk factors tend to cluster together within individuals, with patients with several psychological risk factors having an increased risk of poor health outcomes [6, 7]. Therefore, psychological risk factors should be studied in concert rather than using a 'risk factor of the month' approach. In this regard, personality traits play an important role as determinants of substantial individual differences in vulnerability to psychological risk factors.

Another important issue is how and through which pathways psychological factors may exert their deleterious effect on health outcomes. Although accumulating evidence suggests a number of physiological and behavioural pathways that may explain the association between psychological factors and CVD, there are still many unanswered questions. This may in part be attributed to the complex relationships between psychological factors and heart disease, as many different bodily systems and pathways are involved. It is important to increase our knowledge of these pathways as well as factors that may moderate the effect of psychological risk factors on health outcomes. This may help to optimize secondary prevention trials that target psychological risk factors.

In terms of managing and treating psychological risk factors, some information is available from pharmacological, behavioural, and stress management trials. Nevertheless, there still remain several unresolved issues, including: the optimal time point(s) for screening for psychological factors; which screening instrument(s) to use; which treatment to choose; the timing of the intervention to reduce the impact of psychological factors on health outcomes; and which intervention works best for which patient.

This chapter will focus on the psychological impact of heart disease and the ensuing consequences of psychological manifestations for cardiovascular health, with emphasis on depression, anxiety, social isolation, health status, and Type D personality. Mechanisms, both biological and behavioural, that may be responsible for the link between psychological factors and cardiovascular prognosis are discussed together with results of recent behavioural and pharmacological intervention trials that target psychological risk factors. Suggestions are provided as to how clinicians may identify and help patients who have a psychological profile that may increase their risk of adverse cardiovascular health.

Psychological impact of heart disease

The diagnosis and treatment of CVD may have a major psychological impact. This has been documented in patients with coronary artery disease (CAD) (➲Chapter 16 and 17), chronic heart failure (CHF) (➲Chapter 23), and peripheral arterial disease (PAD) (➲Chapter 36), and in the context of invasive cardiac treatment, including percutaneous coronary intervention (PCI) (➲Chapter 16), coronary artery bypass graft surgery (CABG) (➲Chapter 17), heart transplantation, and implantable cardioverter defibrillator (ICD) therapy (➲Chapter 30). Importantly, there are large individual differences in the manifestation of psychological distress and poor health status.

Depression

Depression is one of the most studied psychological factors in CVD [5, 8, 9]. Clinical depression is characterized by the presence of a depressed mood or markedly decreased interest in daily activities (persisting for at least 2 weeks), in combination with at least four of the following additional symptoms: unintentional changes in weight, sleep problems, fatigue, psychomotor retardation or agitation, feelings of guilt or worthlessness, problems concentrating, and suicidal thoughts [10]. Apart from clinical depression as a psychiatric disorder, patients may also experience symptoms of depression without crossing the threshold for depressive disorder. However, typical symptoms of depression such as sadness and guilt are not frequently reported by cardiac patients; rather, they may complain of atypical symptoms like worries or feelings of malaise [11].

The prevalence of clinical depression in CAD is higher than in the general population, ranging between 15–25% [12], and is estimated to be slightly higher (i.e. 30%) for depressive symptoms [13]. Depression is also a common issue in patients with CHF [14]. While depression may be a reactive, transient phenomenon in some patients, it may be more persistent in others. Both standardized interviews and self-report questionnaires can be used to assess depressive disorder and symptoms of depression, respectively [15]. However, two recent reports have formulated opposite recommendations regarding depression screening: one recommends routine screening for depression in patients with CAD [5], whereas the other concludes that there is little evidence to indicate that depression screening would improve cardiovascular outcomes [8].

Apart from depression, vital exhaustion is a related construct that is characterized by feelings of fatigue, irritability, and demoralization, and which may also be associated with adverse clinical outcomes [16]. Within the broad spectrum of depressive symptoms, clinicians should also be aware of the role of specific depressive symptoms, such as feelings of hopelessness [17] and anhedonia, or the relative absence of positive mood states [18]. Both these specific symptoms may impact negatively on cardiovascular health [17, 18].

Recent evidence suggests that depression does not involve a homogeneous diagnostic category in cardiovascular patients, but may comprise distinctly different subtypes. Suggestions have also been made that some manifestations of depression may actually reflect the severity of cardiac disease [19]. Further, recent studies failed to find a relationship between depression and prognosis following MI [20], or found that this relationship may be limited to first-ever depression [21] and somatic symptoms of depression [19], but not to recurrent depression or affective depression symptoms. Depression, as well as CHF, is associated with symptoms of fatigue and malaise, and this overlap in symptoms represents an extra diagnostic challenge. Finally, there is some evidence to suggest that depression in post-MI patients is not accompanied by the distorted depressive cognitions that are typical of psychiatric depressive disorder [22]. As will be discussed later in this chapter, depression does have biological and behavioural effects, such as increased blood platelet reactivity, decreased heart rate variability, and poor adherence to treatment, which may have an adverse effect on prognosis.

Anxiety

In contrast to depression, anxiety in cardiac patients is frequently under-recognized and ignored by healthcare providers [23–26]. Anxiety is a negative emotion that occurs in response to perceived threats and is characterized by a perceived inability to predict or control the threatening situation [23]. Anxious patients are more likely to perceive upcoming situations as threatening, and may fear that they will not be able to control these situations. Although anxiety is a normal reaction to an acute cardiac event and prompts an individual to seek appropriate medical care, persistent anxiety has adverse consequences, including difficulty adhering to treatment [23], and an increase in cardiac symptoms [24]. Anxiety and depression tend to co-occur in post-MI patients [11, 15, 24, 27, 28], and screening for anxiety may help to identify patients at risk for post-MI depression [11].

Anxiety is common among cardiac patients; its prevalence ranges between 70–80% in patients who have experienced an acute cardiac event, and between 20–25% in cardiac patients with persistent anxiety over the long term [23]. More than 30% of patients experience anxiety following an MI [24], and anxiety is also a common negative emotional condition in patients with CHF [14], and in patients treated with ICD therapy [26].

There is some evidence to suggest that the anxious apprehension of some cardiovascular patients may result in physiological arousal and an associated increase in cardiac risk. In patients who survive an acute coronary event (➲Chapter 16), anxiety has been associated with increased in-hospital complications, such as arrhythmias and continued myocardial ischaemia [29], and with rehospitalizations and outpatient visits to cardiologists after discharge from the hospital [25].

Other factors

Panic disorder

Panic disorder is a more specific manifestation of anxiety, and qualifies as a form of mental disorder that is associated with periods of intense anxiety. One study found that panic disorder was prevalent in 9% of outpatients with CHF [30], while another study showed that as many as 38% of patients referred to an outpatient chest pain clinic suffered from panic disorder [31]. Female patients and patients with a lower level of education may be at increased risk of comorbid panic disorder [30, 31]. Panic disorder has a significant adverse effect on quality of life in patients with CHF, also after adjustment for age, gender, and New York Heart Association (NYHA) functional class [30, 31]. After long-term follow-up, panic has also been associated with more chest pain intensity and psychological distress [31].

Post-traumatic stress disorder

Cardiac patients may be prone to develop post-traumatic stress disorder (PTSD). A cardiac event is potentially life threatening and likely involves a psychological response that is characterized by hyperarousal, fear and helplessness, which, together with symptoms of intrusion and avoidance, provide sufficient criteria to qualify for a diagnosis [32]. Not surprisingly, PTSD may evolve in the aftermath of an acute cardiac event such as MI or cardiac arrest [33, 34]. However, a chronic cardiac condition, such as CHF, may also qualify as traumatic because it may incur a *continuous* risk of sudden death, thereby constituting a *chronic* traumatic stressor. Further, treatment with an ICD may also be psychologically traumatic [35]. The prevalence rate of PTSD ranges between 8–32% in patients with MI, 5–38% in survivors of sudden cardiac arrest, and 8–18% following cardiac surgery [32].

Often, these patients experience intrusive and avoidant symptoms, as well as physiological hyperarousal. In fact, sympathetic hyperactivity and reduced parasympathetic cardiac control are hallmarks of PTSD, thus linking PTSD to atherosclerotic progression [32]. Avoidance behaviour, which is a common feature in PTSD, may also induce non-adherence to medication, because ingestion of medication may serve as a reminder of the traumatic cardiac event [36]. This non-adherence to medication, in turn, may increase the risk of adverse clinical events in cardiac patients with comorbid PTSD. Therefore, it is unfortunate that PTSD is generally overlooked in these patients [35].

Social isolation

Social factors that may affect a patient's psychological status include size and frequency of everyday contacts (social networks), the existence and type of relationships (social relationships), and the quality of support provided by others (social support) [37]. Lack of supportive social networks and relationships may lead to social isolation. Several years ago, Ruberman and colleagues noted the potential importance of social isolation for the clinical course of post-MI patients [38].

Social inhibition (the tendency to inhibit self-expression in social interaction) and social avoidance (the tendency to avoid social contact) are personality traits that may predispose to social isolation. Both traits have been linked to an increased cardiovascular risk [39, 40]. The notion that social isolation may have an adverse effect in patients with CAD is supported by animal [41] and human [42] research showing that isolation is associated with increased physiological stress reactivity. Of note, CR may provide an opportunity to offer social interaction and peer support to socially isolated patients [37].

Health status

Health status refers to the impact of disease on patient functioning, as reported by the patient [43]. Given that health status involves a range of manifestations of disease including symptoms, functional limitations, and (discrepancies between actual and desired) quality of life, health status is often used as a patient-centred outcome [44, 45]. Since there is a large discrepancy between physician-rated and patient-rated symptom burden and functional status, physicians need to rely on standardized health status measures in order to accurately estimate patients' health status [43, 46]. An example of a frequently used generic measure is the Short Form Health Survey 36 (SF-36; a measure of overall physical and mental health status) [47]. The Seattle Angina Questionnaire (SAQ), the Kansas City Cardiomyopathy Questionnaire (KCCQ), and the Minnesota Living with Heart Failure Questionnaire (MLHFQ) comprise examples of frequently used disease-specific measures of health status in CAD (SAQ) and CHF (KCCQ, MLHFQ) patients [44, 48].

Standardized assessment of health status has been proposed as a complementary to current cardiac assessment as a means of improving the quality of care of patients [43, 49]. Importantly, health status measures are not merely surrogate markers for standard cardiac diagnostic assessments, but rather comprise important tools for monitoring patients in routine clinical practice, examining outcomes in clinical trials, and, eventually, a means by which to improve medical decision making [44, 50].

The patient-report of subjectively experienced physical and mental health is not only a function of the limitations incurred by the severity of cardiac disorder, but is also closely related to the patient's psychological status. Hence, not surprisingly, depression has been associated with poor health status in cardiac patients [51, 52]. In 2005, the Working Group on Outcomes Research in Cardiovascular Disease of the National Heart, Lung, and Blood Institute in the US stated that the first goal in promoting 'patient-centred' care is to identify determinants of health status [45]. With reference to this issue, the personality of the patient is a major determinant of large individual differences in health status and psychological distress. This will be discussed in more detail in the following sections.

Type D personality

Patients differ substantially in their vulnerability to psychological distress following a cardiovascular event, and personality traits may account for a large part of these individual differences in physical and mental health status. Across the years, various personality traits have been studied in relation to the risk of physical illness [53]. With reference to CVD, research initially focused on the type A behaviour pattern (characterized by time urgency and hostility), but due to mixed findings on type A research it became outdated to study personality types [54]. In the aftermath of type A research, studies on the role of personality mainly focused on specific traits such as hostility [55]. However, with the introduction of the *distressed* personality or *Type D* personality [56] in recent years, there is now a renewed interest in the role of personality [54, 57].

Type D personality construct

Type D personality is defined as the combination of two normal and stable personality traits, with Type D patients characterized by an elevated score on both negative affectivity (tendency to experience negative emotions) and social inhibition (tendency to inhibit self-expression) at the same time (➲Table 35.1). These Type D traits can be assessed with the standardized and validated 14-item Type D Scale (DS14) that consists of seven items measuring negative affectivity (e.g. 'I often feel unhappy') and seven items measuring social inhibition (e.g. 'I am a closed kind of person') [58]. The DS14 is presented in the section on clinical implications (see ➲Table 35.9). Patients with a Type D personality have a score of ≥10 on both traits; they tend to experience increased negative emotions, such as worrying, feeling down in the dumps, and being irritable, while at the same time not sharing these emotions with others due to fear of negative reactions.

The prevalence of Type D ranges from 25–33% across different types of CVDs, including CAD, CHF, PAD, heart transplantation recipients, and patients with life-threatening arrhythmias treated with ICD therapy [59].

Table 35.1 Definition of Type D personality

	Personality trait	
	Negative affectivity	**Social inhibition**
Definition	Tendency to experience negative emotions across time/situations	Tendency to inhibit emotions and behaviours in social interaction
Profile	Often feels unhappy, pessimistic; tends to worry, easily irritated; symptoms of depression and anxiety	Feels insecure in social interaction; tends to be closed and reserved; avoids criticism from others
Assessment	Score ≥10 on the Negative Affectivity subscale of the DS14	Score ≥10 on the Social Inhibition subscale of the DS14
Criteria	Patients who have an elevated score on both negative affectivity as well as social inhibition are classified as having a Type D personality	

Differences between Type D and depression

Type D personality is conceptually different from depression and other measures of negative affect, despite some overlap [59, 60]. The most distinctive features of Type D compared with other measures of negative affect comprise its chronicity, and that social inhibition is embedded within the Type D construct. In other words, the construct also stipulates how patients cope with their negative emotions, that is, that they do not disclose their emotions, whereas this is not contained within depression [58, 59]. In a substudy of the Myocardial INfarction and Depression–Intervention Trial (MIND-IT), 206 out of 1205 post-MI patients (17%) met criteria for depressive disorder, while 224 (19%) had a Type D personality. Of note, only one out of four distressed patients displayed both depression and Type D personality, but as many as 74% displayed one form of distress—depression or Type D—but not the other (➲Fig. 35.1).

Impact of Type D on depression, anxiety, and health status

Psychological risk factors often cluster together within individuals [6], and the Type D construct was specifically designed to identify patients who are at risk of this clustering of risk factors. Accordingly, patients with a Type D

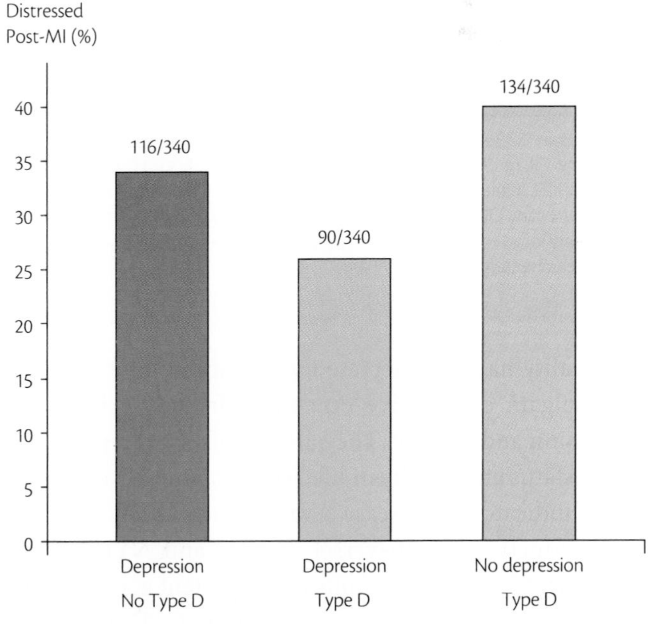

Depression: patients who met ICD-10 criteria for major or minor depressive disorder; Type D: patients with a Type D personality

Figure 35.1 Percentage of distressed post-myocardial infarction patients (n = 340), stratified by depressive disorder and Type D personality. Reproduced from Denollet J, de Jonge P, Kuyper A, *et al.* Depression and Type D personality represent different forms of distress in the Myocardial INfarction and Depression–Intervention Trial (MIND-IT). *Psychol Med* 2009; **39**: 749–56. Copyright (2008), with permission from Cambridge University Press.

Table 35.2 Type D personality and increased risk of poor health status

Authors	Patients	Study design	Adjusted risk
Ischaemic heart disease			
Al-Ruzzeh *et al.* [62]	437 CABG	Cross-sectional	ORs: 2.3–5.5
Denollet *et al.* [63]	319 CAD	Prospective	OR: 2.2
Pedersen *et al.* [70]	692 PCI/SES	Prospective	ORs 1.60–3.99; PF: ns
Pelle *et al.* [101]	368 CAD/CR	Prospective	Independent predictor (p = 0.001)
Chronic heart failure			
Schiffer *et al.* [64]	84 CHF	Cross-sectional	OR: 3.3
Schiffer *et al.* [61]	166 CHF	Prospective	ORs: 3.4-6.0; physical dimensions: ns
Heart transplantation			
Pedersen *et al.* [65]	186 HTX	Cross-sectional	ORs: 3.5–6.1; BP and GH: ns
Implantable cardioverter defibrillator			
Pedersen *et al.* [66]	154 ICD	Prospective	Independent predictor (p <0.001)
Peripheral arterial disease			
Aquarius *et al.* [67]	150 PAD; 150 controls	Case–control	OR: 7.4 (overall QoL)
Aquarius *et al.* [68]	150 PAD	Prospective	ORs: 3.9–8.6
Aquarius *et al.* [69]	203 PAD	Prospective	ORs: 3.7–6.0

BP, bodily pain (SF-36); CABG, coronary artery bypass graft surgery; CHF, chronic heart failure; CR, cardiac rehabilitation; GH, general health (SF-36); HTX, heart transplantation; ICD, implantable cardioverter defibrillator; IHD, ischaemic heart disease; NS, not significant; OR, odds ratio; PAD, peripheral arterial disease; PCI, percutaneous coronary intervention; PF, physical functioning (SF-36); QoL, quality of life; SES, sirolimus-eluting stent.

personality have an increased vulnerability to experience an amalgam of negative outcomes, including increased depression and anxiety. They are also likely to report poor health status and quality of life, which cannot be accounted for by indicators of disease severity, such as left ventricular dysfunction, multi-vessel disease, and NYHA functional class [59]. These results are consistent across studies and cardiovascular diagnosis (including CAD, CHF, and PAD) and despite state-of-the art treatment such as PCI with drug-eluting stenting and ICD therapy [59]. An overview of studies [61–70] on the impact of Type D on health status and quality of life is shown in ➲Table 35.2, indicating that the associated independent risk ranges from two- to sevenfold.

Psychological risk factors for poor prognosis

The influence of psychological factors on cardiovascular mortality and morbidity is well documented, with the associated risk being at least of an equal magnitude to that of demographic and clinical risk factors, and independent thereof [9, 59]. Hence, the addition of psychological factors to traditional biomedical risk factors might help enhance risk stratification in cardiac patients. Nevertheless, there are still several gaps in our understanding and conceptualization of psychological risk factors, including whether they should be viewed as *true* risk factors or as risk markers, the most opportune time to screen, and which interventions might help moderate the effect of these psychological factors on health outcomes [9]. The most pertinent psychological factors influencing cardiovascular health outcomes are discussed in the following sections.

Depression

Depression is a common comorbid disorder of CAD [71] that has been associated with increased mortality, morbidity, rehospitalizations, healthcare consumption, and poor quality of life and adherence [9, 72–77]. Not only major depressive disorder but also subclinical levels of depression may increase the risk of adverse clinical events [9, 19, 77], with the associated risk being twofold [9, 72–77]. In addition, there is accumulating evidence that specific depressive symptoms may exert differential effects on prognosis [17, 19], with the quest for the identification of the most cardio-toxic symptoms currently ongoing. The relative importance of new onset versus persistent depression as a prognostic marker is also as yet undetermined, with results to date being mixed [21, 78–80]. Although it is generally assumed that depression in cardiac patients has the same form as that found in psychiatric patients, preliminary evidence indicates that depression in cardiac patients is both quantitatively and qualitatively different [22]. Post-MI patients with clinical depression seem to report lower mean levels of depressive cognitions and also less cognitive/affective but more somatic symptoms of depression than psychiatric patients with clinical depression [22].

Depression as a prognostic marker in CVD has primarily been studied in patients with MI, but seems to be associated with adverse clinical events across different types of cardiac populations, including unstable angina [77], PCI with drug-eluting stenting [17], CABG [78], PAD [81], and CHF [14, 82]. Depression has also been shown to precipitate ventricular arrhythmias in patients implanted with an ICD [83]. Examples of the most recent reviews and meta-analyses on the impact of depression on prognosis are listed in ➲Table 35.3 [9, 14, 50, 73, 84–86].

Anxiety

Anxiety has received far less attention in cardiovascular research than depression, as also reflected in the paucity of reviews and meta-analyses available on anxiety and prognosis (➲Table 35.3). Findings on the role of anxiety as a prognostic factor are mixed, with most but not all studies confirming a relationship between anxiety and adverse clinical events [14, 24, 25, 28, 86, 87], and with the associated risk being around twofold in the positive studies [86]. In a recent study, anxiety was found to be an independent predictor of mortality following CABG [88]. There is also evidence to show that anxiety is associated with in-hospital ischaemic and arrhythmic complications [29], increased health care consumption [25], poor health status and quality of life [87], and that anxiety may also enhance the detrimental effect of depression on health status [89]. These studies have primarily been conducted in patients with acute coronary syndrome (ACS) (➲Chapter 16) or CHF (➲Chapter 23), whereas there is a lack of studies on the prognostic role of anxiety in ICD patients (➲Chapter 30) and PAD patients (➲Chapter 36).

Table 35.3 Examples of recent reviews and meta-analyses examining the impact of depression, anxiety, and health status on prognosis in CVD

Authors	Year	Patient group	Endpoints
Depression			
Barth *et al.* [84]	2004	CHD	Mortality
van Melle *et al.* [73]	2004	MI	Mortality; cardiovascular events
Rutledge *et al.* [85]	2006	CHF	Mortality; hospitalization; clinical events; healthcare costs; healthcare use
Nicholson *et al.* [9]	2006	CHD	Mortality
Pelle *et al.* [14]	2008	CHF	Mortality
Anxiety			
Januzzi *et al.* [86]	2000	CHD	Mortality; clinical events
Pelle *et al.* [14]	2008	CHF	Mortality
Health status			
Mommersteeg *et al.* (50)	2009	CAD and CHF	Mortality; rehospitalization

CAD, coronary artery disease; CHD, coronary heart disease; CHF, chronic heart failure; MI, myocardial infarction.

Other factors

Panic disorder

Beginning evidence shows that panic disorder may also be associated with increased mortality and morbidity in patients with CVD, with results being more convincing for an impact on quality of life [30, 31] than mortality [31]. This was demonstrated in two recent studies of chest pain patients [31] and patients with CHF [30].

Post-traumatic stress disorder

The influence of symptoms of PTSD on cardiovascular prognosis has also received little attention, although available evidence indicates that PTSD is associated with increased morbidity, impaired health status and quality of life, and likely also with a greater risk for mortality [33, 34]. A recent study of ICD-treated cardiac event survivors provides more definite evidence that PTSD symptoms significantly increase the risk of long-term mortality, independent of disease severity [35].

Social isolation

Several years ago, Ruberman and colleagues noted that post-MI patients who were socially isolated had a poor clinical course as compared to patients with low levels of isolation [38]. In more recent years, social isolation has been associated with poor prognosis among patients with heart disease in some, but not all studies [37, 90]. On balance, social isolation incurs a two- to threefold risk of mortality, although the impact seems to be greatest in those patients who are most isolated [37]. A recent meta-analysis showing that having a partner increases the chance of participating in CR [91] provides evidence that this may comprise one of the pathways through which social isolation influences cardiovascular health.

Health status

Patient-rated health status is becoming an increasingly important outcome measure in cardiovascular research and a performance measure in clinical practice [45]. Cumulative evidence also shows that poor patient-rated health status predicts prognosis both in CAD and CHF [50], and in patients treated with ICD therapy [92]. This risk is independent of traditional biomedical risk factors [50, 92]. The evidence for an impact of health status is stronger for physical health status than for mental health status in both CAD and CHF [50]. Health status assessed with a disease-specific questionnaire seems to have greater prognostic value compared to health status assessed with a generic measure [50]. Given this evidence and that there

Table 35.4 Type D personality and adverse clinical events

Study authors	Year	Index event	Follow-up	Primary endpoint	Adjusted OR/HR
Denollet *et al.* [56]	1996	CAD	6–10 years	Cardiac mortality	3.8
Denollet *et al.* [63]	2000	CAD	5 years	Cardiac mortality, MI	8.9
Denollet *et al.* [147]	2006	CAD	9 months	All-cause mortality, MI, PCI, or CABG	2.9
Denollet *et al.* [93]	2008	CAD	5–10 years	All-cause mortality, MI	4.6
Pedersen *et al.* [94]	2004	CAD	9 months	All-cause mortality, MI	5.3
Pedersen *et al.* [95]	2007	CAD	2 years	All-cause mortality, MI	2.5
Denollet *et al.* [27]	1998	CHF	6–10 years	Cardiac mortality, MI	8.2
Denollet *et al.* [96]	2007	HTX	5.4 years (mean)	All-cause mortality, early or more severe rejection	6.8
Aquarius *et al.* [97]	2008	PAD	4 years	All-cause mortality	3.5

CABG, coronary artery bypass graft surgery; CAD, coronary artery disease; HR, hazard ratio; HTX, heart transplantation; MI, myocardial infarction; OR, odds ratio; PAD, peripheral arterial disease; PCI, percutaneous coronary intervention.

is often a discrepancy between the physician's evaluation of patients' health status compared to patients' own report [46], assessment of patient-rated health has incremental value in clinical practice and may help in risk stratification and enhance secondary prevention [44].

Type D personality

Personality characteristics have been shown to explain individual differences in health outcomes in patients with somatic disease, including the onset and course of heart disease [53, 59]. Although findings associating global type A behaviour with mortality have been inconsistent, there is some evidence that facets of type A behaviour, in particular hostility, exerts an adverse effect on cardiovascular health and helps accelerate the atherosclerotic process [53]. Especially, with the introduction of the Type D personality construct in recent years, there is a renewed interest in the role of personality in CVD [57] 35.1.

Type D personality is associated with increased mortality and morbidity [27, 39, 56, 63, 93–97], with the mortality risk being around fourfold (➲Table 35.4). As shown in a substudy of the Rapamycin-Eluting Stent Evaluated At Rotterdam Cardiology Hospital (RESEARCH) registry that included PCI patients treated with sirolimus-eluting versus bare metal stenting, Type D personality was associated with mortality and non-fatal MI already at 9 months (i.e. 15 months post index PCI), despite optimal treatment using state-of-the-art in interventional cardiology (➲Fig. 35.2) [94]. A later RESEARCH registry substudy showed that the impact of Type D on prognosis can be attributed to the combination of the two subcomponents of Type D,—*negative affectivity* and *social inhibition*—rather than the single traits [39]. The risk incurred by Type D is independent of standard risk factors, including left ventricular dysfunction and multi-vessel disease, indicating that the increased risk of mortality and morbidity in patients with this personality disposition cannot be attributed to these patients having more severe underlying cardiac disease [56, 59].

Recently, Type D was also shown to have incremental value above and beyond other, single personality traits, such as neuroticism, in predicting mortality: 'This raises the possibility that perhaps this type [i.e. referring to Type D personality] embodies unique intra-individual information relevant to health that is not captured by multiple trait ratings' [98]. Importantly, Type D personality has also been shown to have incremental value above depression as a predictor of poor prognosis [99].

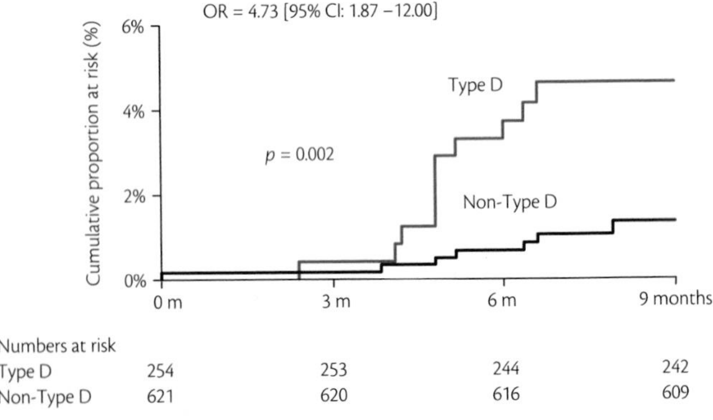

OR: odds ratio; CI: confidence interval

Figure 35.2 Type D and 9 months' cumulative risk of death or myocardial infarction after percutaneous coronary intervention. Reproduced from Pedersen SS, Lemos PA, van Vooren PR, *et al.* Type D personality predicts death or myocardial infarction after bare metal stent or sirolimus-eluting stent implantation: a Rapamycin-Eluting Stent Evaluated at Rotterdam Cardiology Hospital (RESEARCH) registry substudy. *J Am Coll Cardiol* 2004; **44**: 997–1001. Copyright 2004, with permission from Elsevier.

Independent risk or confounding by somatic symptoms?

Despite an association between psychological factors and mortality and morbidity in CAD, there is some debate whether these factors exert an independent effect [9], or whether their influence may be confounded by somatic symptoms, including indices of disease severity such as left ventricular dysfunction. If this is true, the implication is that psychological factors predict prognosis largely due to their overlap with the underlying cardiac disease, and that some of these psychological manifestations (e.g. depression) may arise secondary to CAD due to these patients experiencing a more severe disease burden.

The results to date are somewhat mixed, with preliminary evidence showing that, in particular, depression may be confounded by somatic symptoms [19, 100–102], whereas personality factors, such as Type D, seem to be less prone to such confounding [100, 102, 103]. What is puzzling, however, is that generally psychological factors predict cardiac prognosis despite adjustment for measures of disease severity. One plausible explanation is that despite confounding there is a unique psychological component that incurs an increased risk of adverse health outcomes that is independent of disease severity and somatic symptoms [19].

A related issue pertains to whether psychological factors fulfil the criterion of being risk factors for the progression of CAD in the true sense of the word, or whether they constitute risk markers that lie on the causal pathway between a third variable and cardiac prognosis. To be a risk factor, a psychological factor would at a minimum have to satisfy the following criteria [59, 104]:

1) To confer an independent risk on prognosis, with an increase in the risk factor being associated with an increased risk of mortality in a dose-response fashion.
2) The dose–response relationship must be confirmed across different studies either within a country or across countries.
3) Basic and clinical research must have established the pathway through which the risk factor operates.
4) It must be shown that a reduction in the risk factor, using a randomized controlled trial design, would also lead to a concomitant improvement in survival.

Given these criteria, even depression, the psychological factor that has received the most attention in cardiovascular research, does not warrant risk factor status, in particular given that randomized controlled behavioural and pharmacologic intervention trials, such as the Enhancing Recovery in Coronary Heart Disease clinical trial (ENRICHD) and Sertraline AntiDepressant Heart Attack Randomized Trial (SADHART), have not been able to modify the impact of depression on survival despite some reduction in depressive morbidity [105, 106].

Mechanisms linking psychological factors to adverse prognosis

Mechanisms linking psychological factors such as (chronic) stress, depression, anxiety, and Type D personality to cardiac prognosis are not yet well understood. However, a number of plausible mechanisms, both biological and behavioural, have been identified that may explain the link between psychological factors and prognosis.

The multiple biological and behavioural mechanisms that may serve as candidate intermediaries between psychological factors and progression of cardiac disease are for a large part shared between the psychological factors—although most studies have been done on depression. Therefore, each following section will discuss the individual plausible mechanisms successively, instead of dealing with each psychological factor separately. An overview of all suggested mechanisms is given in ➲Fig. 35.3.

Biological mechanisms

Cortisol

Cortisol, the end-product of the hypothalamus–pituitary–adrenal (HPA) axis, is an important steroid hormone in the regulation of normal physiology, and plays a pivotal role in the body's stress response. In depression, or as a consequence of continued exposure to stress, the HPA axis may become deregulated, resulting in a chronically excessive secretion of cortisol. A number of studies have implicated HPA axis dysregulation as a potential mechanism for explaining the link between depression and poor prognosis in CAD, as HPA axis dysregulation is associated with cardiovascular risk factors such as coronary artery stenosis, visceral obesity, high blood pressure and heart rate, and hypercholesterolemia [107]. Studies in CAD have shown that depressed patients have impaired feedback control and consequent HPA axis hyperactivity [108]. Similar findings of HPA axis hyperactivity have been found in cardiac patients with a Type D personality [109, 110].

Autonomic balance

Current literature testifies to the importance of autonomic nervous system imbalance, favouring sympathetic activation,

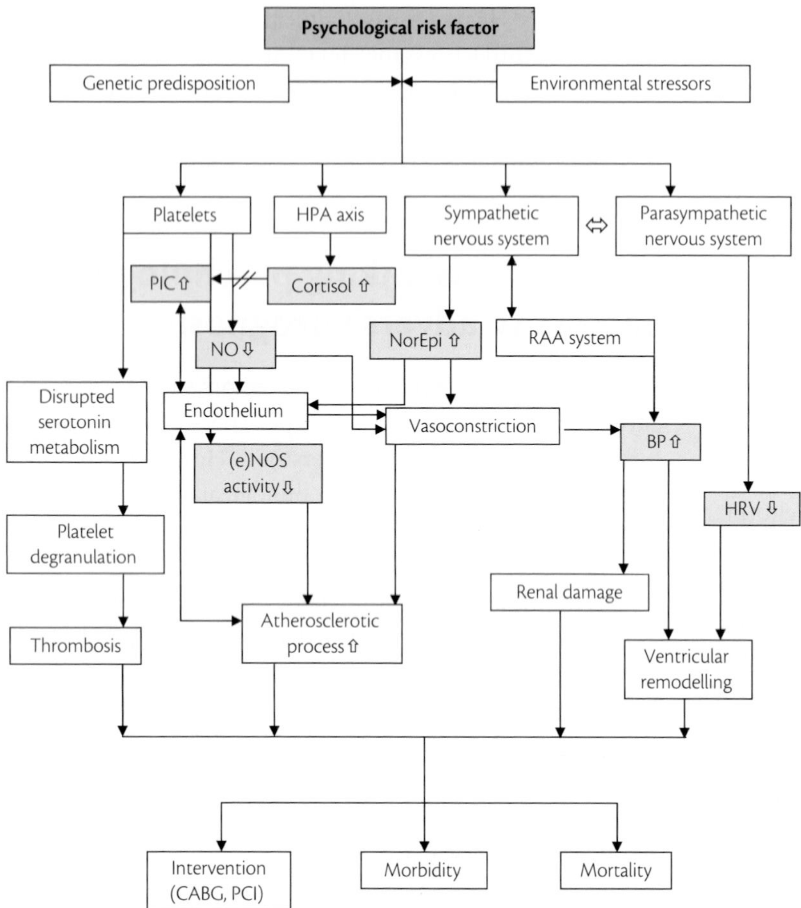

Figure 35.3 Candidate mechanisms explaining the link between psychological risk factors and progression in cardiovascular disease. BP, blood pressure; (e) NOS, (endothelial) nitric oxide synthase; HRV, heart rate variability; NO, nitric oxide; NorEpi, norepinephrine; PIC, pro-inflammatory cytokine; RAA, renin–angiotensin–aldosterone.

as a risk factor for cardiac prognosis and death (e.g. 111). One of the reasons that depression increases the risk for cardiovascular morbidity and mortality may be decreased heart rate variability, due to vagal withdrawal, which in turn may increase the risk for ventricular arrhythmias. Similarly, sympathetic hyperactivity has been implicated in inducing high blood pressure and myocardial ischaemia, due to coronary vasoconstriction [112]. Depressed post-MI patients are characterized by decreased heart rate variability [113, 114], with one study suggesting heart rate variability to be one of the mediating mechanisms between depression and mortality [115]. More research is needed for a more complete understanding, as a recent study specified that heart rate variability is only related to somatic symptoms but not cognitive symptoms of depression [114]. Another measure of vagal control, baroreceptor sensitivity, was found to be associated with high levels of anxiety, but not depression in one study of post-MI patients [116].

Both anxiety and depression have been linked to abnormalities in the duration of ventricular repolarization (i.e. long QT intervals) and QT variability (QTV), which also have been associated with increased risk of sudden death in cardiac patients (see also ➲Chapter 30). Hypertensive patients with anxiety have been shown to have longer QT intervals, corrected for heart rate, as compared to hypertensive patients without anxiety [117]. Furthermore, there is consistent evidence that links depression to larger QT intervals and QTV in post-MI patients [118] and psychiatric populations [119]. People characterized by high levels of neuroticism also seem to have longer QT intervals [120], placing them at increased risk for life-threatening arrhythmias. Increased arrhythmic activity, i.e. 24-hour ventricular ectopy, has been related to increased levels of state anxiety and self-reported stress in post-MI patients during routine daily activities [121].

Platelet function

Another explanation for the increased morbidity and mortality in patients with comorbid CAD and depression concerns platelet abnormalities, such as increased platelet activation, or a disturbed serotonin metabolism in the platelet, which leaves the platelet more likely to degranulate to certain triggers, in turn leading to thrombosis [122]. Experimental research has shown that depressive and anxious symptoms are related to increased platelet P-selectin expression in response to acute stress, and a delayed recovery [123].

Decreased nitric oxide synthase (NOS) activity and plasma levels of nitric oxide (NO) comprise other abnormalities found in depressed cardiac patients. These abnormalities may contribute to increased platelet aggregation and coronary vasoconstriction, thereby increasing the risk of angina and ischaemia [124]. There is also pre-clinical data to suggest that brain NO is markedly increased in stress, anxiety and anxiety-related disorders [125]. No information to date is present on plasma NO levels in patients with comorbid anxiety and CAD.

Endothelial function

Endothelial dysfunction, comprising vasoconstriction, leucocyte adhesion, thrombosis and cellular proliferation of the vessel wall, is a hallmark of early atherosclerosis development [126] (➲Chapter 16). Depression seems to be associated with endothelial dysfunction, as several studies have reported impaired arterial flow-mediated dilatation in depressed psychiatric patients [127] as well as in CAD patients with depressive symptomatology [128]. Furthermore, increased levels of biomarkers for endothelial dysfunction such as soluble tissue factor, von Willebrand factor, and soluble intercellular adhesion molecule-1 have been associated with PTSD [129].

Immune function

Atherosclerosis has been identified as an inflammatory process [130], with cardiac patients with increased levels of pro-inflammatory cytokines, such as tumour necrosis factor (TNF)-α and interleukin (IL)-6, having an increased risk of adverse clinical events [131]. Increased pro-inflammatory cytokine levels are also found in CHF patients, which have been suggested to be due to cardiac remodelling. CAD and CHF patients with depression [108], Type D personality [132], or PTSD [34] have all been characterized by an increased pro-inflammatory state. Although increased inflammation is linked to adverse prognosis, it is yet elusive whether this mediates the association between the psychological factors and prognosis.

Mental stress ischaemia

A significant percentage of CAD patients experience myocardial ischaemia in response to mental stress and in a small portion of patients, mental stress-induced ischaemia may occur in the absence of exercise- or adenosine-induced ischaemia. Mental stress-induced ischaemia is an independent predictor of poor prognosis in CAD patients, related to incident MI and mortality [133]. Anxiety has been related to an increased incidence of in-hospital complications after acute MI, including myocardial ischaemia [29]. Future studies should examine whether stress-related constructs such as depression and Type D personality are also associated with mental stress-induced ischaemia.

Emotional stress may also lead to a specific type of cardiomyopathy, i.e. the Takotsubo cardiomyopathy (TC) (➲Chapter 18), also referred to as the apical ballooning syndrome. TC is a reversible cardiomyopathy that is precipitated by acute emotional stress, such as the death of a family member, fierce argument, or natural disaster, and is characterized by symptoms of ACS and transient apical and midventricular wall motion abnormalities in the absence of obstructive CAD. TC is most common in older postmenopausal women [134]. Research findings reveal several possible pathophysiologic mechanisms such as multivessel coronary vasospasm, elevated plasma catecholamine levels, elevated sympathetic tone, and impaired coronary microcirculation, although the exact aetiology and pathophysiology remain unknown [135].

Common genetic vulnerability

From a genetic perspective, diseases such as CAD and factors like depression or personality are all considered to be genetically complex, influenced by multiple genes exerting small effects, as well as by interactions between genes, and between genes and the environment. Behavioural genetics studies have indicated moderate to substantial heritability for Type D personality [136], depression, and anxiety [137]. Whether common genetic mechanisms underlie the co-occurrence of heart disease and psychological factors has only been tested for depression, as a large twin study revealed that shared genetic factors contribute substantially to the covariation of depression and CAD [138].

Behavioural mechanisms

In addition to the biological mechanisms reviewed in earlier sections, there are several behavioural mechanisms linking psychological factors to morbidity and mortality in cardiac patients. These include poor self-management, poor compliance with treatment and CR, and lifestyle factors such as continued smoking, unhealthy eating habits, and lack of physical exercise. The most prominent findings are presented in the following sections, and summarized in ➲Fig. 35.4.

Non compliance

World Health Organization (WHO) statistics show that in patients with chronic conditions, about 50% of patients are not compliant with recommendations on prevention or treatment. Patients may be non compliant for multiple

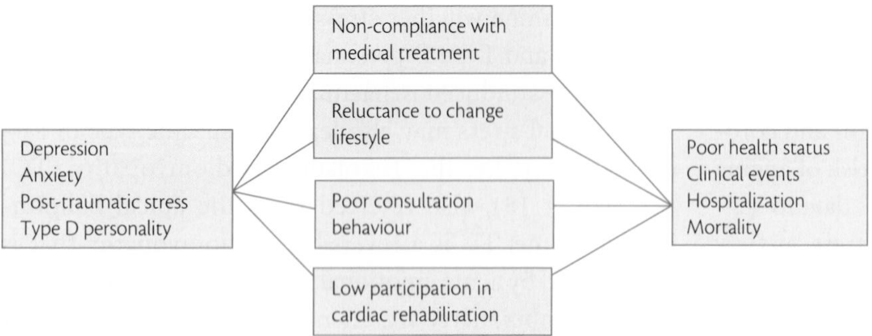

Figure 35.4 Potential behavioural mechanisms explaining the link between psychosocial risk markers and prognosis in heart disease.

reasons, including side effects of medication, but psychological factors such as depression, anxiety, phobias, or inhibition may also interfere with adherence. It is essential for a patient's compliance to have positive expectations and beliefs in the benefits of treatment. Depression may have an adverse effect on these expectations and beliefs. Evidence shows that depression is associated with a threefold increased risk of non compliance to treatment and with a low participation rate in CR [139]. PTSD has also been associated with poor adherence to treatment in acute MI patients, resulting in an increased risk of rehospitalization [36]. In patients with obstructive sleep apnoea (a risk factor for CVD), adherence to treatment was significantly lower in Type D patients compared to non-Type D patients [140]. Hence, non compliance is an important behavioural mechanism for patients with combined cardiac disease and one of these psychological factors.

Reluctance to make life style changes

Common means of behavioural secondary prevention in CAD include lifestyle modifications (➲Chapter 17), such as smoking cessation and dietary intervention, but also the targeting of psychological risk factors. It is often difficult to implement the appropriate lifestyle changes after a cardiac event. Reasons for reluctance to make these changes may include lack of social support and educational support [141]. Changes in mental health due to the medical illness, i.e. increased symptoms of anxiety and depression, may add to the unwillingness or inability to make lifestyle adjustments [139] (see also ➲Table 35.5).

Poor consultation behaviour

Type D patients experience negative emotions, which they refrain from sharing with others. A recent study showed that these characteristics negatively affect consultation behaviour of CHF patients. Even though patients with a Type D personality experienced more cardiac symptoms and appraised these symptoms as more worrisome compared to non-Type D patients, they were less likely to consult their cardiologist or heart failure nurse for these symptoms, potentially leading to under-treatment [142]. Poor consultation behaviour has only been examined in relation to Type D personality, and not anxiety or depression.

Low participation in cardiac rehabilitation

Benefits of CR are undisputed, although only a minority of eligible patients seem to attend. There may be multiple reasons for this non-attendance, including: socio-demographic factors, like low income, living alone, and living far away from CR facilities; lifestyle factors, such as lack of regular exercise habits; and clinical factors, such as more severe illness and lack of active physician endorsement [143, 144].

Table 35.5 Why patients and high-risk people find it hard to make lifestyle changes

Factors that make lifestyle changes more difficult
Low socio-economic status (SES)
Campaigns and lifestyle change programmes are less effective in people with low SES
Social isolation
People who live by themselves are more prone to indulge in an unhealthy lifestyle. In addition, support from a significant other or social network is important for changing lifestyle factors
Stress
Chronic stress (e.g. work stress, marital stress, or post-traumatic stress) leads people to neglect their health, making them less likely to quit smoking, temper alcohol use, and adopt dietary changes
Negative emotions
Depression, anxiety, hostility, post-traumatic stress, and Type D personality all have a negative impact on lifestyle changes, but appropriate treatment may facilitate lifestyle modifications

Adapted with permission from the 2007 European guidelines on CVD prevention (Graham I, Atar D, Borch-Johnsen K, *et al.* (2007). European guidelines on cardiovascular disease prevention in clinical practice: executive summary. Fourth Joint Task Force of the European Society of Cardiology and other societies on cardiovascular disease prevention in clinical practice (constituted by representatives of nine societies and by invited experts). *Eur J Cardiovasc Prev Rehabil* 2007; **14**(Suppl.2): E1–E40).

Psychological factors are also involved, as research shows that patients who experience more symptoms of depression and anxiety are less likely to participate in rehabilitation [143]. Hence, in clinical practice, it would be advisable to discuss patient barriers to participation in rehabilitation with the patient, as these may include psychological motives.

Pharmacological and behavioural interventions

Pharmacological interventions aim to treat psychiatric disorders such as depression, while behavioural interventions encompass various forms of psychotherapy and behavioural therapy to treat, for example, depressed mood, stress or anxieties. Lifestyle interventions often take place in the context of cardiac rehabilitation and target eating habits, smoking, alcohol consumption and exercise (see ➲Chapter 25). Below, a short overview is given of the effects of these interventions on psychological and cardiovascular health. ➲Table 35.6 summarizes all clinical trials that are discussed in this section.

Pharmacological interventions

Among the available antidepressant agents, tricyclic antidepressants (TCAs) and selective serotonin reuptake inhibitors (SSRIs) are used most often to treat depression. In cardiac patients, however, TCAs are not well tolerated at a cardiovascular level, and therefore should be avoided. SSRIs on the other hand do not have undesirable cardiovascular effects in MI, unstable angina, and CHF, and have been used in several clinical trials to examine their effect on depression in these patient groups. An overview of these trials and their main results are summarized in ➲Table 35.6. In general, the two SSRI trials (SADHART and CREATE) show that although SSRI treatment is safe, it is not very efficacious in treating depression in cardiac patients [106, 145]. MIND-IT is another pharmacological trial that evaluated the effects of mirtazapine, a non-tricyclic antidepressant, on adverse clinical events and long-term depression post-MI. The findings of MIND-IT were essentially similar to those of SADHART and CREATE; although mirtazapine was shown to be safe in cardiac patients, it had no effect on recurrent cardiac events, nor were there significant differences between patients assigned to the intervention versus usual care with respect to depressive and somatic symptoms, or quality of life [146].

Behavioural interventions

During the past decades, it became apparent that psychological factors may have a negative impact on cardiac prognosis. More recently, a number of clinical trials have also examined whether behavioral treatment of these factors would lead to an improvement in cardiac prognosis.

Depression and vital exhaustion

Two behavioural intervention trials have examined the effects of cognitive behavioural therapy (CBT) or interpersonal psychotherapy (IPT) on depressive symptoms and adverse cardiac events or death in cardiac patients [105, 145]. The results of these trials are mixed at best. In the ENRICHD trial [105], the intervention significantly reduced depression, while in the CREATE trial [145] interpersonal therapy was not superior to clinical management in terms of reducing depression. Both trials failed to positively affect the incidence of major adverse cardiac events or death (see ➲Table 35.6 for an overview).

Vital exhaustion, characterized by a triad of symptoms, i.e. feelings of excessive fatigue, irritability, and demoralization, has been targeted in the Exhaustion Intervention Trial (EXIT) with the intervention focusing on stress reduction and hostility treatment. Results showed that vital exhaustion and the occurrence of de novo lesions were reduced in the treated PCI patients without a history of CAD, but not in patients with a previous history. There were no treatment effects on new coronary events [148].

Anxiety

Intervention studies that have focused on the treatment of anxiety have primarily been conducted in ICD patients, employing either CBT, CR, or telephone support as the mainstays of treatment or in combination. These intervention studies were small scale and only focused on patient-centred outcomes, with no data available to show whether the intervention also had an effect on hard medical outcomes. All anxiety interventions in ICD patients seem to be successful in reducing anxiety, although CBT and CR have shown the strongest and most stable reductions [149].

In summary, behavioural interventions seem to be somewhat effective in reducing the level of psychological symptoms, such as depression and exhaustion. Although the interventions do not seem to affect cardiac outcomes in the overall group, recent subgroup analyses do reveal some significant relations between, for example, more severe, persistent depression and mortality [150]. It is therefore important to learn from these trials, instead of discarding them because of unexpected findings.

Table 35.6 Clinical trials for evaluation of treatment of psychosocial factors in heart disease*

Trial name	Patients Inclusion criteria	Intervention	Primary endpoints/main results	Secondary endpoints/main results
Pharmacological (or mixed)				
SADHART [106]	N = 369 ACS patients with confirmed MDD diagnosis	Sertraline (SSRI) in flexible dosages (50–200mg/day) (n = 186) or placebo (n = 183) for 24 weeks	LVEF No significant change in LVEF	Cardiac measures (QT distance, %PCV), depression No change in secondary cardiac measures No difference between sertraline and placebo in reducing depression
CREATE [145]	N = 284 CAD patients with a current MDD diagnosis	IPT directed at treating depression and social support vs. clinical management and citalopram (SSRI) vs. placebo	Reduction in depression, serious adverse events Treatment with citalopram significantly reduced depression (ES = 0.33). Not sufficient adverse events to analyse	Reduction in social support Treatment with citalopram significantly increased perceived social support
MIND-IT [146]	N = 190 post-MI patients vs. 130 post-MI controls, with confirmed MDD DSM-IV diagnosis	Mirtazapine vs. placebo + care as usual for 24 weeks In case of refusal or non-response: open treatment with citalopram	Cardiovascular events, cardiac functioning No significant effects of treatment on incidence of cardiac events	Depressive symptomatology, health complaints, quality of life No significant differences between patients assigned to intervention or care as usual with respect to depressive symptoms, health complaints, disability, and quality of life
Behavioural				
EXIT [148]	N = 710 exhausted (MQ ≥7) PCI patients	Weekly group sessions (first 10 weeks) followed by 4 monthly sessions of focusing on stress reduction, and hostility treatment	Vital exhaustion, new cardiac events and de novo lesions Exhaustion was reduced in patients without a history of CAD (OR = 0.44), as well as occurrence of de novo lesions (RR = 0.34). No treatment effects on new coronary events	–
CREATE [145]	N = 284 CAD patients with a current MDD diagnosis	IPT directed at treating depression and social support vs. clinical management and citalopram (SSRI) vs. placebo	Reduction in depression, serious adverse events IPT was not superior to clinical management in reducing depression, not sufficient adverse events to analyse	Reduction in social support No differences between treatment and control groups were found for social support
ENRICHD [105]	N = 2481 patients recovering from acute MI, diagnosis of MDD, minor depression, lifetime MDD, or dysthymia, and/or the ENRICHD criteria for LPSS.	CBT directed at depression and LPSS vs. usual care	Composite endpoint of death or recurrent non-fatal MI No differences in event free survival between treatment and control group	Change in depression or social support Treatment improved depression and social support compared to control group ($p < 0.001$), although this effect diminished over time as at 30 months the benefit of the intervention has disappeared

* Only studies after 2000 have been displayed. For a full overview of these studies, please see this recent meta-analysis [151]. ACS, acute coronary syndrome; CCR, comprehensive cardiac rehabilitation; ES, effect size; HRQL, health-related quality of life; IHD, ischaemic heart disease; IPT, interpersonal therapy; LPSS, low perceived social support; MDD, major depressive disorder; MQ, Maastricht questionnaire for vital exhaustion; PCI, percutaneous coronary intervention; PMR, progressive muscle relaxation; SSRI, selective serotonin reuptake inhibitor; WMA, wall motion abnormalities.

Stress management

Stress management uses specific cognitive behavioural strategies to help patients reduce stress levels. Strategies include relaxation training, cognitive techniques and cognitive challenge, and/or consideration of specific coping strategies to be used at times of stress. Stress management may be applied on its own, or in the context of CR, and aims to improve patients' morale and functioning, and decrease suffering.

Multiple studies have examined the efficacy of relaxation therapy, and these are comprehensively reviewed in several reviews and meta-analyses [151, 152]. Results of these meta-analyses show that, if an intervention is successful in reducing psychological stress, the risk of <2-year mortality is reduced by 28%. However, when taking sex differences into account, there was only a significant benefit for men, not women. Increasingly, stress management programmes are tracking markers of cardiovascular risk, showing that stress management reduces cardiac risk by reducing heart rate and stress-induced wall motion abnormalities, and by increasing heart rate variability, and flow-mediated dilatation [e.g. 153]. Blood pressure seems not to be affected by stress reduction [151].

Biofeedback is increasingly used in addition to stress management programmes in CR. Essentially, biofeedback tries to regulate the input of the autonomic nervous system to the heart. There have not yet been any randomized controlled trials assessing the effectiveness of biofeedback to reduce psychological stress and cardiovascular risk [154].

A multi-factorial CR programme that also included psychological intervention has been shown to be successful in improving both emotional functioning and long-term prognosis at 9-year follow-up [155]. This intervention programme focused on stress reduction, coping with stress, assertiveness training, and, depending on the needs of the patient, individual psychological therapy, using CBT to deal with chronic stress and tension, depression, anxiety, non-expression of emotions, hostility and irritability, and partner issues.

Clinical implications

The role of psychological factors in patients with CAD has implications for clinical practice and the management of patients. We may as yet be dealing with a number of unknown factors, with the two most important being: 1) psychological factors may not be risk factors in the true sense of the word, but risk markers that lie on the causal pathway between other variables and major adverse cardiac events; and 2) psychological factors may be difficult to modify, at least to the extent of influencing survival, as shown from mixed results from clinical trials targeting depression [105, 106, 145]. In addition, evidence is mixed as to the usefulness of performing routine screening for depression in patients with CAD, at least when it comes to improving cardiovascular outcomes [5, 8]. Irrespectively, there is sufficient and sound evidence to show that psychological factors are related to a wide range of adverse health outcomes in patients with CAD (➲Table 35.7). In addition, disorders such as depression and anxiety are serious and debilitating, and influence quality of life, which comprise sufficient reasons for warranting that psychological factors be taken seriously and managed in clinical practice.

Despite the fact that anxiety is common among cardiovascular patients and may have adverse health consequences if untreated, it is infrequently assessed or managed appropriately [23]. It has been estimated that among post-MI patients, only one out of three anxious patients are asked about such symptoms [24]. Importantly, treatment of anxiety with anxiolytic medication may protect against the triggering of arrhythmias [156]. Hence, there is an urgent need to detect anxiety in these patients, and to improve patients' outcomes by placing anxiety in the forefront of clinical cardiac practice [23].

Screening for psychological factors can easily be made an integral part of patient clinical care, with the use of brief, standardized, and validated measures. Recently, an advisory of a consortium of councils of the American Heart Association advocated routine screening for depression of

Table 35.7 Reasons for assessing and managing psychological factors in clinical practice

Highly prevalent in cardiac patients
Linked to behavioural and cardiovascular risk factors
May trigger acute events
Incur an increased risk of mortality and morbidity that is independent of traditional biomedical risk factors
The associated prognostic risk is at least of an equal magnitude to that of traditional biomedical risk factors
Impact adversely on quality of life
Moderate the effects of medical interventions
Impede the adoption of lifestyle changes
There is a poor match between physician-evaluated and patient-rated psychological states and health status
Psychological factors tend to cluster together within individual patients, increasing the risk of adverse health outcomes compared to single factors

Table 35.8 The Patient Health Questionnaire 2 (PHQ-2)*

Over the last 2 weeks, how often have you been bothered by any of the following problems?				
0 = not at all; 1 = several days; 2 = more than half the days; 3 = nearly everyday				
1. Little interest or pleasure in doing things	0	1	2	3
2. Feeling down, depressed, or hopeless	0	1	2	3

* Score range from 0–6; the questionnaire can also be used with the answer categories 'yes' and 'no'. As recommended by the American Heart Association, if the answer is 'yes' to either question on the PHQ-2, patients should be referred for more comprehensive evaluation.

PHQ-2 is adapted from PRIME MD today, developed by Drs Robert L. Spitzer, Janet B.W. Williams, Kurt Kroenke, and colleagues, with an educational grant from Pfizer Inc. For research information, contact
Dr Spitzer at rls8@columbia.edu. Use of the PHQ-2 may only be made in accordance with the terms of use available at http://www.pfizer.com. PRIME MD today is a trademark of Pfizer Inc.

all cardiac patients seen in clinical practice, using the two-item Patient Health Questionnaire (PHQ) followed by the nine-item PHQ if screening positive on one or both items of the PHQ-2 [5]. Depending on the score on the PHQ-9, patients may subsequently be referred to a mental health professional for a more thorough evaluation [5]. However, this two-stepped approach seems to have no greater value in terms of identifying major depression in cardiac patients compared to the use of the PHQ-2 or PHQ-9 alone [157]. Hence, given its brevity, the PHQ-2 may be the preferred instrument to use in clinical practice (➲Table 35.8).

There are other viable alternatives to the PHQ-2 and the PHQ-9 as screening instruments for depression in clinical practice, including the 21-item Beck Depression Inventory [158] and the 14-item Hospital Anxiety and Depression Scale [159]. The Hospital Anxiety and Depression Scale provides the opportunity to identify not only symptoms of depression but also anxiety. Patients with a Type D personality disposition can be identified with the Type D Scale (DS14), a brief 14-item standardized and validated measure that is easy to administer (➲Table 35.9) [58]. Following an update of the European guidelines on CVD prevention in clinical practice by the Third Joint Task Force of European and other Societies on Cardiovascular Disease Prevention [1], an international committee provided recommendations for the assessment of psychosocial risk factors, and included the Beck Depression Inventory, the Hospital Anxiety and Depression Scale, and the Type D Scale (DS14) among the measures to use in clinical cardiology practice to identify high-risk patients [160]. Personality measures may comprise particularly good candidates as screening tools in clinical cardiology practice, as they assess

Table 35.9 The 14-item Type D Scale (DS14)

Name: .... **Today's date:**					
Below are a number of statements that people often use to describe themselves. Please read each statement and then **circle** the appropriate **number** next to that statement to indicate your answer. There are no right or wrong answers: your own impression is the only thing that matters.					
0 = False; 1 = Rather false; 2 = Neutral; 3 = Rather true; 4 = True					
1 I make contact easily when I meet people	0	1	2	3	4
2 I often make a fuss about unimportant things	0	1	2	3	4
3 I often talk to strangers	0	1	2	3	4
4 I often feel unhappy	0	1	2	3	4
5 I am often irritated	0	1	2	3	4
6 I often feel inhibited in social interactions	0	1	2	3	4
7 I take a gloomy view of things	0	1	2	3	4
8 I find it hard to start a conversation	0	1	2	3	4
9 I am often in a bad mood	0	1	2	3	4
10 I am a closed kind of person	0	1	2	3	4
11 I would rather keep other people at a distance	0	1	2	3	4
12 I often find myself worrying about something	0	1	2	3	4
13 I am often down in the dumps	0	1	2	3	4
14 When socializing, I don't find the right things to talk about	0	1	2	3	4
Scoring of Negative Affectivity and Social Inhibition					
The Negative Affectivity and Social Inhibition scales can be used as continuous variables to assess these two traits in their own right. Scores on both scales range from 0–28, and can be calculated as follows:					
Negative Affectivity = sum of scores on items 2 + 4 + 5 + 7 + 9 + 12 + 13					
Social Inhibition = sum of scores on items 1 [reversed] + 3 [reversed] + 6 + 8 + 10 + 11 + 14					
Assessment of Type D personality					
With reference to assessment of Type D personality, 10 is the cut-off for both scales. Subjects are classified as Type D if both Negative Affectivity is greater or equal to 10 and Social Inhibition is greater or equal to 10.					

Reproduced with permission from Denollet, J. (2005). DS14: Standard assessment of negative affectivity, social inhibition, and Type D personality. *Psychosom Med* 2005; **67**: 89–97. J. Denollet © 2005, American Psychosomatic Society.

a predisposition to experience a wide variety of emotions across time and situations. Due to the stability of personality characteristics, such measures may also be less prone to be influenced by acute events, such as MI, and the underlying disease severity [100].

Currently, there is no consensus as to the most optimal time point for screening for psychological factors. Evidence from the depression literature indicates that assessment close to an acute cardiac event may be more likely to tap the physical ill health associated with the acute event than actual depression [9, 161]. Evidence on the importance of new onset versus persistent depression as a prognostic marker is also conflicting [21, 78–80]. Hence, pending further research, it seems better to screen patients at serial time points when patients are seen in clinical practice at follow-up visits.

Conclusion

Despite unanswered questions in relation to the role of psychological factors in patients with heart disease, these factors should be taken into account in the clinical management of patients. When seeing patients in clinical practice, it is important that cardiologists take the time to listen carefully to patients, use clear and succinct communication, and make specific and simple recommendations. It may be necessary to spend some time on investigating whether the patient is adhering to his/her medication and goals set for lifestyle changes, in which case involving and questioning the partner may provide added information. When setting goals for lifestyle changes, the chance of success is likely to be enhanced, when the patient is involved in setting the goals rather than the cardiologist dictating what the patient should do [6]. However, the cardiologist can help the patient develop personal, and preferably emotional, reasons for changing behaviour, set goals that are specific and sufficiently small such that they are realistic, and promote self-management and autonomy in terms of looking into, together with the patient, which barriers (e.g. stress) may impede attainment of the set goals and how to deal with these barriers (e.g. engaging in physical exercise or relaxation training to deal with stress) [6]. If the results from screening for psychological factors indicate that these risk indicators are present, it may be necessary to refer the patient to other healthcare professionals, such as a medical psychologist or a psychiatrist, as the patient may then require more intensive monitoring and treatment of a behavioural and psychological nature [160].

Personal perspective

Identification of psychological risk factors in patients with heart disease is important for secondary prevention, as they are associated with a wide range of adverse health outcomes, including mortality, morbidity, and poor quality of life, and also serve as barriers for treatment adherence and the adoption of more healthy lifestyles. Given that psychological factors have been shown to impact on cardiovascular health independent of standard risk factors and cannot be inferred from any other measures available in clinical cardiology practice, there is a need for assessing these factors in their own right.

Hence, patients should be screened for psychological risk factors at clinical follow-up visits as part of standard clinical practice, using validated and standardized screening tools, in order to monitor and prevent that psychological symptoms become chronic. Repeated assessments of health status should also be undertaken, as deterioration in health status may indicate an aggravation in the severity of the patient's disease, helping the cardiologist pinpoint subgroups of patients who may need more aggressive treatment and adjustment of their medication.

The cardiologist plays a pivotal role in the entire process of identifying, monitoring, and, if necessary, referring patients to other healthcare professionals, if the psychological profile of patients places them at risk for poor cardiovascular health. Management of the patient's disease is best achieved by using a multidisciplinary approach, with the knowledge of a multidisciplinary team of healthcare professionals likely being more than the sum of its parts. Interventions should be tailored to the individual patient, with multifactorial CR offering several learning opportunities to patients. These include: experiencing that exercising is possible and safe despite having heart disease; targeting of standard risk factors, such as hypercholesterolemia and smoking, by means of increasing the motivation for adopting more healthy lifestyles; CR also has a beneficial impact on the patient's level of distress, thereby enhancing quality of life and perhaps also cardiovascular health.

The field of cardiac psychology is faced with several unresolved issues that are likely to be the subject of research over the next 5–10 years. These include the following:

- Are psychological factors *really* risk factors or *merely* risk markers of poor prognosis?
- Are some psychological factors more cardio-toxic than others?
- Through which pathways do psychological factors exert a pathological influence on prognosis?

- Are there factors that moderate the influence of psychological factors on cardiovascular health, e.g. do patients with a Type D personality who have a partner have a better prognosis than Type D patients without a partner?
- Can we reduce the influence of psychological risk factors on cardiovascular health, such that a reduction in the psychological risk factor leads to a concomitant beneficial influence on survival?
- Which intervention works for which patient?
- When, how many times, and with which instruments should we screen patients in clinical practice?

Irrespective of how these issues will be settled, heart disease has a psychological impact on patients' lives in general and their quality of life and health status in particular, and also serve as barriers for treatment adherence and the adoption of healthy lifestyles. In addition, there are large individual differences in the manifestation of psychological distress, health status, and prognosis between patients, with identification of the high-risk patients being cost effective, as this will serve to optimize treatment in those patients that need it the most. For this reason, psychological factors are here to stay both in the guidelines for the secondary prevention of CVD but also as pertinent variables to be included in cardiovascular research. In particular, the continuous advances in the field of cardiology and medicine in general to optimize the treatment of patients with heart disease necessitate that psychological factors be considered.

Remote monitoring of patients with a device is an example of a technological advance that is increasingly being used as an alternative to or in combination with clinical follow-up visits. The majority of patients may welcome such an advance, as it reduces time spent in hospital for follow-up visits and may facilitate patients getting on with life rather than being continuously placed in the 'sick role'. However, in a subgroup of patients this may give rise to concerns and feelings of insecurity. These patients might prefer to come in for clinical follow-up visits, as these visits also provide an opportunity to discuss concerns with the device nurse and other healthcare professionals. In other words, advances in cardiology and medicine need to be tested in terms of their psychological impact and whether these advances may interact with psychological factors to affect cardiovascular health.

From a clinical practice point of view, routine assessment of health status is likely to be incorporated as a performance measure of high quality care in the future, with such initiatives currently being supported in parts of the US. With routine assessment of health status, patients whose health status deteriorate can be identified and treatment options be reconsidered, as a deterioration in health status may be indicative of aggravation of the underlying disease. Health status measures can also serve to guide treatment, as indicated in the recent Clinical Outcomes Utilizing Revascularization and Aggressive Drug Evaluation (COURAGE) trial of patients with stable coronary artery disease randomized to a combination of PCI and medical therapy compared to medical therapy alone [162].

Further reading

Molinari E, Compare A, Parati G (eds.) *Clinical psychology and heart disease*, 2006. Milan: Springer-Verlag.

Sher E (ed.) *Psychological factors and cardiovascular disorders: The role of psychiatric pathology and maladaptive personality features*, 2008. New York: Nova Science Publishers Inc.

Additional online material

35.1 Discussion by the author, 'Type D personality — a new risk factor: fact or fiction?'.

For full references and multimedia materials please visit the online version of the book (http://esctextbook.oxfordonline.com).

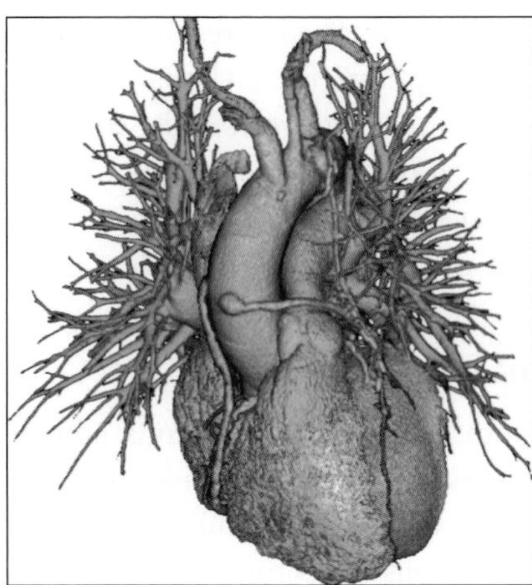

CHAPTER 36

Peripheral Arterial Occlusive Disease

Alberto Cremonesi, Nicolas Diehm, Andrea Stella, Mauro Gargiulo, Gianluca Faggioli, Estêvão Carvalho de Campos Martins, and Fausto Castriota

Contents

Summary

Peripheral arterial occlusive disease (PAD) is a disorder of the peripheral arteries comprising all human arterial beds except for the coronary circulation. The interest in detection and dedicated treatment options for PAD patients has increased substantially during recent years. Given that PAD is a powerful indicator of systemic atherosclerosis and, independent of symptoms, is associated with an increased risk of myocardial infarction and stroke as well as a six times greater likelihood of death, the prevalence and demographic distribution of measurable PAD becomes relevant.

The management of patients with PAD—wherever the disease is located—has to be planned in the context of natural history, epidemiology of disease, risk factors predicting deterioration, and clinical presentation. Setting the correct indication for different treatment options (medical, endovascular, surgical, hybrid) in patients affected by PAD is a condition where the principles of multi-disciplinary integration between all the specialties involved in that specific field find a paradigmatic application.

An objective evaluation of benefits and risks related to different therapeutic strategies is still difficult and sometimes controversial. Reliable information on clinical outcome or symptom relief is weak and illustrates discrepancies between published reports of specific treatment from centres of excellence and what happens to patients routinely treated in communities around the world. However, a continuing shift away from surgical revascularization towards the less invasive endovascular procedures for PAD patients is being witnessed. Endovascular interventions have greatly changed the current therapeutic spectrum and many indications such as for renal, pelvic, and femoro-popliteal arteries are today regarded as standard practice. Currently, controversy exists regarding whether carotid artery stenting should be accepted as an alternative to the surgical approach for the treatment of obstructive carotid artery disease.

Peripheral arterial disease

Key points

- Measurement of the ankle–brachial index (ABI) is the most effective, widely-applicable, and accurate method to gauge the severity of PAD and assess cardiovascular disease burden.
- Decisions regarding reconstructive surgery versus endovascular options for peripheral obstructive disease are centred on clinical presentation and vascular examination. Appropriate patient selection is critical for successful decision making.
- Endovascular options have developed rapidly since the first balloon angioplasty in 1977. Percutaneous revascularization therapy is progressively replacing surgical therapies as the initial treatment of choice for lower extremity vascular disease.
- Despite substantial improvements in stent design and application of drug-coated angioplasty balloons, restenosis remains the major drawback of femoro-popliteal and below-the-knee angioplasty. Further technical developments will likely expand endovascular treatment options in PAD patients in the near future.

Introduction

PAD is a disorder of the peripheral arteries comprising all human arterial beds except for the coronary circulation. In clinical practice, it is the circulation of the lower limb that is most frequently involved. The interest in detection and dedicated treatment options for PAD patients has increased substantially during recent years and a continuing shift away from surgical revascularization towards the less invasive endovascular procedures for PAD patients is being witnessed [1, 2].

Epidemiology and risk factors

Besides the local symptoms of lower limb ischaemia, atherosclerotic vascular disease is a diffuse progressive condition that simultaneously affects multiple vascular territories. Its main clinical manifestations are coronary heart disease (CHD) (➲Chapters 16 and 17), cerebrovascular disease (CVD), and PAD, which, taken together, have been the leading causes of death in adults for many years [3].

In recent years, our understanding of PAD has undergone a profound change. Besides its direct clinical implications related to lower limb ischaemia it is now perceived as an indicator disease for generalized atherosclerosis. This is due to the fact that a number of prospective studies have shown the considerable co-prevalence of PAD and the other manifestations of atherosclerosis [1]. Depending on the study population, concomitant CHD has been diagnosed in up to 90% and concomitant CVD in about 50% of patients with PAD [4]. Interestingly, only 5% of patients with PAD have a history of any cerebrovascular event. Intermittent claudication (IC) and critical limb ischaemia (CLI) are differentiated from a symptomatic and prognostic standpoint (➲Table 36.1).

Early epidemiologic studies have indicated that total disease prevalence based on objective testing is in the

Table 36.1 Classification of chronic PAD

Fontaine		Rutherford		
Stage	**Clinical description**	**Grade**	**Category**	**Objective description**
Stage I	Asymptomatic	Stage 0		Asymptomatic, normal treadmill test
Stage IIa	IC, pain-free walking distance >200m	Stage I	Grade 1	Mild IC, treadmill exercise limited to 5min; ankle pressure after exercise >50mmHg, but at least 20mmHg lower than at rest
Stage IIb	IC, pain-free walking distance <200m		Grade 2	Moderate IC, between Rutherford 2 and 3 disease
Stage II (complicated)	Trophic lesions with IC but without critical leg ischaemia		Grade 3	Severe IC, treadmill exercise limited to <5min; ankle pressure after exercise <50mmHg
Stage III	Rest pain	Stage II	Grade 4	Rest pain, ankle pressure <40mmHg and/or great toe pressure <30mmHg; pulse volume recording barely pulsatile of flat*
Stage IV	Ischaemic lesion (ulcer, gangrene, necrosis)	Stage III	Grade 5	Limited ischaemic lesion, ankle pressure <30mmHg; pulse volume recording barely pulsatile or flat*
			Grade 6	Extended ischaemic lesion (above metatarsal level)*

IC, intermittent claudication; *chronic critical limb ischaemia.

range of 3–10%, increasing to 15–20% in people aged over 70 years [5, 6]. In a large German cross-sectional population study, PAD as defined by presence of an ABI <0.9 was shown to be 19.8% in men and 16.8% in women in primary care [7]. In that study, the presence of PAD was shown to be an independent predictor of increased mortality and rate of cardiovascular events at 3 years [8].

Although PAD is progressive in the pathophysiological definition, the natural course of IC is comparatively benign: the Basle study, a large population-based trial, has found significant angiographic progression in 63% of PAD patients after 5 years, although 66% did not exhibit disabling or lifestyle-limiting claudication [9]. Only one-quarter of patients with IC deteriorates and ultimately requires revascularization, with a total of only 5% progressing to CLI [1]. Major amputation is necessary in only 1–3% of claudicants over a 5-year period [1]. Independent predictors of disease progression are multi-level PAD, low ABI, renal insufficiency (➲Chapter 15), diabetes mellitus, and heavy smoking (➲Chapter 14).

In contrast, presence of CLI is associated with excessive morbidity and mortality rates. Lepantalo has reported 1-year mortality and amputation rates of 54% and 46%, respectively, for CLI patients not amenable for arterial reconstruction. Our group has experienced a cumulative 1-year mortality rate of 30.4% in CLI patients partly amenable for endovascular or surgical revascularization [10]. In the latter series, age and renal insufficiency were independent predictors of higher mortality, whereas arterial revascularization was independently associated with lower mortality [10].

PAD of atherosclerotic origin is typically encountered in elderly males [1]. Cigarette smoking is the most important modifiable risk factor that increases both the risk of development and the progression of PAD [1, 11]. PAD is diagnosed 10 years earlier in smokers than in non-smokers and amputation is more common in heavy smokers. Diabetes mellitus is associated with a 1.5- to sixfold increase in PAD prevalence. Moreover, IC is two to four times more common in diabetics than in non-diabetics and the incidence of amputation is increased tenfold [1]. Moreover, in patients with diabetes (➲Chapter 14), a 26% increased risk of PAD has been found for every 1% increase in haemoglobin A1c [12]. Arterial hypertension (➲Chapter 13) is associated with a 2.5-fold increase in PAD incidence in men and a 3.9-fold increase in women [1]. Dyslipidaemia is a further independent risk factor for the development and progression of PAD [1]. In the Framingham study, a fasting cholesterol level >7mmol/L (270mg/dL) was associated with a twofold increase of the incidence of IC [13].

The prevalence of hyperhomocysteinaemia is high in the vascular disease population, compared with 1% in the general population. Hyperhomocysteinaemia may thus be an independent risk factor for atherosclerosis and it may be a stronger risk factor for PAD than for CAD [1]. Of note, distribution pattern of lower limb PAD is clearly affected by patient risk factor profile [14]. Iliac disease is associated with younger age, male gender,and cigarette smoking, whereas infrageniculate disease is associated with higher age, male gender, and diabetes mellitus [14].

Diagnostic strategy

Physical examination in PAD patients should include the entire circulatory system consisting of measurement of bilateral blood pressures; assessment of cardiac murmurs, gallops, and arrhythmias; examination of carotid, aortic, iliac, and femoral bruits; as well as abdominal palpation for aortic aneurysm (➲Chapter 31) [1]. Moreover, changes in lower limb skin colour and temperature, muscular atrophy, decreased hair growth, and presence of hypertrophied, slow-growing nails should be evaluated. Specific lower limb vascular examination comprises palpation of femoral, popliteal, dorsalis pedis, and posterior tibial artery pulses. These pulses should be assessed bilaterally and pulse abnormalities correlated with lower limb symptoms. Finally, patients with a history or examination suggestive of PAD should undergo objective diagnostic testing such as ABI, oscillometric measurement, and duplex ultrasound.

Since the prevalence of abdominal aortic aneurysms (➲Chapter 31) in patients with PAD has been shown to be significantly higher than that reported in the general population [15], we recommend that an abdominal ultrasound quick-screen be routinely included in the study of patients with PAD [16]. Doppler ultrasound measurement of ankle artery pressures and its relation to brachial pressure remains the most effective, accurate, and practical non-invasive test for the detection of PAD and for assessment of haemodynamic efficacy after revascularization [1, 17–19]. A resting ABI <0.9 approaches 95% sensitivity for presence of PAD and 99% specificity in excluding individuals without impairment of arterial perfusion [20] (➲Fig. 36.1).

Exercise testing should be performed in claudicants with normal pulses and normal ABI at rest. Patients with IC and relevant arterial obstruction will typically exhibit a >20mmHg drop in post-exercise ankle pressure. Of note, isolated affection of the internal iliac artery which can result in buttock claudication and impotence in males will not result in diminished peripheral pulses and decreased ABI.

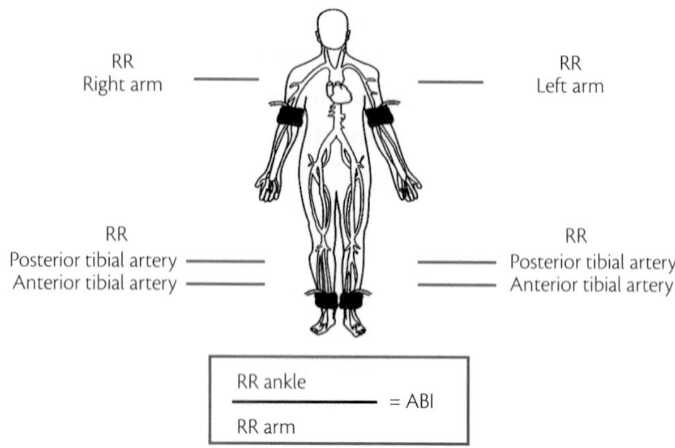

Figure 36.1 Measurement of ankle–brachial index (ABI).

Presence of medial arterial calcification as frequently found in patients with diabetes mellitus and renal disease can result in falsely elevated ABI which independently predicts adverse outcomes [21]. In case of falsely elevated ABI, toe pressure measurements of photoplethysmographic and oscillometric measurements are necessary for the diagnosis of PAD.

In cases of pathologic results from ABI or toe pressure and oscillometric measurements, colour-coded duplex sonography is warranted for assessment of the amenability for surgical or endovascular revascularization— the lower extremity arterial tree can thereby be visualized, with the extent and degree of lesions accurately assessed and arterial velocities measured. Moreover, the common femoral arteries should be analyzed by sonography prior to obtaining arterial access for endovascular therapy. In patients with renal insufficiency scheduled for endovascular intervention, use of duplex ultrasound can help minimize contrast doses.

In many centres, magnetic resonance angiography (MRA) (➲Chapter 5) has become the preferred imaging technique for the diagnosis and treatment planning of patients with PAD [1, 22]. The advantages of MRA include its safety and ability to provide high-resolution three-dimensional imaging of the entire abdominal and lower limb vasculature in one setting. Moreover, pre-interventional use can help to minimize use of iodinated contrast material and exposure to radiation.

Multidetector computed tomography angiography (➲Chapter 6) (MDCTA) is being widely used for diagnostic evaluation and treatment planning of PAD [22] (➲Chapter 6). It enables rapid imaging of the entire lower extremity and abdomen in one breath-hold at very high spatial resolution. The major limitations of MDCTA include the need for iodinated contrast and radiation exposure.

Intra-arterial digital subtraction angiography using iodine contrast is currently considered the 'gold standard' for morphological evaluation of PAD patients despite a certain morbidity risk associated with the invasiveness of the procedure [23]. Intravascular ultrasound (IVUS) is used to quantify the extent of arterial obstructions in study settings [23].

In summary, if a patient qualifies for endovascular or surgical revascularization, angiographic depiction of the arterial tree will ultimately be required in most cases. Although digital subtraction angiography (DSA) is still technically superior to other non-invasive methods, the technique has no real place anymore in the standard pre-treatment work-up in patients with PAD. However, the risks and benefits of either imaging method must be carefully weighed up and tailored to the individual patient's needs. Which non-invasive method (CTA, MRA, etc.) to use mainly depends on the local situation.

Clinical classification of chronic peripheral arterial disease

In patients with PAD the first symptom is IC, i.e. limited walking ability with discomfort of the lower limbs (muscle fatigue or cramping) produced by exercise and relieved by rest. During exercise, leg muscles require a higher blood flow but the presence of PAD limits this increase; the consequence is that the muscle becomes hypoxic and this causes claudication. Discomfort is usually localized distally to the level of arterial obstruction. Symptoms involve the buttocks if the occlusive disease is localized in the abdominal aorta and/or common and internal iliac arteries; the thigh if there is an occlusive disease of external iliac and/or common femoral arteries; or the calf if the arterial disease involves superficial femoral, popliteal, and tibial arteries. IC coincides with stage II of the Fontaine classification and categories 1–3 of the Rutherford classification (➲Table 36.1); it can be classified based on patient walking distance using a graded treadmill test. In sedentary patients and in diabetic patients with peripheral neuropathies, PAD of this stage can be asymptomatic and claudication may not occur. The diagnosis of IC should include patient history and physical examination; differential diagnosis comprises spinal stenosis, hip, foot, and ankle arthritis, Baker's cyst, venous claudication, and nerve root compression.

Although PAD is progressive in the pathological aspects, only 25% of patients with IC deteriorate in terms of clinical stage characterized by ischaemic rest pain and/or ischaemic skin lesions (ulcers or gangrene) with an incidence of 7–9% during the first year after diagnosis [1]. The term CLI describes patients with chronic ischaemic rest pain and/or tissue loss for more than 2 weeks. Recognizing the importance of objectively diagnosing such degrees of ischaemia the diagnosis of CLI should be confirmed by haemodynamic criteria; CLI occurs below an ankle pressure <50mmHg, a toe pressure <30mmHg, and a transcutaneous oxygen partial pressure <20–30mmHg. In patients with CLI the risk of major limb amputation is more than 35% without revascularization [1].

Diabetic foot

The presence of diabetes (➲Chapter 14) increases the frequency of PAD with IC threefold in males and eight-fold in females [24]. An Italian study [25] has shown a prevalence of PAD in the diabetic population of 21.1% and a prevalence of symptomatic PAD (IC) of 7.3%. In patients aged 65–74 years, diabetes increases the limb amputation risk by 20-fold [24].

In the past, there has been some speculation that ischaemia in the diabetic foot is a result of an obstruction in the microcirculation; anatomic studies showed, however, that there was no evidence of a small artery or arteriolar occlusive process in diabetic foot but only a thickening of the capillary basement membrane [26].

The most distinguishing feature of atherosclerosis in diabetes is the more rapid progression, the high incidence of the calcification of the media, and the pattern in which it occurs in the lower extremity arteries (the occlusive process tends to involve the infragenicular arteries, whereas the foot arteries are relatively spared) [27–29].

Peripheral neuropathy is a common complication of diabetes; it leads to sensory loss, atrophy of intrinsic muscle with the development of foot deformities and build-up of pressure points. It makes the foot more susceptible to ulceration even at lesser degrees of ischaemia that would not cause ulceration in the non-diabetic and in the presence of normal arterial circulation. Therefore diabetic foot ulcerations can be divided into three broad categories: ischaemic, neuro-ischaemic, and neuropathic. In diabetic patients all foot ulcers should be classified according to the aetiology and infection complication [30] (➲Table 36.2). In diabetic patients with peripheral neuropathy PAD is usually asymptomatic; therefore in these patients the first clinical symptom is frequently skin ulcers.

In diabetic patients with PAD and tibial arteries calcification, the incompressibility of distal arteries causes a falsely elevated ABI; in these cases measurement of toe pressure or transcutaneous oxygen partial pressure should be implemented. In patients with forefoot gangrene and infection, the last two investigations are oftentimes impossible to take; therefore, frequently, in diabetic patients it is impossible to define CLI by means of haemodynamic criteria but only with clinical definition.

End-stage renal disease

PAD is very common in patients affected with chronic renal insufficiency (➲Chapter 15). From the results of the National Health and Nutrition Examination Survey 1999–2000 [12] the prevalence of PAD in patients >40 years with creatinine clearance <60mL/min (1.73m^2) is 24% as compared to 3.7% of the population with normal renal function. Moreover, chronic renal insufficiency seems to be associated with PAD in women in the postmenopausal period [31]. Histologically, atherosclerotic occlusive disease is characterized by heavy calcification while the occlusive process tends to involve tibial and foot arteries [32].

Therapeutic strategy

The aim of IC therapy is to remove patients' symptoms, improve patients' walking ability, and slacken the clinical and anatomo-pathological progression of PAD. In patient with CLI, instead, the aim is to relieve pain, heal skin lesions, and save limbs—an improvement of quality of life and a decrease in mortality. Therefore, the therapy consists of risk factor control, exercise rehabilitation, medical therapy, and endovascular and/or conventional surgical revascularization.

Modification of atherosclerotic risk factors

Among smokers, the risk of developing PAD is two to three times higher than for non-smokers [33]. Abolition of

Table 36.2 Wound classification: University of Texas Wound Classification System

	Grade 0	Grade I	Grade II	Grade III
Stage A	Pre- or post-ulcerative lesion	Non-infected, non-ischaemic, superficial ulceration	Non-infected, non-ischaemic ulcer that penetrates to capsule or bone	Non-infected, non-ischaemic ulcer that penetrates to bone or deep
Stage B	With infection	With infection	With infection	With infection
Stage C	Without infection, with ischaemia	Without infection, with ischaemia	Without infection, with ischaemia	Without infection, with ischaemia
Stage D	With infection, with ischaemia	With infection, with ischaemia	With infection, with ischaemia	With infection, with ischaemia

smoking is the most important accomplishment in patients affected by PAD [34]; subjects that keep smoking exhibit a significantly increased probability of progression of atherosclerosis including limb loss, myocardial infarction, stroke, and death [33, 34].

Diabetes is associated with PAD and with its progression [35]. An appropriate control of the disease includes glycaemia values between 80–120mg/dL before meals, 180mg/dL after meals, with haemoglobin A1c <7% [36].

Different studies have shown the stabilization or the regression of femoral atherosclerotic lesions and the reduction of the risk of development or worsening of ICs through the control of hyperlipidaemia [37–39]; however, in further studies this effect was not confirmed [40, 41]. Therefore, lipid-lowering therapy in PAD patients with LDL cholesterol values >125mg/dL is recommended with a LDL target value of <100mg/dL. Hypertension must be controlled to reduce the risk for stroke, myocardial infarction, and cardiovascular death.

Exercise rehabilitation

Rehabilitation (➲Chapter 38) has a fundamental role in claudicants. However, this therapy only offers best results when performed under medical supervision and three times per week [42–44]. A recent meta-analysis of various studies has highlighted a 122% increase in maximum walking capacity as evaluated with a treadmill test [45].

Pharmacotherapy (➲Chapter 11)

Different studies on aspirin (ASA) and ticlopidine indicate their effectiveness in reducing myocardial infarction, stroke, and death from cardiovascular disease (ASA 25%, ticlopidine 29%) [46, 47]. While the effectiveness of antiplatelet agents in reducing the incidence of complications in atherosclerotic disease is well known, there is no evidence as to functional improvements in symptoms for PAD; all patients with evidence of PAD (with or without clinical signs) should be treated with antiplatelet agents (except those with specific contraindications) to reduce the incidence of cardiovascular mortality and morbidity.

Anticoagulation is suitable only in patients affected by atrial fibrillation, hypercoagulable state, or valvular prosthesis. For patients with IC, sufficient evidence supporting the routine use of drugs such as pentoxifylline, vasodilators (alpha-blocking, Ca-antagonists), buflomedil, defibrotide, and prostaglandins is lacking [1]. Because of their antiplatelet and vasodilatory effects, prostaglandins have been administrated either intravenously or intra-arterially in advanced stages of PAD. Treatment with prostanoids is indicated only in patients with CLI unsuitable for revascularization and in those with revascularization failures, where the alternative is a major amputation.

Pain control in PAD is necessary to improve quality of life. Narcotics can be used for a short period even during the post-operative period. Epidural single shot or continuous epidural analgesia represent a valid choice for pain control before and after revascularization. An adequate ischaemic pain control is basic for CLI patients; analgesia, however, must not postpone the definitive treatment of the arterial lesions.

Therapeutic angiogenesis is a new area in cardiovascular medicine that has received attention in recent years. Isner's group has proposed intramuscular injection of naked plasmid-expressing vascular endothelial growth factor in order to stimulate collateral growth in PAD [48]. Preliminary studies in patients with CLI have shown improvement in rest pain and ulcer healing [49].

Treatment of skin lesions

In patients with PAD and at stage IV according to the Fontaine classification (➲Fig. 36.2 and ➲Table 36.1), the treatment of ischaemia must be associated with the treatment of the skin lesions and must be contemporary or immediately after limb revascularization. In forefoot lesions the treatment of choice is minor amputation; for lesions localized on dorsal and plantar sites of the foot and heel it is necessary to remove the necrotic and/or infected tissues, followed by dressing. In cases of infection (➲Fig. 36.3) a broad-spectrum antibiotic therapy is necessary; a culture exam is indispensable to define the source of the infection and to commence a specific antibiotic therapy.

Other treatments

Hyperbaric oxygen must be exclusively used as an adjunctive therapy of revascularization in CLI patients and skin

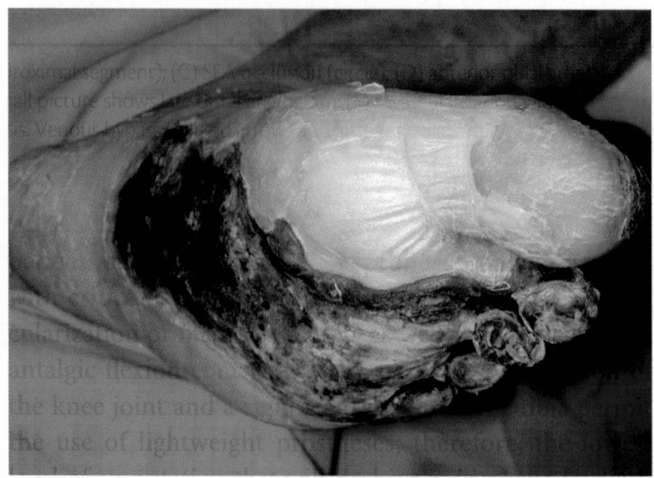

Figure 36.2 Critical limb ischaemia (CLI): gangrene of the forefoot and plantar surface of the foot.

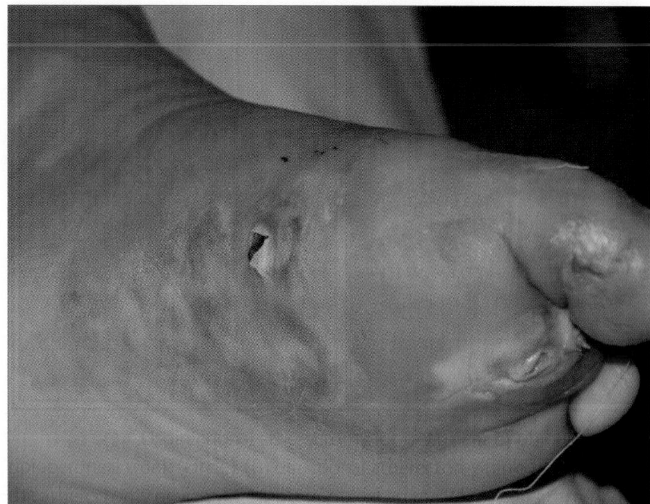

Figure 36.3 Foot infection in diabetic patient with peripheral arterial occlusive disease.

lesion with infection. That is particularly recommended in diabetic patients [50]; at present, there is no evidence supporting the use of hyperbaric oxygen in CLI patients unsuitable for revascularization. Spinal cord stimulation can be used in patients with CLI not suitable for revascularization clinically characterized by rest pain (Fontaine stage III, Rutherford category 4) or little skin lesions (Rutherford category 5) [51].

Revascularization management

In the management of patients with IC, revascularization should be considered only if regular exercise and other non-interventional therapies fail and if a patient's handicap is severe. However, in a patient with CLI the revascularization strategy should be considered as the first treatment in conjunction with control of pain and foot infection, prevention of progression of thrombosis, and optimization of cardiac and respiratory function.

Limb revascularization can be achieved by using endovascular techniques or arterial surgery. The choice between an endovascular and surgical procedure depends largely on the exact level (aorto-iliac, femoro-popliteal, and infrapopliteal disease) and the extent (stenosis, occlusion, length of the lesion) of the PAD. If the both techniques are equally feasible with a similar success rate and medium-term outcome, the technique associated with lower morbidity and mortality is indicated—the endovascular procedure. Endovascular techniques include balloon angioplasty, stents, stent-grafts, and plaque debulking procedures; surgical options include bypass (with autogenous, synthetic, or cryopreserved grafts), endarterectomy, or a hybrid procedure.

In order to apply the correct treatment option for aorto-iliac, femoro-popliteal, and tibial arteries in a specific patient, the TransAtlantic Inter-Society Consensus (TASC) introduced a morphological classification in 2000 [52], recently updated for aorto-iliac and femoro-popliteal segments [1]. TASC classifications regarding aorto-iliac, femoro-popliteal, and infrapopliteal disease are shown in ➲Tables 36.3–36.5 [1, 52].

On the basis of the results of the last 15 years on surgical and endovascular treatment of PAD [53–83], it is possible to assert that for type A lesions the first treatment is

Table 36.3 TransAtlantic Inter-Society Consensus classification of aorto-iliac lesions

Type A lesions	Unilateral or bilateral stenosis of CIA Unilateral or bilateral single short (≤3cm) stenosis of EIA
Type B lesions	Short (≤3cm) stenosis of infrarenal aorta Unilateral CIA occlusion Single or multiple stenosis totalling 3–10cm involving the EIA not extending into the CFA Unilateral EIA occlusion not involving the origins of internal iliac or CFA
Type C lesions	Bilateral CIA occlusions Bilateral EIA stenoses 3–10cm long not extending into the CFA Unilateral EIA stenosis extending into the CFA Unilateral EIA occlusion that involves the origins of internal iliac and/or CFA Heavily calcified unilateral EIA occlusion with or without involvement of origins of internal iliac and/or CFA
Type D lesions	Infrarenal aorto-iliac occlusion Diffuse disease involving the aorta and both iliac arteries requiring treatment Diffuse multiple stenoses involving the unilateral CIA, EIA, and CFA Unilateral occlusions of both CIA and EIA Bilateral occlusions of EIA Iliac stenoses in patients with AAA requiring treatment and not amenable to endograft placement or other lesions requiring open aortic or iliac surgery

AAA, abdominal aortic aneurysm; CFA, common femoral artery; CIA, common iliac artery; EIA, external iliac artery.

Table 36.4 TransAtlantic Inter-Society Consensus classification of femoral-popliteal lesions

Type A lesions	Single stenosis ≤10cm in length Single occlusion ≤5cm in length
Type B lesions	Multiple lesions (stenoses or occlusions) each ≤5cm Single stenosis or occlusion ≤15cm not involving the infrageniculate popliteal artery Single or multiple lesions in the absence of continuous tibial vessels to improve inflow for a distal bypass Heavily calcified occlusion ≤5cm in length Single popliteal stenosis
Type C lesions	Multiple stenoses or occlusions totalling >15cm with or without heavy calcification Recurrent stenoses or occlusions that need treatment after two endovascular interventions
Type D lesions	Chronic total occlusions of CFA or SFA (>20cm, involving the popliteal artery) Chronic total occlusion of the popliteal artery and proximal trifurcation vessels

CFA, common femoral artery; SFA, superficial femoral artery.

endovascular therapy while for type D lesions it is surgery; type B lesions offer sufficiently good results with endovascular therapy; and type C lesions should be addressed with open revascularization, reserving endovascular therapy only for surgical high-risk patients.

Aorto-iliac revascularization

Iliac artery obstructions have been traditionally treated by open interventions, e.g. aorto-femoral or aorto-bifemoral bypass grafting. This treatment is highly effective with a high patency rates: in patients with Fontaine's clinical stage II the patency rate is 91% (90–94%) at 5 years and 86.8% (85–92%) at 10 years; in patients with critical ischaemia patency is 87.5% (80–88%) at 5 years and 81.8% (70–85%) at 10 years, with a mortality rate of 3.3% and systemic morbidity of 8.3% [84]. This treatment is generally performed with a transperitoneal approach; alternative choices have been suggested such as a retroperitoneal approach and, more recently, a laparoscopic approach [85–87].

Interest in the aortic endoarterectomy has gradually declined because of the excellent results with bypass and currently is mostly reserved to young patients, patients with short lesions unsuitable for endovascular treatment, and patients at high risk for infection; the patency at 5 years varies between 60–94% [88–90]. In patients at high surgical risk or with hostile abdomen an extra-anatomical bypass can be performed. The subclavian artery, the descending thoracic aorta or the contralateral iliac and femoral arteries can be used as donor vessels. The patency after 5 years varies from 30–79% in axillo-femoral bypass; from 33–85% for the axillo-bifemoral bypass; around 80% in toraco-femoral bypass; and between 55–92% in femoro-femoral crossover [91–103].

Percutaneous transluminal angioplasty (PTA) is a less invasive alternative and in the last few years has proven to be an effective technique for the treatment of focal iliac artery lesions (type A and type B iliac lesions) (➲Fig. 36.4; 36.1–36.12). In our experience, in most cases iliac artery lesion can be treated using ipsilateral retrograde access but, in total occlusions, antegrade recanalization using a cross-over or left brachial approach is recommended. The reported success rate is 85–99% (mean 95%); adjunctive stent implantation has even increased the primary success rate to 95–100% (mean 99%) [82]. The current indications for iliac arteries stenting are elastic recoil, dissection and thrombosis after PTA, chronic occlusion, restenosis and complex lesions; balloon-expandable stents should be chosen for implantation in short lesions of common iliac artery while self-expanding stents may be considered for long, less calcified, non-ostial lesions in the external iliac artery. The patency rate after 5 years for endovascular treatment of iliac artery stenosis is 80–90%; the long-term patency for PTA of complete iliac occlusion is reported to be 20% lower than that for iliac stenosis [69, 82] (➲Fig. 36.5; 36.13–36.20).

Table 36.5 Classification of infrapopliteal lesions

Type A lesions	Single stenoses <1cm in the tibial or peroneal vessels
Type B lesions	Multiple focal stenoses of the tibial or peroneal vessel, each <1cm in length One or two focal stenoses, each <1cm long, at the tibial trifurcation Short tibial or peroneal stenoses in conjunction with femoropopliteal PTA
Type C lesions	Stenoses 1–4cm in length Occlusions 1–2cm in length of the tibial or peroneal vessels Extensive stenoses of the tibial trifurcation
Type D lesions	Tibial or peroneal occlusions >2cm Diffusely diseased tibial or peroneal vessels

PTA, percutaneous transluminal angioplasty.

Femoro-popliteal revascularization

The low morbidity and mortality of endovascular technique such as PTA makes it the preferred choice of treatment in limited disease such as type A and type B femoro-popliteal lesions. A key issue for successful endovascular intervention is selection of the appropriate vascular access. Two standard approaches are available for femoral, popliteal, and tibial artery interventions: the cross-over and the antegrade approach. Other possibilities are the transpopliteal and the pedal approaches. The cross-over approach from the common femoral artery is considered in many centres

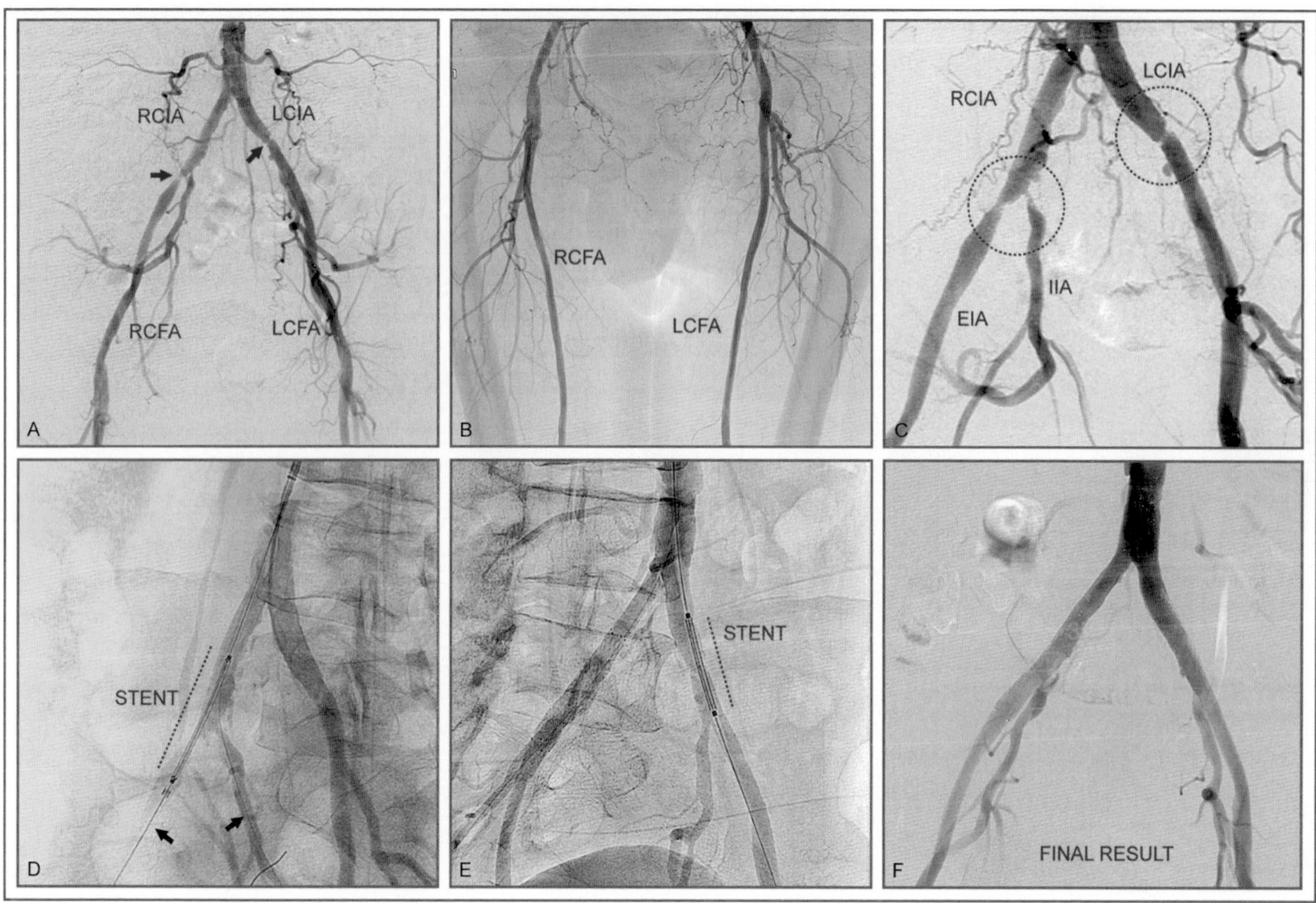

Figure 36.4 Focal iliac artery lesions endovascular treatment. Bilateral iliac artery angioplasty and stenting: (A) angiogram showing bilateral iliac artery stenosis (arrows); (B) femoral arteries free of disease; (C) iliac angiogram revealing a bifurcation stenosis on the RCIA and a focal stenosis on the LCIA; (D) using the kissing-wire technique (arrows) a stent is positioned at the bifurcation level (stent length represented by dotted line); (E) angiogram showing good result of the bifurcation angioplasty and the stent positioning at the LCIA stenosis (stent length represented by dotted line); (F) final angiographic result. EIA, external iliac artery; IIA, internal iliac artery; LCFA, left common femoral artery; LCIA, left common iliac artery; RCFA, right common femoral artery; RCIA, right common iliac artery. Also see 36.1–36.12.

to be the standard access technique for femoro-popliteal interventions. Some interventionalists prefer the antegrade approach because it provides more direct access to many lesions in the medial and distal femoro-poplital segment and the infrageniculate arteries; it may be helpful for crossing very calcified lesions. Antegrade puncture is technically more challenging in obese patients.

The technical success rate of PTA of femoro-popliteal artery stenoses and occlusions exceeds 95% and 85% respectively. There is general agreement that for acute failure of PTA (thrombosis, flow-limiting dissections, and residual stenosis >30%) of a femoral artery lesion and restenosis, stent placement is indicated. Based on the study of Schillinger *et al.* [104] we know that primary stent placement of superficial femoral artery (SFA) lesions has a better outcome than PTA plus optional stent placement. Only self-expanding stents should be used in the SFA—an artery that is subject to compression, elongation, shortening, and distortion over its whole length. The stent should always cover the whole lesion, and preferably extend for a few millimetres into the healthy vessel (➲ Fig. 36.6; 36.21–36.31). The occlusion of side-branches after stenting is rare. The diameter of self-expanding nitinol stents should be 1–2mm larger than the reference vessel; post-dilatation for adaptation of the stent is necessary in the majority of cases. Fracture can occur in self-expanding nitinol stents in the SFA. The primary patency rate at 12 months is significantly lower for patients with stent fracture [105].

In patients with long occlusion of the femoro-popliteal axis (TASC type C lesion) with an indication of endovascular treatment, stent-graft can be used [106, 107]. Surgery is the treatment of choice in patients with TASC type D lesions. The surgical intervention more frequently used in femoro-popliteal lesions is bypass.

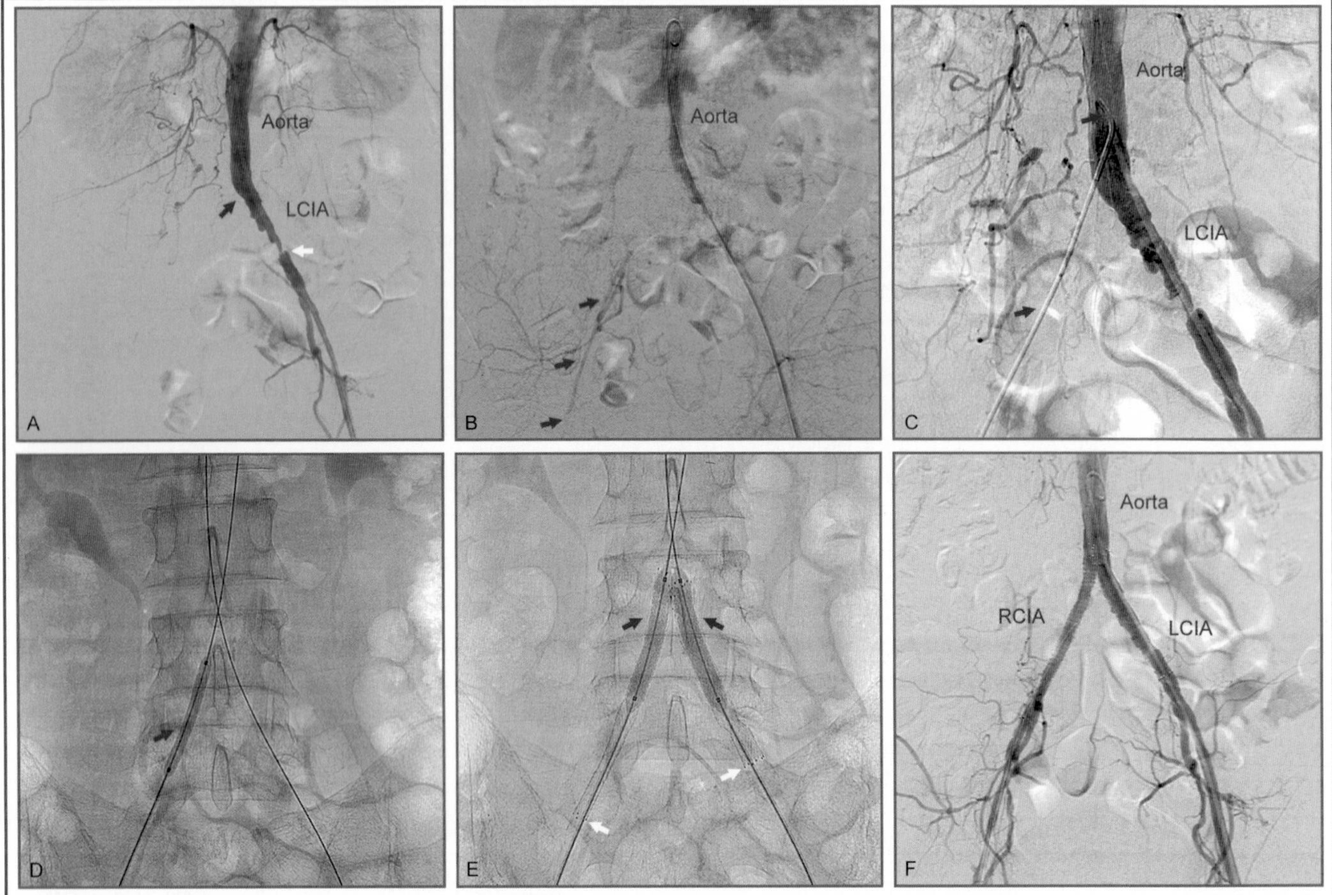

Figure 36.5 Complete iliac occlusion endovascular treatment. Chronic total iliac occlusion recanalization: (A) distal aorta angiogram (pigtail catheter from left femoral access). Note the occlusion at the origin of RCIA (red arrow) and a severe stenosis in the LCIA; (B) prolonged angiogram revealing opacification of the distal right iliac artery (arrows) by collateral vessels; (C) crossing the occlusion (arrows) from right femoral access; (D) lesion pre-dilatation with balloon angioplasty (arrow); (E) final kissing balloon angioplasty (red arrows) after bilateral stenting. Note the distal end of both stents (white arrows); (F) final angiographic result. LCIA, left common iliac artery; RCIA, right common iliac artery. Also see 36.13–36.20.

The above-knee bypass in patients with IC performed with autologous veins has a primary patency rate after 5 years of 80%, the rate is 75% in polytetrafluoroethylene (PTFE) bypass [108]; in patients with critical ischaemia the primary patency after 5 years is 66% with autologous vein and 47% with PTFE [108]. The results of a recent meta-analysis on femoro-distal bypass performed with saphenous vein and PTFE in patients with critical ischaemia and IC [109] underline the role of the saphenous vein as first graft choice. In recent publications there is no statistical significant differences between the results of the two prosthetic materials; as a logical consequence, in order to save the autologous vein for any subsequent surgical infrapopliteal revascularization, PTFE can be proposed as the first-choice prosthetic material in above-the-knee femoro-popliteal bypass. Saphenous vein has better long-term patency than prosthetic in below-the-knee bypass (➲Fig. 36.7). In its absence, other venous tissue (contralateral long saphenous vein, lesser saphenous vein, arm veins) or prosthetic bypass graft with adjunt procedures (arterio-venous fistula, cuff) have been suggested.

In patients with IC, stenosis or short occlusion of the origin of the profunda femoris artery, long occlusion of SFA, and excellent collateral flow to the tibial arteries, an isolated profundoplasty is recommended; the use of these technique in patients with CLI appears to be controversial.

Infrapopliteal revascularization

The therapeutic recommendations proposed by TASC for this district are oriented to endovascular treatment in type A and surgery in type D lesions. In spite of these clear recommendations, many recent publications report very promising clinical results of endovascular treatment applied to infrapopliteal type D lesions in patients with CLI [110–113].

Endovascular treatment of infrapopliteal arteries is mainly indicated in patients with CLI (➲Fig. 36.8; 36.32–36.37); restoration of straight-line flow to the pedal arch by angioplasty in one or more tibial arteries is

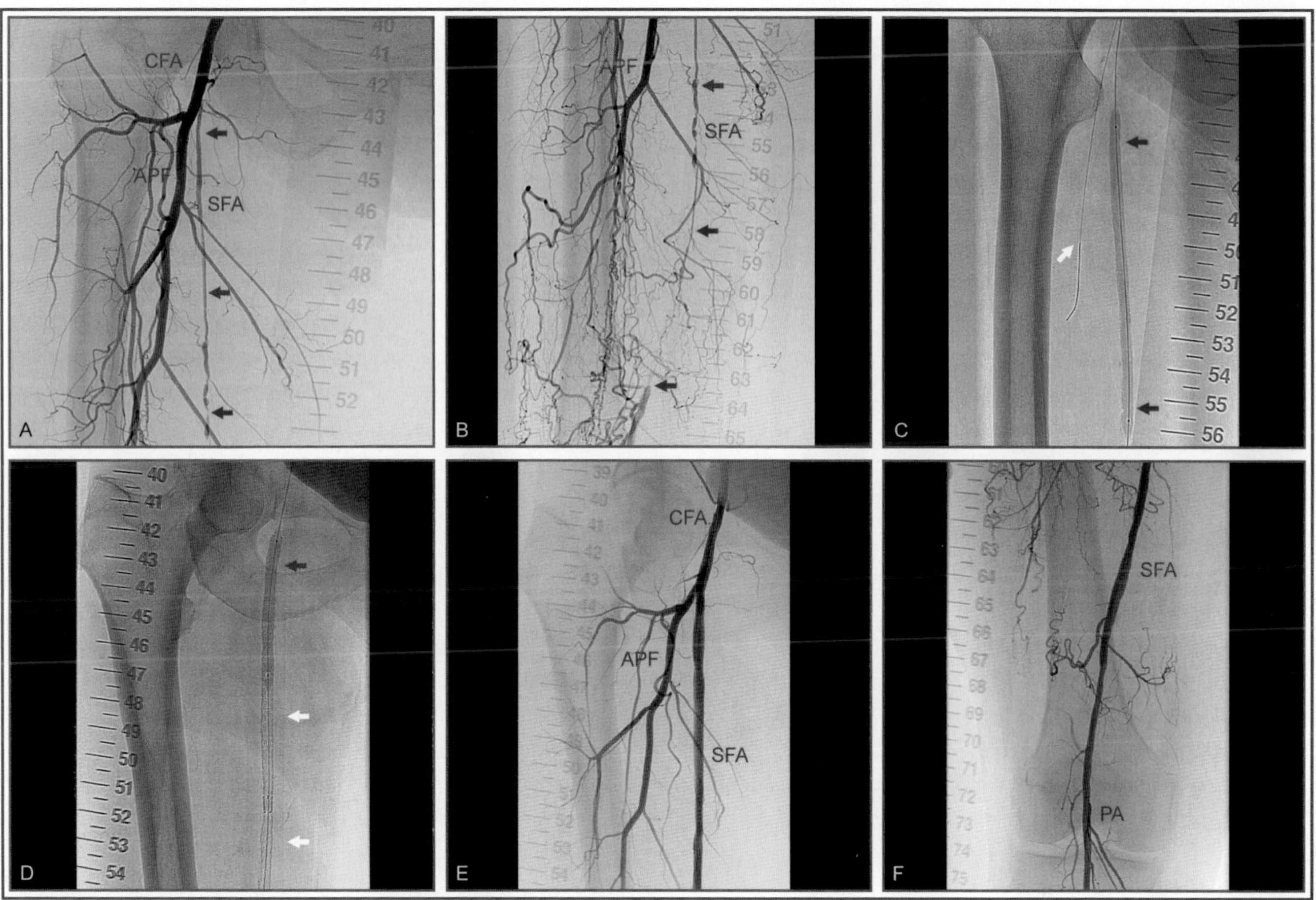

Figure 36.6 Angioplasty and stenting of femoral artery diffuse disease and occlusion. Right SFA diffuse disease and occlusion. (A) severe and diffuse disease on the proximal segment of right SFA (arrows); (B) vessel occlusion in the mid portion of the SFA; (C) lesion pre-dilatation with angioplasty balloon (red arrow). Note: a 'protection' 0.014-inch (0.35mm) guidewire left in the arteria profunda femoris (white arrow); (D) stent post-dilatation (red arrow). Note that two long stents were overlapped to cover the lesion (white arrows); Final angiographic result of (E) proximal and (F) distal segments of the SFA. APF, arteria profunda femoris; CFA, common femoral artery; PA, popliteal artery; SFA, superficial femoral artery. Also see 36.21–36.31.

necessary for clinical success. In most cases, below-the-knee stenoses and occlusions can be treated using an ipsilateral antegrade approach; alternatively, the intervention can be performed using cross over technique. Only low-profile balloons should be used to dilate infrapopliteal vessels; in cases of long occlusions or multiple vessel stenoses, long balloons (≥10cm) have been demonstrated to be the best option. The technical success rate of infrapopliteal artery PTA is >90% while limb salvage has been reported to be ≥80% at 2 years [25, 110, 114]. Negative prognostic factors for technical success and early and long-term clinical outcome include long occlusion, calcified lesion, poor run off, chronic renal disease, and posterior tibial artery angioplasty [1, 112, 115–117].

Stent implantation in below-knee arteries should be limited to recoil and any post-procedural complications (thrombosis, flow-limiting dissections). One limitation of conventional recanalization techniques remains the partial inability to cross total occlusions. As an alternative, laser ablation can be used in a step-by-step manner where the guidewire and then a laser catheter are sequentially advanced and activated until the occlusion or stenosis is crossed.

Pedal bypass grafting with autologous vein is indicated in patients with CLI, long occlusions of tibial arteries or tibial lesions unsuitable for endovascular therapy, and patent foot arteries (➲ Fig. 36.9); this technique is safe, effective, and durable. The limb salvage success rate has been reported to be ≥80% at 2 years [118].

Post-procedural treatment

After surgical or endovascular limb revascularization, adjuvant therapy is required. Antiplatelet agents must be proposed indefinitely in all patients who undergo limb revascularization. In patients with bypass at high risk of thrombosis (poor run off, vein bypass with suboptimal graft, and so on) the recommendation is antiplatelet agents and anticoagulants. In patients submitted to endovascular

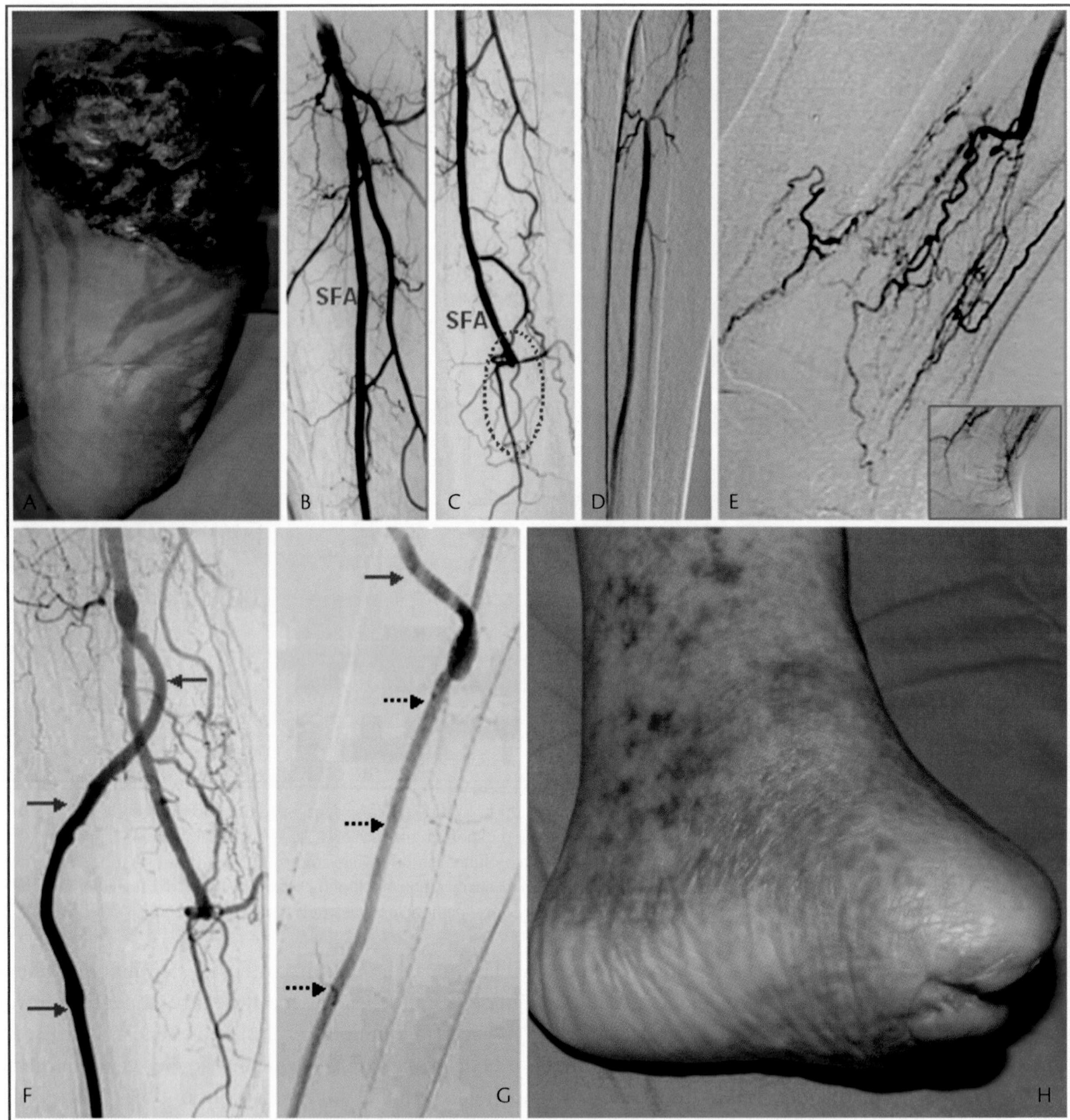

Figue 36.7 CLI surgical treatment. (A) forefoot gangrene; (B) SFA angiogram (proximal segment); (C) SFA occlusion (circle); (D) anterior tibial artery patency; (E) posterior and peroneal artery occlusion with reduced distal flow. Small picture shows late distal angiogram; (F) revascularization with femoro-distal (anterior tibial artery) bypass (arrows); (G) bypass distal anastomosis. Venous bypass (full red arrow) and anterior tibial artery (dotted black arrow); (H) clinical result after 12 months.

treatment for total occlusion or stent implantation (high risk of reocclusion) antiplatelet therapy can be associated with low-molecular-weight heparin for 4 weeks.

Primary amputation

Primary amputation is defined as major amputation (amputation above the ankle) without an antecedent attempt at revascularization. Primary amputation of the lower limb in patients suffering from PAD is proposed only in patients with critical ischaemia unsuitable for any form of revascularization or medical therapy, as well as in patients with antalgic flexion contractures of the limb. Preservation of the knee joint and a significant length of the tibia permit the use of lightweight prostheses; therefore, the lowest level of amputation that will heal is the ideal site for limb transaction.

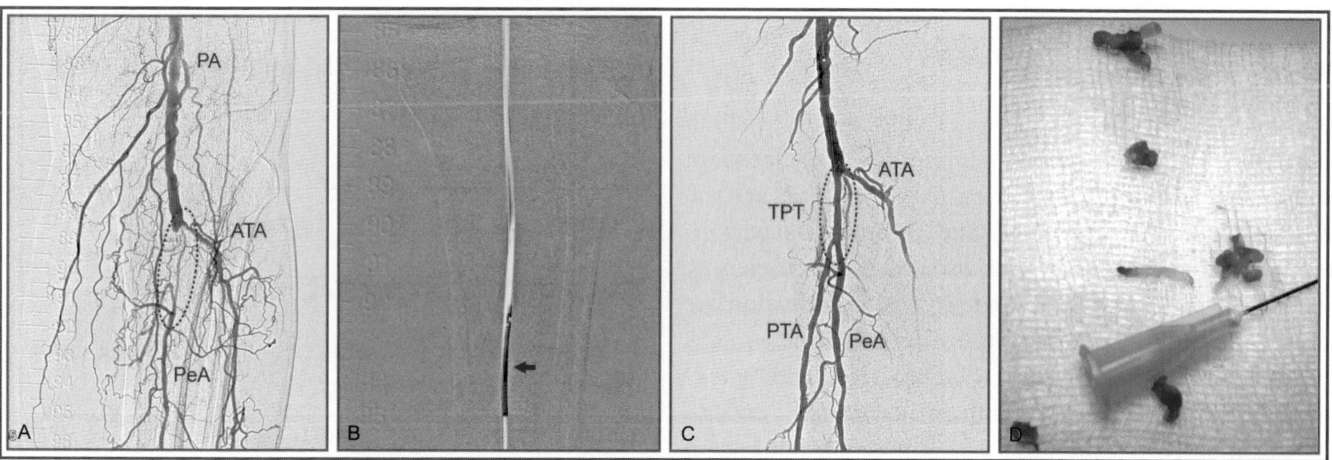

Figure 36.8 CLI: directional atherectomy for treatment of tibio-peroneal trunk occlusion. Tibio-peroneal trunk occlusion: (A) occlusion of the tibioperoneal trunk (circle). (B) directional atherectomy (arrow) after lesion pre-dilatation; (C) final angiographic result. (D) specimens retrieved from the atherectomy device. ATA, anterior tibial artery; PA, popliteal artery; TPT, tibio-peroneal trunk; PeA, peroneal artery; PTA, posterior tibial artery; SFA, superficial femoral artery. Also see 36.32–36.37.

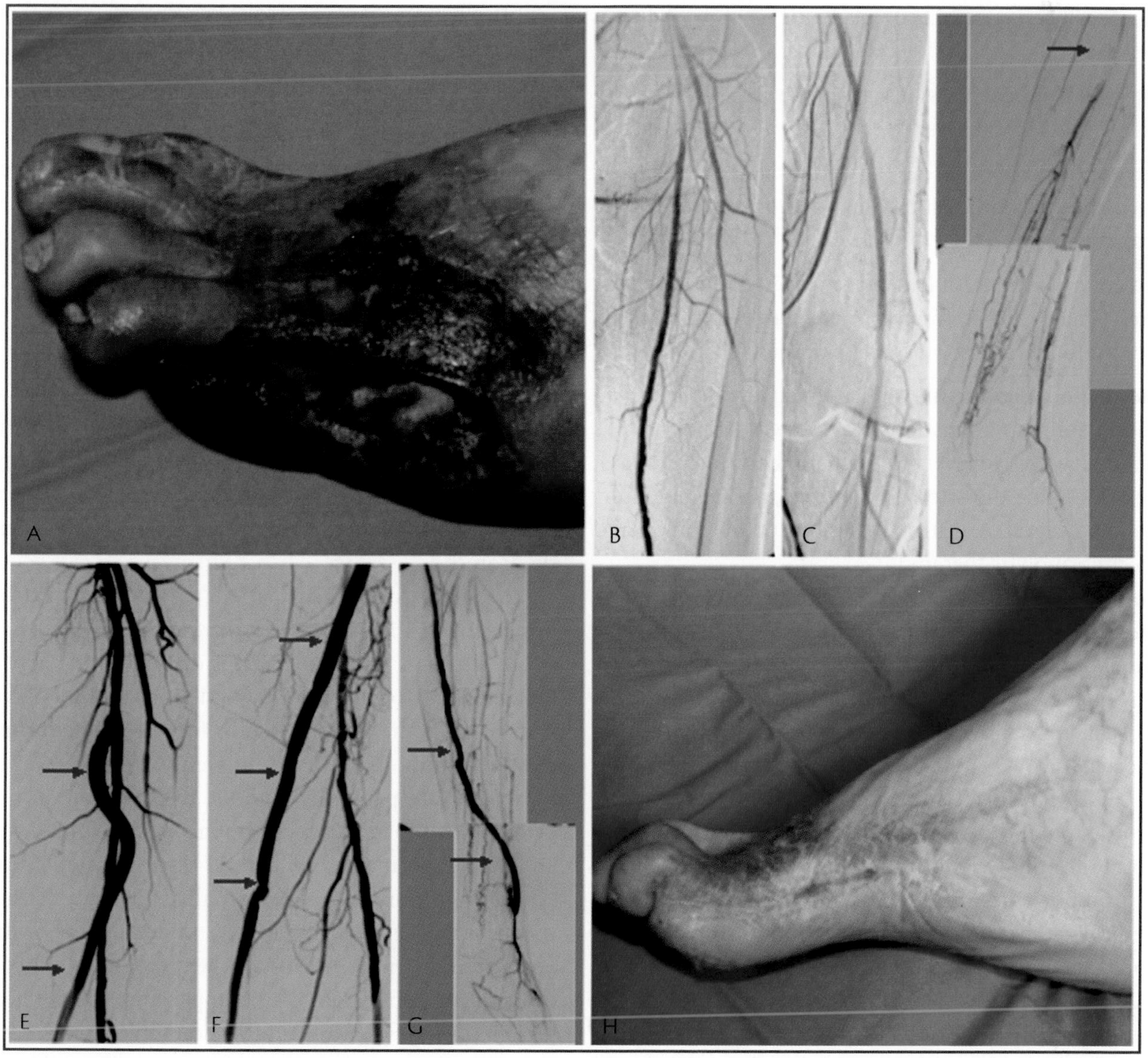

Figure 36.9 Anterior tibial artery bypass grafting for critical limb ischaemia in diabetic patient. (A) foot gangrene; (B) SFA angiogram; (C) angiogram at the level of the knee; (D) below-the-knee angiogram. Note the long occlusion of three tibial arteries (arrow); (E,F) This patient was submitted to arterial revascularization with composite autologous vein bypass between the superficial femoral artery (G) and the anterior tibial artery at the ankle; (H) clinical result after 6 months.

Acute limb ischaemia

Acute limb ischaemia is defined as a sudden decrease in limb perfusion with a risk of limb damage. The most frequent causes are arterial embolization (heart disease, arterial atheroma, arterial aneurism) and thrombosis (peripheral arterial aneurism, arterial dissection, atherosclerotic plaque). A patient's history and physical examination are often sufficient to frame the cause of acute ischaemia.

Patients with acute limb ischaemia refer with unexpected pain often associated with an alteration of sensitivity and motility. At the physical examination findings of acute limb ischaemia may include the '5Ps' in the ischaemic area: pain, pulselessness, pallor, paresthesia (abnormal sensitivity), and paralysis. In acute limb ischaemia the alteration of sensitivity and motility influences the prognosis. Acute ischaemia is clinically classified on limb vitality in 3 categories:

- Category I: presence of vital signs of the limb—no sensory loss or muscle weakness.
- Category II: risk of losing the limb—moderate sensory loss associated with rest pain, mild-to-moderate muscle weakness.
- Category III: irreversible damage of nerve/muscle structures—major tissue loss or permanent nerve damage, with profound sensory loss and paralysis.

The diagnosis of acute limb ischaemia is clinical; in addiction some investigations may be performed such as continuous wave Doppler (to evaluate the Winsor index), duplex (to define the arterial occlusion), and angiography (to define the level of obstructive lesion and the run off and to inject fibrinolytic therapy).

Prompt reconstruction of perfusion is the most effective treatment in terms of maintaining a viable limb. The first goal of the therapy is to prevent thrombosis propagation by giving intravenous heparin. The aetiology of acute limb ischaemia allows the most appropriate therapy to be chosen (thrombolysis or surgery)—surgical therapy is proposed in category I and II; for patients in category III a major amputation is indicated; thrombolysis (intra-arterial local thrombolysis) is proposed in limb ischaemia due to a thrombotic origin. Endovascular techniques include thrombolysis, percutaneous aspiration thrombectomy, and percutaneous mechanical thrombectomy. The surgical technique used to treat acute limb ischaemia includes the use of the Fogarty catheter balloon that offers better results in arterial embolization; intraoperative angiography should be performed to define surgical result. In acute, severe, and prolonged limb ischaemia a fasciotomy must be performed that should cover all the compartments.

Cerebral vascular disease

Key points (also see ➲Chapter 15)

- Cerebrovascular disease is the second leading cause of death in Western countries.
- Risk factors for supra-aortic trunk occlusive disease include systemic hypertension, diabetes, hyperlipidaemia, smoking, and concomitant coronary and PAD.
- Recognition of clinical presentation, associated to rapid and early recanalization of severe carotid stenosis, is critically important for stroke prevention.
- Up to now, no systematic evidence exists to support the preferential use of carotid endarterectomy over carotid stenting, or vice versa.
- Carotid stenting with emboli protection performed by an experienced operator should be viewed as a valid alternative to surgery for patients at high risk for endarterectomy.

Definition

Occlusive disease involving the supra-aortic vessels is common, but symptomatic lesions are relatively infrequent. Most clinically significant lesions are caused by atherosclerosis followed by fibromuscular dysplasia, Takayasu's arteritis, post-traumatic lesions, and external compression syndromes.

A detailed history of the patient's symptoms is extremely important and is a key factor for establishing the diagnosis. In addition, the history helps distinguishing asymptomatic lesions from symptomatic lesions and this division is most often the deciding factor for selecting appropriate treatment options. It is also imperative to ascertain if the symptoms are primarily embolic or ischaemic in origin. Common complaints depend on the specific vessel involved and in the specific case of carotid disease include cerebral symptoms of vertigo, headache, gait disturbances, syncope, transient ischaemic attacks (TIAs), minor and major stroke. Less specific symptoms like a slowly progressive shortness of memory, and tremor of the upper limbs or the head in patients over 60 years old and without other evident disease should induce the generalist to initiate a diagnostic process to exclude the presence of a carotid artery disease.

A significant (>50%) stenosis of the internal carotid artery may account for 5–10% of all strokes [119]. The prevalence of carotid disease increases with age. Even though half of men over 75 years of age may have evidence of carotid atherosclerosis, stenoses of >50% are detected in only approximately 5% [120]. The highest prevalence (12.5–28%) of carotid stenosis is found in patients with PAD, whereas carotid stenosis among unselected patients with coronary disease is rare (<5%) [121]. Conversely, even in the absence of cardiac symptoms, patients with carotid disease frequently (25–60%) have significant coronary artery disease [122]. The risk of stroke in patients with carotid disease is predicted by recent neurological symptoms and the degree of stenosis. In asymptomatic patients it is estimated to be <2% per year but may increase to as high as 5.5% per year among individuals with stenosis >75% [123]. In patients with severe carotid stenosis presenting with TIAs, the risk of subsequent stroke is approximately 10% at 1 year and 30–35% at 5 years [124].

Diagnostic strategy

The diagnostic tool of choice for assessing carotid stenosis is duplex ultrasonography (DUS). A systematic review of the literature addressing the efficacy of DUS in discriminating between severe (70–99%) and moderate (<70%) stenosis compared with DSA yielded a pooled sensitivity and specificity of 87% and 86% respectively [125]. In the same analysis, the sensitivity and specificity of MRA was 95% and 90% respectively. Although currently somewhat less reliable, CTA may be used as an alternative, non-invasive imaging modality in addition to DUS [126]. Improvements in non-invasive carotid diagnostics have lowered the need for DSA, which remains the gold standard for the diagnosis of carotid stenosis. Since DSA even in experienced hands carries a risk of stroke (< 1%), diagnostic angiography should be performed only in selected cases [127].

As previously mentioned, duplex ultrasound is the most practical non-invasive test in the diagnostic algorithm. Ultrasound provides both anatomic and physiologic information regarding a lesion and is the best initial test to establish the haemodynamic and functional significance of a stenosis.

- Indications for echo colour Doppler:
  - patients with a recent TIA or stroke;
  - patients with evidence of vascular disease in other territories;
  - patients with coronary artery disease;
  - patients with multiple risk factors for vascular disease.
- Quantitative assessment:
  - intimal thickening (<0.8mm) disease >1.5;
  - mild stenosis (up to 40% of the vessel area);
  - moderate stenosis (50–70% of the vessel area);
  - critical stenosis (>70% of the vessel area);
  - normal velocity of systolic–diastolic flow (up to 1.3 ± 0.5m/sec);
  - pathologic flow velocity (>1.3 ± 0.5m/sec);
  - critical flow velocity (>2.0 ± 0.7m/sec).
- Qualitative assessement:
  - Stable carotid plaque (➲Fig. 36.10):
    - fibrotic;
    - fibrolipidic;
    - fibrocalcific.
  - Unstable carotid plaque (➲Fig. 36.11):
    - lipid cores;
    - protein cores;
    - mucopolysaccharide cores;
    - subintimal haemorrhages;
    - thrombotic lesions.

For complete and updated information regarding the indications and clinical competence of new techniques of vascular imaging with CT and MR, we refer the reader to the recently published document of consensus of the ACCF/AHA [128].

From surgical trials to daily practice: risk–benefit assessment in symptomatic and asymptomatic patients

The role of carotid artery disease therapy in the prevention of stroke has been debated for many years in the literature. In the early 1990s, the results from two large randomized surgical trials, comparing medical management with carotid endarterectomy lead to set the therapeutic recommendations still valid today [129, 130].

Risk–benefit assessment is an objective process, based on the best scientific evidence, oriented to the identification of the optimal treatment options in different categories of patients with carotid disease, according to grade of carotid stenosis, neurological symptoms, and clinical conditions. Of paramount importance in this setting is the method of carotid stenosis grading: the NASCET method is the one used in this chapter, and correspond to the arteriographic

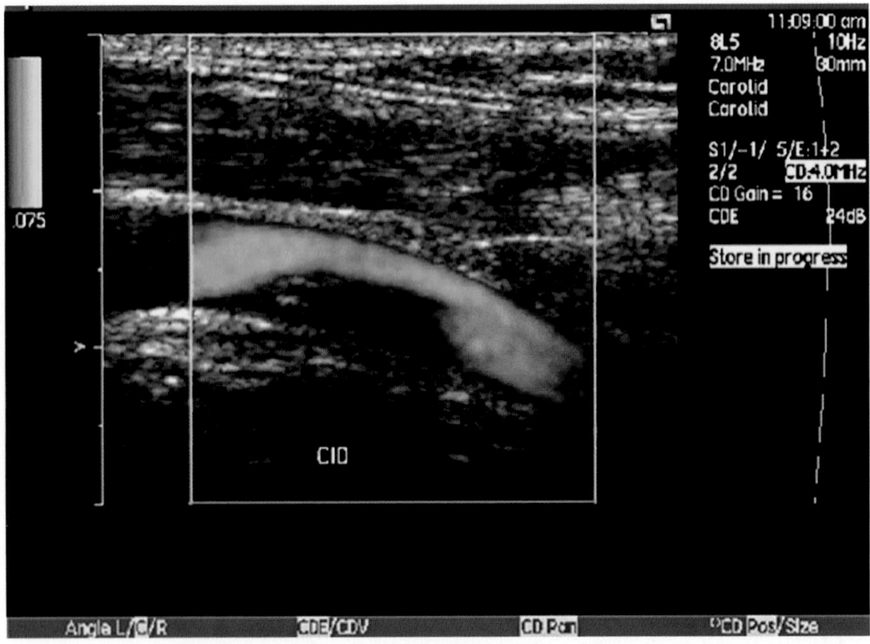

Figure 36.10 Example of stable fibrotic plaque.

diameter reduction calculated as the minimum residual lumen at the point of maximum stenosis referenced to the diameter of the distal lumen of the internal carotid artery at the first point at which the arterial walls became parallel [129].

Symptomatic patients are defined as patients who have experienced transient cerebral ischaemia, non-disabling stroke, transient monocular blindness, or retinal infarction in the last 6 months [129, 130].

Low-grade carotid stenosis (<50% in symptomatic patients and <60% in asymptomatic patients)

A review of the available randomized trials [131] and the results from two large randomized controlled trials (RCTs), NASCET and ECST [129, 130], showed that in patients with low-grade carotid stenosis, medical therapy is superior to surgery, since the risk of stroke or death in patients submitted to carotid endarterectomy increased by 20% compared with patients treated medically. Best medical therapy was assessed by the guidelines of the American Heart Association issued in 2006 and should aim to lower blood pressure below 120/80mmHg, control glucose in diabetic patients to near-normoglycaemic levels (target haemoglobin A1c <7%), and change lifestyle to lower low-density lipoprotein cholesterol in patients with coronary artery disease, symptomatic peripheral atherosclerotic disease, or multiple risk factors. Smokers should achieve cessation. Antiplatelet therapy such as aspirin (50–325mg/day) or clopidogrel should be administrated to patients with history of ischaemic stoke or TIA [132].

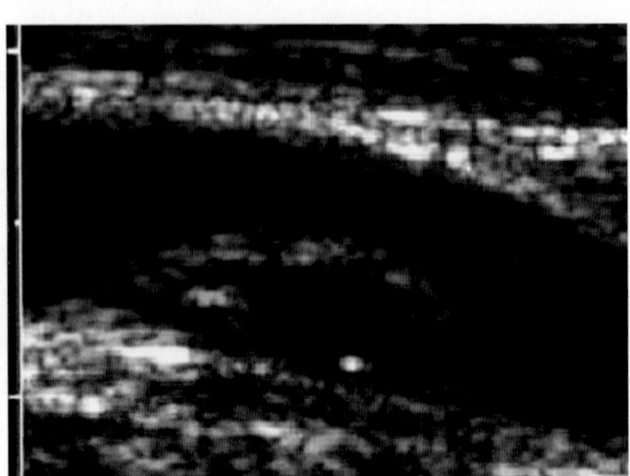

Figure 36.11 Example of unstable plaque with necrotic core.

Moderate or severe carotid stenosis (>50%) in symptomatic patients

Symptomatic patients with carotid stenosis greater than 50% have a clear benefit from surgery. Carotid endarterectomy is therefore recommended in these patients. The pooled data from the major carotid surgery trials have shown that even if great care is taken to optimize the medical risk factors, patients with carotid stenosis greater than 50% have a 5-year cumulative risk of 21.2% for ipsilateral ischaemic stroke if treated medically alone [133, 134]. In contrast, although the risk of stroke and death within 30 days after endarterectomy was 5.8% in NASCET and 7.5% in ECST, the subsequent rate of stroke in surgically treated patients with severe stenosis was only 1–2% per annum [133, 134]. Thus a stroke can be prevented in every 15 patients treated by carotid endarterectomy. Patients with more severe stenosis (70–99%) had a greater benefit from surgery (ipsilateral stroke rate at 2 years was 9% versus 26% in the medical arm), leading to one stroke prevented every nine patients treated [129].

Similar results were obtained in the ECST where surgery leads to a 3-year risk of stroke of 2.8% versus 16.8% of medical therapy at 3 years. Disabling stroke or death occurred in 6.0% of patients in the surgical arm versus 11.0% in medical therapy; thus seven patients should undergo surgery to prevent one stroke [130].

However, there is no conclusive evidence for the effectiveness of carotid endarterectomy in patients with symptoms from the posterior cerebral circulation or with acute stroke and internal carotid occlusion. Also, other subgroups of patients, such as those aged over 80 with a life expectancy of <5 years were excluded from NASCET; consequently, although many studies are supporting the benefit of carotid endarterectomy in these specific settings, no definitive recommendation can be given. Similarly, the best management of ulcerated symptomatic plaques with low-grade stenosis is uncertain [135].

Asymptomatic patients with moderate or severe carotid stenosis (>60%)

The efficacy of carotid revascularization in asymptomatic patients has been debated more aggressively in the literature; however, there is clear evidence that surgery is significantly more beneficial than best medical therapy in asymptomatic patients with carotid stenosis greater than 60% according to NASCET criteria. Three RCTs with appropriate study design and consistent results showed reduction of the postoperative incidence of perioperative stroke, death and subsequent stroke in the surgical arm [135–137].

However, it has to be emphasized that, given the small although significant benefit in the surgical arm of the studies in asymptomatic patients, surgery should be performed with a complication rate (combined stroke and mortality) equal or inferior than that reported in the studies (3%). These results are usually easily achieved in most vascular surgery centres worldwide [138].

Medical therapy

Antiplatelet drugs, lipid-lowering agents, and antihypertensive therapy are the mainstays of medical treatment in patients with carotid disease. The efficacy of antiplatelet therapy has not been specifically addressed in this patient population. Nonetheless, based on the efficacy of these agents in both stroke and coronary prevention, they should be administered in all patients with carotid [122]. Similarly, the clinical benefit of statins has not been studied in patients with significant carotid disease. A histological analysis performed on endarterectomy specimens has suggested that statin therapy may have a beneficial effect on carotid plaque stabilization [139]. Aggressive lipid management is indicated based on the high-risk status for cardiovascular events in this patient population [122].

Medical management versus endarterectomy

Large-scale randomized trials have compared carotid endarterectomy and medical management in patients with carotid stenosis. Overall, the benefit of surgery in terms of stroke prevention has been greater among patients with symptomatic disease than among asymptomatic individuals. In symptomatic disease, endarterectomy is superior to medical management in the presence of carotid stenosis >50%, and particularly if the luminal narrowing is >70% [140]. Among asymptomatic patients, clinical trials detected a moderate but significant benefit for patients with stenosis >60% [141]. Recent results of the ACST study clearly indicate that in asymptomatic patients under 75 years of age with an internal carotid stenosis of 70%, immediate carotid endarterectomy, taking into account a 3% perioperative hazard, halved the net 5-year stroke risk from about 12% to about 6% [136].

Revascularization management

Surgical treatment

Technical aspects of surgical carotid revascularization are well known and standardized worldwide. Anaesthesia can be performed by general or locoreregional techniques [142, 143], according to the surgeon's preference and clinical surgical risk to the patient. While general anaesthesia is usually preferred in patients with difficult exposures (obese patients, high carotid lesions), locoregional anaesthesia give the advantage of a simple and reliable neurological monitoring. Standard endarterectomy is performed through a longitudinal arteriotomy of the carotid bulb by identifying a sub-adventitial plane in the proximal part of the plaque in the common carotid. The plaque is then everted from the external carotid artery and dissection is subsequently performed internally until a non-diseased segment of the intima is reached. Shunting to maintain cerebral vascularization can be performed selectively in the awake patient or on the basis of cerebral perfusion monitoring techniques (EEG, infrared spectroscopy, evoked potential, transcranial Doppler) or routinely, although there is no evidence on the superiority of one method over others [143]. Arteriotomy closure is performed by a direct running 6-0 or 7-0 suture or, more commonly, with the use of a synthetic (Dacron, PTFE) or autologous vein patch.

In case of internal carotid redundancy, coiling or kinking, or simply as an alternate method to avoid patch closure, eversion endarterectomy can be performed by sharply dividing the internal carotid artery from the bifurcation and everting the plaque through a sub-adventitial plane until its distal end. The internal carotid is then re-sutured back on the bifurcation, possibly shortening it in case of necessity [144].

Endovascular treatment

Endovascular carotid interventions (➲ Fig. 36.12; 36.38–36.46) have been increasingly used as an alternative treatment for carotid disease, particularly in patients at high risk for surgery. Over the last few years, neurological complications associated with angioplasty and stenting have decreased. Putative explanations include greater experience of the operators, optimization of antiplatelet therapy, and better equipment. Specifically, the introduction of neuroprotective devices, such as filters and distal or proximal occlusion devices, has been a major breakthrough [145, 146]. Although no randomized study has been performed to compare 'protected' and 'unprotected' carotid stenting, there is substantial evidence that the use of emboli protection devices reduces neurological events associated with percutaneous carotid intervention [147].

Carotid stenting: some technical concepts to improve procedural outcomes

Tailored-approach concept

To achieve high procedural success the carotid artery stenting (CAS) strategy involves a 'tailored-approach' in the application of endovascular techniques to a specific patient with a specific lesion and vascular anatomy. This requires an in-depth knowledge of neuro-assessment, carotid plaque characteristics, vascular anatomy (➲ Fig. 36.13), and technical features of endovascular materials—guiding-catheters and sheaths, guide-wires, embolic protection devices (EPDs), balloons, and stents (➲ Figs. 36.14 and 36.15).

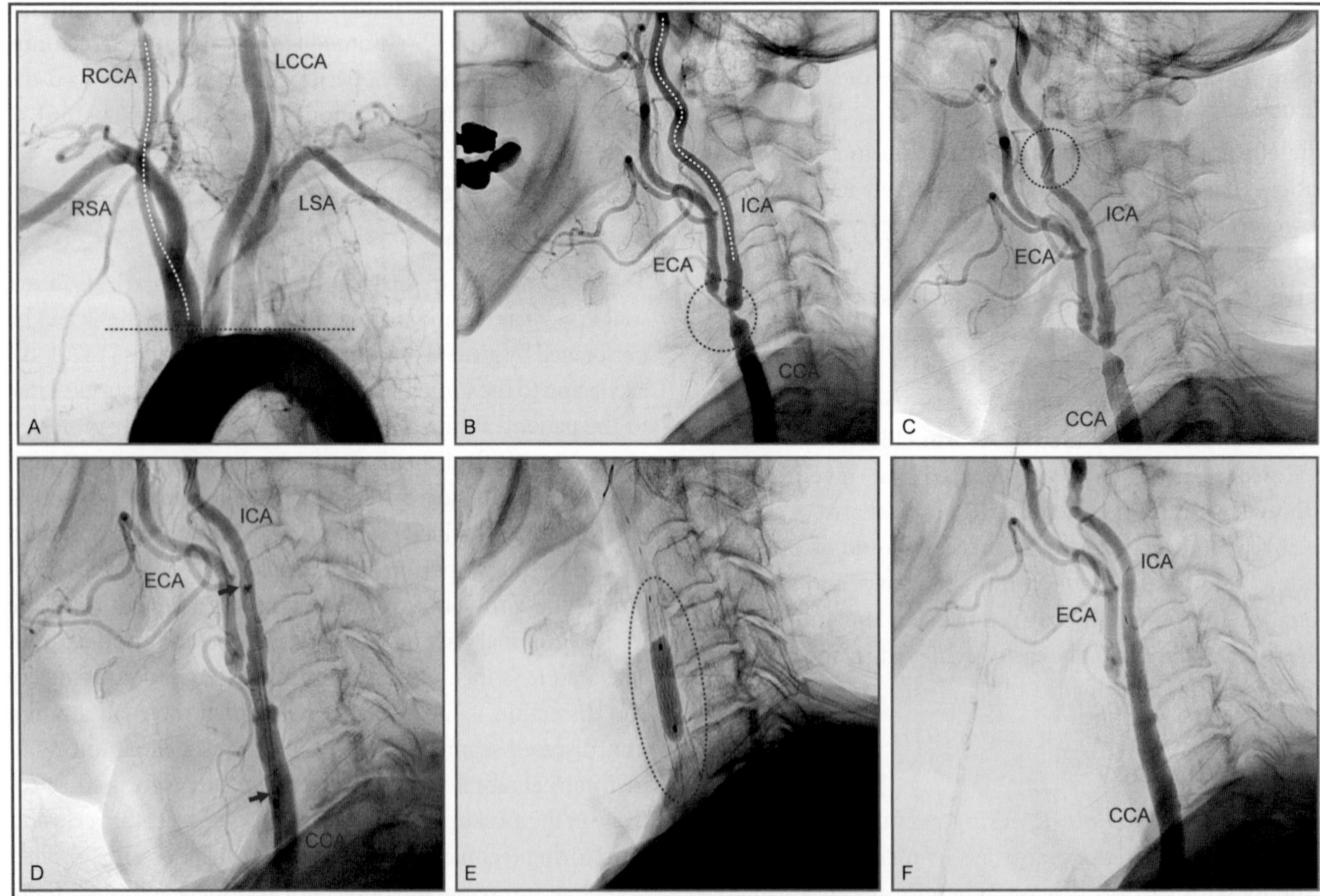

Figure 36.12 Protected carotid artery stenting. Simple case of carotid artery angioplasty: (A) simple aortic arch (red line) associated to mild proximal tortuosity of RCCA (white line); (B) severe stenosis at carotid bifurcation (circle) and mild distal tortuosity of ICA (white line); (C) distal filter positioned at the landing zone (circle); (D) stent positioning (arrows pointing distal and proximal stent edges); (E) stent post-dilatation (circle delimitating stent length); (F) final angiographic result. CCA, common carotid artery; ECA, external carotid artery; ICA, internal carotid artery; LCCA, left common carotid artery; LSA, left subclavian artery; RCCA, right common carotid artery; RSA, right subclavian artery. Also see 36.38–36.46.

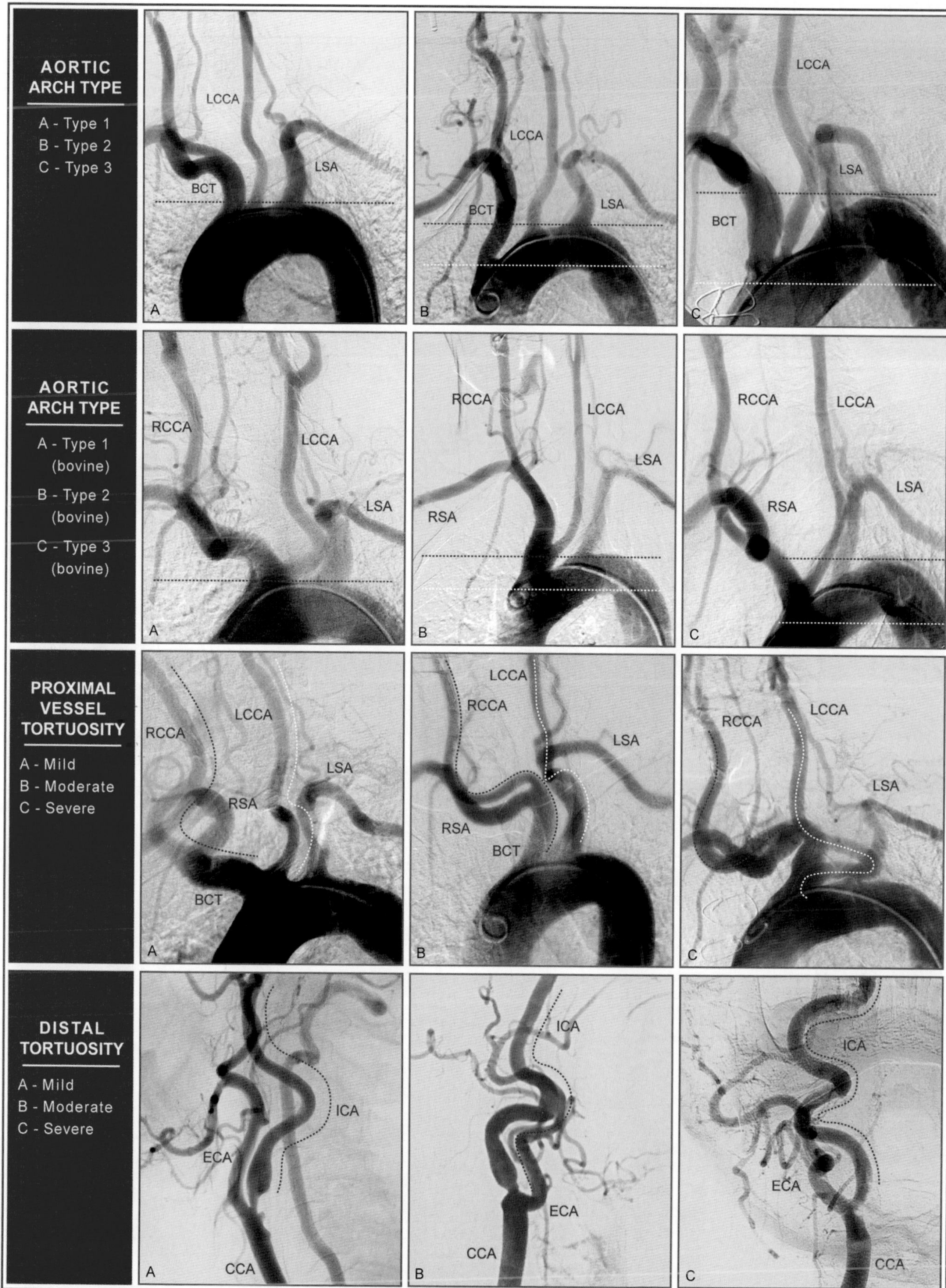

Figure 36.13 Supra aortic trunk anatomy: what is important for carotid stenting? Aortic arch type: classification defined by the distance between the line at the top of the aortic arch (red line) to the line at the origin of the brachiocephalic trunks (white line). Bovine aortic arch is defined as LCCA arising from brachiocephalic trunk. Proximal vessel tortuosity (of CCA): represented by red line (right common carotid artery) and white line (left common carotid artery). Distal vessel tortuosity: ICA tortuosity (red line). BCT, brachiocephalic trunk; CCA, common carotid artery; ECA, external carotid artery; ICA, internal carotid artery; LCCA, left common carotid artery; LSA, left subclavian artery; RCCA, right common carotid artery; RSA, right subclavian artery.

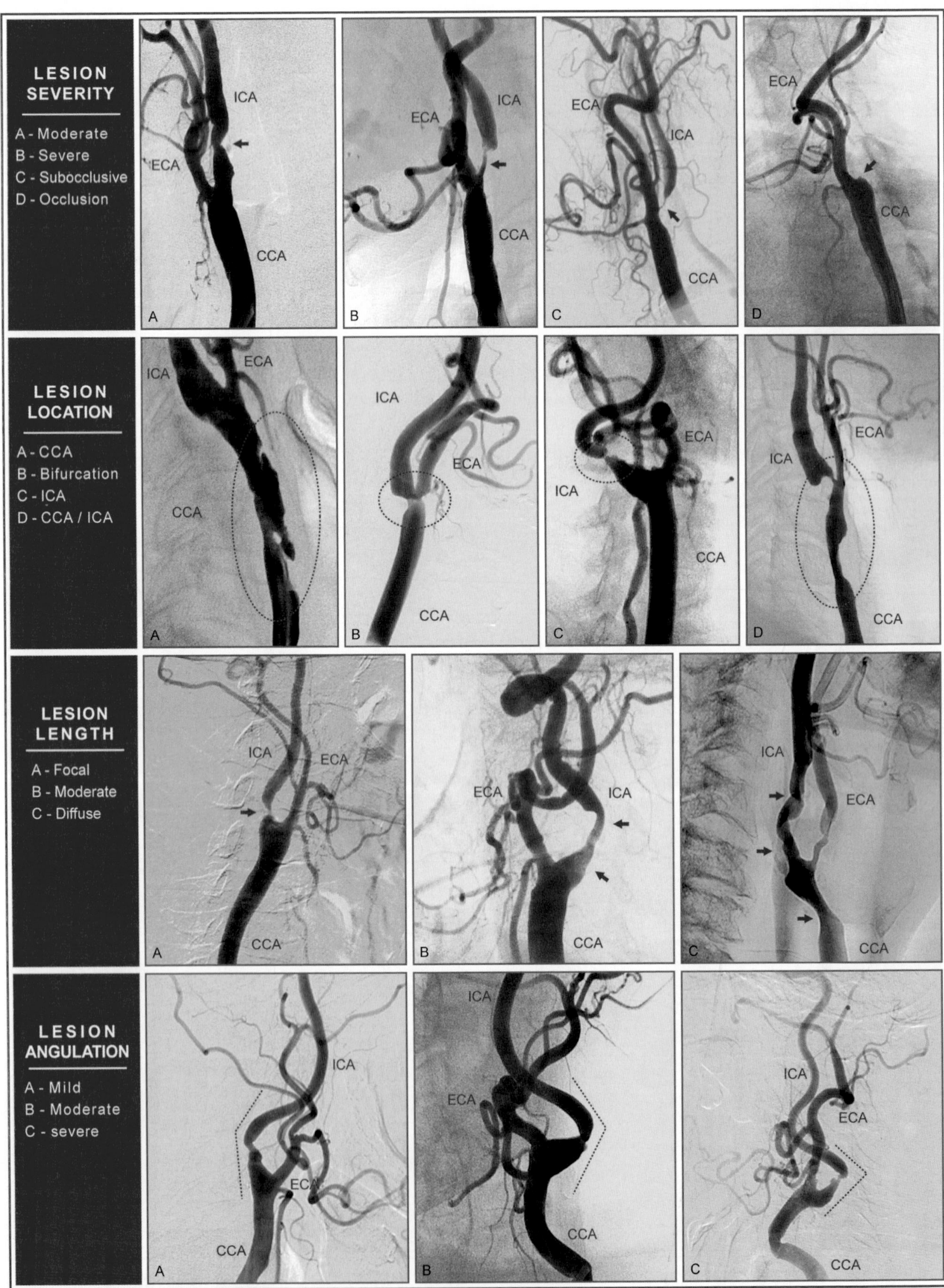

Figure 36.14 Carotid lesion morphology. Lesion severity: arrows point to lesions. Lesion location: lesions are surrounded by circles. Lesion length: arrows point to lesions. Lesion angulation: lesion angle is represented by dotted lines. CCA, common carotid artery; ECA, external carotid artery; ICA, internal carotid artery.

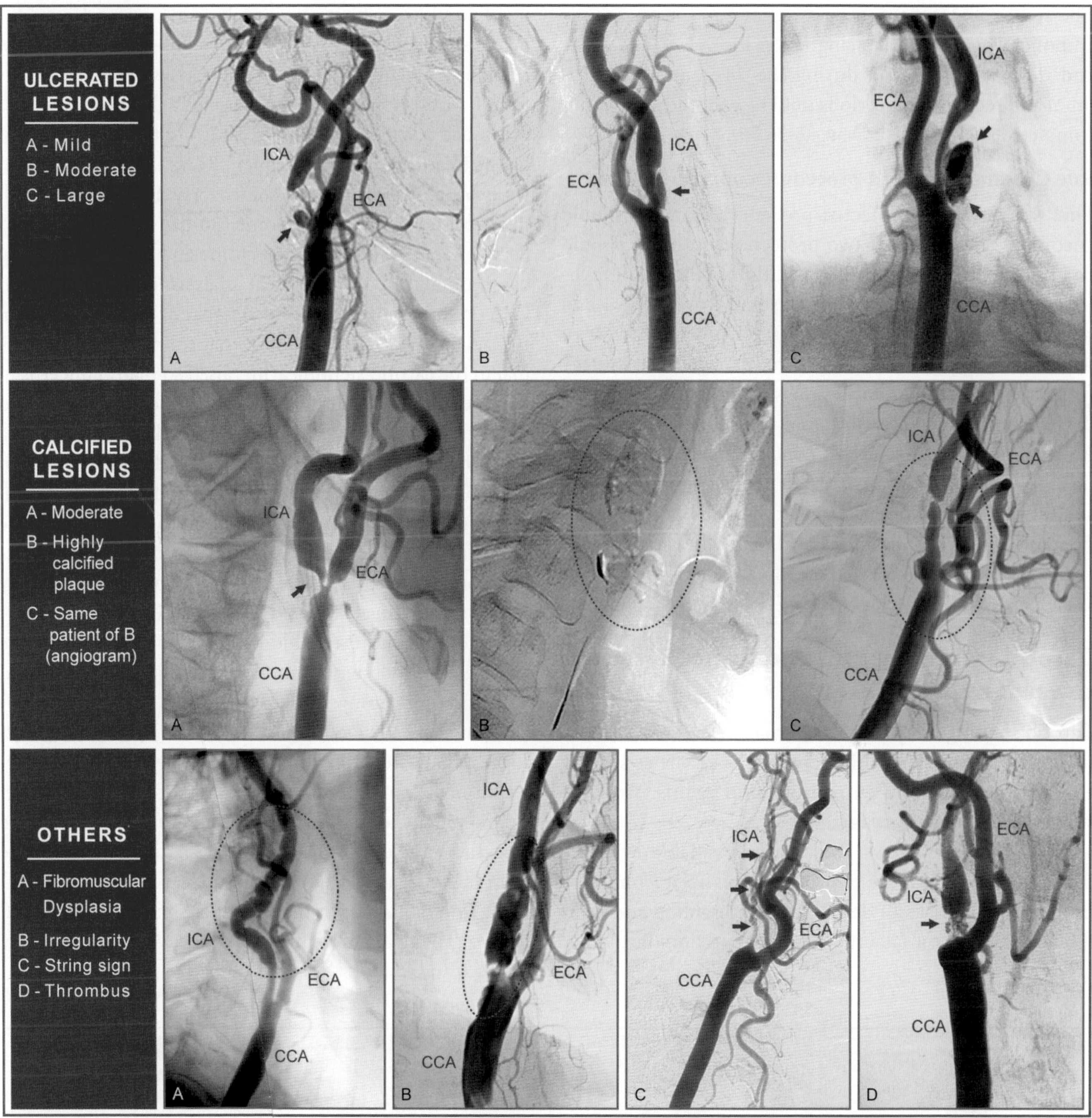

Figure 36.15 Carotid lesion complexity. Ulcerated lesion: arrows point at lesions. Calcified lesions: (A) arrows point to calcified plaques; (B) and (C) calcified plaque is surrounded by dotted circles. Others: (A) angiographic aspect of fibromuscular dysplasia is shown by the circle, (B) irregular lesion (circle), (C) ICA lesion with string sign (arrows), (D) thrombus containing lesion (arrow). CCA, common carotid artery; ECA, external carotid artery; ICA, internal carotid artery.

Stent intrinsic anti-embolic property concept

The major source of complications related to CAS is distal embolization, either intraprocedural or postprocedural. For effective reduction of intraprocedural risk great emphasis is placed on the use of neuroprotective devices (EPDs). An important concept to consider is the view that in the presence of an EPD, the type of stent implanted may not significantly impact on the risk of intraprocedural complications but may subsequently play a vital part in preventing neurological events due to plaque prolapse. It is appreciated that whereas in the open surgical techniques the atheroma and thrombus burden are excised, the stent-protected angioplasty technique compacts this material to the wall, retaining it with its supporting scaffolding and wall-coverage properties.

The stent-cell geometry may thus have an 'intrinsic anti-embolic property' influencing the risk of plaque prolapse and distal embolization during the 24-hour postprocedural and recuperative periods until re-endothelialization is completed (➲Fig. 36.16; 36.47–36.56).

Safe CAS and protected-procedure concept

The 'safe CAS and protected-procedure' concept should encompass the idea that two protection-positions should be implemented in practice. In addition to the use of high-tech devices to contain plaque (stents) or capture and remove embolic debris (EPDs), the implementation of the tailored-approach to the entire management strategy from appropriate patient/lesion selection to meticulous device choice and interventional techniques is essential. An important element of this concept is that the recognition of high-risk cases for CAS depends primarily on the skill of the interventional vascular specialist. This is considerably more relevant in this field than other areas of percutaneous interventions (➲Fig. 36.17; 36.57–36.66 and ➲Fig. 36.18; 36.67–36.80).

Carotid stenting versus endarterectomy: towards a consensus

Carotid stenting is a potential alternative to carotid endarterectomy but whether this technique is as safe as surgery and whether the long-term protection against stroke is similar to that of surgery is still unclear.

In 2005, in a review [148] of the available evidence derived from RCTs, the two procedures were compared in terms of the risks of death, stroke (disabling and non-disabling), and non-fatal myocardial infarction. Five trials, involving 1269 patients, were included (Cavatas, Kentucky, Leicester, SAPPHIRE, Wallstents). In this systematic review, no significant difference in the major risks of treatment was found, but the substantial heterogeneity between the trials precluded any possibility to exclude a difference in favour of one treatment. Two subsequent RCTs (EVA 3-S, SPACE) were not able to clarify the controversy. In EVA 3-S [149], the reported primary endpoint (30-day risk of stroke or death) was 3.9% for endarterectomy and 9.6% for stenting based on an intention-to-treat analysis. Unfortunately, in EVA-3S the various levels of experience of the interventional physicians, with clear evidence that training was suboptimal in the carotid stenting arm, raised so many concerns in the scientific community that we are objectively unable to judge the real safety of CAS from this trial. Not even data from the SPACE trial [150] solved the debate. In spite of the substantial equivalence in the rate of death or ipsilateral ischaemic stroke from randomization to 30 days after the procedure (6.8% for carotid stenting versus 6.3% for endarterectomy), the SPACE trial failed to prove non-inferiority of carotid stenting compared with endarterectomy.

Something more reliable has come recently from the analysis of middle-term results of carotid stenting compared with endarterectomy: both in SPACE (2 years' follow-up) [151] and in EVA 3-S (4 years' follow-up) [152] the results suggest that carotid stenting is as effective as carotid endarterectomy for middle-term prevention of ipsilateral stroke. In this still unclear and conflicting situation, where data are sometimes useless or misleading, and many criticisms have been levied against trial designs, a clear consensus is difficult to established. In the lack of absolute evidence, and in favour of a patient-centred approach, we can summarize

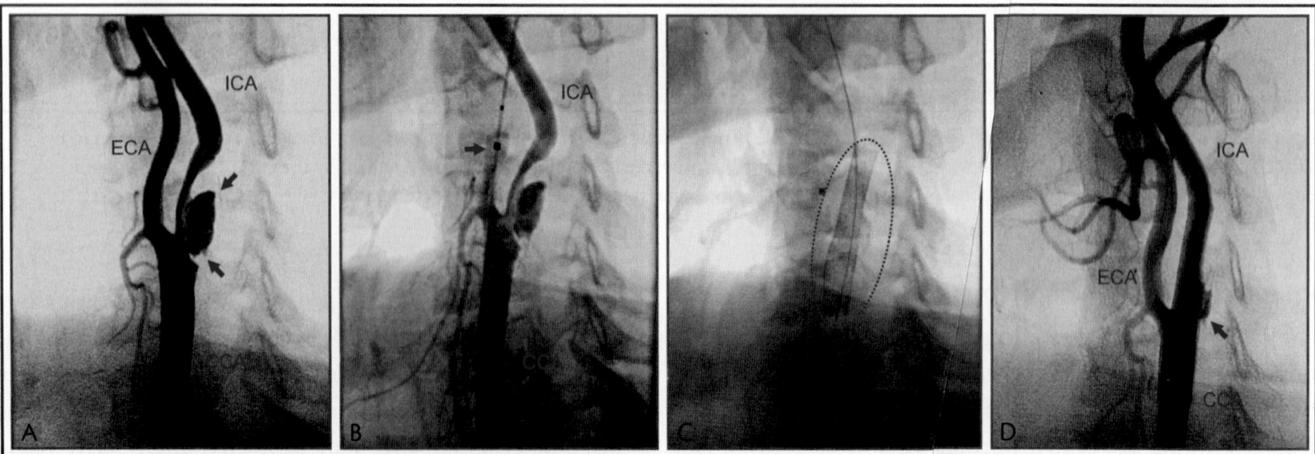

Figure 36.16 Endovascular treatment of carotid ulcerated lesion. Stent intrinsic anti-embolic properties. (A) severe carotid stenosis with a large ulcer (arrows); (B) proximal cerebral protection device, note the distal balloon inflation (arrow) in the ECA; (C) closed cell carotid stent (circle) (D); final angiographic result, note a small residual ulcer (arrow). CCA, common carotid artery; ECA, external carotid artery; ICA, internal carotid artery. Also see 36.47–36.56.

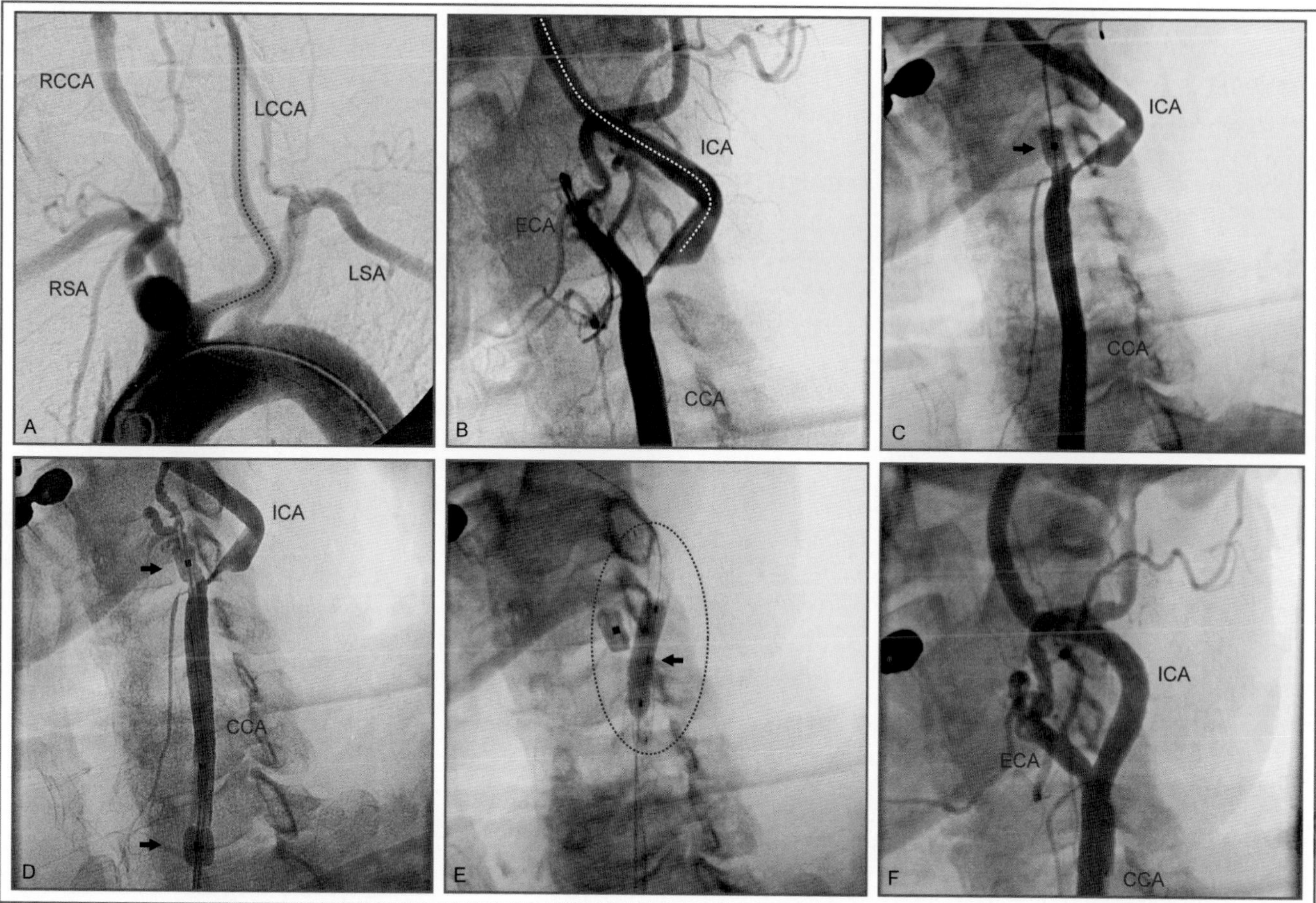

Figure 36.17 Endovascular treatment of soft carotid plaque. Complex case of carotid artery angioplasty. (A) bovine aortic arch with moderate proximal tortuosity of LCCA (red line); (B) severe stenosis with large plaque burden associated to ICA tortuosity (white line); (C) proximal cerebral protection device, note the distal balloon (arrow) inflated in the ECA; (D) complete proximal flow blockage, note the distal and proximal balloons inflation (arrows) and contrast injection through the protection device lumen; (E) stent post-dilatation with 5.5 × 20mm angioplasty balloon (arrow); (F) final result. CCA, common carotid artery; ECA, external carotid artery; ICA, internal carotid artery; RCCA, right common carotid artery; RSA, right subclavian artery; LCCA, left common carotid artery; LSA, left subclavian artery. Also see 36.57–36.66.

the role of endarterectomy and carotid stenting in the following concepts:

- The sole incentive for the treatment of carotid artery stenosis is stroke prevention.
- In symptomatic as well asymptomatic lesions, the stroke risk associated with any type of prophylactic intervention should not exceed the risk inherent in the natural course of carotid atherosclerosis.
- There is currently insufficient evidence to support a widespread change in clinical practice away from recommending carotid endarterectomy as the treatment of choice for suitable carotid artery stenosis.
- Carotid stenting with emboli protection performed by an experienced operator should be viewed as a valid alternative to surgery for patients at high risk for endarterectomy.
- The results of ongoing randomized trials should be awaited before expanding the indications for carotid stenting to a lower-risk population.

Renal artery stenosis

Key points (also see ➲Chapter 13)

- The incidence of renovascular hypertension (➲Chapter 13) is about 4% in the general population; in specific subsets, such as patients with recognized coronary artery disease, the incidence can be as high as 15–30%.
- In patients with renovascular hypertension, both clinical presentation and response to therapy can be different depending on the stages of renal artery stenosis.

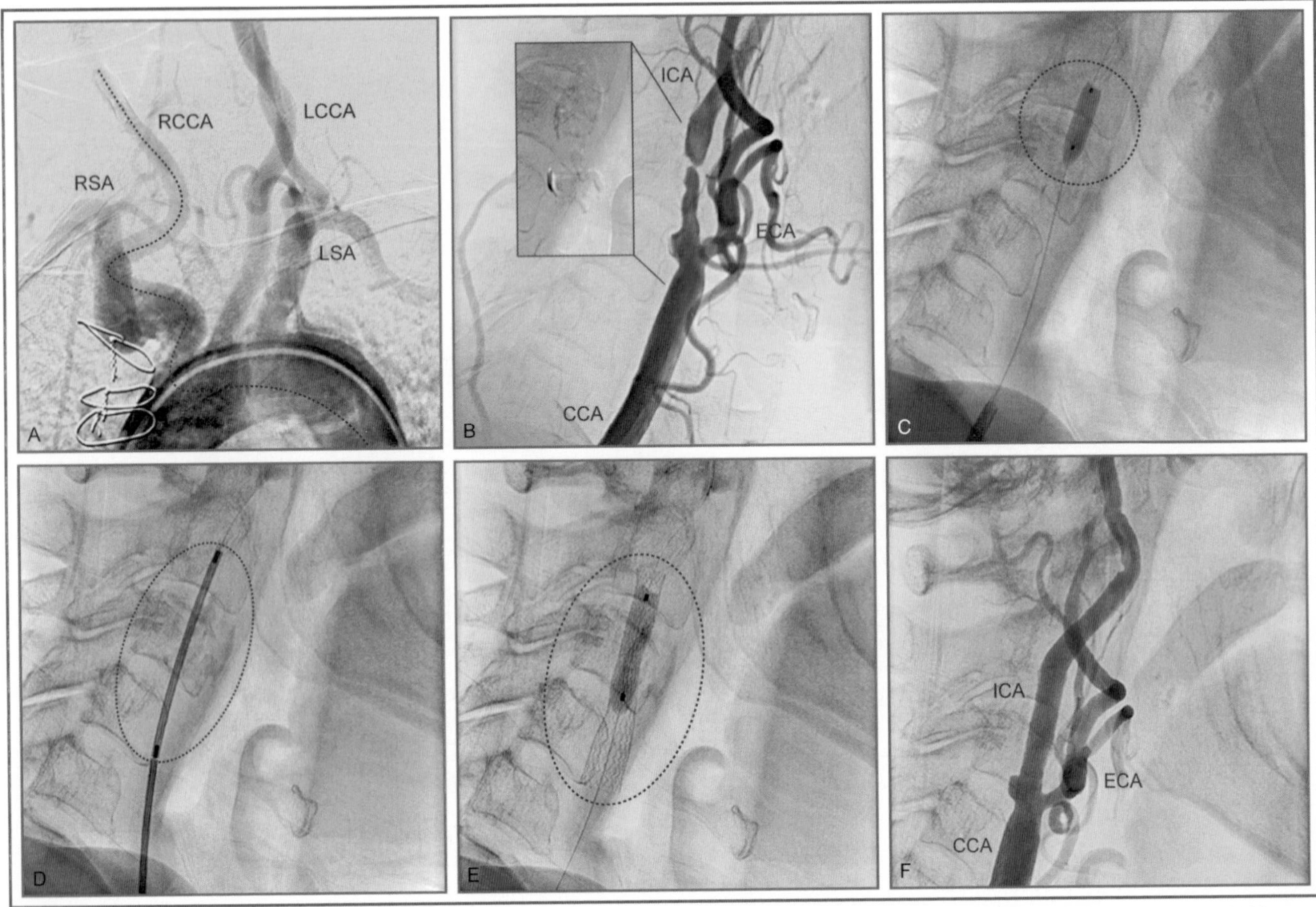

Figure 36.18 Endovascular treatment of calcified carotid plaque. Complex case of carotid artery angioplasty. (A) severe proximal tortuosity (red line); (B) severe carotid stenosis, the small picture shows in detail the highly calcified plaque component; (C) lesion pre-dilatation with coronary cutting balloon (circle); (D) stent positioning (circle); (E) stent post-dilatation (circle); final angiographic result. CCA, common carotid artery; ECA, external carotid artery; ICA, internal carotid artery; RCCA, right common carotid artery; RSA, right subclavian artery; LCCA, left common carotid artery; LSA, left subclavian artery. Also see 36.67–36.80.

- The technique of catheter revascularization (stent-assisted renal angioplasty) has greatly improved, especially with the introduction of low-profile instruments and stents.
- Hypertension with significant renal artery stenosis (RAS) may respond well (cure or improvement) in two-thirds of patients with atherosclerosis and in 80% of those with fibromuscular dysplasia.
- Renal insufficiency may be improved by renal artery revascularization. Rapid deterioration prior to intervention but with GFR >10mL/min is a positive predictive factor.

Epidemiology and risk factors

RAS is the cause of arterial hypertension in 1–5% of patients (renovascular hypertension). The majority of RAS is a consequence of atherosclerotic disease of the aortic wall, with progression in the renal arterial lumen giving the typical appearance of ostial, eccentric stenosis; <10% of renal stenosis has a different aetiology, usually represented by fibromuscular dysplasia or vasculitis, both of which are usually found in younger patients (<40 years old) [153] and mainly affecting the middle portion of the renal artery.

In older patients, atherosclerotic RAS is prevalent and is often associated with multiple cardiovascular risk factors (smoking, diabetes, dyslipidaemia) and with atherosclerotic disease in other vascular districts: in one series, coronary artery disease was present in 71% of patients with atherosclerotic RAS, peripheral arterial disease in 41%, carotid artery disease in 38%, abdominal aortic aneurysm in 13%, and involvement of both renal arteries in 16% [154].

Pathophysiology of renal artery stenosis

The presence of a functionally significant RAS activates several pathophysiological mechanisms which, in turn, can lead to the occurrence of both cardiovascular and renal events. Renal ischaemia is a trigger for neuroendocrine activation, with increased production of renin, angiotensin II, and sympathetic activation; together with salt retention, this sustains arterial hypertension and damage at the heart (left ventricular hypertrophy), brain (stroke), blood vessels (accelerated atherosclerosis), and kidney (nephrosclerosis). Based on pathophysiology of renovascular hypertension the different clinical presentations can be grouped into three stages:

- Phase I:
  - increased renin and angiotensin II levels;
  - blood pressure tends to be angiotensin-converting enzyme inhibitor (ACE-I) responsive.
- Phase II:
  - renin and angiotensin II levels return towards normal;
  - increased extracellular fluid volume is present;
  - blood pressure tends to be not as responsive to ACE-I.
- Phase III:
  - hypertension is not reversible by correction of renal artery stenosis.

From a therapeutic stand point, it is crucial to understand which stage of renovascular hypertension the patient is in. By definition, phase I and II are therapy responsive and the administration of antihypertensive drugs and/or the correction of RAS can improve the hypertensive status and prevent the deterioration of renal function. The irreversible renal damage which occurs in the late stages (phase III) may render renovascular hypertension untreatable. At this point, correction of RAS does not cure or ameliorate the hypertension: blood pressure elevation is maintained by mechanisms other than those triggered by the initial aetiology of the disease and analogous to those of hypertension in chronic renal failure of any cause. The progressive renal damage we can detect in the non-stenosed kidney is attributable to the effect of chronic sustained hypertension.

From a more clinical appraisal, it is important to highlight that left ventricular hypertrophy, stroke, accelerated atherosclerosis, and nephrosclerosis are not just the causes of hypertension, but also derive from direct effects of angiotensin II, endothelin, transforming growth factor β, platelet-derived growth factor β, and reactive oxygen species (smooth muscle cell proliferation, plaque rupture, endothelial dysfunction, inhibition of fibrinolysis, cardiac myocite hypertrophy) [155, 156]. Indeed, myocardial hypertrophy occurs when angiotensin II is present, even when blood pressure is controlled [157]. Not surprisingly, renal artery disease represents a negative prognostic factor, both for general survival and 'renal-related' survival. The risk of cardiovascular morbidity and mortality is substantial, with a 6-year survival free of cardiovascular events of 53%; moreover, up to 27% of patients develop chronic renal failure within 6 years, and 18% of stenotic renal arteries progress to occlusion within 5 years [158, 159]. For all these reasons, treatment of RAS has been proposed to interrupt the 'vicious circle' of renal ischaemia and to achieve three main results:

1) better control of blood pressure, reducing the need for multiple drugs and preventing left ventricular hypertrophy;
2) preservation of renal function;
3) prevention of episodes of congestive heart failure ('flash' pulmonary oedema).

Diagnosis of renal artery stenosis

Clinical presentation

Patients with RAS may present with hypertension, renal insufficiency, or acute pulmonary oedema. Clinical examination often shows bruits over major vessels—including the abdominal aorta—although lateralizing bruits over the renal arteries are uncommon. RAS can be predicted on the basis of the following clinical parameters:

- advanced age;
- recent onset of hypertension;
- female gender;
- presence of atherosclerosis;
- smoking;
- abdominal bruits;
- elevated creatinine;
- hypercholesterolemia.

From a clinical stand point, RAS should be suspected in any patient with vascular disease who has significant hypertension.

Blood tests

To assess for RAS serologically, some blood tests have been proposed:

- the simplest test is to observe for an increase in serum creatinine with ACE-inhibitor treatment;
- plasma renin levels can be measured, especially by assessing captopril-augmented plasma renin activity;
- selective renal vein renin sampling for lateralization has been used, mostly for study purposes.

However, we have to stress that none of these tests has a sufficient sensitivity or specificity to advocate their routine use.

Diagnostic tests

Investigative tests include colour DUS, captopril renography, magnetic resonance arteriography (MRA), spiral CT, and selective renal arteriography. Compared to selective renal arteriography (diagnostic gold standard), CT A and gadolinium-enhanced MRA can obtain the highest diagnostic accuracies. Ultrasonography is simple, reliable, and comparatively inexpensive, but demonstrates considerable variability in sensitivity and specificity, reflecting the fact that the technique is operator and centre dependent.

Management of renal artery stenosis

Medical management

Appropriate medical management is an important part of the care of a RAS patient. This includes tight blood-pressure control with the use of ACE inhibitors or angiotensin blockers as long as these medications do not cause significant azotaemia. Salt restriction and diuretic use may improve the effectiveness of angiotensin blockade in controlling blood pressure. Advanced RAS lesion morphologies (severe bilateral RAS, critical RAS in patients with a single kidney) deserve particular attention since ACE inhibition may aggravate hyper-azotaemia, and these conditions represent a relative contraindication to angiotensin II blockade/inhibition. Aggressive risk factor modification (tight control of lipids and smoking cessation) is mandatory in these patients at high risk for other cardiovascular events, including coronary artery disease and myocardial infarction. Strict vigilance for concomitant coronary or peripheral vascular disease is also indicated.

Revascularization strategies

Options available for renal artery revascularization include surgery (endarterectomy, aorto-renal bypass) and percutaneous transluminal angioplasty with or without stent placement (➲Fig. 36.19; 36.81–36.88). Initially, the

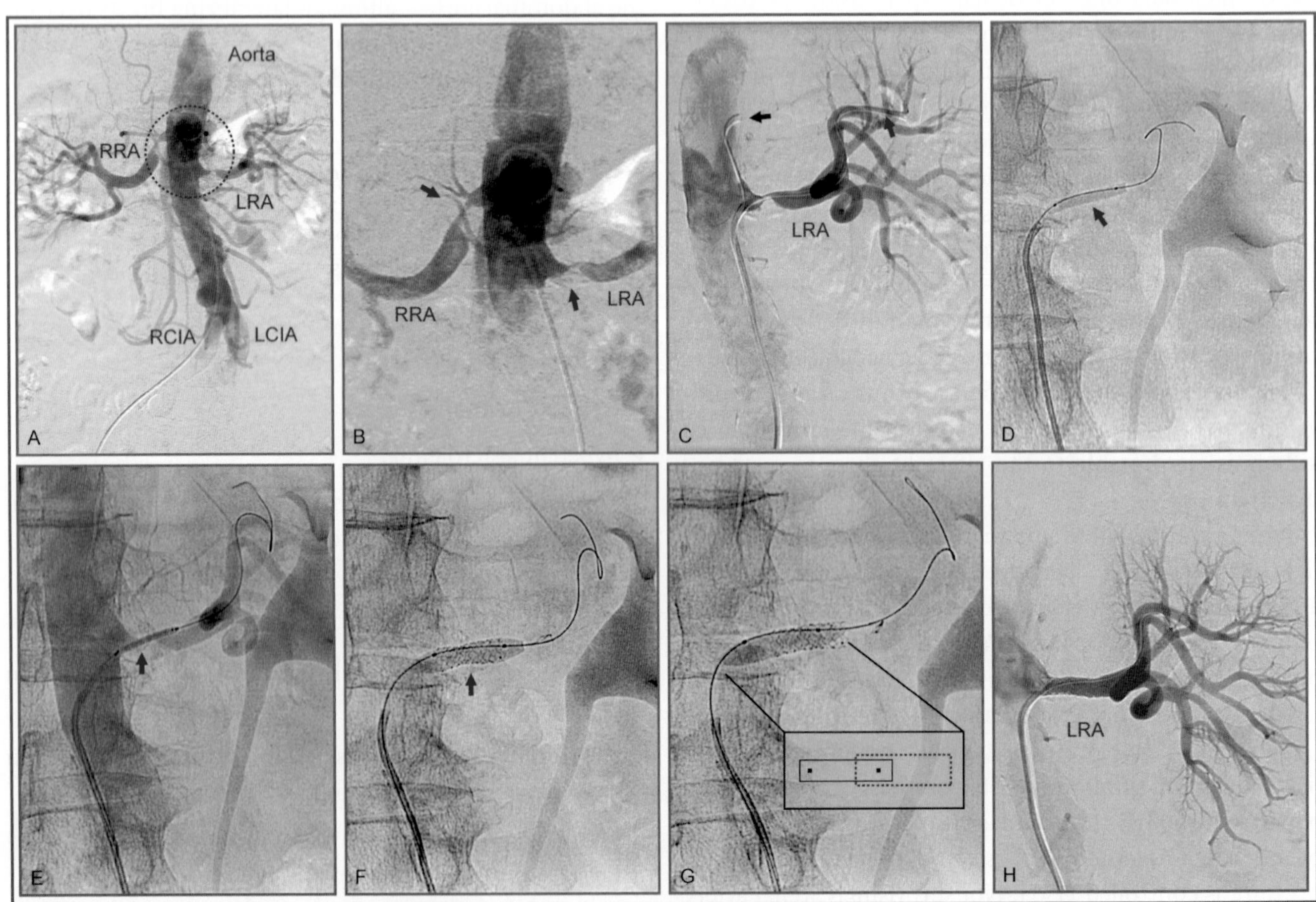

Figure 36.19 RAS endovascular treatment. Case of renal angioplasty and stenting. (A) abdominal aorta angiogram revealing bilateral renal artery stenosis (circle); (B) stenosis in detail (arrows); (C) using the 'no-touch' technique (black arrow points to the 0.035-inch (0.89mm) guidewire left on the aorta) the lesion was crossed using a 0.014-inch (0.35mm) guidewire (red arrow); (D) pre-dilatation with conventional angioplasty balloon (arrow); (E) stent positioning (arrow); (F) stenting (arrow); (G) stent post-dilatation. The picture illustrate the ostial dilatation of the stent performed by positioning the proximal half of the balloon inside the aorta; (H) final angiographic result. LCIA, left common iliac artery; LRA, left renal artery; RCIA, right common iliac artery; RRA, right renal artery. Also see 36.81–36.88.

treatment was open surgery, which has now been replaced by percutaneous endovascular interventions (percutaneous transluminal renal angioplasty (PTRA) with stenting and, more recently, distal filters to avoid periprocedural atheroembolization) [160, 161]. Nevertheless, evidence clearly showing the clinical efficacy of renal artery stenting is still lacking. Hopefully, this issue will be solved by several ongoing randomized clinical trials, such as the CORAL trial which will enrol >1000 patients and will determine the incremental value of stent revascularization in addition to best medical therapy [162]. Based on the previously discussed physiopathological considerations, two relevant issues should be considered for evaluating and understanding the real benefit related to the endovascular intervention:

1) effect of renal stenting on blood pressure control, antihypertensive drugs, and renal function;
2) restenosis rates after renal stenting.

Renal stenting and blood pressure control

Blockage of the renin–angiotensin–aldosterone system is highly effective in controlling blood pressure. In renovascular hypertension, the activation of this system can be reduced by restoring normal blood flow to the kidney with renal artery stenting. A meta-analysis of three randomized trials comparing balloon angioplasty with medical therapy showed a moderate effect on blood pressure, with a reduced need for antihypertensive drugs [163]. However, these trials were conducted on a limited number of patients and medical treatment was not optimal as some classes of drugs (e.g. ATII receptor blockers) were not available at the time. The lack of an impressive effect of renal artery stenting on blood pressure may be attributed to the fact that hypertension may be sustained by secondary processes, such as long-standing ischaemic damage to the stenotic kidney and hypertensive injury to the non-stenotic kidney.

The effect of renal artery stenting on left ventricular hypertrophy is another important issue under investigation for a better understanding of the potential benefits related to renal revascularization. Indeed, left ventricular mass index, a measure of ventricular hypertrophy which, in turn, is a well-known risk factor for cardiovascular events in both the presence and absence of hypertension, has been show to decline after renal artery revascularization [164].

Renal stenting and renal function improvement

In clinical practice the main indication for revascularization of RAS has recently changed from hypertension to renal insufficiency. Nonetheless, the efficacy of renal artery stenting in slowing the decrease of renal function and the progression to end-stage renal disease is still a matter of debate. Despite some observational studies showed that kidney function may stabilize or improve in some subjects, this may not be achieved if renal parenchymal disease is already present, and a detrimental effect may even ensue due to contrast nephropathy or atheroembolic disease.

There are clear data on transplanted or single-kidney RAS which indicate marked improvement with PTRA and/or stenting. The situation with kidney insufficiency in the presence of two kidneys and one-sided RAS is more complex. However, several studies addressing this problem showed that in patients with moderately elevated serum creatinine, stabilization or improvement of renal insufficiency may be achieved in >70% of patients [165–168]. Even in a group of patients with severely impaired renal function, catheter revascularization achieved functional improvement or at least prevention of deterioration in 50% [167] (➲Fig. 36.20). Even when renal function is rapidly deteriorating prior to intervention, as long as the glomerular filtration rate (GFR) remains >10mL/min, revascularization has a positive effect [167, 168]. In case of pronounced damage of renal parenchyma as indicated by a GFR <10mL/min or a Doppler flow velocity resistance index >0.80 [169], revascularization of RAS comes too late to achieve functional improvement.

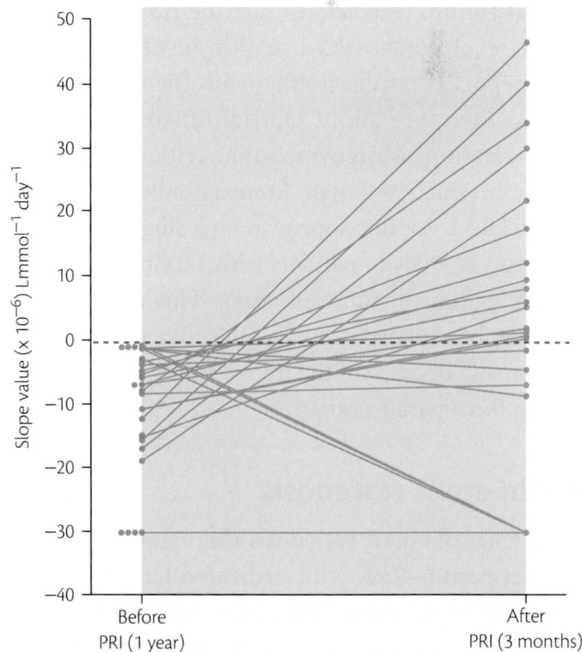

Figure 36.20 Change in slope of reciprocal serum creatinine (creatinine clearance analogue) 1 year before and 3 months after renal artery stenting in 22 patients with renal insufficiency (serum creatinine >300micromol/L) undergoing renal artery stenting. Negative slopes indicate decreasing values over 2 years previously, zero slope indicates stabilization and positive slopes indicate increasing values of serum creatinine after intervention. Reproduced with permission from Korsakas S, Mohaupt MG, Dinkel HP, *et al.* Delay of dialysis in end-stage renal failure: prospective study on percutaneous renal artery interventions. *Kidney Int* 2004; **65**: 251–8.

Recent unpublished data from the ASTRAL (angioplasty and stent for renal arterial lesions) trial deserve a specific mention [170]. The ASTRAL trial was designed to address the issue of whether renal arterial revascularization with balloon angioplasty and/or endovascular stenting can safely prevent progressive renal failure among a wide range of patients with atherosclerotic renovascular disease (ARVD). Patients with significant RAS were randomized to percutaneous renal artery revascularization (angioplasty and/or stenting) plus medical therapy (n = 403) or medical therapy alone (n = 403). The principal findings can be easily summed up as follows:

- cardiovascular mortality occurred in 7.4% of the revascularization group and 8.2% of the medially treated group (p = ns);
- hospitalization for fluid overload or heart failure occurred in 12% of the revascularization group and 14% of the medially treated group (p = ns);
- there was no difference in serum creatinine, systolic blood pressure, time to first renal event, or overall vascular event during follow-up (p = ns for all outcomes).

The ASTRAL investigators interpreted these data as lack of evidence regarding significant benefit for renal artery revascularization. Needless to say, the ASTRAL trial data raised a lot of controversy, mainly justified by the fact that the reported results conflict with the vast majority of published literature about clinical outcomes after renal revascularization. Moreover, some criticisms have been levied against the trial design. From a methodological stand point, ASTRAL doesn't appear to be a single trial; actually it is a group of trials in patients with varying clinical problems and significant other illnesses. This methodological issue inevitably underpowers the objective value of the trial results, mostly because of the impossibility of meaningfully analyzing the separate scenarios.

Renal in-stent restenosis

The incidence of binary restenosis after renal artery stenting ranges between 6–23% with dedicated bare metal stents. In the Great trial, comparing a bare metal to a sirolimus-eluting Genesis peripheral stent, the reported rate of restenosis was 6.7% for patients treated with sirolimus-eluting stents and 14.6% in patients receiving bare metal stents [171]. Predictors for restenosis include vessel diameter (it rarely occurs in vessels ≥6mm in diameter), body mass index, and history of smoking. Clinically, the diagnosis of in-stent renal artery restenosis is elusive, since the only finding may be an increase in blood pressure 6–8 months after the procedure.

Several imaging techniques can be used for detection of renal in-stent restenosis. Angiography, although considered the gold standard, can not be proposed as a screening tool due to its invasiveness. Gadolinium-enhanced MR angiography has become more popular in the last decade, because it is non-invasive, the contrast agent is generally safe regarding renal function, and MR allows the measurement of pressure gradient [172]. Nevertheless, recent data report that contrast agent gadolinium may be involved in developing nephrogenic systemic fibrosis (NSF) in patients with severe renal disease [173]. Multi-slice spiral CT angiography offers high-resolution three-dimensional vessel reconstruction with fewer stent artefacts as compared to MRI; however, its use as a serial routine follow-up procedure is limited by the need of iodinated contrast agents [174]. Duplex ultrasound, being non-invasive and less expensive, is probably the best imaging technique for screening of restenosis after RAS.

Among the different duplex parameters available, peak systolic flow velocity >200cm/sec or a renal aortic flow velocity ratio >3.5 are correlated to a 50–60% angiographic diameter restenosis, whereas a side difference of the renal resistive index [(peak systolic velocity – end diastolic velocity)/peak systolic velocity × 100] of ≥0.05 has a highly specific correlation reflecting an at least 70% angiographic diameter stenosis [175].

Current indications for renal artery stenting

Endovascular revascularization of RAS is controversial. If it can be agreed that a patent renal artery is better than an occluded one, the scientific debate is focused on whether opening the artery is clearly associated with any significant change in clinical outcome. Available literature data are not useful to clarify several areas of uncertainty regarding the indications for renal revascularization in patients with renovascular disease. Despite this, many renal stenting procedures are still performed in the Western world, often without clear indications, probably forgetting that these procedures may carry, even in so called 'simple cases', a significant risk of morbidity, and a distinct risk of mortality.

Summing up the current understanding on renal revascularization techniques, we can conclude that:

- Hypertension with significant RAS may respond well (cure or improvement) in two-thirds of patients with atherosclerosis and in 80% of those with fibromuscular dysplasia.

- Renal insufficiency may be improved by renal artery revascularization. Rapid deterioration prior to intervention but with GFR >10mL/min is a positive predictive factor.
- Revascularization should be performed as soon as haemodynamically significant stenosis has been documented to avoid progression to full occlusion.

Based on the previously mentioned published data, the accepted indications to renal artery stenting of severe ostial and proximal artery stenoses have been restricted to some specific pathological conditions:

- Mono or bilateral RAS (>70%) with:
  - mild, moderate, or severe hypertension or in presence of poly-vasculopathy (especially CAD);
  - mild, moderate, or severe renal insufficiency or acute/sub-acute renal failure or anuria;
  - recurrent flash pulmonary oedema.
- RAS (>70%) in patients with occlusion of contralateral renal artery (also asymptomatic).

Personal perspective

The problems connected with the treatment of PAD represent a major matter of debate in cardiovascular medicine. In this chapter we point out not only the strong/weak results of existing scientific evidence, but also many objective biases regarding the methodological quality of several studies and, consequently, the difficulty related to their transferability to different clinical settings.

In the field of treatment options for PAD, in spite of the lack of strong scientific evidence, the rapidly evolving technical improvements over the last few years have produced not only dramatic changes in therapeutic strategies, but also substantial shifts in the perception and socio-political evaluation of the disease. A few years ago, for example, CLI was considered a more-or-less fatal illness without real prospects of medical treatment, the only alternative being vascular surgery in selected cases and end-stage disease. Nowadays, using sophisticated non-invasive techniques, it is possible to determine the extent and severity of the disease without any serious risk to the patient. Moreover, endovascular options opened the doors to less invasive therapeutic techniques, enabling reconsideration of risks and benefits in a considerably ageing population, who have the right to receive optimal medical care that should include improvements not only in life expectancy, but also in quality of life.

With regard to the treatment of different forms of PAD, we have seen that a real inter-disciplinary consensus is still lacking. Currently, controversy exists regarding whether carotid artery stenting should be accepted as an alternative to carotid endarterectomy for the treatment of obstructive carotid artery disease. If in surgical high-risk patients the endovascular techniques of stenting with neuroprotection is demonstrated to be not inferior to vascular surgery, we have no conclusive data regarding the indication for the endovascular treatment in asymptomatic patients with high-degree carotid stenosis. Specifically for carotid stenting, recent randomized evidence highlighted the importance of physicians' qualifications to perform protected carotid angioplasty and stent placement, including training, acceptable complication rates, and certification. In the near future, intensive education and strict guidelines for certification are mandatory.

It is generally accepted that angioplasty and stenting is the treatment of choice for atherosclerotic renal artery occlusive disease. However, physicians should cast a very cold eye to current scientific evidence on renal stenting, reconsidering a crucial non-technical issue: the clinical indication. As the clinical effectiveness of the intervention is still not well defined, the interventional community should recognize the need to generate solid scientific evidence.

With regard to the pelvic region, the new recanalization techniques, in combination with excellent balloon-expandable and self-expandable stents with or without the support of lythic therapy, guarantee extremely high success rates with long-term results comparable with surgical series, so that the number of inaccessible iliac lesions is no higher than 10%. This is the reason why endovascular solutions for aorto-iliac obstructive disease are going to be considered the first choice approach in our daily practice.

The situation is different in the infrainguinal region. Recanalization techniques have been demonstrated to be highly effective, with primary success rates in excess of 90%, including very long and calcified lesions. However, the long-term results are still not satisfactory in this extremely complex conduit that is subject to the continuously changing forces of compression, distortion, and elongation. The improvements achieved with nitinol stents in stabilizing the primary intervention may be overshadowed by the stent fracture. Improvements in the mechanical properties of the stent, particularly for the treatment of long lesions, are today considered absolutely mandatory. The broad application of drug-eluting stents in the femoro-popliteal tract needs further scientific evaluation. Below-the-knee endovascular treatment is becoming one of the most promising challenges for the near future. The use of low-profile materials, in combination with other new options (debulking techniques, eluting stents) has changed the scenario completely, permitting unexpected results in tibial vessels and, generally, in the field of diabetic foot treatment.

The final comment has to be dedicated to the 'team approach' concept: all treatment options should always be decided according to the best balance between the benefits and risks to the patient that emerge from a multidisciplinary objective evaluation. It means that a prerequisite for an optimal care strategy is strict collaboration of the different disciplines (diabetologists, neurologists, vascular surgeons, and interventionalists). Moreover, centres specifically dedicated to the treatment of the vascular patients should be intensively supported.

Acknowledgement

A special thanks to Barbara Spagnolo, PhD, for the manuscript revision.

Further reading

Abela GS. Peripheral vascular Disease—Basic Diagnostic and Therapeutic Approach, 2004. Philadelphia, PA: Lippincott Williams & Wilkins.

Bates ER, Babb JD, Casey DE, Jr., *et al.* ACCF/SCAI/SVMB/SIR/ASITN 2007 clinical expert consensus document on carotid stenting: a report of the American College of Cardiology Foundation Task Force on Clinical Expert Consensus Documents (ACCF/SCAI/SVMB/SIR/ASITN Clinical Expert Consensus Document Committee on Carotid Stenting). *J Am Coll Cardiol* 2007; **49**(1): 126–70.

Brancherau A, Jacobs M. *Open surgery versus endovascular procedures*, 2007. Oxford: Paris Consultants Ltd.

Cremonesi A, Setacci C, Bignamini A, *et al.* Carotid artery stenting: first consensus document of the ICCS-SPREAD Joint Committee. *Stroke* 2006; **37**(9): 2400–9.

Greenhalgh RM. *Vascular and endovascular consensus update*, 2008. London: Biba Publishing.

Management of peripheral arterial disease TransAtlantic Inter-Society Consensus (TASC). *Eur J Vasc Endovasc Surg* 2000; **19**(Suppl.A): S1–S250.

Norgren L, Hiatt WR, Dormandy JA, *et al.* Inter-Society Consensus for the Management of Peripheral Arterial Disease (TASC II). *J Vasc Surg* 2007; **45**(Suppl.1):S5–S67.

Sangiorgi G, Holmes Jr DR, Rosenfield K, *et al. Carotid Atherosclerotic Disease—Pathologic Basic for Treatment*, 2008. UK: Informa Healthcare.

Additional online material

- 36.1–36.12 Focal iliac artery lesions endovascular treatment.
- 36.13–36.20 Complete iliac occlusion endovascular treatment.
- 36.21–36.31 Angioplasty and stenting of femoral artery diffuse disease and occlusion.
- 36.32–36.37 Critical limb ischaemia: directional atherectomy for treatment of tibio-peroneal trunk occlusion.
- 36.38–36.46 Protected carotid artery stenting.
- 36.47–36.56 Endovascular treatment of carotid ulcerated lesion.
- 36.57 –36.66 Endovascular treatment of soft carotid plaque.
- 36.67–36.80 Endovascular treatment of calcified carotid plaque.
- 36.81–36.88 Renal artery stenosis endovascular treatment.

For full references and multimedia materials please visit the online version of the book (http://esctextbook.oxfordonline.com).

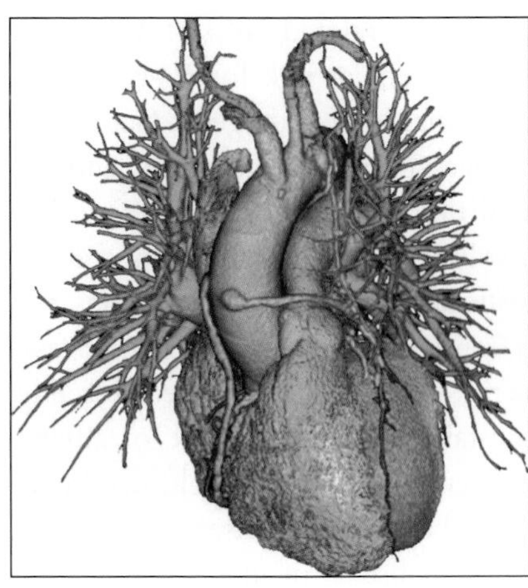

CHAPTER 37

Venous Thromboembolism

Sebastian M. Schellong, Henri Bounameaux, and Harry R. Büller

Contents

Summary

In this chapter, deep vein thrombosis (DVT) and pulmonary embolism (PE) are discussed as manifestations of the same disease process. Despite the steadily growing use of medical thromboprophylaxis, PE remains the third most frequent cause of cardiovascular mortality.

The current concept of venous thromboembolism (VTE) is that of a multifactorial disease. Besides age, several transient and permanent risk factors have been recognized. The strongest in the former group are surgery and trauma, whereas the latter is dominated by active cancer and thrombophilia. However, a substantial proportion of cases present without an identifiable risk factor and are therefore classified as 'idiopathic' or 'unprovoked' episodes. In those patients, or in the presence of a permanent risk factor, VTE is a chronic relapsing disease.

The diagnosis of a current episode has to be based on the result of an imaging procedure. During the last 10 years, compression ultrasound and helical computed tomography have turned out to be the most powerful diagnostic tools. However, strategies have been developed to safely exclude the disease on the basis of clinical pre-test probability and D-dimer testing alone in one-third of all suspected cases.

For most patients anticoagulation is the only acute treatment modality. Subcutaneous low-molecular-weight heparins or fondaparinux represent the current standard of care. The post-thrombotic syndrome as the long-term sequela of DVT can be effectively prevented by compression therapy. Haemodynamic instability in PE requires systemic thrombolysis according to the risk of fatal right heart failure. Vitamin K antagonists remain the standard treatment for maintenance therapy, the duration of which has to be balanced between the risk of recurrence and the potential for major bleeding.

Natural history

Venous thrombosis results from the presence of a clot in the venous circulation. Signs and symptoms of the disease are caused by obstruction of the respective vein(s) and/or by embolization of parts of the clot into the pulmonary circulation. This definition applies only for lower and upper extremity veins. Thrombosis of cerebral and visceral veins is beyond the scope of this chapter.

PE is not a rare complication but occurs regularly in patients with DVT. If searched for meticulously, asymptomatic PE can be detected in up to 70% of patients with proximal DVT. For this reason, DVT and PE are considered as two manifestations of the same disease: venous thromboembolic disease or VTE. As they share most aspects of natural history, diagnosis and treatment, DVT and PE will be discussed together.

Aetiology

Venous thrombus formation is due to an imbalance between local and systemic procoagulant—anticoagulant and profibrinolytic—antifibrinolytic activity. According to Virchow, all pathogenic factors responsible for this imbalance can be classified into three categories: disturbances of venous flow, disturbances of vessel wall and disturbances of blood components. ➲Table 37.1 gives a sample of pathogenic factors of the respective categories.

There are distinct subject-related or setting-related constellations placing a patient at risk for VTE. Almost all of them involve more than one pathogenic factor. The constellations with the biggest impact are age, cancer, and surgery. ➲Table 37.2 gives the most frequent constellations, listing the mechanisms involved and the magnitude of risk [1]. With regard to prognostic and therapeutic implications, risk factors are classified as transient or permanent. In most cases of VTE, more than one risk factor can be identified. Recently, similarities have been established between risk for atherothrombotic diseases and venous thromboembolic disease [2] pointing to a link between both vascular disease groups [3]. According to the presence or absence of an identifiable transient risk factor, the current episode of VTE is referred to as 'provoked' ('triggered') or 'unprovoked' ('idiopathic').

Epidemiology

Combining the results of incidence studies from different countries with different methodologies, the annual incidence of VTE, if standardized for age and sex distribution in the US, is 71–117 cases per 100,000 population [4]. On clinical grounds, the ratio between PE and DVT is 1:3 to 2:3; if the information is mainly autopsy based, the ratio is 0.5:0.5. The largest impact on VTE incidence is age (➲Fig. 37.1), with incidences of <5/100,000 in childhood to >500/100,000 in persons >80 years of age. Between males and females there seems to be no clear difference in VTE

Table 37.1 Pathophysiological mechanisms underlying venous thromboembolism, according to Virchow's triad

Impairment of blood flow (venous stasis)	Vessel wall impairment	Impairment of blood constituents
External compression of proximal veins	Malignant infiltration	Dehydration
Solid tumour	Inflammatory infiltration	Polyglobulinaemia
Arterial aneurysm	Surgery	Polycytosis
Tourniquet	Venous puncture	Hyperfibrinogenaemia
(Lympho)coele	Other trauma	Inherited thrombophilia
Baker's cyst	Hyperhomocysteinaemia	Antiphospholipid antibodies/lupus-like anticoagulant
Pregnancy	Antiphospholipid antibodies/lupus-like anticoagulant	Heparin-induced thrombocytopenia
Internal obstruction	Heparin-induced thrombocytopenia	Tumour procoagulant
Residual thrombus from previous DVT	Residual thrombus from previous DVT	Pregnancy, puerperium
Catheter		Drugs
Immobilization		Hypofibrinolysis
Impaired respiratory movements		Alien body (catheter, pacemaker cable, caval filter)
Obesity		
Congestive heart failure		
Varicose veins		

Table 37.2 Clinical risk factors for venous thromboembolism

Clinical risk factor	Category
Surgery	
Fracture (hip or leg)	Strong
Hip or knee replacement	Strong
Major general surgery	Strong
Arthroscopic knee surgery	Moderate
Laparoscopic surgery	Weak
Trauma	
Major trauma	Strong
Spinal cord injury	Strong
Medical illness	
Malignancy	Moderate
Congestive heart or respiratory failure	Moderate
Paralytic stroke	Moderate
Previous venous thromboembolism	Moderate
Bed rest > 3 days	Weak
Iatrogenic factors other than surgery	
Central venous line	Moderate
Chemotherapy	Moderate
Oral contraceptive therapy	Moderate
Hormone replacement therapy	Moderate
Non-disease-related conditions	
Pregnancy/postpartum	Moderate
Pregnancy/antepartum	Moderate
Increasing age/decennium	Weak
Varicose veins	Weak
Prolonged sitting (air or car travel)	Weak
Obesity	Weak
Thrombophilia	
Antiphospholipid syndrome	Strong
Severe antithrombin deficiency	Strong
Severe protein C deficiency with family history	Strong
Severe protein S deficiency with family history	Strong
Factor V Leiden mutation, homozygous	Strong
Factor V Leiden mutation, heterozygous	Moderate
Prothrombin 20210 mutation	Moderate
Elevated factor VIII and IX levels	Moderate
Hyperhomocysteinaemia	Moderate

Categories: Strong = odds ratio >10; moderate = odds ratio 2–9; weak = odds ratio <2. Risk factors are weighted within each section and within each category.

Data from Anderson FA, Spencer FA. Risk factors for venous thromboembolism. *Circulation* 2003; **107**: 19–116.

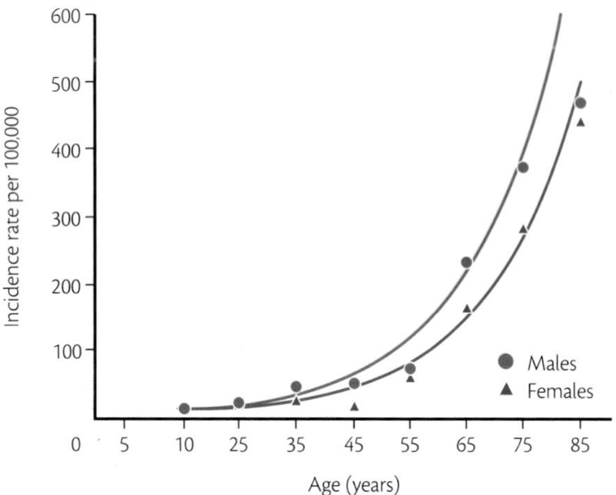

Figure 37.1 Age dependency of VTE incidence. Reproduced with permission from Anderson FA, Wheeler HB, Goldberg RJ, *et al.* A population-based perspective of the hospital incidence and case-fatality rates of deep vein thrombosis and pulmonary embolism. The Worcester DVT Study. *Arch Intern Med* 1991; **151**: 933–8.

incidences. For aetiological constellations, approximately 20% of cases are due to cancer, and surgery, trauma, and immobilization account for around 50% of cases. The remaining 30% (ranging from 26–47% in different studies) have to be classified as 'idiopathic' or 'unprovoked'. When tested systematically for thrombophilia, a large proportion (25–50%) of patients with VTE will show one or more of the established conditions, such as factor V Leiden mutation, prothrombin 20210 mutation, deficiency of antithrombin, of protein C or S, or antiphospholipid syndrome [5, 6].

Types of acute deep vein thrombosis (➲ Fig. 37.2)

By far the most common type of DVT is ascending leg DVT. It originates in calf muscle veins or in the paired calf veins. Owing to a persisting thrombogenic stimulus, and precipitated by the presence of the thrombus itself, the clot grows from distal to proximal by apposition of new thrombotic material. In every stage of thrombus propagation the process can be aborted by a change of balance between thrombogenic and antithrombotic mechanisms. If not, the clot may grow from calf muscles to iliac veins within days or even hours. In other cases propagation to femoral or iliac veins may take weeks.

With actively propagating thrombus, proximal parts of the clot may break off and move via the right heart to the lungs. As long as the thrombus is confined to the paired calf veins, the risk for embolization is very low. If the thrombus extends beyond the paired calf veins into popliteal veins or above, and in particular in the case of a fast-growing thrombus, the risk for PE becomes considerably high. The length

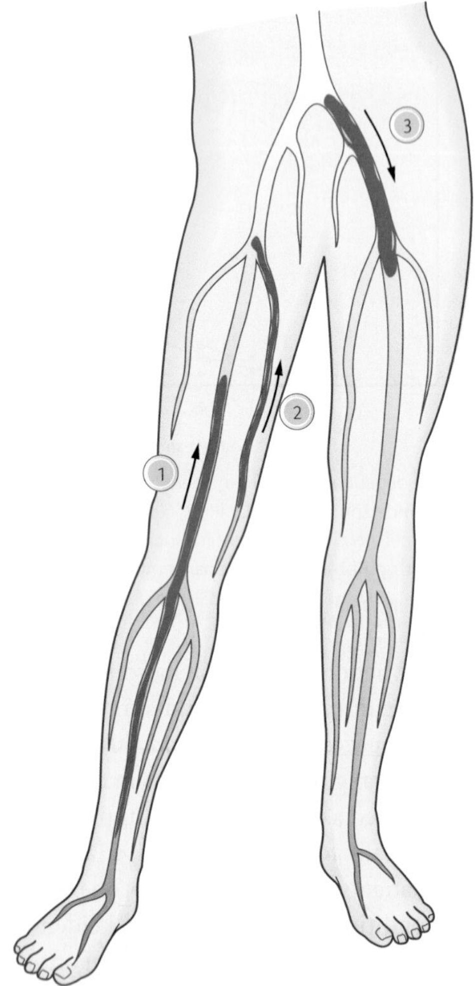

Figure 37.2 Types of deep vein thrombosis. 1, ascending DVT; 2, transfascial DVT; 3, descending iliofemoral DVT.

of the embolus may vary from millimetres to dozens of centimetres.

Less frequent but clinically more impressive is the descending type of leg DVT. It originates from the iliac veins. In 90% of cases the left iliac vein is primarily involved. The reason for this uneven side distribution is the so-called venous spur, named after May and Thurner. It is a fibrous obstructive lesion within the left common iliac vein as a response to the chronic microtraumatization of this venous segment by the pulse movements of the right common iliac artery crossing the left iliac vein. Among the trigger factors for left-sided iliac vein thrombosis are pregnancy and recent onset of oral contraceptive use. Thrombotic obstruction of the iliac vein by thrombus can develop within hours, leading to rapid and massive leg swelling, pain, and discoloration.

There are rare patients in whom the venous return of the leg is completely blocked due to an overwhelming thrombotic obstruction of the entire venous circulation. Oedema may increase to an extent that tissue pressure compromises arterial inflow and fully obstructs microcirculation (phlegmasia coerulea dolens). Viability of the leg is threatened as long as revascularization of at least the iliac veins cannot be accomplished [7]. Precondition, however, is a massive prothrombotic disease like metastatic cancer or heparin-induced thrombocytopenia (HIT).

The third type of leg DVT is transfascial thrombosis. The site of origin is the greater or lesser saphenous vein. Superficial phlebitis with thrombosis in varicose as well as in non-varicose veins has the potential to propagate proximally. Once approaching the inflow segment into the deep venous system it crosses the fascia at the inguinal (greater saphenous vein) or popliteal level (lesser saphenous vein), thereby turning from superficial into DVT. The deep vein part of the clot is prone to embolization.

Upper extremity DVT usually is segmental subclavian and/or axillary vein thrombosis. Trigger factors are either a central venous line or heavy shoulder/arm muscular exercise ('thrombose par effort', Paget–von Schrötter syndrome). In some cases thrombosis is precipitated by an anatomic narrowing formed by the clavicle and the first rib or a neck rib ('thoracic inlet syndrome'). Also, upper extremity DVT may be the first sign of mediastinal malignancy, mostly lymphoma or bronchus carcinoma. PE from upper extremity DVT has been documented [8].

Without PE, DVT alone does not have a mortality of itself. However, 10–20% of patients will die in the first year owing to underlying diseases, mostly cancer.

Pulmonary embolism

Every clot in the venous circulation has a tendency to grow. Speed and extent of thrombus growth are defined by the presence and the strength of the underlying risk factor(s). Fresh appositional thrombus is prone to be dislodged from its original site. From there it will be transported by the venous blood flow and, after having passed the right heart, it will embolize into the pulmonary circulation. The impact of this event on the clinical condition of the patient depends exclusively on the size of the embolus. Millimetre-sized emboli will go entirely asymptomatic, whereas large thrombotic masses corresponding to the volume of the iliofemoral veins may result in shock or sudden death. In the case of a patent foramen ovale and increased pulmonary artery pressure (e.g. previous PE or Valsalva manoeuvre), small clots may be pushed across to the left atrium and cause central or peripheral arterial occlusion (paradoxical embolization); larger clots may stick within the foramen ovale (transit thrombus or straddling thrombus). Sometimes the embolus or parts of it will be caught by the tricuspid valve.

At this site it may cause further thrombus accumulation with relapsing embolization.

Three categories of sequelae of pulmonary embolization have to be considered (➲Fig. 37.3): local alterations of lung and pleural tissue, functional impairment of respiration and impairment of cardiac function. The first will occur preferably with subsegmental and segmental emboli (peripheral PE), the last two in lobar or main stem pulmonary artery occlusion (central PE). Subsegmental and segmental emboli cause a local imbalance between pulmonary arterial blood flow for gas exchange and systemic arterial nutritional blood flow in subpleural areas of the lung. Lung infarction results in pleural irritation with pleuritic chest pain, alveolar haemorrhage, and infarction pneumonia. As long as VTE is untreated, relapses may occur, producing a changing pattern of multiple peripheral pulmonary infiltrates.

Larger emboli exclude a number of segments or even lobes of the lung from perfusion, although ventilation of these parts is preserved. The resulting perfusion–ventilation mismatch impairs gas exchange significantly, leading to hypoxia, which may be mild or life threatening. Mismatch and hypoxia lead to vasoconstriction of the pulmonary circulation, thereby contributing to an increase in pulmonary artery pressure. In about one-third of patients, shunting of deoxygenated blood via a patent foramen ovale directly into the systemic circulation will increase hypoxemia.

More importantly, however, right ventricular afterload is increased by massive thromboembolic obstruction of the pulmonary vessels itself [9]. As the right heart of a previously healthy person is only adapted to an invariably low mean pulmonary artery pressure of about 25mmHg, the sharp increase in afterload is a critical challenge. An increase to >40mmHg will lead to right ventricular dysfunction, right heart failure, or sudden death due to irreversible right ventricular dilatation. In many cases, the first arrival of a large embolus in the main stem of the pulmonary artery causes right heart failure, which resolves several heart beats later when the embolus is fragmented and pushed to more peripheral parts of the pulmonary circulation. As left ventricular load depends on right ventricular output, this sequence of events will clinically manifest as syncope.

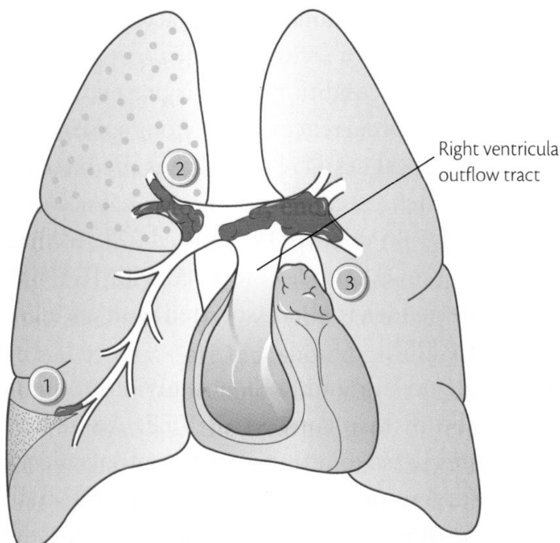

Figure 37.3 Elements of pathophysiology in pulmonary embolism. 1, Haemorrhagic pulmonary infarction with or without pneumonia in subsegmental pulmonary embolism; 2, significant perfusion/ventilation mismatch in segmental or lobar pulmonary embolism; 3, massive pulmonary artery obstruction of > 50% with right heart failure.

Based on this pathophysiological concept, three different haemodynamic presentations of PE may be differentiated [10]. They are directly related to early mortality, defined as in-hospital or 30-days' mortality. Therefore, diagnostic and therapeutic strategies for PE are based on the concept of three different risk classes [50]:

- PE is called *high risk* if accompanied by hypotension or shock. Early mortality in this patient group is >15%. If hypotension or shock are absent, patients belong the non-high-risk group, i.e. intermediate risk or low risk.
- PE is called *intermediate risk* if the systemic circulation is unaffected but the right ventricle shows signs of dysfunction as indicated by echocardiographic criteria or elevated brain natriuretic peptide (BNP) or NT-proBNP (N-terminal prohormone BNP) levels, and/or shows signs of myocardial injury with may be detected by positivity for troponin I or T. Short-term mortality in this patient group is 3–15%.
- PE is called *low risk*, if the systemic circulation is unaffected and there are no signs of right ventricular dysfunction or myocardial injury. Early mortality in this patient group does not exceed 1–3%.

A particular type of PE is chronic relapsing embolization of small clots from persisting DVT. Both every single pulmonary event and the underlying—often limited—DVT remain clinically silent for months or years. Fresh emboli will steadily add to older ones and to fibrous scarring of pulmonary arteries. In this case the right ventricle is able to adapt to the slowly increasing afterload. Patients will be diagnosed only late in the course of the disease, with fixed pulmonary artery pressures of 60–80mmHg or higher. In New York Heart Association (NYHA) classes III and IV of chronic thromboembolic pulmonary hypertension (CTPH), intermediate-term prognosis is poor [11].

Chronic sequelae of venous thromboembolism

Once the acute VTE has been overcome, endogenous repair mechanisms will be activated. Fibrinolysis will dissolve fresh thrombus material, whereas occlusive peripheral thrombi will be organized by granulation tissue and will be recanalized during the following weeks and months. Although patency can be restored, venous function may remain impaired due to destruction of the venous valves. Reflux causes chronic venous hypertension of the leg, leading to secondary varices with venous volume overload, which further enhances venous hypertension. Corresponding clinical symptoms are pain and swelling with leg dependency. Mediated by backwards damage of the microcirculation, venous hypertension leads to trophic disturbance of the skin with the extreme of venous ulcer. Without any measure to counteract venous hypertension, about 50% of patients with DVT will suffer from some degree of the post-thrombotic syndrome (PTS), 20% having severe signs or symptoms. Venous ulcer will occur in <5%. With every relapse of ipsilateral DVT the risk of severe PTS will increase [12, 13].

Iliac DVT of the descending type will resolve completely without PTS in most patients owing to either endogenous recanalization or, more frequently, collateralization. However, venous claudication will develop in some of them. This may be caused by insufficient transport capacity of collaterals or by spinal irritation, in the case when lumbar collaterals within the vertebral canal are used.

Upper extremity DVT is collateralized within days or weeks. However, some patients will persistently suffer from exertion-driven symptoms such as pain, swelling, and discoloration [14].

Owing to the significantly more powerful fibrinolytic capacity of the pulmonary circulation, pulmonary hypertension is rare after a single episode of PE and is seen in not >4% of cases [15, 16].

Venous thromboembolism as a chronic relapsing disease

Even in adequately treated patients with acute VTE, relapses will occur. For DVT it has been established that after having received 3 months of anticoagulation the cumulative incidence of recurrent VTE is 5% after 3 months, 18% after 2 years, and 30% after 8 years. Of these recurrences, 45% were ipsilateral, 36% contralateral, and 19% were PE. Factors that increase the risk of recurrence are age and body mass index [17]. Recurrence rates for PE are at least as high as for DVT. Interestingly, 80% of recurrences of DVT will again be a DVT, and 80% of the recurrences in patients with PE will again be a PE. Mortality of both types of recurrence differs largely, being 5% in DVT and 25% in PE.

The most important determinant of recurrence is the presence or absence of a transient risk factor as the trigger factor for the index event [18]. In general, with a transient risk factor present the risk of recurrence is as low as 0–4% in the first 2 years. If no transient risk factor can be identified ('idiopathic' or 'unprovoked' VTE) or if the identified risk factor is permanent (cancer, thrombophilia), the risk of recurrence is as high as 20% or more (➲Fig. 37.4).

For thrombophilia an overall hazard ratio of 1.44 for the risk of recurrence has been established. However, considerable differences exist within the group of thrombophilias. On the one hand, it has become clear that the heterozygous factor V Leiden mutation as well as the heterozygous prothrombin 20210 mutation do not increase or minimally increase the risk of recurrence. On the other hand, individuals with a severe antithrombin deficiency or those from VTE families with severe protein C or protein S deficiencies have such a high risk for a first event that, only under the assumption of the persistence of this predisposition, their risk of recurrence may be considered to be much higher than for most of all other patients with idiopathic VTE, even though solid data are lacking. The same high level of risk has to be anticipated in patients with a lupus-like anticoagulant and/or with antibodies against cardiolipin. In between these two groups, various thrombophilic conditions may be rated, such as: a persistent elevation of factor VIII or factor IX; hyperhomocysteinaemia and combined thrombophilias, such as factor V Leiden mutation plus factor II mutation or the homozygous form of factor V Leiden.

A 'thrombophilic' condition per se is present if the index event is already the recurrence of a previous episode of VTE. Prandoni and colleagues [17] found that the hazard ratio for recurrence after a second episode was 1.7; accordingly, the Austrian AUREC cohort [19] showed 22% recurrences 2 years after a second episode compared with 10.5% after a first one. Male gender is also associated with an increased recurrence rate [20].

With these data in mind, a dichotomy has to be introduced into the disease concept of VTE. An acute VTE episode as a response to a transient thrombogenic stimulus such as surgery or trauma will very likely remain the only episode during life. Conversely, in the absence of such a stimulus, or with an identifiable permanent risk factor present, VTE becomes a lifelong chronic relapsing disease.

Recently, two markers that may help to identify individual patients with increased risk of recurrence have

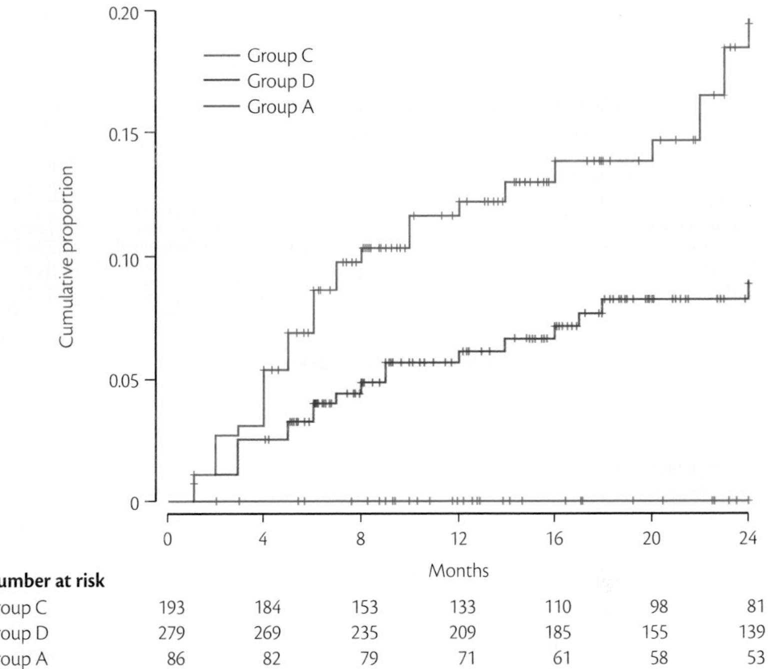

Number at risk							
Group C	193	184	153	133	110	98	81
Group D	279	269	235	209	185	155	139
Group A	86	82	79	71	61	58	53

Figure 37.4 Risk of recurrence in venous thromboembolism according to precipitating factor [13]. Group A, recent surgery; group C, idiopathic VTE; group D, non-surgical trigger factors.

been validated. A persistently elevated D-dimer level after cessation of anticoagulant treatment is a clear marker of increased risk of recurrence. Conversely, a low D-dimer level 1 month after cessation of at least 3 months' anticoagulation after a first VTE event has a 60% risk reduction for VTE recurrences in the following 2 years [21, 22]. Similarly, persistent residual vein thrombosis, as detected by serial compression ultrasound of the common femoral and popliteal veins, defines a likelihood of recurrent VTE events with a factor between 2 and 3 compared with those without residual vein thrombosis [23].

Diagnosis

Venous thromboembolic disease places a person at risk for an acute life-threatening illness or even death, and for a chronic disabling condition in the long term. For this reason, a reliable and quick diagnosis is warranted in every case of clinical suspicion. As the disease is common, and signs and symptoms are equivocal, suspicion should be raised frequently in daily practice. Under these circumstances a cohort of patients with suspicion of VTE will contain not >20% of positive cases. This, in turn, means that the diagnostic work-up has to be as non-invasive and as cost-effective as possible in order not to harm the subjects without the disease, and not to inappropriately increase the burden for the health system.

History, signs, and symptoms

Suspicion of DVT may be founded on every one-sided leg symptom such as discomfort, pain, oedema, discoloration, and warmth. According to pathophysiology, suspicion of PE should be raised in every patient with pleuritic chest pain, with dyspnoea, with syncope, and with sudden haemodynamic instability. As in all clinical reasoning, the possibility of VTE has to be weighed against alternative diagnoses according to the individual risk profile and medical history. VTE is more likely in patients with recent surgery or trauma, with recent immobilization, with cancer, with a previous episode of VTE, and with a positive family history.

Once suspicion of VTE has been raised a diagnostic work-up has to be performed, which should lead to a clear-cut 'yes' or 'no' answer. Physical examination is unable to provide enough evidence against or in favour of the diagnosis to dispense from objective testing. The same is true for the basic diagnostics of PE, for example, electrocardiogram (ECG), chest radiograph, or arterial blood gases analysis. However, all of these diagnostic elements may contribute to a categorization of the patient regarding his probability of having the disease. This probability definitely helps to guide the diagnostic work-up.

Today, a broad variety of diagnostic tools for VTE are available. The rest of this section will discuss them separately. In a second step they will be combined into diagnostic

Table 37.3 Clinical pre-test probability in DVT according to Wells

Criterion	Score
Active cancer (patient receiving treatment for cancer within the previous 6 months or currently receiving palliative treatment)	1
Paralysis, paresis or recent plaster immobilization of the lower extremities	1
Recently bedridden for 3 days or more, or major surgery within the previous 12 weeks, requiring general or regional anaesthesia	1
Localized tenderness along the distribution of the deep venous system	1
Entire leg swollen	1
Calf swelling at least 3cm larger than that on the asymptomatic side (measured 10cm below tibial tuberosity)	1
Pitting oedema confined to the symptomatic leg	1
Collateral superficial veins (non-varicose)	1
Previously documented DVT	1
Alternative diagnosis at least as likely as DVT	−2

A score of 2 or higher indicates that the probability of DVT is likely; a score of <2 indicates that the probability of deep vein thrombosis is unlikely. In patients with symptoms in both legs, the more symptomatic leg is used for scoring.

pathways (algorithms) that have been proven to be safe and resource saving.

Diagnostic tools

Assessment of clinical (pre-test) probability

The most quick and simple way to categorize patients with suspected VTE is to add up basic clinical information into a qualitative assessment of probability for either DVT or PE. This can be done by a formal scoring system that ascribes a certain number of points to predefined clinical features, and which defines thresholds for different categories of probability. Alternatively, the evaluation can be undertaken by an experienced physician who integrates the clinical information intuitively. In any case, the result of clinical or pre-test probability assessment has to be given in two or three categories (high vs. intermediate vs. low; high vs. non-high; high vs. low), and it has to be documented explicitly as with any result of other diagnostic tests. ➲Table 37.3 and ➲Tables 37.4 and 37.5, present scores for DVT and PE, respectively [24–26]. Validation of scores demonstrated that they discriminate reliably between groups with low (2–5%), intermediate (10–20%), and high (>40%) prevalence of the disease.

Table 37.4 Revised Geneva score for suspected PE

Variable	Points
Risk factors:	
Age >65 years	+ 1
Previous DVT or PE	+ 3
Surgery (under general anaesthesia) or fracture (of the lower limbs) within 1 month	+ 2
Active malignancy (solid or haematological malignancy, currently active or considered as cured since <1 year)	+ 2
Symptoms:	
Unilateral lower limb pain	+ 3
Haemoptysis	+ 2
Clinical signs:	
Heart rate:	
75–94bpm	+ 3
≥95bpm	+ 5
Pain on lower limb deep vein palpation and unilateral oedema	+ 4
Clinical probability:	**Total no. of points:**
Low	0–3
Intermediate	4–10
High	≥11

D-dimer testing

D-dimers are degradation products of cross-linked fibrin. They are generated by the action of the fibrinolytic enzyme plasmin. As any thrombotic process in the circulation is accompanied by increased endogenous fibrinolysis, a rise in plasma D-dimer levels indicates some kind of thrombotic activity. The more extensive the thrombotic process, the higher plasma D-dimer levels can be measured. For technical

Table 37.5 Clinical pre-test probability in pulmonary embolism according to Wells

Criterion	Score
Clinical signs and symptoms of DVT (minimum of leg swelling and pain with palpation of the deep veins)	3.0
An alternative diagnosis is less likely than pulmonary embolism	3.0
Heart rate greater than 100 beats/min	1.5
Immobilization or surgery in the previous 4 weeks	1.5
Previous DVT/pulmonary embolism	1.5
Haemoptysis	1.0
Malignancy (at treatment, treated in the last 6 months or palliative)	1.0

Note: ≤ 2.0 points indicates a low probability of pulmonary embolism; 2.0–5.5 points indicates a moderate probability; and ≥ 6.0 points indicates a high probability.

as well for practical reasons, the result of D-dimer testing is given as 'positive' vs. 'negative' by defining a threshold plasma level. The threshold is chosen according to sensitivity and specificity of the test, and to its purpose. In general, specificity of D-dimer testing for VTE is low, as many other conditions and disorders (e.g. infection, inflammatory disease, trauma, surgery, pregnancy) may be accompanied by fibrin generation and lysis. Therefore, thresholds have been chosen to allow for excluding VTE in case of a concentration below the threshold (so-called negative results).

For DVT there is a sensitivity gap of different extent with all available test systems. This means that the combination with other diagnostic tools is required in order to safely exclude the disease. For PE there is evidence that the disease can safely be excluded by means of D-dimer testing alone, except perhaps in the patients categorized as having high clinical probability. D-dimer test systems should only be used in clinical practice if they have been validated in methodologically sound studies with sufficient patient samples [27].

Different test systems are being used at present. Latex-enhanced ELISA (enzyme-linked immunosorbent assay) systems require full laboratory equipment and provide continuous values for plasma D-dimer levels. Card ELISA tests are able to present results in categories of plasma levels. Bedside test systems give only the positive/negative type of result and have the lowest sensitivity of the available systems. On the other hand, only bedside tests and rapid ELISA test systems are suitable for a quick work-up (within 1 hour) of patients in an office, an outpatient department or in the emergency room. In fact, despite their lower sensitivity, bedside tests are efficient tools if used in combination with clinical probability assessment (see Diagnostic algorithms in venous thromboembolism, p.1346).

Venous ultrasound

Venous ultrasound is able to detect deep venous thrombosis by means of different diagnostic criteria: direct visualization of intravascular thrombus using B-mode, or alteration or lack of the flow signal using pulsed wave (PW) or colour Doppler. The most simple and unequivocal modality, however, is compression ultrasound (CUS) using the B-mode technique. Since the 1980s, venous ultrasound has been tested against venography in numerous studies with differing protocols. In 1998, a meta-analysis showed that sensitivity is high enough to exclude the disease in ultrasound-negative patients in symptomatic proximal DVT. However, sensitivity was much lower in symptomatic distal DVT and did not allow ruling out of the diagnosis. This led to the conclusion that CUS should be performed only on proximal veins. As virtually all symptomatic proximal DVTs are detectable either in the groin or in the popliteal region, examination of these two regions should suffice [28]. Because of the low emboligenic potential of isolated calf DVT, it has been demonstrated that it is safe to withhold anticoagulation in patients with a negative CUS for proximal veins, which remains negative when repeated after 1 week [29]. However, this approach is not cost effective as 80% of patients require a repeat CUS.

Alternatively, more extensive CUS protocols have been developed which systematically examine all veins of the leg including the calf veins (complete or comprehensive compression ultrasound, CCUS; ➲Fig. 37.5). It has been demonstrated that a single CCUS examination of all leg veins is safe in excluding DVT when used as the only diagnostic test in all patients [30]. Such a protocol is not time consuming but requires in-depth training of sonographers. In addition, the single complete ultrasound strategy helps identifying alternative diagnoses in DVT-negative patients, such as ruptured Baker's cyst, calf haematoma, or muscle fibre rupture. Theoretically, using CCUS for diagnosis of DVT might lead to overtreatment: first, the rate of false-positive distal DVT findings generated by CCUS is not known, even though the magnitude of this problem seems to be limited. Second, as distal DVT in many cases has a self-limited course it might not be indicated to treat every distal DVT detected by CCUS. Data to solve the latter problem are not available yet. Thus, some experts argue that a single negative proximal CUS might also rule out the diagnosis of DVT in these patients, as the 3-month thromboembolic risk is similar to the risk observed in patients with a negative venogram.

Venous ultrasound is not only useful for diagnosing patients with symptoms of DVT but also for the work-up of patients with clinically suspected PE. If a DVT can be demonstrated by ultrasound in a patient with signs and symptoms suggestive of PE, the diagnostic process can be stopped, as treatment of the—proven—DVT is almost equal to that of the—yet unproven—PE [30].

Venography

It is the historic privilege of venography to set the gold standard for the diagnosis of DVT. As a matter of fact, a negative venography reliably excludes DVT [31]. However, there are clear drawbacks of this method: radiation burden, adverse effects of contrast media such as allergic reactions or hyperthyroidism, and discomfort for the patient. A widely under-recognized problem is that—similar to the situation with venous ultrasound—different venography protocols may yield different quality levels of results, as has been demonstrated by a comparison of the elaborate long leg method with the standard ascending venography by

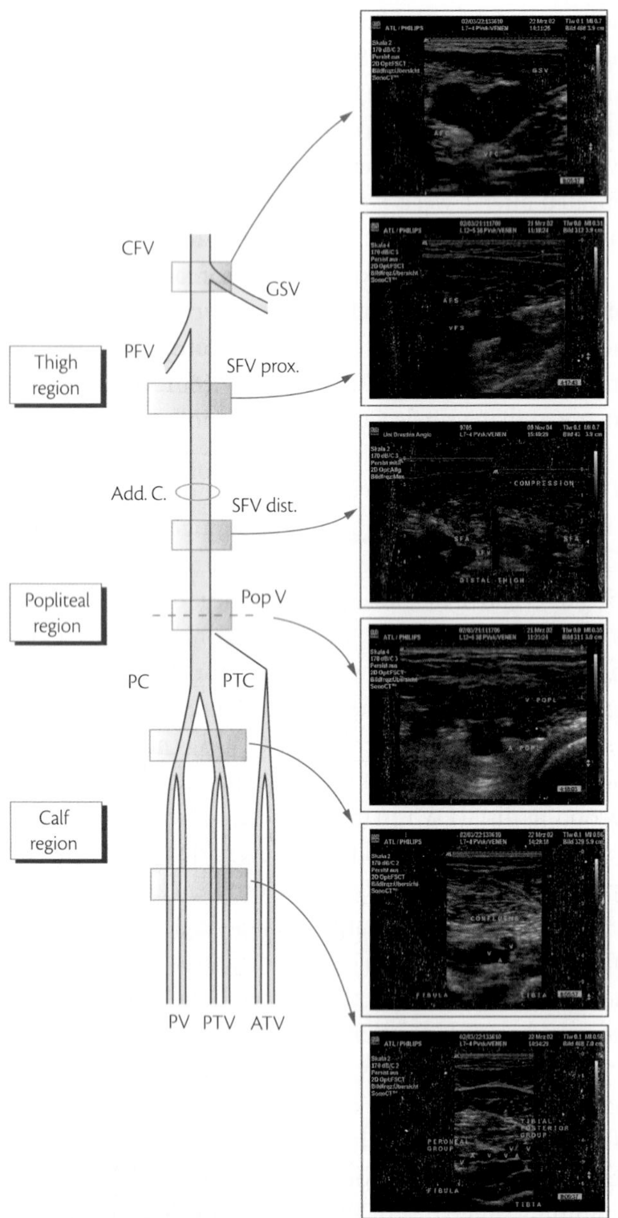

Figure 37.5 Visualization of all regions of the leg veins in transverse planes for complete compression ultrasound (CCUS). CFV, common femoral vein; GSV, greater saphenous vein; PFV, profound femoral vein; SFV, superficial femoral vein; prox., proximal; dist., distal; Add. C., adductor canal; Pop V, popliteal vein; PC, peroneal confluens; PTC, posterior tibial confluens; PV, peroneal veins; PTV, posterior tibial veins; ATV, anterior tibial veins.

Paulin Rubinov [32]. Furthermore, with sharply declining numbers of venograms performed, experience of radiologists fades away, giving rise to an overall quality problem of the procedure. Thus, with the emergence of ultrasound venography has changed its role from gold standard to a back-up procedure.

Lung scan

From a pathophysiological point of view, lung scan provides the most direct information about a patient with suspected PE, i.e. a perfusion defect in an otherwise healthy part of the lung. The advantages of the method include the low radiation burden and the huge amount of scientific data having evaluated its diagnostic efficacy. A clear-cut positive examination has such a high specificity that further therapy can be based on this result. Furthermore, a definitely normal scan excludes PE. No further testing will be needed in order to withhold anticoagulation [33]. However, the problem with lung scan is the high proportion (50–60%) of indeterminate test results, i.e. results that do not allow for an unequivocal diagnosis [34]. The efficacy of the procedure can be enhanced by applying the SPECT (single photon emission computed tomography) technique instead of planar imaging [35]. Of utmost importance for appropriate utilization of the method is that the result of each individual examination is given in categories ('positive', 'negative', or 'indeterminate') rather than in great anatomic detail. As a matter of fact, lung scan has been largely replaced by spiral computed tomography (CT). However, it remains a valuable option for patients with contraindication to X-ray contrast media.

Spiral computed tomography

Spiral CT offers a very elegant way to visualize clots in the pulmonary circulation. This may be achieved within body cross-sections only or by means of digital reconstruction of the pulmonary arterial tree (CT pulmonary angiography, CTPA) [36]. Specificity seems to be not a significant problem. However, sensitivity depends critically on the technical equipment. First-generation single-row detector CTs were able to reliably detect thrombi down to a size of segmental pulmonary arteries. The overall sensitivity of 70% compared with pulmonary angiography precluded this test from being used as the only test for exclusion of PE [37]. Sensitivity of CTPA has significantly increased with second- or third-generation scanners, i.e. 4-row or 16-row multislice detectors (➲Fig. 37.6) [38]. While single-row detector CT is required to be combined with lower limb venous CUS, it has been recently demonstrated that this is no longer the case if multi-row detector CT is used, due to the improved sensitivity of this new generation of CT [39]. Among the pros for CTPA are the increasing global availability and the short duration of the examination procedure, making it suitable even for patients with cardiorespiratory instability. Drawbacks of the method are the need for contrast media and the high radiation burden exceeding that of perfusion lung scanning by four- to sixfold.

It has been demonstrated that by means of CT angiography the peripheral venous circulation can be visualized

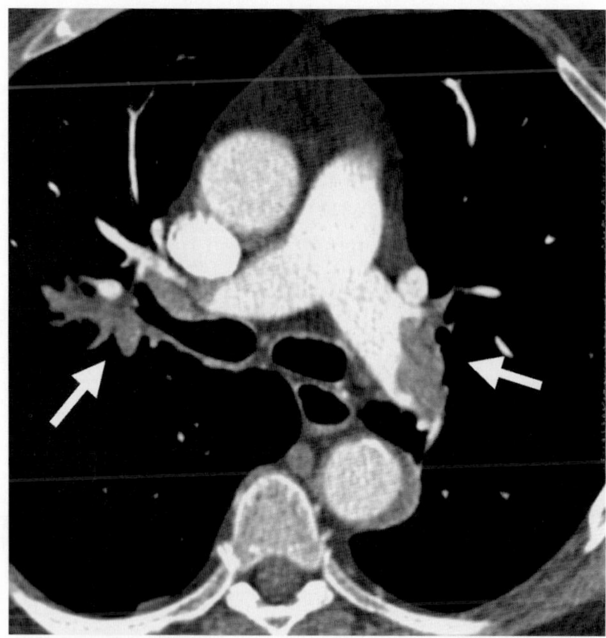

A

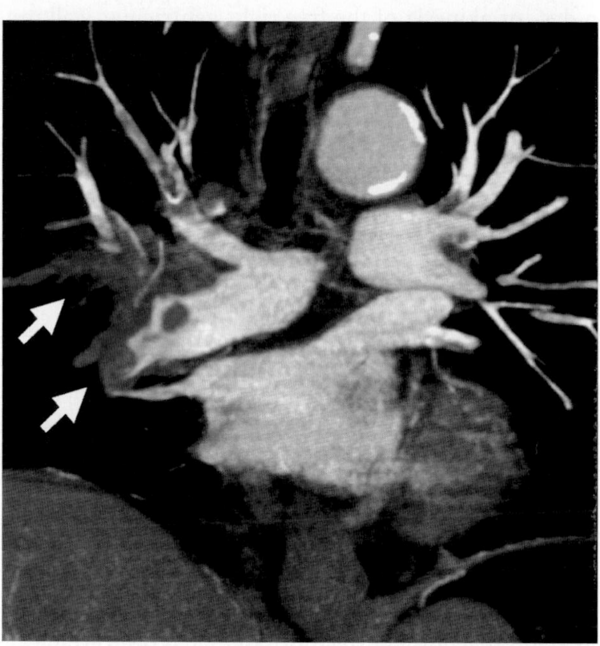

B

Figure 37.6 Helical computerized tomography for diagnosis of pulmonary embolism. (A) Transverse plane with massive bilateral embolization. (B) Coronal plane from CT pulmonary angiography with predominant right-sided embolization. (Courtesy of Dr J. Leonhard, Institute of Diagnostic and Interventional Radiology, University Hospital Dresden.)

as well. Even if the radiology literature reports almost ideal sensitivity and specificity figures for detection of DVT, the clinical need for this procedure is at least questionable. However, CT is a valuable method in detecting isolated iliac vein and inferior or superior caval thrombosis. The advantage is the exact visualization not only of its extent but also of possibly causal pathologies in the surrounding anatomic region (pelvic mass, retroperitoneal mass, mediastinal mass) [40].

Pulmonary angiography

All that has been said about venography applies to pulmonary angiography as well. However, some issues make this procedure even more problematic. First, pulmonary angiography is an entirely invasive procedure that bears the highest procedural risk among all diagnostic tests for VTE. Second, imaging quality of pulmonary angiography has significantly been impaired by the almost complete transition from classic X-ray film angiography to the digital subtraction angiography (DSA) technology. Third, even more than for venography, radiologists' personal experience and skills with this method have been reduced to very few centres, the number of which is declining steadily. Today, pulmonary angiography serves as a back-up procedure in clinical diagnostic studies rather than in real-life healthcare.

Magnetic resonance imaging

Different imaging modalities of magnetic resonance imaging (MRI) provide a clear visualization of clots in both the peripheral venous and the pulmonary artery circulation. The use of contrast agents enhances image quality and reduces examination time [41]. As for CT, radiologists report excellent accuracy data for MRI in comparison with standard diagnostic procedures [42]. However, availability of MRI, and in particular with VTE adopted protocols, is limited and resource utilization is high. In addition, the optimal place of MRI in the diagnostic work-up of a patient with suspicion of VTE has never been investigated consistently. At present, MRI is a promising imaging alternative for VTE, which may have advantages over standard tests in specific clinical situations, e.g. detection of isolated iliac or caval DVT in a patient with contraindications to X-ray contrast agents, or in pregnancy [43]. Nevertheless, the technique awaits validation in methodologically sound outcome studies with sufficient patient samples.

Echocardiography

There are three types of echocardiographic findings linked to PE: direct visualization of thrombembolic material, increased tricuspid pressure gradient as a measure of increased pulmonary artery pressure, and signs of right ventricular dysfunction.

Thrombotic masses my be found in the pulmonary main stem, as a transit or 'straddling' thrombus caught in a patent foramen ovale, or as a free-floating thrombus in the right atrium and/or ventricle caught in the tricuspid valve (➲ Fig 37.7).

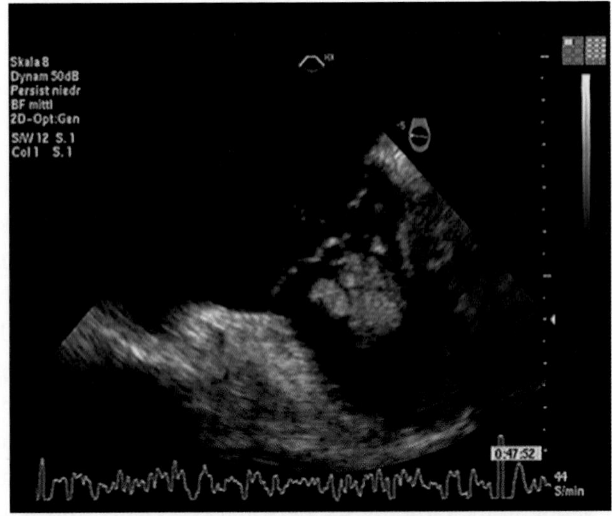

A

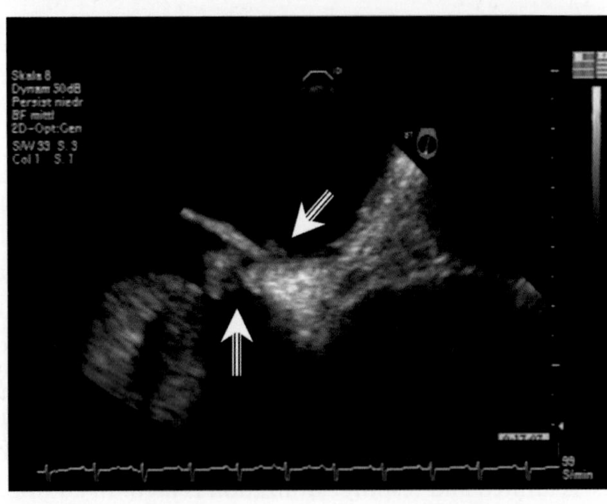

B

Figure 37.7 Thrombus visualization by echocardiography. (A) Large right atrial thrombus caught by the tricuspid valve. (B) Straddling thrombus in transit from the right to the left atrium (see arrows). (Courtesy of Dr M. Weise, Medical Clinic, University Hospital Dresden.)

The latter one is indicative of a worse prognosis due to its potential for immediate and substantial re-embolism. The pulmonary artery pressure may be accurately estimated by measurement of the tricuspid valve pressure gradient. A decrease of the acceleration time supports the finding of increased PA pressure. However, it has to be noted that PA pressure does not correlate to right ventricular strain. Obviously, the higher the PA pressure the better the right ventricular performance. Signs of right ventricular dysfunction include:

- an end-diastolic diameter of the right ventricle of >30mm or an right ventricle/left ventricle ratio >1 (➲Fig. 37.8);
- the paradoxical, i.e. systolic outwards movement or systolic flattening of the interventricular septum;

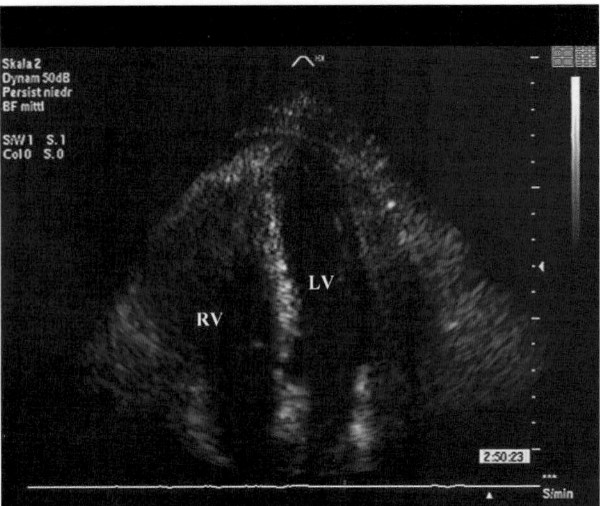

Figure 37.8 Acute right ventricular dysfunction: massive enlargement of the right ventricle with lack of filling of the left ventricle due to decreased preload. (Courtesy of Dr M. Weise, Medical Clinic, University Hospital Dresden.)

- a dys- or akinesia of the free right ventricular wall in the presence of normo- or hyperkinesias of its apical portion.

None of these echocardiographic findings, or a combination of them, has a sensitivity high enough to refute the diagnosis of PE if absent. This excludes echocardiography from being part of the primary diagnostic process in patients with suspected PE. The only exception is the patient with haemodynamic instability. If in such a patient no sign of PE, in particular right ventricular dysfunction, can be found, an alternative diagnosis must be made. On the other hand, if a patient presents with sudden onset instability, and right ventricular dysfunction can be seen in bedside echocardiography PE is the most likely cause. Indeed, if the condition is life threatening and an immediate treatment decision is needed, echocardiography may suffice to justify thrombolytic treatment for suspected PE.

Nevertheless, echocardiography should be performed in all patients in whom the diagnosis of PE has been established. As right ventricular dysfunction is the most reliable predictor of short-term mortality, echocardiography provides an ideal tool for assessing the prognosis of an individual patient [44]. Important treatment decisions can be based on the right ventricular dysfunction assessment. Again, it has to be stressed, that pulmonary artery pressure correlates neither to right ventricular dysfunction nor to early mortality.

Diagnostic algorithms in venous thromboembolism

According to the immediate risk of the patient, the first distinction that has to be made is whether a patient with

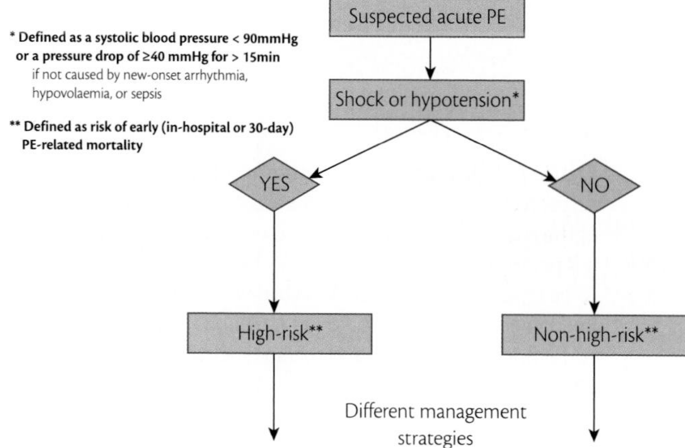

Figure 37.9 Initial risk stratification of patients with suspicion of PE.

suspicion of PE is haemodynamically stable or unstable (➲Fig 37.9). Shock or hypotension in this regard is defined as a systolic pressure <90mmHg or a pressure drop of 40mmHg and more within the last 15min. If one of these criteria applies and is not attributable to new onset arrhythmia, hypovolaemia, or sepsis, the patient with suspicion of PE has to be managed according to their high-risk status (➲Fig 37.10): CT is preferable to echocardiography if the condition of the patient allows for performing it, and if it is available immediately. If not, bedside echocardiography is the test of choice. If no other test is available, demonstration of right ventricular dysfunction by echocardiography justifies acute treatment of PE such as thrombolysis or embolectomy.

The non-high-risk patient with suspicion of VTE will be managed differently. In order to enhance the diagnostic effectiveness and to reduce the burden for both patients and healthcare resources, the diagnostic tools should be combined in a structured work-up of all patients under suspicion of VTE. The goal is to safely diagnose a maximum number of patients by simple and non-invasive tests [45].

For both entities, DVT and PE, the first diagnostic step should be the combination of pre-test probability and D-dimer. The combination of a non-high pre-test probability and a negative D-dimer reliably excludes VTE, so that the patient can be left without anticoagulant treatment [46]. This situation applies to approximately one-third of outpatients clinically suspected of DVT or PE, when using a rapid ELISA test. A positive D-dimer in a patient with a non-high pre-test probability will prompt further testing, as well as a high pre-test probability regardless of the D-dimer result.

For patients with clinically suspected DVT, the next step is compression ultrasound (➲Fig. 37.11) [47]. The need for further testing depends on the comprehensiveness of the ultrasound protocol. If the sonographer has been trained for a complete ultrasound protocol and states that they have imaged the entire leg vein system and that it was negative, the patient can be left untreated without further testing. If the proximal veins were negative and the examination of distal veins was equivocal or not examined at all then the patient should have a repeat ultrasound for proximal veins after 1 week or proceed to venography if the final diagnosis is warranted immediately.

Non-high-risk patients, i.e. haemodynamically stable patients with suspicion of PE, the next step is multidetector helical CT if available (➲Fig 37.12) [48]. Currently, the result will confirm or exclude the diagnosis. If only a single detector CT is available the combination with a negative proximal CUS is required to leave the patient untreated. If there is concern regarding deterioration of impaired renal function by administration of contrast media, the patient may undergo CUS of proximal leg veins first. If positive,

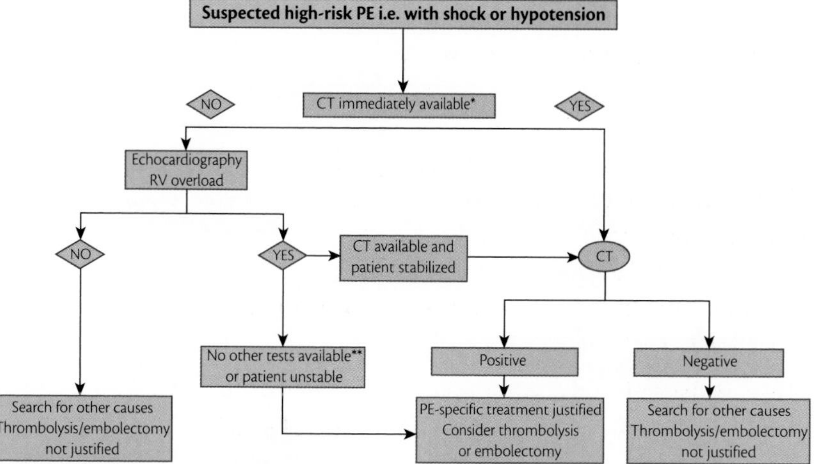

Figure 37.10 Diagnostic algorithm for high-risk patients with suspicion of PE.

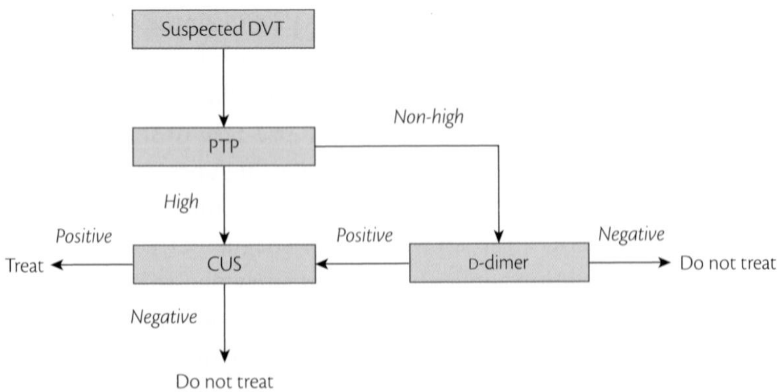

Figure 37.11 Diagnostic algorithm for the diagnosis of suspected DVT. If CUS is performed as complete examination of the entire leg the negative test results in 'Do not treat'. If it is performed as proximal CUS only the negative test has to be repeated after 1 week. Modified with permission from Bounameaux H, Righini M, Perrier A. Venous thromboembolism: contemporary diagnostic and therapeutic aspects. *Vasa* 2008, **37**: 211–26.

treatment decisions can be based on this finding. If negative, lung scanning is appropriate: a normal as well as a high probability scan allows for the correct treatment decision. In case of an intermediate probability lung scan the combination with a negative CUS suffices to exclude PE. Only if clinical pre-test probability was high additional tests may be warranted.

In general, if there is suspicion of VTE, diagnostic work-up has to be carried out straight away without delay. If any of the tests or their results is not available, and the patient is stable, subcutaneous injections of low-molecular-weight heparin (LMWH) should be given in therapeutic dosages to minimize the risk of immediate (relapsing) PE. The period of 'blind' treatment should not exceed 24–36 hours, i.e. two or three injections in order to minimize the risk of bleeding complications.

Treatment

Treatment of VTE is composed of three periods: the acute phase (days), the intermediate (weeks to months), and the long-term period (months to years). According to the natural history of the disease, treatment comprises three components (➲Fig. 37.13):

1) control of thrombus progression during acute disease in order to clear away the risk of an immediate, possibly fatal PE;
2) control of acute and chronic pulmonary and peripheral venous hypertension;
3) control of relapsing disease in the intermediate and long-term course.

The pivotal measure for the first and the third component is anticoagulation. For the purpose of this chapter, therapeutic anticoagulation of VTE will be referred to as 'initial anticoagulation' (acute phase), 'early maintenance therapy' (intermediate), or 'long-term maintenance therapy'. The term 'maintenance therapy' corresponds to the concept of VTE as a chronic relapsing disease, and avoids an inaccurate use of the term 'secondary prevention'. All therapeutic aspects of VTE are covered by the most recent American College of Chest Physicians (ACCP) consensus [49] and by the ESC guidelines on the diagnosis and management

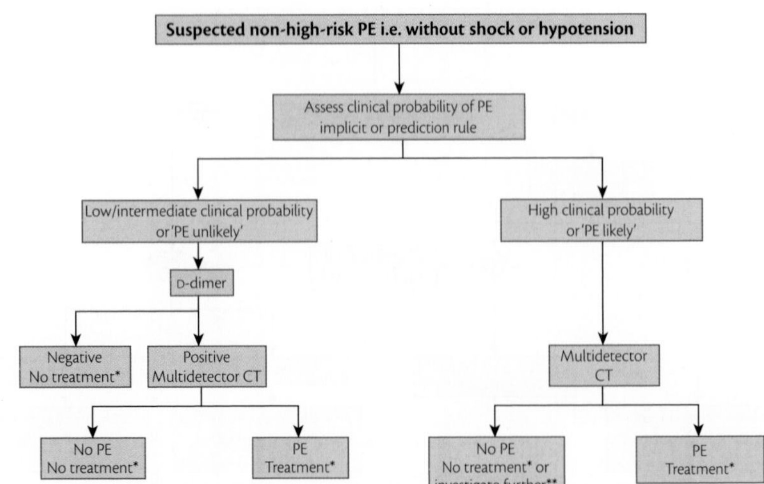

Figure 37.12 Diagnostic algorithm for non-high-risk patients with suspicion of PE.

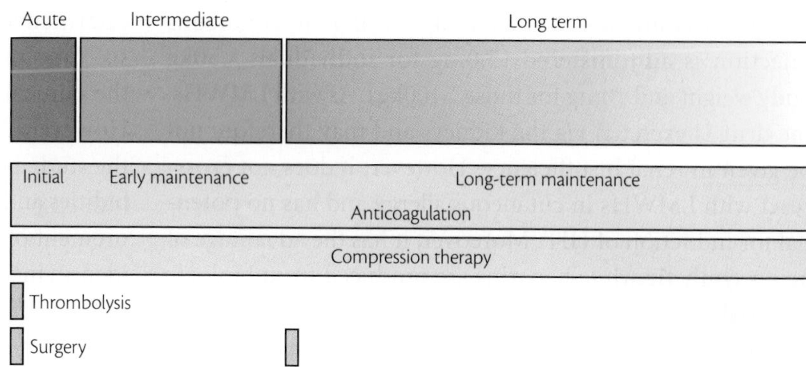

Figure 37.13 Treatment elements of VTE.

of acute PE [50], both issued in 2008 and both based on the available evidence. The present chapter follows these recommendations and suggestions in all major topics. The very few deviations will be discussed.

Treatment modalities of the acute phase

More than 90% of patients with VTE will be treated by anticoagulation alone, for DVT in conjunction with compression therapy. Alternatives or add-ons out of the full spectrum of treatment options may be considered only in a few patients with specific conditions. Most of them are related to contraindications against anticoagulation, to haemodynamic instability, or to decompensation of the leg circulation.

Initial anticoagulation

At present, therapeutic dosages of heparins are the standard for initial anticoagulation. In the high-risk PE patient unfractionated heparin (UFH) has to be administered in order to allow for subsequent interventions with high bleeding risk. In non-high-risk patients, almost all available LMWH preparations have been tested against UFH. Several meta-analyses have pooled these trials, with the overall result that fixed-dose subcutaneous LMWHs without laboratory monitoring are at least as safe and efficacious as intravenous UFH with activated partial thromboplastin time (aPTT) monitoring [51]. One trial demonstrated this explicitly for PE [52]. Regarding major bleeding, some meta-analyses showed superiority of LMWHs. These results apply for patients with preserved renal function. Thus, LMWHs have to be considered as the actual standard for the initial anticoagulation of patients with VTE, i.e. both DVT and PE. The different preparations with their respective dose regimens are listed in ➲Table 37.6. Patients with impaired renal function and patients with cutaneous allergy against LMWHs should be treated with intravenous UFH or fondaparinux. Dose adjustments according to aPTT measurements should follow a nomogram to enhance performance of UFH administration. In order to facilitate the diagnosis of emerging HIT, platelet counts have to be performed at day 1 of heparin treatment and should be repeated during administration beyond day 7, and at regular intervals thereafter.

The synthetic pentasaccharide fondaparinux has been evaluated in two large trials for the initial anticoagulation of DVT and PE [53, 54]. It showed non-inferiority compared with LMWH in patients with DVT, and in PE compared with UFH infusion. The drug is registered in most

Table 37.6 Anticoagulants for initial treatment of acute venous thromboembolism

Preparation	Brand name	Manufacturer	Dose	Regimen
Certoparin	MonoEmbolex	Novartis	8000aXaU	BID
Dalteparin	Fragmin	Pfizer	100aXaU/kg BW	BID
Enoxaparin	Lovenox/Clexane	Sanofi-Aventis	1.0mg/kg BW	BID
Enoxaparin	Lovenox/Clexane	Sanofi-Aventis	1.5mg/kg BW	OD
Nadroparin	Fraxiparin	GlaxoSmithKline	85aXaU/kg BW	BID
Nadroparin	Fraxiforte/Fraxodi	GlaxoSmithKline	171aXaU/kg BW	OD
Tinzaparin	Innohep	Leo	175aXaU/kg BW	OD
Fondaparinux	Arixtra	GSK	7.5mg (5.0mg <50kg BW) (10mg <100kg BW)	OD

Note: aXaU, anti factor Xa units; BW, body weight; OD, once daily; BID, twice daily.

European countries. A once-daily 7.5-mg subcutaneous injection is administered (5.0mg for individuals <50kg body weight and 10mg for those >100kg). As with LMWHs, the drug is excreted via the kidneys and may therefore not be given in renal insufficiency. However, it does not cross-react with LMWHs in cutaneous allergy and has no potential for induction of HIT. Moreover, it has the advantage of being synthetic while heparins are produced from biologic material.

Initial anticoagulation with heparin or fondaparinux has to be administered for at least 5 days. After this period early maintenance therapy will follow. The present standard is to switch to therapy with vitamin K antagonists (VKAs). As it takes 5–7 days to accomplish therapeutic anticoagulation with VKAs, the first doses can be given simultaneously with the initial anticoagulation, in most patients on the day of diagnosis. The initial anticoagulant will be stopped when the intended stable therapeutic intensity of VKAs has been achieved.

Systemic thrombolysis

Systemic thrombolysis in VTE is able to reduce thrombus mass more rapidly and more comprehensively than anticoagulation alone. This holds true when given for PE as well as for DVT. On the other hand, bleeding complications will occur at a significantly increased frequency compared with anticoagulation alone. The figures for major haemorrhage, intracranial haemorrhage, and fatal haemorrhage approximate 15%, 1.5%, and 1% respectively [55].

In PE the goal of thrombolysis is short term. Reduction of thrombotic obstruction of the pulmonary artery bed enables the right ventricle to recover from severe dysfunction or frank failure. Obviously, the advantage is present only if right ventricular function is critically challenged. This is the case in all patients with hypotension or shock, i.e. in all high-risk patients. A recent meta-analysis of all randomized trials comparing thrombolytic therapy with heparin revealed that only in haemodynamically unstable patients was thrombolysis associated with a reduction of recurrence and death. If those patients were excluded, no benefit could be found [56]. The preferable regimen is intravenous infusion of 100mg of recombinant plasminogen activator (rtPA) within 2 hours; a loading dose of 10mg may be given upfront. Under cardiopulmonary resuscitation (CPR), the 100mg may be given as a fractionated bolus injection. Alternative regimens consist of either high-dose urokinase or high-dose streptokinase. By contrast, there is definitely no indication for thrombolysis in low-risk patients. However, it is currently under debate whether intermediate-risk patients will benefit from thrombolysis. One randomized controlled trial demonstrated that the clinical course of the disease may be improved [57]. However, there was no impact on mortality. In addition, the study population was highly selected regarding comorbidities and bleeding risk. Besides echocardiography, measurement of cardiac troponins and of pro-BNP may help in identifying patients in whom thrombolysis should be considered [58, 59]. A stratified treatment concept of systemic thrombolysis in PE is given in ➲Table 37.7 [50, 60, 61].

In DVT the goal of thrombolysis is exclusively long term, i.e. reduction of frequency and severity of PTS. It is anticipated that removal of the clot decreases venous outflow resistance and prevents the venous valves from scarring; thereby, venous haemodynamics would be preserved. From retrospective and prospective cohorts there is some indication that this concept is durable; however, a prerequisite seems to be complete early lysis of the entire clot. This result will be achieved at best only in one-third of the patients. Given the low rate of clinically severe cases of PTS of approximately 10% under standard treatment and the potentially life-threatening complications of systemic thrombolysis there seems to be little room for a benefit of thrombolysis. As a matter of fact, the very few randomized controlled trials reporting long-term outcomes are small, have methodological flaws, and do not prove that systemic thrombolysis is superior to the current standard therapy

Table 37.7 Treatment concept for pulmonary embolism stratified by the haemodynamic situation

Haemodynamic situation	Treatment modalities
Cardiac arrest	Cardiopulmonary resuscitation (even extended) Intubation, ventilation Immediate (bolus) systemic thrombolysis without regard to any bleeding risk Therapeutic anticoagulation (UFH)
Unstable systemic haemodynamics	Catecholamines Intubation, ventilation when needed Early systemic thrombolysis (2 hours) with regard to only life-threatening bleeding risk Therapeutic anticoagulation (UFH)
Systemic haemodynamics stable; right ventricular dysfunction in echocardiography; positive cardiac troponins	Therapeutic anticoagulation (LMWH, fondaparinux) Consider elective systemic thrombolysis (2 hours) in patients without any increased bleeding risk
Systemic haemodynamics stable; no right ventricular dysfunction in echocardiography	Therapeutic anticoagulation (LMWH, UFH, fondaparinux)

consisting of anticoagulation and compression stockings for at least 2 years [62]. The only indication might be the exceptionally rare condition of phlegmasia coerulea dolens because even incomplete lysis with partial recanalization of the iliac veins might overcome the acute critical haemodynamics.

Catheter-based procedures

Several authors have convincingly demonstrated that pulmonary artery thrombus burden can be reduced by mechanical thrombus fragmentation, thereby allowing for rapid right ventricular recovery. Transfemoral, transjugular, or transbrachial catheter devices with or without local thrombolysis are used [63]. There are no data as to whether this approach is more efficacious than systemic thrombolysis. However, it certainly requires more logistics, equipment and trained personnel. It seems very likely that no prospective study will systematically investigate the potential value of this regimen. Still, it may be argued that mechanical thrombus fragmentation can be beneficial in haemodynamically unstable patients with severe contraindications against systemic thrombolysis, such as early postoperative patients, particularly after brain surgery, or in the immediate postpartum period.

Over the last years, there is increasing interest among interventionists in applying catheter-based therapies to DVT. The most common procedure is distal cannulation of the vein with intrathrombal administration of thrombolytic agents. If the clot is successfully removed, remaining stenoses, in particular in the iliac segments, are subjected to recanalization by balloon angioplasty, with or without stenting [64]. There is a registry with increasing numbers of treatment episodes. Most of the patients have the descending type of DVT [65]. However, the target criterion of success, i.e. frequency and severity of PTS in treated patients, is not consistently reported. Before a recommendation for catheter-based therapy in VTE can be given, the long-term benefit has to be clearly established by appropriately designed randomized controlled trials [66].

Caval filters

Caval filters have been widely used in the past. with a sharply declining frequency in the last decade. The rationale for caval filter insertion is to lower the chance of (recurrent) PE originating from a proven proximal DVT. Several types of filter devices have been developed. In addition to technical details of filter insertion and placement, the main differences are related to long-term durability and complications such as filter fragmentation, perforation, migration, embolization, or filter thrombosis [67]. After decades of obvious overuse, a randomized controlled trial established that in proximal DVT the frequency of early PE could be lowered by insertion of a caval filter in addition to standard anticoagulation, even although mortality was not affected. However, in the long term, the caval filter group had significantly more episodes of recurring DVT than the standard treatment group [68]. Today, the only indications for insertion of a caval filter include early recurrence of PE despite appropriate anticoagulation or absolute contraindications against any type and intensity of anticoagulation. However, these patients not only have a high risk of filter thrombosis and subsequent PE; most of them will turn out to have advanced cancer. Whatever rare reason for filter insertion is made plausible in a specific patient, temporary filters should be favoured over permanent filters.

Surgery

Emergency open-lung pulmonary thrombectomy, a procedure with a history of >150 years, is of no distinctive value in today's medicine. In a remarkable prospective comparison with systemic thrombolysis, no advantage of heart–lung machine-assisted thrombectomy could be found [69]. It requires even more logistics than mechanical thrombus fragmentation. Theoretically, it could be an option for a patient under CPR who cannot be stabilized by systemic thrombolysis; however, to substantiate this concept at least a couple of such cases resulting in full recovery should be reported [70].

In DVT, scientific support for the validity of the thrombectomy approach is even less than for thrombolysis. Only one randomized controlled trial including 30 patients with incomplete follow-up and non-standardized treatment in the control arm evaluated the target criterion, i.e. development of PTS [71]. The main consistent finding in larger cohort studies is a procedure-related mortality of approximately 3% [72]. An additional problem is the high rate of early and late re-occlusions. As with the catheter-guided approach, surgery is a treatment concept—if at all—for descending iliac DVT of recent onset in young and otherwise healthy individuals [73].

Logistics of initial treatment

By tradition in some European countries, bed rest was a treatment modality for DVT. Two randomized controlled trials, even though of limited sample size, demonstrated that under the condition of therapeutic anticoagulation, bed rest does not reduce the embolic potential of acute DVT [74, 75]. In addition, immediate ambulation under graduated compression therapy offers a benefit regarding relief of symptoms.

The emergence of LMWHs has brought outpatient treatment of DVT into perspective. Two randomized controlled trials demonstrated that, at least in selected patients, home treatment with subcutaneous LMWH is as safe and effective as in-hospital treatment with intravenous UFH [76, 77]. Subsequent feasibility studies revealed that several prerequisites have to be met for outpatient treatment of DVT. Patient-related factors are a low acute bleeding risk and full compliance. Institution-related factors are personnel capacity for individual patient education at diagnosis, 24-hour accessibility, and ability to provide or organize professional home care if needed. DVT characteristics and comorbidities seem to be less important. With these requirements fulfilled, 80–90% of outpatients with acute proximal DVT can be treated primarily at home [78]. As the short-term prognosis of the patient with acute PE but without any haemodynamic compromise is as well as for the patient with DVT alone, home treatment or early discharge may be considered for these patients. The prerequisite, however, is a comprehensive risk stratification including echocardiography [79].

Maintenance therapy

Once the acute embolic risk has been tempered down by immediate and adequate anticoagulation, maintenance therapy is required to overcome the risk of recurrence. According to the natural history of VTE, early- and long-term maintenance therapy have to be differentiated.

Early maintenance therapy

As early recurrences are triggered by the presence of the clot and its endogenous repair rather than by patient-related or circumstantial risk factors, the duration of early maintenance therapy should reflect the extent of the clot, i.e. thrombus mass. There is evidence that for isolated calf vein thrombosis a course of 6 weeks of therapy is sufficient, and that a 3-month course is appropriate for femoropopliteal DVT [80]. It seems plausible to assume this period to be 6 months for massive DVT involving iliac veins or the inferior caval vein. The standard therapy regimen for this period is VKA, with an intensity international normalized ratio (INR) of 2.0–3.0. ➲Table 37.8 gives the main features of the most widely used VKAs.

Given the high endogenous fibrinolytic potential of the pulmonary circulation, pulmonary emboli will subside within 3 months of maintenance therapy. Therefore, the presence or absence of PE gives no reason for prolonging the period of early maintenance therapy. Any additional consideration taking into account the higher case fatality rate of a PE recurrence has to be handled as part of the long-term maintenance therapy issue.

These durations are the minimal therapy of any VTE episode that may not be reduced. However, only patients with a first triggered episode of VTE will receive early maintenance therapy alone. Once this period is over, the current VTE episode and the patient in whom it occurred have to be assessed with regard to whether to prolong maintenance therapy for a limited or an indefinite period of time. Making a decision about long-term maintenance therapy has to balance the risk of recurrence of VTE against the bleeding risk of the planned treatment regimen in the patient. Decision-making will also include the preferences of the informed patient.

Bleeding risk associated with standard vitamin K antagonist treatment

Determinants of haemorrhagic complications in patients on VKA therapy are intensity of anticoagulation, patient characteristics, length of therapy, and the use of concomitant drugs. Particularly for intracranial haemorrhage, the most important risk factor is the intensity of anticoagulation [81].

For secondary prophylaxis of VTE with the standard intensity INR of 2.0–3.0, there are two sources of data regarding the frequency of haemorrhagic complications. Data quality is high from randomized controlled trials. However, due to selection bias the frequencies of complications may be considerably lower than in registries of patients in standard care [82]. In randomized trials, the incidence of major bleeds within the first 3 months is about 1%. For prolonged anticoagulation, the annual frequencies are 0.2–0.6% for fatal bleeds, 2–3% for major bleeds, and 5–15% for minor bleeds. A retrospective cohort of unselected patients on standard intensity VKA treatment in an outpatient setting reported a monthly incidence of major haemorrhage of 0.82% for the first 3 months decreasing to 0.36% for the months thereafter, amounting to an annual incidence of 4.3%. These figures may reflect the everyday standard of

Table 37.8 Vitamin K antagonists

Generic name	Brand name	Half-life (S-/R-Enantiomer)	Average maintenance dose	Loading dose
Acenocoumarol	Sintrom	1–12 hours	4mg	No
Warfarin	Coumadin	25–47 hours	5mg	No
Phenprocoumon	Marcumar/Falithrom	125–160 hours	3mg	Yes

care situation more closely. By contrast, Prandoni and colleagues [83] reported an annual incidence for major bleeds of 0.5% for a cohort of well-selected patients on indefinite VKA treatment after a second VTE in an outpatient setting of a highly specialized institution.

Comorbid conditions have a strong impact on bleeding complications. The most common are history of gastrointestinal bleeding with a hazard ratio of 2.7, history of stroke (HR 2.6), and the presence of recent myocardial infarction, renal insufficiency, severe anaemia, or diabetes (HR 2.2). Active cancer has a higher risk of bleeding as well.

Net clinical benefit

When comparing different regimens of secondary prophylaxis the criterion for a treatment decision should be the net clinical benefit of the available alternatives. This benefit is mostly considered to be the sum of recurrent VTE events prevented at the cost of all major bleeding episodes provoked by anticoagulation. In order to integrate both components, a given regimen can be characterized by its 'net clinical harm', i.e. the sum of VTE events plus major bleeds compared with the respective sum of the alternative regimen. However, it should be kept in mind that the nature of a VTE recurrence and a major bleed differ substantially. On the basis of all randomized controlled trials on VTE treatment between 1966–1997, Douketis and colleagues [84] established that the risk of fatal PE after start of treatment of a VTE episode was low, with incidences of 0.4% per year for DVT patients and 1.5% per year for patients with PE during the anticoagulation period. After anticoagulation, it was 0.3% per year in DVT patients; for patients with PE there was no such event. Based on substantially the same trial data, Linkins [85] and colleagues were able to define the clinical impact of major bleeding episodes in VTE patients. They found a case fatality rate of major bleedings of 13.4% for all patients and 9.1% for those receiving anticoagulation for >3 months. This rate is about twice as high as the case fatality rate of a recurrent VTE episode in DVT patients. Probably even more meaningful are the figures for intracranial haemorrhage. The overall rate of intracranial haemorrhage was 1.15% per year and 0.65% per year for those on long-term anticoagulation. This comparison indicates that assessment of the risk:benefit ratio of long-term maintenance therapy has a component that is subjected to highly individual judgements and preferences.

Duration of long-term maintenance therapy with vitamin K antagonist

The basic fact in the search for optimal duration of maintenance therapy is that the recurrence rate for VTE is very low (<1%) as long as VKA with a target INR of 2.0–3.0 is given [86]. A second fact that may safely guide the decision is that the risk of recurrence in secondary VTE, i.e. after an episode with a transient risk factor, is too low to justify anticoagulation beyond the required minimum duration of early maintenance therapy. Conversely, for all identifiable and strong permanent risk factors it is now generally accepted to prolong maintenance therapy indefinitely after a first VTE event. This is true for the antiphospholipid syndrome [87] and for active cancer [88], and it is common practice by tradition for inherited thrombophilias, such as severe symptomatic antithrombin deficiency or severe protein C or S deficiencies in patients with VTE and a positive family history.

For recurrent disease as well as for unprovoked episodes, randomized controlled trials were performed in order to establish an optimal duration of maintenance therapy [89, 90]. However, these studies only confirmed the basic facts mentioned earlier: the rate of recurrence is very low during anticoagulation, and the number of bleeding episodes does increase steadily with prolongation of anticoagulation. However, subgroup analyses pointed to a relative additional benefit for patients with thrombophilias. In addition, two studies—one for DVT and another for PE—found consistently that there seems to be a kind of 'catch-up' phenomenon after cessation of prolonged maintenance therapy [91, 92]. This observation supports the view that the period ideally should be indefinite in a patient who needs prolonged therapy.

Based on these findings and considerations, the ACCP consensus made the following recommendations: patients with a first idiopathic episode of VTE with or without thrombophilia should receive maintenance therapy for 3 months. After that period, patients should be re-evaluated. If bleeding risks are absent and good anticoagulant monitoring is available, indefinite treatment should be given. Patients with two documented VTE episodes should receive indefinite treatment. In all patients with indefinite treatment the risk:benefit ratio should be reassessed at periodic intervals. It was stated that these recommendations and suggestions ascribe a higher value to preventing recurrences than on bleeding and costs [49].

Intensity of long-term maintenance therapy with vitamin K antagonist

Recently, two trials tested the efficacy and safety of a low-intensity VKA regimen with a target INR of 1.5–2.0 as long-term maintenance therapy in patients with unprovoked or recurrent VTE. The PREVENT trial compared it to placebo [93], and the ELATE trial to the standard intensity of

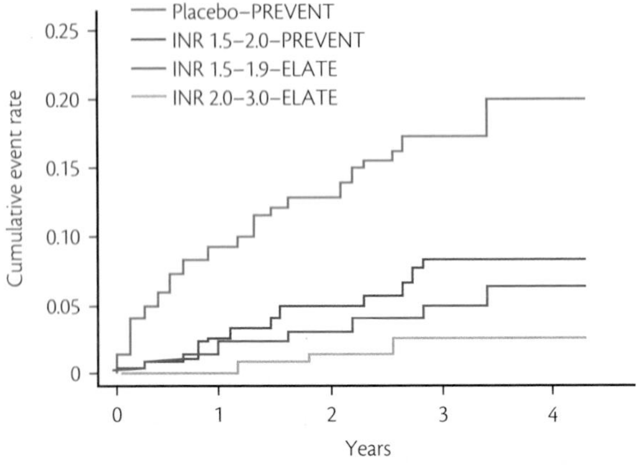

Figure 37.14 Combined results of the PREVENT and the ELATE trial showing the gain in prevention of recurrences achieved by three different regimens (placebo/no treatment vs. VKA INR 1.5–2.0 vs. VKA INR 2.0–3.0. Data from Ridker PM, Goldhaber SZ, Danielson E, *et al.* Long-term, low-intensity warfarin therapy for the prevention of recurrent venous thromboembolism. *N Engl J Med* 2003; **348**: 1425–34.

INR 2.0–3.0 [94]. The relative efficacy is shown in ➲Fig. 37.14 [95]. The major advantage over placebo is achieved by the low-intensity regimen with a considerably smaller surplus benefit of the standard intensity regimen. Not surprisingly, major bleeding rates in the low-intensity arms of both studies (1% per year) were lower than those in standard intensity arms in previous studies (2–4% per year), even though neither study was powered to detect a significant difference in bleeding rates. However, in direct comparison with the ELATE study, the rate of major bleeds in the standard VKA arm was found to be as low as in the low-intensity arm. Thus, the recommendation for clinical practice now depends on how this low bleeding rate can be generalized. As long as the bleeding risk in a given patient is estimated to be as low as 1% per year, the higher efficacy of the standard intensity regimen should be offered. Since the PREVENT trial established that the less intensive INR-target of 1.5–2.0 can be hit with less frequent INR-testing, patients may choose this option if they strongly prefer longer testing intervals.

Alternatives to vitamin K antagonist in maintenance therapy

Since 1994, a couple of randomized controlled trials have been performed to evaluate the efficacy and safety of LMWHs compared with VKA in early maintenance therapy of DVT, i.e. for 3–6 months. The most comprehensive meta-analysis included >1300 patients [96]. Regarding efficacy, there was an insignificant trend in favour of LMWHs; regarding safety, LMWHs showed a statistically significant reduction in major bleeds by 55%; total mortality did not differ. Different dosages of LMWHs have been used as a substitute for standard intensity VKA treatment varying from high-dose prophylactic to full therapeutic dosages. No direct comparison is available. However, at least the half-therapeutic dose should be chosen. In cancer patients, a large randomized trial demonstrated superior efficacy of 75% of therapeutic dose LMWH over standard intensity VKA [97]. For this reason, cancer patients should receive LMWH instead of VKA for the first months of maintenance therapy.

Regarding practical issues, the cost of long-term LMWH use has to be considered. Given the relatively weak data basis for a real advantage of LMWHs—at least in the non-cancer population—standard VKA treatment remains the first choice for most patients after an acute episode of VTE. In patients with difficult access to laboratory monitoring or in those with poor compliance to VKA dose adjustments, LMWHs may be considered as a feasible, effective, and safe alternative.

A large patient group that clearly benefits from this alternative consists of those patients who need to interrupt their VKA long-term maintenance therapy in order to undergo any kind of invasive or surgical procedure. For feasibility reasons, LMWHs may be considered as the first option for the bridging period between cessation and full re-institution of VKA medication [98]. There are no randomized controlled trials to establish the relative efficacy and safety of LMWH bridging regimens in comparison with dose-adjusted UFH. Moreover, there are no consistent data allowing for an estimate of thrombotic and/or bleeding complications in bridging episodes with UFH. Thus, it is of great value that the number of prospective cohorts of bridging episodes with LMWH is growing, indicating that LMWHs—albeit not approved—are safe and effective in this indication [99].

New anticoagulants are being developed at present with the explicit goal to create an alternative to VKA for secondary as well as long-term maintenance therapy. The long-acting pentasaccharide idraparinux has been evaluated in initial anticoagulation and early- and long-term maintenance therapy of VTE. The 5-day half-life of the parenteral compound allows for a once- weekly dosing schedule without laboratory monitoring [100]. However, the van Gogh study failed to demonstrate non-inferiority of idraparinux compared to standard therapy in patients with PE [101]. Large phase III study programmes are evaluating other novel oral anticoagulants for initial and maintenance treatment in acute VTE. These novel drugs include dabigatran etexilate (a direct thrombin inhibitor), rivaroxaban, and apixaban (two factor Xa inhibitors).

Chronic sequelae of venous thromboembolism

These present as post-thrombotic syndrome and chronic thromboembolic pulmonary hypertension, the details of which are given in the following sections.

Post-thrombotic syndrome

As chronic venous hypertension is the pivotal factor in the pathophysiology of this condition, compression therapy is the appropriate measure to counteract post-thrombotic syndrome. Randomized controlled trials demonstrated the effect of graduated elastic compression stockings compared with no treatment. When administered from the beginning of DVT treatment, compression therapy will almost halve the overall incidence of PTS. The effect is evenly distributed throughout the different degrees of severity of PTS [102, 103]. Below-knee stockings will be appropriate for almost all patients. The pressure at ankle level has to be between 30–40mmHg.

Only half of all patients with DVT will develop PTS. As these patients can reliably be identified only at 2 years after the index event, compression therapy must be recommended for all of them in the initial treatment phase. After 2 years the patient must be re-evaluated clinically. If they show signs and symptoms of PTS when not using the stockings, they are likely to need them permanently for symptom control in order to avoid progression of PTS. If no symptoms occur, compression therapy may be stopped [104].

Once PTS has developed as a clinically relevant condition, compression therapy is the mainstay of treatment. This is particularly true in patients with venous ulcer. The local and surgical measures to treat venous ulceration are not within the scope of this chapter.

Chronic thromboembolic pulmonary hypertension

At diagnosis, almost all patients with CTPH have had a period of months or years with clinically silent, repetitive PE from undetected DVT. Only a few patients will develop the condition as consequence of a single symptomatic PE episode. However, in order not to miss those cases, all patients with PE who have had any degree of right ventricular dysfunction during acute illness should undergo echocardiography 1 year after the acute event. If there is still some degree of pulmonary hypertension they must be subjected to close surveillance with control examinations at regular intervals. Deteriorating pulmonary hypertension should prompt a thorough re-evaluation for DVT and may require lifelong anticoagulation.

If CTPH clinically progresses to NYHA class III or IV, or if the patient has already reached this stage when being diagnosed for the first time, pulmonary thromboendarterectomy (PTEA) should be considered. The procedure itself is technically demanding. Even more taxing, however, is the immediate postoperative period, which can be managed only by a team of specialists dedicated to this specific problem. Thus, PTEA for CTPH is confined to a very few centres. Still, perioperative mortality has been reported to be in the range of 5–25%. Following PTEA, permanent anticoagulation is required. In addition, most surgeons will insert a permanent caval filter as part of the procedure.

Other manifestations of venous thromboembolism

Minimal disease

All therapeutic considerations so far are related to proximal DVT and to PE. There are only very few data that help to guide therapy of minimal thromboembolic disease, i.e. DVT confined to single segments of the calf veins or even isolated calf muscle vein thrombosis. Today, maintenance therapy for 3 months is the upper end of the spectrum of therapeutic recommendations. At the other end, several authors suggest not even looking for minimal disease as it does not require therapy at all [105]. Given the undisputable potential of minimal disease to progress to proximal DVT and PE [106], there is a real gap in the present knowledge that has to be filled by reliable data. The most important issue is to identify in advance those patients in whom minimal disease will propagate. While awaiting these data, a reasonable compromise could be to administer anticoagulation, for example by LMWH, for a limited period of time (1–4 weeks) in conjunction with compression therapy for 3 months. Prolongation of these measures may be tailored according to the individual course of the disease. An alternative would be to not administer anticoagulants and to perform follow-up with repeated ultrasound.

Superficial thrombophlebitis

Unfortunately, knowledge of therapy is confounded by the fact that the two distinct entities headed under the term ‘superficial thrombophlebitis’ have not been consistently differentiated in current literature [107]. Based on natural history, circumscript phlebitis in varicose veins has to be discriminated from ascending saphenous phlebitis for the purpose of diagnosis as well as of therapy.

As long as superficial thrombophlebitis is locally confined to venous segments with varicosity, the risk of progression into the deep venous system via the inguinal or popliteal junctions of the greater or the lesser saphenous vein is low. Progression into the deep venous system via perforator veins at the level of the inflammatory lesion may occur in 10–20% of cases, but does not seem to place the patient at risk for clinical manifest DVT or PE [108]. Thus, in most cases of varicose vein thrombophlebitis, local measures such as percutaneous incision thrombectomy, cooling and compression therapy, in conjunction with systemic non-steroidal anti-inflammatory drugs (NSAIDs), are sufficient to control the actual episode. In the interval, varicophlebitis as a complication of varices should prompt the evaluation of the patient as a candidate for varicosectomy.

By contrast, with the ascending type of saphenous vein thrombosis there is a substantial probability of progression into the popliteal or the femoral vein, respectively, leading to DVT and even PE. Therapeutic anticoagulation for a minimum duration of 10–20 days, preferably with LMWH, is effective in preventing thrombus propagation into the deep venous system. Compression therapy may be added. Up until now, the question is unanswered as to whether maintenance therapy should be given in order to counteract the risk of recurrence [109].

Upper extremity deep vein thrombosis

As the upper extremity is a potential source of PE and has a high rate of symptoms seriously affecting activities of daily living, even in the long term the same sequence of therapeutic elements has to be applied as for DVT of the leg. No randomized controlled data about treatment modalities are available [8]. By analogy, initial anticoagulation, preferably with LMWHs in therapeutic dosage, will be followed by early maintenance therapy. Most authors suggest a duration of 3 months. Catheter-guided thrombolysis is technically feasible, with a low procedural complication rate. Successful recanalization has been documented in many cases. However, the effect on long-term course remains unclear. Given the high rate of temporary risk factors, long-term maintenance therapy plays no role in upper extremity DVT. However, in the rare case of thoracic inlet syndrome surgical decompression may be indicated.

Almost all patients with long-term symptoms have not received adequate compression therapy. Similar to stockings for the leg, DVT compression 'sleeves' are available and should be prescribed from the very beginning of therapy. They have to be fitted carefully to the individual patient and closely quality controlled.

Heparin-induced thrombocytopenia

The immunological type of HIT is a complication of heparin administration and in itself a cause of venous as well as arterial thromboembolism. All aspects of pathophysiology, clinical course, diagnosis, and therapy have been reviewed extensively during the past 10 years and several comprehensive monographs are readily available [110]. Therefore, only a very few clinical considerations will be presented here.

Unlike in other diseases, diagnosis and therapy of HIT are simultaneous processes. The clinical suspicion is derived from the laboratory finding of thrombocytopenia fulfilling the diagnostic criterion of a rapid, >50% drop compared with the baseline value. The absolute platelet count does not provide the same information. Thrombocytopenia may occur with or without symptomatic thromboembolic events. However, there must be ongoing heparin therapy for at least 5–7 days. In case of suspicion of HIT, heparin therapy has to be stopped and replaced with alternative anticoagulation. Three compounds with explicit approval in Europe are the high-sulphated heparinoid danaparoid, the recombinant hirudin analogue lepirudin, and the peptidomimetic direct thrombin inhibitor argatroban (➲Table 37.9). The dosage has to be chosen according to the previous heparin dose (prophylactic vs. therapeutic). With a thromboembolic event present, therapeutic regimens have to be applied.

Having established alternative anticoagulation, the diagnosis has to be examined carefully in order to definitely confirm or refute it. Results of HIT antibody tests (ELISA or heparin-induced platelet activation, HIPA) will be available with a delay of only around 2 days. A negative result of both tests excludes the diagnosis. In this case, heparin can be restarted. A positive antibody test supports the diagnosis; however, it is far from proving it. In this case, the alternative anticoagulation has to be continued. For confirmation of the diagnosis, an increase of platelet count must occur after 4 days to 2 weeks. If thrombocytopenia persists, any differential diagnosis is more likely than HIT. In general, validation of the diagnosis is more difficult in thrombocytopenia alone than in an episode of arterial or VTE with thrombocytopenia.

A firmly established diagnosis of HIT has to be discussed with the patient to enable them to avoid re-exposure

Table 37.9 Alternative anticoagulants in HIT

Generic name	Drug class	Route of administration	Half-life	Prophylactic dose regimen	Therapeutic dose regimen	Monitoring
Danaparoid	Heparinoid	IV, SC	25 hours (prolonged in renal impairment)	750IU, BID or TID	2250IU bolus; infusion of 400 to 150U/hours with dose adjustment	aXa activity; therapeutic level 0.5–0.8U/mL
Lepirudin	Recombinant hirudin analogue (peptidic)	IV, SC	1.3 hours (~200 hours in renal failure)	15mg BID	0.40mg/kg bolus; infusion of 0.15mg/kg/hours with dose adjustment	aPTT 1.5–2.5-fold (alternative: ECT)
Argatroban	Synthetic direct thrombin inhibitor (peptidomimetic)	IV	40–50min (four- to fivefold in liver impairment)	Not tested	No bolus; infusion of 2mcg/kg/min with dose adjustment	aPTT 1.5–3.0-fold (< 100 s)

Note: BID, twice daily; ECT, ecarin clotting time; IV, intravenous; SC, subcutaneous; IU, international units; TID, three times daily. For special dose regimens, see [110].

to heparin in future treatment settings. Some sort of emergency document may be helpful. A patient with a history of confirmed HIT must not receive either UFH or LMWH, in particular during the period of elevated HIT antibody titres. Thromboprophylaxis as well as VTE treatment may be provided by danaparoid or fondaparinux, even though one isolated case of HIT has been reported with this compound. Titres will return to normal within months after the acute illness. A patient with a history of HIT may safely undergo open-heart surgery with an UFH-anticoagulated heart–lung machine if the test is negative for HIT antibodies. Obviously, the short period of re-exposure to UFH is not sufficient to reactivate the immune mechanism.

Personal perspective

In the past 15 years, fundamental changes have occurred regarding both the conception and the management of VTE. The most challenging discovery was the elucidation of a broad variety of thrombophilic conditions, which formed the concept of a widespread genetic susceptibility for the disease. However, the translation of individual genetic findings into clinical practice turned out to be more difficult than anticipated in the enthusiasm of the first few years. By contrast, the identification of patients who suffer from VTE as a chronic relapsing disease by clinical evaluation only has been firmly established, confirming the unprovoked and the relapsing episode as strongest indicators for a high risk of recurrence.

Management of VTE switched from the hospital-only setting to a primarily out-patient-based patient care. The stimulus for this development was the proof that LMWHs in therapeutic dosage are at least as efficacious and safe as UFH in the initial anticoagulation, thereby allowing for subcutaneous administration without laboratory monitoring. At the other end of the disease spectrum, i.e. in the field of life-threatening PE, recent progress has been made in validating the fundamental distinction between 'high-risk' and 'non-high-risk' PE, and to build it into all major guideline recommendations on this topic.

The field has now moved to address one major unresolved issue, i.e. the individualization of the risk:benefit ratio of long-term maintenance therapy after initial- and intermediate-term anticoagulation. Major progress has been made with the concept that lack of a transient risk factor or presence of a permanent risk factor makes the patient a candidate for indefinite maintenance therapy. Most thrombophilias are no longer regarded as permanent risk factors. The determinants for recommending indefinite maintenance therapy, however, are not only the risk of disease recurrence, for which new markers are being assessed, but also the features of new anticoagulants that are currently under development. If new drugs turn out to be associated with a lower bleeding risk than VKAs then the current trend towards longer periods of maintenance therapy will increase.

It is noteworthy that previously underestimated issues are now being subjected to thorough scientific investigation, like minimal disease, upper extremity DVT, the post-thrombotic syndrome, or compression therapy.

Further reading

Bounameaux H, Righini M, Perrier A. Venous thromboembolism: contemporary diagnostic and therapeutic aspects. *Vasa* 2008, **37**: 211–26.

Kearon K, Kahn SR, Agnelli G, *et al.* Antithrombotic therapy for venous thromboembolic disease. American College of Chest Physicians Evidence-Based Clinical Practice Guidelines (8th edition) *Chest* 2008; **133**: 454S–545S.

Kyrle PA, Eichinger S. Deep vein thrombosis. *Lancet* 2005; **365**: 1163–74.

Tapson V. Acute pulmonary embolism. *N Engl J Med* 2008; **358**: 1037–52.

Torbicki A, Perrier A, Konstantinides S, *et al.* Guidelines on the diagnosis and management of acute pulmonary embolism. *Eur Heart J* 2008; **29**: 2276–315.

➲ For full references and multimedia materials please visit the online version of the book (http://esctextbook.oxfordonline.com).

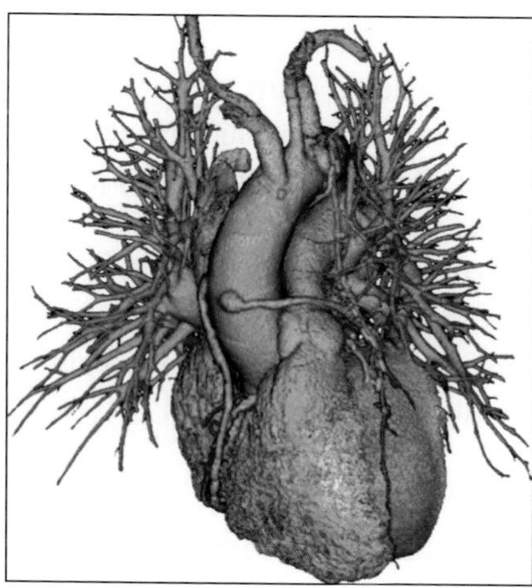

CHAPTER 38

Occupational and Regulatory Aspects of Heart Disease

Demosthenes G. Katritsis and Michael M. Webb-Peploe

Contents

Summary

This chapter deals with socioeconomic aspects of heart disease. First, the recent evidence linking occupational factors and heart disease is discussed. Subsequent sections review guidelines and regulations governing the socio-economic integration of patients following cardiac events or procedures. These guidelines and regulations—published by cardiology societies and other authorities—aim to assist the physician in determining the ability of patients to safely resume normal activities and return to work, particularly when that work impacts public safety. Main issues discussed are private and professional driving and ability of the cardiac patient to travel by air. Guidelines on driving published by the European Society of Cardiology are compared with the comprehensive recommendations put forward by the Canadian Society of Cardiology, and recent modifications of previous guidelines of the American Heart Association. Guidelines on air travel have been published by the Canadian Society of Cardiology and the US Aerospace Medical Association. Guidelines are presented relating to different cardiac conditions and controversial issues are discussed. Regulations for medical licensing of professional pilots have been published by national authorities, the European Joint Aviation Authorities and the European Aviation Safety Agency, and, most recently, the International Civil Aviation Organization.

Occupational risk factors for heart disease

Introduction

The relationship between socioeconomic status and heart disease is well established. Low socioeconomic status and social deprivation are associated with an increased risk of heart disease which itself may jeopardize career prospects and social success [1–5]. Cardiovascular disease contributes most to socioeconomic inequalities in mortality in European countries [6]. Recognition of the social dimension of heart disease is important because poor socioeconomic status is not only a potentially reversible risk factor, but also influences access to and development of modern, high-cost cardiac care.

The reasons for the observed socioeconomic inequalities in health are not clear. Plausible explanations that have received attention in recent years include job characteristics and, especially, education. Educational attainment, occupational status, and adverse physical working conditions have been associated with an increased incidence of myocardial infarction [7] and heart failure [4], and low socioeconomic status is associated with reduced exercise capacity in patients with known coronary artery disease [5]. Low employment and income grade are also associated with the feeling of unfairness at work and vital exhaustion, both identified as predictors of ischaemic heart disease [8]. The postulated underlying biological mechanisms in these conditions include: increased prevalence of metabolic syndrome [9, 10]; psychological factors [11]; impaired autonomic function [12]; elevated fibrinogen levels [13]; and low-grade inflammation [14].

Hazardous working conditions

Work stress

There is now considerable evidence supporting the role of job strain (a combination of high work demands and low job control) as a risk factor for heart disease [15–18], despite negative previous studies from the USA [19, 20] and Japan [21]. Observational data suggest an average 50% excess cardiovascular risk among employees with work stress [16], and, particularly in younger male populations (19–55 years), job strain carries a 1.8 times higher age-adjusted risk of incident ischaemic heart disease [22]. The feeling of unfairness at work has recently been identified as an independent predictor of increased coronary events and impaired health [8].

Shift work

Shift work is an emerging practice in many industries worldwide, with approximately 22% of the population in industrialized countries performing some type of shift work [23]. There is strong evidence favouring an association between shift work and heart disease, mainly coronary artery disease [23, 24]. The desynchronization of circadian rhythms due to altered sleep cycles predisposes to heart disease by provoking hypertension, dyslipidaemia, insulin resistance, and obesity [25].

Hazardous working environments

Several occupational environments and physical factors have been associated with heart disease.

Exposure to passive smoking

The adverse effects of exposure to environmental tobacco smoking are well established. There is a reduction in the total number of hospital admissions both among active and passive smokers for acute coronary syndrome (➲Chapter 17) after the enactment of legislation banning smoking in public places [26].

Exposure to air pollutants

Increased levels of air pollutants that occur in several manufacturing and mining industries as well as in heavily polluted inner cities have been associated with increased cardiovascular morbidity and mortality. Inhalation of air pollutants affects heart rate, heart rate variability, blood pressure, vascular tone, blood coagulability, and the progression of atherosclerosis [27]. Ambient fine particulate matter and black carbon are particularly dangerous, especially the first month after a previous myocardial infarction (➲Chapter 17) [28] Potential mechanisms of inhalation-mediated cardiovascular toxicity include activation of pro-inflammatory pathways and generation of reactive oxygen species as well as translocation of ultrafine particles into the circulation where they can induce cardiac arrhythmias and decrease cardiac contractility and coronary flow [27].

Other factors

➲Table 38.1 presents factors for which there has been evidence of a causative relationship with heart disease [29, 30].

Regulations concerning individual risk and public safety

Introduction

Risk stratification, i.e. estimation of the probability of a future cardiac event, is the mainstay of proper management

Table 38.1 Professions and work environments that have been associated with heart disease—in bold are conditions for which the evidence is stronger. Previous concerns about exposure to low frequency magnetic fields have not been substantiated

Exposure to passive smoking
Exposure to air pollutants—fine particulate matter and black carbon
Professional driving—especially bus drivers in heavy traffic
Fishing in arctic waters
Plastic and paper industry
Firefighting
Slaughterhouse
Intense industrial noise
Cold weather (<18°C) for individuals >50 years old
Chronic exposure to carbon monoxide (CO)
Chronic exposure to carbon disulfide (CS_2)
Chronic exposure to carbon dioxide (CO_2)

of patients with heart disease. It is also important in safe re-integration of the patient in society and employment following a serious cardiac event or procedure. First, it allows the physician to appreciate the ability of the patient to safely resume normal activities and return to work. Second, it is particularly useful when considering employment in jobs that impact public safety. Patients with disturbed cardiac function—arrhythmias in particular—may experience complete or partial loss of consciousness threatening their own safety and that of the general public when engaged in certain personal or professional activities. Driving is an obvious example.

The issue of patient recovery and recuperation is usually addressed by guidelines, i.e. systematically developed statements by national and international cardiology societies aimed at assisting decisions about appropriate healthcare for specific clinical circumstances. Individual and public safety matters are dealt with by regulations issued by appointed committees as well as cardiology societies and carry greater authority than guidelines. Regulations and laws concerning the eligibility for a private or commercial driving licence are also issued by Government Departments and Agencies at a national level. An example is the guide to medical standards issued every 6 months by the UK Driver and Vehicle Licensing Agency (DVLA) (see ➲ Online resources, p.1369).

Probably the most common questions concern the advisability of driving and flying, in either a private or commercial capacity. Rarely, with other demanding jobs related to public safety, e.g. operating heavy machinery in a factory, similar recommendations to those for commercial driving may be applicable.

Driving regulations

The frequency with which medical causes contribute to motor vehicle accidents is not precisely known. Data on arrhythmias as a cause of motor vehicle accidents is hard to obtain due to the difficulty of documenting such events in the general population. However, the proportion is believed to be small. Data from Canada and the USA suggest that <5% of accidents involving commercial vehicles can be attributed to cardiovascular disease [31–33]. Experience in Europe also suggests that the impact of arrhythmia-induced loss of consciousness is a relatively minor factor in road accidents. Approximately 0.1% of reported road accidents are attributed to medical causes, and only 10–25% of these are due to cardiac events [31, 33].

In the European Society of Cardiology (ESC) reports [33, 34] two groups of drivers are defined. Group one comprises drivers of motorcycles, cars, and other small vehicles with and without a trailer. Group two includes drivers of vehicles >3500kg or passenger-carrying vehicles exceeding eight seats excluding the driver. Drivers of taxicabs, small ambulances, and other vehicles form an intermediate category between the ordinary private driver and the vocational driver. The Canadian Cardiovascular Society (CCS) [32] distinguishes a private driver from a commercial driver on the basis of number of kilometres driven per year (<36,000); hours per year behind the wheel (<720); weight of the vehicle (<11,000kg); and whether or not the vehicle is used to earn a living. Case fatality rates for accidents involving commercial vehicles (large goods and passenger carrying vehicles) are three to four times greater than those involving ordinary private motor cars [35].

In general, regulations define as acceptable risk for driver incapacity an event rate at or below 20% per annum for ordinary licences and 2% for vocational licences [35]. However, in most countries, drivers in their late 70s may hold a vocational licence by which age their annual death rate from coronary disease exceeds 2%. Driving guidelines applied to particular heart conditions are discussed in later sections in this chapter.

It should be noted that physicians have different legal responsibilities in different countries in Europe. In the UK the physician is legally required to notify the DVLA regarding a patient's condition that is not compatible with driving privileges. It is then the DVLA's responsibility to decide further action.

Table 38.2 Cardiovascular contraindications to commercial airline flight

1. Uncomplicated myocardial infarction within 2–3 weeks*
2. Complicated myocardial infarction within 6 weeks
3. Unstable angina
4. Congestive heart failure, severe, decompensated
5. Uncontrolled hypertension
6. CABG within 10–14 days
7. CVA within 2 weeks
8. Uncontrolled ventricular or supraventricular tachycardia
9. Eisenmenger syndrome**
10. Severe symptomatic valvular heart disease

*Stable patients successfully revascularized by primary angioplasty can be allowed air travel as early as 1 week after discharge.

**There is recent evidence that patients with cyanotic congenital heart disease, however, may tolerate cabin hypoxia well, with or without oxygen [38, 39].

Aviation regulations

Recommendations for travellers by air

Hypobaric hypoxia (i.e. hypoxia due to lowered oxygen pressure at high altitude) is the main concern for airline travellers with cardiovascular disease. Commercial aircraft are pressurized up to 8000 feet (2438m). The standard barometric pressure at sea level is 760mmHg and the inspired partial pressure of oxygen 149mmHg which gives an arterial PaO_2 of about 103mmHg (13.7kPa) when breathing air. At 2438m, the inspired partial pressure of oxygen falls to 108mm Hg with a consequent arterial PaO_2 of 65mmHg (8.7kPa). The dissociation curve of normal haemoglobin allows for 90% saturation of arterial blood at the cabin pressures normally encountered unless the haemoglobin is abnormal or air introduced into the chest during heart surgery has not been resorbed (usually 10–14 days). The normal person responds to hypobaric hypoxia with a mild tachycardia that increases myocardial oxygen demand. Patients with significant heart disease (➲Table 38.2) may become symptomatic during the flight. Conditions that constitute contraindications to commercial airline flight have been summarized by the Aerospace Medical Association (AsMA) in the USA [36]. If the journey is unavoidable in such cases, medical oxygen may be required. In general, however, patients with stable heart disease who are symptom-free at rest and who can climb a flight of stairs are fit to fly [37].

Medical licensing for pilots

A scheduled jet aircraft transportation accident due to a medical cause is extremely uncommon [40]. The last airline accident in Europe in which a cardiovascular event was a contributory cause was 36 years ago. Since that time the world airlines have flown approximately 0.75 billion hours. In Europe, the aviation environment was regulated by the Joint Aviation Authorities (JAA) which now exists as a liaison office only, legal competency being in transition to the European Aviation Safety Agency (EASA) (see ➲Online resources, p.1369).

Medical standards for aircrew are laid down by the International Civil Aviation Organization (ICAO) in chapter 6 to ICAO Annex 1 [41]. They were first promulgated in 1947. The JAA interpretation of these basic rules was published in 1996 as part of the European harmonization process in Joint Aviation Requirements (JAR) FCL Part 3 MEDICAL, sub-parts A, B, and C, as Requirements (including Appendices) and advisory material [42]. It is likely that the new EASA standard which will be derived from this material will be implemented by 2012. The international target for (fatal) large passenger-aircraft hull loss from any cause is one such event in 10^7 flying hours. The target event rate for medical cause of one such an accident is <1% of the total (i.e. <1 in 10^9 hours). If an incapacitating event in a member of a multi-crew (as opposed to a single-crew) operation occurs at a rate not exceeding 1%/annum (1/100 years) this theoretical objective can be achieved. It is known as the 1% rule and is calculated as follows: there are 8760 hours in a year and an event rate of 1%/annum implies a rate of 1/876,000 hours. This may be rounded up to $1/10^6$ hours. If 10% of the flight is critical (take-off, descent, approach) and 1/100 incapacitating events in the critical phase result in an accident (simulator data) then the fatal multi-pilot aircraft accident rate due to cardiovascular cause should not occur more frequently than in 10^9 hours. This has symmetry with the cardiovascular mortality of a West European male aged 65 years (the age of retirement under the JAR), but has been considered too rigorous [43]. The same does not apply to single-crew operations where the whole mission is critical and the accident rate will equal the event rate. Mathematical modelling of a target event rate (the 1% rule) emerged from the two UK and two European Workshops in Aviation Cardiology [44–48]. These workshops represent the first attempt, worldwide, to make certificatory judgement evidence-based and were copied by the USA, Australia, and Canada. Thus, a standard risk, professional pilot should be granted an unrestricted licence (JAA Class 1). A pilot with degraded medical fitness may be permitted to fly if their perceived risk of cardiovascular event is <1% annum, but they will be restricted to fly as or with a co-pilot—an operational multi-crew limitation (Class 1(OML)). For single-crew professional operations (e.g. with the carriage of fare-paying passengers) in which the fatal accident rate is likely to equal the serious incapacitation rate, ideally the medical cause accident rate should not exceed $1/10^7$ flying hours (the cardiovascular event rate of a 45-year-old male). For private flying (JAA Class 2) the all cause fatal accident rate is 10 to 20 times worse than that for scheduled airlines (approximately 1/50,00 flying hours versus 1/<1 million flying hours). In view of the higher overall event rate in Class 2 operations there is commonality between Class 1 (OML) and Class 2. The UK Civil Aviation Authority has produced algorithms for common cardiac conditions setting out the requirements for certification in the context of specific problems (medicalweb@srg.caa.co.uk). In 2006 and more recently in 2008, the ICAO updated its cardiology standards and guidance material (see ➲ Online resources, p.1369).

Specific cardiac conditions

In the following sections, available guidelines have been summarized according to specific cardiac conditions (for driving—ESC 1998 [33], updated on syncope in 2004 [34]; American Heart Association on patients with arrhythmias 1996 [31] and with ICD 2007 [49]; CCS 2004 [32]. For air travel—CCS 2004 [50]; US Aerospace Medical Association 2003 [36]).

Ischaemic heart disease

Stable coronary artery disease (also see ➲ Chapter 17)

Currently available models for risk stratification in patients with diagnosed ischaemic heart disease utilize clinical evaluation, quantification of ventricular function, assessment of ischaemia, and the extent of coronary disease on angiography [51, 52]. There are several methodology problems with risk stratification schemes [53] and even the threshold for defining 'high risk' is not unanimous. The ESC guidelines [50] consider predicted annual cardiovascular mortality of >2% as high risk; of <1% as low risk; and of 1–2% as intermediate risk. The American College of Cardiology/American Heart Association (ACC/AHA) guidelines [52] accept as high risk predicted mortality >3% per annum. For comparison, in asymptomatic subjects the SCORE (Systematic Coronary Risk Evaluation) system defines high risk a calculated annual event rate >0.5% [54].

Patients with treated, stable coronary artery disease are allowed both private and commercial driving (➲ Table 38.3). There is also no contraindication to air travel with chronic stable angina pectoris provided regular medication continues at the right intervals despite changes in time zones. According to the CCS recommendations [32], patients with a successful angioplasty are allowed private and commercial driving 48 hours and 7 days, respectively, after the procedure. Airline travel is allowed immediately after the procedure. In the case of coronary artery bypass grafting (CABG), the time taken for air to resorb from the pleural cavity (10 days to 2 weeks) and the stability of the sternal wound are major factors when contemplating air travel. Air trapped in the chest cavity after surgery will expand by 25% at altitude of 2438m and can cause barotrauma. The AsMA [37] suggested at least 10 days should elapse before allowing air travel following CABG, whereas the CCS [34] recommended that short flights (<2 hours) are safe as early as 4 days following operation provided the patient's haemoglobin is >90g/L.

Acute coronary syndromes (also see ➲ Chapter 16)

Following a ST-elevation myocardial infarction (MI), patients are at risk for arrhythmic sudden death over the next 1–2 years, particularly when early thrombolysis or primary angioplasty has not been administered. The risk of sudden cardiac death/cardiac arrest in patients with a recent MI is highest in the first 30 days after infarction [55]. Unfortunately, there are no tests with sufficient positive

Table 38.3 Driving guidelines for patients with ischaemic heart disease (European Society of Cardiology 1998)

Diagnosis	Disqualifying criteria: group 1	Disqualifying criteria: group 2
Angina pectoris (stable or unstable)	Symptoms at rest or at the wheel; driving may be recommended once symptoms are controlled	Any history of and/or treatment for. If asymptomatic and requiring no anti-anginal medication (re-)licensing may be permitted subject to regular exercise evaluation
Myocardial infarction, CABG, PTCA	None, once clinical recovery has taken place, usually 4 weeks following MI or CABG, and 1 week following PTCA	Not permitted until at least 6 weeks have elapsed from the index event. If asymptomatic and requiring no anti-anginal medication (re-) licensing may be permitted subject to regular exercise evaluation

Group 1 (private drivers) and group 2 (vocational drivers): exercise evaluation shall be performed on a bicycle or treadmill. Drivers should be able to complete 3 stages of the Bruce protocol or equivalent safely, without anti-anginal medication for 48 hours and should remain free from signs of cardiovascular dysfunction, such as angina pectoris, syncope, hypotension, ventricular tachycardia, and/or electrocardiographic ST segment shift (usually >2mm horizontal or down-sloping) which accredited medical opinion interprets as being indicative of myocardial ischemia. In the presence of established coronary heart disease, exercise evaluation shall be required at regular intervals, usually annually. If drug treatment for any cardiovascular condition is required then any adverse effect which may affect driver performance will disqualify them. CABG, coronary artery bypass grafting; MI, myocardial infarction; PTCA, percutaneous transluminal coronary angioplasty.

Reproduced from Petch MC. Driving and heart disease. *Eur Heart J* 1998; **19**: 1165–77.

predictive value (>30%) that allow identification of patients prone to ventricular arrhythmias and sudden death [56] and routine ICD implantation 8–40 days after MI has not been found beneficial [57]. Prognosis and recovery time following myocardial infarction or unstable angina have greatly improved in recent years due to implementation of aggressive medical and invasive therapy. After the acute phase patients should be fully investigated for risk stratification, and decisions about socioeconomic integration will depend on test results and subsequent management. Return to work after MI may be difficult to influence because it depends on a variety of socioeconomic and psychological factors such as job satisfaction, financial stability, and patient perceptions of their own disability [58]. Cardiac rehabilitation programmes (➲Chapter 25) aiming to improve both physical and psychological well-being contribute to reductions of mortality and improved physical and emotional status, and encourage an early return to normal living [58]. Daily walking is allowed immediately and in stable patients without complications, sexual activity with the usual partner can be resumed within 7–10 days. The exact timing of return to work depends on the clinical condition of the patient and the job demands. In PAMI (primary angioplasty in myocardial infarction)-II, a study of primary angioplasty in low-risk patients with MI, patients were encouraged to return to work at 2 weeks and no adverse events occurred as a result of this strategy [59]. The implementation of early invasive approaches in patients with unstable angina has also allowed quicker mobilization. Patients with unstable angina who are revascularized and otherwise stable may return to work, driving, air travel, and other normal activities often within a few days.

Private driving is allowed 1 month after an uncomplicated acute event (➲Table 38.3), although in stable patients treated by primary angioplasty driving could be allowed earlier. For patients who have experienced a complicated MI (one that required cardiopulmonary resuscitation or was accompanied by hypotension, serious arrhythmias, high-degree block, or heart failure), driving should be delayed for 3–4 weeks after symptoms have resolved. According to the CCS [32], patients with unstable angina and/or non-ST elevation MI who have been treated with successful angioplasty can resume private and commercial driving as early as 48 hours and 7 days, respectively, post-procedure. There is no unanimous international consensus regarding return to work for drivers of commercial and public transport vehicles following MI. One approach (evaluated in Canadian bus drivers post-MI) [60] is to test each individual in the stress laboratory using graded exercise and to compare MET levels achieved in the exercise laboratory with those required for driving duty. Cardiac stress values during driving in the Canadian bus drivers were on average only half those achieved in the stress laboratory. Satisfying the CCS guidelines allowed a return to work sometimes as early as 1 week after hospital discharge, and the observed risk of sudden cardiovascular incapacity causing injury or death to passengers, other road users and the drivers themselves was 1 in 50,000 driving years. This would suggest that, subject to local laws, commercial driving can begin as early as 1 week after hospital discharge provided certain exercise test standards are met. This would not be acceptable in several European countries. In the UK for example, there has to be a 6-week wait before satisfactory exercise evaluation may lead to restoration of the licence. Air travel in stable patients who had successful percutaneous revascularization may not be contra-indicated as early as 1 week after discharge, whereas complicated cases may fly 6 weeks after the event.

Arrhythmias

Patients with brady- (➲Chapter 27) or tachyarrhythmias (➲Chapters 28 and 30) may experience sudden impairment or loss of consciousness. Ventricular tachycardia or fibrillation is the most common cause of out-of-hospital cardiac arrest, accounting for approximately 75% of cases, the remaining 25% being caused by bradyarrhythmias or asystole [61]. Although ventricular arrhythmias are the most common cause of sudden cardiac death, conducting system failure and the usually more benign supraventricular arrhythmias may also rarely lead to syncope and interfere with the ability of a patient to drive or operate in a safety critical environment. ➲Table 38.4 presents the ESC recommendations for driving in patients with arrhythmias.

Bradyarrhythmias and conducting system disorders (also see ➲ Chapter 27)

Symptomatic bradyarrhythmias usually constitute an indication for permanent cardiac pacing. Patients without symptoms usually do not need a pacemaker and can drive as long as they are symptom free. Bundle-branch and fascicular blocks do not constitute an indication for pacing but should prompt a search for evidence of intrinsic cardiac abnormality or higher degree of block in the absence of which private or commercial driving is permissible.

Permanent pacemakers (also see ➲ Chapter 27)

Patients who have cardiac pacemakers are unlikely to have further symptomatic bradycardia and if symptoms recur they are rarely due to pacemaker malfunction. For patients treated with permanent pacing a period of time should pass to ensure stable lead function before they return to driving. This may be 1 day to 1 week for non-commercial drivers

Table 38.4 Driving guidelines for patients with arrhythmias (European Society of Cardiology 2004)

	Group 1 (private drivers)	Group 2 (vocational drivers)
Cardiac arrhythmias		
Cardiac arrhythmias, medical treatment	Until successful treatment is established	Until successful treatment is established
Pacemaker implant; successful catheter ablation	Within 1 week	For pacemaker, until appropriate function is established. For ablation, until long-term success is confirmed, usually 3 months
ICD implant	Low risk, controversial opinions, tendency to shorten the time of restriction	Permanent
Neurally-mediated syncope		
(a) Vasovagal:		
–Single/mild	No restrictions	No restriction unless it occurred during high-risk activity
–Severe	Until symptoms controlled	Permanent restriction unless effective treatment has been established
(b) Carotid sinus:		
–Single/mild	No restrictions	No restriction unless it occurred during high-risk activity
–Severe	Until symptoms controlled	Permanent restriction unless effective treatment has been established
(c) Situational:		
–Single/mild	No restrictions	No restriction unless it occurred during high-risk activity
–Severe	Until appropriate therapy is established	Permanent restriction unless effective treatment has been established
Syncope of uncertain cause		
Single/mild	No restrictions unless it occurred during high risk activity*	Until diagnosis and appropriate therapy is established
Severe	Until diagnosis and appropriate therapy is established	Until diagnosis and appropriate therapy is established

*Neurally-mediated syncope is defined as severe if it is very frequent, or occurring during the performance of a 'high-risk' activity, or recurrent or unpredictable in 'high-risk' patients.

Adapted from Brignole M, Alboni P, Benditt DG, *et al.* Task Force on Syncope, European Society of Cardiology. Guidelines on management (diagnosis and treatment) of syncope-update 2004. Executive Summary. *Eur Heart J* 2004; **25**: 2054–72.

and until appropriate pacemaker function has been established (up to 4 weeks) for commercial drivers (➲Table 38.4). These patients may also travel by air travel 1 week after pacemaker implantation, or battery change.

Supraventricular tachycardias (also see ➲Chapter 28)

There are no data documenting the frequency with which syncope related to supraventricular tachycardia causes motor vehicle accidents, but it is probably very rare. Patients with atrial fibrillation and flutter should be evaluated for underlying cardiac abnormality and appropriately treated. Driving may be permitted when adequate rate control without any evidence of impaired consciousness is achieved. Multifocal atrial tachycardia is usually associated with serious underlying metabolic or pulmonary disease. Patients with this arrhythmia should not be considered fit for professional driving at least until the underlying disease is assessed and treated.

Although the life expectancy in patients with Wolff–Parkinson–White syndrome and other supraventricular tachycardias is generally favourable, at least one single episode of syncope is reported in approximately 25% of patients referred to electrophysiology laboratories for assessment [62]. There is evidence that catheter ablation should be recommended in all patients with symptomatic pre-excitation [63]. Patients with atrioventricular re-entrant tachycardia due to an accessory pathway or atrioventricular nodal re-entrant tachycardia that appear to have been successfully ablated may drive after recovery from the procedure since the risk of arrhythmia recurrence causing injury is low.

Ventricular tachycardia and fibrillation (also see ➲Chapter 30)

Patients susceptible to life-threatening ventricular arrhythmias do not comprise a homogeneous group. They span a wide range of underlying pathology from cardiomyopathies to apparent normality as seen in a number of inherited conditions and 'channelopathies' that usually present as idiopathic ventricular fibrillation or unexplained cardiac arrest. However, most patients (>90%) with a cardiac arrest have demonstrable coronary artery disease, although less than half (20–30%) seem to have suffered an acute myocardial infarction [61]. Patients presenting with ventricular tachyarrhythmias are at considerable risk of recurrence, but, with the exception of left ventricular ejection fraction, there are no tests with sufficient positive predictive value to allow identification of patients prone to sudden death [56]. Thus, the modern therapy of most cases of sustained ventricular tachycardia and ventricular fibrillation is implantation of an implantable cardioverter defibrillator (ICD). A notable exception is probably patients who have idiopathic ventricular tachycardia and who do not have symptoms of impaired consciousness with their presenting arrhythmia. If such patients have normal ventricular function, normal coronary arteries, and no evidence of arrhythmogenic right ventricular cardiomyopathy or other cardiac pathology, prognosis is favourable and catheter ablation is often successful. Accordingly, it is likely that if the patient has not had symptoms of impaired consciousness with the presenting arrhythmia, future episodes will be equally well tolerated. Thus, in selected individuals, a shorter period of driving restriction may be appropriate following catheter ablation and initiation of treatment with beta-blockers or calcium-channel blockers.

In the Antiarrhythmics Versus Implantable Defibrillators (AVID) [64] trial of patients who had previously been resuscitated from near-fatal ventricular tachyarrhythmias, all survivors were sent a driving questionnaire a median of 9 months after enrolment. Eighty-three per cent replied, and of these 758 patients 627 had driven in the year prior to their index ventricular tachyarrhythmia and were sent further questionnaires every 6 months. Fifty-seven per cent of these patients resumed driving within 3 months of trial randomization, 78% within 6 months, and 88% within 12 months, and 25% were driving >100 miles per week. While driving, 2% had a syncopal episode, 11% had dizziness or palpitations that necessitated stopping the vehicle, and 22% had dizziness or palpitations that did not necessitate stopping the vehicle. Eight per cent of the 295 patients with an ICD received a shock while driving. Fifty patients reported having had at least one accident for a total of 55 accidents during 1619 patient years of follow-up after resumption of driving (3.4% per patient-year). Only 11% of these accidents were preceded by symptoms of possible arrhythmia (0.4% per patient-year). Thus, although these high-risk patients commonly had symptoms of possible arrhythmia while driving, accidents were uncommon and occurred with a frequency lower than the annual accident rate in the general US driving population (7.1%).

Syncope (also see ➲ Chapter 26)

Syncope as such is a rare cause of traffic accidents. In an anonymous survey, 3% of patients with syncope reported ever having had syncope while driving, but only 1% reported having had a car crash; only 9% of those banned from driving stopped driving because of syncope [65]. Syncope due to documented arrhythmias has been discussed in the previous section. In the case of neurally-mediated syncope, the decision to allow a patient to resume driving should be based on the severity and nature of the presenting event (➲Table 38.4). Patients who have syncope in the context of congenital long QT syndrome (➲Chapter 9), Brugada syndrome (➲Chapter 9), or other forms of channelopathy associated with ventricular fibrillation are usually treated with ICD implantation (➲Chapter 30). For patients with long QT syndrome who are asymptomatic or who have a history of symptoms but are asymptomatic on treatment, the AHA 1996 guidelines recommend regaining of driving privileges after a 6-month symptom-free interval [31]. The CCS allows commercial driving when the annual risk of sudden incapacitation in the context of these conditions is believed to be 1% or less [32]. The ESC 2004 guidelines [35] concerning fitness to drive are presented in ➲Table 38.4.

Implantable cardioverter defibrillators (also see ➲ Chapter 30)

In 1996 and 1998, the AHA [31] and the ESC [33] respectively, published scientific statements with recommendations about driving for patients treated with an ICD due to a previous episode of life-threatening arrhythmia, i.e. *secondary prevention* therapy. According to these recommendations, driving should be prohibited for the first 6 months after ICD implantation. This recommendation was based on the fact that the risk for another event is a descending exponential curve, with the greatest chance for another arrhythmia in the period immediately after an event. After 3 months the curve flattens significantly, and at 6 months it is flat. In 2007 the AHA/Heart Rhythm Society [50] updated these recommendations for patients treated with ICD because they are at risk for life-threatening ventricular arrhythmias, i.e. *primary prevention* of sudden cardiac death (➲Table 38.5). Recommendations for patients treated with ICD for secondary prevention were not changed. Patients receiving ICD for primary prevention should be restricted from driving a private automobile for at least 1 week to allow for recovery from implantation of the defibrillator. Thereafter, in the absence of symptoms potentially related to an arrhythmia, these driving privileges can be restored.

Table 38.5 Driving guidelines for patients with ICD (American Heart Association/Heart Rhythm Society, 2007)

Type of driving	Indication	Driving restriction
Private	Primary prevention	Recovery from implantation (at least 1 week)
	Secondary prevention	6 months
Commercial	Primary prevention	Cannot be certified to drive
	Secondary prevention	Cannot be certified to drive

Patients who have received an ICD for primary prevention who subsequently receive an appropriate therapy for VT or VF, especially with symptoms of cerebral hypoperfusion, should then be considered to be subject to the driving guidelines previously published for patients who received an ICD for secondary prevention.

Reproduced from Epstein AE, Baessler CA, Curtis AB, *et al.* American Heart Association; Heart Rhythm Society. Addendum to 'Personal and public safety issues related to arrhythmias that may affect consciousness: implications for regulation and physician recommendations: a medical/scientific statement from the American Heart Association and the North American Society of Pacing and Electrophysiology.' Public safety issues in patients with implantable defibrillators: a scientific statement from the American Heart Association and the Heart Rhythm Society. *Circulation* 2007; **115**: 1170–6.

However, when highway (high-speed) or long-distance travel is anticipated, patients should be encouraged to have an adult companion driver. If ICD discharge occurs after implantation, either with or without associated syncope or presyncope, patients should be advised not to drive for the next 6 months. For commercial drivers who spend a much greater proportion of their time driving or who tend to carry passengers, the risk of causing harm to other road users as a consequence of syncope or presyncope in association with ICD discharge is substantially increased, hence the recommended that all commercial driving be prohibited permanently after ICD implantation. In the forthcoming guidelines of the ESC Working Group Report for Driving of Patients with ICDs similar recommendations are made. However, driving after ICD implantation for primary prevention is allowed after 4 weeks provided that proper functioning of the system is verified, and driving after ICD implantation for secondary prevention is restricted for 3 months after the index arrhythmia. For patients refusing ICD implantation, no restriction of private driving is recommended in case of primary prevention as opposed to 7 months' restriction when the ICD is indicated for secondary prevention. Professional driving is not allowed in any case. The forthcoming recommendations of the European Heart Rhythm Association Task Force on ICD and Driving are summarized in ➲Table 38.6 [66].

Most of these recommendations, however, are hampered by a lack of good data regarding the actual risk of an ICD discharge during driving. Although no published data exist on symptoms at the time of shocks in patients enrolled in trials of ICD for primary prevention, the frequency of appropriate or inappropriate shocks can be used as a surrogate marker of risk of driving in patients with ICD. In early trials on patients with ICD device discharge rates were high. In the CABG-Patch Trial [67] 50% of patients received a discharge during 1 year of follow-up; in MADIT I [68] 60% of patients had a shock during 2 years of follow-up. The rate of ICD discharges is considerably lower in current practice. ➲Table 38.7 presents trials that have published information on the rate of shocks in patients with an ICD for primary prevention. A significantly lower rate has been invariably documented. In the subgroup of patients in the AVID trial [64] fitted with an ICD, 8% reported receiving a shock while driving. Recently, the TOVA (Triggers of Ventricular Arrhythmias) study [70] investigators analyzed data on driving habits and ICD discharges in 1188 patients.

Table 38.6 European Heart Rhythm Association recommendations for driving with an ICD

	Restriction for private driving	Restriction for professional driving
ICD implantation for secondary prevention	3 months	Permanent
ICD implantation for primary prevention	4 weeks	Permanent
After appropriate ICD therapy	3 months	Permanent
After inappropriate ICD therapy	Until measures to prevent inappropriate therapy are taken	Permanent
After replacement of the ICD	1 week	Permanent
After replacement of the lead system	4 weeks	Permanent
Patients refusing ICD for primary prevention	No restriction	Permanent
Patients refusing ICD implantation for secondary prevention	7 months	Permanent

Reproduced with permission from Vijgen J, Botto G, Camm AJ, *et al.* Consensus Statement of the European Heart Rhythm Association: Updated Recommendations for Driving of Patients with Implantable Cardioverter Defibrillators. Europace 2009; in press.

Table 38.7 ICD discharge rates in primary prevention trials

Trial/ reference	Patients with ICD	F-U (months)	Annual Mortality (%)	Discharge rate Patients (%) per year	
				Appropriate	Inappropriate
MADIT II [69]	719	20	8.5	14.1*	6.9*
DEFINITE [70]	229	29	4	7.4	8.8
SCD-HeFT [71]	829	45	5.8	5.1	2.4

*Disclosed in later reports.

Table 38.8 Driving guidelines for patients with various cardiac conditions (European Society of Cardiology, 1998)

Diagnosis	Disqualifying criteria Group 1	Disqualifying criteria Group 2
Hypertension (➲Chapter 13)	None (provided that there is no other disqualifying condition)	If the blood pressure at rest consistently exceeds 180mmHg systolic and/or 100mmHg diastolic
Aortic aneurysm including Marfan syndrome (➲Chapter 31)	None (provided that there is no other disqualifying condition)	If aortic transverse diameter >5.0cm. (Re-)licensing may be permitted following satisfactory repair and provided that there is no other disqualifying condition
Heart failure (➲Chapter 23)	Symptoms at rest or at wheel. Driving may be permitted once symptoms are controlled	Any persisting symptoms. If asymptomatic (re-)licensing may be permitted provided that the LV ejection fraction is >0.40 on contrast angiography (or equivalent), there is no disqualifying arrhythmia (see below), and the exercise requirements can be satisfied
Heart and/or lung transplantation (see Heart failure) (also see ➲Chapter 23)	Persisting symptoms If asymptomatic (re-)licensing may be permitted provided that the exercise and arrhythmia requirements can be met	
Valve disease including valve surgery (➲Chapter 21)	None (provided that there is no other disqualifying condition)	Persisting symptoms If asymptomatic (re-)licensing may be permitted provided that there is no other disqualifying condition and no history of systemic embolism. Following cerebral or systemic embolism whilst receiving anti-coagulant treatment (re-)licensing is not permitted
Congenital heart disease (➲Chapter 10)	None (provided that there is no other disqualifying condition)	Any complex or sever disorder Minor disorders and those which have been successfully corrected may be (re-)licensed provided that there is no other disqualifying condition
Hypertrophic cardiomyopathy (➲Chapter 18)	None (provided that there is no other disqualifying condition)	Persisting symptoms If asymptomatic (re-)licensing may be recommended for those with no family history of sudden cardiomyopathic death, no ventricular tachycardia on ambulatory electrocardiography, and no hypotension on exercise testing

Reproduced from Petch MC. Driving and heart disease. *Eur Heart J* 1998; **19**: 1165–77.

Of these, 80% reported driving their car at least once per week (as did 75% within 6 months after implantation); over a median follow-up period of 562 days there were 193 ICD shocks for ventricular tachycardia/ventricular fibrillation based on data from driving in relation to ICD shock. This showed that an ICD shock for ventricular tachycardia or ventricular fibrillation within 1 hour of driving was around 1 episode per 25,116 person-hours spent driving. Interestingly, among 7 patients who received an ICD shock for ventricular tachycardia or ventricular fibrillation during driving, only 1 resulted in a motor vehicle accident. This underlines the relative uncertainty about the actual validity of guidelines and perhaps allows physicians to consider certain cases on an individual basis. The inability to drive places significant limitations on an individual, greatly reducing their employment, educational, and recreational opportunities. Fifty-nine per cent of the AVID participant drivers [64] considered inability to drive a severe hardship and 39% were the only driver in the household. Decisions to withdraw driving privileges should not be taken without careful consideration. Perhaps not surprisingly, it has been documented in several studies that many patients refuse to comply with medical advice that is not enforceable by law and continue or resume driving following conditions such as implantation of a defibrillator for documented ventricular arrhythmias.

Patients with ICD are at low risk for airline travel once medically stable, although the CCS recommends air travel 1 month from last device discharge associated with severe presyncope/syncope. Interaction with airline electronics or airport security devices is highly unlikely. Recently, the rare possibility of ICD software reset by cosmic radiation that is denser at high altitudes and near the poles, has also been noted [73].

Heart failure, valve disease, and other conditions

➲Table 38.8 summarizes the ESC regulations for patients with heart failure, cardiomyopathies, valve disease, and other cardiac conditions. Patients with most of these conditions are allowed private driving and air travel with or without supplementary oxygen (➲Table 38.2). Commercial driving is allowed in patients with LVEF >40%, although a value of 35%

Personal perspective

There is now considerable evidence in support of the causative relationship between socioeconomic factors and cardiovascular disease. Heart disease, the leading cause of mortality and morbidity in European populations, inevitably has a strong social dimension and this should not be overlooked in planning prevention and management strategies. Job strain, shift work, and work in polluted environments are associated with increased risk of cardiac disorders. Regulations and guidelines addressing issues of social integration following a major cardiac event and/or cardiac interventions have been published by national and international cardiology societies, including the ESC. However, most of them vary considerably from country to country, are not comprehensive, and become outdated in the light of emerging new evidence. Systematic, practical, and constantly updated guides that balance patient well-being with public safety, such as the JAA/EASA recommendations in aviation and the ESC guidelines for driving, are much needed in Europe. Two important considerations apply. First, it is recognized that a goal of a zero risk is unattainable, nor does the controlling legislation require it. Second, what constitutes an acceptable risk cannot always be answered by scientific evidence and may have to be a matter of consensus. Individual rights include acceptance of personal risk but compete with the right of society to protect itself from harm. Such policy must seek to be fair to all persons, recognizing that restriction in the public interest may limit personal freedom, job security, and feelings of well-being. Several published recommendations on driving and flying have a level of evidence C, i.e. consensus of opinion of experts and/or small studies and registries. Thus, dogmatic approaches are not scientifically justified. The balance between individual freedom and protection of the public is not easily achieved and requires ongoing review and update.

(a usual cut-off for ICD indication) might now be more reasonable. According to the CCS [32] patients with heart transplantation deserve (re-)licensing for commercial driving 6 months after discharge if the LVEF is >35% and there are no signs of ischaemia. Patients fitted with a left ventricular assist device (LVAD) are not considered suitable to drive [32].

Acknowledgement

We are grateful to Dr Mark Anderson for having critically reviewed the manuscript.

Further reading

Brignole M, Alboni P, Benditt DG, *et al*. Task Force on Syncope, European Society of Cardiology. Guidelines on management (diagnosis and treatment) of syncope-update 2004. Executive Summary. *Eur Heart J* 2004; **25**: 2054–72.

Epstein AE, Baessler CA, Curtis AB, *et al*. American Heart Association; Heart Rhythm Society. Addendum to 'Personal and public safety issues related to arrhythmias that may affect consciousness: implications for regulation and physician recommendations: a medical/scientific statement from the American Heart Association and the North American Society of Pacing and Electrophysiology': public safety issues in patients with implantable defibrillators: a scientific statement from the American Heart Association and the Heart Rhythm Society. *Circulation* 2007; **115**:1170–6.

Joy M. The application of evidence based medicine to employment fitness standards: the transportation industries with special reference to aviation. In Yusuf S, Cairns JA, Camm AJ, *et al*. (eds.) *Evidence Based Cardiology*, 3rd edn., in press. Oxford: Wiley-Blackwell.

Petch MC. Driving and heart disease. *Eur Heart J* 1998; **19**: 1165–77.

Schnall P, Belkic K, Landsbergis P, Baker D. The Workplace and Cardiovascular Disease. In Belkic K, Landsbergis PA, Schnall P, *et al*. (eds.) *Occupational Medicine: State of the Art Reviews*, vol. 15, 2000. Philadelphia, PA: Hanley and Belfus, Inc.

Vijgen J, Botto G, Camm J, *et al*. Consensus Statement of the European Heart Rhythm Association: Updated Recommendations for Driving of Patients with Implantable Cardioverter Defibrillators. *Europace* 2009; in press.

Online resources

- European Aviation Safety Agency (EASA): http://www.easa.eu
- International Civil Aviation Organization (ICAO) publications: http://www.icao.int/icao/en/m_publications.html
- Joint Aviation Authorities (JAA): http://www.jaat.eu
- UK Driver and Vehicle Licensing Agency (DVLA): http://www.dvla.gov.uk/medical/ataglance.aspx

➲ For full references and multimedia materials please visit the online version of the book (http://esctextbook.oxfordonline.com).

Index

Note: Page numbers in *italics* refer to figures and/or tables